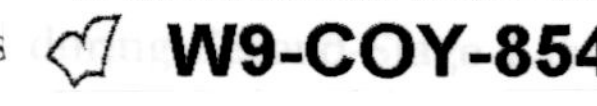

Warning Signs

Emergencies

Research Highlights

Fifth Edition

MATERNITY & GYNECOLOGIC CARE

The Nurse and the Family

Fifth Edition

MATERNITY & GYNECOLOGIC CARE

The Nurse and the Family

Irene M. Bobak, RN, MS, PhD, FAAN

Professor Emerita
San Francisco State University,
San Francisco, California

Margaret Duncan Jensen, RN, MS

Professor Emerita
San Jose State University,
San Jose, California

Associate Editor

Deitra Leonard Lowdermilk, RNC, PhD

Clinical Associate Professor
University of North Carolina
School of Nursing
Chapel Hill, North Carolina

with 1168 illustrations and 18 color plates

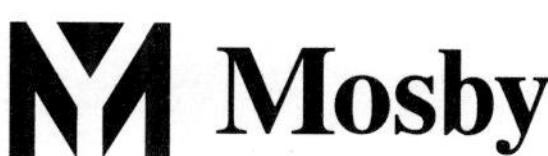

St. Louis Baltimore Boston Chicago London Philadelphia Sydney Toronto

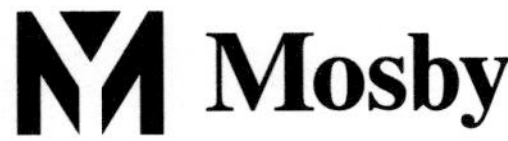

Dedicated to Publishing Excellence

Managing Editor: Susan R. Epstein
Developmental Editor: Beverly J. Copland
Project Manager: Karen Edwards
Production Editor: James W. Russell
Manuscript Editor: Sylvia Barnard
Designer: David Zielinski
Production Assistants: Ginny Douglas, Jeanne Genz

Great care has been used in compiling and checking the information in this book to ensure its accuracy. However, because of changing technology, recent discoveries, and research and individualization of prescriptions according to patient needs, the uses, effects, and dosages of drugs may vary from those given here. Neither the publisher nor the authors shall be responsible for such variations or other inaccuracies. We urge that before you administer any drug you check the manufacturer's dosage recommendations as given in the package insert provided with each product.

FIFTH EDITION

Printed in the United States of America.

Mosby–Year Book, Inc.
11830 Westline Industrial Drive
St. Louis, Missouri 63146

Library of Congress Cataloging in Publication Data

Bobak, Irene M.
Maternity and gynecologic care: the nurse and the family / Irene M. Bobak, Margaret Duncan Jensen: associate editor, Deitra L. Lowdermilk.—5th ed.
p. cm.
Includes bibliographical references and index.
ISBN 0-8016-6663-5
1. maternity nursing. 2. Gynecologic nursing. I. Jensen, Margaret Duncan, 1921- . II. Lowdermilk, Deitra L. III. Title.
[DNLM: 1. Family—nurses' instruction. 2. Gynecology—nurses' instruction. 3. Infant, Newborn—nurses' instruction. 4. Obstetrical Nursing. 5. Pregnancy—nurses' instruction. WY 157.3 B663m]
RG951.B667 1992
610.73'678—dc20
DNLM/DLC
for Library of Congress **92-48711 CIP**

93 94 95 96 97 CL/VH/VH 9 8 7 6 5 4 3 2 1

Contributors

Kathryn Rhodes Alden, RN, MSN
Clinical Instructor-Obstetrics
School of Nursing
University of North Carolina at Chapel Hill
Chapel Hill, North Carolina

M. Lucille Boland, RNC, MSN
Assistant Clinical Professor
School of Nursing
George Mason University
Fairfax, Virginia

Ruth E. Davidhizar, RN, DNS, CS
Assistant Dean and Chairperson of Nursing
Bethel College
Mishawaka, Indiana

Carol Fowler Durham, RN, MSN
Clinical Assistant Professor
School of Nursing
University of North Carolina
Chapel Hill, North Carolina

Ruth Holmes Ferguson, RN, MS
Associate Professor
Tidewater Community College
Portsmouth, Virginia

Cynthia Garrett, RNC, MSN
Perinatal Clinical Nurse Specialist
Duke University Medical Center
Durham, North Carolina

Bonnie K. Gensch, RN
Certified Death Educator/ADEC
RTS Counselor and Coordinator
Lutheran Hospital-LaCrosse
LaCrosse, Wisconsin

Joyce Newman Giger, RN, EdD, CS
Professor and Chair
Department of Nursing
Columbus College
Columbus, Georgia

Jayne Haberman-Cohen, RN, DNSc
Associate Professor
San Jose State University
San Jose, California

Cheryl Hall Harris, RN, BSN
Director, Nursing Community Ethics Project
Midwest Bioethics Center
Kansas City, Missouri

Phyllis A. Johnson, RN, PhD
Associate Professor
School of Nursing
Georgia State University
Atlanta, Georgia

Sue A. Joines, RN, MSN
Assistant Nurse Manager
Stanford University Hospital
Stanford, California

Cheryl Pope Kish, RN, MSN, EdD
Associate Professor
School of Nursing
Georgia College
Milledgeville, Georgia

Dorothy Lemmey, RNC, MSN
Assistant Professor
Maternity Nursing
Lakeland Community College
Mentor, Ohio

Rana K. Limbo, RN, MS, MSN
Outpatient Therapist
Lutheran Hospital-LaCrosse
LaCrosse, Wisconsin

Deitra Leonard Lowdermilk, RNC, PhD
Clinical Associate Professor
School of Nursing
University of North Carolina at Chapel Hill
Chapel Hill, North Carolina

Susan Mattson, RNC, PhD, CTN
Associate Professor
California State University at Long Beach
Long Beach, California

Carolyn F. McCain, RN, MSN
(Former) Asst. Professor
School of Nursing
University of North Carolina
Chapel Hill, North Carolina

Mary Courtney Moore, RN, RD, MSN, PhD, CNSN
Vanderbilt University
Nashville, Tennessee

Shannon E. Perry, RN, PhD, FAAN
Professor and Vice Chair, Graduate Program
Department of Nursing
San Francisco State University
San Francisco, California

Judy Poole, RNC, MN, ACCE
Perinatal Outreach Education Coordinator
Carolinas Medical Center
Department of Obstetrics-Gynecology
Charlotte, North Carolina

Edna B. Quinn, RN, PhD, CNM
Professor of Nursing
Salisbury State University
Salisbury, Maryland

Mary M. Reeve, RN, EdD,
Associate Professor
San Jose State University
San Jose, California

Jane R. Starn, RNC, DrPH, ACCE
Associate Professor
School of Nursing
University of Hawaii
Honolulu, Hawaii

Helen Stetson, RN, EdD, ACCE
Emerita
San Francisco State University
Associate Professor
University of San Francisco
San Francisco, California

Karen A. Stevens, RN, MSN, FNP, PhD
Assistant Professor
Catholic University
Washington, DC

Cecilia Tiller, RN, DSN
Assistant Professor
Department of Parent-Child Nursing
Medical College of Georgia
Augusta, Georgia

Susan M. Tucker, RN, MSN
Director of Nursing, MCH
Kaiser Permanente Medical Center
Panorama City, California

Joyce H. Vogler, RN, MS, ACCE
Assistant Professor
School of Nursing
University of Hawaii
Honolulu, Hawaii

Sara Wheeler, RN, MSN
Associate Professor
Lakeview College of Nursing
Danville, Illinois
Certified Grief Consultant, Grief, Ltd.
Covington, Indiana

Philomena Whelan, RNC, MS
Nurse Manager
Stanford University Hospital
Stanford, California

Susan C. Wieczorek, RN, MSN
Assistant Professor
Department of Nursing
Columbus College
Columbus, Georgia

Rhea P. Williams, RN, PhD
Associate Professor
California State University
Los Angeles, California

PREVIOUS EDITIONS

Iris E. Campbell, RN, SCM, MTD, MN
Assistant Professor
Faculty of Nursing
University of Alberta
Edmonton, Canada

Diane S. Charsha, RNC, MSN
MCH Clinical Specialist
Shore Memorial Hospital
Somers Point, New Jersey

Debra I. Craig, RN, MSN
Assistant Professor of Nursing
Point Loma Nazarene College
San Diego, California

Barbara A. Derwinski-Robinson, RN, MSN
Associate Professor
Montana State University
Billings, Montana

Cheryl Harris, RN, BSN
Staff Nurse
Neonatal Intensive Care Unit
Children's Mercy Hospital
Kansas City, Missouri

Charlotte D. Kain, RNC, EdD
Professor of Nursing
Montgomery County Community College
Blue Bell, Pennsylvania

Susan Weiner, RNC, MSN
Perinatal Nurse Clinician
Thomas Jefferson University Hospital
Philadelphia, Pennsylvania

Joan Edelstein, RN, PNP, DrPH
Associate Professor
San Jose State University
San Jose, California

Beverly Gaglione, RN, PhD
Chairperson, Director of Nursing
Professor of Parent Child Nursing
East Stroudsburg University
East Stroudsburg, Pennsylvania

Carla D. Harris, RNC, MSN
Nurse Practitioner, Associate Professor of Nursing
California State University
Instructional Design Associate
Huntington Beach, California

Beverly Horn, RN, PhD
Associate Professor, School of Nursing
University of Washington
Seattle, Washington

Linda Lee Miller, RN, MS
Instructor, San Jose State University
San Jose, California

Barbara Petree, RN, MA
Clinical Nursing Coordinator, Delivery Room
Stanford University Hospital
Stanford, California

Celeste Phillips, RN, EdD
Director of Nursing Education, Maternity Nursing Instructor
Cabrillo College
Aptos, California

M. Colleen Stainton, RN, DNS
Assistant Dean
Research and Development Professor, Faculty of Nursing
The University of Calgary
Alberta, Canada

Lucille Whaley, RN, EdD
Professor Emeritus, San Jose State University
San Jose, California
University of Southern California
Los Angeles, California

Consultant Panel

Marilyn Abraham, BSN
Instructor, Department of Nursing
University of South Dakota
Vermillion, South Dakota

Bernadine Adams, BSN, MN
Associate Professor
School of Nursing
Northeast Louisiana University
Monroe, Louisiana

Maria Alvarez Amaya, RN, PhD
Associate Professor
College of Nursing and Allied Health
University of Texas at El Paso
El Paso, Texas

Claudia Beckman, RN, PhD
Associate Professor
University of Wisconsin
Milwaukee, Wisconsin

Eleanor (Lee) Brown, RNC, MSN
Assistant Professor
Macon College
Macon, Georgia

Sandra Godman Brown, RN, DSN
Assistant Professor
College of Nursing
Medical University of South Carolina
Charleston, South Carolina

Iris E. Campbell, RN, SCM, MTD, MN
Assistant Professor
Faculty of Nursing
University of Alberta
Edmonton, Alberta, Canada

Jacquelyn Campbell, RN, PhD, FAAN
Associate Professor
College of Nursing
Wayne State University
Detroit, Michigan

Penny Cass, RN, PhD
Dean
College of Nursing
University of Wisconsin Oshkosh
Oshkosh, Wisconsin

Nancy L. Chapman, BSN, MSN
Nursing Faculty
Trident Technical College
Charleston, South Carolina

Carol Cobb, MSN
Department of Nursing
Pensacola Junior College
Pensacola, Florida

Patricia Collier, MS, CRN, NP
Assistant Professor of Nursing
SUNY School of Nursing
Stony Brook, New York

Joan Corder-Mabe, RN, MS, OGNP
Instructor
Medical College of Virginia
Richmond, Virginia

Maxine Dine, RN, BNSc, BA, BAEd
Professor, Nursing Program
Durham College
Oshawa, Ontario, Canada

Barbara Doetsch, RN, MA
Associate Professor
Orange County Community College
Middletown, New York

Mary Kay Fallon, RNC, MS, MAEd
Perinatal Clinical Nurse Specialist
Barnes Hospital
St. Louis, Missouri

Ruth Holmes Ferguson, RN, MS
Associate Professor
Tidewater Community College
Portsmouth, Virginia

Elaine Gebhart, RNC, PhD
Maternal/Child Specialist
University of Texas
Arlington, Texas

Winifred M. Gordon, RN, SCM
Professor, Nursing Programs
Durham College
Oshawa, Ontario, Canada

Kristine Henderer, RNC, EdD
Assistant Professor
School of Nursing
University of Portland
Portland, Oregon

Pearl Herbert, RN, SCM, BN, MSc
Assistant Professor
Nursing Department
Memorial University of Newfoundland
St. John's, Newfoundland, Canada

Phyllis Johnson, RN, PhD
Associate Professor
School of Nursing
Georgia State University
Atlanta, Georgia

Pamela Jordan, RN, PhD
Associate Professor
School of Nursing
University of Washington
Seattle, Washington

Joan Keller-Maresh, RNC, MSN
Associate Professor
Department of Nursing
Viterbo College
LaCrosse, Wisconsin

Cheryl Pope Kish, RN, MSN, EdD
Associate Professor and Coordinator
Maternal-Child Nursing
School of Nursing
Georgia College
Milledgeville, Georgia

Phyllis M. Klein, RN, MSN
Clinical Specialist
Maternal-Infant Nursing
Fairfax, Virginia

Muriel Larson, BA, RN
Instructor of Nursing
University of South Dakota
Vermillion, South Dakota

Maureen Laryea, SRN, SCM, BA, MPhiL
Associate Professor
School of Nursing
Memorial University of Newfoundland
St. John's, Newfoundland, Canada

Shirley M. Lund, BSN, MSN
Nursing Instructor
University of South Dakota
Vermillion, South Dakota

Nancy McKee, RN, DNS
Professor and Chair,
Undergraduate Nursing Studies
Indiana State University
Terre Haute, Indiana

M. Kay Matthews, BN, MN, SCM
Assistant Professor
School of Nursing
Memorial University of Newfoundland
St. Johns, Newfoundland, Canada

Janice Mirecki, RN, MN
Instructor, Perinatal Nursing
Red River Community College
Winnipeg, Manitoba, Canada

Gwen Lynn Nelson, RN, BSN, CNOR
Perioperative Staff Development Instructor
Pennsylvania Hospital
Philadelphia, Pennsylvania

Theresa L. Piekut, RNC, MSN
Professor/Dept. Head of Nursing
Comm. College of Allegheny County/South Campus
West Mifflin, Pennsylvania

Karen A. Piotrowski, RNC, MSN
Assistant Professor
Division of Nursing
D'Youville College
Buffalo, New York

Victoria L. Poole, RN, DSN
Assistant Professor
School of Nursing
University of Alabama at Birmingham
Birmingham, Alabama

Carol A. Rusin, RN, EdD
Professor
Trocaire College
Buffalo, New York

Edith C. Sanchez, RNC, MEd, MSN
Instructor, Associate Degree in Nursing
South Suburban College
South Holland, Illinois

Kathleen Rice Simpson, RNC, MSN
Perinatal Clinical Nurse Specialist
St. John's Mercy Medical Center
St. Louis, Missouri
Clinical Instructor, School of Nursing
University of Missouri-St. Louis
St. Louis, Missouri

Rachel Spector, RN, CTN, PhD
Associate Professor
Boston College School of Nursing
Chestnut Hill, Massachusetts

Susan Speraw, RN, PhD
Clinical Assistant Professor of Nursing
University of Southern California
Los Angeles, California

Karen Stevens, RN, MSN, CFNP, PhD
Assistant Professor
School of Nursing
Catholic University
Washington, DC

Margaret C. Taylor, RN, PhD
Associate Professor,
School of Nursing and Allied Health
University of Guam
Guam

Judy Van Schoiak, BSN, PNP
Instructor
Columbia Basin College
Pasco, Washington

Tina Weitkamp, RNC, MSN
Assistant Professor of Clinical Nursing
University of Cincinnati
Cincinnati, Ohio

Sarah E. Whitaker, RNC, MSN, DNSc
Lecturer
University of Texas-El Paso
El Paso, Texas

To the memory of my parents, Susan and Joseph Bobak, who
provided a good beginning;
to my family and friends who encourage me and cheer me on;
to my colleagues who supply the professional inspiration;
to my students who motivate me.

I.M.B.

To my husband, Emil Nicholai Jensen, whose love, support,
and encouragement have given meaning to my life.

M.D.J.

Preface

Maternity and gynecologic nursing offers a unique combination of challenge and opportunity. Nurses are challenged to assimilate a tremendous, ever-growing body of scientific knowledge and to develop the technical and analytic skills necessary to apply that knowledge to practice. Each client presents a new challenge, for individual needs must be identified and met. The opportunities, however, are sufficiently extraordinary to make this one of the most fulfilling specialties in nursing practice.

The goal of nursing education is to prepare today's student to meet tomorrow's challenge. This preparation must extend beyond mastery of facts and skills. Nurses must be able to combine competence with caring. They must address both physiologic and psychosocial needs. Above all, they must look beyond the condition and see the client as an individual with specialized needs.

Maternity and Gynecologic Care: The Nurse and the Family was developed to provide students with the knowledge they need to become competent nurses and the sensitivity they need to become caring nurses. This fifth edition has been revised and refined in response to comments and suggestions from both students and educators. It includes the most accurate, current, and clinically relevant information available; it presents that information in a clearly written, visually appealing, logical format.

■ APPROACH

Professional nursing practice continues to evolve and adapt to society's changing health priorities. Nursing education must also reflect these changes, as well as the needs of nursing students. This fifth edition of *Maternity and Gynecologic Care* was designed to meet the unique needs of clients and students in the 1990s.

Today's students are challenged to learn more than ever before and often in less time than their predecessors. We have, therefore, refined the focus of this revision, clearly and succinctly presenting the content most relevant to current practice. Particular attention has been given to the *reading level* to ensure that students in all types of nursing programs would readily understand the material.

To ensure a logical and consistent presentation of material, the five-step *nursing process* has been used as the organizing framework. Each step is specially highlighted throughout the text for emphasis and clarity. Boxed case studies with related nursing care plans reinforce the problem-solving approach for client care.

Health care today emphasizes *wellness*. This focus is an integral part of our philosophy that pregnancy and childbirth are part of the natural developmental process. We therefore present the entire normal childbearing cycle before discussing potential complications. Likewise, the developmental changes a woman experiences throughout her life are considered to be natural and normal. In women's health care the goal is promotion of wellness for the woman through knowledge of her body and its normal functioning throughout her life span, while developing an awareness of conditions that require professional intervention. We believe that students need to thoroughly understand and recognize the normal processes and conditions before they can identify complications and comprehend their implications for care. Content on common gynecologic problems has been expanded and a new chapter on women's health promotion and screening has been added to emphasize the wellness focus of this aspect of nursing.

Teaching for self-care has become an essential component of nursing care. A new chapter on home care after childbirth discusses the nurse's role in teaching self-care and in providing follow-up care after today's shorter hospital stays. The chapter on women's health promotion and screening emphasizes teaching for self-care to promote wellness and encourage preventive care. Special boxed elements highlight client teaching topics throughout the text.

In order to implement *preventive* care, perinatal and gynecologic nurses must be able to recognize signs and symptoms of emergent problems. Throughout the discussions of assessment and care we alert the nurse to signs of potential problems and provide references to pertinent content in the complications unit. Boxes throughout the text highlight warning signs as well as emergency situations.

Today's perinatal and women's health nurses will encounter clients from many diverse ethnic backgrounds. *Cultural implications* are integrated throughout the text to emphasize the wide range of ethnic diversity and its impact on maternity and gynecologic care. The newly revised culture chapter focuses on specific customs related to childbearing and women's health and stresses the importance of assessing both the nurse's *and* the client's cultural beliefs.

To truly meet the specific needs of each client, the nurse must include family members and significant others in the plan of care. *Family dynamics* are rarely more prominent than in pregnancy and childbirth, and the nurse is often the family's primary advocate. Three separate chapters on the family, including grandparents and siblings, as well as integrated considerations throughout, stress the importance of the entire family.

Nursing research has become an integral part of nursing education as well as practice. The chapter on nursing research has been revised to focus on current research methods and the application of research to maternity and gynecologic nursing. In addition, boxed research highlights throughout the text demonstrate the relevance of research to practice.

■ FEATURES

The contemporary new design features larger, bolder print and a more spacious presentation. Students will find that the logical, easy-to-follow headings and *attractive two-color design* highlights important content and increases visual appeal. A *new full-color insert* features photographs of childbirth and newborn assessment. Hundreds of photographs and drawings illustrate important concepts and techniques to further enhance comprehension.

Student learning aids in each chapter include objectives, key terms bold-faced and defined in the narrative, and a Chapter Review. These new Chapter Reviews include key concepts, key terms followed by references to the page in the chapter where the definition is located, **critical thinking exercises**, and questions for nursing research. The key concepts and key terms help students evaluate what they have learned; the critical thinking exercises and questions for nursing research guide them in applying that knowledge.

Nursing process is presented in narrative discussion as well as in case studies and care plans. The narrative discusses client care within the nursing process framework. Case studies illustrate how to apply each of the 5 steps to a specific client with a unique set of problems. Each case study is accompanied by a care plan that is based on the nursing diagnoses derived in the case study. Care plans include client-centered goals, interventions with rationales, and evaluative criteria.

Special boxed elements highlight nursing research, client teaching topics, and emergency situations. Each of the boxed elements has a unique treatment for easy visual identification. *Teaching* boxes supplement the narrative and emphasize the importance of teaching for self-care. *Emergency* boxes alert students to the signs and symptoms of various emergency situations and provide immediate nursing interventions. *Research Highlights* have been expanded to include abstracts, implications for practice, and questions for related nursing research to stress the relevance of both current and future research to practice.

Although childbearing is a normal process, complications can and do occur. During assessment the nurse must always be alert for *signs of potential problems*. We have, therefore, included signs of potential problems in the assessment sections in the normal units, and refer students to relevant content in complications units.

New to this edition is the *Quick Reference for Maternity and Gynecologic Nursing* that is complimentary with each copy of the text. This informative, pocket-sized booklet will be invaluable to students in the clinical setting. Also new is the *Student Learning Guide,* which provides exercises and activities to enhance learning and understanding.

■ ORGANIZATION

The fifth edition of *Maternity and Gynecologic Care* comprises eight units organized to enhance understanding and learning and to facilitate easy retrieval of information.

Unit 1, *"Foundations for Contemporary Practice,"* begins with an overview of contemporary perinatal and women's health nursing practice, then addresses the family as a unit of care. The cultural beliefs relevant to childbearing and women's health are presented and the importance of assessing both the nurse's and the client's beliefs is stressed. Legal and ethical issues and nursing research in maternity and gynecologic nursing are also discussed. The unit concludes with an overview of the reproductive system.

Unit 2, Normal Pregnancy, describes nursing care of the woman and her family from conception through preparation for childbirth. A separate chapter on maternal and fetal nutrition emphasizes this important aspect of care, highlighting the impact of cultural variations on diet and the importance of early recognition of nutritional problems.

Unit 3, Normal Childbirth, focuses on the collaboration among physician, nurse, woman, and family during the process of labor and delivery. Separate chapters deal with the nurse's role in the pharmacologic relief of discomfort and fetal monitoring. These chapters familiarize students with the modalities currently in use and focus on interventions to support and educate the woman and her family.

Unit 4, Normal Newborn, addresses the immediate assessment and care of the newborn. Information on the nutritional needs of the newborn and nursing care associated with breast-feeding and formula-feeding is highlighted in a separate chapter.

Unit 5, Normal Postpartum, deals with a time of significant change for the entire family. The mother requires both physical and emotional support as she adjusts to her new role. A separate chapter discusses family dynamics in response to the birth of a child. A new chapter on home care discusses the nurse's role in providing follow up care after today's shorter hospital stays.

Unit 6, Complications of Childbearing, reviews in detail the maternal conditions that place the mother, fetus, and newborn at risk. Nursing interventions focus on achieving the best possible outcome, as well as supporting the woman and her family when their expectations are not met. A separate chapter discusses adolescent sexuality, pregnancy, and parenthood.

Unit 7, Newborn Complications, has been expanded and reorganized to address the trend of caring for the moderately compromised newborn in the normal nursery. The unit presents general care of the newborn with complications and then details the most common developmental and acquired conditions. A separate chapter on loss and grief discusses nursing care of the family experiencing a maternal, fetal, or neonatal loss.

Unit 8, Women's Health, discusses preventive, curative, and rehabilitative nursing care of women throughout the life span. The unit opens with a new chapter on health promotion and screening, then presents fertility management and violence against women. The chapter on neoplasia has been expanded and includes both benign and malignant conditions.

The text concludes with a glossary of all important terms, appendices that provide valuable resource information, and a detailed, cross-referenced index.

■ TEACHING AND LEARNING PACKAGE

A number of ancillaries to this textbook have been developed to assist instructors and students in the teaching and learning process. These include an *Instructor's Resource Manual* and *Test Bank, a Student Learning Guide,* a computerized test bank, a set of overhead transparency acetates, and a *Quick Reference for Maternity and Gynecologic Nursing.*

The *Instructor's Resource Manual and Test Bank* is keyed chapter by chapter to the text to help coordinate course objectives to chapter content. Each chapter includes an outline of content with course guidelines, suggested learning activities, and student worksheets. These worksheets can be copied and used as a handout to reinforce learning and evaluate comprehension. The worksheets are also reproduced in the *Student Learning Guide,* which can be purchased separately or packaged with the text. The test bank includes more than 500 questions that parallel the new NCLEX format. The answer key provides page references and coding of questions according to the NCLEX test plan categories of nursing process and client needs, as well as level of difficulty.

CompuTest, a *computerized test bank,* is also available and aids instructors using computers in test construction. All questions on the disks are printed in the Instructor's Resource Manual.

The *overhead transparency* set of 50 two-color illustrations provides an additional resource for instructors. These illustrations were selected for their instructional value in lectures and classroom discussions.

The NEW *Quick Reference for Maternity and Gynecologic Nursing* is a valuable resource for students in the clinical setting. This pocket-size reference features assessment guides, nursing interventions for various complications and emergency situations, and guidelines for medications commonly used in the perinatal and gynecologic settings. This handy resource is complimentary with each copy of the text.

■ ■ ■

We are fully aware of the increasingly important contribution men are making to the nursing profession, as well as the growing number of women entering the medical profession. However, the construction of the English language sometimes makes it awkward to totally eliminate the feminine and masculine pronouns. Therefore to present material clearly and consistently, we have occasionally used the feminine pronoun to refer to the nurse and the masculine pronoun to refer to the physician.

Over the years we have received many comments and suggestions regarding our texts. We have incorporated many of these suggestions in the organization and development of this edition. We welcome comments from instructors, students, and practitioners who use this text so that we may continue to be responsive to the needs of the profession.

Irene M. Bobak

Acknowledgments

I wish to thank everyone whose comments and suggestions contributed to this collaborative effort, especially the reviewers who provided such valuable feedback in their evaluation of the manuscript.

A special "thank you" is offered for the shared expertise and/or photographs to the staffs of Stanford University Medical Center, Stanford, California; Swedish Hospital and Medical Center, Seattle, Washington; Kaiser-Permanente Hospital and Santa Clara Valley Medical Center, Santa Clara, California; St. Luke's Hospital, Kansas City, Missouri; Jewish Hospital and Barnes Hospital, St. Louis, Missouri; Mills Memorial Hospital, San Mateo, California; Mt. Zion Medical Center, San Francisco, California; Young People Young Parents, St. Louis, Missouri; Resolve Through Sharing, Lutheran Hospital-La Crosse, La Crosse, Wisconsin; Vogler/Perinatal Health Care Consultants, Kailua, Hawaii; Victoria Kepler Didato, Child Sexual Abuse Institute of Ohio; Cynthia J. Evans, Seattle, Washington; Doris Hisey, CareLink, Home Perinatal Services, Saratoga, California; Barbara J. Limandri, Portland, Oregon; Lisa Livingston, Maternal Child Health Education, Community Birth Center, Community Hospital, Santa Cruz, California.

I would like to thank the following photographers: Judith Bamber, San Jose, California; Joan Edelstein and Ralph Levy, San Jose, California; Chris Cowing and son, San Mateo, California; Paul and Janet Ho and their children Shubert and Candice, Milpitas, California; Ralph Johnson, Pam Lesser and Hillary, St. Louis, Missouri; Capt. Barbara Kalmen and family, Edwards AFB, California; Sarah Keating and family, Mill Valley, California; Dottie Kauffmann, Goshen, Indiana; Jonas McKoy, Chapel Hill, North Carolina; Casey Mowry, Wanda Martin, and Michelle Reid and their families, Denver, Colorado; Nancy Mason and family, Palo Alto, California; Claudia Miller and family, El Granada, California, and her mother, Victoria Chiofalo, San Francisco, California; Hollie Stephens and family, New Jersey; Jack and Judi Teng and son, San Mateo, California; Vivian Wahlberg, Karolinska, Stockholm, Sweden; M. Colleen Stainton, Calgary, Alberta, Canada; and the Yorde family, Marshall, Minnesota.

I am indebted to these families who embody the philosophic basis for this text—family-centered nursing care.

Others have also made contributions of value. Two nursing students in particular have shared their knowledge and insights: Judi Regan Rudis, Parkland College, Champaign, Illinois, and Cynthia Navarro, San Francisco State University, San Francisco, California. Kathy Aderhold, CNM, Adolescent Pregnancy Project, Presbyterian/St. Luke's Medical Center, Denver, Colorado, and Kathy Hanold, RN, MS, Birth Place, Barnes Hospital at Washington University Medical Center, St. Louis, Missouri, found time in their respective practices to obtain hard-to-get photographs. Shannon Perry, San Francisco State University, San Francisco, California, provided the Research Highlights that appear throughout the text.

This edition contains artwork by George Wassilchenko, Broken Arrow, Oklahoma, whose precise, detailed anatomic drawings have made a substantial contribution to the study of complex theory. I look forward to a continuing association with this outstanding medical illustrator.

Special words of gratitude are extended to Nancy Coon, Suzi Epstein, Beverly Copland and Jim Russell of Mosby for their encouragement, inspiration, and assistance in the preparation and production of this text, I acknowledge the assistance of my family, both concrete and supportive, I thank Deitra Leonard Lowdermilk for her major role in this revision and we thank each other for the stimulation, support, and mutual respect generated by this collaboration. To Margaret Duncan Jensen, with whom I co-authored the first four editions of this text, I owe a special debt of gratitude; the thirteen years of collaboration have left me with many fond memories of her and her husband, Emil.

Irene M. Bobak

Contents in Brief

CONTENTS

Unit 3 NORMAL CHILDBIRTH

Unit 4 NORMAL NEWBORN

Fifth Edition

MATERNITY & GYNECOLOGIC CARE

The Nurse and the Family

unit

Foundations for Contemporary Practice

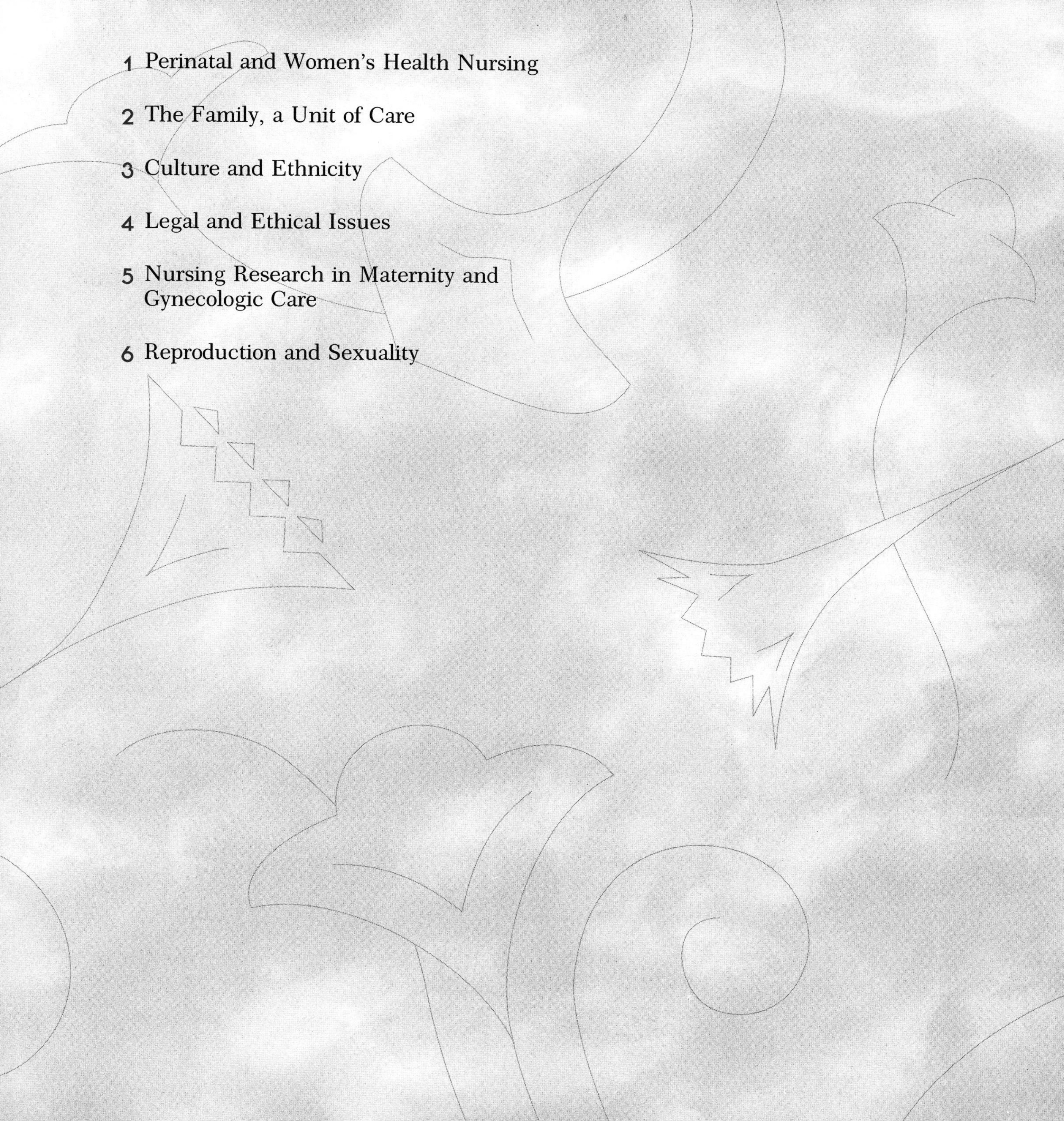

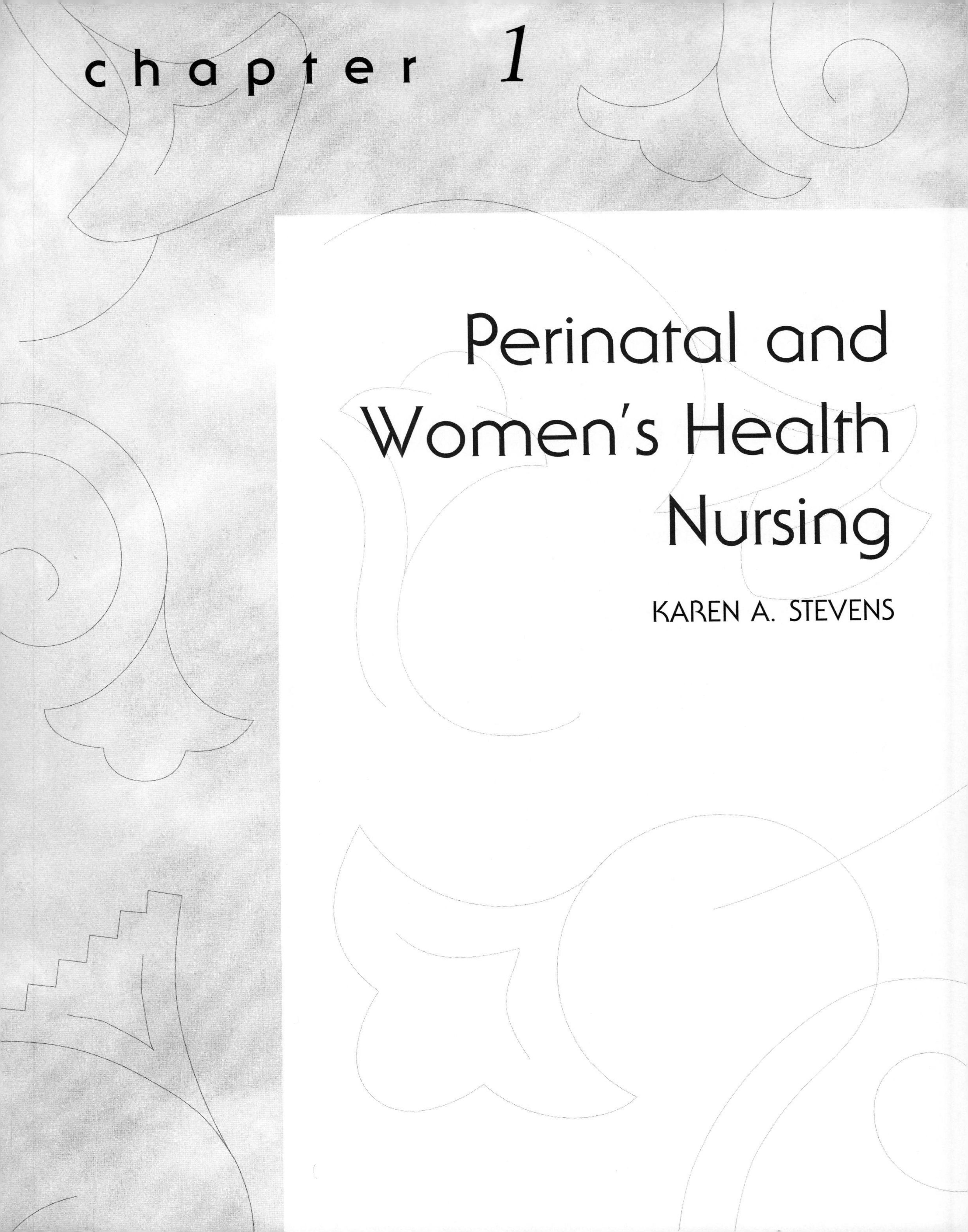

chapter 1

Perinatal and Women's Health Nursing

KAREN A. STEVENS

LEARNING OBJECTIVES

- Define key terms.
- Describe the scope of perinatal and women's health nursing.
- State the settings in which perinatal and women's health nurses work.
- Describe the roles of the perinatal and women's health nurse.
- Describe the professional options in perinatal and women's health nursing.
- Explain certification for perinatal and women's health nurses.
- State the contemporary issues and trends of perinatal and women's health nursing.
- Define important statistical terms.
- Cite several nursing models that may be particularly useful to perinatal and women's health nurses.
- Cite other compatible theories useful to perinatal and women's health nurses.
- Describe the use of critical thinking through the use of the nursing process in perinatal and women's health nursing.
- Describe wellness nursing diagnoses.
- Identify topics for nursing research related to perinatal and women's health nursing.

According to the standards of **NAACOG**: The Organization for Obstetric, Gynecologic, and Neonatal Nurses, "obstetric, gynecologic, and neonatal nursing practice addresses the health-care needs of women and infants in a holistic approach designed to meet the physical, psychological, and spiritual needs of individuals and families" (NAACOG Standards, 1991, p. 3). Obstetric and neonatal nursing focuses on the perinatal period (the time from the beginning of the pregnancy through the first 4 weeks of the infant's life) (Ouimette, 1986). The **perinatal nurse** therefore cares for childbearing families through all stages of pregnancy, birth, and early parenting. During the prenatal period, the nurse monitors the course of pregnancy, evaluates the well-being of the fetus, and prepares the family for childbirth. During labor and birth, the nurse assesses the progress of labor, monitors the status of the mother and baby, assists with comfort measures, and supports the family. After birth, the nurse enhances the mother-baby relationship, aids in the mother's recovery, and teaches newborn care. The neonatal nurse cares for healthy newborns through assessment and maintenance of the transition to extrauterine life as well as through counseling and education of parents. Some neonatal nurses work in neonatal intensive care units that provide highly technical nursing care to high-risk newborns (NAACOG Women's Health Nurse Practitioner, 1990; NAACOG OGN Nursing, Shaping the Future, 1991; NAACOG Standards, 1991).

Gynecologic nursing focuses on the special physical, psychologic and social needs of women throughout their life spans (NAACOG Standards, 1991). In the past, gynecologic nurses predominantly intervened in serious reproductive health problems or in surgery requiring in-hospital or ambulatory care. Now gynecologic nurses also educate women about health as well as counsel about sexuality issues, healthy aging, osteoporosis prevention, exercise, nutrition, and diet (NAACOG Women's Health Nurse Practitioner, 1990; NAACOG Standards, 1991; NAACOG OGN Nursing, Shaping the Future, 1991).

There was a time when care during childbearing and for reproductive problems was the mainstay of "women's health." Today the health care system has broadened its focus to include not only perinatal nursing but also an expanded, more diverse consideration of women's health issues. As a result of influences from the women's movement and changes in society, women's health now means being concerned about the overall experience of women, not only women's diseases or childbearing functions, but also women's general physical and psychologic well-being. Thus **women's health nursing** incorporates not only concern and investigation of conditions unique to women (such as certain reproductive malignancies and menopause), but also sociocultural and occupational factors that may be related to the health problems of women (such as poverty, lower wages, rape, incest, sexual harassment, and family violence) (Boeke, 1991). Nurses caring for women have played an active role in shaping the health care system so that it is more responsive to the needs of contemporary women (Boeke, 1991), and nurses have been "critically important" (Styles, 1990, p. 347) in developing strategies to improve the well-being of women and their infants (Styles, 1990).

The focus of this book is perinatal and women's health nursing, and this chapter presents a general overview of the subject. First, the scope of practice and roles of perinatal and women's health nurses are described. Second, other professional options in this specialty are discussed. Third, issues and trends in perinatal and women's health are cited. Finally, the conceptual and theoretic bases of perinatal and women's health nursing practice are mentioned.

■ PERINATAL AND WOMEN'S HEALTH NURSES

Nurses in the perinatal or women's health specialties are registered nurses who have graduated from a diploma, associate's degree, or baccalaureate educational program. In addition, they have successfully completed the state's licensure examination and are licensed to practice in that state. Perinatal and women's health nurses work in a variety of settings. Probably the most common setting is the hospital, where nurses may work in prenatal clinics, labor and delivery units, antepartum units, nurseries, neonatal intensive care units, postpartum units, women's health clinics, or as childbirth educators. In addition, nurses may work in birthing centers, physicians' offices, community health agencies, or government agencies (such as a community health department). Finally, perinatal and women's health nurses may also work in schools or within their own practices.

Perinatal and Women's Health Nursing Roles

Perinatal and **women's health nursing** roles include caregiver, teacher/educator, advocate, manager, researcher, political activist, and change agent.

CAREGIVER. The nurse practicing in perinatal and women's health uses the nursing process to maximize the health of women and newborns. Nursing care typically involves preventive, curative, and rehabilitative aspects of women's health care during childbearing and throughout their lives (Menard, 1987; Kelly, 1991).

TEACHER/EDUCATOR. The perinatal and women's health nurse is especially active as an educator. Assessing a client's educational needs is based on information obtained from assessing the client's learning needs. Both individual and group teaching programs in childbearing and women's health/illness are provided to enhance the health of women and their newborns (Menard, 1987; Kelly, 1991).

ADVOCATE. A nurse often acts as a liaison, or advocate, between the client and the health care delivery system by encouraging client awareness of health care rights and responsibilities and by helping the client make informed decisions. Because the nurse emphasizes holistic care, it is possible to recognize the client's various needs and explain the options and services available to the client (Kelly, 1991).

MANAGER. In a sense, all nurses are managers when they prioritize client needs and organize care so that the client receives the greatest benefit with the least expense of time and material. Total client care requires more formal management skill in coordinating and facilitating services. Team leaders or charge nurses also manage when they direct the care of client groups and nursing personnel. The role of manager also involves minimizing costs and enhancing and evaluating the quality of care in relation to established nursing standards (Menard, 1987; Kelly, 1991).

RESEARCHER. More nurses are becoming involved in nursing research, either as participants or consumers. Particularly important is research that investigates the effectiveness of nursing interventions, clinical methods, or protocols. Nurses also evaluate current research findings for application to practice (Menard, 1987; Kelly, 1991).

POLITICAL ACTIVIST. Nurses are encouraged to play an active role in the political arena. This may mean merely becoming active in one's professional organizations and/or keeping current about legislative issues affecting childbearing and women's health, or it may mean writing letters to legislators about women's health issues. It is clear, however, that nurses need to have a voice in the political arena in order to advocate, influence, and advance the promotion of women's health (Kelly, 1991; Mason et al 1991; NAACOG Newsletter, 1991). The political participation behaviors of nurse-midwives have been studied (see Research Highlight, p. 6).

CHANGE AGENT. The nurse works within the health care setting to effect change that ensures women's access to quality health care throughout their lives (Papenhausen, 1990; NAACOG Standards, 1991). A nurse can stimulate awareness, concern, and subsequent change by working on utilization, quality assurance, or peer reviews committees; becoming active in professional organizations; or sharing pertinent articles and research findings. Careful action based on scientific facts and approached in a professional manner may cause change that enhances the quality of health care provided to women and their infants (Menard, 1987).

Other Professional Options

Many professional options are possible for nurses in the perinatal and women's health specialty.

CLINICAL NURSE SPECIALIST. According to Menard (1987, p. 15), a **clinical nurse specialist** is "an expert in a specialized area of nursing" who "serves as a role model of excellence in nursing knowledge and clinical practice." Specialists in perinatal and women's health therefore have increased their knowledge and skill in the perinatal or women's health area of nursing (Kelly, 1991; Zukowsky, Coburn, 1991). The expert knowledge and skill of a specialist is gained by formal education as well as experiential career ladders. Most typically, the title of clinical nurse specialist refers to a nurse who has completed a master's degree in perinatal or women's health. The clinical nurse specialist in perinatal and women's health nursing provides high-quality individualized care to women and newborns. In addition, the clinical specialist participates in educating health care professionals and paraprofessionals in the specialty area and participates in research that will improve client care. The clinical nurse specialist promotes cost effectiveness through discharge planning and utilization reviews and also consults with others in the health care system (Menard, 1987; Elder, Bullough, 1990; Kelly, 1991).

NURSE PRACTITIONER. According to NAACOG, the obstetric/gynecologic **nurse practitioner** is a registered professional nurse "who has successfully completed a formal obstetric/gynecologic women's health nurse practitioner program" (NAACOG Guidelines, 1990, p. 1). "The practitioner has acquired specialized knowledge and skills in health promotion and

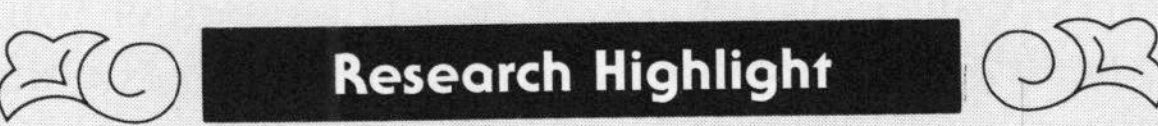

Political Participation Behaviors of Nurse-Midwives

RESEARCH ABSTRACT

A random sample of 600 certified nurse-midwives was surveyed by mailed questionnaire to ascertain political participation activities of this group of health care providers. The survey yielded 364 responses from midwives in 43 states. The majority were Caucasian and held master's degrees. Data were collected using a questionnaire that asked about political attitudes, political participation, organizational activities, women's issues and support activities, and general demographic information (age, education, etc.). Most of the midwives sampled were liberal, were Democrats, and had some interest in political affairs. Voting was the major political activity reported by the midwives. They also reported attending political meetings, working for a political candidate and sending letters to political leaders occasionally. They "rarely" or "never" engaged in protest activities. Since becoming midwives, more than half of the sample increased their professional organization activities, more than one third participated in voluntary community activities, and three fourths of the sample have worked for or actively supported women's issues.

IMPLICATIONS FOR PRACTICE

Leaders often emerge through professional organization activities. Participating in professional organizations and political activities often provides a training ground for leadership and therefore has the potential to influence health policy. Most of the midwives in this study were supportive of women's issues and could therefore become active in supporting legislation to promote women's health or in educating women about health issues. Midwives and other nurses should be encouraged to become active in organizations that promote the best interests of health care, nursing, and the clients they serve.

RELATED RESEARCH QUESTIONS

1. Do the political participation behaviors of nurse-midwives differ from other nurse specialists working in perinatal or women's health?
2. Does a professional nursing education program increase the participation of nurses in political action?
3. To what extent do perinatal and women's health nurses influence health policy?
4. Does a voter registration campaign increase the registration and voting behavior of nurses?

REFERENCE

Gesse T: Political participation behaviors of nurse-midwives, *J Nurse Midwifery* 36(3)184:1991.

maintenance, disease prevention, physical and psychosocial assessment, and management of health and illness in the primary care of women" (NAACOG Guidelines, 1990, p. 1). There is an emphasis on independent physical assessment as well as diagnosis and treatment of minor, stable conditions. In addition, health education and consideration of holistic care is stressed. Clients with complex, unstable conditions are usually referred to physicians or handled in consultation with a physician. The formal practitioner program may be either a master's degree or continuing education program (Kelly, 1991; Zukowsky, Coburn, 1991). There is a trend toward graduate educational programs for the nurse practitioner, however (Kelly, 1991; Zukowsky, Coburn, 1991). Although nurse practitioner care occurs in all settings, ambulatory care settings are the most common (NAACOG Women's Health Nurse Practitioner, 1990; Kelly, 1991; Zukowsky, Coburn, 1991).

NEONATAL NURSES. The National Association of Neonatal Nurses (NANN) defines the **neonatal nurse** practitioner as "a registered nurse with clinical expertise in neonatal nursing who has received formal education with supervised clinical experience in the management of sick newborns and their families" (National Association of Neonatal Nurses, 1989). Responsibilities may include "managing patient care in an intensive care unit, conducting normal newborn assessments and physical examinations, and providing high-risk follow-up visits" (NANN, 1989, p. 128). There are two tracks for becoming a neonatal nurse practitioner: a hospital-based continuing education program (the nurse receives a certificate upon completion) and a university-based master's degree program (Zukowsky, Coburn, 1991). The certificate program is usually a relatively short-term, intense program (typically about 9 months) covering physical assessment, diagnosis, and management skills, with varying amounts of teaching and counseling information. The master's preparation is longer (typically 1 to 2 years) and provides a broader foundation in nursing theory, advanced sciences, initial research skills, and leadership strategies. Those with a master's degree are prepared to be leaders and change agents as well as care providers. Neonatal nurse practitioners are employed in a physician group or may work in neonatal intensive care units, normal newborn nurseries, neonatal follow-up clinics, or in transporting the sick neonate (Zukowsky, Coburn, 1991).

CERTIFICATION. **Licensure** as a registered nurse is mandatory, is granted by the state, and signifies that the nurse has met the minimum requirements for general nursing practice. **Certification,** on the other hand, is voluntary. It signifies that the nurse has met minimum standards as established by professional peers in the nursing specialty (Menard, 1987). NAACOG: The Organization for Obstetric, Gynecologic, and Neonatal Nurses supports the certification programs of the National Certification Corporation (NCC)* for obstetric, gynecologic, women's health, and neonatal nursing specialties. It administers the following certification examinations in perinatal and women's health:

- Obstetric/gynecologic nurse practitioner
- In-hospital obstetric nurse
- Neonatal intensive care nurse
- Neonatal nurse practitioner
- Low-risk neonatal nurse
- Reproductive endocrinology/infertility
- Ambulatory women's health (slated to be available in 1992)

All nurses taking these certification examinations must have graduated from a program acceptable to the NCC but need not have a master's degree. Experience eligibility requirements must be met, however. Upon satisfactory completion of the certification examination, the designation of Registered Nurse Certified (RNC) in that subspecialty can be used by the nurse (The National Certification Program, 1992).

NURSE-MIDWIFE. According to Lops (1988), a **nurse-midwife** is a registered nurse, usually with a bachelor's degree, who has typically taken a midwifery educational program at the master's level. Nurse-midwives provide relatively independent care for women during normal childbearing and for women with minor gynecologic conditions. Settings for care include primary care settings in health maintenance organizations, community health programs, alternative birth centers, private practice, and medical center teams. Most are employed by hospitals, especially public hospitals where midwives provide a cost-effective alternative to physician care (Lops, 1988). High-risk clients as well as those experiencing unexpected complications are referred to physicians (American College of Nurse Midwives, 1987). The American College of Nurse Midwives is the official accrediting agency for educational programs in nurse-midwifery. It defines qualifications, delineates professional roles and functions, and establishes standards of practice (American College of Nurse Midwives, 1987). In addition, it administers the National Certification Examination to graduates of accredited programs. Thus a certified nurse-midwife is "an individual educated in the two disciplines of nursing and midwifery, who possesses evidence of certification according to the requirements of the American College of Nurse Midwives" (Lops, 1988, p. 402).

*645 N. Michigan Avenue, Chicago, Illinois 60611; 312-952-0207.

■ CONTEMPORARY ISSUES AND TRENDS

In this section, various trends and issues regarding perinatal and women's health nursing will be addressed.

Statistical Basis

Analyzing vital statistics is necessary to recognize trends that reveal the use and effectiveness of health care services to women during childbearing and throughout life. Data obtained from health surveys provide a method of determining particular needs and problems. Statistical data concerning trends may also be used to analyze relationships between particular factors influencing health, to evaluate the success of specific nursing interventions, to determine priorities of care, or to estimate staffing needs. Table 1-1 defines statistical terminology useful in analyzing perinatal and women's health care.

TRENDS IN BIRTHRATE, FERTILITY, AND AGE AT TIME OF BIRTH. Particularly important to the perinatal and women's health specialty are fertility and birthrate trends. The most recent statistics available come from 1988 and indicate that since 1970 the birthrate has varied little (ranging from 15.5 to 15.9) (US Department of Health and Human Services, 1990).

Birthrates are typically analyzed by age of the woman at the time of birth. Birthrates for women in their twenties increased only slightly, remaining essentially the same from the middle 1970s until 1988. Teenagers and women age 35 to 44 had the largest increase in births. The birthrate for young teens (age 15 to 17) increased 6%, reaching its highest level since 1977. For older teens (age 18 to 19), the rate increased 2%, but remained within the same narrow range since 1976. Because of shifts in the birthrate by age and because of changes in the age distribu-

TABLE 1-1 Perinatal and Women's Health Biostatistical Terminology

Term	Definition
Abortus	An embryo/fetus that is removed or expelled from the uterus at 20 weeks' gestation or less, or weighing 500 g or less, or measuring 25 cm or less
Birthrate	Number of live births in one year per 1000 population
Fertility rate	Number of births per 1000 women between the ages of 15 and 44 (inclusive), calculated on a yearly basis
Infant mortality rate	Number of deaths of infants under 1 year of age per 1000 live births
Maternal mortality rate	Number of maternal deaths from births and complications of pregnancy, childbirth, and the puerperium (the first 42 days after termination of the pregnancy) per 100,000 live births
Neonatal mortality rate	Number of deaths of infants under 28 days of age per 1000 live births
Perinatal mortality rate	Number of stillbirths and the number of neonatal deaths per 1000 live births
Stillbirth	An infant who, at birth, demonstrates *no* signs of life such as breathing, heartbeat, or voluntary muscle movements

tion of childbearing women, the actual proportion of births to teens fell while the proportion for women age 35 and older rose (US Department of Health and Human Services, 1990).

For women 30 to 44 years of age, there was a steady increase in the birthrate since 1975 (it rose 41%). The birthrate for women age 35 to 39 also increased markedly to its highest level since 1972 (it increased 43% since 1975). Women age 40 to 44 had the greatest increase (the birthrate was 20% higher in 1988 than in 1985). Even though the birthrate for women age 40 to 44 increased substantially, it was still relatively low (4.8 births per 1000). Thus it seems that more women delayed childbearing (indicated by the increase in birth rate for women in their thirties and forties). Even though this has been the trend, the birthrate for women in their thirties and forties is still well below that of women in their twenties (US Department of Health and Human Services, 1990).

The birthrate for African-American women was higher than the rate for Caucasian women in every age group except for women age 30 to 34 (in this age group, Caucasian women had a 10% higher birthrate than African-American women). For African-American women under the age of 25, the birthrate was substantially higher than for Caucasian women of the same age, but for African-American women age 25 to 29 and 35 to 39, the birthrates were only 1% to 2% higher than the rates for Caucasian women of the same age (US Department of Health and Human Services, 1990).

The number of births to Hispanic mothers increased between the years 1983 and 1988. Hispanic births were highly concentrated geographically in 30 states and Washington, D.C. About one in six Hispanic-origin births were to teens, as compared to one in ten Caucasian non-Hispanic births and one in four African-American non-Hispanic births. Hispanic mothers-to-be were less likely than Caucasian mothers-to-be to begin prenatal care in the first trimester. The proportion of low-birth-weight babies born to this group resembled the incidence of low-birth-weight infants born to Caucasian women rather than to African-American women. This is thought to be related to the fewer number of infants born to teens in this cultural group than in the African-American cultural group (Centers for Disease Control, 1989; US Department of Health and Human Services, 1990).

The **fertility rate** (or number of births to women of childbearing age) rose 2% in 1988 (67.2 live births/1000 women age 15 to 44), which was the highest it had been since 1982 (US Department of Health and Human Services, 1990).

TRENDS IN BIRTHS TO UNMARRIED WOMEN. The data indicate that childbearing by unmarried mothers reached an all-time high in 1988, continuing a trend of substantial increases. At the same time, childbearing to married women declined. Because of these two divergent trends, the proportion of all births to unmarried women rose dramatically, from 18.4% in 1980 to 25% in 1988. This increase in nonmarital childbearing was true for both African-American and Caucasian women, but increases were the greatest for Caucasian women (in 1988), which continued a pattern of recent years. However, the rates of childbearing and the proportion of births to unmarried women continued to be substantially higher for African-American than for Caucasian women. Births to unmarried women are frequently related to less favorable outcomes because there are typically a large number of teenagers in the unmarried group. Although the birth rate for younger unmarried women increased from 1980 to 1988, the impact of this on overall levels of nonmarital births was minimal because the number of these women in the population declined (US Department of Health and Human Services, 1990).

NUMBER OF LOW-BIRTH-WEIGHT INFANTS. Babies with low birth weight (less than 5 pounds 8 ounces) are at increased risk for morbidity and mortality. Therefore the health care system strives to reduce the number of low-birth-weight infants born. African-American babies are more than twice as likely as Caucasian babies to be low birth weight and to die in the first year of life. For African-American births, the incidence of low birth weight increased from 12.7% to 13.0% from 1987 to 1988, whereas the rate for Caucasian births fell from 5.7% to 5.6%. It is thought that the number of low-birth-weight infants has not declined because of the large number of preterm births (US Department of Health and Human Services, 1990).

For preterm infants, the percentage of low-birth-weight infants is 12% higher for African-American babies than for Caucasian babies. For term and post-term babies, low birth weight seems to be associated with the mother's age as well; babies born to teenagers or older mothers are more likely to be low birth weight (the least likely ages are 25 to 29 and 30 to 34) (US Department of Health and Human Services, 1990). Even though lifesaving techniques after birth have been perfected to give low-birth-weight infants a better chance of surviving, the number of low-birth-weight infants born has not decreased substantially enough. Therefore further decreases can only be accomplished by reducing risk factors associated with low birth weight (National Commission, 1990; Poland, 1990).

INFANT MORTALITY TRENDS/ISSUES. A common indicator of the adequacy of prenatal care as well as the health of a nation as a whole is the **infant mortality rate.** The lowest rate ever occurred in 1987 (10.1 per 1000 live births). The infant mortality rate continues to be higher for African-American babies than for Caucasian babies (17.6 vs 8.5); the African-American rate continues to be about twice that for Caucasian babies (National Commission, 1990; US Department of Health and Human Services, 1990). Fig. 1-1 cites the trend in infant mortality over the years. Some studies have found factors such as limited maternal education, young maternal age, unmarried status, poverty, and lack of prenatal care to be associated with the higher African-American infant mortality rate (Brecht, 1989). However, an investigation of disadvantaged African-Americans in Washington, D.C., which has the highest infant mortality rate in the country, has found that factors other than socioeconomic status and demographic characteristics contribute more significantly to the higher infant mortality rate of African-Americans. Instead, lack of prenatal care, poor nutrition, smoking and alcohol use, as well as maternal conditions such as poor health or hypertension, were found to be more important contributors. Considered to be particularly important, then, in reducing the gap between African-Americans and Caucasians in infant mortality is better access to health care programs that emphasize nutrition education and support, health and parenting education, smoking cessation, drug and alcohol abuse treatment, pediatric care, immunizations, and accident prevention education (Boone, 1982; National Commission, 1990). A shift from the current emphasis on high-technology medical interventions to a focus on improving access to preventive care for low-income families is necessary. Future improvement in infant mortality and pregnancy outcomes must come from access to care that emphasizes health care as well as changing socioeconomic and behavioral factors that place infants at risk (Wise et al, 1988; National Commission, 1990).

INTERNATIONAL INFANT MORTALITY TRENDS. In comparing the United States with other industrialized nations, it is significant to note that the United

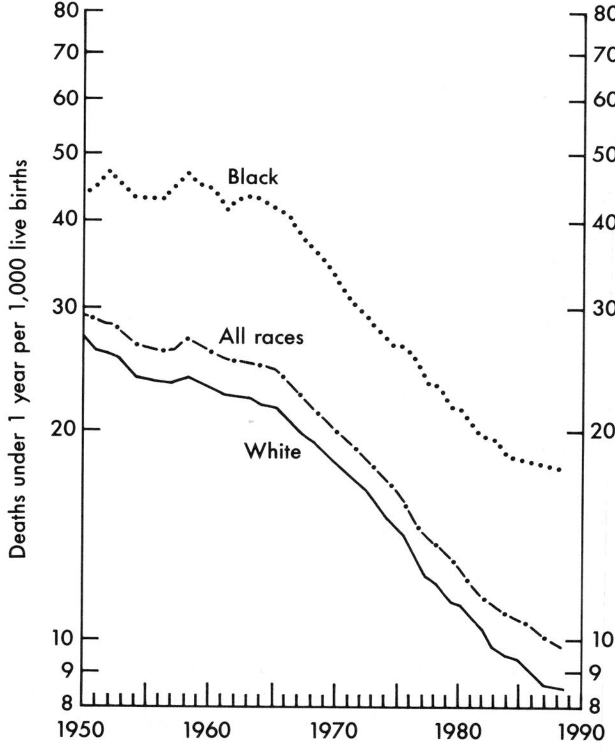

Fig 1-1 Infant mortality rates 1950-1988.
From US Department of Health and Human Services: *Monthly Vital Statistics Report* 39(7):10, 1990.

States ranked 19th in 1985. Even though infant mortality decreased some in the United States, we did not keep pace with other industrialized countries. In fact, the situation worsened; the United States now ranks 21st. Some suggest that the root of the problem in the United States rests with economic barriers and inadequate access to prenatal care, as well as poor financial and social benefits for childbearing women (National Commission, 1990).

MORTALITY TRENDS. In 1987, 251 U.S. women died from complications of pregnancy, childbirth, and the puerperium, indicating a **maternal mortality rate** of 6.6 deaths per 100,000 live births. The maternal mortality rate was 27% higher in 1988 than in 1987 (8.4 vs. 6.6). And, African-American women were 3.3 times more likely to die of causes associated with pregnancy, childbearing, and the puerperium than were Caucasian women in 1988 (US Department of Health and Human Services, 1990).

MORTALITY TRENDS FOR WOMEN. In general, death rates for women have been declining since 1950. Recently, women's mortality has been associated with HIV infections. Overall, HIV was ranked as the 15th leading cause of death for women in 1988, but it ranked higher (in the top ten leading causes of death) for four age-groups (ages 1 to 4, 15 to 24, 25 to 44, and 45 to 64). Drug and alcohol use has also contributed to women's mortality. The rate of deaths resulting from drug use increased 35% from 1983 to 1988 (this does not include accidents or homicides indirectly related to drug use), and was greater for African-American than Caucasian women (2.2 times greater). However, alcohol-induced deaths decreased overall by 14% from 1979 to 1988 (US Department of Health and Human Services, 1990). There were decreased deaths resulting from heart disease, cardiovascular accidents, atherosclerosis, and suicide (between 1987 and 1988), but there were increased deaths caused by pneumonia, influenza, chronic obstructive pulmonary disease, diabetes, and septicemia (US Department of Health and Human Services, 1990).

TRENDS OF CONSUMER INVOLVEMENT, SELF-CARE, AND FOCUS ON HEALTH CARE. In the later 1960s, consumers began to demand information about medical technology and their medical care. A movement toward self-help and toward assuming responsibility for wellness also occurred. No longer do consumers passively accept and comply with advice of health care providers. Consumers demand information and take an active role. Self-care has been appealing not only to consumers but also to the health care system because of its potential to reduce health care costs. Perinatal and women's health care is especially suited to self-care because childbearing is essentially health focused, clients are usually well when they enter the system, and gynecologic visits can present the opportunity for health as well as illness interventions. The literature indicates that prenatal and women's health care needs to help women improve health and reduce risks associated with poor pregnancy outcomes and illness. Areas such as nutrition education, stress management, smoking cessation, alcohol and drug treatment, improvement of social supports, and parenting education have been suggested. In addition, education about conditions important to women (such as depression, anxiety, osteoporosis, reproductive malignancies, and hormone replacement therapy) also needs to be addressed (Griffith-Kenney, 1986; Stotland, 1990; Meacham and Kelley, 1991; Queenan, 1991).

TREND TO HIGH-TECHNOLOGY CARE. Advances in scientific knowledge as well as the large number of high-risk pregnancies have contributed to a health care system that emphasizes high-technology care. Obstetrics has branched out to preconception counseling, more and better scientific techniques to monitor the mother and fetus, more definitive tests for hypoxia and acidosis, and neonatal intensive care units. Gynecology has expanded to emphasize care of older women, newer cancer screening techniques, advances in the diagnosis and treatment of breast cancer, and work on an AIDS vaccine. In general, high-technology care has flourished while "health" care has become relatively neglected. These technologic advances have also contributed to higher health care costs (Queenan, 1990).

HOME HEALTH CARE FLOURISHES. A shift in settings from acute care institutions to the home has been occurring. Even high-risk childbearing women are increasingly cared for in the home. New technology previously available only in the hospital is now found in the home. This has affected the organizational structure of care, the skills required in providing such care, and the costs to consumers (deLissovoy, 1991).

HIGH-RISK PREGNANCIES ESCALATE. High-risk pregnancies have increased, which means that a greater number of pregnant women are at risk for poor pregnancy outcomes. Escalating drug use (11% to 27% of pregnant women, depending on the geographic location) has contributed to higher incidences of prematurity, low birth weight, congenital defects, learning disabilities, and withdrawal symptoms in infants (National Commission, 1990). Alcohol use in pregnancy has been associated with miscarriages (spontaneous abortions), mental retardation, low birth weight, and fetal alcohol syndrome. Syphilis, which contributes to congenital defects and infant deaths, increased 40% between 1980 and 1987. In addition, other sexually transmitted diseases during pregnancy (which can be associated with defects and diseases in the newborn) also increased, as did the incidence of AIDS in childbearing women and children. The rate of unmarried mothers giving birth is high (a large number of whom are teenagers), and neonates born to unmarried mothers are twice as likely to die as those born to married mothers. Teens also are twice as likely to have a low-birth-weight infant. It is now well documented that this need not be the case; adequate prenatal care focusing on health and reduction of risk factors can improve pregnancy outcomes (National Commission, 1990).

HIGH COST TRENDS AND ISSUES. Health care costs have risen dramatically. From 1970 to 1978, expenditures for health care increased at an annual rate of 17%, with only an average of 11% of this increase accounted for by inflation (Letach, 1987). A shift in demographics, an increased emphasis on high-cost technology, and liability costs of a litigious society have created the cost crisis (Queenan, 1991). Most agree that the costs of caring for the increased number of low-birth-weight infants in intensive care units have also contributed significantly to the overall health care costs, especially since 19% of all uninsured women gave birth to a low-birth-weight infant (National Commission, 1991; Queenan, 1991).

Many women are unable to pay for health care. According to Miller (1989), 35% of women of childbearing age are without public or private health insurance. In addition, 25% of the women of childbearing age with some insurance do not have maternity coverage. Thus a large number of women remain uninsured (Health Insurance Institute, 1989). In fact, women and children are disproportionately represented in the group with limited access to care as the result of inability to pay (Health Insurance Institute, 1989; National Commission, 1991). Nursing is making some impact on cost containment by providing midwife care to pregnant women, but the lack of direct access to reimbursement for nurse practitioners and clinical nurse specialist services as direct care providers continues to be a problem (RN, 1989; Papenhausen, 1990; Nursing News, 1991). Nursing data need to be identified and placed in a data base system in order to be included in public policy decisions; nursing variables need to become part of the national data-gathering system. Nurses also need to deal with the politics involved in cost containment health care policies, since they are knowledgeable experts who can provide solutions to many of the health care problems at a relatively low cost (Lang, Marek, 1991; Mason et al, 1991; Queenan, 1991).

ACCESS PROBLEMS CONTINUE. Access to prenatal care continues to be an issue in the 1990s. Between 1980 and 1987, there was an increase in the number of women not receiving any prenatal care (a 26% increase for African Americans and a 17% increase for Caucasians). In addition, many women with access to prenatal care entered the health care system late or came only sporadically. Thus one in three pregnant women received inadequate prenatal care (care beginning after the first 3 months and with less than 13 total visits). Although 79% of Caucasian mothers began prenatal care in the first trimester, only 61% of African-American women did so (National Commission, 1990). The emphasis of the health care system has been on curtailing costs. Access and care actually has been cut back, with the length of hospital stays reduced. Often this has resulted in minimal recovery time or education about health needs and newborn care (Queenan, 1991).

Barriers to access need to be removed so that pregnancy outcomes can be improved (National Commission, 1990; Queenan, 1991). The most significant barrier to access is the inability to pay. In addition to a lack of insurance and high costs, there is a lack of providers for low-income women, since many physicians refuse to take medicaid clients or take only a few. This presents a significant problem because one in six births are to medicaid mothers. Cited as reasons were low reimbursement rates as well as cumbersome processes for clients in obtaining reimbursement (National Commission, 1990; Scupholme et al, 1991). The National League for Nursing (NLN) as well as the Organization of Obstetric, Gynecologic, and Neonatal Nurses have supported the right of childbearing women to receive prenatal care and have encouraged legislation to promote improved access (Executive Board, NAACOG, 1990; Maraldo, 1991; NAACOG Newsletter, 1991; NAACOG Standards, 1991; NLN, 1991).

LEGAL ISSUES IN THE DELIVERY OF CARE. Nursing standards of practice in perinatal and women's health nursing have been described by several organizations, including the American Nurses Association (ANA) (which publishes standards for maternal-child health nursing) and NAACOG: The Organization of Obstetric, Gynecologic, and Neonatal Nurses. These standards reflect current knowledge and represent levels of practice agreed on by leaders in the specialty. Because nursing practice, society, and the health care system are dynamic rather than static, standards have changed and will change over time. In addition to these more formalized standards, agencies often have policy and procedure books that operate, in a sense, as standards to be followed. In determining legal negligence, the care given is compared to standards of care. If the standard was not met, negligence occurred. The number of legal suits in the perinatal area has typically been high. As a consequence, malpractice insurance costs have risen dramatically for physicians as well as nurses (Rhodes, 1989; Pellegrino, 1991; Lang, Marek, 1991). Legal issues are discussed in detail in Chapter 4.

ETHICAL ISSUES. Advances in the science of perinatal and women's health have contributed to ethical dilemmas. Advances such as intrauterine fetal surgery, artificial insemination, surrogate childbearing, infertility surgery, and fetal research have resulted in questions about informed consent as well as allocation of resources. Regulations, guidelines, and ethical committees have become commonplace. Ethical experts are increasingly consulted to examine the array of theories useful for ethical decision making, to assist in applying abstract theories to concrete situations, and to educate the public about methods for making moral decisions. Nursing can play a constructive role in this area by providing rational, knowledgeable, and experienced voices (Styles, 1990; Kaiser Permanente, 1991; Pellegrino, 1991). Legal and ethical issues are discussed in Chapter 4.

CHANGING CHILDBIRTH PRACTICES. Perinatal and women's health has changed dramatically. Women can choose either a physician or a nurse-midwife as their primary care provider. In addition, women can now give birth in a hospital labor room (rather than a delivery room), a birthing room, a birthing center, or at home (see Birth Plan in Index). The method of anesthesia and positions for labor and delivery are also varied, depending on the condition and choice of the mother. No longer are laboring mothers and fathers separated; family-centered nursing care is practiced. Newborns are not whisked away to the nursery, mothers typically do not have general anesthetics, parents are not restricted from nurseries or neonatal intensive care units, and siblings are no longer restricted from visitation. Today fathers take an active part in the birth and are often present even for cesarean births (Stotland, 1990; Boeke, 1991). Parent (childbirth) education classes have become relatively common (see Chapter 13). These include encouraging participation of a support person, breathing/relaxation techniques, and general information about birth. Most recently, nursing care organization has changed to "mother-baby" nursing, a system in which one nurse cares for both the mother and baby after delivery (instead of one nurse caring for the baby and another nurse caring for the mother). In an attempt to control costs and emphasize the healthy, normal aspects of birth, "early discharge" is now a common practice. Mothers no longer stay 3 to 4 days after a vaginal birth, but are discharged anywhere from 6 to 24 to 48 hours after delivery. This creates heavy responsibilities for the nurse to complete education about newborn care and postpartum recovery when mothers may not be physically or emotionally ready. Therefore a growing need for follow-up or home care is becoming evident (Stotland, 1990; NAACOG, 1991) (see Chapter 26).

TRENDS IN NURSING PRACTICE. Since the need for health promotion is prominent, it has been suggested that the curriculums in nursing schools emphasize health education and counseling. To this end, the former division of Maternal Child Health of the Public Health Service funded the March of Dimes Birth Defects Foundation to investigate and develop core competencies in maternal-infant health for basic educational programs (Sherwen, 1987).

The increasing complexity of care for perinatal and women's health clients has contributed to specialization of nurses working with these clients. This specialized knowledge is being gained through experience, advanced degrees, and certification programs.

The North American Nursing Diagnosis Association (NANDA) and other specialty groups such as NAACOG are working on establishing and expanding the classification of nursing diagnoses used by nurses. Diagnoses particularly relevant to perinatal and women's health nursing have been incorporated into this system. Research and development of these diagnoses continues (Starn, Niederhauser, 1990).

Research is vital in establishing a perinatal and women's health science. Nurses need to promote research funding and conduct research concerning perinatal and women's health, especially concerning the effectiveness of nursing strategies for these groups of clients. For example, although it is clear that prenatal care is related to healthier babies, the exact interventions by nurses that affect particular outcomes is unknown (Wise, 1988; Baldwin, 1989; Peoples-Sheps, 1989). Research can validate that nursing care makes a difference. In the past, women have not been included in much of the medical research conducted (Schroeder, 1991). Research in women's health is therefore mandatory. NAACOG has identified research priorities in perinatal, women's, and neonatal nursing. Research is discussed in Chapter 5.

■ CONCEPTUAL THEORETIC BASES FOR PERINATAL AND WOMEN'S HEALTH

Perinatal and women's health nursing operates from a sound scientific base of knowledge. Fawcett and Downs (1986) define a **conceptual model** as abstract and general concepts and propositions used as a frame of reference for the profession. In particular, a nursing conceptual model guides the nurse working with perinatal and women's health clients in appropriate observations, judgments, and strategies for care because it focuses attention on particular aspects of pregnancy and women's health. The nurse is thereby guided by the conceptual "map" of the model, focusing on "essential" aspects, and ignoring other nonessential aspects (Meleis, 1985; George, 1990). Other terms that have been used for a conceptual model are paradigm, conceptual framework, or theoretic model (Meleis, 1985).

Nursing has several conceptual models, each emphasizing different aspects of reality. The choice of a model is determined by the nurse or institution, depending on purposes, beliefs, and the specialty (Meleis, 1985). Models particularly relevant to perinatal and women's health are Dorothea Orem's Self-Care and Sister Callista Roy's Adaptation Theory.

The theory of **self-care** emphasizes activities that individuals perform on their own behalf to encourage health and well-being. Many factors influence the individual's ability for self care, including age, developmental state, life experiences, health, and available resources. Nursing interventions are required when an individual is incapable or limited in effecting self care. Since this theory's focus is on health promotion and maintenance, it is especially relevant for the care of women during childbearing and throughout life (Orem, 1971; Meleis, 1985).

Sister Callista Roy's **adaptation theory** has the adaptation of individuals, families, groups, community, or society as its goal. According to this theory, humans are in constant interaction with a changing environment and therefore need to respond continually to changing demands (Meleis, 1985). Adaptations, or effective healthy responses, are encouraged so that ineffective responses and outcomes are avoided. According to the model, there are four main modes in which the individual must adapt, the physiologic, self-concept, role function, and interdependence modes. Since this theory considers social and psychologic, as well as physiologic functioning, it seems particularly relevant to nursing in the perinatal and women's health specialty (Roy, 1984).

George (1990) states that a concept is composed of words that describe objects, properties, or events that are the basic components of a theory. A theory is defined as a "systematic way of looking at the world in order to describe, explain, predict, or control it" (George, 1990, p. 5). Propositions state relationships between concepts. Both concepts and propositions are therefore components of a theory. Because nursing is holistic, many concepts and theories are necessary to describe all the phenomena with which nurses deal (Roy, 1984).

Nursing conceptual models provide a direction for nursing care. Within these models, other compatible concepts and theories concerning the phenomena with which nurses work are linked and related, depending on their "fit." These "other" theories are visualized through the nursing conceptual model. They are not merely "borrowed" and applied. Instead, a new integration, or merging, of perspectives evolves and is adapted to unique nursing situations (George, 1990). Particularly relevant for nursing in perinatal and women's health are family, crisis, stress, transcultural care, learning, attachment/bonding, and maternal role attainment theories.

The family is one of the most vital considerations for the perinatal and women's health nurse since it is the social institution that has the greatest effect on each person's development. It is within the context of the family that development and maintenance of health and well-being occur. Family is discussed in Chapter 2.

A **crisis** is an anxiety-provoking event or situation that challenges the individual to change. Usual mechanisms of coping are often ineffective in lowering anxiety or restoring equilibrium. The crisis situation therefore threatens to overwhelm, but it is also an opportunity to learn new coping patterns. Through crisis intervention, nurses help the person to reestablish equilibrium and to cope. The event of childbirth requires change and adjustment and therefore is considered to be a maturational crisis by some. Likewise, a diagnosis of a sexually transmitted disease, AIDS, or reproductive malignancy may also be considered a crisis (Dixon, 1979; Aguilera, Messick, 1982).

Stress is an emotional, psychologic, physiologic state that occurs when anxiety and fear are present. It is subjective and unique for each person, differing in duration and intensity. What is stressful for one may not be for another. When demands are placed on an individual, resources are used to avoid the detrimental consequences of stress (Holmes, Masuda, 1974; George, 1990). Detrimental physiologic changes and actual illness have been linked to the inability to cope with stress effectively (Selye, 1973; Griffith-Kenney, 1986). Stress may be encountered in responding to childbirth and parenting as well as in the ongoing situations of women within the family or marketplace (Griffith-Kenney, 1986).

Over the years, Leininger has developed a **transcultural care** theory that emphasizes the fact that varying cultures perceive, know, and practice lifestyle behaviors and view health in different ways. Awareness of these cultural differences and similarities assists and guides nursing interventions. Beliefs and practices about childbirth and parenting as well as about the role of women are highly variable depending on the cultural group (Leininger, 1985).

Learning involves not only gaining information, but also a readiness to learn and to attend. It also requires that the learner have the ability to perform any skills involved in the learning. There are numerous theories concerning the teaching/learning process (Patterson, 1973; Redman, 1988). From parent education classes during pregnancy to teaching mothers to feed and care for their newborns, to education about treatments for reproductive malignancies or prevention of a sexually transmitted disease, it is an everyday, essential activity of the perinatal and women's health nurse. In addition to education about illnesses or treatments, information about healthy lifestyle behaviors is critical for promoting health in pregnancy and throughout a woman's life (Speers, 1989).

Attachment theory, developed originally by Bowlby and Ainsworth, indicates that an affectional tie between parent and infant develops to ensure nurturance and care of the infant and child. It develops and changes over time, with attachment behavior also varying. Trust, separation, and individuation of the parent and child occurs as a result of attachment within the parent-child relationship (Bowlby, 1960; Ainsworth, 1969). Confusion often occurs over similarities and differences between bonding and attachment theories. **Bonding** is described as a unique relationship between two people that endures over time, and the term is used most often to refer to a rapid process (typically occurring immediately after birth) that reflects attachment (Klaus, Kennell, 1982).

According to Rubin (1984), **maternal role attainment** is a process involving progressive cognitive operations of the mother that are linked to achieving maternal tasks. Through achievement of these increasingly complex maternal tasks, the mother "binds" into a maternal identity in relation to her child. Although the process begins in pregnancy, most of the process occurs after birth (Rubin, 1984). Lederman (1984) envisions maternal role attainment to involve changes in the mother's thinking that moves from a single self to a mother-infant unit. This change in thinking is influenced by motivation for motherhood, preparation for it (in daydreams, night dreams, life experiences, conflict resolution, and role rehearsal), and the mother's past and ongoing relationship with her own mother.

■ CRITICAL THINKING AND THE NURSING PROCESS

Perinatal and women's health care is based on critical thinking through the application of the nursing process. **Critical thinking** is reasonable, reflective thinking to decide what to believe or do (Ennis, 1989). It comprises deduction, induction, and informal and practical reasoning, and it is characterized by identifying, analyzing, and evaluating assumptions underlying actions, decisions, and judgments (Bandman, Bandman, 1988; Ennis, 1989). Critical thinking is elaborated further in the following discussion of each step of the nursing process and in the chapter on nursing research (Chapter 5). The nursing process is a "series of interventions to fullfill the purposes of nursing, i.e., to maintain the client's optimal wellness, and, if this state changes, to provide the amount and quality of nursing care the situation demands to direct the client back to wellness" (Yura, Walsh, 1988, p. 105).

There are five components of the nursing process: assessment, analysis with formulation of nursing diagnosis, planning, implementation, and evaluation.

The *assessment* stage involves data collection and then the formulation of inferences. During data collection, the nurse takes a history and performs a health assessment. After this the nurse "sorts, orga-

TABLE 1-2 Typical "Problem" Diagnoses in Maternity with Accompanying Examples of Wellness Diagnoses

Typical "Problem" Diagnosis	Wellness Diagnosis
Alteration in parenting	Progress in parenting
Impaired home maintenance management	Progressive home maintenance management
Disturbance in self-concept, maternal role performance	Progressive, positive self-concept, mothering role performance
Disturbance in self-concept, body image	Progressive, positive self-concept, body image
Anxiety with mothering role	Minimal anxiety with mothering role

nizes, groups, categorizes, compares, analyzes, and synthesizes" (Yura, Walsh, 1988, p. 126) data in order to formulate nursing diagnoses. A *nursing diagnosis* is "the judgment or conclusion reached by the nurse based on assessment data that indicate the potential for or actual human need fulfillment alteration" (Yura, Walsh, 1988, p. 120). It is a two-part statement, the first usually taken from the current North American Nursing Diagnosis Association (NANDA) list of nationally accepted nursing diagnoses and the second part specifying the related etiologic or contributing factors. This diagnosis serves to provide direction for nursing interventions (Yura, Walsh, 1988).

Since childbirth is a normal process and since nurses emphasize health promotion during pregnancy and in caring for women, "wellness" nursing diagnoses are especially helpful. These nursing diagnoses, rather than focusing on "problems" or abnormalities, emphasize normal, healthy processes. To state a healthy diagnosis, a positive word can be substituted for the negative word typically used in a "problem" diagnosis. Identifying positive wellness diagnoses allows strengths to be used to maintain healthy functioning or even to cause a "healthier" state. Several examples cited in Table 1-2 illustrate the typical wellness diagnoses in perinatal and women's health settings. Common maladaptive, "problem" nursing diagnoses are also included (Stevens, 1988).

During *planning,* the nurse designates actions or interventions, prioritizes and formulates nursing diagnoses and client-centered measurable goals, and identifies interventions to achieve the stated goals. Goal setting should be as collaborative as possible between the client and nurse in order to enhance compliance. Nursing interventions include providing direct care, counseling, referring, role-modeling, and teaching. The nurse may select actions from known strategies or may specifically design actions for a particular problem. Specific client information obtained until this point is then formed into a nursing care plan and systematically and concisely communicated (Yura, Walsh, 1988).

During *implementation,* the plan of care is put into action. Planned nursing interventions are carried out either by the nurse directly, by other health professionals and paraprofessionals, or by the family (Yura, Walsh, 1988).

Evaluation involves appraising the changes, or client outcomes, experienced by the client in relation to goals. The nurse considers how the client responded to the nursing interventions and determines progress toward, or attainment of, the goals. The client's behavior and status are compared with the specified outcome criteria cited in the goal (Yura, Walsh, 1988).

■ SUMMARY

Perinatal and women's health nursing is a diversified specialty that cares for women during childbearing as well as throughout their lives. Examining recent trends indicates that a new approach to women's health is critical to improving the overall health and well-being of women and their infants. Perinatal and women's health nurses have a unique opportunity to play an important role in this process (Styles, 1990).

REFERENCES

Ainsworth M: Object relations, dependency, and attachment: a theoretical view of the infant-mother relationship, *Child Dev* 40:969, 1969.

Aguilera DC, Messick JM: *Crisis intervention: theory and methodology*, St Louis, 1982, Mosby–Year Book.

American College of Nurse Midwives: *Today's certified nurse midwives*. Washington, DC, 1987, The American College of Nurse Midwives.

Baldwin KA, Chen SC: The effectiveness of public health services to prenatal clients: an integrated review, *Public Health Nurs* 6(2):80, 1989.

Bandman EL, Bandman B: *Critical thinking in nursing*, Norwalk, Conn, 1988, Appleton & Lange.

Boeke A: Beyond reproduction: a paradigm shift in women's health, *JOGNN* 20(1):12, 1991.

Boone MS: A socio-medical study of infant mortality among disadvantaged blacks, *Hum Org* 41(3):227, 1982.

Bowlby J: *Attachment and loss*, New York, 1969, Basic Books.

Brecht M: The tragedy of infant mortality, *Nurs Outlook* 37(1):18, 1989.

Centers for Disease Control: Postponed childbearing: United States, 1970-1987, *MMWR 1989* 38(47):810, 1989.

deLissovoy G, Feustle JA: Advanced home health care, *Health Policy* 17:227, 1991.

Dixon SL: *Working with people in crisis: theory and practice*, St Louis, 1979, Mosby–Year Book.

Elder RG, Bullough B: Nurse practitioners and clinical nurse specialists: are the roles merging? *Clinical Nurse Specialist* 4(2):78, 1990.

Ennis RH: Critical thinking and subject specificity: clarification and headed research, *Educ Researcher* 18(3):4, 1989.

Executive Board, NAACOG: *Access to health care statement*, Washington, DC, 1990, NAACOG.

Fawcett J, Downs F: *The relationship of theory and research*, Norwalk, Conn, 1986, Appleton-Century-Crofts.

George JB: *Nursing theories: the base for proper nursing practice*, ed 3, Norwalk, Conn, 1990, Appleton & Lange.

Griffith-Kenney J: *Contemporary women's health*, Menlo Park, Calif, 1986, Addison Wesley.

Health Insurance Institute: *Source book of health insurance data*, New York, 1989, Health Insurance Institute.

Holmes TH, Masuda M: *Stressful life events: their virtue and effects*, New York, 1974, Wiley.

Kaiser Permanente, *Health care raises ethical dilemmas*, Fall: 1-2, 1991.

Kelly LY: *Dimensions of professional nursing*, ed 6, New York, 1991, Pergamon Press.

Klaus M, Kennell J: *Parent-infant bonding*, ed 2, St Louis, 1982, Mosby–Year Book.

Lang NM, Marek KD: The policy and politics of patient outcomes, *Journal Nursing Quality Assurance* 5(2):7, 1991.

Leininger M: Transcultural care diversity and universality: a theory of nursing, *Nurs Health Care*, 6:209, 1985.

Lederman RP: *Psychosocial adaptation in pregnancy*, Englewood Cliffs, NJ, 1984, Prentice-Hall.

Letach SW, Levit KR, Waldo DR: National health expenditures, 1987: health care financing funds, *Health Care Train Rev* 10:109, 1988.

Lops VP: Midwifery: past to present, *J Prof Nurs* 4(6):402, 1988.

Maraldo PJ: *National health: prognosis poor*, Executive Wire, July/August: 1991, National League for Nursing.

Mason DJ, Backer BA, Georges CA: Toward a feminist model for the political empowerment of the nurse, *Image* 23(2):72, 1991.

Meachan SE, Kelley SDM: Special issues in prenatal care outreach, *J Health Soc Policy*, 2(3):53, 1991.

Meleis AI: *Theoretical nursing: development and progress*, Philadelphia, 1985, JB Lippincott.

Menard SW: The clinical nurse specialist perspectives and practice, New York, 1987, John Wiley & Sons.

Miller CL et al: Barriers to implementation of a prenatal care program for low income women, *Am J Public Health* 79(1):62, 1989.

NAACOG: NAACOG endorses health care reform plan, *NAACOG Newsletter* 18(9):1, 1991.

National Association of Neonatal Nurses: Press release, *Advance practice role definitions*, Petaluma, Calif, 1989, The National Association of Neonatal Nurses.

National League for Nursing: Nursing introduces the national health strategy to the public, *Public Policy Bulletin* March: 1, 1991.

Nursing News: Drug-enforcement regs could curb prescribing by RNs, *Am J Nurs* July 11, 1991.

Nurses Association of the American College of Obstetricians and Gynecologists: *The obstetric-gynecologic women's health nurse practitioner: role definition, competence, and educational guidelines,* ed 3, Washington, DC, 1990, NAACOG.

Orem DE: *Nursing concepts of practice,* New York, 1971, McGraw-Hill.

Ouimette J: *Perinatal nursing,* Boston, 1986, Jones & Bartlett Publishers, Inc.

Papenhausen TL, Beecroft PC: Nursing's role in the health care crisis, *Clinical Nurse Specialist* 4(37):119, 1990.

Pellegrino ED, Siegler M, Singer PA: Future directions in clinical ethics, *J Clin Ethics* 2(1):5, 1991.

Peoples-Sheps MD, Efird D, Miller A: Home visiting and prenatal care: a survey of practical nursing, *Public Health Nurs* 6(2):74, 1989.

Poland ML et al: Quality of prenatal care: selected social, behavioral, and biomedical factors, and birth weight, *Obstet Gynecol* 75(4):607, 1990.

Queenan JT: Bullish on the 90s, *Contemp OB/GYN* 35(2):9, 1990.

Queenan JT: Ultrasound images from the world at large, *Contemp OB/GYN* 35(12):8, 1990.

Queenan JT: Transient stays, *Contemp OB/GYN* 36(5):8, 1991.

Queenan JT: White House action on US health care, *Contemp OB/GYN* 36(6):8, 1991.

Redman BK: *The process of patient education,* ed 6, St Louis, 1991, Mosby–Year Book.

Rhodes AM: Minimizing the liability risk of genetic counseling, *MCN* 14:313, 1989.

RN: More hospital newborns greeted by nurse midwives, *RN* August: 10, 1989.

Roy SC: *An adaptation model,* ed 2, Englewood Cliffs, NJ, 1984, Prentice-Hall.

Rubin R: *Maternal identity and the maternal experience,* New York, 1984, Springer Publishing.

Schroeder P: Schroeder censures lack of women's health research conducted in the US, *NAACOG Newsletter* 18(8):1, 1991.

Scupholme A, Robertson EG, Kamons AS: Barriers to prenatal care in a multi-clinic urban sample, *J Nurse Midwifery* 36(2):111, 1991.

Selye H: *The stress of life,* New York, 1973, McGraw-Hill.

Sherwen LN: *The maternal infant care competency project,* White Plains, NY, 1987, March of Dimes Birth Defects Foundation.

Speers AT: Patient education: theory and practice, *J Nurs Staff Development* May/June:121, 1989.

Starn J, Niederhauser V: An MCN model for nursing diagnosis to focus intervention, *MCN* 15 (May/June):180, 1990.

Stevens KA: Nursing diagnosis in wellness childbearing settings, *JOGNN* 17(5):329, 1988.

Stotland NL: Social change and women's reproductive health care, *Social Change and Reproductive Health Care* 1(1):4, 1990.

Styles MM: Challenges for nursing in this new decade, *MCN* 15(6):347, 1990.

The National Certification Corporation (NCC): *Certification examinations for the specialty nurse,* Chicago, 1991, NCC.

The National Commission to Prevent Infant Mortality: *Troubling trends: the health of America's next generation.* Washington, DC, 1990.

The Organization for Obstetric, Gynecologic and Neonatal Nurses: *NAACOG standards for the nursing care of women and newborns,* ed 4, Washington, DC, 1991, NAACOG.

The Organization for Obstetric, Gynecologic and Neonatal Nurses: *OGN nursing, commitment to care,* Washington, DC, 1991, NAACOG.

The Organization for Obstetric, Gynecologic and Neonatal Nurses: *Shaping the future,* Washington, DC, 1991, NAACOG.

US Department of Health and Human Services: *Monthly Vital Statistics Report* 39(4):1, 1990.

US Department of Health and Human Services: *Monthly Vital Statistics Report* 39(7):1, 1990.

Wise PH et al: Infant mortality increase despite high access to tertiary care: an evolving relationship among infant mortality, health care and socioeconomic change, *Pediatrics* 81(4):542, 1988.

Yura H, Walsh MB: *The nursing process,* ed 5, Norwalk, Conn, 1988, Appleton & Lange.

Zukowsky K, Coburn CE: Neonatal nurse practitioners, who are they? *JOGNN* 20(2):128, 1991.

BIBLIOGRAPHY

Brookfield S: The development of critical reflection in adulthood: foundations of a theory of adult learning, *New Education* 13(1):39, 1991.

chapter 1 review

Key Concepts

- Caring is the essence of nursing.
- Individuals have the capability to make decisions about their health and affect their health by the choices they make.
- Health and illness behaviors are influenced by cultural values and beliefs, personal definition of health, and personal preferences.
- Nursing practice requires knowledge and skill to help women maintain psychologic and physiologic health as changes occur throughout the life span.
- In developing a professional relationship, the nurse works within the personal and social context of the woman as well as the relationships that pattern the woman's health practice.
- The nurse needs technical and interpersonal competence, social consciousness, commitment to health care for all, health policy and planning ability, and political skills.
- The nursing process involves both client and nurse in all five stages: assessment, nursing diagnosis, planning, implementation, and evaluation.
- Client teaching is directed toward enabling individuals to make informed choices regarding health-related behaviors.
- Through advocacy, nurses can influence the health and well-being of present and future generations.
- Knowledgeable consumers no longer merely comply with the power base of professionals; they wish to be participants in health care.

Key Terms

- adaptation theory (p. 13)
- attachment (p. 14)
- birthrate (p. 7)
- bonding (p. 14)
- certification (p. 7)
- clinical nurse specialist (p. 5)
- conceptual model (p. 13)
- crisis (p. 13)
- critical thinking (p. 14)
- fertility rate (p. 8)
- infant mortality rate (p. 9)
- learning (p. 14)
- licensure (p. 7)
- maternal role attainment (p. 14)
- maternity mortality rate (p. 10)
- NAACOG (p. 4)
- neonatal nurse (p. 6)
- nurse-midwife (p. 7)
- nurse practitioner (p. 5)
- nursing process in perinatal and women's health nursing (p. 14)
- perinatal nurse (p. 4)
- self-care (p. 13)
- stress (p. 13)
- transcultural care (p. 14)
- women's health nursing (p. 4)
- women's health nursing roles (p. 4)

Critical Thinking Exercises

1. After client assignments are made at morning report, the licensed practical (vocational) nurse asks you, the nursing student, "Why do you have to go to school so long? It seems to me that there isn't any difference between what the RN and the LPN (LVN) does."
   a. What assumptions do you think the LPN (LVN) is making? List as many as you can. What are your assumptions about the differences in roles?
   b. Which assumptions can be checked out by simple research or inquiry?
   c. How would you respond to the LPN's (LVN's) statement? What are your reasons for your beliefs and conclusions? How could you evaluate your conclusions?
2. "Data about nursing need to be included in public policy decisions regarding health care and cost containment."
   a. Justify this assumption.
   b. If you agree with this assumption, identify nursing needs to include in the national data gathering system and to be considered in cost containment health care policies.
   c. If you disagree with this assumption, defend your position.

Topics for Nursing Research

- Identify the impact of home health care on (1) a consumer's perception of the adequacy of health care, (2) a consumer's expressed satisfaction with health care, (3) nursing skills required in providing such care, and (4) costs to consumers.
- Identify additional barriers to prenatal care so that the delivery of nursing care can be restructured.
- Refine nursing diagnoses in perinatal and women's health nursing.
- Expand specific nursing interventions that are effective for typical diagnoses in perinatal and women's health nursing.
- Investigate the use of nursing theories in perinatal and women's health nursing.

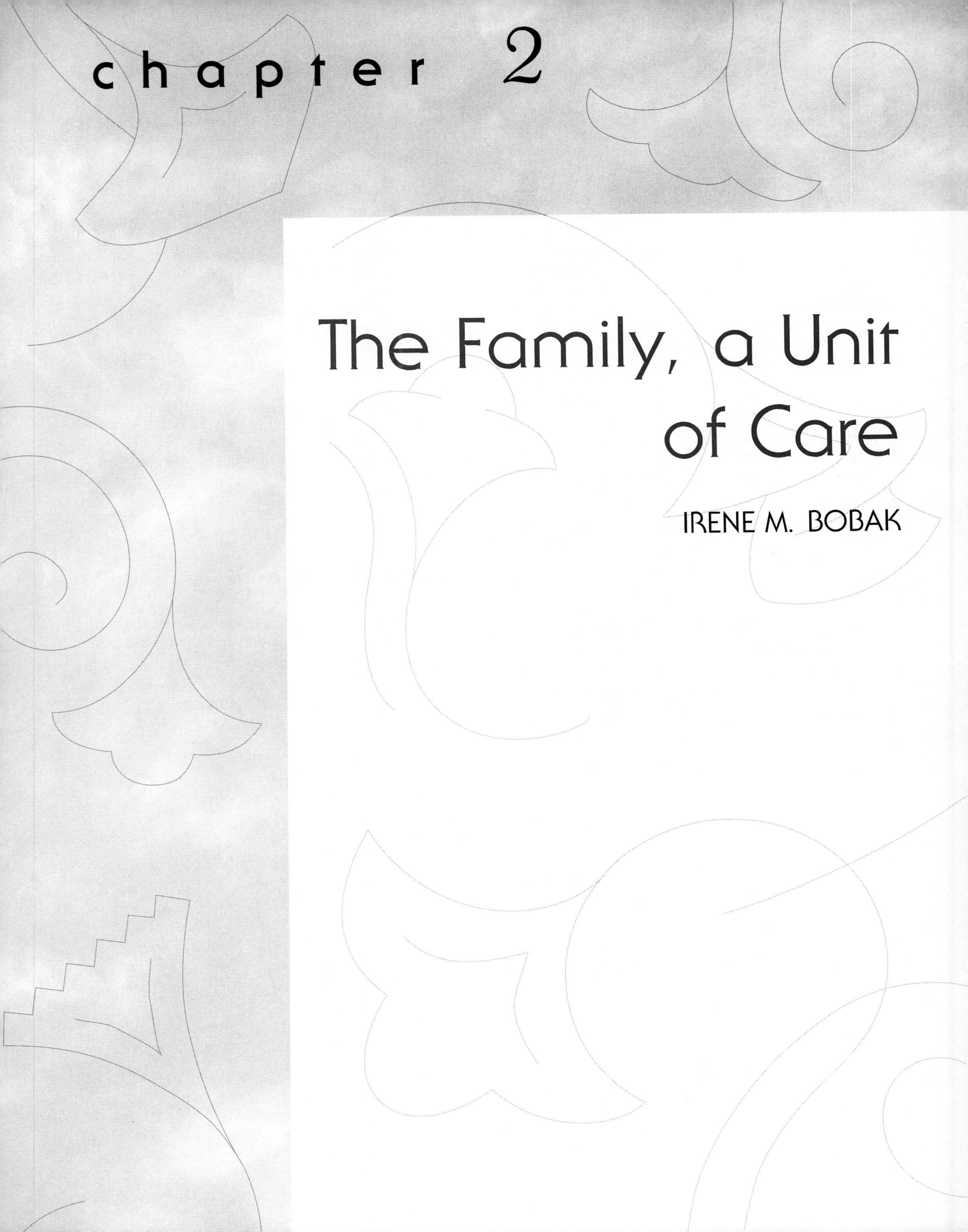

chapter 2

The Family, a Unit of Care

IRENE M. BOBAK

LEARNING OBJECTIVES

- Define the key terms listed.
- Identify key factors in determining the quality of family health.
- Explain the functions carried out by a family for the well-being of its members.
- Distinguish the properties of family dynamics and the criteria for family decision making.
- List three major family theories. Evaluate the components and implications for nursing of each theory.
- Define and give examples of maturational and situational crises.
- Identify factors that can alter one's perceptions of an event.
- Differentiate between constructive and destructive coping mechanisms.
- Relate the role of culture in the nursing care of individuals and families during the childbearing and child-rearing periods.
- Outline important components of a family care plan.
- Identify topics for nursing research related to the family.

Every newborn comes into this world surrounded by a family, be it a single-parent family or a large extended family. Regardless of the family structure, the maternity nurse is in a unique position to influence the care and well-being of these childbearing families. In doing so, the nurse acknowledges the family unit as the focus of care.

As one of society's most important institutions, the family represents a primary social group that influences and is influenced by other people and institutions. It is recognized as the fundamental social unit because most people have more continuous contact with this social group than with any other. The family assumes major responsibility for introducing and socializing persons. It serves to transmit to members the fundamental cultural background of a given family. Despite the stresses and strains to which it now is subject, the family forms a social network that acts as a potent support system for its members.

To deliver safe, comprehensive, and holistic care within the context of the nursing process, nurses working with childbearing families need a clear understanding of the family as an institution in society.

■ DEFINING THE FAMILY

Families are defined in many ways. Definitions of the family involve delineation of family *structure, functions, composition,* and *affectional ties.* A household is composed of the person or persons who occupy a housing unit. Although a majority of households consist of a family type of living arrangement, many do not. Two major categories of households are identified by the U.S. Bureau of the Census as family and non-family. A *family* or *family household* requires the presence of at least two persons: the householder and one or more additional family members related to the householder through birth, adoption, or marriage. A *nonfamily household* is composed of a householder who either lives alone or with persons who are not related to the householder.

The concept of household encompasses not only traditional forms of family structure but also other designated groups: (1) the never-married, (2) one parent and children living together as a one-parent family, (3) two homosexuals living together in a stable union, and (4) stable consensual unions, with or without children (WHO, 1978).

Friedman (1986) offers a broad definition of family, emphasizing the importance of emotional involvement as a necessary characteristic. She says, "the family is composed of people (two or more) who are emotionally involved with each other and live in close geographic proximity."

Various family forms have been defined. Descriptions of these forms follows.

Within the **nuclear family** there are two subgroups: the family of orientation, into which one is born, and the family of procreation, into which people enter as adults and become parents. The nuclear family group consists of parents and their dependent children. The family lives apart from either the husband's or wife's family of origin, and is usually economically independent.

The nuclear family has long represented the traditional American family. In this family group, parents are expected to play complementary roles of husband-wife and father-mother in giving emotional and physical support to each other and their children. Recent trends in contemporary society, however, have caused many variations in this often considered ideal family structure. The "idealized" two-parent, two-child nuclear family where the father is the sole provider and the mother is the homemaker may be a myth of the past (Fig. 2-1). In fact, reporting on a recent family conference, Libman (1988), states that today, couples in an intact first marriage with two children and the mother at home represent only 8% of the nation's families.

Binuclear family is a term used to describe the situation that allows parents to continue the parenting role while terminating the spousal unit (e.g., divorce) (Ahrons, 1979). The degree of cooperation between households and the time the child spends with each can vary. In *joint custody* the court assigns divorcing

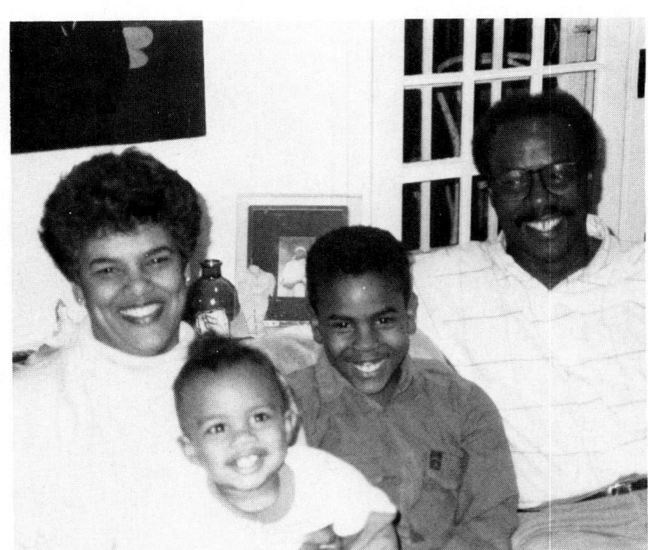

Fig. 2-1 A nuclear family.

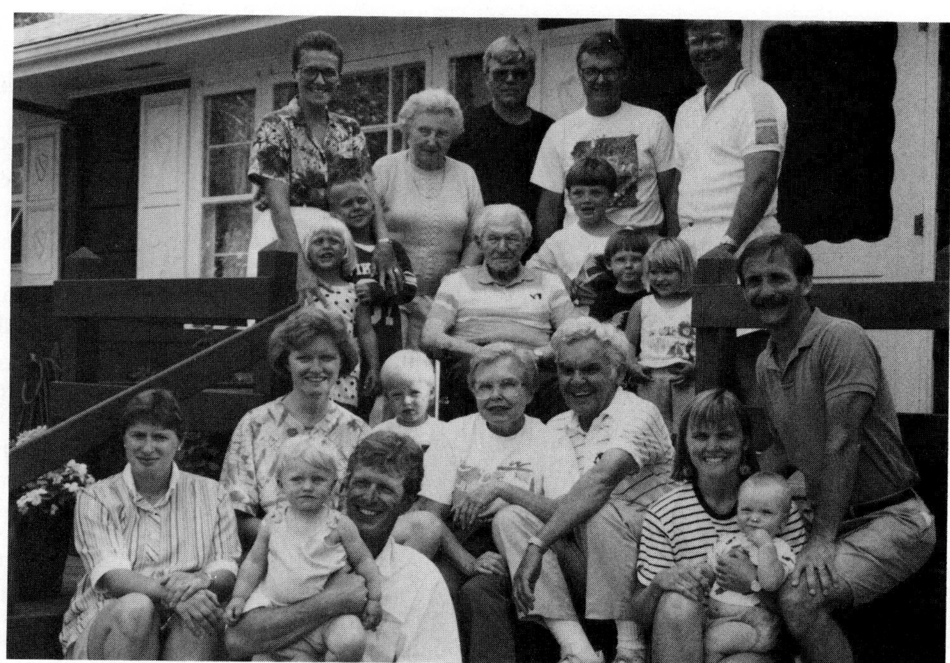

Fig. 2-2 An extended family in the 1990s.

parents equal rights and responsibilities to the minor child or children. These alternate family forms are efforts on the part of those concerned to view divorce as a process of reorganization and redefinition of a family rather than as a family dissolution.

By definition the **extended family** includes three generations (Fig. 2-2). The family is a central focus for all members who live together as a group. Through its kinship network it provides supportive functions to all members. This family structure serves to prescribe the responsibilities and actions of family members.

Variations of the traditional nuclear and extended families have always existed. Until recently, most of these *alternative family forms* have been considered deviations from the norm. Parents outside of matrimony were pressured to conform by either marrying or releasing the newborn for adoption (Evans et al, 1989).

The **single-parent family** is becoming an increasingly recognized structure in our society. The single-parent family may result from loss of a spouse by death, divorce, separation, or desertion; from the out-of-wedlock birth of a child; or from the adoption of a child. The 1986 U.S. Bureau of the Census reveals that there were 8.9 million one-parent family groups in 1986 compared with 3.8 million in 1970. Of all children 17 years old or younger, 26% live in a family with a single parent, another relative, or a nonrelative. It is estimated that of all children born in the 1980s, 35% will have experienced living in single-parent families twice by 1990 (Libman, 1988).

The single-parent family tends to be vulnerable economically and socially. Unless buttressed by a concerned society, it may create an unstable and deprived environment for the growth potential of children (Norton, Glick, 1986).

Today, single parenthood, unintentional or planned, is becoming an acceptable option in many communities within the United States. For adults the single-parent family is a chosen life-style that provides a free and open system for development of parents and children. In these families, decision making and communication are seen as joint commitments between parent and child, and the parent-child relationship is considered a major source of life fulfillment.

Single parenthood can be a voluntary choice that does not result in rejection by family, ostracism by society, or loss of job. In addition, biologic and adoptive parenthood is becoming a socially acceptable option for women and men who do not choose to marry; lesbian and gay parenthood by artificial insemination is another alternative (Evans et al, 1989). The emergence of single parenthood as a planned choice reflects a belief that one has the "right" to choose to be a parent.

The **blended family** includes stepparents and stepchildren. The terms *reconstituted* or *combined* families are sometimes used. Separation, divorce, and remarriage are common phenomena in our society, in which approximately 50% of marriages end in divorce. Divorce and remarriage may occur at any time in the family life cycle and therefore will have different impacts on family function. Whatever the timing, effort is required to restabilize old family groups and constitute and stabilize new family groups (Espinoza, Newman, 1979). This emotional work must be accomplished before family and individual development can proceed (Glick, 1979).

Homosexual families are being recognized increasingly in Western society. A same-sex, or homosexual or gay, family is one in which there is a marital or common-law tie between two persons of the same sex who have adopted children or in which one or both partners have natural children from a heterosexual mating. When one or both partners are parents, one or the other risks losing their children by custody courts biased by the individual parent's sexual orientation. This bias may prejudice the courts, causing them to overlook the best interests of the children or the homosexual parent's ability to parent effectively. Lesbian couples who decide to have children through natural or artificial insemination worry about discrimination in prenatal and childbirth care. Male and female homosexual families risk the censure of their extended families, neighbors, and religious groups and mistreatment by health care professionals and law enforcement agents (Poverny, Finch, 1988; Harvey, Carr, Bernheine, 1989; Wismont, Reame, 1989).

Unfortunately, little research is available on the spousal unit in same-sex relationships or on the effects on children growing up in these households.

Communal family groupings vary from the highly formalized structure of the Amish community in Lancaster County, Pennsylvania, to the loosely knit groups found in the Santa Cruz Mountains near Boulder Creek, California. These latter communities are formed for specific ideologic or societal purposes. They are considered an alternative life-style for people who feel alienated from a predominantly economically oriented society. Some communes consist of nuclear groups living in an extended or expanded family community and are envisioned as persisting over time. Others may provide temporary shelter. In some communes all parents participate in caregiving activities for all children. In many of these groups the combination is fluid; individuals and families are free to come and go as their needs dictate.

Family Unit

Despite the difficulty of defining the family precisely, members of a family can readily describe its composition, who is kin and who is not, how the family has affected their lives, and what family style they believe in.

However the family is defined, the *family unit* is incomplete without an adult. From an adult's perspective the family can be composed of persons of any age or sex bound by a blood or love relationship. From the child's perspective, the family is a set of relationships between the child's dependent self and one or more protective adults.

Regardless of the form it assumes or the society in which it is found, the family possesses enduring characteristics that have far-reaching personal and societal effects. According to Blehar (1979):

> Despite disagreement about the state of the family and its definition, a consensus might be reached on three points: (1) the family is currently in a state of flux precipitated by economic and social pressures; (2) imperfect though it may be, it is difficult to imagine substituting an alternative that could perform all its functions as well; and (3) it is more desirable to bolster families than to attempt to supplant them with untried structures.*

What then are the functions that families must perform, and how can nurses best bolster families facing economic and social pressures?

■ FAMILY FUNCTIONS

As the family progresses through its life cycle (see Table 2-1) from young adulthood to the commitment of two people to share a life and ending with the dissolution of the family through death or other separations, it carries out certain functions for the well-being of its members. The **family functions** extend over five basic areas: biologic, economic, educational, psychologic, and sociocultural (WHO, 1978). The interdependent functions depend on the physical and mental health of family members. As a supportive structure for these functions, each family develops certain common *beliefs, values,* and *sentiments* that are used as criteria in the choice of alternative actions.

Biologic functions include reproduction, care and rearing of children, nutrition, maintenance of health, and recreation. The ability to carry out such functions implies certain prerequisites: a healthy genetic inheritance, fertility management, care during the maternity cycle, good dietary behavior, intelligent use of health services, companionship, and nurturing of its members.

*From Blehar MC: Families and public policy. In Corfman E, editor: *Families today,* vol 2, National Institute of Mental Health, Division of Scientific and Public Information, Science Monograph No 1, Washington, DC, 1979, US Government Printing Office.

TABLE 2-1 Stages of the Family Life Cycle

Family Life Cycle Stage	Emotional Process of Transition: Key Principles	Second-Order Changes in Family Status Required to Proceed Developmentally
Leaving home: single young adults	Accepting emotional and financial responsibility for self	Differentiation of self in relation to family of origin Development of intimate peer relationships Establishment of self regarding work and financial independence
The joining of families through marriage: the new couple	Commitment to new system	Formation of marital system Realignment of relationships with extended families and friends to include spouse
Families with young children	Accepting new members into the system	Adjusting marital system to make space for child(ren) Joining in child-rearing, financial, and household tasks Realignment of relationships with extended family to include parenting and grandparenting roles
Families with adolescents	Increasing flexibility of family boundaries to include children's independence and grandparents' frailties	Shifting of parent-child relationships to permit adolescent to move in and out of system Refocus on midlife marital and career issues Beginning shift toward joint caring for older generation
Launching children and moving on	Accepting a multitude of exits from and entries into the family system	Renegotiation of marital system as a dyad Development of adult-to-adult relationships between grown children and their parents Realignment of relationships to include in-laws and grandchildren Dealing with disabilities and death of parents (grandparents)
Families in later life	Accepting the shifting of generational roles	Maintaining own and/or couple functioning and interests in face of physiologic decline; exploration of new familial and social role options Support for a more central role of middle generation Making room in the system for the wisdom and experience of the elderly; supporting the older generation without overfunctioning for them Dealing with loss of spouse, siblings, and other peers and preparation for own death; life review and integration

From Carter B, McGoldrick M: *The changing family life cycle: a framework for family therapy*, ed 2, New York, 1988, Gardner Press.

Economic functions include earning enough money to carry out the other functions, determining the allocation of resources, and ensuring the financial security of family members. To accomplish these tasks, the family must have the necessary skills, opportunities, and knowledge.

Educational functions include the teaching of skills, attitudes, and knowledge relating to the other functions. To be able to do this, family members must have knowledge, skills, and experience.

The family is expected to provide an environment that promotes the natural development of personality, offers optimum psychologic protection, and promotes the ability to form relationships with people outside the family circle. These tasks require stable emotional health, common bonds of affection between individuals, and the ability to be mutually supportive, to tolerate stress, and to cope with crises.

Sociocultural functions are associated with the socialization of children. The socialization of children includes the transfer of values relating to behavior, tradition, language, religion, and prevailing or previous social mores. It results in the conditioning of family members to a variety of behavior norms appropriate to all stages of adult life. To be able to do this, the family must possess accepted standards and be sensitive to the varying social needs of children according to their ages. It must also accept and exemplify behavioral norms and be willing to explain, defend, and promote them. Although certain functions are relegated to or emphasized more in one phase of the family's life cycle than another (e.g., the care and socialization of children are part of the childbearing and child-rearing phase of the cycle), many of the functions are continuous for the survival and progress of the family.

■ FAMILY DYNAMICS

Families work cooperatively to accomplish family functions. Through **family dynamics,** family members assume appropriate social roles. Social roles are learned in the family, the first social group, and are learned in pairs (e.g., mother-father, parent-child, and brother-sister). A social role does not exist by itself but is designed to mesh with that of a role partner. Pairing of roles enables social interactions to take place in an orderly, predictable manner—the roles are said to be complementary. Some families maintain a traditional pairing of roles, whereas other families have changed the behavior patterns to suit a change in family lifestyle. The process by which paired roles are brought into a new alignment is known as *negotiation*. Negotiation is essential if family equilibrium is to be maintained. Negotiation occurs among family members as well as among outsiders.

From the time it is formed, the family sets up *boundaries* between itself and the outside. People are extremely conscious of those considered members of their family and those who rank as outsiders—those who do not have kinship status. Some families isolate themselves from the outside community. Others have a wide community network to help in times of stress. Although boundaries exist for every family, family members set up *channels* through which they mediate external forces and attempt to protect the family from disturbances. The channels also ensure that the family receives its share of social resources.

Ideally the family uses its resources to provide a safe, intimate environment for the biopsychosocial development of children and its adult members. The family provides for the *nurturing* of the newborn and the gradual *socialization* of the growing child. It is the source of first relationships with others. The relationships children form with parents (or parenting persons) are the earliest and closest and persist throughout a lifetime. For better or worse, parent-child relationships influence a person's concepts of self-worth and ability to form later relationships. The family also interprets and mediates the child's perceptions of the complex outside world. The family provides the growing child with an identity that possesses both a past and a sense of the future. The family transmits cultural values and rituals from one generation to the next (Friedman, 1986).

Through everyday interactions the family develops and uses its own patterns of verbal and nonverbal *communication*. These patterns give insight into the feeling exchange within a family and act as reliable indicators of interpersonal functioning. Family members not only react to the communication or actions of other family members but also interpret and define them.

Over time the family develops protocols for *problem solving*, particularly regarding decisions deemed important to the family, such as having a baby, buying a house, or sending children to college. The criteria used in making decisions are based on *family values* and *attitudes* concerning the appropriateness of the behavior of its various members and the moral, social, political, and economic events of the wider social system. The *power* to make critical decisions is conferred on a family member through tradition or negotiation. This power may be overt or covert and reflects the family's concepts of male or female dominance and cultural practices, social customs, and community norms. As a result, family members are positioned into certain *statuses* or *hierarchies* and play out these statuses by assuming various *roles*. Most families have a member who "takes charge" or "is supportive" or "can't be expected to do anything."

■ FAMILY THEORIES

Many academic disciplines have studied the family and have developed theories that provide differing perspectives for assessing it. Knowledge of these theories provides the nurse with guides to understanding family functioning and dynamics. They provide a basis for planning the day-to-day care of families and help predict certain future events that may necessitate a modification of care. A brief discussion of three **family theories** (structural-functional, developmental, and interactional) is presented here.

Structural-Functional Theory

The **structural-functional theory** originated with the work of social anthropologists Malinowski (1945) and Radcliffe-Brown (1952), who documented the interrelation and interdependence of the national social system and all subsocial systems. According to this theory the family is a social system with components (family members) with specific roles and role behaviors, such as the father role or the mother role. Family dynamics are directed toward maintaining *equilibrium* between complementary roles to permit family functioning within the family unit and in relation to society. Family structure is culturally determined. The United States represents a pluralistic culture in which varying family forms are recognized and accepted in differing degrees. Classification of families according to their structure provides insight into stresses that families may experience as they differ from the normative structures supported by the society.

IMPLICATIONS FOR MATERNITY-GYNECOLOGIC NURSING. The structural-functional approach allows the nurse to examine relationships between the family and other social systems. According to Friedman (1986):

> The structural-functional perspective is a very useful framework for assessing family life because it enables the family system to be examined holistically (as a unit), in parts (as subsystems or dimensions), and interactionally (as a system interacting with other institutions, such as the educational and health system, the family's reference group[s], and the wider society).*

Insights gained from the structural-functional approach can help the nurse become aware of family relationships. First the nurse can recognize the family's *relationship to the larger social system*. Some families establish rigid boundaries, outsiders are kept at a distance, and input from the community is curtailed. Other families are isolated, and when crisis strikes, they often find their inner resources inadequate as coping mechanisms. A third group of families maintains open boundaries through work, school, or community involvement. Energy can flow in both directions, and assistance often is given and accepted.

Second, noting the *internal relationships* of the family may reveal sources of strength or weakness. Commonly the socially conceptualized roles, such as husband and wife, may not fit reality. Hence people establishing or attempting to maintain the so-called normal family roles often face frustration. The interplay of traditionally designed complementary roles may be a source of role conflict. In many families today the husband's and wife's roles are interchangeable; that is, the wife assumes some instrumental functions (earning an income) and the husband assumes some expressive functions (caring for an infant). The ability to negotiate such exchanges is necessary to maintain equilibrium.

Third, the nurse needs to be aware of the development of *reciprocal relationships* within a family that can stunt a person's growth. Some families mold a family member to act as scapegoat; others designate a member to be forever dependent. As an example of the latter, the child born prematurely may always be treated as a sick child.

The major drawback of the structural-functional theory is that its rigid adherence to roles and associated tasks requires a constant updating of the tasks assigned. In addition, this approach tends to "freeze the family in time," minimizing the importance of growth, change, and disequilibrium.

*From Friedman MM: *Family nursing theory and assessment*, New York, 1986, Appleton-Century-Crofts.

Developmental Theory

The **developmental theory** approach to the study of the family incorporates ideas from a number of theoretical and conceptual approaches to the study of society and the individual (social systems approach, structural-functional approach, life cycle concepts of developmental needs and tasks, and concepts of interacting personalities). Familiar proponents of the life cycle concept are Duvall (1977), Wright and Leahey (1984), and Carter and McGoldrick (1988). The central theme in the developmental theory is noting "the changes in the process of internal development with the dimensions of time as central" (Bower, Jacobson, 1978). The family is described as a *small-group, semiclosed* system that engages in interactive behavior within the larger cultural social system. The significant unit in this theory is the *person* rather than the role. The family process is one of *interaction* over the *life cycle* of the family.

Family members pass through phases of growth, from dependence through active independence to interdependence. The family also demonstrates variations in structure and function over time. Together these constitute the *family life cycle*. Stages and tasks of the family life cycle as outlined by Carter and McGoldrick are found in Table 2-1.

Mercer (1989) summarizes the essence of the developmental approach in family nursing:

> Developmental concepts include movement to a higher level of functioning. This implies continuous, unidirectional progression. However, during transitional periods from one stage or phase to the next, disequilibrium occurs, during which time the individual may revert to an earlier level of developmental responses. Families face normative and unexpected transitions that also create a period of disorganization, during which the family functions at a lower level than usual. Resolution of the disequilibrium or crisis has potential to lead to a higher level of family functioning.*

IMPLICATIONS FOR MATERNITY-GYNECOLOGIC NURSING. The developmental theory has provided many useful insights into family functioning. Knowing types of problems, identified during certain phases of the life cycle, can assist nurses in providing anticipatory guidance for families. For example, helping childbearing families prepare for the birth of a

*From Mercer RT: Theoretical perspective on the family. In Gillis CL et al, editors: *Toward a science of family nursing*, Menlo Park, Calif, 1989, Addison-Wesley Publishing.

newborn may minimize the development of crisis situations.

Because the family as a group and the family as individuals are simultaneously engaged in developmental tasks (Erikson, 1968; Duvall, 1977), disharmony (dissonance) is possible if the developmental task of the family is not synchronous with the developmental task of the person. There are many examples of such dissonance. The adolescent father grappling with his need to break from his family ties is expected to establish monetary and other support for the new family he has created. A toddler learning socially acceptable behaviors who is introduced to a new sibling may revert to more infantile behavior. Awareness of the implications of situations such as these can be useful in helping the family develop appropriate coping mechanisms.

The developmental approach presents a concept of family that is fluid and changing and thus more in tune with reality. It is less difficult to plot the phases of the life cycle in the nuclear family than in an extended family. The extended family may involve many generations. Sometimes it is difficult to document the life cycle of a family. Often only glimpses of it are seen; it changes or disintegrates before its significance is grasped.

Interactional Theory

The major theme of the **interactional theory,** also known as action theory or role theory, conceives of the family as a *unit of interacting personalities,* not bound necessarily by legal or contractual agreements, that exists as long as the interaction is taking place. The significant unit is *the individual.* The family process is one of *role taking.* This process is dynamic: family members are constantly testing the concept they have of the role of another and adjusting their own self-concept. The process is accomplished through *symbolic communication,* and all family behaviors stem from family members playing their many roles.

IMPLICATIONS FOR MATERNITY-GYNECOLOGIC NURSING. The interactional theory is particularly useful as a basis for nurse-family interactions. It is broad enough and inclusive enough to encompass various insights into human nature. It transcends family configuration and cultural, ethnic, or social class boundaries of families, such as nuclear family or extended family, and emphasizes *communication* as a central process. It helps the nurse understand how family members relate to one another. For example, the communication or interaction between mother and child on issues of discipline can give the nurse insight about the family's functioning. The interactional approach to working with families does have some limitations, however. For example, it does not consider the consequences of family-environment influence and interaction. Friedman (1986) asserts "Since the family actively and constantly interacts with its environment, that family-environmental interface must be included in an assessment if comprehensive family nursing care is to be provided."

All three of the theories presented here provide the nurse with a useful view of the family. Nurses use the knowledge from family theories to assist in establishing working relationships with families. When nurses question "who is doing what work," they are using knowledge from the structural-functional theory. When they ask about the significance of events such as birth, children leaving home, or death, they are using family developmental approach. When they assess the effect the birth of a child may have on a husband-wife relationship, they are using interactional family theory.

All three theories offer the maternity-gynecologic nurse a basis for understanding the family unit and an approach for using the nursing process to promote family health among childbearing families.

Exchange Theory

Exchange theory, one of the most current theories, provides a rationale to explain human interactions and to advance propositions for predicting behaviors. It is based on two assumptions: individuals interact through the give-and-take of a broad range of commodities, resources, or skills, and all individuals have needs, the fulfillment of which constitutes a reward. Also, individuals attempt to maximize rewards and minimize costs in their exchanges in order to obtain the most profitable outcomes. Behavior is positively reinforced when it is associated with reward and negatively reinforced when it is associated with punishment (Singelmann, 1972). Therefore knowledge of a person's needs, anticipations, and expectations is important if the appropriate reinforcement is to be employed. Because of their repetitiveness and emotional ties, interactions in the family cannot be viewed as merely responses to a reward (Bower, Jacobson, 1978). The feelings and interactions are much more complex. Exchange theory gives little attention to the social, ecologic, or situational aspects of family interactions.

Systems Theory

According to systems theory the family is defined as a group of individuals of at least two generations with ties of affection and responsibility who live in proximity and who share mutual goals (Sargent, 1983). A system has organization, purpose, and a feedback mechanism. Living systems are open systems that exchange energy and information with their environment. Viewed as an open system, the family follows the principles derived from general systems theory. These principles recognize that (Carter, McGoldrick, 1980):

1. A change in one family member creates a change in other members which, in turn, results in a new change in the original changed member.
2. The family as a whole is different from the sum of the individual attributes of its members—"the whole is greater than the sum of its parts."
3. The outcome of any family problem or task depends to a large extent on the current family organization.
4. Interpersonal (communication) messages, transmitted verbally or behaviorally, by a family member precipitate a response from other members.
5. Recurrent patterns of interaction become rules that determine role behaviors by which family members are governed.
6. The family maintains homeostasis of the family life cycle, fluctuating between periods of stability and change while maintaining its integrity through direct responses to deviation.*

Conflict Theory

Grounded in the Marxist philosophy of class conflict, conflict theory is based on the assumption that conflict is natural and inevitable in all human interaction and should not be viewed as bad or disruptive (Eshleman, 1981). When family members are in conflict, the goal is how to manage and resolve the conflict, not how to avoid it. Family situations involve perpetual give-and-take, and harmony can be satisfactorily maintained only through negotiation (Sprey, 1979).

Conflict arises from a variety of sources but the most frequent is a perceived unequal exchange between marriage partners. The outcome can be continued conflict, dissolution of the relationship, or resolution of the conflict. Resolution of the conflict requires three ingredients (Beckman, 1978): (1) open communication, (2) accurate perceptions regarding the degree and nature of conflict, and (3) constructive efforts to resolve conflict. Efforts include a willingness on the part of each member to consider the point of view of the other, alternative solutions, and a willingness to compromise if necessary.

*From Carter E, McGoldrick M: The family life cycle and family therapy: an overview. In Carter E, McGoldrick M, editors: *The family life cycle: a framework for family therapy*, ed 2, New York, 1988, Gardner Press.

■ CULTURAL CONTEXT OF THE FAMILY

The family process in its **cultural context** is a central concern in nursing (for an extensive discussion of culture and ethnicity, see Chapter 3). The reproductive beliefs and practices of a culture are embedded in its economic, religious, kinship, and political structures. Concepts focus on four components of a cultural system: (1) the moral and value system, (2) the kinship system, (3) the knowledge and belief system, and (4) the ceremonial and ritual system. Because of cultural pluralism in North America and the rapid expansion of international nursing, nurses are becoming increasingly aware of the need to focus on cultural variations in perceptions of life events and use of health care systems. Clients have a right to expect that their cultural needs relative to health care will be met, as well as their physiologic and psychologic needs. Social customs need to be maintained and supported that help comfort or make more meaningful the reproductive events that occur to women and their families.

Culture has many definitions. Spradley (1981) defines culture as the "acquired knowledge people use to interpret experience and generate behavior." Each cultural group passes this knowledge to its members from generation to generation. Cultural knowledge includes beliefs and values about each facet of life from birth to death. A person's worldview results from one's cultural knowledge and provides rules for interaction with others, with nature, and with the supernatural (Powers, 1982). These rules have been tested over time and relate to food, language, religion, art, health and healing practices, kinship relationships, and all other systems of behavior. Within each culture may be found many subcultures.

Subculture refers to a group within a larger cultural system that retains its own characteristics; individuals identify themselves as members of the group. A subculture may be an ethnic group or a group organized in other ways. For example, there is a subculture of nursing and a subculture of medicine.

Each subculture has rich and complex traditions, including health practices that have proven effective over time. These traditions vary from group to group. In a pluralistic society, these traditions and practices are subject to the influences from many groups. As cultural groups become associated with each other, the processes of acculturation and assimilation may occur.

Acculturation refers to changes that take place in one or both groups when people from different cultures come in contact with one another. People may retain some of their own culture and also reformulate cultural elements. This familiarization among cultural groups results in much overt behavioral similarity. Individuals exchange and adopt mannerisms, styles, and practices of the other group. Changes are evident when one observes such things as dress, language patterns, food choices, and health practices among cultural groups within the society. An example of acculturation would be the adoption of food practices of ethnic groups in the United States. For example, the original recipe for pizza, which is of Italian origin, has been accepted and adopted by many other groups.

Assimilation, on the other hand, occurs when a cultural group loses its identity and becomes a part of the dominant culture. According to Friedman (1986), "Assimilation denotes the more complete and one-way process of one culture being absorbed into the other." Assimilation is the process by which groups "melt" into the mainstream, thus accounting for the notion of a "melting pot," a phenomenon that has been said to occur in the United States. Spector (1979), however, asserts that in the United States, the "melting pot," with its dream of a common culture "has proved to be a myth and faded; it is now time to identify and both accept and appreciate the differences among people."

Nurses must recognize that a wide range of cultural diversity may exist within a society. Assessment of the beliefs and practices of a group and those within the group is essential for the health care provider striving to provide culturally sensitive health care. The nurse must also be aware of factors that may prevent some individuals from providing this optimum care. Understanding the concepts of ethnocentrism and cultural relativism may be helpful to nurses caring for families in a pluralistic society.

Ethnocentrism is "being centered in one's own ethnic or cultural system, judging the world in general by the standards established in that particular system" (Downs, 1971). Essentially it supports the notion that "my group is the best." Socialization into the profession of nursing occurs within the framework of the Western health care system. This system emphasizes the biomedical model, which in the United States is based primarily on the white, middle-class value system. The biomedical model presents pregnancy and childbirth as phenomena with inherent risks, most appropriately managed through specific knowledge and technology. The nurse encountering behavior in women incongruent with this model may become perplexed and label the women's behavior inappropriate and in conflict with good health practices. If the Western health care system provides the only standards for judging, the behavior of the nurse is termed *ethnocentric.*

Cultural relativism, the opposite of ethnocentrism, involves learning about and applying the standards of another person's culture to activities within that culture. To be culturally relativistic means the nurse recognizes that people from different cultural backgrounds actually see the same objects and situations differently. There are reasons why people behave the way they do, and these reasons are for the most part culturally determined.

Cultural relativism does not require nurses to accept the beliefs and values of another culture; rather, nurses recognize that the behavior of others may be based on a system of logic different from their own. Cultural relativism is an affirmation of the uniqueness and value of every culture. Spector (1979) sees this as mandatory for health professionals. Spector states that ". . . because health care providers learn from their culture the why and the how of being healthy or ill, it behooves them to treat each client with deference to his own cultural background."

■ FAMILY AND CRISIS

We live in a stressful society. For the family system, stress can arise internally or externally. Although many families cope with stress, the situation may become acute and take on the characteristics of a crisis. Crisis may be defined as a disturbance of habit: a disruption in a family's or an individual's usual means of maintaining control over a situation. If faced with a crisis, the family or person attempts to resolve it using customary values and behaviors. If the family's usual behaviors are inadequate to resolve the crisis, new behavior patterns must be developed through crisis intervention.

One of the goals of crisis intervention is to help the client learn new ways of dealing with conflicts or problems. Although the client may seek help for a specific problem, the strategies learned may be applied to future difficulties. Crises can be centered around maturational or situational events.

The experience of childbearing is accompanied by both maturational and situational events that make it a significant turning point in the life of a family. Indeed, childbearing is often considered a time of crisis. Maternity nurses who understand crisis theory can readily assist those families who are unable to cope with the stress of these events.

Maturational Crisis

Maturational crises develop as a result of normal growth and development. They characteristically evolve over time and involve *role* and *status* changes. They include events such as birth, infancy, childhood, adolescence, adulthood, and old age. Each phase of the family life cycle produces characteristic crises or events capable of creating stress of such severity that it can affect the health of one or more family members.

The birth of a child represents one of the most important events in the life of a family. Births and the subsequent care of the children require parental, intellectual, and psychologic maturity, and this may account for periods of crisis in a family.

Nurses assist with the birth of children and can provide support as the adults undertake active parenting roles. Nurses can provide knowledge of human psychosocial development, which will help parents see their children realistically and establish appropriate criteria for children's behavior. Nurses may use this unique relationship with a family to promote birth as a family-centered happening with great growth potential for all participants.

Menopausal concerns often affect the entire family. Few opportunities are available to counsel women regarding normal changes, however, since nurses may not see these women except during an illness. A woman 65 years of age or older is likely to be the concern of the nurse working in acute care, long-term care, and the community (Griffith-Kenney, 1986).

Situational Crisis

Situational crises include such events as preterm birth, mental or physical illness, loss of financial or social support, changed body image, experience of violence or serious illness, divorce, death, and grief. These crises involve a threat to a person's sense of integrity, or an actual or potential loss or deprivation of some kind. Anxiety and depression are characteristic responses. If the situational crisis causes severe strain, it can result in health impairment.

Response to Crisis

In both maturational and situational crises, the family plays a critical role in the alleviation of distress, successful adaptation, and healthy rehabilitation. The nurse's knowledge of a family's reactions to crisis prompts a more rational assessment of the family's ability to withstand the stress. The nurse can help the family mobilize its problem-solving abilities to deal with the problem.

Aguilera and Messick (1990) have devised a stratagem for assessing a family's or an individual's potential or actual response to a crisis. They maintain that three key areas or components act as balancing factors affecting equilibrium: (1) the client's perception of the crisis event, (2) the client's coping mechanisms, and (3) the client's support system. The interplay between these three areas is critical for the outcome or resolution of a problem. A brief discussion of each of the three areas follows.

PERCEPTION OF EVENT. What one person considers a crisis may or may not be perceived as a crisis by someone else. Factors such as *age* and *prior experience* can alter perception. For example, an event viewed as a crisis by an adolescent may not be seen as a crisis by a 30-year-old adult. *Emotional states, anxiety,* or *hostility* may color a person's perception. The highly anxious young mother of a firstborn child may become disorganized by her infant's crying, whereas a mother of four may accept the crying as normal.

Nursing intervention relative to a client's perception of a crisis-provoking event may be limited to helping the client state "what the problem is." However, if the event can have a negative effect on the client, the infant, or the family, more intervention is required.

In some cultures pregnancy is seen as such a natural event that no medical or nursing supervision is considered necessary. Since complications of pregnancy can arise with detrimental effects for mother and child, the nurse should encourage the family to participate in ongoing health care.

Cultures define gynecologic conditions that are acceptable and those that are not. Menopause elevates a woman's status in some cultures (Chapter 41). In others, reproductive cancers are considered "dirty," and the women with these cancers are to be avoided. The nurse in such a situation could act as nurturer, information giver, or organizer.

COPING MECHANISMS. Coping mechanisms can be defined as patterns of behavior that people or families have developed for dealing with threats to their sense of well-being (Stuart, Sundeen, 1991). Coping mechanisms may be constructive or destructive. *Constructive coping mechanisms* lead to a resolution of a problem. They vary with the level of anxiety being experienced. For mild anxiety the individual may resort to crying, sleeping, eating, exercise, or smoking and drinking. In interpersonal situations, avoiding eye contact or limiting close relationships to those who cause no anxiety may be successful.

If the threat and consequent level of anxiety become severe, people will resort to the use of task-oriented reactions or ego-oriented reactions. Task-oriented behaviors are aimed at relieving the stress situations. They are consciously directed and have been objectively appraised by the person using them. Ego-oriented reactions are also known as ego-defense mechanisms. They include repression, projection, and displacement. These reactions protect the person from feelings of inadequacy and worthlessness. However, such responses can be used to the person's detriment. They can distort reality, interfere with interpersonal relationships, and limit working ability. If misused they become *destructive coping mechanisms*.

Nurses use knowledge of human coping mechanisms to assess the type of defense mechanism the person or family uses and the success of the mechanism in ameliorating problems. Attempts are made to substitute more beneficial behaviors, while supporting and reinforcing constructive coping, if the defense is recognized as destructive. However, coping mechanisms, whether constructive or destructive, appear to be essential for all individuals and groups if they are to maintain emotional stability.

SUPPORT SYSTEMS. **Support systems** refer to the support that people may expect from others in their environment during a time of crisis. Caplan (1959), one of the developers of crisis intervention, maintains that the successful resolution of a crisis often depends on the client's support system. If a client's support system is strong, only minimum intervention may be necessary to resolve a crisis and help the client recover. If the client's support system is not strong, disorganization may occur and the client may not recover without considerable intervention from health care professionals.

A client's support system may include family, friends, and significant others in the environment. Other people who function as part of support systems are health personnel, or "community caretakers" (Caplan, 1959). Community caretakers are people in the various agencies that represent the organized health resources of a community. These individuals are knowledgeable and experienced. They may be able to assist those who are unable to handle crises on their own or with the help of family and friends. Maternity nurses are in an ideal position to offer help throughout the maternity cycle. The assistance may take the form of teaching or counseling, or it may involve helping the client learn the procedures for enlisting the aid of other community agencies. For example, nurses have developed *parent education programs* to provide women and men with mechanisms for coping with the stress of labor. These programs also help parents learn about their infants' needs and about child care activities so that the parents are better able to cope with the changing needs of a growing child and to understand the impact of a newborn on the family.

These key factors, family dynamics, socioeconomic status, cultural patterns, and coping responses viewed from a theoretic perspective should all be considered as nurses formulate nursing care plans for the childbearing family.

In addition to professionally led groups, *peer support groups* are now available to clients (e.g., Mothers of Twins, PMS [premenstrual syndrome]). Peer groups encourage interactions between people with similar problems. The groups promote interaction, encourage acceptance and support among members, and serve as a resource. Nurses and social workers have been leaders in originating such groups in the hospital and in the community. They have worked with others in planning and establishing the groups.

■ KEY FACTORS IN FAMILY HEALTH

Family patterns, attitudes, and responses to change play a determining part in the health of individual family members and their use of health services. Because the family acts as a primary force in generating support for clients, an understanding of this unit is essential to the formation of a nursing care plan.

Certain factors have proved important in determining the quality of family health. *Culture patterning* in areas such as childbearing, child rearing, or use of health services determines many health-related responses. *Family dynamics,* which encompass coordination of intrafamilial roles, distribution of power in the family, and the process of decision making, affects the use of health services. *Family responses to crisis,* including coping behaviors and the quality of personal responses and mutual concern, affect the level of support afforded family members. *Family socioeconomic characteristics* are important. Social class affects expectations, obligations, and rewards, all of which affect use of health services. In addition, the family acts as the primary economic unit in which incomes may be pooled, expenditure decisions taken jointly, and services rendered internally.

A healthy family is one characterized by functional communication, parental unity, flexible family roles, and the ability to function during periods of stress (e.g., the illness of one of its members or the addition of a new member) (Reidy, Thibedeau, 1984). Family health can be determined by assessment of nine dimensions (Reidy, Thibedeau, 1984). These include:

- Present health habits
- Knowledge of health and illness

- Attitudes toward health and health care services
- Ability to cope effectively with health problems and complications
- Ability to cope with stressful situations
- Life patterns; life-styles
- Interaction with the environment
- Participation in community life
- Knowledge and use of community and health resources

The family must be viewed as a whole to determine its level of health.

Friedman (1986) considers a family's social class as a prime molder of family life-style. Social class, she says, along with cultural background:

> . . . Exerts the greatest overall influence on family life, influencing our early socialization, the role expectations we hold, the values we stress, the types of behavior we consider acceptable or deviant, or the world experiences we have.*

The Family and Poverty

Family poverty is not synonymous with family dysfunction. Many economically impoverished families have been able to fulfill the developmental needs of their members. Many families learn to adapt creatively to their situation. There is infinite variation among families, cultures, and ethnic groups that contend on a daily basis with an impoverished and hostile environment. However, poverty does exert a pronounced negative force on a family's structure and function. In addition, many of these families are composed of cultural and ethnic minorities (Hines, 1988). Impoverishment and minority status expose individuals and families to major stressors (Hines, 1988): community agencies and officials who frequently intrude in their daily lives; discriminatory attitudes; a multitude of events that constantly bombard them and over which they have no control (e.g., continual exposure to violence in the neighborhood); crucial interdependence of family members financially and emotionally; and unrelenting stress and change.

Hines (1988) described the life cycle of African-American families who exist at the poverty level. Although written with these families in mind, many of the observations may be relevant to other families in similar economic straits. The nurse is cautioned not to make generalizations; individual family assessment is necessary.

Often, impoverished families face many situational crises but have few resources available to cope with them. Adolescents or unattached young adults need time to establish themselves as persons. Young people from these families may be pushed into adult role expectations too early (e.g., they may be forced to leave the home or may be relied on to support the family). They often have difficulty finding legitimate work and so may be drawn into an unlawful "underground" economy. During this developmental stage (see Chapter 8 for more discussion about developmental stages across the life span), impoverished youths may experience difficulty with intimate sexual relationships. Females may view motherhood as one route to achieving an identity; males, finding few economic opportunities, may move from one relationship to another.

The family with children faces other tasks. A stable union may be difficult in light of continual stress and conflicts over the use of time and finances. Taking on the parental role may be difficult for the young person who is still identifying with single peers. For a family to be eligible for Aid to Families with Dependent Children (AFDC) (also known as "welfare"), the father may be pushed into a peripheral role (i.e., the aid is not given if there is an adult male living with the family).

Many become grandparents at an early age. However, if the son or daughter is a young adolescent, the new baby may be brought into the home and be raised as a sibling of her or his parent. Many grandparents find that they may need to take over the parenting roles of their grandchild(ren) if their son or daughter cannot (e.g., is drug-addicted, imprisoned, or dies). An "empty nest" may never occur; women may not ever be able to move out of the child care role (Hines, 1988).

The Nursing Process

To plan for the care of a family or particular family member, the nurse must remember that a family operates as a system. That is, no one family member has a problem; if a problem exists, the whole family has a problem. Solutions to problems can evolve best through family participation.

ASSESSMENT

Data Collection Process

The *process* of an assessment in planning family care is often more difficult and complicated than that involved in assessing the physical health of individual clients. It requires adept skill in communication and the ability to establish a trusting relationship with each member of the family simultaneously. In

*From Friedman MM: *Family nursing theory and assessment*, New York, 1986, Appleton-Century-Crofts.

every family group, areas of openness and privacy exist, and all groups resent interrogation by an outsider. The reasons for obtaining information must be explained clearly to family members.

Information such as the address, marital status, and family members' ages can be obtained readily because it is generally given freely. Other information is attained by (1) *observing* and noting relationships, attitudes, and stress responses (who is doing what), (2) *listening* to conversation about community and family involvements or hopes and aspirations, and (3) *being aware* of cultural and socioeconomic factors that might affect the family's behaviors.

As previously discussed, cross-cultural variations in reproductive and gynecologic practices can greatly influence the family's response to care. It is therefore important that the nurse include cultural considerations when assessing families.

The model developed by Stern (1980) for improving communication between individuals and families from a variety of ethnic and cultural backgrounds and Western health care providers can be useful for nurses when doing family assessment. This model identifies barriers in communication that exist on three levels: approach, custom, and language.

Approach includes numerous factors one considers in interpersonal relationships. The American approach to most issues in health care is to address the problem directly. With many cultures (Stern, 1980) engaging in small talk is vital before a serious discussion. Commenting on flowers or pictures and having tea or a cold drink are equated with showing respect. To begin talking to an expectant mother about the need for prenatal care before commenting on the other children, the pretty chair, or the weather might set up an atmosphere of distrust. In some cultures, women prefer a caregiver of the same sex. Therefore it may be critical that the initial encounter be with a woman. Showing respect and patience is essential in building trust.

Custom includes practices and behaviors characteristic of a culture. Understanding that a cultural reason exists for all behaviors and making a sincere effort to ascertain the person's rationale for behavior are important steps in establishing trust. The clients themselves may be the most helpful to the nurse trying to understand their cultural logic and individual differences. Assessing health beliefs and practices is essential for the health care professional who is striving to achieve a holistic approach to care. For the client, adherence to a particular cultural custom provides a sense of constancy with one's cultural heritage.

Language is an important factor. Stern (1980) emphasizes the use of clear, jargon-free English. When the family does not speak English, a bilingual nurse is ideal for assessing the family. If such a nurse is not available, an interpreter, either a family member or a member of the same cultural group, may be used. When an interpreter is being used, it is important to address questions and responses to the client and not to the interpreter.

LEGAL CONCERNS. For the nurse working with blended and communal families, issues arise about how these families are working at fulfilling their basic family functions. The nurse must be careful to ascertain who is related to whom and who may be the biologic parents, custodial parents, stepparents, and communal parents. The nurse must ascertain who has legal custody of whom and who can sign permits to provide health care.

Analysis, Synthesis, Validation

Following the data-gathering phase, the nurse analyzes and synthesizes the findings. Inferences about the data are formulated. The nurse formulates inferences about the data by asking herself questions, such as, what aspects of family theories are represented by this family: structural-functional, developmental, or interactional? What are the significant stressors influencing this family? Do the family's beliefs reflect myth or old wives' tales? Do these beliefs promote physical or emotional well-being or might they be harmful to the family? Is this family's immediate support system adequate for their coping with potential crises during childbearing? Does family communication respect all family members in light of the individual's developmental stage? Does the family perceive itself to be healthy or in difficulty?

A checklist can assist a nurse in gathering data needed for a plan of care and can act as a tool for validating information with the client. One example of a checklist is found in the box on p. 35.

Because inferences are subjective and based not only on the nurse's competence level but also on individual values and beliefs, the nurse needs to validate the interpretation of the data with the client. Validation of inferences is followed by the development of nursing diagnoses.

NURSING DIAGNOSES

Nursing diagnoses are formulated to reflect the family's perception of its needs, as well as the nurse's perception. *It is important to determine the family's perception of its nursing care needs rather than the perception of any one family member.*

FAMILY COPING ABILITIES/CONTRACT RECORD

Family ID# ____________
Family Name ____________

Coping Scale:	1=Very rarely coping	4=Mostly coping	HV Home Visit
	2=Minimal coping	5=Completely coping	OV Office Visit
	3=Moderately coping—or insufficient information to evaluate		TV Tele. Visit

	Date/Member#						
	Type of Visit (*circle*)	HV OV TV		HV OV TV		HV OV TV	
1. PHYSICAL INDEPENDENCE: Family's ability to move from one place to another in order to obtain what it needs.	Coping Scale Rating:						
		Stat	Inter	Stat	Inter	Stat	Inter
a. Food preparation							
b. Transportation for medical care							
c. Obtaining prescriptions, finances							
d. Other: (*specify*)							
2. THERAPEUTIC COMPETENCE: Family's ability to *apply* prescribed care procedures.	Coping Scale Rating:						
a. Therapeutic treatments							
b. Drugs, diet, activity							
c. Other: (*specify*)							
3. KNOWLEDGE OF HEALTH CONDITION: Family's knowledge of facts about the particular health condition and the principles underlying recommendations for care.	Coping Scale Rating:						
a. Effects of condition/bodily changes of pregnancy							
b. Rationale of therapy							
c. Signs of complications/need for medical care							
d. Facts about developmental change							
e. Other: (*specify*)							
4. APPLICATION OF PRINCIPLES OF GENERAL HYGIENE: Family's actions/practices that promote health	Coping Scale Rating:						
a. Habits of personal hygiene							
b. Balance of exercise, work, sleep, and recreation							
c. Food habits appropriate to age/health status							
d. Parenting							
e. Other: (*specify*)							
5. HEALTH ATTITUDES: Family's expressions of feelings about health care in general	Coping Scale Rating:						
a. Preventive health services							
b. Care of illness, emergency							
c. Other: (*specify*)							

PROBLEM STATUS			INTERVENTION		
N—New	I—Improved	W—Worsened	A—Assess	S—Support	Pl—Plan
R—Resolved	M—Maintained		T—Teach	Ps—Problem Solve	

NOTE: Use asterisk in Intervention Column when making additional entry on Progress Notes.

Continued.

	Date/Member#						
	Type of Visit *(circle)*	HV OV TV		HV OV TV		HV OV TV	
	Coping Scale Rating:	Stat	Inter	Stat	Inter	Stat	Inter
6. EMOTIONAL COMPETENCE: Family's psychologic resourcefulness in coping with daily problems, stress, and change including individual member's inadequate competence.							
a. Meets demands regarding member's developmental health status							
b. Problem solving							
c. Other: *(specify)*							
7. FAMILY LIVING: The ability with which each family member fulfills his/her role within the family system, including decision-making about individual member's roles.	Coping Scale Rating:						
a. Intrafamily cooperation							
b. Role fulfillment (e.g., affection, protection, economics)							
c. Assistance to members regarding meeting societal demands							
d. Other: *(specify)*							
8. PHYSICAL ENVIRONMENT: The quality of the home and community environment as it affects the physical or mental health of each family member and their risk for injury.	Coping Scale Rating:						
a. Sanitation							
b. Safety							
c. Comfort, stimulation							
d. Other: *(specify)*							
9. USE OF COMMUNITY FACILITIES/RESOURCES: Family's ability to seek and appropriately use available community resources according to the family's need for services.	Coping Scale Rating:						
a. Selects/secures needed resources							
b. Utilizes/participates in services responsibly							
c. Other: *(specify)*							
	Total Rating:						
	Nurse Signature:						

Examples of nursing diagnoses (Christensen, Kenney, 1990) commonly encountered with childbearing families include:

- Altered parenting related to
  - —Impaired parent-infant attachment
- Altered family processes related to
  - —Birth of a child with a defect
- Anxiety related to
  - —Expectations of parenting experience
- High risk for ineffective individual coping related to
  - —Knowledge deficit regarding infant care activities
- Social isolation related to
  - —Lack of interaction with peers
- Spiritual distress related to
  - —Conflict between ideal and personal religious practices associated with childbearing

Once the nursing diagnoses are established, the nurse takes time to explore personal value judgments about the family that may affect and impede nursing interventions. It is also essential for the nurse to validate the diagnoses. In addition to direct validation with the family, a review of the literature, an analysis of norms within a cultural context, and discussion with other persons involved in the family are means of validation.

PLANNING

Setting Goals

The next step is to set goals and outcome criteria related to each diagnosis. These are established as a joint enterprise between nurse and family. They are evaluated for realism and acceptance by family members. Goals for care are both short- and long-term. Once agreed on, the goals are assessed to determine priority. Certain health needs require immediate attention (e.g., unexplained vaginal bleeding). Other health needs require more time to resolve (e.g., anger over birth of a child of undesired sex or spiritual distress over diagnosis of breast cancer).

Selecting Nursing Actions

Working with the available data, the nursing diagnoses, and the health goals, the nurse proceeds to organize a plan for implementing the most appropriate interventions. The nurse identifies the nursing role, that is, whether the role is teacher, direct care provider, or referrer.

Teaching must be at a level that is understandable and supportive to individual family members. Different strategies may be necessary for different family members. As a direct care provider, the nurse promotes activities that will lead to the family's own self-care and independence. The nurse plans for the best use of resources available to the family, both internal and community support systems. The nurse must determine whether the resources are appropriate and whether the family is able or willing to use them.

Goals are stated in client-centered terms; for example:

1. The family will support the parent(s) in learning child care activities.
2. The family will use community support groups to cope with one member's breast cancer.

IMPLEMENTATION

The selected nursing actions are implemented, tailored to the individual needs of the family and its members. Nurses may also use their knowledge and skills in guiding family members who will actually implement the interventions.

Maternity-gynecologic nursing involves actions that can be designated as preventive, curative, or rehabilitative in nature (ANA, 1980). It spans the lifetime of an individual from preconceptional planning for children through pregnancy and birth and the early adjustment of the family to a newborn child through middle and late adulthood. These activities may be carried out in the home, clinic, or hospital.

The **preventive actions** of nursing care include health promotion and prevention of disease states. Efforts are made to increase and strengthen the individual's ability to withstand the stress of everyday living. Nursing actions associated with these efforts represent many of the nurse's independent functions. The nurse who teaches good nutrition, personal hygiene, safer sex, and beneficial exercises to a pregnant woman is promoting the health of the woman and her developing fetus. The nurse who encourages a teenager to seek care for pregnancy or who discusses sexual adjustment with pregnant or older couples is acting to promote health and to prevent possible complications.

Curative actions are interventions such as teaching good body mechanics to relieve muscle strain, administering antibiotics or anticancer chemotherapeutics, treating postpartum hemorrhage, providing oxygen to a mother in labor whose fetus is showing signs of distress, and maintaining life-support therapies for the ill preterm infant.

Rehabilitative actions are directed toward returning an individual to her or his previous state with an equal or greater ability to function. The care given a pregnant teenager illustrates the rehabilitative aspects of maternity care. Nurses hope that the physical and emotional support provided these young people will enable them to complete their development toward responsible adulthood. Nurses have provided the impetus to founding teenage clinics, high school programs for pregnant teenagers, and follow-up care to help teenagers give their children the mothering needed.

After a mastectomy or hysterectomy, women (and their partners/families) require sensitive and skillful care. Rehabilitative actions help a woman maintain or regain self-esteem, positive family processes, and sexuality and also help avoid social isolation.

EVALUATION

Evaluation is a joint process between nurse and family. Mutually determined goals and outcome criteria need to be stated precisely and in behavioral terms so that the degree to which goals are met can be determined. The criteria need to be realistic and flexible enough to permit modification as circumstances change.

Friedman (1986) suggests six questions that should be asked when evaluating the nursing process with the family.

1. Were family expectations set in relative and accurate terms?
2. Is there a consensus between the family and other health team members on the evaluation?
3. What additional data need to be collected to evaluate progress?
4. Were the nursing diagnoses, goals, and approaches realistic and accurate?
5. If the family's behavior and perception indicate that the problem has not been satisfactorily resolved, what are the reasons?
6. Were there any unforeseen outcomes that need to be considered?

SUMMARY

The family is the fundamental social unit of every society and it has many functions. One function is to serve as a crucial support system for the individual. Family dynamics are complex. There are many types of families and family dynamics; each family structure has both strengths and potential shortcomings. Family theories provide guides to understanding family functioning and its developmental stages and tasks. The family faces and must cope with maturational and situational crises. Families function within a cultural context. All of the components of the nurse and individual client relationship and of the nursing process are used when the client-family unit is the focus of care.

REFERENCES

Aguilera DC, Messick JM: *Crisis intervention: theory and methodology,* ed 5, St Louis, 1990, Mosby–Year Book.

Ahrons CR: The binuclear family: two households, one family, *Altern Lifestyles* 2:499, 1979.

Allen WR: Black family research in the United States: a review, assessment, and extension, *J Compar Fam Stud* 9:301, 1978.

American Nurses Association: *Nursing: a social policy statement,* Kansas City, Mo, 1980, American Nurses Association.

Beckman LJ: Couples' decision-making processes regarding fertility. In Tauber KE, Burgess LL, Sweet JA, editors: *Social demography,* New York, 1978, Academic Press.

Belsky J: Early human experience: a family perspective, *Dev Psychol* 17:3, 1981.

Blehar MC: Families and public policy. In Corfman E, editor: *Families today,* vol 2, National Institute of Mental Health, Division of Scientific and Public Information, Science Monograph No 1, Washington, DC, 1979, US Government Printing Office.

Bower F, Jacobson M: Family theories: frameworks for nursing practice. In Archer S, Fleshman R, editors: *Community health nursing: patterns and practice,* N Scituate, Mass, 1978, Duxbury Press.

Caplan G: *Concepts of mental health and consultation,* Children's Bureau, US Department of Health, Education and Welfare, Washington, DC, 1959, US Government Printing Office.

Carrington BW: The Afro-American. In Clark AL, editor: *Culture/child-bearing/health professionals,* Philadelphia, 1978, FA Davis.

Carter E, McGoldrick M, editors: *The family life cycle,* New York, 1980, Gardner Press.

Carter E, McGoldrick M: The family life cycle and family therapy: an overview. In Carter E, McGoldrick M, editors: *The family life cycle: a framework for family therapy,* ed 2, New York, 1988, Gardner Press.

Christensen P, Kenney S: *Nursing process: application of theories, frameworks, and models,* ed 3, St Louis, 1990, Mosby–Year Book.

Chung HQ: Understanding the oriental maternity patient, *Nurs Clin North Am* 12:67, March, 1977.

Downs JF: *Cultures in crisis,* Beverly Hills, Calif, 1971, Glencoe Publishing.

Duvall ER: *Marriage and family development,* ed 5, Philadelphia, 1977, JB Lippincott.

Erikson EH: *Identity: youth and crisis,* New York, 1968, WW Norton & Co.

Eshleman JR: *The family: an introduction,* ed 3, Boston, 1981, Allyn & Bacon.

Espinoza R, Newman Y: *Step-parenting,* DHEW Publication No. (ADM)78-579, Washington, DC, 1979, US Government Printing Office.

Evans MI et al: *Fetal diagnosis and therapy: science, ethics, and the law,* Philadelphia, 1989, JB Lippincott.

Friedman MM: *Family nursing theory and assessment,* New York, 1986, Appleton-Century-Crofts.

Glick PC: Children of divorced parents in demographic perspective, *J Soc Issues* 35:170, 1979.

Griffith-Kenney J: Contemporary women's health, Menlo Park, Calif, 1986, Addison-Wesley Publishing.

Harvey S, Carr C, Bernheine S, Lesbian mothers: health care experiences, *J Nurse Midwifery* 34:3, May-June 1989.

Hines PM. The family life cycle of poor black families. In Carter B, McGoldrick M, editors: *The changing family life cycle,* ed 2, New York: Gardner Press, 1988.

Kay MA: The Mexican-American. In Clark AL, editor: *Culture/child-bearing/ health professionals,* Philadelphia, 1978, FA Davis Co.

Libman J: The American ideal is kin through thick and thin, *Los Angeles Times,* November 20, 1988.

Malinowski B: *The dynamics of cultural change,* New Haven, Conn, 1945, Yale University Press.

McAdoo HP: Factors related to stability in upwardly mobile black families, *J Marr Fam* 40:761, 1978.

Mercer RT: Theoretical perspective on the family. In Gillis CL et al, editors: *Toward a science of family nursing,* Menlo Park, Calif, 1989, Addison-Wesley Publishing.

Norton A, Glick P: One parent families: a social and economic profile, *Fam Relations* 35(1):9, 1986.

Perkins TF, Kahan JP: An empirical comparison of natural-father and stepfather family systems, *Fam Process* 18:175, 1979.

Poverny L, Finch W: Gay and lesbian domestic partnerships: expanding the definition of the family, *Soc Casework* Feb 1988.

Powers BA: The use of orthodox and Black-American folk medicine, *Adv Nurs Sci* 4:35, 1982.

Radcliffe-Brown A: *Structure and function in a primitive society,* New York, 1952, Free Press.

Reidy M, Thibedeau M: Evaluation of family functioning: development of a scale which measures family competence in matters of health, *Nurs Papers* 16:42, 1984.

Sargent AJ: The family: a pediatric assessment, *J Pediatr* 102:973, 1983.

Singelmann RB: Exchange as symbolic interaction: convergences between two theoretical perspectives, *Am Soc Rev* 37:414, 1972.

Spector RE: *Cultural diversity in health and illness,* New York, 1979, Appleton-Century-Crofts.

BIBLIOGRAPHY

Doenges M, Kenty J, Moorhouse M: *Maternal/newborn care plans: guidelines for client care,* Philadelphia, 1988, FA Davis.

Farber N: The significance of race and class in marital decisions among unmarried adolescent mothers, *Soc Probl* 37:1 Feb 1990.

Friedemann ML: The concept of family nursing, *J Adv Nurs* 14, 1989.

Friedemann, ML: Closing the gap between theory and mental health practice with families. Part 2: The control-congruence model for mental health nursing of families, *Arch Psych Nurs* 3:1, Feb 1989.

Friedemann ML et al: Advanced family nursing with the control-congruence model, *Clinical Nurse Specialist.* 3:4, 1989.

Gillis C: Family nursing in research. In Gillis C et al, editors: *Toward a science of family nursing,* Menlo Park, Calif, 1989, Addison-Wesley.

Hochschild A, Machung A: *Second shift: inside the two-job marriage,* New York, 1989, Viking Press.

Kulin J: Childbearing Cambodian refugee women, *Can Nurse,* p 46, June 1988.

Lee RV: Understanding Southeast Asian mothers-to-be, *Childbirth Educ* 8(3):32, 1989.

Lee RV et al: Southeast Asian folklore about pregnancy and parturition, *Obstet Gynecol* 71:243, 1988.

Lewis J: *The birth of the family: an empirical inquiry,* New York, 1989, Brunner/Mazel.

London K: Cohabitation, marriage, marital dissolution, and remarriage: United States, 1988, *Advance Data* 194:Jan 1991.

NPA Bulletin: *Increasing culturally relevant practice with Hispanic clients* 3(4):23, 1988.

Olsen D, McCubbin H et al: *Families: what makes them work,* New York, 1989, Sage Publications.

Schnaiberg A, Goldenberg S: From empty nest to crowded nest: the dynamics of incompletely launched young adults, *Soc Probl* 36:3, June 1989.

Spradley BW: *Community health nursing,* Boston, 1981, Little, Brown & Co.

Sprey J: Conflict theory and the study of marriage and the family. In Burr WR et al, editors: *Contemporary theories about the family,* vol 2, New York, 1979, Free Press.

Stern PN et al: Culturally-induced stress during childbearing: the Filipino-American experience, *Issues Health Care Women* 2(3-4):67, 1980.

Stuart GW, Sundeen SJ: *Principles and practice of psychiatric nursing,* ed 4, St Louis, 1991, Mosby–Year Book.

US Bureau of the Census: *Households, families, marital status and living arrangements,* Washington, DC, 1989, US Government Printing Office.

Williams RP: Issues in Women's Health Care. In Johnson BS, editor: *Psychiatric mental health nursing: adaptation and growth,* Philadelphia, 1989, JB Lippincott.

Wismont JM, Reame NE, The lesbian childbearing experience: assessing developmental tasks, *Image J Nurs Sch* 21(3):137, 1989.

Wright LM, Leahey M: Nurses and families: a guide to family assessment and intervention, Philadelphia, 1984, FA Davis.

World Health Organization: *Health and the family: studies in the demography of family life cycles and their health implication,* Geneva, 1978, The Organization.

Schorr L: *Within our reach: breaking the cycle of disadvantage,* New York, 1989, Anchor Books.

Sidel R: *Troubling trends: the health of America's next generation,* Washington, DC, 1990, The National Commission to Prevent Infant Mortality.

US Bureau of the Census: *Statistical abstract of the United States: 1989,* ed 109, Washington, DC, 1988, US Government Printing Office.

Bibliography—Nursing Research

Bozett FW: Social control of identity by children of gay fathers, *West J Nurs Res* 10(5):550, 1988.

Friedemann ML: An instrument to evaluate effectiveness in family functioning, *West J Nurs Res* 13:2, 1991.

Glanz D, Ganong L, Coleman M: Client gender, diagnosis, and family structure, *West J Nurs Res* 11:6, 1989.

Loveland CC et al: A psychometric analysis of the family environment scale, *Nurs Res* 5:38, 1989.

Maurin JT, Russell L, Memmott RJ: An exploration of gender differences among the homeless, *Res Nurs Health* 12(5):315, 1989.

Mercer R, Ferketich S, DeJoseph J: Effects of stress on family functioning during pregnancy, *Nurs Res* 37(5):268, 1989.

Pitzer MS, Hock E: Employed mothers' concerns about separation from the first- and second-born child, *Res Nurs Health* 12(2):123, 1989.

Richards E: Self-reports of differentiation of self and marital compatibility as related to family functioning in the third and fourth stages of the family life cycle, *Scholarly Inquiry for Nursing Practice: An International Journal* 3(3):163, 1989.

Uphold C, Strickland O: Issues related to the unit of analysis in family nursing, *West J Nurs Res* 11(4):405, 1989.

Wismont JM, Reame NE: The lesbian childbearing experience: assessing developmental tasks, *Image J Nurs Sch* 21(3):137, 1989.

chapter 2 review

Key Concepts

- The family forms a social network that acts as a potent support system for its members.
- Ideally, the family provides a safe, intimate environment for the biopsychosocial development of children and its adult members.
- Family theories provide the nurse with useful guides in understanding family function.
- Sometimes it is difficult to document the life cycle of a family; often we can only catch glimpses of it.
- The reproductive beliefs and practices of a culture are embedded in its economic, religious, political, and kinship structures.
- Differences between the dominant culture of North America and other cultures in general are reflected in how the roles of parents are expressed and how children are viewed.
- North American culture is a pluralistic one in which varying family forms are recognized and accepted in differing degrees.
- In both maturational and situational crises the family plays a critical role in the alleviation of distress, successful adaptation, and healthy rehabilitation.
- Balancing factors affecting equilibrium in a family include the client's perception of the crisis event, the client's coping mechanisms, and the client's support system.
- Maternity-gynecologic nursing involves actions that can be called preventive, curative, or rehabilitative.

Key Terms

- blended family (p. 23)
- communal family (p. 24)
- coping mechanisms (p. 31)
- cultural context (p. 29)
- curative actions (p. 37)
- developmental theory (p. 27)
- extended family (p. 23)
- family dynamics (p. 26)
- family functions (p. 24)
- family theories (p. 26)
- homosexual family (p. 24)
- interactional theory (p. 28)
- maturational crises (p. 30)
- nuclear family (p. 22)
- preventive actions (p. 37)
- rehabilitative actions (p. 37)
- single-parent family (p. 23)
- situational crises (p. 31)
- structural-functional theory (p. 26)
- support systems (p. 32)

Critical Thinking Exercises

Select a family unit that is different from your own. Interview an adult member of that family regarding their values and beliefs about family functions, roles, and dynamics.

1. Analyze your findings based on this chapter's content. Determine which family theory (theories) best fits your data, and state evidence that justifies your conclusions.
2. Analyze your findings in relation to your values and beliefs about family functions, roles, and dynamics. Do they differ significantly? What assumptions did you hold that proved to be in error?
3. Using one false assumption, examine the effect this might have had on your nursing plan of care for that family unit.

Topics for Nursing Research

- Replicate study of family theories as frameworks for nursing practice for the 1990s.
- Research the spousal unit in same-sex relationships.
- Research the effects of growing up as a child in any of the family units (e.g., blended [reconstituted], same-sex [homosexual or gay], or communal).

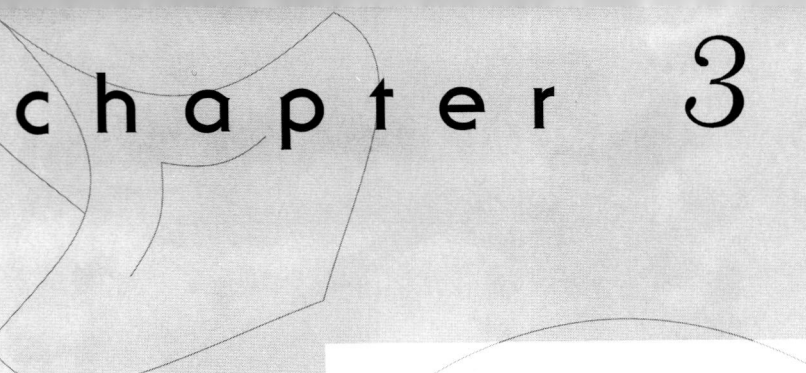

chapter 3

Culture and Ethnicity

JOYCE NEWMAN GIGER
RUTH E. DAVIDHIZAR
SUSAN C. WIECZOREK

LEARNING OBJECTIVES

- Define key terms listed.
- Describe the communication problems encountered when giving nursing care to childbearing families from diverse cultural backgrounds.
- Identify how orientation to time and space may affect nursing care needs of the childbearing family.
- Describe how cultural behavior is acquired in a social setting.
- Identify types of health care practices that may have significant impact on wellness, illness, and health-seeking behaviors of persons in various cultural groups.
- Describe biologic differences that may occur among individuals in childbearing families from diverse racial groups.
- Identify topics for nursing research related to culture and ethnicity.

TRANSCULTURAL NURSING

Before transcultural nursing can be understood adequately, one must have a basic understanding of key terminology such as culture, cultural values, and culturally diverse nursing care. **Culture** refers to a particular group's norms and practices that are learned and shared and that guide thinking, decisions, and actions (Leininger, 1985a). Leininger (1985a) further defines the term **cultural values** as an individual's desirable or preferred way of acting or knowing something that is often sustained over time and that governs actions or decisions. **Culturally diverse nursing care,** an optimal mode of health care delivery, refers to the variability of nursing approaches needed to provide culturally appropriate care.

Cultural Assessment

In a multicultural, pluralistic society, nurses are likely to encounter clients from diverse settings. In order to provide culturally diverse health care, nurses must understand factors that influence individual health and illness behaviors (Tripp-Reimer, Brink, Saunders, 1984). This is especially true when the nurse is providing care to the childbearing family. Childbearing is a critical life experience and as such is often fraught with traditional beliefs and practices. According to Affonso (1979), cultural assessment can add meaning to behaviors that might otherwise be judged negatively. If cultural beliefs and practices are not appropriately identified, the significance of certain behaviors will confuse the nurse and may result in inappropriate care.

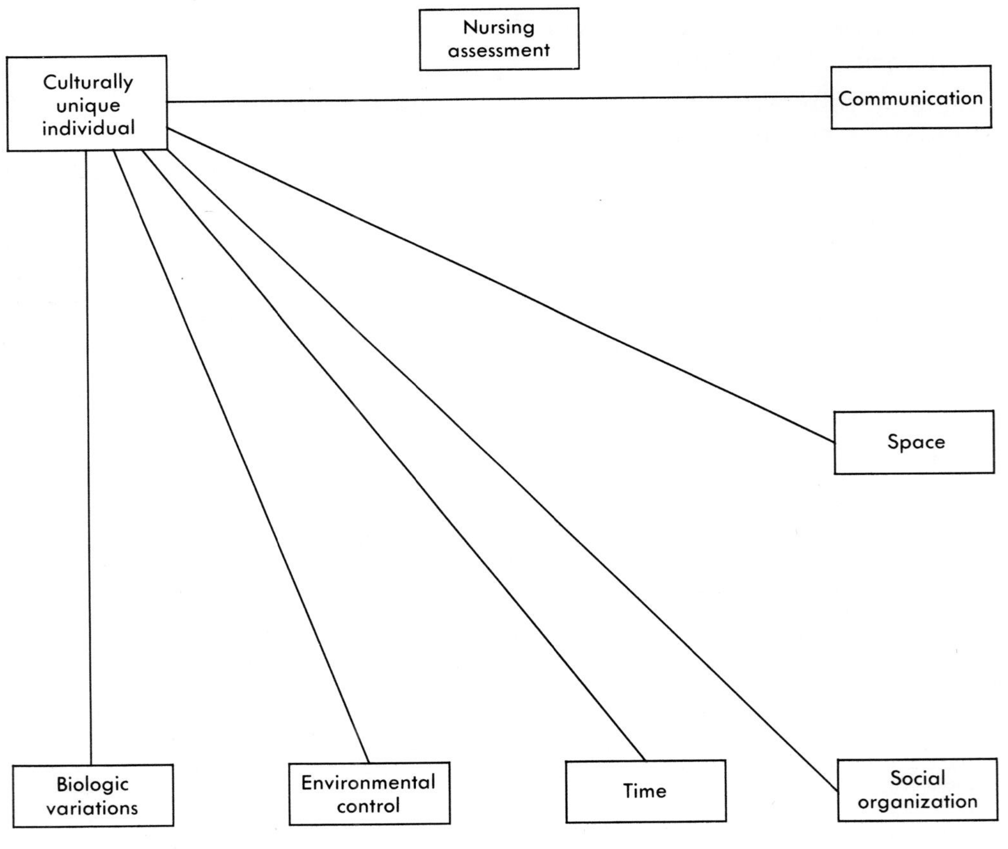

Fig. 3-1 Application of cultural phenomena to nursing care and nursing practice.
From Giger JN, Davidhizar RE: *Transcultural nursing: assessment and intervention,* St Louis, 1991, Mosby–Year Book.

In recent years, transcultural nursing theories have appeared in nursing literature (Affonso, 1979; Leininger, 1985b); however, adequate nursing assessment tools have not accompanied these theories. One of the most comprehensive tools for nursing cultural assessment was developed by Murdock (1971). Murdock's "Outline of Cultural Material" was developed primarily for anthropologists who were concerned with ethnographic descriptions of cultural groups. Although the tool contains 88 major categories and appears comprehensive, it was not designed for nursing practitioners, and it does not provide for systematic use of the nursing process. Another assessment tool is found in Brownlee's *Community, Culture and Care: A Cross-Cultural Guide for Health Care Workers* (1978). Brownlee's work is devoted to the process of practical assessment of a community with specific attention to areas most relevant to health. Brownlee focused on three aspects of assessment: what to find out, why it is important, and how to do it. This tool also has received criticism for being too comprehensive, too difficult, and too detailed to use with individual clients, but, again, Brownlee's tool was not developed for use in nursing assessment. In response to the need for a practical assessment tool for evaluating cultural variables and their effects on health and illness behavior, a model for assessing clients has been developed using six cultural phenomena (Fig. 3-1).

These phenomena, which appear in all cultural groups, are: (1) communication, (2) space, (3) social organization, (4) time, (5) environmental control, and (6) biologic variations. Although these six cultural phenomena are evident, they vary with application and use across cultures. Thus an individualized assessment approach to these six areas is indicated when working with clients from diverse cultural groups. In this chapter, the six cultural phenomena are presented individually along with specific data to be collected in each area (Fig. 3-2). The nurse must

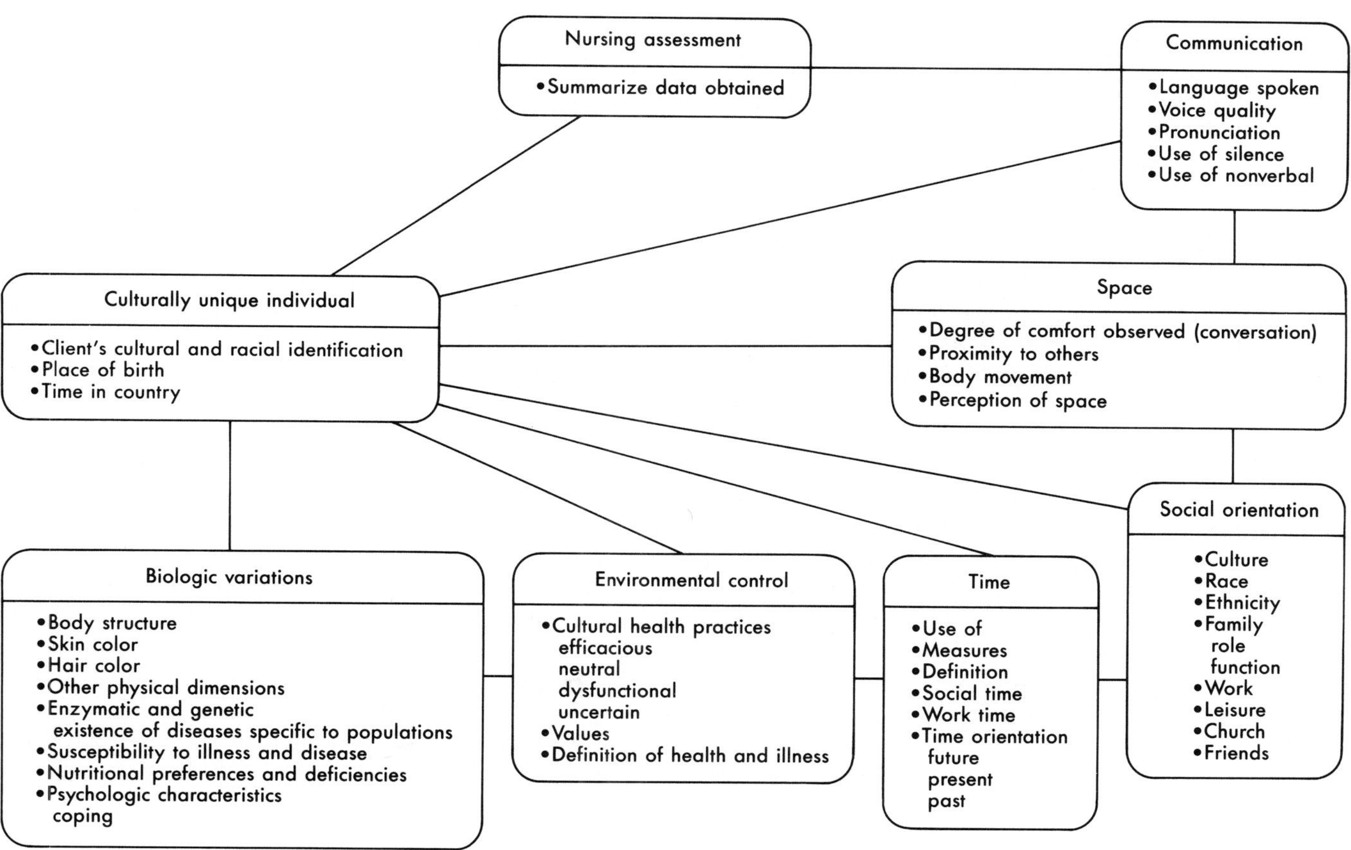

Fig. 3-2 Transcultural assessment model.
From Giger JN, Davidhizar RE: *Transcultural nursing: assessment and intervention*, St Louis, 1991, Mosby–Year Book. Developed by Geneva Turner, PhD, RN, CFLE, associate professor of nursing, Columbus College, Columbus, Georgia.

keep in mind that a comprehensive nursing assessment is necessary for both the nursing practitioner and researcher in order to provide culturally appropriate nursing care for the childbearing family from a multicultural setting (see box on p. 47).

COMMUNICATION

Communication is the factor that often creates what appears to many health care professionals to be the most insurmountable problem when working with childbearing families from diverse cultures. Communication patterns are formed and patterned indelibly by culture (Foster, 1989). People learn to think, feel, believe, and strive for what their culture considers proper (Porter, Samovar, 1985). Culture not only determines appropriateness of the message but also influences all the components of communication. An assessment of communication requires an evaluation of:

1. Dialect
2. Style (language and social situation)
3. Volume (silence)
4. Touch
5. Context of speech (emotional tone)
6. Kinesics (gestures, stances, and eye behavior)

Dialect

Dialect is a communication variable that differs between and among cultural and ethnic groups. Dialect is also influenced by geographic location; for example, persons of the same culture living in Florida may sound different from those living in New York.

Language Styles

Language styles also vary among people of different cultures. Words may have different meanings; for example, when the nurse is interacting with an African-American client, the word "bad" used by the client may actually mean "good" to that client. It is important for the nurse to appreciate that language styles vary not only between and among various cultures but also within cultures.

Negative interrogatives are also associated with language styles. Some Oriental Americans use positive responses in answer to negative interrogatives when replying to a question. For example, the nurse says "Will you not get up without assistance?" and the client responds "yes." The nurse may become confused and repeat the directions, and the client may continue to respond in a manner that appears to convey misunderstanding. Some Chinese Americans and Vietnamese Americans will avoid the word "no" because it is believed that it conveys disrespect. Nevertheless, "yes" may not always indicate understanding or the desire to comply with directions. When interacting with clients, it is essential to clarify the meaning of the word "yes" (Chung, 1977). It is also a common misconception that persons of the same culture can understand each other because of cultural similarity.

Volume of Speech

Volume of speech is also influenced by culture. Such factors as loudness, softness, shouting, and use of silence should be interpreted in a cultural context. For example, Irish people are frequently perceived as using high volume to communicate, not because of anger but rather as a part of their cultural background (Greeley, 1981). On the other hand, some Jewish people are expressive when communicating and may frequently use low volume to place emphasis on what is being communicated (Novak, Waldoks, 1981).

Silence has more significance in some cultures than in others. The nurse who encounters silence when interacting with a client from another culture should determine what can be learned from the silence and the value the silence may have as a form of communication. Cultural influences may inhibit a client from questioning a physician or nurse about health or illness conditions. In such cases, the nurse needs to assume a more active role in order to ensure that the client obtains necessary information. On the other hand, the cultural significance of silence may be related to gender. For example, a Chinese-American client in labor may rely on her husband to communicate her needs even when capable of communicating fluently.

Touch

Persons in some cultures use touch to assist communication. By virtue of some people's cultural values and/or beliefs, touch may be interpreted as intrusive or having sexual connotation and consequently may be perceived as negative. Some cultural groups are characterized by a "do not touch me" way of life. People in these cultures may view kissing and embracing in public as embarrassing. When cultures are considered as a group, the Spanish, Italian, French, Jewish, and South American cultures are considered more tactile, and the English and German cultures are generally considered less tactile (Montagu, 1971). However, in the United States, the mainstream culture generally tolerates hugs and em-

A Transcultural Assessment Model

CULTURALLY UNIQUE INDIVIDUAL

1. Place of birth
2. Cultural definition
   What is . . .
3. Race
   What is . . .
4. Length of time in country

COMMUNICATION

1. Voice quality
   A. Strong, resonant
   B. Soft
   C. Average
   D. Shrill
2. Pronunciation and enunciation
   A. Clear
   B. Slurred
   C. Dialect
3. Use of silence
   A. Infrequent
   B. Often
   C. Length
      (1) Brief
      (2) Moderate
      (3) Long
      (4) Not observed
4. Use of nonverbal
   A. Hand movement
   B. Eye movement
   C. Moves entire body
   D. Kinesics (gestures, expressions, or stances)
5. Touch
   A. Startles or withdraws when touched
   B. Accepts touch without difficulty
   C. Touches others without difficulty
6. Ask these and similar questions:
   A. How do you get your point across to others?
   B. Do you like communicating with friends, family, and acquaintances?
   C. When asked a question, do you usually respond (in words or body movement, or both)?
   D. If you have something important to discuss with your family, how would you approach them?

SPACE

1. Degree of comfort
   A. Moves when space invaded
   B. Does not move when invaded
2. Distance in conversations
   A. 0 to 18 inches
   B. 18 inches to 3 feet
   C. 3 feet or more
3. Definition of space
   A. Describe degree of comfort with closeness when talking with or standing near others
   B. How do objects (e.g., furniture) in the environment affect your sense of space?
4. Ask these and similar questions:
   A. When you talk with family members, how close do you stand?
   B. When you communicate with co-workers and other acquaintances, how close do you stand?
   C. If a stranger touches you, how do you react or feel?
   D. If a loved one touches you, how do you react or feel?
   E. Are you comfortable with the distance between us now?

SOCIAL ORGANIZATION

1. Normal state of health
   A. Poor
   B. Fair
   C. Good
   D. Excellent
2. Ask these and similar questions:
   A. How do you define social activities?
   B. What are some activities that you enjoy?
   C. What are your hobbies, or what do you do when you have free time?
   D. Do you believe in a Supreme Being?
   E. How do you worship that Supreme Being?
   F. What is your function (what do you do) in your family unit/system?
   G. What is your role in your family unit/system (father, mother, child, advisor)?
   H. When you were a child, what or who influenced you most?
   I. What is/was your relationship with your siblings and parents?
   J. What does work mean to you?
   K. Describe your past, present, and future jobs.
   L. What are your political views?
   M. How have your political views influenced your attitude toward health and illness?

TIME

1. Orientation to time
   A. Past-oriented
   B. Present-oriented
   C. Future-oriented

Developed by Geneva Turner, PhD, CFLE, from Giger JN, Davidhizar RE: *Transcultural nursing: assessment and intervention,* St Louis, 1991, Mosby–Year Book.

Continued.

2. View of time
   A. Social time
   B. Clock-oriented
3. Physiochemical reaction to time
   A. Sleeps at least 8 hours a night
   B. Goes to sleep and wakes on a consistent schedule
   C. Understands the importance of taking medication and other treatments on schedule
4. Ask these and similar questions:
   A. What kind of timepiece do you wear daily?
   B. If you have an appointment at 2 PM, what time is acceptable to arrive?
   C. If a nurse tells you that you will receive a medication in "about a half hour," realistically, how much time will you allow before calling the nurses' station?

ENVIRONMENTAL CONTROL

1. Locus-of-control
   A. Internal locus-of-control (believes that the power to affect change lies within)
   B. External locus-of-control (believes that fate, luck, and chance have a great deal to do with how things turn out)
2. Value orientation
   A. Believes in supernatural forces
   B. Relies on magic, witchcraft, and prayer to affect change
   C. Does not believe in supernatural forces
   D. Does not rely on magic, witchcraft, or prayer to affect change
3. Ask these and similar questions:
   A. How often do you have visitors at your home?
   B. Is it acceptable to you for visitors to drop in unexpectedly?
   C. Name some ways your parents or other persons treated your illnesses when you were a child.
   D. Have you or someone else in your immediate surroundings ever used a home remedy that made you sick?
   E. What home remedies have you used that worked? Will you use them in the future?
   F. What is your definition of "good health"?
   G. What is your definition of illness or "poor health"?

BIOLOGIC VARIATIONS

1. Conduct a complete physical assessment noting:
   A. Body structure
   B. Skin color
   C. Unusual skin discolorations
   D. Hair color and distribution
   E. Other visible physical characteristics (e.g., keloids, chloasma)
2. Ask these and similar questions:
   A. What diseases or illnesses are common in your family?
   B. Describe your family's typical behavior when a family member is ill.
   C. How do you respond when you are angry?
   D. Who (or what) usually helps you to cope during a difficult time?
   E. What foods do you and your family like to eat?
   F. Have you ever had any unusual cravings for:
      (1) White or red clay dirt?
      (2) Laundry starch?
   G. When you were a child what types of foods did you eat?
   H. What foods are family favorites or are considered traditional?

NURSING ASSESSMENT

1. Note whether the client has become culturally assimilated or observes own cultural practices.
2. Incorporate data into plan of nursing care:
   A. Encourage the client to discuss cultural differences; people from diverse cultures who hold different worldviews can enlighten nurses.
   B. Make efforts to accept and understand methods of communication.
   C. Respect the individual's personal need for space.
   D. Respect the rights of clients to honor and worship the Supreme Being of their choice.
   E. Identify a clerical or spiritual person to contact.
   F. Determine whether spiritual practices have implications for health, life, and well-being (e.g., Jehovah's Witnesses may refuse blood and blood derivatives; an Orthodox Jew may eat only Kosher food high in sodium and may not drink milk when meat is served).
   G. Identify hobbies, especially when devising interventions for a short or extended convalescence or for rehabilitation.
   H. Honor time and value orientations and differences in these areas. Allay anxiety and apprehension if adherence to time is necessary.
   I. Provide privacy according to personal need and health status of the client (NOTE: the perception and reaction to pain may be culturally related).
   J. Note cultural health practices
      (1) Identify and encourage efficacious practices.
      (2) Identify and discourage dysfunctional practices.
      (3) Identify and determine whether neutral practices will have a long-term ill effect.
   K. Note food preferences
      (1) Make as many adjustments in diet as health status and long-term benefits will allow and that dietary department can provide.
      (2) Note dietary practices that may have serious implications for the client.

braces among those well acquainted with each other and a pat on the shoulder as a gesture of camaraderie.

Most cultures give touch different rules and meanings depending on the sex of the person involved. Touch practices may vary culturally in relation to health situations. In some cultures, taboos about touch between sexes persist even in the physician's office. Mexican-American females report "feeling hot" because of the embarrassment of a pelvic examination even when done by a female doctor or nurse practitioner (Brownlee, 1978).

Customs that involve touch also vary in cultures. In the Navajo culture, the mother massages the newborn baby as a "bonding" experience (Hanley, 1991). In some cultures, touch is considered magical, and thus casual or common touching is considered taboo. Some Mexican Americans and some Native Americans view touch as symbolic of "undoing" of an evil spell, as a means of preventing harm, or as a method of healing. In some cultural groups, handshaking has a cultural significance and symbolism and is therefore a learned behavior. Italian, Spanish, and French people generally view a firm, hearty handshake as symbolic of good character and a sign of strength (Montagu, 1971). On the other hand, some Native Americans such as the Navajo may regard lengthy, vigorous handshaking as aggressive (Hanley, 1991).

Context of Speech

The context of speech refers to the use of emotion in communication and also varies with culture. Other verbal and nonverbal forms of communication, including "small talk," should also be considered for their effect on communication. When some Mexican Americans are interviewed, they may engage in "small talk" before approaching the business of the interview. "Small talk" will often facilitate accomplishing objectives for the interview and is therefore not necessarily a waste of time (Kuipers, 1991). Laughter also serves as an important mode of communication that varies in significance between cultural groups. In the Navajo culture, when the baby laughs for the first time, small gifts are given, and a small feast is prepared in celebration of the occasion (Hanley, 1991).

Kinesics

Kinesics refers to gestures, stances, and eye behavior used when relating to others. A nurse may be able to bridge an interaction by certain gestures or by posture. For example, in the United States, an attentive posture is communicated by leaning towards the individual. However, the meaning of gestures differs from culture to culture. Although palms up usually indicates acquiescence in the United States, in certain cultural groups this gesture may have sexual implications (Mehrabian, 1981).

In the United States, a commonly accepted behavior when communicating with others is to look directly in the eyes of the person. This practice may be perceived as foreign to persons in some cultural groups, even those living in the United States (McKenzie, Christman, 1977; Roberts, 1981; Giger, Davidhizar, 1990). Persons from India may be acculturated to avoid direct eye contact with persons in higher or lower socioeconomic groups (Sue, 1981; Miller, Supersad, 1991). In India, certain eye behavior is restricted with persons of the opposite sex (Sue, 1981). Blinking is another eye movement with different meaning in different cultures, for example, Alaskan Eskimos may use blinking to indicate agreement (Davidhizar, 1988c).

Implications for Nursing Care

Communication is a product of culture and thus must be considered in a cultural context. Personal beliefs, values, and mores affect communication and consequently may influence health. Personal communication must be modified to meet cultural needs. When the client and/or family do not speak the same language as the nurse, special approaches must be used that will allow the family's health care needs to be addressed and culturally appropriate nursing care to be administered. Such approaches include using interpreters to convey not only the client's and family's needs, but also culturally specific health care instructions. However, communication through a third party can also compound the problem of sending a message clearly. It is helpful to have a translator with transcultural sensitivity who can assist in the role of client advocacy and who translates not only the words but also their implications.

■ SPACE

All communication takes place in the context of **space.** Personal space is the area that surrounds a person's body. A discussion of personal space must consider the distances between persons as well as objects that may be present. Territoriality involves feelings or an attitude toward an area. Territoriality can become an important nursing issue when an individual's comfort boundaries are encroached. The concepts of personal space and territoriality should be both understood in relation to interpersonal zones and interpreted in the context of culture.

Interpersonal Zones

According to Hall's (1966) classic work on interpersonal zones, four zones can be delineated: (1) intimate zone, (2) personal zone, (3) social consultative zone, and (4) public zone. The intimate zone involves interactions closer than 18 inches and is reserved for comforting, protecting, and lovemaking by persons who have close relationships. The personal zone ranges from 18 inches to 4 feet and is usually space that is maintained between family members and between friends. The personal zone is often involved in health-related actions with the childbearing family. The social-consultative zone ranges from 4 to 12 feet and is maintained in business situations by people who are working together or in casual gatherings. The public zone ranges from 12 feet and beyond and is outside the sphere of personal involvement.

Territoriality

Territoriality refers to a feeling state characterized by possessiveness, control, and authority over an area of physical space. If the need for territoriality is to be met, the person must be in control of some space and be able to establish rules for that space. Roberts (1978) suggests that the need for territoriality cannot be fully met unless individuals defend their space against misuse by others. Territoriality serves four functions: security, privacy, autonomy, and self-identity (Orland, 1978). Individuals who feel in control of their personal space will have a sense of security and privacy, feelings of autonomy and identity; they will feel safer, less threatened, and less anxious than those who lack feelings of control over their personal space.

Space and Culture

Personal space needs and feelings of territoriality are developed in a cultural setting. Although personal space is an individual matter and varies with the situation, dimensions of personal space comfort zones vary from culture to culture. **Preferred distance** in the United States commonly falls between the intimate and personal zones at approximately 2 or 3 feet. Preferred distance for cultural groups varies; for example, for French Americans 2 to 3 feet is perceived as distant and is generally unacceptable, but African Americans may have great difficulty when their personal space is invaded (Evans, Howard, 1973; Watson 1980).

Implications for Nursing Care

Personal space is important to consider when providing nursing care to the childbearing family. Actions such as touching the client, placing the client in proximity to others, taking away personal possessions, and making decisions for the client can decrease personal security and heighten anxiety. On the other hand, when the need for distance is respected, control is maintained over personal space and personal autonomy is supported, thereby increasing the sense of security. Although use of space varies with the individual, cultural heritage often has some bearing on certain aspects of a person's use of space. Most individuals in the United States have the Western need to be territorial; however, this has traditionally not been a value of the American Eskimo (Orland, 1978). Instead, Eskimo people value sharing. Although acculturation has weakened this particular value system, family rights still take precedence over individual rights (Lefever, Davidhizar, 1991). Individual values and values shared by an entire cultural group vary and may consequently affect individual needs (Lefever, Davidhizar, 1991).

Adjustment to unfamiliar spaces is another factor that may be affected by cultural heritage. Some Navajo clients may have difficulty adapting to spaces that are not familiar to them, particularly the unfamiliar hospital settings.

The client's reaction to close contact with others may also be related to culture. For example, since Chinese Americans have traditionally been a noncontact group, some Chinese Americans may associate closeness, increased eye contact, and touch as being offensive or impolite. Misunderstandings can be reduced by providing explanations when performing these tasks (Chang, 1991). Arab women value modesty. This modesty is defined by dress as well as actions. Bashfulness, humility, diffidence, and shyness are considered proper modest behaviors. In a nursing situation, special care should be taken with Arab-American women so that unnecessary exposure is avoided (Meleis, Sorrell, 1981; Miller, Supersad, 1991). Respect must be shown for the client's culturally based beliefs and values.

■ SOCIAL ORGANIZATION

Family structure and organization, religious values and beliefs, and ethnicity and culture relate to role and role assignment within the group setting and consequently can affect nursing care. Knowledge of the family structure and organization, religious values and beliefs, role, and role assignments can all provide valuable information in assisting the family in achieving goals.

Family Systems and Cultural Significance

Social organization refers to whether a cultural group organizes itself around the **family** unit. For some cultural groups the family unit becomes the single most important social organization. Many Chinese, Mexican, Vietnamese, and Puerto Rican Americans believe the family unit to be supreme to other social organizations. Family causes take on more significance than personal, cultural, or national causes (Giger, Davidhizar, 1990). Some cultural groups (for example, Italian Americans) extend their family beyond normal blood lines and have large extended families. The Vietnamese concept of family and extended family has existed across generations as a "super organic unit" and is profoundly different from the individualization of the nuclear family concept common in the United States (Stauffer, 1991). Many Appalachian people rely heavily on the family for advice and help and are skeptical and even suspicious of newcomers. On the other hand, some Caucasian Americans are quite individualistic and want control of their own lives. Although advice from the family unit is important, personal choice and autonomy take precedence.

Family Roles

Family roles are patterns of wants, goals, feelings, attitudes, and actions that family members have for themselves and others in the family. Roles are related to social class and cultural norms. Certain roles for men and certain roles for women may be stressed. For example, East Indian Hindu women rank far below men in social status. Traditionally, the belief has been held by East Indian Hindus that the role of the woman is faithfulness and servility to her husband. Because East Indian Hindu women are deprived of inheritance, the birth of a son is essential in order to have a male descendant to continue the family name and maintain economic status (Reddy, 1986).

The Role of Men in the Childbearing Family and Cultural Significance

The active or passive role that a man plays in pregnancy and childbirth experiences is profoundly affected by culture and may have significant implications. In some Arab-American families, the birthing experience is a female affair. During labor and delivery some Arab-American women prefer to be surrounded by female relatives and close personal friends.

For the Arab-American family, the absence of the male during the birthing experience should not be interpreted as neglect or disinterest. Rather, the birthing experience is considered a feminine experience (Meleis, 1981).

Impact of Immigration and Acculturation on the Transcultural Childbearing Family

Immigration to the United States and acculturation by many families into the mainstream of American life has resulted in varying degrees of modification of cultural behavior (Fig. 3-3). Patterns of cultural behavior are modified to fit into the dominant culture. Prenatal care in the United States is based on the premise that pregnancy is a condition that requires medical attention to ensure health. In many cultures, pregnancy is considered a normal state, and a woman will only seek help if problems arise. Thus women from other cultures often present themselves for prenatal care late in pregnancy because they regard their condition as only requiring self-care.

Religion and Religious Views and Cultural Significance

Religion is a social phenomenon of major importance (Giger, Davidhizar, 1991). Generally religious structures fall into two basic types: the church type and the withdrawal-group type. The church-type structure is broadly based and represents the normative spiritual values of the society that most people adhere to by virtue of their membership in the society, such as Hinduism in India, or Catholicism in Spain. The church-type structure is a comprehensive system that allows for individual variations and generally does not make rigid demands on members. Individual churches may be identified with an ethnic group rather than with a social class (for example, the African-American church or the Amish church as representations of the African-American and Amish life experiences).

The second type of religious structure is the withdrawal group, which expresses beliefs of those for whom personal commitment and experience are more important than the family and the community functions of religion. In the case of withdrawal

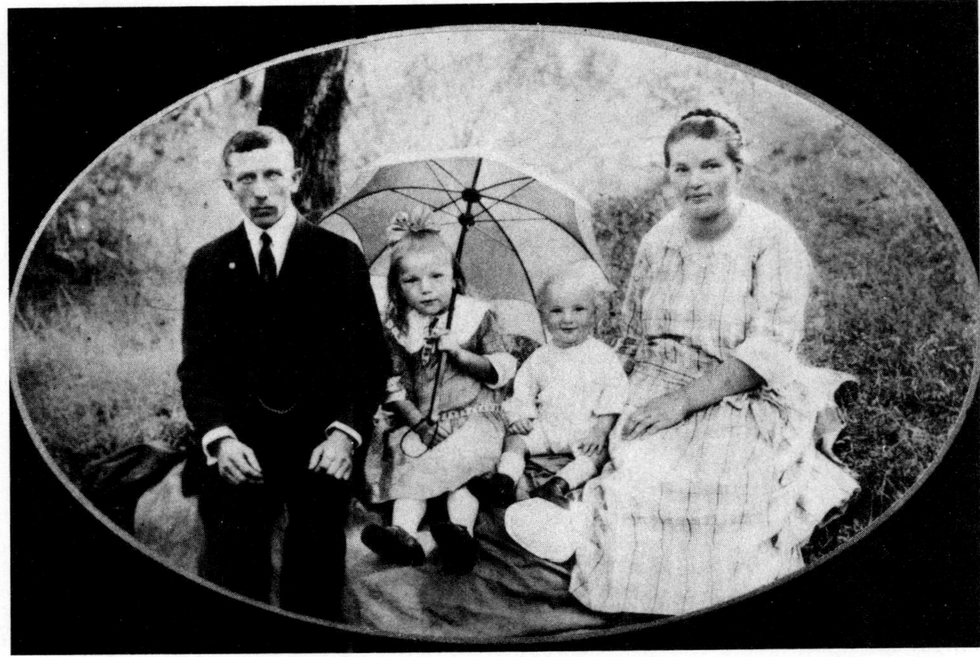

Fig. 3-3 European immigrant nuclear family.

groups, individuals make a choice and place that choice above the family or community functions of religion. This is evidenced in groups such as Jehovah's Witnesses or Amish and represents a more intense or unbending commitment than that held by the average person.

Religion and religious practices have a profound effect on sexual relationships and childbirth experiences. Strict Orthodox Jews observe customs that are basic to Judaism such as "Taharat Hamisishpachia," and other Family Purity Laws. These laws are based on the need to practice sexual discipline within families. For example, during menstruation, sexual relationships must cease and must not begin again for 7 days after the cessation of menstruation. For approximately 12 days, a Jewish woman must observe a state of "niddus" (separation). After this period, the Jewish woman must immerse herself in a special ritually approved pool of water (Mikvah). Upon her return from Mikvah, sexual relationship with her husband may resume (Bash, 1980).

Circumcision is another traditionally practiced ritual observed by many Jewish Americans. This practice is based on the "covenant of circumcision," or "Brit Milah" in Hebrew from the book of Genesis 17:10-14. To keep the covenant with God, it is believed that every Jewish male must be circumcised on the eighth day after birth (Bash, 1980). In the United States, this ritual is performed by a Mohel (a religious person specially trained to perform circumcisions).

Implications for Nursing Care

When one family member is receiving care, the family represents the environment in which care is given. The family also has needs that should be addressed. Although one family member may be the identified client, the client and family should be regarded and treated as a whole (Fig. 3-4). Whether the family is viewed as an environment or as the client, it is essential to incorporate cultural considerations when using the nursing process in developing a plan of care. In a study of psychosocial predictors of pregnancy outcomes in low-income African-American, Hispanic, and Caucasian women, it was noted that social networks might reinforce negative health practices for the Caucasian women studied (i.e., substance use was found to be related to high social support). On the other hand, this study suggested the value of social support in decreasing complications for African-American women lacking partner or mother support (Norbeck, Anderson, 1989).

When the extended family is considered important by a cultural group, it is essential for the nurse to be considerate of this value. Variables in gender role behaviors according to culture is another important

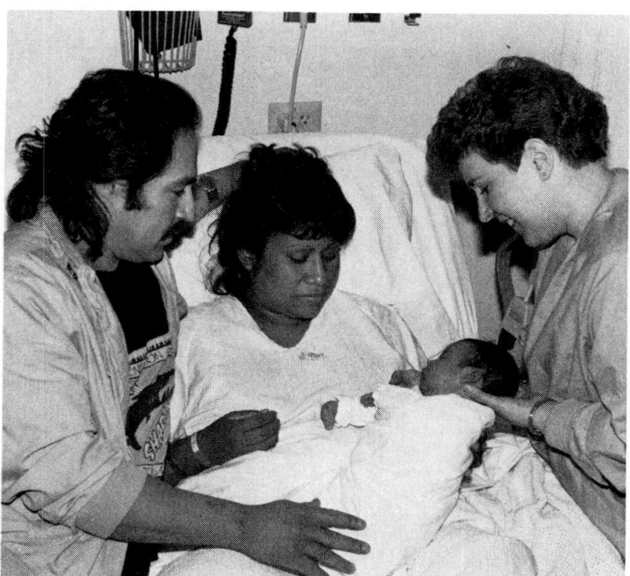

Fig 3-4 While mother and newborn recover physically from birth, attachment and bonding within the new family is progressing.
Courtesy Dottie Kauffmann.

consideration. For example, the nurse needs to be aware that in a matriarchal culture, the wife or mother is responsible for many family decisions, including when to seek health care.

■ TIME

The Concept of Time

Since early civilization, the concept of **time** has been the greatest mystery of all. The concept of time is familiar regardless of cultural heritage. Human beings are cognizant of the fact that the days and nights come and go and that with each passing day, aging occurs. In this sense, time is perceived as real, concrete, and having direct effects. However, time can also be perceived as being "not real," since it is also an abstract concept (i.e., it cannot be touched, seen, smelled, or heard).

Scientific Definition

Various scientific disciplines have attempted to define the concept of time. For example, the mathematic and physical sciences have defined time as a dimension with a function only for location or reference. In contrast, scientists in the biologic sciences have defined time as an essential ingredient in many life processes such as gestation, healing, and metamorphosis.

Time has two distinct although related meanings. One way that time may be viewed is in terms of duration. In this sense, duration is an interval of time. On the other hand, the concept of time may be seen as that of specified instances and points in time. These two meanings are related because a point in time is identified as being the end of a time interval that starts at an arbitrary or fixed reference point such as the "birth of Christ," or the "founding of Rome." Time can also be defined as either "social time" or "clock time." **Social time,** which evolves as a function of interaction, includes patterns and orientations that relate to social processes and to the conceptualization and ordering of social life without respect to any specific hour on the clock or specific time of day (Giger, Davidhizar, 1991). In essence, social time is consensually validated by those persons involved in the interaction.

Clock time, on the other hand, includes precisely measured increments that are cumulative and bear some relationship to a clock. For example, the time 8 AM means 8 hours after midnight as measured on the clock. These hours accumulate into a 24-hour day, days accumulate into weeks, etc. Clock time is standardized against a standard clock and is precise.

Differentiation Between Past-, Present-, and Future-Oriented Cultures

Persons in cultural groups may be either past-, present-, or future-oriented. People who focus on the past strive to maintain tradition and have little motivation for formulating future goals. Although some Appalachians are viewed as presented-oriented individuals, many Appalachians hold to traditions and values that have been passed down from generation to generation (Tripp-Reimer, 1982). In addition, old-order Amish may be viewed as past-oriented individuals (Wenger, 1989). Although some Navajo Americans may be viewed as present-oriented individuals, many Navajo Americans hold a past-time orientation and tend to cling to traditional values and beliefs (Hanley, 1991).

Some people who focus on the present neither save for the future nor appreciate the past. In fact, present-oriented individuals do not necessarily adhere to a strict time-structured schedule. Some present-oriented individuals adopt a view that an acceptable lateness can include up to 30 minutes after the scheduled time. Such individuals are frequently late since the present task is viewed as more significant. For individuals with a present-time orientation, time may be viewed as elastic. This perception of time may be traced back to West Africa, where time encompassed events that had already taken place, as well as those that were about to take place (Mbiti, 1970).

Cultural groups that may be viewed as present time-oriented include African Americans, Puerto Rican Americans, Chinese Americans, and Mexican Americans. A nurse presenting a speech to Jamaican Americans who may be present-time oriented should not be surprised if the program is some hours late in starting. In this case there may be a deep appreciation for the subject of the presentation, but a deeper appreciation for the present interpersonal activity. Some Appalachian people also live in the present, viewing the future as unpredictable and the past as irrelevant (Tripp-Reimer, 1982).

Levine and Wolff (1985) conducted a study to compare the time sense of male and female students in Niteroi, Brazil, and students at California State University at Fresno. The students sampled were asked about their perception of time in specific situations, including what they would consider early or late for a hypothetical lunch appointment with a friend. The analysis of the data indicated the Brazilian students defined lateness as 33½ minutes after the scheduled lunch. In sharp contrast, the Fresno students defined lateness as precisely 19 minutes after the scheduled lunch. One reason cited by the Brazilian students for the lateness was unforeseen circumstances that could not be controlled without prior knowledge. On the other hand, their American counterparts noted that in this scenario a reason for being late was lack of sensitivity about another person's feelings.

People who have a future-time orientation use the present to achieve future goals. A person oriented toward the future may appear cold because future tasks may appear more important than people (Giger, Davidhizar, 1990). Time perception may be related to both socioeconomic status and religious orientation. For example, although some African and Mexican Americans are viewed as present-time oriented, others have been assimilated into the dominant culture, and are very time conscious and take pride in punctuality. These African and Mexican Americans may very likely be future-time oriented and therefore more likely to save and plan for important future events. These individuals may also be well educated and hold professional positions. However, this may not always be the case, since some African and Mexican Americans who are not well educated and do not hold professional positions do value time and have future hope for themselves and their children.

Religious orientation has a profound impact on time orientation. For example, some Native Americans, Mexican Americans, and African Americans hold very strong religious beliefs and are thus more future-time oriented (Giger, Davidhizar, 1991). These individuals share a common belief that life on earth coupled with all the pain and suffering is only bearable if one holds firm to the belief in the afterlife (Giger, Davidhizar, 1991).

Time Orientation and Significance of Compliance and/or Noncompliance with Specific Regimens During Pregnancy and/or Postpartum

Persons with a present-time orientation are often not compliant with medical regimens. For example, since Arabic time orientation is primarily on the present and dictated by need, Arab-American women are often late for or miss scheduled prenatal appointments (Meleis, Sorrell, 1981). This is also true for Chinese-American women (Yeun, 1987; Kim, 1988). Present-time orientation also may result in nonadherence to feeding schedules, visiting hours, and follow-up appointments.

Implications for Nursing Care

The time orientation of the childbearing family system has important implications for nursing care. For example, in talking to a family about an infant's feeding schedule, the nurse may find that a family that has many things going on simultaneously and focuses on the present is comfortable with demand feedings. On the other hand, a family with a future-oriented sense of time, where events are planned in advance, may be much more comfortable with a fixed schedule for the infant's meals (Foster, 1989).

■ ENVIRONMENTAL CONTROL

The Concept of Environmental Control

The term **environmental control** refers to the ability of an individual or persons representing a particular cultural group to plan activities that control nature. At the same time, environmental control refers to the individual's perception of ability to direct factors in the environment (Giger, Davidhizar, 1991).

The definition of environmental control implies that the concept of environment is broader than just the place where an individual resides or merely where treatment occurs (Giger, Davidhizar, 1991). Environment encompasses relevant systems and processes that affect all individuals (Haber et al, 1987). Systems may be viewed as organized structures that affect and influence the individual. Individuals and the environment enjoy a reciprocal relationship in the sense that there is a continuous exchange of matter and energy between the two. This exchange may be purposeful and goal-directed, since the exchange process is functional. On the other hand, the exchange may be viewed as dysfunctional when the exchange has no purpose and lacks goal direction. When this occurs, a dyssynchronous relationship develops (Giuffra, 1987).

In its broadest sense, health and health status reflect a balance between the individual and the environment. For example, in the United States, people are becoming more health conscious. Health practices such as eating nutritiously, exercising, and subscribing to preventive health care services available in the community are emerging as high-profile concerns.

Distinction Between Illness and Disease

Over the last 10 years, scientists, physicians, and anthropologists have begun to make a distinction between the concepts of illness and disease. Individual experiences relating to illness do not necessarily correlate with the biomedical interpretation of disease. Illness can and does occur in the absence of disease. Approximately 50% of visits made by individuals to physicians are for complaints without a definite medical basis. Illness is culturally shaped in the sense that culture influences expectations and perceptions of illness and disease (Kleinman, Eisenberg, Good, 1978). Thus culture shapes the labeling of sickness, and how, when, and to whom communication of health problems occurs.

Cultural Health Practices Versus Medical Health Practices

Culture can and does influence individual health care behavior. Moreover, definition and interpretation of health may be profoundly affected by culture and ethnicity. Nevertheless, the term health care behavior is inclusive. Health is defined as the social and biologic activities of an individual that are related to maintaining acceptable health status or manipulating and/or altering unacceptable conditions (Bauwens, Anderson, 1988).

In the broadest sense, **cultural health practices** may be categorized as efficacious, neutral, dysfunctional, or uncertain (Pillsbury, 1982). By Western medical standards, efficacious cultural health practices are viewed as beneficial to health status. This is even so when these practices differ greatly from modern Western scientific practices (Giger, Davidhizar, 1991). For example, some Chinese Americans subscribe to the theory of "Yin and Yang," and some Mexican Americans hold beliefs that are very similar about "hot and cold" illnesses and/or conditions. Persons holding these beliefs may, for example, avoid hot foods in the presence of a stomach condition such as an ulcer. This practice is consistent with Western medical treatment (i.e., bland diet for ulcer treatment).

Another practice that could be considered efficacious is found in the Chinese culture. To restore balance after birth, some Chinese Americans believe that the mother should not leave her bed and should be protected from wind (Lee, 1989). During this period, the woman should avoid cold food, drink, and medication (Fig. 3-5). Another efficacious belief held by some Chinese Americans is that for a successful birth with the least amount of trauma to the infant, the woman must lie on her side with a pillow supporting the head (Lee, 1989). This practice has some positive effects on the unborn fetus because it may increase placental perfusion and at the same time increase renal perfusion in the mother.

Efficacious practices are also found among Navajo women. Navajo women believe that the unborn fetus has no mind of its own and that the only link to the external world is through the umbilical cord. Therefore Navajo women during pregnancy are encouraged to exercise regularly and to bear in mind the

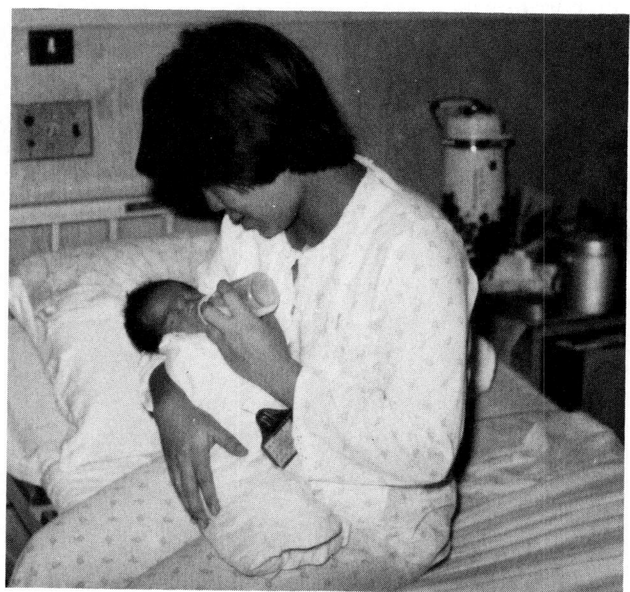

Fig. 3-5 Mother feeds newborn son while proud father takes photo. Note thermos of boiled water and pot of chicken soup on bedside stand. Courtesy Jack and Judy Teng.

link between the fetus, mother, and the umbilical cord (Phillips, Lobar, 1990).

In contrast to efficacious practices, neutral cultural health practices have no effect on the health status of the individual. Neutral health care practices may have no direct physiologic effect on the individual, nevertheless, they should not be dismissed as irrelevant. Pillsbury (1982) noted that such practices may be extremely important because they are often linked to beliefs that are integrated into individual behavior. Greene and Johnston (1980) cited several examples of neutral health care practices in the childbearing family including "the ritual disposal of the placenta and cord," "interpretation of signs in the cord," "avoidance of sexual activity during various stages of pregnancy," certain hygiene practices, and avoidance of exposure to rays of the moon during lunar eclipse.

A neutral health care practice found among traditional Africans occurs during the birthing process, when the woman is expected to sit on her haunches (squatting) with her back against the wall. The infant is delivered directly onto the floor which has been covered with a blanket. The afterbirth is not permitted to leave the hut; instead it is buried in the floor of the hut (Setiloane, 1988). These practices do not necessarily require planned nursing interventions; however, the nurse must recognize their significance and recognize the client's right to subscribe to such practices and beliefs (Table 3-1).

Health care practices that are termed dysfunctional are viewed as harmful to the individual. In the United States, an example of dysfunctional health care practices is found among Americans who consume too much refined flour and sugar. For example, some Orientals believe that the new mother should stay in bed for 10 to 40 days, avoid showering, and avoid contact with persons from the "unclean outside world" (Chung, 1970). These practices may prove dysfunctional, particularly the practice of extended bed rest, because the mother is in a pregnancy-induced hypercoagular state. It is thought that the risk for blood clots is greatly increased (Bobak, 1991).

Williams and Jelliffe (1972) developed a cultural assessment system that included a category of cultural health practices with unknown effects. For the most part, these practices have an uncertain effect on the individual. Included in this category are such practices as swaddling a newborn infant to maintain body temperature and using an abdominal binder for the newborn infant and for the mother to prevent umbilical hernias.

TABLE 3-1 Categories of African-American Health Care Practices

Categories/Effect	Example	Nursing Measures
Efficacious (beneficial)	Hot or cold foods to treat illnesses Avoid sexual activity during menstrual cycle	Encourage practice
Neutral (no effect but no harm)	Red yarn on great finger Copper band around arm or ankle Prayer cloth placed on the bed or gown of an ill person	Gives hope; to discourage could be harmful for the believer Observe for constriction caused by yarn or band Encourage small prayer cloth when placed on bed
Dysfunctional (may cause harm)	Eating white dirt Avoid bath when menstruating	Encourage proper nutrition Assess eating pattern and examine nutritional value of cultural preferences Explain benefits of proper hygiene during menstrual cycle
Uncertain (unknown benefit; may or may not cause harm)	Not allowing baby to look at its image in a mirror Penny around neck	May contribute to delay in development Will wear as a necklace Advise to observe for tightening of string or other item used to make necklace Advise to sterilize coin before using

From Giger JN, Davidhizar RE, Turner G: Categories of black health care practices, *The ABNF Journal* 3(2):45, 1992.

Values and Their Relationship to Health Care Practices

Values may be defined and viewed as individualized sets of rules by which individuals live and are governed. At best, values serve as the cornerstone for beliefs, attitudes, and behaviors. Cultural values are often acquired unconsciously as a direct result of efforts exerted as an individual assimilates into the dominant culture. In the classic work of Kluckhohn and Strodtbeck (1961), value orientations were defined as "complex but definitely patterned principles . . . which give order and direction to the ever-flowing stream of human acts and thoughts as they relate to the solution of common human problems." It is possible for an individual to hold a different value orientation from the mainstream of the cultural group. However, despite differences in value orientation within a cultural group, dominant value orientations can be identified for most persons of a particular cultural group (Kluckhohn and Strodtbeck, 1961).

Locus-of-Control Construct as a Health Care Value

The **locus-of-control** construct originated in the social learning theory area and is defined as follows:

> When a reinforcement is perceived as following some action but not being entirely contingent upon (personal) action, then in our culture it is typically perceived as a result of luck, chance, and fate, as under the control of powerful others, or unpredictable because of the great complexity of the forces surrounding [the individual]. When the event is interpreted in this way by an individual, we have labeled this belief in external control. If a person perceives that the event is contingent upon his own behavior or his permanent characteristics, we have termed this a belief in internal control.*

This definition presupposes that individuals who believe that a contingent relationship exists between actions and outcomes subscribe to a belief based on internal feelings of control. For example, persons who subscribe to beliefs based on internal locus of control and who believe that there is a correlation between lung cancer and smoking may elect not to smoke. Individuals who hold beliefs related to internal locus of control are likely to act to influence future behaviors and situations. In the United States, many middle-class Caucasian Americans are viewed as having an internal locus of control.

*From Rotter JB: Generalized expectancies for internal versus external control of reinforcement, *Psychological Monographs* 80(1):1, 1966.

Individuals who believe that outcomes are controlled by fate, chance, or luck, rather than individual actions, subscribe to feelings of external locus of control. These individuals are likely to believe that their actions are subjugated to and dictated by nature and the environment. Individuals who believe that efforts and rewards are uncorrelated, and who have an external locus of control, are less likely to take action to change the future. Some Navajo Americans, Appalachian Americans, African Americans, Chinese Americans, and Mexican Americans have an external locus of control (Kluckhohn, Strodtbeck, 1961; Tripp-Reimer, 1984). For example, an Appalachian American might say "If I am going to get cancer, I am going to get it" (Giger, Davidhizar, 1991).

Folk Beliefs and the Significance of Cultural Beliefs

Some people in some cultural groups subscribe to a system of folk beliefs. In Western medical practices, folk medicine may be referred to as "third world beliefs." Some health care professionals who are unfamiliar with these beliefs and practices view these beliefs as "strange" or "weird."

Distinction between Natural and Unnatural Illnesses

Some cultural groups view illness and/or disease as natural or unnatural events. Natural events keep balance between nature and humankind and as such are thought to be designed by God. Natural laws are thought to give life predictability (Snow, 1981).

Unnatural events are thought to upset the balance of nature and at their worst represent forces of evil and the Devil. Unnatural events lack predictability because they exist beyond the parameters of nature and are beyond the control of "mere mortals." Some individuals believe that illness is a result of witchcraft. People who supposedly possess supernatural power are thought to be able to alter the health status of others. Cultural groups that may subscribe to this belief include Mexicans and Mexican Americans, African Americans, Haitians, Trinidadians, and some Southern Caucasians (Snow, 1981).

Natural illnesses may be related to dangerous agents such as cold air or impurities in the air, food, or water. Individuals subscribing to the belief of natural illnesses attribute the cause of natural illnesses to the fact that everything in nature is connected. As such, most natural events can be both interpreted and controlled by manipulation of these reciprocal relationships. An example of a natural illness in the professional medical system is cancer. Health care professionals generally link cancer to common environmental hazards such as smog, cigarette smoking, and toxic waste and other chemical irritants. In a gynecologic setting, cervical cancer may be linked to early sexual activity or multiple sexual partners. However, in the African-American folk medicine system, cancer is viewed as an unnatural illness because it may be perceived as a punishment from God or a spell cast by an evil person who is assigned to do the work of the Devil (Snow, 1974).

Implications for Nursing Care

Variations in health care beliefs and practices cross not only ethnic and cultural boundaries but social boundaries as well.

Health care providers must strive to develop health care systems that remove barriers to health care (see Research Highlight below).

Culture influences an individual's expectations and perceptions regarding health, illness, disease, and symptoms related to disease. Cultural beliefs and values can also influence how one copes with illness, disease, or stress (Bauwens, Anderson, 1981).

Individuals from all aspects of society may use folk medicine either alone or in conjunction with a scientifically based medical system. The importance of folk medicine, and the level of practice, varies among the different ethnic and cultural groups depending on education and socioeconomic status (Bullough, Bullough, 1982). In contrast to the scientifically based health care system in the United States, folk medicine is characterized by a belief in either supernatural powers or external forces of some kind. Snow (1983) postulated that it does not matter whether an individual comes from a rural background or not when it becomes necessary to select health care providers. For example, African American folk medicine is still used widely in the African-American community in the United States because of humiliation that may be encountered in the mainstream health care system, lack of money, and lack of trust in health

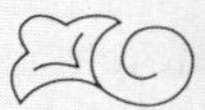 **Research Highlight** 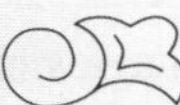

Barriers to Prenatal Care in a Multiethnic, Urban Sample

RESEARCH ABSTRACT

The study was conducted to determine: (1) why women with low socioeconomic backgrounds did not use any prenatal care system, (2) whether ethnicity was a factor in this decision, and (3) the effects of no prenatal care on low birth weight. The study was conducted at a tertiary-level referral center that accepts for delivery women who have had no prenatal care and delivers 16,000 babies per year. During the 3 months of the study, 3028 women gave birth to infants weighing more than 500 g. All nonresidents were excluded. This left 2987 women; 227 had no prenatal care. These 227 women were the study group, and the rest were the comparison group. The questionnaire addressed three main groups of variables: client, system, and financial. Of the 227 women who received no prenatal care, 157 were interviewed for the study during their postpartum stay. The main barriers to care were with the system: location of clinic, inconvenient hours, and lack of transportation. The majority of women thought prenatal care was important. Fifty-seven women did not have clinic fees, and 29 were turned away because they sought care too late in pregnancy. Women who did not receive prenatal care had a higher percentage of low-birth-weight babies. Being single and African American increased the chance of having a low-birth-weight baby. Age and education did not affect the rate of low birth weight. Immigrant women obtained prenatal care more than African-American and Caucasian women, possibly because refugee populations came from countries that emphasize prenatal care.

IMPLICATIONS FOR PRACTICE

There is a need for provision of services that meet sociocultural needs of an urban society. Clinic front desk personnel must provide an environment that encourages prenatal care. Efforts to educate women about the importance of prenatal care must continue.

RELATED RESEARCH QUESTIONS

1. Will an educational program directed at the clinic's front-desk personnel increase the number of women obtaining prenatal care?
2. What types of incentives will influence women to seek prenatal care?
3. Will the use of a mobile prenatal screening van increase the number of women obtaining prenatal care?
4. Will providing child care at the clinic site increase the number of women seeking prenatal care?

REFERENCE

Sculpholme A, Robertson EG, Kamons AS: Barriers to prenatal care in a multiethnic, urban sample, *J Nurse Midwifery* 36(2):111, 1991.

care workers (White, 1977). Even today, some African Americans go to physicians simply for access to medicines and not because they feel the physician is superior in knowledge or training (Murray, 1987). According to McKenzie and Christman (1977), belief in witchcraft, voodoo, and magic has always been an integral aspect of folk medicine systems.

Biologic Variations

Biologic differences exist between individuals in different racial groups. In general, **biologic variations** are less understood than other cultural and racial variations. However, knowledge is developing rapidly in this area. The body of scientific knowledge that exists about biologic racial differences is part of the emerging field known as biocultural ecology.

Biocultural ecology explores the biologic differences between individuals of various racial and cultural groups, and the biologic adaptive efforts necessary for homeostasis (Bennett, Osborne, Miller, 1975). While biocultural ecology concepts have existed in disciplines such as sociology and medical anthropology, it is only recently that the nursing literature has begun documenting this field for nursing practitioners. While the emergence of transcultural nursing is a phenomenon of the last two decades, nursing research on the impact of biologic variations on culturally sensitive nursing care remains an area yet to be explored.

There is a direct relationship between race and body structure, skin color, other visible physical characteristics, enzymatic and genetic variations, physiologic jaundice, twinning, electrocardiographic patterns, susceptibility to disease, and nutritional deficiency. Noting these variables is essential when caring for persons from diverse cultural backgrounds.

Body Structure

One of the obvious differences among racial groups is body size and structure. Variations of body structure are present before birth. Overfield (1985) reported that there are variations even in newborn body proportions. Body proportions of the newborn are genetically programmed to conform to the pelvis of the mother (Overfield, 1985).

Body Size and Gestational Differences

Dimensions of the bony pelvis, newborn size and weight, and length of gestation vary among racial groups. At birth, the average African-American infant weighs 8.5 oz (240 g) less than Caucasian infants. This fact is taken into account when estimating gestational age. Previously, an infant below 5.5 lb was considered "preterm." Today, however, other physical characteristics are evaluated in determining gestational age. Pound for pound, African-American infants exhibit more physiologic maturity than do Caucasian infants (Overfield, 1985). During the first 35 weeks of gestation, the growth rate for African-American fetuses is more rapid. Intrauterine growth in African-American infants is thought to slow after 35 weeks' gestation. The gestational period for African-American fetuses is an average of 9 days shorter than for Caucasians (Pratt, Jones, Seigal, 1977). Puerto Ricans, Japanese, Chinese, and Filipino infants also exhibit lower birth weights than Caucasian infants (Morton, 1977).

Facial Features

When considering body size and structure, the face is one of the most fascinating areas of the body. The face allows people to be categorized by race. For example, when assessing the eyelids of clients, the eyelids vary from racial group to racial group. In some racial groups, eyelids droop over the cartilage plate, and in other racial groups the eyelids do not droop. An example is the presence of epicanthic folds that are found predominantly in individuals of Oriental descent and are postulated to have evolved as a defense against snow or sandstorms (Bleibtreu, Downs, 1971). Filipino Americans have almond-shaped inner eye folds. Nguyen (1988) reports that the eyelids of Vietnamese people usually have an epicanthic fold and a slight droop over the cartilage plate. According to Godsby (1971), "true" Haitians have brown to black eyes with almost square orbits, set widely apart.

Ears, Nose, and Teeth

Racial differences are present in the ears, nose, and teeth. For example, ear lobes can be free and floppy, or attached and close to the head. Noses, on the other hand, come in all sizes and shapes. The size and shape of the nose is directly related to environmental adaptations. For example, small noses are thought to have occurred because of an adaptation to colder climates; high-bridge noses are thought to be an adaptation to living in dry climates, while broad, flat noses may be the result of living in moist, hot climates (Overfield, 1985).

When assessing the teeth, it is essential to note the differences that may be present between races. For example, Orientals, African Americans, and Australian Aborigines have large teeth and tend to have the jaws projecting beyond the upper portion of the face (Overfield, 1985).

Hair Distribution

Variations between races may also be found in hair texture and distribution. For example, the hair of Mexican Americans may be dark and curly or woolly, or straight or wavy. Most Chinese persons have thick, straight, black hair, and Chinese men are reported to have little facial hair. Filipino Americans have coarse scalp hair, and males have very scant body hair. The incidence of male pattern baldness in Filipino males is rare (Giger, Davidhizar, 1991).

Skin Color

Variations also occur in skin color between races. For example, it is difficult to assess the presence of jaundice in persons of Oriental or African descent based upon skin color alone. The sclera of some African-American individuals has a yellowish tint in the normal state because of the presence of subconjunctival fat deposits (Giger, Davidhizar, 1991). Variations in skin color are significant and must be acknowledged by the nurse in order to avoid potentially devastating misinterpretations.

Other Visible Physical Characteristics

The presence of mongolian spots, blue bruiselike discolorations of the skin commonly found on the lower back and buttocks, is well documented in nursing literature and is common in newborns in 90% of African Americans, 80% of Orientals and Native Americans, and 9% of Caucasians (Jacob, Walton, 1976; Overfield, 1985; Boyle, Andrews, 1989). These marks are also noted in Mexican Americans (Monroy, 1983) and American Eskimos (Lefever, Davidhizar, 1991).

Chloasma, or the "mask of pregnancy," a dark discoloration of the skin of the faces and upper chests of pregnant women, is exaggerated in dark-haired and dark-skinned individuals. The increased deposition of melanin is related by an unknown mechanism to pregnancy and/or the use of birth control pills. When the underlying cause is related to pregnancy, the discoloration fades over time after delivery, but may persist permanently if caused by the use of oral contraceptives.* There is no correlation between the amount of areolar pigmentation and the incidence of nipple cracking (Overfield, 1985).

*Newer lower-dose preparations of oral hormonal birth control pills seem to have lesser effect on the deposition of melanin.

Enzymatic and Genetic Variations

From the moment of conception, the basic genetic make-up of an individual is determined. The genetic conceptual map is drawn, more or less, from conception, and cannot be altered or manipulated. For example, growth and development cannot be manipulated beyond what the genes make possible. Although controversial, it must be noted that the intelligence level of an individual is directly related to genetic structure (Burt, 1966; Lorton, Lorton, 1984). Regardless of the amount and type of special tutoring, genes and genetic structure influence intelligence (Burt, 1966; Lorton, Lorton, 1984).

PHYSIOLOGIC JAUNDICE. Physiologic jaundice is present in more than half of Oriental and Native American infants. The bilirubin level peaks in Oriental infants on the fifth and sixth days of life, as opposed to the second and third day of life for Caucasian infants (Overfield, 1985). As many as 40% of Chinese infants have bilirubin levels higher than 12 mg/dL, and up to 23% have levels above 15 mg/dL (and levels are increased by breast-feeding) (Boyle, Andrews, 1989). The effect of breast-feeding on raising bilirubin levels is more pronounced in Oriental and Native American infants, but it does not appear to be associated with a higher level of kernicterus in these two groups (Overfield, 1985; Boyle, Andrews, 1989).

INCIDENCE OF TWINNING. Dizygotic twinning is thought to occur more frequently in African Americans, or in about 4% of African-American births. In contrast, it is thought to occur only in about 2% of Caucasians and 0.25% of Orientals (Overfield, 1985)

HYPERTENSION. Among African Americans, the incidence of hypertension is reported to be significantly higher than among their Caucasian American counterparts. In African Americans, the onset by age is reported to be earlier, more severe, and associated with higher mortality. The incidence of hypertension among African Americans is approximately 35% for those over age 40 (Tipton, 1974). In a study conducted with a random sample of adults between the ages of 18 and 79, 20% of African Americans as compared to 9% of others were found to be hypertensive (Boyle, 1970). Other supporting studies have suggested that there is an equal prevalence of hypertension among both sexes in the African-American race and that there is increased incidence with advancing age (Merck, Sharp, Dohme, 1974). However, there are contrasting opinions that might suggest that hypertension can and does occur more often in men than in women (Phipps, Long, Woods, 1991).

SUSCEPTIBILITY TO DISEASE. Racial groups differ in susceptibility to disease. The increased or decreased incidence of a particular disease may be genetically linked. Although many differences exist, those with particular relevance to the childbearing family will be examined, including blood groups and Rh factors, diabetes, sickle cell anemia, and systemic lupus erythematosus.

BLOOD GROUPS AND RH FACTORS. Racial groups can also be differentiated by blood groups. For example, a prevalence of Type O blood has been found among some Native Americans, with some incidence of Type A, and virtually no incidence of Type B (Jick, 1969; Overfield, 1985). Prevalence of Types A, B, and O in equal incidences has been reported among Japanese and Chinese people. However, Type AB is found in only about 10% of Japanese and Oriental populations. The prevalence of Type A, B, and O blood groups is not differentiated between African Americans and Caucasian Americans. However, the predominant types of blood groups found among these two groups are Types A and O, with fewer incidences of Types AB and B reported.

There is evidence to support the hypothesis that women who have Type O blood have a diminished incidence of thromboembolic disease when taking oral contraceptive pills. The negative Rh factor in blood is reported to be most common among Caucasians and is much more rare in other racial groups (apparently absent altogether in Eskimos) (Lewis, 1942; Overfield, 1985; Lefever, Davidhizar, 1991).

DIABETES. Diabetes mellitus has an incidence in certain Native American tribes, including the Seminoles, Pima, and Papago. On the other hand, diabetes is quite rare among Alaskan Eskimos (Westfall, 1971; Lefever, Davidhizar, 1991). Diabetes is considered a major health problem in the United States, with more than six million diagnosed cases. For every diagnosed case of diabetes there is another case that has gone undiagnosed and therefore untreated (Carter Center, Emory University, 1985). There are three type of diabetes mellitus, including insulin-dependent (IDDM), non–insulin-dependent (NIDDM), and gestational diabetes (GDM). The peak incidence of IDDM is reported to occur between ages 10 and 14; it is reported to have a higher incidence in boys and a higher frequency in Caucasians, and it accounts for approximately 10% to 20% of all diagnosed cases of IDDM (Krolewski, Warram, 1985). On the other hand, NIDDM is reported to increase dramatically with age, have a higher frequency in women, and have a higher incidence in non-Caucasians, particularly Hispanics and Native Americans. NIDDM is said to account for approximately 80% to 90% of all diagnosed cases of diabetes mellitus (Carter Center, Emory University, 1985).

Rifkin (1984) reported that GDM occurs in 20% of all pregnant women and apparently increases with maternal age; however, it does not appear to be affected by race or culture. In contrast to this view, Landen et al (1991) indicated that GDM is more common among Native American women than it is among other women in the general U. S. population. Data from a study of Navajo women at Shiprock Hospital suggested that the prevalence of maternal diabetes during pregnancy is 4.6%. Even when a control was made for women with preexisting diabetes or previous GDM, the data indicated 3.4% of the sampled population had GDM (Landen et al, 1991).

Gestational diabetes mellitus (GDM) may have serious consequences for the fetus because the offspring of mothers who experience GDM are at risk for fetal macrosomia with a significant potential for injury during delivery, and for hypoglycemia, hypocalcemia, polycythemia, and hyperbilirubinemia (Summary of the Second International Workshop-Conference on Gestational Diabetes Mellitus, 1985).

SICKLE CELL ANEMIA. Sickle cell anemia is the most common genetic disorder in the United States. Sickle cell anemia or the trait for sickle cell anemia occurs predominantly in the African-American population. It has been projected that approximately 50,000 African Americans have sickle cell anemia (Wyngaarden, Smith, 1985). Sickle cell anemia or the trait for sickle cell anemia has also been reported in people from Asia Minor, India, the Mediterranean, and the Caribbean. The incidence for this condition among these populations is less than the incidence reported for African Americans. Pregnancy usually results in a worsening of most aspects of sickle cell anemia (Scott et al, 1990). When working with clients with sickle cell anemia, it is important for the nurse to teach the client to recognize symptoms of sickle cell crises. Ongoing surveillance of signs and symptoms of sickle cell crises can potentially promote appropriate treatment and perhaps can decrease early death as a result of sickle cell crises.

SYSTEMIC LUPUS ERYTHEMATOSUS. Systemic lupus erythematosus (SLE) is a chronic disease of unknown cause that affects organs and systems individually or in a variety of combinations. The disease is reported to affect women 8 to 10 times more often than it affects men. The age distribution for this disease is said to span anywhere from 2 to 97 years of age. Once SLE was thought to be a rare disease; however, because of sophisticated detection procedures, researchers now postulate that this is not a rare disease. The incidence for SLE has been estimated to be 2.6 per 100,000 population, although it appears to be more frequent in African Americans than in others, and it is reported to be extremely rare among the Asian population (Giger, Davidhizar, 1991).

NUTRITIONAL DEFICIENCIES. Racially related nutritional deficiencies include lactose intolerance and G6PD (glucose-6-phosphate dehydrogenase) deficiency. Lactose intolerance is an intolerance to milk sugar and is relatively common in many ethnic groups. Lactose intolerance is found in 66% of Mexican Americans and is very common in African-American adults (90%), Native Americans (79%), Orientals (94%), and Ashkenazic Jews (79%) (Kisch, 1953; Bayless, 1975; Burns, Neubort, 1984; Bayless, 1985; Overfield, 1985). About 90% of the population of the world is lactose intolerant (Overfield, 1985).

G6PD is an enzyme deficiency that is thought to be common in certain racial or ethnic groups. There are two types of G6PD deficiencies that have been noted. Williams (1975) noted that the Type A variety of this condition, which moves rapidly on starch-gel electrophoresis, is commonly found in 35% of African Americans who have this deficiency. On the other hand, the slower-moving Type B variety is found in 65% of African Americans and in nearly all others who have this deficiency. Regardless of the type, this condition affects males more than females because the genetic inheritance is carried on the X chromosome. The Canton-Chinese type has an incidence of 2% to 5%. However, it is thought that the most clinically severe type is the Mediterranean variety, which affects approximately 50% of male Greek Sardinians, and 50% of Sephardic Jews (Williams, 1975).

CULTURAL PSYCHOLOGIC REACTIONS TO PAIN AND STRESS. Culture has a profound impact on perceptual and behavioral reaction to pain (see Table 17-1). Weisenberg and Caspi (1989) noted that the perception of pain associated with childbirth is rated high by most women regardless of race, culture, or ethnicity. However, differences were noted both in pain ratings and pain behaviors as a distinctive function of ethnocultural grouping. Findings from the study suggest that during childbirth, the family of origin and level of education may have a profound impact on reaction to and tolerance for pain. The study also indicates that education decreases the influence of the family of origin on the reaction to pain.

Implications for Nursing Care

Knowledge of biologic variations can aid the nurse in giving culturally appropriate nursing care. It is essential for the nurse who cares for people from other cultures and races to know that certain biologic concepts can create variations in assessment findings between and among people. Important biologic variations are related to body structure and skin color. Other biologic variations that may affect the childbearing family include enzymatic and genetic differences and susceptibility to disease. The extent of the impact that biologic variations between racial groups can have upon the childbearing process should be a foremost consideration for culturally appropriate care.

■ SUMMARY

It is essential to understand differences in individuals as they relate to cultural heritage. It is also important to appreciate that each client and family are culturally unique and bring this uniqueness to the care environment. In addition, the nurse who gives care also brings to the client-nurse relationship a personal cultural heritage. It is essential to refrain from imposing personal values and beliefs on the client and to respect the uniqueness and differences each brings to the care environment.

One of the most important roles of the nurse caring for any client, regardless of the client's cultural heritage, is that of teacher. Teaching should begin with assessing the client's ability to communicate and to understand what is being said. To give culturally appropriate nursing care, and to teach people to care for themselves, the nurse needs to understand the importance of cultural and racial variables, including communication, space and spatial relationships, social organization, time, environmental control, and biologic variations. Culture affects the manner in which nursing care is planned and implemented. No nurse can give culturally appropriate nursing care without knowing the cultural and racial factors that affect the client and family.

CASE STUDY

Chinese-American Woman in First Pregnancy

Kim Liu, a 23-year-old Chinese-American university student, has come to the student health pavilion. Averting her eyes, she informs you in broken English that she has missed two menstrual periods, her breasts are tender, and the last few mornings she has felt nauseated.

ASSESSMENT

Through interview, the nurse learns that Kim lives with her husband Woo, a graduate student at the university. Woo and Kim work part time in the family grocery store. They live with Woo's mother, who speaks only Mandarin. Woo speaks fluent English. Kim's mother-in-law made her some herbal tea this morning for her nausea and has been giving her ginseng. Kim shyly asks if she must be examined by a male physician and if it will hurt. The Liu family eats traditional Chinese foods. A nutritional assessment is completed and the nurse determines that Kim does not eat much meat, and her foods are high in sodium as a result of the preparation method. Kim is afraid of how her husband will react to the news of her pregnancy. She has not used birth control because her husband and mother-in-law do not want her to use anything "unnatural." They have no health insurance other than the student policy, which pays 80% of the hospital costs.

Physical examination was performed by the nurse and the certified nurse-midwife (female). Kim's height is 5 feet 4 inches, and her weight is 115 lb. Her vital signs are: BP 110/72, P 84, R 26, T 98.8° F (37.1° C). The CNM confirms an intrauterine pregnancy of 10 to 12 weeks' gestation.

Laboratory tests reveal that Kim's hemoglobin is 11.7 and her hematocrit is 38.8. Her urine is negative for glucose and ketones.

Kim's pregnancy progresses uneventfully, and she is admitted to the perinatal unit in active labor. Following an uneventful labor, Kim gives birth to a female infant. She plans to breast-feed her infant. Kim and Woo are rooming-in with their baby. The baby is noted to have mongolian spots on her lower back. Kim stays in the hospital for 24 hours postpartum and is discharged home with instructions to return in 1 week for PKU and bilirubin testing of the baby.

NURSING DIAGNOSES

Because Mandarin is the primary language of this couple and Kim speaks English haltingly, the nursing diagnosis *Impaired communication, verbal, related to language differences*, can be identified. The nutritional assessment yields information relative to low complete protein consumption and high sodium consumption in a traditional Chinese diet. Additionally, because Chinese are relatively intolerant of lactose, a potential exists for insufficient calcium and phosphorus intake. Sufficient data exist for the nursing diagnosis *Alteration in nutrition: less than body requirements, related to cultural difference, increased requirements of pregnancy, and inability to digest nutrients*.

The nursing diagnosis *Alteration in comfort related to physical changes of pregnancy* is determined from the complaint of breast soreness and nausea. The nursing diagnosis *Alteration in health maintenance related to cultural folk practices and lack of information about pregnancy and birth control* can be supported from the initial assessment information.

Because of the preference in Chinese culture for male infants and the presence of mongolian spots, the nursing diagnosis *Anxiety related to potential nonacceptance of infant and presence of mongolian spots* is made.

PLANNING

The plan of care is developed with Kim and her husband. Careful attention is paid to identifying their cultural values and norms, and *goals* are mutually agreed upon (e.g., Kim and her family will establish a satisfactory communication pattern, and Kim's nutrient intake will be sufficient to support growth and maintain health as measured by adequate fetal and maternal weight gain). *Expected outcomes* set by the nurse should demonstrate consonance between Western medical and nursing practices and deeply held culture-bound medical practices (e.g., Kim will learn to use foods and herbs acceptable to her cultural heritage [and to her mother-in-law], will gain the weight necessary for her and her fetus' well-being, and will not develop associated problems such as pregnancy-induced hypertension).

IMPLEMENTATION

Interventions are derived from the goals and expected outcomes and should be agreeable to Kim and Woo (and the mother-in-law). A translator is provided as needed; graphics, pictures, and demonstration/return demonstration are used. Kim's nutrient intake for 1 week is determined and analyzed; foods acceptable to meet the deficiencies within their budget and preferences are identified; a month's supply of prenatal vitamins are issued. Since Kim refused to take iron supplementation ("iron will get in my bones"), foods to supply the element are suggested.

EVALUATION

Evaluation focuses on the degree that the goals are attained and on the expected outcomes identified during mutual goal setting. The following plan of care demonstrates those principles for the five nursing diagnoses identified.

CARE PLAN Chinese-American Woman in First Pregnancy

GOALS	IMPLEMENTATION	RATIONALE	EVALUATION
Nursing diagnosis 1: Impaired communication, verbal, related to language differences			
Kim and family will establish satisfactory communication pattern.	Provide translator in communication with family, or include Woo in planning since he speaks fluent English. Use graphics, pictures, and demonstration/return demonstration to assess understanding of information.	Visual aids and demonstrations are likely to be effective when a language conflict exists. 1. Include Woo in planning, since he has a fluent command of both English and Mandarin. 2. Information transmitted by a person of the same culture may be better understood and received. 3. It is common among the Chinese people to allow the husband to speak for the wife, even if she speaks fluent English.	Kim and her husband establish an effective communication pattern.
Nursing diagnosis 2: Alteration in nutrition, less than body requirements related to cultural differences, increase in requirements for pregnancy, and inability to digest nutrient			
Kim's nutrient intake will be sufficient to support growth and maintain health as measured by adequate fetal and maternal weight gain.	Identify nutrient intake for a 1-week period; perform a nutrient analysis. Counsel about need to control intake of food high in sodium and to limit intake of "folk herbs" until she has consulted with the nurse. Encourage Kim to eat food high in calcium but low in lactose (tofu, bean curds, lactose-free milk substitute, etc). Encourage food high in iron. Measure fundal height and weight each visit. Encourage Kim to eat dry toast in the mornings and to eat several small meals daily to control nausea.	1. A nutritional assessment of a week of typical foods is likely to identify any major deficiencies. 2. Chinese food is often high in sodium because of the monosodium glutamate used to enhance flavor. 3. Some Chinese do not like to eat meat and will not take supplemental iron. Lactose intolerance is prevalent in Orientals, and identifying culturally acceptable foods is necessary to ensure adequate nutrient intake. 4. Fundal height and maternal weight gain are indicators of maternal and fundal nutritional status	Kim's weight gain and fundal height changes are adequate. At next visit, Kim reports that she is no longer experiencing nausea.

CARE PLAN Chinese-American Woman in First Pregnancy—cont'd

GOALS	IMPLEMENTATION	RATIONALE	EVALUATION
Nursing diagnosis 3: Alteration in comfort related to changes of pregnancy			
Kim will be free from pain after nursing interventions.	Refer to store selling good maternity bras. Encourage Kim to wear support bra 24 hours a day. Have Kim place a warm wash cloth on her breasts at intervals, or take a warm bath or shower.	1. Increase in breast size and weight during pregnancy and lactation can result in increased tension upon support structures. 2. Heat promotes drainage of lymphatic channels, thereby alleviating engorgement and pain.	At next visit, Kim wears a good support bra and is free from pain.
Nursing diagnosis 4: Alterations in health maintenance related to folk practices and lack of information about birth control			
Kim achieves an acceptable balance between current health practices and cultural specifications.	Use graphics and pictures to discuss health maintenance, fetal development, etc. Discuss natural methods of birth control (cervical mucus or Billings method) Explore with Kim and Woo their cultural value system and correlate nursing interventions with deeply held values.	1. Pictures and graphics are universal and cross language barriers. 2. Natural means of birth control (cervical mucus method, Billings method, etc.) may not affront cultural standards and are apt to have a high compliance rate.	Kim does not try home remedies without consulting the nurse or midwife to determine if such practices are efficacious, neutral, or dysfunctional. Kim and her husband achieve an acceptable balance between culturally valued health practices and Western health practices.
Nursing diagnosis 5: Anxiety related to birth of female infant and presence of mongolian spots			
Kim's anxiety is controlled, and parent-child bonding is promoted.	Provide support and feedback during the rooming-in experience. Allow time for ventilation of feelings. Observe bonding behavior between parents and child. Reinforce positive behaviors. Explain presence of mongolian spots to parents, and suggest that the parents inform the day-care providers of their presence. Instruct parents to bring infant in after 1 week for PKU and bilirubin testing.	1. Rooming-in allows family to preserve control and test parenting skills in a safe environment. 2. Bonding between parents and child progresses through a series of observable steps. 3. Mongolian spots are common in dark-skinned individuals and disappear by 3 to 4 years of age. 4. PKU tests are unreliable before 3 days of milk feedings and may not be reliable before 1 week of breast-feeding. Elevation of bilirubin may not occur before 1 week of age in Oriental infants.	Kim, her husband, and their newborn's bonding progresses normally, and they obtain follow-up care on a timely basis for mother and infant. Parents state they understand presence of mongolian spots. The newborn is tested for PKU and bilirubin at 8 days after birth.

REFERENCES

Affonso D: Framework for cultural assessment. In *Childbearing: a nursing perspective,* ed 2, edited by Bauwens E, Anderson S. Social and cultural influences on health care. In Stanhope M, Lancaster J, editors: *Community health nursing: Process and practice for promoting health,* ed 2, 1988, St Louis: Mosby–Yearbook, pp 89-108.

Bash DM: Jewish religious practices related to childbearing, *J Nurse Midwifery* 25(5):39, 1980.

Bauwens E, Anderson S: *Chronic health problems: concept and applications,* St Louis, 1981, Mosby–Year Book.

Bayless T: Lactose and milk intolerance: clinical implications, *N Engl J Med* 292(5):1156, 1975.

Bennett K, Osborne R, Miller R: *Biocultural ecology: annual review of anthropology,* Palo Alto, Calif, 1975, Annual Reviews.

Bleibtreu HK, Downs JF: *Human variations: readings in physical anthropology,* Beverly Hills, Calif, 1971, Glencoe Press.

Bobak IM, Jensen MD: *Essentials of maternity nursing,* ed 3, St Louis, 1991, Mosby–Year Book.

Boyle E: Biological patterns in hypertension by race, sex, body weight, and skin color, *JAMA* 213:1637, 1970.

Boyle JS, Andrews MM: *Transcultural concepts of nursing care,* Glenview, Ill, 1989, Scott, Foresman.

Brownlee AT: *Community, culture, and care: a cross-cultural guide for health workers.* St Louis, 1978, Mosby–Year Book.

Bullough V, Bullough B: *Health care for the other Americans,* New York 1982, Appleton-Century-Crofts.

Burns E, Neubort S: 1984 Sodium content of koshered meat, a letter to the editor of *JAMA,* 1984.

Burt C: The genetic determination of differences in intelligence: a study of monozygote twins reared together and apart, *Br J Psychol,* 57, 137, 1966.

Chang K: Chinese Americans. In Giger J, Davidhizar R, editors: *Transcultural nursing assessment and interventions,* St Louis, 1991, Mosby–Year Book.

Chung HJ: Understanding the Oriental maternity patient, *Nurs Clin North Am* 12(1):67, 1977.

Davidhizar R: Personal communication, 1988.

Evans G, Howard R: Personal space, *Psychol Bull* 80:335, 1973.

Foster R: *Family-centered nursing care of children,* Philadelphia, 1989, WB Saunders.

Giger J, Davidhizar R: *Transcultural nursing: assessment and intervention,* St Louis, 1991, Mosby–Year Book.

Giger J, Davidhizar R: Transcultural nursing assessment: a method of advancing nursing practice, *Int Nurs Rev* 37(1):1990.

Giger JN, Davidhizar RE, Turner G: Black health care beliefs and practices, unpublished manuscript.

Giuffra M: Sociocultural issues. In Haber J, et al, editors: *Comprehensive psychiatric nursing,* ed 3, New York, 1987, McGraw-Hill.

Godsby R: *A race and races,* New York, 1971, MacMillan.

Greeley A: *The Irish Americans,* New York, 1981, Harper & Row.

Haber J, et al: *Comprehensive psychiatric nursing,* New York, 1987, McGraw-Hill.

Hall E: *Hidden dimension,* New York, 1966, Doubleday Inc.

Hanley C: Navajo Indians. In Giger J, Davidhizar R: *Transcultural nursing: assessment and intervention,* St Louis, 1991, Mosby–Year Book.

Hypertension handbook for clinicians. Westpoint, Penn, 1974, Merck, Sharp, & Dohme.

Jacob A, Walton R: Incidences of birthmarks in the neonate, *Pediatrics* 58:218, 1976.

Jick H, et al: Venous thromboembolic disease and ABO blood type, *Lancet* 1:539, 1969.

Kim YY: Intercultural personhood: an integration of Eastern and Western perspectives. In Samovar LA, Porter RE, editors: *Intercultural communication: a reader,* ed 5, Belmont, Calif, 1988, Wadsworth, 344.

Kisch B: Salt poor diet in Jewish dietary laws, *JAMA* 153(16):1472, 1953.

Kleinman A, Eisenberg L, Good B: Culture, illness, and care, *Ann Intern Med* 88:251, 1978.

Kluckhohn F, Strodtbeck F: *Variations in value orientation,* Elmsford, NY, 1961, Row, Peterson.

Krolewski A, Warram G: Epidemiology of Diabetes Mellitus in Marble A, editor *Joslin's Diabetes Mellitus,* ed 12, Philadelphia, 1985, Lea & Febiger.

Kuipers J, Mexican Americans. In editors: *Transcultural nursing: assessment and intervention,* Giger J, Davidhizar R, St Louis, 1991, Mosby–Year Book.

Lee RV: Understanding Southeast Asian mothers-to-be, *CBE* 8(3):32, 1989.

Leininger M: *Qualitative research methods in nursing,* New York, 1985a, Grune & Stratton.

Leininger M: Transcultural care diversity and universality: a theory of nursing, *Nurs Health Care* 6(4):1985b.

Lefever D, Davidhizar R: American Eskimos. In Giger J, Davidhizar R: *Transcultural nursing: assessment and intervention,* St Louis, 1991, Mosby–Year Book.

Lewis J: *The biology of the negro* (Chicago University monographs in medicine), Chicago, 1942, University of Chicago Press.

Lorton J, Lorton E: *Human development through the lifespan,* Belmont, Calif, 1984, Brooks & Cole.

Mbiti SS: *African religions and philosophies,* New York, 1970, Anchor Press.

McKenzie J, Christman N: Healing herbs, gods, and magic, *Nurs Outlook* 25(5):325, 1977.

Mehrabian A: *Silent messages: implicit communication of emotion and attitude,* Belmont, Calif, 1981, Wadsworth Publishing Company.

Meleis A: The Arab American in the health care system, *Am J Nurs* 81(6):1180, 1981.

Meleis A, Sorrell L: Arab American women and their birth experiences, *MCN* 6:171, 1981.

Miller SW, Supersad Nerala J: East Hindu Americans. In Giger J, Davidhizar R, editors:*Transcultural nursing: assessment and intervention,* St Louis, 1991, Mosby–Year Book.

Montagu A: *Touching: the significance of the human skin,* New York, 1971, Columbia University Press.

Morton NE: Genetic aspects of prematurity. In Reed DM, Stanley FJ, editors: *The epidemiology of prematurity,* Baltimore, 1977, Urban & Schwarzenburg.

Murdock G, et al: *Outline of cultural materials,* ed 4, New Haven, Conn, 1971, Human Relations Area Files.

Murray R: *Psychiatric/mental health nursing,* East Norwalk, Conn, 1987, Appleton-Lange.

Novak W, Waldoks M: *The big book of Jewish humor,* Philadelphia, 1981, Harper & Row.

Orland L: The need for territoriality. In Yura H, Walsh MB editors: *Human needs and the nursing process,* New York, 1978, Appleton-Century Crofts, 97.

Overfield T: *Biologic variation in health and illness,* Reading, Mass, 1985, Addison-Wesley.

Phillips S, Lobar S: Literature summary of some Navajo child health beliefs and rearing practices within a transcultural nursing framework, *J Transcultural Nurs* 1(2):13, 1990.

Phipps W, Long B, Woods N: *Medical-surgical nursing: concepts and clinical practice,* St Louis, 1991, Mosby–Year Book.

Pillsbury B: Doing the month: confinement and convalescence of Chinese women after childbirth. In Kay M, editor: *Anthropology of human birth,* Philadelphia, 1982, FA Davis.

Porter RE, Samovar LA: Approaching intercultural communication. In Samovar LA, Porter RE, editors: *Intercultural communication: a reader,* ed 4, Belmont, Calif, 1985, Wadsworth Publishing, 15.

Pratt MW, Jones ZL, Seigal NL: National variations in prematurity (1973-1974). In Reed DM, Stanley FJ, editors: *The epidemiology of prematurity.* Baltimore 1977, Urban & Schwarzenberg, 53.

Reddy G: Women's movement: the Indian scene, *The Indian J Social Work* 46(4):507, 1986.

Rifkin H, editor: *The physician's guide to type II diabetes (NIDDM): diagnosis and treatment,* New York, 1984, The American Diabetes Association.

Roberts SL: *Behavioral concepts and nursing throughout the life span,* Englewood Cliffs, NJ, 1978, Prentice Hall.

Rotter JB: Generalized expectancies for internal versus external control of reinforcement, *Psychol Monographs* 80(1):1, 1966.

Scott JR et al: *Danforth's obstetrics and gynecology,* ed 6, Philadelphia, 1990, JB Lippincott.

Setiloane GM: African views on birth, *Nursing BSA Verpleging* 3(7):43, 1988.

Snow LE: Folk medical beliefs and their implications for care of patients: A review based on studies among Black Americans, *Ann Intern Med* 81:82, 1974.

Snow L: Folk medical beliefs and their implications for the care of patients: A review based on studies among Black Americans. In Henderson G, Primeaux M, editors: *Transcultural health care,* Reading, Mass, 1981, Addison-Wesley.

Snow L: Traditional health beliefs and practices among lower class Black Americans, *West J Med* 139(6):820, 1983.

Stauffer R: Vietnamese Americans. In Giger J, Davidhizar R, editors: *Transcultural nursing: assessment and intervention,* St Louis, 1991, Mosby–Year Book.

Sue D: *Counseling the culturally different: theory and practice:* New York, 1981, John Wiley & Sons.

Tipton D: Physiological assessment of black people. In *Care of black patients (X428.1),* A group of papers, sponsored by Continuing Education in Nursing, University of California, San Francisco, May 1974.

Tripp-Reimer T, Brink P, Saunders J: Cultural assessment: content and process, *Nurs Outlook* 32(2), 1984.

Weisenberg M, Caspi Z: Cultural influence on pain and childbirth, *J Pain Symptom Management* 4(1):13, 1989.

Wenger F: President's address, *Transcultural Nursing Society Newsletter* 9(1):3, 1989.

Westfall D: Diabetes mellitus among the Florida Seminoles, *HSMHA Health Reports,* 86:1037, 1971.

White EH: Giving health care to minority patients, *Nurs Clin North Am* 12:27, 1977.

Williams RA, editor: *Textbook of black related disease,* New York, 1975, Mcgraw-Hill.

Wyngaarden JB, Smith LH, editors: *Cecil textbook of medicine,* Philadelphia, 1985, WB Saunders.

Yeun J: Asian Americans, *Birth Defects Original Article Series* 23(6):164, 1987.

References—Nursing Research

Carter Cancer Center of Emory University: Closing the gap: the problem of diabetes mellitus in the United States, *Diabetes Care* 8:391, 1985.

Greene L, Johnston F: *Social and biological predictors of nutritional status, growth, and development,* New York, 1980, Academic Press.

Landen M, et al: Screening criteria for gestational diabetes among Native Americans, *The IHS Primary Care Provider* 16(8):125, 1991.

Levine R, Wolff E: Social time: the heartbeat of culture, *Psychology Today* 29, 1985.

Nguyen NB: Culture shock: a study of Vietnamese culture and the concept of health and disease, *The Journal of the Associates of Vietnamese Medical Professionals in Canada* 98(Sept):26, 1988.

Norbeck J, Anderson N: Psychosocial predictors of pregnancy outcomes in low-income black, Hispanic, and white women, *Nurs Res* 38(4):204, 1989.

Tripp-Reimer T: Barriers to health care: variations in interpretation of Appalachian client behavior by Appalachian and non-Appalachian health professionals, *West J Nurs Res* 4(2):179, 1982.

Tripp-Reimer T: Research in cultural diversity, *West J Nurs Res* 6(3):353, 1984.

Watson M: *Proxemic behavior: a cross-cultural study,* The Hague, Netherlands, 1980, Moutons.

Williams C, Jelliffe D: *Mother and child health: delivering the services,* London, 1972, Oxford University Press.

BIBLIOGRAPHY

Ahumada LS: Multicultural perinatal health care, *Maternal and Child Health Ed Resources* 6(2): Spring 1991.

Increasing culturally relevant practice with Hispanic clients, *NPA Bulletin* 3(4):23, 1988.

Kulin J: Childbearing Cambodian refugee women, *Can Nurs* p 46, June 1988.

Lee RV: Understanding Southeast Asian mothers-to-be, *Childbirth Educ* 8(3):32, Spring 1989.

Lee RV, et al: Southeast Asian folklore about pregnancy and parturition, *Obstet Gynecol* 71:243, 1988.

Leininger M: A new generation of nurses discover transcultural nursing, *Nurs Health Care* 8(5):1987.

Monroy L: Nursing care of Raza-Latina patients. In Orque M, Bloch B, Monroy L, editors: *Ethnic nursing care: a multi-cultural approach,* St Louis, 1983, Mosby–Year Book, 115.

National Center for Health Statistics: Final natality statistics (1978), *Monthly Vital Stats Rep* 29(1):1, 1980.

Overfield T: Biological variations, *Nurs Clin North Am* 12(1):19, 1977.

Webster's Ninth New Collegiate Dictionary, Springfield, Mass, 1984, Merriam-Webster.

Bibliography—Nursing Research

Lee PA: Health beliefs of pregnant and postpartum Hmong women, *West J Nurs Res* 8(1):83, 1986.

Tipton D: Physiological assessment of black people. In *Care of Black Patients (X428.1),* a group of papers, sponsored by Continuing Education in Nursing, University of California, San Francisco, May 1974.

Tripp-Reimer T, Friedl M: Appalachians: a neglected minority, *Nurs Clin North Am* 12(1):1977.

Tripp-Reimer T: Retention of a folk-healing practice (Matiasma) among four generations of urban Greek immigrants, *Nurs Res* 32(2):97, 1983.

Tripp-Reimer T, Dougherty MC: Cross-cultural nursing research, *Annu Rev Nurs Res* 3:77, 1985.

chapter 3 review

Key Concepts

- Individuals are culturally unique and bring cultural values and beliefs to nurse-client interaction.
- Childbearing as a process is valued uniquely by each cultural group and requires the nurse to blend traditional beliefs and values with safe nursing practice to make childbirth a positive experience.
- Six cultural phenomena appear in all cultural groups: (a) communication, (b) space, (c) social organization, (d) time, (e) environmental control, and (f) biologic variations.
- Communication is evaluated most effectively by evaluating (a) dialect, (b) style (language in social situations), (c) volume (silence), (d) touch, (e) context of speech (emotional tone), and (f) kinesics.
- Space is the environment surrounding an individual's body and includes perception of interpersonal zones and territoriality.
- Social organization includes family structures and organization, religious values and beliefs, ethnicity and cultural roles, and role assignment.
- Individuals have a past, present, or future time orientation affecting prioritizing and decision making. Time may be conceptualized as social time (consisting of periodicity), tempo, timing, duration and sequence, or strict clock time.
- Environmental control refers to the ability of an individual from a particular cultural group to plan activities that control and direct nature.
- Biologic variations include differences existing among various racial groups. Biologic variations must be thoroughly assessed in order to plan nursing care for clients from diverse cultural backgrounds.

Key Terms

- biologic variations (p. 59)
- clock time (p. 53)
- communication (p. 46)
- cultural health practices (p. 55)
- cultural values (p. 44)
- culturally diverse nursing care (p. 44)
- culture (p. 44)
- environmental control (p. 54)
- family (p. 51)
- family roles (p. 51)
- locus of control (p. 57)
- personal space (p. 50)
- preferred distance (p. 50)
- religion (p. 51)
- social organization (p. 51)
- social time (p. 53)
- space (p. 49)
- territoriality (p. 50)
- time (p. 53)

Critical Thinking Exercises

Select a family from a culture different from your own. Interview an adult member regarding values and beliefs about pregnancy and childbirth. Pay particular attention to taboos.

1. Compare your values and beliefs with those of the family, noting differences and similarities.
2. Choose one topic, such as exercise or diet, for a prenatal teaching activity. Formulate a teaching plan, justifying your decisions and actions.
3. Analyze your teaching plan to identify whether your values and beliefs have influenced your assessment, diagnosis, plan, implementation, or evaluation.
4. Exchange your teaching plan and analysis with another student for feedback regarding your sensitivity to the identified cultural variations.

Topics for Nursing Research

- Are there significant and profound racial biologic differences in the childbearing family that necessitate developing culturally appropriate processes to facilitate optimal care?
- To what extent do culture, ethnicity, and race affect the development of health, health-seeking, wellness, and illness behaviors?
- If culturally appropriate nursing techniques were not included in the plan of care, to what extent would the client from a diverse, multicultural background be affected?
- How may a nurse most effectively assess the impact of cultural diversity on a normal experience such as pregnancy?
- To what extent should the nurse include family members in the nursing plan of care for clients from diverse cultural backgrounds?
- When disparity exists between Western medical beliefs and deep-seated cultural beliefs, how can compliance be maximized?

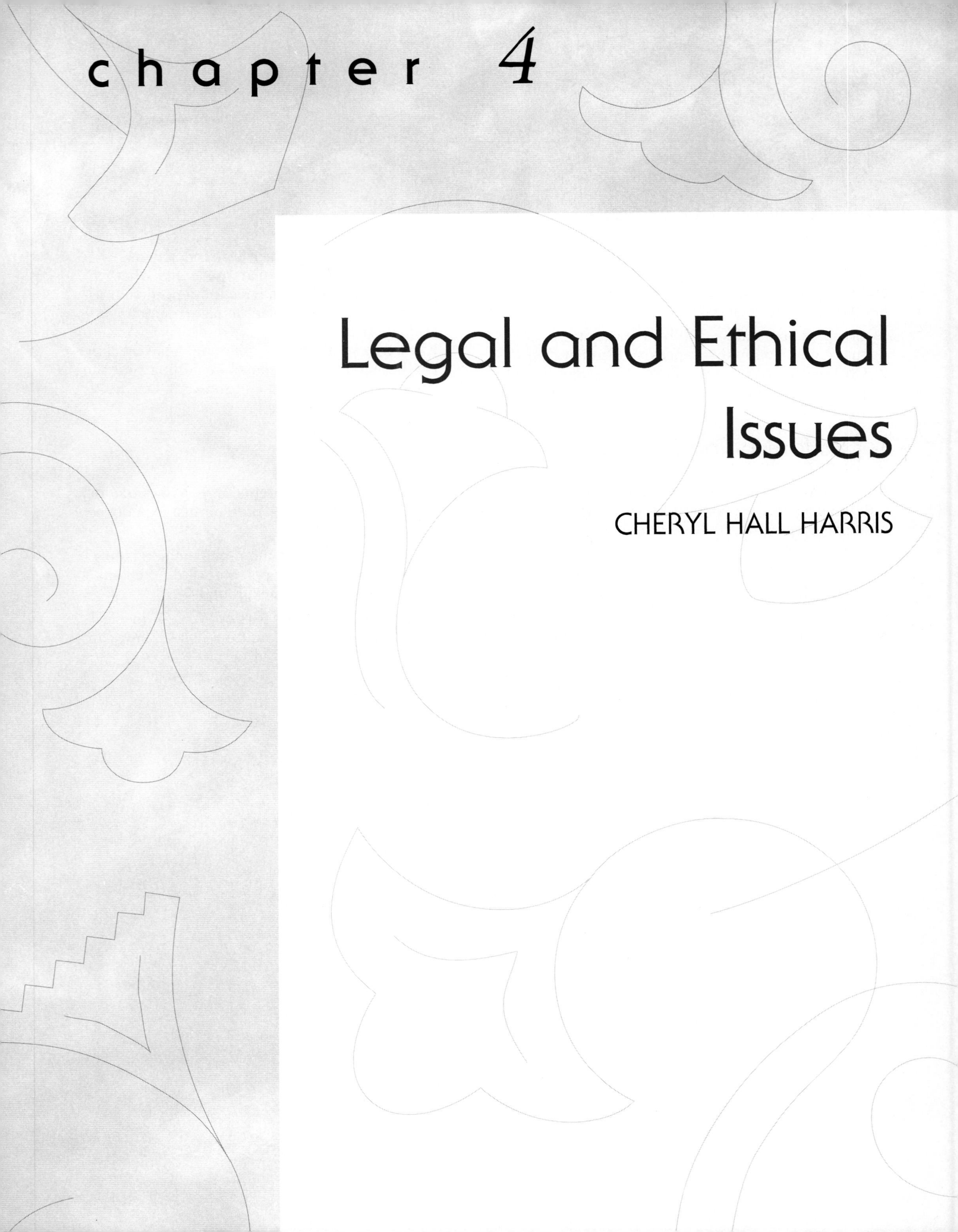

chapter 4

Legal and Ethical Issues

CHERYL HALL HARRIS

LEARNING OBJECTIVES

- Define the key terms listed.
- Identify examples of duty: the standard of care.
- List three ways in which a nurse may commit professional malpractice.
- Describe examples of liability and causation.
- Summarize the independent practice of nursing.
- Assess risk management through practices of prevention and appropriate reporting, and discovery procedures.
- Discuss two purposes for maintaining accurate client records.
- Explore ethical dilemmas in relation to in vitro fertilization and embryo transplantation, elective abortion, neonatal intensive care, and AIDS.
- Identify topics for nursing research related to legal and ethical issues.

The field of maternity and newborn care (perinatal nursing)—in which birth and death, life, and the capacity to make life are encountered on a daily basis—perhaps offers more legal and ethical challenges to the professional nurse than does any other area of nursing.

This chapter introduces the nurse to basic legal and ethical issues that influence women's health care and suggests nursing practices that promote quality professional care. The chapter contains three major divisions: (1) *legal issues,* a broad overview of the legal responsibilities and potential liabilities incurred by perinatal nurses, (2) *risk management*, a system of nursing behavior designed to improve the quality of nursing care and to minimize the risk of legal liability, and (3) *ethical issues,* a discussion of some ethical dilemmas that may be encountered by the perinatal nurse. Reading material suggested for further investigation is listed in the bibliography.

■ LEGAL ISSUES

Laws affect nursing in many ways. Activities required of the nurse by law include eye prophylaxis for the newborn and the reporting of sexually transmitted disease and child abuse. Criminal law affects nursing when the professional nurse exceeds the scope of nursing and practices medicine without a license or aids and abets an unlicensed individual to practice medicine. This discussion, however, is concerned with **civil law** that seeks to compensate parties who have been injured or damaged by the negligence of a professional nurse. This civil law has been termed the *law of torts*. A **tort** is a civil offense.

The sequence of events preceding a legal claim for damages caused by negligence is as follows:

1. The state licenses a professional nurse to practice nursing according to the guidelines established by the state's nurse practice act.
2. A member of the general public enters into a relationship with a professional nurse in which the nurse offers and delivers health care services.
3. By virtue of the license to practice, the nurse has certain duties and obligations. These duties and obligations are called the standards of care.
4. The nurse fails to fulfill these duties and obligations and breaches a standard of care. The nurse need not *intend* to do harm. Harm may be inflicted unintentionally through negligence.
5. As a direct or indirect but foreseeable result of that breach, an actual injury is sustained. The injury must be actual rather than potential or "at risk for" injury. Actual injury includes both physical harm and emotional distress.
6. The client or client's family may be compensated for the injury by monetary damages assessed against the nurse. "General damages" include the cost of health care and rehabilitation, income lost from absence from work, and income lost from the impaired ability to work. "Special damages" include pain and suffering experienced by the injured party.

NOTE: This chapter's content relates only to the United States.

Duty: the Standard of Care

The standard of care, or external code of behavior or expected performance, for a professional nurse is that average degree of skill, care, and diligence exercised under similar circumstances by the reasonably prudent nurse with similar background, training, and experience (Black, 1979). Major points of the American Nurses Association Standards of Maternal-Child Health Nursing are presented in the box on p. 73.

The Organization for Obstetric, Gynecologic, and Neonatal Nurses (NAACOG) has published standards that are presented as recommendations and general guidelines (NAACOG, 1986). Examples of standards for obstetric nursing, neonatal nursing, and gynecologic nursing are in Table 4-1 (pp. 74 and 75).

Standard of care is measured and applied by the courts in the form of verdicts in lawsuits or settlements. To be successful in a lawsuit against a nurse, the plaintiff must first define the nurse's duty or standard of care and then prove that the nurse failed to conform to that standard of care. Standards of care reflect minimum requirements for performance.

To determine the standard of care for professional nursing, the appropriate starting point is the state's **nurse practice act** and the state regulations pertaining to nursing practice. These laws and regulations define the scope of nursing practice, standards for nursing education, and the point of articulation between the profession of nursing and the profession of medicine. To exceed the legal base of nursing practice is, by definition, to violate the standard of care and to be negligent. For instance, if a particular state declares it illegal for the nurse to dispense medication without a physician's order and the professional nurse hands a woman a month's supply of birth control pills, that action is a violation of the standard of care. If there are no written policies or procedures to permit such nursing interventions, the nurse's actions are negligent.

Standards of care are determined by the nursing profession in its definition of nursing practice, poli-

ANA Standards of Maternal-Child Health Nursing

Standard I: The nurse helps children and parents attain and maintain optimum health.
Standard II: The nurse assists families to achieve and maintain a balance between the personal growth needs of individual family members and optimum family functioning.
Standard III: The nurse intervenes with vulnerable clients and families at risk to prevent potential development and health problems.
Standard IV: The nurse promotes an environment free of hazards to reproduction, growth and development, wellness, and recovery from illness.
Standard V: The nurse detects changes in health status and deviations from optimum development.
Standard VI: The nurse carries out appropriate interventions and treatment to facilitate survival and recovery from illness.
Standard VII: The nurse assists clients and families to understand and cope with developmental and traumatic situations during illness, childbearing, childrearing, and childhood.
Standard VIII: The nurse actively pursues strategies to enhance access to and utilization of adequate health care services.
Standard IX: The nurse improves maternal and child health nursing practice through evaluation of practice, education, and research.

From American Nurses Association: Standards of maternal and child health nursing practice, Kansas City, Mo, 1983, American Nurses Association.

cies and procedures for nursing practice, standards of nursing education, and proscription of activities considered outside of nursing. Standards of care are further delineated by nursing specialist organizations and joint boards of medicine and nursing who define appropriate behavior in special and specific circumstances.

Other standards of care established by the profession are the policies and procedures governing nursing practice in a particular agency or unit of an institution. These policies and procedures define behavior expected of all professionals within their domain. They may act to expand behavior expected in a particular situation beyond the customary practice of nursing and into the practice of medicine. For instance, special or standardized procedures may permit a nurse in an intensive care unit to initiate drug therapy if a client displays a particular symptom. They may also permit a nurse to dispense birth control pills under special circumstances where otherwise that behavior would be illegal (Calif. Bus. and Prof. Code).

Professional nurses have a legal obligation to know and understand the standard of care or duty imposed on them. Ignorance of a policy or procedure will not be accepted as an excuse for failure to follow it. This is one reason why it is critical that nurses maintain a current knowledge base in their areas of practice.

Some recent cases have established the duty of the nurse to oversee the behavior of other professionals and to report situations in which other professionals' behavior fails to conform with an established standard of care.

Labor and delivery room nurses occasionally deal with this situation when they call for physician assistance and fail to get it. They must continue to request physician assistance until they do get it. The nurse's responsibility extends beyond the care of clients directly assigned to her or him and encompasses the behavior of other professionals functioning in the same area.

BREACH: FAILURE TO CONFORM TO THE STANDARD OF CARE. In a court of law the standard of care is established by the testimony of expert witnesses who generally are leaders in their fields. Their credentials include administrative responsibility, teaching, and research in addition to clinical competence. These expert witnesses are presented with the actual situation or with a hypothetical situation that is an exact duplicate of the case under consideration. They are then asked to state what behavior is required of the nurse and what behavior would fail to conform to the standard of care. The judge or jury makes the final determination regarding whether the defendant-nurse in the actual situation had breached the standard of care.

When the standard of care is breached and that breach is a cause of injury to the client, the nurse may be guilty of professional malpractice. The legal definition of **malpractice** is "professional misconduct, improper discharge of professional duties, or failure to meet the standard of care of a professional which resulted in harm to another" (Black, 1979). Professional malpractice is a form of **professional negligence.** The legal definition of *negligence* is "carelessness, failure to act as an ordinary, prudent person, or action contrary to what a reasonable person would have done" (Black, 1979). These definitions state the three ways in which a nurse might commit professional malpractice:

1. By performing a duty carelessly or improperly
2. By failing to perform a duty when it is indicated
3. By performing an unauthorized act

TABLE 4-1 Standards for Obstetric, Gynecologic, and Neonatal Nursing

	Nursing Practice	Health Education
CLINICAL AREA	Comprehensive obstetric, gynecologic, and neonatal (OGN) nursing care is provided to the individual, family, and community within the framework of the nursing process.	Health education for the individual, family, and community is an integral part of obstetric, gynecologic, and neonatal nursing practice.
OBSTETRIC NURSING	*Examples:*	*Examples:*
Antepartum	Assessments for risk, need for referrals, maternal and fetal well-being, administers medications, and provides emotional support.	Teaching of maternal adaptations, both physical and psychologic, nutrition, hygiene, and family dynamics.
Intrapartum	Assessments and interventions for maternal and fetal well-being, progress of labor (physical and psychologic), and care and comfort of newborn immediately following birth.	Teaching of labor process, health care during the intrapartum period, control of discomfort, and participation of family.
Postpartum	Assessments and interventions for postdelivery recovery, family interaction, and integration of newborn into family unit.	Teaching of involutional process, parenting skills, family dynamics, infant care, and fertility management.
NEONATAL NURSING		
Normal/low-risk newborn	Assessment and interventions for respirations, temperature, maturity level, infection, family contact, and nutrition.	Teaching of newborn care, protection and safety, nutrition, family dynamics, parenting skills, and newborn characteristics and responses.
High-risk newborn	Assessment and interventions for respirations, temperature, maturity level, infection, and family-newborn interaction.	Teaching of neonatal pathophysiologic processes and care needs, family dynamics, and parenting skills.
GYNECOLOGIC NURSING		
Ambulatory	Assessment and intervention for gynecologic conditions, nutritional status, sexual concerns, and self-care.	Teaching of reproductive anatomy and physiology and health promotion and maintenance.
In-hospital	Assessment for intervention for gynecologic conditions, nutritional status, sexual concerns, self-care, and altered health patterns.	Teaching of content specific to condition, health maintenance and promotion related to a specific condition.

Modified from *Standards for obstetric, gynecologic, and neonatal nursing,* ed 3, Washington, DC, 1986, The Organization for Obstetric, Gynecologic, and Neonatal Nurses (NAACOG).

TABLE 4-1 Standards for Obstetric, Gynecologic, and Neonatal Nursing—cont'd

Policies and Procedures	Professional Responsibility	Personnel
The delivery of obstetric, gynecologic, and neonatal care is based on written policies and procedures.	The OGN nurse is responsible and accountable for maintaining knowledge and competency in individual nursing practice and for being aware of professional issues.	Obstetric, gynecologic, and neonatal staff are provided to meet client-care needs.
Examples:	*Examples:*	*Examples:*
Policies and procedures for scope of practice, nursing orders and standards of care, health education, and monitoring.	Current concepts, trends, and scientific advances for the care of the antepartum client and her family.	Orientation program addresses skills and knowledge needs and quality assurance. Staffing is appropriate.
Policies and procedures for above actions, and for nurse's role regarding informed consents and implementation of independent nursing actions in emergency situations.	Current concepts, trends, and scientific advances for the care of the intrapartum client and her family.	Orientation program addresses skills and knowledge needs for the unit and quality assurance. Staffing is appropriate.
Policies and procedures for above actions, and for postdelivery recovery and nursing research.	Current concepts, trends, and scientific advances for the care of the postpartum client and her family.	Orientation program addresses skills and knowledge needs for the unit and quality assurance. Staffing is appropriate.
Policies and procedures for scope of practice and standard of care, health education, research, and emergency care.	Current concepts, trends, and scientific advances for the care of the normal/low-risk neonate and her/his family.	Orientation program addresses skills and knowledge needs for the unit and quality assurance. Staffing is appropriate.
Policies and procedures for special assessment and interventions of the high-risk newborn and her/his family.	Current concepts, trends, and scientific advances for the care of the high-risk newborn and her/his family.	Orientation program addresses skills and knowledge needs for the unit and quality assurance. Staffing is appropriate.
Policies and procedures for assessment and intervention for the ambulatory client.	Current concepts, trends, and scientific advances for the care of the ambulatory gynecologic client.	Orientation program addresses skills and knowledge needs for the unit and quality assurance. Staffing is appropriate.
Policies and procedures for assessment and intervention for the in-hospital client.	Current concepts, trends, and scientific advances for the care of the hospitalized gynecologic client.	Orientation program addresses skills and knowledge needs for the unit and quality assurance. Staffing is appropriate.

LIABILITY AND CAUSATION. Professional nurses are liable for the consequences of their actions. The best synonym for *liable* is *responsible*. Nurses are responsible for both the direct and indirect results caused by their actions. If a client falls out of bed as a consequence of the nurse's failure to put up the side rails, the nurse is responsible for the harm to the client directly caused by that failure to act. If the nurse fails to report the improper behavior of another health care professional and a client is injured by that other person, the nurse is responsible for that injury indirectly caused by the failure to act.

In current health practice, nurses are viewed as autonomous health care providers who practice independently in certain clearly defined situations. Recent cases have found nurses to be independently liable and did not assign the liability to physicians and hospitals where nurses were acting outside of the direction of physicians and hospitals (Black, 1979).

It is important for the professional nurse to understand the distinction between the dependent practice of nursing, which is the implementation of the physician-directed management of care, and the independent practice of nursing. Based on the California Nurse Practice Act, the California Nurses' Association's definition of the *independent practice of nursing* is:

1. Direct and indirect client care services that ensure the safety, comfort, personal hygiene, and protection of clients and the performance of disease prevention and restorative measures.
2. The performance of skin tests and immunization techniques and the withdrawal of human blood from veins and arteries.
3. The observation of signs and symptoms, reactions to treatment, and general behavior or physical condition and the determination of whether such observations exhibit abnormal findings and the appropriate reporting and referral of such abnormalities (Calif. Bus. and Prof. Code).

The independent practice of nursing encompasses those decisions and actions taken by the nurse based on nursing judgment and a nursing management plan rather than on a management plan directed by the physician. The independent practice of nursing may theoretically become the basis for future independent liability of the nurse.

■ RISK MANAGEMENT

Risk management is an evolving process that identifies risks, establishes preventive practices, develops reporting mechanisms, and delineates procedures for managing a lawsuit once it has been filed. Nurses should be familiar with the concepts of risk management and their implications for nursing practice. Effective risk management minimizes the risk of a lawsuit against the nurse.

Practices involved in risk management also lead to improved nursing care. The nurse should view these concepts as a system of checks and balances that ensures a high quality of client care.

Preventive Practices

QUALITY ASSURANCE. **Quality assurance** is an umbrella term used to encompass those activities that review and evaluate actual client care and institute remedial actions to bring client care into conformity with the standard of care (ACOG, 1980). Quality assurance includes chart review, chart audit, peer review, and performance evaluations.

The first step in quality assurance is to establish the acceptable standard of care. For example, one standard might be taking and recording vital signs once during every 8-hour shift. Another example might be requiring a minimum of graduate-level nursing education for a clinical nurse specialist. A third example might be a rate statement, such as no more than 10 minutes' delay in administering a timed medication. These standards often take the form of policies and procedures.

The second step in quality assurance is to construct a test of the standard. Examples of testing procedures include the following:

1. Review of case management of all clients who develop decubiti.
2. Chart review of all women admitted to labor and delivery room for adequacy of nursing history.
3. Chart audit of random sample of charts of postpartum women to determine frequency of entry of vital signs.
4. Quarterly performance evaluation of all labor and delivery nursing personnel using the job description as a standard of performance.

After the test has been constructed and administered, its results are reviewed and compared with the standard of care. If the results show a failure to conform to the standard of care, remedial action is defined, and a repeat evaluation is scheduled. The goal of quality assurance is to establish that all professional conduct meets the applicable standard of care.

INFORMED CONSENT. The concept of **informed consent** is also a form of risk management and originates with the right of persons to consent to all forms of touching. Violation of that right is called **battery.** Informed consent is established by law and includes the right to consent to or to refuse diagnostic and therapeutic measures (Calif. Adm. Code). Informed consent includes the provision of information about the procedure, its risks, its anticipated results, and any alternatives to it. It is usually the responsibility of the person performing the procedure to obtain informed consent.

Many problems have arisen from the process of informed consent (Cushing, 1984). The major problem for providers is that the only test for informed consent is the client's assertion that she or he understands and agrees. If at a later date the client denies that she or he understood, the provider may have to prove that the consent process was adequate. Unfortunately the only documentation of the procedure may be a short "informed consent obtained" statement on the chart.

The professional nurse should be aware of these issues regarding informed consent:

1. Responsibility for obtaining informed consent rests with the person performing the procedure and is usually not delegated to the nurse. The nurse may, however, contribute to the education process by providing background information about the procedure or by witnessing the signature process.
2. Consent must be obtained from a competent individual. The client must not be a minor and must be in a state of mind unaffected by drugs or injury. There are special considerations if the client is a minor or mentally incompetent or if the nurse is obtaining consent during an emergency.
3. The information process must be geared to the client's level of understanding. It must be done in the language and with the words that the client is capable of understanding.
4. Blanket consents (I consent to everything) and blanket releases (I release everyone from liability) are traditionally disregarded by the courts. They may be seen as an effort to misinform or deceive the client.
5. The consent is only as good as its documentation. The best documentation is by the client in her or his own handwriting included in the chart. Oral consents are also legal and binding. They are, however, difficult to prove several years later in the process of a lawsuit.
6. Client's refusal should be carefully documented and thereafter respected.

As with any surgical procedure, an informed consent is required for voluntary sterilization.

PROFESSIONAL LIABILITY INSURANCE. **Professional liability insurance** is a risk management concept because it may prevent nurses from incurring large losses that result from a legal settlement or judgment against them. Insurance is provided by contract based on the periodic payment of a premium. Coverage is limited by a ceiling amount per lawsuit or settlement and by an aggregate total per year. The insurance policy should be investigated carefully for the type of coverage, limits of coverage, and exceptions to coverage. Some policies do not cover nurses in expanded roles. Others do not cover independent nurses or self-employed nurses.

PROFESSIONAL COMPETENCY AND CURRENCY. Maintaining **professional competency and currency** is a critical issue in risk management and in prevention of liability risk. The standard of care for a professional is conduct required of the average member of the profession with a similar background under similar circumstances. The average member of the profession maintains a level of competency that does not incorporate ignorance of the standard of care. When **expert witnesses** establish the standard of care, it is implied that the average professional is informed and competent in that standard. Ignorance may not be claimed as a defense.

Occasionally nurses are placed in situations in which their professional competency is impeded by an outside factor. Two common situations are "short staffing" and "floating." Professional nurses have a duty to report situations in which the standard of care is breached by circumstances inherent in the situation (Horsley, 1981). The duty extends to the point that communication is clearly given to a person who has the power to remedy the situation. The duty may require the nurse to ask for assistance, supervision, and orientation. Ultimately the nurse may have to try to reject the assignment. Unfortunately the professional nurse may be caught in a conflict with another professional duty, that of not abandoning the client. In trying to resolve this situation the nurse should make these points clear:

1. The breach of the standard of care was reported to a supervisor who was potentially able to remedy the situation.
2. Rejection of the assignment would have placed the client in greater danger from **abandonment.**

One further issue that relates to the nurse's competency is that of mental impairment from excessive fatigue, drugs, or alcohol. A nurse must never endanger a client's condition through the nurse's use of such substances or extreme lack of sleep.

QUALITY OF NURSE-CLIENT RELATIONSHIP. A final concept of prevention is the *quality of the relationship* between the nurse and the client. Many studies suggest that when health care clients feel angry, frustrated, or depersonalized by their caregivers, they are more prone to sue if injury occurs. In addition, people who are ill may experience anger, frustration, and a sense of helplessness as part of their disease. Although nurses are not expected to make every client happy all the time, increased sensitivity to these issues may help reduce a client's inclination to sue.

Documentation of Care

A major aspect of risk management is appropriate *documentation of client care* and effective communication of those incidents that may give rise to a malpractice suit. Documentation of client care is accomplished by charting occurrences and observations on the client record. Incident reports help communicate information about problem situations. It is critical to be aware of the differences between the client record and incident reports.

The two main purposes for keeping client records are (1) to produce a clear and accurate history of the client in relation to the illness or problem and the management plan and (2) to enhance communication between the many health care providers who may provide services in any given situation. Therefore charting must be accurate, objective, and comprehensive.

ERRORS. A major issue in accuracy is the method of correcting *errors*. Here are some guidelines to follow:

1. Never change someone else's charting. If it is clearly inaccurate, place a note in the chart signed by you with the correct information. Do not state that "Ms. X charted in error." Merely make the correct observation. Bring the inaccuracy to the attention of the professional who made it so that the needed correction may be made.
2. To change an error in your own charting, draw one line clearly through the error and write ERROR over it. Do not obliterate the error. Make the necessary correction and sign and date it in a separate notice that is *legibly* written.
3. Never make accusations of error directly in the chart. The appropriate place for those notations may be in an incident report.
4. Always sign your full professional name and title.

OBJECTIVITY. Objectivity in charting may be problematic when conclusions rather than observations are charted. The most troublesome conclusions are those that cast aspersions on the character or reputation of the client, such as alcoholism, substance abuse, violent nature, or irresponsibility. Those conclusions may be appropriate in charting when they represent a confirmed diagnosis or when they are items in a differential diagnosis. Otherwise it is far more accurate and objective to chart the actual behavior observed. Those observations are then available to support a subsequent diagnosis should it be appropriate. For instance, instead of charting that the client was drunk, chart that the client was unsteady, unable to walk, and had an odor of alcohol on his breath.

COMPREHENSIVENESS. No nurse completes client assignments with charts tucked under one arm for immediate recording. There is delay in virtually all charting. Delay may contribute to gaps and omissions in charting, resulting in charting that is not comprehensive. Here are some guidelines to follow:

1. Never chart out of sequence or try to squeeze a note between two other notes. Place the accurate time and date next to the note currently being made, and chart the circumstances accounting for delay in the charting.
2. Chart significant observations or changes immediately. Make sure the time and date are accurate.
3. Never chart that something is done before it is done, especially with medications.
4. When the nurse is too involved with client care to chart, such as in emergency situations, have a recorder note events and changes. This should include accurate times and names of persons giving care. The recorder should not be a member of the family or a casual observer but rather a person with professional responsibility for charting.
5. Omissions in charting may be interpreted to mean that the care did not occur. When vital signs are not charted and the client claims the vital signs were not taken, there is no evidence that they actually were taken (Cushing, 1982). Therefore it is critical to chart all observations to avoid omitting essential information.

In the event of a lawsuit, the client record is the only piece of evidence created at the time the nursing care took place that documents the actual circumstances and chain of happenings surrounding that care. Because the chart is compiled by health care providers, inaccuracies such as lack of comprehensiveness or objectivity in the chart would imply defects in the quality of care given. Health care providers can only fall back on their recollections of the event, which may be hazy or absent with the passage of time. Providers' allegations of quality care tend to sound self-serving on the witness stand when their recollections are contested by the word of the injured client. There is simply no substitute for a careful, accurate, objective client record.

INCIDENT REPORTS. **Incident reports** document situations in which the health care professional and the institution may incur liability. These reports are submitted only to hospital or agency administrators, specifically to risk managers and insurance claims agents. They may document errors or omissions in care that breach the standard of care, irresponsible or negligent professional behavior, and unfortunate outcomes in client care such as injury, disability, or death.

Here are some guidelines for the use of incident reports (Cushing, 1985):

1. Never write "An incident report has been filed" in the client's record or place a copy of the report in the client's record.
2. The report should be written accurately and clearly, giving all the essential facts. Accusations and admissions should be avoided.
3. The report should be submitted to the appropriate member of the hospital administration. The more copies distributed, the weaker the assertion that the report is confidential and privileged. In some states, incident reports are available for *discovery* in a lawsuit.

The complexities of nursing practice in today's health care setting require the nurse to be aware of not only the medicolegal issues of care but also the ethical implications of nursing actions, which are almost a daily occurrence when considered within the context of nurse-to-client, nurse-to-physician, and nurse-to-colleague relationships.

■ ETHICAL ISSUES

Ethical Dilemmas

Ethical dilemmas occur in every field of nursing practice; perinatal nursing is not immune. Technical advances in the medical field have proceeded at a breakneck pace, often outstripping society's ability to consider the ethical implications of these new techniques. Fetal experimentation, neonatal intensive care, amniocentesis resulting in a recommendation for abortion, genetic engineering, and the humane treatment of persons with AIDS are just a few areas in which nurses must determine an ethical stance. For this reason, it is important for nurses to develop a rational, systematic, well-considered **ethical perspective** from which they may analyze these ethical questions. This section will not address all of the ethical decisions a nurse must make, but it should help nursing students develop this aspect of their practice.

During their early years, nurses begin to develop individual values—their system of beliefs about people, objects, and ideas—as a part of their self-identities. These **value systems** are influenced by their families, religious affiliations, and society as a whole. In their educational process, nurses begin to develop their professional identity with values relating to nurse-client relationships, nurse colleagues, physicians, and employing institutions. Problems arise when a nurse's personal values and professional values conflict. To minimize such clashes as they face the ethical dilemmas of nursing practice, many nurses have become involved in peer discussions concerning professional values.

Values Clarification

Across the country, groups of nurses are meeting to engage in **values clarification** activities. Such exercises are a dynamic examination of the individual's own value system compared with those of colleagues. Since nurses are often confronted with alternatives in client care, discussions of values have become increasingly important.

Values clarification may begin with each nurse assigning a rank to his or her values and then discussing those rankings and exploring the values of the group as a whole. If there is no absolute right or wrong answer to a dilemma, this ranking of priorities becomes essential to decision making. For example, a values conflict may arise between two nurses when one believes that life is sacred at all costs, regardless of any pain or suffering that may occur, and the other feels strongly about quality-of-life issues. Through a discussion to clarify values, the nurses may reach an understanding of each other's beliefs and values.

There are many models for ethics decision making, but most are basically problem-solving models that also involve discussing values (Omery, 1989). Thompson and Thompson (1985) have presented a bioethical model for a logical reasoning process that nurses may use to make ethical decisions (see box, p. 80). Through the 10 steps described in this bioethical model, the nurse will be able to analyze critically ethical situations as they arise. Thompson and Thompson suggest that nurses and other professionals form small discussion groups to address ongoing ethical problems within their area of practice.

Ethics Committees

In the late 1970s, a movement began to establish **ethics committees** in many hospitals. These committees generally educate staff about the ethical aspects of health care; serve as a clearinghouse for disagreements among staff, clients, and families; and may offer advice in the decision-making process for

A Bioethical Decision Model

Step One	Review the situation to determine health problems, decision needed, ethical components, and key individuals
Step Two	Gather additional information to clarify situation
Step Three	Identify the ethical issues in the situation
Step Four	Define personal and professional moral positions
Step Five	Identify moral positions of key individuals involved
Step Six	Identify value conflicts, if any
Step Seven	Determine who should make the decision
Step Eight	Identify range of actions with anticipated outcomes
Step Nine	Decide on a course of action and carry it out
Step Ten	Evaluate/review results of decision/action

From Thompson JE, Thompson HO: *Ethics in Nursing,* New York, 1981, Macmillan Publishing.

difficult ethical dilemmas. Murphy (1989) suggests that nurses are valuable members of ethics committees because of their ability to communicate the questions and viewpoints of clients and their families. The nurse may be the one health care team member who is familiar with all of those involved in potential conflicts, and thus the nurse's input becomes critical.

Several different professional associations, including The American Nurses Association, have developed codes of ethics for nurses to follow (see box, top right). These frameworks for ethical conduct are helpful when applied to a given client circumstance in which ethical questions have arisen.

Within the practice of perinatal nursing, many ethical issues arise. From questions surrounding reproductive issues to rights of privacy for AIDS clients to the emotionally charged issues of elective abortions and neonatal dilemmas, nurses in the perinatal setting are beset by ethical questions. This section presents some ethical issues that may confront students in their future practice.

Code for Nurses

1. The nurse provides services with respect for human dignity and the uniqueness of the client unrestricted by considerations of social or economic status, personal attributes, or the nature of health problems.
2. The nurse safeguards the client's right to privacy by judiciously protecting information of a confidential nature.
3. The nurse acts to safeguard the client and the public when health care and safety are affected by the incompetent, unethical, or illegal practice of any person.
4. The nurse assumes responsibility and accountability for individual nursing judgments and actions.
5. The nurse maintains competence in nursing.
6. The nurse exercises informed judgment and uses individual competence and qualifications as criteria in seeking consultation, accepting responsibilities, and delegating nursing activities to others.
7. The nurse participates in activities that contribute to the ongoing development of the profession's body of knowledge.
8. The nurse participates in the profession's efforts to implement and improve standards of nursing.
9. The nurse participates in the profession's efforts to establish and maintain conditions of employment conducive to high quality nursing care.
10. The nurse participates in the profession's effort to protect the public from misinformation and misrepresentation and to maintain the integrity of nursing.
11. The nurse collaborates with members of the health professions.

Reprinted with permission of the International Council of Nurses.

Reproductive Issues

INFERTILITY. The incidence of infertility has increased in recent years. In response to this problem, several medical technologies have been developed to address the problem. The first live birth of an infant after using the techniques of *in vitro fertilization* and *embryo transplantation* occurred in 1978. Since then, many other infants have been born as a result of this technique, but ethical questions have been raised. For example, since these are costly procedures, questions of allocation of scarce financial resources have been introduced. The disposal of fertilized eggs not transplanted has also posed questions of disrespect for human life.

Another response to infertility, the controversial use of *surrogate mothers,* has led to new ethical questions. There are legal complications in some cases, but the ethical implications of parents paying a woman to bear a child for them lead to charges of commercial surrogacy, which Annas (1986) considers dehumanizing to infants and exploitive of women.

ELECTIVE ABORTION. Rarely has the United States encountered the level of debate raised by the dramatic issue of elective abortion. In the years following the landmark Supreme Court decision *Roe vs. Wade,* which legalized abortion in the United States, "pro-life" and "pro-choice" groups have fiercely argued this issue.

As members of health care teams involved in perinatal practice, nurses are often personally and professionally confronted with ethical questions. For this reason, nurses should consider getting involved in values clarification activities to define their own response to elective abortion within the context of providing care for these women. Davis (1990) suggests that although nurses may choose to refuse assignment to provide care during an elective abortion, they should review their response to caring for the woman before and after the procedure.

Prenatal diagnostic tests such as amniocentesis and chorionic villus biopsy, which reveal birth defects as well as fetal gender, raise the specter of abortion for sex selection. This rationale for elective abortion raises serious ethical questions for those health care providers faced with these situations.

Summarizing the abortion controversy is difficult, but basically the pro-choice proponents believe that the mother's rights take precedence and that she should have freedom of choice and privacy. Many pro-choice advocates believe that abortions should be used only as a last resort, with contraception and adoption being other alternatives. Most pro-life proponents believe that the fetus is human from the moment of conception and as such should be protected from abortion, which ends life.

At this writing, the U.S. Supreme Court seems poised to possibly overturn *Roe vs. Wade,* and there are "pro-choice" requests for legislative action by the U.S. Congress to ensure a woman's right to choose to terminate a pregnancy. The advent of other technologic advances such as improved contraceptive techniques (e.g., Norplant) and methods of oral pharmacologic agents to prevent embryonic implantation (RU 486) raises additional ethical questions.

Another technology with ethical implications is the use of *fetal tissue transplantation.* Current research suggests that fetal neurologic, liver, and pancreatic tissues transplanted into adults with Parkinson's disease, metabolic disorders, or head and spinal cord injury could hold promise of recovery for those adults. The important ethical issue is to reduce any pressure for fetal tissues on a mother who is contemplating an elective abortion (Council on Scientific Affairs, 1990).

Elective abortion continues to be a controversial issue, with many ethical issues yet to be resolved. Some states have passed legislation modifying *Roe vs. Wade* in an effort to decrease the incidence of pregnancy by 15- to 17-year-old women (see Research Highlight, p. 82).

Neonatal Intensive Care

Hundreds of neonatal intensive care units (NICUs) are available throughout the United States. They are confronted with many difficult ethical questions and legal problems.

Some of the ethical dilemmas in decision making are ironically caused by the dramatic advances in neonatal-perinatal care. The medical and nursing knowledge base has increased rapidly in a relatively short time. Infants who certainly would have died 10 years ago now have a good chance to survive with few undesirable consequences. In essence, the joint disciplines of perinatology and neonatology have pushed back the point of viability to unimagined degrees. A preterm infant of less than 1500 g (3 lb, 5 oz) and less than 32 weeks of gestation had a slim chance of survival in 1965, whereas an infant of 1000 g (2 lb, 3 oz) has a good chance today. The advances in neonatal surgery have significantly improved the outcome for many infants born with heart defects or other congenital anomalies. This section will explore some of the issues faced by nurses who work in an NICU.

COSTS OF TREATMENT. One ethical problem that arises not only in the NICU but in all areas of perinatal care involves societal pressures about money. Newborn intensive care and fetal surgery are costly. Considering the dwindling public funds available for health care, many persons question the appropriateness of diverting monies from preventive programs (such as prenatal care and immunization programs for the poor) to the care of one critically ill infant. The hospitalization cost for one NICU baby can easily exceed $100,000. Federal, state, and local funds used for this type of care will not be available for other health care programs.

In a thought-provoking article, Young and Stevenson (1990) raise several important ethical questions about "heroic" treatment for extremely preterm, low-birth-weight infants (500 to 750 g). These authors hope to stimulate discussion within the bioethics and health care communities on issues such as **cost-containment** and the cost-effectiveness of preventive measures as opposed to expenditures required to treat a single extremely preterm infant within this

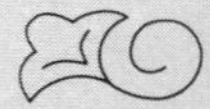 **Research Highlight** 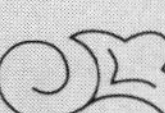

Impact of the Minnesota Parental Notification Law

RESEARCH ABSTRACT

The law in Minnesota requires women who are minors to notify both parents at least 48 hours before an abortion or to seek court approval for the abortion. This study assessed the effects of that law on the rate of abortion and birth, the ratio of abortions to births, and the ratio of early to later abortions. Data on abortion and birth incidence obtained from the Minnesota Center for Health Statistics were examined. After the law was enacted, the yearly abortion rate rose for women 20 to 44 years of age, while the rate declined for women between ages 15 and 17 and ages 18 and 19. Birthrates in all age groups decreased after the law was enacted. The decrease was greater in the 15- to 17-year-old and 18- to 19-year-old groups than in the 20- to 44-year-old group. The ratio of abortions to births dropped in the 15- to 17-year-olds. The late abortion rate declined most for this same group. Enacting the law apparently helped avoid pregnancy in 15- to 17-year-old women.

IMPLICATIONS FOR PRACTICE

The age group affected by this law has limited access to abortion outside the home state. The possibility of having to inform parents before having an abortion apparently motivated these young women to decrease sexual activity or to use effective contraceptives. The study needs to be replicated in other states to determine whether these findings hold true with other populations and higher teenage pregnancy rates. Nurses must continue their efforts to educate teenagers to abstain from sexual relations until they are mature and in stable relationships and to use effective contraceptives if they choose to be sexually active.

RELATED RESEARCH QUESTIONS

1. What are the effects of parental notification laws on abortion rate and birthrate in large states as compared to small states?
2. What are the attitudes of 15-year-old females and males toward parental notification laws?
3. What are the effects of an education program on teenager-parent communication related to sexuality?
4. Do attitudes toward parental notification differ between teenage boys and teenage girls?

REFERENCE

Rogers JL et al: Impact of the Minnesota parental notification law on abortion and birth, *Am J Public Health* 81(3):294, 1991.

weight category. They also raise questions about when it is appropriate to discontinue treatment once it has been initiated. In reviewing overall health care dollar allocations, Young and Stevenson suggest that evaluation is needed to ensure the most appropriate use of health care funds. Storch (1990) suggests that funding is available but that careful review and planning is necessary within U.S. political and economic arenas to ensure care for all.

UNPREDICTABLE PROGNOSES. Many infants who receive care in the NICU have an unpredictable prognosis, which presents ethical dilemmas for all personnel. For example, neonatal asphyxia has a variable outcome depending on the severity of the original episode. If the infant suffers a subsequent cardiac arrest, the appropriate care might be in question. Is resuscitation of the infant ethically correct? How long should resuscitation efforts be continued? Is there an ethical imperative to save all infants?

The NICU is designed to facilitate diagnosis and treatment of infants with immediate and acute but essentially life-threatening problems, such as aspiration pneumonia or respiratory distress syndrome. Proper care can result in a dramatic reduction in morbidity and mortality in these infants. However, an ethical question arises as to whether it is appropriate to use equipment and intensive care skills to keep an infant with a poor prognosis alive while "neglecting" an infant with a better prognosis.

Silverman (1981) suggests that many parents may believe that producing an infant with severe handicapping conditions is worse than having an infant who dies. Furthermore, he deplores the "rescuer" role of many health professionals. In this role, providers make unrestrained heroic efforts to prolong even the most fragile life with no concern for the parents' wishes. Silverman asserts that because parents will have the day-to-day responsibilities for consequences of neonatal intensive care, they should be among the primary decision makers regarding the care of their infant.

There are many ethical debates inherent in the care of medically fragile infants. As issues arise surrounding drug-affected infants whose mothers abused drugs and/or alcohol during pregnancy, further discussion of the economic factors and total resource allocation of newborn intensive care, as well as discussion of right-to-die issues in the NICU, will become increasingly important. Not only do nurses need to determine their own values-based ethical stance on these questions, but they also must realize that the nursing perspective is vital to discussions on the whole.

AIDS

Acquired immunodeficiency syndrome (AIDS) has become an epidemic with broad legal and ethical ramifications. By the beginning of the 1990s between 800,000 and 1.2 million individuals in the United States were infected with the AIDS virus. The lethal nature of this infectious disease has heightened the seriousness of ethical debate and added unique dimensions to the discussions.

Although confidentiality in a nurse-client relationship is a basic ethical tenet, a quandary is presented in considering whether or not to notify sexual or IV-needle partners placed at risk by an HIV-positive client. Monroe (1990) suggests guidelines for ethical decision making in these cases that first requests the client to notify potential at-risk individuals. Some suggest that if confidentiality is not maintained, the spread of the virus may increase because individuals who should be tested for HIV might refuse if the consequences seem unbearable (i.e., loss of job or having medical treatment denied). This question requires careful values clarification and discussion.

Grady (1989) suggests that other ethical issues exist, such as a client's right to health care access, the nurse's obligation to maximize client autonomy in decision making about health care, and the client's right to impartial caregivers who are nonjudgmental.

Because AIDS is a highly charged emotional issue, nurses must carefully examine their individual and professional response to clients with AIDS.

■ SUMMARY

A wide range of ethical and legal issues arise in maternity and newborn nursing. Many of the ethical dilemmas are a result of new medical technology and expanded roles for nurses. Because maternity health care raises monumental ethical and legal questions, it is essential to understand these issues.

REFERENCES

American College of Obstetricians and Gynecologists: *Quality assurance in obstetrics and gynecology,* Washington, DC, 1980, The College.

American Nurses Association: *Standards of maternal-child health nursing practice,* Kansas City, Mo, 1983, American Nurses Association.

Black HC: *Black's law dictionary,* St Paul, 1979, West Publishing.

California Administrative Code, Section 70707; California Business and Professions Code, section 2725. California Administrative Code, section 1470 et seq.

Council on Scientific Affairs and Council on Ethical and Judicial Affairs: Medical Applications of Fetal Tissue Transplantation, *JAMA* 263(4):565 1990.

Cushing M: Gaps in documentation, *Am J Nurs* 82:1899, Dec 1982.

Cushing M: Informed consent—an MD responsibility? *Am J Nurs* 84:437, April 1984.

Driscoll ME: AIDS: legal aspects of occupational exposure, *Calif Nurs Review* 10(3):10, 1988.

Erlen JA, Holzman IR: Anencephalic infants: should they be organ donors? *Pediatr Nurs* 14(1):60, 1988.

Ethics Grand Rounds: When refusing treatment jeopardizes another life, *Nurs '88* 18(5):145, 1988.

Grady C: Ethical issues in providing nursing care to human immunodeficiency virus—infected populations, *Nurs Clin North Am* 24(2):523, June 1989.

Horsley JE: Short-staffing means increased liability for you, *RN* 44(2):73, 1981.

Melroe NH: "Duty to warn" vs. "patient confidentiality": the ethical dilemmas in caring for HIV-infected clients, *Nurse Pract* 15(2):59, Feb 1990.

Murphy P: The role of the nurse on hospital ethics committees, *Nurs Clin North Am* 24(2):551, June 1989.

NAACOG: *Standards for obstetric, gynecologic and neonatal nursing,* ed 3, Washington, DC, 1986, NAACOG.

Omery A: Values, moral reasoning, and ethics, *Nurs Clin North Am* 24(2):499, June 1989.

Silverman WA: Mismatched attitudes about neonatal death, *Hastings Center Rep* 11(6):12, 1981.

Storch TG: The unkindest cut, *Am J Dis Child* 144:533, May 1990.

Thompson JE, Thompson HO: *Ethical decision making for nurses,* Norwalk, Conn, 1985, Appleton-Century-Crofts.

Young EWD, Stevenson DK: Limiting treatment for extremely premature, low-birth-weight infants (500 to 750 g), *Am J Dis Child* 144:549, May 1990.

BIBLIOGRAPHY

Erlen JA: Anencephalic infants as sources of organs: issues and implications for nurses, *JOGNN* 19(3):249, May/June 1990.

Gero E, Giordano J: Ethical considerations in fetal tissue transplantation, *J Neurosci Nurs* 22(1):9, Feb 1990.

Rhodes AM: Major legal initiatives in MCH, *MCN* 16:45, Jan/Feb 1991.

Ryan KJ et al: Patient choice: maternal-fetal conflict: committee opinion from the Committee on Ethics: ACOG, *WHI* 1(1):13, Fall 1990.

Sweeney RN: Your role in informed consent, *RN* 55, Aug 1991.

Wold JL: AIDS testing, an ethical question, *J Neurosci Nurs* 22(4):258, Aug 1990.

chapter 4 review

Key Concepts

- The conduct of all legally competent individuals is held to a standard of care—that degree of care exercised by a reasonably prudent person under similar circumstances.
- Professional nurses are liable for the consequences of their actions.
- The independent practice of nursing encompasses those decisions and actions taken by nurses based on *nursing judgment* and *nursing management* plan.
- Risk management is designed to minimize losses by establishing preventive practices and appropriate reporting practices.
- In the event of a lawsuit, the client record is the only piece of evidence created at the time of client care.
- Ethical dilemmas occur in every field of nursing practice.
- Nurses have responsibilities and commitments to use ethical conduct in relationships with clients, other nurses, physicians, and their employers.
- Inherent in the values of most nurses are beneficence and nonmalfeasance.

Key Terms

Legal Terms

- abandonment (p. 77)
- battery (p. 76)
- breach (p. 73)
- civil law (p. 72)
- duty: standard of care p. 72)
- expert witnesses (p. 77)
- incident reports (p. 79)
- informed consent (p. 76)
- liability and causation (p. 76)
- malpractice (p. 73)
- nurse practice act (p. 72)
- professional competency and currency (p. 77)
- professional liability insurance (p. 77)
- professional negligence (p. 73)
- quality assurance (p. 76)
- risk management (p. 76)
- tort (p. 72)

Ethical Terms

- cost-containment (p. 81)
- ethical dilemmas (p. 79)
- ethical perspective (p. 79)
- ethics committee (p. 79)
- value systems (p. 79)
- values clarification (p. 79)

Critical Thinking Exercises

The following is an excerpt from nursing notes:
3:15 AM—E.L. arrived on the unit. She was drunk and too uncooperative to obtain a history. Client ~~fell~~ ~~going~~ fell coming from bathroom but did not act injured. JK, RN

8:30 AM—Client fall charted incorrectly by night nurse. Incident report filed in chart, and copy sent to nursing office. AS, RN

1. Has the nurse included any assumptions in the notes? If so, what are they, and what information is needed to support or negate these assumptions?
2. How can the reasonably prudent nurse chart these kinds of assessments to meet the standard of care?
3. Evaluate the legal implications of the nursing notes in relation to objectivity, comprehensiveness, management of errors, and incident reports.

An amniocentesis has been performed for your client, who is pregnant with twins. The results indicate that one fetus is normal, but the other twin has Down syndrome. The physician tells the family they have the option of continuing both pregnancies or choosing a selective abortion for the twin diagnosed with Down syndrome. Critically analyze this ethical dilemma.

chapter 5

Nursing Research in Maternity and Gynecologic Care

SHANNON E. PERRY

LEARNING OBJECTIVES

- Define the key terms listed.
- Describe the scope of nursing research in maternity and gynecologic care.
- Discuss the problem of bias in health research.
- List and discuss the steps in the research process.
- Explore the role of the nurse as a consumer of nursing research.
- Identify at least one resource available to practicing nurses to use in evaluating published research studies.
- Examine the value of nursing research in nursing practice.
- Assess the role of the nurse as a clinical researcher.

Clinical nursing research is essential for improving client care, improving the outcomes of care, and advancing the profession. The nurse at the bedside (the clinician) is in the best position to identify researchable clinical problems, to collect research data as a part of practice, and to implement clinically significant findings (Zalar, Welches, Walker, 1985).

With the assistance of an experienced researcher, practicing maternity-gynecologic nurses can learn to translate clinical problems into researchable problems (Nichols, 1989), design research protocols (Tornquist, Funk, 1990), analyze findings, critique research reports, implement research projects, and use findings of research studies (Perry, 1990). Practicing nurses may never wish to become full-time nurse researchers, but they can be extremely helpful in answering the innumerable questions encountered in clinical nursing.

This chapter describes the need for nursing research in maternity and gynecologic care, discusses biases in health research, defines the research process, delineates priorities for nursing research, describes the role of nurses in research, explicates guidelines for critiquing research, and explains the use of research in practice.

Throughout the chapters of this text, research highlights are incorporated. The research highlights include an abstract (summary) of studies that are pertinent to chapter topics, implications of the research for the clinician, and research questions that arise from the studies. The research highlights provide an example of how the research literature can be used to gain additional science-based information about a topic. The highlights may assist nurses in developing a spirit of inquiry in their approach to client care and informing them of current research findings. Two research highlights are included in this chapter: one illustrates a quantitative approach to research (see box on p. 89), and the other illustrates a qualitative approach (see box on p. 90). Topics for nursing research are found at the end of each chapter.

■ RESEARCH PROCESS

The **research process** is a systematic way of arriving at an answer to a question and is an example of critical thinking (see Chapter 1). There are a number of steps (see box above). There are quantitative and qualitative approaches to answering research questions. In a **quantitative approach,** data that are collected can be quantified; that is, numbers can be attached and analyzed (see box, p. 89). In a **qualitative approach**, data are obtained from interviews or observations and are nonnumeric (see box, p. 90). Research texts provide thorough explanations of the steps in the process. For the purposes of this chapter, a brief explanation of the steps follows.

Steps in the Research Process

1. Formulate the research problem.
2. Review the literature.
3. Select a theoretic framework.
4. Formulate hypotheses.
5. Select a design.
6. Identify data collection methods.
7. Formulate a sampling plan.
8. Collect the data.
9. Analyze the data.
10. Report and interpret the results.
11. Disseminate the findings.

Formulate the Research Problem

The research problem is based on an area of concern and addresses unanswered questions about a phenomenon. For example, an area of concern is "preterm labor," and an unanswered question is "What are the responses of women in preterm labor to the medical therapy to treat preterm labor?"

Review the Literature

A literature review is a critical examination of publications related to a topic of interest. The review should be comprehensive and evaluative. For the topic preterm labor and women's responses to medical therapy, the literature on "preterm labor," "medical therapy to treat preterm labor," "women's responses to medical therapy," and "women's responses to medical therapy to treat preterm labor" should be reviewed. The studies identified should be critiqued, and gaps in knowledge should be identified.

Select a Theoretic Framework

The theoretic framework provides a foundation for suggestions for relationships among variables. The framework may come from a nursing theory or a theory from a related field. Roy's adaptation model could be used as a theoretic framework to understand the variables affecting women's responses to medical therapy to treat preterm labor.

Formulate Hypotheses

Hypotheses are statements of expected relationships among variables. The researcher might hypothesize that "women who respond positively to medical therapy to treat preterm labor will carry their infants closer to term than women who respond negatively to the medical therapy." Hypotheses are usually omitted in qualitative research studies or may be generated from the findings.

Select a Design

A research design is a plan for answering the research question. Designs may be exploratory, descriptive, correlational, quasiexperimental, or experimental. For the above hypothetical study using a quantitative approach, a correlational design could be used in which women's positive or negative response to medical therapy is measured and correlated statistically to the length of pregnancy in weeks. A qualitative approach using nonnumeric data could be used to discover women's subjective responses to their experience of being treated for preterm labor.

Identify Data Collection Methods

Methods of collecting data include interviews, questionnaires, observation, and physiologic measurements. Valid and reliable means of measuring the variables of interest must be identified. These may be data collection instruments (tests, surveys, etc.) with established validity and reliability. In other instances, the researcher must develop and test instruments. For the above hypothetical study, the data collection instruments are a demographic (vital statistics) tool, the questionnaire "Women's Responses to Therapy" designed by the researcher, and a chart review form for identifying complications of pregnancy and recording the length of pregnancy and its outcome (e.g., live birth or congenital anomalies). For a qualitative approach, the data would be collected through interviews, observations, diaries, or case studies.

Formulate a Sampling Plan

The population of interest in the hypothetical study is women at risk for preterm labor. The sample is a subset of women at risk for preterm labor who are registered for care in a preterm labor clinic that agreed to participate in the study. For the hypothetical quantitative study, 100 women who were at least 18 years of age, experiencing a second or later preg-

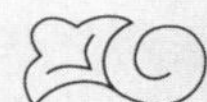

Research Highlight

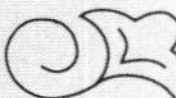

Quantitative Approach
Head Coverings for Newborns under Radiant Warmers

RESEARCH ABSTRACT

The study was conducted to compare heat loss in newborns under radiant warmers when the newborns were using one of three head treatments: no cover for the head, a stockinette hat, or a fabric-insulated bonnet. Three treatment groups of 30 infants each were formed by random assignment. Rectal temperatures were measured at 5, 15, and 30 minutes after birth. The researcher found that the bonnet and no head covering resulted in less heat loss than the stockinette hat.

IMPLICATIONS FOR PRACTICE

Stockinette caps are routinely used in many nurseries to prevent heat loss. In this study, the researcher found that wearing the bonnet or no hat produced less heat loss than wearing a single-layered stockinette cap. This might suggest that infants should not wear stockinette caps under radiant warmers. However, in examining the research more closely, the range of decrease in temperatures of all neonates in the study was from 0.65° F to 1.2° F, remaining within normal limits for newborn infants. Thus, although there were statistically significant differences between groups, the differences were not clinically significant. Until further research is conducted, no changes in practice are warranted.

QUESTIONS FOR FURTHER RESEARCH

1. Is a double-layered stockinette cap more effective in reducing heat loss than a single-layered stockinette cap?
2. How long does the decrease in temperature after delivery continue?
3. Does the route of temperature measurement (rectal, axillary, or skin) make a difference?
4. Would similar results be found if preterm infants were studied instead of term infants?

REFERENCE

Greer PS: Head coverings for newborns under radiant warmers, *JOGNN* 17(4):265, 1988.

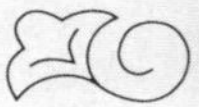 **Research Highlight** 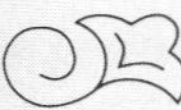

Qualitative Example
Neonatal Death: A Study of Fathers' Experiences

RESEARCH ABSTRACT

The loss of a baby affects the father as well as the mother. This study explored the experiences of fathers of infants who died in a newborn intensive care unit and compared their experiences with the experiences of mothers reported in other studies. The researcher interviewed eight fathers for 30 to 45 minutes each. Fathers were married Caucasians with a mean age of 31.7 years. Infants had lived less than 3 days. The interviews were conducted from 8 months to 20 months after the infant's death. Subjects were asked to tell about the infant's death and the effect the death had on them. When information that was significant for mothers in other studies was not reported by fathers, the researcher asked direct questions on those topics. Fathers said they consented to be interviewed because they wanted something positive to come from their loss. The symptoms of grief experienced included feelings, physical responses, and reactions and behaviors. Fathers expressed feelings by crying and displaying anger and sadness, and they also experienced feelings of guilt, powerlessness, helplessness, and vulnerability. Three fathers reported feeling relieved when the infant died after a problem pregnancy. Fathers reported physical responses of restlessness, difficulty in concentrating, and sleep disturbances. Six fathers reported fatigue and feeling tired or lazy. Reactions and behaviors reported included loneliness and depression, time confusion, social withdrawal, and avoidance. Two fathers considered leaving their marriages, and six fathers reported the relationship was stronger after the stress of the death. They found few supportive persons and felt overwhelmed with having to complete tasks of making funeral arrangements and notifying others of the death. This study confirms that fathers experience intense grief and supports findings of other investigations of loss and grief.

IMPLICATIONS FOR PRACTICE

Fathers as well as mothers become attached to a fetus and the newborn. In spite of roles for which men are socialized (e.g., the rational protector), they feel and express grief at the loss of an infant. Nurses must include fathers as well as mothers in their interventions to help their clients cope with loss. They can provide emotional support and allow expression of feelings in a safe environment.

RELATED RESEARCH QUESTIONS

1. Are there cultural variations in the expression of a father's grief?
2. Does the resolution of grief differ in fathers and mothers?
3. Does the grief response differ when the infant dies after a problem pregnancy as compared to when the death occurs unexpectedly?
4. To what extent does an early and intense grief response facilitate grief resolution?

REFERENCE

Kimble DI: Neonatal death: a descriptive study of fathers' experiences, *Neonatal Network* 9(8):45, 1991.

nancy, and diagnosed as at risk for preterm labor comprised the sample. Subjects were selected through convenience sampling; that is, the first 100 women who came to the clinic, met the selection critieria, and agreed to be in the study were selected. Selection of these women was convenient and accessible for the researcher. In a qualitative approach, the same sample selection process may be used, but because of the richness and volume of data collected, approximately 25 subjects will be included.

Collect the Data

The data collection plan includes when, where, how, and by whom the data will be collected. In the quantitative study example, the data were collected by a research assistant in a private office adjoining the waiting room of the clinic, and the women interviewed were waiting to be seen by the health care provider. In the qualitative study example, the women were interviewed in their homes, observed in the clinic, and interviewed following their examinations. In addition, each woman kept a diary of her feelings about the therapy she was receiving.

Analyze the Data

The data are analyzed to answer the research questions. In the quantitative instance, descriptive statistics will be used to describe the sample (mean age and education, percent of various racial or ethnic categories, etc.), and a correlation of the positive or negative response to therapy with the length of pregnancy will be calculated. Other statistics may be calculated to answer additional questions. For the qualitative approach, a content analysis of the interviews, the diaries, and notes on the observations will be completed. **Content analysis** is a system of examining the data for word meanings and feeling tone. Responses are categorized, and inferences of meaning are developed.

Report and Interpret the Results

Results of the analyses are reported in relationship to the research questions. Since some results may differ from expectations, the researcher may interpret the findings in light of characteristics of the sample or limitations of the data collection instruments or other factors that may have affected results.

Disseminate the Findings

Research is not completed until the findings are disseminated (that is, shared with others). **Dissemination** may occur through presentation at professional meetings and through publication. It is also desirable for the researcher to report findings to personnel at the place where data collection occurred.

THE NEED FOR NURSING RESEARCH IN MATERNITY AND GYNECOLOGIC CARE

There are many areas of concern in maternity and gynecologic care. The following paragraphs describe a number of problems that exist for childbearing women and their families and the types of studies that can be conducted to address the problems.

High Infant Mortality Rate

The infant mortality rate in the United States is 10.2 per 1000 births. Twenty-one countries have lower infant mortality rates than the United States (Driscoll et al, 1990). The infant mortality rate is high even though Americans spent more than $700 billion for health care in 1990 (Barber-Madden, Kotch, 1990). Many pregnant women in the United States have limited or no access to prenatal care. Other pregnant women abuse drugs and alcohol and do not seek prenatal care. And, in spite of having regular prenatal care, some women experience preterm labor and give birth to previable infants. The high infant mortality rate may be related to lack of access to prenatal care, low socioeconomic status, abuse of alcohol and other drugs, and preterm labor. Studies are needed to examine ways to: (1) improve access to care, (2) deliver services effectively to underserved populations, (3) help women remain drug and alcohol free during pregnancy, and (4) develop coping and parenting skills to care for their infants after birth. Continued research into the cause, treatment, responses to therapy, and nursing care of women in preterm labor is needed.

Smoking during Pregnancy

Almost 25% of pregnant women in the United States smoke throughout pregnancy (Centers for Disease Control, 1990). Many women stop smoking when they learn they are pregnant but resume smoking within a year after childbirth. Studies are needed that identify effective interventions to help new mothers remain smoke free. Other studies are needed to examine effects of secondhand smoke on the newborn and other children in the home.

Teenage Sexuality

The proportion of adolescent women who have had premarital intercourse is increasing. In 1988, 51.8% of women surveyed reported having premarital intercourse (Centers for Disease Control, 1991). Early initiation of sexual activity is associated with more sex partners and an increase in sexually transmitted diseases. New ways of educating teenagers about sexuality and sexually transmitted diseases and interventions to change behaviors are needed.

Cesarean Birth

Cesarean birth is the most frequently performed major surgical operation in the United States (Flamm et al, 1990). Approximately 25% of all births are cesarean. This is a higher rate than in many other countries that have lower infant mortality rates. The safety of vaginal birth after cesarean birth has been documented (Flamm et al, 1990). Research is warranted that documents reasons for mothers' requests for cesarean birth rather than a trial of labor, childbirth education that addresses effective coping mechanisms during labor after a previous cesarean birth, and sequelae of cesarean births including potential problems with mother-infant attachment.

Perinatal HIV/AIDS

In the United States, there have been 2374 cases of AIDS in children younger than age 13; the majority of the infections were transmitted by the mother to her infant. Of these children, only 48% are still alive (HIV/AIDS Surveillance, February 1991). In Canada, 43 cases of infants with AIDS have been reported and only 33% of these children are still alive (Federal Centre for AIDS, 1991). In the United States, 14,231 women of childbearing age have been diagnosed with HIV/AIDS (HIV/AIDS Surveillance Report, February 1991). In Canada, 169 cases of HIV/AIDS in adult females of childbearing age have been reported; 37% of these women are still alive. Investigations of parenting a child with AIDS, enhancing growth and development of children with terminal illnesses, caring for people with AIDS, and caregivers' responses to caring for people with AIDS are appropriate topics for nursing research.

The clinician can identify other problems in the health and health care of women and infants. Nurses, through research, can make a difference for these clients.

BIAS IN HEALTH RESEARCH

Bias against women exists in health research. This **research bias** has recently been recognized and publicized. The bias encompasses several areas: excluding women from clinical trials, not analyzing results of studies by gender, inadequate funding of research on diseases of women, and inadequate numbers of female researchers (Society for the Advancement of Women's Health Research, 1991). Two of these areas, excluding women from clinical trials and inadequate funding of research on diseases of women, will be discussed.

Excluding Women from Clinical Trials

Women are systematically excluded from studies. Their exclusion is an effort to obtain a homogenous sample and to avoid introducing variables related to monthly hormonal fluctuations. For example, in a 1990 study at the Harvard School of Public Health, researchers concluded that drinking coffee did not increase the likelihood of people developing heart disease. The study population included 45,589 men and no women (Society for the Advancement of Women's Health Research, 1991). Thus, in applying the findings to "people," the researchers concluded that women could be treated the same as men are treated and yet had eliminated women from participating in the research because they were different.

A study funded by the National Institute on Aging, the Baltimore Longitudinal Study of Aging, started in 1958 but did not include women until 1978. The 1984 report of the study, "Normal Human Aging," is considered to be a definitive study even though there are no data on women contained in the report (Society for the Advancement of Women's Health Research, 1991). However, the results are applied to women.

Inadequate Funding of Research on Diseases of Women

In a 1991 report, the Society for the Advancement of Women's Health Research stated that research on menopause, osteoporosis, breast cancer, ovarian cancer, and postpartum depression is underfunded. The report noted that although menopause is a normal life event, we have limited knowledge of why some women have few symptoms and others may be disabled. In addition, little research has been conducted on the possible consequences of menopause, such as incontinence and osteoporosis. Since only $17 million was spent last year (1990) on breast cancer, a disease that will affect one in nine women, an inadequate proportion of resources is devoted to this disease.

To remedy the underrepresentation of women in research and the underfunding of research on diseases of women, the Women's Health Equity Act (WHEA) of 1991 was introduced into the U.S. Congress (NAACOG, 1991). The WHEA is a comprehensive package of 22 bills that requires inclusion of women and minorities in studies, authorizes $25 million for research on breast cancer, and provides funding for AIDS research on women and the study of ovarian cancer and osteoporosis (Women's Health, 1991).

PURPOSE OF MATERNITY AND GYNECOLOGIC RESEARCH

Maternity and gynecologic nursing research is conducted to (1) gain a better understanding of biopsychosocial responses of women, families, and newborn infants to pregnancy and childbirth, (2) address reproductive issues of women, (3) improve quality and decrease cost of nursing care, (4) describe factors associated with childbirth and problems of childbearing, (5) improve nursing interventions, and (6) test nursing theories. The following examples of nursing research will demonstrate how maternity-gynecologic nurses have fulfilled these purposes of nursing research.

Understanding Biopsychosocial Responses

Stainton (1990) explored parents' awareness of their fetus during the third trimester by interviewing mothers and fathers in their homes. She found four different levels of awareness of the unborn infants. Parents were aware of their infant as an *idea* and described appearance, size, and family similarities. Parents also perceived the infant as a *presence* and referred to the infant as "he" or "she." They reported talking to the fetus and differentiated fetal movements from uterine contractions. Parents were aware of *specific behavior* such as sleep-wake cycles, patterns of activity, and responses to sounds and movement. Some parents also described *interactive abilities* of the fetus and reported touching the maternal abdomen and eliciting a response from the fetus. The findings of this study suggest that parents have a great deal of knowledge about their unborn infants. This sensitivity to the infant indicates that attachment begins prenatally. Nurses can use this information in providing care to pregnant families by recognizing the fetus as real to the parents and speaking in personal ways about the fetus. In working with parents who have suffered a prenatal loss, nurses can acknowledge early attachment, describe fetal appearance and activity, and discuss with parents their perceptions of the fetus. Parents can be counseled that their grief response is real, to be expected, and may last for a considerable time.

A group of researchers (Heitkemper et al, 1991) studied gastrointestinal (GI) symptoms and function and physiologic arousal in dysmenorrheic women. Fifty women recorded stool characteristics, GI symptoms, and anxiety level daily in a diary. Urine catecholamine assays and serum ovarian hormone and cortisol levels were determined at menses and at follicular and luteal phases of the menstrual cycle. The researchers found cycle-related changes and differences in symptoms between dysmenorrheic and nondysmenorrheic women. Dysmenorrheic women had higher levels of GI symptoms and anxiety and changes in the hormonal assays. Clinicians can use this information to further their understanding of dysmenorrhea and to assure dysmenorrheic women that their perceptions of menstrual-related symptoms are valid.

Reproductive Issues of Women

Stress urinary incontinence (involuntary leakage of urine) is a common problem of women in later life. Childbirth may have long-range effects on urinary continence. Sampselle (1990) studied stress urinary incontinence and changes in pelvic muscle strength associated with childbirth. She measured pelvic muscle strength and observed incontinence and interruption of urine flow. She found that postpartum pelvic muscle strength declined from prenatal levels following vaginal birth. Those women who had greater pelvic muscle strength before delivery maintained a higher level of pelvic muscle strength in the postpartum period. Those women who had stress urinary incontinence had less pelvic muscle strength. This knowledge can be used by nurses in assessing urine loss and in teaching clients about the importance of exercise of the pelvic muscles (Kegel exercises).

Quality and Cost of Care Issues

Brooten et al (1986) conducted a randomized trial of early discharge and home follow-up of very low-birth-weight infants. Infants were randomly assigned to two groups. Infants in one group were discharged home according to routine criteria. Infants in the other group were discharged earlier when they met a standard set of criteria. Education, counseling, home visits, and on-call availability of a nurse specialist were provided for 18 months for infants discharged early. The researchers found that infants in the early-discharge group went home an average of 11 days earlier at a weight of 200 g less and 2 weeks younger than the infants who were discharged according to routine criteria. The average hospital charge for the early discharge group was 27% less, or $47,520, compared to $64,940 for the routinely discharged infants. Physician charges were 22% less for early discharge infants ($5933) than for routinely discharged infants ($7649). The home care cost was $576, which resulted in a savings of $18,560 for each infant. There was no difference in the two groups in the number of acute care visits and rehospitalizations or in measures of mental and physical growth of the infants. The authors noted that if only half of the 36,000 very low-birth-weight infants born each year in the United States were discharged under the study protocol, as much as $334 million could be saved annually. This study is a dramatic example of nursing research affecting quality of care with resulting cost savings.

Factors Associated with Childbirth and Problems of Childbearing

There is a disparity in childbirth outcomes between African-American and Caucasian women. There are twice as many low-birth-weight babies born to African-American women as there are born to Caucasian women (Institute of Medicine, 1985). In a replication of the Arizmendi and Affonso (1987) study of the frequency and intensity of stressors related to childbearing in a group of 221 middle-class Caucasian women, Green (1990) interviewed 50 African-American women. The findings of this study were compared to the findings of the original study. In both studies, physical symptoms were the most frequent stressor. Among the African-American sample, external events (lack of money, issues with the mate or family, career, job, and school) were the most frequent causes of stress. In contrast, Arizmendi and Affonso found that, in their Caucasian sample, internal events such as anticipatory concerns or fears caused the most anxiety. African-American women experienced a higher level of stressors. Future studies need to address stress in the African-American family to determine whether stress is a significant factor in the increased incidence of preterm and low-birth-weight infants in this population.

Improving Nursing Interventions

"Gas pains" are common following cesarean delivery. Some new mothers describe these pains as more uncomfortable than incisional pain. Thomas et al (1990) validated a nursing observation that mothers who rocked in a rocking chair following cesarean delivery complained less of intestinal gas pain. They tested the effectiveness of rocking, decrease in ingestion of gas-forming food, and antiflatulent medications in the prevention and relief of gas pains. The researchers found that rocking was an effective intervention in reduction of gas pains but that rocking was most effective in combination with medications and the dietary therapeutic regimen. Based on their findings, rocking after cesarean delivery has become part of standard care at their institution.

Seideman (1990) studied the effects of an educational program on premenstrual symptomatology. Participants were 47 women who scored in the moderate-to-severe range on a menstrual symptomatology questionnaire. Women were randomly assigned to experimental or control groups. The experimental group received an educational program. Participants in both groups recorded symptoms of anxiety, appetite, edema, and depression in a diary. Women in the experimental group had fewer anxiety and appetite symptoms and fewer depression and edema symptoms than did women in the control group. The researcher concluded that the educational program was effective, since symptoms were fewer in the group that received the program. Nurses can use the findings in educating women about ways to control premenstrual symptoms.

Test Nursing Theories

Theories in nursing are used to explain nursing phenomena. Nurses often use theories borrowed from other disciplines (LoBiondo-Wood and Haber, 1990), since theory development in nursing is in its infancy.

In 1963, Rubin described her observations of postpartum mothers handling their newborn infants. Rubin reported that the mothers initially used their fingertips when handling their newborn; only after several days did they use their palms, and later they used their arms and upper torsos. This has been described as a theory of maternal touch. Tulman (1985) tested this theory by studying the pattern of newborn handling by 36 newly delivered women during their infants' first postpartum bedside visit and the pattern of newborn handling by 36 female nursing students at the beginning of their first clinical day in a hospital's normal newborn nursery. The sequence of use of fingers, palms, arms, and trunk was different for mothers and students. Although the mothers did not follow the sequence of handling reported in the literature, the students did, thus casting doubt on the specificity of a pattern of maternal handling of the newborn infant as a means of assessing maternal attachment.

These differences in findings may be attributed to differences in nursing care practices and opportunities of mothers to handle their babies that occurred between 1963 and 1985. The findings from this study demonstrate the importance of testing theories. The findings from one study cannot confirm or negate a theory; however, they do provide the direction for future study.

These examples of research illustrate the variety of maternity and gynecologic care problems that nurses have studied. Nurses can use the information from such studies to strengthen the scientific basis of their nursing practice.

■ PRIORITIES FOR NURSING RESEARCH IN MATERNITY AND GYNECOLOGIC CARE

National Center for Nursing Research

Using expert panels, the National Center for Nursing Research (NCNR) has identified seven **research priorities** for nursing (Hinshaw, Heinrich, Bloch, 1988). Of relevance to maternity nurses is the first priority, "low birth weight: mothers and infants." Maternity and gynecologic nurses may also do research in other priority areas: clients who test positive for human immunodeficiency virus (HIV), their partners and families, symptom management, information systems, health promotion, and technology dependency across the life span.

NAACOG

NAACOG: The Organization for Obstetric, Gynecologic, and Neonatal Nurses has developed research priorities for research in specialty areas. The priorities include both research in studies of the "nursing process, interventions, and outcomes of care" and in "the professional role of maternity, women's health and neonatal nurses in delivery of care" (NAACOG, 1988). The priorities in maternity nursing, women's health nursing, and neonatal nursing are listed in the box to the right.

■ MATERNITY AND GYNECOLOGIC NURSES AS CONSUMERS OF RESEARCH

The clinician, as a **consumer of research** contemplating using research in clinical practice, should examine the study for **scientific merit** and **clinical relevance.** Topham and DeSilva (1988) developed a guide for evaluating research articles for use in clinical practice (see box on p. 96). The guidelines include criteria for **critiquing** a research article and for applying the results to clinical practice. Both types of criteria are essential in determining whether the research findings can be applied to practice.

If the study is lacking scientific merit (that is, if there are serious flaws in the design, method, sampling, analysis, or findings), the research should not be applied to practice. If the study is too costly, has no relevance for the clinical setting in question, takes an undue amount of the clinician's time to implement, used subjects with few characteristics in common with the clinician's practice, or involves significant risk to clients, the findings should not be used in clinical practice.

A final caution concerns **replication** of findings. Practice should not be changed based on the findings of one study. The study should be replicated (duplicated or repeated) in different settings with different subjects. The same or similar findings should be apparent in a number of studies before the findings are applied to clinical practice.

Replicating a study is an appropriate research activity for clinicians and graduate students and should be encouraged as a means to improve practice and to advance the science of nursing. In the process of replications, applicability (**generalizability**) of the interventions, instruments, or findings of previous studies to a particular setting or population can be determined.

The guidelines for **evaluating research** findings provide a valuable tool for busy clinicians to review nursing research as a basis for maternity and gynecologic nursing practice.

NAACOG Research Priorities (NAACOG, 1988)*

MATERNITY NURSING

- Prenatal care
- Low birth weight
- HIV-positive mothers and infants
- Adolescent pregnancy and pre-pregnancy counseling/care
- Drug abuse and other substance abuse during pregnancy
- Stressors and their effects during pregnancy
- Utilization of care by pregnant population

WOMEN'S HEALTH NURSING

- Prevention of sexually transmitted diseases (STDs) in women, particularly the prevention of HIV/AIDS, and care and support of women and families with STDs
- Psychosocial and physical experience of women in midlife and later years
- Behavioral and environmental factors influencing the health of minority women, including ethnic and cultural minorities, social minorities such as the homeless, and other vulnerable groups
- Women's adaption to multiple roles and related health outcomes
- Impact of reproductive technology and reproductive pharmacology on women's health throughout life

NEONATAL NURSING

- Low-birth-weight infants and infants in families known to experience high rates of disease, dysfunction, and death
- Promotion of growth and development in all settings, hospital and home
- Short- and long-term consequences of care and parenting
- Evaluation of current and evolving models of home care in terms of cost and quality of client outcomes

*NOTE: NAACOG is anticipating a name change in 1993.

■ USE OF RESEARCH IN CLINICAL PRACTICE

The combined efforts of clinicians, administrators, managers, and researchers are necessary to conduct clinical research and to use findings in the clinical setting. The nursing administrator plays an important role in facilitating clinical research by legitimizing clinicians' research activities. The nurse manager plays a key role in both the conduct of research and

Guide for Evaluating Research Articles for Use in Clinical Practice

PART A: CRITIQUING THE RESEARCH ARTICLE

1. Is the title reflective of the hypotheses, including identification of key variables and the study design?
2. What theoretic framework is suggested by the review of literature?
3. Are the hypotheses related to the theoretic framework?
4. Is the design appropriate to the theoretic framework and hypotheses?
5. Given the design and the hypotheses, is the sampling method justified?
6. Are the instruments appropriate for testing the hypotheses? Additionally, do the instruments have established reliability and validity?
7. Are the reported statistics relevant to the design and hypotheses?
8. Do the results address the hypotheses?
9. In the conclusions, are the results related back to the review of literature?
10. Based on the results, are the conclusions and implications justified?

Strengths:

Weaknesses:

PART B: APPLYING THE RESULTS TO CLINICAL PRACTICE

1. How do the results compare with existing knowledge and research?
2. Can the results be generalized to the clinician's practice population?
3. What is the clinical significance of the findings?
4. How much client risk is involved if the findings are implemented in clinical practice?
5. What is the cost of the implementation in time and money?
6. Do the potential benefits of implementing the findings in clinical practice outweigh the cost of implementation?

Modified from Topham DL, DeSilva P: *Clin Nurse Spec* 2(2):97, 1988.

utilization of research findings. A manager who is committed to research as an integral component of practice encourages staff nurses on the unit, arranges scheduling so staff nurses can attend research courses, is actively involved in the identification of practice-relevant research problems, and facilitates policy and procedure changes when indicated by the research findings.

The American Nurses Association Commission on Nursing Research (1981) published "Guidelines for the Investigative Function of Nurses." They stated that nurses at all levels have a role in developing scientific knowledge and incorporating knowledge into practice. The **role of nurses in research** was outlined by the Commission on Nursing Research in relation to academic preparation (see box on p. 97). This outline should be viewed as a guideline. It should not limit nurses who have attained additional education, knowledge, and experience but do not have the degree listed. Conversely, having a degree does not mean that a nurse has the interest or expertise to conduct research.

Research can be used in practice in a variety of ways. For example, a women's health nurse practitioner who works in a setting where many women describe problems with stress urinary incontinence could review research to find studies describing methods of reducing stress incontinence. The nurse could use the information in client teaching, in idenidentifying causative factors and in planning treatment.

Studies can be examined to identify effective interventions and to locate tools that can be incorporated into assessment. A postpartum maternity nurse who is concerned about finding an improved intervention for reducing breast pain and engorgement in non–breastfeeding mothers could review research comparing interventions. The nurse would select the intervention that was determined to be most effective and use it with clients.

Studies can be read to increase conceptual understanding of a phenomenon. A nursing student during the maternity rotation who wants to learn more about fetal attachment could read the report of a study of the daily experiences of parents' awareness of the fetus during pregnancy (Stainton, 1990).

Protocols and procedures can be based on research findings. For example, a clinician questions the necessity of wearing cover gowns in the newborn nursery. The nurse could review the literature comparing infection rates with and without gowns. If a number of studies report that wearing gowns makes no difference in infection rates, practice in the nursery can be changed.

Whether results are generalizable to other populations and settings is an important question for the maternity-gynecologic nurse. There must be some degree of certainty that clients will respond to the treatment in the same way as the subjects in the reported study. This certainty is gained through locating a number of studies with similar findings.

Guidelines for the Investigative Function of Nurses

ASSOCIATE DEGREE IN NURSING

A. Demonstrates awareness of the value or relevance of research in nursing.
B. Assists in identifying problem areas in nursing practice.
C. Assists in collection of data within an established structured format.

BACCALAUREATE IN NURSING

A. Reads, interprets, and evaluates research for applicability to nursing practice.
B. Identifies nursing problems that need to be investigated and participates in the implementation of scientific studies.
C. Uses nursing practice as a means of gathering data for refining and extending practice.
D. Applies established findings of nursing and other health-related research to nursing practice.
E. Shares research findings with colleagues.

MASTER'S DEGREE IN NURSING

A. Analyzes and reformulates nursing practice problems so that scientific knowledge and scientific methods can be used to find solutions.
B. Enhances the quality and clinical relevance of nursing research by providing expertise in clinical problems and by providing knowledge about the way in which these clinical services are delivered.
C. Facilitates investigations of problems in clinical settings through such activities as contributing to a climate supportive of investigative activities, collaborating with others in investigations, and enhancing nursing's access to clients and data.
D. Conducts investigations for the purpose of monitoring the quality of the practice of nursing in a clinical setting.
E. Assists others to apply scientific knowledge in nursing practice.

DOCTORAL DEGREE IN NURSING OR RELATED DISCIPLINE

A. Graduate of a practice-oriented doctoral program
   1. Provides leadership for the integration of scientific knowledge with other sources of knowledge for the advancement of practice.
   2. Conducts investigations to evaluate the contribution of nursing activities to the well-being of clients.
   3. Develops methods to monitor the quality of the practice of nursing in a clinical setting and to evaluate contributions of nursing care activities to the well-being of clients.
B. Graduate of a research-oriented doctoral program
   1. Develops theoretical explanations of phenomena relevant to nursing by empirical research and analytical processes.
   2. Uses analytical and empirical methods to discover ways to modify or extend existing scientific knowledge so that it is relevant for nursing.
   3. Develops methods for scientific inquiry of phenomena relevant to nursing.

From American Nurses Association Commission on Nursing Research: *Guidelines for the investigative function of nurses,* Kansas City, Mo, 1981, Author.

■ RESEARCH-RELATED ACTIVITIES

Clinicians can engage in a number of activities related to research. These activities may increase the knowledge and understanding of the clinician and ultimately improve client care. Several research-related activities are discussed below.

Identify Problems. The clinician is uniquely qualified to identify relevant and important problems in practice. The clinician may collaborate with a researcher who might carry out the actual study of the problem identified. The clinician can identify appropriate subjects and facilitate data collection in the setting.

Serve on Research Committees. Many agencies have created nursing research committees. The purpose of the committees encompasses reviewing and critiquing research reports, providing a forum for discussion of research and the research process, judging the scientific merit of research proposals , and determining the clinical relevance and feasibility of proposed research. The clinician serving on the committee can learn about research and the research process, identify relevant clinical topics for study, teach peers about research, and facilitate the conduct of research in the setting.

Nurse as Researcher. Guidelines for evaluating research findings are valuable for busy clinicians to review nursing research as a basis for practice. A review of the literature, however, may not yield adequate studies to provide the necessary basis for changing practice. Therefore the nurse may need to replicate a study or conduct a new study.

Data Gatherer. Clinicians are often requested to collect data in the course of their daily work. This may be limited to ensuring that usual assessments are systematically and conscientiously recorded. It may entail filling out additional forms, asking additional questions, or collecting specimens. Other clinicians may be employed by the researcher as data gatherers.

■ SUMMARY

Clinical research as an integral component of nursing care provides a mechanism for making changes in care. Nurse faculty, nurse administrators, and nurse-researchers must provide assistance for nurses to base practice on sound scientific information.

REFERENCES

American Nurses Association Commission on Nursing Research: *Guidelines for the investigative function of nurses,* Kansas City, Mo, 1981, Author.

Arizmendi T, Affonso D: Stressful events related to pregnancy and postpartum, *J Psychosom Res* 31:743, 1987.

Barber-Madden RA, Kotch JB: Maternity care financing: universal access or universal care? *J of Health Politics, Policy and Law* 15(4):797, 1990.

Brooten D et al: A randomized clinical trial of early hospital discharge and home follow-up of very low-birth-weight infants, *N Engl J Med* 315:934, 1986.

Centers for Disease Control: The surgeon general's 1990 report on the health benefits of smoking cessation, *MMWR* 39(RR-12):1, 1990.

Centers for Disease Control: Premarital sexual experience among adolescent women—United States 1970-1988, *MMWR* 39(51&52):929, 1991.

Chez BF et al: Interpretations of nonstress tests by obstetric nurses, *JOGNN* 19(3):227, 1990.

Diers D: Finding clinical problems for study, *J Nurs Adm* 1(15):15, 1971.

Driscoll M et al: Prevention of preterm labor project in a public hospital: breaking down barriers to prenatal care, *J Perinat Neonatal Nurs* 4(3):44, 1990.

Federal Centre for AIDS: *Adult females cases by year of diagnosis,* March 20, 1991, Canada, Health and Welfare.

Federal Centre for AIDS: *Perinatal cases by year of diagnosis,* March 20, 1991, Canada Health and Welfare.

Flamm BL et al: Vaginal birth after cesarean delivery: results of a 5-year multicenter collaborative study, *Obstet Gynecol* 76(5), Part 1:750, 1990.

Green NL: Stressful events related to childbearing in African-American women: a pilot study, *J Nurs Midwifery* 35(4):231, 1990.

Greer PS: Head coverings for newborns under radiant warmers, *JOGNN* 17(4):265, 1988.

Heitkemper M et al: GI symptoms, function, and psychophysiological arousal in dysmenorrheic women, *Nurs Res* 40(1):20, 1991.

Hinshaw AS, Heinrich J, Bloch D: Evolving clinical nursing research priorities: a national endeavor, *J Prof Nurs* 4(6):398, 1988.

HIV/AIDS Surveillance: *Table 7: AIDS cases by sex, age at diagnosis, and race/ethnicity, reported through January 1991,* United States, Feb 1991, Author.

Institute of Medicine, Committee to study the prevention of low birth weight: *Preventing low birth weight,* Washington, DC, 1985, National Academic Press.

Jordan PL: Laboring for relevance: expectant and new fatherhood, *Nurs Res* 39(1):11, 1990.

LoBiondo-Wood G, Haber J: *Nursing research methods, critical appraisal, and utilization,* ed 2 St Louis, 1990, Mosby–Year Book.

NAACOG: *Research Priorities,* Washington, DC, 1988, Author.

Nichols FH: Translating clinical problems into research projects, *NAACOG Newsletter* 16(3):9, 1989.

Perry SE: Research utilization: science-based practice, *NAACOG Newsletter* 17(4):4, 1990.

Rubin R: Maternal touch, *Nurs Outlook* 11:828, 1963.

Rush J et al: A randomized controlled triad of a nursery ritual: wearing cover gowns to care for healthy newborns, *Birth* 17(1):25, 1990.

Sampselle C: Changes in pelvic muscle strength and stress urinary incontinence associated with childbirth, *JOGNN* 19(5):371, 1990.

Seideman RY: Effects of a premenstrual syndrome education program on premenstrual symptomatology, *Health Care for Women International* 11:491, 1990.

Society for the Advancement of Women's Health Research: *Women's health research: prescription for change,* Washington, DC, 1991, Author.

Stainton MC: Parents' awareness of their unborn infant in the third trimester, *Birth* 17(2):92, 1990.

Thomas L et al: The effects of rocking, diet modifications, and antiflatulent medication on postcesarean section gas pain, *J Perinat Neonatal Nurs* 4(3):12, 1990.

Topham DL, DeSilva P: Evaluating congruency between steps in the research process: A critique guide for use in clinical nursing practice, *Clin Nurse Specialist* 2(2):97, 1988.

Tornquist EM, Funk SG: How to write a research grant proposal, *Image J Nurs Sch* 22(1):44, 1990.

Tulman LJ: Mothers' and unrelated persons' initial handling of newborn infants, *Nurs Res* 34(4):205, 1985.

Women's Health Equity Act introduced, *NAACOG Newsletter* 18(9):15, 1991.

Zalar MK, Welches LJ, Walker DD: Nursing consortium approach to increase research in service settings, *J Nurs Adm* 17(7):36, 1985.

BIBLIOGRAPHY

Thomas BS: *Nursing research: an experiential approach,* St Louis, 1990, Mosby–Year Book.

Woods NF, Catanzaro M: *Nursing research: theory and practice,* St. Louis, 1988, Mosby–Year Book.

chapter 5 review

Key Concepts

- The more nursing practice is based on nursing research, the higher the quality of the practice.
- The nurse at the bedside is in the best position to identify researchable clinical problems.
- Biases against women exist in research.
- National bodies have delineated nursing research priorities.
- As consumers of research, clinicians read research reports to determine the scientific merit and clinical utility of the studies and apply research findings where appropriate.
- Evaluating research findings provides a valuable tool for busy clinicians to review nursing research as a basis for maternity and gynecologic nursing practice.
- There are a variety of ways clinicians can use research in clinical practice.

Key Terms

- clinical relevance (p. 95)
- consumer of research (p. 95)
- content analysis (p. 91)
- dissemination (p. 91)
- evaluating research (p. 95)
- generalizability (p. 95)
- qualitative approach (p. 88)
- quantitative approach (p. 88)
- replication (p. 95)
- research bias (p. 92)
- research priorities (p. 94)
- research process (p. 88)
- role of nurses (in research) (p. 96)
- scientific merit (p. 95)
- utilization (p. 96)

Critical Thinking Exercises

Select a nursing diagnosis and:

1. Identify an area for a potential research study.
2. Review the literature to learn if the identified area has been researched.
3. If studies have been done, select one of the studies and evaluate it.

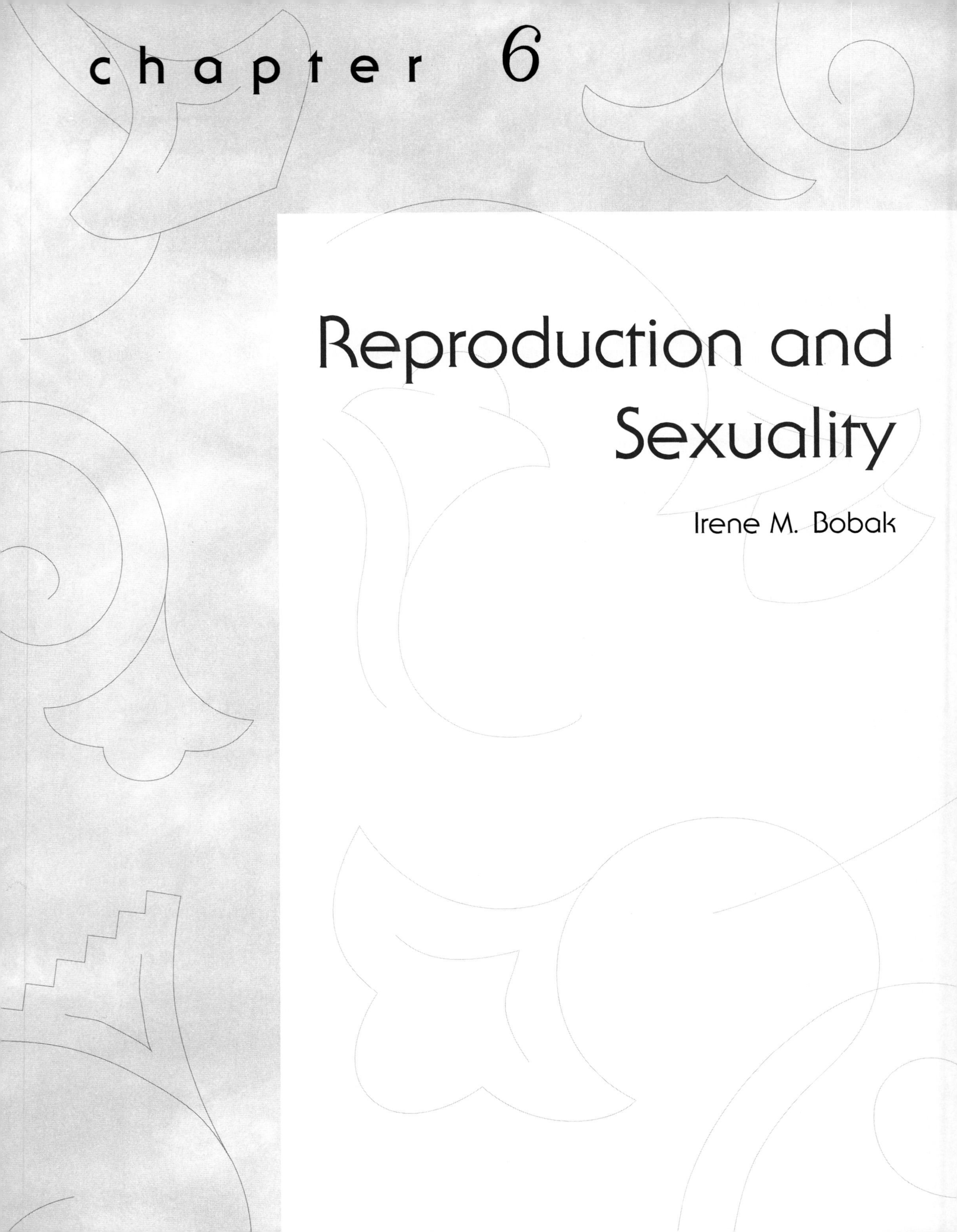

chapter 6

Reproduction and Sexuality

Irene M. Bobak

LEARNING OBJECTIVES

- Define the key terms listed.
- Identify the internal, external, and accessory structures of both the female and male reproductive systems.
- Explain the functions of the structures of both the female and male reproductive systems.
- Summarize the menstrual cycle in relation to hormonal response, ovarian response, and endometrial response.
- Discuss the clinical significance of human sexual response.
- Relate the nurse's role in parental counseling regarding sex education.
- Discuss developmental tasks of adolescence and adulthood according to Erikson.
- Differentiate expected behaviors in the three phases of adolescence.
- List the developmental tasks of Johnson's three phases of adulthood.
- Assess personal belief system regarding sexuality and the impact such beliefs have on one's ability to counsel and teach sexually related material.
- Explain immunologic benefits of colostrum and breast milk to the newborn.
- Compare active and passive immunity using the Rh factor as an example.
- Explain helper, suppressor, and killer cells using AIDS as an example.
- Describe the action of vaccination using rubella as an example.
- Discuss the effect on the functioning of the immune system of factors such as age, life-style, environment, and nutrition.
- Identify topics for nursing research related to the reproductive system, human sexuality, and immune system functioning.

The purposes of this chapter are threefold: (1) to review sexual and reproductive anatomy and physiology, (2) to trace the psychosocial development of sexuality from birth through adulthood, and (3) to present an overview of the immune system.

Nurses providing health care to women require a greater depth and breadth of knowledge of female and male anatomy and physiology than is usually taught in general courses. Often the reproductive system, including the breasts, is the last system taught, and only if there is time. Knowledge of the anatomy and physiology of female and male structures involved in reproduction is basic to planning for, implementing, and evaluating nursing care of the maternity client and her family.

Although the female and male reproductive systems differ markedly in appearance, their structures are homologous (having the same embryonic origin) (Figs. 6-1 and 6-2). Each structure performs a vital role in continuing the human species and generating and maintaining secondary sexual characteristics. Through hormonal influences, the genitals, pelvis, and breasts acquire the unique adaptations necessary to childbearing. Both female and male reproductive systems consist of the following four principal components:

1. External genitals
2. A pair of primary sex glands (gonads)
3. Ducts leading from the gonads to the body's exterior
4. Secondary (accessory) sex glands

■ FEMALE REPRODUCTIVE SYSTEM

The female reproductive system consists of internal organs, located in the pelvic cavity and supported by the pelvic floor, and external genitals, located in the perineum. The female's internal and external reproductive structures develop and mature in response to estrogens and progesterones, starting in fetal life and continuing through puberty and the childbearing years. The reproductive structures **atrophy** (decrease in size) with age or a drop in ovarian hormone production. An extensive and complex innervation and a generous blood supply support the functions of these structures. The appearance of the external genitals varies greatly from woman to woman, since the size, shape, and color are determined by heredity, age, race, and the number of children a woman has borne.

External Structures

The external female genitals (vulva and pudenda) are located in the perineum. The external structures are presented in the following order (from anterior to posterior): Mons pubis (mons veneris), labia majora and minora, clitoris, prepuce of clitoris, vestibule, fourchette, and perineum. The external genitals are illustrated in Fig. 6-3.

MONS PUBIS. The mons pubis, or mons veneris, is the rounded, soft fullness of subcutaneous fatty tissue and loose connective tissue over the symphysis pubis. It contains many sebaceous (oil) glands and develops coarse, dark, curly hair at **pubarche,** about 1 to 2 years before the onset of the menses. **Menarche** (the onset of menses) occurs on the average at 13 years of age. Characteristics of pubic hair vary from sparse and fine among Oriental women to thick, coarse, and curly among African-American women. The functions of the mons are to play a role in sensuality and to protect the symphysis pubis during coitus. During the climacterium the amount of fatty tissue decreases, and pubic hair thins.

LABIA MAJORA. The labia majora are two rounded lengthwise folds of skin-covered fat and connective tissue that merge with the mons. They extend from the mons downward around the labia minora, ending in the perineum in the midline. The labia majora function as protection for the labia minora, urinary meatus, and vaginal introitus. In the woman who has never experienced vaginal childbirth, the labia majora lie close together in the midline, covering the underlying structures. Some labial separation and even gaping of the vaginal introitus follow childbirth and perineal or vaginal injury. During the climacterium, labia majora atrophy.

On their lateral surfaces the labial skin is thick, usually pigmented darker than the surrounding tissues, and covered with coarse hair (similar to that of the mons) that thins out toward the perineum. The medial (inner) surfaces of the labia majora are smooth, thick, and without hair. They contain an abundant supply of sebaceous glands and sweat glands and are highly vascular. The extreme sensitivity of the labia majora to touch, pain, and temperature is caused by the extensive network of nerves; thus they function during sensual arousal.

LABIA MINORA. The labia minora, located between the labia majora, are narrow, lengthwise folds of hairless skin extending downward from beneath the clitoris and merging with the fourchette. Whereas the

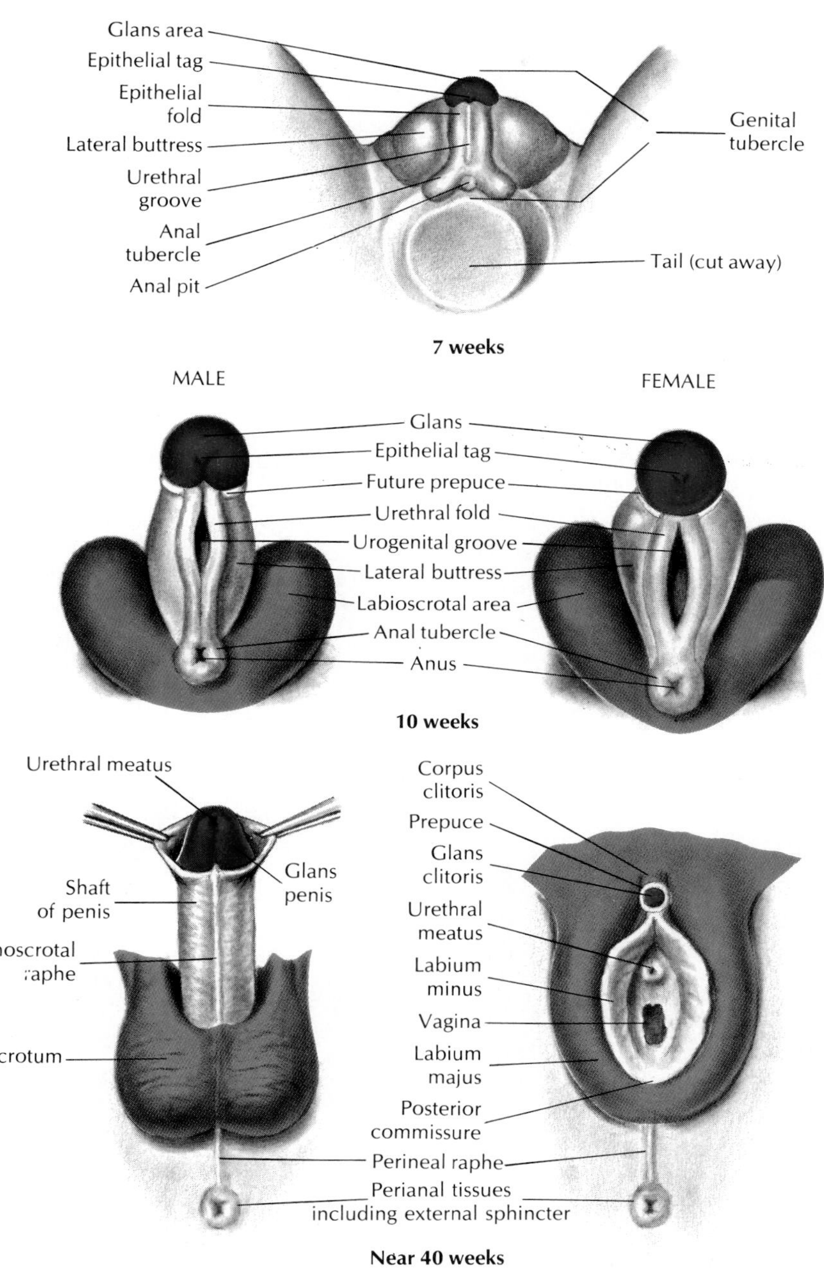
UNDIFFERENTIATED
Glans area
Epithelial tag
Epithelial fold
Lateral buttress
Urethral groove
Anal tubercle
Anal pit
Genital tubercle
Tail (cut away)
7 weeks
MALE
FEMALE
Glans
Epithelial tag
Future prepuce
Urethral fold
Urogenital groove
Lateral buttress
Labioscrotal area
Anal tubercle
Anus
10 weeks
Urethral meatus
Shaft of penis
Glans penis
Penoscrotal raphe
Scrotum
Corpus clitoris
Prepuce
Glans clitoris
Urethral meatus
Labium minus
Vagina
Labium majus
Posterior commissure
Perineal raphe
Perianal tissues including external sphincter
Near 40 weeks

Fig. 6-1 Homologues of external genitals.

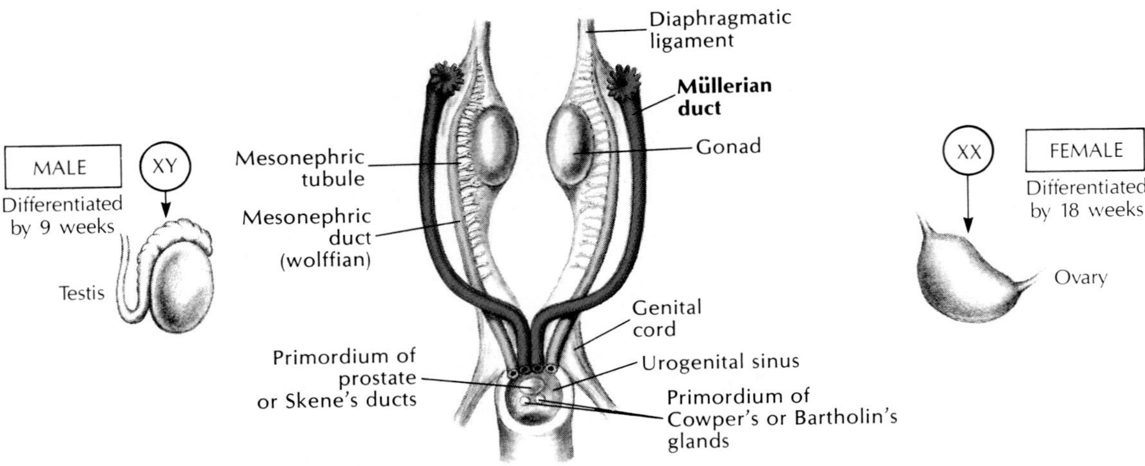

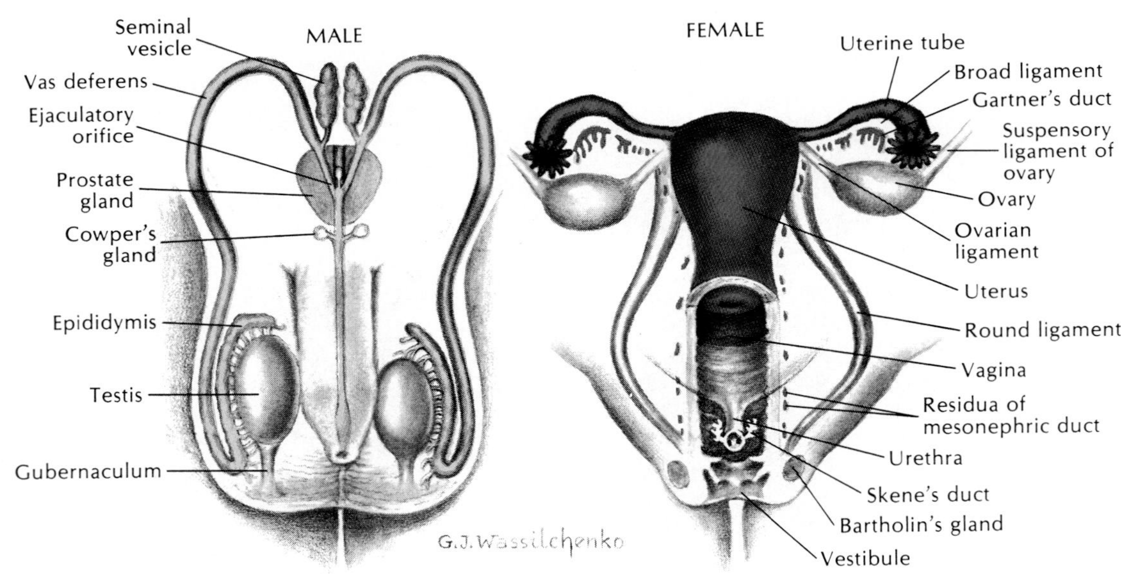

Fig. 6-2 Homologues of internal genitals.

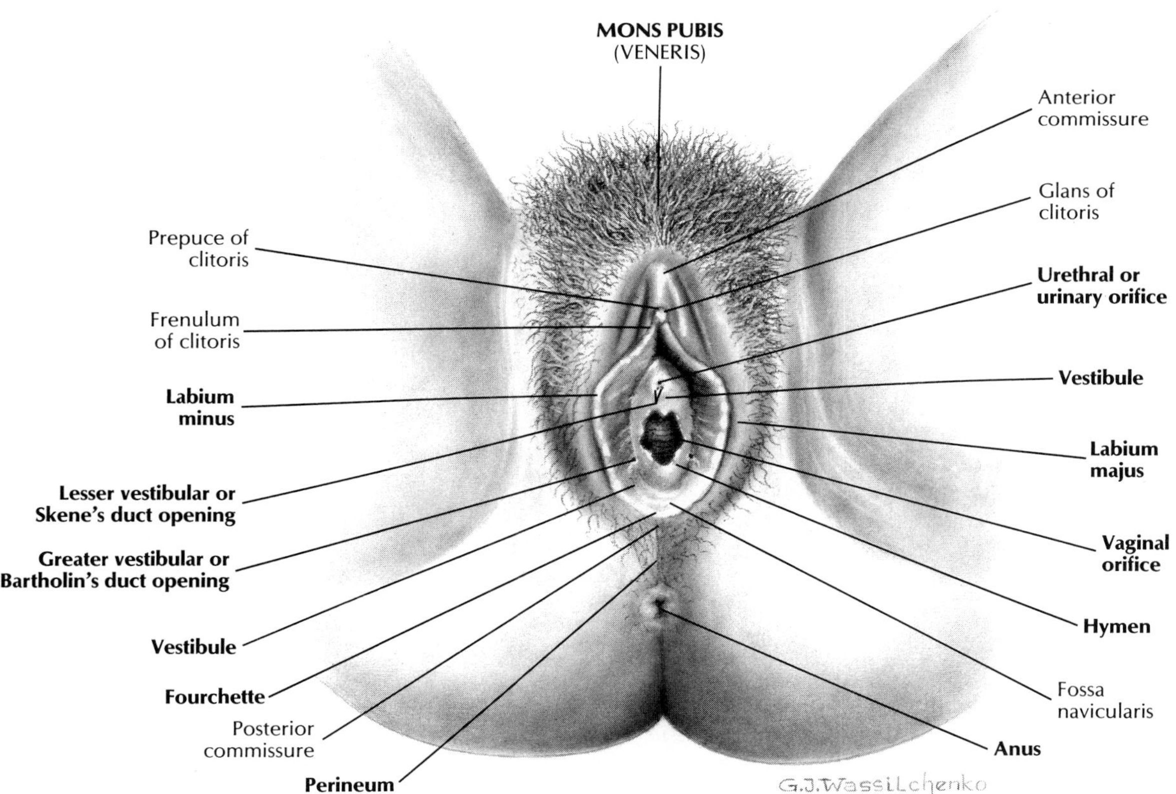

Fig. 6-3 External female genitals.

lateral and anterior aspects of the labia are usually pigmented, their medial surfaces are similar to vaginal mucosa: pink and moist. Their rich vascularity gives them a reddish color and permits marked turgescence (swelling) of the labia minora with emotional or physical stimulation. The glands in the labia minora also lubricate the vulva. A rich nerve supply makes them sensitive, enhancing their erotic function. The space between the labia minora is called the vestibule.

CLITORIS. The clitoris is a short, cylindric, erectile organ fixed just beneath the arch of the pubis; the visible portion is about 6 × 6 mm or less in the unaroused state. The tip of the clitoral body is called the glans and is more sensitive than its shaft. In healthy women the length of the clitoral body varies from 2 mm to 1 cm, and the width is usually estimated at 4 to 5 mm. When sexually aroused, the glans and shaft increase in size.

Sebaceous glands of the clitoris secrete smegma, a cheeselike fatty substance with a distinctive odor that serves as a pheromone (an organic compound that provides communication with other members of the same species to elicit a certain response, which in this case is erotic stimulation of the human male). The term *clitoris* comes from a Greek word meaning "key," because the clitoris was seen as the key to female sexuality. Its rich vascularity and innervation make the clitoris highly sensitive to temperature, touch, and pressure sensation. Its main function is to stimulate and elevate levels of sexual tension.

PREPUCE OF CLITORIS. Near the anterior junction the right and left labia minora separate into medial and lateral portions. The lateral portions unite above the clitoris to form its prepuce, a hoodlike covering; the medial portions unite below the clitoris to form its frenulum. Sometimes the prepuce covers the clitoris. As a result this area has the appearance of an opening that can be mistaken for the urethral meatus if the nurse does not identify vulvar structures carefully. Attempts to insert a catheter into this sensitive area can cause considerable discomfort.

VESTIBULE. The vestibule is an ovoid or boat-shaped area formed between the labia minora, clitoris, and fourchette. The vestibule contains the openings to the urethra, paraurethral (lesser vestibular or Skene's) glands, the vagina, and the paravaginal (greater vestibular, vulvovaginal, or Bartholin's) glands. The thin, almost mucosal, surface of the vestibule is easily irritated by chemicals (feminine deodorant sprays, bubble bath salts), heat, discharges, and friction (tight jeans).

Although not a true part of the reproductive system, the *urinary* (urethral) *meatus* is considered here because of its closeness and relationship to the vulva. The meatus is a pink or reddened opening of varying shapes, often with slightly puckered margins. The meatus marks the terminal, or distal, part of the urethra. It is usually about 2.5 cm (1 inch) below the clitoris.

The *lesser vestibular* (paraurethral or Skene's) *glands* are short tubular structures situated posterolaterally just inside the urethral meatus, at about the 5 and 7 o'clock positions around the meatus. They produce a small amount of mucus, which functions as lubrication.

The *hymen* (see Fig. 6-3) is a partial, rarely complete, elastic but tough mucosa-covered fold around the *vaginal introitus* (opening to the vagina). In virginal females the hymen may be an impediment to vaginal examination, insertion of menstrual tampons, or coitus. The hymen may be elastic and allow distension, or it may be torn easily. Occasionally the hymen covers the orifice completely, resulting in an imperforate hymen that prevents passage of menstrual flow, instrumentation (e.g., with a speculum), or coitus. A hymenotomy may be necessary in some cases. After instrumentation, use of tampons, coitus, or vaginal delivery, residual tags of the torn hymen (hymenal caruncles or carunculae myrtiformes) may be seen.

One common myth is that one can tell by the condition of the hymen whether a female is a virgin. Sexually active and even parous females may have intact hymens. For other women the hymen may be torn during strenuous physical work or exercise, masturbation, or use of tampons. Some cultural groups cleanse the female infant so vigorously that the hymen is torn, leaving only hymenal tags in its place. Therefore the "test for virginity"—evidence of bleeding following sexual intercourse—is an unreliable criterion.

The *greater vestibular* (vulvovaginal or Bartholin's) *glands* are two compound glands at the base of the labia majora, one on either side of the vaginal orifice. Each gland is drained by several ducts, about 1.5 cm long. Each opens into the groove between the hymen and the labia minora. Usually the gland openings are not visible or palpable. The glands secrete a small amount of clear, viscid mucus, especially during coitus. The alkaline pH of the mucus is supportive of sperm.

FOURCHETTE. The fourchette is a thin, flat, transverse fold of tissue formed where the tapering labia majora and minora merge in the midline below the vaginal orifice. A small depression, the fossa navicularis, lies between the fourchette and the hymen.

PERINEUM. The perineum is the skin-covered muscular area between the vaginal introitus and the anus. The perineum forms the base of the perineal body (see Fig. 6-15, p. 116). The terms *vulva* and *perineum* occasionally but inaccurately are used interchangeably.

Internal Structures

The internal reproductive organs are discussed in the order that reflects the path of the ovum. Supportive tissues are discussed along with the internal reproductive organs they support. Internal organs include the ovaries, uterine (fallopian) tubes, uterus, and vagina. A brief description of the bony pelvis follows.

OVARIES. One ovary is located on each side of the uterus, below and behind the uterine tubes. The ovaries are held in place by two ligaments, the mesovarian portions of the uterine *broad ligament,* which suspend them from the lateral pelvic side walls at about the level of the anterosuperior iliac crest, and the *ovarian* ligaments (see Figs. 6-5 and 6-9), which anchor them to the uterus. The ovaries are movable with palpation.

The ovaries are similar in origin (homologous) to the testes in the male. Each ovary resembles a large almond in size and shape (Fig. 6-4). Each is whitish and rounded but flattened, weighs about 3 g, and measures approximately 3 × 2 × 1 cm. At the time of ovulation, ovarian size may double temporarily. The oval-shaped ovaries are firm in consistency and slightly tender. The surface of the ovary is smooth before menarche. After sexual maturity, scarring from repeated ruptures of follicles and ovulation roughens the nodular surface.

The two functions of the ovaries are **ovulation** and hormone production. At birth the normal female's ovaries contain countless thousands of primordial (primitive) ova. At intervals during the reproductive life (generally monthly), one or more ova mature and undergo ovulation. The ovary is also the major site of production of steroid sex hormones (estrogens, progesterone, and androgens) in amounts required for normal female growth, development, and function.

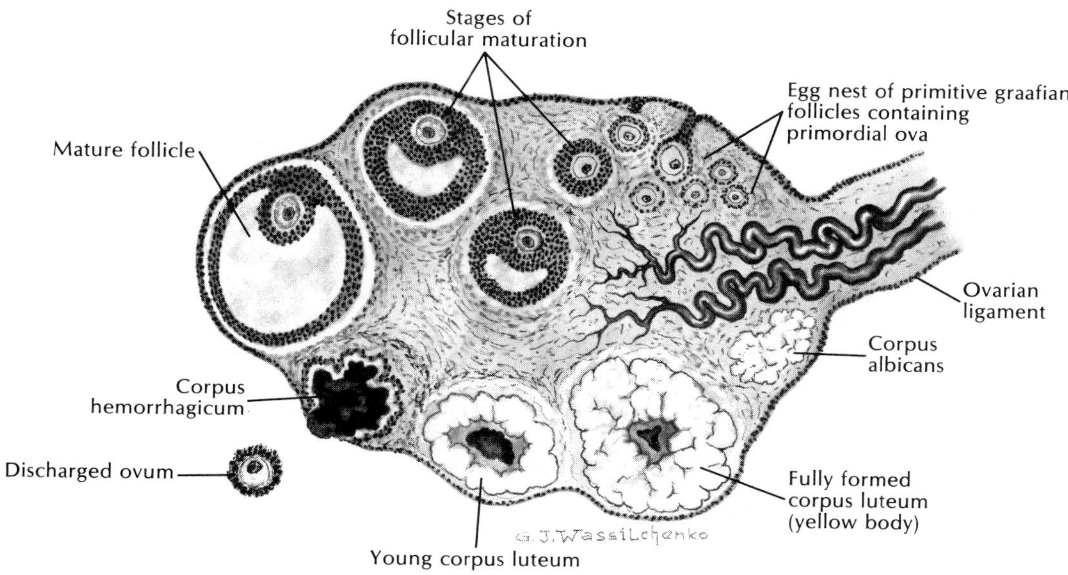

Fig. 6-4 Cross section of ovary.

UTERINE TUBES (OVIDUCTS). The paired uterine (fallopian) tubes are attached to the uterine fundus (Figs. 6-5, 6-6, and 6-9). The tubes extend laterally, enter the free ends of the broad ligament, and curl around each ovary.

The tubes are approximately 10 cm (4 inches) long and 0.6 cm (¼ inch) in diameter. Each tube has an outer coat of peritoneum, a middle, thin muscular coat, and an inner mucosa. The mucosal lining consists of columnar cells, some of which are ciliated and others of which are secretory. The mucosa is at its thinnest during the time of menstruation. Each tube, along with its mucosa, is continuous with the mucosa of the uterus and of the vagina.

The structure of the uterine tube changes along its length. Four distinctive segments can be identified (Figs. 6-5 and 6-6): (1) the infundibulum, (2) the ampulla, (3) the isthmus, and (4) the interstitial part. The *infundibulum* is the most distal portion. Its funnel, or trumpet-shaped opening, is encircled with fimbriae. The fimbriae become swollen, almost erectile, at ovulation. The *ampulla* makes up the distal and middle segment of the tube. It is in the ampulla that the sperm and the ovum unite and fertilization occurs.

The *isthmus* is proximal to the ampulla. It is small and firm, much like the round ligament. The *interstitial* (or intramural) portion passes through the myometrium between the fundus and the body of the uterus and has the smallest lumen. Before the fertilized ovum can pass through this lumen, or tunnel, measuring less than 1 mm in diameter, it has to discard its crown of granulosa cells.

The uterine tubes provide a passageway for the ovum. The fingerlike projections (fimbriae) of the infundibulum pull the ovum into the tube with wavelike motions. The ovum is propelled along the tube, partially by the cilia but primarily by the peristaltic movements of the muscular coat, toward the uterine cavity. Peristaltic motion is influenced by estrogen and prostaglandins. Peristaltic activity of the uterine tubes and the secretory function of their mucosal lining are greatest at the time of ovulation. The columnar cells secrete a nutrient to sustain the ovum while it is in the tube.

UTERUS. Between birth and puberty the uterus descends gradually into the true pelvis from the lower abdomen. After puberty the uterus is usually located in the midline in the true pelvis posterior to the symphysis pubis and urinary bladder and anterior to the rectum.

For most women, with the urinary bladder empty, the uterus is anteverted (tipped forward) and slightly anteflexed (bent forward), with the corpus lying over the top of the posterior wall of the bladder. The cervix is directed downward and backward toward the tip of the sacrum so that it is usually at approximately a right angle to the plane of the vagina. For other women the uterus may be in the midposition or tipped backward (retroverted). A uterus that is bent more than usual so that the fundus is closer to the

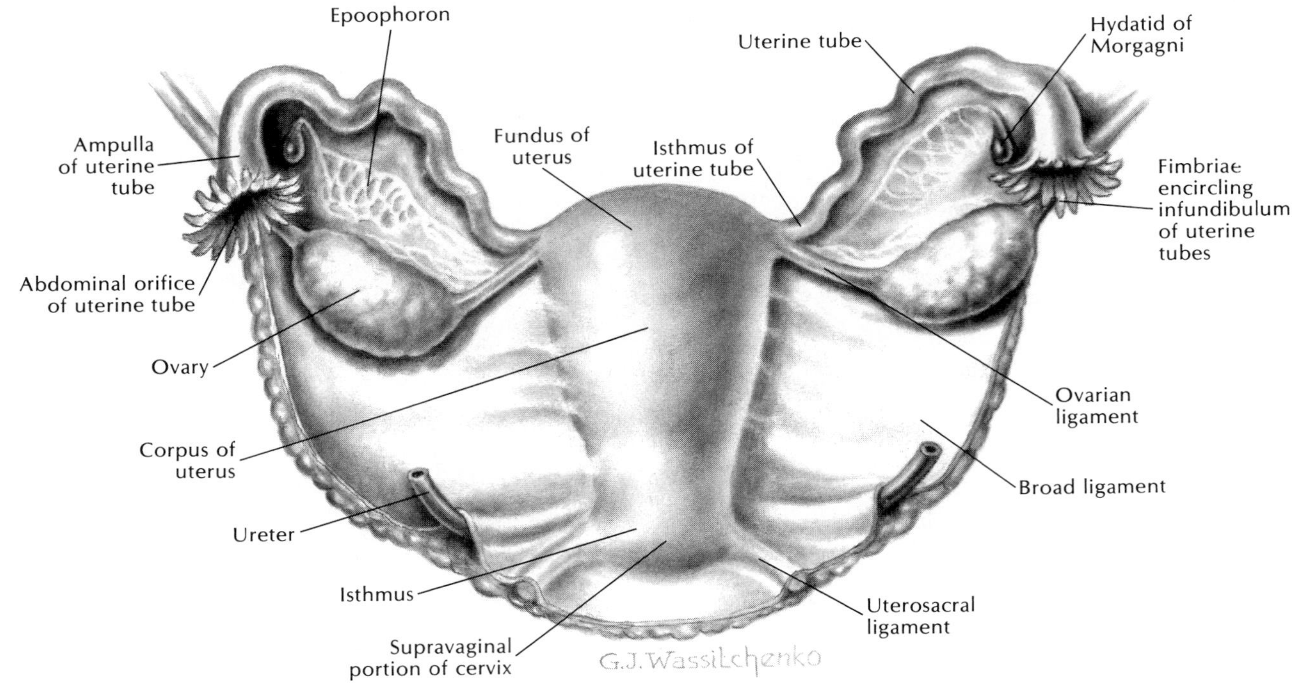

Fig. 6-5 Uterus and adnexa, posterior view.

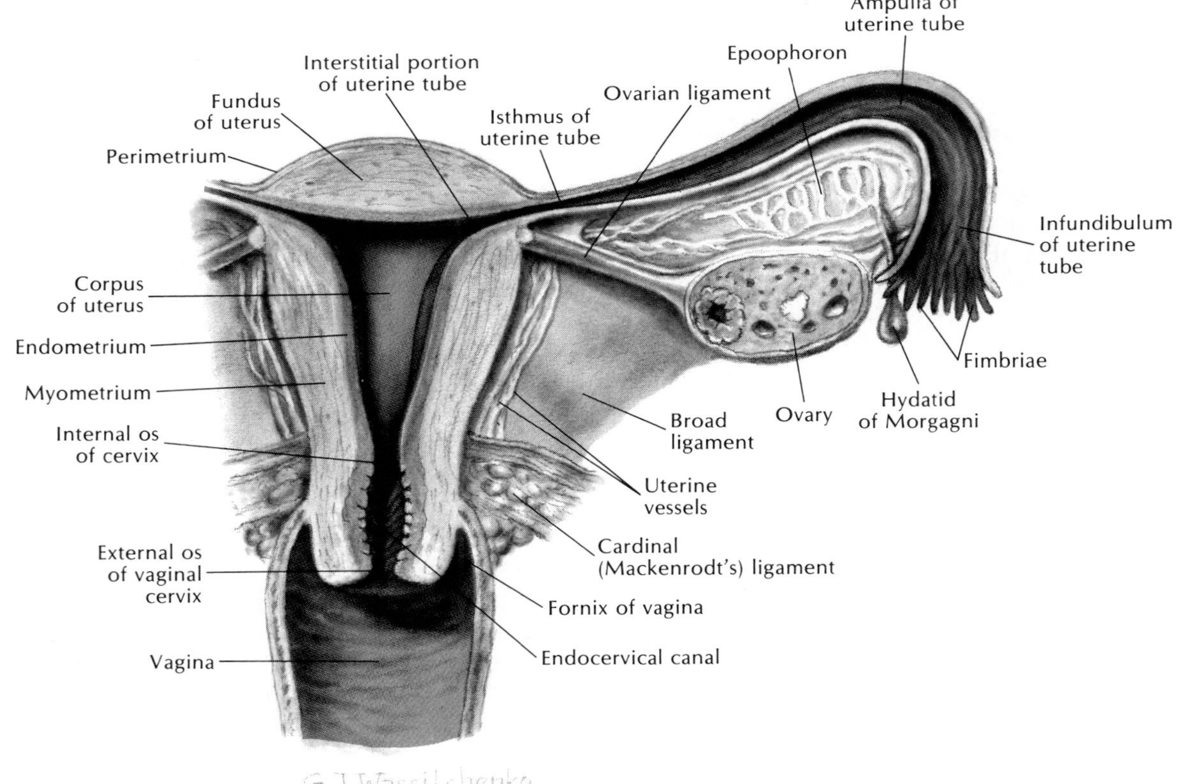

Fig. 6-6 Cross section of uterus, adnexa, and upper vagina.

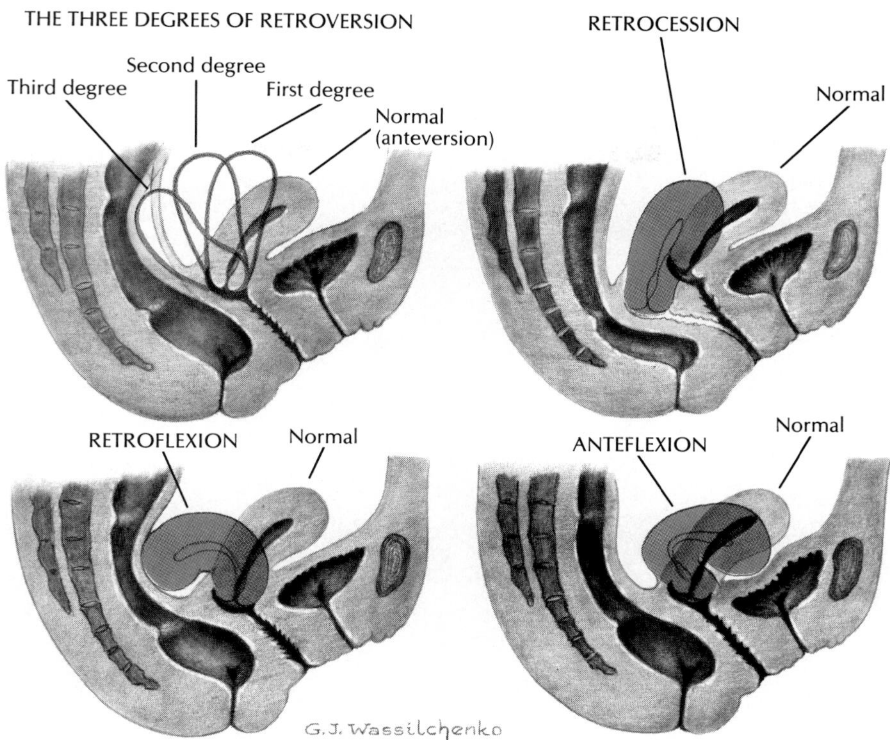

Fig. 6-7 Uterine positions.

cervix is said to be anteflexed, or retroflexed (Fig. 6-7).

A full bladder pushes the uterus back toward the rectum. A full rectum moves the uterus forward against the bladder. Uterine position also changes depending on the woman's position (e.g., lying supine, prone, on her side, or standing), her age, and pregnancy. The free mobility permits the uterus to rise slightly during the sexual response cycle (p. 128) so that the cervix is placed in a position to increase the likelihood of fertilization.

The uterus is supported by ligaments and by muscles of the pelvic floor, including the perineal body. A total of 10 ligaments stabilize the uterus within the pelvic cavity (see Figs. 6-5, 6-6, and 6-9): four paired ligaments—broad, round, uterosacral, and cardinal (transverse or Mackenrodt's); and two single ligaments—anterior (pubocervical) and posterior (rectovaginal). The posterior ligament forms the deep rectouterine pouch known as the *cul-de-sac of Douglas* (Figs. 6-8 and 6-15).

The uterus is a flattened, hollow, muscular, thick-walled organ that looks somewhat like an upside-down pear (Fig. 6-8). Its length, width, and thickness vary averaging about 7.5 × 3.5 × 2 cm (3 × 1½ × ¾ in). In the adult woman who has never been pregnant the uterus weighs 60 g (2 oz). The uterus normally is symmetric in shape and nontender, smooth, and firm to the touch. The degree of firmness varies with several factors; for example, it is spongier during the secretory phase of the menstrual cycle, softer during pregnancy and firmer after menopause.

The uterus has three parts (see Figs. 6-5 and 6-6): the *fundus*, which is the upper, rounded prominence above the insertion of the uterine tubes; the *corpus*, or main portion, encircling the intrauterine cavity; and the *isthmus*, which is the slightly constricted portion that joins the corpus to the cervix and is known during pregnancy as the lower uterine segment.

The three functions of the uterus include cyclic menstruation with rejuvenation of the endometrium, pregnancy, and labor. These functions are essential to reproduction, but they are not necessary for a woman's physiologic survival.

UTERINE WALL. The uterine wall comprises three layers: the endometrium, the myometrium, and a partial outer layer of parietal peritoneum (see Fig. 6-6).

The highly vascular *endometrium* is a lining of mucous membrane composed of three layers: a com-

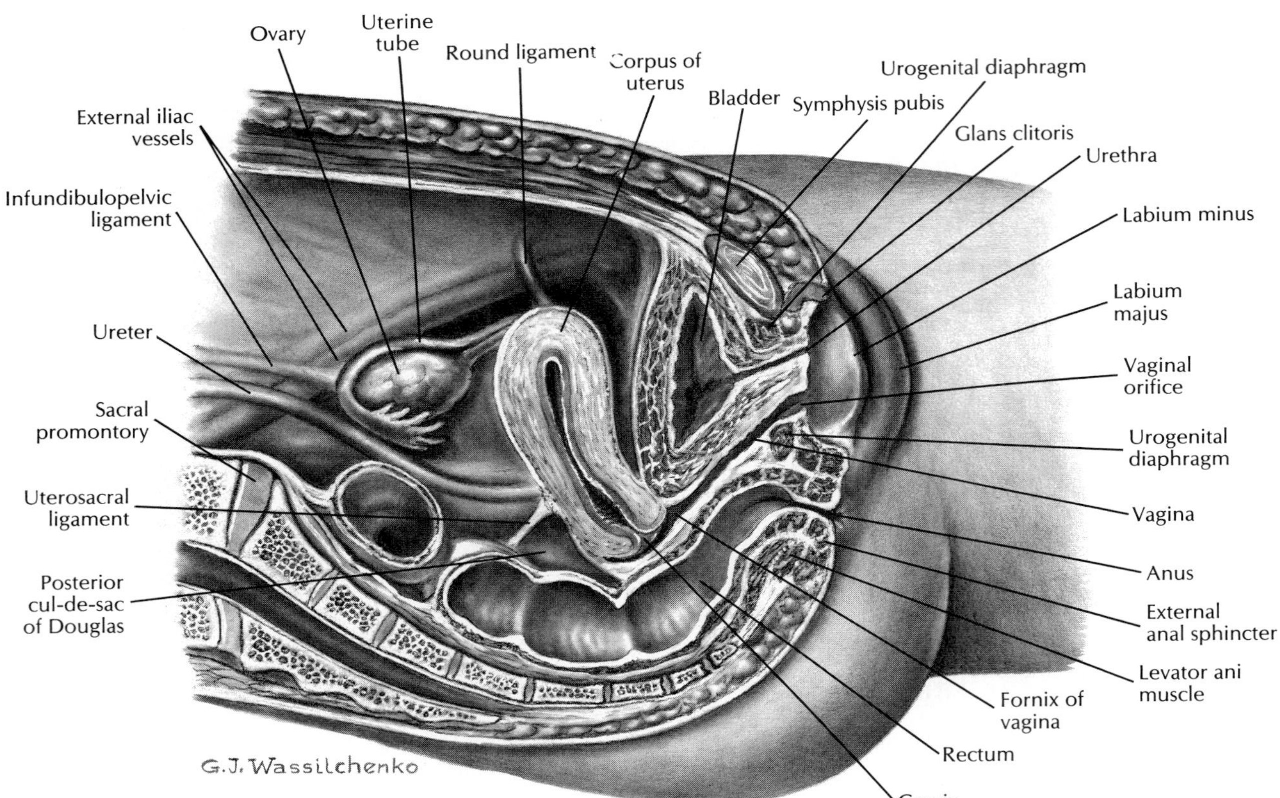

Fig. 6-8 Midsagittal view of female pelvic organs, with woman lying supine.

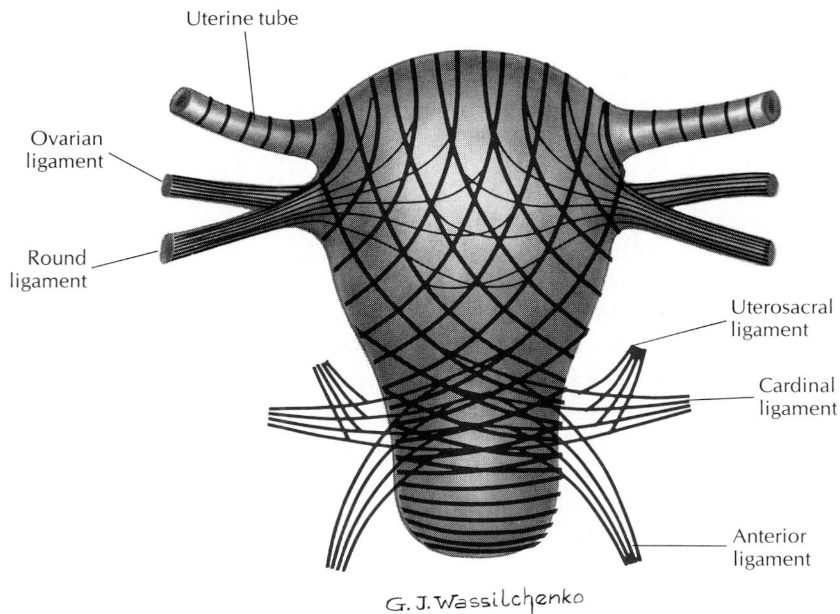

Fig. 6-9 Schematic arrangement of directions of muscle fibers. Note that uterine muscle fibers are continuous with supportive ligaments of uterus.

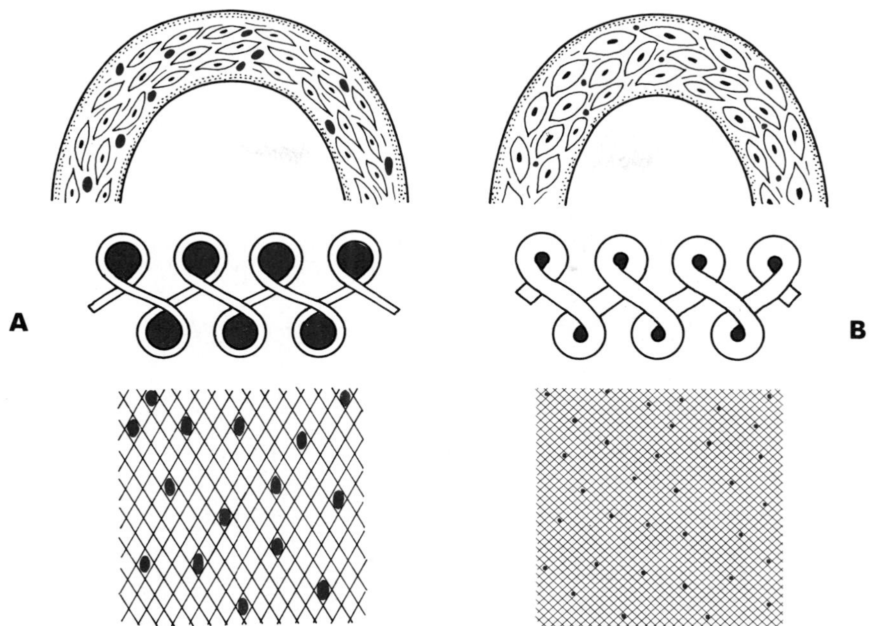

Fig. 6-10 The living ligature: interlacing smooth muscle fibers of the thick middle myometrium. Color denotes blood vessels. A, Relaxed muscle fibers. B, Contracted muscle fibers ligating the blood vessels.

pact surface layer, a spongy middle layer of loose connective tissue, and a dense inner layer that attaches the endometrium to the myometrium. (The upper two layers are also referred to as the functional layer, and the inner layer as the basal layer.) During menstruation and following delivery, the compact surface and middle spongy layers slough off. Just after menstrual flow ends, the endometrium is 0.5 mm thick; near the end of the endometrial cycle, just before menstruation begins again, it is about 5 mm (less than ¼ inch) thick.

Layers of smooth muscle fibers that extend in three directions (longitudinal, transverse, and oblique) make up the thick *myometrium* (Fig. 6-9). The smooth muscle fibers interlace with elastic and connective tissues and blood vessels throughout the uterine wall and blend with the dense inner layer of the endometrium. The myometrium is particularly thick in the fundus, thins out as it nears the isthmus, and is thinnest in the cervix.

The *outer* myometrial layer, found mostly in the fundus, is made up of longitudinal fibers and is therefore well suited for expelling the fetus during the birth process. In the thick *middle* myometrial layer the interlaced muscle fibers form a figure-eight pattern encircling large blood vessels. Contraction of the middle layer produces a hemostatic action (Fig. 6-10). Only a few circular fibers of the *inner* myometrial layer are found in the fundus. Most of the circular fibers are concentrated in the cornua (the place where the uterine tubes join the uterine body) and around the internal os. The sphincter action of this layer prevents the regurgitation of menstrual blood out of the uterine tubes during menstruation. Their sphincter action around the internal cervical os helps retain the uterine contents during pregnancy. Injury to this sphincter can weaken the internal os and result in an incompetent internal cervical os (for further discussion, see Chapter 31).

For clarity and interest, each muscle layer and its function were described individually. It must be remembered that the myometrium works as a whole. The structure of the myometrium, which gives strength and elasticity, presents an example of adaptation to function:

1. To thin out, pull up, and open the cervix and to push the fetus out of the uterus, the fundus must contract with the most force.
2. Contraction of interlacing smooth muscle fibers that surround the blood vessels controls blood loss after abortion and childbirth. Because of their ability to close off (ligate) blood vessels between them, the smooth muscle fibers of the uterus are referred to as the **living ligature** (Fig. 6-10).

The *parietal peritoneum,* a serous membrane,

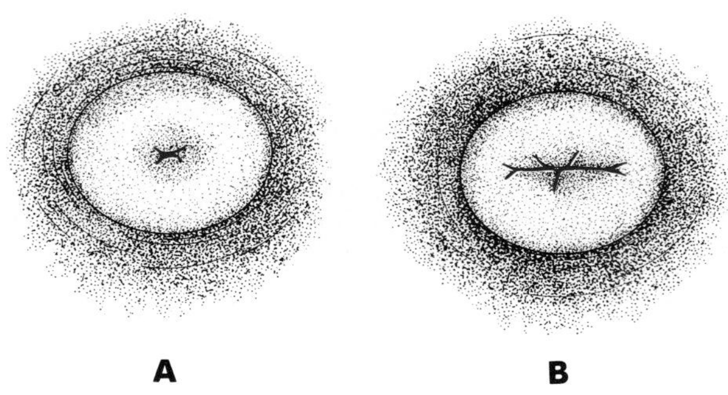

Fig. 6-11 External cervical os as seen through speculum. **A**, Nonparous cervix. **B**, Parous cervix.

coats all of the uterine corpus except for the lower one fourth of the anterior surface, where the bladder is attached, and the cervix. Because parietal peritoneum does not completely cover this organ, it is possible for diagnostic tests and surgery involving the uterus to be performed without entering the abdominal cavity.

CERVIX. The lowermost portion of the uterus is the cervix, or neck. The attachment site of the uterine cervix to the vaginal vault divides the cervix into the longer supravaginal (above the vagina) portion (see Fig. 6-5) and the shorter vaginal portion (see Fig. 6-6). The length of the cervix is about 2.5 to 3 cm, of which about 1 cm protrudes into the vagina in the nonpregnant woman.

The cervix is composed primarily of fibrous connective tissue with some muscle fibers and elastic tissue. The cervix of the nulliparous woman is a rounded, almost conical, rather firm, spindle-shaped body approximately 2 to 2.5 cm in external diameter. The narrowed opening between the uterine cavity and the endocervical canal (canal inside the cervix that connects the uterine cavity with the vagina) is the *internal os*. The narrowed opening between the endocervix and the vagina is the *external os*. The external os is a small circular opening in women who have not borne children. Childbirth changes the circular os to a small transverse opening dividing the cervix into an anterior and a posterior lip (Fig. 6-11).

When the woman is not ovulating or is not pregnant, the tip of the cervix feels firm, much like the end of one's nose, with a dimple in the center. The dimple marks the site of the external os.

The most significant characteristic of the cervix is its ability to stretch during vaginal childbirth. Several factors contribute to cervical elasticity: high connective tissue and elastic fiber content, numerous infoldings in the endocervical lining, and a muscle fiber content of about 10%.

CANALS. There are two cavities within the uterus, which are known as the uterine and cervical canals (see Fig. 6-6). The uterine canal in the nonpregnant state is compressed by thick muscular walls so that it is only a potential space, flat and triangular. The base of the triangle is formed by the fundus. The uterine tubes open into either end of the base. The apex of the triangle points downward and forms the internal os (opening) of the cervical canal.

The endocervical canal with its many infoldings has a surface layer of tall, columnar, mucus-producing cells. *Columnar epithelium* is beefy red, deeper, and rougher looking than the epithelial outer covering of the cervix. After menarche (the start of menstruation) *squamous epithelium* covers the outside of the cervix (ectocervix). This external covering of flat cells gives a glistening pink color to the cervix. A deeper bluish-red color is seen when the woman is ovulating or pregnant. A reddened (hyperemic) cervix may indicate inflammation.

The two types of epithelium meet at the **squamocolumnar junction.** This junction line is usually just inside the external cervical os but may be found on the ectocervix in some women. The squamocolumnar junction is the most common site of neoplastic cellular changes. Therefore cells for cytologic study, the Papanicolaou smear, are scraped from this junction.

The columnar epithelial cells produce odorless and nonirritating mucus in response to ovarian endocrine hormones—estrogen and progesterone.

BLOOD VESSELS. The abdominal aorta divides at about the level of the umbilicus and forms the two iliac arteries. Each iliac artery divides to form two arteries, the major one of which is the hypogastric artery. The uterine arteries branch off from the *hypogastric arteries*. The closeness of the uterus to the aorta ensures an ample blood supply to meet the needs of the growing uterus and conceptus.

In addition the ovarian artery, a direct subdivision of the aorta, first supplies the ovary with the blood and then proceeds to join the uterine artery, thus further adding to the blood supply (Fig. 6-12).

In the nonpregnant state the uterine blood vessels are coiled and tortuous. With advancing pregnancy and an enlarging uterus, these blood vessels straighten. The uterine veins follow along the arteries and empty into the internal iliac veins.

INNERVATION. The internal genitals have a rich supply of afferent and efferent autonomic nerves, both motor and sensory.

Parasympathetic fibers from the sacral nerves are probably responsible for producing vasodilation and inhibiting muscular contraction. Efferent sympathetic motor nerves arise from the ganglia of T-5

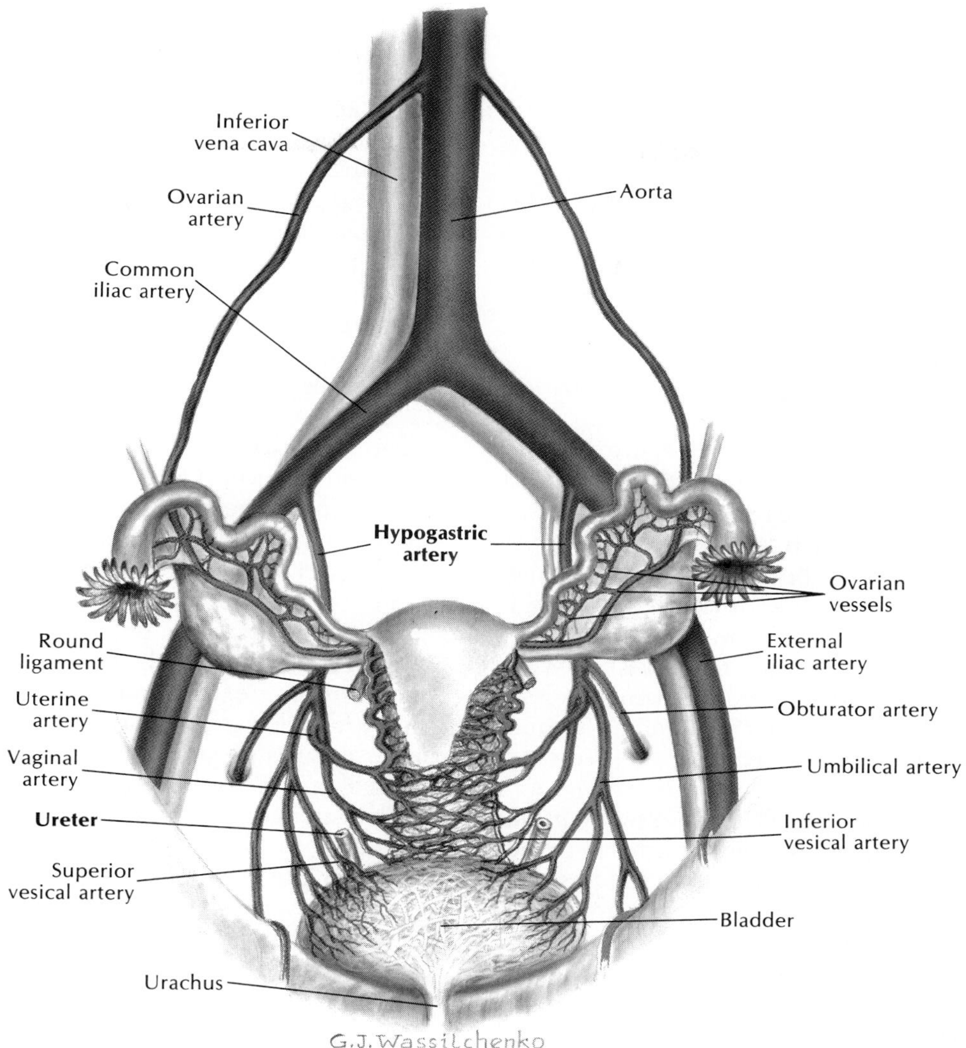

Fig. 6-12 Pelvic blood supply.

(thoracic 5) to T-10, come together over the sacrum, and reach the uterus through ganglia that lie near the base of the uterosacral ligaments. These efferent sympathetic motor nerves are believed to cause vasoconstriction and muscular contraction. The autonomic nerves just described (parasympathetic and efferent sympathetic motor) regulate the action of the uterus, but the uterus has an intrinsic motility (i.e., it can contract and relax even if the nerves to it are cut). This means that even if a woman suffers an accident that injures the spinal cord at or above T-5, she may still be able to have uterine contractions sufficient to deliver an infant vaginally (see spinal cord injury, p. 981).

Sensory fibers carrying pain sensation from the uterus come together in the paracervical areas and proceed upward to pass just below the division (bifurcation) of the aorta, and then travel to the spinal cord at the level of T-11 and T-12. Because of this arrangement, pain that originates in the ovary or in the ureters may mimic pain that originates in the uterus, any of which may be felt in the flank and down to the inguinal and vulvar areas.

VAGINA. The vagina is a tubular structure located in front of the rectum and behind the bladder and urethra (see Fig. 6-8). The vagina extends from the introitus (the external opening in the vestibule between the labia minora of the vulva) to the cervix. When the woman is standing, the vagina slants backward and upward. It is supported mainly by its attachments to the pelvic floor musculature and fascia.

The vagina is a thin-walled, collapsible tube capable of great distension. Because of the way the cervix protrudes into the uppermost portion of the vagina, the length of the anterior wall of the vagina is only about 7.5 cm, while that of the posterior wall is about 9 cm. The recesses formed all around the protruding cervix are called fornices: right, left, anterior, and posterior. The posterior fornix is deeper than the other three (see Figs. 6-6 and 6-15).

The smooth muscle walls are lined with glandular mucous membrane. During the reproductive years this mucosa is arranged in transverse folds called *rugae*.

The vaginal mucosa responds promptly to estrogen and progesterone stimulation. Cells are lost from the mucosa, especially during the menstrual cycle and pregnancy. Cells scraped from the vaginal mucosa can be used to estimate steroid sex hormone levels.

Vaginal fluid is derived from the lower or upper genital tract. The fluid should be slightly acidic. Acidity is maintained by an interaction between vaginal lactobacilli and glycogen. If the pH rises above 5, the incidence of vaginal infection increases. The continuous flow of fluid from the vagina maintains relative cleanliness of the vagina. Therefore *vaginal douching in normal circumstances is not necessary, nor recommended.*

A *Papanicolaou (Pap) smear,* used throughout the world for cancer detection by cell examination (cytology), is a spread of vaginal mucus from the posterior vaginal fornix and a scraping from the squamocolumnar junction of the cervix fixed in ethyl ether and alcohol and then treated with trichrome nucleocytoplasmic stain (see Chapter 41).

The copious blood supply to the vagina is derived from the descending branches of the uterine artery, the vaginal artery, and the internal pudendal arteries (see Fig. 6-12).

The vagina is relatively insensitive. There is some innervation from the pudendal and hemorrhoidal nerves to the lowest one third. Because of this minimal innervation and lack of special nerve endings, the vagina is the source of little sensation during sexual excitement and coitus and causes less pain during the second stage of labor than if this tissue were well supplied with nerve endings.

The *G-spot* is an area on the anterior vaginal wall beneath the urethra defined by Graefenberg as analogous to the male prostate gland. During sexual arousal it may be stimulated to the point of orgasm with ejaculation into the urethra of fluid similar in nature to prostatic fluid (Herbst, 1992).

The vagina functions as the organ for coitus and as the birth canal.

PELVIC FLOOR AND PERINEUM. The pelvic floor and perineum are composed of the pelvic diaphragm, the urogenital diaphragm or triangle, and the muscles of the external genitals and anus. The perineum is sometimes defined as including all the muscles, fascia, and ligaments of the upper (pelvic) and lower (urogenital) diaphragms. The perineal body adds strength to these structures.

The *upper pelvic diaphragm,* composed of muscles and their fascia and ligaments, extends across the lowest part of the pelvic cavity like a hammock (Fig. 6-13). The largest and most significant portion of the diaphragm is formed by the pair of broad, thin *levator ani muscles* that extend sheetlike between the ischial spines and coccyx, and the sacrum. The levator ani group of muscles is made of three muscle pairs: puborectalis, iliococcygeus, and pubococcygeus muscles. The pubococcygeus muscle is particularly significant for women. It plays a role in sexual sensory function, in bladder control, in controlling perineal relaxation during labor, and in expulsion of the fetus during birth.

The second paired muscles of the upper pelvic diaphragm are the closely joined *coccygeus muscles.* These muscles extend from the ischial spines to the coccyx and lower sacrum. The several parts of the pelvic diaphragm provide a slinglike support to abdominal and pelvic viscera.

The strength and resilience of this sling are derived from the way in which the layered parts of this sling are interwoven and interlaced. *The layers are not fixed; that is, they slide over each other.* This unique arrangement strengthens the supportive capacity of the pelvic diaphragm, allows for dilation of the vagina during the birth process and for its closure after delivery, and assists with constriction of the urethra, vagina, and anal canal, which pass through the diaphragm.

The *lower pelvic diaphragm* is located in the hollow of the pubic arch and consists of the transverse perineal muscles, which originate at the ischial tuberosities and insert into the perineal body. The strong muscle fibers provide support to the anal canal during defecation and to the lower vagina during delivery. The deep transverse perineal muscles join to form a central seam, or raphe. Some of their fibers encircle the urinary meatus and vaginal sphincters.

The *perineum* is located below the upper and lower pelvic diaphragm. Its muscles and fascia reinforce the strength of the pelvic diaphragm and aid in constricting the urinary, vaginal, and anal openings. The *bulbocavernosus muscle* (Fig. 6-14) fibers originate in the perineal body and surround the vaginal opening as the muscle fibers pass forward to insert into the pubis.

The *ischiocavernosus muscles* originate in the tuberosities of the ischium and continue at an angle to insert next to the bulbocavernosus muscles (see Fig.

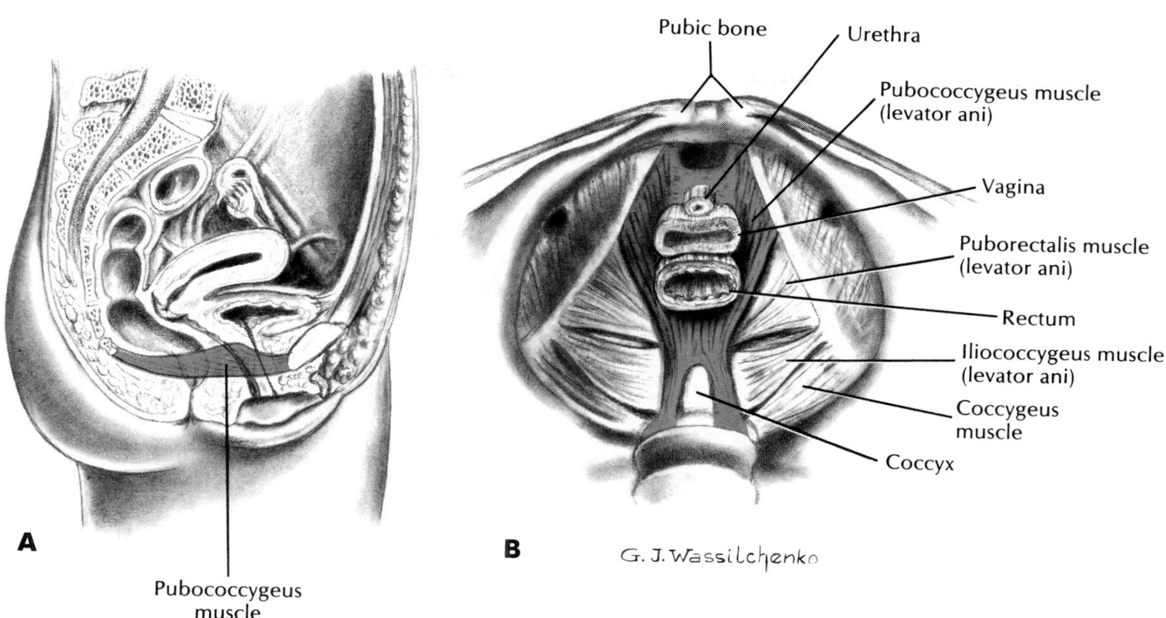

Fig. 6-13 Upper pelvic diaphragm. **A**, Pubococcygeus portion of the levator ani muscles, midsagittal view. **B**, View from above.

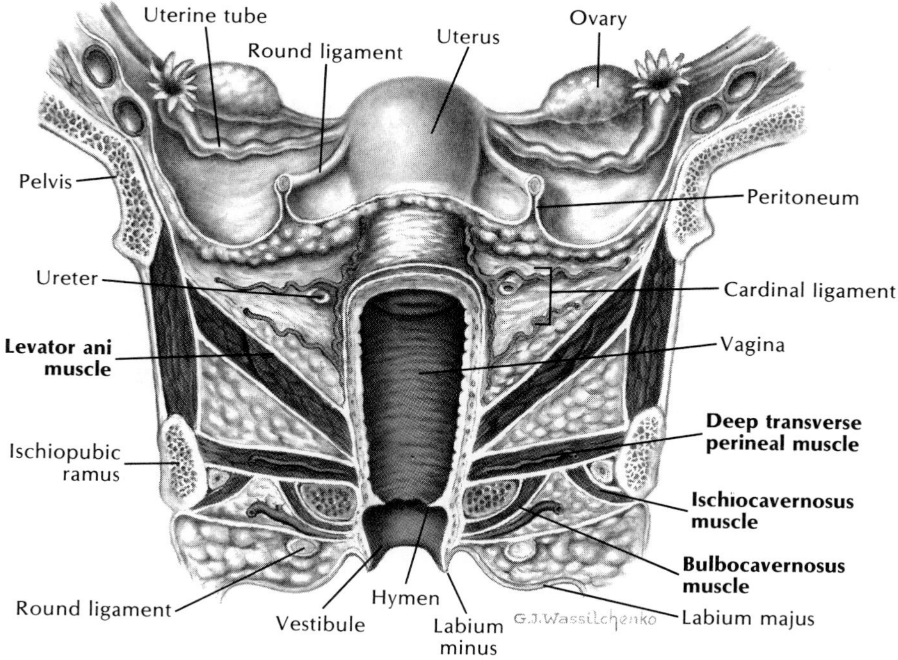

Fig. 6-14 Levator ani muscles of upper pelvic diaphragm and urogenital (lower pelvic) diaphragm, anterior view.

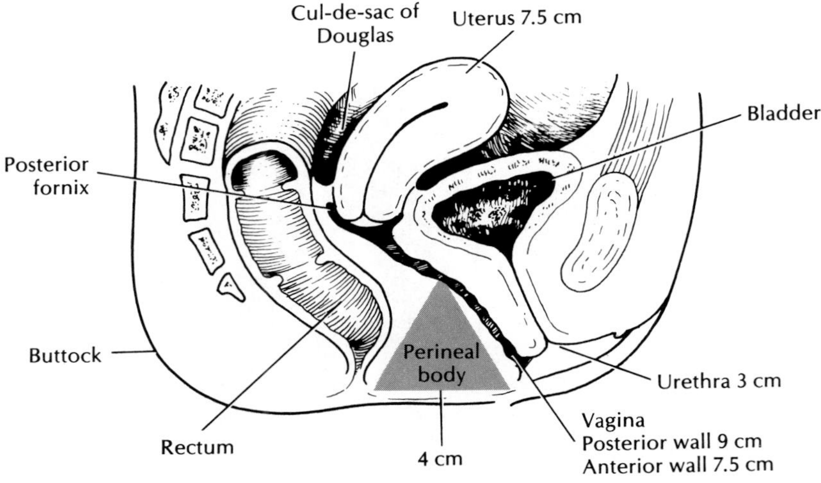

Fig. 6-15 Perineal body. Location and size relative to surrounding tissues, with woman sitting.

6-14). These muscle fibers contract to cause erection of the clitoris.

Anal sphincter muscle fibers originate at the coccyx, separate to pass on either side of the anus, fuse, and then insert into the transverse perineal muscles.

The bulbocavernosus, transverse perineal, and anal sphincter muscle fibers can be strengthened through Kegel exercises (for a description of Kegel exercises, see Chapter 11).

The *perineal body,* the wedge-shaped mass between the vaginal and anal openings, serves as an anchor point for the muscles, fascia, and ligaments of the upper and lower pelvic diaphragms (Fig. 6-15). The skin-covered base of the body is known as the perineum. The perineal body, about 4 cm wide by 4 cm deep, is continuous with the septum between the rectum and vagina. This tissue is flattened and stretched as the fetus moves through the birth canal.

BONY PELVIS. The nurse needs to be thoroughly familiar with the bony pelvis to understand the female reproductive tract and perineum (for an additional discussion of the pelvis related to childbirth, see Chapter 14.) The pelvis serves three primary purposes: (1) Its bony cavity produces a protective cradle for pelvic structures. (2) Its architecture is of special importance in accommodating a growing fetus throughout pregnancy and during the birth process. (3) Its strength provides stable anchorage for the attachment of supportive muscles, fascia, and ligaments.

In a study of the bony pelvis, the following structures and *landmarks* are especially important (Fig. 6-16): iliac crest and superior, anterior iliac spine; sacral promontory; sacrum; coccyx; symphysis pubis; subpubic arch; ischial spines; and ischial tuberosities.

The pelvis (Fig. 6-16, *A*) is made of four bones: (1) and (2) the right and left innominate bones, each of which comprises the right or left pubic bone, ilium, and ischium, which fuse after puberty; (3) the sacrum; and (4) the coccyx. The two *innominate bones* (hip bones) form the sides and front of the bony passage, and the *sacrum* and *coccyx* form the back.

Below the *ilium* is the *ischium,* a heavy bone terminating posteriorly in the rounded protuberances known as the *ischial tuberosities* (see Fig. 6-16, *B*). The tuberosities bear the body's weight in the sitting position. The *ischial spines,* the sharp projections from the posterior border of the ischium into the pelvic cavity, may be blunt or prominent.

The *pubis,* forming the front portion of the pelvic cavity, is located beneath the mons. In the midline the two pubic bones are joined by strong ligaments and a thick cartilage to form the joint called the symphysis pubis. In the female the angle formed by the subpubic arch optimally measures slightly more than 90 degrees.

The *sacrum* is formed by five fused vertebrae. The upper anterior portion of the body of the first sacral vertebra, the promontory, forms the posterior margin of the pelvic brim.

The *coccyx* (tailbone), composed of three to five fused vertebrae, articulates with the sacrum. The coccyx projects downward and forward from the lower border of the sacrum.

The pelvis is divided into two sections, the shallow

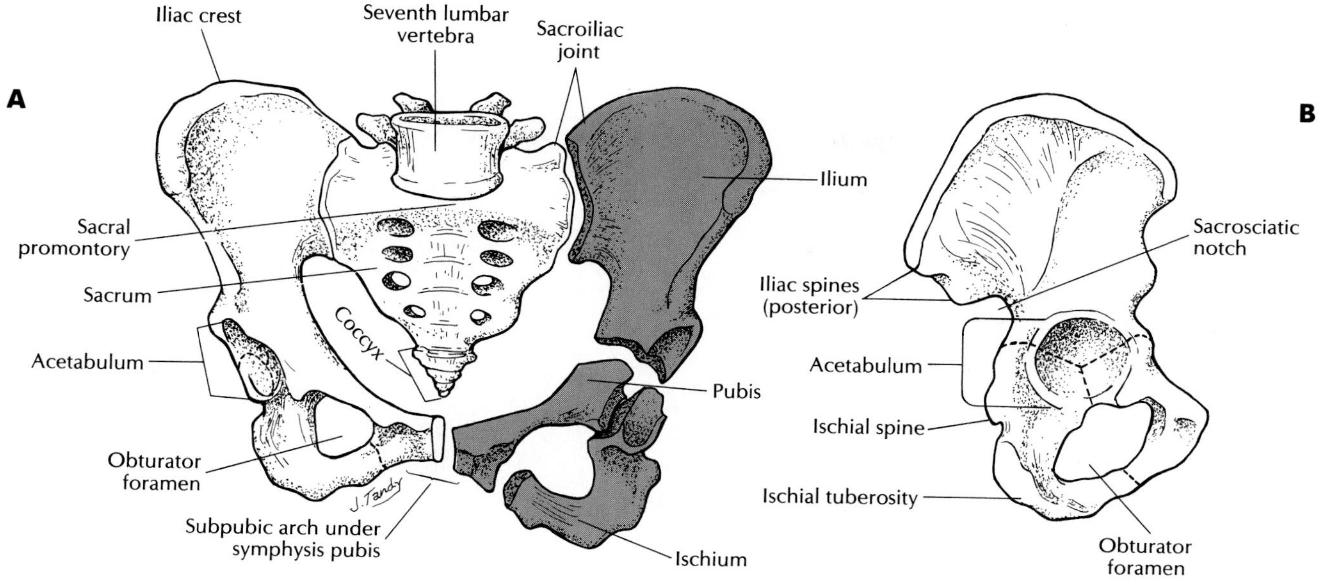

Fig. 6-16 Adult female pelvis. **A,** Anterior view. The three embryonic parts of the left innominate bone are lightly shaded. **B,** External view of right innominate bone (fused).

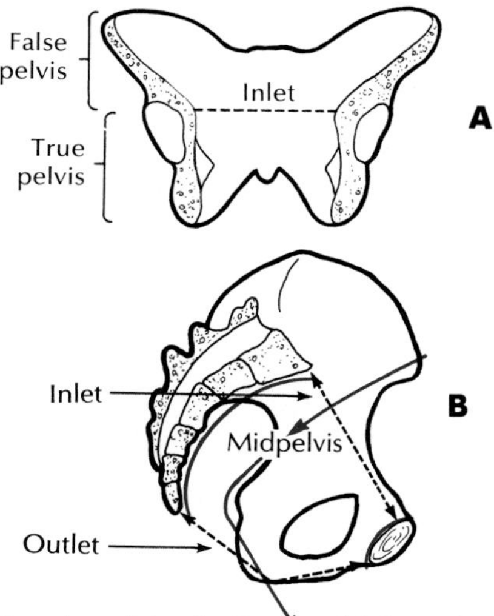

Fig. 6-17 Female pelvis. **A,** Cavity of false pelvis is shallow basin above inlet; true pelvis is deeper cavity below inlet. **B,** Cavity of true pelvis is an irregularly curved canal *(arrows)*.

upper basin, or false pelvis, and the deeper lower, or true, pelvis (Fig. 6-17, *A*). The *false pelvis* lies above the linea terminalis (brim or inlet) and varies considerably in size in different women. The *true pelvis* consists of the brim, or inlet, and the area below.

Pelvic planes include those of the *inlet,* the *midpelvis,* and the *outlet*. The cavity of the (true) mid pelvis resembles an irregularly curved canal (Fig. 6-17, *B*) with unequal anterior and posterior surfaces. The anterior surface is formed by the length of the symphysis (4.5 cm). The posterior surface is formed by the length of the sacrum (12 cm).

Age, sex, and race are responsible for the greatest variations in pelvic shape and size. There is considerable change in the pelvis during growth and development. Pelvic ossification is complete at about 20 years of age or slightly later. Smaller people have smaller, lighter bones than larger people. (Osteoporosis is discussed in Chapter 41.)

Breasts

The breasts are paired mammary glands located between the second and sixth ribs (Fig. 6-18). About two thirds of the breast overlies the pectoralis major muscle, between the sternum and midaxillary line, with an extension to the axilla referred to as the tail of Spence. The lower one third of the breast overlies the serratus anterior muscle. The breasts are attached to the muscles by connective tissue or fascia.

The breasts of healthy mature women are approximately equal in size and shape but are often not absolutely symmetric. The size and shape vary depending on the woman's age, heredity, and nutrition. However, the contour should be smooth with no retractions, dimpling, or masses.

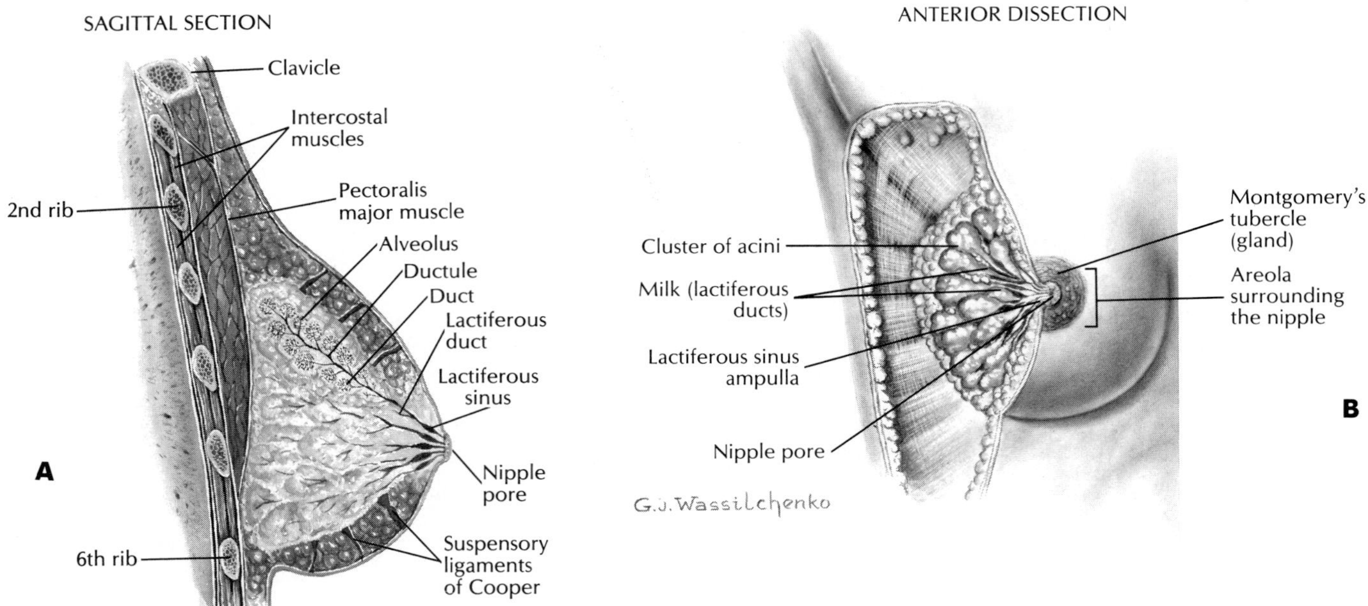

Fig. 6-18 Position and structure of mammary gland. **A,** Sagittal section. **B,** Anterior dissection.
A, Sagittal section from Seidel et al: *Mosby's guide to physical assessment,* ed 2, St Louis, 1991, Mosby–Year Book.

True glandular tissue is called *parenchyma;* supporting tissues, the fat, and fibrous connective tissue are called *stroma.* It is the relative amount of stroma that determines the size and consistency of the breast.

Estrogen stimulates growth of the breast by inducing fat deposition in the breasts, development of stromal tissue (i.e., increase in its amount and elasticity), and growth of the extensive ductile system. Estrogen also increases the vascularity of breast tissue.

Once ovulation begins in puberty, progesterone levels increase. The increase in progesterone causes maturation of mammary gland tissue, specifically the lobules and acinar structures. During adolescence fat deposition and growth of fibrous tissue contribute to the increase in the size of the gland. Full development of the breast is not achieved until after the end of the first pregnancy or in the early period of lactation.

Each mammary gland is made of 15 to 20 lobes, which are divided into lobules. Lobules are clusters of acini. An acinus is a saclike terminal part of a compound gland emptying through a narrow lumen or duct. In discussions of mammary glands the correct anatomic term *(acinus)* is often used interchangeably with *alveolus.* The acini are lined with epithelial cells that secrete colostrum and milk. Just below the epithelium is the myoepithelium (*myo,* or muscle), which contracts to expel milk from the acini (Fig. 6-19).

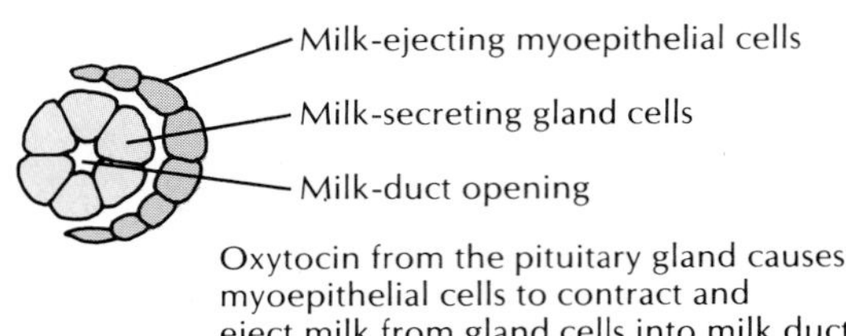

Fig. 6-19 Acinus in cross section.

The ducts from the clusters of acini that form the lobules merge to form larger ducts draining the lobes. Ducts from the lobes converge in a single nipple (papilla) surrounded by an areola. Just as the ducts converge, they dilate to form common lactiferous sinuses, which are also called ampullae. The lactiferous sinuses serve as milk reservoirs. Many tiny lactiferous ducts drain the ampullae and exit in the nipple.

The glandular structures and ducts are surrounded by protective fatty tissue and are separated and supported by fibrous suspensory *Cooper's ligaments.* Cooper's ligaments provide support to the mammary glands while permitting their mobility on the chest wall.

The round nipple is usually slightly elevated above the breast. On each breast the nipple projects slightly upward and laterally. It contains 15 to 20 openings from lactiferous ducts. The nipple (mammary papilla) is surrounded by fibromuscular tissue and covered by wrinkled skin. Except during pregnancy and lactation, there is no discharge from the nipple.

The nipple and surrounding areola are usually more deeply pigmented than the skin of the breast. The rough appearance of the areola is caused by sebaceous glands, *Montgomery tubercles* (see Fig. 6-18), directly beneath the skin. These glands secrete a fatty substance that is thought to lubricate the nipple. Smooth muscle fibers in the areola contract to stiffen the nipple to make it easier for the breastfeeding child to grasp.

The vascular supply to the mammary gland is abundant. In the nonpregnant state the skin does not have an obvious vascular pattern. The normal skin is smooth without tightness or shininess.

The skin covering the breasts contains an extensive superficial lymphatic network that serves the entire chest wall and is continuous with the superficial lymphatics of the neck and abdomen. In the deeper portions of the breasts the lymphatics form a rich network as well. The primary deep lymphatic pathway drains laterally toward the axillae.

Besides their function of lactation, breasts function as organs for sexual arousal in the mature adult.

The breasts change in size and nodularity in response to cyclic ovarian changes throughout reproductive life. Increasing levels of both estrogen and progesterone in the 3 to 4 days before menstruation increase vascularity of the breasts, induce growth of the ducts and acini, and promote water retention. The epithelial cells lining the ducts proliferate in number, the ducts dilate, and the lobules distend. The acini become enlarged and secretory, and lipid (fat) is deposited within their epithelial cell lining. As a result, breast swelling, tenderness, and discomfort are common symptoms just before the onset of menstruation. After menstruation, cellular proliferation begins to regress, acini begin to decrease in size, and retained water is lost.

After breasts have undergone changes numerous times in response to the ovarian cycle, the proliferation and involution (regression) are not uniform throughout the breast. In time, after repeated hormonal stimulation, small persistent areas of nodulations may develop. This normal physiologic change must be remembered when breast tissue is examined. Nodules may develop just before and during menstruation, when the breast is most active. The physiologic alterations in breast size and activity reach their minimum level about 5 to 7 days after menstruation stops. Therefore breast self-examination is best carried out during this phase of the menstrual cycle (Fig. 6-20).

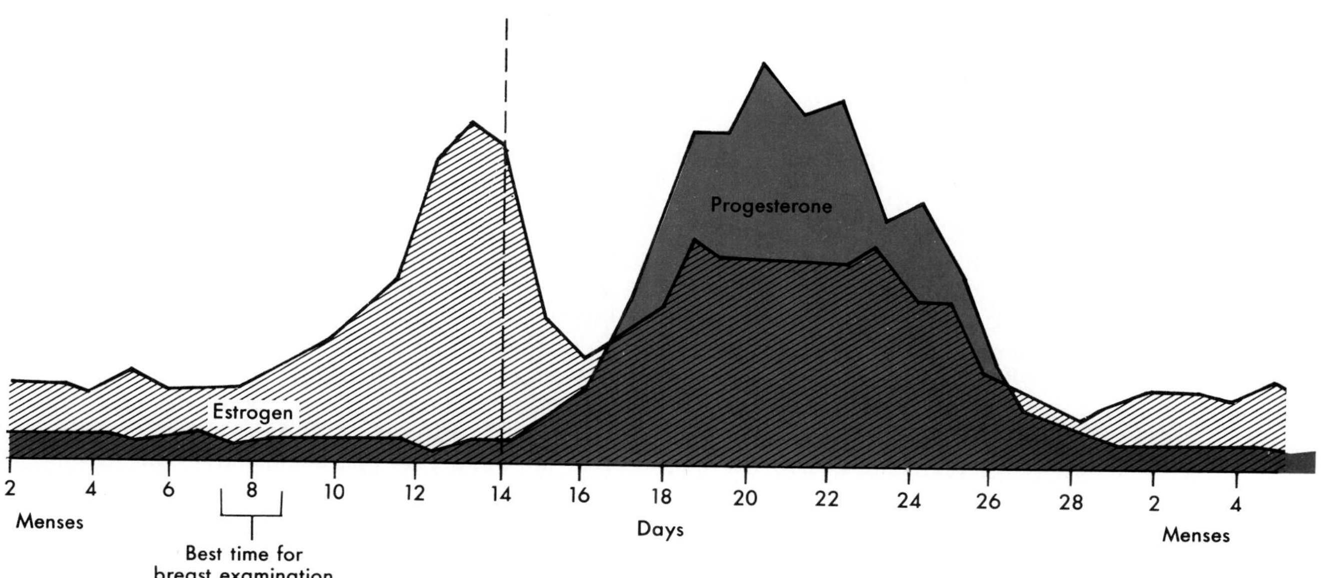

Fig. 6-20 Breast tissue changes in response to hormonal levels of menstrual cycle. Breast self-examination is done when hormonal stimulation is lowest.

Menstrual Cycle

Knowledge of the menstrual cycle is important for nurses providing care to women across the life span. Nurses should be knowledgeable about menstrual myths, menarche, the endometrial cycle, the hypothalamic-pituitary cycle, the ovarian cycle, other cyclic changes, and the climacterium.

MENSTRUAL MYTHS. Many myths have their origin in the mystery that surrounded the woman, her hidden reproductive organs, and her uniqueness in adding new members to society. As a consequence a vast store of folklore, fancies, and superstitions has evolved. Because of their recurring nature and similar sequence, menstrual cycles were thought to be under the control of the moon. Before the discovery of ovulation in humans, it was thought that an egg was produced during menstruation only when fruitful intercourse had occurred. Not until the nineteenth century was knowledge available about the existence of the human egg, ovulation, and ovarian functioning.

An awareness of some myths about menstruation is necessary to use the nursing process effectively with both female and male clients. The menstruating woman is seen as being vulnerable to physical and psychologic stress. Recall some of the myths you may have heard: "Don't wash your hair," "Don't take a bath," "Watch out, you'll catch cold," "That's too heavy for you to carry now."

As late as the second half of this century the many behavioral changes falsely attributed to women during their menstrual cycles have been used to argue, for example, why it would be unwise to have a woman for president of the United States. Historical literature contains many references to dangers attributed to menstruating women. Should a menstruating woman walk through a farmer's fields, the crops would not grow and the flowers would wilt; if she tried to bake bread, the dough would not rise. The danger also exists for her husband so that physical contact, especially sexual intercourse, was and in some places still is prohibited. In many cultures the menstruating woman is kept in a separate menstrual hut or in separate quarters. Following a ritualized "cleansing" the woman returns to her place in her family.

MENARCHE. Although young girls secrete small, rather constant amounts of estrogen, a marked increase occurs between 8 and 11 years of age. Moreover, increasing amounts and variations in gonadotropin and estrogen secretion develop into a cyclic pattern at least a year before menarche or the first menstrual period. This occurs in most girls in North America at about 13 years of age.

Initially periods are irregular, unpredictable, painless, and anovulatory in the majority of young girls. After one or more years a hypothalamic-pituitary rhythm develops, and adequate cyclic estrogen is produced by the ovary to mature a number of graafian follicles. Approximately 14 days *before* the beginning of the next menstrual period, pituitary follicle-stimulating hormone (FSH) rises, a surge of luteinizing hormone (LH) is released by the anterior pituitary, and ovulation (extrusion of the ovum) occurs.

Ovulatory periods tend to be regular, monitored by progesterone. In some women ovulatory periods are associated with *dysmenorrhea* (painful uterine cramping), which may be an effect of progesterone or prostaglandins or both (for further discussion, see Chapter 41). This discomfort is rarely serious and is readily relieved by a hot water bottle, exercise, or simple analgesics. When viewed in its proper perspective, slight cramping may be reassuring to the girl and her parents as an indication of normal ovulatory function.

Although pregnancy may occur in exceptional cases of true (constitutional) precocious puberty, most pregnancies in young girls occur well after the normally timed menarche. *However, all girls would benefit from knowing that pregnancy can occur at any time after the onset of menses.*

ENDOMETRIAL CYCLE. **Menstruation** is periodic uterine bleeding that begins with the shedding of secretory endometrium approximately 14 days after ovulation. The first day of the menstrual discharge has been designated as *day 1* of the **endometrial cycle** (Fig. 6-21). The average duration of menstrual flow is 5 days (range of 3 to 6 days), and the average blood loss is approximately 50 mL (range of 20 to 80 mL), but there is great variation. During menstruation the average daily loss of iron is 0.5 to 1 mg. If the woman's usual blood loss is over 80 mL, she will most likely need iron supplementation to prevent secondary anemia.

For about 50% of women, menstrual blood does not appear to clot. The menstrual blood clots within the uterus, but the clot is liquefied before it is discharged from the uterus. If the discharge leaves the uterus too rapidly, liquefaction may not be complete so that clots will appear in the vagina. Uterine discharge includes mucus and epithelial cells in addition to blood.

The purpose of the menstrual cycle is to prepare the uterus for pregnancy. When pregnancy does not occur, menstruation follows. The individual's age, physical and emotional status, and environment in-

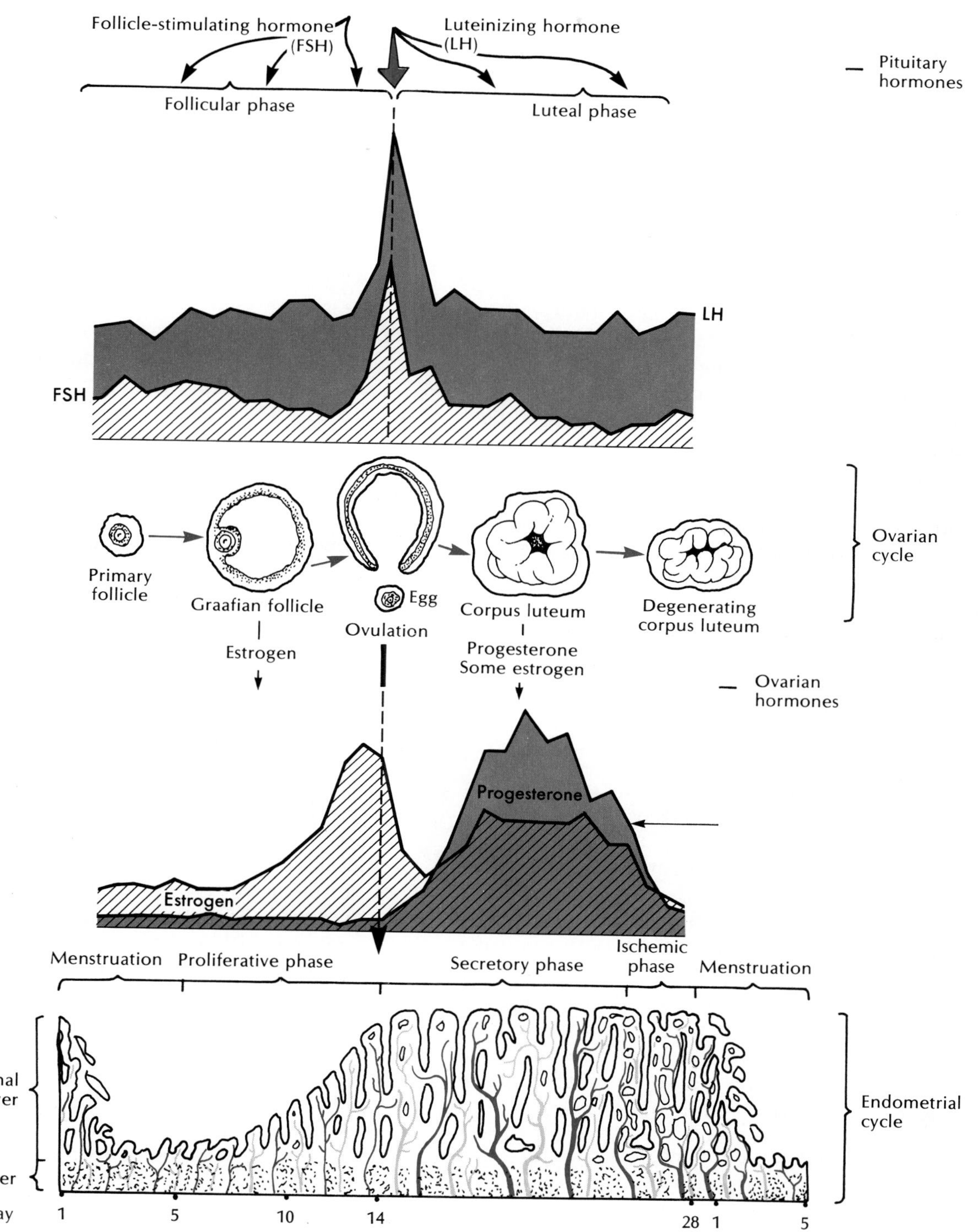

Fig. 6-21 Menstrual cycle: hypothalamic-pituitary, ovarian, and endometrial.

fluence the regularity of her menstrual cycles.

The four phases of the menstrual cycle are (1) the menstrual phase, (2) the proliferative phase, (3) the secretory phase, and (4) the ischemic phase. During the *menstrual phase*, shedding of the functional two thirds of the endometrium (the compact and spongy layers) is initiated by periodic vasoconstriction of the spiral arterioles most marked in the upper layers of the endometrium. The basal layer is always retained, and regeneration begins near the end of the cycle from cells derived from the remaining glandular remnants or stromal cells in the basalis.

The *proliferative phase* is a period of rapid growth that extends from about the fifth day to the time of ovulation, which would be, for example, day 10 of a 24-day cycle, day 14 of a 28-day cycle, or day 18 of a 32-day cycle. The endometrial surface is completely restored in approximately 4 days or slightly before bleeding ceases. From this point on an eightfold to tenfold thickening occurs, with a leveling off of growth at ovulation. Early in the proliferative phase the functional layer is moderately dense and only slightly vascular. Three or four days before ovulation the glands develop and vascularity is increased. The proliferative phase depends on estrogen stimulation derived from ovarian (graafian) follicles.

The *secretory phase* extends from the day of ovulation to about 3 days before the next menstrual period. After ovulation, larger amounts of progesterone are produced. This hormone causes the glands to become tortuous, serrated, and widened. An edematous, vascular, functional endometrium is now apparent. The cells lining the glands secrete a thin, glycogen-containing fluid.

At the end of the secretory phase the fully matured secretory endometrium reaches the thickness of heavy, soft velvet. It becomes luxuriant with blood and glandular secretions, a suitable protective and nutritive bed for a fertilized ovum, should one be available.

Implantation (nidation) of the fertilized ovum generally occurs about 7 to 10 days after ovulation. If fertilization and implantation do not occur, the corpus luteum (yellow body) regresses. With the rapid fall in progesterone and estrogen levels the spiral arteries go into a spasm. During the *ischemic phase* the blood supply to the functional endometrium is blocked and necrosis develops. The functional layer separates from the basal layer, and menstrual bleeding begins, marking day 1 of the next cycle.

HYPOTHALAMIC-PITUITARY CYCLE. Toward the end of the normal menstrual cycle, blood levels of estrogen and progesterone fall (Fig. 6-20). Low blood levels of these ovarian hormones stimulate the hypothalamus to secrete gonadotropin-releasing hormone (Gn-RH). Gn-RH in turn stimulates anterior pituitary secretion of FSH. FSH stimulates development of ovarian graafian follicles and their production of estrogen. Estrogen levels begin to fall, and hypothalamic Gn-RH triggers the anterior pituitary release of LH. A marked surge of LH and a smaller peak of estrogen (day 12, Fig. 6-20) precede the expulsion of the ovum from the graafian follicle by about 24 to 36 hours. LH peaks about the thirteenth or fourteenth day of a 28-day cycle. If fertilization and implantation (nidation) of the ovum have not occurred by this time, regression of the corpus luteum (yellow body) follows (for a discussion of fertilization and implantation, see Chapter 7). Therefore the levels of progesterone and estrogen decline, menstruation occurs, and the hypothalamus is once again stimulated to secrete Gn-RH. This is called the **hypothalamic-pituitary cycle.**

OVARIAN CYCLE. The primitive graafian follicles contain immature oocytes (primordial ova; see Fig. 6-4). Before ovulation, from 1 to 30 follicles begin to mature in each ovary under the influence of FSH and estrogen. The preovulatory surge of LH affects a selected follicle. Within the chosen follicle the oocyte matures, ovulation occurs, and the empty follicle begins its transformation into the corpus luteum. This *follicular phase* (preovulatory phase; Fig. 6-21) of the ovarian menstrual cycle varies in length from woman to woman. *Almost all variations in* **ovarian cycle** *length are the result of variations in the length of the follicular phase.* On rare occasions (1 in 100 menstrual cycles), more than one follicle is chosen and more than one oocyte matures and undergoes ovulation (see discussion of twins, Chapter 7).

After ovulation, estrogen levels drop. For 90% of women, only a small amount of **withdrawal bleeding** occurs so that it goes unnoticed. In 10% of women there is sufficient bleeding for it to be visible, resulting in what is known as *midcycle bleeding*.

The *luteal phase* begins immediately after ovulation and ends with the start of menstruation. This postovulatory phase of the ovarian cycle usually requires *14 days* (range of 13 to 15 days). The corpus luteum (yellow body) reaches its peak of functional activity 8 days after ovulation, secreting both of the steroids estrogen and progesterone. Coincident with this time of peak luteal functioning, the fertilized egg is implanted in the endometrium. If no implantation occurs, the corpus luteum regresses, and steroid levels drop. Two weeks after ovulation, if fertilization and implantation do not occur, the functional layer of the uterine endometrium is shed through menstruation.

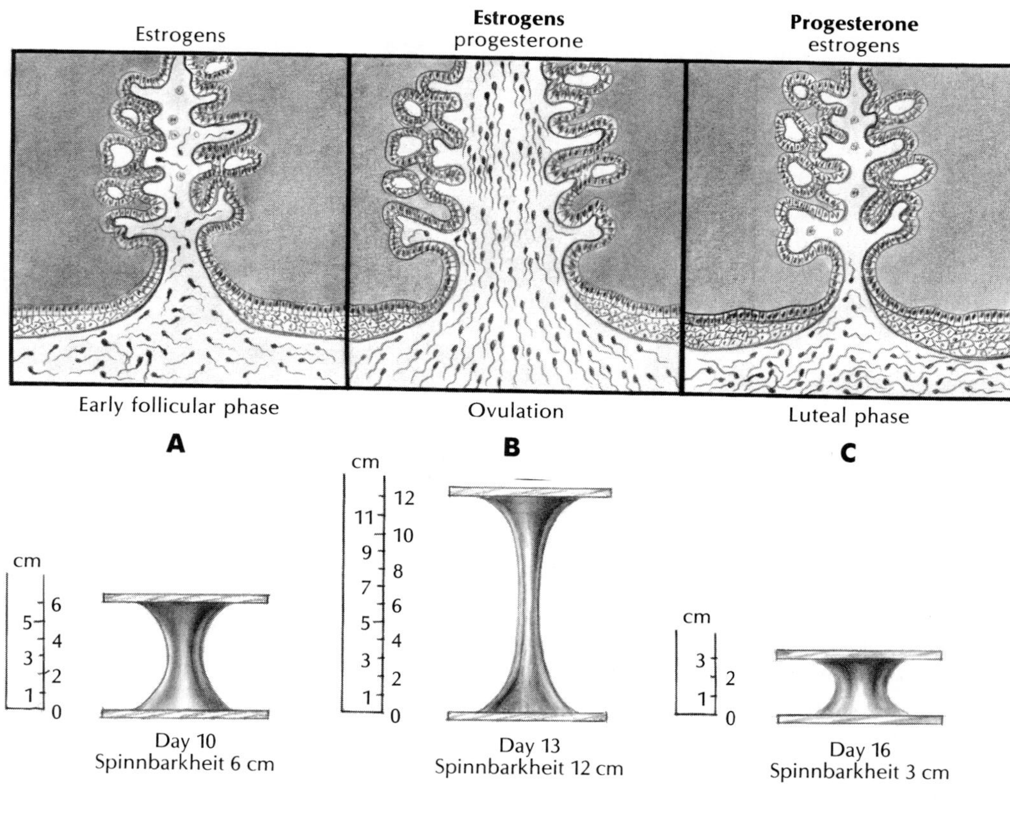

Fig. 6-22 Changes in cervix and in cervical mucus during menstrual cycle. **A**, Changes in opening of the cervix that facilitate sperm migration. **B**, Characteristic stretchable quality of cervical mucus demonstrated between two glass slides.

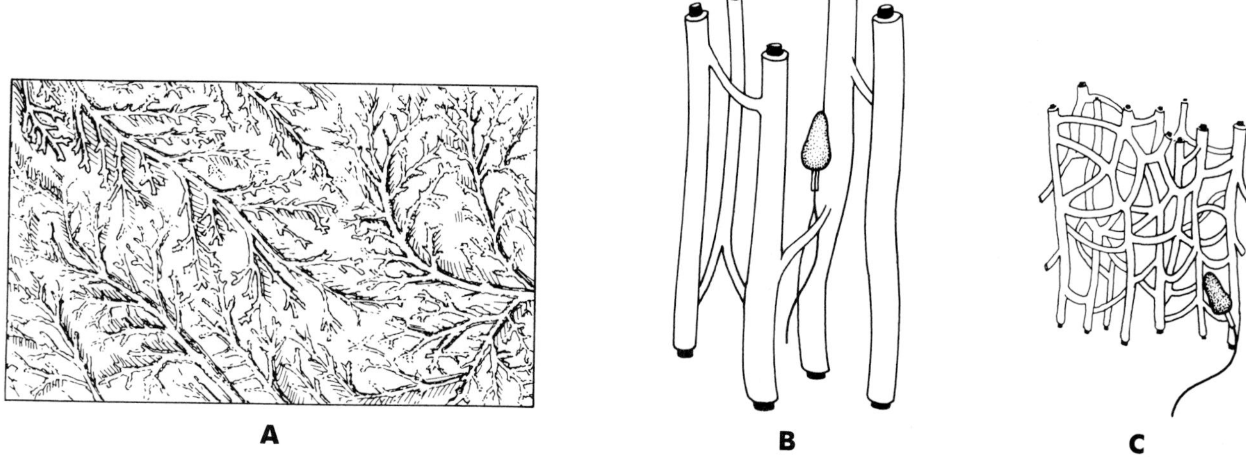

Fig. 6-23 Cervical mucus changes during menstrual cycle. **A**, Fern pattern under estrogen influence. **B**, Mucus receptive to sperm passage under estrogen influence. **C**, Mucus nonreceptive to sperm passage under progesterone influence.
From Fogel CI, Woods NF: *Health care of women: a nursing perspective*, St Louis, 1981, Mosby–Year Book.

OTHER CYCLIC CHANGES. When the hypothalamic-pituitary-ovarian axis is functioning properly, other tissues undergo predictable responses. Before ovulation the woman's basal body temperature (BBT) is lower, often below 98.6° F (37° C); after ovulation, with rising progesterone levels, her BBT rises (see also Chapter 42). Changes in the cervix and cervical mucus follow a generally predictable pattern (Figs. 6-22 and 6-23). Preovulatory and postovulatory mucus is viscous (sticky) so that sperm penetration is discouraged. At the time of ovulation, cervical mucus is thin and clear. It looks, feels, and stretches like egg white. This stretchable quality is termed **spinnbarkheit** (Fig. 6-22). Some women experience localized lower abdominal pain called **mittelschmerz** that coincides with ovulation.

These and other cyclic changes enhance fertility awareness and form the basis for the symptothermal method used for conception and contraception. The subjective and objective signs are biologic markers of the phases of the menstrual cycle (Table 6-1). Examination of women with impaired fertility includes a thorough documentation of the presence or absence of these biologic markers (Chapter 42).

CLIMACTERIUM. The **climacterium** (perimenopause) is a transitional phase during which ovarian function and hormone production are declining. This phase spans the years from the onset of premenopausal ovarian decline to the postmenopausal time when symptoms stop. **Menopause** (from the French *meno,* menstruation, and *pause,* stop) refers only to the last menstrual period. However, unlike menarche, menopause can be dated with certainty only at 1 year after menstruation ceases. The average age at natural menopause is 51.4 years, with an age range of 35 to 60 years. Menopause is an unmistakable biologic marker for the end of reproductive function.

■ MALE REPRODUCTIVE SYSTEM

The male reproductive system consists of external genitals and internal organs located in the pelvic cavity. The male's reproductive system begins to develop in response to testosterone during early fetal life. Essentially no testosterone is produced during childhood. Resumption of testosterone production at the onset of puberty stimulates growth and maturation of reproductive structures and secondary sex characteristics.

External Structures

The structures that make up the external genitals are presented in the following order: mons pubis, penis, and scrotum.

At maturity, pubic hair is long, dense, coarse, and curly, forming a diamond-shaped pattern from the umbilicus to the anus. The area over the symphysis pubis is referred to as the *mons pubis.*

The *penis,* an organ of urination and copulation, consists of the shaft, or body, and the glans (Fig. 6-24). The shaft of this external male reproductive organ, which enters the vagina during coitus, is composed of three cylindric layers and erectile tissue, two lateral *corpora cavernosa* and a *corpus spongiosum,* which contains the urethra. These corpora terminate distally in the smooth, sensitive *glans penis,* which is the counterpart of the female glans clitoris.

Skin and fascia loosely envelop the penis to permit enlargement during erection. The glans is the enlarged end of the penis that contains many sensitive nerve endings and a urethral meatus at the tip (usually). The *prepuce* (foreskin), an extended fold of skin, covers the glans in uncircumcised males (Fig. 6-25). In the newborn the foreskin is generally not retractable and may not be retractable for 4 to 6 months or even as long as 13 years. It is easily retractable in the adolescent and the adult. With sexual arousal, neurocirculatory factors cause considerable increase in blood flow to the erectile tissue of the corpora, and enlargement and erection of the penis occur.

The *urethra* is a common passageway for both urine and semen (see Figs. 6-24 and 6-25).

The *scrotum,* a wrinkled pouch of skin, muscles, and fascia (see Fig. 6-25), is divided internally by a septum, and each compartment normally contains one *testis, epididymis,* and *vas deferens* (seminal duct). The left side of the scrotum hangs somewhat lower (about 1 cm) than the right side. The skin is abundantly supplied with sebaceous and sweat glands and is sparsely covered with hair. Under the skin are found the *cremaster* fascia and thin smooth muscle layer. Contraction and relaxation of this smooth muscle result in retraction of the testes to protect them from external trauma and cold. During hot external (environmental) or internal (fever) temperature the cremaster muscle relaxes, lowering the testes away from the body. Conversely, cold external temperature stimulates contraction of the cremaster muscle to bring the testes close to the body.

TABLE 6-1 Signs and Symptoms of the Phases of the Menstrual Cycle

Sign	Preovulation	Ovulation	At Least 2 Days After Ovulation up to Menses
SUBJECTIVE SIGNS			
Physical discomfort			
Breasts	Unreported	Unreported	Heaviness, fullness; enlarged, tender*
Abdomen	Dysmenorrhea: uterine cramping; nausea, vomiting, and diarrhea; dizziness	Intermenstrual pain (mittelschmerz) occurs 1.7 days after peak of cervical mucus and 2.5 days before increase in BBT	Premenstrual syndrome: backaches; feeling of increasing pelvic fullness
General	Increased weight; feeling of heaviness	Unreported	Headache†; acne
Affective changes‡			
Moods	Some depression may persist from premenses	Sense of well-being	Premenstrual syndrome (PMS): increased irritability, passivity, depression
Libido	Unreported	Increases sexual desire	Unreported
Energy levels	Unreported	Unreported	Spurt of energy, followed by fatigue
OBJECTIVE SIGNS			
BBT	Individualized, often below 98.6° F (37° C)	Slight drop in BBT	Rise of about 0.4°-0.8° F (0.2-0.4° C)
Respiration	Unreported	Unreported	Hyperventilation with decrease in alveolar P_{CO_2}
Heart rate	Unreported	Unreported	Increased slightly
Breasts	Time of least hormonal effect and smallest breast size	Increased nipple erectility; increased areolar pigmentation	Increased nodularity; enlarged
Cervix (see Figs. 6-22 and 6-23)			
Mucus characteristics	"Dry" (no mucus) progressing to viscous, opaque; no ferning	Abundant, thin, clear (egg-white) mucus with spinnbarkheit (4 cm, often up to 10 cm) that dries in a fern pattern (arborization); facilitates sperm transport	Cloudy, sticky, impenetrable to sperm; dries in granular pattern (no ferning)
Mucus pH	About 7.0	7.5	Unreported
Os	Gradual, progressive widening	Open, with mucus seen spilling out	Gradual closing of os
Color of exocervix	Pink	Hyperemic (red)	Gradual return to pink
Body	Firm to touch (like tip of nose)	Soft (like earlobe)	Gradual return to firm

*Sociocultural influences may affect symptoms reported by women. Breast tenderness is rarely reported by Japanese women.

†Headaches reported with greater frequency by Nigerian women.

‡NOTE: Literature usually attributes negative premenstrual symptoms to biology, while good moods and rational behavior are not. When men and women are compared in activity patterns, mood changes, and symptoms, similar variability has been found in *both* men and women even though the changes in women are given more attention by society.

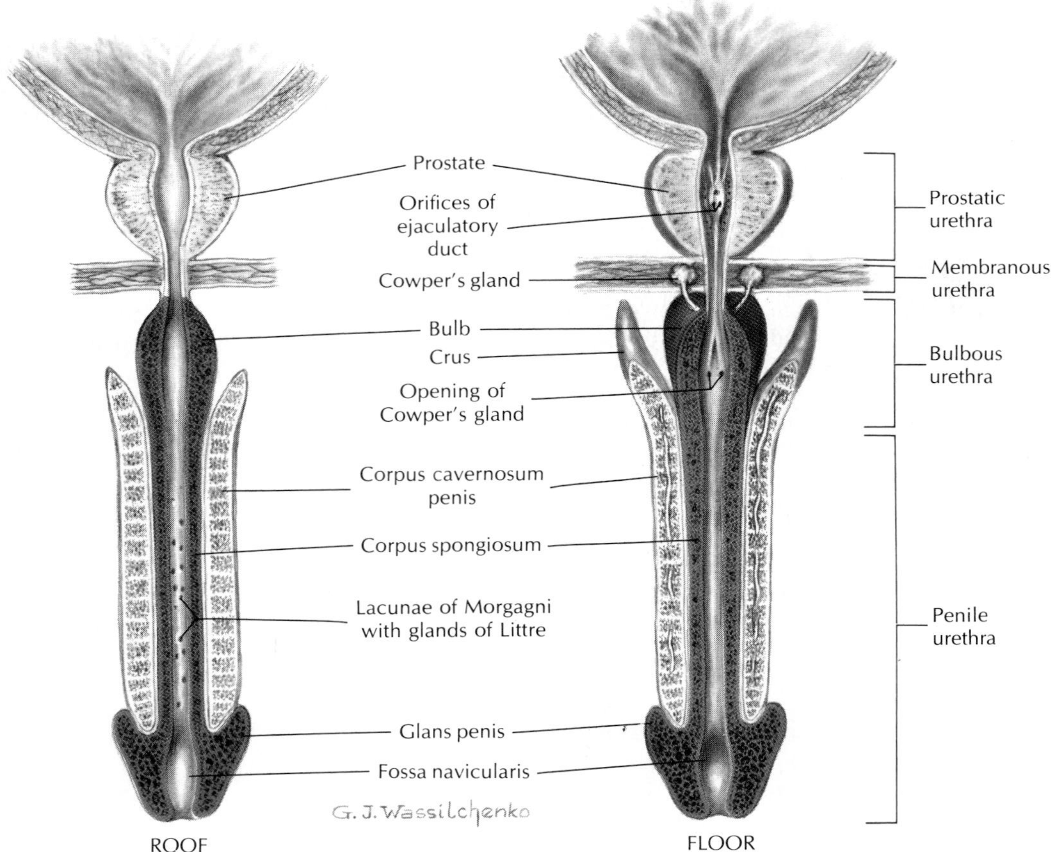

Fig. 6-24 Anatomy of urethra and penis.

The purpose of this mobility is to maintain the testes within an optimum temperature range for the production and viability of sperm. Hot tubs, tight underwear (jockey shorts) and pants, and long-term sitting (long-distance truck drivers) present too hot an external environment or prevent testicular mobility so that spermatogenesis and sperm are jeopardized.

Internal Structures

Internal structures (see Figs. 6-24 and 6-25) include: testes, ducts of the testes, and accessory reproductive tract glands.

TESTES. The testes are two small ovoid glands located within the scrotal sac. Both are suspended by attachment to scrotal tissue and the spermatic cord. Originally located in the abdomen, the testes descend through the inguinal canal by the end of the seventh lunar month of fetal life. At term birth one or both of the testes may still be within the inguinal canals with final descent into the scrotal sac occurring in the early postnatal period. The testes must be within the scrotum for spermatogenesis to occur.

The testes are similar in origin (homologous) to the ovaries in the female. Each testis is whitish, somewhat flattened from side to side, measures about 4 or 5 cm in length, and weighs 10 to 15 g. White fibrous tissue encases each testis and divides it into several lobules. Within each lobule are one to three long (about 75 cm), narrow, coiled *seminiferous tubules* and clusters of *interstitial cells* (Leydig's cells). Spermatids attach to the germinal epithelium (Sertoli cells) within the seminiferous tubules and develop into sperm. The interstitial cells are large connective and supportive tissue (stromal) cells responsible for the production of the androgen hormone testosterone.

The two principal functions of the testes are spermatogenesis and hormone production. Primitive sex cells (spermatogonia) are present in the seminif-

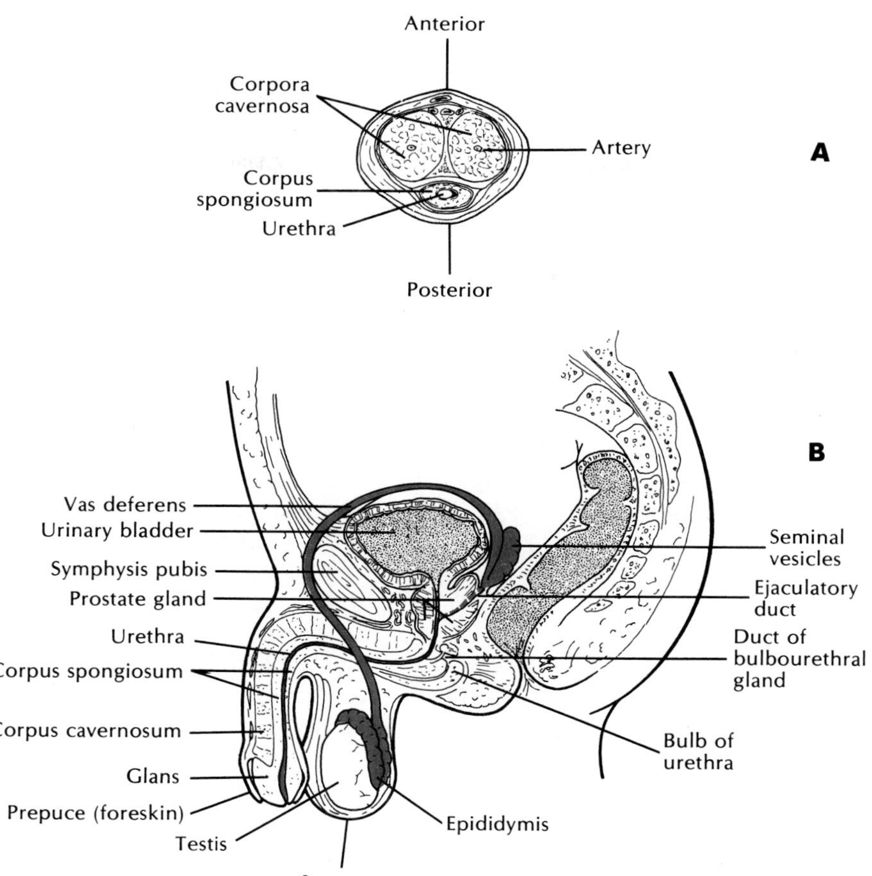

Fig. 6-25 Fascial planes of male lower genitourinary tract. **A,** Transverse section of penis. **B,** Relationship of bladder, prostate, seminal vesicles, penis, urethra, and scrotal contents.

erous tubules of the male newborn. Spermatogenesis, the maturation process that results in sperm, begins during puberty and normally continues throughout a man's lifetime. The testes secrete the steroid sex hormone testosterone in the amounts that are required for normal male growth, development, and function.

DUCTS (CANALS) OF THE TESTES. For sperm to exit the body they must travel the full length of the duct system in succession: seminiferous tubules, epididymides (pl.), vasa deferentia (pl.), ejaculatory ducts, and the urethra. The seminiferous tubules are mentioned earlier. Each testis has one tightly coiled tube, about 6 m (20 ft) in length. This tube, the *epididymis,* (see Fig. 6-25) lies along the top and side of each testis. The epididymides are storage sites for maturing sperm and produce a small part of the seminal fluid (semen). Seminiferous tubules are continuous with the epididymides, which in turn connect to the vasa deferentia.

ACCESSORY REPRODUCTIVE SYSTEM GLANDS. Accessory reproductive glands secrete fluids that support the life and function of sperm. These glands include the paired *seminal vesicles,* located along the lower posterior surface of the bladder; the *prostate gland,* which surrounds the prostatic urethra; and the *bulbourethral* (or Cowper's) *glands,* located below the prostate, one at either side of the membranous urethra (see Figs. 6-24 and 6-25).

SEMEN. Semen is the fluid ejaculated at the time of orgasm. It contains sperm and secretions from the seminal vesicles, prostate gland, and bulbourethral glands. An average volume per ejaculate is 2.5 to 3.5 mL (range: 1 to 10 mL) after several days of continence (no ejaculations). The volume of semen and sperm count decrease rapidly with repeated ejaculations. Semen contains constituents that provide nourishment, support and enhance sperm motility, and buffer the acidic environment of the cervical and vaginal fluids.

Semen is white to opalescent with a specific gravity of 1.028. The pH is alkaline, ranging from 7.35 to 7.5. Sperm count averages 100 million/mL with fewer than 20% abnormal forms. About 60% of the total fluid is derived from the seminal vesicles, about 20% from the prostatic glands. Some fluid is secreted by the bulbourethral glands and probably the urethral glands.

Less than 5% of the ejaculate consists of sperm and fluid from the testes and epididymides. Since vasectomy affects only the production of this portion of the ejaculate, there is no noticeable change in volume, even after sperm are no longer available for transport through the remaining canal system.

A high concentration of prostaglandin is produced by the seminal vesicles, but their function in semen production is not fully understood (Ganong, 1987). Prostaglandins are discussed on pp. 132 and 133.

■ SEXUAL RESPONSE PATTERNS

The hypothalamus and anterior pituitary gland in females and males regulate the production of FSH and LH. The target tissue for these hormones is the gonad: an ovary or testis. In the female the ovary produces ova and secretes estrogen and progesterone; in the male the testis produces sperm and secretes testosterone. A *feedback mechanism* between hormone secretion from the gonads, hypothalamus, and anterior pituitary aids in the control of the production of sex cells and steroid sex hormone secretion (Figs. 6-21 and 6-26).

Physiologic Response to Sexual Stimulation

Although the first outward appearance of maturing sexual development occurs at an earlier age in females, both females and males achieve physical maturity at about the age of 17. However, great variation is possible between individuals' rates of development. Anatomic and reproductive differences notwithstanding, women and men are more alike than different in their physiologic response to sexual excitement and orgasm. For example, the glans clitoris and the glans penis are homologues (see Fig. 6-1). Not only is there little difference between female and male sexual response, but it is also now accepted that the physical response is essentially the same whether the source of stimulation is coitus, fantasy, or mechanical or manual masturbation.

Currently there are two theories to explain the physiologic response to sexual stimulation. The first and most widely used theory is the four-phase response cycle described by Masters and Johnson. The second is Helen Kaplan's biphasic sexual response cycle.

FOUR-PHASE RESPONSE. Physiologically, sexual response, according to Masters and Johnson (1966), can be analyzed in terms of two processes: vasocongestion and myotonia.

Sexual stimulation results in vasocongestion reflex dilation of penile blood vessels (erection in the male) and circumvaginal blood vessels (lubrication in the

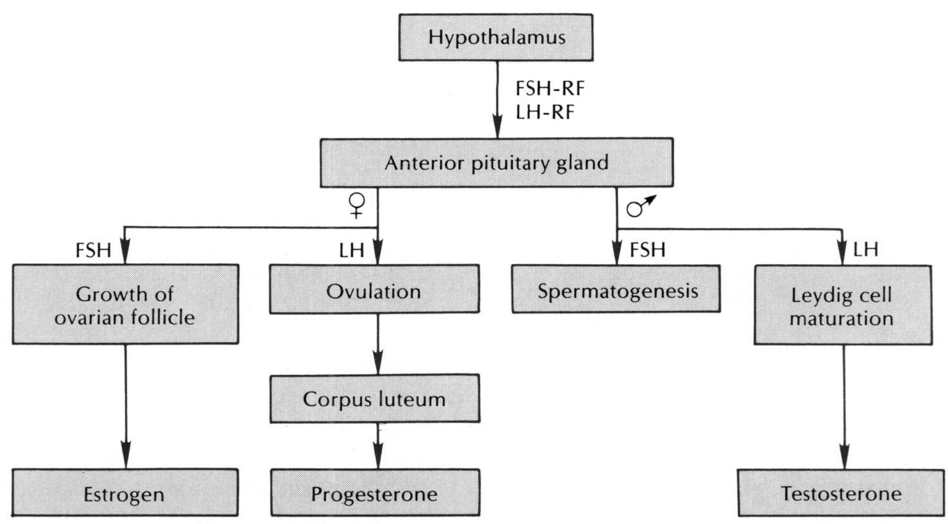

Fig. 6-26 Hypothalamic-pituitary-gonadal axis; comparison of female and male. *RF*, Releasing factor.

female), causing engorgement and distention of the genitals. Venous congestion is localized primarily in the genitals, but it also occurs to a lesser degree in the breasts and other parts of the body.

Arousal is characterized by **myotonia** (increased muscular tension), resulting in voluntary and involuntary rhythmic contractions. Examples of sexually stimulated myotonia are pelvic thrusting, facial grimacing, and spasms of the hands and feet (carpopedal spasms).

The response cycle is arbitrarily divided into four phases: excitement phase, plateau phase, orgasmic phase, and resolution phase. One moves through the four phases progressively, and there is no sharp dividing line between any two phases. However, there are specific body changes that take place in sequence. The time, intensity, and duration for cyclic completion also vary for individuals and situations.

1. EXCITEMENT PHASE. The woman's first observable reaction to sexual stimulation is vaginal lubrication, which has the biologic function of preparing the vagina for penile penetration. The inner two thirds of the vaginal barrel lengthen and distend. The cervix and fundus are pulled upward. The external genitals become congested and darker in color. The clitoris increases in diameter and in tumescence (vascular congestion and swelling).

The man's first observable reaction to sexual stimulation is erection of the penis (increase in length and diameter). The scrotal skin becomes congested and thick. The testes elevate because of contraction of the cremasteric musculature.

2. PLATEAU PHASE. In the woman, the wall of the outer one third of the vagina becomes greatly engorged, along with the labia minora, forming the "orgasmic platform." The clitoris retracts under the clitoral hood to protect the clitoris from intense, direct stimulation.

In the man, preorgasmic emission of two or three drops of mucoid substance is released from the Cowper's glands. The testes continue to elevate until they are situated close to the body to facilitate ejaculatory pressure.

3. ORGASMIC PHASE. Strong, rhythmic (every 0.8 second) muscular contractions occur in the woman's orgasmic platform. The number of contractions ranges from 3 to 15. The uterus also contracts rhythmically.

This phase may be subjectively described as follows:

Stage 1: sensation of "suspension," followed by "intense sensual awareness, clitorally oriented and radiating upward into the pelvis"

Stage 2: "suffusion of warmth" especially in the pelvic area

Stage 3: "pelvic throbbing" located in the vagina and lower pelvis

In men, the testes are held at maximum elevation. Rhythmic contractions of the penis and rectal sphincter occur at 0.8-second intervals for the first three to four major responses.

This phase may be subjectively described as follows:

Stage 1: point of "inevitability," which occurs just before ejaculation and lasts 2 or 3 seconds; awareness of presence of fluid in the urethra

Stage 2: ejaculation with rhythmic contractions capable of expelling semen up to 60 cm (24 in)

4. RESOLUTION PHASE. Blood returns from the engorged walls of the woman's vagina, and the labia majora and minora rapidly return to their unexcited state. The clitoris rapidly returns from under the hood; however, return to normal size may take longer. The uterus descends, and the cervix dips into the seminal pool.

In the first stage of the man's resolution phase 50% of erection is lost rather rapidly. The second stage can last much longer, depending on the maintenance of physical condition.

The *refractory* period is the time necessary to complete the cycle again. The time varies from a few minutes to a few days, depending on the age and state of physical and emotional health.

BIPHASIC RESPONSE. Kaplan (1974) has presented an alternative to the four-phase sexual response cycle of Masters and Johnson. She believes clinical and physiologic evidence suggests that sexual response is biphasic, with the following two distinct and relatively independent components:

1. Genital vasocongestive reaction—produces vaginal lubrication and swelling in the female and penile erection in the male
2. Reflex clonic muscular contractions—constitute orgasm in both sexes

1. VASOCONGESTIVE REACTION. Erection in the male is a local vasocongestive response. During erection the corpora cavernosa become engorged with blood. Special valves in the penile veins are closed by reflex action, preventing loss of blood. This mechanism is regulated by the parasympathetic division of the autonomic nervous system. This system controls the diameter and valves of the penile blood vessels, thus causing erection or loss of erection. Once erection has occurred, excitement can be maintained for some time. Men are physically capable of losing and regaining several erections during love play.

Kaplan calls the vasocongestive reaction in females the "lubrication-swelling" phase. During this phase, dilation of the circumvaginal venous plexus causes a transudate on the walls of the vagina, which results in lubrication. The tissues become the "orgasmic platform" (analogous to erection in the male). In addition the uterus becomes engorged and begins to rise slightly out of the pelvic cavity so that the cervix is placed in a position to increase the likelihood of fertilization.

2. REFLEX CLONIC MUSCULAR CONTRACTIONS. The visceral aspects of the ejaculatory reflex are under control of the sympathetic division of the autonomic nervous system, as opposed to the parasympathetic division that is involved with erection. Male orgasm has two phases: *emission* and *ejaculation*. Emission comprises contractions of the vasa deferentia, the prostate, the seminal vesicles, and the internal part of the urethra. Masters and Johnson (1966) have called the subjective response to emission "ejaculatory inevitability." Ejaculation is the external mechanism that causes spurts of semen to be forced outward from the penis.

The biphasic nature of the response cycle is dramatically explained by the impact of aging on the refractory period. For example, a man's frequency of ejaculation may be reduced, but his ability to have erections may remain relatively the same.

The woman, like the man, has orgasms consisting of a series of reflex, involuntary rhythmic contractions of the orgasmic platform.

CLINICAL SIGNIFICANCE. There are four important findings from the research of Masters and Johnson that have significance for nurses working with women and their families. These findings concern (1) multiple orgasm, (2) simultaneous orgasm, (3) total body response to sexual stimulation and (4) variations in orgasmic patterns.

Since women never physically have a refractory period, they are capable of having one orgasm after another until exhausted. *Multiple orgasms* are most commonly reported by women in their late thirties and early forties. Some women have reported being multiply orgasmic for the first time during the second trimester of pregnancy. The reason is that because of the increased vasocongestion of pregnancy, total completion of the resolution phase never occurs.

Many couples have considered *simultaneous orgasm* the ultimate goal of sexual bliss. The findings of Masters and Johnson and of others show the illogic of such goals, because many couples progress through the response cycle at different rates. The myth of the desirability of simultaneous orgasm has harmed many relationships because of the difficulty of achieving this goal. Although possible, simultaneous orgasm is the exception rather than the rule and is achieved when the woman reaches orgasm easily.

Masters and Johnson demonstrated that an orgasm is a *total body response to sexual stimulation*, with the most intense response located in the pelvic area. The response is essentially the same regardless of whether it is experienced through coitus, masturbation, or mechanical stimulation.

There are many response patterns for both women and men. These patterns vary in both intensity and duration.

PROSTAGLANDINS. **Prostaglandins** (PGs) are oxygenated fatty acids now classified as hormones. The different kinds of PGs are distinguished by letters (PGE, PGF), numbers (PGE_2), and letters of the Greek alphabet ($PGF_{2\alpha}$).

PGs are produced in most organs of the body but most notably by the prostate and the endometrium. Therefore semen and menstrual blood are potent prostaglandin sources. PGs are metabolized quickly by most tissues. They are biologically active in minute amounts in the cardiovascular, gastrointestinal, respiratory, urogenital, and nervous systems. They also exert a marked effect on metabolism, particularly on glycolysis. Prostaglandins play an important role in many physiologic, pathologic, and pharmacologic reactions. $PGF_{2\alpha}$, PGE_1, and PGE_2 are most commonly used in reproductive medicine.

Prostaglandins affect smooth muscle contractility and modulation of hormonal activity. Indirect evidence supports PGs' effects on: ovulation; fertility; changes in the cervix and cervical mucus that affect receptivity to sperm; tubal and uterine motility; sloughing of endometrium (menstruation); onset of abortion (spontaneous and induced); and onset of labor (term and preterm).

After exerting their biologic actions, newly synthesized PGs are rapidly metabolized by tissues in such organs as the lungs, kidneys, and liver.

PGs may play a key role in ovulation. If PG levels do not rise along with the surge of LH, the ovum remains trapped within the graafian follicle. After ovulation, PGs may influence production of estrogen and progesterone by the corpus luteum.

The introduction of PGs into the vagina or into the uterine cavity (from ejaculated semen) increases the motility of uterine musculature, which may assist the transport of sperm through the uterus and into the oviduct. High concentration of PGs in the semen (about 55 $\mu g/mL$) may be necessary for normal fertility in males.

PGs produced by the woman cause regression (return to an earlier state) of the corpus luteum, regression of the endometrium, and sloughing of the endometrium, which results in menstruation. PGs increase myometrial response to oxytocic stimulation, enhance uterine contractions, and cause cervical dilation. They may be one factor in initiating or maintaining of labor or both. In addition, prostaglandins may be involved in the following pathologic states: male infertility, dysmenorrhea, hypertensive states, preeclampsia-eclampsia, and anaphylactic shock. Further discussion of PGs relevant to abortion may be found in Chapter 30; for a discussion of PGs' role in pregnancy and childbirth, see Chapter 35.

■ PSYCHOSOCIAL ASPECTS OF HUMAN SEXUALITY

The nurse is expected to provide counseling and guidance to sexually maturing and sexually active individuals as well as expectant and new parents. New parents often need information about the expected behavioral and physical growth and development of the individuals within their family. This information helps the nurse individualize nursing plans of care. Family members are the first significant others in the child's sexual, cognitive, and personality development. As the child matures and ventures into the wider world, peer, educational, and other social groups provide environments that affect development.

Myths

In a culture characterized by a rapid increase in knowledge and technology, many people still are misinformed about human sexuality. Listed below are common myths about reproduction and birth control (Stuart, Sundeen, 1991):

1. A couple must have simultaneous climaxes (orgasms) if conception is to take place
2. A woman can become pregnant only through penile penetration or artificial insemination
3. Urination by the woman after coitus or having sexual intercourse in a standing position will prevent pregnancy
4. The woman determines the sex of the child
5. Excessive masturbation is harmful
6. Sex during menstruation is unclean and harmful
7. Advancing age means the end of sex

Cognitive Development

Innate intellectual ability and the quality of the environment are decisive factors in **cognitive development.** Piaget (1950), a Swiss scientist, developed theories about how the process of thought develops from birth through adulthood. Table 6-2 summarizes cognitive and personality development across the life span. Reflex activity dominates the beginning of the *sensorimotor stage* (birth to 2 years). It gives way to repetitive and finally to imitative behavior. Any problem solving is the result of trial and error, but a sense of "what causes what" begins to emerge. During the *preoperational stage* (2 to 7 years), children are extremely self-centered, or egocentric. As Whaley and Wong (1990) expressed it, "they are unable to see things from any perspective other than their own; they cannot see another's point of view, nor can they see any reason to do so." They live in a well-defined world comprising what they see, hear, or otherwise experience. The *concrete operations stage* (7 to 12 years) is characterized by a gradual increase in problem-solving ability. The method of reasoning used is inductive. Solutions to problems are not based on abstractions but are derived from what has been perceived and categorized. The "social self" appears. Children are no longer exclusively egocentric but can relate to the feelings and thoughts of others. Progress through the *formal operations stage* (starting about age 12) may be erratic and difficult for the adolescent. By the end of this stage, successful adults can consider hypotheses and analyze scientifically. They should be able to deduce conclusions from a set of observations, consider alternatives, and assess risks. In short, they are capable of reasoning logically by using abstractions and also capable of assuming responsibility for the actions taken as solutions to their problems.

Personality Development

Erikson (1959) proposed a theory of **personality development** that defines the process in stages. Each stage focuses on a central conflict and depends on the ones before it. *Basic trust (birth to 1 year)* develops as a response to being loved and cared for by a giving and concerned adult. If such care makes up the bulk of the infant's experiences, trust takes precedence over mistrust. A sense of *autonomy (1 to 3 years)* develops with the gradual unfolding of the child's control of body, self, and people in the immediate environment. If those who provide care applaud the child's efforts toward self-control and increasing motor skills, autonomy will result. The stage of *initiative vs. guilt (3 to 6 years)* ushers in a phase of active exploring and achieving a balance between daring and caution. The children learn much from their world by playing games and asking endless questions. They show more evidence of being guided by an inner conscience: the parent has been increas-

TABLE 6-2 Summary of Cognitive and Personality Development

Stage	Significant Others	Cognitive Development (Piaget)	Personality Development (Erikson)
Infancy (birth to 18 months)	Maternal (Parental) person ↓	Sensorimotor: reflex→repetition→imitation	Trust vs. mistrust
Toddlerhood (18 months to 3 yrs)	Parental persons and other family members ↓	Preoperational, direct experience	Autonomy vs. shame and doubt
Early childhood (3 to 6 years)	Parental persons and other family members ↓	Preoperational, direct experience	Initiative vs. guilt
Middle childhood (6 to 12 years)	Neighborhood and school ↓	Concrete thinking (not abstract)	Industry vs. inferiority
Adolescence (12 to 18 years)	Peer groups and models of leadership ↓	Formal thinking (deductive and abstract reasoning) may be limited up to 15 years	Identity vs. identity confusion, role diffusion
Early adulthood	Partners in friendship, sex, competition, and cooperation ↓	Formal thinking includes problem solving and separation of fantasy and fact	Intimacy and solidarity vs. isolation
Young and middle adulthood	Divided labor and shared household ↓	Formal thinking	Generativity vs. self-absorption, stagnation
Later adulthood (after climacterium)	Humankind, family, and friends	Formal thinking	Ego integrity vs. despair

ingly internalized. This is a time for fears and phobias. During the period of *industry vs. inferiority (6 to 12 years),* children develop a sense of being productive workers. They need opportunities to complete activities and be rewarded for their efforts. Introduction to formal schooling takes place now. The central conflict of the next phase is *identity vs. identity confusion (12 to 18 years).* The period of adolescence comes after a period of relative calm. During this time of transition between childhood and adulthood, adolescents have certain tasks to perform: they must establish sexual roles, select an occupation, become independent of the family, and develop a social rather than egocentric response to people and the wider society. The adolescent must accept a new body image that includes the ability to reproduce. Successful mastery of these tasks helps adolescents develop a sense of self and identity that both they and society can accept. Inability to master this phase results in identity confusion. Once people have a sense of identity (early adulthood), they can move toward *intimacy.* This can be expressed on a personal level as friendship or sexual intimacy, or the intimacy of parent-child relationships. On a social level love of fellow humans is expressed in concern for the welfare of others. Without this sense of freedom to love and be loved, people may develop a sense of alienation from family, friends, and society. During the period of *generativity vs. self-absorption* (young and middle adulthood), people are concerned with creating the next generation and providing the necessary nurturing and caregiving. The tasks in this stage include preparation for assuming the role of parent, participating in the birth of children, and adapting to the reality of parenthood.

The tasks of this stage may also be accomplished in a variety of ways: adopting children, being friends to adolescents, teaching, or nursing. Growth of the personality, as a person seeks balance between commitment to self and commitment to others, leads to a sense of productiveness and fulfillment. Staying productive and involved in the welfare of others increases the satisfaction, or ego integrity, of people during late adulthood (arbitrarily, after the climacterium or around the age of 65 years in the United States). In many cases the older adult's physical and mental abilities gradually decline, imposing limitations and curtailing the sphere of activity. As people confront the limitations, they must balance acceptance against despair. Wisdom and a sense of satisfaction in their accomplishments come to those who succeed in the search for personal meaning. Table

6-2 summarizes cognitive and personality development.

DEVELOPMENT OF SEXUAL IDENTITY

Sexual identity begins at conception. At that time, through the chance combination of an ovum and a sperm, a person's biologic sex is determined. Thereafter, intrauterine and extrauterine environmental influences both play their part in the realization of each person's sexual potential. Biophysical, psychologic, sociocultural, and ethical factors all contribute to the molding of an individual's **sexuality.**

We are born into a sexually oriented world, and from birth onward we assume socially defined sexual roles that reflect the basic pattern prescribed by the society. These roles are learned informally through being part of a social group. Development of a concept of sexual roles and sexual identity begins at an early age and continues as a series of developmental tasks throughout a person's life span.

Infancy and Childhood

One of the first questions parents ask when their child is born is "Is it a boy or a girl?" The answer sets in motion a series of social influences that will be reflected in the child's concept of "who I am" and "what I can do." The **developmental tasks** relative to forming a sexual identity include developing core gender identity, acquiring prescribed sex role standards, identifying with the parent of the same sex, and establishing gender preference.

Core gender identity is the earliest and most stable form of gender identity. From the child's perspective, knowing oneself as either a girl or a boy begins before full realization of the implications of sexual identity. The infant's gender identity is largely accomplished by acceptance of parental labeling; for example, "Be a good boy," "That's my girl," and "That is my big boy." By 2 years of age children can differentiate between girls and boys through awareness of dissimilarities in hair and clothing and some awareness of anatomic differences. Core gender identity is developed in normal children by the time they have reached 3 or 4 years of age.

The term **sex role standards** refers to the various behaviors, attitudes, and attributes that differentiate the roles. Even 2-year-olds are exposed to this conditioning, because parents choose for them the kinds of clothing, toys, and activities that reflect the parents' expectations of sex role standards.

The feelings children develop about themselves as people in general and as sexual people in particular are directly related to their experiences with their bodies and the attitudes and values they derive from many sources. One of the most important ways children learn about their bodies is through exploratory sexual behavior (sex play). *Sex play* is defined by Kinsey et al (1948, 1953) as "actual genital play." There are four categories of sex play: self-exploration and self-manipulation, same-sex comparison, coital play, and exhibitionism. *Self-exploration and self-manipulation* begin by 2 to 3 months of age. As they grow, infants discover they are able to experience sexual pleasure through self-stimulation. Parents who feel masturbation is harmful will rebuke even young children and forbid them to "play with themselves." *Same-sex comparisons* provide children with reassurance that their genitals are similar in size and shape to those of other children. *Coital play* (e.g., when a boy lies on top of a girl) is largely experimental, imitative, and exploratory. Children become aware of parental sleeping arrangements, bathing, and privacy. They begin differentiating sex role behaviors and will play at being "Mommy" and "Daddy." *Exhibitionism* consists of showing and handling genitals in public, especially in the presence of companions. Most children engage in sex play activities only sporadically, especially when these activities are ignored by adults.

In Western society the adjectives used to describe a female predominantly express a mothering capacity, that is, "gentle, loving, submissive, patient, warm, and concerned." These qualities suit a person whose central reason for being is assumed to be the care and nurturing of the young. Those adjectives used to describe the male, namely, "dominant, aggressive, impatient, objective, and ambitious," portray a person capable of independent, decisive action. These are seen as the qualities needed in the marketplace and the basis for career orientation.

In reality, people of both sexes possess these qualities in common. Some personalities lean more toward the socially defined concept of either female or male; others have no clear demarcation of roles. These latter people, termed *androgynous personalities,* use those qualities most needed at the moment without feeling guilty about usurping another's role. A male nursing student made the following comment during a discussion of mothering:

> It is not a case of one or the other, it is what the time calls forth. The most nurturing behavior of "mothering," if you want to call it that, that I've ever seen was in Vietnam when a man was trying to get a wounded friend out of range of fire. He protected him, covering him with his own body, gave him his food and water. No mother could have shown more devotion.

A common way children prepare for a future parenting role is through sibling caregiving. Older children from either the nuclear or extended family care for younger children. Older children are used to provide role flexibility for mothers and for the development of caregiving skills by children.

As a child comes to identify with the parent of the same sex, the child internalizes the values, attitudes, and ideals of that parent. The exact method by which the process of identification is accomplished is not yet known.

Gender preference implies not only a knowledge of one's gender and the appropriate sex role but also a liking for it. Development of gender preference involves three elements: (1) success in the role, (2) liking the same-sex parent, and (3) reinforcement from family, ethnic group, and social institutions as to the value of the role (Newman, Newman, 1975).

Deep-seated sex preferences on the part of parents can affect initial parent-child relationships if the child is not of the preferred sex. The parenting lag that results can last a day or a lifetime, depending on whether the parent succeeds or fails in resolving conflicting emotions. Certain ethnic groups have welcoming rituals for one sex and not for the other. These seemingly innocuous societal and personal preferences eventually lead a person to make value judgments about the worthiness of her or his sex. As a result the individual's self-esteem is either increased or diminished.

By the time puberty occurs the person has completed most of the developmental tasks of early childhood. Acceptance of childhood sexual identity will have consequences for self-esteem, peer relations, and selection of skills and interest.

IMPLICATIONS FOR NURSING. A nurse has many opportunities to help young parents provide a supportive environment for their children's sexual development. Nurses and parents must be careful not to ascribe adult motives to the sexual behaviors of children. To do so would be like calling a child who believes in ghosts and fairies delusional or mentally ill (Katchadourian, Lunde, 1972). Parents may project contradictory messages about the body. For example, parents tell their children to "wash behind your ears" and then remind them to "wash down there." Parents and many health professionals respond to their own insecurities about sex when confronted by the overt but innocent sexuality of children.

Adolescence

Adolescence, the transitional period between childhood and adulthood, begins with puberty. Biologically the first visible signs of puberty are the development of the secondary sexual characteristics. Menstruation can be a first indication of puberty. Shortly thereafter most teenagers experience a rapid increase in linear growth. Concomitantly, emotional changes such as moodiness, tearfulness, or withdrawal are suddenly noticeable in a previously serene youngster. It is not until adolescence that the socially and parentally defined sex role is openly questioned. In recent years changes in the concepts of what constitutes female and male roles have had great impact on teenagers. Conflict can result when the teenager chooses standards consistent with the peer group's attitude rather than with parental expectations.

DEVELOPMENTAL TASKS. Erikson (1959) has described the adolescent stage of development as the one in which the major task is achieving identity vs. identity confusion. A person's identity has many dimensions, including intellectual, interpersonal, and sexual. It is now recognized that the adolescent developmental process proceeds in sequence through three phases. These phases—early, middle, and late adolescence—put a characteristic stamp on the manner of accomplishing the developmental tasks. The developmental tasks of adolescence may be defined as follows (adapted from Havighurst, 1972):

1. *Achieving awareness and acceptance of body image.* The body image is well established by about 15 years of age. Adolescents must cope with normal but rapid changes in physical appearance and alterations in functional capacity. They must accept their physique and learn to use their bodies effectively. Deviations from the "norm" are a source of stress and may or may not be incorporated into the adolescent's body image.
2. *Achieving emotional independence of parents and other adults.* The movement away from dependence on parents that was begun with the school years is completed in this period of development. Successful accomplishment results in affection and respect for one's parents without a childish dependence on them.
3. *Achieving new and more mature relations with age mates of both sexes.* Adolescents accomplish a satisfactory social adjustment through social activities and experimentation with the peer group. Here they learn to behave as adults as they create, on a small scale, the society of their elders. The influence of the peer group increasingly takes precedence over that of the family.
4. *Achieving a feminine or masculine social role.* Although sex is biologically determined, the feminine and masculine roles are culturally established behavior sets that must be learned.

5. *Establishing a life-style that is personally and socially satisfying.* This includes the choice of a career, as well as contemplation of sexual relationships, marriage, family interdependence, and parenthood.
6. *Acquiring a set of values and an ethical system as a guide to socially responsible behavior.* This includes assuming responsibility for her or his own behavior and recognizing the effect that behavior may have on another's welfare.

EARLY ADOLESCENCE. Early adolescence begins approximately between 11 and 13 years and merges with midadolescence at 14 or 15 years (Johnson, 1983). It is characterized by an increase in height and the appearance of the secondary sexual characteristics.

Young adolescents tend to see the world around them only in relation to the effect it has on *them*. As their capacity for abstract thought increases, they become intensely interested in themselves, their thoughts, ideas, and fantasies, and what effect they have on others. As a result they are introspective, self-conscious, and easily hurt by real or imagined slights. They feel that everyone is looking at them critically, so they demand privacy. The slamming of the bedroom door, the NO ADMITTANCE signs put on retreats, and the long periods of self-enforced isolation from the family are typical of this phase.

The major task of early adolescence is acceptance of a new body image. The rapid changes in appearance cause adolescents to spend much time thinking about their bodies and comparing their physiques with those of others. Girls are interested in their developing breasts and often want to wear brassieres before they are needed. They tend to idealize body structure and feel depressed when their skin, hair, and legs do not compare favorably with the "ideal."

Parents are still in control, and the young adolescent is aware of vulnerability and need for dependence. However, parents and brothers and sisters notice a beginning of the critical appraisal to which they will be increasingly subjected. The adolescent becomes aware of the status of the family in the community and is anxious that her or his family measure up to certain standards. This is the time of intense relationships with members of the same sex, and these relationships are used primarily for support and mutual understanding.

MIDADOLESCENCE. Midadolescence begins around 14 or 15 years and merges with late adolescence at about age 17. Almost all adolescents have reached their growth peak by midadolescence. Many aspects of the body have attained their adult form. For example, in boys the development of the lower jaw alters the contour of the face from the round, childish one to that of the adult. Both boys and girls generally accept their bodies, although this acceptance is tempered by a desire to look otherwise. As a result the interest in their bodies is expressed through efforts to improve themselves. Grooming, makeup, and the right clothes become all important. Stabilizing the body image is important in developing a sense of identity.

The midadolescent phase is characterized by increasing competence in abstract thought (Johnson, 1983). The adolescent is capable of perceiving future implications of current acts and decisions. The ability to think in this manner fluctuates. In times of stress the adolescent reverts to concrete operations.

The major task during this phase is emancipation from the family. Adolescents vacillate between acting like responsible adults and acting like dependent children. Their ability to step into the adult role, even if briefly, increases their resentment of being considered children. Role experimentation becomes a central process in the search for identity.

There is a definite movement away from the family. Midadolescents are critical of their parents, and the parents' appearance, behavior, dress, and social manners are all subjected to intense scrutiny and disparagement. Brothers and sisters are considered a nuisance, and adolescents see themselves as being treated unfairly in terms of other members of the family. An adult outside the family group—a nurse, a physician, a coach, or a school counselor, for example—may be taken as a role model. There is increased participation in the adult world. Adolescents become advocates of various ideologies and enjoy debating the merits of current ideas. Many show evidence of leadership potential as they engage in developing their cognitive skills. Rebellion is usually couched in verbal terms rather than physical ones and is more destructive than constructive. Running away is a common phenomenon for adolescents between the ages of 15 and 17 years as an attempt to solve problems and to prove they are not children.

Peer relationships now dominate over family ones. The adolescent looks to the peer group for definitions of the behavioral code. There is a strong need to affirm the newly developed self-image through the affirmation of peers. Most conflicts with parents reflect this change, and communication patterns that were once open may become closed.

There is a change from relationships with members of the same sex to heterosexual relationships (**heterosexuality**). Adolescents test their ability to attract the opposite sex. They continue to define the parameters of femininity and masculinity.

LATE ADOLESCENCE. The late adolescent phase extends from age 17 through 21. The upper limit of the phase depends on cultural, economic, and educational factors. The late adolescent is physically mature. Most late adolescents have achieved a stable body image, and the agonizing over this or that real or fancied disability is largely over. They have established abstract thought processes. They are future oriented and capable of perceiving and acting on long-range options.

One of the major tasks confronting the late adolescent is to become a fully *independent* productive citizen. They become self-supporting or begin their professional education. They have become socially functioning adults. Late adolescents are capable of forming stable relationships. They are ready for mutuality and reciprocity in caring for another, in contrast to the former self-centered orientation. Although young women are now assuming the right to choose careers rather than early marriage, many still suspend the final shaping of a career until after commitments to parenthood are fulfilled.

Adolescent Sexuality

The adolescent's heightened sexual awareness brings sexual concerns to the surface. These include myths about masturbation and concerns about possible homosexuality, sexual activity, and the presence, frequency, and content of sexual fantasies and dreams. Although physically sexually mature, adolescents are trying to cope with emerging sensations and social situations while they are still psychologically immature.

MASTURBATION. Young adolescents may fear that any variation from normal, particularly of the genitals, has resulted from masturbation. The adolescent needs to learn that **masturbation** is a normal, universal behavior that causes neither physical nor mental harm. It is a natural part of learning about human sexuality and can be a useful means of relieving sexual tension (Brookman, 1983).

Masturbation is also a common mode of discharge of tension for adolescents, particularly when alone, unhappy, or frustrated. It serves to fuse psychologic and physical sexuality. It is not always associated with sexual fantasies. The value of masturbation may be lessened by the shame and guilt that accompany it. Adolescent boys often fear discovery of evidence of ejaculation, and girls often fear changes in their genitals as a result of masturbation. Fears are not limited to discovery by others but also are caused by the expansive experience of orgasm, with the resulting feelings of loss of ego boundaries. If masturbation is used as a continual source of comfort or with inappropriate exposure (exhibitionism), it is indicative of disturbance (Stuart, Sundeen, 1991).

HOMOSEXUALITY. Homosexual experience to some degree is part of the psychosexual development of many individuals. The adolescent who is overly affectionate with same-sex peers or adults may cause considerable parental concern. This is a result of society's unresolved position on the meaning or acceptance of homosexuality. Fantasies about sexual encounters with members of the same sex can be very disturbing to the adolescent. Memories of early same-sex explorations compound the adolescent's fear of becoming homosexual. The fear is probably a reaction to society's negative valuation of homosexuality.

For many years the medical profession, including psychiatry, has searched for causes of **homosexuality.** The message in looking for the cause of a condition is that it is a maladaptive state that can be treated or cured. Today emphasis is placed on learning more about homosexuality and viewing it as a sexual preference or mode of sexual expression (Kinsey, 1948).

Marmor (1980) defined the homosexual person as "one who is motivated in adult life by a definite preferential erotic attraction to members of the same sex and who usually (but not necessarily) engages in overt sexual relations with them." Marmor's definition excludes transitory incidental homosexual activity in adolescence and in primarily heterosexual persons.

The incidence of homosexuality in the United States today has been conservatively estimated at 10% to 15% of the population (APA, 1987). If these estimates are accurate, nurses come into contact with homosexuals on a daily basis. Despite this incidence of homosexuality, nurses generally know little about homosexuality and almost always assume that all clients are heterosexual (Stuart, Sundeen, 1991).

SEXUAL ACTIVITY. Adolescents are surrounded by mixed messages. Parents, religious groups, teachers, health professionals, and others tell them to refrain from sexual contact, to control sexual impulses, and to keep away from temptation. Many of these same adults are asking adolescents to refrain from activities they themselves openly practice. At the same time books, movies, music, and advertisements are laden with sexually stimulating messages.

Questions about whether and when to be sexually active and whether one needs to have sex to be popular become a major part of the lives of adolescents. Sexual decision-making in five young African-American adolescent girls was studied (see Research Highlight, below.) They express confusion about love and how one expresses love and concern about sexual adequacy. Pajama parties and locker room discussions are often the only outlets adolescents have to discuss some of these concerns and to obtain information—and a great deal of misinformation—about sex.

Interest in dating stems from the adolescent's need for companionship and emotional and physical closeness. Intimacy includes hand-holding, kissing, embracing, petting, and sexual intercourse. Approximately two thirds of all teenage boys and one half of all teenage girls have had intercourse at least once (Brookman, 1983; MMWR, 1991). Many younger adolescents may use intercourse as a means of conforming to peer group expectations, as a challenge to parents, as experimentation, or as a means of relieving loneliness or stress. Some adolescents develop sincere commitments to one another that may persist and lead to marriage. Many have "a series of close, committed, single-partner relationships, each lasting weeks, months, or longer" (Brookman, 1983). Few adolescents are **promiscuous;** that is, they do not have multiple partners with little or no commitment.

Adolescents are hesitant to talk to adults, especially parents, because the adult often discounts or invalidates their feelings. Some parents are threatened by their adolescent's budding sexuality. They (and some nurses) deal with their own uncertainty about sex by ignoring the reality of adolescent sexuality or by becoming hostile and punitive. At times little attention is given to the teenager who is reluctant to engage in dating at all. The young person who fails to show any interest may need careful evaluation.

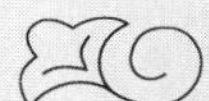 **Research Highlight** 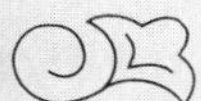

Sexual Decision Making in Young African-American Adolescent Girls

RESEARCH ABSTRACT

The aim of the study was to obtain a broad, detailed view of factors leading to initial sexual activity and the decision to maintain the pregnancy of young African-American adolescents. The participants were five 14-year-old teenagers. The data were gathered through open-ended interviews that lasted 2 to 3 hours. The factors that led to the first sexual activity included establishing a trust relationship with their partners, believing they could not get pregnant, relying on their partner for contraception, and lacking knowledge about contraception. Family relationship also was a factor and included elements such as much unsupervised time, inconsistency in mother's wishes and daughter's behavior, lack of maternal authority, and inability to discuss sex. The critical factors in the decision to maintain the pregnancy included accepting the diagnosis of pregnancy and being aware of available alternatives. The adolescents denied the pregnancy for several months, which narrowed the choices about maintaining the pregnancy. Although none of the girls married, all received support and involvement from the fathers. All of the girls had friends their age who were pregnant or were parents. Four of the girls had financial and emotional support from their families.

IMPLICATIONS FOR PRACTICE

1. What factors influence early sexual involvement?
2. Will a community center with planned activities for adolescents reduce unsupervised time and the pregnancy rate?
3. Will an educational program reduce the number of second pregnancies in adolescent African-American girls?
4. Will a sex education program for mothers of adolescents increase the communication about sex between mothers and adolescents?

REFERENCE

Pete JM, DeSantis L: Sexual decision making in young black adolescent females, *Adolescence* 25(97):145, 1990.

IMPLICATIONS FOR NURSING. Health professionals need to be knowledgeable and comfortable with their own sexuality to work effectively with adolescents. Glossing over important issues and making broad generalizations about sexual concerns can be more confusing than helpful. Nurses who counsel young people about specific sexual issues need (1) knowledge of sexual anatomy, physiology, and behavior; (2) recognition of the importance of local peer influences; and (3) understanding of the adolescent's family and ethnocultural background. The approach to adolescents is based on their intellectual and psychosocial maturation. Provision of privacy and reassurance of confidentiality are essential to building trust and confidence between adolescent and nurse. The adolescent usually is willing to express concerns if the discussions are held in a comfortable and nonjudgmental setting.

The increased incidence of adolescent pregnancy and the increased number of adolescents with sexually transmitted diseases, including AIDS, make sex education and sex counseling a major task for nurses working with adolescents (see Chapter 34). Information about their bodies' sexual responses, contraception, pregnancy, and sexually transmitted disease can be made available to adolescents to help them become sexually responsible adults.

It is important for nurses working with adolescents to be aware of adolescents' concern about masturbation and homosexuality. Factual information about masturbation can be given to adolescents, but it is not appropriate for the counselor to advocate masturbation. The decision should be made by each person and includes personal values, such as religious belief.

It is important to note that some adult homosexuals report awareness of their homosexuality as early as adolescence. Nurses counseling such adolescents need to be accepting and comfortable in communicating with people who exhibit a sexual preference that may differ from their own. The incidence of sexually transmitted diseases and other infections encountered in sexual relationships makes it essential to secure appropriate medical and counseling sources for all individuals. Nurses who are not comfortable with these clients need to refer them to other professionals or agencies who can help them.

Adult Sexuality

Adulthood encompasses the period from adolescence to a person's death. Three phases are discernible: early, middle, and late adulthood.

EARLY ADULTHOOD. Early adulthood encompasses that portion of the life cycle devoted to parenting, consolidation of relationships whether marital or nonmarital, and commitment to a life work. The young adult has attained physical and intellectual maturity. Stature and reproductive growth are virtually complete.

Body image remains a concern for the young adult, particularly in terms of body contour and size (Woods, 1984). Nonacceptance of one's body may inhibit the establishment of sexual relationships.

Cognitive powers include the ability to think abstractly, to be future oriented, and to act on long-range options (Piaget, 1950). Personality development is related to the task of developing intimacy and solidarity as opposed to existing in isolation (Erikson, 1959). Intimacy involves learning to give and receive love, choosing whether to marry, and choosing a sexual partner or partners (Duvall, 1977).

Family ties are important, but the relationship of parent and child takes on an adult quality. The young adult is expected to be moving toward financial and social independence from the family. She or he is also expected to choose a vocation and obtain the necessary education for it. Establishing a career and advancing in it are major concerns throughout this part of the life cycle.

Social groupings include varying age levels and are often based on similar interests. The need for strong friendships with peers diminishes as individual friendships assume permanence.

Early adulthood has been described as a period of maximum sexual self-consciousness (Offer, Simon, 1976). There is social acceptance and legitimization of sexual experiences. The tasks of sexual development for the young adult include maintaining a long-term commitment to a sexual relationship, practicing responsible reproductive health care, and making rational decisions about childbearing.

Commitment to a relationship is strengthened by the need to give and receive pleasure. Commitments vary in length and type. For example, some couples remain monogamous throughout their marriage. Others have open marriages, in which the couple agrees that one or both may participate in other sexual encounters. Some couples remain in relationships without formal marriage. Relationships can be terminated by divorce or death. Finally, **serial monogamy** is practiced by many people in the United States. Serial monogamy is characterized by repeated marriages and divorces. The person is married to only one person at a time but is married a number of times throughout her or his life.

Responsible reproductive health care includes such actions as women having a Papanicolaou smear at prescribed intervals and both women and men avoiding sexually transmitted diseases.

Rational decisions about childbearing are important to ensure that every child is a wanted child. The couple is responsible for using reliable contraceptive means when pregnancy is not desired. Unwanted and unplanned children often become targets of abuse and neglect.

MIDDLE AND LATE ADULTHOOD. These phases of the life cycle represent the greatest maximizing of early potential and then a gradual lessening of biopsychosocial attainment through the normal process of aging. Changes in family structure from events such as children leaving home, death of a spouse, or role reversal in dealing with aging parents necessitate major changes in life-style. The critical task for these years is maintaining feelings of self-esteem vs. despair. The need to love and be loved, to be successful, and to feel meaningful prompts involvement in community service and in leisure pursuits.

Cognitive powers continue unabated until physical insults such as Alzheimer's disease or cerebrovascular accident cause a decline. Body image remains an important concern. Western society's accent on health and youth make grooming, weight, nutrition, and exercise a continuous part of an adult's daily life.

The sexual developmental tasks of middle and late

adulthood focus primarily on adapting to the physical and emotional changes in sexual performance caused by the aging process. The childbearing years are coming to an end. This is a relief for many couples because the possibility of pregnancy can be removed from their lovemaking. Others may mourn the loss of the chance for another child.

The fear of growing older in a youth-oriented society can be a source of depression and anxiety. Bodily changes, lower hormone production, and menopause may contribute to anxiety and depression.

The research of Masters and Johnson (1966) has shown that aging does not decrease libido or the capacity to be orgasmic. Men and women are capable of sexual activity well into their old age. Disinterest and abstinence are probably caused by loss of a partner, boredom, ill health, or cultural attitudes about the appropriateness.

Many older people do not understand the impact of aging on their physical response to sexual stimulation. They see these changes as an indication that they should terminate sexual activity rather than merely as a need to make minor adaptations. For example, vaginal lubrication in women is slower and decreased in amount; in men, erection is slower and erectile firmness decreased. Love play will probably need to be extended, with more direct genital stimulation to produce lubrication and erection. Women have a shortened orgasmic phase and men's need to ejaculate decreases, resulting in decreased force and volume of ejaculation. These physiologic changes require adaptations in sexual behavior and not cessation of sexual activity.

Mims and Swenson (1980) have stated:

> Sexual fulfillment throughout adulthood and into old age is not only possible but likely. The feeling that older people are not interested in sex (except if they are abnormal—the "dirty old man" syndrome) is largely caused by our inability to imagine our parents or our grandparents as sexually active people. The greatest danger of such attitudes is that they tend to comprise a "self-fulfilling prophecy": if people believe that sexual interest ceases with advancing age, they will find that it does cease. Or, if sexual interest persists, people may believe themselves to be abnormal, sinful, or psychologically sick.

IMPLICATIONS FOR NURSING. The nurse is in a unique position to help adults with health maintenance and detection of problems concerning sexuality. The role of sex educator is an important one for nurses working with families during the childbearing and child rearing years. Parents often need help with teaching their children about sex because adults commonly are misinformed about many aspects of reproduction and how their bodies function. Parents therefore need accurate sex information to teach their children to be healthy, responsible sexual beings.

Besides helping with childhood and adult sexuality, the nurse can help prepare clients for the sexual problems and changes occurring with age. Many nurses have not been aware of the importance of sex education for older people because of the myth that the elderly are no longer interested in sex.

Sexual dysfunction problems often begin after children are born. The mother especially may become so involved with child rearing that her relationship with her husband suffers. At the same time, the husband may be actively involved in career establishment, thereby leaving little energy for home life. The nurse needs to be aware of how the demands of parenting can adversely affect the marital relationship. Simple counseling provided during these early years may prevent serious marital problems in later years.

The older woman in particular who has been able to move gracefully into old age and who continues to recognize herself as a sexual being is probably better able to accept the sexuality of the young. The pregnancy of a daughter then may be accepted as a continuation of her own sexuality rather than as a threat or reminder of her lost youth.

A knowledgeable, nonjudgmental nurse who recognizes personal sexual biases can contribute a great deal to the sexual health of young families. The nurse can recognize potential problems within the marriage and either intervene or refer the couple for further counseling.

■ IMMUNOLOGY

Immunology is defined as the study of the molecules, cells, organs, and systems responsible for the recognition and disposal of foreign (nonself) material as well as of how the human body defends itself against this material. The human immune system is necessary for survival. Nonself substances can be as diverse as life-threatening infectious microorganisms or a lifesaving organ transplant. The desirable consequences of immunity include natural resistance, recovery, and acquired resistance to infectious diseases. A deficiency or dysfunction of the immune system can cause many disorders. Undesirable consequences of immunity include allergy, rejection of a transplanted organ, or an autoimmune disorder (a condition in which the body's own tissues are attacked, as if they were foreign material). In medical science, the immune system can be advantageously manipulated to protect against a disorder such as hemolytic disease of the newborn.

Body Defenses

The first barrier to infection is unbroken skin and mucosal membrane surfaces. These surfaces are of utmost importance in forming a physical barrier against many microorganisms. Secretions such as mucus or those produced in the process of eliminating liquid and solid wastes (e.g., the urinary and gastrointestinal processes) are also important as nonspecific mechanisms for removing potential pathogens from the body. The acidity and alkalinity of the fluids of the stomach and intestinal tract, as well as the acidity of the vagina, can destroy many potentially infectious microorganisms. These fluids can also have chemical properties that are of value in defending the body. Lysozyme is an enzyme found in tears and saliva. This enzyme attacks the cell wall of susceptible bacteria, particularly certain gram-positive bacteria, and destroys the organism. Another chemical of importance in tears and saliva is immunoglobulin A (IgA) antibody.

The body has a wide variety of barrier-assisting defenses that initially protect the body against disease. Although these barriers vary between individuals, they do assist in the general resistance to infectious organisms. When barrier-assisting defenses break down, the potential for disease increases. The nurse is frequently faced with such situations. For instance, when the new mother's skin integrity is impaired (e.g., through episiotomy or lacerations) or when she has drying or cracking of the nipples, she is at increased risk for infection. In the older woman, the pH and amount of vaginal fluid are altered, resulting in the increased risk of yeast infection (i.e., *Candida albicans*).

NATURAL IMMUNITY. Natural (innate or inborn) resistance is one of the two ways that the body resists infection after microorganisms have penetrated the first line of resistance. The second form, adaptive or acquired resistance, specifically recognizes and selectively eliminates exogenous (or endogenous) agents.

Natural immunity is characterized as a nonspecific mechanism. If a microorganism penetrates the skin or mucosal membranes, cellular and humoral defense mechanisms become operational. The elements of natural resistance are phagocytic cells, complement, and the acute inflammatory reaction. Despite their relative lack of specificity, these components are essential, because they are largely responsible for natural immunity to many environmental microorganisms.

Cellular Components	Humoral Components
Mast cells (tissue basophils)	Complement
Neutrophils	Lysozyme
Macrophages	Interferon

ADAPTIVE IMMUNITY. If a microorganism overwhelms the body's natural resistance, another form of defensive resistance, acquired or **adaptive immunity,** allows the body to recognize, remember, and respond to a specific stimulus—an antigen. Adaptive immunity can eliminate microorganisms, and it commonly leaves the host with specific immunologic memory. This condition of memory or recall, *acquired resistance,* allows the host to respond more effectively if reinfection with the same microorganism occurs. Adaptive immunity, like natural immunity, is composed of cellular and humoral components.

Cellular Components	Humoral Components
T lymphocytes	Antibodies
B lymphocytes	Lymphokines
Plasma cells	

The major cellular component of this mechanism is the lymphocyte; the major humoral component is the antibody. Lymphocytes selectively respond to nonself materials—antigens—which leads to immune memory and a permanently altered pattern of response or adaptation to the environment. The two categories of the adaptive response are humoral-mediated and cell-mediated immunity. Humoral-mediated immunity is the primary defense against bacterial infection. Cell-mediated immunity is the primary defense against viral and fungal infections, intracellular organisms, tumor antigens, and graft rejections.

ANTIBODY-MEDIATED IMMUNITY. If specific antibodies have been formed to antigenic stimulation, they are available to protect the body against foreign substances. The recognition of foreign substances and subsequent production of antibodies to these substances is the specific meaning of immunity. Antibody-mediated immunity to infection is *acquired* if the antibodies are formed by the host or received from another source. These two types of acquired immunity (Table 6-3) are called *active* and *passive* immunity, respectively.

Active immunity can be acquired by natural exposure in response to an infection or natural series of infections, or it may be acquired by an injection of an antigen. This intentional injection of antigen, called **vaccination,** is an effective method of stimulating antibody production and memory (acquired resistance) without suffering from the disease. The se-

TABLE 6-3 Types of Acquired Immunity

Type	Mode of Acquisition	Antibody Produced by Host	Duration of Immune Response
ACTIVE			
Natural	Infection	Yes	Long*
Artificial	Vaccination	Yes	Long*
PASSIVE			
Natural	Transfer in vivo or through colostrum (maternal antibodies)	No	Short
Artificial	Infusion of serum/ plasma (Rh_oIG)	No	Short

*In the immunocompetent host.

lected antigenic agent should produce the antibodies without the clinical signs and symptoms of the disease in an **immunocompetent** host (a person whose immune system is able to recognize a foreign antigen and build specific antigen-directed antibodies) and produce permanent antigenic memory. Booster vaccinations may be needed in some cases to expand the pool of memory cells.

Artificial **passive immunity** is achieved by infusion of serum or plasma containing high concentrations of antibody. This provides immediate antibody protection against microorganisms such as hepatitis A or antigens such as Rh-positive (fetal) red blood cells. The antibodies have been produced by another person or animal that has been actively immunized, but the ultimate recipient has not produced them. The recipient will only temporarily benefit from passive immunity for as long as the antibodies persist in his or her circulation. Passive immunity can also be acquired naturally by the fetus through the transfer of antibodies by the maternal circulation in utero. Maternal antibodies are also transferred to the newborn after parturition in the prelactation fluid called colostrum. For the newborn to have lasting protection, active immunity must occur.

HYPERSENSITIVITY REACTIONS. Immediate hypersensitivity comprises a subset of the body's antibody-mediated effector mechanisms. This subset consists of the reactions primarily mediated by immunoglobulin E (IgE).

Atopic diseases are processes mediated by or related to IgE-immediate hypersensitivity. The most dramatic and devastating systemic manifestation of immediate hypersensitivity is **anaphylaxis.** Anaphylaxis is an immediate hypersensitivity reaction characterized by local reactions such as *urticaria* (hives) and *angioedema* (redness and swelling), or by systemic reactions in the respiratory tract, cardiovascular system, gastrointestinal tract, and skin. This type of reaction can be fatal. Other types of atopic diseases include allergic rhinoconjunctivitis, asthma, gastrointestinal allergy, and atopic dermatitis, an eczematous skin eruption.

Although antihistamines have a role to play in the treatment of mild allergic phenomena, they cannot be effective in situations of severe manifestations of allergy such as anaphylaxis. In these cases epinephrine (Adrenalin) is the drug of choice (by injection) to reverse the pathophysiologic condition by dilating the bronchi; by constricting the blood vessels, causing an increase in blood pressure; and by increasing the rate and strength of the heartbeat (and therefore the circulation of oxygen through the body).

Some clients have developed a sensitivity to certain foods, soaps, or drugs as allergens. Although it should be standard procedure for the nurse to assess all clients for sensitivity to foods, drugs, and substances (including adhesive tape), occasionally the nurse is involved in producing an inadvertent allergic reaction in a client. Such an incident may even occur while the nurse is administering a protective immunization to a client (as the rubella vaccine), since the vaccine is derived from duck egg or human (foreign protein) culture.

CELL-MEDIATED IMMUNITY. Cell-mediated immunity consists of immune activities that differ from those of antibody-mediated immunity. Cell-mediated immunity is moderated by the link between T lymphocytes and phagocytic cells (i.e., monocyte-macrophage cells). Lymphocytes (T cells) do not recognize the antigens of microorganisms or other living cells, such as *allografts* (a graft of tissue from a genetically different member of the same species [e.g., a human kidney]), directly, but do so when the antigen is present on the surface of an antigen-presenting cell—the macrophage. Lymphocytes are immunologically active through various types of direct cell-to-cell contact and by the production of soluble factors, such as *lymphokines,* for specific immunologic functions. These include the recruitment of phagocytic cells to the site of inflammation. The term *delayed hypersensitivity* is often used synonymously with the term *cell-mediated immunity. Delayed hypersensitivity,* however, refers to the slow appearance of a secondary response in the skin. The term dates back to the time when antibody responses were detected by immediate hypersensitivity and reflected the subtle difference in the length of time that it took for a delayed response to occur (e.g., tuberculin skin test). The process of cell-mediated immunity can be seen in the sequence of events resulting in poison ivy dermatitis caused by binding of the substance to the skin.

Under some conditions, the activities of cell-mediated immunity may not be beneficial. Suppression of the normal adaptive immune response *(immunosuppression)* by drugs or other means is necessary in conditions such as organ transplantation, hypersensitivity, and autoimmune disorders.

CELLS AND CELLULAR ACTIVITIES. The entire leukocytic cell system is designed to defend the body against disease. Each cell type, however, has a unique function and behaves both independently and in many cases in cooperation with other cell types. Leukocytes can be functionally divided into the general categories of granulocyte, monocyte-macrophage, and lymphocyte-plasma cell. The primary phagocytic cells are the polymorphonuclear neutrophilic (PMN) leukocytes and the mononuclear monocyte-macrophage cells. The lymphocytes participate in body defenses primarily through the recognition of foreign antigen and production of antibody. Plasma cells are antibody-synthesizing cells.

In normal circulating blood, the following types of leukocytes can be found in order of frequency: neutrophils, lymphocytes, monocytes, eosinophils, and basophils. The lymphocytes participate in defending the body against disease through recognition of foreign antigens and antibody production. Several major categories of lymphocytes are recognized as functionally active. These categories are the *T cells, B cells,* and the *natural killer (NK)* and *K-type* lymphocytes.

T cells are responsible for cellular immune responses and are involved in the regulation of antibody reactions either by helping or suppressing the activation of B lymphocytes. Sensitized T lymphocytes protect humans against infection by mediating intracellular pathogens that are viral, bacterial, fungal, or protozoan. These cells are responsible for chronic rejection in organ transplantation. T cells are divided into two subsets: the *helper/inducer* (CD_4 [T_4]) and the *suppressor/cytotoxic* (CD_8 [T_8]). Functionally, the helper T cells signal B cells to generate antibodies, control production and switching of types of antibodies formed, and activate suppressor cells. The normal functioning of **helper cells** and **suppressor cells** in the immune response can be reversed under certain conditions, such as autoimmune disorders, and acquired immunodeficiency syndrome (AIDS). The normal ratio of helper cells and suppressor cells (approximately 2:1) can be reversed under certain conditions.

B cells serve as the primary source of cells responsible for humoral (antibody) responses. Participation of B cells in the humoral immune response is accomplished by their maturation into plasma cells with subsequent synthesis and secretion of immune antibodies (immunoglobulins). Stimulation of B cells to produce antibodies is a complex process usually requiring interactions between macrophages (that phagocytize, process, and present antigens to T cells), T cells, and B cells. B lymphocytes aid in the body's defense against encapsulated bacteria, such as streptococci. The condition of hyperacute rejection of transplanted organs is mediated by the B cell.

Lymphocytes that lack the recognizable surface markers of mature T or B lymphocytes include the natural killer (NK) cells and **killer (K) cells.** The NK and K cells destroy target cells through an extracellular nonphagocytic mechanism referred to as a *cytotoxic reaction.* NK cells have the ability to nonspecifically attack certain types of tumor cells and cells infected with a number of different viruses. NK cells are stimulated by interferon (an antiviral substance) released by an intracellular virus. NK cells will actively kill the virally infected target cell and if this is completed before the virus has time to replicate, they will combat viral infection. NK cells are classified as a population of effector lymphocytes that produce such mediators as *interferon* and *interleukin*-2 (IL-2). K cells exhibit a different kind of cytotoxic mechanism than NK cells; the target cell must be coated with low concentrations of IgG antibody. This is referred to as an antibody-dependent cell-mediated cytotoxicity (ADCC) reaction. An ADCC reaction may be exhibited by both K cells and phagocytic and nonphagocytic myelogenous type leukocytes. K cells are capable of lysing tumor cells.

ANTIBODY CLASSES. Five distinct classes of **immunoglobulin** molecules are recognized in most higher mammals: IgM, IgG, IgA, IgD, and IgE. Production of antibodies is induced when the host's immune system comes into contact with a foreign antigenic substance.

The major immunoglobulin in normal serum is IgG. This immunoglobulin diffuses more readily into the extravascular spaces than other immunoglobulins and neutralizes toxins or binds to microorganisms in extravascular spaces. It is capable of crossing the placenta. IgG accounts for 70% to 75% of the total immunoglobulin pool.

IgM accounts for about 10% of the immunoglobulin pool. It is largely confined to the intravascular pool because of its large size. This antibody is produced early in an immune response and is largely confined to the blood. IgM is effective in agglutination and cytolytic reactions. In humans, it is found in smaller concentrations than IgG or IgA.

IgA represents 15% to 20% of the total circulatory immunoglobulin pool. It is the predominant immunoglobulin in secretions, such as tears, saliva, colostrum, breast milk, nasal fluids, and intestinal secretions. Secretory IgA is of critical importance in protecting body surfaces against invading microorganisms. It provides external surfaces of the body with protection from microorganisms because of its presence in seromucous secretions.

IgD is found in very low concentrations in plasma. It accounts for less than 1% of the total immunoglobulin pool and is very susceptible to proteolysis. This immunoglobulin is primarily a cell membrane immunoglobulin found on the surface of B lymphocytes in association with IgM.

IgE is of major importance because it mediates some types of hypersensitivity (allergic) reactions, allergies, and anaphylaxis. It is generally responsible for an individual's immunity to invading parasites. The IgE molecule is unique because it mediates the release of histamines and heparin.

Immunologic Conditions in Maternity and Gynecologic Nursing

Immunologic problems have an impact in every area of nursing practice, including maternity and gynecologic nursing. The nurse must be knowledgeable about the nature of these problems to provide competent care. Hemolytic disease of the newborn, rubella, and AIDS are of particular concern to the maternity nurse. Infertility and neoplasias are frequently encountered by the gynecologic nurse. These conditions may also relate to immunologic problems.

HEMOLYTIC DISEASE OF THE NEWBORN. **Hemolytic disease of the newborn** (HDN), formerly called erythroblastosis fetalis, results from excessive destruction of fetal red blood cells by maternal antibodies. In HDN, the erythrocytes of the fetus become coated with maternal antibodies that correspond to specific fetal antigens (for further discussion of HDN, see Chapter 38).

The following procedures are generally employed in prenatal testing under various conditions. These procedures are ABO blood grouping; Rh testing for D and D^u; alloantibody screening (if negative, it should be repeated again at 34 weeks of gestation); alloantibody identification, if the antibody screening test is positive; antibody titer, if an alloantibody is present; and amniocentesis. Amniocentesis is an analysis of fluid from the amniotic cavity that is obtained by the transabdominal insertion of a needle into the amniotic cavity (see Chapter 27). Amniotic fluid is analyzed to determine whether fetal red blood cells are being hemolyzed (for further discussion, see Chapter 38).

In addition to the procedures listed as prenatal assays, various laboratory procedures are also helpful. These procedures may be useful in determining the presence and assessment of the severity of hemolytic disease of the newborn, or quantitating the extent of fetal-maternal hemorrhage. Postpartum testing of umbilical cord or infant blood includes hemoglobin and hematocrit determination, serum bilirubin assay, ABO and Rh grouping, direct antiglobulin test (DAT), or Coombs' test, and antibody elution and identification. If the DAT is positive, a peripheral blood smear for determining the number of immature erythrocytes in the infant's blood is performed. An exchange transfusion removes bilirubin and circulating maternal antibodies from the infant's plasma and replaces antibody-coated erythrocytes with compatible Rh-negative red blood cells.

Advances in technology in immunology have resulted in decreasing the risk for hemolytic disease of the newborn. Administration of Rh immune globulin (Rh IgG) to the pregnant woman at 28 weeks of gestation (antenatal) has decreased the incidence of primary immunization in Rh_o (D)-negative women to 0.07%. The use of Rh IgG after conditions such as abortion, ectopic pregnancy, or hemorrhage during pregnancy has also contributed to the decreased incidence of D antigen immunization.

For prophylactic treatment using Rh IgG to be effective, appropriate amounts must be administered to previously unsensitized (Coombs' negative) Rh (D)-negative women within 72 hours after delivery or obstetric intervention. Administration of immune prophylaxis is performed after delivery of an Rh (D)-positive infant; following amniocentesis, abortion, or ectopic pregnancy; or before delivery in selected cases (antenatal) (p. 1154). Requirements include the following: the mother must be D and D^u negative, the screening (Coombs') test for alloantibodies must be negative for anti-D antibody, the infant must be D or D^u positive (in cases where the Rh cannot be determined, it must be assumed that this criterion has been met), and the Coombs' test (or DAT). on cord cells or infant's cells, if available, must be negative. These criteria must be met *each time* an Rh-negative mother is pregnant, delivers, or undergoes obstetric intervention.

RUBELLA INFECTION. The rubella virus was first isolated in 1962. Acquired rubella, also known as German or 3-day measles, is caused by a ribonucleic acid (RNA) virus. Because the virus is endemic to humans, the disease is highly contagious and is transmitted through respiratory secretions. Before widespread rubella immunization in the United States and Canada, rubella infections occurred in epidemic proportion at 6- to 9-year intervals. In 1964, more than 20,000 cases of **congenital rubella syndrome** and an unknown number of stillbirths occurred in the United States as the result of an epidemic that year. In countries where vaccination is uncommon, the incidence of rubella infection continues to be high, and epidemics are frequent. Contracting the infection and receiving a vaccination against rubella are the only routes to developing immunity (American College of Obstetricians and Gynecologists, 1981).

It is critical to continue to determine the rubella immune status of women of childbearing age and to vaccinate those who are not immune. Other individuals requiring rubella immune status determination include preschool and school-age children, all women at or just before childbearing age, women who are about to be married, married women, pregnant women, and health care personnel. If a woman is not rubella immune, she should be vaccinated. She is advised not to become pregnant for 3 months because there is a remote possibility that the vaccination could lead to an infected fetus. In pregnant women, a positive test confirms immunity, but to rule out any possibility of unsuspected current infection, an IgM screening procedure may also be ordered. If the pregnant woman is not rubella immune, she should be cautioned to avoid exposure to rubella infection. Vaccination is contraindicated in a pregnant woman. However, the woman should be vaccinated immediately after termination of the pregnancy (for a discussion of fetal/neonatal effects of rubella infection, see Chapter 39).

Because IgG antibody is capable of crossing the placental barrier, there is no way of distinguishing between IgG antibody of fetal origin and IgG antibody of maternal origin in a neonatal blood specimen. Testing for IgM antibody is invaluable in the diagnosis of congenital rubella syndrome in the neonate. IgM does not cross an intact placental barrier, therefore demonstration of IgM in a single neonatal specimen is diagnostic of congenital rubella syndrome.

ACQUIRED IMMUNODEFICIENCY SYNDROME. In 1983, researchers at the Pasteur Institute in Paris isolated a retrovirus (see glossary) from a homosexual man with lymphadenopathy. In 1984, an American team was able to demonstrate conclusively through virologic and epidemiologic evidence that human immunodeficiency virus (HIV) was the cause of **acquired immunodeficiency syndrome (AIDS).**

The AIDS pandemic is still in its early stages, and its ultimate dimensions are difficult to assess accurately. HIV has been isolated from blood, semen, vaginal secretions, saliva, tears, breast milk, cerebrospinal fluid (CSF), amniotic fluid, and urine. To date, however, only *blood, semen, vaginal secretions,* and possibly *breast milk* have been implicated in transmission of HIV. Pediatric AIDS cases are usually related to the receipt of unscreened blood or blood products, or to the mother being infected with HIV during pregnancy.

HIV has a marked preference for the helper-inducer subset of lymphocytes. It displays an affinity for these cells because the CD_4 (T_4) surface marker protein on these cells serves as a receptor site for the virus. The extensive destruction of T cells leads to the gradual depletion of helper/inducer and suppressor/cytotoxic subsets of T lymphocytes. This abnormality exists in the lymph nodes as well as in circulating T cells. Normally, this ratio is 2:1 in heterosexuals and 1.5:1 in homosexuals. A reversal of these subsets is evident in, but *not* diagnostic of, AIDS. In people with AIDS, the lymphocyte subset ratio is usually less than 0.5:1. A diminished ratio can also be seen in individuals with other disorders, such as cutaneous T cell lymphoma, systemic lupus erythematosus (SLE), and acute viral infections. This disease additionally demonstrates defective NK cell activity.

After initial infection, the body mounts a vigorous immune response against the viremia. Immunologic activities include the production of different types of antibodies against HIV. Some antibodies neutralize it, others prevent it from binding to cells, and others stimulate cytotoxic cells to attack HIV infected cells. A *"window" period* of seronegativity exists from the time of initial infection to 6 or 12 weeks or longer thereafter. Increased production of core antigen is believed to be associated with a burst of viral replication and host cell lysis. A detectable antibody response appears about 6 weeks after the time of infection.

GYNECOLOGIC CONDITIONS. The immune system plays a vital role in several gynecologic conditions. Some problems with impaired fertility may be attributed to immunologic factors. For example, some women develop antibodies against their husband's sperm. For further discussion of impaired fertility, see Chapter 42. Neoplasia, especially malignant conditions and their therapy, are best understood if the nurse has some knowledge of immunology. For further discussion of malignant neoplasms, see Chapter 44.

Factors Associated with Immunologic Disease

Factors such as general health and the age of an individual are important considerations in the functioning of the immune system in defense against infectious disease. In the case of noninfectious diseases or disorders, however, additional factors may be of importance.

In the maternity and gynecologic setting, the nurse must consider the development of the immune system in the fetus and newborn, environmental factors, nutritional status, and life-style considerations.

IMMUNITY IN THE NEWBORN. Although nonspecific and specific body defenses are present in the unborn and newborn infant, many of these defenses are not completely developed in this group. A healthy newborn does not sweat, has no tears, and is not born with "normal" skin or intestinal microbial flora. Young children are at greater risk for diseases, particularly infectious diseases. If the integrity of the skin is broken, the newborn is predisposed to tissue and blood invasion by foreign cells such as bacteria. Infants who are preterm, small for gestational age, or postterm have different skin qualities that increase their susceptibility to invasive agents.

Full-term infants usually have passively acquired natural immunity because of the presence of maternal IgG antibodies. These antibodies are transferred from mother to infant through the placental circulation and provide short-term resistance to the specific antigens to which the mother produced antibodies. The preterm infant may be deficient in this type of immunity, especially if born before the thirty-sixth week of gestation. The other antibody type that a newborn can acquire passively is IgA. This class of antibody is present in *colostrum* and can be acquired in the newborn by *breast-feeding*.

The fetus is capable of forming IgM antibodies in response to an intrauterine infection. The newborn can also develop IgM antibodies as the initial humoral response to exposure to an antigenic substance (e.g., bacteria or viruses). In addition, a healthy newborn usually demonstrates the presence of IgA in tears and mucous secretions within a few months after birth.

ENVIRONMENT. The environment of each person is significant in determining the challenges posed to one's immune system. The various component factors of one's environment—the quality of air, water, and food and the ventilation, refrigeration, crowding, and cleanliness in the setting—contribute to the risks that a person encounters from microorganisms and substances. With the infectious diseases of tuberculosis and toxoplasmosis, one can readily appreciate the influence of environment in acquisition and transmission. Not every person is exposed to the tubercle bacillus or to the parasite that causes toxoplasmosis (for a discussion of these infections, see Chapter 29). However, if one lives in a setting in which tubercle bacillus is endemic (e.g., an urban, overcrowded area with poor ventilation), then the risks of exposure are much greater. The cat owner whose pet harbors the toxoplasmosis parasite is at increased risk of acquiring the disease, especially if the person has contact with the cat's feces (i.e., through emptying the litter pan). It is recognized that the infection can be transmitted from mother to fetus via placental transfer.

The environment of the newborn in a hospital setting is a factor over which a nurse can exert some control to effect fewer challenges to the neonate's immune defense system. Persons who harbor infectious diseases should be barred from the nursery, and the medical aseptic technique employed in the nursery environment should be meticulous (Chapter 21). This is not to suggest that the normal newborn should have a sterile environment but that there is no reason to overtax a relatively meager set of immune defense mechanisms. An overwhelming systemic infection, such as that caused by herpes virus in the neonate, can not only interfere with healthy growth and development of the parent-child relationship because of prolonged separation but can also threaten the newborn's life. For this reason the environment into which a fetus will be born must be assessed for its risk potential in posing harm to the newborn.

NUTRITIONAL STATUS. The importance of good nutrition to good health has always been emphasized. Good nutrition is known to be important to growth and development, and it is now suggested that a healthy diet is of importance in the aging process and in the *triad of nutrition, immunity, and infection*. The consequences of diet, however, in multiple aspects of the immune response have been documented in many disorders. Every constituent of body defenses, including phagocytosis and humoral and cellular immunity, appears to be influenced by nutritional intake. Deficient or excessive intake of some dietary components, such as vitamins and minerals, can exert negative effects on the immune response. Therefore a healthy diet is important to the maximum functioning of the immune system.

Malnutrition caused by extremely reduced caloric intake or a deficiency (complete or partial) of a specific nutrient can produce abnormal immune function. Protein deficiency is an example of a disorder that compromises the immune system. Individuals with such a deficiency have altered immune defenses, such as decreased levels of IgA in secretions and decreased total levels and abnormal ratios of lymphocytic white cells. Imbalanced intake of minerals can also cause immunologic abnormalities.

Breast milk is supportive of the body's immune defense system because it favors the growth of *Lactobacillus bifidus* in the infant's intestinal system. This microorganism converts lactose into lactic acid. Lactic acid diminishes the growth of pathogenic organisms in the intestinal tract. Breast milk also provides the necessary amounts of nutrients, such as proteins and essential minerals, that support the healthy functioning of the immune system.

LIFE-STYLE. Certain infectious diseases are associated with the patterns of living that people establish for themselves. For instance, the sexually transmitted diseases of syphilis and gonorrhea are more likely to be acquired by people with multiple sex partners. Many other aspects comprise the concept of *life-style* besides sexual preference patterns and sexual behavior. These factors include the numerous health behaviors that people practice—such as their patterns of rest, exercise, food and drug intake, relaxation, work performance, self-care, and use of health care professionals. It is important for the nurse to assess carefully the numerous details about clients' lifestyles because these factors affect the clients' susceptibility to invasion by harmful substances. For instance, a pattern of heavy *alcohol consumption* is associated with certain nutritional deficiencies (notably the B vitamin complex) that decrease the individual's immune responsiveness to vaccines and depress the cell-mediated and humoral lymphocytic activity (Whitney, Cataldo, 1983). Individuals who assume responsibility for their health and who practice health maintenance and preventive strategies (such as acquiring artificial active immunity) are more likely to enjoy a competent immune defense system.

Nursing Implications

When clients have any degree of compromised immune responsiveness, the nurse must take steps to ensure their protection from sources of infection in the hospital and the home environment. Scrupulous attention must be given to practicing medical asepsis by all caregivers who come in contact with the client to prevent superimposed iatrogenic nosocomial infections. In some cases reverse or protective isolation should be instituted to further protect the client.

To devise an individualized plan the nurse assesses for factors that place a person at risk, such as the client's age, overall health status, environment, and lifestyle. The client requires supportive therapy to maintain good fluid and nutritional status and to maintain the integrity of this first-line defense mechanism. In some situations the client is further protected with passive immunity support via IgG antibody injections. Clients who have a poor prognosis (such as those with AIDS) and their families also need to have supportive psychosocial care and opportunities to discuss and design their own future. Specific care needs that are indicated for clients with problems of immune responsiveness are discussed in Chapter 29.

It is essential that nurses appreciate the complexity of the immune system. It is important to fully understand how to:

1. Support the healthy defense mechanisms of clients
2. Protect clients whose immune responsiveness is impaired
3. Avoid the unintentional stimulation of potentially dangerous (allergic) defense mechanisms

■ SUMMARY

Basic knowledge of the female and male reproductive systems is a prerequisite to understanding the process of conception. A systematic investigation of the human reproductive system provides the nurse with a firm foundation for gaining insight into the client's needs and health concerns.

Basic concepts of the psychosocial nature of human sexuality provide guidelines for anticipatory guidance of the childbearing family. Each individual's cognitive and personality development influences his or her mastery of developmental tasks from infancy through adulthood. The atmosphere in which the child is raised will affect future attitudes and behaviors. Sexual identity begins early and is shaped by societal expectations. Mixed messages about sexuality, peer pressures, and confusion about the relationship of love and sex may cause conflicts. During adulthood childhood potential is realized and key social roles are assumed. The importance ascribed to the roles of man-woman, husband-wife, and parent-child reflect society's concern with the biopsychosocial nature of adult sexuality. Nurses need to understand that everyone's feelings and values regarding sexuality are not going to match their own feelings and values.

Immunologic conditions of importance in maternity and gynecologic nursing include hemolytic disease of the newborn, rubella, AIDS, and infertility.

Factors such as general health and the age of an individual are important considerations in the functioning of the immune system in defense against infectious disease. In the case of noninfectious diseases or disorders, additional factors may be of importance. These factors can include genetic predisposition to many disorders, nutritional status, environment, and life-style. It is essential that nurses be familiar with the complexity of the immune system in order to support the healthy defense mechanisms of clients, protect immunologically impaired clients, and avoid unintentional stimulation of allergic reactions.

REFERENCES

American College of Obstetricians and Gynecologists: Rubella-A clinical update, *ACOG Technical Bulletin* 62:7, 1981.

American Psychiatric Association: *Diagnostic and statistical manual of mental disorders,* ed 3, revised, (DSM-III-R), Washington, DC, 1987, The American Psychiatric Association.

Brookman R: Adolescent sexuality and related health problems. In Hoffman A, editor: *Adolescent medicine,* Menlo Park, Calif, 1983, Addison-Wesley Publishing.

Duvall ER: *Family development,* ed 5, Philadelphia, 1977, JB Lippincott.

Erikson E: Identity and the life cycle; selected papers. In *Psychological issues,* New York, 1959, International Universities Press.

Ganong WE: *Review of medical physiology,* ed 13, Norwalk, Conn, 1987, Appleton & Lange.

Havighurst RJ: *Developmental tasks and education,* ed 3, New York, 1972, David McKay.

Herbst AL: *Comprehensive gynecology,* ed 2, St Louis, 1992, Mosby–Year Book.

Johnson R: Adolescent growth and development. In Hoffman A, editor: *Adolescent medicine,* Menlo Park, Calif, 1983, Addison-Wesley Publishing.

Kaplan HS: *The new sex therapy,* New York, 1974, Brunner/Mazel.

Katchadourian HA, Lunde DT: *Fundamentals of human sexuality,* New York, 1972, Holt, Rinehart and Winston.

Kinsey AC et al: *Sexual behavior in human male,* Philadelphia, 1948, WB Saunders.

Kinsey AC et al: *Sexual behavior in human female,* Philadelphia, 1953, WB Saunders.

Marmor J, editor: *Homosexual behavior: a modern reappraisal,* New York, 1980, Basic Books.

Masters WH, Johnson VE: *Human sexual response,* 1966, Little, Brown & Co.

Mims FH, Swenson M: *Sexuality, a nursing perspective,* New York, 1980, McGraw-Hill.

Premarital sexual experience among adolescent women—United States 1970-1988, *MMWR* 39(51,52):929, 1991.

Newman B, Newman R: *Development through life: a psychosocial approach,* Homewood, Ill, 1975, The Dorsey Press.

Offer D, Simon W: Sexual development. In Sadock B, Kaplan H, Freedman A, editors: *The sexual experience,* Baltimore, 1976, Williams & Wilkins.

Piaget J: *The psychology of intelligence,* Boston, 1950, Routledge & Kegan Paul.

Stuart GW, Sundeen SJ: *Principles and practice of psychiatric nursing,* ed 4, St Louis, 1991, Mosby–Year Book.

Whaley LF, Wong DL: *Nursing care of infants and children,* ed 4, St Louis, 1990, Mosby–Year Book.

Whitney EN, Cataldo CB: *Understanding normal and clinical nutrition,* New York, 1983, West Publishing.

Woods NF: *Human sexuality in health and illness,* ed 3, St Louis, 1984, Mosby–Year Book.

BIBLIOGRAPHY

Anthony CP, Thibodeau GA: *Textbook of anatomy and physiology,* ed 12, St Louis, 1987, Mosby–Year Book.

Brown Y et al: Female circumcision, *Can Nurse* p 19, April 1989.

Froberg JH: The anemias: causes and courses of action, *RN* p 42, May 1989.

Gallo RC, Montagnier L: AIDS in 1988, *Sci Amer* 259(4):40, 1988.

Ganong WF: *Review of medical physiology,* ed 14, Norwalk, Conn, 1989, Appleton & Lange.

Groër M: Psychoneuroimmunology: an emerging discipline gives new theoretical support to nursing care of the 'bodymind', *Am J Nurs* 91(8):33, 1991.

Malasanos L et al: *Health assessment,* ed 4, St Louis, 1989, Mosby–Year Book.

Nossal GJ: Current concepts: immunology, the basic components of the immune system, *N Engl J Med,* 316(21):1320, 1987.

Phipps WJ, Long BC, Woods NF: *Medical-surgical nursing: concepts and clinical practice,* ed. 4, St Louis, 1991, Mosby–Year Book.

RN Update: Measles outbreak: implications for nurses, *RN* 53(3):10, 1990.

Sarrel PM: Sexuality and menopause, *Obst Gynec* 75(4):26(suppl), 1990.

Scott JR et al: *Danforth's obstetrics and gynecology,* ed 6, Philadelphia, 1990, JB Lippincott.

Seidel HM et al: *Mosby's guide to physical examination,* ed 2, St Louis, 1991, Mosby–Year Book.

Smith DH et al: Sexuality and changes with aging, *Contemp Ob/Gyn* 31(6):88, 1988.

Taylor DL: Immune response: physiology, signs, and symptoms, *Nursing 84* 14(5):52, 1984.

Thompson JM et al: *Mosby's manual of clinical nursing,* ed 2, St Louis, 1989, Mosby–Year Book.

Thornton NG, Dewis M: Multiple sclerosis and female sexuality, *Can Nurse,* p 16, April 1989.

Turgeon ML: *Clinical hematology,* Boston, 1988, Little, Brown & Co.

Turgeon ML: *Fundamentals of immunohematology,* Philadelphia, 1989, Lea & Febiger.

Ungvarski P: Coping with infections that AIDS patients develop, *RN* p 53, Nov 1988.

US Department of Health and Human Services: Universal precautions for prevention of transmission of HIV, hepatitis B virus, and other blood borne pathogens in health care settings, *MMWR* 37:377, 1988.

US Department of Health and Human Services: Update: acquired immunodeficiency syndrome and HIV infection among health care workers, *MMWR* 37:229, 1988.

Uvnäs-Moberg K: The gastrointestinal tract in growth and reproduction, *Sci Am* p 78, July 1989.

Wiley K, Grohar J: Human immunodeficiency virus and precautions for obstetric, gynecologic, and neonatal nurses, *JOGN Nurse* 17(3):165, 1988.

Wilkin TJ: Receptor autoimmunity in endocrine disorders, *N Engl J Med* 323(19):1318, 1990.

Zacharin RF: Functional anatomy of the pelvic floor, Contemp *Ob/Gyn* 34(4):111, 1989.

chapter 6 review

Key Concepts

- The myometrium of the uterus is uniquely designed to expel the fetus and promote hemostasis after birth.
- The uterus has an intrinsic motility allowing uterine contractions even after spinal cord injury.
- Normal feedback regulation of the menstrual cycle depends on an intact hypothalamic-pituitary-gonadal mechanism.
- The female's reproductive tract structures and breasts respond predictably to changing levels of sex steroids across the life span.
- Prostaglandins play an important role in reproductive functions by their effect on smooth muscle contractility and modulation of hormones.
- Nurses need to be aware of their own feelings and values regarding sexuality before they can adequately and competently help clients meet their needs for information or refer them for further counseling.
- Responsible sexuality includes commitment to a relationship, responsible reproductive health care, and rational decisions about childbearing.
- The desirable consequences of immunity include natural resistance, recovery, and acquired resistance to infectious diseases.
- With medical science, the immune system can be advantageously manipulated to protect against disorders of the newborn, as well as many environmental microorganisms.
- Vaccination is an effective method of stimulating antibody production and memory.
- IgA, the predominant immunoglobulin in secretions (including colostrum and breast milk), is of critical importance in protecting body surfaces (internal and external) against invading microorganisms.
- Factors such as fetal/neonatal development, lifestyle, environment, and nutrition affect the functioning of the immune defense system.

Key Terms

- acquired immunodeficiency syndrome (AIDS) (p. 144)
- active immunity (p. 140)
- adaptive immunity (p. 140)
- anaphylaxis (p. 141)
- atrophy (p. 102)
- climacterium (p. 124)
- cognitive development (p. 131)
- congenital rubella syndrome (p. 144)
- core gender identity (p. 133)
- developmental tasks (p. 133)
- endometrial cycle (p. 120)
- gender preference (p. 134)
- helper cells (p. 142)
- hemolytic disease of the newborn (p. 143)
- heterosexuality (p. 134)
- homosexuality (p. 136)
- hypothalamic-pituitary cycle (p. 122)
- immunocompetent (p. 141)
- immunoglobulin (p. 142)
- immunology (p. 139)

- killer cells (p. 142)
- living ligature (p. 111)
- masturbation (p. 136)
- menarche (p. 102)
- menopause (p. 124)
- menstruation (p. 120)
- mittelschmerz (p. 124)
- myotonia (p. 131)
- natural immunity (p. 140)
- ovarian cycle (p. 122)
- ovulation (p. 106)
- passive immunity (p. 141)
- personality development (p. 131)
- promiscuous (p. 137)
- prostaglandins (p. 130)
- pubarche (p. 102)
- serial monogamy (p. 138)
- sex role standards (p. 133)
- sexuality (p. 133)
- spinnbarkheit (p. 124)
- squamocolumnar junction (p. 112)
- suppressor cells (p. 142)
- vaccination (p. 140)
- withdrawal bleeding (p. 122)

Critical Thinking Exercises

The local high school has asked your clinical group to teach some classes to high school seniors. The subjects to be covered are male and female anatomy, sexuality, and the immune system. One third of group is teaching each class.

1. The first group is to develop an outline of essential content on the anatomy and physiology of the male and female reproductive systems and to select appropriate teaching methods. Justify the selection of content and teaching methods.
2. The second group is to develop an outline of essential content on human sexual response and to identify appropriate teaching methods. Justify the selection of content and teaching methods.
3. The third group is to develop an outline of essential content on the functioning of the immune system in relation to age, life-style, environment, and nutrition. Appropriate teaching methods should be identified. Justify the selection of content and teaching methods.

Topics for Nursing Research

- How do nurses perceive their role in parental counseling regarding sex education?
- What is the relationship between nurse's sex knowledge and attitudes and comfort in providing parental counseling regarding sex education?
- What is the relationship between therapeutic touch and immunity?

unit 2

Normal Pregnancy

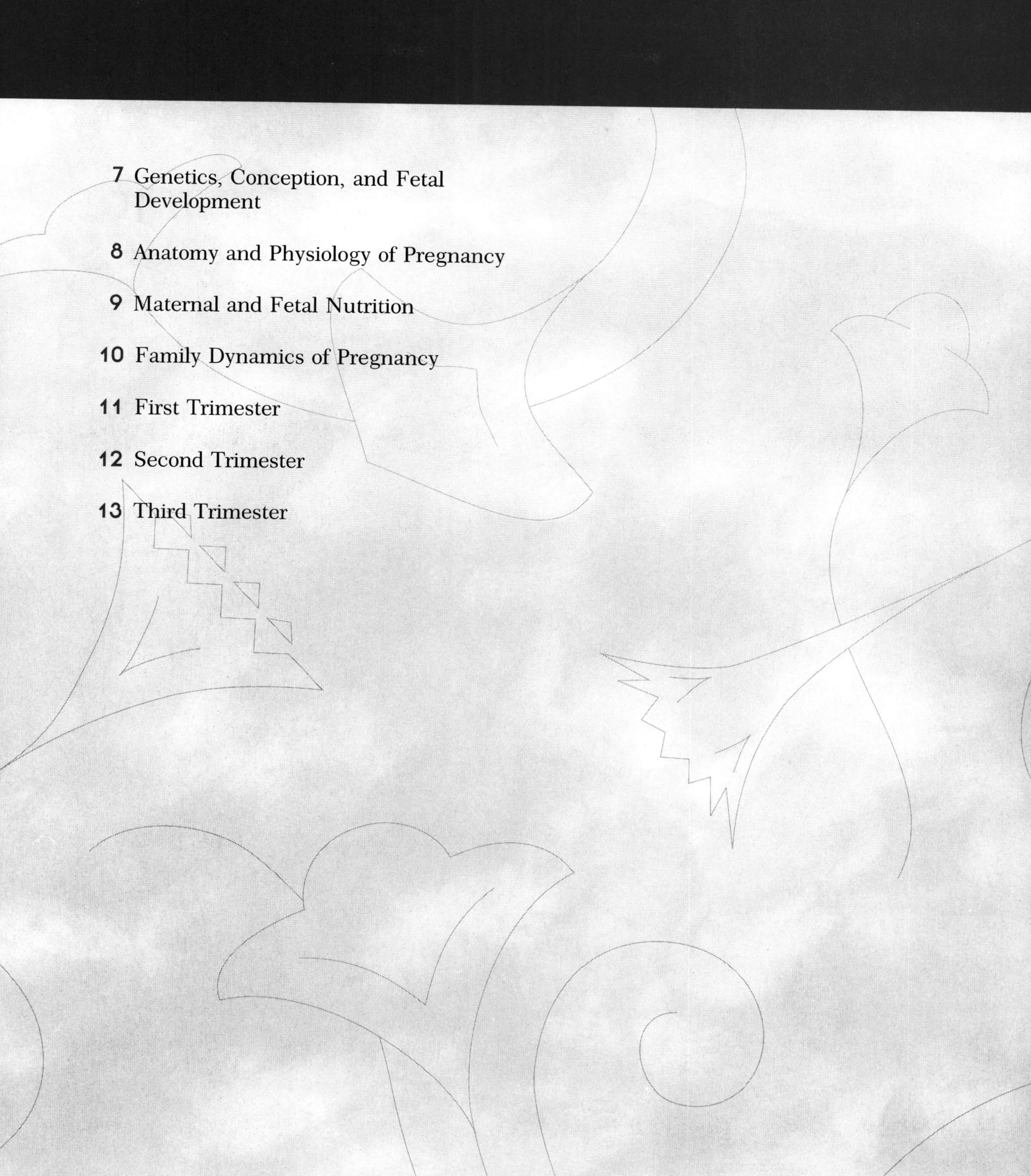

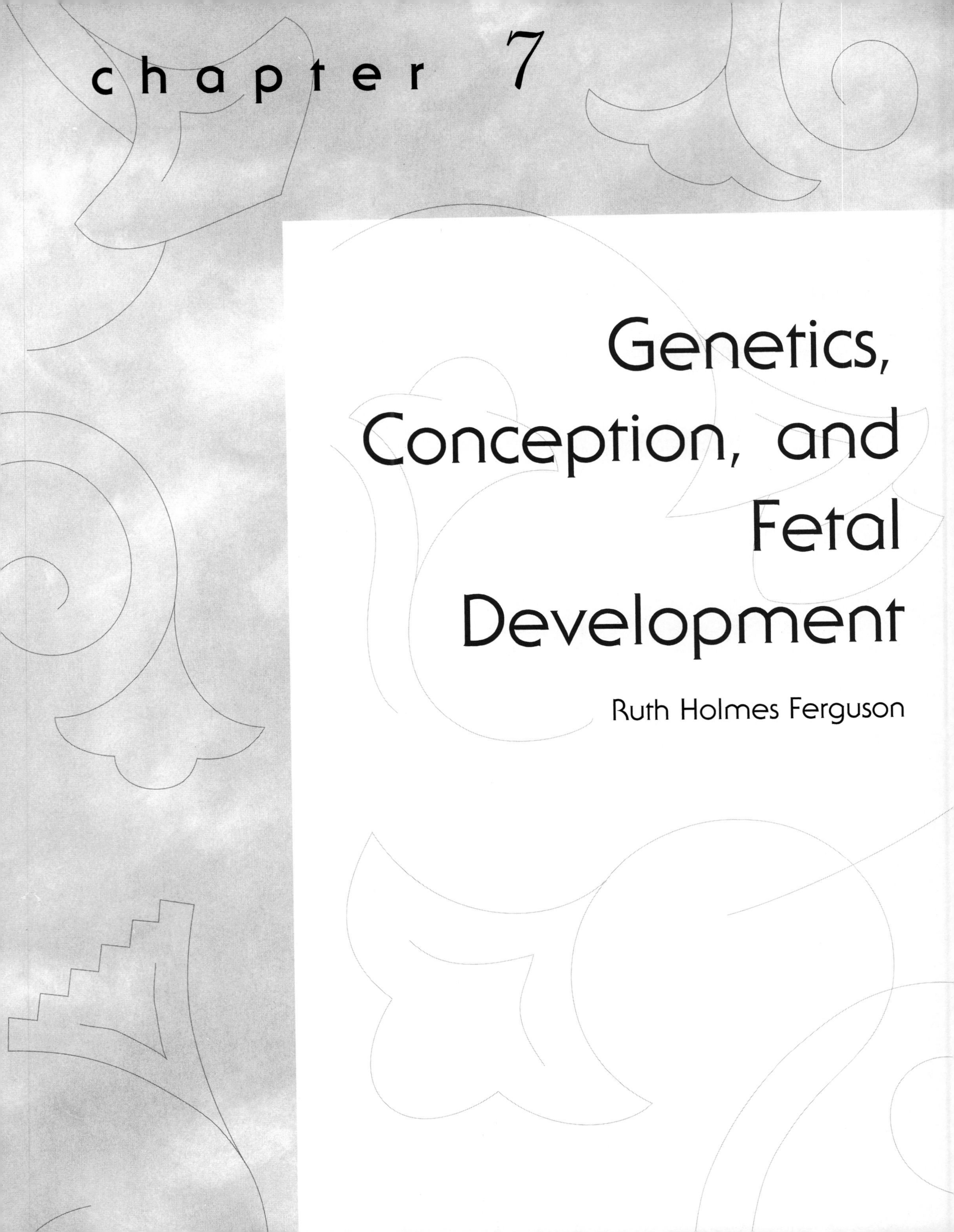

chapter 7

Genetics, Conception, and Fetal Development

Ruth Holmes Ferguson

LEARNING OBJECTIVES

- Define the key terms listed.
- Explain the difference between mitosis and meiosis.
- Summarize the process of fertilization.
- Explain the basic principles of genetics.
- Describe the development, structure, and functions of the placenta.
- Describe the composition and functions of the amniotic fluid.
- Identify three organs or tissues arising from each of the three primary germ layers.
- Summarize the significant changes in growth and development of the embryo and fetus.
- Identify the potential effects of teratogens during the vulnerable periods of embryonic and fetal development.
- Identify topics for nursing research related to conception and fetal development.

This chapter presents a brief overview of the genetic basis of inheritance and the origin of common genetic disorders. The main focus is on the physical process of fertilization and the development of the normal embryo and fetus.

■ GENETICS

Human development is a complicated process that depends on the systematic unraveling of instructions found in the genetic material of the united egg and sperm. Although the progress from conception to birth of a normal, healthy baby occurs without incident in most cases, occasionally some anomaly in the genetic code of the embryo creates a birth defect or disease. Parents are then left to wonder what went wrong, which parent might be "responsible," or, most significantly, what are the chances of the problem recurring with the next pregnancy. The science of genetics seeks to explain the underlying causes of congenital disorders (disorders present at birth) as well as the patterns in which inherited disorders are passed from generation to generation. A basic understanding of genetics will help the professional nurse assist new families in locating the right sources (often genetics counselors) to help them cope with the questions and fears surrounding birth defects.

Genes and Chromosomes

An individual's physical characteristics are determined by the hereditary material carried in the nucleus of every one of his or her somatic (body) cells. This material, called deoxyribonucleic acid (DNA), forms threadlike strands known as **chromosomes.** Each chromosome is composed of many smaller segments of DNA referred to as **genes.** Genes or combinations of genes contain coded information that determines the person's unique characteristics. The "code" is found in the specific linear order of the molecules that combine to form the strands of DNA.

All human somatic cells contain 46 chromosomes arranged as 23 pairs of homologous (matched) chromosomes, one of each pair inherited from each parent. There are 22 pairs of **autosomes,** which control most traits in the body, and one pair of **sex chromosomes,** which, in addition to some other traits, control sex determination. The large female chromosome is called the X; the tiny male chromosome is the Y. Generally the presence of a Y chromosome causes an embryo to develop as a male; in the absence of a Y chromosome, the individual develops as a female. Thus in a normal female the homologous pair of sex chromosomes would be XX, and in a normal male the homologous pair would be XY.

Because each gene occupies a specific chromosome location, and because chromosomes are inherited as homologous pairs, each person has two genes for every trait. In other words, if an autosome has a gene for hair color, its partner will also have a gene for hair color—in the same location on the chromosome. However, although both genes code for hair color, they may not code for the *same* hair color. Different genes coding for different variations of the same trait are called alleles. An individual having two copies of the same allele for a given trait is said to be homozygous for that trait; with two different alleles, the person is heterozygous for the trait.

Some genes are **dominant,** and their characteristics are expressed even if another allele is present on the other chromosome. Other genes are **recessive,** and their characteristics will be expressed only if they are carried by both homologous chromosomes. For example, the gene for brown eyes is dominant over the gene for blue eyes. Thus a person with one brown eyes gene and one blue eyes gene will have brown eyes. When an egg and a sperm unite, the combination of alleles becomes that individual's entire genetic makeup, or genotype, which includes all of the genes that the person carries and that can be passed to offspring. The genotype determines the person's physical appearance, or phenotype, but this is affected by the nature of the dominant or recessive allele. To continue the above example, an individual with two brown eyes alleles at the gene for eye color will have the same phenotype as one with one brown eyes and one blue eyes allele.

The pictorial analysis of the number, form, and size of an individual's chromosomes is known as a **karyotype.** It can be obtained from a blood sample specially treated and stained to make the replicating chromosomes visible under a microscope. The photographed chromosomes are cut out and arranged in a specific numeric order according to their length and shape. Fig. 7-1 illustrates the chromosomes in a body cell. Karyotypes can be used to determine what sex a child will be and whether any gross chromosomal abnormalities are present.

Cell Division

Cells are reproduced by two different methods: mitosis and meiosis. Mitosis is the process by which body cells replicate to yield two cells with the same genetic makeup as the parent cell. First the cell makes a copy of its DNA; then it divides, and each daughter cell receives one copy of the genetic mate-

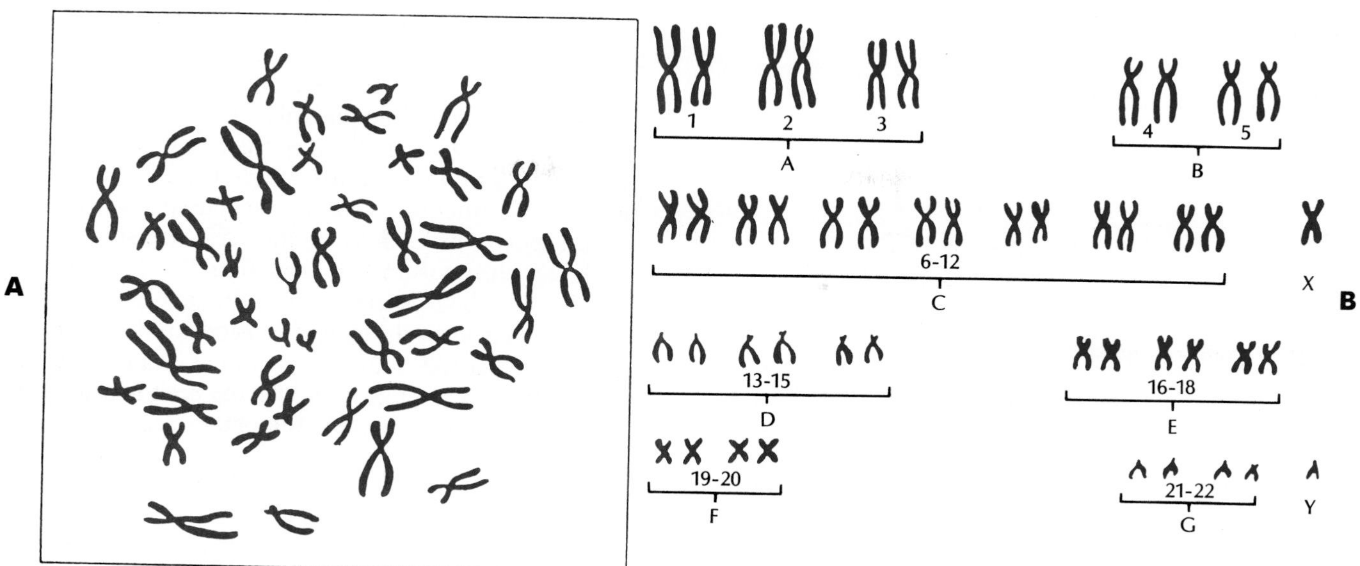

Fig. 7-1 Chromosomes during cell division. **A,** Example of photomicrograph. **B,** Chromosomes arranged in karyotype; female and male sex-determining chromosomes.
From Whaley LF and Wong DL: Nursing care of infants and children, ed 4, St Louis, 1991, Mosby–Year Book.

rial. The purpose of mitotic division is for growth and development or cell replacement.

Meiosis is the process by which **gametes** (eggs and sperm) are produced. When you recall that for each homologous pair of chromosomes one is received from the mother and one from the father, it is easy to understand that meiosis must result in cells that contain one of each of the 23 pairs of chromosomes. Because these germ cells contain 23 single chromosomes, half of the genetic material of a normal somatic cell, they are said to be haploid. This halving of the genetic material is accomplished by replicating the DNA once and then dividing twice. In mitosis, the DNA is replicated once followed by a single cell division. When the female gamete (egg or ovum) and the male gamete (spermatozoan) unite to form the **zygote,** the diploid number of human chromosomes (46 or 23 pairs) is restored.

The process of DNA replication and cell division in meiosis allows different alleles for genes to be distributed at random by each parent and then rearranged on the paired chromosomes. The chromosomes then separate and proceed to different gametes. Because parents have genotypes derived from four different grandparents, many combinations of genes on each chromosome are possible. This random mixing of alleles accounts for the variation of traits seen in the offspring of the same two parents.

Gametogenesis

When a male reaches puberty, his testes begin the process of spermatogenesis. The cells that undergo meiosis in the male are called spermatocytes. The primary spermatocyte, which undergoes the first meiotic division, contains the diploid number of chromosomes. Remember, however, that the cell has already copied its DNA before division, so four alleles for each gene are actually present. Because the copies are bound together—one allele plus its copy on each chromosome—the cell is still considered diploid. During the first meiotic division, two haploid secondary spermatocytes are formed, each containing 22 autosomes and one sex chromosome; one contains the X chromosome (plus its copy), and the other the Y chromosome (plus its copy). During the second meiotic division, the male produces two gametes with an X chromosome and two gametes with a Y chromosome, all of which will develop into viable sperm (Fig. 7-2).

Oogenesis, the process of egg (ovum) formation, begins in the fetal life of the female. All of the cells that may undergo meiosis in a woman's lifetime are contained in her ovaries at birth. The majority of the estimated 2 million primary oocytes (the cells that undergo the first meiotic division) degenerate spontaneously. Only 400 to 500 ova will mature during the

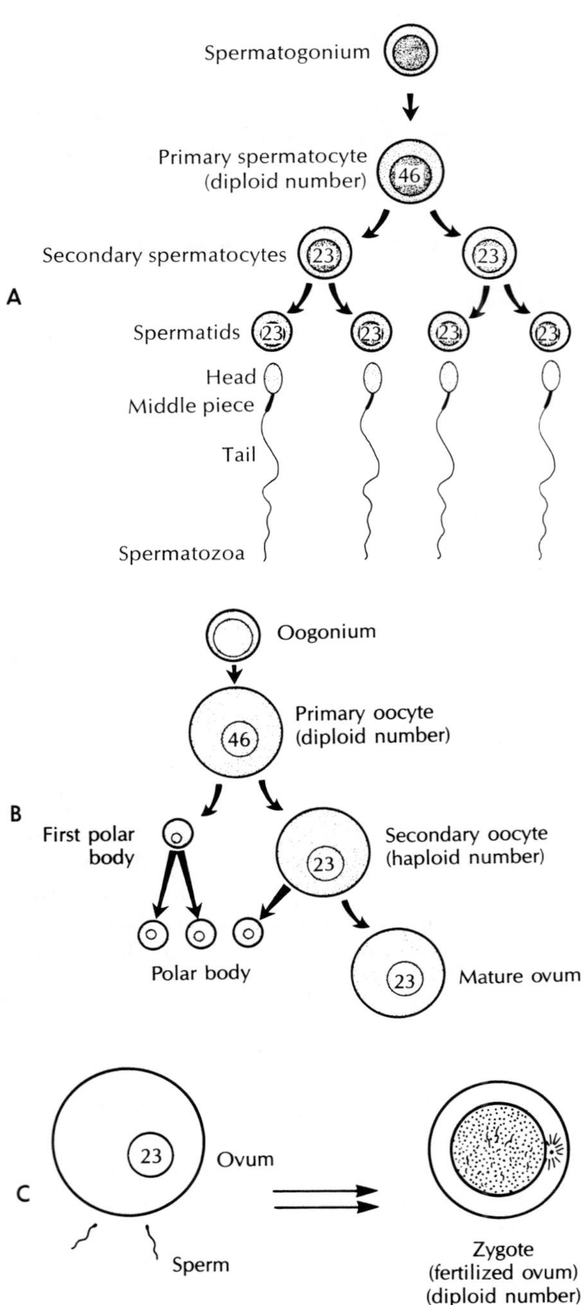

Fig. 7-2 **A**, Spermatogenesis. Gametogenesis of the male produces four mature gametes, the sperm. **B**, Oogenesis. Gametogenesis in the female produces one mature ovum and three polar bodies. Note the relative difference in overall size between the ovum and sperm. **C**, Fertilization results in the single-cell zygote and the restoration of the diploid number of chromosomes.

approximately 35 years of a woman's reproductive life. The primary oocytes begin the first meiotic division (i.e., they replicate their DNA) during fetal life but remain suspended at this stage until puberty (Fig. 7-2). Then, usually monthly, one primary oocyte matures and completes the first meiotic division, yielding two unequal cells: the secondary oocyte and a small polar body. Both contain 22 autosomes and one X sex chromosome. At ovulation, the second meiotic division begins. However, the ovum does not complete the second meiotic division unless fertilization occurs. At this time, a second polar body and the zygote (the united egg and sperm) are produced. If fertilization does not occur, the ovum degenerates.

Chromosomal Abnormalities

Errors resulting in chromosomal abnormalities can occur in either mitosis or meiosis. These occur in either the autosomes or the sex chromosomes and exist as abnormalities of number or of structure. Even small deviations in chromosomes without the presence of obvious structural malformations can cause problems in fetal development.

AUTOSOMAL ABNORMALITIES. Autosomal abnormalities involve differences in the number or structure of chromosomes resulting from unequal distribution of the genetic material during gamete formation. Some of the causes and clinical effects of these genetic problems are discussed below.

ABNORMALITIES OF CHROMOSOME NUMBER. Abnormalities of chromosome number, aneuploidy, are most often caused by nondisjunction. Nondisjunction occurs during meiosis when a pair of chromosomes fails to separate and one resulting cell contains both chromosomes while the other contains none. The product of the union of a normal gamete with a gamete containing an extra chromosome is a trisomy. The resulting individual has 47 chromosomes in each cell.

The most common trisomal abnormality is **Down syndrome,** or trisomy 21. The affected individual has an extra chromosome 21 (with a total of 47 chromosomes). The clinical characteristics include a broad, small skull; flat facial profile; epicanthal folds with slanted palpebral fissures in the eyes; flat, low-set ears (Fig. 7-3, *A*); protruding tongue; short neck with fat pads at the nape; short, broad hands with a single transverse (simian) crease (Fig. 7-3, *B*); and hypotonic muscles with hypermobility of joints. Mental retardation is the major limitation, although there are also increased incidences of congenital heart disease, infectious diseases, and acute childhood leukemia in individuals with Down syndrome. The inci-

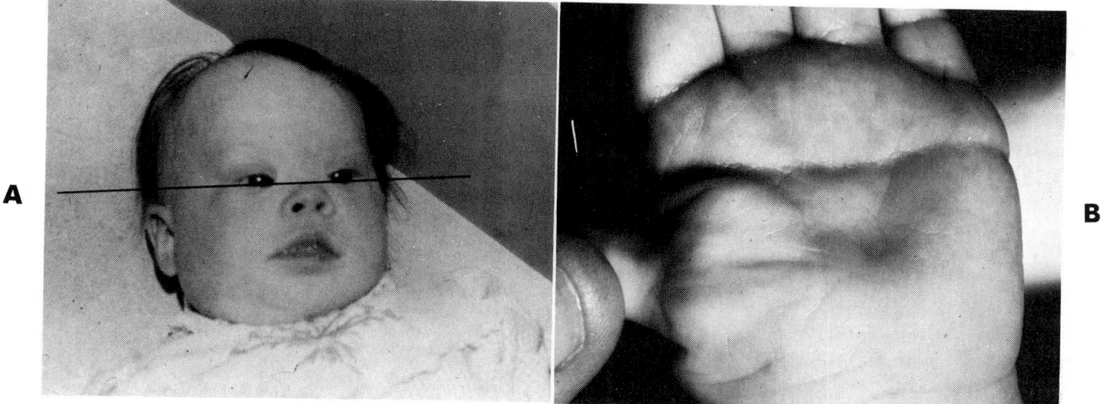

Fig. 7-3 Trisomy 21 (Down syndrome). **A**, Low-set ears. **B**, Simian crease.

dence of Down syndrome increases with maternal or paternal age (Carothers, 1987). Many affected embryos are spontaneously aborted, and some affected fetuses are stillborn.

Other autosomal trisomies that have been diagnosed are trisomy 18 and trisomy 13. Both conditions have a very poor prognosis, with most affected children dying from cardiac or respiratory complications within 6 months of birth.

The product of the union of a normal gamete (ovum or sperm) with a gamete missing a chromosome is a monosomy. The individual would have only 45 chromosomes in each cell. Missing an autosomal chromosome always results in death of the embryo.

Nondisjunction can also occur during mitosis. If this occurs early in development when cell lines are forming, then the individual has a mixture of cells, some with a normal number of chromosomes and others either missing a chromosome or containing an extra chromosome. This condition is known as mosaicism. Mosaicism in the autosomes is most commonly seen as another form of Down syndrome. Depending on when the nondisjunction occurs during development, different body tissues will have different numbers of chromosomes. The clinical characteristics of Down syndrome may be present mildly or with varying degrees of severity depending on the number and location of the abnormal cells. However, an individual with mosaic Down syndrome may have normal intelligence.

ABNORMALITIES OF CHROMOSOME STRUCTURE. Abnormalities of chromosome structure involve chromosome breakage usually resulting from one of two events: (1) translocation and (2) additions and/or deletions. Translocation occurs when genetic material is transferred from one chromosome to another different chromosome. Thus, instead of two normal pairs of chromosomes, the individual contains one normal chromosome of each pair, plus a third chromosome that is a fusion of the other two. As long as all genetic material is retained in the cell, the individual is unaffected but is a carrier of what is known as a balanced translocation. Problems may arise for offspring, however, if such an individual's genetic material is divided unequally during meiosis.

When a balanced translocation carrier produces ova or sperm, chances are significant that the chromosomes will not be separated equally in the gametes. If a gamete receives only the two normal chromosomes *or* the single fused version of the two chromosomes, the resulting offspring will be clinically normal. (In the latter case, of course, the offspring would also be a carrier.) If the gamete receives a normal chromosome *plus* the fused version, however, the resulting offspring will have an extra copy of one of the chromosomes. This condition, called an *unbalanced translocation,* often has serious clinical effects.

Like autosomal mosaicism, this also occurs most commonly with Down syndrome. The extra chromosome 21 becomes attached to chromosome 14. When the translocation carrier gamete containing a normal chromosome 21 plus the fused 14/21 chromosome unites with a normal gamete, the resulting offspring has a trisomy of chromosome 21 and all of the characteristics of Down syndrome.

Whenever a portion of a chromosome is deleted from one chromosome and added to another, the gamete produced may contain either extra copies of genes or too few copies. The clinical effects produced may be mild or severe depending on the amount of genetic material involved. Two of the more common conditions that have been described are the deletion of the short arm of chromosome 5 *(cri du chat syndrome)* and the deletion of the long arm of chromosome 18. Cri du chat syndrome, so named after the typical mewing cry of the affected infant, causes severe mental retardation with microcephaly and unusual facial appearance. Deletion of the long arm of chromosome 18 causes severe psychomotor retardation with multiple organ malformations.

SEX CHROMOSOME ABNORMALITIES. Several sex chromosome abnormalities have been identified that are caused by nondisjunction during gametogenesis in either parent. The most common deviation in females is *Turner's syndrome,* or monosomy X. The affected female is missing an X chromosome and exhibits juvenile external genitalia with undeveloped ovaries. She is usually short in stature with webbing of the neck. Intelligence may be impaired. Most affected embryos abort spontaneously.

The most common deviation in males is *Klinefelter's syndrome,* or trisomy of the sex chromosomes XXY. The affected male has an extra X chromosome and exhibits poorly developed secondary sexual characteristics and small testes. He is infertile, usually tall, and effeminate. Males mosaic for Klinefelter's syndrome may be fertile. Subnormal intelligence is usually present.

Males with XYY syndrome have an extra Y chromosome. They are apparently normal males, but some have exhibited overly aggressive or criminal behavior.

Females with XXX syndrome are fertile and normal in appearance. Some are mildly mentally retarded, but they can bear normal children.

Abnormalities in individuals with two extra sex chromosomes (XXXX or XXXY) tend to be severe. A zygote with monosomy Y missing the X chromosome is nonviable.

Patterns of Genetic Transmission

Heritable characteristics are those that can be passed on to offspring. The patterns by which genetic material is transmitted to the next generation are affected by the number of genes involved in the expression of the trait. Although many phenotypic characteristics result from two or more genes on different chromosomes acting together (referred to as multifactorial inheritance), others are controlled by a single gene (unifactorial inheritance).

Unlike chromosomal abnormalities, defects at the gene level cannot be determined by conventional laboratory methods such as karyotyping. Instead, genetic counselors predict the probability of the presence of an abnormal gene from the known occurrence of the trait in the individual's family and the known patterns by which the trait is inherited.

UNIFACTORIAL INHERITANCE. If a particular trait, disease, or defect is controlled by a single gene, its pattern of inheritance is referred to as unifactorial mendelian, or single-gene inheritance. The number of unifactorial abnormalities far exceeds the number of chromosomal abnormalities. This is understandable considering that 50,000 to 100,000 genes in the haploid number (23) of chromosomes are passed on to an offspring from each parent.

Unifactorial or single-gene disorders follow the inheritance patterns of dominance, segregation, and independent assortment described by Mendel and include autosomal dominant, autosomal recessive, and X-linked recessive and dominant modes of inheritance.

AUTOSOMAL DOMINANT INHERITANCE. Autosomal dominant inheritance disorders are those in which the abnormal gene for the trait is expressed even when the other member of the pair is normal. The abnormal gene may appear as a result of a **mutation,** a spontaneous and permanent change in the normal gene structure, in which case the disorder occurs for the first time in the family. However, an affected individual usually comes from multiple generations having the disorder. An affected parent who is heterozygous for the trait has a 50% chance of passing the abnormal gene to each offspring. Males and females are equally affected.

Autosomal dominant disorders are not always expressed with the same severity of symptoms. The parent may have a minor abnormality that had not been diagnosed until the birth of a more severely affected child. There is no way to predict whether an offspring will have a minor or a severe abnormality.

Examples of common autosomal dominantly inherited disorders are achondroplasia (dwarfism), polydactyly (extra digits), Huntington's chorea, and polycystic kidney disease.

AUTOSOMAL RECESSIVE INHERITANCE. Autosomal recessive inheritance disorders are those in which both genes of a pair must be abnormal for the disorder to be expressed. Heterozygous individuals have only one abnormal gene and are unaffected clinically because their normal gene overshadows the abnormal gene. They are known as carriers of the recessive trait. Because these recessive traits are inherited by generations of the same family, an increased incidence of the disorder occurs in consanguinous matings (closely related parents). In order for the trait to be expressed, two carriers must each contribute the abnormal gene to the offspring (Fig. 7-4, C). There is a 25% chance of the trait occurring in each child. A clinically normal offspring may be a carrier of the gene. Males and females are equally affected.

Most recessive disorders tend to have severe clini-

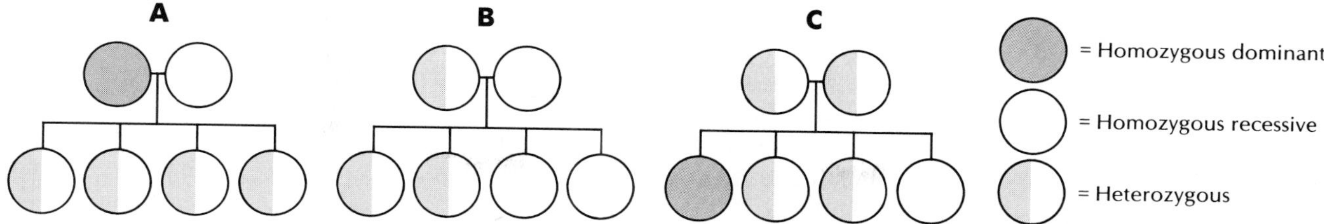

Fig. 7-4 Possible offspring in three types of matings. **A,** Homozygous-dominant parent and homozygous-recessive parent. Children all heterozygous, displaying dominant trait. **B,** Heterozygous parent and homozygous-recessive parent. Children 50% heterozygous display dominant trait; 50% homozygous display recessive trait. **C,** Both parents heterozygous. Children 25% homozygous-dominant trait; 25% homozygous-recessive; 50% heterozygous display dominant trait.

cal manifestations, and affected offspring do not often reproduce. If they do, all of their offspring will be carriers for the disorder.

Most inborn errors of metabolism, such as phenylketonuria (PKU), galactosemia, maple syrup urine disease, Tay Sachs disease (Chapter 38), sickle cell anemia, and cystic fibrosis, are all autosomal-recessive inherited disorders.

X-LINKED RECESSIVE INHERITANCE. Abnormal genes for **X-linked recessive inheritance** disorders are carried on the X chromosome (Fig. 7-5). Females may be heterozygous or homozygous for traits carried on the X chromosome because they have two. Males are hemizygous because they have only one X chromosome carrying genes with no alleles on the Y chromosome. Therefore X-linked recessive disorders are most commonly manifested in the male with the abnormal gene on his single X chromosome. The male receives the defective gene from his carrier mother on her affected X chromosome. Female carriers (those heterozygous for the trait) have a 50% probability of transmitting the abnormal gene to each offspring. An affected male can pass the abnormal gene only to his daughters on the X chromosome, but not to his sons. The daughters will be carriers of the trait if they receive a normal gene on the X chromosome from their mother. They can be affected only if they receive an abnormal gene on the X chromosome from their mother also.

Hemophilia, color blindness, and Duchenne muscular dystrophy are all X-linked recessive disorders.

X-LINKED DOMINANT INHERITANCE. X-linked dominant inheritance disorders occur both in males and heterozygous females. Because the females also have a normal gene, the effects are more severe in affected males. Affected males transmit the abnormal gene only to their daughters on the X chromosome. Heterozygous females have a 50% chance of transmitting the abnormal gene to each offspring.

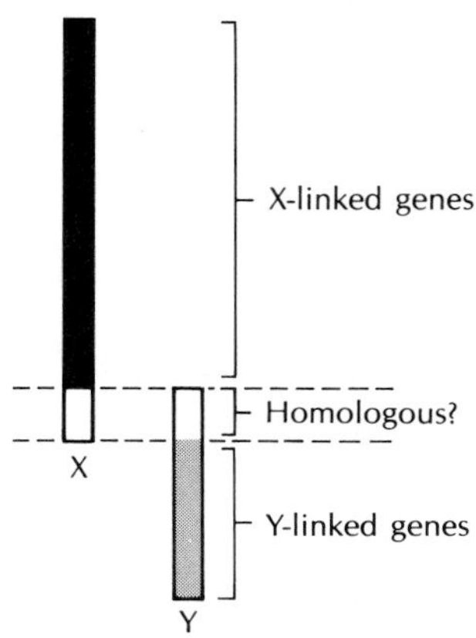

Fig. 7-5 X and Y chromosomes.

An example of these extremely rare disorders is vitamin D–resistant rickets.

Fragile-X syndrome is a relatively new diagnosis. The "fragile site" on the X chromosome was identified in a central nervous system disorder affecting males and also seen in heterozygous carrier females. Affected individuals are mentally handicapped.

INBORN ERRORS OF METABOLISM. Disorders of protein, fat, or carbohydrate metabolism reflecting absent or defective enzymes generally follow a recessive pattern of inheritance. Enzymes, the actions of which are genetically determined, are essential for all the physical and chemical processes that sustain body systems. Defective enzyme action interrupts the normal series of chemical reactions from the affected point onward. The result may be an accumulation of a damaging product such as phenylalanine or the absence of a necessary product such as thyroxin or melanin (see Appendix F for screening tests for inborn errors of metabolism).

Phenylketonuria (PKU) is an uncommon disorder

caused by autosomal recessive genes. Heterozygous carriers and affected infants may be identified by genetic screening methods. A deficiency in the liver enzyme phenylalanine hydroxylase results in failure to metabolize the amino acid phenylalanine, allowing its metabolites to accumulate in the blood. The incidence of this disorder is 1 per every 10,000 to 20,000 births. The highest incidence is found in Caucasians (from northern Europe and the United States). It is rarely seen in Jewish, African, or Japanese populations.

Tay-Sachs disease, inherited as an autosomal recessive trait, results from a deficiency of hexosaminidase. It occurs primarily in Jewish families. Until 4 to 6 months of age, infants appear normal; in fact, their facial features are considered very beautiful. Then the clinical symptoms appear: apathy and regression in motor and social development and decreased vision. Death occurs between 3 and 4 years of age. There is as yet no known treatment for Tay-Sachs disease. In subsequent pregnancies amniocentesis may be performed on women who have delivered infants with this condition.

Cystic fibrosis (mucoviscidosis or fibrocystic disease of the pancreas) is inherited as an autosomal recessive trait characterized by generalized involvement of exocrine glands. Clinical features are related to the altered viscosity of mucus-secreting glands throughout the body. It is a serious chronic disease occurring primarily in Caucasians but can appear in those of mixed ancestry. Overall incidence is 1 per every 2000 births. It is thought that the carrier state is 1:20 to 25. Advances in diagnosis and treatment have improved the prognosis so that now many affected individuals live to adulthood. Some affected women have borne children, but men generally are sterile (MacMullen, Brucker, 1989). If the mother has cystic fibrosis and the father has no family history, offspring have a 50% chance of inheriting the gene for cystic fibrosis (MacMullen, Brucker, 1989).

Meconium ileus occurs in about 10% of newborns with cystic fibrosis. Although an initial stool may be passed from the rectum with none thereafter, no meconium is usually passed during the first 24 to 48 hours, the abdomen becomes increasingly distended, and eventually the newborn requires a laparotomy for diagnosis and treatment of the condition.

MULTIFACTORIAL INHERITANCE. Most of the common congenital malformations result from multifactorial inheritance: a combination of genetic and environmental factors. Examples are cleft lip, cleft palate, congenital heart disease, neural tube defects, and pyloric stenosis. Each malformation may range from mild to severe, depending on the number of genes present for the defect or the amount of environmental influence. A **neural tube defect** may range from spina bifida, a bony defect in the lumbar region of the vertebrae with little or no neurologic impairment, to anencephaly, absence of brain development, which is always fatal. Some malformations occur more often in one sex or the other. For example, pyloric stenosis and cleft lip are more common in males, and cleft palate is more common in females. Multifactorial disorders also tend to occur in families.

NEGATIVE FACTORS INFLUENCING DEVELOPMENT. Not all congenital disorders are inherited. Congenital simply means that the condition was present at birth. Some congenital malformations may be the result of **teratogens,** defined as environmental substances or exposures that cause adverse effects (for additional

Human Teratogens

DRUGS AND CHEMICALS

Alcohol
Androgens
Anticoagulants (warfarin and dicumarol)
Antithyroid drugs (propylthiouracil, iodide, and methimazole)
Chemotherapeutic drugs (methotrexate and aminopterin)
Diethylstilbestrol (DES)
Lead
Lithium
Organic mercury
Phenytoin
Polychlorinated biphenyls (PCBs)
Isoretinoin*
Streptomycin
Tetracycline
Thalidomide
Trimethadione paramethadione
Valproic acid

INFECTIONS

Cytomegalovirus
Rubella
Syphilis
Toxoplasmosis
Varicella

EXPOSURES (e.g., radiation)

MATERNAL CONDITIONS

Diabetes mellitus
Phenylketonuria

From Reed GB, Claireaux AE, Bain AD, editors: *Diseases of the fetus and newborn: pathology, radiology, and genetics, St Louis,* 1989, Mosby–Year Book.

*Trade name: Accutane, a synthetic derivative of vitamin A.

information, see Chapter 27). Although teratogens are not genetic material per se, they frequently produce their ill effects by altering the normal expression of the embryonic genome in some fashion. Known human teratogens are drugs and chemicals (for embryonic fetal effects, see Appendix E) (Thomson, Cordero, 1989; Brown, Bellinger, Matthews, 1990), infections, exposure, and certain maternal conditions (see box on p. 160). A teratogen has the greatest effect on the organs and parts of an embryo during its periods of rapid differentiation. This occurs during the embryonic period, specifically from days 15 to 60. During the first 2 weeks of development, teratogens either have no effect on the embryo, or their effects are so severe that they cause spontaneous abortion. Brain growth and development continue during the fetal period, and teratogens can severely affect mental development throughout gestation (Fig. 7-6).

Besides the genetic makeup and the influence of teratogens, the adequacy of maternal nutrition also influences development. The embryo and fetus must obtain the nutrients they need from the mother's diet; they cannot tap the maternal reserves. Malnutrition during pregnancy produces low-birth-weight newborns who are more susceptible to infection. It also affects brain development during the latter half of gestation, resulting in learning disabilities in the child.

■ CONCEPTION

Conception, formally defined as the union of a single egg and sperm, is the benchmark of the beginning of a pregnancy. But this event does not occur in isolation. A series of events surround it, including gamete (egg and sperm) formation, ovulation (release of the egg), union of the gametes, and implantation of the embryo in the uterus. Only after all of these events are successfully completed can the process of embryonic and fetal development begin.

Ovum

As discussed previously, the result of meiosis in the female is the production of an egg, or ovum. This process occurs in the ovaries, specifically in the ovarian follicles. Each month one ovum matures with a host of surrounding supportive cells.

At the time of ovulation, the ovum bursts from the ruptured ovarian follicle. High estrogen levels have increased the motility of the uterine tubes so that their cilia will be able to capture the ovum and propel

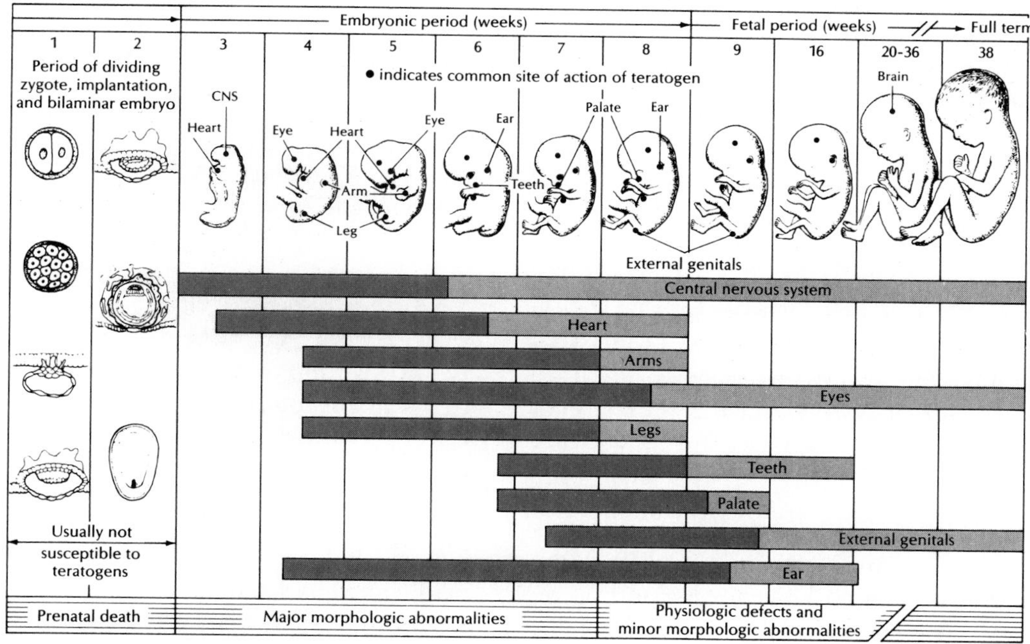

Fig. 7-6 Sensitive, or critical, periods in human development. Dark color denotes highly sensitive periods; light color indicates stages that are less sensitive to teratogens.
From Moore KL: *The developing human: clinically oriented embryology*, ed 2, Philadelphia, 1977, WB Saunders.

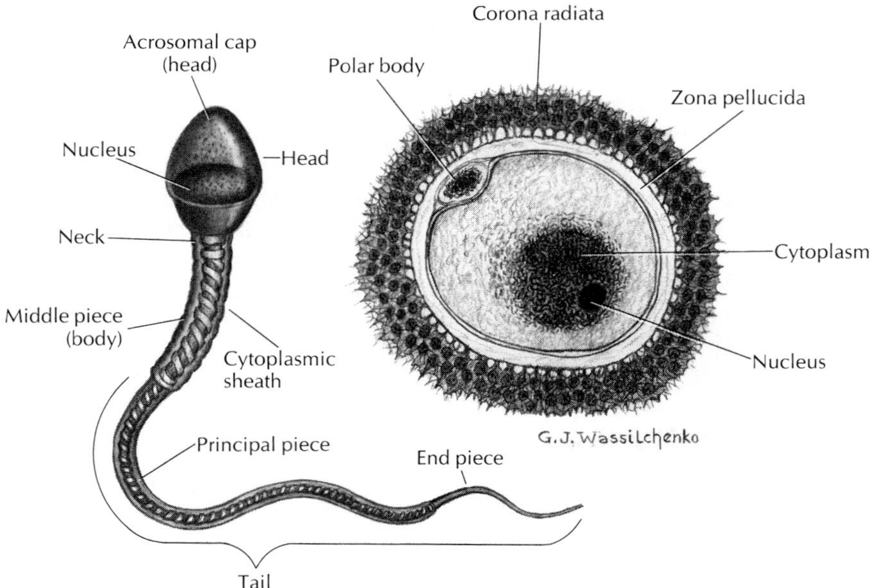

Fig. 7-7 Sperm and ovum.

it through the tube toward the uterine cavity. The ovum cannot move by itself.

The ovum is surrounded by two protective layers of tissue (Fig. 7-7). The first is a thick, shapeless membrane, the zona pellucida. The outer ring, the corona radiata, is composed of elongated cells held together by hyaluronic acid.

Ova are considered fertile for about 24 hours after ovulation. If unfertilized by a sperm, the ovum degenerates and is reabsorbed.

Sperm

Ejaculation during sexual intercourse normally propels less than a teaspoon of semen containing as many as 200 to 500 million sperm into the vagina. The sperm swim with the flagellar movement of their tails. Some sperm can reach the site of fertilization within 5 minutes, but average transit time is 4 to 6 hours. *Sperm remain viable* within the woman's reproductive system for 2 to 3 days. Most sperm are lost in the vagina, within the cervical mucus, in the endometrium, or enter the tube that contains no ovum. As the sperm travel through the uterine tubes, enzymes produced there aid in capacitation of the sperm. *Capacitation* is a physiologic change that removes the protective coating from the heads of the sperm (the acrosomes). Then, small perforations form in the acrosome, allowing enzymes (e.g., hyaluronidase) to escape. These enzymes are necessary for the sperm to penetrate the protective layers of the ovum before fertilization.

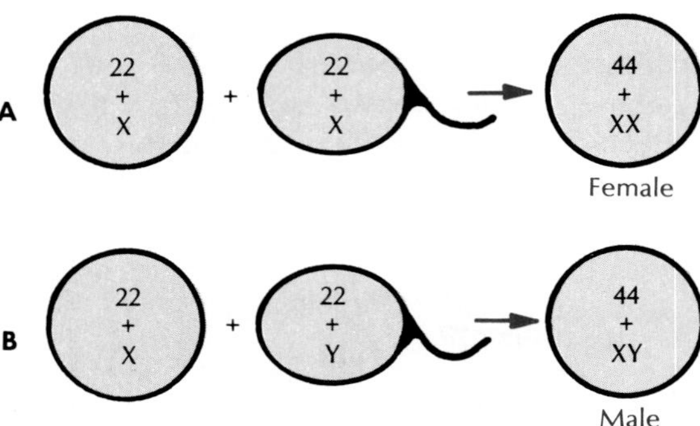

Fig. 7-8 Fertilization. **A,** Ovum fertilized by X-bearing sperm to form female zygote. **B,** Ovum fertilized by Y-bearing sperm to form male zygote.

Fertilization

Fertilization takes place in the ampulla (outer third) of the uterine tube. When a sperm successfully penetrates the membrane surrounding the ovum, both sperm and ovum are enclosed within the membrane, and it is rendered impenetrable to other sperm. This is termed the zona reaction. The second meiotic division of the oocyte is completed, and the ovum nucleus becomes the female pronucleus. The head of the sperm enlarges to become the male pronucleus, and the tail degenerates. The nuclei fuse and the chromosomes combine, restoring the diploid number (46) (Fig. 7-8). Conception, the formation of the zygote (the first cell of the new individual), has been achieved.

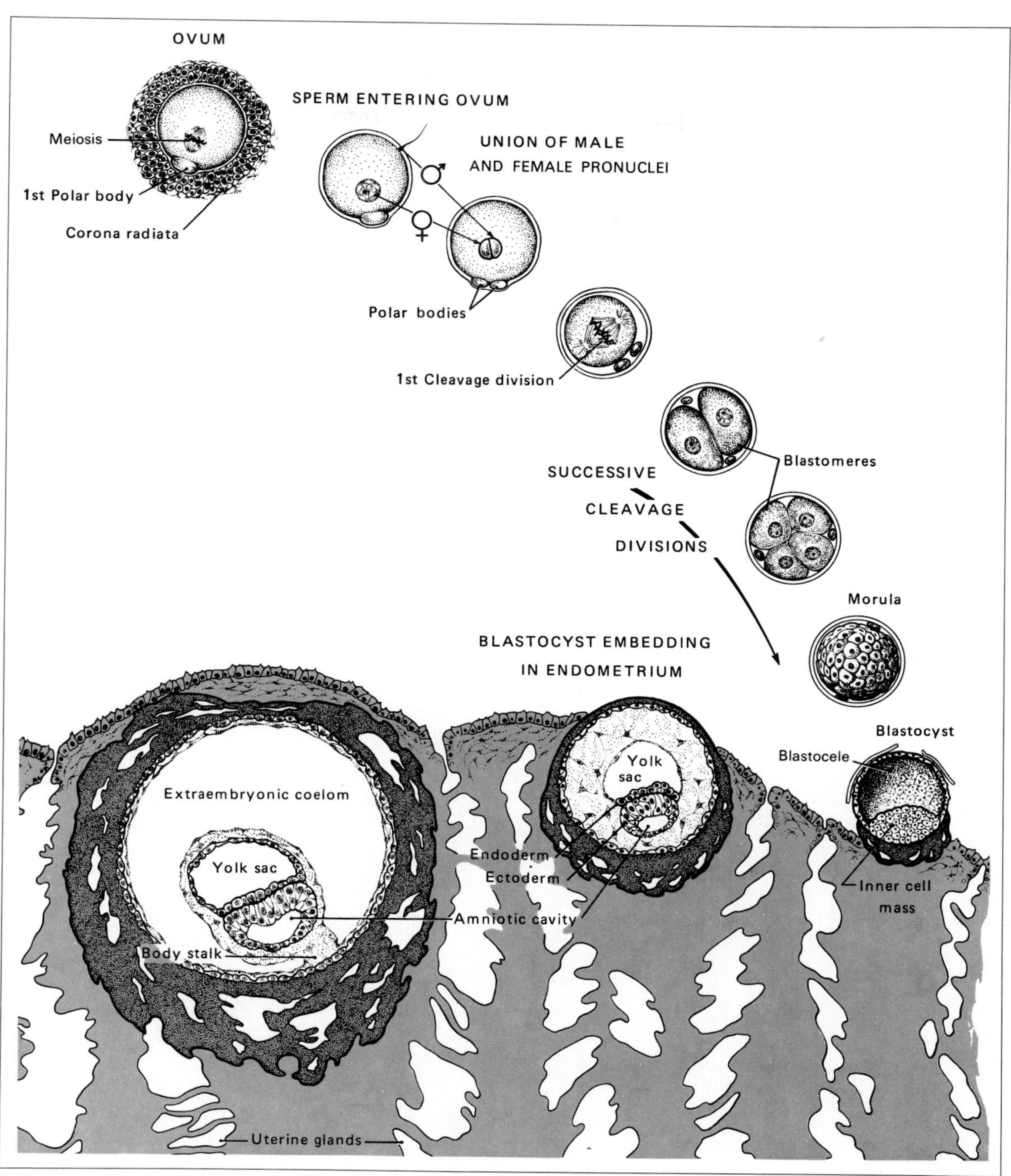

Fig. 7-9 First week of human development. *Top, left to right,* oocyte immediately after ovulation. Fertilization approximately 12 to 24 hours after ovulation. Stage of male and female pronuclei. Spindle of first meiotic division. Two cell stages (approximately 30 hours old). Morula containing 12 to 16 blastomeres, then advanced morula stage reaching uterine lumen (approximately 3 days old). Early blastocyst stage (approximately 4½ days old); zona pellucida has disappeared. Early phase of implantation. Formation of germ layers.

From Langley LL, Tefford IR, Christensen JB: *Dynamic human anatomy and physiology,* ed 5, New York, 1980, McGraw-Hill; copyright Mosby–Year Book.

Mitotic cellular replication, called cleavage, begins as the zygote travels the length of the uterine tube into the uterus. This voyage takes 3 to 4 days. Because the fertilized egg divides rapidly with no increase in size, successively smaller cells, blastomeres, are formed with each division. A 16-cell **morula,** a solid ball of cells, is produced within 3 days (Fig. 7-9). It is still surrounded by the protective zona pellucida. Further development occurs as the morula floats freely within the uterus. Fluid passes through the zona pellucida into the intercellular spaces between the blastomeres. A cavity forms within the cell mass as the spaces come together, forming a structure called the **blastocyst.** Formation of the blastocyst signals the first major differentiation of the embryo. The inner solid mass of cells develop into the embryo and the embryonic membrane called the *amnion*. The outer layer of cells surrounding the cavity is the trophoblast, from which develops the other embryonic membrane, the chorion, and the embryonic part of the placenta.

Implantation

The zona pellucida degenerates, and the trophoblast attaches itself to the uterine endometrium, usually in the anterior or posterior fundal region. Between 7 and 10 days after conception, the trophoblast secretes enzymes that enable it to burrow into the endometrium until the entire blastocyst is covered. This is known as **implantation.** Endometrial blood vessels are eroded, and some women experience slight implantation bleeding. **Chorionic villi,** fingerlike projections, develop out of the trophoblast and extend into the blood-filled spaces of the endometrium. These villi are vascular processes that obtain oxygen and nutrients from the maternal bloodstream and dispose of carbon dioxide and waste products into the maternal blood.

After implantation, the endometrium is called the decidua. The portion directly under the blastocyst, where the chorionic villi tap the maternal blood vessels, is the **decidua basalis.** The portion covering the blastocyst is the decidua capsularis, and the portion lining the rest of the uterus is the decidua vera (Fig. 7-10).

■ EMBRYONIC AND FETAL DEVELOPMENT

Pregnancy is calculated to last 10 lunar months, 9 calendar months, 40 weeks, or 280 days. *Length of*

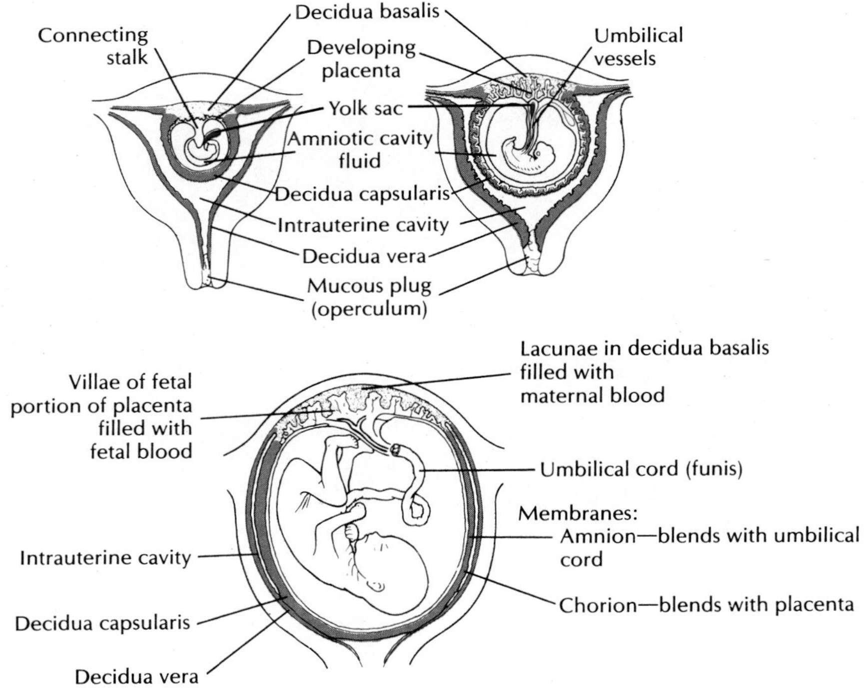

Fig. 7-10 Development of fetal membranes. Note gradual obliteration of intrauterine cavity as decidua capsularis and decidua vera meet. Also note thinning of uterine wall. Chorionic and amniotic membranes are in apposition to each other but may be peeled apart.

pregnancy is computed from the first day of the last menstrual period (LMP) until the day of delivery* (see discussion of Nägele's rule, and adjustment for longer and shorter cycles, p. 269). However, conception is calculated to occur 2 weeks after the first day of the LMP. Thus the postconception age of the fetus is 2 weeks less for a total of 266 days or 38 weeks. For the discussion of fetal development, postconceptional age will be used.

Intrauterine development is divided into three stages: ovum, embryo, and fetus. Table 7-1 summarizes this development. The stage of the ovum lasts from conception until day 14. This period covers cellular replication, blastocyst formation, initial development of the embryonic membranes, and establishment of the primary germ layers.

Embryonic Development

The stage of the **embryo** lasts from day 15 until approximately 8 weeks after conception or until the embryo measures 3 cm (1.2 inches) from crown to rump. This stage is the most critical time in the development of the organ systems and the main external features. Developing areas with rapid cell division are the most vulnerable to malformation by environmental teratogens. At the end of the eighth week, all organ systems and external structures are present, and the embryo is unmistakably human (Fig. 7-11).

MEMBRANES. At the time of implantation, two **fetal membranes,** which will surround the developing embryo, begin to form. The chorion develops from the trophoblast and contains the chorionic villi on its surface. The villi burrowing into the decidua basalis increase in size and complexity as the vascular processes develop into the placenta. The chorion becomes the covering of the fetal side of the placenta. It contains the major umbilical blood vessels as they branch out over the surface of the placenta. As the embryo grows, the decidua capsularis becomes stretched. The chorionic villi on this side atrophy and degenerate, leaving a smooth chorionic membrane.

The inner cell membrane, the amnion, develops from the interior cells of the blastocyst. The cavity that develops between this inner cell mass and the outer layer of cells (trophoblast) is the amniotic cavity (Fig. 7-9). As it grows larger, the amnion forms on the side opposite to the developing blastocyst (Fig. 7-10). The developing embryo draws the amnion around itself, forming a fluid-filled sac. The amnion becomes the covering of the umbilical cord and covers the chorion on the fetal surface of the placenta. As the embryo grows larger, the amnion enlarges to accommodate both the embryo-fetus and its surrounding **amniotic fluid.** The amnion eventually comes in contact with the chorion all around the fetus.

AMNIOTIC FLUID. Initially, the amniotic cavity derives its fluid by diffusion from the maternal blood. The amount of fluid increases weekly, so that, at term, there is normally between 800 and 1200 mL of transparent, slightly yellow liquid. The amniotic fluid volume changes constantly. The fetus swallows fluid, and fluid flows into and out of the fetal lungs. The fetus urinates into the fluid, greatly enhancing its volume. Having less than 300 mL of amniotic fluid (oligohydramnios) is associated with fetal renal abnormalities. Having greater than 2 L of amniotic fluid (hydramnios) is associated with gastrointestinal and other malformations.

There are many functions served by amniotic fluid for the embryo-fetus. It cushions the fetus from trauma by blunting and dispersing the forces. It allows freedom of movement for musculoskeletal development. It keeps the embryo from tangling with the membranes, which facilitates symmetric growth of the fetus. If the embryo does intersect with the membranes, extremity amputations or other deformities can occur from constricting amniotic bands (Reed, Claireaux, Bain, 1989). Amniotic fluid helps maintain a constant body temperature. It serves as a source of oral fluid as well as a waste repository.

Amniotic fluid contains albumin, urea, uric acid, creatinine, lecithin, sphingomyelin, bilirubin, fructose, fat, leukocytes, proteins, epithelial cells, enzymes, and lanugo hair. Study of the amniotic fluid via amniocentesis (Chapter 27) yields much information about the fetus. Genetic studies (karyotyping) provide knowledge about the sex and normality of chromosome number and structure. Other studies determine the health or maturity of the fetus.

YOLK SAC. At the same time as the amniotic cavity and amnion are forming, another blastocyst cavity has formed on the other side of the developing embryonic disk (Fig. 7-9). This cavity becomes surrounded by a membrane, forming the yolk sac. This aids in transferring maternal nutrients and oxygen, which have diffused through the chorion to the embryo. Blood vessels form to aid transport. By the third week, blood cells and plasma are manufactured in the yolk sac. At the end of the third week, the primitive heart begins to beat to circulate the blood

*The first day of the last menstrual period refers to the first day of menstrual flow. For a discussion of the menstrual cycle, see Chapter 6.

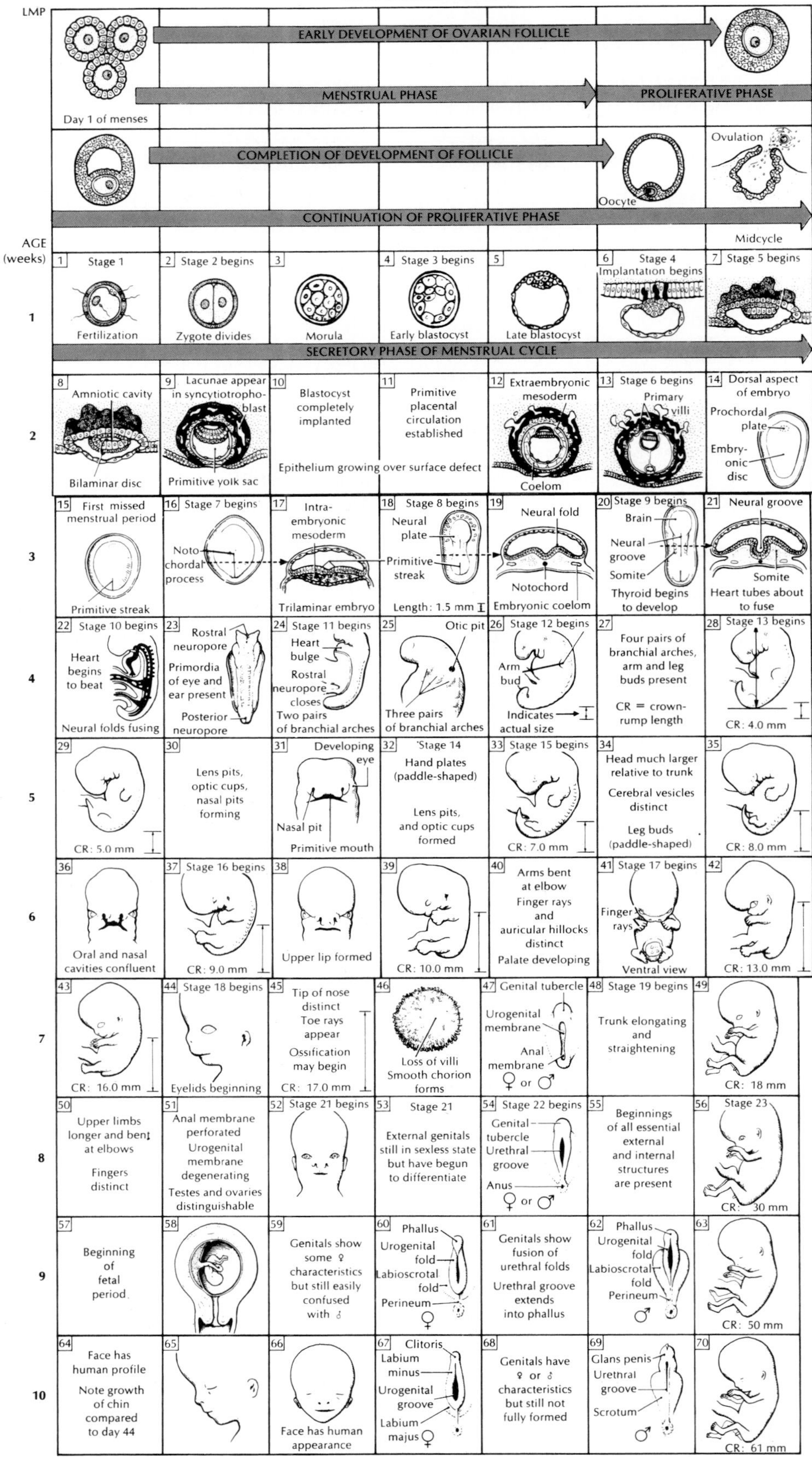

Fig. 7-11 Timetable of human prenatal development from LMP and weeks 1 to 10 following fertilization. Within large boxes are small boxes with numbers in upper left corner. These numbers refer to days since fertilization.

From Moore KL: *The developing human: clinically oriented embryology*, ed 2, Philadelphia, 1977, WB Saunders.

through the embryo, connecting stalk, chorion, and yolk sac.

The folding in of the embryo during the fourth week results in part of the yolk sac being incorporated into the embryo's body as the primitive digestive system. Primordial germ cells arise in the yolk sac and migrate into the embryo. The shrinking remains of the yolk sac degenerate (Fig. 7-10). By the fifth or sixth week, the remnant has separated from the embryo.

PRIMARY GERM LAYERS. During the second week after conception, the embryonic disk differentiates into three primary germ layers: the ectoderm, mesoderm, and endoderm or entoderm (Fig. 7-9). From these three layers develop all tissues and organs of the embryo.

The *ectoderm,* the upper layer of the embryonic disk, gives rise to the epidermis, glands, nails and hair, the central and peripheral nervous systems, eye lens, tooth enamel, and the floor of the amniotic cavity.

The middle layer, the *mesoderm,* develops into the bones and teeth, muscles (skeletal, smooth, and cardiac), dermis, and connective tissue, the cardiovascular system and spleen, and the urogenital system.

The lower layer, the *endoderm,* gives rise to the epithelium lining the respiratory tract and digestive tract, including the oropharynx, the liver and pancreas, urethra, bladder, and female vagina. The endoderm forms the roof of the yolk sac.

UMBILICAL CORD. By day 14 after conception, the embryonic disk, amniotic sac, and yolk sac are attached to the chorionic villi by the connecting stalk. During the third week, the blood vessels develop to supply the embryo with maternal nutrients and oxygen. During the fifth week, after the embryo has curved inward on itself from both ends, bringing the connecting stalk to the ventral side of the embryo, the connecting stalk becomes compressed from both sides by the amnion forming the narrower **umbilical cord** (Fig. 7-10). Two arteries carry blood from the embryo to the chorionic villi, and one vein returns blood to the embryo. One percent of umbilical cords contain only two vessels, one artery and one vein. This occurrence is sometimes associated with congenital malformations.

The cord rapidly increases in length. At term, the cord ranges from 30 to 90 cm long (average 55 cm) and is 2 cm in diameter. It twists spirally on itself and loops around the embryo-fetus. A true knot is rare, but false knots occur as folds or kinks in the cord. Connective tissue called Wharton's jelly prevents compression of the blood vessels to ensure continued nourishment of the embryo-fetus. Compression can occur if the cord lies between the fetal head and the pelvis or is twisted around the fetal body. When the cord is wrapped around the fetal neck, it is called a *nuchal cord.*

As the placenta develops from the chorionic villi, the umbilical cord is usually located centrally. A peripheral location is less common and is known as a battledore placenta (Fig. 7-12). The blood vessels are arrayed out from the center to all parts of the placenta.

PLACENTA

STRUCTURE. During the third week after conception, the trophoblast cells of the chorionic villi continue to invade the decidua basalis. As the uterine capillaries are tapped, then the endometrial spiral arteries, the spaces formed fill with maternal blood. The chorionic villi grow into the spaces with two layers of cells: the outer syncytium and the inner cytotrophoblast. A third layer develops into anchoring septa, dividing the projecting decidua into separate areas called cotyledons. In each of the 15 to 20 cotyledons, the chorionic villi branch out with a complex system of fetal blood vessels forming. Each cotyledon is a functional unit. The whole structure is the **placenta.** The maternal-placental-embryonic circulation is in place by day 17, when the embryonic heart starts beating. By the end of the third week, embryonic blood is circulating between the embryo and the chorionic villi. In the intervillous spaces (between the villi), maternal blood is supplying oxygen and nutrients to the embryonic capillaries in the villi (Fig. 7-13). Waste products and carbon dioxide are diffusing into the maternal blood. The placenta is functioning as a means of metabolic exchange. Exchange is minimal at this time because the two cell layers of the villous membrane are too thick. Permeability increases as the cytotrophoblast thins and disappears by the fifth month, leaving only the single layer of syncytium between the maternal blood and the fetal capillaries. The syncytium is the functional layer of the placenta. By the eighth week, genetic testing may be done by obtaining a sample of chorionic villi by aspiration biopsy (Chapter 27). The structure of the placenta is complete by the twelfth week. The placenta continues to grow wider until 20 weeks when it covers about one half of the uterine surface. It then continues to grow thicker. The branching villi continue to develop within the body of the placenta, increasing the functional surface area.

FUNCTIONS. One of the early functions of the placenta is as an endocrine gland with the production of four hormones necessary to maintain the pregnancy and support the embryo-fetus. The hormones are produced in the syncytium.

The protein hormone, **human chorionic gonado-**

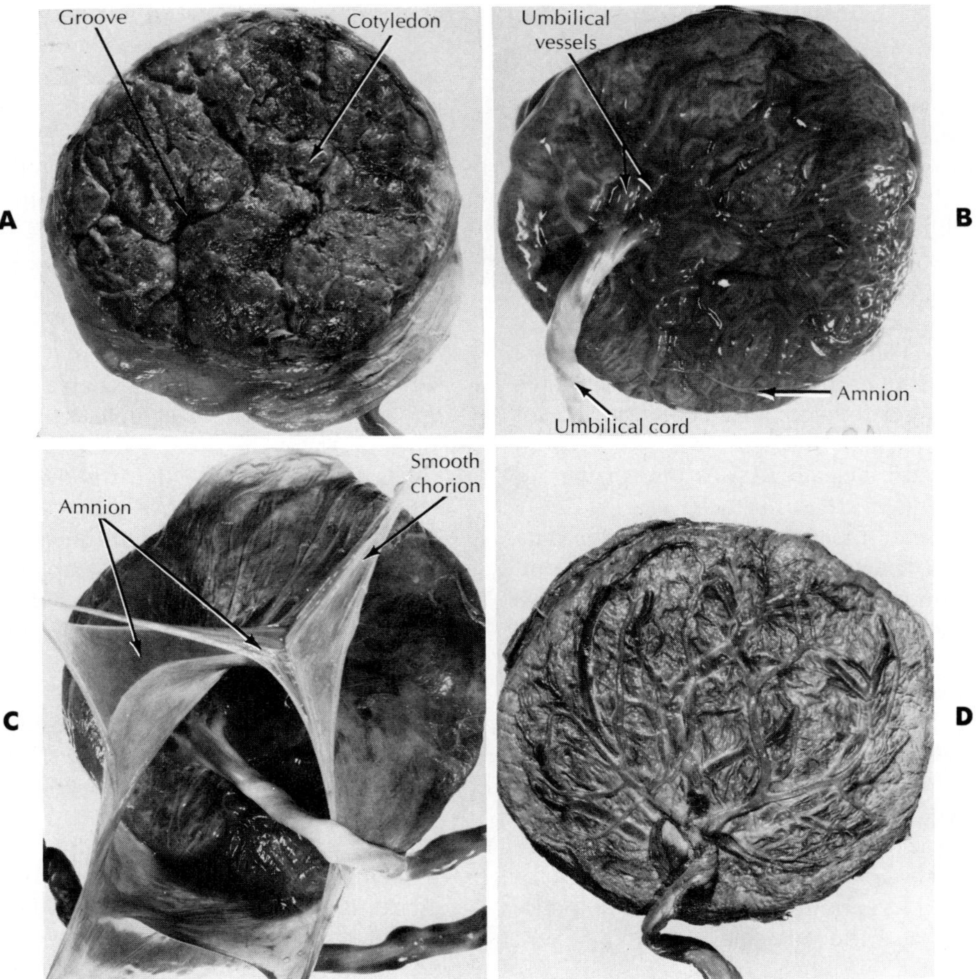

Fig. 7-12 Photographs of full-term placentas. **A,** Maternal (or uterine) surface, showing cotyledons and grooves. **B,** Fetal (or amniotic) surface, showing blood vessels running under amnion and converging to form umbilical vessels at attachment of umbilical cord. **C,** Amnion and smooth chorion are arranged to show that they are (1) fused and (2) continuous with margins of placenta. **D,** Placenta with a marginal attachment of the cord, often called a battledore placenta because of its resemblance to bat used in medieval game of battledore and shuttlecock.
From Moore KL: *The developing human: clinically oriented embryology,* ed 2, Philadelphia, 1977, WB Saunders.

tropin (hCG) is detected in the maternal serum by 8 to 10 days after conception, shortly after implantation. It is the basis for pregnancy tests (for a discussion of pregnancy tests, see Chapter 8). The hCG preserves the function of the ovarian *corpus luteum,* ensuring a continued supply of estrogen and progesterone needed to maintain the pregnancy. Spontaneous abortion occurs if the corpus luteum stops functioning before 11 weeks, when the placenta is producing sufficient estrogen and progesterone. The hCG reaches its maximum level at 50 to 70 days, then begins to decrease.

The other protein hormone produced by the placenta is *human placental lactogen (hPL).* This is a growth hormone-like substance that stimulates maternal metabolism, to supply needed nutrients for fetal growth. It facilitates glucose transport across the placental membrane and stimulates breast development to prepare for lactation.

The placenta eventually produces more of the steroid hormone *progesterone* than the corpus luteum does during the first few months of pregnancy. Progesterone maintains the endometrium and decreases the contractility of the uterus. It stimulates develop-

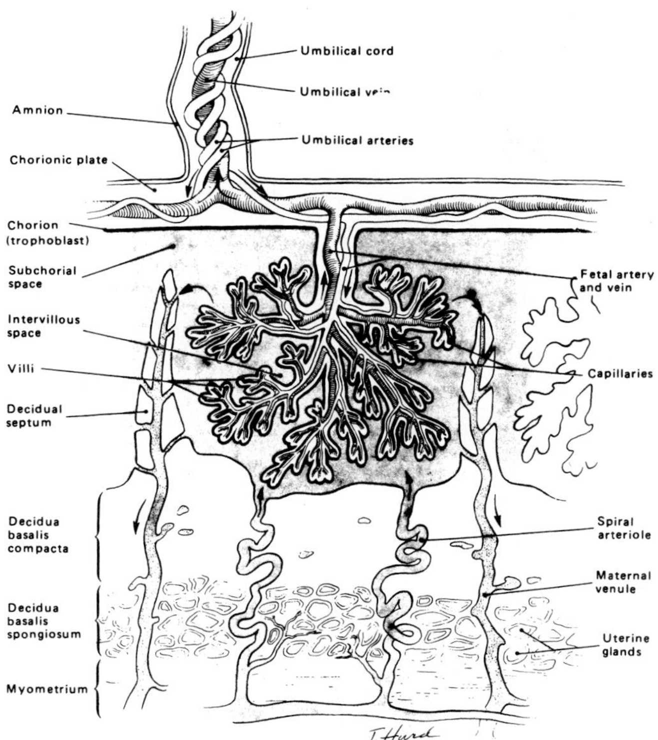

Fig. 7-13 Cross section through placenta. Arrows indicate direction of blood flow.
From Langley LL, Telford IR, Christensen JB: *Dynamic human anatomy and physiology,* ed 5, New York, 1980, McGraw-Hill; copyright Mosby–Year Book.

ment of breast alveoli and maternal metabolism.

By 7 weeks, the placenta is producing most of the maternal *estrogens,* another steroid hormone. The major estrogen secreted by the placenta is estriol, while the ovaries produce mostly estradiol. Measuring estriol levels is a clinical assay for placental functioning. Estrogen stimulates uterine growth and uteroplacental blood flow. It also causes a proliferation of the breast glandular tissue. Estrogen stimulates myometrial contractility. Placental estrogen production increases markedly toward the end of pregnancy. One theory for the cause of the onset of labor is the decrease in circulating levels of progesterone and the increased levels of estrogen.

The metabolic functions of the placenta may be summarized as respiration, nutrition, excretion, and storage. Oxygen *diffuses* from the maternal blood across the placental membrane into the fetal blood, and carbon dioxide diffuses in the opposite direction. In this way, the placenta functions as the fetal lungs.

Water, inorganic salts, carbohydrates, proteins, fats, and vitamins pass from the maternal blood supply across the placental membrane into the fetal blood supplying nutrition. Water and most electrolytes with a molecular weight less than 500 readily diffuse through the membrane. Hydrostatic and osmotic pressures aid the bulk flow of water and some solutions. *Facilitated and active transport* assist in the transfer of glucose, amino acids, calcium, iron, and substances with higher molecular weight. Amino acids and calcium are transported against the concentration gradient between the maternal blood and fetal blood. The fetus requires a higher level of these nutrients as well as glucose. The fetal concentration of glucose is lower than the glucose level in the maternal blood because of its rapid metabolism by the fetus. This requires transport of larger amounts of glucose from the maternal blood than would be supplied by diffusion alone.

Pinocytosis is a mechanism used for transferring large molecules, such as albumin and gamma globulins, across the placental membrane. This mechanism conveys the maternal immunoglobulins that render early passive immunity to the fetus.

Metabolic waste products cross the placental membrane from the fetal blood into the maternal blood. The maternal kidneys then excrete them.

Many viruses can cross the placental membrane and infect the fetus. Some bacteria and protozoa first infect the placenta and then infect the fetus (see Chapter 29).

Drugs can also cross the placental membrane and may harm the fetus. Caffeine, alcohol, nicotine, carbon monoxide and other toxic substances in cigarette smoke, and prescription and recreational drugs such as cocaine and marijuana readily cross the placenta. More examples of these drugs are listed in Appendix E.

Although there is no direct link between the fetal blood in the vessels of the chorionic villi and the maternal blood in the intervillous spaces, only one cell layer separates them. Breaks in the placental membrane occasionally occur. Fetal erythrocytes then leak into the maternal circulation, and the mother may develop antibodies to the fetal red blood cells. This is often how the Rh-negative mother becomes sensitized to the erythrocytes of her Rh-positive fetus (see Chapter 39).

Carbohydrates, proteins, calcium, and iron are stored in the placenta for ready access to meet fetal needs.

Even though the placenta and fetus are living tissue transplants, they are not destroyed by the host mother (Cunningham, MacDonald, Gant, 1989). The immunologic response is suppressed by the placental hormones, or the tissue evokes no response (Willson, Carrington, 1991). For further discussion of the immune system, see Chapter 6.

Placental function depends on the maternal blood

pressure supplying circulation. Maternal arterial blood, under pressure in the small uterine spiral arteries, spurts into the intervillous spaces. As long as rich arterial blood continues to be supplied, pressure is exerted on the blood already in the intervillous spaces, pushing it toward drainage by the low-pressure uterine veins. At term gestation, 10% of the maternal cardiac output goes to the uterus. If there is interference with the circulation to the placenta, the placenta cannot supply the embryo-fetus. Uterine blood flow is diminished by vasoconstriction, such as that caused by hypertension. Decreased maternal blood pressure or cardiac output also diminishes uterine blood flow, such as occurs when the woman lies on her back with the pressure of the uterus compressing the vena cava, diminishing blood return to the right atrium (for discussion of supine hypotension, see p. 203). Excessive maternal exercise that diverts blood to the muscles away from the uterus compromises placental circulation. Optimum circulation is achieved when the woman is lying at rest on her left side. It is also believed that Braxton Hicks contractions (see p. 195) enhance the movement of blood through the intervillous spaces, aiding placental circulation. However, prolonged contractions or too-short intervals between contractions during labor reduce blood flow to the placenta.

Fetal Maturation

The stage of the **fetus** lasts from 9 weeks until the pregnancy is terminated. Changes in the fetal period are not as dramatic, since refinement of structure and function are taking place. The fetus is less vulnerable to teratogens except for those affecting central nervous system functioning.

Viability refers to the capability of the fetus to survive outside the uterus. In the past, 28 weeks after conception was determined to be the earliest age at which fetal survival could be expected. With modern technology and advancements in maternal and neonatal care, viability has now been delimited at 20 weeks after conception (22 weeks since LMP; fetal weight $\geq$ 500 g). The limitations on survival outside the uterus are based on central nervous system functions and oxygenation capability of the lungs.

FETAL CIRCULATORY SYSTEM. The cardiovascular system is the first organ system to function in the developing human. Blood vessel and blood cell formation begin in the third week to supply the embryo with oxygen and nutrients from the mother. By the end of the third week, the tubular heart begins to beat and the primitive cardiovascular system links the embryo, connecting stalk, chorion, and yolk sac. During the fourth and fifth weeks, the heart develops into the four-chambered organ. By the end of the embryonic stage, the heart is developmentally complete.

Because the fetal lungs do not function for respiratory gas exchange, a special circulatory pathway exists that bypasses the lungs.

Oxygen-rich blood from the placenta flows rapidly through the umbilical vein into the fetal abdomen (Fig. 20-3).

When the umbilical vein reaches the liver, it divides into two branches. One circulates some oxygenated blood through the liver. Most of the blood passes through the ductus venosus into the inferior vena cava. There it mixes with the deoxygenated blood from the fetal legs and abdomen on its way to the right atrium. Most of this blood passes straight ahead through the right atrium and through the **foramen ovale,** an opening into the left atrium. There it mixes with the small amount of blood returning deoxygenated from the fetal lungs through the pulmonary veins. The blood flows into the left ventricle and is squeezed out into the aorta. Here, the arteries supplying the heart, head, neck, and arms receive the major part of the oxygen-rich blood. This pattern, supplying the highest levels of oxygen and nutrients to the head, neck, and arms, enhances the **cephalocaudal** (head-to-toe) **development** of the embryo-fetus. Deoxygenated blood returning from the head and arms enters the right atrium through the superior vena cava. This blood is directed downward into the right ventricle, where it is squeezed into the pulmonary artery. A small amount of blood circulates through the resistant lung tissue, but the majority follows the path with less resistance through the **ductus arteriosus** into the aorta, distal to the point of egress of the arteries supplying the head and arms with oxygenated blood. The oxygen-poor blood flows through the abdominal aorta into the internal iliac arteries where the umbilical arteries direct most of it back through the umbilical cord to the placenta. There the blood gives up its wastes and carbon dioxide in exchange for nutrients and oxygen. The blood remaining in the iliac arteries flows through the fetal abdomen and legs, ultimately returning through the inferior vena cava to the heart.

There are three special characteristics that enable the fetus to obtain sufficient oxygen from the maternal blood:

1. Fetal hemoglobin carries 20% to 30% more oxygen than maternal hemoglobin.
2. The fetal hemoglobin concentration is about 50% greater than that of the mother.
3. The fetal heart rate (FHR) is 120 to 160 beats per minute, making the fetal cardiac output per unit of body weight higher than that of an adult.

HEMATOPOIETIC SYSTEM. **Hematopoiesis** is the formation of blood, which occurs in the yolk sac (Fig. 7-10) beginning in the third week. Hematopoietic stem cells seed the fetal liver during the fifth week and hematopoiesis begins there during the sixth week, accounting for its relatively large size between the seventh and ninth weeks. Stem cells seed the fetal bone marrow, spleen and thymus, and lymph nodes between weeks 8 and 11.

The antigenic factors that determine blood type are present in the erythrocytes soon after the sixth week. For this reason, the Rh-negative woman is at risk for isoimmunization after any pregnancy that lasts longer than 6 weeks after fertilization (see Chapter 39).

RESPIRATORY SYSTEM. The respiratory system begins development during embryonic life, continues through fetal life and into childhood. The development of the lungs is divided into four overlapping stages:

1. Pseudoglandular period (5 to 17 weeks): formation of trachea, bronchi, and lung buds. Respiration is not possible.
2. Canalicular period (16 to 24 weeks): enlargement of bronchi and terminal bronchioles and formation of vascular structures and primitive alveoli. Respiration is possible toward the end of this period. Infants born then have a chance of survival with intensive care.
3. Terminal sac period (24 weeks to term birth): formation of many more primitive alveoli with blood supply. Specialized alveolar cells secrete pulmonary **surfactants** (wetting agents) to line the interior of the alveoli. Surfactants facilitate expansion of the alveoli at birth by counteracting surface tension forces. Fetuses born between 24 and 32 weeks may survive. After 32 weeks, sufficient surfactant is present in developed alveoli and infants have a good chance of survival.
4. Alveolar period (late fetal period to about 8 years): increase in number of immature alveoli, formation of mature alveoli, increased size of alveoli.

PULMONARY SURFACTANTS. The detection of the presence of pulmonary surfactants, surface-active phospholipids, in amniotic fluid has been used to determine the degree of fetal lung maturity, or the ability of the lungs to function after birth. Lecithin is the most critical alveolar surfactant required for postnatal lung expansion. It increases in amount after the twenty-fourth week. Another pulmonary phospholipid, sphingomyelin, remains constant in amount. Thus the measure of **lecithin** (L) in relation to **sphingomyelin** (S), or the **L/S ratio** of 2:1, is used to determine fetal lung maturity. This occurs at approximately 35 weeks of gestation (Creasy, Resnek, 1989).

Certain maternal conditions alter the development of the fetal lungs. Those conditions that accelerate lung maturity generally cause decreased maternal placental blood flow. The resulting fetal hypoxia apparently stresses the fetus, increasing blood levels of corticosteroids that accelerate alveolar and surfactant development. Conditions such as maternal hypertension, placental dysfunction, infection, or corticosteroid use accelerate maturity. Conditions such as gestational diabetes and chronic glomerulonephritis can retard fetal lung maturity.

The recent approval of the use of intrabronchial synthetic surfactant in the treatment of respiratory distress syndrome in the newborn has greatly improved the chances of survival of preterm infants (Paynton, 1991) (see Chapter 37).

Fetal respiratory movements have been seen on ultrasound as early as the eleventh week. They may aid in development of the chest wall muscles and regulate lung fluid volume. The fetal lungs produce fluid that expands the air spaces in the lungs. The fluid drains out into the amniotic fluid or is swallowed by the fetus. Before birth, secretion of lung fluid decreases. The normal birth process squeezes out approximately one third of the fluid. Infants of cesarean births do not benefit from this squeezing process; thus they have more respiratory difficulty at birth. The fluid remaining in the lungs at birth is usually reabsorbed by the infant's bloodstream within 2 hours of birth.

RENAL SYSTEM. The permanent kidneys form during the fifth week. Urine formation is present during the third month. Urine is excreted into the amniotic fluid and forms a major part of the amniotic fluid volume. *Oligohydramnios,* an abnormally small amount of amniotic fluid, is indicative of renal dysfunction. Because the placenta acts as the organ of excretion and maintains fetal water and electrolyte balance, an infant does not need functioning kidneys during fetal life. However, at birth, they are required immediately for excretory and acid-base regulatory functions.

A fetus who has a renal malformation can be diagnosed in utero. This can be treated successfully with fetal surgery, either corrective or palliative, or plans can be made for treatment immediately after birth.

At term, the fetus has fully developed kidneys. However, the glomerular filtration rate (GFR) is low, and the kidneys lack the ability to concentrate urine. This makes the newborn more susceptible to both overhydration and dehydration.

Most newborns void within 24 hours of birth. With the loss of the swallowed amniotic fluid and the metabolism of placenta-provided nutrients, voidings for the first days of life are scanty until fluid intake increases.

NEUROLOGIC SYSTEM. The nervous system originates from the ectoderm at 18 days after fertilization. The open neural tube forms during the fourth week. It initially closes at what will be the junction of the brain and spinal cord, leaving both ends open. The embryo folds in on itself lengthwise at this time, forming a head fold in the neural tube at this junction. The cranial end of the neural tube closes, then the caudal end. During week 5, different growth rates cause more flexures in the neural tube that delineate three brain areas: the forebrain, midbrain, and hindbrain.

The forebrain develops into the eyes (cranial nerve II) and cerebral hemispheres. The development of all areas of the cerebral cortex continues throughout fetal life and into childhood. The olfactory system (cranial nerve I) and thalamus also develop from the forebrain. Cranial nerves III and IV (oculomotor and trochlear) form from the midbrain. The hindbrain forms the medulla, pons, cerebellum, and the remainder of the cranial nerves. Brain waves can be recorded on an electroencephalogram by week 8.

The spinal cord develops from the long end of the neural tube. Another ectodermal structure, the neural crest, develops into the peripheral nervous system. By the eighth week, nerve fibers traverse throughout the body. By week 11 or 12, the fetus makes respiratory movements, moves all extremities, and changes position in utero. The fetus can suck his or her thumb and swim in the amniotic fluid pool, turning somersaults and possibly tying a knot in the umbilical cord. When the movements are strong enough to be perceived by the mother as "the baby moving," **quickening** has occurred. For the nullipara, this occurs after 16 weeks. For the multipara, the perception occurs earlier. The mother becomes aware of the sleeping and waking cycles of the fetus.

SENSORY AWARENESS. Purposeful movements of the fetus have been demonstrated in response to a firm touch transmitted through the mother's abdomen. Invasive procedures to be done on a fetus require anesthesia.

Fetuses have been shown to respond to sound by 24 weeks. Different types of music evoke different movements. The fetus can be soothed by the sound of the mother's voice. Acoustic stimulation can be used to evoke an FHR response (see Chapter 27). The fetus does become accustomed to noises heard repeatedly.

The fetus is able to distinguish taste. By the fifth month, when the fetus is swallowing amniotic fluid, a sweetener added to the fluid causes the fetus to swallow twice as fast (Poole, 1986). The fetus also reacts to temperature changes. A cold solution placed into the amniotic fluid can cause fetal hiccups.

The fetus is able to see. Eyes are developed with both rods and cones in the retina by the seventh month. A bright light shone on the mother's abdomen in late pregnancy causes abrupt fetal movements. During sleep time, rapid eye movements (REMs) have been observed similar to those occurring in children and adults while dreaming (Poole, 1986).

At term, the fetal brain is approximately one fourth the size of an adult brain. Neurologic development continues. Stressors on the fetus and neonate, such as chronic poor nutrition or hypoxia, drugs, environmental toxins, trauma, or disease cause damage to the central nervous system long after the vulnerable embryonic time for malformations in other organ systems. Neurologic insult can result in cerebral palsy, neuromuscular impairment, mental retardation, and learning disabilities (see Chapter 37).

GASTROINTESTINAL SYSTEM. During the fourth week, the embryo changes from almost straight to a "C" shape as both ends fold in toward the ventral surface. A portion of the yolk sac is incorporated into the body from head to tail as the primitive gut (digestive system).

The foregut produces the pharynx, part of the lower respiratory tract, the esophagus, the stomach, the first half of the duodenum, the liver, the pancreas, and the gallbladder. These structures evolve over the fifth and sixth weeks. The malformations that occur in these areas are esophageal atresia, hypertrophic pyloric stenosis, duodenal stenosis or atresia, and biliary atresia.

The midgut becomes the distal half of the duodenum, the jejunum and ileum, the cecum and appendix, and the proximal half of the colon. The midgut loop projects into the umbilical cord between weeks 5 and 10. A malformation (omphalocele) results if the midgut fails to return to the abdominal cavity, and intestines protrude from the umbilicus. Meckel's diverticulum is the most common malformation of the midgut: attached to the ileum is a remnant of the yolk stalk that has failed to degenerate, leaving a blind sac.

The hindgut develops into the distal half of the colon, the rectum and parts of the anal canal, the urinary bladder, and urethra. Anorectal malformations are the most commonly occurring abnormalities of the digestive system.

The fetus swallows amniotic fluid beginning in the fifth month. Gastric emptying and intestinal peristalsis occur. Fetal nutrition and elimination needs are taken care of by the placenta. However, as the fetus nears term, fetal waste products have accumulated in the intestines as dark green to black, tarry **meconium.** Normally, this substance is passed through the rectum within 48 hours of birth. Sometimes with a breech birth or fetal hypoxia, meconium is passed in utero in the amniotic fluid (for further discussion, see Chapter 27). The failure to pass meconium after birth could be indicative of atresia somewhere in the digestive tract, an imperforate anus, or a meconium ileus with a firm meconium plug blocking passage. This is seen in infants with cystic fibrosis.

The metabolic rate of the fetus is relatively low, but the infant has great growth and development needs. Beginning in week 9, the fetus synthesizes glycogen for storage in the liver. Between 26 to 30 weeks, the fetus begins to lay down stores of brown fat in preparation for extrauterine cold stress. Thermoregulation in the neonate requires increased metabolism and adequate oxygenation.

The gastrointestinal system is mature by 36 weeks. Digestive enzymes are present in sufficient quantity except pancreatic amylase and lipase. The neonate cannot digest starches or fats efficiently. Little saliva is produced.

HEPATIC SYSTEM. The liver and biliary tract develop from the foregut during the fourth week of gestation. Hematopoiesis begins during the sixth week, requiring that the liver be large. The embryonic liver is prominent and occupies most of the abdominal cavity. Bile formation begins in the twelfth week. Bile is a constituent of meconium.

Glycogen is stored in the fetal liver beginning at week 9 or 10 and continuing for extrauterine needs. At term, glycogen stores are twice those of the adult. Glycogen is the major source of energy for the fetus and neonate who is stressed by in utero hypoxia or by extrauterine loss of the maternal glucose supply, by the work of breathing, or by cold stress.

Iron is stored in the fetal liver. If the maternal intake is sufficient, enough iron can be stored to last for 5 months after birth.

During fetal life, the liver does not have to conjugate bilirubin for excretion because the unconjugated bilirubin is cleared by the placenta. Therefore the fetal liver has less glucuronyl transferase enzyme needed for conjugation than is required after birth. This predisposes the neonate to hyperbilirubinemia.

Coagulation factors II, VII, IX, and X cannot be synthesized in the fetal liver because of the *lack of vitamin K synthesis* in the sterile fetal gut. This coagulation deficiency persists after birth for several days and is the rationale for the prophylactic administration of vitamin K to the newborn.

ENDOCRINE SYSTEM. The thyroid gland develops with structures in the head and neck during the third and fourth weeks. The secretion of thyroxine begins during the eighth week. Maternal thyroxine does not readily cross the placenta; therefore the fetus who does not produce thyroid hormones will be born with congenital hypothyroidism. If untreated, this can result in severe mental retardation. All neonates are screened for hypothyroidism with a blood test after birth.

The adrenal cortex is formed during the sixth week and is producing hormones by the eighth or ninth week. As term approaches, the fetus produces more cortisol. This is believed to aid in initiation of labor by decreasing the maternal progesterone and stimulating production of prostaglandins.

The pancreas forms from the foregut during the fifth through eighth weeks. The islets of Langerhans develop during the twelfth week. Insulin is produced by the twentieth week. In infants of diabetic mothers, maternal hyperglycemia produces fetal hyperglycemia, stimulating hyperinsulinemia and islet-cell hyperplasia (for more discussion, see Chapters 31 and 39). This results in a macrosomatic fetus. The hyperinsulinemia also blocks lung maturation, placing the neonate at risk for respiratory distress and hypoglycemia when the maternal glucose source is lost at delivery. Control of the maternal glucose level during pregnancy minimizes the problems for the infant.

REPRODUCTIVE SYSTEM. Until the seventh week, there is no gender differentiation in the embryo. Then the Y chromosome in the male dictates the formation of testes. By the end of the embryonic period, testosterone is being secreted and causes formation of the male genitalia. By week 28, the testes begin descending into the scrotum. After birth, low levels of testosterone continue to be secreted until the pubertal surge.

The lack of a Y chromosome in the female brings about the formation of ovaries and female external genitalia. Female and male external genitalia are indistinguishable until after the ninth week. By the sixteenth week, oogenesis has been established. At birth, the ovaries contain the female's lifetime supply of ova. The female lacks most female hormone production until puberty. However, the fetal endometrium responds to the maternal hormones, and withdrawal bleeding or vaginal discharge may occur at birth when these hormones are lost.

IMMUNOLOGIC SYSTEM. During the last trimester, albumin and globulin are present in the fetus. The only immunoglobulin that crosses the placenta is IgG, providing passive acquired immunity to specific bacterial toxins. IgM immunoglobulins are produced by the fetus by the end of the first trimester. These are produced in response to blood group antigens, gram-negative enteric organisms, and some viruses. IgA immunoglobulins are not produced by the fetus. However, colostrum, the precursor to breast milk, contains large amounts and can provide passive immunity to the neonate.

The normal neonate can fight infection, but not as effectively as an older child. The preterm infant is at much greater risk for infection.

MUSCULOSKELETAL SYSTEM. Bones and muscles both develop from the mesoderm by the fourth week of embryonic development. The cardiac muscle is already beating. The mesoderm beside the neural tube forms the vertebral column and ribs. The parts of the vertebral column grow toward each other to enclose the developing spinal cord. Ossification or bone formation begins. If there is a defect in the bony fusion, spina bifida may occur. A large defect affecting several vertebrae may allow the membranes and spinal cord to pouch out from the back, producing neurologic deficits as well as the skeletal deformity.

The flat bones of the skull develop during the embryonic period, and ossification continues through childhood. At birth, connective tissue sutures exist where the bones of the skull meet. The areas where more than two bones meet, called *fontanelles,* are especially prominent. The sutures and fontanelles allow the bones of the skull to mold, or move during birth, enabling the head to pass through the birth canal. The larger fontanelle remains open until the second year of life.

The bones of the shoulders, arms, hips, and legs appear in the sixth week as a continuous skeleton with no joints. Differentiation occurs, producing separate bones and joints. Ossification will continue through childhood to allow growth.

Beginning during the seventh week, muscles contract spontaneously. Arm and leg movements are visible on ultrasound, although the mother does not perceive them until the sixteenth to the twentieth week.

INTEGUMENTARY SYSTEM. The epidermis begins as a single layer of cells derived from the ectoderm at 4 weeks. By the seventh week, there are two layers of cells. The superficial layer cells are sloughed and become mixed with the sebaceous gland secretions to form the white, greasy vernix caseosa, the material that protects the skin of the fetus. The vernix is thick at 24 weeks but becomes scant by term. The basal layer of the epidermis is the germinal layer, which replaces the lost cells. Until 17 weeks, the skin is very thin and wrinkled, with blood vessels visible underneath. The skin thickens, and all layers are present at term. After 32 weeks, as subcutaneous fat is deposited under the dermis, the skin is less wrinkled and red in appearance.

By 16 weeks, the epidermal ridges are present on the palms of the hands, the fingers, the bottom of the feet and the toes. This makes the hand and footprints unique to that individual infant.

Hairs form from hair bulbs in the epidermis, which project into the dermis. Cells in the hair bulb keratinize to form the hair shaft. As the cells at the base of the hair shaft proliferate, the hair grows to the surface of the epithelium. The very fine hairs, called *lanugo,* appear first at 12 weeks on the eyebrows and upper lip. By 20 weeks, they cover the entire body. At this time, the eyelashes, eyebrows, and scalp hair are beginning to grow. By 28 weeks, the scalp hair is longer than the lanugo, which is thinning and may disappear by term gestation. The amount of lanugo remaining is one of the criteria used to assess gestational age of a newborn (see Chapter 37).

The fingernails and toenails develop from thickened epidermis at the tips of the digits beginning during the tenth week. They grow slowly. Fingernails usually reach the fingertips by 32 weeks, and toenails reach toetips by 36 weeks.

Multifetal Pregnancy

TWINS. The woman who produces two mature ova in one ovarian cycle has the potential for both to be fertilized by separate sperm. This results in two zygotes or **dizygotic twins.** (Fig. 7-14). There are always two amnions, two chorions, and two placentas that may be fused together. These fraternal twins may be the same sex or different sexes and are genetically no more alike than siblings born at different times. Dizygotic twinning occurs in families and more often among African-American women than Caucasian women and least among Asian women. It increases in frequency with maternal age up to 35 years, with parity, and with the use of fertility drugs.

Identical twins develop from one fertilized ovum, which then divides (hence the term **monozygotic twins**) (Fig. 7-15). They are the same sex and have the same genotype. If division occurs soon after fertilization, two embryos, two amnions, two chorions,

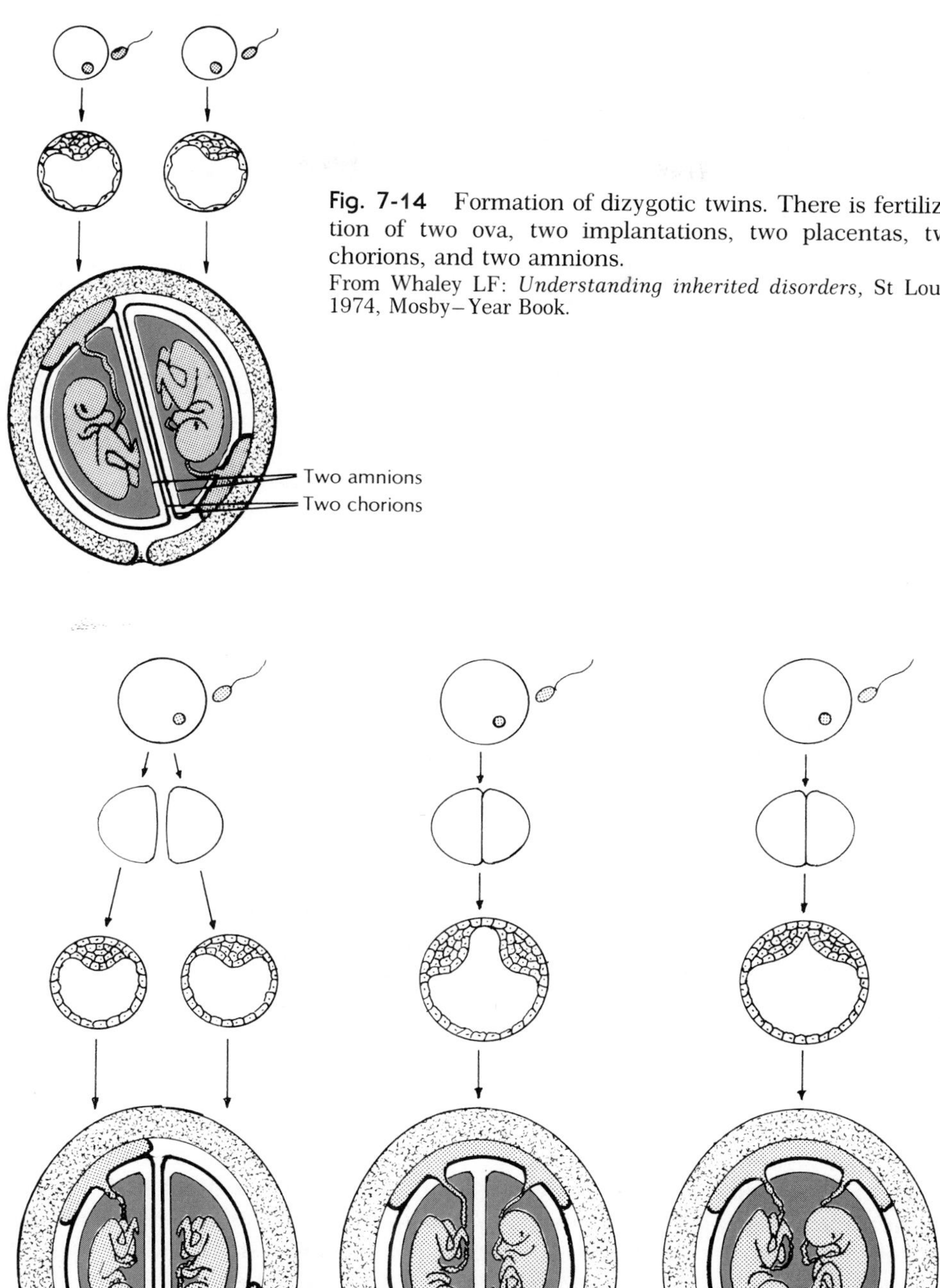

Fig. 7-14 Formation of dizygotic twins. There is fertilization of two ova, two implantations, two placentas, two chorions, and two amnions.
From Whaley LF: *Understanding inherited disorders,* St Louis, 1974, Mosby–Year Book.

Fig. 7-15 Formation of monozygotic twins. **A,** One fertilization: blastomeres separate, resulting in two implantations, two placentas, and two sets of membranes. **B,** One blastomere with two inner cell masses, one fused placenta, one chorion, and separate amnions. **C,** Later separation of inner cell masses, with fused placenta and single amnion and chorion.
From Whaley LF: *Understanding inherited disorders,* St Louis, 1974, Mosby–Year Book.

and two placentas that may be fused will develop. Most often, division occurs between 4 and 8 days after fertilization, and there are two embryos, two amnions, one chorion, and one placenta. Rarely, division occurs after the eighth day after fertilization. In this case, there are two embryos within a common amnion and a common chorion with one placenta. This commonly causes circulation problems because the umbilical cords tangle together, and one or both fetuses may die. If division occurs very late, cleavage may not be complete, and conjoined or "Siamese" twins could result.

Monozygotic twinning occurs in approximately 1 of 250 births (Cunningham, MacDonald, Gant, 1989). There is no association with race, heredity, maternal age, or parity. Fertility drugs do increase the incidence (Deron et al, 1987).

OTHER MULTIFETAL PREGNANCIES. The occurrence of multifetal pregnancies with three or more fetuses has increased with the use of fertility drugs and in vitro fertilization. Triplets occur once in about 7600 pregnancies. They can occur from the division of one zygote into two, with one of the two dividing again, producing identical triplets. Triplets can also be produced from two zygotes, one dividing into a set of identical twins and the second zygote a single fraternal sibling, or from three zygotes. Quadruplets, quintuplets, sextuplets, and so on, likewise, have similar possible derivations.

Genetic Counseling

Rapid expansion in the identification, understanding, and diagnosis of genetic disease has been accompanied by effective medical or surgical therapies in a small number of cases; however, for the majority of genetic conditions therapeutic or preventive measures are nonexistent or disappointingly limited. Consequently the most useful means of reducing the incidence of these disorders is by preventing their transmission. With the accumulation of knowledge about genetic disease the probability of recurrence in any given situation can be predicted with increased accuracy. Providing families, through health professionals, with genetic information and services is at present the best means for reducing the number of children born with genetic defects.

CLIENTS. The reasons that persons seek genetic counseling are varied. The persons may or may not be affected themselves. Persons seeking counseling commonly fall into the following categories:

1. Persons who want to know if they have a genetic disease or if they are carriers of a genetic disease
2. Persons who are concerned whether they are at risk for producing a child with a specific genetic disease
3. Persons who are planning parenthood and who want to know the implications (prognosis and treatment) of a genetic disease afflicting one or both partners
4. Persons seeking help in making a decision about prenatal diagnosis, selective abortion, artificial insemination by donor, or adoption
5. Persons seeking help for a child affected with a genetic disease

For all pregnancies, it is standard practice to assess for heritable disorders to identify potential clients (Creasy, Resnik, 1989). The interviewer inquires about the health status of family members, abnormal reproductive outcomes, history of maternal disease (e.g., diabetes, PKU, and cystic fibrosis), drug exposures, and illness (Fanaroff, Martin, 1992). Advanced maternal and paternal ages are determined.

Ethnic origin should be recorded, since some disorders appear more frequently in some groups (Creasy, Resnik, 1989). Examples include: Tay-Sachs disease in Jewish individuals of Ashkenazic or Sephardic descent, β-thalassemia in Italians and Greeks, sickle cell anemia in African Americans, α-thalassemia in Southeast Asians and Filipinos, and tyrosinemia in French Canadians from the Lac St. Jean-Chicoutimi region of Quebec (Fanaroff, Martin, 1992).

GOALS. Counseling for any situation is a process of communication involving a mutual exchange of ideas and opinions that provides the basis for mutual problem solving.

There are three major goals of genetic counseling. The *first* is to provide families with accurate information regarding recurrence risks when a member of the family has a disorder that might be genetically determined. The risk in their particular situation should be presented in language the clients can understand and should be placed in the proper perspective in relation to a random risk situation. The *second* goal of genetic counseling is to alert health professionals to the possibility of a genetic disease in a family. This increases the likelihood that the disease will be detected and treatment initiated earlier. Clues to this possibility are the presence of an affected sibling or parent or environmental factors that may have been operating during a pregnancy. The *third* goal of genetic counseling is to reduce the numbers of children affected with a hereditary condition by prenatal detection of a disorder, heterozygote testing in families and populations at risk, and providing information about recurrence risks as a basis for judicious family planning in families at risk.

COUNSELING SERVICES. The most efficient counseling facilities are associated with the larger universities and major medical centers where support services are available (e.g., biochemical and cytology laboratories) and consist of a group of specialists under the leadership of a physician trained in medical genetics. Many of these regional centers maintain satellite clinics or services in more remote areas to provide contact with both consumers and health professionals. A number of specialized groups provide clinics and services for persons with a specific genetic disorder such as cystic fibrosis, muscular dystrophy, hemophilia, and diabetes. Health professionals should become familiar with persons who provide genetic counseling and places in which counseling services are available to clients in their area of practice.

All nurses, and particularly those involved in the care of mothers and children, need to (1) have an understanding of genetic theory and the nature of more common genetic disorders to recognize cues that may indicate a genetically related problem, (2) be able to help families obtain counseling services, and (3) augment the counseling process (Stringer, Librizzi, Weiner, 1991). They assist with preparation of clients for procedures and counseling and with diagnostic procedures and therapeutic programs, interpret and reinforce counseling, maintain follow-up care, support the family's coping capacities, and assist them in their problem solving. To provide supportive care for families involved in genetic counseling, nurses need an understanding of the process and some of the procedures the family will experience.

MANAGEMENT OF GENETIC DISEASE. At this time there is no cure for genetic disease, although remedies can be implemented to prevent or reduce the harmful effects of a few disorders. Structural defects can sometimes be modified to produce normal or near-normal function. Research is continually being carried out in the hope that methods can be devised to influence or change the genes directly, thereby preventing the disease process. However, at this time the major thrust in therapy is modification of the internal or external environment to minimize the effects of the disease.

Some therapy is available. Surgical therapy is employed for congenital heart defects and cosmetic defects such as cleft lip. Advances in fetal surgery are occurring. Other conditions are treated with product replacement (thyroid for hereditary cretinism), diet modification (low phenylalanine diet for PKU), and corrective devices for missing limbs.

Persons with some diseases, such as glucose-6-phosphate dehydrogenase (G6PD) deficiency or the porphyrias can prevent the disease simply by avoiding the specific chemical agent that precipitates the symptoms. Avoiding circumstances that reduce tissue oxygenation can reduce the sickling of red blood cells in sickle cell anemia.

Researchers continue to develop therapies for heritable diseases. Some possible methods of future management include replacement or stabilization by pills, injections, or other methods, altering intracellular DNA, and other projected feats of genetic engineering. Rapid progress is evident in the field of genetic engineering (Barber, 1991). Molecular techniques provide infinite possibilities for altering human genes through gene splicing, for example. Thus altered, genes in ova and sperm can be used for in vitro fertilization (see Chapter 42).

COUNSELING PROCESS. The counseling process begins with an accurate diagnosis and a careful, detailed family history. The diagnosis is frequently made on the basis of clinical manifestations but may require special biochemical or cytologic tests, especially in very rare or unusual cases. The correct diagnosis is essential, because there are a number of diseases that have similar manifestations but different modes of inheritance. The mode of inheritance determines the recurrence risks and sometimes the prognosis. For example, the X-linked form of Duchenne's muscular dystrophy has a much more ominous outlook than either of the forms with a dominant or a recessive inheritance pattern.

ESTIMATION OF RISK. The risks are determined by the mode of inheritance. The risk of recurrence for disorders caused by a factor that segregates during cell division (genes and chromosomes) can be estimated with a high degree of accuracy by application of the mendelian principles. In a dominant disorder the risk is 50%, or one in two, that a subsequent offspring will be affected; an autosomal-recessive disease carries a one-in-four risk of recurrence; and an X-linked disorder is related to the sex of the child as described in X-linked inheritance. Translocation chromosomes present a high risk of recurrence.

Disorders in which a subsequent pregnancy would carry no more risk than there would be for pregnancy (estimated at 1 in 30) include those resulting from isolated incidences not likely to be present in another pregnancy, such as maternal infections (e.g., rubella or toxoplasmosis), maternal ingestion of drugs, most chromosomal abnormalities, and a disorder determined to be the result of a fresh mutation.

The risk of recurrence for multifactorial conditions can be estimated empirically. An *empiric* risk is not based on genetic theory, but on experience and observation of the disorder in other families. Recurrence risks are determined by applying the frequency of a similar disorder in other families to the case under consideration.

INTERPRETATION OF RISK. Counselors explain the risk estimates to clients without making recommendations or decisions and avoid allowing their own biases to interfere. The counselor provides appropriate information about the nature of the disorder, the extent of the risks in the specific case, the probable consequences, and (if appropriate) alternative options available, but the final decision must be left to the family. An important nursing role is reinforcing the information the clients are given and continuing to interpret this information on their level of understanding.

Since most clients do not have an adequate knowledge of genetics and human biology, the complex concepts of cell division, segregation, and recombination are often difficult to comprehend. However, most persons have an adequate understanding of games of chance and have had experience with flipping coins, lotteries, and various other games based on probabilities. These are effective devices for illustrating monogenic disorders; weather forecasts and horse-racing handicaps are excellent examples of empiric-risk estimates.

The most important concept that must be emphasized to families is that each pregnancy is *an independent event*. For example, in monogenic disorders in which the risk factor is one in four that the child will be affected, the risk remains the same no matter how many affected children are already in the family. It is not uncommon for families to maintain the erroneous assumption that the presence of one affected child ensures that the next three will be free of the disease. However, "chance has no memory." The risk is one in four for each pregnancy.

On the other hand, in a family in which there is a child affected with a disorder caused by multifactorial causes, the risk increases with each subsequent child born with the disorder.

ROLE OF NURSE IN GENETIC COUNSELING. Nurses are assuming an increasingly important role in counseling persons regarding genetically transmitted or genetically influenced conditions. Diagnosis and treatment of genetic disorders require medical skills; the complexities of determining risk factors for many diseases and for individual circumstances require the expertise of a geneticist. Nurses who are actively involved in counseling require a minimum of a master's degree in genetics and related subjects. However, nurses without advanced preparation in genetics can be productive members of a counseling service. Nurses are usually the persons who provide follow-up care and maintain contact with the clients. They are persons who are in the best position to sustain a close relationship (e.g., community health nurses who have already established a rapport with many families) and for whom interviewing and counseling skills are an integral part of their professional practice.

The following are some of the experiences that are usually part of the counseling and diagnostic processes. It is the responsibility of the nurse to have a beginning understanding of these processes and the impact that they may have on the family. In this way they will be better prepared to provide supportive care to these families.

PREPARATION FOR COUNSELING. The circumstances surrounding the counseling determine the type of preparation needed by the clients. They must first be aware that there is a genetic problem or a potential genetic problem and either seek counseling on their own initiative or be referred for counseling by a physician or another knowledgeable person.

The initial interview or intake visit is often conducted by a nurse. At this time a detailed family history is obtained. The family is told what to expect during the counseling process, procedures to be performed, and the personnel with whom they will be involved. The interview serves as an opportunity to assess the client or family's needs and reduce their anxiety. Most persons who come for genetic counseling are nervous and apprehensive, not only because they are concerned about a genetic condition, but also because they know that the outcome of the counseling and the decisions that will be made may significantly alter their lives. Therefore an atmosphere should be provided that is free from distractive elements. This may require care for small children whose restlessness and behavior can divert attention from what is being said. An ample amount of time is allotted to reduce their clients' anxiety and provide them with as much information as possible. In this way they can gain more from the counseling session.

In addition to the medical and genetic facts that the family are able to provide, the interviewer can obtain information about the social aspects of their lives and the meaning that disorder has for this particular person or family. It is a time for clarification about what counseling does and does not provide and for answering the clients' questions and listening to their concerns. They need to know that they have the freedom to talk about their fears and concerns with a sympathetic and nonjudgmental listener. It is more effective for the nurse to discuss with the family the issues they raise before discussing issues of concern with the counselor.

The persons involved need to know where and how the service is conducted and structured, including such things as the number and timing of visits, how many members should come, and some concept of what they can expect during the process. Most families have only vague ideas of what the service will do for them. Some have unrealistic expectations; many are confused about the service and what it might provide for them. Instructions should be clear and specific and may need to be repeated. If there is something they should bring, such as records or photographs, this should be explained. The counselor will also need to be provided with some information about the family, their needs, and any pertinent aspects of the case that may facilitate the counseling process.

It is not uncommon for families to be sensitive about or even ashamed of their genetic problem. They may avoid keeping appointments. Part of their preparation is reassurance, which may require several calls or visits before the family feels secure enough to follow through.

DIAGNOSTIC TESTS AND PROCEDURES. The family and persons directly involved with diagnostic procedures need to know the purpose of each test, what they can expect, and what they can do to facilitate the process. They may be concerned about whether or not the test will be painful, if they will be required to undress, and if they can be accompanied by a family member. Nurses can do a great deal to allay fears and to supply support and reassurance.

The tests are not usually performed at the time of the initial interview but at a subsequent visit or visits. This gives the client and family time to assimilate any information and explanations presented during the first visit. These visits provide an opportunity to obtain any additional information, clarify misconceptions, and explore some of the thoughts generated by information from the previous visit. It may require several visits before a definitive diagnosis can be made.

The pregnant woman who submits to chorionic villus sampling or amniocentesis for detection of genetic disease in a fetus is particularly anxious (Stringer, Librizzi, Weiner, 1991; Nyhan, 1991). Although the physical risk to fetus and mother is almost negligible (approximately 1%), the procedure may be fraught with emotional issues and sequelae. When the fetus is found to be free of the disorder for which the test is carried out, the parents need only a thorough explanation of the procedure and support during the test (see Chapter 27).

FOLLOW-UP CARE. Maintaining contact with the family after genetic counseling, testing, or therapy is one of the most important nursing responsibilities, since *the success of counseling is measured by the way the family uses the information that is presented to them.* Most counseling services try to schedule at least one postdiagnostic or postcounseling visit to assess how well the family is beginning to incorporate this new information into their lives and value systems. Follow-up visits to the counseling service or visits to the home provide additional opportunities to reexplore all aspects of the situation and to answer any questions that may have occurred to the family since the previous contacts. At the first counseling session all clients have some anxiety, which is a block to effective assimilation of information. Therefore much of the counseling information may require repetition under less stressful circumstances. If possible, the nurse should contact the counseling service to determine the pertinent information that has been conveyed to the family. Clarifying information and misunderstanding of information are important nursing functions.

A newly diagnosed disorder often implies the implementation of a therapeutic regimen. For example, the disorder in question may be an inborn error of metabolism, such as PKU or galactosemia, that requires consistent and rigid adherence to a diet. The family may need help to secure the necessary formula and counseling from dietetic services. The importance of maintaining the diet, especially keeping an adequate supply of special preparations and avoiding unauthorized substitutions, must be impressed on the family.

Referral to appropriate agencies is another essential part of the follow-up management. Many organizations and foundations help to provide services and equipment for affected children, for example, the Cystic Fibrosis Foundation and the Muscular Dystrophy Association. Early Infant Stimulation Foundation programs are available for a child born with Down syndrome. There are also numerous parent groups with whom the family can share experiences and derive mutual support from other families with a similar problem. Nurses should become familiar with services available in their community that provide assistance and education to families with these special problems.

EMOTIONAL SUPPORT. Probably the most important of all nursing functions is providing emotional support to the family during all aspects of the counseling process. Feelings that are generated under the real or imagined threat posed by a genetic disorder are as varied as the persons being counseled. Responses may include all stress reactions, such as apathy, denial, anger, hostility, fear, embarrassment, grief, and loss of self-esteem (for a discussion of loss and grief, see Chapter 40).

Guilt and self-blame are universal reactions. Many look on the disorder as a stigma—especially if the disorder is visible to others. Persons involved with the family are often able to dispel fears and even absolve the family from guilt simply by explaining the random nature of cell division and segregation and the comforting fact that everyone carries defective genes, which, when combined with the same genes in a partner, can produce undesirable consequences. Old wives' tales, supersititions, and long-held misconceptions are all factors that may influence a client's reaction to a genetic disorder.

The attitude of other family members and relatives can have a significant impact on some persons—especially in situations where the blame can be pinpointed (such as a dominant or an X-linked disorder). Recessive disorders are less likely to cause blaming, since both partners carry the defective gene. Unfortunately most families tend to view a genetic disorder as a cause for shame, and its presence in a family may be cause to alter plans for marriage or childbearing even when the probability of recurrence is no more than a random risk. The way a family views the probability of recurrence varies tremendously. For example, one family will consider a 10% risk as reassuring, whereas another may consider it too great a risk to contemplate marriage or childbearing.

The nature of a genetic condition also influences the way families respond to a disorder. Factors such as the severity or chronicity of a disease, the age of onset, the threat of early death, a lengthy period of deterioration, presence or absence of pain, mental retardation, or cosmetic disfiguration all determine the impact that a condition will produce in a family. One family may risk a child with a disorder that produces a minor defect or even an early death but will not risk having a child with a lifelong physical or mental disability.

Obstacles such as religious beliefs, intellectual

TABLE 7-1 Milestones in Human Development Before Birth Since LMP

	4 Weeks	8 Weeks	12 Weeks	16 Weeks
EXTERNAL APPEARANCE	Body flexed, C-shaped; arm and leg buds present; head at right angles to body	Body fairly well formed; nose flat, eyes far apart; digits well formed; head elevating; tail almost disappeared; eyes, ears, nose, and mouth recognizable	Nails appearing; resembles a human; head erect but disproportionately large; skin pink, delicate	Head still dominant; face looks human; eyes, ears, and nose approach typical appearance on gross examination; arm-leg ratio proportionate; scalp hair appears
CROWN-TO-RUMP MEASUREMENT (cm), WEIGHT (g)	0.4-0.5, 0.4	2.5-3, 2	6-9, 19	11.5-13.5, 100
GASTROINTESTINAL SYSTEM	Stomach at midline and fusiform; conspicuous liver; esophagus short; intestine a short tube	Intestinal villi developing; small intestines coil within umbilical cord; palatal folds present; liver very large	Bile secreted; palatal fusion complete; intestines have withdrawn from cord and assume characteristic positions	Meconium in bowel; some enzyme secretion; anus open

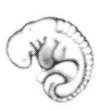

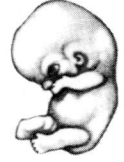

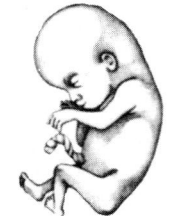

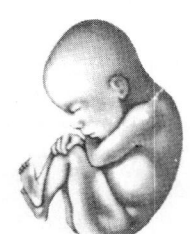

Modified from Whaley LF, Wong DI: *Nursing care of infants and children*, ed 4. St Louis, 1991, Mosby–Year Book.

level, and prior attitudes toward the disease affect the way in which families respond to counseling information. Sometimes counselors and other health personnel create barriers through their own attitudes toward a specific disease. It is often difficult to be nonjudgmental and objective in all instances, and nurses may intentionally or unintentionally influence families in making decisions. This is especially true when the client's intellectual level makes it difficult or impossible for that person to comprehend the ramifications of a situation. Even persons who can repeat information accurately often fail to grasp its significance in their case. Families may pressure the nurse to make decisions for them with questions such as, "What would you do if you were me?"

Families and individuals need education, guidance, and support throughout the counseling process. They should be given the facts and possible consequences and all of the assistance they need in problem solving, but the final decision regarding a course of action must be their own.

■ SUMMARY

A basic knowledge of genetic concepts and heredity is necessary for the nurse dealing with prospective parents and new parents. The desire for a "perfect" baby and the need to know what went wrong when that end is not achieved often leads to discussion with the nurse. Knowledge of conception and normal fetal development is shared with expectant parents since that knowledge determines when their baby is due and what their baby looks like throughout pregnancy. Table 7-1 summarizes embryonic and fetal development.

20 Weeks	24 Weeks	28 Weeks	30-31 Weeks	36 Weeks	40 Weeks
Vernix caseosa appears; lanugo appears; legs lengthen considerably; sebaceous glands appear	Body lean but fairly well proportioned; skin red and wrinkled; vernix caseosa present; sweat glands forming	Lean body, less wrinkled and red; nails appear	Subcutaneous fat beginning to collect; more rounded appearance; skin pink and smooth; has assumed delivery position	Skin pink, body rounded; general lanugo disappearing; body usually plump	Skin smooth and pink, copious vernix caseosa; moderate to profuse hair; lanugo on shoulders and upper body only; nasal and alar cartilage apparent
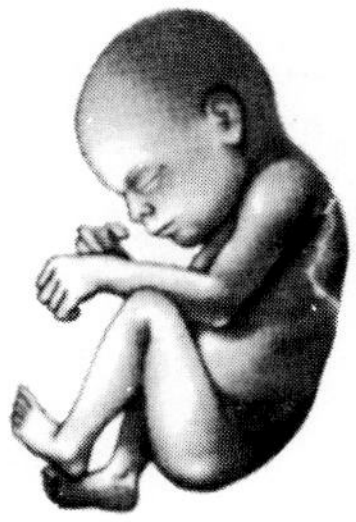	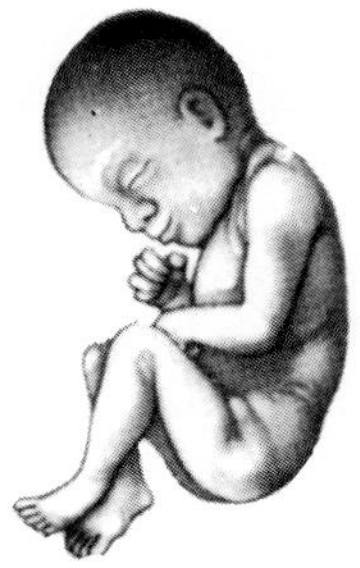		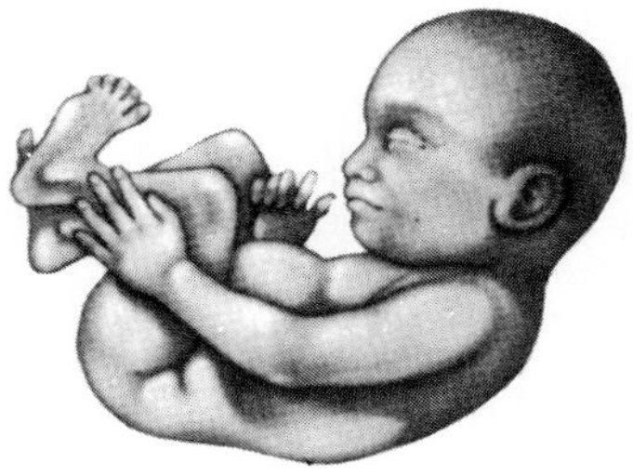		
16-18.5, 300	23, 600	27, 1100	31, 1800-2100	35, 2200-2900	40, 3200+
Enamel and dentine depositing; ascending colon recognizable					

Continued.

TABLE 7-1 Milestones in Human Development Before Birth Since LMP—cont'd

4 Weeks	8 Weeks	12 Weeks	16 Weeks
MUSCULOSKELETAL SYSTEM			
All somites present	First indication of ossification—occiput, mandible, and humerus; fetus capable of some movement, definitive muscles of trunk, limbs, and head well represented	Some bones well outlined, ossification spreading; upper cervical to lower sacral arches and bodies ossify; smooth muscle layers indicated in hollow viscera	Most bones distinctly indicated throughout body; joint cavities appear; muscular movements can be detected
CIRCULATORY SYSTEM			
Heart develops, double chambers visible, begins to beat; aortic arch and major veins completed	Main blood vessels assume final plan; enucleated red cells predominate in blood	Blood forming in marrow	Heart muscle well developed; blood formation active in spleen
RESPIRATORY SYSTEM			
Primary lung buds appear	Pleural and pericardial cavities forming; branching bronchioles; nostrils closed by epithelial plugs	Lungs acquire definite shape; vocal cords appear	Elastic fibers appear in lungs; terminal and respiratory bronchioles appear
RENAL SYSTEM			
Rudimentary ureteral buds appear.	Earliest secretory tubules differentiating; bladder-urethra separates from rectum	Kidney able to secrete urine; bladder expands as a sac	Kidney in position; attains typical shape and plan
NERVOUS SYSTEM			
Well-marked midbrain flexure; no hindbrain or cervical flexures; neural groove closed	Cerebral cortex begins to acquire typical cells; differentiation of cerebral cortex, meninges, ventricular foramens, cerebrospinal fluid circulation; spinal cord extends entire length of spine	Brain structural configuration roughly complete; cord shows cervical and lumbar enlargements; fourth ventricle foramens developed; suckling present	Cerebral lobes delineated; cerebellum assumes some prominence
SENSORY ORGANS			
Eye and ear appearing as optic vessel and otocyst	Primordial choroid plexuses develop; ventricles large relative to cortex; development progressing; eyes converging rapidly; internal ear developing	Earliest taste buds indicated; characteristic organization of eye attained	General sense organs differentiated
GENITAL SYSTEM			
Genital ridge appears (fifth week)	Testes and ovaries distinguishable; external genitals sexless but begin to differentiate	Sex recognizable; internal and external sex organs specific	Testes in position for descent into scrotum; vagina open

20 Weeks	24 Weeks	28 Weeks	30-31 Weeks	36 Weeks	40 Weeks
Sternum ossifies; fetal movements strong enough for mother to feel		Astragalus (talus, ankle bone) ossifies; weak, fleeting movements, minimum tone	Middle fourth phalanxes ossify; permanent teeth primordia seen; can turn head to side	Distal femoral ossification centers present; sustained, definite movements, fair tone; can turn and elevate head	Active, sustained movement; good tone; may lift head
	Blood formation increases in bone marrow and decreases in liver				
Nostrils reopen; primitive respiratory-like movements begin	Alveolar ducts and sacs present; lecithin begins to appear in amniotic fluid (weeks 26-27)	Lecithin forming on alveolar surfaces	L/S ratio = 1.2:1	L/S ratio $\geq$ 2:1	Pulmonary branching only two thirds complete
				Formation of new nephrons ceases	
Brain grossly formed; cord myelination begins; spinal cord ends at level S-1	Cerebral cortex layered typically; neuronal proliferation in cerebral cortex ends	Appearance of cerebral fissures, convolutions fast appearing; indefinite sleep-wake cycle; cry weak or absent; weak suck reflex		End of spinal cord at level (L-3); definite sleep-wake cycle	Myelination of brain begins; patterned sleep-wake cycle with alert periods; cries when hungry or uncomfortable; strong suck reflex
Nose and ears ossify	Can hear	Eyelids reopen; retinal layers completed, light receptive; pupils capable of reacting to light	Sense of taste present; aware of sounds outside mother's body		
	Testes at inguinal ring in descent to scrotum		Testes descending to scrotum		Testes in scrotum; labia majora well developed

REFERENCES

Barber HRK: Ethics, morals, and gene control, *The Female Patient* 16(10):13, Oct 1991.

Brown MJ, Bellinger D, Matthews J: In utero lead exposure, *MCN* 15(2):94, March/April 1990.

Carothers GP: Down syndrome and maternal age: the effect of erroneous assignment of parental origin, *Am J Hum Genet* 40:147, 1987.

Creasy RK, Resnik JR, editors: *Maternal-fetal medicine: principles and practice,* ed 2, Philadelphia, 1989, WB Saunders.

Cunningham FG, MacDonald PC, Gant NF: *Williams obstetrics,* ed 18, Norwalk, Conn, 1989, Appleton & Lange.

Derom C et al: Increased monozygotic twinning rate after ovulation induction, *Lancet* 1:1237, 1987.

Dickason EJ, Schultz MO, Silverman BL: *Maternal-infant nursing care,* St Louis, 1990, Mosby–Year Book.

Fanaroff AA, Martin RJ, editors: *Neonatal-perinatal medicine: diseases of the fetus and infant,* ed 5, St Louis, 1992, Mosby–Year Book.

MacMullen NJ, Brucker MC: Pregnancy made possible for women with cystic fibrosis, *MCN* 14(3):196, May/June 1989.

Moore KL: *The developing human: clinically oriented embryology,* ed 4, Philadelphia, 1988, WB Saunders.

Nyhan WL: Diagnosing inborn errors of metabolism antenatally, *Contemp Ob/Gyn* 36(11):62, Nov 1991.

Paynton A: Synthetic surfactant: giving premature infants a better chance for survival, *Nursing 91,* 21(3):64, 1991.

Poole RM editor: *The incredible machine,* Washington, DC, 1986, National Geographic Society.

Reed GB, Claireaux AE, Bain AD, editors: *Diseases of the fetus and newborn: pathology, radiology and genetics,* St Louis, 1989, Mosby–Year Book.

Stringer M, Librizzi R, Weiner S: Establishing a prenatal genetic diagnosis: the nurse's role *MCN* 16(3):152, May/June 1991.

Thomson EJ, Cordero JF: The new teratogens: accutane and other vitamin-A analogs, *MCN* 14(4):244, July/Aug 1989.

Whaley LF, Wong DL: *Nursing care of infants and children,* ed 4, St Louis, 1991, Mosby–Year Book.

Willson JR, Carrington ER: *Obstetrics and gynecology,* ed 9, St Louis, 1991, Mosby–Year Book.

BIBLIOGRAPHY

Copper RL et al: Catecholamine secretion in fetal adaptation to stress, *JOGNN* 19(3):223, 1990.

England MA: *Color atlas of life before birth: normal fetal development,* St Louis, 1990, Mosby–Year Book.

Jones KL: *Smith's recognizable patterns of human malformation,* ed 4, Philadelphia, 1988, WB Saunders.

Manning FA: The fetal biophysical profile score: current status, *Obstet Gynecol Clin North Am* 17(1):147, 1990.

Moore KL: *Essentials of human embryology,* Philadelphia, 1988, BC Decker.

Polin RA, Fox WW: *Fetal and neonatal physiology,* vols 1 and 2, Philadelphia, 1991, WB Saunders.

Rayburn WF: Fetal body movement monitoring, *Obstet Gynecol Clin North Am* 17(1):95, 1990.

Rhodes AM: Legal alternatives for fetal injury, *MCN* 15(2):111, 1990.

Sarno Jr AP et al: Fetal acoustic stimulation in the early intrapartum period as a predictor of subsequent fetal condition, *Am J Obstet Gynecol* 162(3):762, 1990.

Shaw KJ et al: Fetal response to external stimuli, *Obstet Gynecol Clin North Am* 17(1):235, 1990.

Sparling JW et al: Developing a taxonomy of fetal movement: the first step in a longitudinal collaborative study, *Phys Occup Ther Pediatr* 10(1):43, 1990.

Twomey Jr JG: The ethics of in utero fetal surgery: a possible threat to the autonomy of pregnant women? *Nurs Clin North Am* 24(4):1025, 1989.

Williams JK: Screening for genetic disorders, *J Pediatr Health Care* 3(3):115, 1989.

Williams SR: *Basic nutrition and diet therapy,* ed 8, St Louis, 1988, Mosby–Year Book.

Bibliography—Nursing Research

Stainton MC: Parents' awareness of their unborn infant in the third trimester, *Birth: Issues in Perinatal Care and Education* 17(2):92, 1990.

TABLE 8-1 Gravidity and Parity Using Five-digit and Two-digit Systems

	Five-digit System					Two-digit System
Condition	Pregnancies	Term birth	Preterm birth	Abortions	Living children	Gravidity/ Parity
Judith is pregnant for the first time.	1	0	0	0	0	I/O
She carries the pregnancy to term, and the neonate survives.	1	1	0	0	1	I/I
She is pregnant again.	2	1	0	0	1	II/I
Her second pregnancy ends in abortion.	2	1	0	1	1	II/I
During her third pregnancy, she delivers preterm twins.	3	1	1	1	3	III/II

Gravidity: Times uterus has been pregnant; *parity:* number of full-term deliveries; *abortions:* spontaneous or elective.

ovulation are thereby suppressed during pregnancy. Menstrual cycles cease. Although the majority of women experience **amenorrhea** (absence of menses), at least 20% have some slight, painless spotting during early gestation for unexplained reasons; implantation bleeding and bleeding following intercourse related to cervical friability may account for some instances. A great majority of these women continue to full term and have normal infants. However, all instances of bleeding should be reported and evaluated.

After implantation, the fertilized ovum and the chorionic villi produce human chorionic gonadotropin (hCG), which maintains the corpus luteum's production of estrogen and progesterone for the first 8 to 10 weeks of pregnancy until the placenta takes over their production (Scott et al, 1990) (for further discussion of hCG, see Chapter 7).

PREGNANCY TESTS. Human chorionic gonadotropin (hCG) is the biologic marker on which pregnancy tests are based. Human chorionic gonadotropin can be measured by radioimmunoassay and detected in the blood as early as 6 days after conception, or about 20 days since the last menstrual period (LMP). Its presence in the urine in early pregnancy is the basis of the various laboratory tests for pregnancy, and it can sometimes be detected in the urine as early as 14 days after conception (Ganong, 1989). Less specific tests may not be accurate until 4 to 10 days after the missed menstrual period or 3 weeks after conception.

A first-voided morning urine specimen contains levels of hCG approximately the same as those in serum, whose levels increase exponentially between days 21 and 70 (counting from the first day of the LMP). Random urine samples usually have lower levels. The ability to recognize the beta subunit of hCG is the newest innovation in the evolution of endocrine tests for pregnancy. The wide variety of tests precludes discussion of each; however, several categories of tests are described here. The nurse should read the manufacturer's directions for the test to be used.

Latex agglutination inhibition (LAI) tests are easy to do and give results in 2 minutes. They are accurate from 4 to 10 days following missed menses. Examples of this type of test include the Gravindex slide, Pregnosticon slide, and UCG Beta slide.

Hemagglutination inhibition (HAI) tests are more sensitive than LAI tests but require 1 to 2 hours to obtain results. Except for one test, Neocept, which gives accurate results at or before missed menses, all HAI tests are accurate about 4 days following missed menses. Also on the market is "e.p.t." (early pregnancy test), an HAI in-home test available for consumer purchase (Doshi, 1986).

The *radioreceptor assay* is a 1-hour serum test that requires fairly sophisticated equipment. Radioreceptor assays are usually accurate at the time of missed menses (14 days after conception) (Brucker, MacMullen, 1985). Biocept G is an example of this type of test.

Radioimmunoassay pregnancy tests for the beta subunit of hCG use radioactively labeled markers, which require the testing to be done in a laboratory. Depending on the degree of sensitivity required, the test time ranges from 1 to 48 hours. Radioimmunoassays are the most sensitive pregnancy tests available today (Brucker, MacMullen, 1985). Pregnancy can be diagnosed 8 days after ovulation or 6 days before missed menses.

Enzyme immunoassays use complex monoclonal

anti-hCG with enzymes.* A visible color change makes the results easy to read. This new test holds promise for the future. Confidot is an immunoenzymatic assay **home pregnancy test.** The manufacturers of Confidot claim that this self-administered test confirms pregnancy approximately 10 days after fertilization, or about 4 days before missed menses.

Enzyme-linked immunosorbent assay (ELISA) testing is the most popular testing procedure for pregnancy (Batzer, 1985; Scott et al, 1990). It uses a specific **monoclonal antibody** produced by hybrid cell-line technology (News, 1985). An enzyme rather than a radioactive compound identifies the antigen of the substance to be measured. The enzyme induces a simple color-change reaction. The endpoint of the test can be read with either the eye or a spectrometer.

ELISA testing has many advantages. The antigen enzyme conjugate and test reagents are stable, the equipment needs are simple, and there are no nuclear waste products. As an office or home procedure it requires minimal time and offers results in 5 minutes coupled with sensitivities from 25 to 50 mIU/mL of hCG in the specimen. ELISA technology is the basis for the new over-the-counter home pregnancy tests. The manufacturer provides directions for collection of specimen (serum, plasma, or urine), care of specimen, testing procedure, and reading of results.

Interpreting the results of pregnancy tests requires some judgment. The type of pregnancy test and its degree of *sensitivity* (ability to detect low levels of a substance) and *specificity* (ability to discern the absence of a substance) are interpreted in conjunction with the woman's history, which includes the date of the last normal menstrual period (LNMP), usual cycle length, and results of previous pregnancy tests. It is important to know if the woman is a substance abuser. Interactions with other drugs can give false results. Improper collection of the specimen, hormone-producing tumors, and laboratory errors may be responsible for false reports (Doshi, 1986). Where there is any question, serial testing may be the answer (Batzer, 1985). Speed and convenience need to be weighed against sensitivity and specificity.

*Read package inserts for a description of "monoclonal anti-hCG with enzymes."

Uterus

The phenomenal uterine growth in the first trimester occurs in response to the hormonal stimulus of high levels of estrogen and progesterone. **Uterine enlargement** results from (1) increased vascularity and dilation of blood vessels, (2) hyperplasia (production of new muscle fibers and fibroelastic tissue) and hypertrophy (enlargement of preexisting muscle fibers and fibroelastic tissue), and (3) development of the decidua (Fig. 8-1). By 7 weeks, the uterus is the size of a large hen's egg; by 10 weeks, the size of an orange (twice its nonpregnant size); by 12 weeks, the size of a grapefruit. Table 8-2 compares uterine measurements for the nonpregnant and pregnant uterus at 40 weeks' gestation. After the third month uterine enlargement is primarily the result of mechanical pressure of the growing fetus (Seidel et al, 1991). In the nonpregnant woman, the uterine cavity holds about 10 mL of fluid; during pregnancy, its ca-

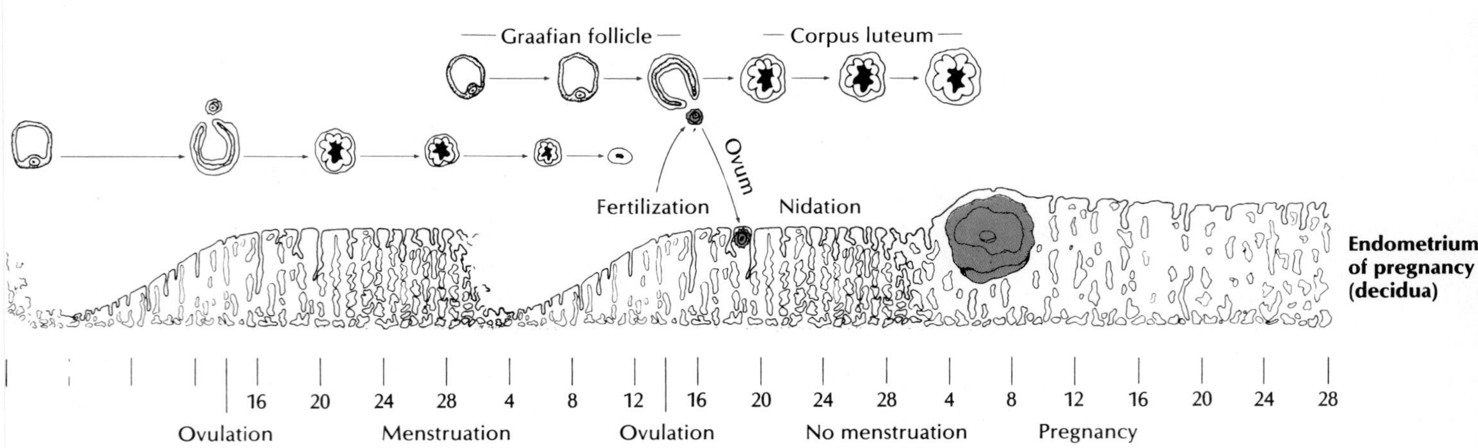

Fig. 8-1 Changes in endometrium and corpus luteum if pregnancy occurs (in days). Nidation refers to implantation.

TABLE 8-2 Comparison of Measurements for Nonpregnant and Pregnant Uterus at 40 Weeks*

Measurement	Nonpregnant	Pregnant (40 Weeks)
Length	6.5 cm (2½ in)	32 cm (12½ in)
Width	4 cm (1½ in)	24 cm (9½ in)
Depth	2.5 cm (1 in)	22 cm (8½ in)
Weight	60-70 g (2½ oz)	1100-1200 g (2½ lb)
Volume	≥10 mL	5000 mL

*Note that references vary as to the exact values, but all references agree on the magnitude of the growth the uterus undergoes during pregnancy.

pacity increases to 5 to 10 L or more (Cunningham, MacDonald, Gant, 1989).

As the uterus increases in size, it also changes in weight, shape, and position. The muscular walls strengthen and become more elastic. At conception the uterus is shaped like an upside-down pear. During the second trimester it is spherical or globular. Later, as the fetus lengthens, the uterus becomes larger and more ovoid, and it rises out of the pelvis into the abdominal cavity.

The pregnancy may "show" after the fourteenth week, although this depends to some degree on the woman's height and weight. Abdominal enlargement may be less apparent in the primigravida with good abdominal muscle tone (Fig. 8-2). Posture also influences the type and degree of abdominal enlargement seen. In normal pregnancies, the uterus enlarges at a predictable rate. This measurement is used to estimate the duration of pregnancy. Uterine enlargement is determined by measuring fundal height. (Measurement of fundal height is described and il-

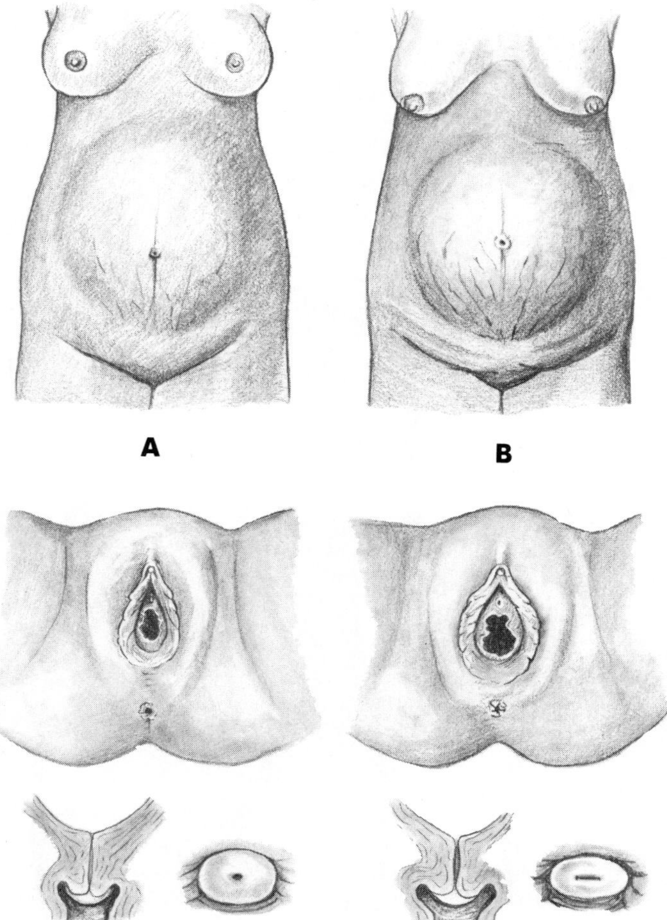

Fig. 8-2 Comparison of abdomen, vulva, and cervix in **A**, nullipara, and **B**, multipara, at the same stage of pregnancy.

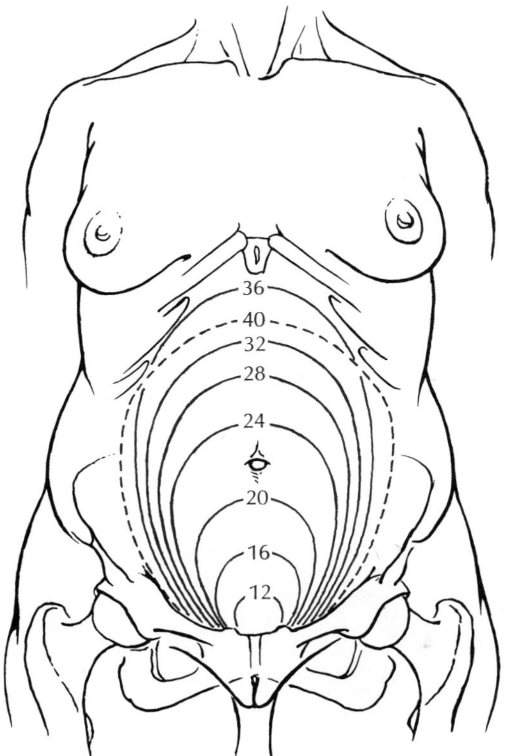

Fig. 8-3 Height of fundus by weeks of normal gestation with a single fetus. Dotted line indicates height after lightening.

From Malasanos L et al: *Health assessment*, ed 4, St Louis, 1990, Mosby–Year Book.

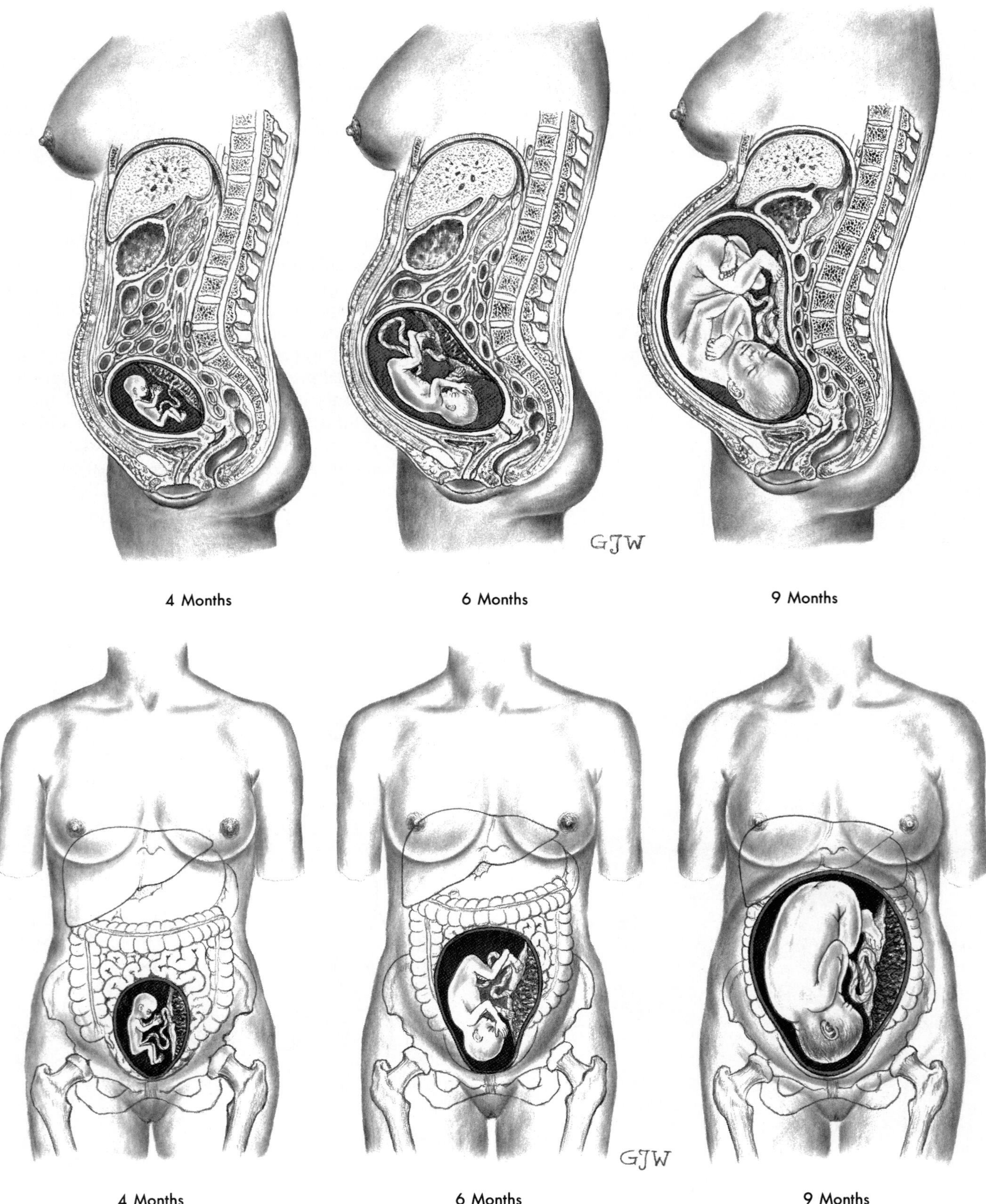

Fig. 8-4 Displacement of internal abdominal structures and diaphragm by the enlarging uterus at 4, 6, and 9 months of gestation.

lustrated in Chapter 12.) Variation in the positions of the fundus or the fetus, variations in the amount of amniotic fluid present, the presence of more than one fetus, and maternal obesity reduce the accuracy of this estimation of the duration of pregnancy.

As the uterus grows it is elevated out of the pelvic area and may be palpated above the symphysis pubis sometime between the twelfth and fourteenth weeks of pregnancy (Fig. 8-3). The uterus rises gradually to the level of the umbilicus at about 22 to 24 weeks and nearly reaches the xiphoid process at term. Between weeks 38 and 40, fundal height drops as the fetus begins to descend and engage in the pelvis (**lightening**) (Fig.8-3, see dotted lines). Generally, lightening occurs in the nullipara about 2 weeks before the onset of labor and at the start of labor in the multipara.

Generally the uterus is rotated to the right as it elevates, probably because of the presence of the rectosigmoid colon on the left side. However, the extensive **hypertrophy** (enlargement) of the round ligaments keeps the uterus in line. Eventually the growing uterus touches the anterior abdominal wall and displaces the intestines to either side of the abdomen (Fig. 8-4). When a pregnant woman stands, the major part of her uterus rests against the anterior abdominal wall and contributes to altering her center of gravity.

During the early weeks of pregnancy an increase in uterine blood flow and lymph causes pelvic congestion and edema. As a result, the uterus, cervix, and isthmus soften perceptibly and progressively, and the cervix takes on a bluish color (**Chadwick's sign**).

At about the seventh to eighth week the following patterns of uterine softening are noted: lower uterine segment (the uterine isthmus) softening and compressibility (**Hegar's sign;** Fig. 8-5), cervical softening (**Goodell's sign**), easy flexion of the fundus on the cervix (**McDonald's sign**), softening and slight fullness of the fundus near the area of implantation (**Braun von Fernwald's sign**), or a soft lateral bulge with cornual implantation (**Piskacek's sign**). After the eighth week, general enlargement and softening of the uterine corpus and cervix are likely.

Some believe that the nonsteroid ovarian hormone relaxin may act along with progesterone (Cunningham, MacDonald, Gant, 1989; Scott et al, 1990). Relaxation occurs not only in the uterus but throughout various parts of the body, such as the joints, walls of blood vessels and gastrointestinal and renal system structures.

Soon after the fourth month of pregnancy, uterine contractions can be felt through the abdominal wall. These contractions are referred to as the **Braxton Hicks sign,** a probable sign of pregnancy (for a discussion of possible, probable, and positive manifestations of pregnancy, see Chapter 11). Braxton Hicks contractions are a continuation of the irregular, painless contractions that occur intermittently throughout each menstrual cycle. The contractions are felt as uterine firmness through the abdominal wall or are evident because they raise and push the uterus forward. Contractions facilitate uterine blood flow through the intervillous spaces of the placenta and thereby promote oxygen delivery to the fetus. Although Braxton Hicks contractions are not ordinarily painful, some women do complain that they are annoying. After the twenty-eighth week, contractions become much more definite, especially in slender women. Generally these contractions cease with walking or exercise. Rarely are they perceived as painful and they do not progress in intensity, duration, and frequency as true labor contractions would. They may become strong enough during the last few weeks to be confused with the contractions of beginning labor.*

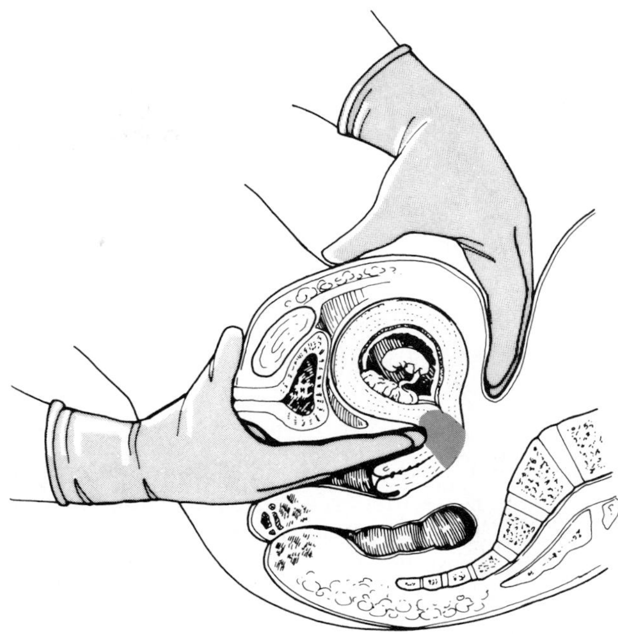

Fig. 8-5 Hegar's sign. Bimanual examination for assessing compressibility, softening of isthmus (lower uterine segment) while the cervix is still firm.

*Some authors warn that any contractions should be taken seriously. This reflects concern that preterm labor contractions may be confused with "normal" Braxton Hicks contractions, thereby missing the opportunity for early diagnosis with the possibility of suppressing preterm labor.

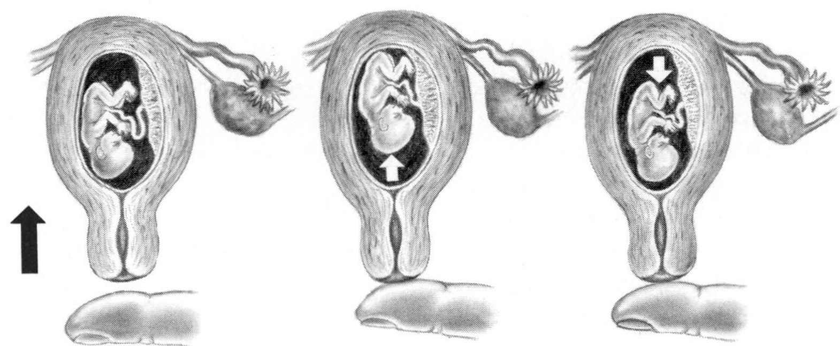

Fig. 8-6 Internal ballottement (18 weeks).

Blood flow increases rapidly as the uterus increases in size. Although uterine blood flow increases twentyfold, the size of the conceptus grows more rapidly. Consequently, more oxygen is extracted from the uterine blood during the latter part of pregnancy (Ganong, 1989). In a normal term pregnancy, one sixth of the total maternal blood volume is within the uterine vascular system. The rate of blood flow through the uterus averages 500 mL/min, and oxygen consumption of the gravid uterus averages 25 mL/min. Maternal arterial pressure, contractions of the uterus, and maternal position are three factors known to influence blood flow (see p. 199). Estrogens also play a role in uterine blood flow.

Using an ultrasound device or a fetal stethoscope, the physician or nurse may hear (1) the **uterine souffle,** or bruit, a rushing or blowing sound of maternal blood flowing through uterine arteries to the placenta that is synchronous with the maternal pulse, (2) the **funic souffle,** which is synchronous with the fetal heart rate and caused by fetal blood coursing through the umbilical cord, and (3) the **fetal heart rate** *(FHR).* For further discussion, see Chapter 16.

Passive movement of the unengaged fetus is called **ballottement.** Ballottement can be identified generally between the sixteenth and eighteenth week. Ballottement is a technique of palpating a floating structure by bouncing it gently and feeling it rebound. The examiner's finger within the vagina taps gently upward; the fetus rises. Then the fetus sinks, and a gentle tap is felt on the finger (Fig. 8-6). Internal ballottement of a fetus within a uterus is a probable objective sign of pregnancy.

The first recognition of fetal movements, or "feeling life," by the multiparous woman may occur as early as the fourteenth to sixteenth week. The nulliparous woman may not notice these sensations until the eighteenth week or later. **Quickening** is commonly described as a flutter and is difficult to distinguish from peristalsis. Gradually, fetal movements increase in intensity and frequency. Noting the week in which quickening occurs provides a tentative clue in dating the duration of gestation.

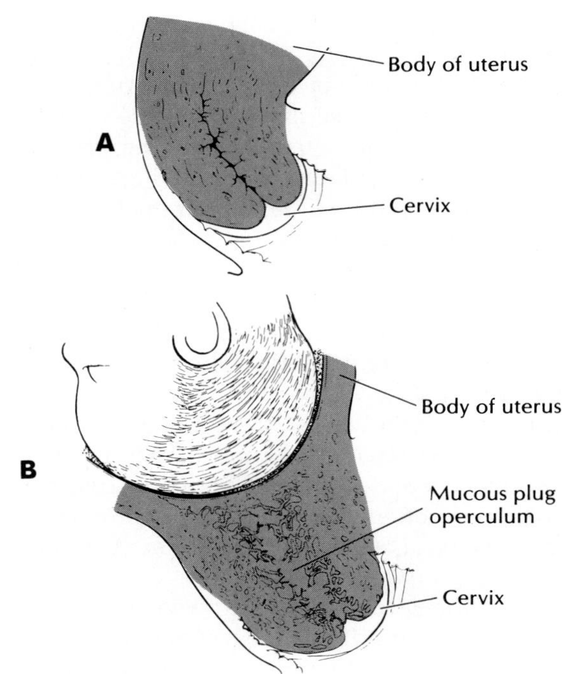

Fig. 8-7 **A,** Cervix in nonpregnant woman. **B,** Changes in cervix during pregnancy.

A softening of the cervical tip may be observed about the beginning of the sixth week in a normal, unscarred cervix. The softening of the cervix during pregnancy (Goodell's sign) is brought about by increased vascularity, slight hypertrophy, and **hyperplasia** (increase in number of cells) of the muscle and its collagen-rich connective tissue, which becomes loose, edematous, highly elastic, and increased in volume. The glands near the external os proliferate beneath the stratified squamous epithelium, giving the cervix the velvety consistency characteristic of pregnancy. The changes in the cervix as well as those of the vagina help prepare the birth canal for the fetus' passage through it (Fig. 8-7). **Friability** is increased; that is, the cervix bleeds easily when scraped or touched. Increased friability is the cause of the few drops of blood seen after coitus with deep penetration or vaginal examination. These few drops are usually within normal limits.

The cervix of the nullipara is rounded. Lacerations of the cervix almost always occur during the birth process. With or without lacerations, following childbirth the cervix becomes more oval in the horizontal plane, and the external os appears as a transverse slit (see Fig. 8-2).

Vagina and Vulva

Pregnancy hormones prepare the vagina for distention during labor by producing a thickened vaginal mucosa, loosened connective tissue, hypertrophied smooth muscle, and an increase in the length of the vaginal vault. Increased vascularity results in a violet-bluish color of the vaginal mucosa and cervix. The deepened color, termed *Chadwick's sign* or *Jacquemier's sign,* may be evident as early as the sixth week, but is easily noted at the eighth week of pregnancy. Desquamation (shedding of cells, or exfoliation) of the vaginal, glycogen-rich cells occurs under estrogen stimulation. The cells that are shed contribute to the thick, whitish vaginal discharge, leukorrhea.

Leukorrhea is a white or slightly gray mucoid discharge with a faint musty odor. Increased estrogen and progesterone stimulation of the cervix produces copious mucoid fluid. The fluid is whitish because of the presence of many exfoliated vaginal epithelial cells caused by normal pregnancy hyperplasia. This vaginal discharge is never pruritic or blood stained. Because of the progesterone effect, **ferning** (see Fig. 6-23, *A*) does *not* occur in the dried cervical mucous smear. The mucus fills the endocervical canal, resulting in the formation of the mucous plug (**operculum**) (Fig. 8-7). The operculum acts as a barrier against bacterial invasion during pregnancy.

During pregnancy, the pH of vaginal secretions becomes less acidic. The pH changes from about 4 to 5 to about 5.5 to 6.5. *The rise in pH makes the pregnant woman more vulnerable to vaginal infections,* especially yeast infections.

The increased vascularity of the vagina and other pelvic viscera results in a marked increase in sensitivity. The *increased sensitivity may lead to a high degree of sexual interest and arousal,* especially during the second trimester of pregnancy. The increased congestion plus the relaxed walls of the blood vessels and the heavy uterus may result in edema and varicosities of the vulva. The edema and varicosities usually resolve during the postpartum period.

External structures of the *perineum* are enlarged during pregnancy because of an increase in vasculature, hypertrophy of the perineal body, and deposition of fat (Fig. 8-8). The labia majora of the nullipara approximate and obscure the vaginal introitus; those of the parous woman separate and gape after childbirth and perineal or vaginal injury. Torn resid-

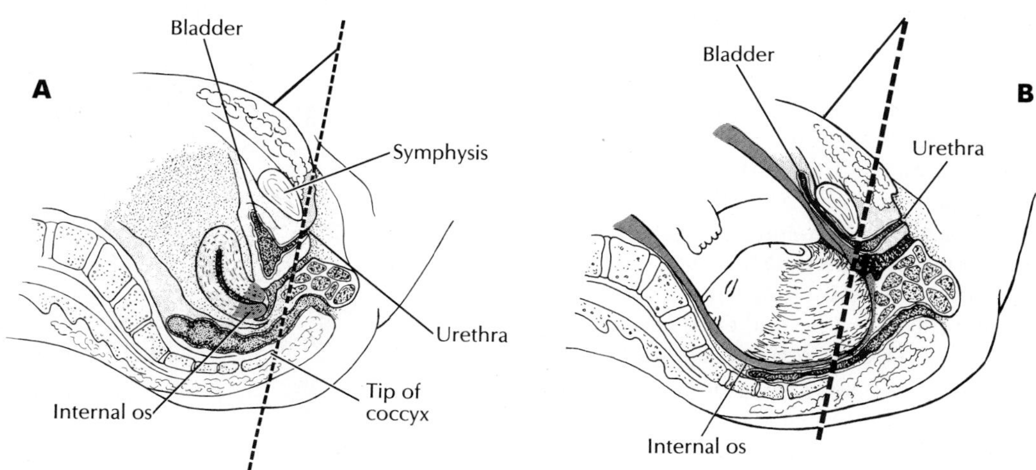

Fig. 8-8 A, Pelvic floor in nonpregnant woman. B, Pelvic floor at end of pregnancy. Note marked hypertrophy and hyperplasia below dotted line joining tip of coccyx and inferior margin of symphysis. Note elongation of bladder and urethra as a result of compression. Fat deposits are increased.

ual tags of the hymen remain after tampon use, coitus, and vaginal delivery. Fig. 8-2 compares the perineum of the nullipara and the multipara.

Breasts

Fullness, heightened sensitivity, tingling, and heaviness of the breasts begin as early as the sixth week of gestation as a result of increased levels of estrogen and progesterone. Breast sensitivity varies from mild tingling to frank pain (mastodynia). Nipples and areolae become more pigmented, secondary pinkish areolae develop, extending beyond the primary areolae, and nipples become more erectile. Hypertrophy of the sebaceous (oil) glands embedded in the primary areolae, called **Montgomery's tubercles** (see Fig. 6-18, *B*), may be seen around the nipples. These sebaceous glands may have a protective role in that they keep the nipples lubricated. Suppleness of the nipples is jeopardized if the protective oils are washed off with soap.

The richer blood supply dilates the vessels beneath the skin. Once barely noticeable, the blood vessels now become visible, often appearing in an intertwining blue network beneath the surface of the skin. Venous congestion in the breasts is more obvious in primigravidas. Striae gravidarum may appear at the outer aspects of the breasts.

During the second and third trimesters, growth of the mammary glands accounts for the progressive increase in breast size. The high levels of luteal and placental hormones in pregnancy promote proliferation of the lactiferous ducts and lobule-alveolar tissue, so that palpation of the breasts reveals a generalized, coarse nodularity. The increase in glandular tissue displaces connective tissue, and as a result the tissue becomes softer and looser. Overstretching of the fibrous, suspensory Cooper's ligaments (Fig. 6-18, *A*) supporting the breasts may be reduced with a well-fitted maternity brassiere.

Although development of the mammary glands is functionally complete by midpregnancy, lactation is inhibited until a drop in estrogen level occurs after delivery of the fetus and placenta. A thin, clear, viscous precolostrum secretion, however, may be expressed from the nipples by the end of the sixth week (Seidel et al, 1991).* This secretion thickens as term approaches and is then known as **colostrum.** Colostrum, the creamy, white-to-yellowish premilk fluid, may be expressed from the nipples during the third trimester. See discussion of pituitary prolactin in this chapter.

*References differ as to the gestational week during which precolostrum can be expressed. Some references cite week 16 as the earliest time at which fluid may be expressed from the breasts.

■ GENERAL BODY SYSTEMS

Cardiovascular System

Maternal adjustments to pregnancy involve extensive changes in the cardiovascular system, both anatomic and physiologic. Cardiovascular adaptations protect the woman's normal physiologic functioning, meet the metabolic demands pregnancy imposes on her body, and provide for fetal developmental and growth needs.

Slight cardiac hypertrophy (enlargement) or dilation is probably secondary to increased blood volume and cardiac output. This enlargement is reversed after childbirth. As the diaphragm is displaced upward, the heart is elevated upward and rotated forward to the left (Fig. 8-9). The apical impulse (PMI) is shifted upward and laterally about 1 to 1.5 cm (½ inch). The degree of shift depends on the duration of pregnancy and the size and position of the uterus.

Auscultatory changes accompany the changes in heart size and position. Increases in blood volume

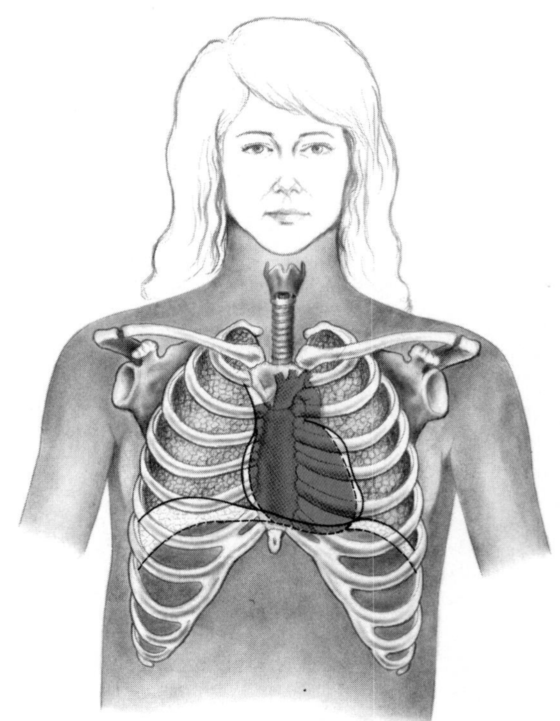

Fig. 8-9 Changes in position of heart, lungs, and thoracic cage in pregnancy. *Broken line,* Nonpregnant; *solid line,* change that occurs in pregnancy.

and cardiac output also contribute to auscultatory changes common in pregnancy. There is more audible splitting of S_1 and S_2, and S_3 may be readily heard after 20 weeks of gestation. Additionally, grade II systolic ejection murmurs may be heard over the pulmonic area.

Between 14 and 20 weeks, the *pulse* increases slowly up to 10 to 15 beats per minute, which then persists to term. Palpitations may occur.

The cardiac rhythm may be disturbed. The pregnant woman may experience sinus arrhythmia, premature atrial contractions, and premature ventricular systole. In the healthy woman with no underlying heart disease, no therapy is needed.

BLOOD PRESSURE. *Arterial blood pressure* (brachial artery) varies with age, activity level, and presence of health problems. Additional factors must be considered. These factors include maternal position, maternal anxiety, and size of cuff. *Maternal position* affects readings. Brachial blood pressure is highest when the woman is sitting, lowest when she is lying in the left lateral recumbent position, and intermediate when she is supine. Therefore the same maternal position and the same arm are used at each visit. The position and arm used are noted along with the reading.

Maternal anxiety can elevate readings. If an elevated reading is found, the woman is given time to rest, and the reading is repeated.

The *proper size cuff* is absolutely necessary for accurate readings. The cuff should be 20% wider than the diameter of the arm around which it is wrapped: about 12 to 14 cm (about 6 in) for average-sized individuals and 18 to 20 cm (about 8 in) for obese persons. Too small a cuff yields a false high reading; too large a cuff yields a false low reading.

During the second trimester of pregnancy, there is a decrease in both systolic and diastolic pressure of 5 to 10 mm Hg. The decrease in blood pressure is probably the result of peripheral vasodilation from hormonal changes during pregnancy. During the third trimester, maternal blood pressure should return to the values obtained during the first trimester (for a discussion of hypertensive states in pregnancy, see Chapter 28).

The **mean arterial pressure (MAP)** increases the diagnostic value of the findings. The MAP is estimated by adding one third of the *pulse pressure* to the diastolic pressure. Pulse pressure is the difference between the systolic and diastolic values.

Example

Blood pressure: 106/70
Pulse pressure (106 − 70): 36 ÷ 3 = 12
MAP: (diastolic) 70 + 12 = 82

Some degree of compression of the vena cava occurs in all women who lie on their back during the second half of pregnancy (see Fig. 27-10). Some women experience a fall of ≥30 mm Hg systolic. After 4 to 5 minutes a reflex bradycardia is noted, cardiac output is reduced by half, and the woman feels faint (see *hypotensive syndrome,* Chapter 11).

Other women will show an increase in blood pressure in the supine position (see **roll-over** or **supine pressor test,** Chapter 13) (Cunningham et al, 1989).

Compression of the iliac veins and inferior vena cava by the uterus causes increased venous pressure and reduced blood flow in the legs (except when the woman is in the left lateral position). These alterations contribute to the dependent edema, varicose veins in the legs and vulva, and hemorrhoids experienced by women in the latter part of term pregnancy.

BLOOD VOLUME AND COMPOSITION. The degree of blood volume expansion varies considerably (Cunningham, MacDonald, Gant, 1989). Blood volume increases by approximately 1500 mL* (normal value: 8.5% to 9% of body weight). The increase is composed of 1000 mL *plasma* plus 450 mL *red blood cells* (RBCs) (Fig. 8-10). The increase in volume starts about the tenth to twelfth week, peaks at about 25% to 45% above the nonpregnant levels at the thirty-second to thirty-fourth week, then decreases slightly at the fortieth week. The increased volume is a protective mechanism. It is essential for (1) the hypertrophied vascular system of the enlarged uterus, (2) adequate hydration of fetal and maternal tissues when the woman assumes an erect or supine position, and (3) fluid reserve for blood loss during the delivery and puerperium. Peripheral vasodilation maintains a normal blood pressure despite the increased blood volume in pregnancy.

During pregnancy there is an accelerated production of RBCs (normal 4 to 5.5 million/mm^3). The percentage of increase depends on the amount of iron available. The RBC mass increases by 30% to 33% by term if an iron supplement is taken. It increases by only 17% in some women if no supplement is taken. For the discussion of iron therapy, see Chapter 9.

Despite an increase in RBC production, there is an apparent decrease in normal *hemoglobin* values (12 to 16 g/dL blood) and *hematocrit* values (37% to 47%). This condition is referred to as **physiologic anemia.** The decrease is more noticeable during the second trimester, when rapid expansion of blood volume takes place faster than red blood cell production. If the hemoglobin value drops to 10 g/dL or less or if

*Expansion of blood volume: primigravidas, 1250 mL; multigravidas, 1500 mL; twin pregnancies, 2000 mL.

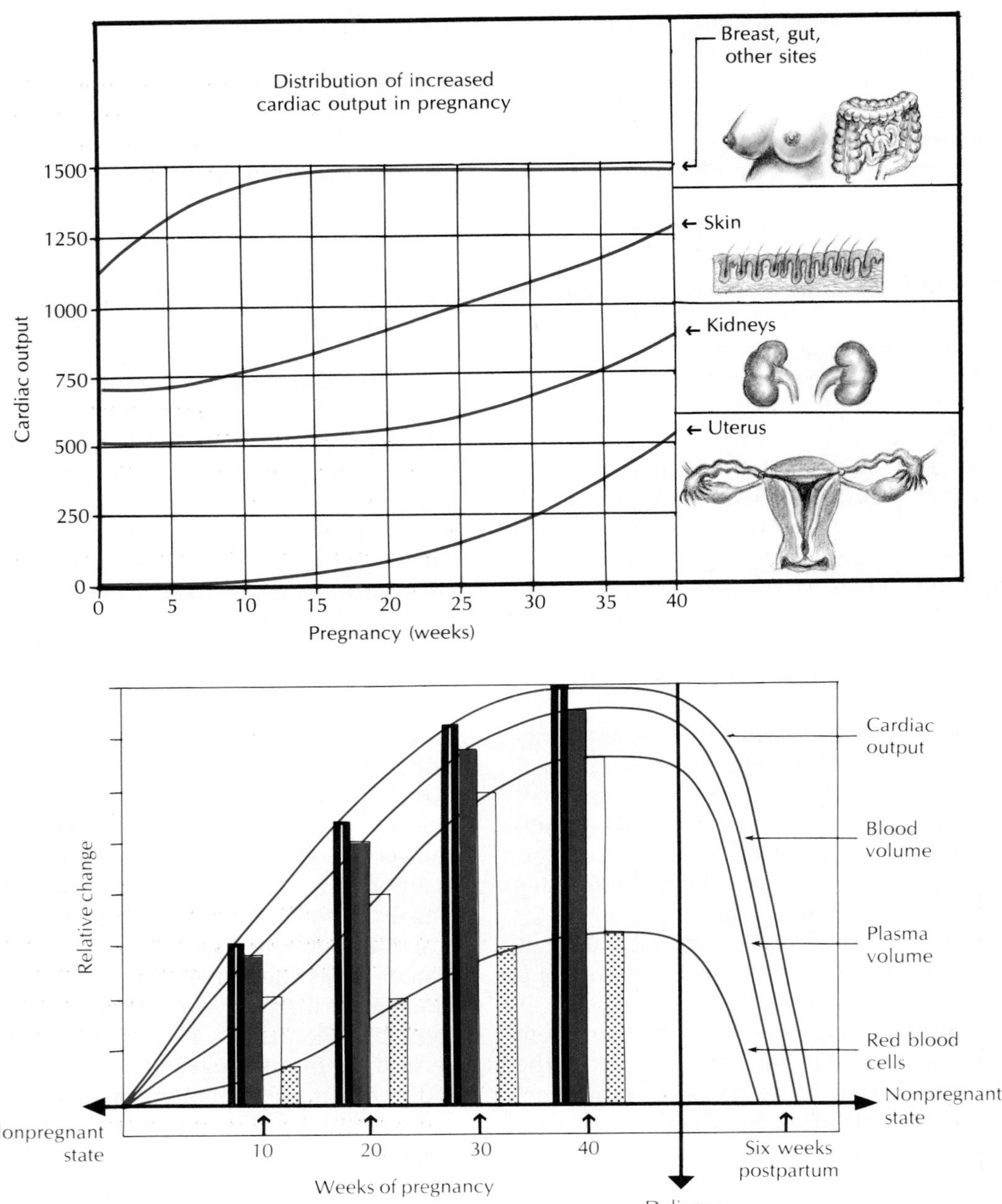

Fig. 8-10 Distribution of increased cardiac output in pregnancy.

the hematocrit drops to 35% or less, the woman is considered anemic (for further discussion of anemia, see Chapter 32).

The total *white cell count* increases during the second trimester and peaks during the third trimester. This increase is primarily in the granulocytes; the lymphocyte count stays about the same throughout pregnancy. See Appendix D for laboratory values during pregnancy.

CARDIAC OUTPUT. Cardiac output increases from 30% to 50% by the thirty-second week of pregnancy; it declines to about a 20% increase at 40 weeks. The elevated cardiac output is largely a result of increased stroke volume and in response to increased tissue demands for oxygen (normal value is 5 to 5.5 L/min) (Fig. 8-10). Cardiac output in late pregnancy is appreciably higher when the woman is in the lateral recumbent position than when she is supine. In the supine position, the large, heavy uterus often impedes venous return to the heart and affects blood pressure (see discussion of blood pressure on p. 199). Cardiac output increases with any exertion, such as labor and delivery.

CIRCULATION AND COAGULATION TIMES. The circulation time decreases slightly by week 32. It returns to near normal near term.

There is a greater tendency for blood to coagulate (clot) during pregnancy because of increases in various clotting factors. Fibrinolytic activity (the splitting up or the dissolving of a clot) is depressed during pregnancy and the postpartum period, making the woman more vulnerable to thrombosis. During the postpartum period, fibrinolytic activity is depressed, and the woman is again more vulnerable to thrombosis.

Respiratory System

Structural and ventilatory adaptations occur during pregnancy to provide for both maternal and fetal needs. Maternal oxygen requirements increase in response to the acceleration in metabolic rate and the need to add to the tissue mass in the uterus and breasts. The fetus requires oxygen and a way to eliminate carbon dioxide.

Elevated levels of estrogen cause the ligaments of the rib cage to relax, permitting increased chest expansion (see Fig. 8-9). The transverse diameter of the thoracic cage increases by about 2 cm (¾ inch), and the circumference increases by 5 to 7 cm (2 to 2¾ inches) (Cunningham, MacDonald, Gant, 1989). The costal angle of approximately 68 degrees before pregnancy increases to about 103 degrees in the third trimester. The lower rib cage appears to flare out. The chest may not return to its prepregnant state after pregnancy (Seidel et al, 1987).

The level of the diaphragm is displaced by as much as 4 cm (1½ inches) during pregnancy. With advancing pregnancy, thoracic breathing replaces abdominal breathing, and descent of the diaphragm with inspiration becomes less possible. Thoracic breathing is primarily accomplished by the diaphragm rather than by the costal muscles (Blackburn, Loper, 1992). At this stage of pregnancy, women complain of being short of breath. They may need to sleep on a number of pillows in order to be comfortable (for a discussion of cardiovascular and respiratory disorders, see Chapter 32).

Increased vascularization in response to elevated levels of estrogen also occurs in the upper respiratory tract. As the capillaries become engorged, edema and hyperemia develop within the nose, pharynx, larynx, trachea, and bronchi. This congestion within the tissues of the respiratory tract gives rise to several conditions commonly seen during pregnancy. These conditions include nasal and sinus stuffiness, epistaxis (nosebleed), changes in the voice, and marked inflammatory response to even a mild upper respiratory infection.

Increased vascularity also swells tympanic membranes and eustachian tubes, giving rise to symptoms of impaired hearing, earaches, or a sense of fullness in the ears.

PULMONARY FUNCTION CHANGES. The pregnant woman breathes deeper (increases *tidal volume*, the volume of gas moved into or out of the respiratory tract with each breath) but increases her respiratory rate only slightly (about two breaths per minute). The increase in respiratory tidal volume associated with the normal respiratory rate results in an increase in respiratory minute volume by approximately 26%. The increase in the respiratory minute volume is the *hyperventilation of pregnancy*, which is responsible for a decreased concentration of carbon dioxide in alveoli. The hyperventilation of pregnancy is apparently caused by the increased levels of progesterone, since it has been mimicked in males given progesterone (Scott et al, 1990).

During pregnancy, changes in the respiratory center result in a lowered threshold for carbon dioxide. Progesterone and estrogen are presumed to be responsible for the increased sensitivity of the respiratory center to carbon dioxide. In addition, pregnant women experience increased awareness of the need to breathe; some may complain of dyspnea at rest.

Although pulmonary function is not impaired by pregnancy, diseases of the respiratory tract may be more serious during gestation (Cunningham, MacDonald, Gant, 1989). One important factor may be the increased oxygen requirements.

BASAL METABOLISM RATE. The basal metabolism rate (BMR) usually rises by the fourth month of gestation. It is increased by 15% to 20% by term. The BMR returns to nonpregnant levels by 5 to 6 days postpartum. The elevation in BMR reflects increased oxygen demands of the uterine-placental-fetal unit as well as oxygen consumption from increased maternal cardiac work. Peripheral vasodilation and acceleration of sweat-gland activity assist in dissipating the excess heat resulting from the increased metabolism during pregnancy. Pregnant women may experience heat intolerance, which is annoying to some women. **Lassitude** and **fatigability** after only slight exertion are described by many women in early pregnancy. These feelings may persist, along with a greater need for sleep. Lassitude and fatigability may be caused in part by the increased metabolic activity (see discussion of thyroid gland later in this chapter).

ACID-BASE BALANCE. By about the tenth week of pregnancy, there is a decrease of about 5 mm Hg in P_{CO_2}. Progesterone may be responsible for increasing the sensitivity of the respiratory center receptors so that tidal volume is increased and P_{CO_2} falls, the base excess (HCO_3, or bicarbonate) falls, and pH rises (becomes more basic). These alterations in acid-base balance indicate that *pregnancy is a state of respiratory alkalosis* compensated by mild metabolic acidosis.

Renal System

The kidneys are vital excretory organs. Their purpose is to maintain the body's internal environment in the relatively constant homeostatic state necessary for the efficient functioning of the body at the cellular level. The kidneys are responsible for maintaining electrolyte and acid-base balance, regulating extracellular fluid volume, excreting waste products, and conserving essential nutrients.

ANATOMIC CHANGES. Changes in renal structure result from hormonal activity (estrogen and progesterone), pressure from an enlarging uterus, and an increase in blood volume. As early as the tenth week of pregnancy, the renal pelvis and the ureters dilate. Dilation of the ureters is more pronounced above the pelvic brim, in part because they are compressed between the uterus and the pelvic brim. Dilation above the pelvic brim is more marked on the right side (see discussion of uterine position, Chapter 6). In most women the ureters below the pelvic brim are of normal size. The smooth-muscle walls of the ureters undergo hyperplasia and hypertrophy and relaxed muscle tone. The ureters elongate, become tortuous, and form single or double curves. In the latter part of pregnancy, the right renal pelvis and ureter dilate more than on the left as a result of the displacement of the heavy uterus to the right by the sigmoid colon.

Because of these changes, a larger volume of urine is held in the pelves and ureters, and urine flow rate is slowed. Urinary stasis or stagnation has several consequences:

1. There is a lag between the time urine is formed and when it reaches the bladder. Therefore clearance test results may reflect substances contained in glomerular filtrate several hours before.
2. Stagnated urine is an excellent medium for the growth of microorganisms. In addition, the urine of pregnant women contains greater amounts of nutrients, including glucose, increasing the pH (making the urine more alkaline). Therefore, during pregnancy, women are more susceptible to urinary tract infection.

Bladder irritability, nocturia, and **urinary frequency** and **urgency** (without dysuria) commonly are reported in early pregnancy. Near term, bladder symptoms may return especially after lightening occurs.

Urinary frequency results from increased bladder sensitivity and later from compression of the bladder (see Fig. 8-8). In the second trimester the bladder is pulled up out of the true pelvis into the abdomen. The urethra lengthens to 7.5 cm (3 inches) as the bladder is displaced upward. The pelvic congestion of pregnancy is reflected in hyperemia of the bladder and urethra. This increased vascularity causes the bladder mucosa to be traumatized and bleed easily. There may be a decrease in bladder tone, which permits distention of the bladder to approximately 1500 mL. At the same time the bladder is compressed by the enlarging uterus, resulting in the urge to void even if the bladder contains only a small amount of urine.

RENAL FUNCTION CHANGES. In normal pregnancy, renal function is altered considerably. Glomerular filtration rate (GFR) and renal plasma flow (RPF) increase early in pregnancy (Cunningham, MacDonald, Gant, 1989). The woman's kidneys must manage the increased metabolic and circulatory demands of the maternal body and also excretion of fetal waste products. Changes in renal function are caused by pregnancy hormones, an increase in blood volume, the woman's posture, physical activity, and nutritional intake.

Renal function is most efficient when the woman

lies in the left lateral recumbent position and least efficient when the woman assumes a supine position. A side-lying position increases renal perfusion, which increases urinary output and decreases edema. When the pregnant woman is lying supine, the heavy uterus compresses the vena cava and the aorta, and cardiac output decreases. The result is a drop in maternal blood pressure and fetal heart rate (vena cava or *hypotensive syndrome*) and a drop in the volume of blood to the kidneys (see Fig. 8-10). When cardiac output drops, blood flow to the brain and heart is continued at the expense of other organs, including the kidneys and uterus.

FLUID AND ELECTROLYTE BALANCE. Selective renal tubular reabsorption maintains sodium and water balance regardless of changes in dietary intake and losses through sweat, vomitus, or diarrhea. From 500 to 900 mEq of sodium is normally retained during pregnancy to meet fetal needs. The need for increased maternal intravascular and extracellular fluid volume requires additional sodium to expand fluid volume and to maintain an isotonic state. To prevent excessive sodium depletion, the maternal kidneys undergo a significant adaptation by increasing tubular reabsorption. As efficient as the renal system is, it can be overstressed by excessive dietary sodium intake or restriction or by using diuretics. *Severe hypovolemia and reduced placental perfusion are two consequences of using diuretics during pregnancy.*

The capacity of the kidneys to excrete water during the early weeks of pregnancy is more efficient than later in pregnancy. Occasionally in early pregnancy the extent of water loss may cause some women to feel thirsty. The pooling of fluid in the legs in the latter part of pregnancy decreases renal blood flow and GFR. The diuretic response to the water load is triggered when the woman lies down, preferably on her left side, and the pooled fluid reenters general circulation. This pooling of blood in the lower legs is sometimes referred to as **physiologic edema,** which requires no treatment.

Normally the kidney reabsorbs almost all of the glucose and other nutrients from the plasma filtrate. In pregnant women tubular reabsorption of glucose is impaired so that *glucosuria* does occur at varying times and to varying degrees. Normal values are 0 to 20 mg/dL. That is, during any one day the urine is sometimes positive and sometimes negative. When it is positive, the amount of glucose varies from 1+ to 4+.

In nonpregnant women, blood glucose levels must be at 160 to 180 mg/dL before glucose is "spilled" into the urine (not reabsorbed). During pregnancy, glucosuria occurs when maternal glucose levels are lower than 160 mg/dL. Why glucose, as well as other nutrients such as amino acids, is wasted during pregnancy is not understood, nor has the exact mechanism been discovered. Although glucosuria may be found in normal pregnancies (indeed 1+ levels may be seen with increased anxiety states), the possibility of diabetes mellitus and gestational diabetes must be kept in mind (Chapter 31).

Proteinuria occurs more frequently during pregnancy (Blackburn, Loper, 1992). The increased amount of amino acids that needs to be filtered may exceed the capacity of the renal tubules to absorb them so that small amounts of protein are lost in the urine. Values of 1+ protein (dipstick assessment) are common; these values do not necessarily mean that there is a renal pathologic condition or pregnancy-induced hypertension (PIH) (see Chapter 28). During pregnancy, proteinuria is not considered abnormal until values exceed 300 mg/24 hr (Blackburn, Loper, 1992). The amount of protein excreted is not an indication of the severity of renal disease, nor does an increase in protein excretion in a pregnant woman with known renal disease necessarily indicate a progression in her disease. However, a pregnant woman with hypertension and proteinuria must be carefully evaluated, since she may be at greater risk for an adverse pregnancy outcome (for further discussion, see Chapter 28).

Integumentary System

Alterations in hormonal balance and mechanical stretching are responsible for several changes in the integumentary system during pregnancy. General changes include increases in skin thickness and subdermal fat, hyperpigmentation, hair and nail growth, accelerated sweat and sebaceous gland activity, and increased circulation and vasomotor activity. There is greater fragility of cutaneous elastic tissues, resulting in striae gravidarum, or stretch marks. Cutaneous allergic responses are enhanced.

Pigmentation is caused by the anterior pituitary hormone melanotropin, which is increased during pregnancy (Chapter 12). Facial melasma, also called **chloasma** or **mask of pregnancy,** is a blotchy, brownish hyperpigmentation of the skin over the malar prominences (cheeks), nose, and the forehead, especially in dark complexioned expectant women. Chloasma appears in 50% to 70% of pregnant women, beginning after the sixteenth week and increasing gradually to delivery. The sun intensifies this pigmentation in susceptible women. Chloasma caused by normal pregnancy usually fades after delivery. Darkening of the nipples, areolae, axillae, and vulva occurs at about the same time.

The **linea nigra** is a pigmented line extending from the symphysis pubis to the top of the fundus in

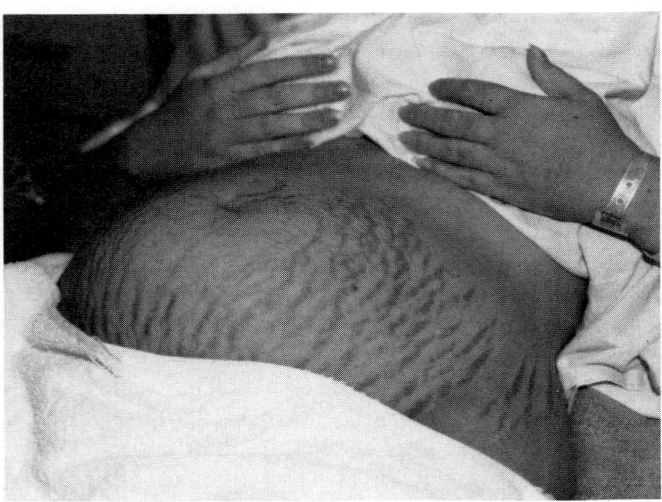

Fig. 8-11 Striae gravidarum, or "stretch marks."

the midline; this line is known as the linea alba before hormone-induced pigmentation. In primigravidas the extension of the linea nigra, beginning in the third month, keeps pace with the rising height of the fundus; in multigravidas the entire line often appears earlier than the third month.

Striae gravidarum, or stretch marks (seen over lower abdomen in Fig. 8-11), which appear in 50% to 90% of pregnant women during the second half of pregnancy, may be caused by action of adrenocorticosteroids. Striae reflect separation within the underlying connective (collagen) tissue of the skin. These slightly depressed streaks tend to occur over areas of maximum stretch (i.e., abdomen, thighs, and breasts). The stretching sometimes causes a sensation that resembles itching. Tendency to the development of striae may be familial. After delivery they usually fade, although they never disappear completely. Color of striae varies depending on the pregnant woman's skin color. The striae appear pinkish on a woman with light skin, and they appear lighter than surrounding skin in dark-skinned women. In the multipara, in addition to the striae of the present pregnancy, glistening silvery lines (in light-skinned women) or purplish lines (in dark-skinned women) are commonly seen. These represent the scars of striae from previous pregnancies.

Angiomas or **telangiectasias** are commonly referred to as **vascular spiders.** They are tiny, star-shaped or branched, slightly raised and pulsating end-arterioles. The spiders, a result of elevated levels of circulating estrogen, are usually found on the neck, thorax, face, and arms. They are also described as focal networks of dilated arterioles radiating about a central core. The spiders are bluish in color and do not blanch with pressure. Striae may be evident on the breasts as a result of stretching as they increase in size. Vascular spiders appear during the second to the fifth month of pregnancy in 65% of Caucasian women and 10% of African-American women. The spiders usually disappear after delivery.

Pinkish-red, diffuse mottling or well-defined blotches are seen over the palmar surfaces of the hands in about 60% of Caucasian women and 35% of African-American women during pregnancy (Cunningham, MacDonald, Gant, 1989). These color changes and **palmar erythema** are related primarily to increased peripheral circulation.

Epulis (gingival granuloma gravidarum) is a red, raised nodule on the gums that bleeds easily. This lesion may develop around the third month and usually continues to enlarge as pregnancy progresses. Treatment by excision is initiated only if it becomes too large, causes pain, or bleeds excessively.

By the sixth week some women notice *thinning and softening of the fingernails and toenails*. Nail polish and nail polish remover may need to be discontinued and the nails kept short to prevent breakage. Oily skin and *acne vulgaris* may occur during pregnancy. For other women the skin clears and looks radiant. *Hirsutism* the excessive growth of hair or growth of hair in unusual places, is commonly reported. An increase in fine hair growth may occur. The fine hair tends to disappear after pregnancy. Growth of coarse or bristly hair does not usually disappear after pregnancy. Some women comment that their hair is thickest and most abundant during pregnancy.

Musculoskeletal System

The gradually changing body and increasing weight of the pregnant woman cause marked alterations in posture (Fig. 8-12) and walking. The great abdominal distention that gives the pelvis a forward tilt, decreased abdominal muscle tone, and increased weight bearing in late pregnancy require a realignment of the spinal curvatures. The woman's center of gravity shifts forward. An increase in the normal lumbosacral curve (lordosis) develops, and a compensatory curvature in the cervicodorsal region (exaggerated anterior flexion of the head) is required to maintain balance. Aching, numbness, and weakness of the upper extremities may result. Large breasts and a stoop-shouldered stance will further accentuate the lumbar and dorsal curves. Walking is more difficult, and the waddling gait of the pregnant woman, called "the proud walk of pregnancy" by Shakespeare, is well known. The ligamentous and muscular structures of the middle and lower spine may be severely

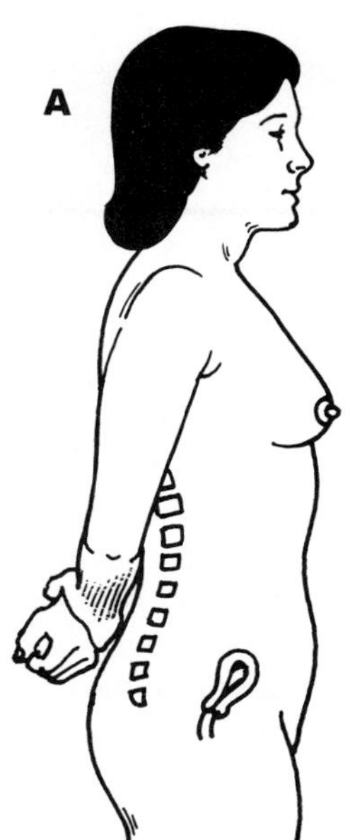

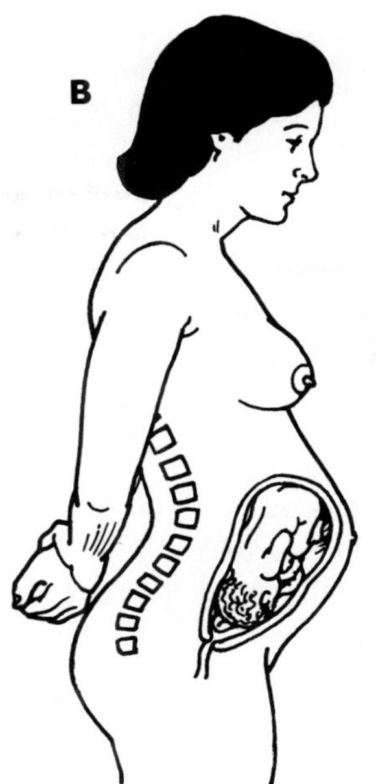

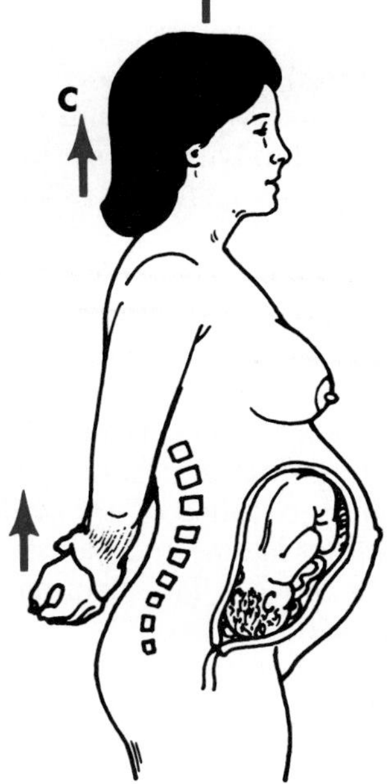

Fig. 8-12 Postural changes during pregnancy. **A,** Nonpregnant. **B,** Incorrect posture. **C,** Correct posture.

stressed. These and related changes often cause musculoskeletal discomfort.

The young, well-muscled woman may tolerate these changes without complaint. However, older women or those with a back disorder or a faulty sense of balance may have a considerable amount of back pain during and just after pregnancy.

Slight relaxation and increased mobility of the pelvic joints are normal during pregnancy. This is secondary to exaggerated elasticity and softening of connective and collagen tissue and is the result of increased circulating steroid sex hormones, especially estrogen. Relaxin, an ovarian hormone, assists in this relaxation and softening. These adaptations permit enlargement of pelvic dimensions to facilitate labor and birth. The degree of relaxation varies, but considerable separation of the symphysis pubis and the instability of the sacroiliac joints may cause pain and difficulty in walking. Obesity and multifetal pregnancy tend to increase the pelvic disability.

The muscles of the abdominal wall stretch and ultimately lose some tone. During the third trimester the rectus abdominis muscles may separate (Fig. 8-13), allowing abdominal contents to protrude at the midline. The umbilicus flattens or protrudes. After delivery, the muscles gradually regain tone. However, separation of the muscles (**diastasis recti abdominis**) may persist. The maternal pelvis is discussed in detail in Chapter 14.

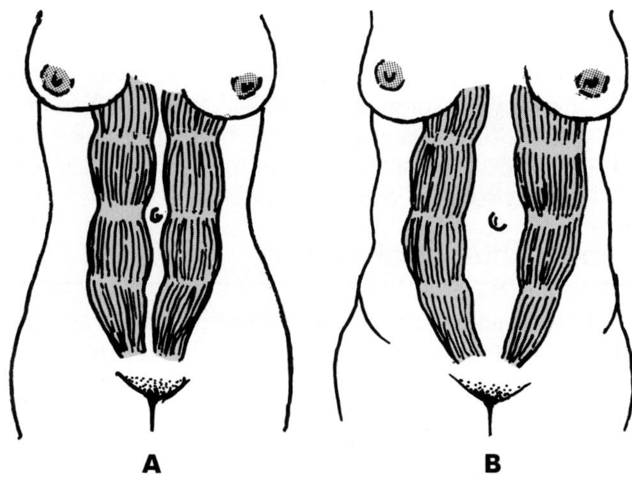

Fig. 8-13 Possible change in rectus abdominis muscles during pregnancy. **A,** Normal position in nonpregnant woman. **B,** Diastasis recti in pregnant woman.

Neurologic System

Little is known regarding specific alterations in function of the neurologic system during pregnancy, aside from hypothalamic-pituitary neurohormonal changes. Specific physiologic alterations resulting from pregnancy may cause the following neurologic or neuromuscular symptoms:

1. Compression of pelvic nerves or vascular stasis caused by enlargement of the uterus may result in sensory changes in the legs.
2. Dorsolumbar lordosis may cause pain because of traction on nerves or compression of nerve roots.
3. Edema involving the peripheral nerves may result in *carpal tunnel syndrome* during the last trimester. The edema compresses the median nerve beneath the carpal ligament of the wrist. The syndrome is characterized by paresthesia (abnormal sensation such as burning or tingling because of a disorder of the sensory nervous system) and pain in the hand, radiating to the elbow. The dominant hand is usually affected most.
4. Acroesthesia (numbness and tingling of the hands) is caused by the stoop-shouldered stance (see Fig. 8-12, *B*) assumed by some women during pregnancy. The condition is associated with traction on segments of the brachial plexus.
5. Tension headache is common when anxiety or uncertainty complicates gestation. However, vision problems such as refractive errors, sinusitis, or migraine may also be responsible for headaches.
6. "Lightheadedness," faintness, and even syncope (fainting) are common during early pregnancy. Vasomotor instability, postural hypotension, or hypoglycemia may be responsible.
7. Hypocalcemia may cause neuromuscular problems such as muscle cramps or tetany.

Gastrointestinal System

The functioning of the gastrointestinal tract during pregnancy presents a curiously interesting picture. The appetite increases. Intestinal secretion is reduced. Liver function is altered, and absorption of nutrients is enhanced. The colon is displaced laterally upward and posteriorly. Peristaltic activity (motility) decreases. As a result bowel sounds are diminished, and constipation, nausea, and vomiting are common. Blood flow to the pelvis increases as does venous pressure, contributing to hemorrhoid formation in later pregnancy.

APPETITE. During pregnancy, the pregnant woman's appetite and food intake fluctuate. Early in pregnancy, in response to increasing levels of hCG, some pregnant women experience "morning sickness." **Morning sickness** refers to nausea with or without vomiting. It appears at about 4 to 6 weeks and subsides by the end of the third month (first trimester) of pregnancy. Severity varies from mild distaste for certain foods to more severe vomiting. The condition may be triggered by the sight or odor of various foods. Taste and smell may be affected as well. Appetite may be reduced during this time secondary to morning sickness or the appetite depressant effect of hCG and altered carbohydrate metabolism. Later, appetite increases in response to increasing metabolic needs. Rarely does morning sickness have harmful effects on the embryo/fetus or the woman. If the vomiting is severe or persists beyond the first trimester, or if it is accompanied by fever, pain, or weight loss, medical intervention is necessary (for more information, see discussion of hyperemesis gravidarum, Chapter 31).

MOUTH. The gums are hyperemic, spongy, and swollen. They tend to bleed easily because the rising levels of estrogen cause selective increased vascularity and connective tissue proliferation (a nonspecific gingivitis). There is no increase in secretion of saliva. Women do complain of ***ptylism*** (excessive salivation). This perceived increase is thought to be caused by the decrease in unconscious swallowing by the woman when nauseated. Epulis and bleeding gums are discussed under "Integumentary System."

TEETH. The pregnant woman requires about 1.2 g of calcium and approximately the same amount of phosphorus every day during pregnancy. This is an increase of about 0.4 g of each of these elements over nonpregnant needs. With a well-balanced diet (Chapter 9), these requirements are satisfied. Serious dietary deficiency, however, may deplete the mother's osseous stores of these elements but does not draw on calcium in her teeth. Demineralization of teeth does not occur during pregnancy. Hence the old adage "for every child a tooth" is untrue. Gingivitis and poor dental hygiene during pregnancy or anytime may contribute to dental caries, which could result in the loss of a tooth.

ESOPHAGUS, STOMACH, AND INTESTINE. Herniation of the upper portion of the stomach (*hiatal hernia*) occurs after the seventh or eighth month of pregnancy in about 15% to 20% of pregnant women. This condition results from upward displacement of the stomach, which causes a widening of the hiatus of the diaphragm. It occurs more often in multiparas and older or obese women.

Increased estrogen production causes decreased secretion of hydrochloric acid. Therefore peptic ulcer formation or flare-up of existing peptic ulcers is uncommon during pregnancy.

Increased progesterone production causes decreased tone and motility of smooth muscles so that there is esophageal regurgitation, increased emptying time of the stomach, and reverse peristalsis. As a result the woman may experience "acid indigestion" or *heart-burn* (**pyrosis**).

In response to increased needs during pregnancy, iron is absorbed more readily in the small intestine. In general, if the individual is deficient in iron, iron absorption is increased.

Increased progesterone (causing loss of muscle tone and decreased peristalsis) results in an increase in water absorption from the colon. **Constipation** may result. In addition, constipation is secondary to hypoperistalsis (sluggishness of the bowel), unusual food choice, lack of fluids, decreased activity level, abdominal distention by the pregnant uterus, and displacement of intestines with some compression. *Hemorrhoids* (varicose veins of the rectum and anus) may be everted or may bleed during straining at stool. Bowel habits and a characteristic type of stool are established early in life. Variations will be noted with concern and may be perceived as a disease process. A mild ileus (sluggishness and lack of movement) that follows delivery, as well as postdelivery fluid loss and perineal discomfort, contribute to continuing constipation.

GALLBLADDER AND LIVER. The gallbladder is quite often distended because of its decreased muscle tone during pregnancy. Increased emptying time and thickening of bile secondary to prolonged retention are typical. These features, together with slight hypercholesterolemia from increased progesterone levels, may account for the common development of *gallstones* during pregnancy.

Hepatic function is difficult to appraise during gestation. However, only minor changes in liver function develop during pregnancy. Occasionally, intrahepatic cholestasis (retention and accumulation of bile in the liver, caused by factors within the liver) in response to placental steroids, occurs late in pregnancy and may result in *pruritus gravidarum* (severe itching) with or without jaundice. Oatmeal baths and lotions help ease the itching. These distressing symptoms subside promptly after delivery.

ABDOMINAL DISCOMFORT. Intraabdominal alterations that can cause discomfort include pelvic heaviness or pressure, round ligament tension, flatulence, distention and bowel cramping, and uterine contractions. In addition to displacement of intestines, pressure from the expanding uterus increases venous pressure in the pelvic organs. Although most abdominal discomfort is a consequence of normal maternal alterations, the physician is constantly alert to the possibility of disorders such as bowel obstruction or an inflammatory process.

Appendicitis may be difficult to diagnose. The *appendix* is displaced upward and laterally, high and to the right, away from McBurney's point (Fig 32-4, B).

Endocrine System

Profound endocrine changes occur that are essential for pregnancy maintenance, normal fetal growth, and postpartum recovery. Metabolic changes and weight gain are discussed in detail in Chapter 9.

THYROID GLAND. During pregnancy there is an increase in gland activity and hormone production. The increased activity is reflected in a moderate enlargement of the thyroid gland caused by hyperplasia of the glandular tissue and increased vascularity (Cunningham, MacDonald, Gant, 1989; Scott et al, 1990). Oxygen consumption and BMR increase secondary to the metabolic activity of the products of conception (for a discussion of changes in thyroid hormone production see Cunningham, MacDonald, Gant, 1989; Scott et al, 1990).

PARATHYROID GLAND. Pregnancy induces a slight secondary hyperparathyroidism, a reflection of increased requirements for calcium and vitamin D.

When the needs for growth of the fetal skeleton are greatest (during the last half of pregnancy), plasma parathormone levels are elevated; that is, the peak level occurs between 15 and 35 weeks' gestation.

PANCREAS. The fetus requires significant amounts of glucose for its growth and development. To meet its need for fuel, the fetus not only depletes the store of maternal glucose but also decreases the mother's ability to synthesize glucose by siphoning off her amino acids. Maternal blood glucose levels fall. Maternal insulin does *not* cross the placenta to the fetus. As a result, in early pregnancy, the pancreas decreases its production of insulin.

However, as pregnancy continues, the placenta grows and produces progressively larger amounts of hormones (i.e., human placental lactogen [hPL], estrogen, and progesterone). Cortisol production by the adrenals also increases. Estrogen, progesterone, hPL, and cortisol collectively decrease the mother's ability to use insulin. Cortisol stimulates increased production of insulin but also increases the mother's peripheral resistance to insulin (i.e., the tissues cannot use the insulin). Insulinase is an enzyme produced by the placenta to deactivate maternal insulin. Decreasing the mother's ability to use her own insulin is a protective mechanism that ensures an ample supply of glucose for the needs of the fetoplacental unit. The result is an added demand for insulin by the mother. The normal beta cells of the islets of Langerhans in the pancreas can meet the demand for insulin that continues to increase at a steady rate until term. See Chapter 31 for further discussion of diabetes mellitus.

PITUITARY PROLACTIN. In pregnancy, serum prolactin begins to rise in the first trimester and increases progressively to term. It is generally believed that although all the hormonal elements (estrogen, progesterone, thyroid, insulin, and free cortisol) necessary for breast growth and milk production are present in elevated concentrations during pregnancy, the high levels of estrogen inhibit active alveolar secretion by blocking the binding of prolactin to breast tissue, thus inhibiting the milk-producing effect of prolactin on the target epithelium (Scott et al, 1990).

ENDOCRINE SYSTEM AND MATERNAL NUTRITION. Progesterone and estrogen cause the deposit of fat in subcutaneous tissues over the abdomen, back, and upper thighs. The fat serves as an energy reserve for both pregnancy and lactation. Estrogen promotes the enlargement of the genitals, uterus, and breasts. It also results in the growth of glandular tissues, ducts, alveoli, and nipples. Estrogen alters metabolism of nutrients by interfering with folic acid metabolism, increasing total body proteins, and promoting retention of sodium and water by kidney tubules. Estrogen may decrease secretion of hydrochloric acid and pepsin, which may be responsible for digestive upsets such as nausea.

Several other hormones affect nutrition. *Aldosterone* conserves sodium. *Thyroxin* regulates metabolism. *Parathyroid hormone* controls calcium and magnesium metabolism. *Human placental lactogen (hPL)* acts as a growth hormone. *Human chorionic gonadotropin (hCG)* is one factor that induces nausea and vomiting in some women in early pregnancy.

■ SUMMARY

The intimate union of mother and fetus is referred to as the fetoplacental maternal unit. Because the maternal organism responds as a total unit to the developing fetus, the intrauterine environment of the fetus is maintained at an optimum nurturing level only to the extent that the mother's systems can adjust to the developing organism.

Adaptation to pregnancy involves all of a woman's body systems. The mother's physical response is assessed in relation to normal expected alterations. Subjective symptoms and objective signs arising from these changes serve as a basis for diagnosis of pregnancy.

REFERENCES

Batzer FR: Guidelines for choosing a pregnancy test, *Contemp Ob/Gyn* 26:37, Oct 1985 (special issue).

Blackburn ST, Loper DL: *Maternal, fetal, and neonatal physiology: a clinical perspective,* Philadelphia, 1992, WB Saunders.

Brucker MC, MacMullen NJ: What's new in pregnancy tests? *JOGN Nurs* 14:353, Sept-Oct 1985.

Cunningham FG, MacDonald PC, Gant NF: *Williams obstetrics,* ed 18, Norwalk, Conn, 1989, Appleton & Lange.

Doshi ML: Accuracy of consumer performed in-home tests for early pregnancy detection, *Am J Public Health,* 76:512, 1986.

Ganong WF: *Review of medical physiology,* ed 13, Norwalk, Conn, 1989, Appleton & Lange.

News: Monoclonals: new frontiers in reproductive medicine in Technology 1986, *Contemp Ob/Gyn* 26:75, Oct 1985.

Scott JR et al: *Danforth's obstetrics and gynecology,* ed 6, Philadelphia, 1990, JB Lippincott.

Seidel HM et al: *Mosby's guide to physical examination,* ed 2, St. Louis, 1991, Mosby–Year Book.

BIBLIOGRAPHY

Austin DA, Davis PA: Valvular disease in pregnancy, *J Perinat Neonat Nurs* 5(2):13, Sept 1991.

Brown Y, Calder B, Rae D: Female circumcision, *Can Nurse* p 19, April 1989.

Capeless E, Clapp J: Cardiovascular changes in early phase of pregnancy, *Am J Obstet Gynecol* 161:1449, 1989.

Chez RA: Advising pregnant women about nutrition *Contemp Ob/Gyn* 36(1):80, Jan 1991.

Creasy R, Resnick R: *Maternal-fetal medicine: principles and practice,* Philadelphia, 1989, WB Saunders.

Elkayam U, Gleicher N: *Changes in cardiac findings during normal pregnancy.* In Elkayam U, Gleicher N, editors: *Cardiac problems in pregnancy,* ed 2, New York, 1990, Alan R. Liss.

Greene GW et al: Postpartum weight change: how much of the weight gained in pregnancy will be lost after delivery? *Obstet Gynecol.* 71:701, 1988.

Groër M: Psychoneuroimmunology, *AJN* 91(8):33, Aug 1991.

Hart JL: Low back pain, radiculopathies, and pregnancy, *Pain Management* p 103, March/April 1990.

Institute of Medicine, National Academy of Sciences, Food and Nutrition Board: *Nutrition during pregnancy. Part I: Weight gain. Part II: Nutrient supplements.* Washington, DC, 1990, National Academy Press.

Malasanos L et al: *Health assessment,* ed 4, St. Louis, 1989, Mosby–Year Book.

Mirales WJ et al: The use of antenatal vitamin K in the prevention of early neonatal intraventricular hemorrhage, *Am J Obstet Gynecol.* 159:774, 1988.

Samples JT et al: The dynamic characteristics of the circum-vaginal muscles, *JOGN Nurs* 17(3):194, 1988.

Terhaar M, Schakenbach L: Care of the pregnant patient with a pacemaker, *J Perinat Neonat Nurs* 5(2):1, Sept 1991.

Uvnäs-Moberg K: The gastrointestinal tract in growth and reproduction, *Sci Am* p 78, July 1989.

Wilson JR, Carrington ER: *Obstetrics and gynecology,* ed 9, St Louis, 1991, Mosby–Year Book.

chapter 8 review

Key Concepts

- The biochemical, physiologic, and anatomic adaptations that occur during pregnancy are profound and return to the nonpregnant state following delivery and lactation.
- Maternal adaptations are attributed to the hormones of pregnancy and to mechanical pressures arising from the enlarging uterus and other tissues.
- The understanding of these adaptations to pregnancy remains a major goal, for without such knowledge it is difficult, if not impossible, to understand the disease processes—pregnancy induced or coincidental—that can threaten women during pregnancy and the puerperium.
- The ability to recognize the beta subunit of hCG through monoclonal antibody technology has revolutionized endocrine tests for pregnancy.
- Adaptations to pregnancy protect the woman's normal physiologic functioning, meet the metabolic demands pregnancy imposes, and provide for fetal developmental and growth needs.
- The rise in pH of the pregnant woman's vaginal secretions makes her more vulnerable to vaginal infections.
- Increased vascularity and sensitivity of the vagina and other pelvic viscera may lead to a high degree of sexual interest and arousal.
- Some adaptations to pregnancy result in discomforts such as fatigue, urinary frequency, nausea, and breast sensitivity.
- Balance and coordination are affected by changes in joints and the woman's center of gravity as pregnancy progresses.

Key Terms

- amenorrhea (p. 191)
- ballottement (p. 196)
- Braun von Fernwald's sign (p. 195)
- Braxton Hicks sign (p. 195)
- Chadwick's sign (p. 195)
- colostrum (p. 198)
- constipation (p. 207)
- diastasis recti abdominis (p. 205)
- chloasma (mask of pregnancy) (p. 203)
- epulis (p. 204)
- fatigability (p. 202)
- ferning (p. 197)
- fetal heart rate (p. 196)
- friability (p. 197)
- funic souffle (p. 196)
- Goodell's sign (p. 195)
- gravida (p. 190)
- gravidity (p. 190)
- Hegar's sign (p. 195)
- hirsutism (p. 204)
- home pregnancy test (p. 192)
- hyperplasia (p. 196)
- hypertrophy (p. 195)
- lassitude (p. 202)
- leukorrhea (p. 197)
- lightening (p. 195)
- linea nigra (p. 203)
- mean arterial pressure (MAP) (p. 199)
- McDonald's sign (p. 195)
- monoclonal antibody (p. 192)

- Montgomery's tubercles (p. 198)
- morning sickness (p. 206)
- multigravida (p. 190)
- multipara (p. 190)
- nulligravida (p. 190)
- nullipara (p. 190)
- operculum (p. 197)
- palmar erythema (p. 204)
- parity (p. 190)
- physiologic anemia (p. 199)
- physiologic edema (p. 203)
- pigmentation (p. 203)
- Piskacek's sign (p. 195)
- primigravida (p. 190)
- primipara (p. 190)
- ptylism (p. 206)
- pyrosis (p. 207)
- quickening (p. 196)
- radioimmunoassay (p. 191)
- striae gravidarum (p. 204)
- urgency (p. 202)
- urinary frequency (p. 202)
- uterine enlargement (p. 192)
- uterine souffle (p. 196)
- vascular spiders (p. 204)
- viability (p. 190)

Critical Thinking Exercises

1. Interview three pregnant women (and partner, if present) at different stages of their pregnancy:
   a. How does each pregnant woman feel about changes in her body related to anatomic and physiologic adaptations?
   b. Which changes do they find pleasant?
   c. Which changes do they find uncomfortable or troublesome?
   d. What is their level of understanding of these adaptations?
   e. What complaints or questions were asked by clients related to anatomic or physiologic changes?

   Analyze your findings. Use your findings in developing a protocol for assessment for the different stages of this pregnancy:
   - Formulate interview questions.
   - Describe the physical examination.
   - List appropriate laboratory or diagnostic tests.

   Justify your decisions.
2. Explore your own emotions and attitudes regarding the changes a woman's body undergoes during pregnancy.
3. Obtain one over-the-counter pregnancy test. Read the instructions. Are they easy to follow? How would you teach woman to use that pregnancy test?

Topics For Nursing Research

- Is there a difference between Braxton Hicks contractions and preterm labor contractions? If so, how can they be differentiated?
- Are there preventive measures, such as exercises or an article of clothing, that can reduce the incidence or severity of diastasis recti abdominis?
- If a pregnant woman assumes the hands-and-knees position for a specified time one or more times a day, will this affect some maternal changes (e.g., physiologic edema, backache, or varicosities)?

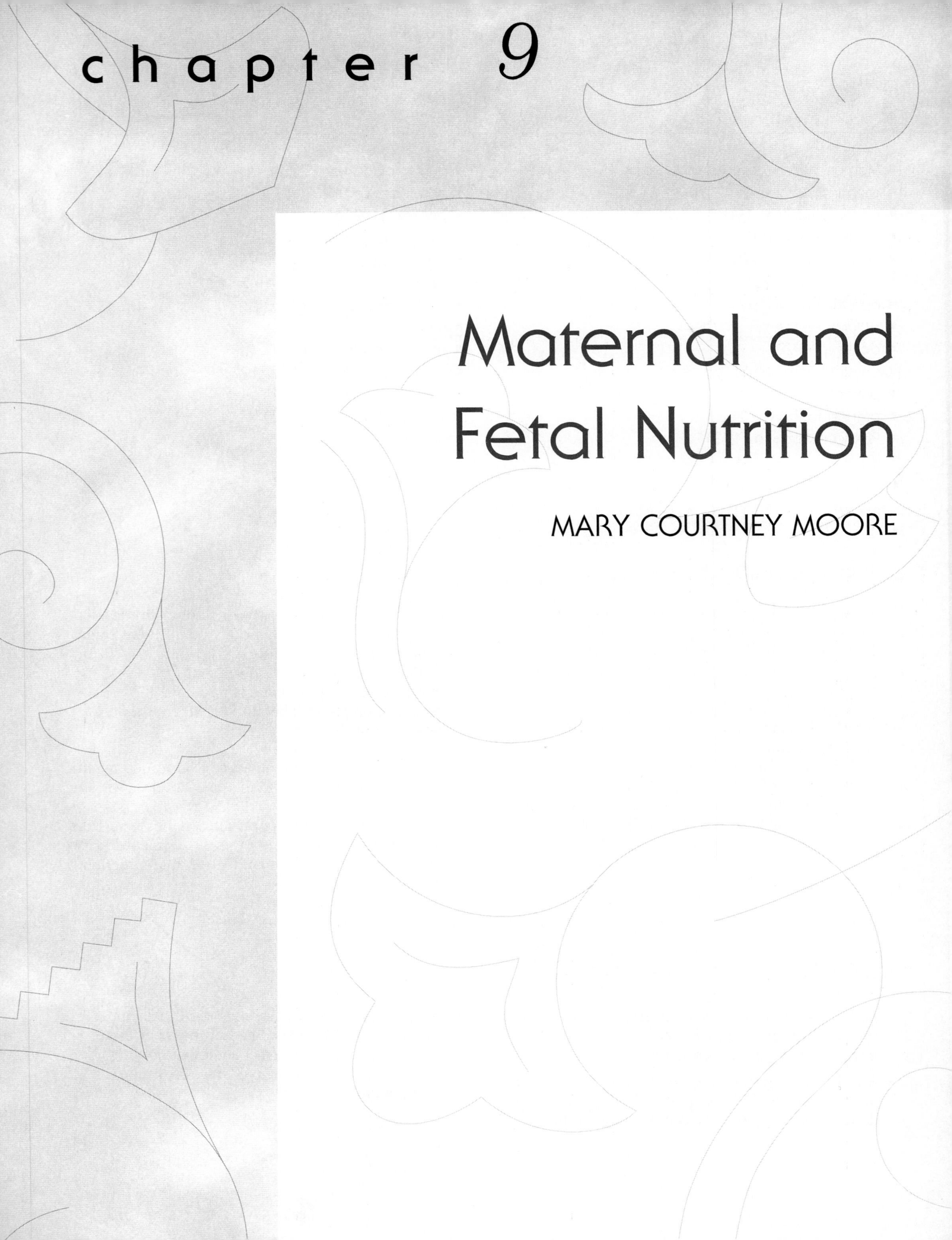

chapter 9

Maternal and Fetal Nutrition

MARY COURTNEY MOORE

LEARNING OBJECTIVES

- Correctly define the key terms listed.
- Explain recommended maternal weight gain during pregnancy (both total amount and rate of gain) based on prepregnancy weight for height.
- State recommended daily allowance (RDA) for kilocalories, protein, vitamins, and minerals during pregnancy.
- Give examples of food sources of the nutrients required for optimum maternal nutrition during pregnancy.
- Examine the role of nutritional supplements during pregnancy.
- List five nutritional risk factors during pregnancy.
- Give examples of cultural food patterns and possible dietary problems for two ethnic groups.
- Evaluate nutritional status during pregnancy.
- Outline and give examples of nursing care related to maternal and fetal nutrition based on the five-step nursing process.
- Identify topics for nursing research related to maternal and fetal nutrition.

The outcome of pregnancy depends to a significant degree on a woman's nutritional status before and during pregnancy. It is therefore important that the nurse have a thorough understanding of nutrient needs during pregnancy and that nutrition assessment, intervention, and evaluation be an integral part of the nursing process for the pregnant woman. See addition at end of chapter regarding the pyramid of five food groups adopted in 1992.

NUTRIENT NEEDS DURING PREGNANCY

Although a balanced diet is needed throughout pregnancy, the required amount of nutrients is determined, at least in part, by the stage of gestation. During the first trimester when the embryo/fetus is very small, needs are only slightly increased over those before pregnancy. In contrast, during the second and third trimesters, the fetus's needs for some nutrients increases greatly (Table 9-1). Factors that contribute to the increase in nutrient needs include the following:

1. *Uterine-placental-fetal unit.* Placentas of poorly nourished mothers often contain fewer and smaller cells. Poorly developed placentas have a reduced ability to synthesize substances needed by the fetus, to facilitate flow of needed nutrients, and to inhibit passage of potentially harmful substances. Therefore it is understandable that the infant of a poorly nourished mother would be poorly nourished and small for gestational age (SGA) (Chapter 37). Fig. 9-1 shows a possible mechanism by which maternal malnutrition may produce **intrauterine growth retardation (IUGR).**
2. *Maternal blood volume and constituents.* Total blood volume is known to increase about 33% above normal during pregnancy. Plasma volume increases 50% in first pregnancies and more in multiparity. Red blood cell (RBC) production is stimulated during pregnancy. The number of RBCs increases gradually; the expansion of plasma volume proceeds rapidly. This rapid increase in plasma volume results in hemodilution and is referred to as *physiologic anemia of pregnancy*. At the same time, a deficiency of iron or of folic acid may contribute to the development of true **anemia.**

Blood levels of many nutrition-related factors, such as albumin, decrease during pregnancy as a result of hemodilution. In contrast, most plasma lipid fractions rise during pregnancy. For example, the total cholesterol level increases from less than 200 mg/dL to 250 to 300 mg/dL.

3. *Maternal mammary changes.* Marked increase of the lactiferous ducts and lobule-alveolar tissue takes place (see Chapters 8 and 22).
4. *Metabolic needs.* Basal metabolism rates (BMRs), when expressed as kilocalories (kcal) per minute, are about 20% higher in pregnant women than in nonpregnant women. This increase includes the energy cost for tissue synthesis. The increased basal energy need plus the energy needed by the new tissue after it is formed brings the energy needs during the second and third trimesters to approximately 300 kcal per day more than prepregnancy needs.

Energy Needs

Energy needs are met by carbohydrate, fat, and protein in the diet. There are no specific recommendations for the amount of carbohydrate and fat in the diet of the pregnant woman. However, intake of these nutrients should be adequate to support the recommended weight gain. Although protein can be used to supply **energy (kcal),** its primary role is to provide amino acids for synthesis of new tissues (see discussion later in chapter).

WEIGHT GAIN. The optimal weight gain during pregnancy is not precisely known. It is known, however, that the amount of weight gained by the mother during pregnancy makes an important contribution to the pregnancy's course and outcome. Although adequate weight gain does not necessarily indicate that

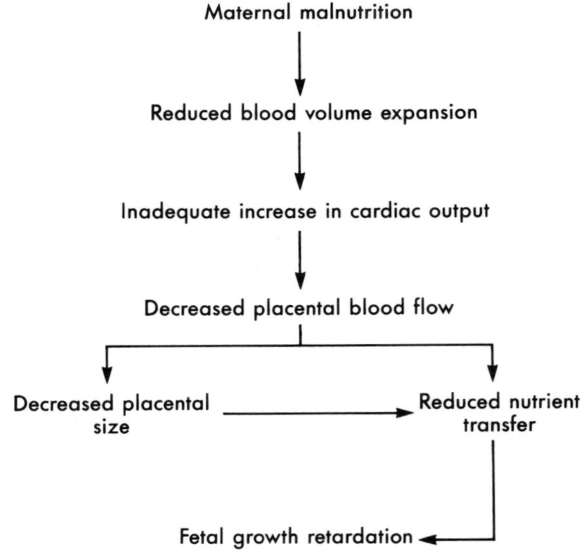

Fig. 9-1 Postulated mechanisms responsible for placental and fetal (intrauterine) growth retardation.
From Rosso P: Placental growth, development, and function in relation to maternal nutrition, *Fed Proc* 39:250, 1980.

TABLE 9-1 Nutritional Recommendations During Pregnancy and Lactation

Nutrient	RDA for Nonpregnant Female (25-50 yr)	RDA During Pregnancy	RDA for Lactation* (first 6 mo/second 6 mo)	Reasons for Increased Need	Food Sources
Calories	2200	2200 (first trimester); 2500 (second and third trimesters)	2700/2700	Increased energy needs for fetal growth and milk production	Carbohydrate, fat, protein
Protein (g)	50	60	65/62	Synthesis of the products of conception: fetus, amniotic fluid, placenta; growth of maternal tissue: uterus, breasts, red blood cells, plasma proteins, secretion of milk protein during lactation	Meats, eggs, milk, cheese, legumes (dry beans and peas, peanuts), nuts, grains
Minerals					
Calcium (mg)	800	1200	1200/1200	Fetal skeleton and tooth bud formation; maintenance of maternal bone and tooth mineralization	Milk, cheese, yogurt, sardines or other fish eaten with bones left in, deep green leafy vegetables except spinach or Swiss chard,† tofu, baked beans
Phosphorus (mg)	800	1200	1200/1200	Fetal skeleton and tooth bud formation	Milk, cheese, yogurt, meats, whole grains, nuts, legumes
Iron (mg)	15	30	15/15	Increased maternal hemoglobin formation, fetal liver iron storage	Liver, meats, whole or enriched breads and cereals, deep green leafy vegetables, legumes, dried fruits
Zinc (mg)	12	15	19/16	Component of numerous enzyme systems; possibly important in preventing congenital malformations	Liver, shellfish, meats, whole grains, milk

RDA, Recommended daily allowance.
*Milk production generally declines during the second 6 mo of lactation as the infant's diet increasingly begins to include other foods. Thus maternal needs for many nutrients decrease.
†Spinach and chard contain calcium but also contain oxalic acid, which inhibits calcium absorption.
‡*RE*, Retinol equivalents. Replaces international units (IU). 1 RE = 5 IU.
§As cholecalciferol. 10 μg cholecalciferol = 400 IU of vitamin D.

Continued.

TABLE 9-1 Nutritional Recommendations During Pregnancy and Lactation—cont'd

Nutrient	RDA for Nonpregnant Female (25-50 yr)	RDA During Pregnancy	RDA for Lactation* (first 6 mo/second 6 mo)	Reasons for Increased Need	Food Sources
Iodine (μg)	150	175	200/200	Increased maternal metabolic rate	Iodized salt, seafood, milk and milk products, commercial yeast breads, rolls, and donuts
Magnesium (mg)	280	320	355/340	Involved in energy and protein metabolism, tissue growth, muscle action	Nuts, legumes, cocoa, meats, whole grains
Selenium (μg)	55	65	75/75	Antioxidant (protects cell membranes), tooth component	Organ meats, seafood, whole grains, legumes, molasses
Fat-soluble vitamins					
A (RE)‡	800	800	1300/1200	Essential for cell development, thus growth; tooth bud formation (development of enamel-forming cells in gum tissue); bone growth	Deep green leafy vegetables, dark yellow vegetables and fruits, chili peppers, liver, fortified margarine and butter
D (μg)§	5	10	10/10	Involved in absorption of calcium and phosphorus, improves mineralization	Fortified milk, fortified margarine, egg yolk, butter, liver, seafood
E (mg)	8	10	12/11	Antioxidant (protects cell membranes from damage), especially important for preventing hemolysis of red blood cells	Vegetable oils, green leafy vegetables, whole grains, liver, nuts and seeds, cheese, fish
Water-soluble vitamins					
C (mg)	60	70	95/90	Tissue formation and integrity, formation of connective tissue, enhancement of iron absorption	Citrus fruits, strawberries, melons, broccoli, tomatoes, peppers, raw deep green leafy vegetables
Folic acid (μg)	180	400	280/260	Increased red blood cell formation, prevention of macrocytic or megaloblastic anemia	Green leafy vegetables, oranges, broccoli, asparagus, artichokes, liver
Thiamin (mg)	1.1	1.5	1.6/1.6	Involved in energy metabolism	Pork, beef, liver, whole or enriched grains, legumes
Riboflavin (mg)	1.3	1.6	1.8/1.7	Involved in energy and protein metabolism	Milk, liver, enriched grains, deep green and yellow vegetables
Pyridoxine (mg)	1.6	2.2	2.1/2.1	Involved in protein metabolism	Meat, liver, deep green vegetables, whole grains
B_{12} (μg)	2.0	2.2	2.6/2.6	Production of nucleic acids and proteins, especially important in formation of red blood cells and prevention of megaloblastic or macrocytic anemia	Milk, egg, meat, liver, cheese
Niacin (mg)	15	17	20/20	Involved in energy metabolism	Meat, fish, poultry, liver, whole or enriched grains, peanuts

TABLE 9-2 Recommended Weight Gain During Pregnancy (Based on Body Mass Index* [BMI] Before Pregnancy)

BMI	Weekly Gain During Second and Third Trimesters: kg (lb)	Total Gain: kg (lb)
<19.8 (underweight)	0.5 (1.1)	12.5-18 (28-40)
19.8 to 26.0 (normal)	0.4 (0.9-1)	11.5-16 (25-35)
26.0 to 29.0 (overweight)	0.3 (0.67)	7-11.5 (15-25)
>29.0 (obese)	Individualize	≥6.8 (15)

Modified from: Institute of Medicine: *Nutrition during pregnancy,* Washington, DC, 1990, National Academy Press.
*See text for explanation of calculating BMI.

the diet is nutritionally adequate (Aaronson, MacNee, 1989), it reduces the risk of delivering an SGA or a preterm infant (Frentzen et al, 1988; Abrams et al, 1989; Abrams, Parker, 1990). The weight gained during a normal pregnancy will vary among individual women. The primary factor is the appropriateness of prepregnancy weight for height, that is, whether the woman is of normal weight, underweight, or overweight. A commonly used method of evaluating the appropriateness of weight for height is the **body mass index (BMI)**. The following formula is used in calculation of BMI:

$$\text{BMI} = \text{Weight/height}^2$$

where the weight is in kilograms and height is in meters. Thus, for a woman who weighed 51 kg (112 lb) before pregnancy and is 1.57 m (62 in) tall:

$$\text{BMI} = 51/(1.57)^2, \text{ or } 20.7$$

BMI can be interpreted as follows: less than 19.8, underweight; 19.8 to 26.0, normal weight; 26.0 to 29.0, overweight; and greater than 29.0, obese (Institute of Medicine, 1990). Table 9-2 shows the **recommended weight gain** for these BMI categories. No recommendations have been made regarding optimal weight gain based on BMI for multifetal gestations. In twin gestations, gains of approximately 20 kg (44 lb) have been reported to be associated with the best outcomes (Pederson et al, 1989).

During the first and second trimesters, growth takes place primarily in maternal tissue, whereas growth occurs primarily in fetal tissues during the third trimester (Fig. 9-2). At term in a pregnancy in which the woman has gained 11 kg (at the upper end of the recommended range for overweight women), increase in the weight of maternal tissues accounts for approximately 6 kg and the fetus, pla-

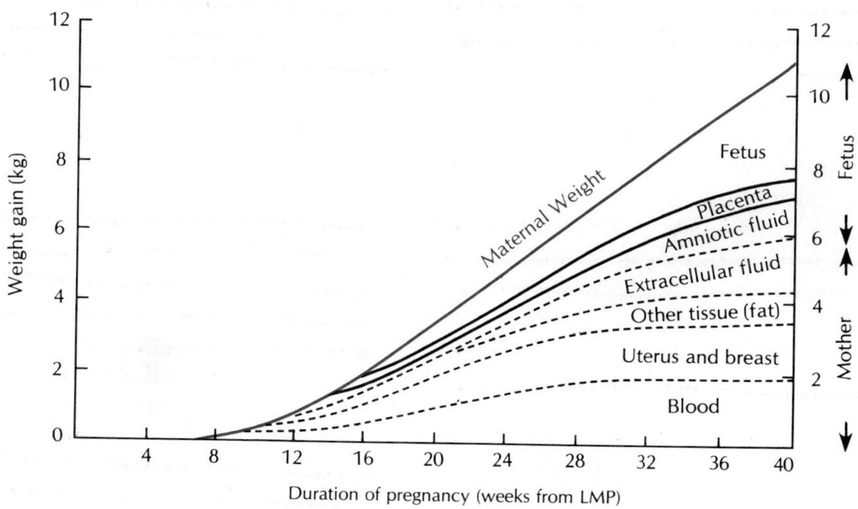

Fig. 9-2 Pattern and components of weight gain throughout course of pregnancy, assuming an 11-kg (24.5 lb) weight gain. *LMP,* last menstrual period.
From Schneider HA et al: *Nutritional support of medical practice,* ed 2, Philadelphia, 1983, JB Lippincott.

centa, and amniotic fluid account for 5 kg of the weight gain (Fig. 9-2).

PATTERN OF WEIGHT GAIN. During the first trimester, there is an average gain of only 1 to 2.5 kg (2 to 5 lb). Thereafter optimal weight gain increases to 0.3 to 0.5 kg (0.66 to 1.1 lb) weekly; the lower rate of gain is preferred for overweight women and the higher rate for those who are underweight (Table 9-2). The recommended caloric intake corresponds to this pattern of gain (Table 9-1). For the first trimester, there is no increment; during the second and third trimesters, an additional 300 kcal per day is recommended.

It is important that weight gain take place throughout pregnancy. Poor weight gain early in pregnancy has been reported to increase the risk of delivering an SGA infant. Inadequate gains during the last half of pregnancy have been observed to increase the likelihood of preterm delivery (Hediger et al, 1989). These risks were found to exist even when the total gain for the pregnancy fell into the recommended range.

HAZARDS OF RESTRICTING ADEQUATE WEIGHT GAIN. Young women in North America enter pregnancy already burdened by cultural obsession with thinness and "dieting." This conscious or unconscious pressure is difficult to dislodge. There are potential hazards, however, for both mother and infant from restricting weight gain during pregnancy. The mother's weight gain and prepregnancy weight are the two strongest influences (except gestational age) on birth weight. **Low birth weight** (LBW) (<2500g) is the greatest risk factor in the infant's survival and also may have adverse effects on development of the central nervous system.

Some persons have advocated restriction of weight gain in obese women so that they conclude pregnancy with a net loss. However, dietary restrictions to limit calories may also result in excessive limitation of other nutrients in the diet. Moreover, dietary restriction results in catabolism of fat stores, which in turn results in increased production of ketones. The long-term effects of mild ketonemia during pregnancy are not known (Rizzo et al, 1990), but ketonuria has been found to be correlated with preterm labor (Frentzen et al, 1987).

On the other hand, pregnancy should not be used as an excuse for uncontrolled dietary indulgence. Excessive weight gained during pregnancy may be difficult to remove after pregnancy, thus contributing to chronic overweight or obesity, an etiologic factor in a host of chronic diseases, including hypertension, diabetes mellitus, and arteriosclerotic heart disease. The woman who gains 18 kg (40 lb) or more is especially at risk (Olsen, Mundt, 1986; Greene et al, 1988; Parham et al, 1990).

Protein

Protein, with its essential constituent, nitrogen, is the nutritional element that is basic to growth. More protein is essential to meet increasing demands in pregnancy. These greater needs result from the rapid growth of the fetus; from the enlargement of the uterus, mammary glands, and placenta; from the increase in maternal circulating blood volume and the subsequent demand for increased plasma protein to maintain colloidal osmotic pressure; and from the formation of amniotic fluid.

Milk, meat, eggs, and cheese are complete protein foods of high biologic value. Protein-rich foods also contribute other nutrients such as calcium, iron, and B vitamins. The amounts of these foods that would supply the quantities of protein needed are indicated in the recommended daily food plan (Table 9-3 and Fig 9–5). Additional protein may be obtained from legumes, whole grains, and nuts.

Water

Water as an essential nutrient is commonly overlooked during assessment. Among its many functions, water assists digestion by dissolving food and aiding its transport. It is essential during the exchange of nutrients and wastes across cell membranes. Water is the main substance of cells, blood, lymph, and other vital body fluids. It also aids in maintaining body temperature. Drinking 6 to 8 glasses (1500 to 2000 mL) of water, milk, and juices every 24 hours is recommended.

It is best to limit intake of caffeine-containing beverages. The effects of caffeine on the fetus are not well defined. On the basis of a review of the available data, Berger (1988) suggested that caffeine intake greater than 300 mg (equivalent to approximately two 6-oz cups of coffee) a day might reduce birth weight and that pregnant women would be well advised to limit their caffeine consumption to this level until more is known. Tea, chocolate, and some soft drinks contain caffeine or related compounds, although the concentration of caffeine in these is generally considerably lower than in coffee. The use of beverages that contain the artificial sweetener saccharin should be discouraged (London, 1988). Saccharin crosses the placenta and is cleared by the fetus only very slowly. It has at least mild carcinogenic effects in adult animals; although its long-term effects on the fetus are not known, it is possible that in

TABLE 9-3 Daily Food Guide for Pregnancy and Lactation

Food Group	Serving Size	Suggested Number of Servings: Nonpregnant, nonlactating woman	Pregnant woman	Lactating woman
Grain products				
Include whole-grain and enriched breads, cereals pasta, and rice.	1 slice bread; ½ bun, bagel, or English muffin; 1 oz ready-to-eat cereal; ½ c cooked grains	6-11	6-11	6-11
Vegetables				
Use dark green leafy and deep yellow often. Eat dry beans and peas often; count ½ c, cooked dry beans or peas as a serving of vegetables or 1 oz from meat group.	1 c raw leafy greens; ½ c of others	3-5	3-5	3-5
Fruits				
Include citrus fruits, strawberries, or melons frequently.	1 medium apple, orange, banana, peach, etc; ½ c small or diced fruit; ¾ c juice	2-4	2-4	2-4
Milk and milk products				
	1 c milk or yogurt; 1½ oz cheese	2-3	3 or more	4 or more
Meat, poultry, fish, dry beans, nuts, and eggs				
Use peanut butter or nuts rarely to avoid excessive fat intake. Limit eggs to reduce cholesterol intake; trim fat from meat, and remove skin from poultry.	½ c cooked dry beans, 1 egg, or 1-½ T peanut butter is equivalent to 1 oz meat	Up to 6 oz total	Up to 6 oz total	Up to 6 oz total

c, cup; *T*, tablespoon.

utero exposure could predispose the individual to later development of cancer. Although aspartame (Nutrasweet, Equal), another artificial sweetener, has not been found to have any adverse effects on the normal mother or fetus, its use should be avoided by pregnant women homozygous for phenylketonuria (London, 1988).

Minerals and Vitamins

In general, the nutrient needs of pregnant women, with the exception of those for iron, can be met through dietary sources. Counseling about the need for a varied diet rich in vitamins and minerals should be a part of every pregnant woman's early prenatal care and should be reinforced throughout pregnancy. However, supplements of certain nutrients (listed in the following discussion) are recommended if the woman's diet is very poor or if significant nutritional risk factors are present. Nutritional risk factors in pregnancy include adolescent pregnancy; multifetal gestation; maternal smoking, drug use, or alcohol abuse; poor knowledge of nutrition; or insufficient funds to allow for an adequate diet.

IRON. The changes in maternal red blood volume and cell mass accompanying pregnancy represent a fundamental physiologic adjustment. Full-term infants whose weight is appropriate for gestational age (AGA) are born with high hemoglobin levels of 18 to 22 g/dL and with a supply of iron stored in the liver to last 3 to 6 months. Thus the maternal organism must transfer about 300 mg of iron to the fetus during gestation.

If dietary iron is not available to meet the needs of the maternal-placental-fetal unit, fetal iron reserves will not be impaired; however, maternal iron stores will be depleted and maternal red cell mass will be reduced. If the mother has no iron reserves, which occurs commonly in young women, especially teenagers, maternal hemoglobin levels will drop more than usual. This may result in iron-deficiency anemia in addition to the physiologic anemia of pregnancy.

The anemic woman has an impaired ability to tolerate a potential hemorrhage at the time of delivery. In addition, she may suffer from lethargy and lack of energy. The Institute of Medicine (1990) recommends that all pregnant women receive a supplement providing 30 mg of ferrous iron daily, starting by 12 weeks of gestation. If iron-deficiency anemia, manifested by low levels of hematocrit or hemoglobin and serum ferritin, is present, increased dosages are required. (Client teaching regarding iron supplementation is discussed on p. 235.)

CALCIUM. Fetal calcification is responsible for most of the increase in calcium needs during pregnancy. Milk is the richest source of calcium, with 1200 mg —precisely the recommended daily amount—in 1 L (approximately 1 quart). Other good sources are listed in Table 9-1. Cottage cheese and ice cream contain less calcium than does milk or cheese. **Lactose** (milk sugar) **intolerance** caused by lack of the lactase enzyme is relatively common in adults, particularly among African Americans, Orientals, Native Americans, and Eskimos. In these individuals, milk consumption may cause abdominal cramping, bloating, and diarrhea. Yogurt, sweet acidophilus milk, buttermilk, cheese, chocolate milk, and cocoa may be tolerated even if fresh fluid milk is not (Chong, Hardy, 1989). Commercial products that contain lactase enzyme (e.g., Lactaid) are available in pharmacies and some large supermarkets. These products hydrolyze or digest the lactose when they are added to milk, making it possible for lactose-intolerant persons to drink milk.

SODIUM. During pregnancy there is a slight increase in the need for sodium, primarily because the body water is expanding (e.g., the expanding blood volume). Sodium is integrally involved in maintaining body water balance. Routine restriction of sodium was practiced in the past, but such a restriction is physiologically unsound and unfounded. In general, sodium restriction is necessary only if a maternal medical condition such as renal or liver failure or hypertension requires the restriction of sodium to control fluid retention and blood pressure.

Excessive intake of sodium is discouraged, however, because it may contribute to fluid retention and edema. High amounts of sodium are found in many canned and processed foods. Products low in nutritive value and excessively high in sodium include pretzels, potato chips, soft drinks, and bouillon cubes. Hidden sources of sodium are present in medications such as bicarbonate of soda. Some people are unaware that table salt contains sodium.

ZINC. The metal zinc is a constituent of numerous enzymes involved in major metabolic pathways. It may be noteworthy that maternal zinc deficiency is highly teratogenic in rats. The incidence of malformations of the central nervous system (CNS) in humans appears to be increased in geographic areas where zinc deficiency is prevalent.

Large intakes of iron and folic acid interfere with absorption of zinc and decrease serum zinc levels (Hambidge et al, 1988). Because iron and folic acid supplements are commonly prescribed during pregnancy, pregnant women should be encouraged to consume good sources of zinc daily (Table 9-1)

FAT-SOLUBLE VITAMINS. Fat-soluble vitamins—vitamins A, D, E, and K—are stored in the body tissues; with chronic overdoses, these vitamins can reach toxic levels. Because of the high potential for toxicity, pregnant women are advised to take fat-soluble vitamin supplements only as prescribed. Deficiencies of vitamins E and K are uncommon in healthy adults. Needed amounts are readily available in the diet or, in the case of vitamin K, by means of synthesis in the gastrointestinal tract. Although infants are born with poor stores of vitamin K and need supplementation at birth, maternal supplementation during pregnancy is of no benefit in increasing vitamin K levels in the fetus. Vitamins A and D deserve special mention.

Adequate intakes of vitamin A are needed to allow the fetus to store sufficient amounts of the vitamin. However, dietary sources can readily supply sufficient amounts. Congenital malformations have occurred in infants of mothers who took excessive amounts of vitamin A during pregnancy, and thus supplements are not recommended during pregnancy (Institute of Medicine, 1990). Vitamin A analogues (e.g., isotretinoin [Accutane]) prescribed for cystic acne are a special concern (Thomson, Cordero, 1989). In addition, sexually active adolescents and women who take these medications should be warned of the risks associated with their use and instructed in reliable methods of contraception.

Vitamin D plays an important role in promoting positive calcium balance in pregnancy. It is present naturally in only a few animal foods such as fish liver oils, eggs, butter, and liver. The main food sources are enriched or fortified foods such as milk and ready-to-eat cereals. It is also produced in the skin by the action of ultraviolet light (irradiation) on dehydrocholesterol. Excessive amounts in the mother may cause hypervitaminosis D expressed as hypercalcemia in infants. Severe deficiency may cause neonatal hypocalcemia and tetany, as well as hypoplasia of the tooth enamel. Because most milk in the United States is fortified with vitamin D at a level of 10 μg per quart, the daily consumption of a quart of milk provides the full allowance of vitamin D and of calcium as well for most pregnant women. For this reason, women who do not drink milk should be encouraged to do so. It is advisable for women with lactose intolerance and those who refuse to include milk in the diet to take a daily supplement providing 10 μg (400 IU) of vitamin D, particularly during the winter months and in northern latitudes where sun exposure is limited (Institute of Medicine, 1990).

WATER-SOLUBLE VITAMINS. Body stores of water-soluble vitamins are much smaller than those of fat-soluble vitamins, and the water-soluble vitamins, in contrast to fat-soluble ones, are readily excreted in the urine. Therefore, good sources of these vitamins must be consumed frequently, and toxicity with overdosage is less likely than with fat-soluble vitamins.

The augmented maternal erythropoiesis of pregnancy requires substantially increased amounts of folic acid (folacin). Moreover, because folic acid is intimately involved in DNA synthesis, requirements are particularly high in rapidly growing cells such as fetal and placental tissues. It has been suggested that folic acid supplementation before and/or just after conception might reduce the prevalence of neural tube defects. There have been no carefully controlled double-blind studies of periconceptual folic acid supplementation, and conflicting conclusions have been derived from surveys (Mills et al, 1989; Milunsky et al, 1989). Until further evidence is available, the Institute of Medicine (1990) does not recommend routine supplementation with folic acid for pregnant women. Instead it emphasizes the need to counsel all pregnant women about the importance of a good diet, with inclusion of green leafy vegetables, whole grains, and meats. A supplement of 300 μg/day is recommended for women at nutritional risk.

Thiamin (vitamin B_1), riboflavin (vitamin B_2), and niacin (vitamin B_3) are involved in release and storage of energy from carbohydrate, fat, and protein in the diet. Needs for these vitamins increase as caloric needs increase in the second and third trimesters of pregnancy and during lactation. However, as caloric intake increases, intake of these vitamins also increases. Thus a deficiency is unlikely in healthy women, although deficiencies are very likely in women with poor diets, such as alcohol abusers. Pyridoxine, or vitamin B_6, is involved in protein metabolism. Although levels of a pyridoxine-containing enzyme have been reported to be low in women with pregnancy-induced hypertension (PIH), there is no evidence that supplementation prevents or corrects the condition. No supplement is recommended routinely, but women with poor diets and those at nutritional risk may need a supplement providing 2 mg/day (Institute of Medicine, 1990).

Vitamin B_{12} is required for synthesis of nucleic acids and thus for synthesis of new tissue. It is found only in animal products such as meat, poultry, eggs, milk products, and fish. Strict vegetarians, who consume no animal products, lack a source of this vitamin and need a supplement of 2 μg/day (Institute of Medicine, 1990). Signs of vitamin B_{12} deficiency include megaloblastic anemia and neurologic deficits in the mother and infant.

Vitamin C has many functions, including participation in synthesis of connective tissue and norepinephrine, enhancement of iron absorption, incorporation of iron into ferritin (a storage form of iron), and maintenance of immune responses. Scurvy, or deficiency of vitamin C, results in excessive bruising, petechiae, and spongy, bleeding gums. Vitamin C needs of most women are readily met by dietary sources, but smokers have an increased need. For women at nutritional risk, a supplement of 50 mg/day is recommended (Institute of Medicine, 1990). Research has failed to provide evidence that ascorbic acid (vitamin C) is effective in prevention of colds. Moreover, if the mother takes pharmacologic doses of the vitamin during pregnancy, scurvy or ascorbic acid deficiency may develop even in the infant who is consuming what would normally be adequate levels of vitamin C.

■ NURSING PROCESS IN NUTRITIONAL CARE

Adequate nutrition is vital throughout the life span. During pregnancy, nutrition plays a key role in achieving an optimum outcome for the mother and her unborn baby. Motivation to learn about nutrition is usually higher during pregnancy, as parents strive to “do what’s right for the baby.” Optimum nutrition cannot eliminate all problems that may arise in pregnancy, but it establishes a good foundation for supporting the needs of the mother and her unborn child.

ASSESSMENT

Assessment is based on information obtained from an interview and review of the woman's health records, physical examination, and laboratory analyses.

Client History and Health Interview

The interview and review of the client's health records provide information about the health and diet history, including the impact of socioeconomic and cultural factors on food intake.

HEALTH HISTORY. Nutritional status is integrally related to health history and practices. In assessing nutritional status, it is especially important to include the following information in the data base.

OBSTETRIC HISTORY. Nutritional reserves may be depleted in the woman with high parity or frequent pregnancies (especially three or more pregnancies during 2 years). A history of preterm delivery or delivery of an LBW or small-for-gestational age (SGA) infant may indicate inadequate dietary intake. PIH may also be a factor in poor maternal nutrition. Delivery of an LGA infant may indicate maternal diabetes mellitus. Previous contraceptive methods also may affect reproductive health. Increased menstrual blood loss often occurs with use of an intrauterine contraceptive device for the first 3 to 6 months of use. Consequently the user may have low iron stores or even iron deficiency anemia. Use of oral contraceptive agents, on the other hand, is associated with decreased menstrual losses and increased iron stores.

MEDICAL HISTORY. Chronic maternal illnesses such as diabetes mellitus, renal disease, liver disease, cystic fibrosis or other malabsorptive disorders, seizure disorders, hypertension, and phenylketonuria (PKU)—and in some instances the medications used to treat these illnesses—may affect nutritional status and dietary needs. In illnesses that have resulted in nutritional deficits or that require dietary treatment (e.g., diabetes mellitus or PKU), it is preferable for nutritional care to begin and for optimal nutritional status to be achieved before conception, if possible.

PERSONAL HEALTH PRACTICES. Exercise patterns should be evaluated because they may influence health not only during pregnancy but also throughout life. Excessive exercise, as well as chronic dieting, can result in a decrease in body fat. In addition, smoking, alcohol intake, drug use, and excessive caffeine intake are personal habits that can adversely affect the fetus. *Smoking* has been shown to reduce birth weight and increase the incidence of fetal and neonatal death. Women who smoke should be strongly encouraged to stop, or if this proves impossible, to reduce their use of smoking materials. Full-blown *fetal alcohol syndrome (FAS),* a group of characteristics that includes abnormal facies, microcephaly, impaired growth, and learning disabilities, is generally seen only with heavy prenatal alcohol use. However, milder evidence of FAS has been reported with more moderate alcohol intake. (For further discussion, see Chapter 39.) At present, a safe level of alcohol intake during pregnancy is unknown, and abstinence is advisable. Illicit or controlled drugs and the life-styles commonly accompanying their use contribute to IUGR and other pregnancy complications (Institute of Medicine, 1990; Lindenberg et al, 1991). (For further discussion, see Chapter 33.) Every effort should be made to convince the pregnant drug user to cease the habit. The effects of *maternal caffeine* usage on the fetus are controversial, but the safest policy at present is to avoid caffeine or at least to limit intake to the equivalent of no more than 12 ounces (360 ml) of coffee daily.

Diet History

To provide a basis for intervention and teaching, the **diet history** should include assessment of both the client's diet and her knowledge and plans regarding feeding her infant. The woman's usual food and beverage intake (Fig. 9-3), adequacy of her income and other resources to meet her nutritional needs, any dietary modifications, food allergies and intolerances, and all medications and nutrition supplements taken should be ascertained. In addition, the pres-

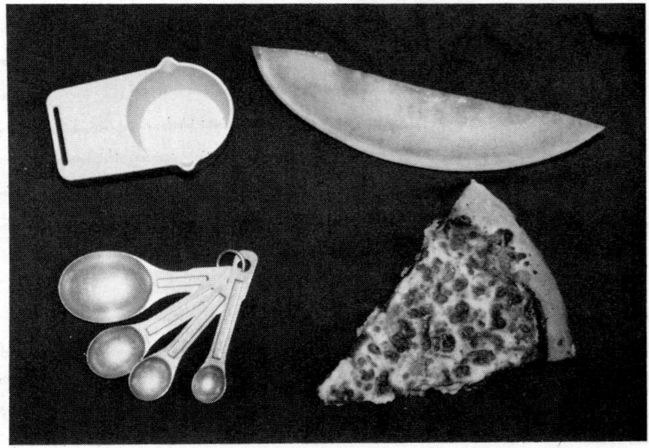

Fig. 9-3 Measuring utensils or sample servings, or both, help the woman to estimate portion sizes accurately.

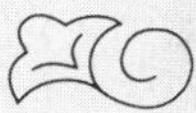 **Research Highlight** 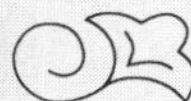

Dietary Practices and Pregnancy Discomforts

RESEARCH ABSTRACT

Discomforts of pregnancy are usually attributed to changes in hormonal and physiologic balance. Some of these discomforts may be due to improper diet. This study investigated the relationship between discomforts of pregnancy and dietary practices in a convenience sample (one easily accessible to the researchers) of 50 African-American women in a clinic population. Data collected were prenatal weight and hemoglobin levels, 24-hour recall of diet, and pregnancy discomforts assessed by a questionnaire. Subjects were interviewed twice: once during the first trimester and once during the third trimester. The researchers found that dietary intake of milk products, fruit and vegetables was low. Most subjects met the RDA for meat and bread/cereal. A number of subjects (20%) reported excessive intake of meat and citrus fruit in the first trimester and of meat, fruit, and bread/cereals in the third trimester. Increased intake of meat, noncitrus fruit, and iron was related to decreased weight gain in the third trimester. Increased intake of vegetables and vitamins and decreased intake of noncitrus fruit, as well as reduced cigarette smoking, were related to higher hemoglobin values in the third trimester. Subjects who had an increased intake of milk, green/yellow vegetables, citrus fruit, and bread/cereal in the third trimester had less nausea, heartburn, and constipation; were less tired; and had less difficulty sleeping. Those who had an increased intake of meat, noncitrus fruit, and vitamin and iron supplements and who smoked cigarettes had more nausea, vomiting, heartburn, and general and total discomfort.

IMPLICATIONS FOR PRACTICE

Food intake is related to discomforts in pregnancy. Nurses can use this information to counsel their clients who experience these discomforts. Counselors need to be aware of cultural variations in food preferences and socioeconomic factors that influence dietary intake.

RELATED RESEARCH QUESTIONS

1. Is there a relation between hemoglobin levels, food intake, and discomforts of pregnancy in other cultural/ethnic groups?
2. Does a nutritional educational program increase the number of women consuming a diet that meets recommended daily allowances of food?
3. Is there a relation between cigarette smoking and consumption of a diet that meets recommended daily allowances of food?
4. Do discomforts of pregnancy vary among cultural/ethnic groups?

REFERENCE

Gulick EE, Shaw V, Allison M: Dietary practices and pregnancy discomforts among urban blacks, *J Perinat* 9(3):271, 1989.

ence and severity of nutrition-related discomforts of pregnancy, such as morning sickness, constipation, and pyrosis, should be determined. The nurse should be alert to any evidence of eating disorders, for example, anorexia nervosa, bulimia, or frequent and rigorous dieting before or during pregnancy.

Cultural (including religious and ethnic) influences on dietary intake are extremely strong, although they may lessen if the woman and her family become more integrated into the dominant culture. Dietary practices of African-American women and pregnancy discomforts have been studied (see Research Highlight). Nutrition beliefs and practices of selected cultural groups are summarized in Table 9-4. **Pica,** the practice of consuming nonfood substances (e.g., clay, laundry starch) or excessive amounts of foodstuffs low in nutritional value (e.g., cornstarch, ice), often is influenced by the woman's cultural background (Lacey, 1990). In the United States it appears to be most common among African-American women, women from rural areas, and women with a family history of pica (Horner et al, 1991). Regular and heavy consumption of low-nutrient products may displace more nutritious foods from the diet, and the items consumed may interfere with absorption of nutrients, especially minerals. The presence of pica, as well as details of the type and amounts of products ingested, is likely to be discovered only by the sensitive interviewer who has developed a relationship of trust with the woman. It has been proposed that pica and **food cravings** (e.g., urge to have ice cream, pickles, pizza) during pregnancy are caused by an innate drive to consume nutrients missing from the diet. However, research indicates that this is not likely (Worthington-Roberts et al, 1989).

Another cultural impact on nutritional status is observing a **vegetarian diet.** It is important to find out from the vegetarian woman exactly what her diet entails. Foods basic to almost all vegetarian diets are

TABLE 9-4 Characteristic Food Patterns of Some Cultures

Ethnic Group	Milk Group	Protein Group	Fruits and Vegetables	Breads and Cereals	Possible Dietary Problems
Native American, (many tribal variations; many "Americanized")	Fresh milk Evaporated milk for cooking Ice cream Cream pies	Pork, beef, lamb, rabbit Fowl, fish, eggs Legumes Sunflower seeds Nuts: walnut, acorn, pine, peanut butter Game meat	Green peas, beans Beets, turnips, squash, peppers Leafy green and other vegetables	Refined bread Whole wheat Cornmeal Rice Dry cereals "Fry" bread Tortillas	Obesity, diabetes, alcoholism, nutritional deficiencies expressed in dental problems and iron deficiency anemia Inadequate amounts of all nutrients Excessive use of sugar
Middle Eastern* (Armenian, Greek, Syrian, Turkish)	Yogurt Little butter	Lamb Nuts Dried peas, beans, lentils Sesame seeds	Peppers, tomatoes, cabbage, grape leaves, cucumbers, squash Dried apricots, raisins, dates	Cracked wheat and dark bread	Fry many meats and vegetables Lack of fresh fruits Insufficient foods from milk group High consumption of sweetenings, lamb fat, and olive oil
African-American	Milk† Ice cream Cheese: longhorn, American	Pork: all cuts, plus organs, chitterlings Beef, lamb Chicken, giblets Eggs Nuts Legumes Fish, game	Leafy vegetables Green and yellow vegetables Potato: white, sweet Stewed fruit Bananas and other fresh fruit	Cornmeal and hominy grits Rice Biscuits, pancakes, white breads	Extensive use of frying, "smothering" in gravy, or simmering Fats: salt pork, bacon drippings, lard, and gravies High consumption of sweets Insufficient citrus Vegetables often boiled for long periods with pork fat and much salt Limited amounts from milk group†
Chinese (Cantonese most prevalent)	Milk: water buffalo	Pork sausage‡ Eggs and pigeon eggs Fish Lamb, beef, goat	Many vegetables Radish leaves Bean, bamboo sprouts	Rice/rice flour products Cereals, noodles Wheat, corn, millet seed	Tendency of some immigrants to use large amounts of grease in cooking

MSG, Monosodium L-glutomate.
*Religious holidays may involve fasting, which is believed to increase the likelihood of premature labor (Kaplan, Fidelman and Aboulafia 1983). Fasting requirement may be waived during pregnancy.
†Lactose intolerance relatively common in adults.
‡Lower in fat content than Western sausage.
§Milk and milk products not eaten with meat; milk may be taken before the meal or 6 hours after meal; different sets of dishes and silverware are used to serve milk and meat products.

TABLE 9-4 Characteristic Food Patterns of Some Cultures—cont'd

Ethnic Group	Milk Group	Protein Group	Fruits and Vegetables	Breads and Cereals	Possible Dietary Problems
Chinese (Cantonese most prevalent)—cont'd		Fowl: chicken, duck Nuts Legumes Soybean curd (tofu)			Limited use of milk and milk products Often low in protein, calories, or both May wash rice before cooking, removing vitamins added in fortification Soy sauce (high sodium)
Polish	Milk Sour cream Cheese Butter	Pork (preferred) Chicken	Vegetables Cabbage Roots Fruits	Dark rye	Sodium in ham, sausages, pickles High consumption of sweets Tendency to overcook vegetables Limited fruits (especially citrus), raw vegetables, and meats
Puerto Rican	Limited use of milk products Coffee with milk (*café con leche*)	Pork Poultry Eggs (Fridays) Beans (*habichuelas*)	Avocado, okra Eggplant Sweet yams Starchy vegetables and fruits (*viandas*)	Rice Cornmeal	Small amounts of pork and poultry Extensive use of fat, lard, salt pork, and olive oil Lack of milk products
Scandinavian: Danish, Finnish, Norwegian, Swedish	Cream Butter Cheeses	Wild game Reindeer Fish (fresh or dried) Eggs	Berries Dried fruit Vegetables: cole slaw, roots	Whole wheat, rye, barley, sweets (cookies and sweet breads)	Insufficient fresh fruits and vegetables High consumption of sweets, pickled, salted meats and fish Liberal use of fat
Southeast Asian: Vietnamese, Cambodian	Generally not taken Coffee with condensed cow's milk Plain yogurt Ice cream (rare) Soybean milk	Fish (daily): fresh, dried, salted Poultry/eggs: duck, chicken Pork Beef (seldom) Dry beans Tofu	Seasonal variety: fresh or preserved Green, leafy vegetables Yams Corn	Rice: grains, flour, noodles French bread "Cellophane" (bean starch) noodles	Fresh milk products generally not consumed Poultry/eggs may be limited Meat considered "unclean" is avoided Preference for a diet high in salt and pepper as well as rice and pork High intake of MSG and soy sauce

Continued.

TABLE 9-4 Characteristic Food Patterns of Some Cultures—cont'd

Ethnic Group	Milk Group	Meat and Alternatives	Fruits and Vegetables	Breads and Cereals	Possible Dietary Problems
Jewish: Orthodox*	Milk§ Cheese§	Meat (bloodless; Kosher prepared): beef, lamb, goat, deer, poultry (all types), no pork Fish with fins and scales only No crustaceans	Wide variety	Wide variety	High intake of sodium in meat products
Filipino (Spanish-Chinese influence)	Flavored milk, milk in coffee Cheese: gouda, cheddar	Pork, beef, goat, deer, rabbit Chicken Fish Eggs, nuts, legumes	Many vegetables and fruits	Rice, cooked cereals Noodles: rice, wheat	Limited use of milk and milk products Tendency to prewash rice Tendency to have only small portions of protein foods
Italian	Cheese Some ice cream	Meat Eggs Dried beans	Leafy vegetables Potatoes Eggplant, tomatoes, peppers Fruits	Pasta White breads, some whole wheat Farina Cereals	Prefer expensive imported cheeses; reluctant to substitute less expensive domestic varieties Tendency to overcook vegetables Limited use of whole grains High consumption of sweets Extensive use of olive oil Insufficient servings from milk group
Japanese (Isei, more Japanese influence; Nisei, more westernized)	Increasing amounts being used by younger generations	Pork, beef, chicken Fish Eggs Legumes: soya, red, lima beans Tofu Nuts	Many vegetables and fruits Seaweed	Rice, rice cakes Wheat noodles Refined bread, noodles	Excessive sodium: pickles, salty crisp seaweed, MSG, and soy sauce Insufficient servings from milk group May use prewashed rice
Hispanic, Mexican-American	Milk Cheese Flan, ice cream	Beef, pork, lamb, chicken, tripe, hot sausage, beef intestines Fish Eggs Nuts Dry beans: pinto, chickpeas (often eaten more than once daily)	Spinach, wild greens, tomatoes, chilies, corn, cactus leaves, cabbage, avocado, potatoes Pumpkin, zapote, peaches, guava, papaya, citrus	Rice, cornmeal Sweet bread, pastries Tortilla: corn, flour Vermicelli (*fideo*)	Limited meats primarily because of cost Limited use of milk and milk products Large amounts of lard Abundant use of sugar Tendency to boil vegetables for long periods

vegetables, fruits, legumes, nuts and seeds, and grains. However, there are many variations in vegetarian diets. *Strict vegetarians or vegans,* consume only plant products. Because vitamin B_{12} is found only in foods of animal origin, deficiency of this vitamin is a potential problem for strict vegetarians unless a supplement is taken or vitamin B_{12}-fortified foods are consumed. Vitamin B_{12} deficiency can result in megaloblastic anemia, glossitis, and neurologic deficits in the mother. Infants born to affected mothers are likely to have megaloblastic anemia and neurodevelopmental delays. *Lactovegetarians* include milk and milk products, and *lacto-ovovegetarians* consume milk, milk products, and eggs, as well as plant products. Fish is included in the *pesco-vegetarian* diet.

In general, the more types of foods included, the more likely the woman is to have an adequate diet. Calcium intake is often low in women who do not use milk products. Protein intake should be assessed especially carefully. Plant proteins tend to be "incomplete," or lacking in one or more amino acid required for growth and maintenance of body tissues. However, combinations of different types of complementary incomplete proteins, in which one protein source will be rich in an amino acid that the other protein source lacks, and vice versa, can provide sufficient amounts of complete protein. Fig. 9-4 demonstrates **complementary protein** combinations. It is probably not essential that complementary proteins be consumed at the same meal; that is, it is sufficient that the woman consume wheat muffins at breakfast and bean cakes at lunch. However, it is an excellent practice to become accustomed to planning meals around complementary proteins to ensure that the diet is balanced and that all types of protein foods are included.

The impact of food allergies and intolerances on nutritional status ranges from very important to almost nil. Lactose intolerance, or inability to digest the carbohydrate in milk, is of special concern during pregnancy and lactation because no other food group equals milk and milk products in calcium content. If lactose intolerance is reported, the interviewer should explore intake of other calcium sources (Table 9-1).

The assessment must include evaluation of the woman's financial status and knowledge of sound dietary practices. The quality of the diet increases with increasing socioeconomic status and educational level. The box on pp. 228 and 229 shows a tool that can be used for obtaining diet history information.

INFANT FEEDING. Many women make the decision to breast-feed or bottle-feed their infants prior to or early in pregnancy (Kaufman, Hall, 1989). Thus it is important to explore the woman's knowledge and opinions about infant feeding as early as possible to provide a basis for correcting any misinformation, supplying additional information, and providing support to the woman in her choice of feeding method.

PHYSICAL EXAMINATION. **Anthropometric** (body) **measurements** provide both short- and long-term in-

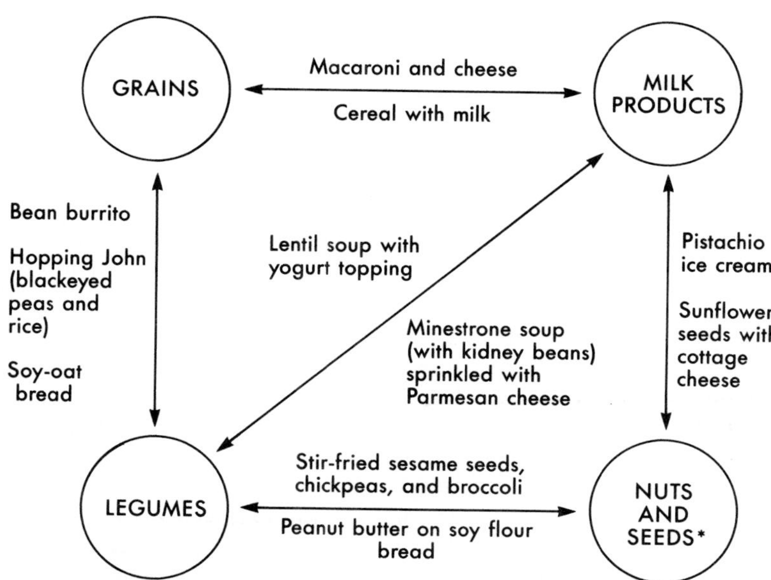

Fig. 9-4 Complementary proteins. The circled items are major types of protein in many vegetarian diets. Items connected by arrows are complementary. Examples of dishes providing complementary proteins are given beside the arrows.

Tool For Diet History

Name____________________________________Age__________Date____________________
Height________Weight before pregnancy________Cultural background____________________
Occupation______________________________Occupation of husband or significant other (if living in the household or providing support)____________________

EXERCISE/ACTIVITY

Does the client obtain regular (at least 3 days/wk) exercise involving rhythmic, repeated movements of large muscle groups? How much activity does her work entail?

DIET

Is the client on any special diet regimen (e.g., low salt, diabetic, low cholesterol, weight reduction)?
Is there any food the client cannot eat? What happens when she eats this food?
Does the client have any food cravings? If so, what foods?
Does the client have cravings for or eat such things as ice, clay, or cornstarch?

GASTROINTESTINAL FUNCTION

Does the client experience nausea and vomiting? If so, when does it usually occur and how often?
Does the client report diarrhea, constipation, or heartburn?

HEALTH HABITS

Does the client smoke? If so, how many cigarettes per day?
Does she drink beer, wine, or other alcoholic beverages? If so, how much and how often?
Does she use illicit or controlled drugs? If so, what and how often?

MEDICATIONS

Does the client take any prescription or over-the-counter drugs? (Ask about vitamin-mineral supplements, if not mentioned by the client.)

WIC, Women, infants, and children.
*Avoid asking about specific meals, for example, "What do you usually eat for breakfast?" This may cue the client to respond with the "right" answer. It is preferable to ask, "On a typical day, what would be the first thing that you would eat or drink?" "When would that be?" "When would you next eat or drink something?"

dications of nutritional status and are thus essential to the assessment. At a minimum, the woman's height and weight must be determined on her first entry into the health care system, and her weight must be measured regularly thereafter (See discussion of BMI, p. 217).

A careful physical examination can reveal objective signs of malnutrition (Table 9-5). It is important to note, however, that some of these signs are nonspecific and that the physiologic changes of pregnancy may complicate the interpretation of physical findings. For example, lower extremity edema often occurs in calorie and protein deficiency, but it may also be a normal finding in the third trimester of pregnancy. Interpretation of physical findings is made easier by a thorough health history and by laboratory testing (where necessary).

SIGNS OF POTENTIAL PROBLEMS. The woman must be monitored throughout pregnancy for complications that may be nutrition-related, and reassessment of the diet and health practices should occur at the first sign of one of these problems. Of particular concern are deviations from the usual values for either prepregnant weight or weight gain during pregnancy. The following categories are considered to be deviations from the norm.

UNDERWEIGHT (PREPREGNANT BMI <19.8). Women who are underweight before pregnancy are more likely than women of normal weight to experience preterm labor and to deliver LBW (<2500 g) infants (Frentzen et al, 1987; Frentzen et al, 1988).

OVERWEIGHT (PREPREGNANT BMI >26.0). Hypertension is an especially common finding among obese pregnant women. Women who weigh

Tool For Diet History—cont'd

HOUSEHOLD AND ECONOMIC CONSIDERATIONS

How much money is spent each week for food in the client's household? How many does this feed? Who does the shopping?

Is the client receiving food stamps or WIC vouchers?

Does the client eat away from home? How often? Where (e.g., fast food restaurant, full service restaurant, vending machines)?

What food preparation and storage equipment is available to the client (refrigerator, hot plate, cooktop, oven)? Who does the cooking?

FOOD INTAKE

What is a typical day's intake for the client?* Include preparation methods and approximate portion sizes of all foods and beverages. (Question client specifically about the following topics if not mentioned: beverage intake, including number of cups of coffee, consumption of soft drinks, use of alcoholic beverages, frequency of water intake; addition of sugar or artificial sweeteners, butter or margarine, cream, dressings, sauces, or gravies to foods and drinks; desserts and snacks—what is consumed and how much.)

	Food Consumed	Amount	How Prepared
Early morning			
Midmorning			
Noon			
Afternoon			
Evening			
Night			

INFANT FEEDING

Does the client plan to breast- or bottle-feed? How did she feed any previous children? If she wishes to breast-feed, are there any family members or friends who have breast-fed who can offer her support and advice? Do her family and friends support her decision to breast-feed? If she chooses to bottle-feed, is she eligible to receive formula through the WIC program?

more than 77.3 kg (170 lb) experience the highest fetal death rates of any weight category (National Center for Health Statistics, 1986).

INADEQUATE GAIN DURING SECOND AND THIRD TRIMESTERS. This includes gain of < 1 kg (2.2 lb) per month by normal-weight or underweight women and gain of < 0.5 kg (1.1 lb) per month by obese women. Maternal weight gain, at least for normal-weight and underweight women, is directly related to infant birth weight and thus to pregnancy outcome (National Center for Health Statistics, 1986; Frentzen et al, 1988; Aaronson, MacNee, 1989; Abrams et al, 1989). Failure to gain adequate weight or actual weight loss can contribute to reduced size of the placenta, IUGR, preterm birth, and increased fetal and neonatal mortality. Inadequate gain is most often the result of inadequate intake. Possible causes of inadequate intake include poverty, lack of understanding of the importance of weight gain during pregnancy or placing a priority on maintaining a slim physique, or both, cultural proscriptions that interfere with following a nutritious diet, nausea and vomiting that continue past the first trimester, alcohol or drug abuse, and concurrent maternal illness (e.g., malignancy, inflammatory bowel disease, or other diseases causing malabsorption). Smoking depresses the appetite and consequently may reduce maternal intake. Young adolescent and African-American mothers are especially likely to deliver LBW infants. Therefore their weight gain goal should be at the upper end of the recommended range for their BMI (Institute of Medicine, 1990).

EXCESSIVE GAIN. This includes a gain of 3 kg

TABLE 9-5 Physical Assessment of Nutritional Status

Signs of Good Nutrition	Signs of Poor Nutrition
General appearance	
Alert, responsive, energetic, good endurance	Listless, apathetic, cachectic, easily fatigued, looks tired
Weight	
Normal for height, age, body build	Overweight or underweight
Posture	
Erect, arms and legs straight	Sagging shoulders, sunken chest, humped back
Muscles	
Well developed, firm, good tone, some fat under skin	Flaccid, poor tone, undeveloped, tender, "wasted" appearance
Nervous control	
Good attention span, not irritable or restless, normal reflexes, psychologic stability	Inattentive, irritable, confused, burning and tingling of hands and feet, loss of position and vibratory sense, weakness and tenderness of muscles, decrease or loss of ankle and knee reflexes
Gastrointestinal function	
Good appetite and digestion, normal regular elimination, no palpable organs or masses	Anorexia, indigestion, constipation or diarrhea, liver or spleen enlargement
Cardiovascular function	
Normal heart rate and rhythm, no murmurs, normal blood pressure for age	Rapid heart rate, enlarged heart, abnormal rhythm, elevated blood pressure
Hair	
Shiny, lustrous, firm, not easily plucked, healthy scalp	Stringy, dull, brittle, dry, thin and sparse, depigmented, can be easily plucked

Modified from Williams SR: Nutritional guidance in prenatal care. In Worthington-Roberts BS, Williams SR: *Nutrition in pregnancy and lactation,* ed 4, St Louis, 1989, Mosby–Year Book.

(6.6 lb) or more per month. Rapid weight gain occurs with tissue fluid retention, possibly indicating the onset of PIH. Signs of PIH include hypertension, proteinuria, and excessive edema, especially edema of the hands and face. The role of diet in the cause of PIH remains unclear. Although poor protein intake was once believed to be the primary nutrition-related factor contributing to development of PIH, deficits in other nutrients, including calcium, sodium, and vitamins E and A, also have been thought to play a role. The relationship between these nutrients and PIH has not been established, but the current belief is that a diet adequate in all nutrients is associated with reduced risk of PIH. (Chapter 28 provides further information.)

Multifetal gestation, which imposes increased nutritional needs on the mother, is another cause of unusually large weight gain. Excessive caloric intake may also be a factor. Undesirably large weight gain contributes to mechanical complications of pregnancy and labor (see discussion of dystocia in Chapter 35). For example, cesarean and forcep-assisted births and vacuum extractions occur more often in women with very high weight gain. Short women < 157 cm or 62 in tall) are especially susceptible to these mechanical problems with excessive weight gain and should have a weight gain target near the lower limits of the recommended range for their BMI (Institute of Medicine, 1990).

OTHER NUTRITION-RELATED COMPLICATIONS. These include severe nausea and vomiting, which compromise nutritional intake, especially if they continue past the first trimester of pregnancy (hyperemesis gravidarum), and anemia. *Iron deficiency anemia* is the most common anemia of pregnancy. Women of childbearing age often have poor

TABLE 9-5 Physical Assessment of Nutritional Status—cont'd

Signs of Good Nutrition	Signs of Poor Nutrition
Skin (general)	
Smooth, slightly moist, good color	Rough, dry, scaly, pale, pigmented, irritated, easily bruised, petechiae
Face and neck	
Skin color uniform, smooth, pink, healthy appearance; no enlargement of thyroid gland; lips not chapped or swollen	Scaly, swollen, skin dark over cheeks and under eyes, lumpiness or flakiness of skin around nose and mouth; thyroid enlarged; lips swollen, angular lesions or fissures at corners of mouth
Oral cavity	
Reddish pink mucous membranes and gums; no swelling or bleeding of gums; tongue healthy pink or deep reddish in appearance, not swollen or smooth, surface papillae present; teeth bright and clean, no cavities, no pain, no discoloration	Gums spongy, bleed easily, inflamed or receding; tongue swollen, scarlet and raw, magenta color, beefy, hyperemic and hypertrophic papillae, atrophic papillae; teeth with unfilled caries, absent teeth, worn surfaces, mottled.
Eyes	
Bright, clear, shiny, no sores at corners of eyelids, membranes moist and healthy pink color, no prominent blood vessels or mound of tissue (Bitot's spots) on sclera, no fatigue circles beneath	Eye membranes pale, redness of membrane, dryness, signs of infection, Bitot's spots, redness and fissuring of eyelid corners, dryness of eye membrane, dull appearance of cornea, soft cornea, blue sclerae
Extremities	
No tenderness, weakness, or swelling; nails firm and pink	Edema, tender calf, tingling, weakness; nails spoon-shaped, brittle
Skeleton	
No malformations	Bowlegs, knock-knees, chest deformity at diaphragm, beaded ribs, prominent scapulas

iron stores; when coupled with the need for increased iron to provide for the increased blood volume of pregnancy, this can result in anemia. Folate deficiency (associated with macrocytic or megaloblastic anemia) also occurs in some pregnant women.

LABORATORY TESTING. The only nutrition-related laboratory testing needed by the majority of pregnant women is a hematocrit or hemoglobin measurement to screen for the presence of anemia. The woman may need additional testing on the basis of her history or physical findings. This includes a glucose tolerance test to rule out gestational diabetes, a complete blood cell count with a differential to identify megaloblastic anemia, and measurement of specific vitamins or minerals believed to be lacking in the diet.

NURSING DIAGNOSES

Nutrition-related nursing diagnoses that commonly arise from the assessment include the following:

- Altered nutrition: Less than body requirements
  —This can be related to a poor understanding of the nutritional needs and optimal weight gain during pregnancy, inadequate income, stress over an unwanted pregnancy, nausea and vomiting (either the mild to moderate effects of morning sickness or the more severe effects of hyperemesis gravidarum), cultural patterns of food intake, adherence to a therapeutic diet regimen, concurrent use of medications, drug or alcohol abuse, failure to take nutritional supplements as prescribed, smoking, multife-

tal gestation, or adolescent pregnancy, in which the increased needs of pregnancy are imposed on a girl whose own needs for growth and maturation are still high and whose eating habits are often poor.

- Altered nutrition: More than body requirements
  —Related factors include a poor understanding of nutritional needs and optimal weight gain during pregnancy, with resultant overeating, cultural patterns that foster overeating, a decline in activity as pregnancy progresses, and use of unneeded dietary supplements (particularly supplements of fat-soluble vitamins).
- Altered nutrition: High risk for more than body requirements
  —Contributing factors are the same as for preceding diagnosis.
- Constipation
  —This problem may be related to a decrease in activity with pregnancy, inadequate fiber or fluid intake, use of an iron supplement, displacement of the intestines by the enlarging uterus, and increased progesterone levels during pregnancy, which decrease the tone and motility of the intestinal musculature.

PLANNING

An individualized nursing care plan based on the nursing diagnoses should be developed in collaboration with the client. Some common nutrition-related goals are for the client to take the following actions:

1. Achieve an appropriate weight gain during pregnancy. An appropriate goal for weight gain takes into account such factors as prepregnancy weight, presence of overweight/obesity or underweight, and whether the pregnancy is single or multifetal.
2. Consume adequate nutrients from the diet and supplements to meet estimated needs.
3. Cope with nutrition-related discomforts associated with pregnancy, such as pyrosis (heartburn), morning sickness, and constipation.
4. Avoid or reduce potentially harmful practices such as smoking, alcohol consumption, and caffeine intake.
5. Make an informed decision about the method of feeding her infant. This decision must be one with which the mother (and usually her family members or other members of her support system) is satisfied, and not necessarily the choice that would seem best to the health care team.
6. Return to prepregnancy weight (or an appropriate weight for height) within 6 months of delivery.

IMPLEMENTATION

Nutritional care and teaching generally involve (1) acquainting the woman with nutritional needs during pregnancy and the characteristics of an adequate diet, if necessary, (2) helping her to individualize her diet so that she achieves an adequate intake while satisfying her personal, cultural, financial, and health needs, (3) acquainting her with strategies for coping with the nutrition-related discomforts of pregnancy, (4) helping her to use nutrition supplements appropriately, (5) discussing with her the advantages and disadvantages of breast-feeding or formula feeding her infant and supporting her in her decision (see Chapter 22), and (6) consulting with and making referrals to other professionals or services as indicated.

Adequate Dietary Intake

Diet teaching can take place in a one-on-one interview or in a group setting. In either case, it should emphasize the importance of choosing a varied diet composed of readily available foods (rather than specialized diet supplements).

PREGNANCY. The pregnant woman must understand what adequate weight gain during pregnancy means, recognize the reasons for its importance, and be able to evaluate her own gain in terms of the desirable pattern. Many women, particularly those who have worked hard to control their weight before pregnancy, may find it difficult to understand why the weight gain goal is so high when a newborn infant is so small. The nurse can explain that maternal weight gain consists of increments in the weight of many tissues, not just the growing fetus (see Fig 9-2 and p. 214). Nutrition intervention is particularly important in twin gestation (see Research Highlight, p. 233).

Dietary overindulgence, on the other hand, which may result in excessive fat stores that persist after delivery, should be discouraged. Nevertheless, it is best not to focus unduly on weight gain, which can result in feelings of stress and guilt in the woman who does not follow the preferred pattern of gain. Teaching regarding weight gain during pregnancy is summarized in the box on p. 233.

POSTPARTUM. The need for a varied diet with representation from all food groups continues throughout lactation. Because of deposition of energy stores, the woman with optimal weight gain during pregnancy is heavier after delivery than at the beginning of pregnancy. A weight reduction diet is not recommended during lactation inasmuch as it may interfere with milk production or impair maternal nutri-

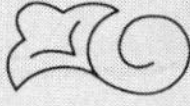
Research Highlight
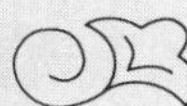

Nutrition Intervention in Twin Pregnancy

RESEARCH ABSTRACT

Pregnancy outcomes of 354 twins treated with the Higgins Nutrition Intervention Program and 686 untreated twins were compared. The Program consists of assessing a pregnant woman's risk profile for adverse birth outcomes and providing an individualized nutrition program based on the profile. Additional calories and protein allowances are provided for each fetus: an additional 1000 kcal and 50 g of protein each day. Data were collected through a review of medical records of twins born at 18 hospitals who had been treated with the nutrition intervention. The untreated group was randomly selected from the same hospitals. The researchers found that the twins in the treated group weighed an average of 80 g more than the untreated twins at birth and that their rate of infants of very low birth weight was 25% lower. The rate of preterm delivery was 30% lower in the treated group, but the rate of intrauterine growth retardation was similar. Both early neonatal mortality and maternal morbidity were lower in the treated group. The authors concluded that a nutritional program significantly improved the outcome of the twin pregnancies.

IMPLICATIONS FOR PRACTICE

Increase in caloric intake is recommended during pregnancy to provide for the needs of the fetus. When there are two or more fetuses, a corresponding increase in caloric and protein intake is necessary. Mothers may not ingest enough calories and protein to compensate for the additional requirements of a multifetal pregnancy. Birth weight and maternal weight gain have a positive relationship, and the incidence of low birth weight and intrauterine growth retardation are higher in twins. Thus, increasing the weight gain of mothers by increasing caloric and protein intake may reduce the incidence of low weight and growth-retarded infants. In their contacts with women whose pregnancies are multifetal, nurses should provide counseling or refer the women to nutritionists so that adequate nutritional intake is ensured.

RELATED RESEARCH QUESTIONS

1. Will an educational program about nutrition increase weight gain in multifetal pregnancies?
2. Is there a relationship between quality of nutritional intake and weight gain in multifetal pregnancies?
3. What is the average weight gain in multifetal pregnancies of women who carried the infants to term?
4. Is there a relation between prepregnancy weight and weight gain during pregnancy?

REFERENCE

Dubois S et al: Twin pregnancy: the impact of the Higgins Nutrition Intervention Program on maternal and neonatal outcomes, *Am J Clin Nutr* 53:1397, 1991.

tional status. As a result of the caloric demands of lactation, however, the mother who avoids dietary excesses and consumes only moderately more (approximately 500 calories) than she did before pregnancy will usually experience a gradual but steady weight loss. The woman who does not breast-feed will lose weight gradually if she consumes a balanced diet but one that provides slightly less than her daily energy expenditure. Fat is the most concentrated source of calories in the diet (9 kcal/g, vs. 4 kcal/g in carbohydrates and proteins), and fat calories are more efficiently converted into fat stores than are calories from carbohydrate or protein. Therefore the first step in weight reduction (or controlling excessive weight gain) is to evaluate sources of fat in the diet and explore with the client ways of reducing them. Even foods such as vegetables that are originally low in fat can become high in fat when fried or sauteed, served with excessive amounts of salad dressing, consumed with high-fat dips or sauces, or seasoned with butter or bacon drippings. A desirable rate of loss for the

TEACHING Weight Gain During Pregnancy

- Progressive weight gain during pregnancy is essential for normal fetal growth and development and for deposition of maternal stores that promote successful lactation.
- Recommended weight gain during pregnancy is determined largely by prepregnancy weight for height.
  Normal-weight women: 11-16.5 kg (25-35 lb)
  Underweight women: 12.5-18 kg (28-40 lb)
  Overweight women: 7-11.5 kg (15-25 lb)
- Weight gain should be achieved through a balanced diet of regular foods chosen from all of the different food groups (Table 9-3).
- The pattern of weight gain is important: approximately 0.4 kg (0.9-1 lb) per week during the second and third trimesters for normal-weight women. 0.5 kg (1.1 lb) per week for underweight women, and 0.3 kg (0.67 lb) per week for overweight women.

nonlactating mother is approximately 1 to 2 pounds per week.

DAILY FOOD GUIDE AND MENU PLANNING. The daily food plan (Table 9-3 and Fig 9-5) can be used as a guide for educating the woman regarding nutritional needs during pregnancy and lactation. This food plan is general enough to be used by individuals from a wide variety of cultures, including those following a vegetarian diet. One of the more helpful teaching strategies is to assist the client to plan daily menus that follow the food plan and are affordable, that are realistic in terms of preparation time, and that are compatible with personal preferences and cultural practices. This activity is often especially difficult for the nurse whose socioeconomic or cultural background is very different from that of the client. Table 9-4 and some of the sources in the bibliography at the end of the chapter provide information regarding dietary practices of different ethnic and cultural groups. U.S. government publications* are one source of sound information and useful teaching materials for the nurse or dietitian working with women from lower socioeconomic groups.

THERAPEUTIC DIETS. Modifications may have to be made in the food plan for women on special therapeutic diets. For instance, the pregnant woman following a low-cholesterol/low saturated fat diet plan for treatment or prevention of heart disease will usually find that three to four servings of milk products and two servings of meat exceed her daily allowance of cholesterol and saturated fat. In this case, she can be advised to substitute plant proteins for meats as often as possible; to avoid liver, brains, and other organ meats; to substitute low-fat fish or skinned turkey or chicken for red meats; to use skim milk products in preference to whole or low fat; to use egg substitutes or egg whites rather than whole eggs (because egg yolk is rich in cholesterol and saturated fat, but egg white contains none; two egg whites equal one whole egg in cooking); and/or to substitute a calcium supplement for all or part of the milk group servings.

Similarly, the woman with diabetes will require a diet tailored to her individual needs. Because fetal deformity and death are more common in pregnancies complicated by hyperglycemia or hypoglycemia, every effort should be made to maintain blood glucose levels in the normal range throughout pregnancy. All pregnant women with diabetes, whether the condition has been diagnosed before pregnancy or develops during pregnancy (gestational diabetes), should meet with a dietitian for diet planning and instruction. The woman with diabetes should have a food plan that includes four to six meals and snacks daily, with the daily carbohydrate intake distributed fairly evenly among those meals and snacks. The complex carbohydrates—fibers and starches—should be well represented in the diet of the diabetic woman, because complex carbohydrates tend to have a reduced "glycemic index" compared with simple carbohydrates such as sucrose (table sugar) and lactose. The glycemic index is an indication of the excursion of the blood sugar after a particular food is eaten. Foods with a lower glycemic index produce a lower peak blood glucose level, partly because they are relatively slowly digested and thus are absorbed gradually. To maintain strict control of blood glucose, the pregnant diabetic woman usually must monitor her own blood glucose daily. Urine glucose and ketone measurements are not sensitive enough to detect hyperglycemia accurately and provide no information about hypoglycemia. The nurse must teach the woman self-monitoring of blood glucose unless the woman has been doing this before pregnancy.

Coping with Nutrition-Related Discomforts of Pregnancy

The most common nutrition-related discomforts of pregnancy are nausea and vomiting, or "morning sickness," constipation, and pyrosis, or heartburn.

NAUSEA AND VOMITING. These symptoms are most common during the first trimester. In most cases, nausea and vomiting cause only mild to moderate problems. The pregnant woman may find the following suggestions helpful.

- Eat dry, starchy foods such as dry toast, Melba toast, or crackers on awakening in the morning and at other times when nausea occurs.
- Avoid excessive amounts of fluids early in the day or when nausea is present (but compensate by drinking fluids at other times).
- Eat small amounts frequently and avoid large meals.
- Avoid skipping meals and thus becoming extremely hungry, which may worsen nausea.
- Decrease intake of fatty foods.
- Avoid cooking odors as much as possible.
- Choose, during periods of nausea, foods served at cool temperature and foods with little aroma.

A sample daily food plan, which follows these guidelines while providing an adequate diet for the pregnant woman, is shown in the box on p. 235.

Occasionally, hyperemesis gravidarum will occur, causing fluid and electrolyte imbalances and seriously impairing nutritional intake. In some instances,

*Available through the Consumer Information Center, P.O. Box 100, Pueblo, CO 81002.

total parenteral nutrition (balanced intravenous feedings of amino acids, carbohydrate, lipid, vitamins, and minerals) has been used to nourish women with hyperemesis gravidarum when nutritional status was severely imperiled.

CONSTIPATION. Improved bowel function generally results from increasing the intake of fiber in the diet, because fiber helps to retain water within the stool, creating a bulky stool that stimulates intestinal peristalsis. An adequate fluid intake serves as an adjunct to the fiber. Making a habit of regular exercise that uses large muscle groups (walking, swimming, cycling) also helps to stimulate bowel motility.

PYROSIS. Reflux from the stomach into the esophagus can be minimized by the consumption of small, frequent feedings, rather than two or three larger meals daily; avoiding fluid intake with meals (but drinking plenty of fluids between feedings) inasmuch as fluids increase the distention of the stomach; avoiding lying down immediately after eating; and making sure that clothing does not bind across the abdomen.

Food Plan for a Woman with Nausea and Vomiting During Early Pregnancy

Breakfast

Toasted oat bran bagel, plain

Midmorning

Blueberry muffin
Skim milk

Lunch

Chickpea-pasta salad
Carrot sticks
Melon balls
Water

Afternoon

Vegetable juice
Rice cake

Dinner

Baked chicken with skin removed
Spinach salad
Butternut squash casserole
Skim milk

After dinner

Wheat bran cereal
Strawberries
Skim milk

Counseling Regarding Iron Supplementation

The nutritional supplement most commonly needed during pregnancy is iron. A variety of dietary factors can affect the completeness of absorption of an iron supplement. If bran, milk, egg yolk, coffee, tea, or oxalate-containing vegetables such as spinach and Swiss chard are consumed at the same time as iron, they inhibit iron absorption. Conversely, iron absorption is promoted by a diet rich in vitamin C sources (e.g., citrus fruits or melons) or "heme iron" (found in red meats, fish, and poultry). Iron supplements are best absorbed on an empty stomach. Thus they can be taken between meals with beverages other than milk, tea, or coffee. Some women have gastrointestinal discomfort when they take the supplement on an empty stomach; a good time for them to take the supplement is just before bedtime. Iron supplements should be kept away from any children in the household because their ingestion could result in acute iron poisoning and even death. The teaching box below summarizes the important points of teaching about iron supplementation.

Referral for Additional Services

The nurse functions as part of a team of health professionals. The registered dietitian (RD) is one member of the team who can be especially valuable

TEACHING Iron Supplementation

- It is difficult to consume enough iron in the diet to meet iron needs and prevent anemia during pregnancy
- Vitamin C (in citrus fruits, tomatoes, melons, and strawberries) and heme iron (in meats) increase iron supplement absorption. Include these in the diet often.
- Bran, tea, coffee, milk, oxalates (in spinach and Swiss chard), and egg yolk decrease iron absorption. Avoid consuming them at the same time as the supplement.
- Iron is best absorbed if it is taken when the stomach is empty; that is, take it between meals with a beverage other than tea, coffee, or milk.
- Iron can be taken at bedtime if abdominal discomfort occurs when it is taken between meals.
- Keep the supplement in a child-proof container out of the reach of any children in the household.

when the nutritional assessment indicates that there is a nutritional alteration or a high risk for such a problem. The RD is also helpful for women who require extensive diet instruction (e.g., women with gestational diabetes or PKU).

Where family income is limited, the nurse can refer the client to the Special Supplemental Program for Women, Infants, and Children (WIC). WIC provides pregnant and lactating women, as well as infants and children at nutritional risk, with vouchers for selected foods and with food stamps.

EVALUATION

In developing the nursing care plan, it is essential to set concrete, measurable goals, to evaluate progress toward these goals regularly, and to revise the plan of care if the goals are not met. Common goals are listed on p. 232.

In evaluating the adequacy of nutritional intake during pregnancy, the client's weight gain can be compared with standardized grids showing optimal patterns (Institute of Medicine, 1990). It is helpful to remember that these grids are based on mean data and do not always account for factors such as ethnic or racial variations. To evaluate the adequacy of the woman's diet it can be compared with the plan in Table 9-3. Again it is essential that individual factors affecting nutritional needs and dietary intake be considered. Physical examination and laboratory testing (see Assessment) can be used to confirm that nutritional status is adequate. For example, a hematocrit greater than 35% and a hemoglobin concentration greater than 11.5 g/dL are indicators that iron intake is adequate to prevent anemia. When weight gain is found to be inadequate or nutritional deficits appear, it is essential that the nurse reassess the client and her understanding of her nutritional needs, reinforce teaching as needed, and continue to reevaluate regularly.

The case study (p. 238) and nursing plan of care (p. 239) provide an example of goal setting, intervention, and evaluation for the pregnant woman with nutrition-related problems.

Food Nutrition Pyramid

In 1992, the United States adopted a pyramid of five food groups (Fig. 9-5). The pyramid places the

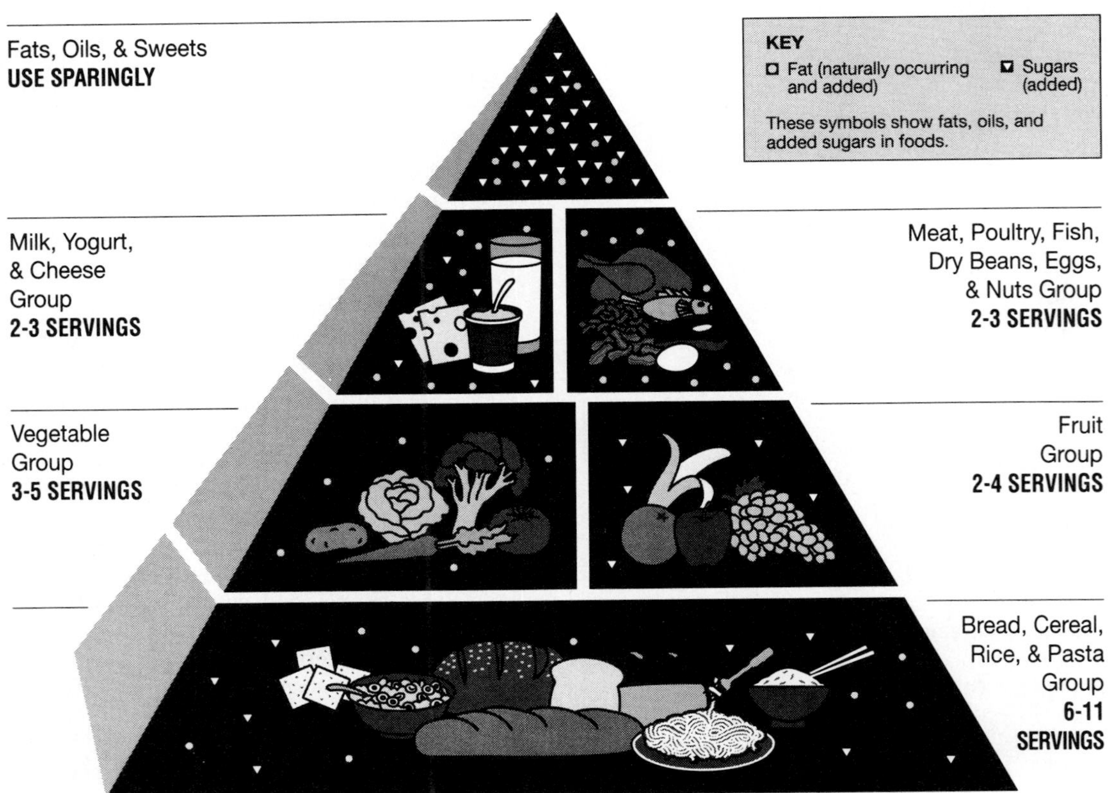

Fig 9-5 Food guide pyramid: a guide to daily food choices.
Courtesy of Department of Agriculture, Washington, DC.

bread, cereal, rice, and pasta group at its base; six to eleven servings are recommended each day. Vegetables (three to five servings) and fruits (two to four servings [now two groups instead of one]) are just above the grains group. The milk, yogurt, and cheese group (two to three servings) and the meat, poultry, fish, dry beans, eggs, and nuts group (two to three servings) form a narrow band near the top of the pyramid. At the apex are fats, oils, and sweets (not considered a food group), which are to be used sparingly. The serving sizes and numbers of servings are not yet specified for pregnancy and lactation.

■ SUMMARY

Maternal nutritional status before and during pregnancy has a major influence on outcome of pregnancy. Nutritional needs of most women can be met through a balanced, varied diet. If maternal diet is poor or significant nutritional risk factors are present, vitamin-mineral supplementation is recommended.

REFERENCES

Abrams B, Parker JD: Maternal weight gain in women with good pregnancy outcome, *Obstet Gynecol* 76:1, 1990.

Abrams B et al: Maternal weight gain and preterm delivery, *Obstet Gynecol* 74:577, 1989.

Berger A: Effects of caffeine consumption on pregnancy outcome: a review, *J Reprod Med* 33:945, 1988.

Chong ML, Hardy CM: Cocoa feeding and human lactose intolerance, *Am J Clin Nutr* 49:840, 1989.

Frentzen BH, Dimperio DL, Cruz AC: Maternal weight gain: effect on infant birth weight among overweight and average-weight low-income women, *Am J Obstet Gynecol* 159:1114, 1988.

Frentzen BH, Johnson JWC, Simpson S: Nutrition and hydration: relationship to preterm myometrial contractility, *Obstet Gynecol* 70:887, 1987.

Greene GW et al: Postpartum weight change: how much of the weight gained in pregnancy will be lost after delivery? *Obstet Gynecol* 71:701, 1988.

Hambidge KM et al: Acute effects of iron therapy on zinc status during pregnancy, *Obstet Gynecol* 70:593, 1988.

Hediger ML et al: Patterns of weight gain in adolescent pregnancy: effects on birth weight and preterm delivery, *Obstet Gynecol* 74:6, 1989.

Horner RD et al: Pica practices of pregnant women, *J Am Diet Assoc* 91:34, 1991.

Institute of Medicine: *Nutrition during pregnancy,* Washington, DC, 1990, National Academy Press.

Kaplan M, Eidelman AI, Aboulafia Y: Fasting and the precipitation of labor; the Yom Kippur effect, *JAMA* 250:1317, 1983.

Lacey EP: Broadening the perspective of pica: literature review, *Public Health Rep* 105:29, 1990.

London RS: Saccharin and aspartame: are they safe to consume during pregnancy? *J Reprod Med* 33:17, Jan 1988.

Mills JL et al: The absence of a relation between the periconceptual use of vitamins and neural-tube defects, *N Engl J Med* 321:430, 1989.

Milunsky A et al: Multivitamin/folic acid supplementation in early pregnancy reduces the prevalence of neural tube defects, *JAMA* 262:2847, 1989.

National Center for Health Statistics: *Maternal weight gain and the outcome of pregnancy, United States 1980* (Vital and Health Statistics, Series 21, No 44), US Department of Health and Human Services Pub No (PHS) 86-1922, Washington, DC, 1986, US Government Printing Office.

Olsen LC, Mundt MH: Postpartum weight loss in a nurse-midwifery practice, *J Nurse Midwife* 31:177, July/Aug 1986.

Parham ES, Astrom MF, King SH: The association of pregnancy weight gain with the mother's postpartum weight, *J Am Diet Assoc* 90:550, 1990.

Pederson AI, Worthington-Roberts B, Hickok DE: Weight gain patterns during twin gestation, *J Am Diet Assoc* 89:642, 1989.

Rizzo T et al: Correlations between antepartum maternal metabolism and newborn behavior, *Am J Obstet Gynecol* 163:1458, 1990.

Thomson EJ, Cordero JF: The new teratogens: accutane and other vitamin A analogs, *MCN* 14:244, 1989.

Worthington-Roberts B et al: Dietary cravings and aversions in the postpartum period, *J Am Diet Assoc* 89:647, 1989.

References—Nursing Research

Aaronson LS, MacNee CL: The relationship between weight gain and nutrition in pregnancy, *Nurs Res* 38:223, 1989.

Kaufman KJ, Hall LA: Influences of the social network on choice and duration of breast-feeding in mothers of preterm infants, *Res Nurs Health* 12:149, 1989.

Lindenberg CS et al: A review of the literature on cocaine abuse in pregnancy, *Nurs Res* 40:69, 1991.

BIBLIOGRAPHY

Carruth BR, Skinner JD: Practitioners beware: regional differences in beliefs about nutrition during pregnancy, *J Am Diet Assoc* 91:435, 1991.

Food and Nutrition Board: *Recommended dietary allowances,* ed 10, Washington, DC, 1989, National Academy of Sciences—National Research Council.

Institute of Medicine (Food and Nutrition Board, National Academy of Sciences): *Nutrition during pregnancy, Part I: Weight gain,* Washington, DC, 1990, National Academy Press.

Institute of Medicine (Food and Nutrition Board, National Academy of Sciences) *Nutrition during pregnancy, Part II, Nutrition Supplements* Washington, DC, 1990, National Academy Press.

Report of a special panel on desired prenatal weight gains for underweight and normal weight women, *Public Health Rep* 105:24, 1990.

Schneck ME et al: Low-income pregnant adolescents and their infants: dietary findings and health outcomes, *J Am Diet Assoc* 90:555, 1990.

Nursing Process: Alterations in Nutrition

Marty Ellis, a 28-year-old woman in week 24 of her first pregnancy, comes to the clinic for a routine prenatal visit.

ASSESSMENT

Marty's height is 157.5 cm (5 ft 2 in) and current weight is 70 kg (154 lb); her prepregnancy weight was 56 kg (123 lb). A review of her records reveals that her rate of weight gain had been high throughout pregnancy. She has no edema or proteinuria, and her blood pressure is 110/76. The nurse interviews Marty to update her diet history. In Marty's cultural group, pregnant women are pampered, and part of the pampering includes urging the woman to eat more to have a strong, healthy baby and to maintain her own strength. Marty states that she especially craves ice cream and eats two or three servings most days. She seems embarrassed, saying, " I never intended to get this heavy. Somehow it just happened. And the more I thought about not eating ice cream or some other food that I wanted, the more I wanted it." In assessing activity patterns, the nurse finds that Marty is a nurse who previously worked on a very busy pediatric unit where she was constantly moving about. Shortly after she became pregnant, Marty took a job in an outpatient clinic because the working hours were better. The new job is very sedentary. Marty was on the swimming team in high school but has not exercised regularly since then.

In addition, Marty complains that she is experiencing the need to defecate but has difficulty in doing so and that her stools have become infrequent (once or twice a week), hard, and small. She also reports that she is having heartburn (pyrosis).

NURSING DIAGNOSIS

On the basis of Marty's weight gain pattern, eating habits, and activity level, the nurse concludes that an appropriate *nursing diagnosis No. 1* is altered nutrition: more than body requirements. In addition, the nurse identifies *nursing diagnosis No. 2,* constipation, and *nursing diagnosis No. 3,* pain related to pyrosis.

PLANNING

Together the nurse and Marty develop a plan of care to address her nutrition-related problems. The *goals* they set are to reduce Marty's rate of weight gain and to alleviate constipation and pyrosis. *Expected outcomes* established by the nurse include reduction of weight gain to no more than 2 kg (4.4 lb) per month for the remainder of pregnancy; elimination of regular, soft, formed stools; and reduction of discomfort related to gastroesophageal reflux.

IMPLEMENTATION

In regard to nursing diagnosis No. 1, altered nutrition: more than body requirements, the nurse discusses with Marty her dietary habits and her weight gain in comparison with the usual pattern but avoids a judgmental attitude or one that would seem to place blame on Marty. The nurse emphasizes that now is not the time to try to lose weight, and together the nurse and Marty identify some of the high-calorie foods and food preparation methods commonly included in her diet. They plan daily menus with nutritious, appealing lower-calorie foods (e.g., fresh fruits, fruit sorbets or ices, angel food cake, or low-fat cookies such as gingersnaps or fruit-filled cookies to replace higher-calorie dessert items such as ice cream). With the nurse's guidance, Marty also plans to begin swimming regularly.

In addressing nursing diagnosis No. 2, constipation, the nurse and Marty review Marty's diet history and identify low-fiber foods that can be replaced with high-fiber alternatives (e.g., bran cereals rather than low-fiber highly processed ones; whole grain wheat, rye, or oat bread rather than white bread; fresh fruits and/or vegetables daily rather than canned ones). They also plan for a daily fluid intake of at least 30 to 40 ml/kg body weight to assist in hydrating the dietary fiber and producing bulky, easy-to-pass stools.

In regard to nursing diagnosis No. 3, pain related to pyrosis, the nurse and Marty plan a daily food intake pattern that provides small, frequent meals or snacks to avoid excessive stomach distention. Dinner is to be several hours before bedtime, and Marty will avoid snacking after dinner so that she does not lie down while her stomach is still full, thus promoting gastroesophageal reflux.

EVALUATION

The expected outcomes were used to evaluate the effectiveness of these interventions and Marty's compliance with the plan of care at the next clinic visit and at each successive visit. Marty's weight was checked at each clinic visit, and she and the nurse recorded her weight gain. Marty also found that it was helpful to record her food intake for 3 days each week to identify (1) particular times of the day when she was especially vulnerable to overeating and (2) foods that were especially likely to tempt her to overeat. She also began swimming laps at a local pool four or five days a week. Although Marty did not quite achieve her weight gain goal the first month (gaining 2.5 kg), she reduced the rate of her weight gain and was eager to continue the diet plan she and the nurse had devised.

Marty was also able to report that the problem of constipation had resolved; she began to have one formed but soft bowel movement daily after she increased her fiber intake and began to exercise regularly. In addition, she had no more symptoms of pyrosis. Therefore the goals related to nursing diagnoses No. 2 and No. 3 were met.

See the related Care Plan that follows.

CARE PLAN Alterations in Nutrition

GOALS	IMPLEMENTATION	RATIONALE	EVALUATION
Nursing diagnosis: Altered nutrition: more than body requirements			
Rate of weight gain will be reduced to no more than 2 kg (4.4 lb)/mo for the remainder of pregnancy.	Discuss optimal weight gain for prepregnant weight. Review principles of a healthful diet.	Knowledge of optimal pattern of gain assists Marty to plan for weight gain during the remainder of pregnancy. A nutritious intake must be maintained, and no weight reduction diet should be begun during pregnancy to avoid ketonemia and to ensure that the diet is not so restricted that it becomes difficult to consume adequate nutrients.	Marty's gain slowed to 2.5 kg (5.5 lb) the first mo; although the goal was not completely achieved. Marty was pleased with her progress and wanted to continue with the plan.
	Review diet history with Marty and assist her to plan lower-calorie menus.	Identification of excesses in her diet, especially excessive intake of fat, a major contributor to weight gain, can assist her to begin to develop new food habits.	
	Assist Marty to plan a regular exercise regimen using large-muscle groups.	Exercise increases energy expenditure.	
Nursing diagnosis: Constipation			
Marty will have regular, soft, formed stools that are eliminated without discomfort.	Review diet history with Marty, identify fiber sources, and help her plan menus with increased raw fruits and vegetables, bran, and whole grains.	Identifies ways that fiber in the diet can be increased to produce bulky stools that stimulate peristalsis.	Marty's constipation resolves; she passes soft, formed stools daily.
	Encourage intake of 30-40 mL of fluid/kg daily (½ oz/lb) in water, fruit juices, decaffeinated tea, and milk.	Fluid helps to produce bulky stools.	
	Help Marty to devise a plan for regular exercise.	Exercise improves muscle tone, stimulates peristalsis.	
Nursing diagnosis: Pain related to pyrosis (heartburn)			
Marty will experience no discomfort related to pyrosis.	Review diet history with Marty, with emphasis on time and type of foods/beverages consumed and the onset of discomfort.	Determining the relationship between food intake and onset of symptoms may assist the nurse and Marty in planning interventions.	Marty reports that pyrosis has resolved.
	Discuss with Marty the factors that can contribute to reflux of gastric fluid into the esophagus.	Understanding the physiologic basis of her discomfort will help Marty plan and implement interventions.	
	Suggest that Marty avoid wearing garments that fit snugly over her abdomen.	This reduces intraabdominal pressure.	
	Recommend that Marty avoid lying down for at least 2 to 3 hours after eating.	The force of gravity helps reduce reflux when Marty is upright.	
	Help Marty plan her diet to include several small, nutritious meals daily, rather than two to three larger meals, and suggest that Marty consume most of her fluids between meals rather than with meals.	Reflux is more likely to occur when the stomach is very full; fluids, especially, can contribute to distention of the stomach.	

chapter 9 review

Key Concepts

- A woman's nutritional status before, during, and after pregnancy contributes, to a significant degree, to her well-being and that of her infant.
- Many physiologic changes occurring during pregnancy influence the need for nutrients and the efficiency with which the body uses them.
- Both the total maternal weight gain and the pattern of weight gain are important determinants of the outcome of pregnancy.
- The recommended weight gain during pregnancy is determined by the appropriateness of the mother's prepregnancy weight for her height.
- Nutritional risk factors include adolescent pregnancy, smoking, alcohol abuse, drug use, multifetal gestation, poor knowledge of nutrition and sound dietary practices, and poverty.
- Iron supplementation is recommended routinely during pregnancy. Other supplements may be warranted when nutritional risk factors are present.
- The nurse and the client are influenced by cultural and personal values and beliefs during nutrition counseling.
- Pregnancy complications that may be nutrition-related include anemia, pregnancy-induced hypertension, preterm delivery, and intrauterine growth retardation.
- Dietary adaptions can be effective interventions for some of the common discomforts of pregnancy, including nausea and vomiting, constipation, and pyrosis.

Key Terms

- anemia (p.214)
- anthropometric measurements (p. 227)
- body mass index (BMI) (p. 217)
- complementary proteins (p. 227)
- diet history (p. 222)
- energy (kcal) (p. 214)
- food cravings (p. 223)
- intrauterine growth retardation (IUGR) (p. 214)
- lactose intolerance (p. 220)
- low birth weight (p. 218)
- pica (p. 223)
- recommended weight gain (p. 217)
- vegetarian diet (p. 223)

Critical Thinking Exercises

1. Describe your own nutritional status and dietary strengths and weaknesses; your positive and negative eating habits; the influence of your culture, religion, and ethnic group on your dietary practices; your attitudes toward overweight and underweight persons; and how your views and beliefs about nutrition may influence women when providing care for prenatal clients.
2. Use the material compiled in exercise 1 above for discussion with peers about their views and beliefs. People of varying backgrounds may be able to offer additional insights into problems with acceptance of clients' varying attitudes and practices.
3. Perform a physical assessment of nutritional status using Table 9-5 as a guide.

Topics for Nursing Research

- Previous research has demonstrated that most women who breast-feed decide to do so either very early in pregnancy or before pregnancy begins. Longitudinal studies need to be done to determine whether educating teenage girls and young women about the advantages of breast-feeding before they begin childbearing will influence them to breast-feed their infants. If early breast-feeding education is effective, strategies for accomplishing this teaching should be tested to determine which are the most successful and cost-effective.
- Effective tools for nutrition education of clients who are illiterate or who do not speak the same language as the members of the health care team need to be designed and tested.
- A weight gain curve for optimal outcome of twin pregnancy has been devised (Pederson et al, 1989), but it was derived from a relatively limited number of women in a single health care setting. Weight gain data from twin pregnancies with both good and poor outcomes should be compiled from different settings and compared with the published data. Ideally, the published weight gain curve also should be tested in a prospective manner.
- Intervention methods effective in helping women to stop smoking, alcohol use, and drug use need to be identified.

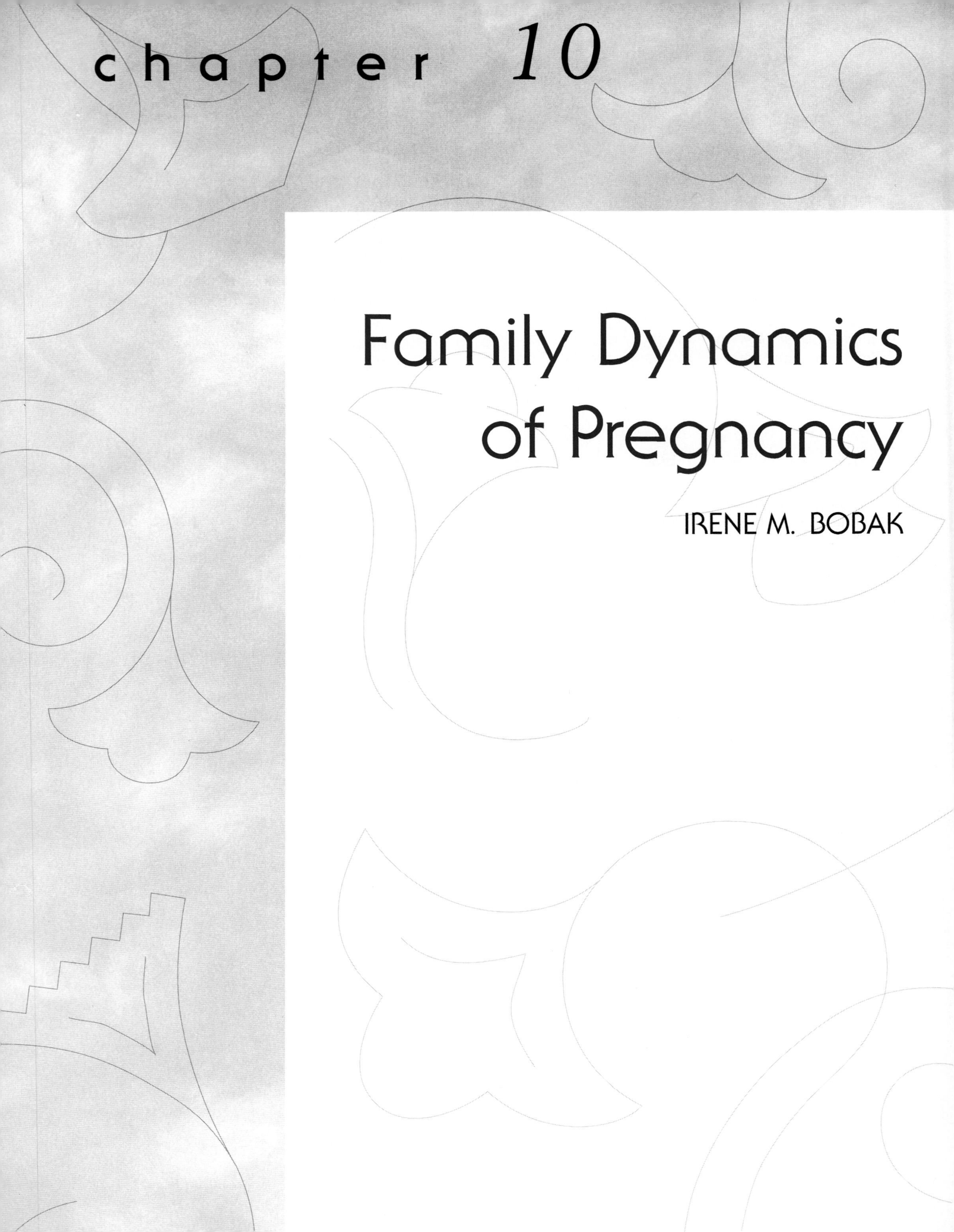

chapter 10

Family Dynamics of Pregnancy

IRENE M. BOBAK

LEARNING OBJECTIVES

- Define the key terms listed.
- Examine maternal adaptation to pregnancy in regard to acceptance, identification with motherhood role, family relationships, and anticipation of labor.
- Examine paternal adaptation to pregnancy in regard to acceptance, identification with fatherhood role, family relationships, and anticipation of labor.
- Discuss sibling adaptation to pregnancy.
- Discuss grandparent adaptation to pregnancy.
- Evaluate pregnancy after age 35.
- Identify cultural beliefs and practices related to pregnancy.
- Identify topics for nursing research related to family dynamics.

Pregnancy involves all family members. Because "conception is the beginning, not only of a growing fetus but also of the family in a new form with an additional member and with changed relationships," each family member must adapt to the pregnancy and interpret its meaning in light of his or her own needs (Grossman et al, 1980).

This process of family adaptation to pregnancy takes place within a cultural environment. There have been dramatic changes in the fabric of Western society in recent years, and the nurse must be prepared to support single-parent families, reconstituted or blended families, homosexual families, and dual-career families in the childbirth experience. Much of the research on family dynamics in pregnancy and childbirth preparation in the United States and Canada has been done with white, middle-class families. As a result, findings may not apply to subcultures, minorities, or families who do not fit the traditional American model. The terms "spouse" or "husband" or "partner" and "wife" are used consistently in the literature. The nurse may have to adapt these terms to apply to corresponding roles in many families. The reality of today's family may differ significantly from the image of the ideal family described by researchers in traditional terms.

The role of women has changed. In most families, women have moved out of the home and participate actively in the economic, social, and political life of their communities. This has resulted in a corresponding role change for many men; the role of father now includes more direct participation in childbirth preparation, the birth process, and in caring for the child. More research is needed to assess the impact of this involvement on the family, but it has been reported that increased involvement of fathers fosters positive attitudes and behaviors toward the mother and child (Jones, 1986; Westney, et al, 1988). Another trend related to the changing role of women is the tendency to postpone childbearing (see discussion, p. 257).

■ MATERNAL ADAPTATION

Women, from teenagers to women in their 40s, use the 9 months of pregnancy to adapt to the maternal role. This is a complex social and cognitive process that is not intuitive but learned (Rubin, 1967a). In becoming a mother, the teenager must shift from being mothered to mothering. The adult must move from "well-established routines to the unpredictable context created by an infant" (Mercer, 1981). The nullipara, "the woman without child," becomes "the woman with child" and the multipara, "the woman with child," becomes the "woman with children" (Lederman, 1984).

Subjective experience of time and space changes during pregnancy as plans and commitments become regulated by the expected date of delivery (EDD) (Rubin, 1984). Early in pregnancy nothing seems to be happening, and there may be a resistance to giving up the full days of social demands and activities for a "burdensome, empty time." A lot of time is spent sleeping. With quickening (feeling of life) in the second trimester, there is a reduction of time and space, both geographic and social, as the woman turns her attention inward to her pregnancy and to relationships with her mother and other women who have been or are pregnant. With the third trimester there is a slower pace and a sense that time is running out as the woman's activities are curtailed (Rubin, 1984).

Pregnancy is a **maturational crisis** that can be stressful but rewarding as the woman prepares for a new level of caring and responsibility. Her self-concept must change in readiness for parenthood as the dynamic interaction between intrapsychic and biologic processes cause her to reassess her "self-image, beliefs, values, priorities, behavior patterns, relationships with others, and problem-solving skills" (Lederman, 1984). Gradually, she moves from being self-contained and independent to being committed to a lifelong concern for another human being. This growth requires mastering certain developmental tasks: accepting the pregnancy, identifying the role of mother, reordering the relationships between mother and daughter and between herself and her partner, establishing a relationship with the unborn child, and preparing for the birth experience (Lederman, 1984; Stainton, 1985a, b). Studies indicate that the partner's emotional support is an important factor in the successful accomplishment of these developmental tasks (Leifer, 1980; Entwistle, Doering, 1981; Mercer, 1981). Even unwed adolescent fathers may provide significant support to young mothers who must master the developmental tasks of pregnancy superimposed on those of adolescence (Westney et al, 1988).

Acceptance of Pregnancy

The first step in adapting to the maternal role is acceptance of the idea of pregnancy and assimilation of the pregnant state into the woman's way of life (Lederman, 1984). The degree of acceptance is reflected in the woman's readiness for pregnancy and her emotional responses.

READINESS FOR PREGNANCY. The availability of birth control means that pregnancy for many women is a joint commitment between responsible partners. Planning a pregnancy, however, does not necessarily ensure acceptance of the pregnancy (Entwistle, Doering, 1981). Other women view pregnancy as a natural outcome of the marital relationship that may or may not be desired, depending on circumstances. For the adolescent, pregnancy can result from sexual experimentation without contraception.

Women prepared to accept a pregnancy are prompted by early symptoms to seek medical validation of the pregnancy, but some women who have strong feelings of "not me," "not now," and "not sure" may postpone seeking supervision and care (Rubin, 1970).

Once pregnancy is confirmed, a woman's emotional response may range from great delight to shock, disbelief, and despair. The reaction of many women is the "someday but not now" response:

> There is a real pleasure in finding oneself functionally capable of becoming pregnant. There is pleasure in learning that others are pleased with the promise of having, and being given, a child. But these feelings exist independently of the question of time. Personally and privately she is not ready, not now.*

Caplan (1959) reports that most of his clients were dismayed initially at finding themselves pregnant. However, eventual acceptance of pregnancy paralleled the growing acceptance of the reality of a child. He cautions against equating nonacceptance of the pregnancy with rejection of the child. A woman may dislike being pregnant but feel love for the child to be born.

EMOTIONAL RESPONSES. Women who are happy and pleased about their pregnancies often view pregnancy as biologic fulfillment and part of their life plan. They have high self-esteem and tend to be confident about outcomes for themselves, their babies, and other family members. Even though a general state of well-being predominates, an **emotional lability** expressed as rapid mood changes is common in pregnant women.

Rapid mood changes and an increased sensitivity to others are disturbing to the mother-to-be and those around her. Increased irritability, explosions of tears and anger, and feelings of great joy and cheerfulness alternate, apparently with little or no reason. According to one father-to-be:

> I sometimes think she is crazy—we're going somewhere she wants to go, out to dinner or a concert. She goes upstairs happy as a lark and in 2 minutes is down again in a regular temper, won't go, and shouts at me. I really feel bewildered by it all.

Many reasons, such as sexual concerns or fear of pain during delivery, have been used to explain this seemingly erratic behavior. Profound hormonal changes that are part of the maternal response to pregnancy may also be responsible for mood changes, much as they are before menstruation or during menopause.

As pregnancy progresses, the woman becomes more open about her feelings toward herself and others (Caplan, 1959). She is willing to talk about matters previously not discussed or discussed only within the family and seems to believe that her thoughts and symptoms will be of interest to the listener whom she views as protective. This openness, coupled with a readiness for learning, makes working with pregnant women a delight and increases the likelihood that supportive care will be effective.

When the child is wanted, the discomforts associated with pregnancy tend to be considered irritations, and measures taken to relieve them are usually successful. Pleasure derived from thinking about the unborn child and a feeling of closeness to the child help the mother adjust to these discomforts.

In some instances the woman who commonly complains about physical discomforts may be asking for help with conflicts regarding the mothering role and its responsibilities. Further assessment of coping measures and tolerance is indicated (Lederman, 1984).

RESPONSE TO CHANGES IN BODY IMAGE. The physiologic changes of pregnancy result in rapid and profound changes in body contour. During the first trimester body shape changes little, but by the second trimester obvious bulging of the abdomen, thickening of the waist, and enlargement of the breasts proclaim the state of pregnancy. The woman develops a feeling of an overall increase in the size of her body and of occupying more space. This feeling intensifies as pregnancy advances (Jessner, 1970). There is a gradual loss of definite **body boundaries** that serve to separate the self from the nonself and provide a feeling of safety: "I looked in the mirror and wondered if it were really me. I had a sudden feeling that I was ballooning outward, there was no end, and I did not know how to bring it together and be myself again." Fawcett (1978) describes this feeling as an awareness of the "perceived zone of separation between self and nonself."

*From Rubin R: Cognitive style in pregnancy, *Am J Nurs* 70:502, 1970.

Men respond in a variety of ways to their partner's changing shape (Fawcett et al, 1986). Some say she is most beautiful when pregnant, whereas others make derisive comments.

Negative feelings may be countered by a "Mother Earth" feeling, one of being a protective shield for the fetus (Colman, 1969; Rubin, 1970), or by exercise. Research on exercise in pregnancy is relatively new and should be examined critically, but it indicates that moderate exercise seems to be beneficial in combating a negative **body image** and reducing anxiety (Reich, 1987). For most women the feeling of liking or not liking their bodies in the pregnant state is temporary and does not cause significant changes in their perception of themselves.

AMBIVALENCE DURING PREGNANCY. Ambivalence is defined as simultaneously conflicting feelings, such as love and hate toward a person, thing, or state of being. Ambivalence is a normal response experienced by persons preparing for a new role. Most women have some ambivalent feelings during pregnancy.

Even women who are pleased to be pregnant may experience feelings of hostility toward the pregnancy or unborn child from time to time. Such things as a partner's chance remark about the attractiveness of a slim, nonpregnant woman or hearing about a colleague's promotion when the decision to have a child means relinquishing a job can give rise to ambivalent feelings. Body sensations, feelings of dependence, or realization of the responsibilities associated with child care can trigger such feelings.

Intense feelings of ambivalence that persist through the third trimester may indicate unresolved conflict with the motherhood role (Lederman, 1984). Upon the birth of a healthy child, memories of these ambivalent feelings are dismissed. If a child with a defect is born, a woman may look back at the times of not wanting the child and feel intensely guilty. She may believe that her ambivalence caused the defect in her child.

Being a self-reliant person, someone in control of her own destiny, has become part of the woman's self-expectations. Pregnancy alters this state: her baby is always with her as part of her body consciousness. She needs nurturing and support from others through birth and child rearing. Adaptation to dependency requires a change in self-image while moving from independence to dependency.

RITE OF PASSAGE. Pregnancy functions as a **rite of passage** that indicates reaching maturity in a society that has no other obvious rituals. In many states the pregnant woman is legally an adult regardless of her age and may give personal consent for any type of care for herself or for her newborn. She is entitled to financial and other aid from a government source if needed and, if unwed, is considered to be the sole legal guardian of her child. As such she has the right to care for the child herself, place the child in a foster home, or give the child up for adoption.

Identification with Motherhood Role

The process of identifying with the motherhood role begins early in each woman's life, with the memories she has of being mothered as a child. Her social group's perception of what constitutes the feminine role can also make her lean more toward motherhood or a career, toward being married or single, or toward being independent rather than interdependent. Stepping-stone roles, such as playing with dolls, baby-sitting, or taking care of siblings, may increase her understanding of what being a mother entails.

Many women have always wanted a baby, like children, and looked forward to motherhood. They are highly motivated to become parents, which affects acceptance of pregnancy and eventual prenatal and parental adaptation (Grossman et al, 1980; Lederman, 1984). Other women apparently have not considered in any detail what motherhood means to them. During pregnancy conflicts such as not wanting the pregnancy or child or career-related decisions need to be resolved.

Mother-Daughter Relationship

The woman's relationship to her mother has proved significant in adaptation to pregnancy and motherhood (Rubin, 1967a, b; Mercer et al, 1982). Lederman (1984) noted the importance of four factors in the pregnant woman's relationship with her mother: the mother's availability (past and present), her reactions to the daughter's pregnancy, respect for her daughter's autonomy, and the willingness to reminisce.

During childhood the availability of the mother was perceived as her being there, loving and supportive. Women with such mothers used them as role models. Other women in the study perceived their mothers as emotionally unavailable. However, during pregnancy, some of these daughters perceived a change in the relationship that promoted emotional support. "With the common bond of motherhood and mutual availability, subjects often described a closeness that appeared to facilitate the development and adaptation of both individuals" (Lederman, 1984).

The mother's reaction to the daughter's pregnancy signified her acceptance of the grandchild and of her daughter. If the mother was supportive, the daughter had an opportunity to discuss pregnancy and labor and her feelings of joy or ambivalence with a knowledgeable and accepting woman. Rubin (1975) noted that if the pregnant woman's mother is not pleased with the pregnancy, the daughter begins to have doubts about her self-worth and the eventual acceptance of her child by others.

Mothers who respected their daughters' autonomy prompted feelings of self-confidence in their daughters. The coming child helped the grandmother-to-be move toward a grandmother role. Some grandmothers used the birth of their grandchildren as a second chance at mothering. Grandparents who had helped their children become independent were seen as being willing to help rather than interfere or dominate.

Reminiscing about the pregnant woman's early childhood and sharing the grandmother-to-be's account of her childbirth experience helped the daughter anticipate and prepare for labor and delivery (Levy, McGee, 1975). Hearing about themselves as young children made the pregnant women feel loved and wanted. They drew closer to their parents and began to feel that in spite of the errors they might make in their own mothering experiences, they would continue to be loved by their children.

Partner Relationship

The most important person to the pregnant woman is usually the father of her child (Richardson, 1983). There is increasing evidence that the woman who is nurtured by her male partner during pregnancy has fewer emotional and physical symptoms, fewer labor and childbirth complications, and an easier postpartum adjustment (Grossman et al, 1980; May, 1982b). Women have expressed two major needs within this relationship during pregnancy (Richardson, 1983). The first need relates to the woman receiving signs that she is loved and valued. The second need relates to the partner's acceptance of the child and willingness to assimilate the infant into the family. Rubin (1975) states that "as the childbearer, it devolves on the pregnant woman to ensure the necessary social and physical accommodation within the family and within the household for a new member."

The marital or committed relationship is not static but evolves over time. The addition of a child changes forever the nature of the bond between partners. Lederman (1984) reported that couples grew closer during pregnancy. In this study pregnancy had a maturing effect on the partners' relationship as they assumed new roles and discovered new aspects of one another. Partners who trusted and supported each other were able to share mutual dependency needs. Women expressed a need for the partner's active involvement in preparation for birth. The father-to-be was seen as a stabilizing influence, a good listener to his mate's expressions of doubts and fears, and a source of physical and emotional reassurance (Grossman et al, 1980). Most women were aware of their partner's developmental needs during pregnancy. They were sympathetic toward his need for reassurance about his importance to his mate and recognized that he could feel jealous of the unborn baby.

CONCERNS ABOUT SEXUAL RELATIONSHIP. Sexual expression is a concern for many couples during pregnancy (Zalar, 1976; Ellis, 1980; Swanson, 1980; Lederman, 1984). It is affected by physical, emotional, and interactional factors, including myths about sex during pregnancy, sexual dysfunction problems, and physical changes in the woman.

Myths about body functions and fantasies about the influence of the fetus as a third party in lovemaking are frequently expressed. Anomalies, mental retardation, and other injuries to the mother and fetus are often attributed to sexual relations during pregnancy. Many couples fear that the woman's genitals will be drastically changed by the birth process. Embarrassment or not wanting to appear foolish often prevents couples from expressing their concerns to the health professional.

Dyspareunia (painful intercourse), differing sexual drives, and erectile problems (impotence) are the three major problems reported. Dyspareunia may be caused by pressure on the woman's abdomen and deep penile thrusting. Postcoital cramping, backache, and even breast tenderness during the first trimester also have been reported.

As pregnancy progresses, changes in body shape, body image, and levels of discomfort influence both partners' desire for sexual expression. During the first trimester the woman is frequently plagued by nausea, fatigue, and sleepiness. As she progresses into the second trimester, her combined sense of well-being and increased pelvic congestion may profoundly increase her desire for sexual release. In the third trimester, fatigue, fetal demands, and physical bulkiness increase her physical discomfort and lower her libido.

Both partners need to feel free to discuss their sexual responses during pregnancy. Sensitivity to each other and a willingness to share concerns can strengthen their sexual relationship. Communication between the couple is important. Partners who do not understand the seemingly rapid physiologic and emotional changes of pregnancy can become confused by the other's behavior. By talking to each other about the changes they are experiencing, couples are able to define problems and offer the needed support.

CONCERNS ABOUT THE FETUS. Parental concern for the health of the child seems to vary during the course of pregnancy (Leifer, 1980). The first concern appears in the first trimester and relates to abortion. One woman expressed her feelings as follows: "I spotted [blood] off and on. The doctor said, 'If you are going to hold it, you will; if you abort it, it is probably just as well.' How could he say 'it'? He was talking about my baby." As the child becomes more of a reality, with movement and an audible heartbeat, parental anxiety focuses on possible defects in the child. Parents talk openly about these anxieties and press for confirmation that the child will be all right. In the later stages of pregnancy fear about the death of the child is less identifiable; this possibility is evidently remote for parents.

Mother-Child Relationship

Emotional **attachment** to the child begins during the prenatal period as women use fantasizing and daydreaming to prepare themselves for motherhood (Rubin, 1975; Stainton, 1983, 1985b). They think of themselves as mothers and imagine maternal qualities they would like to possess. Expectant parents desire to be warm, loving, and close to their child. They try to anticipate changes the child will bring to their lives and wonder how they will react to noise, disorder, less freedom, and caregiving activities. They question their ability to share their love for other children with the unborn child. Rubin (1967a, b) found that women "try on" and test the motherhood role by taking their own mothers or substitute mothers as role models who serve as confidantes, support persons, or sources of information and experience.

The mother-child relationship progresses through pregnancy as a developmental process (Rubin, 1975; Leifer, 1980). Three **developmental tasks** in the evolution of the relationship have been identified by theorists. Phases in the developmental pattern become apparent.

PHASE 1. The woman accepts the biologic fact of pregnancy. She needs to be able to state, "I am pregnant" and incorporate the idea of a child into her body and self-image.

Early in pregnancy the mother's thoughts center around herself and the immediate reality of the pregnancy itself. The child is viewed as "part of one's self," and most women think of their fetus as "unreal" during the early period of pregnancy (Lumley, 1980a, b; 1982a).

PHASE 2. The woman accepts the growing fetus as distinct from the self and as a person to nurture. She can now say, "I am going to have a baby."

During the second trimester, usually by the fifth month, there is a growing awareness of the child as a separate being. This differentiation of the child from the woman's self permits the beginning of the mother-child relationship that involves not only *caring* but also *responsibility*. Researchers have noted that women who planned the pregnancy are pleased with their pregnancy and develop attachment to the child earlier than other women (Leifer, 1980; Lumley, 1982b; Koniak-Griffin, 1988).

With acceptance of the reality of the child (hearing the heartbeat and feeling the child move) and the decline of early symptoms, the woman enters a quiet period and becomes more introspective. A **fantasy child,** or dream child becomes precious to the woman. As she seems to withdraw and to concentrate her interest on the unborn child, her partner sometimes feels "left out," and other children in the family become more demanding in their efforts to redirect the mother's attention to themselves.

Sometimes a pregnant women holds her abdomen and gently rocks it as though rocking the child. Conversation reveals the intensity of this intimate mother-baby relationship as women talk freely about their children and their hopes and aspirations for the children's futures. Pet names may be given: "I called all my babies 'Herman' before they were born." Sexual preferences surface: "I just knew I was going to have a boy this time." Some women even begin to plan the child's career: "I saw her as a ballet dancer."

The child becomes precious to the women, and the feeling that "I am going to have a baby" supersedes all else.

PHASE 3. The woman prepares realistically for the birth and parenting of the child. She expresses the thought "I am going to be a mother" and defines the nature and characteristics of the child.

Although the mother alone experiences "the child within," both parents and siblings believe the unborn child responds in a very individualized, personal manner. Family members may interact a great deal with the unborn child by talking to the fetus and stroking the mother's abdomen, especially when the fetus shifts position (Fig. 10-1).

Most of our ideas about maternal-fetal attachment are based on clinical impressions and theoretic notions rather than empirical, or tested, data. There seems to be support for the theory that attachment is a gradual prenatal developmental process (Gaffney, 1987). However, the growing body of research relating psychologic variables to prenatal attachment has produced "counterintuitive" or conflicting findings.

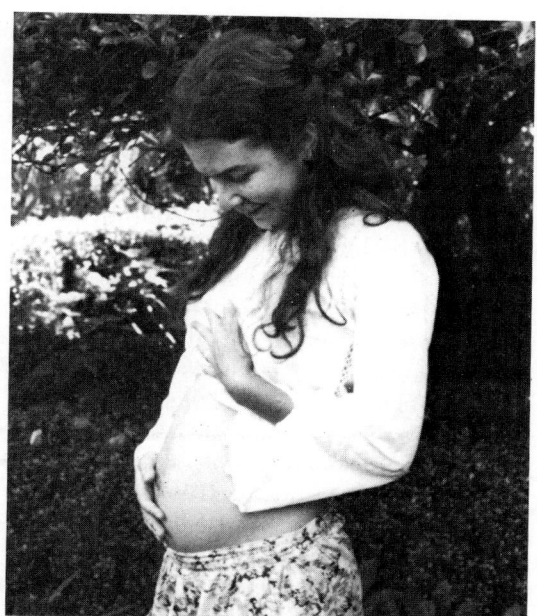

Fig. 10-1 Mother talks to her baby: "How are you doing in there?"

Gaffney (1988) has summarized selected studies that fail to show consistent significant correlations among factors believed to effect maternal-fetal attachment.

Koniak-Griffin's 1988 study of 90 pregnant adolescents representing a variety of ethnic backgrounds failed to show that maternal attachment was related to self-esteem and social support. Although maternal attachment is believed to develop over time, length of pregnancy was not a significant predictor of prenatal attachment (Koniak-Griffin, 1988). Kemp and Page (1987) found no significant relationship between attachment and maternal age, race, whether the pregnancy was planned, or whether the woman had a sonogram. Concepts from theoretic models, such as anxiety, early relationship with the mother, and self-esteem, appear to be only a few of the many factors that shape parental attitudes (Mercer et al, 1988).

Theories may be useful even in the absence of solid empirical support; despite methodologic flaws, studies of maternal-fetal attachment are useful. Nurses become better observers when they test theory and question the assumptions on which their practice is based. They must continue to seek to understand and foster attitudes and behaviors that promote early attachment and reduce the risk of negative long-term effects such as child neglect and abuse. More research relating psychologic variables to prenatal attachment and maternal-fetal interaction with maternal-infant interaction is needed.

NATURE AND CHARACTERISTICS OF THE UNBORN CHILD. Stainton (1985a) found that expectant parents usually agreed on the nature and characteristics of the unborn child, as expressed in five categories: appearance, communication, gender, sleep-wake cycles, and temperament.

The description of *appearance* of the child included features such as color of hair, size and shape of eyes, and size of the infant. For races other than white, color of hair and eyes were taken for granted.

Both fathers and mothers believed there was *communication* with the fetus. The unborn child responded to quiet talking, music, or massage by "settling down" and to loud voices or music by moving or kicking excessively.

Cultural conditioning may color the couple's preference for the *gender* of children. Women frequently defer to their partners' stated preference. If the sex of the child was known by sonogram, the child might be named and referred to by name. If the sex was not known, the parents guessed it on the basis of the size of the baby or type of movement (Stainton, 1985a). Regular movement is associated with fetal well-being.

The *sleep-wake cycles* of the child are described as (1) sleeping: when the unborn child is still and unresponsive to noise, talking, or touch; (2) a quiet but calm state: the child gently rocks or rolls slightly; and (3) an upset or alert state: the child responds readily to touch or noise by kicking, stretching, and, until past 30 weeks' gestation, rolling over (Stainton, 1985a).

The *temperament* of the child was described variously as "calm, cooperative" or "having a temper just like mine." Movements of the child are interpreted as indicating pleasure, discomfort, or playfulness. Some parents reported their newborn's activity, responsiveness, and sleep-wake patterns at 2 months of age to be remarkably similar to their description of the unborn child's behavior at 8 months' gestation (Stainton, 1983).

Preparation for Childbirth

Many women prepare actively for birth. They read books, view films, attend parenting classes, and talk to other women (mothers, sisters, friends, strangers). They will seek the best caregiver for advice, monitoring, and curing (Patterson, 1990). One study was conducted to explore how pregnant women use health care (see Research Highlight, p. 250). Other women tend to recount problems they experienced with deliveries that may frighten the woman in her first pregnancy. The multiparous woman has her own history of labor and delivery that can either comfort her or make her fearful.

Anxiety can arise from concern about a safe passage for herself and her child during the birth pro-

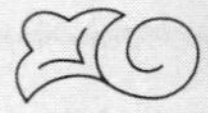 **Research Highlight** 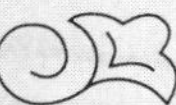

Utilizing Health Care during Pregnancy

RESEARCH ABSTRACT

The study was conducted to explore how pregnant women use health care. Participants were 27 women who had sought prenatal care early, late, or not at all. The women were interviewed at their prenatal care sites or on the postpartum unit. Several phases of seeking safe passage through pregnancy emerged from the data. When a self-diagnosis of pregnancy was made, the next phase was "letting it sink in." Then attention was to maintaining health for the mother and the baby. They then began to search for prenatal care. Women gathered information about care providers by consulting with others; some transferred from private to public care for financial reasons or from one source to another when their expectations were not met. The criteria for selecting care included financial considerations, reputation of the provider, quality of care, and use of existing relationships. A phase of waiting often occurred between diagnosis and searching for care. Contingency planning was an active decision; it involved deciding to seek care when labor occurred or if complications were detected. The women also engaged in self-care to promote safe passage.

IMPLICATIONS FOR PRACTICE

Women do seek safe passage for themselves and their babies. This seeking may consist of a single approach or may combine several approaches. Intrapartal care was seen as necessary, but prenatal care was not considered to be essential. Health care providers need to make the environment as welcoming as possible so that women will be willing to seek prenatal care in public as well as private settings.

RELATED RESEARCH QUESTIONS

1. What factors of private care are appealing to women?
2. How can more choices in prenatal care be offered to women?
3. What parts of prenatal care can women safely manage themselves?
4. Do women who have relatives or friends who experience complications of pregnancy seek care earlier than those who do not?

REFERENCE

Patterson ET, Freese MP, Goldenberg RL: Seeking safe passage: Utilizing health care during pregnancy, *Image* 22(1):27, 1990.

cess. This may not be expressed overtly, but cues are given as the nurse listens to plans women make for care of the new baby and other children in case "anything should happen." These feelings persist despite statistical evidence about the safe outcome of pregnancy for the mother. Many women fear the pain of delivery or mutilation because they do not understand anatomy and the birth process. Women express concern over what behaviors will be appropriate during the birth process and how the persons who will be caring for them will accept them and their actions. Lederman (1984) found women fear loss of control and concomitant loss of self-esteem in labor.

Loss of control was related to the loss of physical control and also to medical decisions regarding care made without the woman's knowledge. Women worried about emotional control—crying or becoming hysterical or hostile to their husbands or the staff. Possible loss of control in labor affected the women's plans for use of analgesics and anesthetics during labor, varying from complete rejection to acceptance. The use of medications during labor was also related to concern about the safety of the child.

Reaching the hospital in time for the birth, arranging for the care of children at home, and being unable to plan specific dates for outside help or the partner's vacation were concerns that made the last few weeks a time of tension; the tension was compounded by a lack of adequate rest. The ability to participate wholeheartedly in situations that result in growth, joy, and pleasure and, conversely, the ability to face pain, separation, disability, or death adequately come in part from the feelings one has about the ability to maintain control, from sharing these critical periods with those who care, and from the nurturing provided by others.

Preparation of a **birth plan** allows the expectant mother/family to state goals for controlling and allowing others to control safe passage for herself and the child during the birth process (Carty, Tier, 1989; Latham, 1990) (see discussion of birth plan, p. 278).

The best preparation for labor was found to be "a healthy sense of the realistic—an awareness of work, pain, and risk balanced by a sense of excitement and expectation of the final reward" (Lederman, 1984).

READINESS FOR CHILDBIRTH. Toward the end of the third trimester, breathing is difficult and movements of the fetus become vigorous enough to disturb the mother's sleep. Backaches, frequency and urgency of urination, constipation, and varicose veins can become troublesome. The bulkiness and awkwardness of her body interfere with the woman's ability to care for other children, perform routine work-related duties, and assume a comfortable position for sleep and rest.

By this time most women become impatient for labor to begin, whether the birth is anticipated with joy or dread, or a mixture of both. A strong desire to see the end of pregnancy, "to be over and done with it," make women at this stage ready to move on to childbirth.

SECOND-TIME MOTHERS. Mothers expecting their second child have different concerns in pregnancy (Merilo, 1988). They may have unresolved feelings about their first labor. They may be so focused on their first child that they are less excited and think less about the second baby than they did about the first. They are concerned about the first child's reaction to separation at the sibling's birth and aware that a change in their relationship with the first child will occur after the new baby is born. These concerns may lead to a sense of loss and sadness. Friends and family, assured of the mother's ability to care for an infant, may offer less attention and help.

The nurse needs to recognize that there are dependency needs with every pregnancy. She can help second-time mothers meet their dependency needs by encouraging them to take time out to focus on the second child and their own needs. They need to set realistic expectations for themselves, arranging for household help and child care and reducing outside commitments. Parent education classes in which second-time mothers are able to share concerns and experiences can help these women recognize that their needs are legitimate and will promote a positive adaption to the many demands of their new role (Merilo, 1988).

■ PATERNAL ADAPTATION

Expectant fathers, like expectant mothers, have been preparing for parenthood through out their lives. Subconsciously or consciously men think about having a wife and children. During courtship and early marriage discussion of future plans may even include the number, spacing, and names of their children-to-be (Bobak, 1968).

The father's beliefs and feelings about the ideal mother and father and his cultural expectation of appropriate behavior during pregnancy will affect his response to his partner's need for him.

One man may engage in nurturing behavior. Another may feel lonely and alienated as the woman becomes physically and emotionally engrossed in the unborn child. He may seek comfort and understanding outside the home or become interested in a new hobby or involved with his work. Some men view pregnancy as a proof of their masculinity and their dominant role. To others, pregnancy has no meaning in terms of responsibility to either mother or child. However, for most men pregnancy is a time of preparation for the parental role, of fantasy, of great pleasure, and of intense learning.

How fathers adjust to the parental role is the subject of increasing contemporary research (Fawcett, 1986a, b; Strickland, 1987). In older societies the man was expected to subject himself to various behaviors and taboos associated with pregnancy and giving birth (Bobak, 1968; May, 1982b). These practices are known as **couvade** (French, "to hatch"). By enacting the couvade, the man's responses are channeled into acceptable modes of expression and this new status is recognized and endorsed. His behavior acknowledges his psychosocial and biologic relationship to the mother and child. In Western societies participation of fathers in childbirth has risen dramatically over the last 20 years, and the father in the role of labor coach is now well established (May, 1982b).

The man's emotional responses to becoming a father, his concerns, and his informational needs change during the course of pregnancy. Phases of the developmental pattern become apparent. May (1982c) describes three phases characterizing the three developmental tasks experienced by the expectant father: the announcement phase, the moratorium phase, and the focusing phase.

The early period, the **announcement phase,** may last from a few hours to a few weeks. The developmental task is to accept the biologic fact of pregnancy. The man needs to be able to state, "She is pregnant and I am the father." Men react to the confirmation of pregnancy with joy or dismay depending on whether the pregnancy is desired or unplanned or unwanted. Realization of the reality of the pregnant state seems to come more slowly for the father who does not experience the early symptoms of pregnancy and sees little physical change in his wife in the first trimester of pregnancy. On seeing a sonograph of his son at 12 weeks, one man remarked, "Until I saw his picture, it was all unreal. I knew intellectually my wife was pregnant, but it didn't mean anything to me. It was amazing—in a few minutes I became a father" (Jordan, 1990).

The second phase, the **moratorium phase,** is the period of adjusting to the reality of pregnancy. The developmental task is to accept the pregnancy and to be able to state, "We are going to have a baby, and we are changing." Men appear to put conscious thought find the alterations in life plans and life-styles difficult to accept and do not necessarily become reconciled to the pregnancy (May, 1982c).

EMOTIONAL RESPONSES. *Styles of involvement* in pregnancy refers to the "general patterns of feelings and behaviors that reflect the way men see themselves in relation to pregnancy" (May, 1980). Their basic personality structure is reflected in this style. May (1980, 1982a) describes three styles characteristic of men studied during their wives' first-time pregnancy: the observer style, the expressive style, and the instrumental style.

Observer style was defined as a detached approach to involvement in the pregnancy. The fathers in this category fell into two major groupings, those who wanted the pregnancy and those who did not. Those who were happy about the pregnancy were supportive of their wives and wanted to be good fathers. However, because of cultural values or shyness, they needed to distance themselves from such activities as parent education classes, decisions about breast-feeding, or choice of professional care. By nature unemotional and matter-of-fact, they appeared to need an "emotional buffer zone," and the pregnancy did not change them (May, 1982a).

The group that was not happy about the pregnancy reported feelings of ambivalence about pregnancy and the role of father (May, 1982c). These men needed time to adjust to the idea of pregnancy and fatherhood; they responded to their ambivalent feelings by becoming involved in careers and resisting their wives' attempts to involve them in preparations for the coming child. "Men established an emotional distance from the pregnancy in relation to the amount of ambivalence they experienced. Women often sensed this distance and attempted to involve their partners more closely. Often the man responded by withdrawing more" (May, 1982c).

Expressive style was defined as a strong emotional response to pregnancy and a desire to be a full partner in the project (Fig. 10-2) These husbands showed awareness of their wives' needs for support and were conscious of the times when they were not able to give that support. They experienced the same emotional lability and ambivalence that characterizes pregnant women. They were excited and pleased about the baby but also worried about their ability to be good fathers. Some of these fathers experienced the discomforts usually associated with women in pregnancy, such as nausea, lassitude, and various aches and pains (Strickland, 1987). **Mitleiden** (suffering along), or psychosomatic symptoms of expectant fathers, has long been recognized as a phenomenon of expectant fatherhood. In 1627 Bacon ob-

of the pregnancy aside for a time. They become more introspective and engage in many discussions about their philosophy of life, religion, childbearing, and child-rearing practices and their relationships with family members and friends. Depending on the man's readiness for the pregnancy, this phase may be relatively short or persist until the last trimester (May, 1982c).

The third phase, the **focusing phase**, begins in the last trimester and is characterized by the father's active involvement in both the pregnancy and his relationship with his child. The developmental task is to negotiate with his partner the role he is to play in labor and to prepare for parenthood. He needs to be able to state, "I know my role during the birth process, and I am going to be a parent." In this phase the man concentrates on "his own experience of pregnancy, and in doing so he feels more in tune with his wife. He begins to redefine himself as a father and the world around him in terms of his future fatherhood" (May, 1982c).

Acceptance of Pregnancy

READINESS FOR PREGNANCY. May (1982c) found that fathers' readiness for pregnancy was reflected in three areas: "(1) a sense of relative financial security, (2) stability in the couple relationship, and (3) a sense of closure to the childless period in their relationship."

Many men express concern for the family's *economic security* (Glazer, 1989). Today most young married women are employed outside the home. Although pregnant women and mothers with young children may continue their employment, many childbearing and child-rearing women have a phase of unemployment. Length of leave from employment is determined by a combination of factors, such as the couple's economic status, the policies of the employer, and the couple's value system. Some men attempt to compensate for anticipated needs by keeping their current jobs even though they had planned a change. They may put more effort into earning rapid promotions by working overtime or by taking on extra work. Some men acquire new or additional insurance at this time (Bobak, 1968).

Those couples who have a *stable relationship* before pregnancy tend to draw closer as a result of their coming parental roles (Lederman, 1984).

The partner's pregnancy brings *to closure the childless period* in men's lives. Many men view having children and being a father as an integral part of their life plan. Couples who plan for pregnancy are more accepting of pregnancy (Lederman, 1984). If pregnancy is unplanned or unwanted, some men

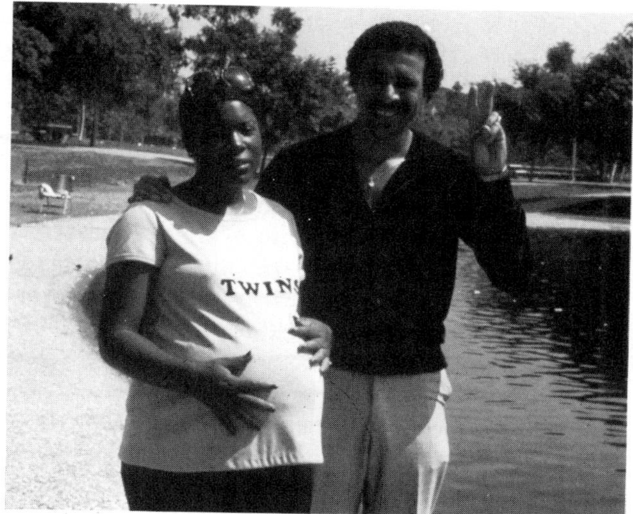

Fig. 10-2 Mother and father walk together. Women respond positively to their partner's interest and concern. Courtesy Marjorie Pyle, RNC, Lifecircle, Costa Mesa, Calif.

served, "That loving and kinde Husbands, have a Sense of their Wives Breeding Childe, by some Accident in their owne Body." And another author in the 1600s commented, "It often falls out, that when the woman is in good health, the husband is sick, yea sometimes being many miles off" (Hunter, Macalpine, 1963). The male partner alone may suffer these discomforts. The symptoms can bring the couple closer together and help the father in becoming more caring.

The **instrumental style** was adopted by men who emphasized tasks to be accomplished and saw themselves as "caretakers or managers of the pregnancy" (May, 1980). They asked questions, became interested in the role of labor coach, and planned for photographs during pregnancy, birth, and the neonatal period. They felt responsible for the outcome of pregnancy and were protective and supportive of their wives.

The three styles of involvement emphasize the different ways men can experience pregnancy. Each needs to feel free to define his role in pregnancy just as the woman does. Because of cultural conditioning or a different supportive style, not all men are able or willing to attend childbirth classes or act as labor coaches. More research is needed to determine if similar styles of involvement occur in partners of multiparous women and in same-sex partners.

Identification with Fatherhood Role

Each father brings to pregnancy attitudes that affect the manner in which he adjusts to pregnancy and the parental role (Cronenwett, Kunst-Wilson, 1981; Kunst-Wilson, Cronenwett, 1981; Lederman, 1984).

The father's memories of fathering by his own father, the experiences he has had with child care, and the perceptions of the male and father roles within his social group will guide his selection of the tasks and responsibilities he will assume. Some men are highly motivated to nurture and love a child. They may be excited and pleased about the anticipated role of father. Men who have reasonable self-esteem and control of financial resources and working conditions seem more able to incorporate fatherhood into their life plans. Identification with the fatherhood role is a crucial developmental step: "It can temporarily reactivate conflicts with his own parents, intensify feelings of separation, heighten dependency needs, and rekindle feelings of sibling rivalry. The husband who can look at these temporary regressions honestly is more likely to effect attachment and bonding with his newborn" (Lederman, 1984).

House (1981) outlined four types of support necessary in preparing for fatherhood:

1. *Emotional support.* The man's primary source of support is his partner (Lein, 1979). This support has to be modified to permit nurturing of the baby and the additional nurturing his partner needs. Therefore the father needs to seek support from family and friends.
2. *Instrumental support.* The father needs to know that he can depend on family or friends for help if necessary.
3. *Informational support.* The father needs to know who is available (e.g., professionals or relatives) to provide "tips" on how to solve immediate problems.
4. *Appraisal support.* The father needs to find others to provide criteria against which he can measure his performance.

A recent study described the experience of becoming a new father (see Research Highlight, p. 254).

Partner Relationship

Ballou (1978) found the male partner's role in pregnancy to be one of nurturance, responding to his partner's feelings of vulnerability in both her biologic state and in her relationship with her own mother. The man's support indicates to his mate his involvement in the pregnancy and his preparation for attachment to their child (Grossman, et al, 1980; Leifer, 1980; Lederman, 1984).

In psychoanalytic literature some aspects of the father's behavior indicates rivalry. Rivalry between the expectant father and his pregnant partner is not new. In Greek legend, Zeus, angered by his wife's superior wisdom after she conceived, swallowed her and later gave birth to Athena, who emerged full grown from his forehead. In the same instant he both punished and replaced his wife. Direct rivalry with the fetus may be evident, especially during sexual activity.

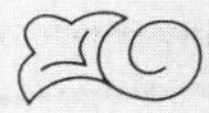
Research Highlight
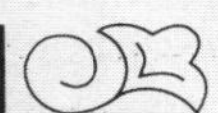

The Experience of Expectant and New Fathers

RESEARCH ABSTRACT

The purpose of this study was to capture the experience of becoming a new father. Participants included 56 expectant and new fathers, 28 of whom were in a longitudinal group (data were collected over time) and 28 in a cross-sectional group (data were collected at one point in time). Audiotaped interviews were conducted at a place and time convenient to the subjects. More than 180 interviews were completed. Subjects in the longitudinal group were interviewed six to seven times during pregnancy and the postpartum period. Subjects in the cross-sectional group were interviewed only once. The researchers defined the experience of becoming a new father in terms of "working for relevance." Working for relevance means (1) dealing with the reality of the pregnancy and the baby, (2) striving for recognition as a parent, and (3) working at making a role as an involved father. Men reported being recognized as helpers or breadwinners but said they felt excluded from the pregnancy experience. They believed they had no models to assist them to become new fathers.

IMPLICATIONS FOR PRACTICE

Health care providers can develop a better understanding of the paternal experience and develop interventions to assist in easing the transition to the role of father. They can use this information to counsel expectant and new fathers.

RELATED RESEARCH QUESTIONS

1. Does a male role model ease the experience of becoming a father?
2. How can males be included more in the pregnancy experience?
3. Does working for relevance change over time during pregnancy?
4. Does working for relevance differ among cultural and ethnic groups?

REFERENCE

Jordan PL: Laboring for relevance: expectant and new fatherhood, *Nurs Res* 39(1):11, 1990.

Husbands may protest that fetal movements prevent sexual gratification, making comments such as, "We can't have sex with 'that' kicking around in there" (Bobak, 1968).

The woman's increased introspection may cause her partner to experience a sense of uneasiness as she becomes preoccupied with thoughts of the child and of her mother, with her growing dependence on her physician, and with her reevaluation of their relationship. He may sense that his partner's support—his key support—is being withdrawn.

Deciding on the infant's feeding method is of concern when the partners' preferences differ or when one partner has intense reactions. Recognized benefits and disadvantages of one method over another appear to be irrelevant. Some men insist that the woman breast-feed; others are adamantly set against breast-feeding. When the male partner refuses to voice an opinion, the woman experiences uneasiness. Inwardly, she may accuse him of disinterest or feel uncertain about choosing the right way. The woman seems to ask for his support for whatever choice is made.

Father-Child Relationship

The father-child attachment can be as strong as the mother-child relationship, and fathers can be as competent as mothers in nurturing their infants (Jones, 1981; Cronenwett, 1982). Paternal behavior toward children does not differ significantly from maternal behavior, with the exception of play with the infants (Field, 1978).

Men prepare for fatherhood in many of the same ways as women do for motherhood—reading, fantasizing, and daydreaming about the baby. They may adjust work commitments to include new responsibilities or plan vacations to enable them to spend time with their new families.

Daydreaming is a form of role playing or anticipatory emotional preparation for the infant most common in the last weeks before delivery. Rarely do men confide their daydreams unless they are reassured that daydreams are normal and fairly common. Questions such as the following help the nurse and the parent in identifying concerns and allow for reality testing:

1. What do you expect the child to look and act like?
2. What do you think being a father will be like?
3. Have you thought about the baby's crying? Changing diapers? Burping the baby? Being awakened at night? Sharing your partner with the baby?

The father may not wish to share his answers with

the nurse at the moment but may need time to think them through or discuss them with his partner.

If an expectant father can imagine only an older child and has difficulty visualizing or talking about the infant, this area needs to be explored. The nurse can give information about the unborn child's ability to respond to light, sound, and touch and encourage the father to feel and talk to the fetus. Plans for seeing, holding, and examining his newborn child can be made.

As the birth day approaches, questions regarding fetal and newborn behaviors increase. "What do they do in there [in utero]?" "Is he hiccuping?" "Does he suck his thumb?" "How is he breathing?" "What does a newborn baby look like?" Some fathers express shock or amazement about the small size of clothes and furniture for the baby. Other fathers protest, "He'll only be real to me when I can hold him in my arms."

Some fathers become involved by picking the child's name and anticipating the child's sex. Some couples select the name of the child as early as the first month of pregnancy. Family tradition, religious customs, and continuation of one's own name or names of relatives and friends are important in the selection process. The names chosen are tried on for fit. For example, the father might emphatically state, "I just can't picture myself as being a father to a boy named John." Armed with several names, one expectant father said he would decide on his final choice only after he saw the baby, pointing out that "to be named Eric, he *must* be blue-eyed and blond" (Bobak, 1968).

At the time of birth, most parents are able to accept the sex of the child born to them, but occasionally disappointment is evident and voiced. The parents may experience a grief reaction and a sense of loss at birth as they release the fantasized child and begin to accept the real child.

Anticipation of Labor

The days and weeks immediately before the expected day of delivery are characterized by anticipation and anxiety. Boredom and restlessness are common as the couple focuses on the birth process.

During the last 2 months of pregnancy, many expectant fathers experience a surge of creative energy, both at home and on the job. They may become dissatisfied with their present living space. If possible, they tend to act on the need to alter the environment. This may be tangible evidence of sharing in the childbearing experience while channeling the anxiety or other feelings experienced during the final weeks before birth. This behavior earns recognition and compliments from friends, relatives, and the wife.

The father's anxieties may be expressed by refusal to think about the birth, by planning other activities during his partner's labor, or by sleeping and resting to the exclusion of all else. The expectant mother may become concerned about the possibility of being deserted physically or emotionally at a time when she is feeling most vulnerable.

The father's major concerns are getting the mother to a medical facility in time for the birth and not appearing ignorant. Many fathers want to be able to recognize labor and to determine when it is appropriate to leave for the hospital or call the physician or midwife. They may fantasize several ridiculously humorous situations and plan what they will do or rehearse the routes to the hospital, timing each route at different times of the day. Suitcase, car, and essential telephone numbers are readied.

Many fathers have questions about the labor suite's furniture, nursing staff, location, and availability of physician and anesthesiologist. Others want to know what is expected of them when their partners are in labor. The father has fears of mutilation and death for his partner and child. While he harbors these fears within, he cannot help his mate with her unspoken or overt apprehension. Words such as "dropped," "rupture of bag of waters," "bloody show," "tears and stitches," and "labor pains" have violent overtones (Bobak, 1968).

With the exception of parent education classes, a father has few opportunities to learn how to be an involved and active partner in this rite of passage into parenthood. Tensions and apprehensions of the unprepared, unsupportive father are readily transmitted and may increase the mother's fears. His own self-doubts and fear of inadequacy may be realized if he is not supported. Self-confidence comes from achieving realistic goals and earning the approval of others.

■ GRANDPARENT ADAPTATION

The definition of "grand" is extensive and includes descriptions such as impressive or imposing; stately, majestic, dignified; highest, or very high, in rank or official dignity; of great importance or distinction; first-rate, very good, splendid; princely, regal, royal, and exalted. A grandparent is an ancestor, one generation more remote—a founder or originator of a family. Grandparents are a vital link between generations (Horn, Manion, 1985).

Every pregnancy affects all family relationships. In particular, a first pregnancy is undeniable evidence that one is now old enough to have a child who is soon to bear a grandchild. Many think of a "grandparent" as old, white-haired, and becoming feeble of mind and body. Being "old" carries a stigma for some in predominantly youth-oriented societies. Some people face grandparenthood when still in their 30s and 40s. A mother-to-be announcing her pregnancy to her mother may be greeted by, "How *dare* you do that to me! *I* am not ready to be a grandmother!" Both daughter and mother may be startled and hurt by the outburst. Some grandparents-to-be not only are nonsupportive but also use subtle means to decrease the self-esteem of the young parents-to-be. Mothers may talk about their terrible pregnancies; fathers may discuss the endless cost of rearing children; and mothers-in-law may describe the neglect of their son as the concern of others is directed toward the pregnant daughter-in-law.

However, most grandparents are delighted with the prospect of a new baby in the family. It reawakens their feelings of their own youth, the excitement of giving birth, and their delight in the behavior of the parents-to-be when they were infants. They set up a memory store of first smiles, first words, and first steps, which can be used later for "claiming" the newborn as a member of the family. Satisfaction comes with the realization that continuity between past and present is guaranteed.

The grandparent is the historian who transmits the history of the family and provides continuity with the present, a resource person who shares knowledge based on experience, a role model, and a support person. The grandparent's presence can strengthen family systems by widening the circle of support and nurturance (Barranti, 1985). Other sources of information cannot replace the unique contribution that grandparents make.

Recent research indicates the importance of the grandparent-grandchild relationship. Grandparents act as a potential resource for families. Their support can strengthen family systems by widening the circle of support and nurturance (Barranti, 1985). The parent acts as negotiator in establishing the grandparent-grandchild relationship (Greene, Polivka, 1985). Many women report that their pregnancies bridged the final gap between them and their own mothers. The estrangement that began in adolescence disappeared as the now-pregnant daughter experienced joys, concerns, and anxieties similar to those her mother had felt before her.

Expectant grandparenthood can be a maturational crisis for the parent of an expectant parent. To be truly *family-oriented,* maternity care must include the grandparent in implementing the nursing process with childbearing families. (See also Chapter 24.) Grandparents' classes represent one method of facilitating the adjustment to the grandparenting role, of incorporating the grandparents into the family system, and of encouraging communication between the generations (Maloni, et al 1987) (see discussion of Parent Education, p. 334).

Grandparents' anxieties and concerns and their relationships with expectant parents and grandchildren should be opened to discussion during courses for expectant parents as well. The expectant parents may use this opportunity to begin to resolve conflicts and perceived differences with their parents, a task that can enhance their ability to relate to their own children.

■ SIBLING ADAPTATION

Sharing the spotlight with a new brother or sister may be the first major crisis for a child. The older child often experiences a sense of loss or feels jealous on being "replaced" by the new baby.(See also Chapters 2 and 24.) Some of the factors that influence the child's response are age, the parents' attitudes, the role of the father, the length of separation from the mother, the hospital's visitation policy, and how the child has been prepared for the change (Honig, 1986).

The mother with other children must devote much time and energy to reorganizing her relationships with existing children. She needs to prepare siblings for the birth of the child and to begin the process of role transition in the family by including the children in the pregnancy and being sympathetic to older children's protests against losing their places in the family hierarchy. No child willingly gives up a familiar position.

Siblings' responses to pregnancy vary with age and dependency needs. The 1-year-old infant seems largely unaware of the process, but the 2-year-old child notices the change in mother's appearance and may comment, "Mommy's fat." The 2-year-old child's need for sameness in the environment makes the child aware of any change. Toddlers may exhibit more "clinging" behavior and revert to dependent behaviors in toilet training or eating.

By the third or fourth year of age children like to be told the story of their own beginning and accept its being compared to the present pregnancy. They like to listen to heartbeats and feel the baby moving in utero. Sometimes they worry about how the baby is being fed and what it wears. Parents often take older children with them to antepartal visits, particularly in the last few weeks (Fig. 10-3). One mother reported, "Near the end [of the pregnancy] he began to kiss my belly. I was surprised by that" (Walz, Rich, 1983). Interference with established routines can

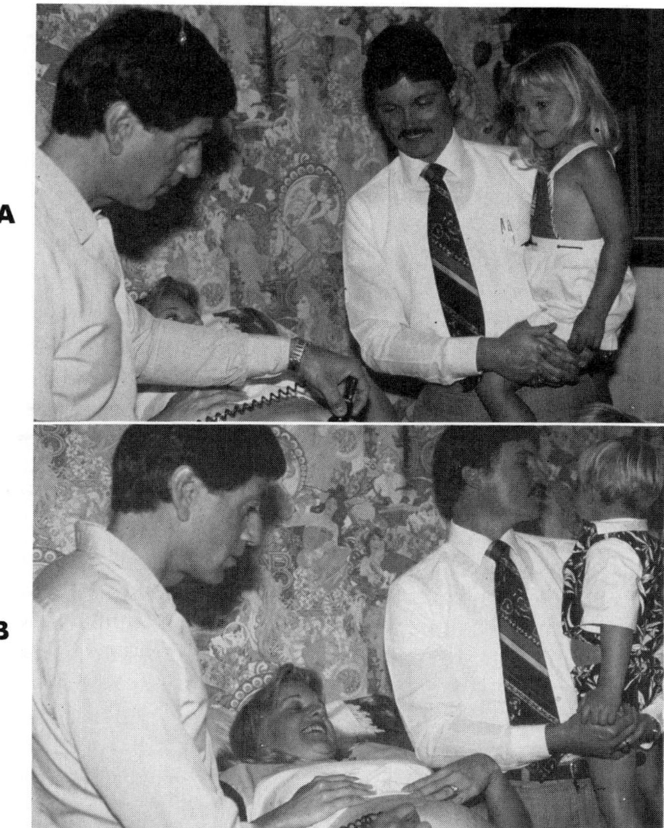

Fig. 10-3 Father and siblings accompany mother on prenatal visit. A. Daughter's attention is focused on nurse listening to baby's heart. B. Son is reluctant to watch as fetal heart rate is assessed.
Courtesy Marjorie Pyle, RNC, Lifecircle, Costa Mesa, Calif.

cause anger. One 4-year-old boy resented not being able to fit on his mother's lap anymore; his father resolved the issue by making the child a small ski he could slide down his mother's bosom and over her abdomen ("over the hump"). He could still sit close by, touch her, and accept her abdomen as part of his life. Sharing possessions with the unborn child is often short-lived, and cribs or toys donated to the coming child are mostly reclaimed.

School-age children take a more clinical interest in their mother's pregnancy. They may want to know in more detail, "How did the baby get in there?" and "How will it get out?" Children in this age group notice pregnant women in stores, churches, and schools and sometimes seem shy if they need to approach a pregnant woman directly. On the whole they look forward to the new baby, see themselves as "mothers" or "fathers," and enjoy buying baby supplies and readying a place for the baby. Because they still think in concrete terms and base judgments on the here and now, they respond positively to their mother's current good health and do not seem to be anxious about a future injury to her or to the unborn child. They need help to cope with any adverse change in the status of the parent or newborn, since they do not anticipate such a change.

Early and middle adolescents preoccupied with the establishment of their own sexual identity may have difficulty accepting the overwhelming evidence of the sexual activity of their parents. They reason that if they are "too young" for such activity, certainly their parents are "too old." They seem to take on a critical parental role and may ask, "What will people think?" or "How can you let yourself get so fat?" Many pregnant women with teenage children will confess that their teenagers are the most difficult factor in their current pregnancy.

On the positive side, parents-to-be may be suddenly confronted by a warm, sensitive person who is able to restore the mother's self-esteem, as illustrated by the following example.

> I came home one day feeling very pregnant, tired, and heavy and dreading the idea of making dinner and being helpful—you know—the mother bit! Mary [aged 15 years] was cooking some hamburger, had the table set for dinner, and even had a flower centerpiece. For some reason I just started to cry. She came to me and hugged me and said, "I think you're doing the loveliest thing in the world, having a baby." I'll always remember that—she was really *my* mother for the moment.

Late adolescents do not appear to be unduly disturbed. They think that they soon will be gone from home. Parents usually report they are comforting and act more as other adults than as children. One mother delivering her tenth baby remarked, "The only complaint my oldest daughter made was, 'Mother, I'm getting married in August, so don't you dare be too pregnant to come to the wedding.' "

Classes to prepare children for the birth of a new brother or sister (see Fig. 13-5) are available in many communities. A general teaching plan parents can use for young children is found in the teaching box on p. 258. The general plan can be modified to fit needs of children of different ages and the needs of children who will be present during the birth.

■ PARENTHOOD AFTER 35

The following discussion relates to the older woman (over 35 years). Adolescent clients, both mother and father, are discussed in Chapter 34.

Two groups of older parents have emerged in the population of women having a child late in their childbearing years. One group consists of women who have many children or who have a child during the menopausal period. The other group of older par-

TEACHING Sibling Preparation

Familiarity with a new environment helps allay anxiety
Have older sibling:
- Visit hospital classroom.
- Dress up in hospital clothing.
- Learn hospital "rules," such as walk slowly and talk quietly.
- Tour maternity area, see and touch telephone that he can use to talk to his mother.
- See naked newborn.

Realistic expectations help in accepting the newborn's behavior.
Have older sibling practice in new role:
- By listening to stories about what newborns can do and how older children react to newborn babies.
- By holding a doll with care to support the head.
- By exploring what to do when the baby cries.

Children need assistance in substituting acceptable behavior for unacceptable behavior.
Have older sibling practice through role playing:
- When parent spends time with the newborn.
- When the child gets angry with the newborn.

Recognizing one's feelings can increase one's ability to cope.
Have older sibling:
- Watch a film depicting jealousy, anger, and being left out (Johnsen, Gaspard, 1985).
- Participate in discussion of film and how to ask for help when needed.
- Draw a picture to show the child's feelings about and understanding of the mother's pregnancy and the coming baby.

ents includes relative newcomers to maternity care. These are women who have deliberately delayed childbearing until their 30s or early 40s.

Multiparous Women

Multiparous women may be those who have never used contraceptives because of personal choice or lack of knowledge concerning contraceptives, or they may be women who have used contraception successfully during the childbearing years. As menopause approaches, women in the latter group may cease to menstruate regularly, stop using contraception, and consequently become pregnant. The older multiparous woman often experiences displacement, feeling that pregnancy alienates her from her peer group and that her age interferes with close associations with young mothers (Hogan, 1979). Other parents welcome the unexpected infant as evidence of continuing maternal and paternal roles.

Including the family in preparation for the birth is important. The other children in the family may be teenagers. Women often welcome the professional person's support and suggestions concerning how to best involve them. Because older siblings often assume aspects of the parental role, the child develops in a "multiparent" household.

Nulliparous Women

The number of first-time pregnancies in women between the ages of 35 and 40 years has increased by 40%. Births in this age-group have increased by 37% over the last 10 years. It is no longer uncommon to see women in their late 30s or even in their early 40s pregnant for the first time. Reasons include advanced education, career priorities, and better contraceptive measures.

These women choose parenthood as opposed to the alternative, a child-free life-style. They often are successfully established in a career and a life-style with a partner that includes time for self-attention, establishment of a home with accumulated possessions, and freedom to travel. When questioned as to why they chose pregnancy late in life, many reply, "because time is running out." Sheehy (1977) points out that age 35 brings a biologic boundary into view. Deutch (1945) refers to the late desire for a child as a biologic "closing of the gates."

The dilemma of choice includes recognition that being a parent will have both positive and negative consequences (Chervenak, Kardon, 1991). Couples need to discuss the consequences of childbearing and child rearing before committing themselves to a lifelong venture. Partners in this group seem to share the preparation for parenthood, the planning for a family-centered birth, and the desire to be loving and competent parents. Robinson et al (1987) determined that older women were less troubled by pregnancy and remained better adjusted as they entered the last trimester of pregnancy. However, the reality of child care may prove difficult for these parents. The mother who is accustomed to the stimulation of and contact with other adults may find the isolation with her infant difficult to accept. Anger and resentment toward the father (or infant) can result, even with "preparation" for these aspects of parenting.

Only one study of the psychologic dimension of older first-time mothers has been reported in the nursing literature. Using grounded theory, Winslow (1987) reported findings from a group of 12 married first-time mothers between the ages of 35 to 40 years. All of these women were white, well-educated, and articulate. Despite its limitations, the study identified important dimensions for consideration in planning care for the first-time mother after 35. The four phases these women worked through can provide a basis for understanding this age-group.

The women in this group approached pregnancy as a project. The early periods (preconception) were characterized by *planning and control*. The "right time" for pregnancy seemed to be influenced by five factors: commitment and love relationship with the father, increasing possibility of infertility or genetic defects with advancing age, presence of a sense of accomplishment and satisfaction with life to date, desire for a baby, and rejection of remaining childless.

Seeking *safe passage* marked the second phase (up to 20 weeks' gestation). The women sought information from books and friends about pregnancy. One learning approach that did not provide them with the greater control they were seeking, however, was parent education courses for parents-to-be (Winslow, 1987) (See discussion of parent education in Chapter 13). They actively sought to rule out fetal disorders, and they were careful in searching for the best possible maternity care.

The *reality of now* refers to the transition period between 24 to 34 weeks' gestation. The women in this group were aware of movement from one role and life-style to another. Overall, they felt a sense of physical well-being. At the same time they noted that they had begun to perceive themselves differently. During this phase they identified sources of stress in their lives at that time, and anticipation of childbirth was the only problem identified that related to pregnancy.

Anticipating the future occupied considerable time and energy during the latter part of pregnancy. The women's concerns centered on issues such as having enough energy and stamina to meet the demands of parenting, fitting a new role into the established role as a working woman, meeting the need to alter their relationships with their partners, and restructuring their lives to include care of the baby.

During pregnancy, both mother and father explore the possibilities and responsibilities of changing identities and new roles. They must prepare a safe and nurturing environment during pregnancy and after birth. They must also integrate the child into an established family system and negotiate new roles (parent roles, sibling roles, grandparent roles) for family members.

■ PREGNANCY IN VARIOUS CULTURES

Nurses working with childbearing families in the United States and Canada care for families from various cultures and ethnic groups. To provide a high level of care to all families, the nurse should be aware of the cultural beliefs and practices that are important to these families. There are countless beliefs and practices that are of either a religious or ethnic derivation and may or may not still be followed by families from diverse cultural backgrounds. (For an extensive discussion of cultural aspects of care, see Chapter 3.)

Childbearing is one facet of health that is related to all aspects of a woman's life. Although most cultures do not regard pregnancy or childbirth as an illness, both conditions are considered times of heightened susceptibility to dangerous elements. Stern et al (1985) noted that "pregnant women seek security measures and court benevolent gods with ritualized behavior, whether anointing their abdomens with herbal oils in an African village or practicing daily yoga in California." Perception of the time of greatest vulnerability varies among cultures, with some groups placing greatest emphasis on the prenatal period and others on labor and delivery, or the postbirth period. Western health care culture places the greatest emphasis on the prenatal and labor and delivery periods and least on the postbirth period.

Childbearing in all cultures is complete with norms and behavioral expectations for each stage of the perinatal cycle. All relate to each culture's view of how a person maintains health and prevents illness. Health practices reflect theories of balance and harmony among opposing forces. The intrinsic factors influencing balance and harmony include heat and cold (Lee et al, 1988; Ahumada, 1991). The intrinsic factors include air and water, food and drink, sleep and wakefulness, movement, exercise and rest, evacuation and retention, and passions of the spirits, or emotions. Thus for pregnant women of many cultures, maintenance of health during childbearing implies a balance and harmony in each woman's relationship to her physical, social, and spiritual environment.

Table 10-1 provides examples of some cultural beliefs and practices surrounding childbearing that may be important to Mexican-Americans, Asians, and African-Americans. Most of these cultural beliefs and customs reflect the traditional culture and are not universally practiced by all members of the cultural group in all parts of the country. Variables such as degree of acculturation, educational and income levels, and amount of contact with the older generations influence the extent to which these customs are practiced. Women from these cultural-ethnic groups may adhere to some, all, or none of the practices listed.

It is important that the nurse become familiar with the woman as an individual and validate which, if

TABLE 10-1 Cultural Beliefs and Practices: Childbearing and Parenting

Pregnancy	Childbirth	Parenting
MEXICAN-AMERICAN (Kay, 1978) Pregnancy desired soon after marriage Expectant mother influenced strongly by mother or mother-in-law Cool air in motion considered dangerous during pregnancy Unsatisfied food cravings thought to cause a birthmark Some pica observed in the eating of ashes or dirt (not common) Milk avoided because it causes large babies and difficult deliveries Many predictions about the sex of the baby May be unacceptable and frightening to have pelvic examination by male doctor Use of herbs to treat common complaints of pregnancy Drinking chamomile tea thought to ensure effective labor	**Labor** Use of "partera" or lay midwife preferred in some places After delivery of baby, mother's legs brought together to prevent air from entering uterus **Postpartum** Diet may be restricted after delivery; for first 2 days only boiled milk and toasted tortillas permitted Bed rest for 3 days after delivery Mother's head and feet protected from cold air—bathing permitted after 14 days Mother often cared for by her own mother Forty-day restriction on sexual intercourse	**Newborn** Breast-feeding begun after the third day; colostrum may be considered "filthy" Olive oil or castor oil given to stimulate the passage of meconium Male infant not circumcised Female infant's ears pierced Belly band used to prevent umbilical hernia Religious medal worn by mother during pregnancy; placed around infant's neck Infant protected from the "evil eye" Various remedies used to treat "mal ojo" and fallen fontanelle (depressed fontanelle)
AFRICAN AMERICAN (Carrington, 1978) Acceptance of pregnancy dependent on economic status Pregnancy thought to be state of "wellness," which often results in delay in seeking prenatal care, especially by lower income Blacks Old wives tales include beliefs that having picture taken during pregnancy will cause stillbirth; reaching up will cause the cord to strangle the baby Craving of certain foods, including chicken, greens, clay, starch, dirt	**Labor** Use of "Granny midwife" in certain parts of the country Stoic behavior exhibited to avoid attracting attention Mother may arrive at hospital in far-advanced labor Emotional support often provided by other women, especially own mother **Postpartum** Vaginal bleeding seen as sign of sickness; tub baths and shampooing of hair prohibited Sassafras tea thought to have healing power Liver thought to cause heavier vaginal bleeding because of its high "blood" content Pregnancy viewed by some African-American men as a sign of their virility Self-treatment for various discomforts of pregnancy, including constipation, nausea, vomiting, headache, and heartburn	**Newborn** Feeding very important: "Good" baby thought to eat well Early introduction of solid foods May breast-feed or bottle-feed; breast-feeding may be considered embarrassing Parents fearful of spoiling baby Commonly call baby by nicknames May use excessive clothing to keep baby warm Belly band used to prevent umbilical hernia Abundant use of oil on baby's scalp and skin Strong feeling of family, community, and religion

Modified from Williams RP: Issues in women's health care. In Johnson BS, editor: *Psychiatric mental health nursing: adaptation and growth,* Philadelphia, 1989 JB Lippincott Co.

TABLE 10-1 Cultural Beliefs and Practices: Childbearing and Parenting—cont'd

Pregnancy	Childbirth	Parenting
ASIAN-AMERICAN (Chung, 1977) Pregnancy considered time when mother "has happiness in her body" Pregnancy seen as natural process Strong preference for female physician Belief in theory of hot and cold May omit soy sauce in diet to prevent dark-skinned baby Prefer soup made with ginseng root as general strength tonic Milk usually excluded from diet because it causes stomach distress	**Labor** Mother attended by other women Father does not actively participate **Postpartum** Protection from Yin (cold forces) for 30 days Ambulation limited Shower prohibited Avoidance of fruits and vegetables (Chinese) **Diet** Some vegetarianism Seaweed soup with rice (Korean) High in hot foods (Chinese)	**Newborn** Concept of the family is important and valued Father is head of the household; wife plays a subordinate role The birth of a boy is preferred

any, cultural beliefs are meaningful to her. The following questions illustrate ways to elicit cultural explanations regarding childbearing.

1. What do you and your family think you should do to keep healthy during pregnancy?
2. What are the things you can do or not do to affect your health and the health of your baby?
3. Who do you want with you during your labor?
4. What things or actions are important to you and your family to do after the baby is born?
5. What do you and your family expect from the nurse or nurses caring for you?
6. How will family members participate in your pregnancy, childbirth, and parenting?

Equipped with this knowledge, the nurse supports and nurtures those beliefs that promote physical or emotional adaptation. However, if certain beliefs are identified that might be harmful, the nurse should carefully explore those beliefs with the client and use them in the reeducation and modification process.

A nurse cannot be expected to know all there is to know about every culture and subculture, as well as their many life-styles. Understanding one's own culture is necessary to come to a better realization of why we believe as we do. Understanding clients' cultures, through interview, study, contact, and a demonstrated sincere interest, is invaluable. This understanding enables nurses to render culturally sensitive and relevant nursing care.

SUMMARY

Pregnancy represents a maturational crisis that requires changes in outlook, role responsibilities, and everyday living of all family members. The ability to respond to changes with new behaviors and new self-concepts is fostered not only by intrinsic strengths but also by extrinsic strengths, such as the love and support of outsiders.

Nurses can act as one source of extrinsic strength. Their knowledge of the responses of all family members to a pregnancy enables them to use those responses as the cornerstones of nursing-care plans. The long-term contact nurses have with clients and their families provides unique opportunities for informed supportive nursing that may have a long-term effect on family life. The nurse encourages the childbearing family to participate in parent education classes. Attendance at such classes permits sharing of experiences with other couples and families. The couple is reassured by knowing that their thoughts, feelings, and concerns are common to others. Classes can increase confidence and self-assurance and help parents develop new coping skills.

Consumers learn about birth-setting choices from a variety of sources. The knowledgeable nurse serves as a valuable resource for couples who want to individualize their childbirth experience.

REFERENCES

Ahumada LS: Multicultural perinatal health care, *Matern Child Health Educ Resources* 6, Spring 1991. (Center for Health Education Resources, 1 W. Campbell Ave, Bldg D, Campbell, CA 95008.)

Ballou JW: *The psychology of pregnancy,* Lexington, Mass, 1978, DC Health & Co.

Barranti C: The grandparent/grandchild relationship: family resource in an era of voluntary bonds, *Fam Relat* 34:3, July 1985.

Caplan G: *Concepts of mental health and consultation,* Washington, DC, 1959, US Department of Health, Education, and Welfare.

Carrington BW: The Afro-American. In Clark AL, editor: *Culture/child-bearing/health professionals,* Philadelphia, 1978, FA Davis Co.

Carty E, Tier T: Birth planning: A reality-based script for building confidence, *Nurse Midwife* 34:3, May/June 1989.

Chervenak JL, Kardon NB: Advancing maternal age: the actual risks, *Female Patient* 16:17, Nov 1991.

Colman AD: Psychological state during the first pregnancy, *Am J Orthopsych* 39:778, 1969.

Deutch H: *The psychology of women,* vol 2, New York, 1945, Bantam Books.

Ellis D: Sexual needs and concerns of expectant parents, *JOGNN* 9, Sept/Oct 1980.

Entwistle DR, Doering SG: *The first birth: a family turning point,* Baltimore, 1981, Johns Hopkins University Press.

Fawcett J: Body image and the pregnant couple, *MCN* 3:227, 1978.

Field T: The three Rs of infant-adult interactions: rhythms, repertoires, and responsitivity, *J Pediatr Psychol* 3:131, 1978.

Gaffney KF: New directions in maternal attachment research, *J Pediatr Health Care* 2:181, 1988.

Greene R, Polivka J: The meaning of grandparent day cards: an analysis of the intergenerational network, *Fam Relat* 34:2, April 1985.

Grossman FK, Eichler LS, Winckoff SA: *Pregnancy, birth, parenthood,* San Francisco, 1980, Jossey-Bass.

Hogan LR: Pregnant again—at 41, *Matern Child Nurs J* 4:174, 1979.

Honig JC: Preparing preschool-aged children to be siblings, *MCN* 11(1):37, 1986.

Horn M, Manion J: Creative grandparenting: bonding the generations, *JOGN Nurs* 14:233, May/June 1985.

House JS: *Work, stress and social support,* Reading, Mass, 1981, Addison-Wesley.

Hunter R, Macalpine I, editors: *Three hundred years of psychiatry: 1535-1860,* London, 1963, Oxford University Press.

Jessner L et al: The development of parental attitudes during pregnancy. In Anthony EJ, Benedek T, editors: *Parenthood,* Edinburgh, 1970, Churchill Livingstone.

Johnsen NM, Gaspard ME: Theoretical foundations of a prepared sibling class, *JOGNN* 14:237, May/June 1985.

Jones LC: A meta-analytic study of the effects of childbirth education on the parent-infant relationship, *Health Care Women Int* 7:357, 1986.

Kay MA: The Mexican-American. In Clark AL, editor: *Culture/child-bearing/health professionals,* Philadelphia, 1978, FA Davis Co.

Lederman RP: *Psychosocial adaptation in pregnancy: assessment of seven dimensions of maternal development,* Englewood Cliffs, NJ, 1984, Prentice-Hall.

Lee RV et al: Southeast Asian folklore about pregnancy and parturition, *Obstet Gynecol* 71:243, 1988.

Leifer M: *Psychological effects of motherhood: a study of first pregnancy,* New York, 1980, Praeger Publishers.

Lein L: Male participation in home life: impact of social supports and breadwinner responsibility on the allocation of tasks, *Fam Coord* 28:489, 1979.

Levy JM McGee RK: Childbirth as a crisis, *J Pers Soc Psychol* 31:171, 1975.

Lumley J: The development of maternal-fetal bonding in first pregnancy. In Zichella LJ, editor: *Emotions and reproduction,* New York, 1980a, Academic Press.

Lumley J: The image of the fetus in the first trimester, *Birth Fam J* 17:5, 1980b.

Lumley J: Attitudes to the fetus among primigravidas, *Aust Pediatr J* 18:106, 1982a.

Lumley J: *Maternal-fetal bonding. II. Implications for the next three months,* unpublished manuscript, Melbourne, 1982b, Monash University.

Maloni JA, McIndoe JE, Rubenstein G: Expectant grandparents class, *JOGNN* 16:26, Jan 1987.

May KA: The father as observer, *MCN* 7:319, 1982a.

May KA: Father participation in birth: fact and fiction, *J Calif Perinat Assoc* 2:41, Fall 1982b.

Mercer RT, Hackley K, Bostrom A: *Factors having an impact on maternal role attainment in the first year of motherhood,* San Francisco, 1982, University of California, San Francisco, Dept of Family Health Care Nursing.

Mercer RT: *First-time motherhood: experiences from teens to forties,* New York, 1986, Springer Publishing Co.

Merilo KF: Is it better the second time around? *MCN* 13:200, 1988.

Reich CL: Exercise in pregnancy: a review for nurse practitioners, *Health Care Women Int* 8:349, 1987.

Richardson P: Women's perceptions of change in relationships shared with children during pregnancy, *Matern Child Nurs J* 12:2, Summer 1983.

Robinson GE et al: Psychological adaptation to pregnancy in childless women more than 35 years of age, *Am J Obstet Gynecol* 156:328, 1987.

Rubin R: Cognitive style in pregnancy, *Am J Nurs* 70:502, 1970.

Rubin R: Maternal tasks in pregnancy, *Matern Child Nurs J* 4: Spring 1975.

Rubin R: *Maternal identity and the maternal experience,* New York, 1984, Springer Publishing Co.

Sheehy G: *Passages: predictable crises of adult life,* New York, 1977, Bantam Books.

Stainton MC: The fetus: a growing member of the family, *Fam Relations* 34:321, 1985a.

Stainton MC: Origins of attachment: culture and cue sensitivity, *Diss Abstr Int* 46:3786-B (University Microfilms No. 8600606), 1985b.

Stern PN, Tilden VP, Maxwell EK: Culturally induced stress during childbearing: the Filipino-American experience, *Health Care Women Int* 6:105, 1985.

Swanson J: The marital sexual relationship during pregnancy, *JOGNN* 9:Sept/Oct, 1980.

Walz B, Rich O: Maternal tasks of taking on a second child in the postpartum period, *Matern Child Nurs J* 12:3, Fall 1983.

Westney OE, Cole OJ, Munford TL: The effects of prenatal education intervention on unwed prospective adolescent fathers, *J Adolesc Health Care* 9:214, 1988.

Williams RP: Issues in women's health care. In Johnson BS, editor: *Psychiatric mental health nursing: adaptation and growth,* Philadelphia, 1989, JB Lippincott Co.

Winslow W: First pregnancy after 35: what is the experience? *MCN* 12(2):92, 1987.

Zalar MK: Sexual counseling for pregnant couples, *MCN* 1(3):176, 1976.

References—Nursing Research

Bobak I: *Fathers,* Unpublished research, 1968.

Broom B: Consensus about the marital relationship during transition to parenthood, *Nurs Res* 33:4, July/Aug, 1984.

Cronenwett LR: Father participation in child care: a critical review, *Res Nurs Health* 5:63, 1982.

Cronenwett LR, Kunst-Wilson W: Stress, social support, and the transition of fatherhood, *Nurs Res* 30:196, 1981.

Fawcett J, York R: Spouses' physical and psychological symptoms during pregnancy and the postpartum, *Nurs Res* 35(4):144, 1986a.

Fawcett J, et al: Spouses' body image changes during and after pregnancy: a replication and extension, *Nurs Res* 35(4):220, 1986b.

Glazer G: Anxiety and stressors of expectant fathers, *West J Nurs Res* 11:1, 1989.

Jones C: Father to infant attachment, effects of early contact and characteristics of the infant, *Res Nurs Health* 4:193, 1981.

Jordan P: Laboring for relevance: expectant and new fatherhood, *Nurs Res* 39:1, Jan/Feb 1990.

Kemp VH, Page CK: Maternal prenatal attachment in normal and high-risk pregnancies, *JOGNN* 16(3):179, 1987.

Koniak-Griffin D: The relationship between social support, self-esteem, and maternal-fetal attachment in adolescents, *Res Nurs Health* 11:269, 1988.

Kunst-Wilson W, Cronenwett L: Nursing care for the emerging family: promoting paternal behavior, *Res Nurs Health* 4:201, 1981.

Latham L: An altered birth script: mother's perceptions of intrapartum transfer from an alternative birth center to a conventional hospital setting, master's thesis, Detroit, 1990, Wayne State University.

May KA: A typology of detachment and involvement styles adopted during pregnancy by first-time expectant fathers, *West J Nurs Res* 2:445, 1980.

May KA: Three phases of father involvement in pregnancy, *Nurs Res* 31:337, 1982c.

Mercer RT: A theoretical framework for studying factors that impact on the maternal role, *Nurs Res* 30:2, March/April 1981.

Mercer RT et al: Further exploration of maternal and paternal fetal attachment, *Res Nurs Health* 11:83, 1988.

Patterson ET, Freese M, Goldenberg R: Seeking safe passage: utilizing health care during pregnancy, *Image* 22(1):27, Spring 1990.

Rubin R: Attainment of the maternal role. I. Processes, *Nurs Res* 16:237, 1967a.

Rubin R: Attainment of the maternal role. II. Models and referents, *Nurs Res* 16:342, 1967b.

Stainton MC: *A comparison of prenatal and postnatal perceptions of their babies by parents.* Paper presented to the First International Congress on Pre- and Peri-natal Psychology, Toronto, July 8, 1983.

Strickland OL: The occurrence of symptoms in expectant fathers, *Nurs Res* 36(3):184, 1987.

BIBLIOGRAPHY

Carter B, McGoldrick M: *The changing family life cycle: a framework for family therapy,* ed 2, New York, 1988, Gardner Press.

Christensen P, Kenney S: *Nursing process: application of theories, frameworks, and models,* ed 3, St Louis, 1990, Mosby–Year Book.

Doenges M, Kenty J, Moorhouse M: *Maternal/newborn care plans: guidelines for client care,* Philadelphia, 1988, FA Davis.

Friedemann M-L: The concept of family nursing, *J Adv Nurs* 14, 1989.

Friedemann M-L et al: Advanced family nursing with the control-congruence model, *Clini Nurse Specialist* 3:4, 1989.

Gay JT et al: Reva Rubin revisited, *JOGNN* 17:394, 1988.

Giblin P, Poland M, Ager J: Effects of social supports on attitudes, health behaviors, and obtaining prenatal care, *J Community Health* 15:1990.

Giger J, Davidhizar R: *Transcultural nursing: assessment and intervention,* St Louis, 1991, Mosby–Year Book.

Hochschild A, Machung A: *Second shift: inside the two-job marriage,* New York 1989, Viking Press.

Mercer RT: Theoretical perspective on the family. In Gillis CL et al, editors: *Toward a science of family nursing,* Menlo Park, Calif, 1989, Addison-Wesley Publishing Co.

Redman BK: *The process of patient education,* ed 6, St Louis, 1988, Mosby–Year Book.

Waxler-Morrison N, Anderson J, Richardson E, editors: *Crosscultural nursing,* Vancouver, 1990, University of British Columbia Press.

Bibliography—Nursing Research

Bozett FW: Social control of identity by children of gay fathers, *West J Nurs Res* 10:550, 1988.

Brown L et al: A sociodemographic profile of families of low birth weight infants, *West J Nurs Res* 11:5, Oct 1989.

Friedemann M-L: An instrument to evaluate effectiveness in family functioning, *West J Nurs Res* 13:2, 1991.

Kulin J: Childbearing Cambodian refugee women, *Can Nurse,* p. 46, June 1988.

Loveland CC et al: A psychometric analysis of the family environment scale, *Nurs Res* 5:38, 1989.

Majewski J: Conflicts, satisfactions, and attitudes during transition to the maternal role, *Nurs Res* 35(I):10, 1985.

Mercer R, Ferketich S, and DeJoseph J: Effects of stress on family functioning during pregnancy, *Nurs Res* 37:268, 1989.

Mercer RT et al: Theoretical models for studying the effect of antepartum stress on the family, *Nurs Res* 35(6):339, 1986.

Pitzer MS, Hock E: Employed mothers' concerns about separation from the first- and second-born child, *Res Nurs Health* 12(2):123, 1989.

Uphold C, Strickland O: Issues related to the unit of analysis in family nursing, *West J Nurs Res* 11:405, 1989.

Wismont JM, Reame NE: The lesbian childbearing experience: assessing developmental tasks, *Image J Nurs Sch* 21(3):137, 1989.

chapter 10 review

Key Concepts

- Pregnancy involves all family members, who react to pregnancy and interpret its meaning in light of their own needs and the needs of the others affected.
- The fetus is a powerful influence in the family system, bringing changes in parental behavior and family functioning.
- The process of family adaptation to pregnancy takes place within a cultural environment.
- Pregnancy presents several developmental tasks to the mother-, father-, grandparent-, and sibling-to-be as they prepare for new levels of caring and responsibility.
- Because pregnancy is a developmental crisis, it is a time of emotional upheaval for both the man and the woman, necessitating adequate communication between them.
- The parent-child, sibling-child, and grandparent-child relationships start during the pregnancy.
- Maternal and familial adaptations to pregnancy generate needs that the nurse-clinician can anticipate and meet by providing support, and teaching/counseling/advocacy.
- The father/partner may take any one of a number of roles during the woman's pregnancy; the important concept is that each partner agrees on the other's role.
- The psychosocial aspects of care are of utmost importance and may well affect the whole course of pregnancy, childbirth, and the adjustment of the new family.
- The expectant family's developmental crisis also presents a developmental opportunity for maturation and growth.

Key Terms

- announcement phase (p. 251)
- attachment (p. 248)
- birth plan (p. 250)
- body boundaries (p.245)
- body image (p. 246)
- couvade (p. 251)
- developmental tasks (p. 248)
- emotional lability (p. 245)
- expressive style (p. 252)
- fantasy child (p. 248)
- focusing phase (p. 252)
- instrumental style (p. 253)
- maturational crisis (p. 244)
- mitleiden (p. 252)
- moratorium phase (p. 251)
- observer style (p. 252)
- rite of passage (p. 246)
- safe passage (p. 249)

Critical Thinking Exercise

1. You are participating in a health screening fair. Melanie B. approaches you and asks, "What can you tell me about pregnancy for a woman past 35?" What assumptions would you make? What further information do you need before responding? Discuss at least four phases experienced during pregnancy by women between ages 35 and 40.
2. Jennifer P., pregnant with her second child, confides in you, "I don't know how my 18-month old will take to a new sister or brother. To make matters worse, the grandparents are trying to outdo each other in telling us what to do!" What assumptions would you make? What further information do you need before responding? Briefly discuss at least two interventions you might consider, and justify your choices.

Topics for Nursing Research

- Compare the concerns in pregnancy of a first-time mother with those of a second-time mother.
- Identify ambivalent feelings experienced throughout the pregnancy when the expectant couple is of the same sex.
- Replicate the study by Richardson (1983) with other populations, such as the first-time mother after age 35.
- Identify significant characteristics of parent-parent support when the expectant couple is of the same sex or from different cultures.
- Replicate studies that relate the psychologic variables of prenatal attachment and maternal-fetal interaction with mother-infant interaction (p. 248).
- Replicate studies to determine if the styles of involvement, identified by May (p. 252), are evidenced by partners of multiparous women and by same-sex partners during pregnancy.

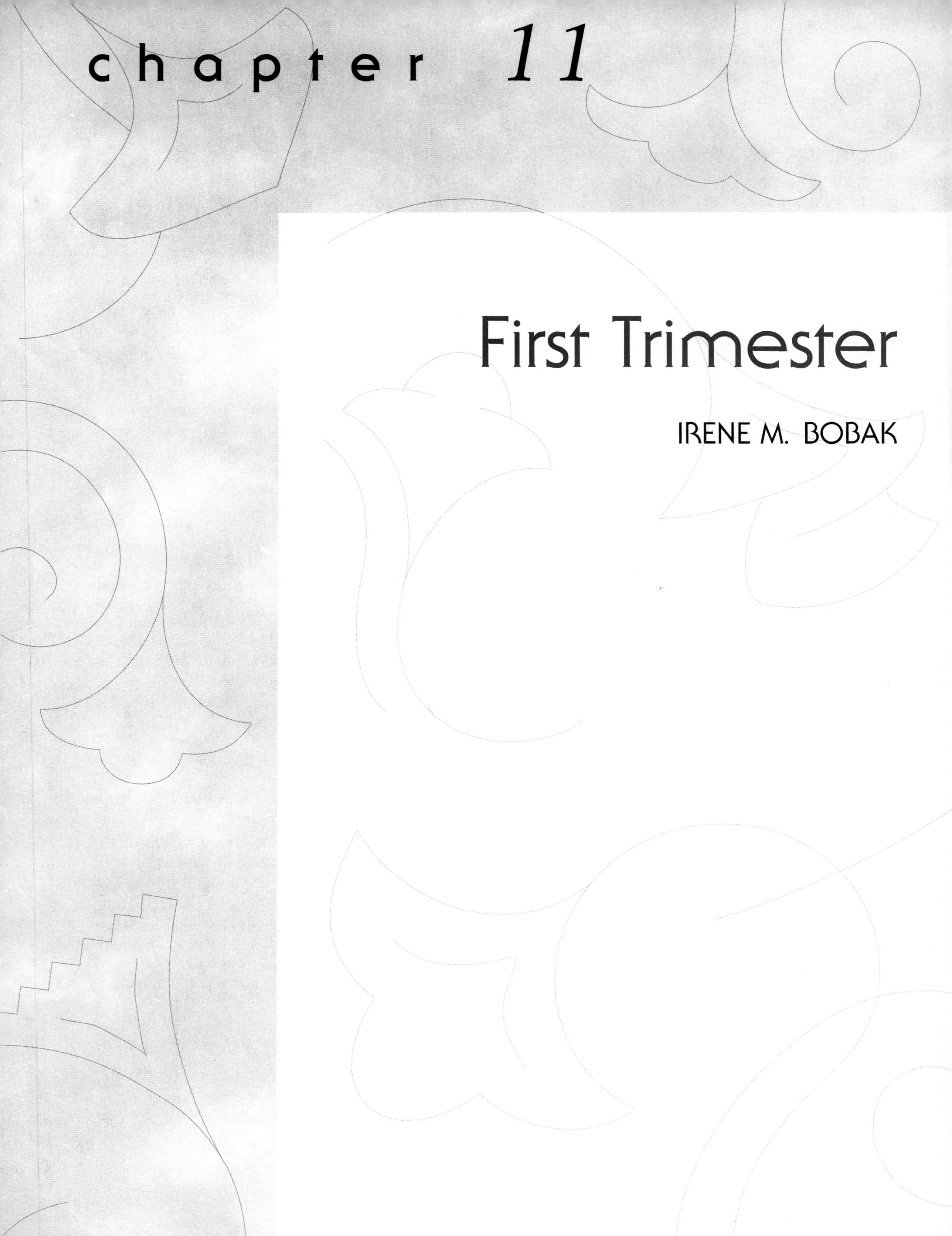

chapter 11

First Trimester

IRENE M. BOBAK

LEARNING OBJECTIVES

- Define the key terms listed.
- Summarize health assessment of the pregnant woman.
- Identify the presumptive, probable, and positive manifestations of pregnancy.
- State the important components of the initial prenatal visit.
- Outline the schedule of visits for the woman during the first trimester.
- Evaluate cultural influences on the woman's/family's response to pregnancy and the use of the health care system.
- List physical warning signs in the first trimester.
- Discuss physiology and self-care of discomforts related to maternal adaptations.
- Explain guidelines for teaching self-care for urinary tract infections, breast self-examination, and Kegel exercises.
- Discuss the benefits of assisting pregnant women/couples to develop a birth plan.
- Formulate possible nursing diagnoses.
- Discuss planning, implementation, and evaluation of nursing care during the first trimester.
- Identify topics for nursing research related to the first trimester of pregnancy.

The prenatal period is a time of physical and psychologic preparation for birth and parenthood. Becoming a parent represents one of the maturational crises of our lives, and as such it is a time of intense learning for parents and for those close to them. The prenatal period provides a unique opportunity for nurses and other members of the health care team to influence family health. During this period, essentially healthy women seek regular care and guidance. The nurse's health promotion interventions can affect the well-being of the woman, her unborn child, and the rest of her family for many years to come.

Regular prenatal visits, ideally beginning soon after the first missed menstrual period, offer opportunities to ensure the health of the expectant mother and her infant. This is achieved by supervising the course of pregnancy. Prenatal health supervision permits diagnosis and treatment of maternal disorders that may have preexisted or may develop during the pregnancy. It is designed to follow the growth and development of the fetus and to identify abnormalities that may interfere with the course of normal labor. The woman and her family can seek support for stress and learn parenting skills.

The professionals who have contact with the pregnant woman and her family will include a cross section of health workers such as nurse, physician, nutritionist, and social worker. It is essential that these persons collaborate to provide holistic care for their clients. The initial visit of the woman to either the physician's office or a maternity clinic is important in setting the tone for her care. The woman needs to feel welcomed and important. The initial visit may include diagnosing the pregnancy and establishing the data base, depending on the duration of gestation. If pregnancy is too early and cannot be verified, her next appointment is scheduled in 2 weeks.

The woman's desire for pregnancy is evaluated. If she is pregnant and does not wish to continue the pregnancy, she is referred for abortion counseling (see Chapter 42). If she is not pregnant and does not wish to be, she is referred for fertility management, if appropriate (see Chapter 42). If the woman is pregnant and plans to carry the pregnancy to term, prenatal health supervision should begin.

Pregnancy spans 9 months, approximately 40 weeks. Pregnancy is divided into three 3-month periods or trimesters. The **first trimester** covers weeks 1 through 13; the second, weeks 14 through 26; the third, weeks 27 through term gestation (38 to 40 weeks).

Once pregnancy is diagnosed, prenatal care is instituted. Nursing care follows the nursing process: assessment, analysis and formulation of nursing diagnoses, planning, implementation, and evaluation.

■ DIAGNOSIS OF PREGNANCY

The clinical diagnosis of pregnancy before the second missed period may be uncertain in at least 25% to 30% of women. Physical variability, lack of relaxation, obesity, or tumors, for example, may make it difficult even for the experienced obstetrician or midwife to diagnose pregnancy. Accuracy is most important, however, because emotional, social, medical, or legal consequences of an inaccurate diagnosis, either positive or negative, can be extremely serious. A correct date for the first day of the **last menstrual period (LMP),** the date of intercourse, or the basal body temperature (BBT) record may be of great value in the accurate diagnosis of pregnancy. Reexamination in 2 to 4 weeks may be required for verifying the diagnosis.

Great variability is possible in the subjective and objective symptoms of pregnancy. The diagnosis of pregnancy is classified as follows: presumptive, probable, and positive.

The nurse is referred to Chapter 8 for an in-depth discussion of the symptoms reflecting maternal adaptations to pregnancy. Many of the signs and symptoms of pregnancy are clinically useful in the diagnosis of pregnancy. However, the **presumptive signs and symptoms** of pregnancy can be caused by conditions other than gestation. Therefore no one manifestation can be relied on for a final impression, nor are combinations of manifestations diagnostic. For example, amenorrhea may be caused by an endocrine disorder; lack of energy and fatigue may signify anemia or infection; and nausea or vomiting may be caused by a gastrointestinal upset or allergy.

Presumptive findings include subjective symptoms and objective signs. Subjective symptoms may include **amenorrhea,** nausea and vomiting **(morning sickness), breast changes** and sensitivity, **urinary frequency,** lack of energy or fatigue, weight gain, and mood swings. "Quickening" may be noted between weeks 16 and 20. Objective signs include a variety of demonstrable anatomic and physiologic changes (see Chapter 8), elevation of BBT; skin changes such as striae gravidarum, deeper pigmentation (chloasma, linea nigra); breast changes; abdominal enlargement; and changes in the uterus and vagina.

Probable subjective symptoms are the same as presumptive symptoms. When combined with probable objective signs, they strongly suggest pregnancy and are called **probable signs and symptoms**. Objective signs include uterine enlargement, Braxton Hicks contractions and souffle (soft, blowing sound of blood in the arteries of the pregnant uterus and synchronous with maternal pulse), ballottement, and positive pregnancy test results from less sophisticated tests.

The **positive signs** of pregnancy are demonstration of fetal heart tones distinct from heart sounds of the mother, verification of fetal movement by someone other than the mother, and visualization of the fetus with a technique such as ultrasound (Scott et al, 1990). The positive signs used to confirm the diagnosis of pregnancy include certain pregnancy tests (see Chapter 8).

Estimated Date of Delivery

After the diagnosis of pregnancy the woman's first question usually concerns when she will give birth. This date has traditionally been termed the estimated date of confinement (EDC). To promote a more positive perception of both pregnancy and delivery, however, the term **estimated date of delivery (EDD)** usually is used. Because the precise date of conception generally must remain inexact, many formulas or rules of thumb have been suggested for calculating the EDD. None of these rules of thumb is infallible, but Nägele's rule is reasonably accurate and is the method usually used.

NÄGELE'S RULE. **Nägele's rule** is as follows: add 7 days to the first day of the LMP, subtract 3 months, and add 1 year. The formula becomes EDD = ([LMP + 7 days] − 3 months) + 1 year. For example, if the first day of the LMP was July 10, 1993, the EDD is April 17, 1994. In simple terms, add 7 days to the LMP and count forward 9 months.

Nägele's rule assumes that the woman has a 28-day cycle and that the pregnancy occurred on the fourteenth day. An adjustment is in order if the cycle is longer or shorter than 28 days. If the menstrual cycle is less than 28 days, subtract that number of days from the EDD; if it is longer than 28 days, add that number of days to the EDD. On the basis of Nägele's rule, only about 4% to 10% of pregnant women will deliver spontaneously on the EDD. Most women will deliver during the period extending from 7 days before to 7 days after the EDD.

■ NURSING PROCESS

ASSESSMENT

The process of assessment continues throughout the prenatal period. It begins when a woman makes contact with health professionals because she suspects she is pregnant. Assessment techniques include the interview, physical examination, and laboratory tests.

A checklist of care needs spanning pregnancy is a valuable tool. A checklist provides the team of care providers with a communication tool to prevent gaps and to identify areas of repeated concern for clients. When shared with clients, the checklist items can provide reassurance to pregnant women and their families that their concerns are common in many pregnancies. Reading the checklist also reminds clients of otherwise forgotten data. A checklist for the first trimester is shown below.

Interview

The initial assessment interview establishes the therapeutic relationship between nurse and client. It

First-Trimester Checklist

- Diagnosis and expected date of delivery
- Schedule and events of visits
- Counseling for self-care:
  - Birth plan
  - Adaptations/discomforts
    - Breast changes
    - Urinary frequency
    - Nausea and vomiting
    - Nasal stuffiness and epistaxis
    - Gingivitis and epulis
    - Leukorrhea
    - Fatigue
    - Psychosocial responses and family dynamics
- Exercise and rest
- Relaxation
- Nutrition
- Sexuality
- Cultural variation
- Warning signs
- Resources
  - Education
  - Dental evaluation
  - Medical service
  - Social service
  - Emergency room
- Diagnostic tests
  - Specify
- Other

is planned, purposeful communication that focuses on specific content. Two sources are usually used in collecting data: the client's subjective interpretation of health status and the nurse's objective observations. During the interview the nurse observes the client's affect, posture, body language, skin color, and other physical and emotional signs. These observations provide important data in the assessment.

Often the client will be accompanied by a family member or members. The nurse builds a relationship with these persons as part of the social context of the client. They also are helpful in recalling and validating information related to the client's health. With the client's permission, those accompanying her can be included in the initial prenatal interview. Wright and Leahey (1984) offer excellent guidance to the nurse in developing skills for interviewing families and assessing the interaction among family members. Observations and information about the client's family are part of the interview. For example, if the client is accompanied by small children, the nurse can inquire about her plans for child care during the forthcoming labor and delivery.

The interview provides information about the client's biopsychosocial status. Although the format for interviewing or recording the client's health history may differ, the information obtained is universal.

REASON FOR SEEKING CARE. The client's description of the purpose for the request for care is quoted verbatim in the record. For example, "I think I am pregnant" or "My legs get so swollen I can hardly walk." This statement does not constitute a diagnosis, because the client's condition needs to be confirmed by the nurse or physician before any care is instituted. Recording the chief purpose of a visit in the client's own words alerts other personnel to the "priority of need" as seen by the client.

MEDICAL HISTORY. The interviewer will record such information as the woman's menstrual history, sexual activity, and previous pregnancies and their outcomes. The conduct of the *present pregnancy* is predicated on the reports of previous pregnancies.

The medical history describes medical or surgical conditions that may affect the course of pregnancy or that may be affected by the pregnancy. For example, the pregnant woman who has diabetes or epilepsy will require special care. Because most clients are anxious during the initial interview, reference to cues such as a Medic-Alert bracelet will help the client explain allergies, chronic diseases, or medications being used (e.g., cortisone, insulin, or anticonvulsants) If the woman is using any medications, she is asked to list them and describe their use.

Previous surgeries are described. Abortion may predispose the woman to incompetent cervix; uterine surgery or extensive repair of the pelvic floor may necessitate cesarean birth; appendectomy rules out appendicitis as cause of right lower quadrant pain; spinal surgery may contraindicate spinal or epidural anesthesia. Any *injury* involving the pelvis is noted particularly.

Often clients who have adapted well to chronic or handicapping conditions forget to mention them because they are so integrated into their life-style. Special shoes or a limp may indicate a pelvic structural defect, which is an important consideration in pregnancy. The nurse who observes these special characteristics and can inquire about them sensitively obtains individualized data that will provide the basis for a comprehensive nursing care plan. Observations are vital components of the interview process because they prompt the nurse and the client to focus on the specific needs of the client and her family.

FAMILY HISTORY. The family history provides information about the client's immediate family, including parents, siblings, and children. This helps identify familial or genetic disorders or conditions that could affect the present health status of the woman. A description of a detailed family history is presented in Chapter 2.

SOCIAL AND EXPERIENTIAL HISTORY. *Situational factors* such as the family's ethnic and cultural background and socioeconomic status are determined in the social and experiential history. *Perception of this pregnancy* is explored. Is this pregnancy wanted or not, planned or not? Is the woman/couple pleased, displeased, accepting, or nonaccepting? Is the pregnancy "hers" or "theirs"? What problems arise because of the pregnancy: financial, career, and living accommodations? The *family support* system is determined (see Chapter 2). What primary support is available to the mother? Are changes needed to promote adequate support for the mother? What are the existing relationships among mother, father, siblings, and in-laws? What preparations are being made for the care of the woman and dependent family members during labor and for the care of the infant after birth? Is community support needed, for example, financial, educational? What are the woman's/couple's ideas about childbearing, expectations of infant's behavior, and outlook on life and the female role? Questions that need to be asked include, What will it be like to have a baby in the home? How is your life going to change by having a baby? What plans do having a baby interrupt? During interviews throughout the pregnancy the nurse remains alert for *potential* *parenting disorders* such as depression, lack of family support, and inadequate living conditions. What is the woman's/couple's attitude toward health care, particularly during childbearing? What is expected of the physician, and how is the relationship between the woman/couple and nurse viewed?

Coping mechanisms and patterns of interacting are identified (see Chapters 2 and 10). Early in the pregnancy the nurse determines the woman's/couple's knowledge of pregnancy, maternal changes, fetal growth, care of self, and care of the newborn, including feeding. It is important to ask about attitudes toward unmedicated or medicated childbirth and about parental knowledge of availability of parenting skills classes. Before planning for nursing care, the nurse needs information about the woman's/couple's decision-making abilities and living habits (e.g., exercise, sleep, diet, diversional interests, personal hygiene, clothing). Common stressors in childbearing have been identified (see Research Highlight, below).

Attitudes concerning the range of *acceptable sexual behavior* during pregnancy are explored. Questions such as the following could be asked: What has your family (partner, friends) told you about sex during pregnancy? *Sexual self-concept* is given more emphasis by employing questions such as, How do you feel about the changes in your appearance? How does your partner feel about your body now? Do maternity clothes make pregnant women attractive?

All women should be assessed for a history or risk of physical abuse. Although visual cues from the client's appearance or behavior may suggest the possibility, if questioning is limited to those who fit the supposed profile of the battered woman, many will be missed (Helton, 1987; Chez, 1989). (See Chapter 43 for a more complete discussion of this issue.)

REVIEW OF SYSTEMS. During this portion of the interview, symptoms that indicate pregnancy are elicited. In addition, preexisting or concurrent problems

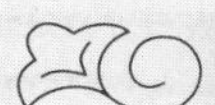 **Research Highlight** 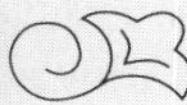

Common Stressors in Childbearing

RESEARCH ABSTRACT

The purpose of this study was to identify common stressors in pregnancy and to measure the intensity of the stressors identified. A group of 221 women who were contacted by the researchers agreed to participate. Participants were in different trimesters of pregnancy: 81, first trimester; 80, third trimester; and 60, postpartum. Data were collected during a 20 to 30 minute interview by two research assistants who used a one-page protocol. Women were asked to identify stressful events and to assign a number rating between 1 and 100 to each event. The women reported 1403 responses that were stress related. The stressors reported most often included physical symptoms, changes in body image, concerns about baby welfare, changes in living patterns, emotional changes, and concerns about the technology of pregnancy. The most intense stressors were the baby's welfare, the labor and birth process, pregnancy, behaviors of the newborn, and the relationship with the baby's father. There were differences in the frequency and intensity of stressors across pregnancy and the postpartum period. Because the same women were not interviewed over time, this study should be replicated using a longitudinal approach (interviewing the same women at all three times).

IMPLICATIONS FOR PRACTICE

Inasmuch as the types of stressors and their intensity were different in the first and third trimesters and in the postpartum period, care providers should tailor prenatal care to different phases of childbearing. People interacting with women in childbearing phases, both care providers and partners, should be aware of the effects of comments about appearance and emotions on the woman and should learn sensitive ways of phrasing such comments.

RELATED RESEARCH QUESTIONS

1. Do the types of stressors a woman experiences during pregnancy and the postpartum period change over time?
2. Does education reduce the number of stressors experienced during pregnancy and the postpartum period?
3. Does education reduce the type of stressors experienced during pregnancy and the postpartum period?
4. Do the types and intensity of stressors differ across cultural and ethnic groups?

REFERENCE

Affonso D, Mayberry LJ: Common stressors reported by a group of childbearing American women, *Health Care Women Int* 11(3)331: , 1990.

are identified and described for all body systems and mental status. The woman is questioned about physical symptoms she has experienced such as shortness of breath or pain. Pregnancy affects and is affected by all body systems (see Chapter 8); therefore knowledge of the present status of body systems is important in planning care. For each sign or symptom expressed, the following additional data should be obtained: body location, quality, quantity, chronology, setting, aggravating or alleviating factors, and associated manifestations (onset, character, course) (Seidel et al, 1991).

BIRTH PLAN. The client's preparation for the childbirth experience is assessed. Is she planning to attend parent education classes (with out without her partner) during the first trimester? Is the couple considering a birth plan? Attendance at parent education classes and the development of a birth plan may vary with the client's culture, usual means of coping (classes and reading material or other), and feelings about the role of the health care givers. Some women may come with a form of birth plan; for example, after the birth of an ill infant, the woman anticipating a second birth may prefer to deliver only at a tertiary care center with a neonatal intensive care unit. A highly dependent woman may allow the health care team to make decisions about birth plans, assuming that its decisions would be the wisest. A more independent, assertive woman may seek health care that is within her philosophy of care and her beliefs and knowledge; she wants her wishes honored during pregnancy, labor and birth, and the postpartum period. The birth plan is discussed later in this chapter.

WOMAN WITH A DISABILITY. Clients with serious and handicapping physical or emotional disorders—the deaf, the blind, the depressed, the physically disabled, the mentally retarded, the brain injured—must all be respected and the assessment approach adapted to their needs. Clients who are emotionally restricted may not be able to give an effective history, but they must be respected, and the history should be obtained from *them* to the extent possible. Their points of view and their attitudes matter. Still, when necessary, the family, other health professionals involved in care, and the client's record must be queried to get the complete story. Each client must be fully respected and fully involved to the limit of her emotional, cognitive capacity or physical handicap.

Physical Examination

The initial physical examination provides the baseline for assessing subsequent changes. The examiner needs to determine the client's needs for basic information regarding the structure of the genital organs and to provide this information, along with a demonstration of the equipment that may be used and an explanation of the procedure itself. The interaction requires an unhurried, sensitive, and gentle approach with a matter-of-fact attitude.

It is important that the examiner ensure the cleanliness of the facilities, equipment, supplies, and hands. All equipment necessary for the procedure should be in place to avoid interrupting the examination (Fig. 11-1).

The woman is ensured of privacy for the examination without unexpected intrusions. She is given a cover gown and drape for modesty. The environment is comfortably warm and pleasant.

The physical examination begins with assessment of vital signs, height and weight, and blood pressure. Because the bladder must be empty before pelvic examination, the urine specimen is obtained.

Each examiner has developed a routine for proceeding with the physical examination; most choose the head-to-toe progression. Heart and breath sounds are evaluated, and extremities are examined. Distribution, amount, and quality of body hair is of particular importance because the findings reflect nutritional status, endocrine function, and general emphasis on hygiene. The thyroid gland is assessed carefully. The typical basic examination is usually completed without much difficulty for the healthy woman.

The examiner needs to remain alert to the woman's clues that give direction to the remainder of the assessment and that indicate possible problems such as supine hypotension (p. 275).

THYROID GLAND. The thyroid gland is the largest endocrine gland in the body and the only one accessible to direct physical examination. Assessment of thyroid function or possible dysfunction includes more than observation and palpation of the area where the thyroid gland is located. Metabolic rates and rhythms, including menstrual regularity in the woman of childbearing age, are governed by the thyroid gland. The effects of thyroid activity are widespread. Therefore observations of behavior, appearance, skin, eyes, hair, and cardiovascular status are important. Several findings require further attention (e.g., enlargement, coarse and gritty consistency, nodules).

BREASTS. The gynecologic examination includes an evaluation of the breasts primarily to establish a data base of normal findings. However, the practitioner needs to be alert to the possibility of carcinoma at all

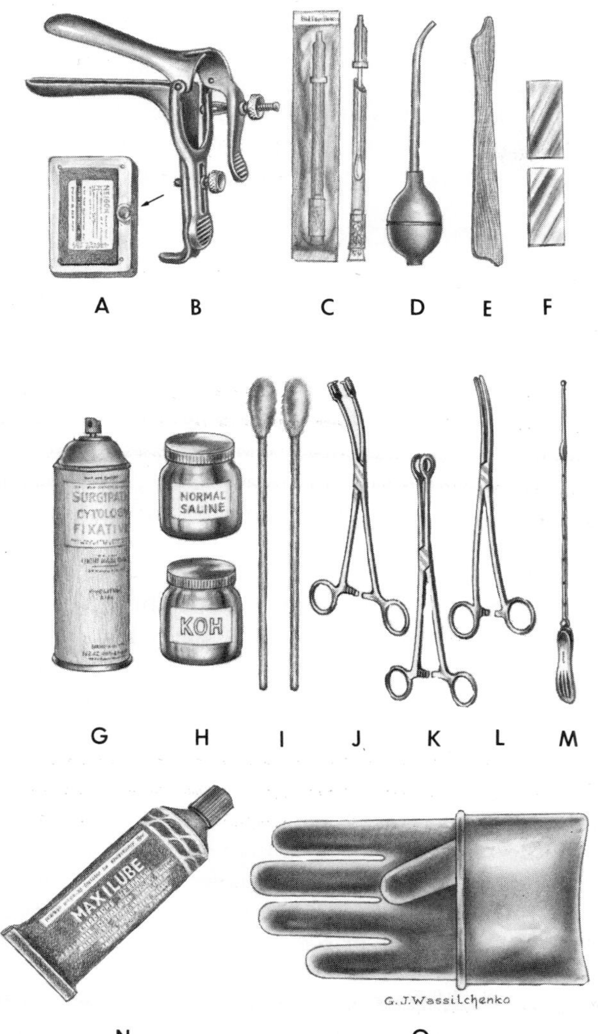

Fig. 11-1 Equipment used for pelvic examination. **A,** Thayer-Martin medium for isolation of *Neisseria gonorrhoeae*. Cylindric container *(arrow)* is for pellet that releases carbon dioxide; medium and specimen are refrigerated until transport to laboratory. **B,** Vaginal speculum. **C,** Culturette, modified Stuart's bacterial transport medium with self-contained sterile swab. **D,** Vaginal pipette with rubber bulb. **E,** Plastic spatula for Papanicolaou smear and cytology specimens. **F,** Slides for cytology specimens (Pap smear) or for wet mounts for diagnosing cause of vaginitis. **G,** Spray can of fixative for slide specimens. When dry, slides are packaged in cardboard for transport to laboratory. **H,** Normal saline and 10% potassium hydroxide (KOH) for wet mounts of vaginal fluids. **I,** Cotton pledget stick. **J,** Tenaculum. **K,** Ring (sponge or stick) forceps. **L,** Tissue forceps. **M,** Uterine sound (slightly curved for insertion). **N,** Sterile lubricant; may be antiseptic. **O,** Glove for vaginal and rectal examinations (sterile for vaginal, clean for rectal).

times. Early detection of potential malignancies has been and continues to be the single most important factor in the successful treatment of this disease. Because professional assessment occurs only periodically, each woman is advised to do a **breast self-examination (BSE)** on a monthly basis at the time when the breast is least affected by menstrual changes, 4 to 10 days after the last menstrual period (see Fig. 6-20).

Anatomy and physiology of the breast are presented in several sections of this text.* As the examiner proceeds through the examination, the woman is taught BSE, or if she already follows a routine for BSE, her knowledge and technique are refreshed.

At the start of the examination, the breasts are observed for symmetry, contour, color, size, and surface characteristics such as vascularity, moles, and nevi. The nipples are checked for areolar pigmentation and discharge and for response to stimulation (i.e., erection, flattening, or inversion). The woman then presses her hands against her waist to cause pectoral contraction and repeats the assessment just described.

When the woman raises her arms above her head, the position of the nipple and any dimpling (localized skin retraction) of the surface are noted. Breasts may appear symmetric at rest, but elevating them may reveal lesions. If the woman's breasts are pendulous, and problems exist, leaning forward to allow the breast to hang loose may reveal dimpling or other irregularities.

For the next part of the examination, the woman lies flat with her arm abducted and her hand under her head to help flatten breast tissue evenly over the chest wall, facilitating inspection and palpation. A pillow placed under the shoulder of the breast to be examined helps position breast tissue. Each breast is examined separately. The examiner can use both hands; however, in self-examination, the woman uses the hand opposite the side being examined. The fingers are held flat against the breast, and the tissue is palpated gently against the chest wall. The examination may be done either by using a circular method, quadrant by quadrant, or a spoke-wheel pattern (Fig. 11-2). The presence of regions of tenderness are distinguished, as are thickened or firm zones. Any masses are noted for location, size, consistency, and mobility or fixation to the skin or chest wall. Palpation of the breast includes glandular tissue, areolar areas, and the nipples. Normally breast tissue is slightly lobular; hard fixed masses are ab-

*Anatomy, physiology, growth, development across the life span, Chapter 6; maternal adaptation to pregnancy, Chapter 8; during the postdelivery period, Chapter 23; during lactation, Chapter 22.

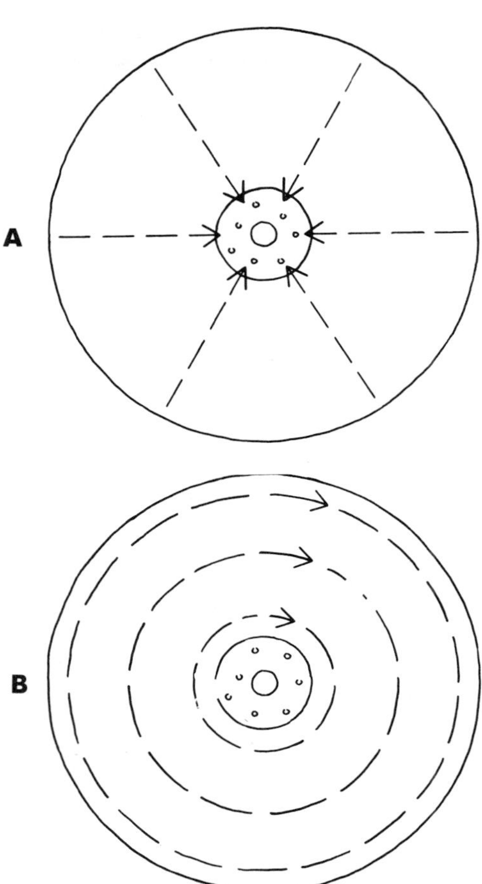

Fig. 11-2 Two methods of systematic breast palpation. **A,** Palpation in wedge sections (spoke-wheel fashion) from breast periphery to center. **B,** Palpation along concentric circles from periphery to center. It usually takes three circles to cover all breast tissue.

From Malasanos L et al: *Health assessment*, ed 4, St Louis, 1990, Mosby–Year Book.

normal. The nipple should be palpated and then compressed to reveal any drainage. No examination is complete without assessing those parts of the breast known as the tail of Spence and the axillary lymph nodes. The lymph nodes are palpated while the woman is in a sitting position. Easy access is gained to the axillary nodes with the woman's arms at her sides and muscles relaxed. To gain the necessary muscle relaxation, the examiner supports the woman's arm. The lymph nodes are assessed by using a rotary motion with two or three fingertips. Although malignancy may occur anywhere in the breast, the most common site is the upper outer quadrant.

ABDOMEN. The examination of the abdomen is done carefully and systematically. The skin is assessed for general condition, color, rashes, lesions, scars, striae, dilated veins, turgor, texture, and hair distribution. Contour, symmetry, and presence of hernias are noted. Bowel sounds are auscultated.

Pelvic Examination

The pelvic examination may be deferred to the next prenatal visit if the woman is anxious, tense, or refuses to have one at this visit. The vagina enlarges, and supporting structures are more relaxed as pregnancy advances. When the examination is performed, the tone of the pelvic musculature and need for and knowledge of Kegel exercises (p. 282) are assessed. During the pelvic examination the nurse remains alert for symptoms of supine hypotension (p. 275).

Many women are intimidated by the gynecologic portion of the physical examination. The nurse in this instance can take an advocacy approach that supports a partnership relationship between the client and the care provider.

The woman is assisted into the **lithotomy position** (Fig 11-3, *A*) for the pelvic examination (see Procedure on p. 275). When she is in the lithotomy position, the woman's hips and knees are flexed with the buttocks at the edge of the table and her feet supported by heel or knee stirrups. Some women prefer to keep their shoes or socks on, especially if the stirrups are not padded.

Many women express feelings of vulnerability and strangeness when in the lithotomy position. During the procedure the nurse assists the woman with relaxation techniques—the physician's and nurse's behavior toward her to this point adds to her ability to relax. One method of helping the woman relax is to have her place her hands on her chest at about the level of the diaphragm, breathe deeply and slowly (in through her nose and out through her O-shaped mouth), concentrate on the rhythm of breathing, and relaxing all body muscles with each exhalation (Malasanos et al, 1990). This breathing technique is particularly helpful for the adolescent or the woman whose introitus may be especially tight or for whom the experience may be new or may provoke tension.

Some women relax when they are encouraged to become involved with the examination with a mirror placed so that the area being examined can be seen by the client. This type of participation helps with health teaching as well. Distraction is another technique that can be used effectively, for example, placement of interesting pictures or mobiles on the ceiling over the head of the table.

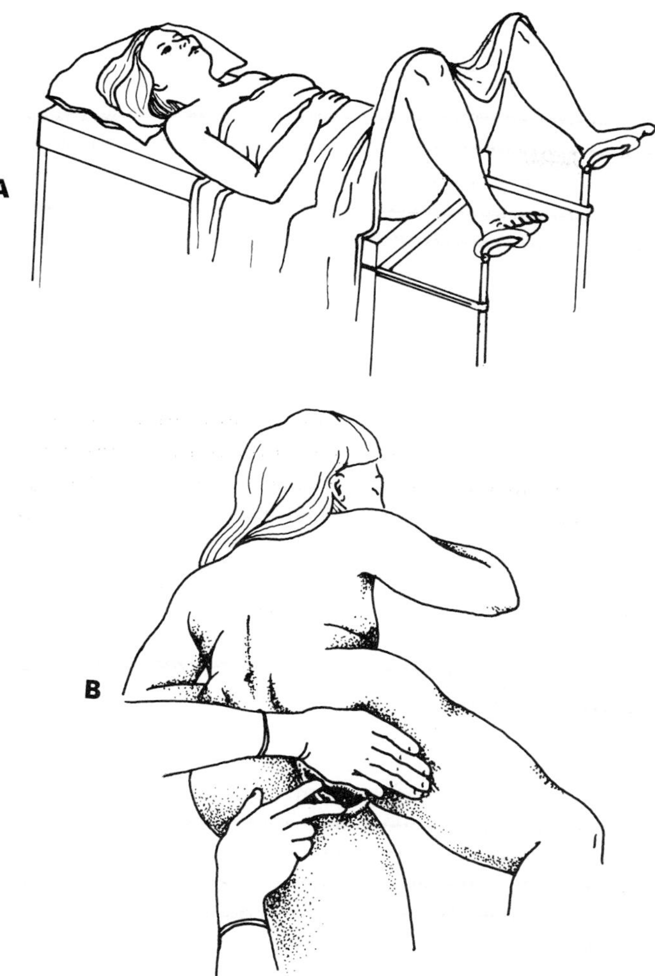

Fig. 11-3 A, Lithotomy position. B, Alternate position examination of genitals, left lateral position.

Procedure—Assisting with Pelvic Examination

Wash hands.
Ask woman to empty her bladder before the examination (obtain clean-catch urine specimen as needed).
Assist with relaxation techniques. Have the woman place her hands on her chest at about the level of the diaphragm, breathe deeply and slowly (in through her nose and out through her O-shaped mouth), concentrate on the rhythm of breathing, and relax all body muscles with each exhalation (Malasanos et al, 1990).
Encourage woman to become involved with the examination if she shows interest. For example, a mirror can be placed so that the area being examined can be seen by the woman.
Remind the woman *not* to squeeze her eyes closed, clench her fists, or squeeze the nurse's hand.
Assess woman for and treat signs of problems such as supine hypotension. (see Emergency Box, p. 276).
Instruct woman to bear down when speculum is being inserted.
Apply gloves and assist examiner with collection of specimens for cytologic examination, such as Pap smear. After handling specimens, remove gloves and wash hands.
Assist woman at completion of examination to a sitting position and then a standing position.
Provide tissues to wipe lubricant from perineum.
Provide privacy for woman while she is dressing.

The nurse is reminded that the woman *must not squeeze her eyes closed or clench her fists;* tightening these muscles permits the tightening of the perineal muscles.

Many women find it distressing to attempt to converse in the lithotomy position. Most women appreciate an explanation of the procedure as it unfolds as well as coaching for the type of sensations they may expect. Generally, however, women prefer not to have to respond to questions until they are again upright and at eye level with the examiner. Questioning during the procedure, especially if they cannot see their questioner's eyes, may make women tense.

SUPINE HYPOTENSION. When a woman is lying in the lithotomy position (Fig 11-3, *A*), the weight of abdominal contents may compress the vena cava and aorta, and result in a drop in blood pressure (**supine hypotension**) (see box on p. 276). If the woman is unable to tolerate the lithotomy position, the left lateral position may be used for genital examination (Fig. 11-3, *B*).

EXTERNAL INSPECTION. The examiner sits at the foot of the table for the inspection of the external genitals and for the speculum examination. To facilitate open communication and to help the woman relax, the woman's head is raised on a pillow and the drape is arranged so that eye-to-eye contact can be maintained. In good lighting, external genitals are inspected for sexual maturity, clitoris, labia, and perineum. After childbirth or other trauma there may be healed scars. Normal findings are discussed in Chapter 6.

EMERGENCY

Hypotension

SIGNS/SYMPTOMS

Pallor
Dizziness, faintness, breathlessness
Tachycardia
Nausea
Clammy (damp, cool) skin; sweating

INTERVENTIONS

Position woman on her left side until her signs/symptoms subside and vital signs stabilize within normal limits (WNL).

EXTERNAL PALPATION. The examiner proceeds with the examination using palpation* and inspection. The examiner wears gloves for this portion of the assessment. The labia are spread apart to expose the structures in the vestibule: urinary meatus, Skene's glands, vaginal orifice, and Bartholin's glands. To assess the Skene's glands, the examiner inserts one finger into the vagina and "milks" the area of the urethra. Any exudate from the *urethra* or the *Skene's glands* is cultured. Masses and erythema of either structure are assessed further. Ordinarily, the openings to the Skene's glands are not visible; prominent openings may be seen if the glands are infected (e.g., with gonorrhea). During the examination, the examiner keeps in mind the findings from the review of systems, such as history of burning on urination.

The *vaginal orifice* is examined. Carunculae myrtiformes (hymenal tags) are normal findings. With one finger still in the vagina, the examiner repositions the index finger near the posterior part of the orifice. With the thumb outside the posterior part of the labia majora, the examiner compresses the area of *Bartholin's glands* located at the 8 o'clock and 4 o'clock positions and looks for swelling, discharge, and pain.

The *support* of the anterior and posterior *vaginal wall* is assessed. The examiner spreads the labia with the index and middle finger and asks the woman to strain down. Any bulge from the anterior wall (urethrocele or cystocele) or posterior wall (rectocele) is noted and compared with the history, such as difficulty to start the stream of urine or constipation.

The *perineum* (area between the vagina and anus) is assessed for scars from old lacerations or episiotomies, for thinning, fistulas, masses, lesions, and inflammation. The *anus* is assessed for hemorrhoids, hemorrhoidal tags, and integrity of the anal sphincter. Occasionally, after traumatic delivery, with lacerations that extended into the anal sphincter, the muscle may not have been correctly repaired; for example, the examiner will see a "dimple" over two ends of separated muscle and the "wink" reflex is incomplete. If the anal sphincter was not repaired correctly, the woman may have given a history of incontinence. The anal area is also assessed for lesions, masses, abscesses, tumors. If there is a history of sexually transmitted disease, the examiner may want to obtain a culture specimen from the anal canal at this time.

Throughout the genital examination, the examiner notes the odor. Odor may indicate infection and poor hygienic practices.

INTERNAL EXAMINATION. When the woman made the appointment for her examination, she was asked to refrain from douching or using vaginal medications for the previous 24 hours. (NOTE: Douching is *not* recommended during pregnancy.) These actions cloud diagnosis based on secretions, cells, and odor. In addition, douching removes vaginal secretions, making insertion of the vaginal speculum more difficult. Some women have difficulty complying with this request; they cannot go to the physician feeling unclean in the genital region.

Vaginal specula consist of two blades and a handle. Specula come in a variety of types and styles (Fig. 11-4). Vaginal specula are used to view the vaginal vault and cervix. (The pelvic examination is detailed in the procedure on p. 275.)

The speculum blades are opened to reveal the cervix and are locked into the open position. The cervix is inspected: position and appearance of os, position, color, lesions, bleeding, and discharge. Cervical findings not within normal limits (e.g., ulcerations, masses, inflammation, excessive protrusion into the vaginal vault), anomalies (e.g., cock's comb [protrusion over cervix that looks like a rooster's comb], hooded, or collared cervix [seen in DES daughters]), and polyps are noted.

Collection of Specimens

Collection of specimens for cytologic examination is an important part of the gynecologic examination.

*As a sign of caring and to assist the woman to feel more at ease, the woman should receive a verbal cue and a cue through touch on a nonemotionally charged body part (e.g., knee) before experiencing touch on her genitals. The back of the hand, lightly touching the inner aspect of the thigh often works well.

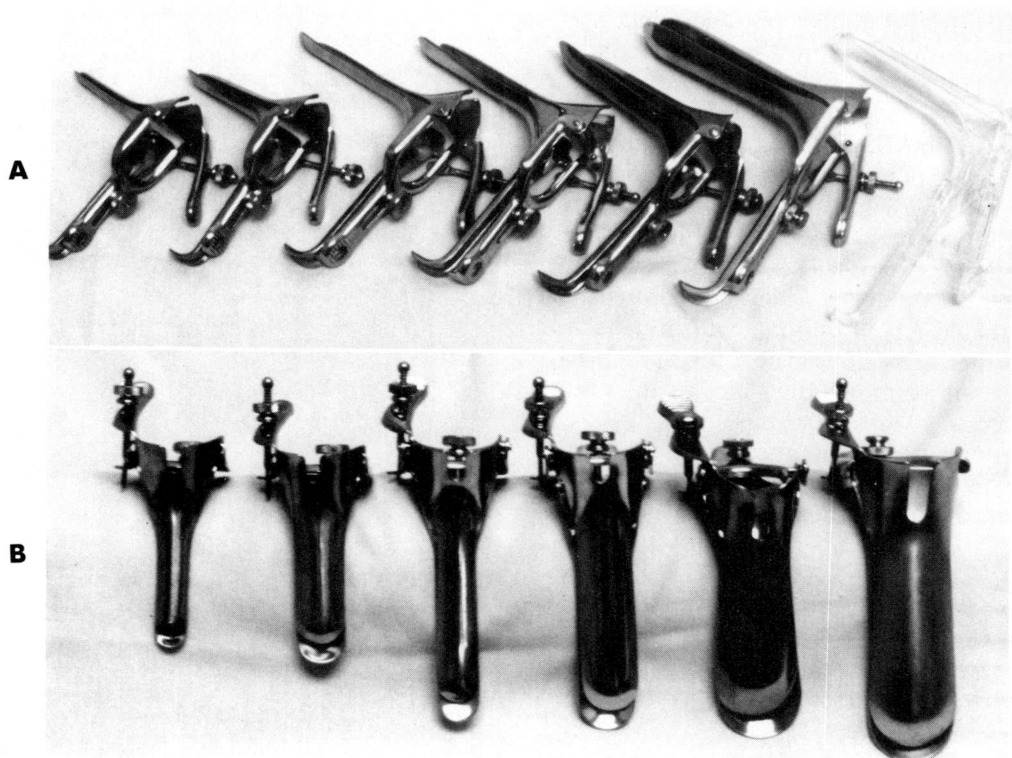

Fig. 11-4 Vaginal specula. From left to right: **A,** Short-billed pediatric, pediatric, small Pederson, Pederson, small Graves, large Graves, plastic Graves. **B,** Short-billed pediatric, pediatric, small Pederson, Pederson, small Graves, large Graves.
From Seidel H et al: *Mosby's guide to physical examination,* St Louis, 1987, Mosby–Year Book.

Infection can be diagnosed through examination of specimens collected during the pelvic examination. These infections include gonorrhea, *Chlamydia trachomatis,* and herpes simplex types 1 and 2. Once the diagnoses have been made, treatment can be instituted.

PAPANICOLAOU SMEAR. *Carcinogenic conditions,* potential or actual, can be determined by examination of cells from the cervix collected during the pelvic examination. The woman needs to know the purpose of the test and what sensations she will feel as the specimen is obtained (i.e., pressure, not pain). The woman is counseled to avoid douching, using any vaginal medications, or engaging in intercourse at least 24 hours before the procedure. In addition, no lubricant is used before obtaining the specimen. These precautions are taken to avoid cell distortion.

The specimen for the **Papanicolaou (Pap) smear** is obtained by placing the **S**-shaped end of the cervical spatula just within the cervical canal at the external os. The blade is rotated 360 degrees so that the surface at the squamocolumnar junction is uniformly scraped. If the junction is inside the cervical canal, a swab may be used to obtain cells. If gross exudate is present, the excess is gently pushed away from the os with the end of the spatula. The specimen is spread on a slide without rubbing or drying, sprayed lightly with fixative, and allowed to dry. Some mucus is obtained from the posterior fornix (vaginal pool) with the rounded end of the spatula, spread on another slide, sprayed, and dried. The specimens are sent to the pathology laboratory promptly for staining, evaluation, and a written report, with special reference to abnormal elements, including cancer cells.

GONORRHEAL CULTURE. A culture specimen for gonorrhea is obtained to screen women for gonorrheal infection that could affect the woman, her fetus if she is pregnant, and her partner. The woman is told the reason for the test (e.g., test for vaginal infection). If she is pregnant, the test is done routinely at the first prenatal visit and repeated toward the end of pregnancy (week 36).

The specimen is obtained at the same time as the Pap smear, and the same precautions regarding use of digital examinations and lubricant are followed. A specimen is obtained from the endocervical canal using a sterile cotton-tipped applicator. The applicator is rolled on a culture plate with a special medium (Thayer-Martin). The plate is then incubated.

CHLAMYDIA TRACHOMATIS SMEAR. Smears of urethral or cervical secretions are collected during the pelvic examination, following the same precautions used for the Pap smear. A fluorescein-conjugated monoclonal antibody test system for the detection of *Chlamydia* antigen is available. Slides containing the smears are incubated for 30 minutes with fluorescein-labeled antibodies. The physician, nurse practitioner, or midwife then examines the slides using a fluorescent microscope.

Tissue cultures are still sometimes used, although they are more expensive and it takes longer to obtain results with them than with the monoclonal tests.

HERPES SIMPLEX, TYPES 1 AND 2 CULTURE*. If an open lesion is present at the time of the initial pelvic examination, a viral culture specimen is obtained from the lesion and is repeated at intervals. A positive Pap smear result may be caused by the presence of herpes simplex, type 2.

Vaginal Examination

For assessing vaginal discharges other than blood, see Chapters 8 and 29. After the specimens are obtained, the vagina around the cervix is viewed by rotating the speculum. The speculum blades are unlocked and partially closed. As the speculum is withdrawn, it is rotated and the vaginal walls inspected for color, lesions, rugae, fistulas, and bulging.

Incontinence of urine during straining is not a normal finding and is noted. A variety of factors can cause incontinence, including pubococcygeal muscles that are weak from lack of exercise (Kegel) or trauma from childbirth (see Kegel exercises, p. 282).

BIMANUAL PALPATION. The examiner stands for this part of the examination. A small amount of lubricant is dropped† onto the fingers of the gloved hand for the internal examination. To avoid tissue trauma and contamination, the thumb is abducted and the ring and little fingers are flexed into the palm (Fig. 11-5).

The vagina is palpated for distensibility, lesions, and tenderness. The cervix is examined for position, shape, consistency, motility, and lesions. The fornix around the cervix is palpated.

*See also Chapter 29.
†If the contaminated glove touches the tube, the tube is discarded.

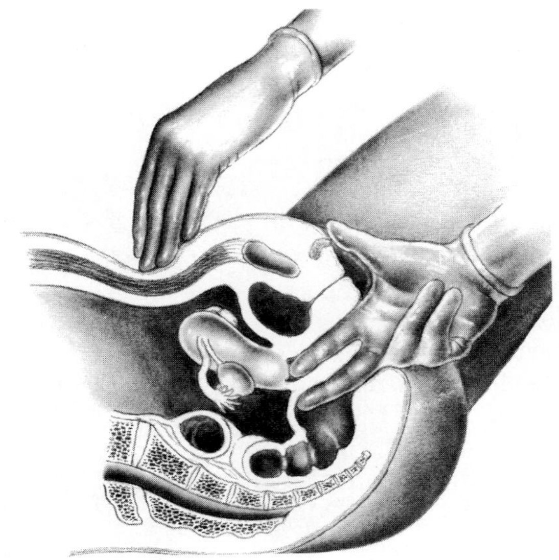

Fig. 11-5 Rectovaginal palpation.
From Seidel H et al: *Mosby's guide to physical examination,* St Louis, 1987, Mosby–Year Book.

The other hand is placed on the abdomen halfway between the umbilicus and symphysis pubis and exerts pressure downward toward the pelvic hand. Upward pressure from the pelvic hand traps reproductive structures for assessment by palpation. The uterus is assessed for position (see Fig. 6-7), size, shape, consistency, regularity, motility, masses, and tenderness.

Moving the abdominal hand to the right lower quadrant and the fingers of the pelvic hand in the right lateral fornix, the adnexa is assessed for position, size, tenderness, and masses. The examination is repeated on the woman's left side.

Just before the intravaginal fingers are withdrawn, the woman is asked to tighten her vagina around the fingers as much as she can. If the muscle response is weak, the woman is assessed for her knowledge about Kegel exercises (see Kegel exercises, p. 282).

RECTOVAGINAL PALPATION. To prevent contamination of the rectum from organisms in the vagina (e.g., gonorrhea) it is best to change gloves, add fresh lubricant, and then reinsert the index finger into the vagina and the middle finger into the rectum (Fig. 11-5). Insertion is facilitated if the woman strains down. The maneuvers of the abdominovaginal examination are repeated. The rectovaginal examination permits assessment of the rectovaginal septum, the posterior surface of the uterus, and the region behind the cervix.

After the pelvic examination, the woman is assisted into a sitting position, given tissues or wipes to cleanse herself, and privacy to dress. The woman often returns to the examiner's office for a discussion of findings, prescriptions for therapy, and counseling.

Laboratory Tests

The data obtained from laboratory examination of specimens add important information concerning the symptoms of pregnancy and health status. Both nursing and medical diagnoses stem from such information.

Specimens are collected at the initial visit so that results of their examination will be ready for the next scheduled visit (Table 11-1). A clean-catch urine specimen is tested. Tine or purified protein derivative of tuberculin (PPD) tests are administered for exposure to tuberculosis. During the pelvic examination cervical and vaginal smears for cytologic study (Pap smear and herpes simplex type 2) and for diagnosis of infection (*Chlamydia* organisms, gonorrhea) are obtained. Blood is drawn to test for a variety of conditions: venereal disease research laboratory (VDRL) test for syphilis; complete blood cell count (CBC) with hematocrit, hemoglobin, and differential values; blood type and Rh factor; antibody screen (Kell, Duffy, rubella, toxoplasmosis, and anti-Rh); sickle cell anemia; and level of folacin when indicated. Urine is tested for glucose, protein, and acetone; culture and sensitivity tests are ordered as necessary. Testing for antibody to the human immunodeficiency virus (HIV) is done with the client's permission, as necessary (Middleton, 1989).

Fetal Development

A summary of the development of the fetus at 13 weeks is presented in the box on p. 280.

Toward the end of the first trimester, before the uterus is an abdominal organ, the fetal heart tones (FHTs) can be heard with an ultrasound fetoscope or an ultrasound stethoscope (see Fig. 16-1, *D* and *E*). The instrument is placed in the midline just anterior

TABLE 11-1 Laboratory Tests in Prenatal Period

Laboratory Test	Purpose
Hemoglobin/hematocrit, WBC, differential	Detects anemia
Hemoglobin electrophoresis	Identifies women with hemoglobinopathies (e.g., sickle cell anemia, thalassemia)
Blood type, Rh, and irregular antibody	Identifies those fetuses at risk for developing erythroblastosis fetalis or hyperbilirubinemia in neonatal period
Rubella titer	Determines immunity to rubella
Tuberculin skin testing; Chest film after 20 weeks' gestation in clients with reactive tuberculin tests	Screens high-risk population
Urinalysis, including microscopic examination of urinary sediment; pH, specific gravity, color, glucose, albumin, protein, RBC, WBC, casts, acetone; hCG	Identifies women with unsuspected diabetes mellitus, renal disease, hypertensive disease of pregnancy; infection; pregnancy
Urine culture	Identifies women with asymptomatic bacteriuria
Renal function tests: BUN, creatinine, electrolytes, creatinine clearance, total protein excretion	Evaluates level of possible renal compromise in women with a history of diabetes, hypertension, or renal disease
Pap smear	Screens for cervical intraepithelial neoplasia and herpes simplex type 2
Vaginal or rectal smear for *Neisseria gonorrhoeae*, *Chalamydia*, HPV	Screens high-risk population for asymptomatic infection
VDRL/FTA-ABS	Identifies women with untreated syphilis
HIV antibody, *hepatitis B surface antigen	Screens high-risk population
1-hour glucose tolerance	Screens for gestational diabetes; done at initial visit for clients with risk factors; done at 28 weeks for all clients
3-hour glucose tolerance	Screens for diabetes in clients with elevated glucose level after 1 hour test; must have elevated fasting or two elevated readings for diagnosis (see Chapter 31)
Cardiac evaluation: ECG, chest x-ray film, and echocardiogram	Evaluates cardiac function in women with a history of hypertension or cardiac disease

BUN, Blood urea nitrogen; *ECG*, electrocardiogram; *FTA-ABS*, fluorescent treponemal antibody absorption test; *hCG*, human chorionic gonadotropin; *HPV*, human papillomavirus.
*With client permission.

Fetal Development at 13 Weeks

Differentiation of tissues complete as period of organogenesis ends
Human appearance
Sex distinguishable
Skeleton ossifying
Tooth buds forming
Respiratory activity evident
Insulin secreted (since eighth week)
Kidneys secreting urine
Intestine returns to abdomen
Head is one third of total length
Length: 9 cm (3½ in)
Weight: 15 g (½ oz)
Fetus less susceptible to malformation from teratogenic agents after 8-10 weeks' gestation

to the symphysis pubis. Firm pressure is needed as the scope is used. The woman and her family can be offered the opportunity to listen to the FHTs.

Signs of Potential Problems

The interview, physical examination, and laboratory tests (see Table 11-1) may yield findings suggesting potential complications.

When the data base is complete, a judgment is made of the woman's risk status and need for referral for specialized care or further evaluation. A variety of assessment tools have been developed to assess the degree of risk. (See Chapter 27 for a full discussion of the diagnosis of risk; see Unit VI for Complications of Childbearing.)

During the course of pregnancy, warning signs (see box on p. 428) may appear. The woman and her family need to be aware of these signs so that they can seek appropriate interventions promptly.

NURSING DIAGNOSES

Each client and family will have a unique set of responses to pregnancy. To attend to these responses the nurse begins by formulating appropriate nursing diagnoses. The following are examples of nursing diagnoses that may arise from analysis of assessment findings during the first trimester:

- Anxiety related to
  —Concern about herself
  —Physical changes with pregnancy
  —Her (or other's) feelings about the pregnancy
- Pain, related to
  —Early discomforts of pregnancy
- Altered family processes related to
  —Family's response to diagnosis of pregnancy
- Anxiety related to knowledge deficit
  —Maternal and familial adaptations to pregnancy
  —Maternal and familial adaptations to EDD
- Altered nutrition: less than body requirements, related to
  —Morning sickness
- Altered sexuality patterns, related to
  —Discomforts of early pregnancy

PLANNING

Planning care for clients during the first trimester is based on the biopsychosocial assessment of the client and her family. For each client a plan is developed that relates specifically to her clinical and nursing problems. The information in this chapter is general; that is, not all women will experience all problems discussed or require all facets of the care described. The nurse selects those aspects of care relevant to the client and the client's family based on the following client-centered goals.

Goals Related to Physiologic Care

1. Client's pregnancy is diagnosed and EDD determined.
2. Client will have pertinent knowledge of the adaptation of the maternal body to a developing fetus as a basis for understanding the rationale and necessity for modalities of care.
3. Client will have knowledge of self-care for nutritional needs, sexual needs, activities of daily living, and discomforts of pregnancy.
4. Client's risk factors are identified, and referral for further evaluation or therapy is initiated promptly if indicated.
5. Client is alerted to symptoms that indicate deviations from normal progress and protocols for reporting them.

Goals Related to Psychosocial Care

1. Client's information needs/readiness for learning are identified.
2. Client and her family become active participants in the woman's care during the first trimester of pregnancy.

3. Client begins to develop a birth plan.
4. Client develops trusting relationship with caregivers.

IMPLEMENTATION

The nurse-client relationship is critical in setting the tone for further interaction. The techniques of listening with an attentive expression, touching, and using eye contact have their place, as does recognition of the client's feelings and her right to express them. The intervention may occur in various formal or informal settings. For certain persons, involvement in goal-directed health groups is neither feasible nor acceptable. Encounters in hallways or clinic examining rooms, home visits, or telephone conversations may provide the only opportunities for contact and can be used effectively. Sometimes women seek information about a particular problem repeatedly, not so much for the advice given but to direct the nurse's attention toward themselves. The nurse can help these women by asking for a client-generated solution and a report of its effectiveness.

In supporting a client one must remember that both the nurse and the client are contributing to the relationship. The nurse has to accept the client's responses as a factor in trying to be of help. An example of one nurse-client relationship follows:

> Mrs.__________________ had been very forthright in saying that this pregnancy was unplanned but had countered this statement with comments such as "All things happen for the best," "We always wanted the boys to have a family to turn to," and "Children bring their own love."
>
> Over a period of time, as our relationship developed to one of *mutual* trust, she complained increasingly of her fear of pain, her hating to wear maternity clothes, and her having to give up helping the family. Finally I ventured to say, "Sometimes when a pregnancy is unplanned, women resent it very much and are angry about it." Her relief was evident. She said, "Oh, you don't know how angry I've been."
>
> As a result the whole tenor of support being offered changed, and the plan was adjusted to meet her real needs.

The nurse also needs to accept the fact that the woman must be a willing partner in a purely voluntary relationship. As such, the relationship can be refused or terminated at any time by the pregnant woman or her family.

Supportive care involves developing, augmenting, or changing the mechanisms used by women and families in coping with stress. An effort is made to promote active participation by the individuals in the process of solving their own problems. Clients are helped to gather pertinent information, explore alternative actions, make decisions as to choice of action, and assume responsibility for the outcomes. These outcomes may be any or all of the following: living with a problem as it is, easing effects of a problem so that it can be accepted more readily, or eliminating the problem by effecting change.

Expectations of success in the area of emotional supportive care must of necessity be flexible. No outsider can ensure another person a rewarding, satisfying experience. The mother and persons significant to her are crucial elements in this process. Many of their problems are beyond the scope or capabilities of any professional worker (Zerwekh, 1991). In describing her work with young and poor persons, Edwards (1973) noted: "They did not usually change their living situation and I was not instrumental in modifying home or drug problems." However, this did not deter her from encouraging clients to use the decision-making process as a means of coping with problems rather than merely complaining about injustice.

At other times a successful outcome can be readily documented. A woman who early in her pregnancy had predicted a severe depressive state in the postdelivery period was elated when such a state did not materialize. She remarked to the nurse who had provided support during the pregnancy and birth, "You're the best nerve medicine I've ever had!"

Education for Self-Care

Health maintenance is an important aspect of prenatal care. Client participation in the care ensures prompt reporting of possible problems. Client assumption of responsibility for health maintenance is prompted by understanding of maternal adaptations to the growth of the unborn child and a readiness to learn. Nurses provide clients with the information necessary for self-care and compliance with health care measures.

The expectant mother needs an overview of the planned prenatal care and information about many other subjects. During the initial health assessment, the woman may have indicated a need to learn self-care activities such as BSE, prevention of urinary tract infection, and Kegel exercises. Guidelines for client teaching for BSE are presented on p. 1248.

PREVENTION OF URINARY TRACT INFECTION. Urinary tract infections may be asymptomatic. Whether symptomatic or not, urinary tract infections present a risk to both mother and fetus. Prevention of these infections is essential. The woman's understanding and use of general hygiene measures are assessed.

Before developing a plan of care, the nurse needs to determine the woman's feelings or ideas concerning cultural, ethnic, religious, or other factors affecting health practices.

The woman may need to learn that every woman should always wipe from front to back after urinating or moving bowels and use a clean piece of toilet paper for each wipe. Wiping from back to front may carry bacteria from the rectal area to the urethral opening and increase risk of infection. Soft, absorbent toilet tissue, preferably white and unscented, should be used because harsh, scented, or printed toilet paper may cause irritation. Nonpregnant women need to change tampons, panty shields, or sanitary napkins often. Bacteria can multiply in menstrual blood or on soiled napkins. Women need to wear underpants and panty hose with a cotton crotch. They should avoid wearing tight-fitting slacks or jeans or panty shields for long periods. A buildup of heat and moisture in the genital area may contribute to the growth of bacteria.

Some women do not have an adequate fluid and food intake. After discovering her food preferences, the nurse should advise the woman to drink 2 to 3 quarts (8 to 12 glasses) of liquid a day. Eight to 10 ounces of cranberry juice may be included because cranberry juice is more acidic than other fluids and can lower the pH of the urinary tract, making it less hospitable to developing bacteria. Yogurt and acidophilus milk may also help prevent urinary tract and vaginal infections.

The nurse should review with the woman healthy urination practices. Women need to maintain fluid intake to ensure frequent urination and not limit fluids to reduce frequency of urination. They should not ignore signals that indicate the need to urinate. Holding urine increases the time bacteria are in the bladder and allows them to multiply. Women should plan ahead in situations that require the delay of urination (e.g., a long car ride). They should always urinate before going to bed at night. Bacteria can be introduced during intercourse. Therefore women are advised to urinate before and after intercourse, then drink a large glass of water to promote additional urination.

The nurse can be reasonably assured that teaching was effective if the woman does not develop a urinary tract infection.

KEGEL EXERCISES. Kegel exercises (exercises for the pelvic floor) strengthen the muscles around the reproductive organs and improve muscle tone.

Many women are not aware of the muscles of the pelvic floor (see Figs. 6-13 and 6-14) until it is pointed out that these are the muscles used during urination and sexual intercourse and are therefore consciously controlled. Inasmuch as pelvic floor muscles encircle the outlet through which the baby must pass, it is important that they be exercised, because an exercised muscle can stretch and contract readily at the time of birth.

To help the pelvic floor muscles return to normal functioning, Kegel exercises should be started immediately after delivery. Kegel exercises can strengthen these muscles and improve muscle tone. If practiced on a regular basis, the exercises help prevent prolapsed uterus and stress incontinence later in life.

The exercise is performed as follows.

A. The muscles that stop the flow of urine are the pubococcygeal muscles. Doing Kegel exercises during urination helps the woman know whether she is doing them correctly. If she can stop the stream of urine, her tone is good.
B. After a woman has located the correct muscles, Kegel exercises can be done in the following ways:
    1. *Slowly:* Tighten the muscle, hold it for the count of three, and relax it.
    2. *Quickly:* Tighten the muscle, and relax it as rapidly as possible.
    3. *Push out–pull in:* Pull up the entire pelvic floor as though trying to suck up water into the vagina. Then bear down as if trying to push the imaginary water out. This uses abdominal muscles also.

This exercise needs to be practiced several times a day to be effective. It must be done every day for the rest of the woman's life.

This exercise can be done 10 times in a row at least three times or more a day. Although some people recommend doing this exercise as many as 100 times in a row, this only fatigues the pelvic floor muscles.

A good time to practice is during trips to the bathroom, but additional practice at other times is even more beneficial.

The nurse can be reasonably assured that teaching was effective if the woman reports increased muscle tone to control urine flow and during sexual intercourse.

ADDITIONAL TEACHING. Other subjects about which clients need information include diet, exercise, sleep, bowel habits, smoking, alcohol ingestion, medication usage, and sexual relations. It is impossible to impart at one visit all the information the woman and her family may need at the time her pregnancy is diagnosed. She can be given printed in-

Warning Signs—First Trimester

SIGNS/SYMPTOMS	POSSIBLE CAUSES
Severe vomiting	Hyperemesis gravidarum (see Chapter 31)
Chills, fever	Infection
Burning on urination	Infection
Diarrhea	Infection
Abdominal cramping; vaginal bleeding	Spontaneous abortion, miscarriage (see Chapter 30)

formation* at this time, such as material prepared by the obstetrician, published pamphlets, or a list of books for lay persons about pregnancy. If the last, the obstetrician, nurse, or nurse-midwife should have read the materials carefully to be certain they supply the kind of information desired.

Nutritional intake is an important factor in the maintenance of maternal health during pregnancy and in the provision of adequate nutrients for embryonic/fetal development. Assessing nutritional status and providing nutritional information are part of the nurse's responsibilities in prenatal care. For detailed information concerning maternal and fetal nutritional needs and related nursing care, see Chapter 9.

Formal classes in childbirth and parenthood education have proved successful for some women and families. "Early bird" classes provide fundamental information to meet the needs of most expectant parents during the first trimester. Allowing the expectant mother or family the opportunity to ask questions and express any anxieties or fears she or they may have is also important.

SCHEDULE FOR CARE. During the initial visit, women appreciate knowing the schedule for return prenatal visits. Most women can expect to return every 4 weeks until the twenty-eighth week of pregnancy, every 2 weeks until the thirty-sixth week of pregnancy, and then every week from week 37 until delivery. More frequent visits may be needed to accommodate the woman's individual needs. The initial prenatal visit is usually lengthy. Women can be reassured by knowing what to expect on subsequent visits.

*The nurse must determine, in a sensitive manner, that the woman can read the material given to her. Some women do not use reading as a means of coping; thus other means may be more appropriate (e.g., videotapes or audio-cassettes).

WARNING SIGNS. One of the first responsibilities of persons involved in the care of the pregnant woman is to alert her to signs and symptoms that indicate a potential complication of pregnancy. The client needs to know how to report such **warning signs** (see box above). When one is stressed by a disturbing symptom, it is difficult to remember specifics. Therefore the woman and her family are reassured if they receive a printed form listing the signs and symptoms that justify an investigation and the telephone numbers to call in an emergency.

DISCOMFORTS OF PREGNANCY. Women pregnant for the first time are confronted with symptoms that would be considered abnormal in the nonpregnant state. Much of prenatal care requested by such women relates to explanations of the causes of the discomforts and what measures can be taken to relieve them. The discomforts are fairly specific to each trimester of pregnancy. Information about the physiology, prevention, and self-care of discomforts experienced during the first trimester are given in Table 11-2.

Nurses can anticipate these symptoms and provide anticipatory guidance for women. Women who understand the physical discomforts of pregnancy are less apt to become overly anxious about their health. Understanding the rationale for treatment promotes participation in their own care. Nurses need to use terminology the woman (or couple) can understand.

EMPLOYMENT. Many women continue to work during pregnancy. Whether the expectant mother can work and for how long depends on the physical activity involved, industrial hazards, and medical or obstetric complications. A prime consideration is the avoidance of a fetotoxic environment (e.g., chemical dust particles or gases such as inhalation anesthesia). Employment during later pregnancy is discussed later in this chapter.

Table 11–2 Discomforts/Concerns Related to Maternal Adaptations to Pregnancy

Discomfort	Physiology*	Teaching For Self-care
Breast changes, new sensations: pain, tingling	Hypertrophy of mammary glandular tissue and increased vascularization, pigmentation, and size and prominence of nipples and areolae caused by hormone stimulation	Supportive maternity brassiere with pads to absorb discharge may be worn at night; wash with warm water and keep dry; see Maternal physiology and sexual counseling
Urgency and frequency of urination	Vascular engorgement and altered bladder function caused by hormones; bladder capacity reduced by enlarging uterus	Kegel exercises; limit fluid intake before bedtime; reassurance; wear perineal pad; refer to physician for pain or burning sensation
Lack of energy; fatigue (early pregnancy, usually)	Unexplained, may be caused by increasing levels of estrogen, progesterone, and hCG or to elevated BBT; psychologic response to pregnancy and its required physical/psychologic adaptations	Reassurance; rest as needed; well-balanced diet to prevent anemia
Nausea and vomiting, morning sickness—occurs in 50% to 75% of pregnant women; starts between first and second missed periods and lasts until about fourth missed period; may occur any time during day; if mother does not have symptoms, expectant father may; may be accompanied by "bad taste" in mouth	Cause unknown (may result from hormonal changes, possibly hCG; may be partly psychologic, reflecting pride in, ambivalence about, or rejection of pregnant state)	Avoid empty or overloaded stomach; maintain good posture—give stomach ample room; stop or decrease smoking; eat dry carbohydrate on awakening; remain in bed until feeling subsides, or alternate dry carbohydrate 1 hour with fluids such as hot tea, milk, or clear coffee the next hour until feeling subsides; eat five to six small meals per day; avoid fried, odorous, spicy, greasy, or gas-forming foods; consult physician if intractable vomiting occurs; reassurance
Ptyalism (excessive saliva)—may occur starting 2 to 3 weeks after first missed period	Appears to have no physiologic basis (Van Dintner, 1991); may be related to reluctance to swallow because of nausea	Use hard candy; chewing gum; support
Gingivitis and epulis (hyperemia, hypertrophy, bleeding, tenderness): condition will disappear spontaneously 1 to 2 months after delivery	Increased vascularity and proliferation of connective tissue from estrogen stimulation	Well-balanced diet with adequate protein and fresh fruits and vegetables; gentle brushing and good dental hygiene; avoid infection
Nasal stuffiness; epistaxis	Hyperemia of mucus membranes related to high estrogen levels	Humidifier; avoid trauma; normal saline nose drops or spray
Leukorrhea: often noted throughout pregnancy	Hormonally stimulated cervix becomes hypertrophic and hyperactive, producing abundant amount of mucus	Not preventable; *do not douche;* hygiene; perineal pads; reassurance; refer to physician if accompanied by pruritis, foul odor, or change in character or color
Psychosocial dynamics (see Chapter 10): mood swings, mixed feelings	Hormonal and metabolic adaptations; feelings about female role, sexuality, timing of pregnancy, and resultant changes in one's life and life-style	Treatment same as prevention; both partners need reassurance and support; support significant other who can reassure woman about her attractiveness, etc.; improved communication with her partner, family, and others; refer to social worker, if needed, or supportive services (financial assistance, food stamps)

*Review Chapter 8 for more extensive discussion of anatomy and physiology of pregnancy.

PHYSICAL ACTIVITY. Many women exercise regularly and strenuously in the nonpregnant state. They are concerned about loss of physical fitness during an enforced period of decreased activity during pregnancy (Culpepper, 1990; Mittelmark, 1991). Women who have led sedentary life-styles need to begin with physical activity of very low intensity and advance activity levels gradually (Fishbein, Phillips, 1990). A number of researchers have recommended moderate exercise during pregnancy (Culpepper, 1990; Mittelmark, 1991) (see box on p. 286). However, activities continued to the point of exhaustion or fatigue compromise uterine perfusion and fetoplacental oxygenation. If the woman is accustomed to jogging, she may continue; however, she should not reach the point of fatigue. Heat stress may also endanger the fetus. Furthermore, as gestation advances, the woman's center of gravity changes, her bony pelvic support loosens, her coordination usually decreases, and she notices a sensation of awkwardness. Connective tissue laxity increases the risk of joint injury; therefore stretches should not be taken to the point of maximum resistance. Deep flexion or extension of joints must be avoided. Any activity such as jumping, jarring motions, or rapid changes in direction are contraindicated because of joint instability (Fishbein, Phillips, 1990). Awkwardness may cause the woman to lose balance and fall, injuring herself.

Exercises such as those depicted in Fig. 12-6 are taught either at prenatal classes or by the nurse in the clinic or the physician's office. The exercises promote comfort and help prepare the woman for labor. Other topics for discussion and demonstration are posture and how to lift and move objects safely to counteract the awkwardness and prevent the discomfort experienced starting in the second trimester of pregnancy.

DENTAL HEALTH. Dental care during pregnancy is especially important. Nausea during pregnancy may lead to poor oral hygiene, and dental caries may develop. No physiologic alteration during gestation can cause dental caries. Calcium and phosphorus in the teeth are fixed in enamel. Therefore the old adage "for every child a tooth" need not be true.

There is no scientific evidence that filling teeth or even dental extraction with the use of local or nitrous oxide–oxygen anesthesia causes abortion or premature labor. Antibacterial therapy should be considered for sepsis, however, especially in pregnant women who have had rheumatic heart disease or nephritis. Extensive dental surgery is postponed for the woman's comfort, if possible, until after delivery (Chenger, 1987).

MEDICATIONS. Although much has been learned in recent years about fetal drug toxicity (Appendix E), the possible teratogenicity of many drugs, both prescription and over-the-counter (OTC), is still unknown. This is especially true for new medications and combinations of drugs. Moreover, certain subclinical errors or deficiencies in intermediate metabolism in the fetus may convert an otherwise harmless drug into a hazardous one. The greatest danger of drug-caused developmental defects in the fetus exists from the time of fertilization through the first trimester. Self-treatment must be discouraged. All drugs, including aspirin, should be limited, and a careful record should be kept of all therapeutic agents used (Dicke, 1989).

IMMUNIZATION. There has been some concern over the safety of various immunization techniques during pregnancy (Barry, Bia, 1989; Cunningham et al, 1989). Immunization with live or attenuated live viruses is contraindicated during pregnancy because of potential teratogenicity. Vaccines with killed viruses may be used. Live virus vaccines include measles (rubeola and rubella) (Burgess, 1990), mumps, and the Sabin (oral) poliomyelitis vaccine. Some women may need immunization against influenza. For immediate protection after exposure, inactivated polio vaccine (IPV) may be used. Immunization against cholera, typhoid, and poliomyelitis may be needed if the woman must travel to endemic areas. Tetanus toxoid or varicella immunoglobulin may be given when necessary.

ALCOHOL, CIGARETTE SMOKE, AND OTHER SUBSTANCES. No safe level of alcohol consumption has yet been established. Although occasional alcoholic beverages *may* not be harmful to the mother or her developing embryo or fetus, complete abstinence is strongly advised. Maternal alcoholism is associated with high rates of spontaneous abortion; the risk for spontaneous abortion is dose-related (three or more drinks per day) in the first trimester (Cook et al, 1990). Fetal alcohol syndrome is discussed in Chapters 33 and 39 (see also Appendix E).

Cigarette smoking or continued exposure to a smoke-filled environment (even if the mother does not smoke) is associated with fetal growth retardation and an increase in perinatal and infant morbidity and mortality. Smoking also increases the frequency of preterm labor, premature rupture of membranes (PROM), abruptio placentae, placenta previa, and fetal death resulting possibly from decreased placental perfusion. Laboratory studies indicate a lowered oxygen pressure (PO_2 level) in both mother and fetus

Exercise Tips for Pregnant Women

Consult your health care provider when you know or suspect you are pregnant. Discuss your medical and obstetric history, your current regimen, and the exercises you would like to continue throughout pregnancy.

Seek help in determining an exercise routine that is well within your limit of tolerance, especially if you have not been exercising regularly.

Consider decreasing weight-bearing exercises (jogging, running) and concentrate on non–weight-bearing activities such as swimming, cycling, or stretching. If you are a runner, starting in your seventh month, you may wish to walk instead.

Because strenuous exercise during the last few weeks of pregnancy increases the risk of low birth weight, stillbirth, and infant death, reduce exercise sharply 4 weeks before your due date.

Avoid risky activities such as surfing, mountain climbing, skydiving, and racquetball. Activities requiring precise balance and coordination may be dangerous. Avoid activities that require holding your breath and bearing down (Valsalva's maneuver). Jerky, bouncy motions also should be avoided.

Exercise regularly at least three times a week, as long as you are healthy, to improve muscle tone and increase or maintain your stamina. Sporadic exercises may put undue strain on your muscles.

Limit activity to shorter intervals. Exercise for 10 to 15 minutes, rest for 2 to 3 minutes, then exercise for another 10 to 15 minutes.

Decrease your exercise level as your pregnancy progresses. The normal alterations of advancing pregnancy, such as decreased cardiac reserve and increased respiratory effort, may produce physiologic stress if you exercise strenuously for a long time.

Take your pulse every 10 to 15 minutes while you are exercising. If it is more than 140 beats/min, slow down until it returns to a maximum of 90. You should be able to converse easily while exercising. If you cannot, you need to slow down.

Avoid becoming overheated for extended periods. It is best not to exercise for more than 35 minutes, especially in hot, humid weather. As your body temperature rises, the heat is transmitted to your fetus. Prolonged or repeated fetal temperature elevation may result in birth defects, especially during the first 3 months. Your temperature should not exceed 38° C (100.4° F).

Limit the time you spend in hot baths. Stay in water at 39.0° C (102.2° F) for less than 15 minutes.

Warm-up and stretching exercises prepare your joints for more strenuous exercise and lessen the likelihood of strain or injury to your joints. No exercise should be performed flat on your back after the fourth month of gestation.

A cool-down period of mild activity involving your legs after an exercise period will help bring your respiration, heart, and metabolic rates back to normal and avoid pooling of blood in the exercise muscles.

Rest for 10 minutes after exercising, lying on your left side. As the uterus grows, it puts pressure on a major vein on the right side of your abdomen, which carries blood to your heart. Lying on your left side removes the pressure and promotes return circulation from your extremities and muscles to your heart, increasing blood flow to your placenta and fetus. Care should be taken to rise gradually from the floor to avoid feeling dizzy or fainting (orthostatic hypotension).

Drink two or three 8-ounce glasses of water after you exercise, to replace the body fluids you lost through perspiration. While exercising, drink water whenever you feel the need.

Increase your caloric intake to replace the calories burned during exercise and to provide the extra energy needs of pregnancy. Choose such high-protein foods as fish, cheese, eggs, or meat.

Take your time. This is not the time to be competitive or train for activities requiring long endurance.

Wear a supportive bra. Your increased breast weight may cause changes in posture and put pressure on the ulnar nerve.

Wear supportive shoes. As your uterus grows, your center of gravity shifts and you compensate by arching your back. These natural changes may make you feel off balance and more likely to fall.

Stop exercising immediately if you experience shortness of breath, dizziness, numbness, tingling, pain of any kind, more than four uterine contractions per hour, decreased fetal activity, or vaginal bleeding, and consult your health care provider.

Modified from Paglone A, Worthington S: Cautions and advice on exercise during pregnancy, *Contemp OB/GYN* 25:160, May 1985 (special issue); Fishbein EG, Phillips M: How safe is exercise during pregnancy? *JOGNN* 19:45, Jan/Feb 1990.

during exposure to cigarette smoke. Smoking may result in a lessened supply of milk during lactation, and harmful substances may be transferred to the infant in the milk.

If the woman is a smoker, the nurse needs to discuss the options she has regarding methods designed to help her quit. If she is resistant to the idea of quitting, the nurse can try to offer ways in which she can cut down (Ershoff et al, 1989).

Most studies of human pregnancy report no association between caffeine consumption and birth defects or low birth weight (Leviton, 1988; Cunningham et al, 1989). However, the stimulant effects of caffeine are increased during pregnancy. A pregnant woman may find she is jittery or has difficulty sleeping after consuming her usual prepregnancy level of caffeine (Aaronson, MacNee, 1989). Other effects are unknown; therefore pregnant women are advised to limit caffeine intake. Possible hazards of a commonly used artificial sweetener are discussed in Chapter 9.

Any mind-altering substance has a harmful effect on the fetus and should not be used (see Chapter 39 and Appendix E). Marijuana, heroin, and cocaine are common examples of such substances.

Parent Education Classes

A typical preparation-for-parenthood program recognizes that expectant parents and their families have different interests and information needs as the pregnancy progresses. Consequently, the program is designed to meet the informational needs of parents at the three major stages of pregnancy and after birth: first-trimester classes, second-trimester classes (p. 313), third-trimester classes (p. 334), and postpartum ("fourth trimester") classes.

First-trimester classes, early pregnancy ("early bird") classes, provide fundamental information. Classes are developed around the following areas: (1) early fetal development, (2) physiologic and emotional changes of early pregnancy, (3) human sexuality, (4) birth settings and types of caregivers, (5) rest, exercise, and relief measures for common discomforts, (6) the nutritional needs of the mother and fetus, and (7) the development of a birth plan. Environmental and workplace hazards have become important concerns in recent years. Even though pregnancy is considered a normal process, exercises, danger signs, drugs, and self-medication are topics of interest and concern.

Throughout the series of classes there is discussion of support systems that are available during pregnancy and after birth. Such support systems help parents function independently and effectively. During all the classes the open expression of feelings and concerns about any aspect of pregnancy, birth, and parenting is welcomed.

Not all pregnant women and support persons attend formal classes in preparation for childbirth. For those who do attend, extensive preparation is possible. Many do not take advantage of classes for a variety of reasons: employment; inaccessibility because of time, cultural/ethnic/religious orientation; cost; lack of knowledge regarding choices in parent education classes; and lack of readiness. Therefore clinicians need to provide this information, as needed.

Birth Plan

The **birth plan** is a natural evolution of the contemporary wellness-oriented life-style (see Chapter 1 for more extensive discussion of contemporary options). It is a tool by which parents can explore their childbirth options and choose those that are most important to them. Many parents have already indicated some of their preferences by the type of health care provider (physician, certified nurse midwife) and birth setting (hospital and the options it offers or free-standing birth center) they have chosen. Some pregnant women enlisted the services of the health care provider only after an interview and a tour of the birth facility. Others have not given conscious thought to the conduct of their pregnancies, labors and birth, recovery, and early parenthood. These women may need help with decision making. After the confirmation of pregnancy, couples tend to focus on the reality of their situation and their emotional responses. However, it is acceptable for the nurse to initiate a discussion of a birth plan during the first and second prenatal visit. Some maternity clinics have printed material describing available options and answers to frequently asked questions. In addition, tours of the birth setting are offered by almost all facilities that provide perinatal services.

Clients' expectations must be reasonable for the resources available in the community. The nurse can provide couples with pertinent information for informed decision-making, alerting them to various options and the advantages and consequences of each. The nurse needs to assess clients' readiness to learn and to avoid overload. Some physicians or clinics provide birth plan lists. A discussion of the printed list serves as a means of starting couples to think about, discuss, and identify what is personally important.

Topics for discussion and decision making may include any or all of the following:

- *Partner's participation.* Attend prenatal visits? parent education classes? Present during labor? during birth? during cesarean birth?

- *Birth setting.* Hospital delivery room or birthing room (if available)? a birthing center?
- *Labor management.* Would you like to walk around during labor? use a rocking chair? use a shower? Jacuzzi (available in many new labor, delivery, recovery, and postpartum [LDRP] rooms)? perineal preparation or enema (if they are still done routinely at that particular setting)? consider an electronic fetal monitor? consider stimulation of labor? consider medication—what kind? be interested in having music or dimmed lighting? older children or other people present?
- *Birth.* Have you considered the various positions for birth—side lying? on hands and knees, kneeling or squatting? or using a birthing bed? or delivery table? Will you be photographing or filming any of the labor or birth? Who would you like to be present—partner, older siblings, other family member(s), or friend(s)? What are your feelings about forceps, episiotomies? Will your partner choose to cut the umbilical cord?

Other relevant topics might best be presented during the second trimester.

The birth plan also can serve as a tool for open communication between the pregnant woman and her partner and between them and health care providers. Early introduction to the idea of a birth plan allows the couple time to think about events or situations that could make their childbearing experience meaningful and those they would prefer to avoid. The nurse-client interaction concerning the birth plan needs to occur in an accepting atmosphere in which clients can see themselves as unique and yet normal.

TEACHING Sexuality in First Trimester of Pregnancy*

- Be aware that maternal physiologic changes, such as breast enlargement, nausea, fatigue, abdominal changes, perineal enlargement, leukorrhea, pelvic vasocongestion, and orgasmic responses, may affect sexuality and sexual expression.
- Discuss responses to pregnancy with your partner.
- Keep in mind that cultural prescriptions (do's) and proscriptions (don'ts) may affect your responses.
- Although your libido may be depressed during the first trimester, it increases during the second and third trimesters.
- Discuss and explore with your partner:
  —Alternative behaviors (e.g., mutual masturbation, foot massage, cuddling)
  —Alternative positions (e.g., female superior, side-lying) for sexual intercourse.
- Intercourse is safe as long as it is not uncomfortable:
  —There is no correlation between intercourse and spontaneous abortion, but observe the following precautions.
  —Abstain from intercourse if you experience uterine cramping or vaginal bleeding; report event to your caregiver as soon as possible.
  —Abstain from intercourse (or any activity that results in orgasm) if you have a history of cervical incompetence, until it is corrected.
- Continue to use "safer sex" behaviors.

*For alterations in sexual practice if one of the sexual partners has human immunodeficiency virus (HIV) antibodies, see Chapter 29.

Sexual Counseling during Pregnancy

Sexual counseling includes countering misinformation, providing reassurance of normality, and suggesting alternative behaviors. The uniqueness of each couple is considered within a biopsychosocial framework.

Counseling couples concerning sexual adjustment during pregnancy demands self-assessment by the nurse as well as a knowledge of the physical, social, and emotional responses to sex during pregnancy (Mueller, 1985; Zalar, 1976). Not all maternity nurses are comfortable dealing with the sexual concerns of their clients. Nurses who are aware of their personal strengths and limitation in dealing with sexual content are in a better position to make referrals when necessary.

A significant number of clients merely need *permission* to be sexual during pregnancy. Many other clients need *information* about the physiologic changes that occur during pregnancy and to have myths associated with sex during pregnancy disproved. Giving permission and providing information are within the purview of the maternity nurse and should be an integral component of providing health care (see Teaching for Self-Care, above).

Some couples must be referred for either *sex therapy* or *family therapy*. Couples with long-standing sexual dysfunction problems that are intensified by pregnancy are candidates for sex therapy. When a sexual problem is a symptom of a more serious interactional problem, the couple would benefit from family therapy.

OBTAINING A HISTORY. The history provides a baseline for sexual counseling. History taking is an ongoing process. Receptivity to changes in attitudes, body image, marital relationships, and physical status are relevant topics throughout pregnancy. When changes occur, unexpected problems may develop that require intervention. The history reveals the client's knowledge of female anatomy and physiology and of attitudes about sex during pregnancy, as well as perceptions of the pregnancy, the health status of the couple, and the quality of their marital relationship. Identification of the couple's subjective experience provides the direction and focus of sexual counseling.

COUNTERING MISINFORMATION. Many myths and much of the misinformation related to sex and pregnancy are masked behind seemingly unrelated issues. For example, a question about the baby's ability to hear and see in utero may be related to the baby's role as an observer in lovemaking. The counselor must be extremely sensitive to questions behind the question when counseling in this highly charged emotional area.

SUGGESTING ALTERNATIVE BEHAVIORS. To date research has not proved conclusively that coitus and orgasm are contraindicated at any time during pregnancy for the obstetrically and medically healthy woman (Cunningham, et al, 1989; Enkin, 1989; Scott et al, 1990). However, a history of more than one spontaneous abortion or a threatened abortion in the first trimester, impending miscarriage in the second trimester, or premature rupture of membranes, bleeding, or abdominal pain during the third trimester warrant precaution against coitus and orgasm. Naeye (1979) suggests that improved genital hygiene and perhaps other actions may reduce the risk of intrauterine infection. Until more data are available, Naeye concludes that "a reasonable policy might be to recommend the avoidance of intercourse and orgasm in the third trimester in women with a poor reproductive history or in those who, on pelvic examination, have premature ripening of the cervix." In an interview Naeye commented further that he "was not prepared to recommend prolonged abstinence during pregnancy, since this can cause serious marital discord."

Solitary and mutual masturbation and oral-genital intercourse may be used by couples as *alternatives to penile-vaginal intercourse*. Men who enjoy cunnilingus may feel "turned off" by the normal increase in amount and odor of vaginal discharges during pregnancy. Couples who practice cunnilingus should be cautioned concerning the blowing of air into the vagina, particularly during the last few weeks of pregnancy. There have been cases reported of maternal death and near-fatal cases from air emboli caused by forceful blowing of air into the vagina (Bernhardt et al, 1988). If the cervix is slightly open (as it may be near term), there is the possibility that air will be forced between the membranes and the uterine wall. Some air may enter the maternal placental lakes, thus gaining entrance into the maternal vascular bed.

The woman or couple also should be cautioned against masturbatory activities when orgasmic contractions are contraindicated (e.g., history of spontaneous abortion). Studies have shown that orgasm is often more intense when induced by masturbation. After being cautioned against orgasm, some women require reassurance if they experience erotic dreams.

Pictures of possible variations of *coital position* are often helpful. The female-superior, side-by-side, and rear-entry positions are possible alternative positions to the traditional male-superior position. The woman astride (superior position) allows her to control the angle and depth of penile penetration as well as to protect her breasts and abdomen. The side-by-side position is the one of choice, especially during the third trimester, because it requires reduced energy and pressure on the pregnant abdomen.

Multiparous women have reported severe *breast tenderness* in the first trimester. A coital position that avoids direct pressure on the woman's breasts and decreased breast fondling during love play can be recommended. The woman should also be reassured that this condition is normal and temporary. *Lactating mothers* lose milk in uncontrolled spurts in response to sexual stimulation. The couple that is forewarned can be prepared for this eventuality.

Some women complain of lower abdominal cramping and backache after orgasm during the first and third trimesters. A back rub can often relieve some of the discomfort, as well as provide a pleasant experience. A tonic uterine contraction, often lasting up to a minute, replaces the rhythmic contractions of orgasm during the third trimester. Changes in fetal heart rate (FHR) without fetal distress have been reported.

The National Family Planning and Reproductive Health Association, Washington, DC, suggests that for some women, *use of the contraceptive condom should be continued* throughout the pregnancy (Goldsmith, 1989). The objective of "safer sex" is prophylaxis against the acquisition and transmission of sexually transmitted diseases (e.g., herpes simplex virus [HSV], gonorrhea, acquired immunodeficiency syndrome [AIDS]).

Well-informed nurses who are comfortable with their own sexuality and the sexual counseling needs of pregnant couples can offer counseling in a valuable but often neglected area. They can establish an open environment in which couples can feel free to introduce their concerns about sexual adjustment and seek support and guidance (Mueller, 1985).

Cultural Variation in Prenatal Care

Prenatal care as we know it is a phenomenon of Western medicine. The Western biomedical model of care encourages women to seek prenatal care as early as possible in their pregnancy by visiting a physician or clinic. Visits are usually routine and follow a systematic sequence, with the initial visit followed by a monthly, then bimonthly, then weekly visits. Monitoring weight and blood pressure; testing blood and urine; teaching specific information about diet, rest, and activity; and preparing for childbirth are common components of prenatal care.

This model not only is unfamiliar but commonly seems strange to many groups (Increasing culturally relevant practice, 1988; Lee et al 1988; Lee 1989; Green, 1990; Kulig, 1990). Many cultural variations in prenatal care exist. Even when the prenatal care described is familiar, some practices may conflict with a subcultural group's beliefs and practices. Because of these and other factors, such as lack of money, lack of transportation, and poor communication on the part of health care providers, many groups do not participate in the prenatal care system. Their behavior may be misinterpreted by nurses as uncaring, lazy, or ignorant.

A concern for *modesty* is also a deterrent for prenatal care for many persons. Exposing one's body parts, especially to a man, is a major violation of modesty. For many women invasive procedures such as vaginal examination may be so threatening that they cannot be discussed, even with one's own husband. Thus many women prefer a midwife over a male physician. Too often health care providers assume women lose this modesty during pregnancy and labor. Most women value and appreciate efforts to maintain modesty.

For numerous cultural groups a physician is

Fig. 11-6 Summary of fetal development and maternal events.
From *Safe passage: a woman's guide to a healthier pregnancy,* McNeil Consumer Products Co, Fort Washington, Penn.

	Week 1	Week 2	Week 3	Week 4	Week 5	Week 6
Baby's Development	The ovum becomes fertilized, divides and burrows into the uterus.	The embryonic disk (ectoderm, entoderm, mesoderm) is formed. These three primitive germ layers will generate every organ and tissue in your baby's body.	The first body segments appear, which will eventually form the primitive spine, brain and spinal cord.	Heart, blood circulation and digestive tract take shape. The embryo is now one-fifth of an inch long, the head one-third of its total length.	The heart starts to pump blood; limb buds appear. Major divisions of the brain can now be discerned.	Eyes begin to take shape; external ears develop from skin folds.
Maternal Events	Ovaries increase production of "pregnancy maintaining" hormone, progesterone.	First missed period	Placenta grows to cover one-fifteenth of the uterine interior. Breast may begin to feel tender. No weight gain.			Exchange of fetal and maternal metabolites begins across the placenta, yet the two circulations are completely separate.

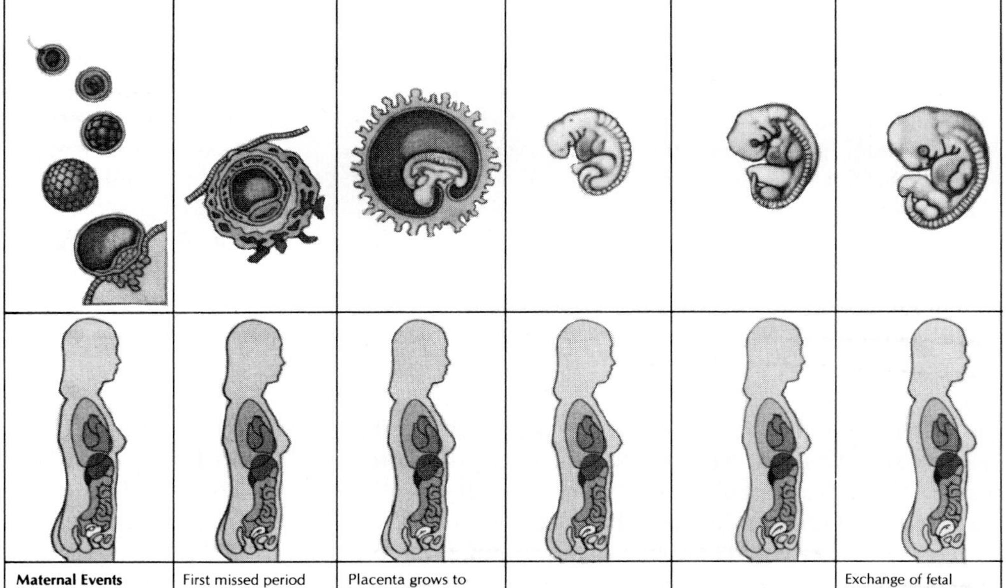

deemed appropriate only in times of illness. The services of a physician are considered inappropriate when pregnancy is considered a normal process and the woman is in a state of health. Even when problems with pregnancy develop according to beliefs of Western medicine, they may not be perceived as problems but may be considered normal.

Although pregnancy is considered normal by many, certain practices are expected of women of all cultures to ensure a good outcome. **Cultural prescriptions** tell women what to do, and **proscriptions** establish *taboos*. The purposes of these practices are to prevent maternal illness from a pregnancy-induced imbalanced state and to protect the vulnerable fetus. Prescriptions and proscriptions are related to emotional response, clothing, activity and rest, sexual activity, and dietary practices.

EMOTIONAL RESPONSE. Virtually all cultures emphasize the importance of a socially harmonious and agreeable environment. Absence of stressful relationships is important for a successful outcome for mother and baby. Harmony with other persons must be fostered. Visits from extended family members may be required to demonstrate continued pleasant and noncontroversial relationships. If discord exists in any relationship with others, it is usually dealt with in culturally prescribed ways.

Imitative magic functions in other proscriptions in addition to food. Many Mexicans advise against pregnant women witnessing an eclipse of the moon because they believe it may cause a cleft palate in the infant. Exposures to an earthquake may result in preterm delivery or miscarriage. A breech presentation may occur if the earthquake was exceptionally strong (Clark, 1970). Snow (1974) notes that in some cultures a pregnant woman must not ridicule someone with an affliction for fear her child might be born

Week 7	Week 8	Week 9	Week 10	Week 11	Week 12	Week 13
Development is proceding rapidly. The face is now complete with eyes, nose, lips and tongue — even primitive milk teeth. Tiny bones and muscles appear beneath the thin skin.	The embryo is now a little more than an inch long, its tiny heart beating at about 40-80 times a minute.	**Baby's Development** Genitalia is now well defined; the baby's sex is determined. Eyelids finish forming and seal shut. The embryo has become a fetus.	The fetus assumes a more human shape as the lower body rapidly develops. Blood and bone cells form. The first movements begin.	Organs begin to function. The pancreas is producing insulin; the kidneys, urine.	The lungs have taken shape; primitive breathing motions begin. The swallowing reflex has been mastered as the fetus sucks its thumb while floating weightlessly in the amniotic fluid.	
No noticeable weight gain.	The placenta now covers about one-third of the uterus lining.	**Maternal Events** Maternal blood volume has increased 30-40%.	The sensation of these first movements has been described by some women as if something were blowing bubbles through a straw in their stomachs.	2-3 lb weight gain. Possible increase in perspiration.	The placenta has reached complete functional maturity, acting as the baby's lungs, kidneys, liver, digestive and immune systems.	

with the same handicap. A mother should not hate a person lest her child resemble that person, and dental work should not be done during pregnancy because it may cause a baby to have a harelip. Carrington (1978) describes a widely held folk belief in many cultures that includes refraining from raising one's arm above one's head and from tying knots, so that the umbilical cord does not wrap around the baby's neck and become knotted.

CLOTHING. Although most cultural groups do not prescribe specific clothing for pregnancy, modesty is an expectation for many (Clark, 1970; Meleis, Sorrell, 1981). Some Spanish-speaking people of the Southwest wear a cord beneath the breast and knotted over the umbilicus. This cord, called a *muneco,* is thought to prevent morning sickness and ensure a safe delivery (Brown, 1976). Amulets, medals, and beads may be worn to ward off evil spirits.

PHYSICAL ACTIVITY AND REST. Norms that regulate physical activity of mothers during pregnancy vary tremendously. Many groups (Carrington, 1978; Horn, 1982; Lee, 1989) encourage women to be active, to walk, and to engage in normal although not strenuous activities to ensure that the baby is healthy and not too large. On the other hand, the Filipino woman may be cautioned that any activity is dangerous, and others willingly take over work (Affonso, 1978; Stern, 1981). The belief among some Filipinos is that inactivity constitutes a protection for mother and child. The mother is encouraged simply to produce the succeeding generation. Health care providers could misinterpret this behavior as laziness or noncompliance with the health regimen desired in prenatal care. Again it is important for the nurse to find out the meaning of activity and rest for each culture.

SEXUAL ACTIVITY. In most cultures sexual activity is not prohibited until the end of pregnancy. Among some cultures sexual relations are viewed as natural because pregnancy is a state of health (Carrington, 1978). Many Mexican-Americans view sexual activity as necessary to keep the birth canal lubricated (Kay, 1982). On the other hand, Vietnamese may have definite proscriptions about sexual intercourse, requiring abstinence as early as the sixth month (Lee, 1989). Sexual taboos are more common after delivery.

DIET. Nutritional information given by Western health care providers may be a source of conflict for many cultural groups. The conflict commonly is not known by the health care providers unless they have an understanding of dietary beliefs and practices of the persons for whom they are caring (see Chapter 9).

EVALUATION

Evaluation of effectiveness of nursing care is based on the degree to which the following goals of care have been achieved.

- The woman's pregnancy is diagnosed and her EDD is calculated.
- She understands maternal adaptations and self-care measures.
- Her risk factors (if present) are identified and referral for further evaluation or therapy is begun promptly.
- She knows the danger signs and to whom to report if they occur.
- She and her family become active participants in her care during the first trimester.
- She develops a trusting relationship with her caregivers.

■ SUMMARY

The prenatal period is one of growth and change in the woman's personal and social context. Achieving a goal of a safe and satisfying pregnancy for a woman and her family requires a mutual effort on the part of the woman and the professionals involved. Practitioner and client need a clear understanding of their objectives, roles, and capabilities. Nursing care provided during this period can act as a stimulus for the continued use of the health care system by the woman and her family. Nursing actions reflect the changes experienced by the woman as she progresses through the first trimester of pregnancy. Fig. 11-6 summarizes maternal events and embryonic/fetal development during the first trimester.

CASE STUDY

Nausea (Morning Sickness), Fatigue, and Altered Sexual Pattern

Ruth Piper is a 36-year-old married woman experiencing her first pregnancy. She has just been diagnosed as being 8 weeks' pregnant.

ASSESSMENT

During her initial prenatal visit she tells the nurse that she is experiencing nausea and dry heaves on awakening in the morning. She states that this prevents her from eating breakfast and is interfering with her morning routine, sometimes making her late to work. Ruth also reports that at 4 PM when she gets home from work, she is so tired that she cannot fix dinner for herself and her husband; all she wants to do is go to bed for the night. She states she misses having sex with her husband. This break in her routine is upsetting her, and she asks for help. A physical examination revealed she is a healthy woman. All findings are within normal limits (WNL). Her urine test result was positive for pregnancy. Other laboratory test results will be available by the next visit.

NURSING DIAGNOSIS

Because Ruth was very concerned about her bouts of morning nausea and dry heaves, the nurse identifies the following nursing diagnosis: Altered nutrition, less than body requirements, related to nausea and dry heaves of early pregnancy.

PLANNING

Ruth and the nurse mutually identify the following *goal:* Ruth will be free of morning nausea and dry heaves and will be able to eat some breakfast. The nurse sets the following *expected outcomes:* Ruth will experience less discomfort, be able to eat so that she can meet the added metabolic needs, increase her ability to cope through self-care, and become an active participant in prenatal health care.

IMPLEMENTATION

The nurse takes a 24-hour diet history and a description of food (or their odors or appearance) that have precipitated nausea and dry heaves. The incidence and possible causes of the discomfort are discussed. Ruth and the nurse discuss the following interventions to try to reduce the discomfort:

- Avoid empty or overloaded stomach.
- Maintain good posture to give stomach ample room
- Stop or decrease smoking
- Eat dry carbohydrate on awakening
- Remain in bed until feeling subsides
- Alternate dry carbohydrate 1 hour with fluids such as hot tea, milk, or clear coffee the next hour until feeling subsides
- Eat five to six small meals per day
- Avoid fried, odorous, spicy, greasy, or gas-forming foods
- If severe or persistent vomiting occurs, Ruth should inform the physician immediately (see discussion of hyperemesis gravidarum, Chapter 31)

Reassure Ruth that "morning sickness" occurs in 50% to 75% of pregnant women; it starts between the first and second missed menstrual period and lasts until about the fourth missed period.

EVALUATION

At the first prenatal visit, Ruth verbalizes that she understands the information. She and her husband state they will try to work out a plan to help her. At the next visit, Ruth reports occasional nausea, no vomiting, and no dry heaves. Ruth has gained 1 pound.

CARE PLAN **Nausea (Morning Sickness), Fatigue, and Altered Sexual Pattern**

GOALS	IMPLEMENTATION	RATIONALE	EVALUATION
Nursing diagnosis: Altered nutrition, less than body requirements, related to nausea and dry heaves of early pregnancy			
Ruth will be free of nausea and dry heaves. Ruth will meet nutritional requirement and gain about 3 lb during the first trimester.	Discuss incidence, causes.	Reassures that this is a common discomfort, can be treated, and is time limited.	Ruth verbalizes understanding of information.
	Take a 24-hour diet history.	Establishes data base to identify foods that cause nausea.	

Continued.

CARE PLAN Nausea (Morning Sickness), Fatigue, and Altered Sexual Pattern—cont'd

GOALS	IMPLEMENTATION	RATIONALE	EVALUATION
	Caution Ruth to avoid eating fried or greasy foods, or other offensive foods, especially before bedtime. Discuss eating small, frequent meals; avoid having an empty stomach. Advise Ruth to keep unsalted crackers (or other dry carbohydrate) at her bedside and to eat some on awakening, before getting out of bed.	Removes potential causes. Food is essential to meet increased metabolic needs; it also helps to fend off fatigue. An empty stomach is associated with nausea. Increases ability to cope through self-care.	At next visit, Ruth reports occasional mild nausea but no dry heaves.
	Advise her that if vomiting occurs and is severe, to call physician immediately.	Severe vomiting may indicate the complication of hyperemesis gravidarum (see Chapter 31).	Ruth reports no incident of vomiting.
Nursing diagnosis: Fatigue related to early pregnancy and possibly to insufficient intake of calories			
Ruth will learn how to deal with the fatigue of early pregnancy. Ruth will be able to increase her activity level and resume activities of daily living without undue fatigue.	Discuss ways to deal with the fatigue of pregnancy: ■ Adequate nutrition ■ Rest periods while at work; nap after work, before supper ■ Husband may be willing to prepare her favorite preferred foods and present them attractively. Discuss resources to help with home maintenance. Reduce work hours for a few weeks.	Adequate nutrition is needed to meet increased metabolic demands and to prevent anemia. Participation in decision making has positive effect by lessening feeling of powerlessness. Increases ability to cope through self-care.	Ruth verbalizes understanding of information. At next visit, Ruth reports a lessening of fatigue and an increase in activity level. Her husband reports satisfaction with his ability to "help out" and "contribute."
Nursing diagnosis: Altered sexuality pattern related to discomforts of early pregnancy			
Ruth will understand how physiology of pregnancy affects intercourse.	Ask appropriate questions and verbalize understanding and acceptance of information discussed. Discuss those symptoms Ruth is experiencing that affect foreplay and intercourse. Discuss sexuality and alternative sexual behaviors and positions that can be used during pregnancy.	Open discussion legitimizes this concern, which is shared by other pregnant couples. Open discussion demonstrates nurse's caring and ability to be a resource person. Alternative behaviors and positions are available for expression of sexuality. Presents possibility for enhancing couple's relationship and family coping.	Ruth verbalizes understanding of information. At the next visit, Ruth states that she and her husband had found mutually acceptable alternative behaviors and patterns. Ruth and her husband verbalize satisfaction with their sexual adaptation to pregnancy.

REFERENCES

Affonso DD: The Filipino American. In Clark AL, editor: *Culture/childbearing/health professionals,* Philadelphia, 1978, FA Davis Co.

Barry M, Bia F: Pregnancy and travel, *JAMA* 261:728, 1989.

Bernhardt TL et al: Hyperbaric oxygen treatment of cerebral air embolism from orogenital sex during pregnancy, *Crit Care Med* 16:729, 1988.

Brown MS: A cross-cultural look at pregnancy, labor, and delivery, *Obstet Gynecol Nurs* 5:35, 1976.

Burgess MA: Rubella vaccination just before or during pregnancy, *Med J Aust* 152:507, 1990.

Carrington BW: The Afro-American. In Clark AL, editor: *Culture/childbearing/health professionals,* Philadelphia, 1978, FA Davis Co.

Chenger P, Korvacek A: Dental hygiene during pregnancy: a review, *Am J Matern Child Nurs* 12:342, 1987.

Chez R: Battered pregnant women, *Genesis* 11:15, Jan 1989.

Clark M: *Health in the Mexican-American culture: a community study,* Berkeley, 1970, University of California Press.

Cook PS, Petersen RC, Moore DT: *Alcohol, tobacco, and other drugs may harm the unborn,* US Department of Health and Human Services, DHHS Pub No (ADM)90-1711, Rockville, Md, 1990, Office for Substance Abuse Prevention.

Culpepper L: Exercise during pregnancy. In Merkatz IR, Thompson JE editors: *New perspectives on prenatal care,* New York, 1990, Elsevier Science Publishing Co.

Cunningham FG, MacDonald RC, Gant NF: *Williams obstetrics,* ed 18, Norwalk, Conn, 1989, Appleton & Lange.

Dicke JM: Teratology: principles and practice, *Med Clin North Am* 73:567, 1989.

Edwards M: *Communications: dimensions in childbirth education,* Pacific Grove, Calif, 1973, M Edwards.

Enkin M et al: *A guide to effective care in pregnancy and childbirth,* New York, 1989, Oxford University Press.

Ershoff DH et al: A randomized trial of a serialized self-help smoking cessation program on pregnant women in an HMO, *Am J Public Health* 79:182, Feb 1989.

Fishbein EG, Phillips M: How safe is exercise during pregnancy? *JOGNN* 19:45, Jan/Feb 1990.

Goldsmith MF: Pregnancy Dx? Rx may now include condoms, *JAMA* 261:678, 1989.

Horn BM: Northwest coast Indians: the Muckleshoot. In Kay, MA, editor: *Anthropology of human birth,* Philadelphia, 1982, FA Davis Co.

Increasing culturally relevant practice with Hispanic clients, *NPA Bull* 3:23, Nov/Dec 1988.

Kay MA, editor: *Anthropology of human birth,* Philadelphia, 1982, FA Davis Co.

Lee RV: Understanding Southeast Asian mothers-to-be, *Childbirth Educ* 8:32, Spring 1989.

Lee RV et al: Southeast Asian folklore about pregnancy and parturition, *Obstet Gynecol* 71:243, 1988.

Leviton A: Caffeine consumption and the risk of reproductive hazards, *J Reprod Med* 33:175, 1988.

Main D, Mennuti M: Neural tube defects: issues in prenatal diagnosis and counseling, *Obstet Gynecol* 67:1, 1986.

Malasanos L et al: *Health assessment,* ed 4, St Louis, 1990, Mosby–Year Book.

Meleis AI, Sorrell L: Bridging cultures: Arab American women and their birth experiences, *MCN* 6:171, 1981.

Mittelmark RA et al, editors: *Exercise in pregnancy,* ed 2, Baltimore, 1991, Williams & Wilkins.

Mueller L: Pregnancy and sexuality, *JOGNN* 14:4, July/Aug 1985.

Naeye RL: Coitus and associated amniotic-fluid infections, *N Engl J Med* 301:1198, 1979.

Paglone A, Worthington S: Cautions and advice on exercise during pregnancy, *Contemp OB/GYN* 25:160, May 1985 (special issue).

Scott JR et al: *Obstetrics and gynecology,* ed 6, Philadelphia, 1990, JB Lippincott Co.

Seidel HM et al: *Mosby's guide to physical examination,* ed 2, St Louis, 1991, Mosby–Year Book.

Snow L: Folk medical beliefs and their implications for care of patients, *Ann Intern Med* 81:82, 1974.

Stern PM: Solving problems of cross-cultural health teaching: the Filipino childbearing family, *Image* 13:47, 1981.

Van Dinter MC: Ptyalism in pregnant women, *JOGNN* 20:206, May/June 1991.

Wright LM, Leahey M: *Nurses and families: a guide to family assessment and interaction,* Philadelphia, 1984, FA Davis Co.

Zalar MK: Sexual counseling for pregnant couples, *MCN* 1:176, May/June 1976.

References—Nursing Research

Aaronson LS, MacNee CL: Tobacco, alcohol and caffeine use during pregnancy, *JOGNN* 18:279, July/Aug 1989.

Green NL: Stressful events related to childbearing in African-American women: a pilot study, *J Nurse Midwife* 35:231, July/Aug 1990.

Helton A et al: Prevention of battering during pregnancy: focus on behavioral change, *Public Health Nurs* 4:166, Sept 1987.

Kulig JC: Childbearing beliefs among Cambodian refugee women, *West J Nurs Res* 12:108, Feb 1990.

Middleton J: Voluntary HIV screening at the first prenatal visit, *J Nurse Midwife* 35:349, Nov/Dec 1989.

Zerwekh JR: At the expense of their souls, *Nurs Outlook* 39:58, March/April 1991.

BIBLIOGRAPHY

Bernhardt JH: Potential workplace hazards to reproductive health: information for primary prevention, *JOGNN* 19:53, Jan/Feb 1990.

Buekens P: Variations in provision and uptake of antenatal care, *Baillieres Clin Obstet Gynaecol* 4:187, 1990.

Jewell D: Prepregnancy and early pregnancy care, *Baillieres Clin Obstet Gynaecol* 4 (1):1, 1990.

Lewallen LP: Health beliefs and health practices of pregnant women, *JOGNN* 18:245, May/June 1989.

Lindell SG: Education for childbirth: a time for change, *JOGNN* 17:108, March/April 1988.

NAACOG: *Standards for the nursing care of women and newborns,* ed 4, Washington DC, 1991, NAACOG.

Petitti D et al: Early prenatal care in urban black and white women, *Birth* 17:1, March 1990.

Starn J, Niederhauser V: An MCN model for nursing diagnosis to focus intervention, *MCN* 15:180, May/June 1990.

Stevens KA: Nursing diagnoses in wellness childbearing settings, *JOGNN* 17:329, Sept/Oct 1988.

Bibliography—Nursing Research

Dawkins C et al: Health orientation, beliefs, and use of health services among minority, high risk expectant mothers, *Public Health Nurs* 5:7, March 1988.

Jacoby A: Mothers' views about information and advice in pregnancy and childbirth: findings from a national study, *Midwifery* 43:103, Sept 1988.

Patterson ET et al: Seeking safe passage: utilizing health care during pregnancy, *Image J Nurs Sch* 22:27, Spring 1990.

chapter 11 review

Key Concepts

- The prenatal period is a preparatory one both physically, in terms of fetal growth and maternal adaptations, and psychologically, in terms of anticipation of parenthood.
- Important components of the initial prenatal visit include detailed and carefully recorded findings from the interview, a comprehensive physical examination, and selected laboratory tests.
- Through assessment, formulation of nursing diagnoses, and planning, mutually derived with the client and her family when appropriate, individualized care may be implemented; evaluation of care is an ongoing process.
- Maternal physical and familial adaptations to pregnancy generate needs that the nurse-clinician can anticipate and meet.
- Discomforts and changes of pregnancy can cause anxiety in the pregnant woman and her family and require sensitive attention and a plan for teaching self-care measures.
- The pregnant woman's readiness to learn is at a high level, making this an excellent time to help her expand her self-care skills.
- The psychosocial aspects of care are of paramount importance and may well affect the whole course of pregnancy, childbirth, and the adjustment of the new family.
- Cultural prescriptions and proscriptions influence responses to pregnancy and to the health care delivery system.
- Even in normal pregnancy the nurse must remain alert to hazards such as supine hypotension, danger signs, and signs of potential parenting disorders and family maladaptations.

Key Terms

- amenorrhea (p. 268)
- birth plan (p. 272)
- breast changes (p. 268)
- breast self-examination (BSE) (p. 273)
- cultural prescriptions and proscriptions (p. 291)
- estimated date of delivery (EDD) (p. 269)
- first trimester (p. 268)
- imitative magic (p. 291)
- Kegel exercises (p. 274)
- last menstrual period (LMP) (p. 268)
- lithotomy position (p.274)
- morning sickness (p. 268)
- Nägele's rule (p. 269)
- Papanicolaou (Pap) smear (p. 277)
- positive signs (p. 269)
- presumptive signs and symptoms (p. 268)
- probable signs and symptoms (p. 269)
- supine hypotension (p. 272)
- urinary frequency (p. 268)
- warning signs (p. 283)

Critical Thinking Exercise

For each activity, justify your claims, beliefs, conclusions, decisions, and actions.

1. In an actual or simulated clinical setting, complete an initial prenatal interview (history, including sexual history) and comprehensive physical examination. Formulate three nursing diagnoses (one physical, one psychosocial, and one growth and developmental) and corroborate with defining characteristics. For each diagnosis, develop one client-centered goal, one intervention specifying rationale, and one evaluative criterion.
2. Discuss how the nurse's role as support person would differ for a woman with a supportive family who was pleased with her pregnancy and for a woman facing pregnancy without such support.
3. In small groups, discuss cultural influences based on data from interviews with clients or from personal experiences.

Topics for Nursing Research

- Strategies to promote early prenatal care
- Nursing interventions to meet the needs of specific cultural groups
- Evaluation of various educational strategies to assist clients with behavioral change
- Effectiveness of worksite health promotion programs
- Effects of assessing for risk factors on maternal anxiety

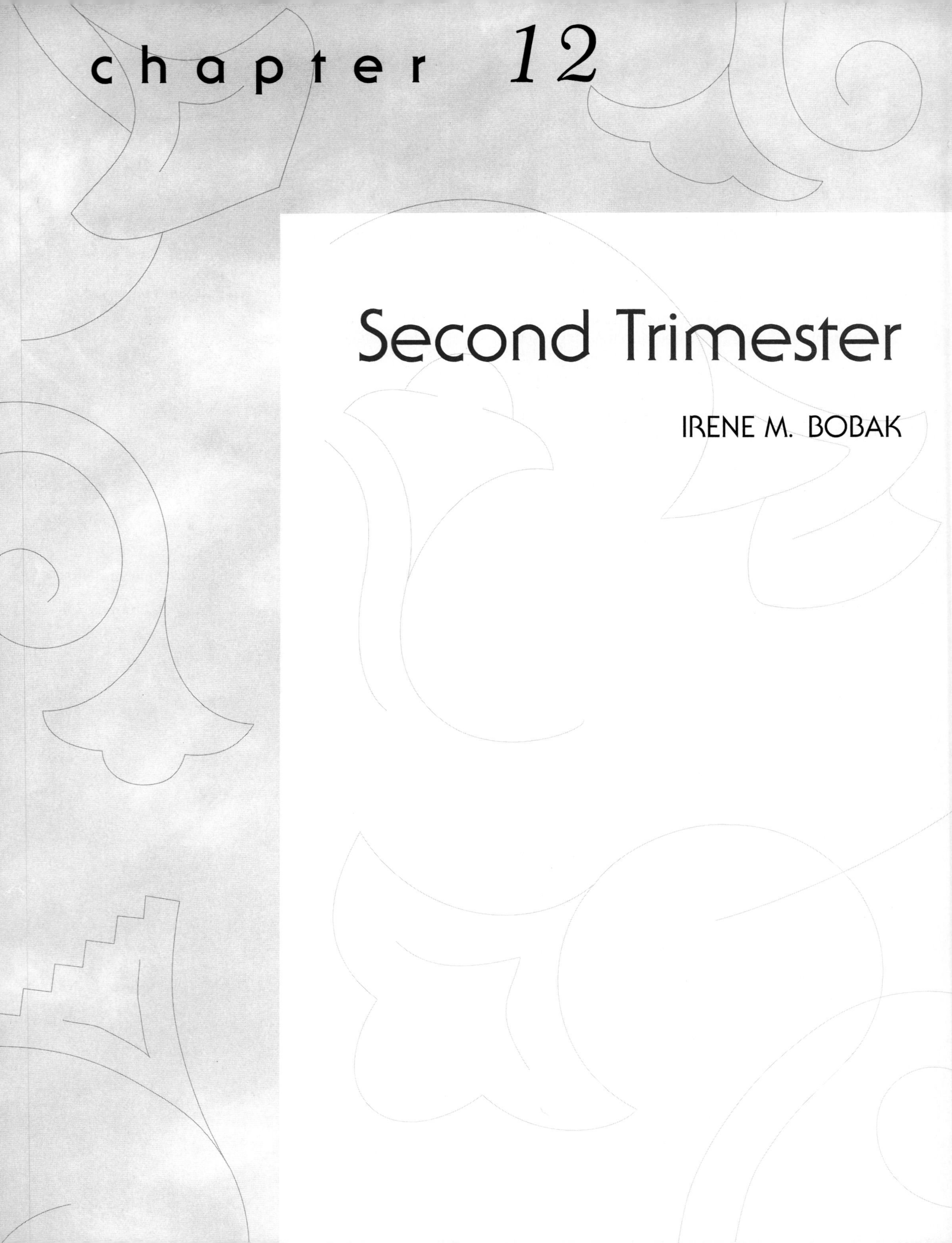

chapter 12

Second Trimester

IRENE M. BOBAK

LEARNING OBJECTIVES

- Define key terms listed.
- Summarize health assessment of the pregnant woman and her fetus.
- Outline the schedule of visits for the woman during the second trimester.
- Discuss the physiology and self-care of discomforts related to maternal adaptations.
- List physical warning signs in the second trimester.
- Discuss the developing birth plan.
- Develop guidelines for exercise tips for pregnant women.
- Formulate possible nursing diagnoses.
- Discuss planning, implementation, and evaluation of a nursing plan of care during the second trimester of pregnancy.
- Identify topics for nursing research related to the second trimester of pregnancy.

The **second trimester** spans weeks 14 through 26 of pregnancy. By the second trimester the pregnancy usually has been verified. The woman and her family have had time to adjust to the pregnancy, and the initial visit or two have been completed. For many women, discomforts common to the first trimester are resolving, but it is still too early to focus on the labor and birth.

Most women have no major problems. For them, a common pattern for return visits is scheduled. Throughout the second trimester, monthly visits are sufficient, although additional visits are warranted should the need arise.

NURSING PROCESS

Ideally, a trusting relationship has been established among the pregnant woman and her family, the nurse, and other health care providers. The nursing plan of care has been initiated, and changes based on ongoing evaluation continue to be addressed. As during the first trimester, health promotion, primary prevention, and secondary prevention remain the focus of nursing care. Continued growth and development of the mother and her fetus and the family unit direct the changes in nursing management during the second trimester of pregnancy.

ASSESSMENT

Maternal Assessment

INTERVIEW. Follow-up visits are less intensive than the initial prenatal visit. At each visit, the woman is asked for a summary of events since the previous visit. She is asked about her general emotional and physiologic well-being, complaints or problems, or questions she may have. Personal and family needs are identified and explored (to review this content, see Chapter 10).

Emotional well-being is assessed at each visit. The woman's emotional state has an impact on her general well-being and on that of her family. Because emotional changes are common during pregnancy, it is reasonable for the nurse to inquire whether she has experienced any mood swings, reactions to changes in her body image, bad dreams, or worries. Positive feelings (her own and those of her family) are also noted. Reactions of family members to the pregnancy and her emotional changes are recorded.

How is she progressing through the developmental tasks of pregnancy (see Chapter 10)? By the beginning of the second trimester, most women have accepted the biologic fact of pregnancy. Usually by the fifth month, pregnant women experience a growing awareness of the child as a separate being, distinct from themselves; women can say, "I am going to have a baby." With quickening, has she turned her attention inward (become introspective) to her pregnancy and to relationships with others (e.g., her mother, partner). Success or failure of self-care measures is discussed, and learning needs and readiness for learning are assessed.

The nurse inquires about parent education classes. Did the woman (with or without her partner) attend Early Bird classes during the first trimester? If so what questions does she have? Is she planning to attend second-trimester classes? If a birth plan is being formulated, what questions does she have and how far has she/the couple come in its development?

A checklist of care needs during the second trimester of pregnancy is a valuable tool. It provides the team of care providers with a communication tool to prevent gaps and to identify areas of concern for clients. A sample checklist for the second trimester is shown in the box below.

Second-Trimester Checklist

- Schedule and events of visits
- Maternal assessment
- Fetal growth and development
- Diagnostic tests
  - Specify
- Counseling for self-care:
  - Birth plan
  - Adaptations/discomforts
    - Skin changes
    - Palpitations
    - Faintness
    - Gastrointestinal distress
    - Varicosities
    - Neuromuscular and skeletal distress
  - Safety (seat belts with shoulder harness and head rest)
  - Exercise and rest
  - Relaxation
  - Nutrition
  - Alcohol and other substances
  - Sexuality
  - Personal hygiene
  - Warning signs
- Other

PHYSICAL EXAMINATION. Reevaluation is constant. Each woman reacts differently to pregnancy. Careful monitoring of pregnancy and reactions to care is vital. A data base updated at each contact with a client reveals patterns in movement and content.

At each visit pulse and respirations are measured; blood pressure (right arm, woman sitting) is taken; weight and the determination of whether weight gain (or loss) is compatible with the overall plan for weight gain are evaluated (for discussion of nursing related to nutrition, see Chapter 9); urinalysis is performed; and presence and degree of edema are noted. Abdominal inspection and palpitation and measurement of fundal height are part of each visit; these are discussed in more detail in the section that follows. While assessing the pregnant woman's abdomen, the nurse must remain alert to the possibility of *supine hypotension* (see Emergency Box, Chapter 11).

The findings from the interview and physical examination reflect the status of maternal adaptations. When the interview or physical examination findings are suspicious, an in-depth examination is performed.

Careful interpretation of blood pressure is important in risk-factor analysis for all pregnant women. Blood pressure is evaluated on the basis of absolute values and length of gestation and is interpreted in the light of modifying factors (see p.199 for an extensive discussion of blood pressure).

Absolute values of a systolic blood pressure ≥140 mm Hg and a diastolic blood pressure ≥90 mm Hg suggest hypertension. A rise in systolic blood pressure ≥30 mm Hg over baseline and/or in diastolic blood pressure ≥15 mm Hg over baseline are also significant regardless of whether absolute values are less than 140/90. For example, if a woman's blood pressure normally is 105/60, a change to 120/75 must be viewed as potential for hypertension.

The mean arterial pressure (MAP) reaches its lowest point in the second trimester at about 22 weeks, then rises slowly to term (Page et al, 1981). MAP readings of 82 at 22 weeks are within the normal range for the length of gestation. An MAP of ≥90 in the second trimester is associated with an increase in the incidence of pregnancy-induced hypertension (PIH) in the third trimester.

LABORATORY TESTS. Routine laboratory tests during the second trimester are limited. A clean-catch urine specimen is used to detect levels of glucose, acetone, albumin/protein, RBCs, and leukocytes. Pregnant women may experience glycosuria (for review, see nutrient excretion, p. 203). Urine for culture and sensitivity, as well as blood samples, are obtained only if signs and symptoms warrant. Hematocrit (HCT) or packed cell volume (PCV) determination is done at each visit in some offices.

SIGNS OF POTENTIAL MATERNAL PROBLEMS. The mother is monitored continuously for potential complications. Persistent and excessive vomiting may lead to hyperemesis gravidarium (see p. 948). Uterine cramping and vaginal bleeding are signs of spontaneous abortion (p. 887). Chills and fever accompany infection (see Chapter 29). Hypertension must be investigated (see Chapter 28).

Fetal Assessment

FUNDAL HEIGHT. During the second trimester the uterus becomes an abdominal organ. Measurement of the height of the uterus above the symphysis pubis is used as one indicator of the progress of fetal growth. It also provides a gross estimate of the duration of pregnancy.

A pliable (not stretchable) tape measure or a pelvimeter may be used to measure **fundal height.** The height of the fundus is measured from the notch of the pubic symphysis over the top of the fundus without tipping the uterus back.

To increase measurement reliability the same person examines the woman at each of her prenatal visits, and one protocol is established for use by all examiners providing care to a group of pregnant women. The protocol must include the woman's position on the table and the measuring device and method used. *The woman's position is supine with the knees slightly bent and the head and shoulders slightly elevated. Early in pregnancy, her bladder should be empty.* If a pliable measuring tape is used, it should be specified whether the measurement is taken with the tape held in contact with the skin from the uterus to the fundus or whether the measurement is read with the palm of the hand at the fundus and the tape elevated between the forefinger and the middle finger (Fig. 12-1). *McDonald's rule* adds precision to the measurement of fundal height during the second and third trimesters. It is calculated as follows:

$$\text{Height of fundus (cm)} \times 2/7 \text{ (or } + 3.5) = \text{Duration of pregnancy in lunar months}$$

$$\text{Height of fundus (cm)} \times 8/7 = \text{Duration of pregnancy in weeks}$$

Because fingers vary in size from person to person, assessing the fundal height with a tape measure is more accurate than the use of fingerbreadths. The umbilicus, which is not in the center of the abdomen for all women, cannot be used as a landmark in measuring fundal height (Engstrom, 1988).

Measurement of fundal height may aid in identifi-

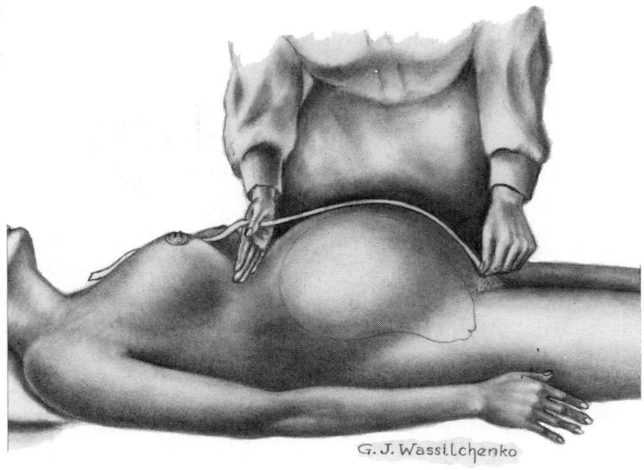

Fig. 12-1 Measurement of fundal height from symphysis.

cation of high-risk factors. A stable or decreased fundal height may indicate intrauterine growth retardation (IUGR), and an excessive increase could mean multifetal gestation or hydramnios (see Unit 7). Among the factors that affect the accuracy of measurement are *obesity* (subtract 1 cm from the measurement if the woman weighs 90 kg [200 pounds] or more), the *amount of amniotic fluid,* multifetal gestation, the fetal size and attitude, and the tilt of the uterus.

GESTATIONAL AGE. In a normal pregnancy, **fetal gestational age** is estimated after determining the duration of pregnancy and the expected date of delivery (EDD) (to review EDD and Nägele's rule, see p. 269). Fetal gestational age is determined from the menstrual history, contraceptive history, pregnancy test, and clinical evaluation:

- Menstrual history
  - First day of last normal menstrual period (LNMP): date, duration, amount
  - Last menstrual period (LMP): date, duration, amount
  - First day of previous menstrual period (before LMP) (PMP): date, duration, amount
  - Menarche: date, interval, duration
  - History of menstrual irregularity
- Contraceptive history
  - Type of contraceptive
  - When stopped
- Pregnancy test
  - Date:
  - Type:
  - Result:
- Clinical evaluation
  - First uterine size estimate: date, size
  - Fetal heart tone (FHT) first heard: date, Dopptone, fetoscope
  - Date of quickening
  - Current fundal height, estimated fetal weight (EFW)
  - Current week of gestation
  - Ultrasound: date, week of gestation, biparietal diameter (BPD)
  - Reliability of dates

Quickening ("feeling life") refers to the mother's perception of fetal movement. It usually occurs between weeks 16 and 20 of gestation.

In some centers ultrasonography is used with all pregnancies, and a more exact estimation of gestational age can be made. Ultrasonography may be used to establish the duration of pregnancy if the woman is unable to give a precise date for her LMP or if the size of the uterus does not conform to the stated date of the LMP (for a discussion of ultrasonography, see Chapter 27). Ultrasonography is not, however, a universally recommended procedure.

HEALTH STATUS. Assessment of **fetal health status** includes consideration of fetal movement, fetal heart rate (FHR), and abnormal maternal or fetal symptoms.

The mother is instructed to note the extent and timing of fetal movements and to report immediately if the pattern changes or if movement ceases. Regular movement has been found to be a reliable determinant of fetal health (Cohen, 1985).

The FHR is checked on routine visits once it has been heard (Fig. 12-2). Early in this trimester, the FHR may be heard with the ultrasound stethoscope (Fig. 12-2, *C*) or the ultrasound fetoscope (see Fig. 16-1). Before the fetus can be palpated by Leopold's maneuvers (see p. 437 and Fig. 17-8), the scope is moved around the abdomen until the FHR is heard. Each nurse develops a set pattern for searching the abdomen, for example, starting first in the midline about 2 to 3 cm (1 in) above the symphysis, followed by the left lower quadrant, and so on. The FHR is counted and the quality and rhythm noted (see Chapter 16). Later in the second trimester, the FHR can be determined with the fetoscope or stethoscope (Fig. 12-2, *A* and *B*). Normal rate and rhythm are other good indicators of fetal health. Absence of FHR, once noted, requires immediate investigation.

The second trimester is a period of rapid growth. The box on p. 303 summarizes fetal development.

SIGNS OF POTENTIAL FETAL PROBLEMS. Intensive investigation of fetal health status is initiated if any maternal or fetal complications arise (e.g., maternal

A

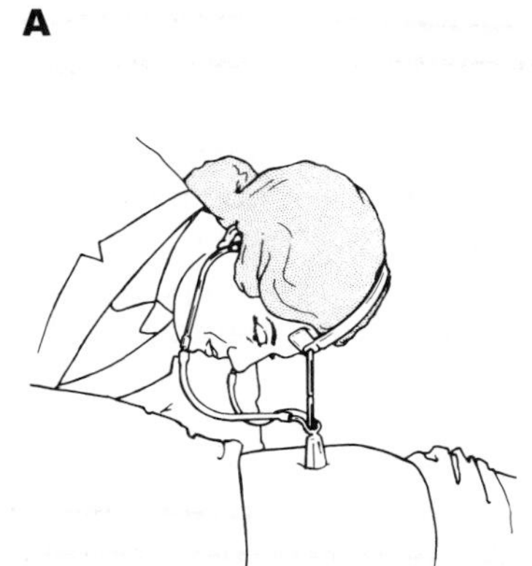

B

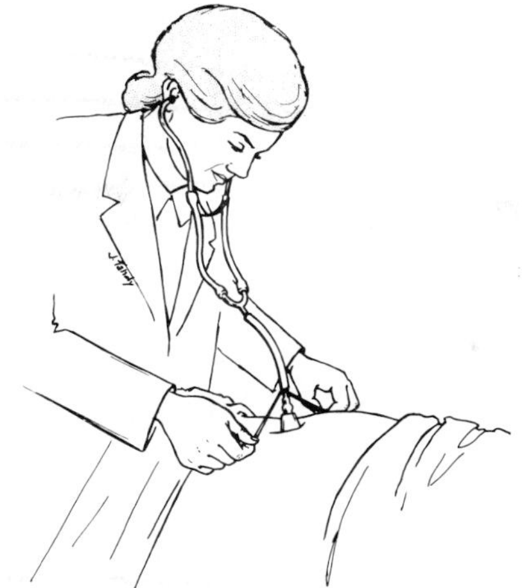

C

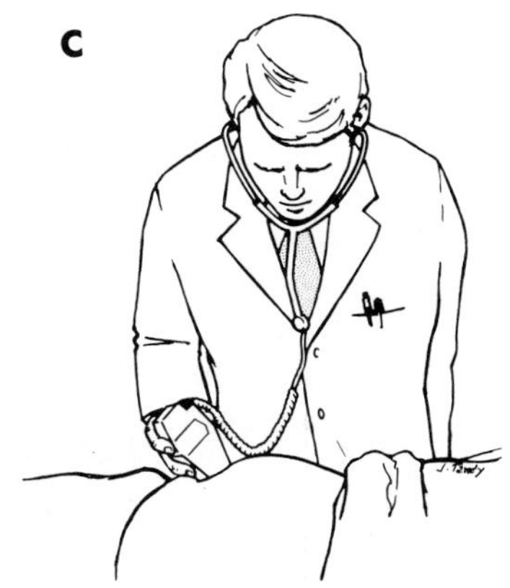

D

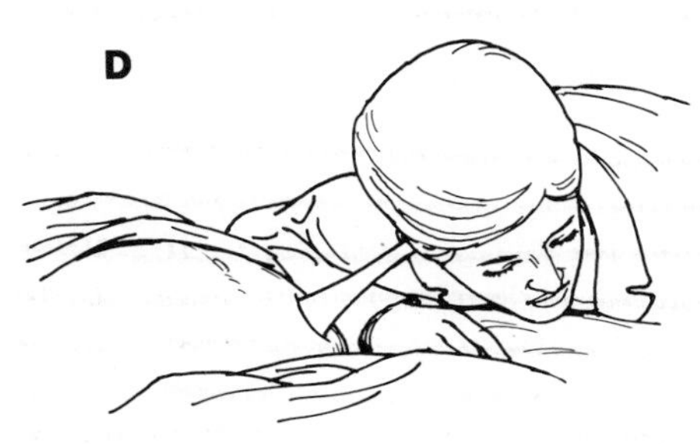

Fig. 12-2 Detecting fetal heartbeat. **A,** Fetoscope. **B,** Stethoscope with rubber band. **C,** Ultrasound stethoscope. **D,** Pinard's stethoscope. NOTE: Hands should not touch stethoscope while listening.

Fetal Development at 26 Weeks

Viable at week 24*
Fetal movements obvious
FHR readily heard
Scalp hair, eyebrows, eyelashes, fine downy lanugo and vernix cover the skin
Eyelids still fused
Skin is red, shiny, and thin
Face is wrinkled, giving an "old man appearance"
Length is 30 cm (12 in)
Weight is 600 g (1¼ lb)
Uterus at or just above level of umbilicus

*In Canada, the fetus achieves viability at 20 weeks' gestation and 500 g in weight.

hypertension, IUGR, premature rupture of membranes, irregular or absent FHR, or absence of fetal movements after quickening). (For a discussion of electronic fetal monitoring, see Chapter 16; for other monitoring techniques of the fetus at risk, see Chapter 27).

Careful, precise, and concise recording of client responses and laboratory results contribute to the continuous supervision vital to the mother and fetus.

NURSING DIAGNOSES

Each individual is affected differently by pregnancy. Careful monitoring of the pregnancy and responses to care are of utmost importance. It is particularly difficult to distinguish discomforts of the second and third trimesters. Women who have given birth before tend to demonstrate some discomforts in pregnancy earlier than first-time mothers do. Continuous assessment, analysis, and formulation of diagnosis are imperative. Common nursing diagnoses during the second trimester may include the following:

- Body image disturbance related to
  —Anatomic and physiologic changes of pregnancy
- Alteration in health maintenance related to knowledge deficit regarding self-care measures
  —Rest and relaxation
  —Personal hygiene (increased sweating, oily skin, leukorrhea)
- Pain related to
  —Discomforts of pregnancy

- High risk for injury related to
  - —Nonuse of safety harness and head rest in automobiles
  - —Exposure to harmful chemicals
- Altered family processes related to
  - —Lack of understanding of second trimester changes
  - —Changing sexual relationship or marital support
- Anxiety related to
  - —Discomforts of pregnancy
  - —Changing family dynamics
  - —Fetal well-being

PLANNING

Planning care for clients during the second trimester of pregnancy is guided by the nursing diagnosis. To the extent possible, the client participates in developing an individualized plan that relates specifically to her needs. The information in this chapter is general; not all women will experience all problems discussed or require all facets of care described. Goals are similar to those for the first trimester.

GOALS RELATED TO PHYSIOLOGIC CARE

1. Woman's EDD is confirmed.
2. Woman and her family have pertinent information about maternal adaptations and fetal development as a basis for understanding the management of care during the second trimester.
3. Woman will have information for self-care.
4. Client's risk factors are identified, and referral for further evaluation or therapy, if indicated, is initiated promptly.
5. Client is alerted to symptoms that indicate deviations from normal progress and protocols for reporting them.

GOALS RELATED TO PSYCHOSOCIAL CARE

1. Client's information needs/readiness for learning are identified.
2. Women and their families are active participants in their care during the second trimester of pregnancy.
3. Client continues to develop a birth plan.
4. Client's trusting relationship continues to progress.

IMPLEMENTATION

The supportive and therapeutic nurse-client relationship grows as the nurse implements the nursing process during the second trimester. The nausea often experienced in the first trimester has resolved. Nutrition counseling is offered at each visit, and the woman is complimented on her progress, as appropriate.

Women experience several new discomforts or changes as maternal adaptations continue in the second trimester. Clear separation of discomforts and changes by trimester is impossible. (See pp. 284 and 326 if a discomfort or change is not found in Table 12-1.)

Counseling about sexuality and exposure to alcohol, cigarette smoke, and other substances is provided as necessary (see Chapter 11). It must be remembered that, although the consumption of three alcoholic drinks a day during the first trimester is associated with spontaneous abortion, only two drinks a day are associated with miscarriage during the second trimester (Cook, 1990). (For nursing care related to substance abuse, see Chapter 33.)

Women who are prepared for the possibility of experiencing emotional changes are more likely to feel reassured that they are not unusual or unnatural and that it is acceptable to talk about their reactions. As pregnancy progresses, women become more open about their feelings toward themselves and others. Active listening by the nurse can help reassure women. If psychologic disturbance is severe, referral for appropriate treatment may be necessary (see Chapter 33).

CLOTHING. Comfortable, loose clothing is best. Washable fabrics (e.g., absorbent cottons) are often preferred. Because maternity clothes are expensive and rarely wear out, hand-me-downs or clothing from garage sales can suffice. Tight brassieres and belts, stretch pants, garters, tight-top knee socks, panty girdles, and other constrictive clothing should be avoided. Tight clothing over the perineum encourages vaginitis and miliaria (heat rash). Impaired circulation in the legs can cause varices.

A well-fitted *maternity* girdle, frequently readjusted, may be used for backache by obese women or those with a multifetal pregnancy. The woman should be cautioned to begin fastening the girdle from the pubic symphysis upward to support the uterus from below. An old, even large, girdle meant for the nonpregnant woman is unsuitable during pregnancy because it pushes the abdomen (uterus) inward. A nonmaternity girdle also may aggravate backache and leg ache.

Maternity brassieres are constructed to accommodate the increased breast weight, chest circumference, and size of breast tail tissue (under the arm).

TABLE 12–1 Discomforts/Concerns Related to Maternal Adaptations to Pregnancy*

Discomfort	Physiology	Teaching for Self-Care
Pigmentation deepens, acne, oily skin	Melanocyte-stimulating hormone (from anterior pituitary)	Not preventable; usually resolved during puerperium; reassurance given to women and their families
Spider nevi (telangiectasias)—appear during trimesters 2 or 3 over neck, thorax, face, and arms	Focal networks of dilated arterioles (end-arteries) from increased concentration of estrogens	Not preventable; reassurance that they fade slowly during late puerperium; rarely disappear completely
Palmar erythema occurs in 50% of pregnant women; may accompany spider nevi	Diffuse reddish mottling over palms and suffused skin over thenar eminences and fingertips may be caused by genetic predisposition or hyperestrogenism	Not preventable; reassurance that condition will fade within 1 week after giving birth
Pruritus (noninflammatory)	Unknown cause; various types as follows:	Keep fingernails short and clean; refer to physician for diagnosis of cause
	Nonpapular; closely aggregated pruritic papules	Not preventable; symptomatic: Keri baths; mild sedation
	Increased excretory function of skin and stretching of skin possible factors	Distraction; tepid baths with sodium bicarbonate or oatmeal added to water; lotions and oils; change of soaps or reduction in use of soap; loose clothing
Palpitations	Unknown; should not be accompanied by persistent cardiac irregularity	Not preventable; reassurance; refer to physician if accompanied by symptoms of cardiac decompensation
Supine hypotension (aorto-vena cava syndrome) and bradycardia (also see Emergency Box, Chapter 11)	Posture induced by pressure of gravid uterus on ascending vena cava when woman is supine; reduces uterine-placental and renal perfusion	Side-lying position or semisitting posture, with knees slightly flexed (see supine hypotension, Chapter 11)
Faintness and, rarely, syncope (orthostatic hypotension); may persist throughout pregnancy	Vasomotor lability or postural hypotension from hormones; in late pregnancy may be caused by venous stasis in lower extremities	Moderate exercise, deep breathing, vigorous leg movements; avoid sudden changes in position† and warm crowded areas; move slowly and deliberately; keep environment cool; avoid hypoglycemia by eating 5 to 6 small meals per day; elastic hose; sit as necessary; if symptoms are serious, refer to physician
Food cravings (see Chapter 9)	Cause unknown; cravings determined by culture or geographic area	Not preventable; satisfy craving unless it interferes with well-balanced diet; report unusual cravings to physician
Heartburn (pyrosis, or acid indigestion): burning sensation in lower portion of chest or upper part of abdomen, occasionally with burping and raising of a little sour-tasting fluid	Progesterone slows GI tract motility and digestion, reverses peristalsis, relaxes cardiac sphincter, and delays emptying time of stomach; stomach displaced upward and compressed by enlarging uterus	Limit or avoid gas-producing or fatty foods and large meals; maintain good posture; sips of milk for temporary relief; hot tea, chewing gum; physician may prescribe antacid between meals, refer to physician for persistent symptoms

GI, Gastrointestinal.

*Review chapter 8 for more extensive discussion of anatomy and physiology of pregnancy.

†Caution woman to rise slowly, to sit on edge of bed or to assume hands-and-knees posture before rising, and to get up slowly after sitting or squatting.

Continued.

TABLE 12-1 Discomforts/Concerns Related to Maternal Adaptations to Pregnancy—cont'd

Discomfort	Physiology	Teaching for Self Care
Constipation—occurs in about 50% of all pregnant women	GI tract motility slowed because of progesterone, resulting in increased resorption of water and drying of stool; intestines compressed by enlarging uterus; predisposition to constipation because of oral iron supplementation	Six glasses of water per day; roughage in diet; moderate exercise; regular schedule for bowel movements; use relaxation techniques and deep breathing; do *not* take stool softener, laxatives, other drugs, or enemas without first consulting physician; *never* ingest mineral oil
Flatulence with bloating and belching	Reduced GI motility because of hormones, allowing time for bacterial action that produces gas; swallowing air	Chew foods slowly and thoroughly; avoid gas-producing foods, fatty foods, large meals; exercise; regular bowel habits
Varicose veins, may be associated with aching legs and tenderness; may be present in legs and vulva; **hemorrhoids** are **varicosities** in the perianal area (Fig. 12-3)	Hereditary predisposition; relaxation of smooth muscle walls of veins because of hormones, causing pelvic vasocongestion; condition aggravated by enlarging uterus, gravity, and bearing down for bowel movements; thrombi from leg varices rare but may be produced by hemorrhoids	Avoidance of obesity, lengthy standing or sitting, constrictive clothing, and constipation and bearing down with bowel movements; moderate exercises; rest with legs and hips elevated (Fig. 12-4); support stockings; thrombosed hemorrhoid may be evacuated; relieve swelling and pain with warm sitz baths, local application of astringent compresses
Headaches (through week 26)	Emotional tension (more common than vascular migraine headache); eye strain (refractory errors); vascular engorgement and congestion of sinuses from hormone stimulation	Emotional support; prenatal teaching; conscious relaxation; refer to physician for constant "splitting" headache after assessing for hypertension
Carpal tunnel syndrome (involves thumb, second and third fingers, lateral side of little finger)	Compression of median nerve from changes in surrounding tissues: pain, numbness, tingling, burning, loss of skilled movements (typing); dropping of objects	Not preventable; elevation of affected arms, splinting of affected hand may help; surgery is curative but has a 1% risk of sympathetic syndrome
Periodic numbness, tingling of fingers (acrodysesthesia); occurs in 5% of pregnant women	Brachial plexus traction syndrome from drooping of shoulders during pregnancy (occurs especially at night and early morning)	Maintain good posture; wear supportive maternity brassiere; reassurance that condition will disappear if lifting and carrying baby does not aggravate it
Round ligament pain (tenderness)	Stretching of ligament caused by enlarging uterus	Not preventable; reassurance, rest, good body mechanics to avoid overstretching ligament; relieve cramping by squatting or bringing knees to chest
Joint pain, backache, and pelvic pressure; hypermobility of joints	Relaxation of symphyseal and sacroiliac joints because of hormones, resulting in unstable pelvis; exaggerated lumbar and cervicothoracic curves caused by change in center of gravity from enlarging abdomen	Maternity girdle; good posture and body mechanics; avoid fatigue; wear low-heeled shoes; conscious relaxation; firm mattress; local heat and back rubs; pelvic rock exercise; rest; reassurance that condition will disappear 6 to 8 weeks after delivery.

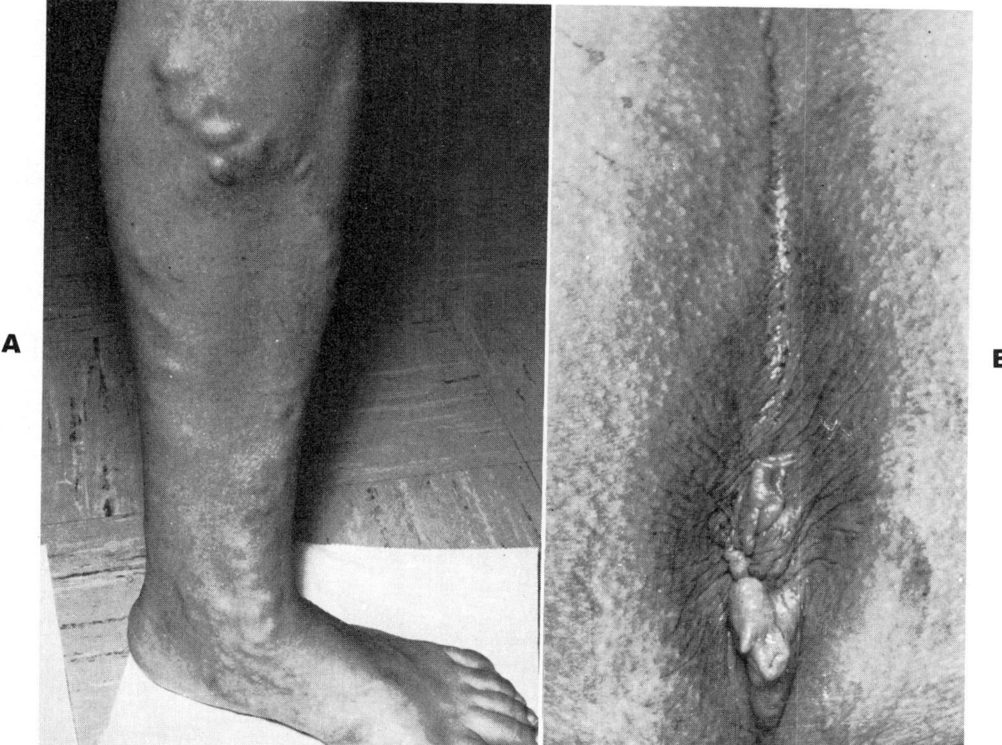

Fig. 12-3 **A,** Varicose veins of lower extremity. **B,** Varicosities of rectal area (hemorrhoids).
Courtesy Mercy Hospital and Medical Center, San Diego, Calif.

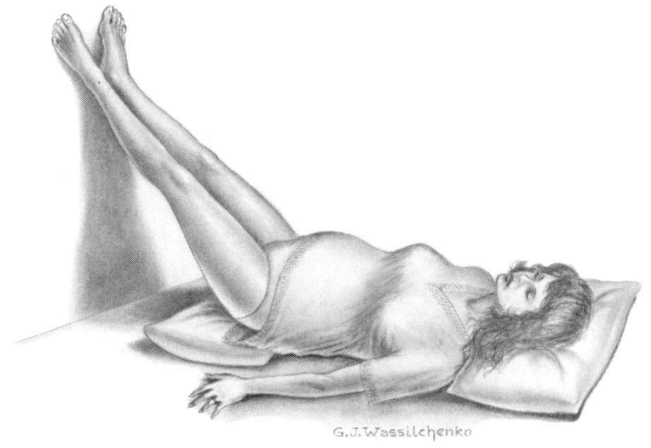

Fig. 12-4 Position for resting legs and reducing swelling, edema, and varicosities. Encourage woman with vulvar varicosities to place pillow under her hips.

These brassieres have drop-flaps over the nipples to facilitate breast-feeding. A good brassiere can help prevent neckache and backache.

Elastic hose or *maternity* leotards may give considerable comfort to women with large varicose veins or swelling of the legs. Comfortable shoes that provide firm support and promote good posture and balance are advisable. Very high heels and platform shoes are not recommended because of the woman's changed center of gravity. She has a tendency to lose her balance. In the third trimester her pelvis tilts forward and her lumbar curve increases. Leg aches and leg cramps (p. 326) are aggravated by nonsupportive shoes.

POSTURE AND BODY MECHANICS. Many maternal adaptations predispose the woman to backache and possible injury. The pregnant woman's center of gravity changes (Fig. 12-5). Pelvic joints soften and relax (see extensive discussion of connective tissue laxity on p. 205). Stress is placed on abdominal musculature (see Figs. 8-10 and 8-13). Poor posture and **body mechanics** contribute to discomfort and potential for injury.

Women can acquire a kinesthetic sense for good body posture. In addition to fostering good posture, the following activities can be used (see box on p. 309).

BATHING AND SWIMMING. Tub bathing is permitted even in late pregnancy because water does not enter the vagina unless under pressure. However, tub bathing is contraindicated after rupture of the membranes. Baths and warm showers can be thera-

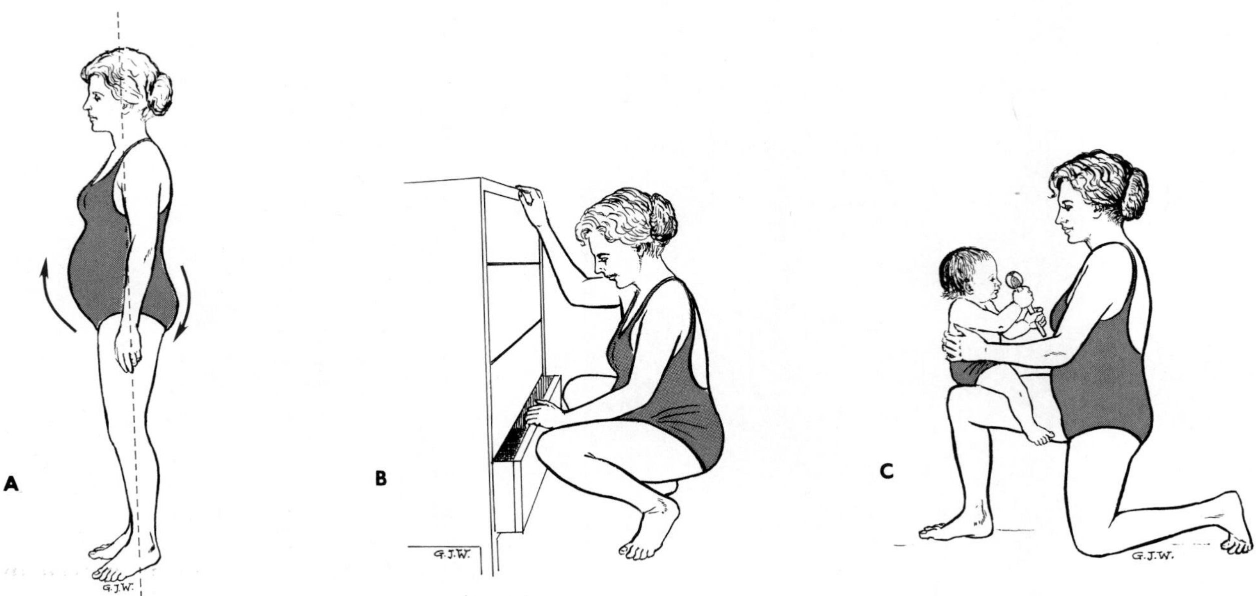

Fig. 12-5 Correct body mechanics. **A**, Standing. **B**, Stooping. **C**, Lifting.

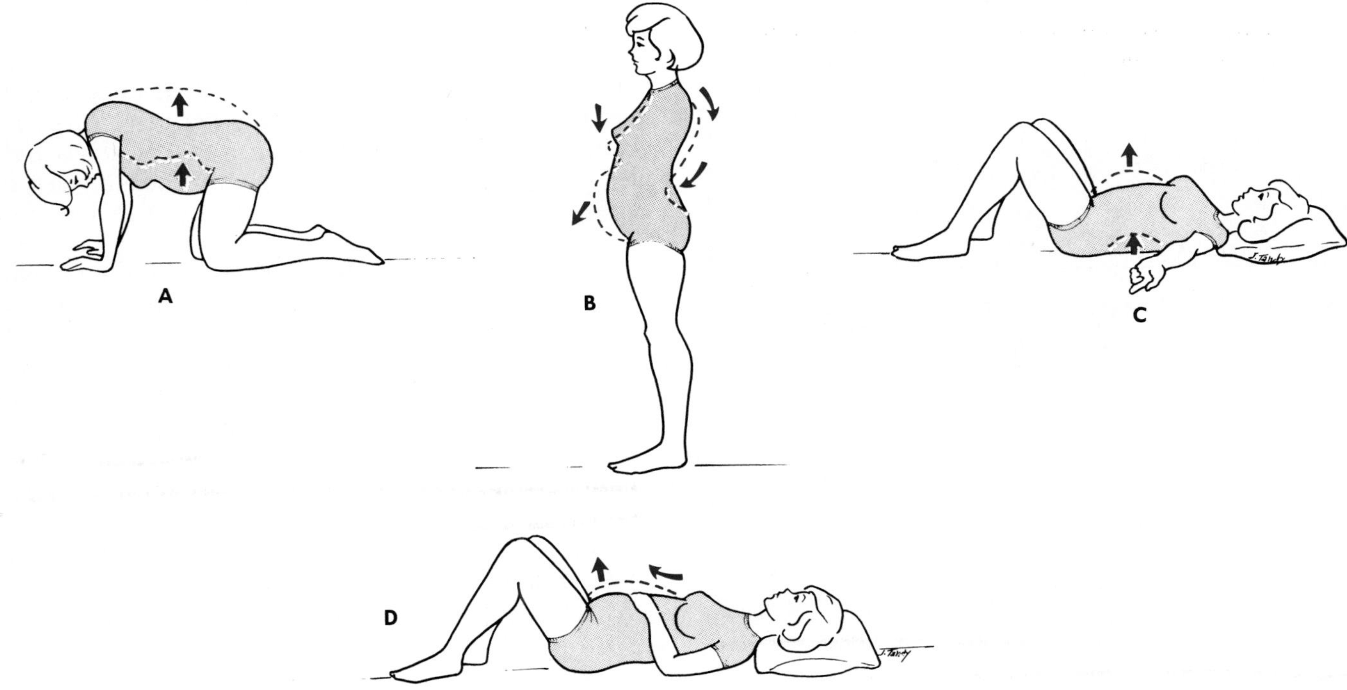

Fig. 12-6 Exercises. **A-C**, Pelvic rocking relieves low backache (excellent for relief of menstrual cramps as well). **D**, Abdominal breathing aids relaxation and lifts abdominal wall off uterus.

TEACHING Posture and Body Mechanics

To *prevent or relieve backache*
- Do pelvic tilt:
  — **Pelvic tilt (rock)** on hands and knees, and while sitting in straight-back chair (Fig. 12-6, *A*).
  —Pelvic tilt (rock) in standing position against a wall, or lying on floor (Fig. 12-6, *B* and *C*).
  —Perform abdominal muscle contractions during pelvic tilt while standing, lying, or sitting to help strengthen rectus abdominis muscle (Fig. 12-6, *D*).
- Use good body mechanics:
  —Use leg muscles to reach objects on or near floor. Bend at the knees, not the back. Knees are bent to lower body to squatting position. Feet are kept 12 to 18 inches apart for a solid base to maintain balance (Fig. 12-6, *B*).
  —Lift with the legs. To lift heavy object (young child), one foot is placed slightly in front of the other and kept flat as woman lowers herself on one knee. She lifts the weight holding it close to her body and never higher than chest high. To stand up or sit down, one leg is placed slightly behind the other as she raises or lowers herself.

To *restrict the lumbar curve:*
- Wear a maternity girdle to support weak abdominal muscles.
- For prolonged standing (e.g., ironing, out-of-home employment), place one foot on low footstool or box; change positions often.
- Move car seat forward so that knees are bent and higher than hips. If needed, use a small pillow to support low back area.
- Sit in chairs low enough to allow both feet on floor and preferably with knees higher than hips.

To *prevent round ligament pain and strain on abdominal muscles*
- Implement suggestions given in Table 12-1.

peutic because they relax tense tired muscles, help counter insomnia, and make the pregnant woman feel fresh. However, physical maneuverability presents a problem (increased chance of falling) late in pregnancy. Swimming is also permitted during normal pregnancy, although diving is discouraged because of possible injury.

PHYSICAL ACTIVITY. Physical activity promotes a feeling of well-being in the pregnant woman. It improves circulation, assists relaxation and rest, and counteracts boredom as it does in the nonpregnant woman. Exercise tips for pregnancy are presented in detail in the box on p. 286. Suggestions for teaching the client Kegel exercises to strengthen the muscles around the reproductive organs and improve muscle tone are found on p. 282.

REST AND RELAXATION. The pregnant woman is encouraged to plan regular rest periods, particularly as pregnancy advances (Fig. 12-7). The side-lying position is recommended to promote uterine perfusion and fetoplacental oxygenation by eliminating pressure on the ascending vena cava and descending aorta (supine hypotension). During shorter rest periods, the woman can assume the position in Fig. 12-4 to promote venous drainage from the legs and relieve **leg edema** and varicose veins. The mother is shown how to rise slowly from a side-lying position to avoid strain on the back and minimize the orthostatic hypotension caused by changes in position common in the latter part of pregnancy. To stretch and rest back muscles at home or at work, the nurse can instruct the woman to perform the following exercises:

Stand behind a chair. Support and balance self using the back of the chair (Fig. 12-8). Squat for

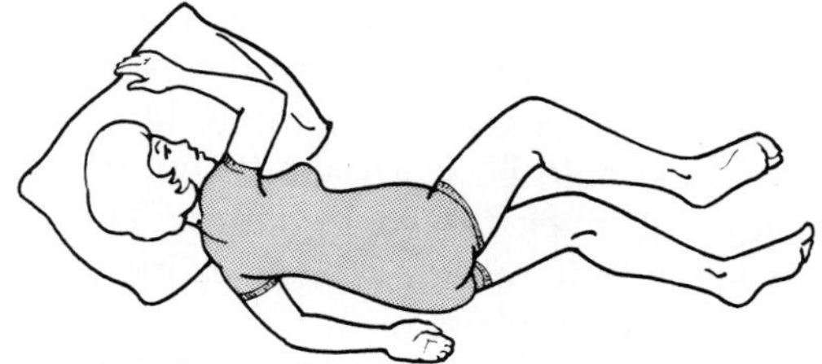

Fig. 12-7 Positions for rest and relaxation. Side-lying position. Some women prefer to support upper part of leg with pillows.

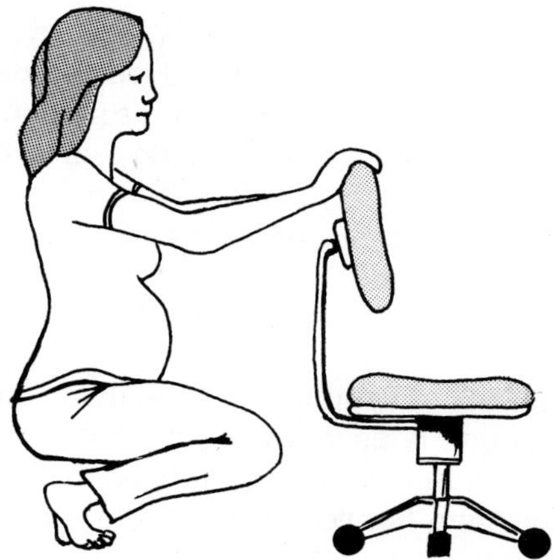

Fig. 12-8 Squatting for muscle relaxation and strengthening and for keeping leg and hip joints flexible.

TEACHING Conscious Relaxation

Preparation: Loosen clothing, assume a comfortable sitting or side-lying position with all parts of body well-supported with pillows.
Beginning: Allow self to feel warm and comfortable. Inhale and exhale slowly, and imagine peaceful relaxation coming over each part of the body starting with the neck and working down to the toes. Often persons who learn conscious relaxation speak of feeling relaxed even if some discomfort is present.
Maintenance: Imagine (fantasize or daydream) to maintain the state of relaxation. With *active imagery* the person imagines herself as moving or doing some activity and experiencing its sensations. With *passive imagery,* one imagines watching a scene, such as a lovely sunset.
Awakening: Return to the wakeful state gradually. Slowly begin to take in the stimuli from the surrounding environment.
Further retention and development of the skill: Practice regularly for some periods of time each day, for example, at the same hour for 10 to 15 minutes each day to feel refreshed, revitalized, and invigorated.

30 seconds; stand for 15 seconds. Repeat six times, several times per day, as needed.
While sitting in the chair, lower head to knees for 30 seconds. Raise up. Repeat six times, several times per day, as needed.

Relaxation is the release of the mind and body from tension through conscious effort and practice. The ability to relax consciously and intentionally can be beneficial for the following reasons:

Relief of normal discomforts related to pregnancy
Reduction of stress and therefore diminished pain perception during the childbearing cycle
Heightened self-awareness and trust in own ability to control one's responses and functions
Coping with stress in everyday life situations, pregnant or not

The techniques for **conscious relaxation** are numerous and varied. The guidelines given in the teaching box (above) can be used by anyone.

EMPLOYMENT. Continued assessment during the prenatal period is necessary to determine if working is causing undue fatigue or stress. With a recommendation from her physician, it may be possible for the woman to change the type of work she does (Bryant, 1985). Some women may lose interest in work as they become more introverted during the second trimester of pregnancy. This response may be difficult to accept for the woman who has always been competent and independent before pregnancy.

Activities that depend on a good sense of balance should be discouraged, especially during the last half of pregnancy. Commonly, excessive fatigue is the deciding factor in the termination of employment. Women in sedentary jobs need to walk around at intervals and should neither sit nor stand in one position for long periods. Crossing the legs at the knees should be avoided. Activity is necessary to counter the usual sluggish circulation in the legs that causes a predisposition to varices and thrombophlebitis. The pregnant woman's chair should provide adequate back support. A footstool can prevent pressure on veins, relieve strain on varices, and minimize swelling of feet. Work breaks are best spent resting in the left lateral side-lying position. It is recommended that employers have an area where women can lie down. Standards for maternity care and employment of mothers in industry have been recommended by the United States Children's Bureau to safeguard the interests of expectant mothers employed in industry.

TRAVEL. If the woman must travel for long distances, she should schedule periods of activity and rest. While sitting, the woman can practice deep breathing, foot circling, and alternating contracting and relaxing different muscle groups. Fatigue should be avoided.

Although travel in itself is not a cause of either abortion or preterm labor, certain precautions are recommended. A woman who does not wear automobile restraints risks injury to herself and her fetus (Krozy et al, 1985). Some women do not use automobile restraints (see Research Highlight, p. 311). Maternal death as a result of injury is the most common cause of fetal death (Crosby, 1983). The next most common cause is placental separation. Body contours change in reaction to the force of a collision. The uterus as a muscular organ can adapt its shape to that of the body. The placenta lacks the resiliency to change, and placental separation can occur (Crosby, 1983). A combination lap belt and shoulder harness is the most effective automobile restraint (Fig. 12-9) (Chang, 1985). Both shoulder and lap belts should be used. The lap belt should be worn low across the pelvic bones and as snug as is comfortable. The shoulder harness should be worn above the gravid uterus and below the neck to avoid chafing. The pregnant woman should sit upright. The headrest should be used to avoid a whiplash injury.

In high-altitude regions, lowered oxygen levels may cause fetal hypoxia, especially if the pregnant woman is anemic (Barry, Bia, 1989). Women who travel extensively expose themselves to the risk of serious accident and may find themselves far removed

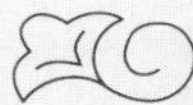 **Research Highlight** 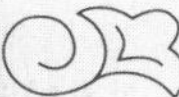

Use of Seat Belts during Pregnancy

RESEARCH ABSTRACT

All pregnant women receiving prenatal care at Wilford Hall U.S. Air Force Medical Center were eligible for participation in a study to evaluate seat belt use by pregnant women. Almost 1200 surveys were distributed, and 725 women completed the survey. The researchers placed a two-page questionnaire in the obstetric record. The women participating in the study completed and turned in the forms as they waited to be seen at their scheduled appointments. The questionnaire was designed by the investigators and consisted of 12 questions. The researchers found that 88% of the women surveyed used seat belts 100% of the time when they were driving, and 90% of the women used seat belts 100% of the time when they were passengers. In addition, 22% of the women asked passengers to use seat belts. Only 42% had been spoken to by an obstetric care provider about the advisability and proper technique for wearing seat belts during pregnancy. Of those who used seat belts, 22% used them incorrectly. Some of the women (14%) believed that wearing a seat belt would increase the risk of injuring the fetus.

IMPLICATIONS FOR PRACTICE

Although the majority of these women used seat belts, a significant proportion used them improperly or thought the fetus was more likely to be injured with their use. Health care providers should routinely include information about the proper use of seat belts in their prenatal teaching and counseling.

RELATED RESEARCH QUESTIONS

1. Will an educational program increase the proportion of health care providers who routinely teach pregnant women about proper use of seat belts?
2. Will an educational program increase the proportion of pregnant women who use seat belts properly?
3. Do women routinely "buckle up" their children?
4. Does the rate of seat belt use differ between men and women?

REFERENCE

Hammond TL et al: The use of automobile safety restraint systems during pregnancy, *JOGNN* 19:339, 1990.

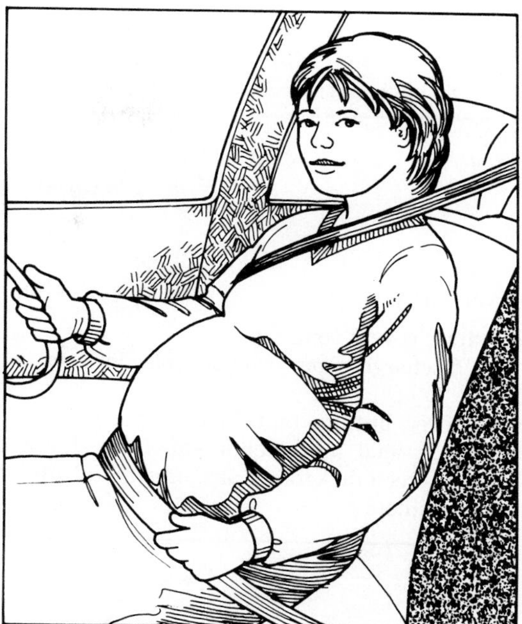

Fig. 12-9 Proper use of seat belt and head rest.

TEACHING Safety during Pregnancy

Maternal adaptations to pregnancy involve relaxation of joints, alteration to center of gravity, faintness, and discomforts. Problems with coordination and balance are common. Therefore the woman should follow these guidelines:

- Use good body mechanics.
- Use safety features on tools/vehicles; safety seat belts, shoulder harnesses, and head rests, goggles, helmets, as specified.
- Avoid activities requiring coordination, balance, and concentration.
- Take rest periods, reschedule daily activities to meet rest and relaxation needs.

Embryonic and fetal development is vulnerable to environmental teratogens. Many potentially dangerous chemicals are present in the home, yard, and workplace: cleaning agents, paints, sprays, herbicides, and pesticides. The soil and water supply may be unsafe. Therefore the woman should follow these guidelines:

- Read all labels for ingredients and proper use of product.
- Ensure adequate ventilation with "clean" air.
- Dispose of wastes appropriately.
- Wear gloves when handling chemicals.
- Change job assignments or workplace as necessary.
- Avoid high altitudes (not in pressurized aircraft), which could jeopardize oxygen intake.

Warning Signs—Second Trimester

SIGN/SYMPTOM	POSSIBLE CAUSE
Persistent, severe vomiting	Hyperemesis gravidarum
Fluid discharge from vagina—bleeding or amniotic fluid	Premature rupture of membranes (PROM); miscarriage
Chills, fever, burning on urination, diarrhea	Infection
Change in fetal movements—absence of fetal movements after quickening, any unusual change in pattern or amount	Fetal jeopardy or intrauterine fetal death

Fig. 12-10 Summary of fetal development and maternal events.
From *Safe passage: a woman's guide to a healthier pregnancy*, McNeil Consumer Products Co., Fort Washington, Penn.

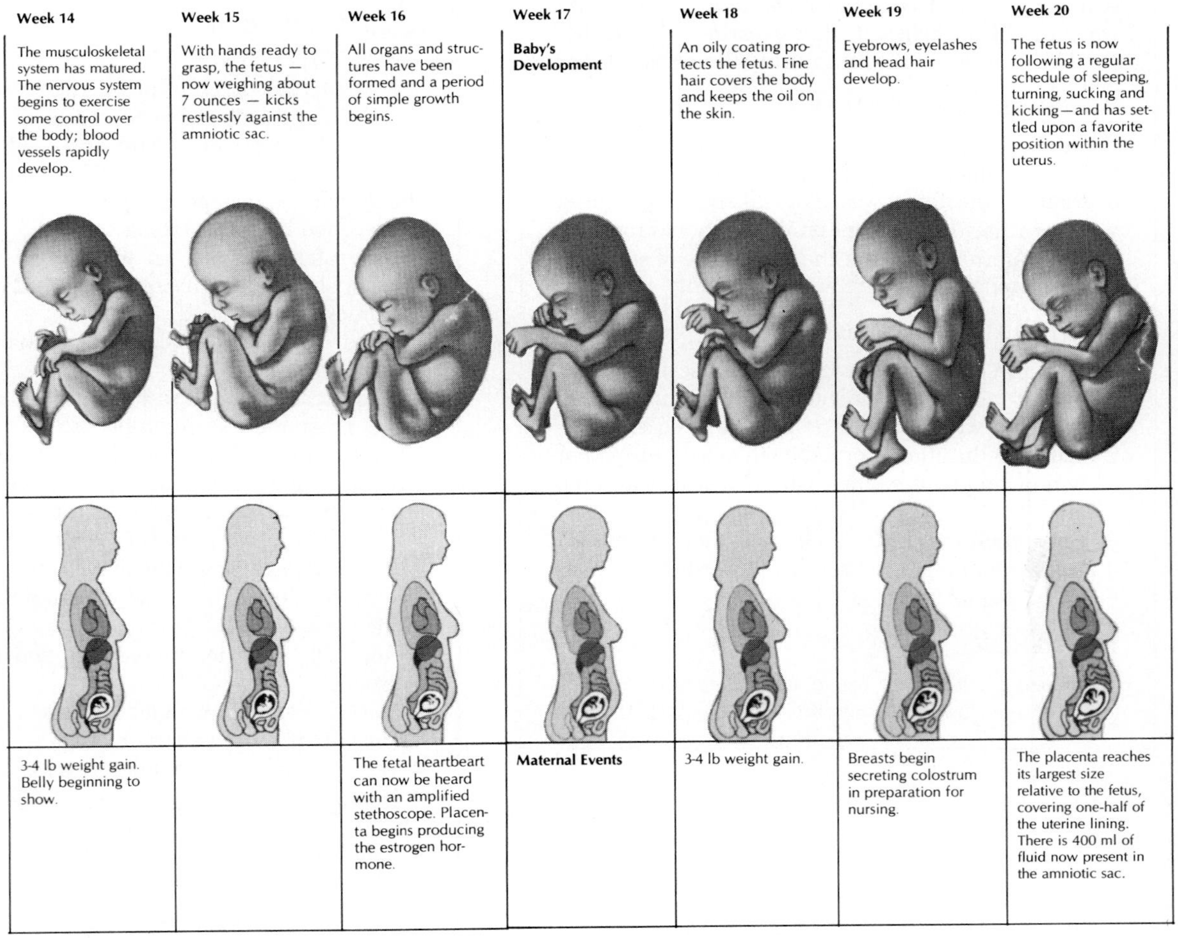

	Week 14	Week 15	Week 16	Week 17	Week 18	Week 19	Week 20
Baby's Development	The musculoskeletal system has matured. The nervous system begins to exercise some control over the body; blood vessels rapidly develop.	With hands ready to grasp, the fetus — now weighing about 7 ounces — kicks restlessly against the amniotic sac.	All organs and structures have been formed and a period of simple growth begins.		An oily coating protects the fetus. Fine hair covers the body and keeps the oil on the skin.	Eyebrows, eyelashes and head hair develop.	The fetus is now following a regular schedule of sleeping, turning, sucking and kicking—and has settled upon a favorite position within the uterus.
Maternal Events	3-4 lb weight gain. Belly beginning to show.		The fetal heartbeart can now be heard with an amplified stethoscope. Placenta begins producing the estrogen hormone.		3-4 lb weight gain.	Breasts begin secreting colostrum in preparation for nursing.	The placenta reaches its largest size relative to the fetus, covering one-half of the uterine lining. There is 400 ml of fluid now present in the amniotic sac.

from good perinatal care. In addition, fatigue or tension, as well as altered regular personal habits and diet during arduous travel, may be detrimental.

If long-distance travel is necessary, the trip should be made by air. Perhaps fortuitously, U.S. flight regulations do not permit pregnant women aboard during the last month without a statement from an obstetrician. Most foreign airlines have a cutoff of 35 weeks' gestation. Many health insurance carriers do not cover delivery in a foreign setting or even hospitalization for preterm labor (Barry, Bia, 1989). Air travel itself carries little risk. Magnetometers (metal detectors) used at airport security checkpoints are not harmful to the fetus. The 8% humidity at which cabins are maintained in commercial airlines may result in some water loss; hydration (with *water*) should be maintained under these conditions (Barry, Bia, 1989). Sitting in a cramped seat of an airliner for prolonged periods may increase the risk of superficial and deep thrombophlebitis. A 15-minute walk around the aircraft for every hour of travel is recommended to minimize this risk. A seat in the nonsmoking section of flights where smoking is permitted is advised to prevent elevated carboxyhemoglobin levels.

Many women experience a sense of uneasiness when traveling by any vehicle. They describe feelings of fear for the safety of their unborn baby (see the box on p. 311).

WARNING SIGNS/SYMPTOMS. The nurse can reinforce teaching about warning signs and symptoms by inquiring about them at each visit (see box, p. 312). A printed list to place by the telephone, along with the telephone number to call, is helpful for quick referral. The woman is reminded about how to describe what is happening, for example, "I can't keep anything down" or "I lost a teaspoonful of blood."

PARENT EDUCATION CLASSES. Parent education classes are available in some communities to meet the needs of parents in the second trimester of preg-

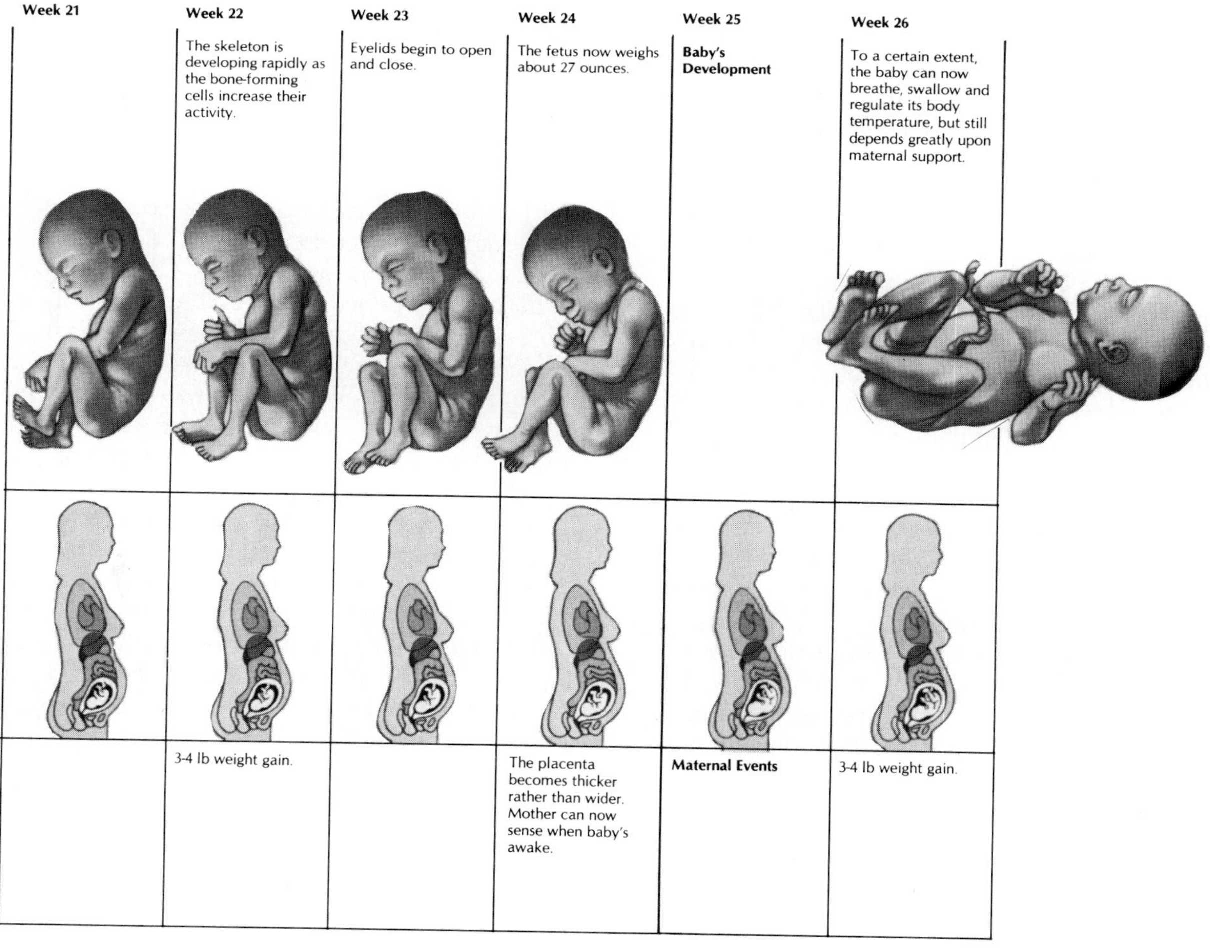
Week 21
Week 22
The skeleton is developing rapidly as the bone-forming cells increase their activity.
Week 23
Eyelids begin to open and close.
Week 24
The fetus now weighs about 27 ounces.
Week 25
Baby's Development
Week 26
To a certain extent, the baby can now breathe, swallow and regulate its body temperature, but still depends greatly upon maternal support.
3-4 lb weight gain.
The placenta becomes thicker rather than wider. Mother can now sense when baby's awake.
Maternal Events
3-4 lb weight gain.

nancy. Second-trimester classes emphasize the woman's participation in self-care. Classes provide information on (1) preparation for breast and formula feeding, (2) basic hygiene, (3) common complaints and simple, safe remedies, (4) continued fetal development, (5) infant health, (6) parenting, and (7) updating and refining the birth plan. Discussion of concerns may touch on topics such as birth choices: labor and birth positions; labor, delivery, recovery, postpartum (LDRP) rooms; medications to stimulate labor; and episiotomy. More extensive discussion on these topics usually occurs in the third-trimester classes when labor and birth are closer. Support systems that expectant parents can use are discussed. Open discussion of feelings and concerns is encouraged. If the expectant parents have not yet begun to think about a birth plan, they are encouraged to do so now.

BIRTH PLAN. During the second trimester, the nurse can answer questions and discuss concerns that arose in the process of formulating a birth plan. The clients need to be reminded that no birth plan can be guaranteed, and alternative plans need to be suggested. That is, what if a cesarean birth is necessary? Does the woman wish to be awake or not, does she wish her partner to be present, and if awake, does she want to hold the baby immediately (if the baby's and mother's conditions warrant it)? Alternative plans serve to reduce disappointment.

Although most pregnant women are more introspective (focused inward) during this time, the nurse can initiate considerations of after-birth events:

- *Immediately after birth* Did you want to hold the baby right away? To breast-feed immediately?
- *Newborn care* What about eye treatment, vitamin K injection, circumcision, for your baby? How will baby be fed—breast, formula, glucose water between feeding, feeding "on demand"?
- *Postpartum care* What kind of care do you anticipate—LDRP, mother-baby coupling, "request" coupling (newborn cared for in nursery while mother rests)? How long do you plan to stay—6 hours, 2 to 3 days? Would you like self-care classes or videotapes? On which subjects?

If older siblings are to be included in the labor and birth process, the possibility needs to be reviewed and cleared with the physician or nurse midwife, as well as the staff at the birth setting. This is done long before the EDD to avoid the stress of this type of negotiation during labor. The client needs to be cautioned that some staff members may be unwilling to participate. The client needs to specify who will be responsible for the sibling during labor and birth because hospital personnel are not available for that purpose.

EVALUATION

Continuous evaluation of effectiveness of interventions is essential to the management of the pregnant woman and her family's care during the second trimester of pregnancy. Evaluation is based on the degree to which goals are met.

- The EDD has been confirmed
- The pregnant woman and her family have verbalized understanding of maternal physical and psychologic adaptations and fetal development
- Any risk factors are identified and referred for further evaluation or therapy
- Any questions or concerns of the woman and her family have been addressed.
- To their desired degree, the woman and her family are active participants in prenatal care during the second trimester.

SUMMARY

Monthly prenatal visits during the second trimester are designed to monitor the individual woman's pregnancy and responses to care. Careful assessment during this period provides the basis for preventive care. A heightened readiness for learning is experienced by the pregnant woman and her family. Counseling for self-care, fetal growth and development, and diagnostic tests is offered. Assessment findings of maternal and fetal physical well-being are evaluated for potential complications. (Fetal development and maternal events are summarized in Fig. 12-10 on p 312.) The pregnant woman and her family are alerted to warning signs that need immediate medical attention. Standards for maternity care and employment are shared with expectant parents. During this time, the relationship between the health care team and the expectant parents progresses and the parents-to-be develop in their roles as active participants in their health care.

REFERENCES

Barry M, Bia F: Pregnancy and travel, *JAMA* 261:728, 1989.

Bryant H: Antenatal counseling for women working outside the homes, *Birth* 12:4, Winter 1985.

Chang A: Auto safety in pregnancy, a neglected area, *Contemp OB/GYN* 25(4):117, 1985.

Cohen A: Movement as a yardstick for fetal well-being, *Contemp OB/GYN* 26:61, Aug 1985.

Cook PS, Petersen RC, Moore DT: *Alcohol, tobacco, and other drugs may harm the unborn,* US Department of Health and Human Services Pub No (ADM)90-1711, Rockville, Md, 1990, Office for Substance Abuse Prevention.

Crosby WM: Traumatic injuries during pregnancy, *Clin Obstet Gynecol* 26:902, 1983.

Engstrom JL: Measurement of fundal height, *JOGNN* 17:172, May/June 1988.

Krozy RE et al: Auto safety, pregnancy and the newborn, *JOGNN* 14:1, Jan/Feb 1985.

Page EW, Villee CA, Villee DB: *Human Reproduction: essentials of reproductive and perinatal medicine,* ed 3, Philadelphia, 1981, WB Saunders.

Stevens KA: Nursing diagnosis in wellness childbearing settings, *JOGNN* 17:329, Sept/Oct 1988.

BIBLIOGRAPHY

Berry L: Realistic expectations of the labor coach (a study of 40 expectant fathers), *JOGNN* 17:354, Sept/Oct 1988.

Bentz JM: Missed meanings in nurse/patient communication, *MCN* 5:55, Jan/Feb 1980.

Chez RA: Why it's important to help patients prepare for pregnancy, *Contemp OB/GYN* 33:64, June 1989.

Commentary: Preconception care: risk reduction and health promotion in preparation for pregnancy, *JAMA* 264:1147, 1990.

Cunningham FG, MacDonald RC, Gant NF: *Williams obstetrics,* ed 18, Norwalk Conn, 1989, Appleton & Lange.

Fast A et al: Low-back pain in pregnancy, *Spine* 12:368, 1987.

Gerlach C, Schmid M: Second-skill educational development of personnel for a single-room maternity care system, *JOGNN* 17:388, Nov/Dec 1988.

Goldsmith MF: Pregnancy Dx? Rx may now include condoms, *JAMA* 261:678, 1989.

Hammond TL et al: The use of automobile safety restraint systems during pregnancy, JOGNN 19:339, July/Aug 1990.

Hart JL: Low back pain, radiculopathies, and pregnancy, *Pain Management,* p 103, March/April 1990.

Helton AS: A buddy system to improve prenatal care, *MCN* 15:234, July/Aug, 1990.

Kulin J: Childbearing Cambodian refugee women, *Can Nurs* p 46, June 1988.

Lee RV: Understanding Southeast Asian mothers-to-be, *Childbirth Educ* 8:32, Spring 1989.

Lee RV et al: Southeast Asian folklore about pregnancy and parturition, *Obstet Gynecol* 71:243, 1988.

Leviton A: Caffeine consumption and the risk of reproductive hazards, *J Reprod Med* 33:175, 1988.

Lewallen LP: Health beliefs and health practices of pregnant women, JOGNN 18:245, May/June 1989.

Lindell SG: Education for childbirth: a time for change, *JOGNN* 17:108, March/Arpil 1988.

Malasanos L et al: *Health assessment,* ed 4, St Louis, 1990, Mosby–Year Book.

Increasing culturally relevant practice with Hispanic clients, *NPA Bull* 3:23, Nov/Dec 1988.

Patterson ET, Freese MP, Goldenberg RL: Seeking safe passage: utilizing health care during pregnancy, *Image J Nurs Sch* 22:27, Spring 1990.

Peterson C: Husbands' and wives' perception of marital fairness across the family life cycle, *Int J Aging Human Dev,* 31(3):179.

Redman BK: *The process of patient education,* ed 6, St Louis, 1988, Mosby–Year Book.

Rosen MG: Preconception care: why it is necessary, *Female Patient* 15:73, May 1990.

Rossavik IK, Fishburne JI: Conceptional age, menstrual age, and ultrasound age: a second-trimester comparison of pregnancies of known conception date with pregnancies dated from the last menstrual period, *Obstet Gynecol* 73:1989.

Scott JR et al: Obstetrics and gynecology, ed 6, Philadelphia, 1990, JB Lippincott.

Seidel HM et al: *Mosby's guide to physical examination,* ed 2, St Louis, 1991, Mosby–Year Book.

Starn J, Niederhauser V: An MCN model for nursing diagnosis to focus intervention, *MCN* 15:180, May/June 1990.

Tucker SM et al: *Patient care standards,* ed 5 St Louis, 1992, Mosby–Year Book.

Watson WJ et al: Fetal responses to maximal swimming and cycling exercise during pregnancy, *Obstet Gynecol* 77:382, 1991.

Bibliography—Nursing Research

Aaronson LS: Perceived and received support: effects on health behavior during pregnancy, *Nurs Res* 38:4, Jan/Feb 1989.

Bliss-Holtz VJ: Primiparas' prenatal concern for learning infant care, *Nurs Res* 37:20, Jan/Feb 1988.

Doering L, Dracup K: Comparisons of cardiac output in supine and lateral positions, *Nurs Res* 37:114, March/April 1988.

Heidrich SM, Cranley MS: Effect of fetal movement, ultrasound scans, and amniocentesis on maternal-fetal attachment, *Nurs Res* 38:81, March/April 1989.

CASE STUDY

Carpal Tunnel Syndrome, Constipation, and Varicose Veins

Ruth Piper, a 36-year old married woman pregnant for the first time, is now at 22 weeks, gestation. She has continued to work as an office manager. She and her husband have attended a second-trimester parent education class and are developing a birth plan.

ASSESSMENT

All health assessment findings of Ruth and her fetus are within normal limits. At work, Ruth divides her time between standing at a counter and sitting in front of a computer. Within the last 2 weeks, she has noted pain, numbness, tingling and burning, some loss of ability to type, and increased tendency to drop objects involving her right (dominant) hand. The physician has diagnosed carpal tunnel syndrome. In addition, she stated she is distressed by constipation, hemorrhoids, and the appearance of varicosities in her legs. She denies discomfort in her legs. She has been "very busy" at work and finds it hard to take her breaks, have a full lunch period, and remember to drink water.

NURSING DIAGNOSIS

All of her discomforts are distressing to Ruth. However, the symptoms of carpal tunnel syndrome take priority because they may result in injury if her hand is numb and she drops things. The following nursing diagnosis is chosen: High risk for pain and injury related to symptoms of carpal tunnel syndrome.

PLANNING

Planning of interventions is derived from the medical diagnosis and accepted therapy. The nurse and Ruth mutually agree on the *goal:* Ruth will experience relief from discomfort. The nurse sets the *expected outcome:* Compression of the median nerve will be decreased.

IMPLEMENTATION

The focus of interventions is to relieve compression from surrounding tissue on the median nerve of her right wrist and hand. The nurse reviews with Ruth her understanding of the physician's explanation of the cause and treatment. Ruth is reminded to elevate her right arm on a pillow while sleeping and whenever she can during the day. Ruth is asked to demonstrate the application of the splint. The nurse asks Ruth if there is a way she can decrease the amount of time she spends at the computer.

EVALUATION

Ruth is able to state the cause, the recommended therapies, and their purposes. At the next visit, Ruth states that there is an appreciable decrease in the severity of symptoms and that she is no longer dropping objects.

CARE PLAN Carpal Tunnel Syndrome, Constipation, and Varicose Veins

GOALS	IMPLEMENTATION	RATIONALE	EVALUATION
Nursing diagnosis: High risk for pain and injury related to symptoms of carpal tunnel syndrome.			
Ruth will experience relief from discomfort.	Review with Ruth her understanding of the physician's explanations of cause and therapy.	Allows opportunity to review information for accuracy and reinforce learning.	Ruth states correct information.
	Advise Ruth to elevate right arm on a pillow while sleeping and whenever possible during the day; reduce work at computer; apply splint appropriately and wear as indicated.	Elevation of extremity permits gravity drainage of fluid, thus reducing compression on nerve. Splinting of extremity and reduction in time spent typing reduces trauma from use of hand.	At the next visit, Ruth describes a reduction in discomfort and a relief from dropping of objects.
Nursing diagnosis: Constipation related to inadequate fluids, foods with roughage, exercise, and regular bowel habits			
Ruth's constipation is resolved with return to healthy habits.	Discuss physiology of adaptations.	Knowledge provides basis for compliance with self-care.	Ruth states correct information.
	Assess Ruth's knowledge regarding prevention of constipation; reinforce her knowledge about fluids, foods with roughage, exercise and regular bowel habits.	Ruth possessed the knowledge but needs to implement it: fluids add moisture, roughage adds bulk, roughage and exercise stimulate bowel movement.	At the next visit Ruth states she has returned to her usual healthy habits and is no longer constipated.
	Suggest that Ruth walk more and stand in one place less; keep a container of water at her work station to sip; take her breaks and full lunch period to eat well.	Avoidance of constipation can bring some relief from hemorrhoids (varicosities in perianal area).	
Nursing diagnosis: High risk for alteration in self-concept related to appearance of varicosities			
Ruth will state she feels better regarding the appearance of varicosities and about being able to do something to slow their development.	Explain the hereditary predisposition to and physiology of varicosities.	Knowledge often aids in reducing anxiety and in motivating self-care.	Ruth states she understands information.
Ruth will not experience aching legs and tenderness often associated with moderate to severe varicosities.	Advise regarding ways to avoid aggravating factors: Standing for long periods Wearing tight, constrictive clothing, e.g., nonmaternity stretch pants, garters, tight-top knee socks or hose. Crossing the legs at the knees	These activities impair circulation to legs as uterus enlarges and gets heavier.	Ruth states she gets most relief from postural drainage, wearing loose clothing and elastic hose.
	Advise regarding positional drainage (Fig. 12-4) as often as possible; possible use of maternity girdle and elastic hose.	Position employs gravity to assist venous drainage. Maternity girdle may aid in supporting uterus; elastic hose may prevent venous congestion in legs.	

chapter 12 review

Key Concepts

- Blood pressure is evaluated on the basis of absolute values and length of gestation and interpreted in the light of modifying factors.
- Normal MAPs during the second trimester are <90 mm Hg.
- In the absence of factors that affect accuracy, measurement of fundal height is one screening tool to assess the progress of fetal growth.
- Auscultation of fetal heart tones is another tool for assessing fetal health status.
- Discomforts and changes of pregnancy can cause anxiety in the pregnant woman and her family.
- Education about healthy ways of using the body (e.g., exercise, body mechanics) is essential given maternal anatomic and physiologic responses to pregnancy.
- Appropriate use of auto seat belts with shoulder harness and head rest is essential for the pregnant woman.
- The pregnant woman's readiness to learn is at a high level, making this an excellent time to help her expand her self-care skills.
- Standards for maternity care and employment have been developed by the U.S. Children's Bureau and by Health and Welfare, Canada, family-centered maternity and newborn care national guidelines.

Key Terms

- body mechanics (p. 307)
- carpal tunnel syndrome (p. 306)
- conscious relaxation (p. 310)
- constipation (p. 306)
- fetal gestational age (p. 302)
- fetal health status (p. 302)
- food cravings (p. 305)
- fundal height (p. 301)
- heartburn (p. 305)
- hemorrhoids (p. 306)
- leg edema (p. 309)
- pelvic tilt (rock) (p. 309)
- quickening (p. 302)
- round ligament pain (p. 306)
- second trimester (p. 300)
- varicosities (p. 306)

Critical Thinking Exercises

1. Answer the following questions based on your recorded observations of two contrasting settings; for example, observe a physician's office and a county welfare clinic or a home health nurse or public health nurse involved in prenatal care.
   a. Did the tone and the information provided to the women and their families differ? If so, how?
   b. Did the women have rights, and were they allowed to assert those rights? Did they?
   c. What questions were asked of the clients, and what were the answers? Were those answers adequate?
   d. Compare the visits you observed with the ideal text book description of client care.
   e. How did each clinical experience make you feel? Which approach would you use? Justify your decisions.
2. Discuss with your peers and instructor the implications that the findings from exercise 1 above have for the following:
   a. The delivery of health care in our society.
   b. The acceptance and use of health care in our society.
3. What physical discomforts or problems might a 15-year-old primigravida in her twentieth week of pregnancy experience when attending her local high school? For one of these problems, role-play how you would provide her with pertinent information. Justify your decisions and actions.
4. What physical discomforts or problems might May P., age 36, a primigravida in her thirty-second week of pregnancy, experience at this time? For one of these problems, role-play how you would provide her with pertinent information. Justify your decisions and actions.

Topics for Nursing Research

- Discomforts of pregnancy and appropriate self-care measures
- Nurse satisfaction in LDRP room versus traditional (separate room) or mother-coupling
- Women's perceptions of body changes in the second trimester of pregnancy.

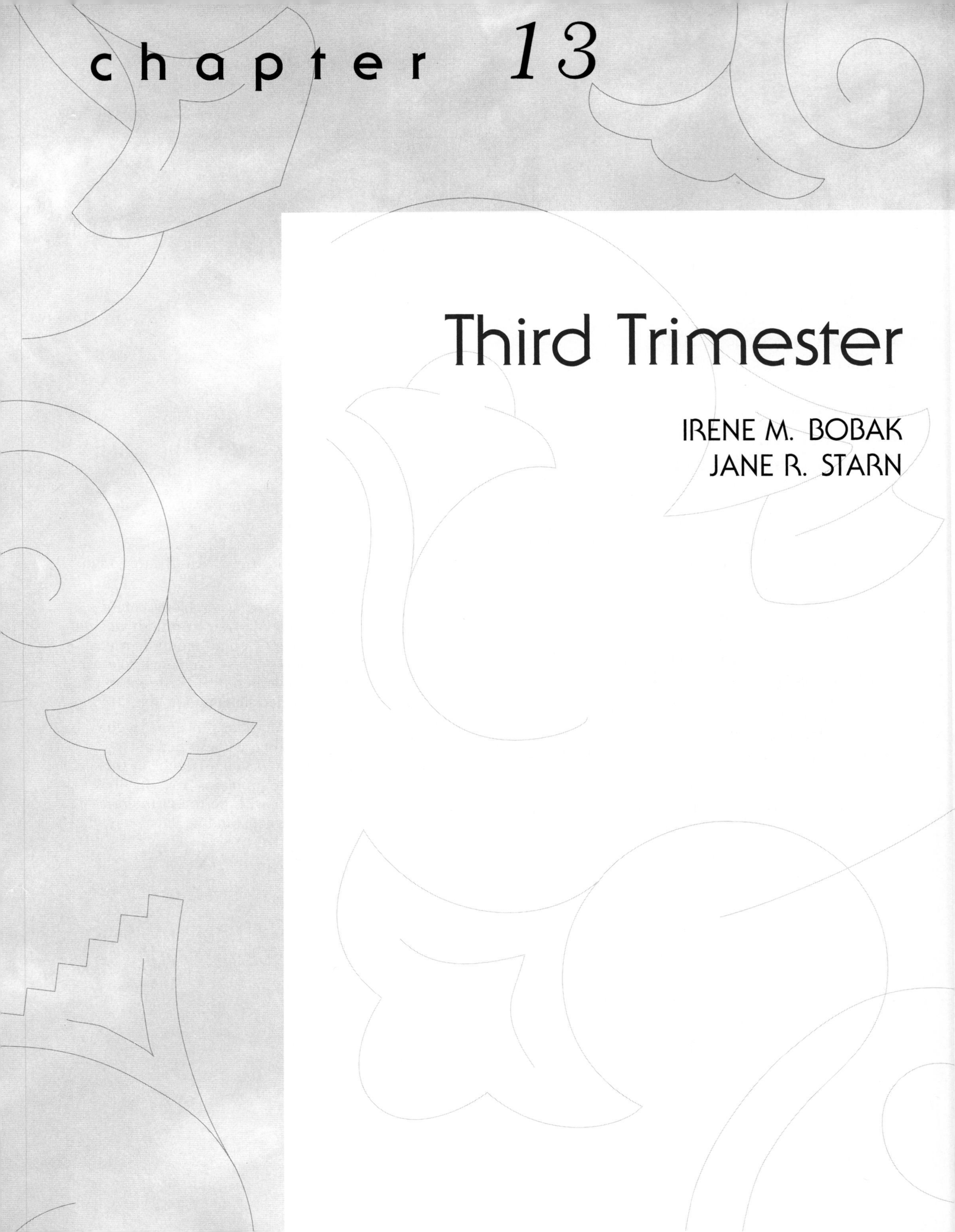

chapter 13

Third Trimester

IRENE M. BOBAK
JANE R. STARN

LEARNING OBJECTIVES

- Define the key terms listed.
- Discuss maternal and fetal assessment.
- Discuss teaching for self-care for discomforts related to maternal adaptations.
- Explain counseling for prenatal warning signs.
- Discuss client teaching for recognizing preterm labor, and identify six warning signs and symptoms of preterm labor.
- Identify the purpose of parent education.
- Compare methods of parent education for childbirth.
- Describe four birth-setting choices.
- Outline a teaching plan to assist women in nipple preparation for breast-feeding.
- Compare the care of a woman carrying one fetus with that of a woman carrying two or more fetuses.
- Explain five supportive strategies learned in parent education classes to help couples cope with labor and birth.
- Discuss finalizing the birth plan.
- List three significant research findings related to the effect of parent education.
- Identify topics for nursing research related to the third trimester of pregnancy.

The quiet period of the second trimester gives way to an active period, a trimester with more emphasis on the practical realities of expectant parenthood. Parental attachment to the fetus grows in the third trimester, a period spanning weeks 27 to 40. Mixed among the daydreams about the "coming baby" are parental anxieties that focus on possible defects in mental and physical abilities of the child. The expectant mother's attention turns to thoughts of a **safe passage** for herself and her child (Patterson et al, 1990). Fears of pain and mutilation and concerns about her behavior and possible loss of control during labor are important issues.

Physical discomforts and fetal movements often interrupt the expectant mother's rest. *Dyspnea,* return of urinary frequency, backache, constipation, and *varicosities* are experienced by most women in late pregnancy. Increased bulkiness and awkwardness affect the woman's ability to perform activities of daily living. Positions of comfort are more difficult to achieve. Increasingly, she becomes more impatient to "get this over with."

Many expectant fathers/partners become more involved with the pregnancy. Activity and energy to create and achieve characterize this phase. Styles of involvement differ according to the man's perception of the male and fathering roles within his social group. Men begin to redefine their relationship to the fetus and themselves as fathers. Role playing through daydreaming is common. The expectant father/partner feels some of the same concerns as the expectant mother. Often, however, he may not share these concerns with anyone.

Expectant families approaching childbirth have many needs. Siblings and grandparents must be considered, too. Clearly the nurse is in a pivotal position within the team of health care providers to assist parents with these needs during the third trimester of pregnancy. The schedule of care reflects the increased need. Starting with week 28, visits are scheduled every 2 weeks until week 36, and then every week until delivery.

■ THE NURSING PROCESS

The nursing process provides a framework for identifying client needs, selecting and ordering interventions, and evaluating the effectiveness of care. The nurse needs a broad knowledge of nursing to meet the physiologic and psychosocial needs of pregnant women and their families. Although pregnancy is essentially a healthy state, the nurse must be constantly on the alert for conditions that potentially place the client and her family at high risk for a less than optimal outcome.

ASSESSMENT

During the third trimester current family occurrences and their effect on the mother are assessed, for example, siblings' and grandparents' responses to the pregnancy and the coming child. In addition, the following questions are addressed:

- What anticipatory planning is in progress concerning new parenting responsibilities, sibling rivalry, recuperation from pregnancy and birth, and fertility management?
- What successes or frustrations is the mother experiencing with diet, rest and relaxation, sexuality, and emotional support?
- What is the mother's understanding of her family's needs in relation to the pregnancy and child?
- How well prepared are the parents in the event of emergency? That is, does the mother know and understand warning signs and how and to whom to report them?
- Does the mother know the signs of preterm and term labor?
- What is the mother's understanding of the labor process and expectations of herself and others during labor; does she know what to bring to the hospital?
- What plans has the mother and her family made for labor (see Birth Plan, p. 314 and Parent Education, p. 334, and Birth Setting Choices, p. 340)?
- What anxieties is the mother or her family experiencing regarding labor or child?
- What does the mother wish to know about control of discomfort during labor?
- Is the mother (and her partner or support person) planning to attend any parent education classes?
- Does the mother have questions about fetal development and methods to assess fetal well-being?

A checklist for third-trimester assessment should be used to ensure that important areas are addressed (see box, p. 323).

Maternal Assessment

INTERVIEW. The initial question in the third-trimester interview is asked with the intent to identify the woman's main concern of the moment. Focusing on the woman takes advantage of her readiness to learn and affirms the caregiver's interest in her as a person. Based on the client's expressed needs, her status to date, and the general needs of most women in late pregnancy, the nurse's clinical judgment guides the content and direction of the interview.

Third-Trimester Checklist

Schedule and events of visits
Fetal growth and development
Teaching for self-care:
Birth Plan
Adaptations/discomforts
- Dyspnea
- Insomnia
- Psychosocial responses and family dynamics
- Gingivitis and epulis
- Urinary frequency
- Perineal discomfort and pressure
- Braxton Hicks contractions
- Leg cramps
- Ankle edema

Safety (balance)
Exercise and rest
Relaxation
Nutrition
Sexuality
Warning signs—general
Warning signs—preterm labor
Preparation for baby
- Feeding method
- Nipple preparation

Preparation for labor
- Recognition: false versus true
- Parent education classes
- Control of discomfort
- Hospital tour
- Provision for other family members
- Preparation for homecoming

Diagnostic tests
- Specify

Other

The nurse determines if clients attended midpregnancy classes. If so, what questions and concerns arose that need to be addressed? Does the couple plan to attend third-trimester parent education classes? Has the birth plan been developed with realistic expectations? Is the plan feasible and flexible?

A review of physical systems is appropriate at each meeting. Any suspicious signs or symptoms are assessed in depth. Discomforts reflecting pregnancy adaptations are identified. Special inquiries are made about possible infections (e.g., genitourinary tract, respiratory tract). Knowledge of and success with self-care measures and prescribed therapy are assessed. Psychosocial responses to the pregnancy and approaching parenthood are assessed.

PHYSICAL EXAMINATION. During the third-trimester physical examination, temperature, pulse, respirations, blood pressure, and weight are assessed and noted. Suspicious signs and symptoms uncovered during the interview are evaluated. Presence, location, and degree of edema are documented carefully. Gestational age is confirmed. Abdominal palpation (Leopold's maneuvers [p. 437]) and measurement of fundal height (p. 301) continue to be performed. Risk assessment continues throughout pregnancy (see Chapter 27).

The **roll-over test** is sometimes used as one predictor of a potential hypertensive problem in the third trimester. This test may be done at each visit after the twentieth week of gestation. The roll-over test can be done as follows (Fanaroff, Martin, 1991; Cunningham, 1989). Position the woman on her side. When the blood pressure (BP) is stable, determine BP level in the upper portion of the arm. "Roll" her over onto her back, checking the pressure again. Wait 5 minutes and check the BP level once again.

An increase of 20 mm Hg in diastolic BP from the side position to the back position indicates a *positive roll test* reaction. The significance of a roll test is that if results are negative, the chances are less than 1 in 100 that preeclampsia will develop (For a discussion of hypertension and pregnancy, see Chapter 28.) If the test reaction is positive, even though the BP level is within normal limits and the woman has no signs of fluid retention, full-blown preeclampsia or pregnancy-induced hypertension (PIH) will develop at least 60% of the time. If the roll-over test is positive, it is imperative that home self-care measures be instituted. The woman should spend more time in bed in the lateral recumbent position to improve perfusion of the uterus and kidneys. Increased perfusion of kidneys leads to diuresis, with a reduction of edema. Stress in the home should be reduced, and her diet should be reviewed (see Chapter 28).

LABORATORY TESTS. At each visit urine is tested for glucose (to assess for diabetes) and albumin protein (to assess for hypertension). A urine culture and sensitivity test is done as necessary. Hematocrit determination by finger stick is made at each visit in some facilities. Blood tests are repeated as necessary: Venereal Disease Research Laboratory (VDRL) test for syphilis; complete blood cell count (CBC) with hematocrit, hemoglobin, and differential values; antibody screen (Kell, Duffy, rubella, toxoplasmosis, anti-Rh, acquired immunodeficiency syndrome [AIDS]); sickle cell; and level of folacin when indicated. If not done earlier in pregnancy, a glucose screen for women over 25 years of age is performed. Glucose challenge is usually done between 24 and 28 weeks (for a discussion of diabetes mellitus, see Chapter 31). Cervical and vaginal smears are repeated at 32 weeks or as necessary to examine for *Chlamydia* organisms, gonorrhea, and herpes simplex, types 1 and 2 (For a discussion of infection, see Chapter 29.).

SIGNS OF POTENTIAL PROBLEMS. The nurse is constantly on the alert for potential problems such as the following:

- *Hemorrhagic condition*—vaginal bleeding; severe abdominal pain
- *Hypertensive conditions*
  - Visual disturbances—blurring, double vision, or spots
  - Swelling of face or fingers and over sacrum
  - Headaches—severe, frequent, or continuous
  - Muscular irritability or convulsions
  - Epigastric pain (perceived as severe stomachache)
- *Infections*—positive laboratory test results
  - Chills, fever
  - Burning on urination, frequency, aching back and side
  - Diarrhea
- *Diabetes mellitus:* glucosuria, positive glucose tolerance test reaction
- *Fluid discharge from vagina*—amniotic fluid
- *Signs of preterm labor* (p. 329)

Fetal Assessment

Beginning at the thirty-second week, identification of fetal presentation, position, and station (engagement), with the aid of Leopold's maneuvers (described in Chapter 17), is done weekly. This period of rapid fetal growth is summarized in the box at right (see also Fig. 13-7).

Fundal height is measured at each visit. The method described on p. 301 is used. Uterine measurements and size (weight) of fetus are compared with supposed duration of pregnancy. Although some clinicians can estimate fetal weight with unbelievable accuracy, estimations are generally inconsistent and unreliable. Accuracy in estimating fetal weight improves with ultrasound determination of biparietal diameter (BPD). Possible intrauterine fetal growth retardation (IUGR), multifetal pregnancy, or inaccuracy of the estimated date of delivery (EDD) may be disclosed by ultrasound. (For an extensive discussion of fetal monitoring, see Chapter 16; for discussion of assessment for risk factors, see Chapter 27.)

SIGNS OF POTENTIAL PROBLEMS. Fetal health status is evaluated at each visit. The mother is requested to describe fetal movements. She is asked if she has warning signs (see p. 329) to report, for example, absence of or change in fetal movements, rupture of membranes. (For a discussion of electronic monitoring, see Chapter 16, for other monitoring techniques, see Chapter 27.) Ultrasound may reveal intrauterine growth retardation (IUGR) or abnormal (e.g., breech) presentation, for example.

Fetal Development at 40 Weeks

Nutrients and maternal immunoglobulins stored
Subcutaneous fat deposited
Dramatic storage of iron, nitrogen, and calcium
In male: testes are within well-wrinkled scrotum
In female: labia are well-developed and cover vestibule
Lanugo shed, except for shoulders, generally
Body contours plump
Decreased vernix
Scalp hair 2 to 3 cm (1 in) long
Cartilage in nose and ears well developed
45 to 55 cm (18 to 22 in) in length
Weighs 3400 g (7½ lb) (average)
Fundal height below xiphoid after lightening

NURSING DIAGNOSES

Each woman and her family respond to and are affected by pregnancy in different ways. Careful monitoring of the pregnancy and responses to care is of the utmost importance. The following are representative of nursing diagnoses that may be formulated in the third trimester from the data base of a "normal" pregnancy.

- Impaired individual coping related to knowledge deficit regarding
  - —Assessment for risks such as preterm labor
  - —Recognizing onset of true versus false labor
  - —Self-care measures
  - —Emergency arrangements
- Altered family processes related to
  - —Inadequate understanding of third-trimester changes and needs
  - —Increased concern about labor
  - —Insomnia or sleep deficit
- Sleep pattern disturbance related to
  - —Discomforts of late pregnancy
  - —Anxiety about approaching labor
- Activity intolerance related to
  - —Increased weight and change in center of gravity
  - —Anxiety
  - —Sleep disturbances

PLANNING

Planning care for clients and their families during the third trimester of pregnancy is given direction from identified nursing diagnoses and from a comprehensive view of the expectant family. A plan is developed mutually with the client to the extent possible. The plan is individualized, relating specifically to the client's needs and the needs of her family. Goals are similar to those of the first and second trimesters.

GOALS RELATED TO PHYSIOLOGIC CARE

1. Woman and her family have pertinent information about maternal adaptations and fetal development as a basis for understanding the management of care during the third trimester.
2. Woman will have knowledge for self-care.
3. Client's risk factors are identified, and referral for further evaluation or therapy, if indicated, is initiated promptly.
4. Client is alerted to symptoms that indicate deviations from normal progress and protocols for reporting them.

GOALS RELATED TO PSYCHOSOCIAL CARE

1. Client's information needs/readiness for learning are identified.
2. Women and their families are active participants in their care during the third trimester of pregnancy.
3. Client finalizes the birth plan.
4. Client's trusting relationship continues to progress.

IMPLEMENTATION

Social Support

Esteem, affection, trust, concern, consideration of cultural and religious responses, and listening are components of emotional support. The woman's feelings of satisfaction with her relationships and support, as well as her feeling of competence and sense of being in control, are important issues to address in the third trimester. A discussion of parental awareness of the unborn child's responses to stimuli, such as sound, light, maternal posture, or tension, and patterns of sleeping and waking can be helpful. Opportunities are also provided to discuss probable emotional tensions related to the following: childbirth experience such as fear of pain, loss of control, and possible birth of child before reaching hospital; responsibilities and tasks of parenthood; mutual parental concerns arising from anxiety for safety of mother and unborn child; mutual parental concerns related to siblings and their acceptance of new baby; mutual parental concerns about social and economic responsibilities; and mutual parental concerns arising from conflicts in cultural, religious, or personal value systems (Starn, 1991).

The father's/partner's commitment to the pregnancy, the couple's relationship, and their concerns about sexuality and sexual expression emerge as issues for many expectant parents. An important support measure is to validate the normality of their responses (if they fall within normal limits). Validation, feedback, and social comparison characterize appraisal support.

Providing opportunity to discuss concerns, providing a listening ear, and validating the normality of responses will meet the mother-to-be's needs in varying degrees. Nurses also need to implement specific "interventions targeted at improving expectant parents' partner support satisfaction, because this support constitutes the majority of their total support" (Brown, 1986, 6a). Referral to childbirth education classes is made as necessary (p. 334).

During the third trimester, the birth plan is finalized. When the plan is ready, it can be written out, signed by the client and primary care practitioner, and added to the prenatal record. The intent is to decrease the possibility of a conflict with staff members over the use of drugs for pain, for example. A pleasant, relaxed atmosphere encourages expectant parents to ask questions and verbalize anxieties and fears without worrying about possible rejection. Thoughtful answers that reflect the nurse's caring can be reassuring. Clients should not feel pressured either to attend parent education classes or to have a birth plan.

Nurses need to recognize that men have increased feelings of vulnerability during pregnancy. Anticipatory guidance and health promotion strategies can help fathers-to-be with their concerns. Nursing intervention may directly help them with such concerns as the need to share intimate feelings or may indirectly do so by education of mothers. Health care providers can stimulate and encourage open dialogue between the couple.

Nursing students especially are cautioned that, despite their knowledge, skill, concern, and caring, some clients will be unable to benefit from their interventions. It is equally important for the nurse to maintain self-esteem and a positive self-concept in the face of a less than optimum client outcome.

Immune System Support

For the woman with Rh negativity, Rh sensitization is possible during pregnancy (see Chapter 38).

For the woman with findings of Rh_OD, D^U, and Coombs' test negativity, Rh immunoglobulin (RhIG) is administered during pregnancy after an amniocentesis (see Chapter 27) and at about 28 weeks' gestation.

A new immunization strategy to protect newborn infants is available through the vaccination of mothers late in pregnancy. In effect, it allows for vaccination of babies before they are born. It works by passing protective antibodies from the mother to the fetus (*San Francisco Chronicle*, 1991). Newborns may be protected from *Haemophilus influenzae* type B, which is a potentially lethal infection that causes meningitis and pneumonia; this bacterium is a leading killer of children. Between 15% to 40% of *Haemophilus* infections occur before 6 months of age. Immunization is given during the third trimester; levels of antibodies in the infant's blood streams last for the first 6 months of life. Vaccinations may not be available for routine use because vaccine manufac-

TABLE 13-1 Discomforts/Concerns Related to Maternal Adaptations During the Third Trimester

Discomfort	Physiology	Teaching for self-care
Shortness of breath and dyspnea—occur in 60% of pregnant women	Expansion of diaphragm limited by enlarging uterus; diaphragm is elevated about 4 cm (1½ in); some relief after lightening	Good posture; flying exercise; sleep with extra pillows; avoid overloading stomach; stop smoking; refer to physician if symptoms worsen to rule out anemia, emphysema, and asthma
Insomnia (later weeks of pregnancy)	Fetal movements, muscular cramping, urinary frequency, shortness of breath, or other discomforts	Reassurance; conscious relaxation; back massage or **effleurage** (Fig. 13-1); support of body parts with pillows; warm milk or warm shower before retiring
Psychosocial responses (Chapter 10): mood swings, mixed feelings, increased anxiety	Hormonal and metabolic adaptations; feelings about impending labor, delivery, and parenthood	Reassurance and support from significant other and nurse; improved communication with partner, family, and others
Return of urinary frequency and urgency	Vascular engorgement and altered bladder function caused by hormones; bladder capacity reduced by enlarging uterus and fetal presenting part; lightening	Kegel's exercises; limit fluid intake before bedtime; reassurance; wear perineal pad; refer to physician for pain or burning sensation
Perineal discomfort and pressure	Pressure from enlarging uterus, especially when standing or walking; multifetal gestation	Rest, conscious relaxation and good posture; maternity girdle; refer to physician for assessment and treatment if pain is present; rule out labor
Braxton Hicks contractions	Intensification of uterine contractions in preparation for work of labor	Reassurance; rest; change of position; practice breathing techniques when contractions are bothersome; effleurage; *rule out labor*
Leg cramps (gastrocnemius spasm)—especially when reclining	Compression of nerves supplying lower extremities because of enlarging uterus; reduced level of diffusible serum calcium or elevation of serum phosphorus; aggravating factors: fatigue, poor peripheral circulation, pointing toes when stretching legs or when walking, drinking more than 1 L (1 qt) of milk per day; cause unclear	Rule out blood clot by checking for Homans' sign; use massage and heat over affected muscle; stretch affected muscle until spasm relaxes (Fig. 13-2); stand on cold surface; physician-ordered oral supplementation with calcium carbonate or calcium lactate tablets; aluminum hydroxide gel, 1 oz, with each meal removes phosphorus by absorbing it
Ankle edema (nonpitting) to lower extremities	Edema aggravated by prolonged standing, sitting, poor posture, lack of exercise, constrictive clothing (e.g., garters), or hot weather	Ample fluid intake for "natural" diuretic effect; put on support stockings before arising; rest periodically with legs and hips elevated (see Fig. 12-4), exercise moderately; refer to physician if generalized edema develops; *diuretics are contraindicated*

Fig 13-1 Pattern for effleurage: a light, rhythmic stroking useful for inducing relaxation. **A**, Self-effleurage. **B**, Effleurage by another.

turers may wish to avoid lawsuits that could be filed by women who give birth prematurely or who have other complications after getting the immunization (whether or not such complications are related to the vaccination). Researchers are investigating whether a whole variety of infections could be prevented in this way: group B streptococcus, whooping cough, pneumococcus, *Escherichia coli,* and *Pseudomonas*.

During the third trimester, some women are retested for sexually transmitted diseases (STDs) such as syphilis, gonorrhea, and chlamydia. (See Chapter 29 for a discussion of these infections and their management.)

Teaching for Self-Care

Not only are some new discomforts seen in the third trimester, but others seen previously in the first trimester (e.g., fatigue) also recur. Pregnant women in the older age-group may experience an aggravation of varicose veins or severe backache from postural changes associated with a heavy, pendulous abdomen and relaxed joints. Such symptoms are frightening and uncomfortable.

In Table 13-1 the physiology, prevention, and self-care of several discomforts are discussed. (Discomforts not found in this Table may be found in Tables 11-2 and 12-1. Relaxation, exercises, body mechanics, safety, and employment issues are described and discussed in Chapter 12. Nutrition is covered in Chapter 9.)

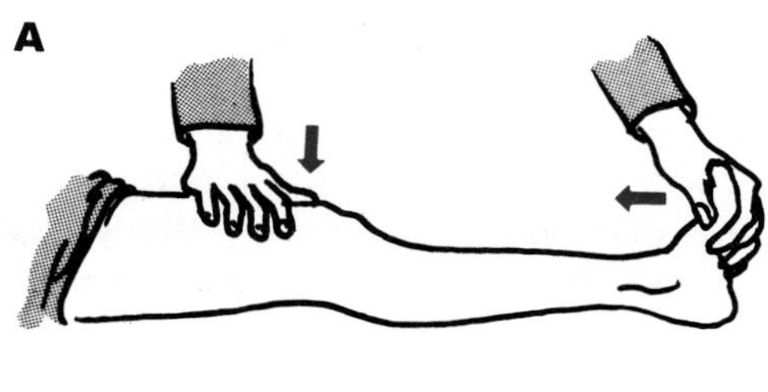

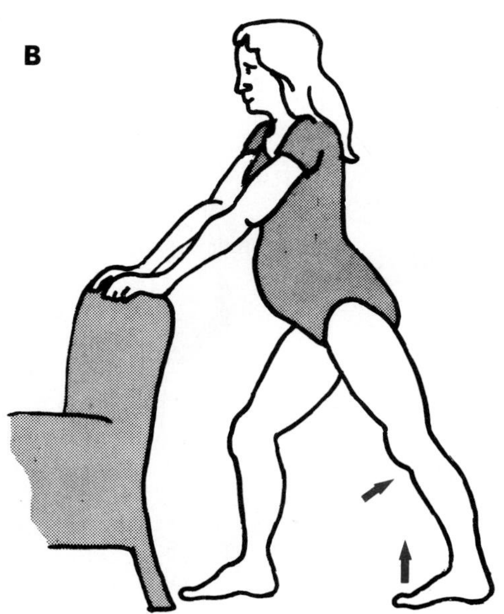

Fig 13-2 Relief of muscle spasm (leg cramps). **A**, Another person dorsiflexes the foot with the knee extended. **B**, Woman stands and leans forward on affected leg.

PREPARATION FOR FEEDING THE NEWBORN. Pregnant women are usually eager to discuss their plans for feeding the newborn. Breast milk is the food of choice, and breast-feeding is associated with a decreased incidence in perinatal morbidity and mortality. However, deep-seated aversion to breast-feeding by mother or father, the mother's need for certain medications, and certain medical complications, such as pulmonary tuberculosis, are contraindications to breast-feeding. The woman and her partner are encouraged to decide which method of feeding is suitable for them. Once the couple has been given information about the advantages and disadvantages of bottle-feeding and breast-feeding, they are in a position to make an informed choice. Nurses need only to support their decisions.

Most women are motivated by the sixth or seventh month of pregnancy to learn about breast preparation and breast-feeding. Each woman is first assessed for risk of preterm labor. Anticipatory guidance during pregnancy contributes to later success in breast-feeding (Nicholson, 1985).

The **pinch test** determines whether the nipple is erectile or retractile (Fig. 13-3). The nurse guides the woman through the pinch test. The woman places her thumb and forefinger on her areola and presses inward gently. This will cause her nipple to stand erect or to retract (invert). Most nipples will stand erect. Inverted nipples need more preparation time. Nipple preparation for these women can start during the last 2 months of pregnancy.

The woman learns that nipples are cleansed with warm water to prevent blocking of the ducts with dried colostrum. Soap is not used because it removes protective oils that keep nipples supple.

The woman who plans to breast-feed should purchase a nursing brassiere that will suffice for the increased size required for the last few months of pregnancy, as well as for lactation. If her breasts are very heavy, or if the woman feels uncomfortable with the weight unsupported, the brassiere can be worn day and night. One of the easiest ways to get the nipples used to tactile stimulation is to leave the flaps on the brassiere open as much as possible during the day and night. This allows the nipples to rub against clothing and gradually desensitizes (toughens) them (Worthington-Roberts, Williams, 1989).

Toughening of nipples can be accomplished in a

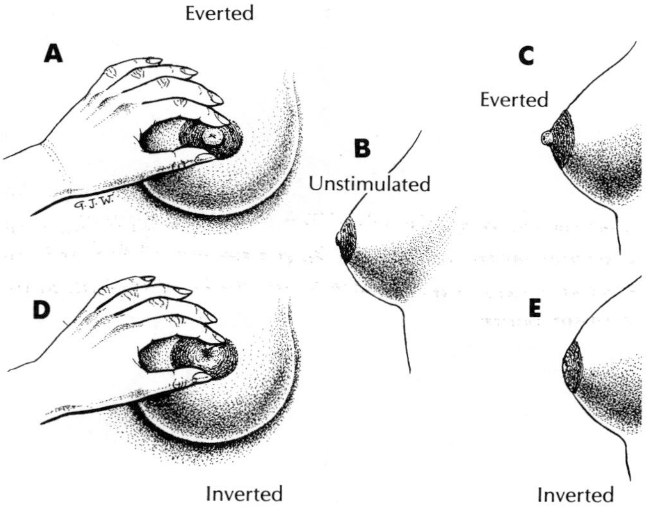

Fig 13-3 A, and C, When stimulated, nipples evert (protract erect). B, Unstimulated, nipples look the same. D, and E, When stimulated, nipples invert (retract).

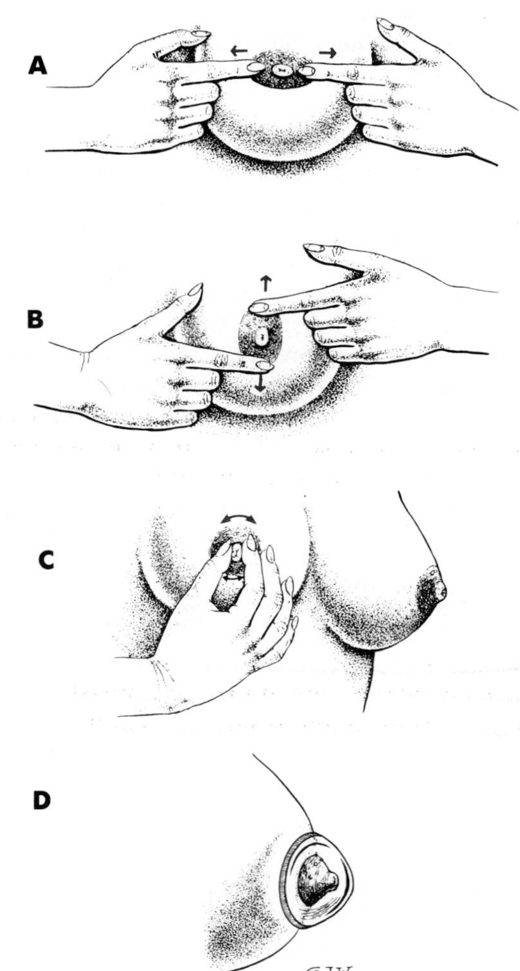

Fig 13-4 A, and B, Nipple stretching. C, Nipple rolling. D, Nipple cup in place. (Some concern has been expressed regarding nipple stimulation and potential for preterm labor.)

variety of ways. After a bath or shower, the woman can towel dry nipples well, but not so hard as to cause irritation or soreness. The woman can grasp the nipple between the thumb and forefinger and roll each nipple gently for a short time each day (Fig. 13-4). *Because this procedure may cause uterine contractions, it may be contraindicated for those women at risk for preterm labor.* Exposing nipples to air and sunlight for short periods of time each day can also toughen nipples, but sunburn must be avoided.

Other techniques can be employed to encourage protraction of inverted nipples. The woman can place four fingers close to the inverted nipple, pressing firmly into the breast tissue, and gradually pull away from areola. Massage is done vertically and horizontally, about five times each day.

Some women obtain *nipple cups* designed specifically for correcting inverted nipples. Plastic doughnut-shaped cups are available for correcting inversions or retractions (Fig. 13-4, *D*). A continuous, gentle pressure exerted around the areola pushes the nipple through a central opening in the inner shield. Nipple cups should be worn during the last two trimesters of pregnancy for 1 to 2 hours daily. The time for wearing them should be increased gradually. Brand names for these cups include Woolwich, Netsy, La Leche League Cups, Nurse-Dri, Free and Dry, and Hobbit Shields. These cups can also be worn after childbirth. However, because body warmth can foster rapid bacterial growth and contamination, milk that collects in the cup should be discarded and not fed to the infant (Riordan, 1983).

Breast stimulation may also produce uterine activity and should be avoided in women at risk for preterm labor if contractions are noted (Iams et al, 1988). However, the assumption that nipple stimulation causes the release of exogenous oxytocin has not been proved. Ross et al (1984) were unable to detect a surge of oxytocin into the plasma of women whose uterus contracted in association with nipple stimulation (Cunningham et al, 1989).

The possibility of contaminants in breast milk concerns many women, both consumers and professionals (Wardlaw, Insel, 1990). Breast milk potentially can be hazardous as illustrated in the following examples. The mother harboring *Salmonella kottbus* transmits this organism through her milk. Environmental pollutants tend to concentrate in humans. The long-term effects of contamination of breast milk with pollutants such as polybrominated biphenyl (PBB) is as yet unknown. Medications that pass through the mother's milk are listed in Appendix G.

REVIEW OF WARNING SIGNS. The nurse needs to answer questions honestly as they arise during pregnancy. It is often difficult for the woman to know when to report signs and symptoms. The mother is encouraged to refer to a printed list of warning signs (see below) and to listen to her body. If she senses that "something is wrong," she should call her primary care practitioner. Several signs and symptoms need to be discussed more extensively. These include vaginal bleeding, alteration in fetal movements, symptoms of preeclampsia or PIH, rupture of membranes, and preterm labor.

If *vaginal bleeding* occurs in the third trimester, it is important to rule out brownish spotting occurring 48 hours after vaginal examination and to rule out "show" of pinkish mucus. The woman is to come to the hospital's emergency area immediately for diagnosis and treatment if bleeding is other than one of the preceding types.

Should the woman notice cessation, noticeable lessening, or acceleration in the amount of *fetal movement,* she is to come to the clinic or the physician's office for evaluation.

Appearance of *edema* of the hands and around the eyes, severe *headaches, visual changes,* or feelings of *jitteriness* require immediate evaluation for hypertension.

A gush or trickle of clear *watery discharge* that appears to come from the vagina may indicate rupture of membranes. The diagnosis requires a visit to the clinic or hospital for evaluation.

RECOGNIZING PRETERM LABOR. Teaching each mother-to-be to recognize preterm labor is necessary (Bonovich, 1990; Herron, 1988; Hill, Lambertz, 1990; Hill, 1989). Preterm labor occurs after the twentieth week but before the thirty-seventh week of pregnancy. It is a condition in which uterine contractions cause the cervix to open earlier than normal. It could result in the birth of a preterm baby. Although certain factors may increase a woman's chances of having preterm labor, such as carrying twins, the specific cause or causes are not known. It may be possible to prevent a preterm birth by knowing the warning signs and symptoms of preterm labor and by seeking care early if warning signs and symptoms should occur. ***Warning signs and symptoms of preterm labor*** include the following:

Uterine contractions that occur every 10 minutes or more with or without other signs

Menstrual-like cramps felt in lower portion of the abdomen constantly or intermittently

Low dull backache felt below the waistline constantly or intermittently

Pelvic pressure that feels like baby is pushing down constantly or intermittently

Abdominal cramping with or without diarrhea

Increase or change in vaginal discharge; more than usual or change in consistency or color.

Hospitals have developed pamphlets to help mothers remember what they learn. (See the box below for teaching preterm labor recognition.) Occasionally, birth occurs before the woman has access to professional attendants. Emergency childbirth is outlined in Chapter 18.

TEACHING Preterm Labor Recognition

Because the onset of preterm labor is subtle and often hard to recognize, it is important to know how to feel your abdomen for uterine contractions. You can feel for contractions in the following way. While lying down, place your fingertips on the top of your uterus. A contraction is the periodic "tightening" or "hardening" of your uterus. If your uterus is contracting, you will actually feel your abdomen get tight or hard and then feel it relax or soften when the contraction is over.

If you think you are having any of the other signs and symptoms of preterm labor, empty your bladder, drink three to four glasses of water for hydration, lie down tilted toward your side, and place a pillow at your back for support.

Check for contractions for 1 hour. To tell how often contractions are occurring, check the minutes that elapse from the beginning of one contraction to the beginning of the next.

It is *normal* to have some uterine contractions throughout the day. They usually occur when a woman changes positions. These usually irregular and mild contractions are called Braxton Hicks contractions. They help with uterine tone and uteroplacental perfusion.

It is *not normal* to have frequent uterine contractions (every 10 minutes or more often for 1 hour).

Contractions of labor are regular, frequent, and hard. They also may be felt as a tightening of the abdomen or a backache. This type of contraction causes the cervix to efface and dilate.

Call your doctor, clinic, or delivery room, or go to the hospital if any of the following signs occur:

- You have uterine contractions every 10 minutes or more often for 1 hour *or*
- You have any of the other signs and symptoms for 1 hour *or*
- You have any bloody spotting or leaking of fluid from your vagina.

It is often difficult to identify preterm labor. Accurate diagnosis requires assessment by the care provider, usually in the hospital or clinic.

Post these instructions where they can be seen by everyone in the family.

PREBIRTH PREPARATION. Not all expectant mothers and support persons attend formal classes in preparation for childbirth. For those who do attend, extensive preparation is possible (see p. 334 and Fig. 13-6). Many do not take advantage of classes for a variety of reasons: employment, inaccessibility because of time, cultural/ethnic/religious orientation, cost, lack of knowledge regarding choices in prenatal education classes or lack of readiness. Therefore clinicians need to provide information that includes the following:

Process of labor: admission, examination, care in labor

Plans to get to hospital (when to go and where); care of other children

Methods to control pain (e.g., analgesia and anesthesia (see Chapter 15) breathing-relaxing techniques (in this chapter)

Supplies to have in a suitcase ready for the trip to the hospital: personal items for grooming, items for labor as desired (e.g., warm socks, focal point), supportive bra, nightgowns, slippers

Responsibilities of the partner, family member, or friend who will be accompanying the woman through the labor and delivery

Care of the newborn (i.e., clothing, feeding, daily hygienic care) and postnatal care (see Chapter 21)

Emergency arrangements (e.g., precipitate delivery) (see Chapter 18)

A nurse needs to be ready to teach when the woman is ready to learn as shown by the following example. One nurse described her intervention with an expectant mother as follows

> I tried to teach her about relaxation and breathing techniques during her pregnancy, but she was not interested. When she phoned to tell me she was at the hospital in labor, she said, "What was all that stuff you were saying about breathing?" In between the next few contractions I repeated the salient points.

Even if the woman/couple has attended parent education classes, the nurse discusses preparation for childbirth. The following topics are discussed:

Symptoms of impending labor (see box on p. 331) and what information to report

Breathing and relaxation techniques (see p. 338)

Involvement of significant other

Provision for needs of other children

Plans to get to hospital

Plans of labor, terminology, and what care to expect

Preparation for baby

Preparation of grandparents and siblings (see Chapter 10)

If a hospital delivery is planned, the woman is of-

Symptoms of Impending Labor

Uterine contractions: The woman is instructed to report the frequency, duration, and intensity of uterine contractions. First-time mothers usually are counseled to remain at home until contractions are regular and 5 minutes apart. Parous women are counseled to remain at home until contractions are regular and 10 minutes apart. If the woman lives more than 20 minutes from the hospital or has a history of rapid labors, these instructions are modified accordingly.

Rupture of the membranes (see Chapter 17).

Bloody "show": The "show" is scant, pink, and sticky (contains mucus).

ten required to preregister at the hospital of choice. Most hospitals now provide pamphlets containing information such as where to report when labor begins and policies pertaining to visitors and visiting hours. Many facilities also conduct tours.

Counseling is provided to relieve emotional tensions, which often relate directly to the childbirth experience (e.g., anxiety about pain or possible delivery of the child before reaching the hospital). Nursing strategies include providing an opportunity for discussing the woman's specific fears or anxieties, helping her make definite plans concerning what she will do when labor starts, repeating instructions willingly, and having "sharing sessions" with mothers who have recently delivered. If possible, involve significant others in preparation for the birth. Arrange to have them participate in a supportive way during labor and delivery. These techniques may be effective in preventing or minimizing anxiety.

Most men whose partners are approaching labor may have their anxieties decreased through intervention before the event. Fantasies can be replaced by knowledge gained through activities such as the following:

A hospital tour to enable visualization of the labor room and waiting areas

A demonstration of helping and supportive measures to comfort the woman during labor

A brief review of what to expect from the woman during the labor process

A description of what to expect of the staff during the woman's labor

A realistic discussion of all known factors helps the father/partner problem-solve more rationally and plan for the event. Such discussions are ego strengthening because they help focus the father's/partner's energies toward more appropriate coping strategies by easing anxieties about the unknown. Today many men/partners elect to participate actively during labor and the delivery of the child. However, some men/partners, because of personal or cultural concepts, neither wish nor intend to participate. *The important concept is that each partner agrees on the other's roles.* For nurses to advocate any changes in these roles may cause confusion or feelings of guilt.

EVALUATION

Evaluation is a continuous process as each intervention is assessed for effectiveness and an alternate intervention is used as necessary. Any change in client condition or concern requires readjustment in the nursing care plan. The degree to which the goals for the mother, couple, or fetus are met is continuously evaluated according to measurable established criteria:

- The woman and her family have sufficient information about maternal adaptations and fetal development to understand the management of care and self-care during the third trimester
- The client's risk factors were identified, and referral for further evaluation or therapy, if indicated, was initiated promptly.
- The client was alerted to symptoms that could indicate deviations from normal progress and protocols for reporting them.
- The client's information needs/readiness for learning were identified and met.
- The women and their families were active participants in their care during the third trimester of pregnancy.
- The client had formalized a birth plan.
- The client's trusting relationship with caregivers continued to progress.

■ MULTIFETAL PREGNANCY

A pregnancy with more than one fetus places the mother and fetuses at risk. Maternal blood volume is increased in multiple gestations, resulting in an increased strain on the maternal cardiovascular system. Anemia often develops because of a greater demand for iron by the fetuses. Marked uterine distention and increased pressure on the adjacent viscera and pelvic vasculature occur in **multifetal pregnancies.** Diastasis of the two recti abdominis muscles (in the midline) may occur. Placenta previa develops more commonly in multifetal pregnancies because of the large size or placement of the placentas (Figs. 7-14 and 7-15; note placement of placentas) (Cunningham et al, 1989; Scott et al, 1990). Premature separation of the placenta may occur before the second and subsequent fetuses are born.

After the thirtieth week the weight of each twin plus placenta usually is less than that of an infant and placenta of a singleton pregnancy. However, their combined weight is almost twice that of a singleton near term. The mean weight of twins in the United States is more than 2270 g (5 lb). Congenital malformations are twice as common in monozygotic twins as in singletons. There is no increase in the incidence of congenital anomalies in dizygotic twins. Two-vessel cords—that is, cords with a single umbilical artery—occur more often in twins than in singletons. This abnormality is most common in monozygotic twins. The most serious problem for the fetus is the local shunting of blood between placentas (twin-to-twin transfusion) (see Fig. 7-15, *B* and *C*). The *recipient* twin is larger. However, congenital heart failure may develop in this twin during the first 24 hours after birth. The *donor* twin will be small, pallid, dehydrated, malnourished, and hypovolemic. Prematurity is a serious problem for the neonates.

Clinical diagnosis of multifetal pregnancy is accurate in only about three fourths of cases. A correct diagnosis of twins may be possible by the twenty-fourth to twenty-sixth week based on the following factors:

- History of dizygous twins in the female lineage
- Abnormally large maternal weight gain (inconsistent with diet or edema)
- Hydramnios
- Palpation of excessive number of small or large parts
- Asynchronous fetal heart beats or more than one fetal electrocardiographic tracing
- Radiographic or ultrasonographic evidence of more than one fetus (see Chapter 27).

Prenatal Care

Prenatal care includes changes in the pattern of care and modifications in other aspects such as weight gain and diet. Prenatal visits by the mother with multifetal pregnancy are scheduled at least every 2 weeks in the second trimester and weekly thereafter.

Diet and weight control are supervised to allow weight gain of about 50% or more than the average woman with a singleton pregnancy (as much as 18 kg [40 lb] above the woman's ideal nonpregnant weight). Iron and vitamin supplementation is desir-

CASE STUDY

Third Trimester: Insomnia, Ankle Edema, and Braxton Hicks Contractions

Ruth Piper, a 36-year-old married woman pregnant for the first time is now at 35 weeks of gestation. She is planning to work one more week as an office manager before taking maternity leave. She and her husband are attending a parent education class to prepare for childbirth and early infant care (p. 334). Their birth plan is being finalized.

ASSESSMENT

Ruth states she is feeling more fatigued, her legs ache (no cramping), her ankles are swollen every afternoon and worsen by bedtime, and the fetus awakens and becomes active as she settles down to sleep. Her fatigue, leg aches, ankle edema, and fetal activity keep her awake. She feels her abdomen tighten periodically and expresses concern that she could give birth to a "premie." Findings from physical examination and laboratory tests are all within normal limits.

NURSING DIAGNOSIS

Analysis of assessment findings supports the nursing diagnosis: Sleep pattern disturbance related to discomforts of late pregnancy.

PLANNING

The nurse and Ruth discuss the goals for her care. They mutually agree on the *goal* that takes priority at this time: Ruth will get at least 7 hours of restful sleep each night. The nurse identifies the *expected outcome:* Ruth will avoid consequences of sleep deprivation, that is, mood alteration, fatigue, and anxiety and will add to her repertoire of self-care measures.

IMPLEMENTATION

The nurse reassures Ruth that insomnia is a common discomfort late in pregnancy. Several comfort measures can be learned for self-care: conscious relaxation, effleurage, support of body parts with pillows during rest periods and at night, warm milk or warm shower or whirlpool bath (jet hydrotherapy) before retiring, and avoidance of caffeine-containing fluids and foods during the late afternoon and evening.

EVALUATION

The nurse can be reasonably assured that interventions have been effective if, at the next visit in 1 week, Ruth reports more restful sleep and less fatigue. Ruth states she feels that self-care comfort measures "work" for her.

CARE PLAN Third Trimester: Insomnia, Ankle Edema, and Braxton Hicks Contractions

GOALS	IMPLEMENTATION	RATIONALE	EVALUATION
Nursing diagnosis: Sleep pattern disturbance related to discomforts of late pregnancy			
Ruth will learn and use self-care comfort measures and get a minimum of 7 hours restful sleep/night.	Reassure that insomnia is a common occurrence during late pregnancy.	Validates normality of her "complaint."	Ruth states she understands but she would feel better is she could sleep.
	Teach rationale, demonstrate and observe return demonstration, (where possible) of self-care measures: conscious relaxation; effleurage; support of body parts with pillows; warm milk or shower before retiring; whirlpool bath (jet hydrotherapy (Chapter 17) before retiring; avoidance of caffeine-containing fluids/foods late in day.	Knowledge and skill increases individual coping, self-esteem, and sense of power over situation. Measures utilize gate-control theory, normal physiologic function, and facilitate relaxation.	At next visit. Ruth states she is sleeping better, feels better, and both she and her husband are benefiting from the relaxation techniques; she states she and her husband are learning these same techniques in the parent education class.
Nursing diagnosis: Leg pain related to ankle edema and compression of blood vessels and nerves supplying lower extremities because of enlarging uterus			
Ruth will experience less ankle edema and leg ache.	Explore possibility of her walking or stair climbing several times each day. Explore possibility of 15-20 min during morning, lunch, and afternoon breaks and after work to rest with legs and hips elevated (see Fig. 12-4) and to support arms and legs with pillows at night while in side-lying position.	Standing and sitting for extended periods impairs peripheral circulation and causes fatigue and leg aches: Walking and climbing stairs stimulates circulation. Position uses gravity to help reduce ankle edema.	At next visit Ruth reports she has noted less ankle edema and leg ache.
	Suggest maternity girdle to help support heavy abdomen. Suggest maintaining water intake up to 8 glasses/day.	Supporting and lifting heavy uterus facilitates venous/lymphatic drainage. Water intake and side-lying position aid in diuresis by improving renal perfusion.	
Nursing diagnosis: Anxiety related to knowledge deficit regarding recognition of preterm labor			
Ruth will learn how to recognize preterm labor today.	Using written instructions* (box on p. 330), teach Ruth how to assess and time contractions.	Knowledge permits Ruth to collaborate in her care; increases self-confidence.	Ruth demonstrates actions and states rationale correctly.
Ruth will put the pamphlet where family can see it, as soon as she gets home. Ruth will telephone her primary care practitioner if she experiences any of the warning signs and symptoms of preterm labor.	Suggest pamphlet/instructions be placed where husband/family can find them easily.	Ruth may be too anxious or unable to use them; family members may need to help with assessment and reporting to primary care practitioner.	At next visit 1 week later, Ruth states she posted instructions on the telephone after reviewing them with her husband/family.

*Nurse has determined that both Ruth and her husband can read the instructions.

able. Attempts are made to prevent preeclampsia/eclampsia (which occurs more frequently during pregnancies with more than one fetus), and vaginitis; if they cannot be prevented, they are treated early and properly.

The considerable uterine distention can cause increase in backache. Elastic stockings or maternity tights may control leg varices.

Abstinence from both coitus and masturbation to the point of orgasm during the last trimester is recommended. This may help prevent preterm labor.

Enforced rest periods, begun as soon as pregnancy is diagnosed, may help avoid untimely early labor. The mother needs to assume the left lateral position.

Untimely early labor should be avoided. Delivery after the thirty-sixth week increases the likelihood of survival of the neonates.

Psychosocial Adjustment

The diagnosis of a twin pregnancy comes as a shock to many expectant parents. They will need support and education to help them cope with the changes they face. The mother will need nutritional counseling to gain more weight, maternal adaptations will probably be more uncomfortable, and she faces the possibility of a preterm birth.

The degree to which parents are overwhelmed was dramatized in the following occurrence. A young couple had known they were to become parents of twins since an early sonogram revealed the presence of two gestational sacs. They had adjusted to the event and were looking forward to twins. At birth, a third baby was born. The father became irate, accused the physician of negligence in not diagnosing triplets, and threatened to sue her. This couple needed additional support during their initial adjustment period.

The additional newborn(s) will strain finances, space, workload, and individual and family coping capability. Life-style changes may be necessary. Parents will need assistance to make realistic plans for the care of the babies, for example, breast-feeding and raising them as "alike" or as separate individuals. Parents should be referred to national organizations such as Parents of Twins, Mothers of Multiples, and the La Leche League.

■ PARENT EDUCATION

The Organization for Obstetric, Gynecologic, and Neonatal Nurses (NAACOG) has defined parent (childbirth) education as "the process designed to assist parents in making the transition from the role of expectant parents to the role and responsibilities of parents of a new baby, which includes the period from the time of conception to approximately three months after birth" (1981). The goal of parent education is to prepare the parents to meet the challenges of childbirth and early parenting, labor, birth, postpartum recovery, and early infancy (Riesch, 1988). Classes focus on preparing families intellectually, emotionally, and physically for childbirth, as well as promoting wellness and improved life-style behaviors during the childbearing year (American Society for Psychoprophylaxis in Obstetrics [ASPO] and Lamaze, 1990). The effect of childbirth classes on obstetric outcomes has been studied (see Research Highlight, p. 335).

History of the Childbirth Movement

Throughout time women have shared information and assisted each other in childbirth. Until the late nineteenth century, childbirth was a family/social event in which women gave birth at home, often with the help of a midwife. The Industrial Revolution, with attendant urban crowding and associated health problems, led to higher and higher rates of maternal and infant death from puerperal fever, sepsis, and/or infant diarrhea (Wertz, 1979). The associated changes of male domination of obstetrics, drugs, and medication for pain and infection control in birth, as well as weakening family bonds brought on by industrialization, moved childbirth from being "women's work" and controlled by nature into the hospital (Lindell, 1988).

During the early twentieth century women accepted centralized and routinized birth practices over which they had no control in the belief that childbirth would be safer for themselves and their babies. Not until midway into the twentieth century did women (fueled by consumer rights, the women's movement, and increased use of certified nurse-midwives) begin to question the rigid policies, medicalization, and routinization of birth. The parent education movement evolved in the 1950s and grew in the 1960s until prepared parent classes are now recommended for all families by most physicians and hospitals, as well as the federally appointed panel on prenatal care (Public Health Service, 1989). The parent education movement evolved simultaneously with family-centered maternity care.

Studies show that parent education "promotes positive attitudes towards labor and delivery and . . . fosters early maternal-infant attachment" (Lindell, 1988). A 1990 study of 800 women in England found that receipt of information and feeling in control were important aspects in women's satisfaction with the birth and in subsequent emotional well-being. Physiologic effects of length of labor and anesthesia/analgesia on mother and infant are varied. Some studies found that formal preparation results in reduced use of analgesia and anesthesia (Lindell, 1988; Hetherington, 1990). However, others do not demonstrate that attendance at parent education classes reduces interventions during labor and delivery (Lindell, 1988; Sturrock, Johnson, 1990). Slager-Earnest et al (1989) demonstrated that combining a multidisciplinary team and comprehensive health services in coordination with parent education resulted in significantly fewer obstetric, postnatal, and neonatal complications for teenagers enrolled in the program. Thus new approaches and classes tailored to the needs of varied groups may be essential for effective outcomes.

Early Methods

An English physician, Grantly Dick-Read, published two books in which he theorized that pain in childbirth is socially conditioned and is caused by a fear-tension-pain syndrome. His first book, *Natural Childbirth,* was published in 1933. Dick-Read's second book, *Childbirth Without Fear,* was published in the United States in 1944. The work of Dick-Read became the foundation for organized programs of preparation for childbirth and teacher training throughout the United States, Canada, Great Britain, and South Africa. In 1960, the nurses prepared through such programs established the **International Childbirth Education Association (ICEA).** This method, referred to as *childbirth without fear,* basically recommends three techniques: deep breathing both in abdominal respirations and thoracic respirations; shallow breathing; and breath holding for the second stage of labor.* Relaxation is an important part of the **Grantly Dick-Read method.** Women are taught to use conscious relaxation methods that involve progressive relaxation of the muscle groups in the entire body. Consequently, during labor the woman is able to relax completely between contractions. Using conscious relaxation techniques, some women are actually able to sleep between contractions.

During the 1960s the **Lamaze method,** also known as the psychoprophylactic method (PPM), gained popularity in the United States. PPM offered new perspectives on preparation for childbirth by emphasizing mind control. Marjorie Karmel introduced

*Breath holding is now discouraged.

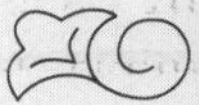 **Research Highlight** 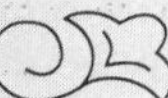

Effect of Childbirth Classes on Obstetric Outcomes

RESEARCH ABSTRACT

The study was designed to assess the effect of childbirth preparation classes on obstetric outcomes. Couples attending classes in a large, inner-city hospital were matched with nonattenders on several variables. Over an 18-month period, 114 women signed up for classes and 83 couples took the entire class series. For this study, 52 couples were eligible; the rest delivered at other hospitals, had cesarean deliveries, or were unable to be matched on the relevant variables. The variables on which groups were matched were age, race, parity, marital status, and client status (public or private). Four matched control subjects were found for each woman. Significant differences between groups were found in use of analgesics and anesthetics during labor and in use of forceps, as well as full-term and preterm births and Apgar scores. Most of the women had an episiotomy. Women accomplished their goals: being in control during labor and birth, using less medication, being better prepared, and enhancing the experience.

IMPLICATIONS FOR PRACTICE

The study demonstrates the effectiveness of childbirth preparation in a clinic population. Previous research has documented its effectiveness in middle-class couples. Efforts should be made to ensure that all women are prepared for childbirth. Significant recruitment efforts may be necessary to convince women of the importance of the classes. Marketing strategies should be devised to promote the classes. In addition, culturally sensitive course content should be included in the classes.

RELATED RESEARCH QUESTIONS

1. What are factors associated with the performance of an episiotomy?
2. What variables are associated with the decision to attend childbirth classes?
3. Are there differences in self-esteem, powerlessness, life stresses, and anxieties between attenders and nonattenders of childbirth education classes?
4. Are couples who attend classes more able to make decisions for themselves than are couples who do not attend classes?

REFERENCE

Hetherington SE: A controlled study of the effect of prepared childbirth classes on obstetric outcomes, *Birth* 17(2):86, 1990.

PPM to the United States in her book, *Thank You, Dr. Lamaze,* which was published in the United States in 1959. PPM combines controlled muscular relaxation and breathing techniques. Active relaxation is an integral part of the Lamaze method (Lamaze, 1970). The woman is taught to relax uninvolved muscle groups (neuromuscular control) while she contracts a specific muscle group. By this process the woman can relax the uninvolved muscles in her body while her uterine musculature contracts. Instead of crying out and losing control during uterine contractions, women are taught to respond with conditioned relaxation and breathing patterns. In 1960 the **American Society for Psychoprophylaxis in Obstetrics (ASPO)** was formed in New York as a national organization to promote use of the Lamaze method and to prepare teachers of the method.

A Denver obstetrician, Robert Bradley, published *Husband-Coached Childbirth* in 1965. In the book he advocates what he calls true "natural" childbirth, without any form of anesthesia or analgesia and with a husband-coach and breathing techniques for labor. The American Academy of Husband-Coached Childbirth (AAHCC) was founded to make the **Bradley method** available and to prepare teachers. This method of partner-coached childbirth uses breath control, abdominal breathing, and general body relaxation. Working in harmony with the body is emphasized (Bradley, 1965). Bradley's technique focuses on environmental variables such as darkness, solitude, and quiet to make childbirth a more natural experience. Women using the Bradley method often appear to be sleeping during labor. However, they are not asleep but simply in a state of deep mental relaxation. The importance of the partner's support is foremost in this method.

Each of these three methods just discussed emphasizes intellectual and physical components. However, the Grantly Dick-Read and Bradley methods emphasize the naturalness of childbirth, whereas Lamaze emphasizes active mental and physical conditioning. Each program educates women to exchange fear of the unknown for confidence and understanding. Adequate prenatal education includes information on maternal adaptation, nutrition, sexuality, and basic hygiene, as well as information on labor and birth. Support for the woman in labor is provided by her husband or another support person chosen by the expectant mother. Specially trained labor attendants termed **monitrices** sometimes provide support for the laboring mother using the Lamaze method.

There is now physiologic evidence that specific breathing techniques (such as breath-holding while pushing) may be harmful to the fetus and have no influence on the progress of the second stage of labor. Fresh approaches to old techniques are being proposed. These emphasize *tuning into the laboring woman's body cues and encouraging her to do what feels natural.* In this holistic approach to childbirth education the emphasis is on how the mind, body, and spirit are related and affect one another.

Recent Trends in Parent Education

A variety of approaches to parent education have evolved as parent educators attempt to meet learning needs (Haire, 1991). In addition to classes designed specifically for pregnant adolescents and their partners and/or parents, classes have begun for other groups with special learning needs such as first-time mothers over 35, single women, adoptive parents, and parents of twins. Refresher classes for parents with children not only review coping techniques for labor and delivery but help couples prepare for sibling reactions and adjustments to a new baby. Cesarean delivery classes are offered for couples who have a scheduled cesarean birth because of breech position or some other predisposing factor. Another specialized class focuses on **vaginal birth after cesarean (VBAC).** This choice is supported by research and clinical trials indicating that many women successfully deliver vaginally after previously giving birth by cesarean (Safrin-Disler, 1990).

Because environmental influences and maternal behavior strongly affect newborn health, many programs encourage women to choose healthy life-styles during pregnancy and early parenting. Preconception and early pregnancy classes (p. 287) support women to adopt nutrition and exercise behaviors that are closely associated with improved pregnancy outcomes and to avoid environmental hazards, smoking, alcohol, and drugs. Women with a developed sense of self-control tend to engage in health-promoting activities during pregnancy (Whitcher, 1989; Lewaller, 1989; Riesch, 1988). Research supports that moderate exercise during the childbearing years has no adverse effects on women otherwise healthy but should be based on ACOG exercise guidelines for pregnancy and the postpartum period (Fishbein, Phillips, 1990). (See box, Chapter 11, p. 286.)

Classes designed to meet the needs of America's growing multiethnic populations are also essential. Classes for new immigrants are particularly effective when taught in native language (i.e., Spanish, Filipino, or Chinese). For classes to be meaningful parent educators must understand the value systems in other cultures and their influence on nutrition, valuing of early prenatal care, maternal weight gain, and infant feeding practices. Parent educators must establish rapport, be understood, and build on cultural

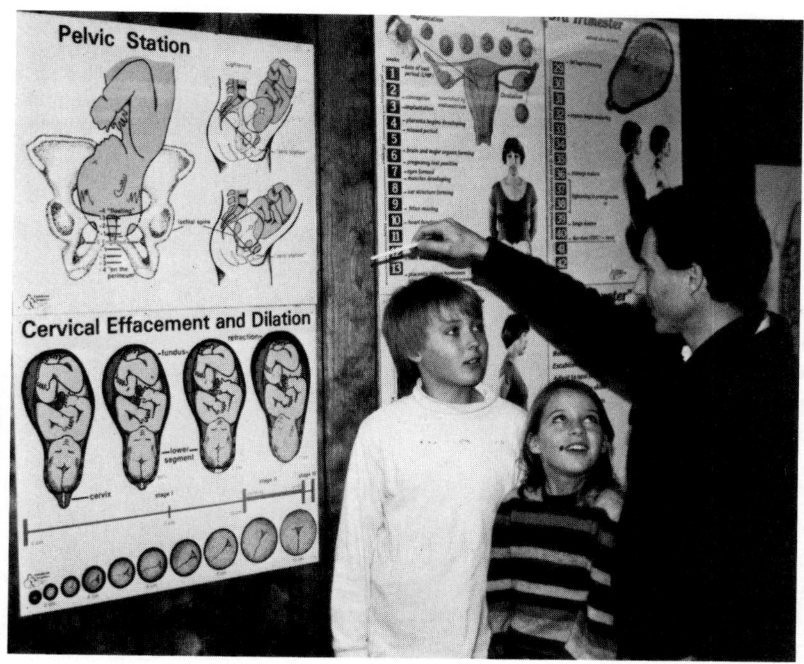

Fig 13-5 Sibling preparation class.
Community Birth Center, Community Hospital, Santa Cruz, Calif.

practices, reinforcing the positive and promoting change only if a practice, such as pica, is directly harmful (USDA, USDHHS, 1990; Waxler-Morrison et al, 1990).

Most parent education classes are attended by the pregnant woman and her partner, although a friend, teenage daughter, or parent may be the designated support person. Because family-centered care has supported the presence of family members at birth, classes have also evolved for grandparents and siblings to prepare them for their attendance at birth and/or the arrival of the baby (Fig. 13-5). Siblings often see a birth film and are helped to learn ways they can help welcome the baby. They also learn to cope with the adjustment, including reduction in parental time and attention (Spadt et al, 1990). Grandparents learn about current child-care practices and how to help their adult children adapt to parenting without being perceived as interfering. Each of these approaches to parent education draws on a variety of strategies for childbirth (discussed in the following section).

Supportive Strategies for Childbirth

PAIN MANAGEMENT. Fear of pain is a key issue for pregnant women and the reason they give for attending parent education classes. Some women do indeed experience childbirth without pain, but most women do not. Although childbirth physicians Dick-Read and Lamaze promised "painless childbirth," numerous studies show that women who have received childbirth preparation report not less pain but less distress from and greater ability to cope with the pain than do unprepared women (Nichols, Humenick, 1988). Physiologic responses to labor pain cause increased respirations and sympathetic nervous system responses that lead to increased cardiac output, elevated blood pressure, and respiratory alkalosis. Increased norepinephrine release blocks oxytocin, decreases contractions, and lengthens labor. Increased anxiety also correlates with increased levels of epinephrine, decreased uterine contractility, and longer labor (Lederman et al, 1978).

Pain management strategies are an essential component of childbirth education. Research is inconclusive on the pros and cons and potential side effects of pain medication during labor. Couples need information about the types of analgesia and regional anesthesia commonly used during labor. There are times when the woman or couple will choose not to cope with labor and will request analgesia or anesthesia (total or partial). Neither partner need feel guilty should pain medication be required during a particular labor experience. However, an emphasis on nonpharmacologic pain management strategies also helps couples manage the labor and birth with dignity and increased comfort. At present, most instructors are teaching a flexible approach, which helps couples learn and master many techniques that can be used with flexibility during labor. Women are encouraged to incorporate their natural responses into coping with the pain of labor and birth. Couples are taught gate-control techniques such as massage, pressure on palms or soles of feet, hot compresses to the perineum, perineal massage, applications of heat or cold, breathing patterns, and focusing as ways to increase coping and decrease the distress from labor pain. For a discussion of **gate-control theory,** see Chapter 15.

Valuable tools the couple can incorporate include vocalization or "sounding" to relieve tension during pregnancy and labor, subdued lighting, and the use of warm water for showers or bathing during labor. Some hospitals have added Jacuzzi bathtubs to good effect (Aderhold, Perry, 1991) (see Chapter 17).

Childbearing couples are also taught to recognize labor's start and to practice coping skills such as relaxation, slow breathing, and other nonpharmacologic strategies.

RELAXATION. Relaxation is a technique promoted by the three major philosophies—those of ICEA, ASPO/Lamaze, and Bradley. The relaxation response counters the effects of sympathetic nervous system arousal. It also produces a balance between the sympathetic and parasympathetic systems, slowed heart and breathing rates, increased uterine contractility, and a sense of security and tranquility. Learning relaxation in prepared childbirth classes can help couples throughout the stresses of pregnancy, labor and birth, and adjustment to parenting, as well as stress management throughout life. To be effective, varied relaxation techniques must be incorporated into every parent education class session. When couples work together to learn relaxation, they also increase communication skills. For example, through massage with a light touch to encourage relaxation, they learn to give each other positive reinforcement, and enhance their sense of being a team (Shrock, 1984). The following are types of relaxation taught (Fig. 13-6).

PACED BREATHING. This is the technique most associated with prepared childbirth. The ASPO/Lamaze, ICEA, and Bradley methods encourage the couple to utilize breathing and relaxation patterns that work best for them. In the 1960s ASPO/Lamaze used a "cookbook" approach in which couples were to learn three breathing patterns, one for each phase of labor. Lamaze teachers still teach the slow-paced, modified, and patterned breathing technique but with the understanding that each labor is different and couples need to adapt breathing techniques to their individual birth (see the box on p. 656). Nurses need to be experienced in guiding couples in the application of breathing and relaxation methods during labor and in using pushing techniques for birth that support moaning or non-breath–holding pushing.

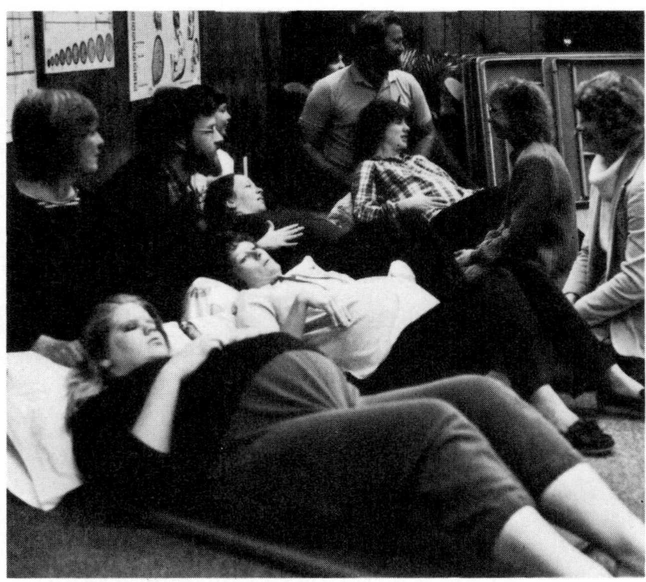

Fig 13-6 Expectant parents attend classes to learn relaxation techniques.
Courtesy Lisa Livingston, Maternal Child Health Education, Community Birth Center, Community Hospital, Santa Cruz, Calif.

BIOFEEDBACK. This technique is often taught in prepared childbirth classes to help couples develop awareness of their bodies and to learn strategies to change the physiologic response. In other words, if the woman responds to pain during a contraction with tightening muscles, frowning, moaning, and breath holding, her partner uses verbal and touch feedback to help her relax. The electronic fetal monitor also can be a tool to help the woman know when a contraction is starting, when the peak is over, and when the contraction has eased so that she can maintain relaxation through all phases of the contraction.

THERAPEUTIC TOUCH. Therapeutic touch is used during labor to decrease anxiety and pain and to increase relaxation. Therapeutic touch requires a subjective, intuitive approach and may be taught by having the partners first experience their own energy field between their palms. Then they learn the phases of centering, assessing differences of energy flow across the body, unruffling the field, and directing energy (usually over the uterus or back) to restore harmony (Nichols, Humenick, 1988).

ACUPRESSURE. This is another relaxation method that is receiving attention in prepared childbirth classes. Acupressure, which consists of applying pressure to various pressure points, has been correlated with relief of dizziness, headaches, back pain, leg cramps, and labor pain (Nichols, Humenick, 1988). A recent controlled clinical trial testing the efficacy of acupressure wrist bands for relief of nausea in early pregnancy found that 75% of subjects felt relief from nausea and its associated anxiety, depression, and other negative effects (Hyde, 1989).

Research on the use of *imagery* is scant, but clinical reports indicate that imagery and visualization can be used to produce a sense of well-being during pregnancy and to assist with cervical dilatation and to decrease the experience of pain and tension during labor. Imagery utilizes techniques such as imagining a walk through a restful garden or breathing in light, energy, and healing color and breathing out worries and tension (Nichols, Humenick, 1988). The woman also can be taught to transform the throbbing or sensation of pain during a contraction into a pleasant, warm feeling while visualizing cervical dilatation during labor. However, no more than two 20-minute sessions a day should be used, and women with psychotic or prepsychotic conditions should not use imagery (Bressler, 1979).

Finally, *music* provides relaxation and has been known for centuries to be therapeutic (Kershner, Schenck, 1991). Research supports the use of music for enhancing relaxation and reducing pain responses during childbirth. Couples who are introduced to music as a strategy often integrate music with other techniques during labor (Clark et al, 1981; Shea, Davis, 1986).

PROMOTING WELLNESS AND FAMILY HEALTH THROUGH PARENT EDUCATION. In addition to preparing families for childbirth, childbirth educators also promote wellness. Pregnancy is a time of growth during which most couples are open to making changes in eating and life-style habits. Infant care, feeding and stimulation, and couple and family adjustments are also incorporated into many prenatal classes.

PRENATAL/POSTNATAL NUTRITION AND LIFE-STYLE MANAGEMENT. Because most families anticipating a birth are motivated to have a healthy baby, childbirth instructors can promote good nutrition and avoidance of smoking, drinking, and taking street drugs. Having couples keep a 24-hour diet and life-style history, choosing a day's food from a menu, and then comparing their choice with recommended foods for pregnancy are ways to simulate and model healthy pregnancy choices. Pregnant couples need to know expected weight gain guidelines and how the weight is distributed (see Figure 9-2). Fathers-to-be can be encouraged to help their partner make healthy choices for meals and snacks, and to avoid smoking, drugs, and alcohol during the pregnancy.

COUPLE RELATIONSHIP AND SEXUALITY. Pregnancy is a time when the couple relationship can be strengthened or stressed (Aaronson, 1989). Pregnancy, birth, and parenthood are major developmental tasks that move the couple from being a twosome to becoming a family. In addition to the physical changes during pregnancy, the pregnant woman and her partner face significant emotional, social, and cognitive changes. Expectant fathers/partners often experience weight gain and nausea. They also are concerned about finances, their role as a father, sexuality, and the child's effect on the couple's relationship. Fathers/partners often worry about their role during childbirth classes, and during labor and delivery, as well as the safety of their partner and baby during the birth (Shapiro, 1987; Nichols, Humenick, 1988). Both the pregnant woman and her partner need an assessment of the symptoms and changes they are experiencing and their individual coping styles (Drake et al, 1988). Helping couples acknowledge the many changes they are experiencing and teaching them exercises and skills to keep the lines of communication open enhance the couple's relationship.

INFANT CARE AND FEEDING. Childbearing couples who have grown up in large families or have had exposure to infants from baby-sitting or careers in nursing, early childhood, or medicine may be aware of the care and feeding demands of a newborn infant. Many couples, however, express concern about learning infant care and feeding techniques (Bliss-Holtz, 1988). Although many women by the third trimester have already chosen a method of feeding, parent education classes provide an opportunity to inform couples of the pros and cons of breast- versus bottle-feeding, the basic techniques of each, and resources for support or information once they are home with the baby. Parent educators also have an opportunity to introduce environmental issues with new families such as the effects of disposable diapers (Primomo et al, 1990). Many communities now have support or new parents' groups that are helpful to couples making the transition to parenthood. Besides the routine mother-baby classes after birth, a few hospitals have begun to offer daddy-baby classes where new fathers spend 1 to 2 hours with their baby and a nurse educator learning about their baby's unique characteristics and the basics of infant care. Fathers introduced to their newborns through the Brazelton assessment scale seem to become more aware of their infant's abilities, which sets the stage for interaction (Beal, 1989).

INFANT STIMULATION AND MASSAGE. Many parents still have outdated beliefs about their infant's capabilities, such as believing that babies do not see and hear until 4 to 6 weeks of age, much like newborn kittens and puppies. Because the senses are the primary source of information for babies during the first 6 months of life, childbirth educators can help parents acquire the knowledge to facilitate successful parenting (Broussard, Rich, 1990). Infant massage is another therapy that parents-to-be can learn to soothe and comfort the infant, to promote relaxation and less irritability and crying, and to provide a mechanism for positive interaction between parent and infant (Chapter 25).

FAMILY ADJUSTMENTS TO PARENTHOOD. The addition of a baby brings change to all members of the family. The workload increases significantly as parents add the demands of the new infant to their other responsibilities. Childbirth educators help parents-to-be anticipate these changes through the family workload exercise, which facilitates dividing the responsibilities after birth (Starn, 1990).

Because so often both partners work outside the home, a discussion about negotiating maternity leave and plans for returning to work is important. Couples who do not have family or friends available for child care need to find a competent sitter. Resource lists of licensed child-care providers and federal and state guidelines regarding rights to maternity leaves are important sources of information. Couples also need information about emotional and physiologic recovery from childbirth, as well as adaptation to parenthood. This knowledge leads to realistic planning rather than the expectation that the mother will be ready to work 1 week after the baby is born.

Siblings (Spadt et al, 1990) and grandparents also experience transitions when a new baby enters the family. Parents need to know about sibling regression and ways to help older children adapt to a new brother or sister. Sibling classes that show a birth film and help the children talk about the changes that are apt to occur, such as Mommy being busy with the baby, offer valuable interventions. Grandparents also benefit from classes that help them learn strategies for assisting the couple's transition to parenthood. Grandparents can be a valuable asset by helping with household chores and the care of older siblings and by providing social support. Grandparents who insist on caring for the baby instead of allowing the new parents time with their baby, who criticize the parents' caretaking, or question whether the baby is being adequately breast-fed undermine the new parents' adjustment. Grandparents can also benefit by learning about infant stimulation and child-rearing practices that have changed since they had young infants.

Parent education is important for families as they prepare for birth and parenting. Nurses certified as parent educators have the background and knowledge to provide excellent instruction in their classes for childbearing couples. Nurses in practice with knowledge of educational strategies can help empower families and reinforce their coping abilities during pregnancy, childbirth, and parenting.

■ BIRTH-SETTING CHOICES

The concept of family-centered maternity care is implemented in birth rooms or **alternative birth centers** (ABCs) in the hospital. Hospital ABCs, as well as freestanding birth centers, are intended to offer families an alternative to home birth, providing a compromise between hospital and home. These **birth-setting choices** have been shown to be safe alternatives to birth in a traditional delivery setting (Mann, 1981; Marieskind, 1980). In addition, they can be designed to ensure quality control and to be cost effective, two significant issues in the delivery of health care today. Women consider a variety of factors in choosing a setting for childbirth (see Research Highlight, p. 341).

Alternative Birth Centers

ABCs usually are located in hospital suites away from the traditional obstetrics department. They are close to the delivery and operating rooms and medical or neonatal intensive care facilities for use when serious problems arise.

ABCs have homelike accommodations, including a double bed for the couple and a crib for the newborn. Emergency equipment and drugs are discreetly stored within cupboards, out of view but easily accessible. Private bathroom facilities are incorporated into each birth center. There may be an early labor lounge or living room and small kitchen. There is careful screening of each applicant so that the ABC can rule out women with risk factors (see Chapter 27). Only low-risk and prepared women or couples are accepted.

The family is admitted to the ABC, labors there, and gives birth there. Members may remain there until discharge if the time interval and requirements for room use permit. If the family has to remain in the hospital for more than 24 hours after delivery, the demand for use of the ABC by other families may require transfer of the first family to a regular postpartum room.

Labor, Delivery, Recovery, Postpartum (Birthing) Rooms

Labor, delivery, recovery (LDR) and **labor, delivery, recovery, postpartum** (LDRP) **rooms** offer families a comfortable, private space for childbirth. Unlike ABCs in hospitals, there are few admission or risk criteria for the use of these rooms.

Some hospitals incorporate labor support by highly trained nurses, or monitrices. Women labor, give birth, and spend the first bonding time with their families in the LDR room. If they are not in an LDRP

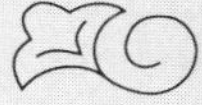 **Research Highlight** 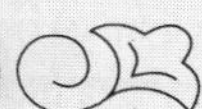

Women's Choice of Childbirth Setting

RESEARCH ABSTRACT

The purpose of this study was (1) to identify reasons for choosing a physician and a hospital for childbirth and for selecting or not selecting a birthing room and (2) to document the results of the decisions. Sixty-one married, multigravid women between 21 and 37 years of age who had been trained in the Lamaze method and who were having a normal pregnancy participated in the study. The women were interviewed twice: at 36 to 38 weeks of gestation while at home and during the postpartum period in the hospital. Data were collected using four data-collection instruments: two semistructured interview guides with questions about choice of caregiver, place of birth, and a description of the childbirth experience; a sociodemographic (vital statistics, e.g., age, education) questionnaire; and an obstetric and infant form. The interviews were tape-recorded, transcribed verbatim, and analyzed. The researcher reported that women gave three reasons for choosing the hospital to give birth: it was the hospital in which their physician practiced, the characteristics of the hospital determined the choice, or it was their place of employment. Physicians were chosen because they were referred by family/friend; by a physician or by a hospital/clinic; or through personal evaluation of the physician. Women chose the birthing room because of its appearance and to avoid transfer to another room, to keep their babies with them, or to allow labor to progress without interference. Other women chose the labor and delivery rooms because of satisfaction with previous births, expectations of complications, or fear of not being checked frequently by the nurses.

IMPLICATIONS FOR PRACTICE

A variety of reasons influence a woman's selection of a hospital, a physician, and the type of birth experience. In this study the reasons women did not choose a birthing room indicated a lack of understanding of the purpose and nature of the birthing room. Some women were influenced by their physician's dislike of the birthing room. To meet the needs of childbearing women, health care providers must be sensitive to the environment women want for childbirth. This may necessitate that hospitals examine their rules and regulations to ascertain whether they are meeting the needs of childbearing women. Unnecessary rules and regulations can be changed to meet the needs of women.

RELATED RESEARCH QUESTIONS

1. Why do physicians dislike birthing rooms?
2. Will an educational program increase understanding of the purpose and nature of a birthing room?
3. Will an educational program increase the use of the birthing room?
4. What type of childbirth environment do women desire?

REFERENCE

Mackey MC: Women's choice of childbirth setting, *Health Care Women Int* 11(2):175, 1990.

room, transfer to a postpartum room is usually the only room change they have to make.

Freestanding Birth Centers

Although most ABCs or LDR/LDRP rooms are located in hospitals, a growing number of **freestanding birth centers** are seen. These units, outside the hospital, are often close to a major hospital so that quick transfer to that institution is possible if necessary.

Most freestanding birth centers are staffed by physicians who have privileges at the local hospital and by certified nurse-midwives who are equipped to attend low risk women through the puerperium. Ambulance service and emergency procedures are readily available. Fees vary with the services provided and the ability of the family to pay (reduced-fee sliding scale). Several insurance companies, as well as Medicaid, recognize and reimburse these clinics.

Services provided by the freestanding birth centers include those necessary for safe management during the childbearing cycle. There are some significant additions, however. Attendance at childbirth and parenting classes is required of all clients. Prenatal supervision of the woman, whose nutritional and health status must be good and who must be experiencing a low-risk pregnancy, begins in the first trimester. All clients must be familiar with situations requiring transfer to a hospital. Each expectant family identifies its *birth plan,* an explanation of practices and procedures they would like to include in or exclude from their childbirth experience.

Birth centers usually have available a lending library, reference files on related topics, recycled maternity clothes and baby clothes and equipment, and supplies and reference materials for childbirth educators. The centers have referral files for community resources that offer services relating to childbirth and early parenting, including support groups (such as single parents, postdelivery support group, parents of twins), genetic counseling, women's issues, and consumer action.

Home Birth

Home birth has always been popular in certain advanced countries, such as Sweden and The Netherlands. In developing countries, hospitals or adequate lying-in facilities often are unavailable to most pregnant women, and home birth is a necessity. In North America home birth is gaining popularity.

National groups supporting home birth are the Home Oriented Maternity Experience (HOME) and the National Association of Parents for Safe Alternatives in Childbirth (NAPSAC). These groups support changes toward more humane childbearing practices at all levels, integrating the alternatives for childbirth to meet the needs of the total population.

The literature on childbirth contains excellent statistics on medically directed home birth services with skilled nurse-midwives and medical back-up.

Selective home birth in uncomplicated pregnancies is feasible. However, those women at high risk must be identified during the prenatal period and referred for hospital delivery. In addition, a transport system should be available for transfer of women with suddenly complicated labors to a nearby adequate medical facility.

Although some physicians and nurses support home births that use good medical and emergency back-up systems, many regard this practice as exposing the mother and the fetus to unnecessary danger.

Fig 13-7 Summary of fetal development and maternal events, From *Safe passage: a woman's guide to a healthier pregnancy,* McNeil Consumer Products Co., Fort Washington, Penn.

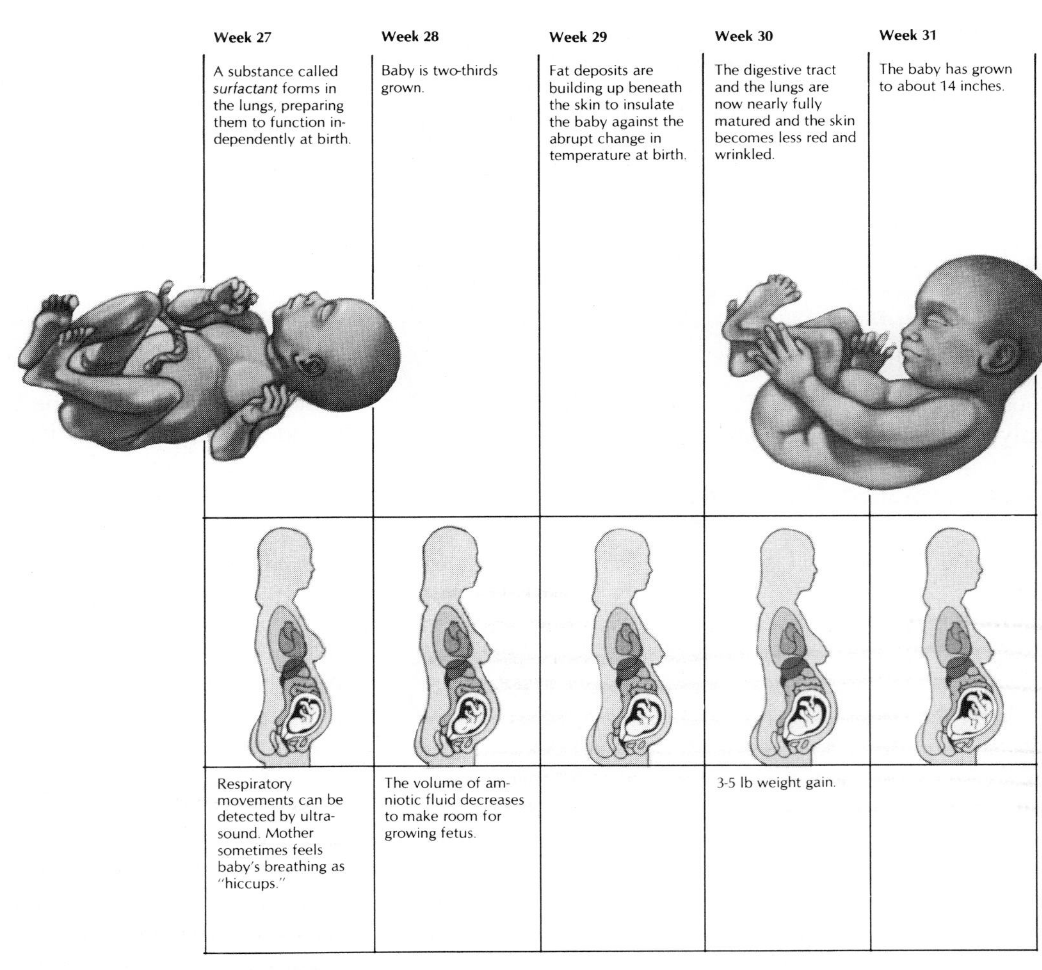

Week 27
A substance called *surfactant* forms in the lungs, preparing them to function independently at birth.
Respiratory movements can be detected by ultrasound. Mother sometimes feels baby's breathing as "hiccups."
Week 28
Baby is two-thirds grown.
The volume of amniotic fluid decreases to make room for growing fetus.
Week 29
Fat deposits are building up beneath the skin to insulate the baby against the abrupt change in temperature at birth.
Week 30
The digestive tract and the lungs are now nearly fully matured and the skin becomes less red and wrinkled.
3-5 lb weight gain.
Week 31
The baby has grown to about 14 inches.

ADVANTAGES. One advantage of home birth is that the birth may be more physiologically natural in familiar surroundings. The mother may be more relaxed than she might be in the impersonal, sterile environment of a hospital. The family can assist in and be a part of the happy event, and mother-father (partner)-infant (and sibling-infant) contact is sustained and immediate. In addition, home birth may be less expensive than a hospital confinement. Serious infection may be less likely, assuming strict aseptic principles are followed. People generally are relatively immune to their own home bacteria.

DISADVANTAGES. Because home births are not generally accepted by the medical community, a family may have difficulty finding a qualified primary care practitioner to give prenatal care and to attend the delivery. Also, back-up emergency care by a physician in a hospital may be difficult to arrange in advance. Further, emergency transfer to a hospital could be life threatening if the hospital were more than a 10-minute distance from the home or if emergency care were not available during the transfer from home to hospital.

CONTRAINDICATIONS. Hospital, not home, birth is indicated for the following women: those with a high-risk pregnancy (fetal or maternal jeopardy) (see Chapter 27), those who cannot be transferred easily to a hospital should the need arise unexpectedly, those who are opposed to home birth, and those women with inadequate home facilities.

FAMILY PREPARATION. If a home birth is planned, it usually will be possible to obtain and store the necessary articles in advance. In contrast, if birth in the home or elsewhere is an emergency or is determined by circumstances beyond control, considerable improvisation may be necessary.

Facilities and supplies can approximate those available in hospitals. The family works closely with the physician, nurse, or midwife to complete prepara-

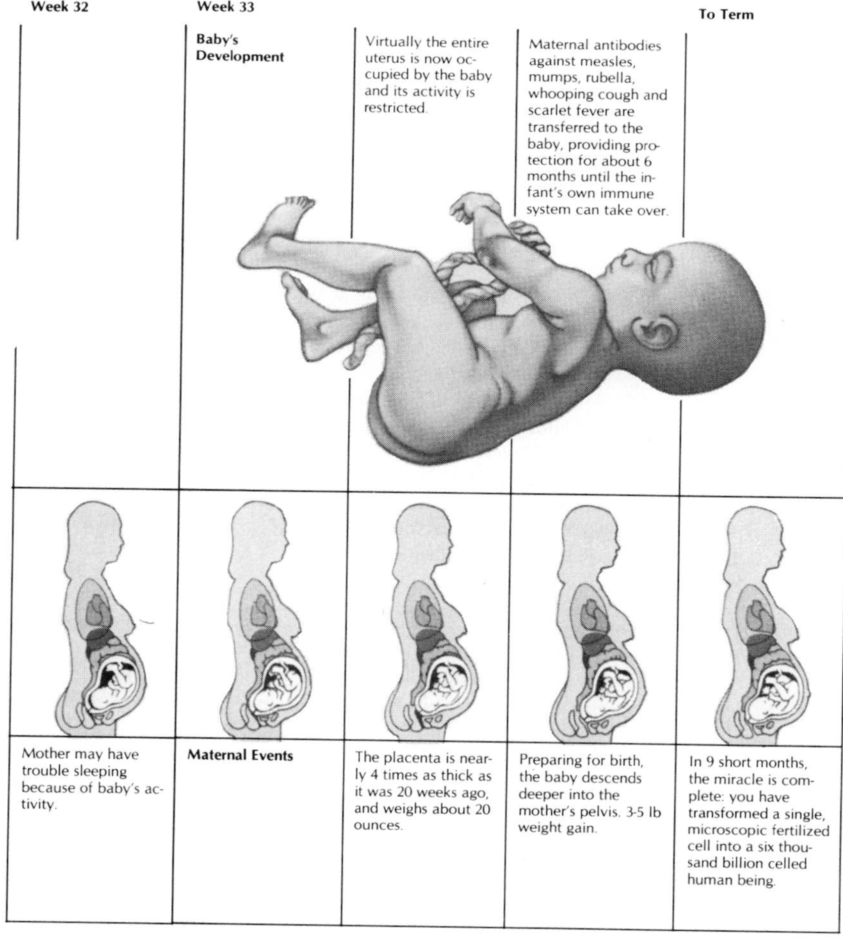
Week 32
Week 33
To Term
Baby's Development
Virtually the entire uterus is now occupied by the baby and its activity is restricted.
Maternal antibodies against measles, mumps, rubella, whooping cough and scarlet fever are transferred to the baby, providing protection for about 6 months until the infant's own immune system can take over.
Mother may have trouble sleeping because of baby's activity.
Maternal Events
The placenta is nearly 4 times as thick as it was 20 weeks ago, and weighs about 20 ounces.
Preparing for birth, the baby descends deeper into the mother's pelvis. 3-5 lb weight gain.
In 9 short months, the miracle is complete: you have transformed a single, microscopic fertilized cell into a six thousand billion celled human being.

tions well in advance of delivery. Attendance by both parents-to-be at parent education classes (prenatal classes for vaginal and abdominal births; instructions about the actual delivery of the child if this should occur before the midwife, physician, or other attendant arrives) adds to the competence and also to the pleasure of the parents and other family members. Classes for siblings and grandparents are recommended.

Detailed descriptions for preparation are required and may be obtained from either the physician's office or from local health agencies. The agencies may provide some of the equipment and supplies.

A visit to the home by the community health nurse is recommended well before the expected date of birth. At that time the process of birth can be discussed, so that all are aware of the characteristics of normal labor and birth, the newborn stage, deviations from normal, and the plan of care for each stage.

Home birth is a selected alternative to hospital birth for some women and couples and a necessity for many. A physically and emotionally safe outcome can be anticipated for most women and couples and their infants, especially if they are prepared and have adequate health care support.

SUMMARY

The prenatal period is one of growth and change in the woman and fetus (Fig. 13-7). The schedule of prenatal visits is designed to monitor the individual woman's pregnancy and responses to care.

During the last trimester, discomforts associated with advancing pregnancy and concerns about the approaching labor preoccupy expectant families.

Assessment for maternal and fetal risk factors continues throughout pregnancy. Prenatal warning signs and recognition of preterm labor are reviewed with each expectant mother and her family. A heightened readiness for learning is experienced by the expectant mother and her family. In addition to individual counseling, parent education classes are available to assist expectant parents as they prepare for transition into parenthood. Consumers learn about birth-setting choices from a variety of sources.

Women experiencing multifetal pregnancy are at risk and require special nursing care to minimize possible complications for themselves and their fetuses.

REFERENCES

Aderhold KJ, Perry L: Jet hydrotherapy for labor and postpartum pain relief, *MCN* 16:97, March/April 1991.

American Society for Psychoprophylaxis in Obstetrics/Lamaze: *Candidate guide: childbirth educator certification program,* Arlington, Va, 1990, The Society ASPO/Lamaze (1840 Wilson Blvd, Arlington, VA 22201).

Beal JA: The effect on father-infant interaction of demonstrating the neonatal behavioral assessment scale, *Birth* 16:22, Jan 1989.

Bonovich L: Recognizing the onset of labor, *JOGNN* 19:141, March/April 1990.

Bradley R: *Husband-coached childbirth,* New York, 1965, Harper & Row.

Bressler D: *Free yourself from pain,* New York, 1979, Simon & Schuster.

Broussard AB, Rich SK: Incorporating infant stimulation concepts into prenatal classes, *JOGNN* 19:381, Sept/Oct 1990.

Clark E, McCorkle R, Williams S: Music therapy–assisted labor and delivery, *J Music Ther* 18:88, 1981.

Cunningham FG, MacDonald RC, Gant NF: *Williams obstetrics,* ed 18, Norwalk, Conn, 1989, Appleton & Lange.

Dick-Read G: *Childbirth without fear,* ed 2, New York, 1959, Harper & Row.

Drake ML, Verhulst D, Fawcett J: Physical and psychological symptoms experienced by pregnant Canadian women and their husbands, *J Adv Nurs* 13(4):439, 1988.

Fanaroff AA, Martin RJ, editors: *Neonatal-perinatal medicine: diseases of the fetus and infant,* ed 5, St Louis, 1991 Mosby–Year Book.

Fishbein EG, Phillips M: How safe is exercise during pregnancy? *JOGNN* 19:47, Jan/Feb 1990.

Haire D: Patient education in childbirth: a long way in forty years, *Int J Childbirth Educ* 6:7, Aug 1991.

Hill WC, Lambertz EL: Let's get rid of the term "Braxton Hicks contractions," *Obstet Gynecol* 75:709, 1990.

Hyde E: Acupressure therapy for morning sickness: a controlled clinical trial, *J Nurse-Midwife* 34:177, July/Aug 1989.

Iams JD, Johnson FF, Creasy RK: Prevention of preterm birth, *Clin Obstet Gynecol* 31:599, Sept 1988.

Johnson FF: Assessment and education to prevent preterm labor, *MCN* 14:157, May/June 1989.

Kershner J, Schenck V: Music therapy–assisted childbirth, *Int J Childbirth Educ* 6:32, Aug 1991.

Lamaze F: *Painless childbirth: the Lamaze method,* Chicago, 1970, Regnery Books.

Lederman R et al: The relationship of maternal anxiety, plasma catecholamines and plasma cortisol to progress in labor, *Am J Obstet Gynecol* 132:495, 1978.

Lewaller LP: Health beliefs and health practices of pregnant women, *JOGNN* 18:246, May/June 1989.

Lindell SG: Education for childbirth: a time for change, *JOGNN* 17:108, March/April 1988.

NAACOG: *Guidelines for childbirth education,* Washington, DC, 1981, NAACOG.

Nichols F, Humenick S: *Childbirth education: practice, research and theory,* Philadelphia, 1988, WB Saunders.

Nicholson W: Midwives, mothers, and breastfeeding, Nunawading, Australia, 1985, Nursing Mothers Association of Australia (5 Glendale St, Nunawading, Victoria 3131, Australia).

Primono J et al: The high environmental cost of disposable diapers, *MCN* 15:279, 1990.

Public Health Service: *Caring for our future: the content of prenatal care.* Washington, DC, 1988, Department of Health and Human Services.

Riesch SK: Changes in the exercise of self-care agency, *West J Nurs Res* 10:272, 1988.

Riordan JM: *A practical guide to breastfeeding,* St Louis, 1983, Mosby–Year Book.

Riesch SK: Changes in the exercise of self-care agency, *West J Nurs Res* 10:272, 1988.

Riordan JM: *A practical guide to breastfeeding,* St Louis, 1983, Mosby–Year Book.

Ross MG et al: Breast stimulation contraction test. Paper presented at the annual meeting of the Society of Perinatal Obstetricians, San Antonio, Feb 2-4, 1984.

San Francisco Chronicle: Immunization strategy to protect newborns: mothers are vaccinated late in pregnancy, Oct 1, 1991.

Scott JR et al: *Danforth's obstetrics and gynecology,* ed 6, Philadelphia, 1990, JB Lippincott Co.

Shapiro JL: *When men are pregnant,* San Luis Obispo, Calif, 1987, Impact Publishers.

Shea E, Davis D: *The perceived effectiveness of music as a relaxation technique in labor,* Unpublished manuscript, 1986.

Shrock P: Relaxation skills: update on problems and solutions, *Genesis* 6:8, 1984.

Spadt SK, Martin KR, Thomas AM: Experiential classes for siblings-to-be, *MCN* 15:184, May/June 1990.

Starn J: Childbirth classroom: labor after birth, *Childbirth Instructor* 1:27, Winter 1991.

Starn JR: Cultural childbearing: beliefs and practices, *Int J Childbirth Educ* 6:38, Aug 1991.

USDA and USDHHS: *Cross-cultural counseling: a guide for nutrition and health counselors,* Washington, DC, 1990, US Government Printing Office.

Wardlaw GM, Insel PM: *Perspectives in nutrition,* St Louis, 1990, Mosby–Year Book.

Wertz R, Wertz D: *Lying in: a history of childbirth in America,* New York, 1979, Schoder Books.

Whitcher S: Preparation for pregnancy: a health promotion program, *Health Values* 13(5):32, 1989.

Worthington-Roberts B, Williams SF: *Nutrition in pregnancy and lactation,* ed 4, St Louis, 1989, Mosby–Year Book.

References—Nursing Research

Aaronson LS: Perceived and received support: effects on health behavior during pregnancy, *Nurs Res* 38:4, Jan/Feb 1989.

Bliss-Holtz VJ: Primiparas' prenatal concern for learning infant care. *Nurs Res* 37:20, Jan/Feb 1988.

Brown MA: Marital support during pregnancy, *JOGNN* 15:475, Nov/Dec 1986a.

Brown MA: Social support, stress and health: a comparison of expectant mothers and fathers, *Nurs Res* 35:72, March/April 1986b.

Herron MA: One approach to preventing preterm birth, *J Perinat Neonat Nurs* 2:33, Jan 1988.

Hetherington S: A controlled study of the effect of prepared childbirth classes on obstetric outcome, *Birth* 17(2):89, 1990.

Patterson ET, Freese MP, Goldenberg RL: Seeking safe passage: utilizing health care during pregnancy, *Image J Nurs Sch* 22:27, Spring 1990.

Safrin-Disler C: Vaginal birth after cesarean, *ICEA Rev* 14(3):9, 1990.

Slager-Earnest SE et al: Effects of a specialized prenatal adolescent program on maternal and infant outcomes, *JOGNN* 16:422, Nov/Dec 1989.

Sturrock WA, Johnson JA: The relationship between childbirth education classes and obstetric outcome, *Birth* 17(2):85, 1990.

BIBLIOGRAPHY

Booth T: Teacher as midwife: facilitating understanding, meaning and mastery in childbirth education, *Int J Childbirth Educ* 6:28, Aug 1991.

Brown S: *Prenatal care: reaching mothers, reaching infants,* Washington, DC, 1988, National Academy Press.

Carter, ER: Quality maternity care for the medically indigent, *MCN* 11:85, March/April 1986.

Chalmers I, Enkin M, Keirse, MJ, (editors): *Effective care in pregnancy and childbirth,* 1989, Oxford, UK, Oxford University Press.

Ericson DL: Territorialism in the health care professions, *Int J Childbirth Educ* 6:31, Aug 1991, (guest editorial).

Gill PJ, Katz M: Early detection of preterm labor; ambulatory home monitoring of uterine activity, *JOGNN* 15:439, Nov/Dec 1986.

Heminki E: Content of prenatal care in the United States: a historic perspective, *Med Care* 26(2):199, 1988.

Honig JC: Preparing preschool-aged children to be siblings, *MCN* 11:37, Jan/Feb 1986.

Horn M, Manion J: Creative grandparents: bonding the generations, *JOGNN* 14:233, May/June 1985.

Increasing culturally relevant practice with Hispanic clients, *NPA Bull* 3:23, Nov/Dec 1988.

Johnson JM: Teaching self-hypnosis in pregnancy, labor, and delivery, *MCN* 5:98, 1980.

Karmel M: *Thank you, Dr. Lamaze,* New York, 1965, Doubleday.

Malasanos L et al: *Health assessment,* ed 4, St Louis, 1990, Mosby–Year Book.

NAACOG: Mother-baby care: *OGN nursing practice resource,* Washington, DC, 1989, NAACOG.

Queenan J, Kimberly L: *Preconception: preparation for pregnancy,* Minneapolis 1989, ICEA Bookcenter, (PO Box 20048, Minneapolis, MI 55420).

Redman BK: *The process of patient education,* ed 6, St Louis, 1988, Mosby–Year Book.

Rooks JP et al: Outcomes of care in birthcenters. The National Birth Center Study, *N Engl J Med* 321:1804, 1989.

Seidel HM et al: *Mosby's guide to physical examination,* ed 2, St Louis, 1991, Mosby–Year Book.

Shapiro JL et al: *The Lamaze ready-reference guide for labor and birth,* Washington, DC, 1989, ASPO Lamaze.

Simchak M: Epidurals still on the rise—is childbirth education necessary anymore? *Int J Childbirth Educ* 6:37, Aug 1991.

Tucker SM et al: *Patient care standards,* ed 4, St Louis, 1988, Mosby–Year Book.

Waxler-Morrison N, Anderson J, Richardson E, editors: *Cross-cultural nursing,* Vancouver, Canada, 1990, University of British Columbia Press.

Bibliography—Nursing Research

Clinton JF: Physical and emotional responses of expectant fathers throughout pregnancy and the early postpartum period, *Int J Nurs Stud* 24:59, Jan 1987.

Cronenwett LR: Network structure, social support, and psychological outcomes of pregnancy, *Nurs Res* 34:93, March/April 1985.

DelGiudice GT: The relationship between sibling jealousy and presence at a sibling's birth, *Birth* 13(4):250, 1986.

Durham L, Collins M: The effect of music as a conditioning aid in prepared childbirth education, *JOGNN* 15:268, 1986.

Fawcett J, Henklein JC: Antenatal education for cesarean birth: extension of a field test, *JOGNN* 16:61, Jan/Feb 1987.

Fawcett J, York R: Spouses physical and psychological symptoms during pregnancy and the postpartum, *Nurs Res* 35:144, July/Aug 1986.

Liu YC: The effects of the upright position during childbirth, *Image J Nurs Schol* 21:14, 1989.

chapter 13 review

Key Concepts

- The quiet period of the second trimester gives way to an active period more oriented to the reality of impending childbirth and parenting responsibilities.
- The psychosocial aspects of care are of paramount importance and may well affect the whole course of pregnancy, childbirth, and the adjustment of the new family.
- The discomforts of pregnancy require sensitive attention and a plan for teaching self-care measures.
- Regardless of the expectant mother's readiness to learn, attention to prebirth preparation is a necessary component of prenatal care.
- Each woman needs to know how to recognize and report preterm labor and other warning signs and symptoms.
- Parent education should be available to all pregnant women and their families in a culturally sensitive format.
- Parent education teaches families stress and pain management strategies that enhance coping during labor and birth.
- Pain and stress management strategies are valuable family tools throughout the life span.
- Parent education strives to promote healthier pregnancies and family life-styles.
- Parent education strives to support and strengthen the couple and family relationships.

Key Terms

- alternative birth centers (ABCs) (p. 340)
- American Society for Psychoprophylaxis in Obstetrics (ASPO) (p. 336)
- birth-setting choices (p. 340)
- Bradley method (p. 336)
- effleurage (p. 326)
- freestanding birth center (p. 341)
- gate-control theory (p. 338)
- Grantly Dick-Read method (p. 335)
- home birth (p. 342)
- International Childbirth Education Association (ICEA) (p. 335)
- labor, delivery, recovery (LDR) room (p. 340)
- labor, delivery, recovery, postpartum (LDRP) room (p. 340)
- Lamaze method (p. 335)
- monitrices (p. 336)
- multifetal pregnancies (p. 331)
- Organization for Obstetric, Gynecologic, and Neonatal Nurses, (NAACOG) (p. 334)
- pinch test (p. 328)
- safe passage (p. 322)
- vaginal birth after cesarean (VBAC) (p. 336)

Critical Thinking Exercises

1. Complete the critical thinking exercise 1 from Chapter 12 with women in their third trimester. Identify similarities and differences, make and check inferences based on data, and evaluate the soundness of your conclusions.
2. Role-play one or more of the following situations and then critique the interactions in a group session:
   a. Assisting an expectant couple in choosing a birth setting (i.e., labor room, home birth).
   b. Teaching a pregnant woman to recognize preterm labor.
3. In a group setting debate the pros and cons of sibling and/or grandparental participation in pregnancy and childbirth. Summarize and critique the conclusions.

Topics for Nursing Research

- How can positive outcomes for childbirth be influenced?
- What is the effect of parent education in strengthening the couple and family relationship?
- What roles of parent educators are the most effective?
- Does knowledge about strategies, options, and choices help expectant parents have a positive birth experience?
- What teaching strategies are the most efficient and for which participants?
- How does attending parent education classes influence early parenting ability?

unit 3

Normal Childbirth

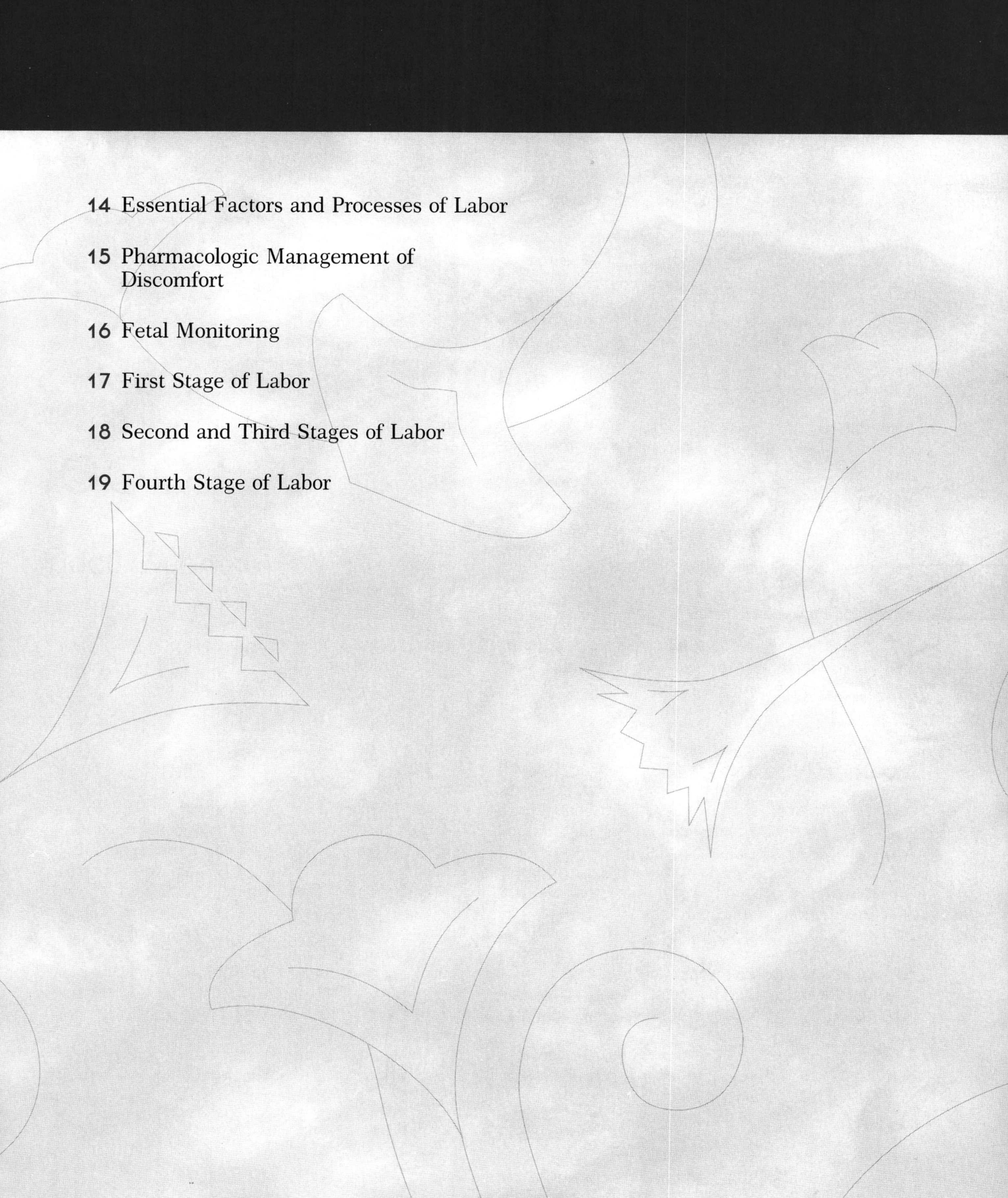

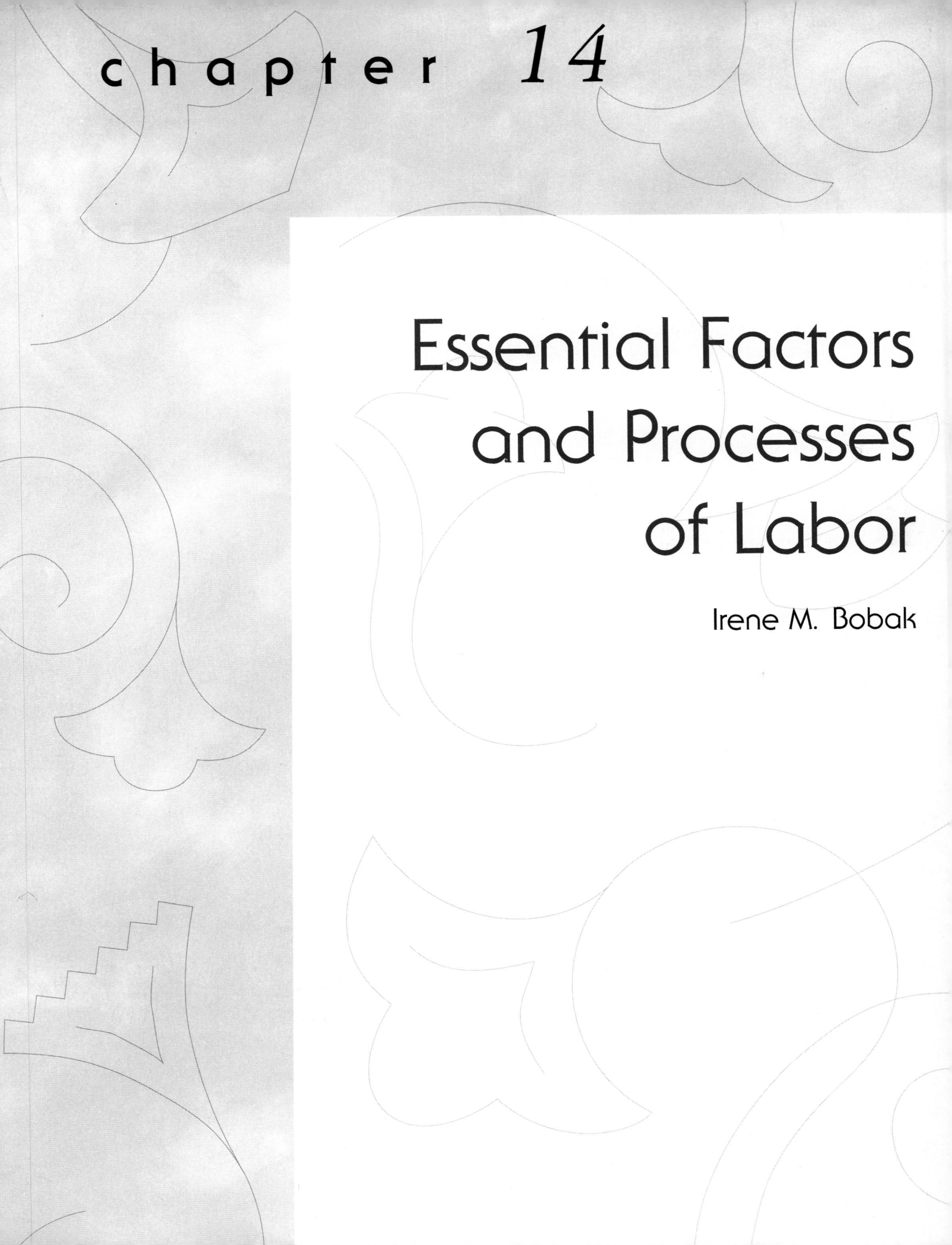

chapter 14

Essential Factors and Processes of Labor

Irene M. Bobak

LEARNING OBJECTIVES

- Correctly define the key terms listed.
- Explain the five essential factors that affect the labor process.
- Describe the anatomic structure of the bony pelvis.
- Differentiate the four types of pelvis.
- Indicate the diameters of the pelvic inlet, cavity, and outlet and also their normal measurements.
- Review the anatomy of the fetal skull and state the normal measurements.
- Summarize the process of molding of the fetal head during labor.
- Describe the cardinal movements of the mechanism of labor.
- Assess the maternal anatomic and physiologic adaptations to labor.
- Describe fetal adaptations to labor.
- Identify topics for nursing research related to essential factors and processes of labor.

During late pregnancy, the mother and the fetus prepare for the labor process. The fetus has grown and developed in preparation for extrauterine life. The mother has undergone various physiologic adaptations during pregnancy that prepare her for the process of birth and the role of motherhood. Labor and delivery represent the end of pregnancy and the beginning of extrauterine life for the newborn infant.

Nurses must understand the essential factors of labor, the process involved, the normal progression of events, and the adaptations made by both the mother and fetus. Once this knowledge is mastered, nurses can proceed to apply the nursing process to each woman and family.

ESSENTIAL FACTORS IN LABOR

Five essential factors affect the process of labor and delivery. These are easily remembered as the five *P*'s: passageway (birth canal), passenger (fetus and placenta), powers, position of the mother, and psychologic response. The first four factors are presented here as the basis of understanding the physiologic process of labor. The fifth factor is discussed in Chapter 10.

Passageway

The **passageway**, or birth canal, is composed of the mother's rigid bony pelvis and the soft tissues of the cervix, pelvic floor, vagina, and introitus (the external opening to the vagina). Although the soft tissues, particularly the muscular layers of the pelvic floor, contribute to delivery of the fetus, the maternal pelvis plays a far greater role in the labor process. The fetus must successfully accommodate itself to this relatively rigid passageway. Therefore the size and shape of the pelvis must be determined before childbirth begins.

BONY PELVIS. The anatomy of the bony pelvis is detailed in Chapter 6. The following discussion focuses on the importance of pelvic configurations as they relate to the labor process. (It may be helpful to refer back to Fig. 6-17.)

The bony pelvis is formed by the fusion of the ilium, ischium, pubis, and sacrum bones. The four pelvic joints are the symphysis pubis, the right and left sacroiliac joints, and the sacrococcygeal joint (Fig. 14-1). The bony pelvis is separated by the brim, or inlet, into two parts: the false pelvis and the true pelvis. The false pelvis is that part above the brim and has nothing to do with childbearing. The true pelvis is divided into three planes: the inlet, or brim; the midpelvis, or cavity; and the outlet.

The pelvic inlet, the upper border of the true pelvis, is formed anteriorly by the upper margins of the pubic bone, laterally by the iliopectineal lines along the innominate bones, and posteriorly by the anterior, upper margin of the sacrum, and the sacral promontory.

The pelvic cavity, or midpelvis, is a curved passage having a short anterior wall and a much longer concave posterior wall. It is bounded by the posterior aspect of the symphysis pubis, the ischium, a portion of the ilium, the sacrum, and the coccyx.

The pelvic outlet is the lower border of the true pelvis. Viewed from below, it is ovoid, somewhat diamond-shaped, bounded by the pubic arch anteriorly, the ischial tuberosities laterally, and the tip of the coccyx posteriorly. In the latter part of pregnancy the coccyx is movable (unless it has been broken in a fall during skiing or skating, for example, and has fused to the sacrum during healing).

The pelvic canal varies in size and shape at various levels. The diameters at the plane of the pelvic inlet, midpelvis, and outlet, plus the axis of the birth canal (Fig. 14-2), determine whether vaginal delivery is possible and the manner by which the fetus may

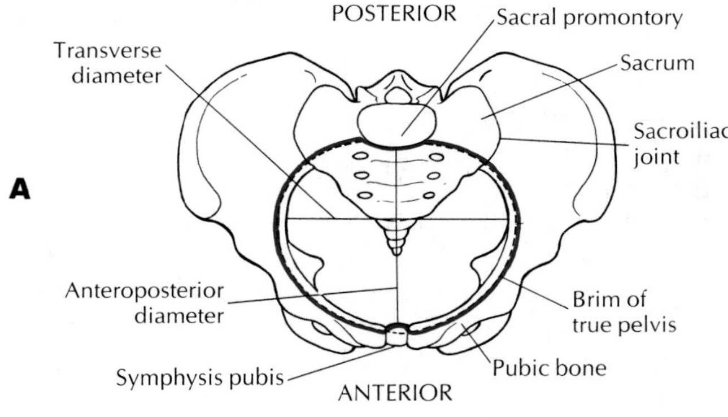

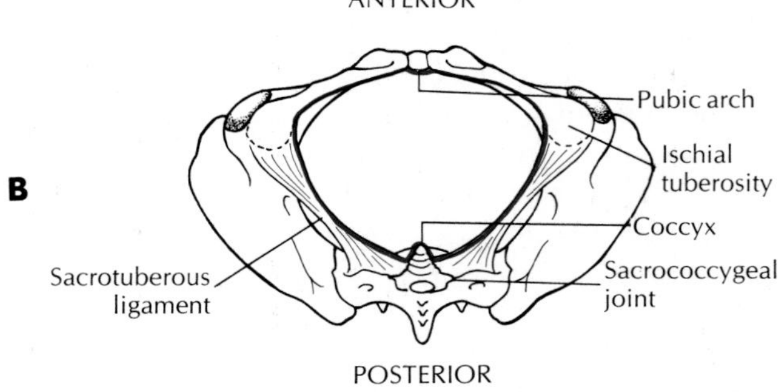

Fig. 14-1 Female pelvis. **A**, Pelvic brim (inlet, linea terminalis, or iliopectineal line) from above. **B**, Pelvic outlet from below.

pass down the birth canal (cardinal movements of the mechanism of labor).

The subpubic angle, which indicates the type of pubic arch, together with the length of the pubic rami and the intertuberous diameter, is of great importance. Because the fetus must first pass beneath the pubic arch, a narrow subpubic angle will be less favorable than a rounded, wide arch. Measurement of the subpubic arch is shown in Fig. 14-3. A summary of obstetric measurements is given in Table 14-1. The most important measurements are depicted in Figs. 14-4 through 14-6, p. 354.

The four basic types of pelvis are classified as follows:

1. Gynecoid (the classic female type)
2. Android (resembling the male pelvis)
3. Anthropoid (resembling the pelvis of anthropoid apes)
4. Platypelloid (the flat pelvis)

The **gynecoid pelvis** is the most common, with major gynecoid pelvic features present in 50% of all women. Significant anthropoid features are present in 24% of women; android configuration occurs in 23%; and the remaining 3% of women have platypelloid pelvic features. Examples of pelvic variations and their effects on mode of delivery are given in Table 14-2 and shown in Fig. 14-7, p. 356. The female and male pelves are compared in Fig. 14-8, p. 356.

Assessment of the bony pelvis may be performed during the first prenatal evaluation and need not be repeated if the pelvis is of adequate size and suitable shape. In the third trimester of pregnancy, the examination of the bony pelvis may be more thorough and the results more accurate because there is relaxation of the pelvic joints and ligaments. The hormones of pregnancy, especially the ovarian hormone progesterone, cause the development of considerable mobility in the pelvic joints. Widening of the joint of the symphysis pubis and instability may cause pain in any or all of the joints.

Because the examiner does not have direct access to the bony structures and because the bones are covered with varying amounts of soft tissue, estimates of size and shape are approximate. Precise bony pelvis measurements can be determined by use of computed tomography, ultrasound, or x-ray films. However, x-ray examination is rarely done because the x-rays may damage the developing fetus (see Appendix E).

SOFT TISSUES. The soft tissues of the passageway include the distensible lower uterine segment, cervix, pelvic floor muscles, vagina, and introitus (external opening to the vagina).

Before labor begins, the uterus is composed of the

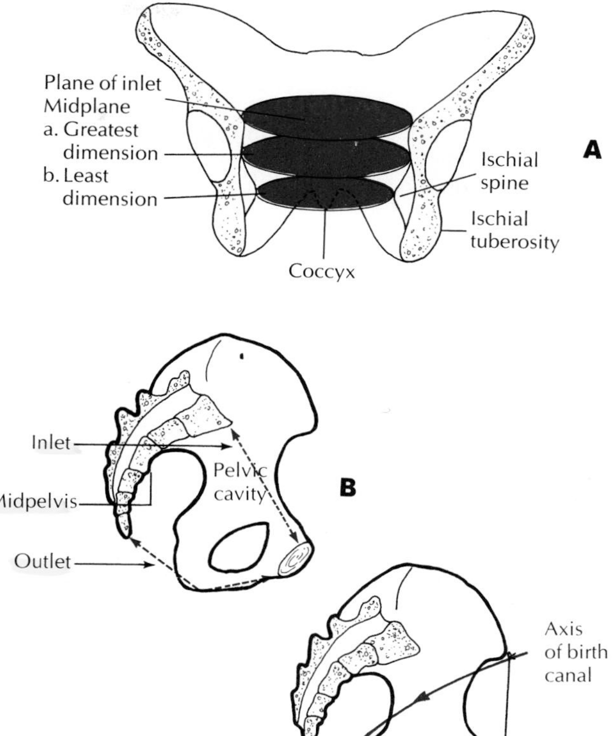

Fig. 14-2 Pelvic cavity. **A,** Inlet and midplane. Outlet not shown. **B,** Cavity of true pelvis. **C,** Note curve of sacrum and axis of birth canal.

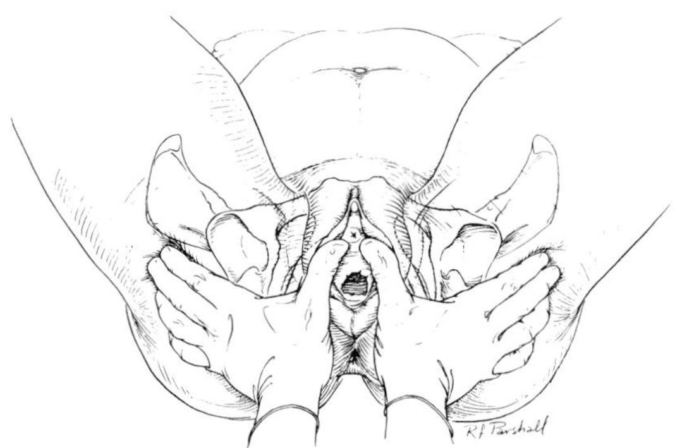

Fig. 14-3 Estimation of angle of subpubic arch. Using both thumbs, examiner externally traces descending rami down to tuberosities.

From Malasanos et al: *Health assessment,* ed 4, St Louis, 1990, Mosby–Year Book.

TABLE 14-1 Obstetric Measurements

Plane	Diameter (cm)	Position
Plane of inlet (superior strait)		
Conjugate diameters		
Diagonal conjugate	12.5-13	From *inferior border* of symphysis pubis to sacral promontory
Obstetric: measurement that determines whether presenting part can engage or enter superior strait	1.5-2 cm less than diagonal (radiographic)	From *posterior surface* of symphysis pubis to sacral promontory (normally ≥ 10 cm)
True (vera) (anteroposterior)	≥11 (12.5) (radiographic)	From *upper margin* of symphysis pubis to sacral promontory
Transverse diameter	≥13	Usually colon obscures this by filling left pelvis
Oblique diameter (right or left)	≥12.75	From sacroiliac joint on one side to opposite iliopectineal prominence
Midplane of pelvis*		
Anteroposterior diameter	≥11.5	From midsymphysis to sacrum (at fused second and third sacral vertebrae)
Transverse diameter (interspinous diameter)	10.5	Narrowest transverse diameter in the midplane
Posterior sagittal diameter	4.5	Segment of anteroposterior diameter dorsal to line between ischial spines; although midplane is comparatively large, critical shortening of interspinous or posterior sagittal diameter of midplane may cause pelvic dystocia
Plane of pelvic outlet†		
Anteroposterior diameter	11.9	From lower border of symphysis pubis to tip of sacrum; coccyx may be displaced posteriorly during labor and is not considered to be a fixed bone
Transverse diameter (intertuberous diameter)	≥8	From inner border of one ischial tuberosity to other
Posterior sagittal diameter	9	Projected from tip of sacrum to a point in space where intertuberous diameter transects anteroposterior projection

*The midplane of the pelvis normally is its largest plane and the one of greatest diameter.
†The outlet presents the smallest plane of the pelvic canal. It encompasses an area including the lower portion of the symphysis pubis, the ischial tuberosities, and the tip of the sacrum.

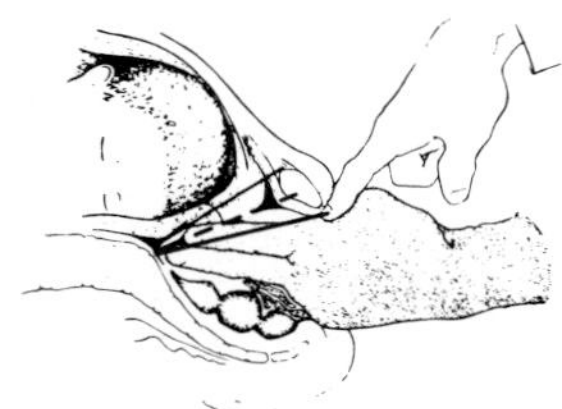

Fig. 14-4 Length of diagonal conjugate *(solid colored line)*, obstetric conjugate *(broken colored line)*, true conjugate *(black line)*.

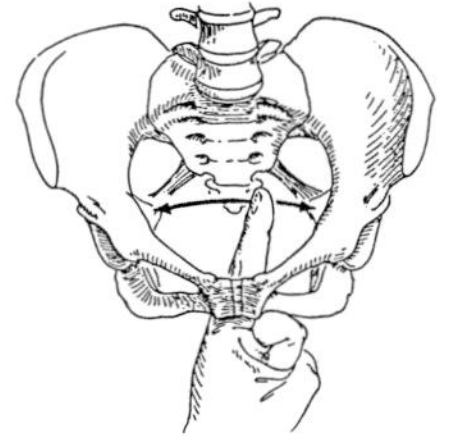

Fig. 14-5 Measurement of interspinous diameter.
From Malasanos et al: *Health assessment*, ed 4, St Louis, 1990, Mosby–Year Book.

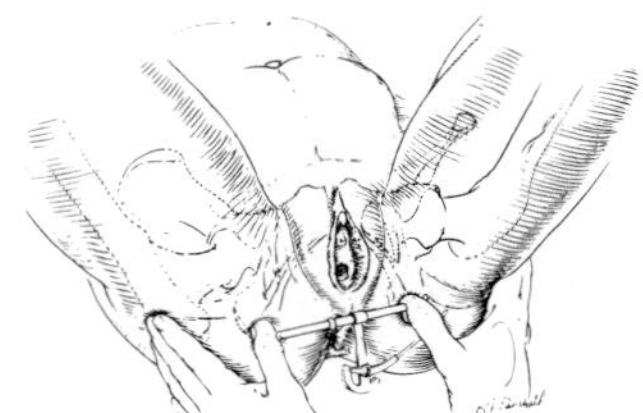

Fig. 14-6 Use of Thom's pelvimeter to measure intertuberous diameter.
From Malasanos et al: *Health assessment*, ed 4, St Louis, 1990, Mosby–Year Book.

TABLE 14-2 Comparison of Pelvic Types

	Gynecoid (50% of Women)	Android (23% of Women)	Anthropoid (24% of Women)	Platypelloid (3% of Women)
Brim	Slightly ovoid or transversely rounded ◯ Round	Heart shaped, angulated ♡ Heart	Oval, wider anteroposteriorly 0 Oval	Flattened anteroposteriorly, wide transversely ⬭ Flat
Depth	Moderate	Deep	Deep	Shallow
Side walls	Straight	Convergent	Straight	Straight
Ischial spines	Blunt, somewhat widely separated	Prominent, narrow interspinous diameter	Prominent, often with narrow interspinous diameter	Blunted, widely separated
Sacrum	Deep, curved	Slightly curved, terminal portion often beaked	Slightly curved	Slightly curved
Subpubic arch	Wide	Narrow	Narrow	Wide
Usual mode of delivery	Vaginal Spontaneous Occipitoanterior position	Cesarean Vaginal Difficult with forceps	Forceps/ spontaneous occipitoposterior or occipitoanterior position	Spontaneous

uterine body (corpus) and cervix (neck). After labor has begun, uterine contractions cause the uterine body to change into a thick and muscular upper segment and a thin-walled passive muscular lower segment. A physiologic retraction ring separates the two segments (Fig. 14-9, p. 357). The lower uterine segment gradually distends to accommodate the intrauterine contents as the wall of the upper segment becomes thick and its accommodating capacity is reduced. Contractions of the uterine body thus exert downward pressure on the fetus, pushing it against the cervix.

The cervix then effaces (thins) and dilates (opens) sufficiently to allow descent of the first fetal portion into the vagina. Actually the cervix is drawn upward and over this first part as it descends.

The pelvic floor is a muscular layer that separates the pelvic cavity above from the perineal space below. This structure helps the fetus rotate anteriorly as it passes through the birth canal. The vagina in turn distends to permit passage of the fetus into the external world. As noted earlier, the soft tissues of the vagina develop throughout pregnancy until at term the vagina can dilate to accommodate the fetus.

Passenger

How the **passenger,** or fetus, moves through the birth canal is a result of several interacting factors: the size of the fetal head, fetal presentation, lie, attitude, and position.

Because the placenta must also pass through the birth canal, it may be considered a passenger along with the fetus. However, the placenta rarely impedes the process of labor in normal delivery. Placenta-related problems are included in the discussion of hemorrhage in Chapter 30.

SIZE OF FETAL HEAD. The fetal head, because of its size and relative rigidity, has a major effect on the birth process. The fetal skull is composed of two parietal bones, two temporal bones, the frontal bone, and the occipital bone (Fig. 14-10, p. 358). These bones are united by membranous sutures: the sagittal, lambdoid, coronal, and frontal. Membrane-filled spaces called **fontanelles** are located where the sutures intersect. During labor, after rupture of membranes, vaginal palpation of fontanelles and sutures identifies fetal presentation, position, and attitude.

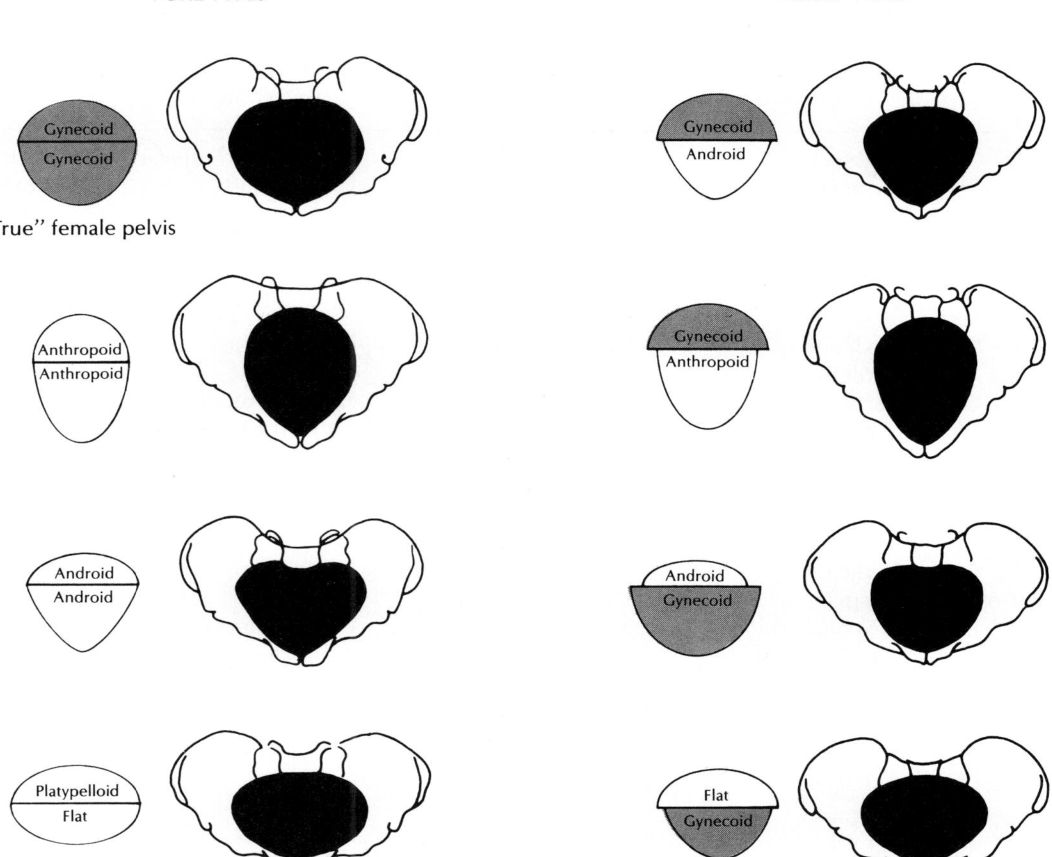

Fig. 14-7 Female pelvis; pure and mixed types. Note differences in shape of inlets.

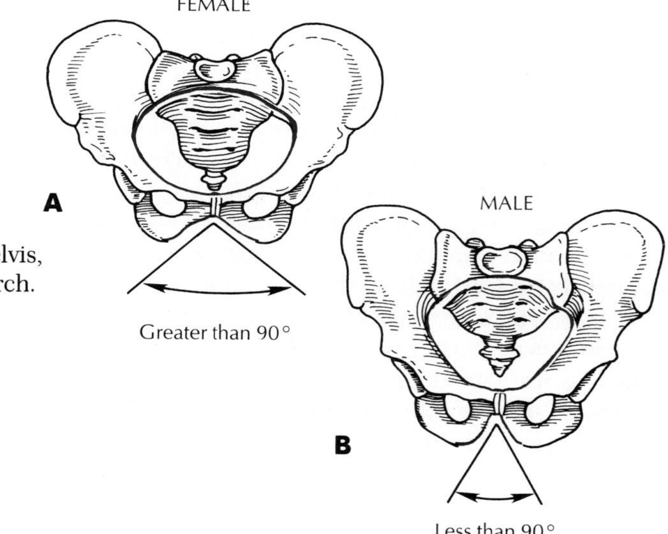

Fig. 14-8 **A**, Gynecoid pelvis, female. **B**, Android pelvis, male. Compare shape of brim and angle of subpubic arch.

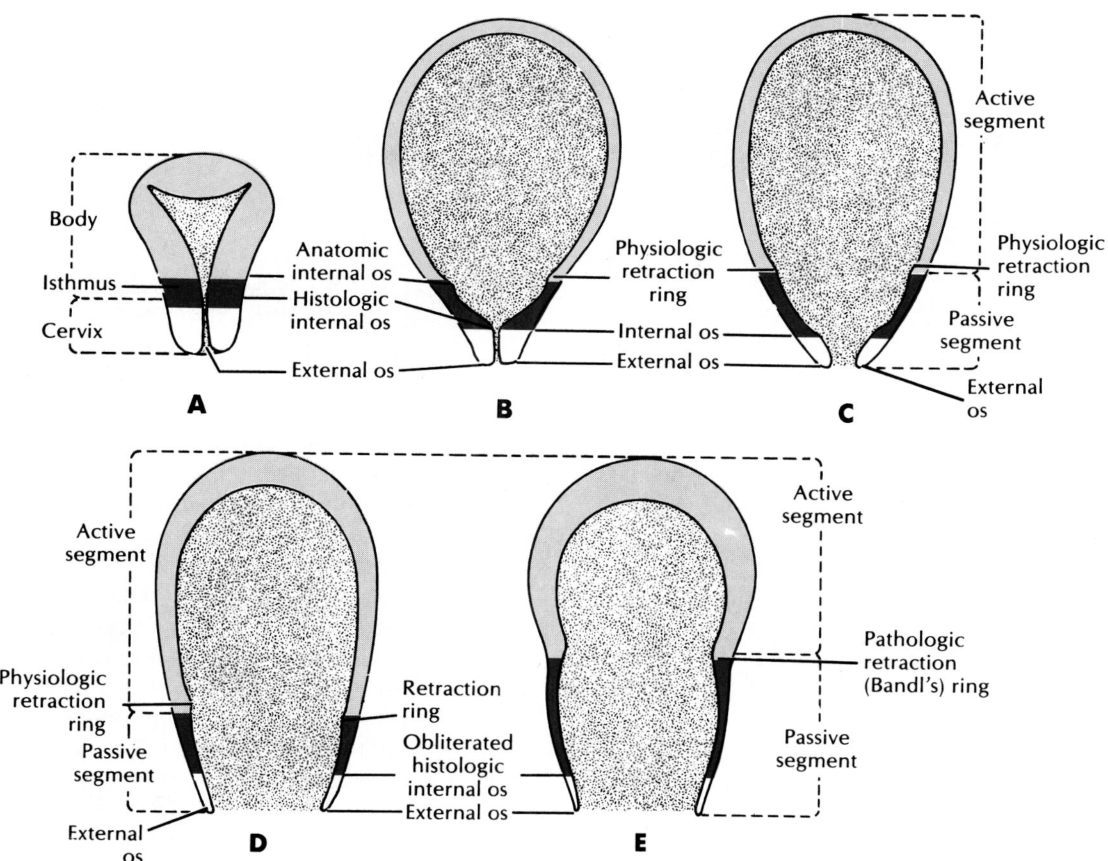

Fig. 14-9 Progressive development of segments and rings of uterus at term. Note differences in (**A**), nonpregnant uterus, (**B**), uterus at term and uterus in normal labor in early first stage (**C**), and second stage (**D**). Passive segment is derived from lower uterine segment (isthmus) and cervix, and physiologic retraction ring is derived from anatomic internal os. **E**, Uterus in abnormal labor in second-stage dystocia. Pathologic retraction (Bandl's) ring that forms under abnormal conditions develops from physiologic ring.
Modified from Willson JR et al: *Obstetrics and gynecology,* ed 9, St Louis 1991, Mosby–Year Book.

Assessment of their size reveals information about the age and well-being of the newborn.

The two most important fontanelles are the anterior and posterior fontanelles. The larger of these, the anterior fontanelle, or **bregma,** is diamond-shaped and lies at the junction of the sagittal, coronal, and frontal sutures. It ossifies by 18 months of age. The posterior fontanelle lies at the junction of the sutures of the two parietal bones and the one occipital bone and is therefore triangular in shape. It closes 6 to 8 weeks after birth.

The presence of sutures and fontanelles gives the skull flexibility to accommodate the infant brain, which continues to grow for some time after birth. Because the bones are not firmly united, however, slight overlapping of the bones, or **molding** of the shape of the head, occurs during labor. Molding can be extensive, but with most newborns the head assumes its normal shape within 3 days of birth. This capacity of the bones to slide over one another also permits adaptation to the various diameters of the maternal pelvis.

Although the size of the fetal shoulders may affect passage, their position can be altered relatively easily during labor, so that one shoulder may occupy a lower level than the other. This creates a smaller shoulder diameter for negotiating the passageway. The circumference of the fetal hips is usually small enough not to create problems.

FETAL PRESENTATION. **Presentation** refers to the part of the fetus that enters the pelvic inlet first and

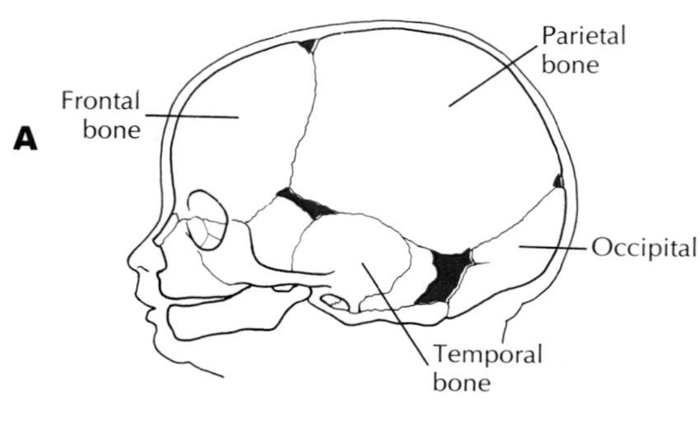

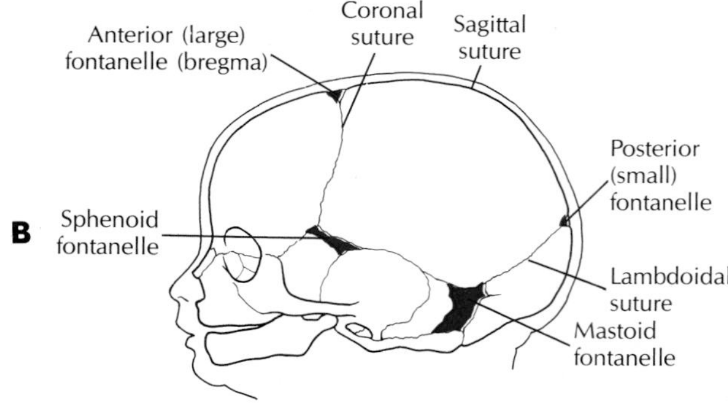

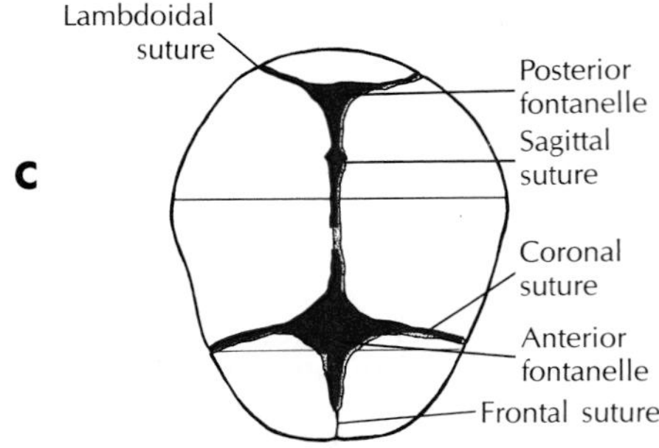

Fig. 14-10 Fetal head at term. **A**, Bones. **B**, and **C**, Sutures and fontanelles.

leads through the birth canal during labor at term. The three main presentations are cephalic (head first), 96% (Fig. 14-11); breech (buttocks first), 3%; and shoulders, 1% (Fig. 14-12, *D*, p. 360). **Presenting part** refers to that part of the fetal body first felt by the examining finger during a vaginal examination. Factors that determine the presenting part include fetal lie, fetal attitude, and extension or flexion or the fetus's head, which are discussed next.

FETAL LIE. **Lie** is the relationship of the long axis (spine) of the fetus to the long axis (spine) of the mother. There are two lies: longitudinal, or vertical, in which the long axis of the fetus is parallel with the long axis of the mother; and transverse, or horizontal, in which the long axis of the fetus is at a right angle to that of the mother (Fig. 14-12, *D*). Longitudinal lies are either cephalic or sacral (breech) presentations, depending on the fetal structure that first enters the mother's pelvis. An oblique or unstable lie converts to a longitudinal or transverse lie early in labor.

FETAL ATTITUDE. **Attitude** is the relationship of the fetal body parts to each other. The fetus assumes characteristic posture (attitude) in utero partly because of the mode of fetal growth and partly because of accommodation to the shape of the uterine cavity. Normally, the back of the fetus is markedly flexed: the head is flexed on the chest, the thighs are flexed at the knee joints, and the arches of the feet rest on the anterior surface of the legs; this attitude is called *general flexion*. The arms are crossed over the thorax, and the umbilical cord lies between the arms and the legs.

Deviations from the normal attitude may cause difficulties in delivery. For example, in a head-first delivery, the fetal head may be extended or flexed in a manner that presents a head diameter unfavorable to the limits of the maternal pelvis. In a cephalic presentation, measurements of the fetal head can be a good way to assess the degree of extension or flexion.

The **biparietal diameter** is the largest transverse diameter (Fig. 14-13, *B*, p. 361). Of the anteroposterior diameters shown, it can be seen that the attitudes of flexion or extension allow diameters of differing sizes to enter the maternal pelvis. With the head in complete flexion, the **suboccipitobregmatic diameter** (the smallest diameter) enters the true pelvis easily, (Figs. 14-13, 14-14, *A*, p. 361).

FETAL POSITION. The presentation or presenting part indicates that portion of the fetus that overlies the pelvic inlet. In a **cephalic presentation,** the presenting part is usually the occiput (O); in a **breech presentation,** it is the sacrum (S); in the transverse lie, the presenting part is the scapula (Sc) of the shoulder. When the presenting part is the occiput, the presentation is noted as **vertex** (Figs. 14-11; 14-13, *A*; and 14-14, *A*).

Position is the relationship of the presenting part (occiput, sacrum, mentum [chin], or sinciput [deflexed vertex], to the four quadrants of the mother's pelvis (Fig. 14-11). Position is described in abbreviated form determined by the first letter of each key word. For example, right occipitoanterior position is written as ROA; right occipitotransverse is abbrevi-

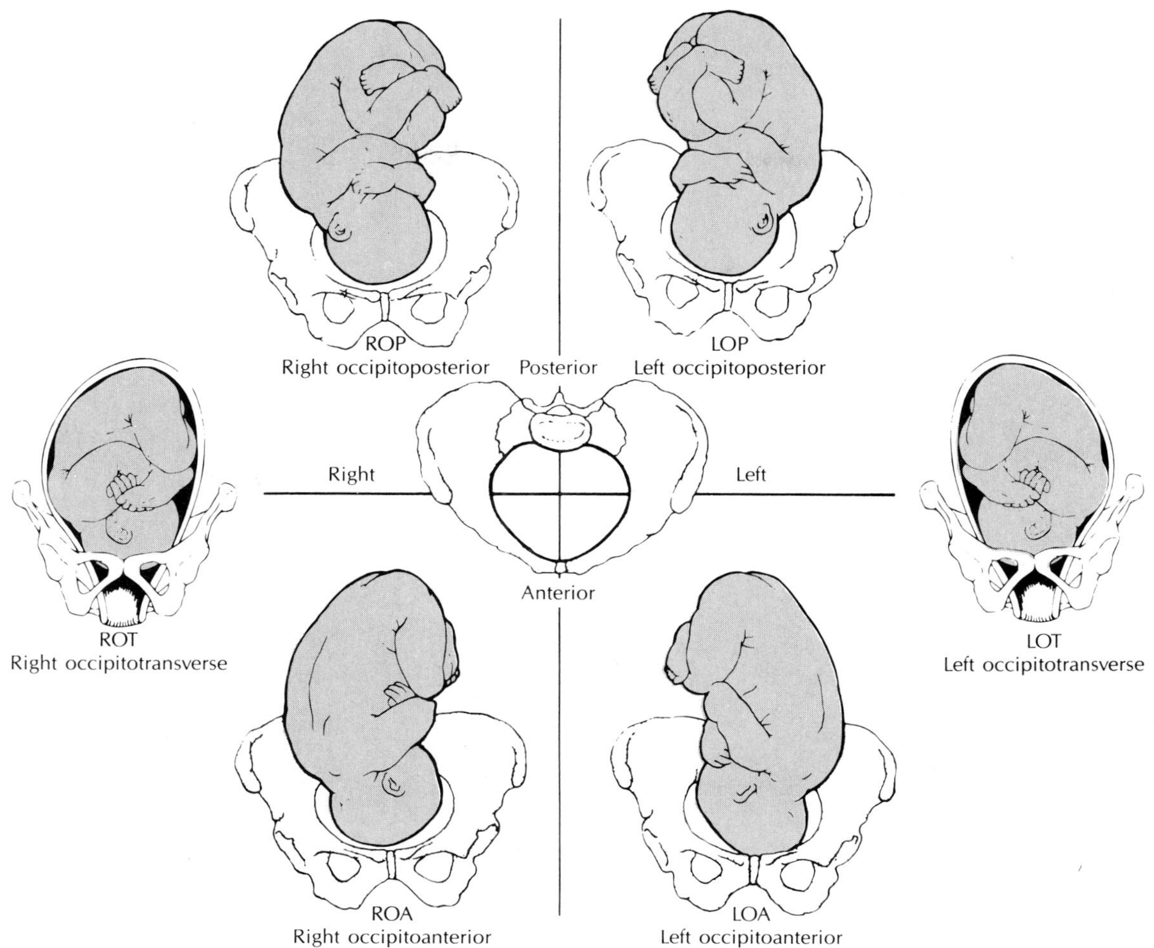

Fig. 14-11 Examples of fetal vertex (occiput) presentations in relation to front, back, or side of maternal pelvis.
Modified from Iorio J: *Childbirth: family-centered nursing,* ed 3, St Louis, 1973, Mosby–Year Book.

ated as ROT (Fig. 14-11).

Engagement indicates that the largest transverse diameter of the presenting part has passed through the maternal pelvic brim or inlet into the true pelvis. In a well-flexed cephalic presentation, the biparietal diameter (9.25 cm) is the widest (Fig. 14-14, *A*). Engagement can be determined by abdominal or vaginal examination.

Station is the relationship of the presenting part of the fetus to an imaginary line drawn between the maternal ischial spines. Station is expressed in terms of centimeters above or below the spines. For example, when the presenting part is 1 cm above the spines, it is noted as being −1 (Fig. 14-15, p. 361). At the level of the spines, the station is referred to as zero.

When the presenting part is 1 cm below the spines, however, the station is said to be +1. Birth is imminent when the presenting part is at +4 to +5 cm. For accurate documentation of the rate of descent of the fetus during labor, the station of the presenting part should be determined when labor begins.

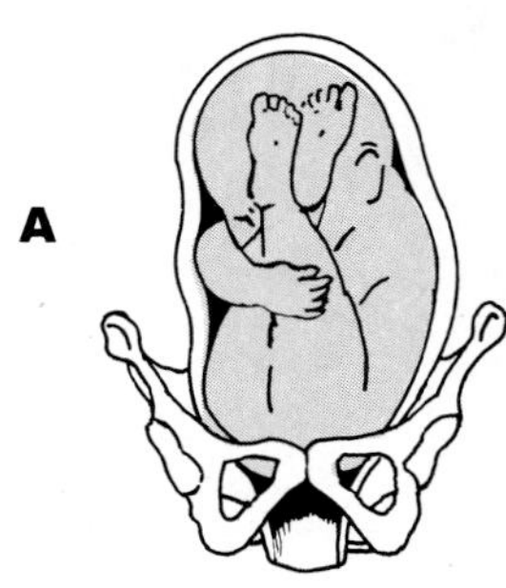

Frank breech

Lie: Longitudinal or vertical
Presentation: breech (incomplete)
Presenting part: sacrum
Attitude: flexion, except for legs at knees

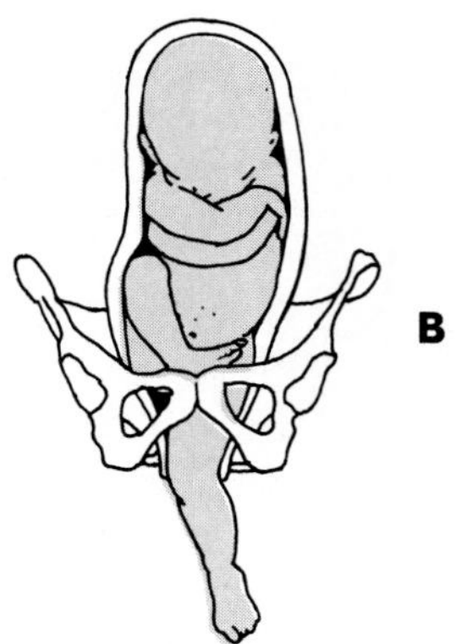

Single footling breech

Lie: Longitudinal or vertical
Presentation: breech (incomplete)
Presenting part: sacrum
Attitude: flexion, except for one leg extended at hip and knee

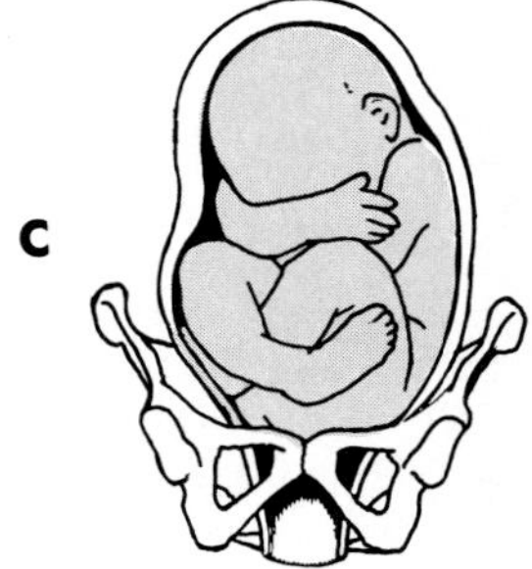

Complete breech

Lie: Longitudinal or vertical
Presentation: breech (sacrum and feet presenting)
Presenting part: sacrum (with feet)
Attitude: general flexion

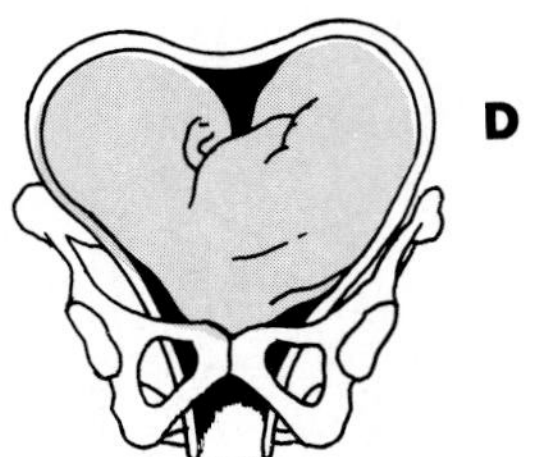

Shoulder presentation

Lie: Transverse or horizontal
Presentation: shoulder
Presenting part: scapula (Sc)
Attitude: flexion

Fig. 14-12 Fetal presentations. **A** to **C**, Breech (sacral) presentation. **D**, Shoulder presentation.

Powers

Involuntary and voluntary contractions by the mother combine to expel the fetus and the placenta out of the uterus. Involuntary uterine contractions, called the *primary* **powers,** signal the beginning of labor. Once the cervix has dilated, voluntary bearing-down efforts, called the *secondary* powers, augment the force of the involuntary contractions.

PRIMARY POWERS. The involuntary contractions originate at certain pacemaker points in the thickened muscle layers of the upper uterine segment. From the pacemaker points, contractions move downward over the uterus in waves, separated by short rest periods. Terms used to describe these involuntary contractions include frequency (the time between contractions—specifically, the time between the beginning of one contraction and the beginning of the next); duration (length of contraction); and intensity (strength of contraction). The following is a description of the primary forces from Willson et al (1991).

> The ultimate effect . . . of a normal labor contraction . . . is a gradient of force directed from the fundus to the least active and weakest area of the uterus, the cervix. This is called *fundal dominance*. The force generated by each contraction is applied to the amniotic fluid and directly against the pole of the fetus that occupies the upper segment. Therefore, each time the muscle contracts, the uterine cavity becomes smaller, and the presenting part of the fetus or the forebag of waters lying ahead of it is pushed downward into the cervix. This tends to force it open, or *dilate* it.

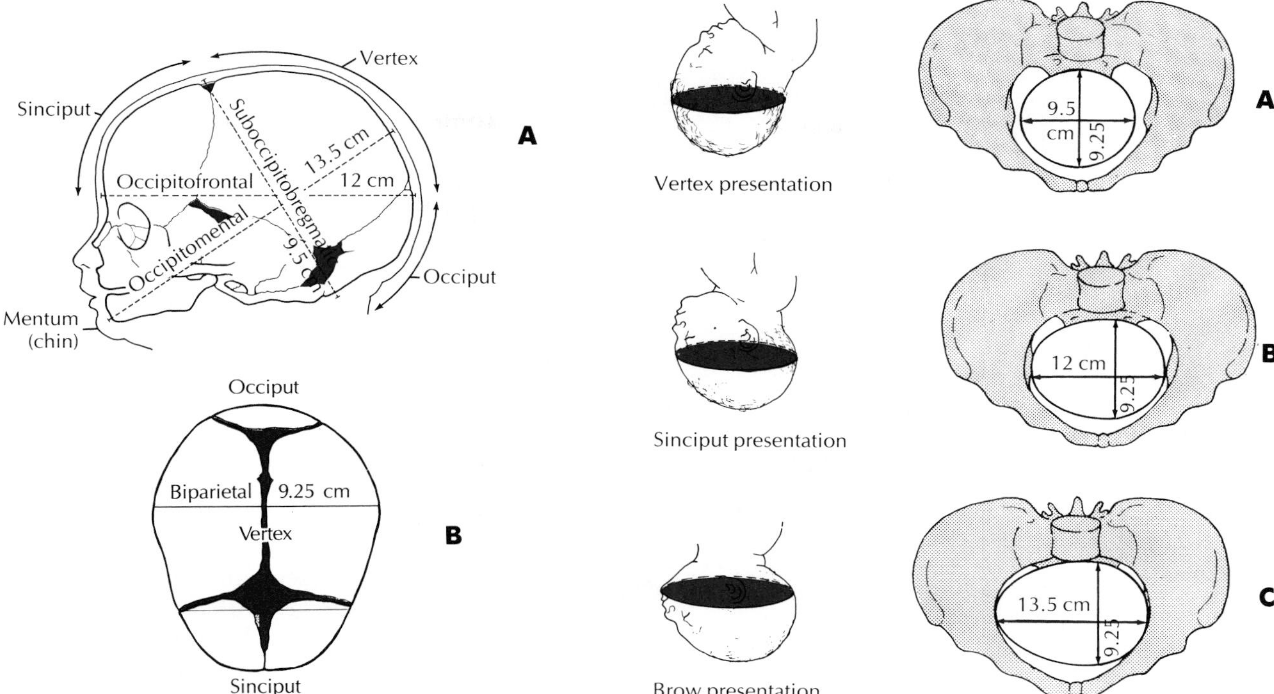

Fig. 14-13 Cephalic landmarks. **A,** Cephalic presentations: occiput, vertex, and sinciput, and cephalic diameters: suboccipitobregmatic, occipitofrontal, and occipitomental. **B,** Cephalic presentations and biparietal diameter.

Fig. 14-14 Head entering pelvis. Biparietal diameter is indicated with a black arrow (9.25 cm). **A,** Suboccipitobregmatic diameter: complete flexion of head on chest so that smallest diameter enters. **B,** Occipitofrontal diameter: moderate extension (military attitude) so that large diameter enters. **C,** Occipitomental diameter: marked extension (deflection) so that largest diameter, which is too large to permit head to enter pelvis, is presenting.

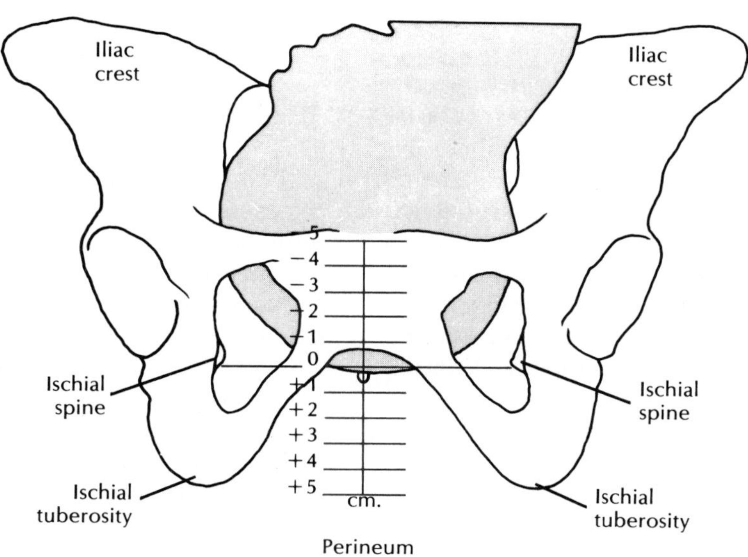

Fig. 14-15 Stations of presenting part, or degree of descent. Silhouette shows head of infant approaching station + 1.
Courtesy Ross Laboratories, Columbus, Ohio.

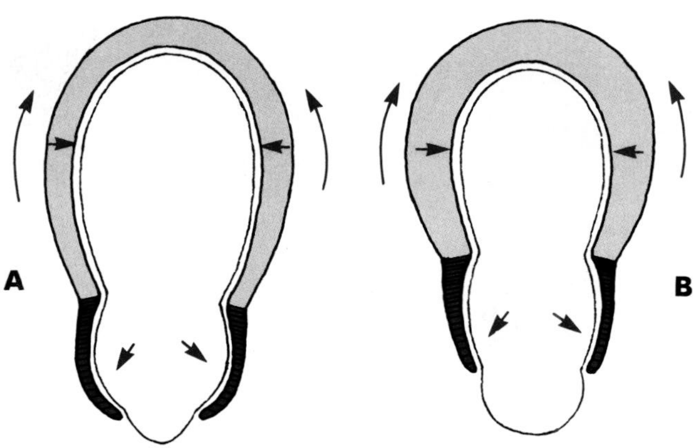

Fig. 14-16 Lower uterine segment and cervix are pulled up (retracted) as the fetus and amniotic sac are pushed downward. **A,** Cervix is effaced and partially dilated. **B,** Cervical dilatation is complete. Cervix is being pulled upward as presenting part descends. Intrauterine space is decreasing.

From Willson JR, Carrington ER: *Obstetrics and gynecology,* ed 8, St Louis, 1987, Mosby–Year Book.

A more potent factor in cervical dilatation, however, is the *retraction of the upper segment.* As this area of the uterus becomes shorter and thicker, it pulls the lower segment and the dilating cervix upward around the presenting part at the same time the uterus contracting directly against the fetus tends to push it through the cervical opening [Fig. 14-16]. The cervix opens or is dilated by a combination of these two factors but retraction is probably more important than the pressure of the presenting part, since dilatation will occur even though the presenting part does not descend into it. A *completely dilated cervix* that will permit a term fetus to pass through it has a diameter of about 10 cm.

The primary powers are responsible for the effacement and dilatation of the cervix and descent of the fetus. **Effacement** of the cervix means the shortening and thinning of the cervix during the first stage of labor. The cervix, normally 2 to 3 cm in length and about 1 cm thick, is obliterated or "taken up" by a shortening of the uterine muscle bundles during the thinning of the lower uterine segment in advancing labor. Eventually only a thin edge of the cervix can be palpated when effacement is complete. Effacement generally is advanced in first-time pregnancy at term before more than slight dilatation occurs. In subsequent pregnancies, effacement and dilatation of the cervix tend to progress together. Degree of effacement is expressed in percentages from 0% to 100% (e.g., a cervix is 50% effaced) (Fig. 14-17).

Dilatation of the cervix is the enlargement or widening of the cervical opening and the cervical canal, which occurs once labor has begun. The diameter increases from perhaps less than 1 cm to full dilatation (approximately 10 cm) to allow delivery of a term fetus. When the cervix is fully dilated (and completely retracted), it can no longer be palpated (Fig. 14-17). Full cervical dilatation marks the end of the first stage of labor.

Dilatation of the cervix occurs by the drawing upward of the musculofibrous components of the cervix with strong uterine contractions. Pressure exerted by the amniotic fluid while the membranes are intact or force applied by the presenting part also encourages cervical dilatation. Scarring of the cervix as a result of prior infection or surgery may retard cervical dilatation.

SECONDARY POWERS. As soon as the presenting part reaches the pelvic floor the contractions change in character and become expulsive in nature. The woman experiences an involuntary urge to push. The **bearing-down effort** (secondary powers) is aided by a voluntary effort similar to that used in the process of defecation. However, a different set of muscles is used bearing down. The mother contracts her diaphragm and abdominal muscles and pushes out the contents of the birth canal. Bearing down results in increased intraabdominal pressure. The pressure compresses the uterus on all sides and adds to the power of the expulsive forces.

The secondary forces have no effect on cervical dilatation, but they are of considerable importance in the expulsion of the infant from the uterus and vagina after the cervix is fully dilated. Any voluntary bearing-down efforts by the woman earlier in labor are counterproductive to cervical dilatation. Straining will exhaust the woman and cause cervical trauma (see discussion in Chapter 17).

Position of the Mother

Maternal position affects her anatomic and physiologic adaptations to labor. An upright position offers a number of advantages. Frequent changes in position relieve fatigue, increase comfort, and improve circulation. Upright positions include standing, walking, and squatting.

In an upright position, gravity can assist in the descent of the fetus. Uterine contractions are generally stronger and more efficient in effacing and dilating the cervix, resulting in shorter labor. In addition, assuming an upright position reduces the incidence of umbilical cord compression.

An upright position is also beneficial to the mother's cardiac output, which normally increases during labor as uterine contractions return blood to the vascular bed. Increased cardiac output improves blood

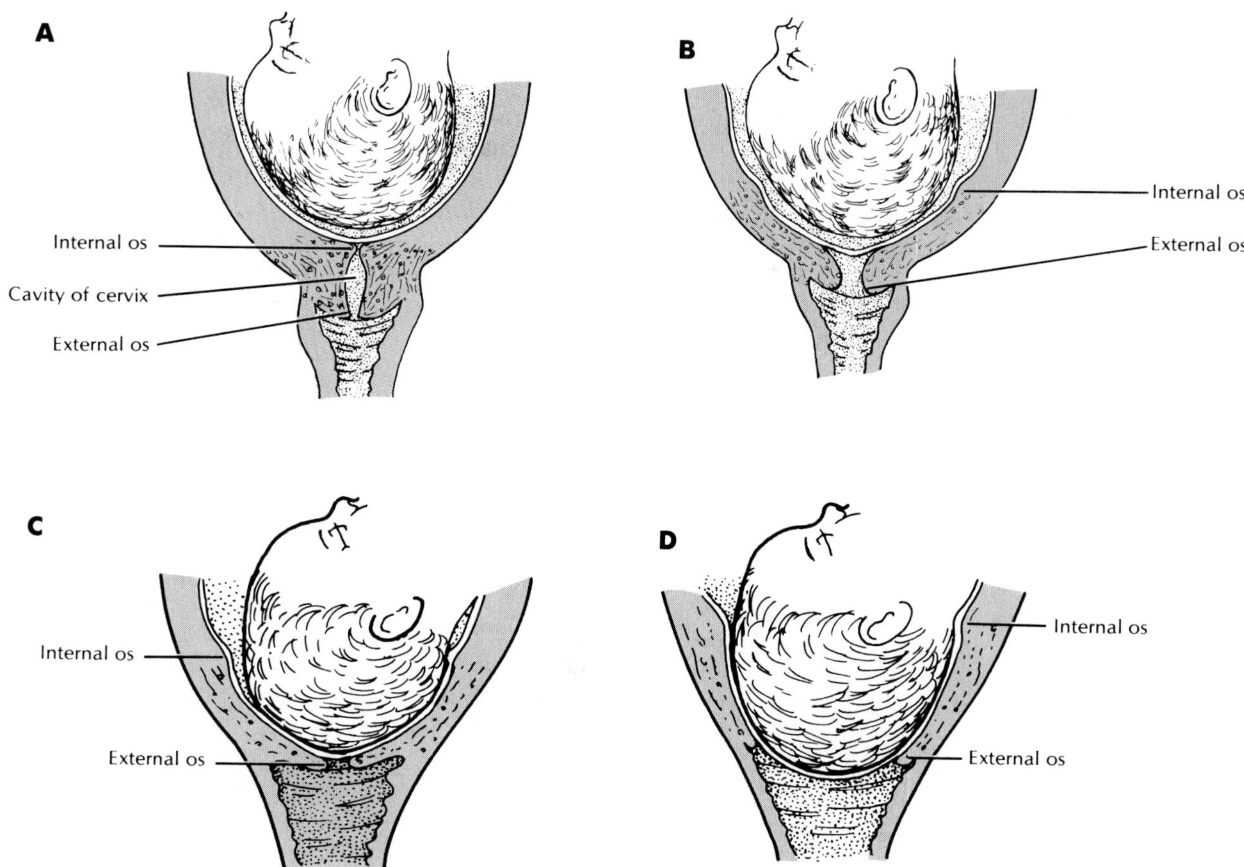

Fig. 14-17 Cervical effacement and dilatation. Note how cervix is drawn up around presenting part (internal os.) Membranes are intact, and head is not well applied to cervix. **A,** Before labor. **B,** Early effacement. **C,** Complete effacement (100%). Head is well applied to cervix. **D,** Complete dilatation (10 cm). Some overlapping of cranial bones. Membranes still intact.

flow to the uteroplacental unit and the maternal kidneys. Cardiac output is compromised if the descending aorta and ascending vena cava are compressed during labor. Compression of these major vessels may result in supine hypotension and fetal heart rate deceleration or in hypertension that decreases placental perfusion. (For further discussion, see p. 275). An upright position helps reduce pressure on the maternal vessels and prevents their compression.

Squatting after fetal presentation moves the uterus forward, thereby straightening the long axis of the birth canal (McKay, 1984). As the fetus descends in the birth canal, the pressure of the presenting part on stretch receptors of the pelvic floor stimulates the woman's bearing-down reflex. Stimulation of the stretch receptors in turn stimulates the release of oxytocin from the posterior pituitary **(Ferguson's reflex)**. Oxytocin increases the intensity of the uterine contractions. In a sitting or squatting position, abdominal muscles work in greater synchronicity with uterine contractions during bearing-down efforts.

■ PROCESS OF LABOR

Labor is the process of moving the fetus, placenta, and membranes out of the uterus and through the birth canal. It is a coordinated sequence of involuntary uterine contractions that result in effacement and dilatation of the cervix and voluntary bearing-down efforts that result in delivery. Various changes take place in the woman's reproductive system in the days and weeks just before labor begins. Labor itself can be discussed in terms of the mechanisms involved in the process and the stages the woman moves through.

Reproductive System Changes

In first-time pregnancies the uterus sinks downwards and forward about 2 weeks before term, when the fetus's presenting part (usually the fetal head) descends into the true pelvis. This settling is called **lightening** or "dropping" and usually happens gradually (Fig. 14-18). After lightening, women feel less congested and breathe more easily. However, there is usually more bladder pressure as a result of this shift and consequently a return of urinary frequency. In multiparous pregnancy, lightening may not take place until after uterine contractions are established and true labor is in progress.

Persistent low backache and sacroiliac distress as a result of relaxation of the pelvic joints may be described. Occasionally the woman may identify strong, frequent, but irregular uterine (Braxton Hicks) contractions.

Prodromal labor events are signs and symptoms experienced before the onset of true labor. The vaginal mucus becomes more profuse in response to the extreme congestion of the vaginal mucous membranes. Brownish or blood-tinged cervical mucus may be passed (**bloody show**). The cervix becomes soft (ripens) and partially effaced and may begin to dilate. The membranes may rupture spontaneously.

Two other phenomena are common in the days preceding labor: (1) loss of 0.5 to 1.5 kg (1 to 3 lb) in weight, caused by water loss resulting from electrolyte shifts that in turn are produced by changes in estrogen and progesterone levels, and (2) a burst of energy. Women speak of a burst of energy that they often use to clean the house and put everything in order. This activity has been described as the "nesting instinct."

The onset of true labor cannot be ascribed to a single cause. Many factors, including changes in the maternal uterus, cervix, and pituitary gland, are involved. Hormones produced by the normal fetal hypothalamus, pituitary, and adrenal cortex probably contribute to the **onset of labor.** Progressive uterine distention, increasing intrauterine pressure, and aging of the placenta seem to be associated with increasing myometrial irritability. This is a result of increased concentrations of estrogen and prostaglandins, as well as decreasing progesterone levels. The mutually coordinated effects of these factors result in strong, regular, rhythmic uterine contractions. Normally, these factors working in concert terminate in the birth of the fetus and the delivery of the placenta. It is still not completely understood how certain alterations trigger others and how proper checks and balances are maintained.

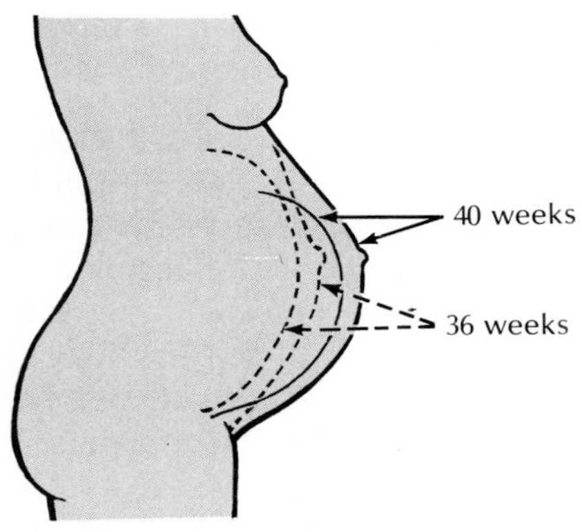

Fig. 14-18 Lightening.

Afferent and efferent nerve impulses to and from the uterus alter its contractility. Although nerve impulses to the uterus will stimulate contractions, the denervated uterus still contracts well during labor because oxytocin in the circulating blood is a regulator of labor. Therefore some women who are paralyzed can still give birth vaginally (for additional discussion of spinal injury and childbirth, see Chapter 32).

Stages of Labor

Labor is considered "normal" when the woman is at or near term, no complications exist, a single fetus presents by vertex, and labor is completed within 24 hours. The course of normal labor, which is remarkably constant, consists of (1) regular progression of uterine contractions, (2) effacement and progressive dilatation of the cervix, and (3) progress in descent of the presenting part. **Four stages of labor** are recognized. These stages are discussed in greater detail, along with nursing care for the laboring woman and family, in Chapters 17 through 19.

The first stage of labor is considered to last from the onset of regular uterine contractions to full dilatation of the cervix. Commonly the onset of labor is difficult to establish; the woman may be admitted to the labor floor just before delivery so that the beginning of labor may be only an estimate. The first stage is much longer than the second and third combined. Great variability is the rule, however, depending on the essential factors discussed earlier. Full dilatation may occur in less than 1 hour in some multiparous pregnancies. In first-time pregnancy, complete dilatation of the cervix is seldom reached in less than 24 hours.

The first stage of labor has been divided into three phases: a *latent phase*, an *active phase*, and a *transition phase*. During the latent phase there is more progress in effacement of the cervix and little increase in descent. During the active phase and the transition phase there is more rapid dilatation of the cervix and descent of the presenting part. If the degree of dilatation and descent is plotted in a graph, it forms an **S** curve. This curve can be used as a basis for assessment of progress in labor (see Figs. 17-6 and 17-7).

The second stage of labor lasts from full dilatation of the cervix to delivery of the fetus. Labor of up to 2 hours is considered within the normal range for the second stage.

The third stage of labor lasts from the birth of the fetus until the placenta is delivered. The placenta normally separates with the third or fourth strong uterine contraction after the infant has been delivered. Then it should be delivered with the next uterine contraction after placental separation. Placental separation usually begins with the contraction that delivers the baby's trunk and is normally completed with the first contraction after the birth of the baby. However, delivery of the placenta within 45 to 60 minutes is generally considered within normal limits.

The fourth stage of labor arbitrarily lasts about 2 hours after delivery of the placenta. It is the period of immediate recovery, when homeostasis is reestablished. It serves as an important period of observation for complications, such as abnormal bleeding.

There are no absolute values for the normal length of the first stage of labor (Willson, Carrington, 1987). Variations may reflect differences in the client population or in clinical practice. The average total length of the first stage in a first-time pregnancy ranges from 3.3 hours to 19.7 hours; in subsequent pregnancies, 0.1 to 14.3 hours. Friedman (1978) provides statistical *upper limits* for the first and second stages of labor:

	Nulliparous	Multiparous
First stage		
Latent phase	20 hr	14 hr
Active phase	1.2 cm/hr	1.5 cm/hr
Second stage	2 hr	1.5 hr

The duration of the third stage will be 15 to 30 minutes or even longer if the physician waits for the mother to expel the placenta herself. When the placental stage is managed actively, its duration can be less than 5 minutes (Willson, Carrington, 1987).

A description of the labor experience of a significant number of women is given in Figs. 17-6 and 17-7. Friedman and Sachtleben (1965) used this information to predict the duration of normal labor for the first and second stages.

Mechanism of Labor

The female pelvis has varied contours and diameters at different levels, and the presenting part of the passenger is large in proportion to the passage. For delivery to occur, the fetus must adapt to the birth canal during the descent. The turns and other adjustments necessary in the human birth process are termed the mechanism of labor (Fig. 14-19). The seven **cardinal movements** of the mechanism of labor that occur in a vertex presentation are **engagement, descent, flexion, internal rotation, extension, external rotation (restitution)**, and finally birth by **expulsion.** Although these phases will be discussed separately, a combination of movements is occurring simultaneously. For example, engagement involves both descent and flexion.

ENGAGEMENT. When the biparietal diameter of the head passes the pelvic inlet, the head is said to be engaged in the pelvic inlet. In most nulliparous pregnancies this occurs before the onset of active labor because the firmer abdominal muscles direct the presenting part into the pelvis. In multiparous pregnancies, in which the abdominal musculature is more relaxed, the head often remains freely movable above the pelvic brim until labor is established. In the majority of cases the head of a normal-sized fetus enters the pelvis with the sagittal suture transverse to the pelvic inlet (see Figs. 14-11 and 17-4, ROT or LOT).

DESCENT. Descent refers to the progress of the presenting part through the pelvis. As **partograms** (labor curves) (see Figs. 17-6 and 17-7) indicate, there is little progress in descent during the latent phase of the first stage of labor. Descent becomes more rapid in the active phase when the cervix has dilated to 5 to 7 cm. It is apparent especially when the membranes have ruptured.

Descent depends on three forces: (1) pressure of the amniotic fluid, (2) direct pressure of the contracting fundus on the fetus, and (3) contraction of the maternal diaphragm and abdominal muscles in the second stage of labor. The effects of these forces are modified by the size and shape of the maternal pelvic planes and the size and capacity of the fetal head to mold.

The degree of descent is measured by the station of the presenting part (Fig. 14-15). The speed of the descent increases in the second stage of labor. In first-time pregnancy this descent is slow but steady; in subsequent pregnancies the descent may be rapid. Progress in the descent of the presenting part is determined by abdominal palpation (Leopold's maneuvers) (see Chapter 17) and vaginal examination until the presenting part can be seen at the introitus.

FLEXION. As soon as the descending head meets resistance from the cervix, pelvic wall, or pelvic floor,

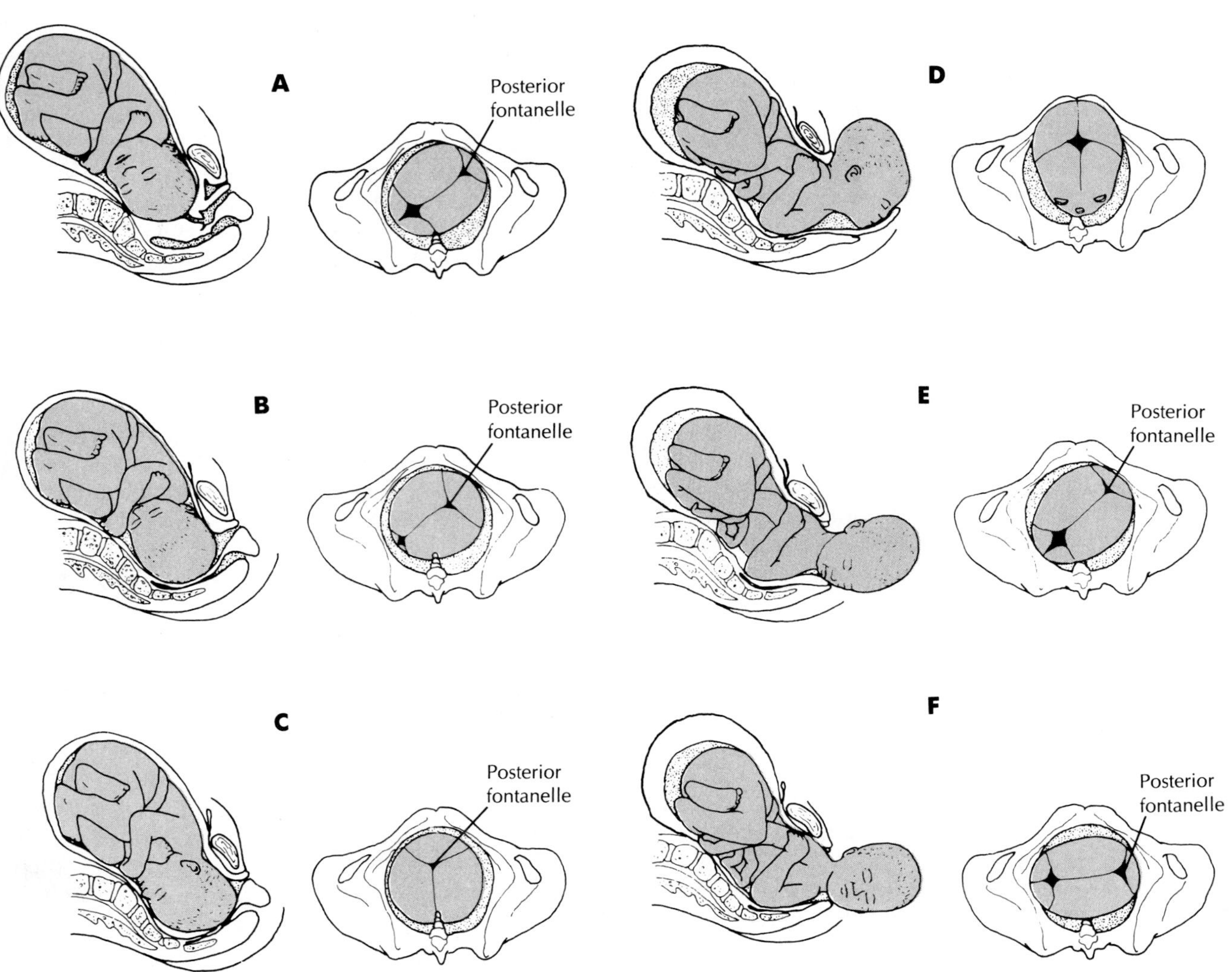

Fig. 14-19 Cardinal movements of the mechanism of labor. Left occipitoanterior (LOA) presentation. **A**, Engagement and descent. **B**, Flexion. **C**, Internal rotation to OA. **D**, Extension. **E**, External rotation beginning (restitution). **F**, External rotation.

flexion normally occurs, and the chin is brought into more intimate contact with the fetal chest (Fig. 14-19, *B*). Flexion permits the smaller suboccipitobregmatic diameter (9.5 cm) rather than the larger diameters to present to the outlet.

INTERNAL ROTATION. The maternal pelvic inlet is widest in the transverse diameter. Therefore the fetal head passes the inlet into the true pelvis in the occipitotransverse position. The outlet is widest in the anteroposterior diameter, however. To exit, the fetal head must rotate. Internal rotation begins at the level of the ischial spines but is not completed until the presenting part reaches the lower pelvis. As the occiput rotates anteriorly, the face rotates posteriorly. With each contraction the fetal head is guided by the bony pelvis and the muscles of the pelvic floor. Eventually the occiput will be in the midline beneath the pubic arch. The head is almost always rotated by the time it reaches the pelvic floor (Fig. 14-19, *C*). Both the levator ani muscles and the bony pelvis are important for anterior rotation. Previous childbirth injury or regional anesthesia compromises the function of the levator sling.

EXTENSION. When the fetal head reaches the perineum for delivery, it is deflected anteriorly by the perineum. The occiput passes under the lower border of the symphysis pubis first, then the head emerges by extension: first the occiput, then the face, and finally the chin (see Fig. 14-19, *D*).

RESTITUTION AND EXTERNAL ROTATION. After delivery of the head, it rotates briefly to the position it occupied when it was engaged in the inlet. This movement is referred to as *restitution* (see Fig. 14-19, *E* and *F*). The 45-degree turn realigns the infant's head with her or his back and shoulders. The head can then be seen to rotate further. External rotation occurs as the shoulders engage and descend in maneuvers similar to those of the head. As noted earlier, the anterior shoulder descends first. When it reaches the outlet, it rotates to the midline and is delivered from under the pubic arch. The posterior shoulder is guided over the perineum until it is free of the vaginal introitus.

EXPULSION. After delivery of the shoulders, the head and shoulders are lifted up toward the mother's pubic bone and the trunk of the baby is delivered by a movement of lateral flexion in the direction of the symphysis pubis. When the baby has completely emerged, birth is complete. *This* is the end of the second stage of labor, and the *time* is recorded on the records.

■ ADAPTATION TO LABOR

The mother and fetus must adapt anatomically and physiologically during the birth process. Accurate assessment of the mother and fetus requires a knowledge of expected adaptations.

Fetal Adaptation

The anatomic adaptations the fetus must undergo to pass through the birth canal have been discussed. Several important physiologic adaptations also occur. The nurse must be aware of what changes to expect in terms of fetal heart rate, fetal circulation, respiratory movements, and other behaviors.

FETAL HEART RATE. Fetal heart rate (FHR) monitoring provides reliable and predictive information about the condition of the fetus related to oxygenation (see Chapter 16). Stresses to the uterofetoplacental unit result in characteristic FHR patterns. It is important that the nurse have a basic understanding of the factors involved in fetal oxygenation and of the fetal responses that reflect adequate fetal oxygenation.

The average FHR at term is 140 beats per minute (beats/min). The normal range is 120 to 160 beats/min. Earlier in gestation the FHR is higher, with an average of approximately 160 beats/min at 20 weeks' gestation. The rate decreases progressively as the maturing fetus reaches term. However, temporary accelerations and slight early decelerations of the FHR can be expected in response to spontaneous fetal movement, vaginal examination, fundal pressure, uterine contractions, and abdominal palpation (for further discussion, see Chapter 16, p.406.

FETAL CIRCULATION. The placenta serves as a link between the fetal and maternal circulation. Uterine spiral arterioles must pass through the full thickness of the myometrium to reach the intervillous space. The maternal blood spurts through these arterioles into the intervillous space. Oxygen, nutrients, and inherent warmth are absorbed by the thin-walled fetal capillaries contained within the chorionic villi of the placenta. These are eventually carried to the fetus by the umbilical vein. Carbon dioxide and fetal waste products circulate back to the placenta through the umbilical arteries and fetal capillaries in the chorionic villi. Here they cross back through the intervillous space to the maternal circulation.

Fetal circulation can be affected by many factors. These include maternal position, uterine contractions, blood pressure, and umbilical cord blood flow. Maternal position is discussed earlier in this chapter and in Chapter 17. Uterine contractions during labor tend to decrease circulation through the spiral arterioles and subsequent perfusion through the intervillous space. Most healthy fetuses are well able to compensate for this stress. Those with adequate uterofetoplacental circulation will respond in fairly predictable ways to stresses. For example, the fetus is exposed to increased pressure while moving passively through the birth canal during labor. Usually umbilical cord blood flow is undisturbed by uterine contractions or fetal position.

FETAL RESPIRATION AND BEHAVIOR. Certain changes prepare the fetus for initiating respirations after birth. During vaginal delivery, 7 to 42 ml of amniotic fluid is squeezed out of the fetal lungs. Normally, fetal oxygen pressure Po_2, falls from 80 to 15 mm Hg, arterial carbon dioxide pressure (Pco_2) rises from 40 to 70 mm Hg, and arterial pH falls below 7.35. The average fetal range is 7.30 to 7.35; the normal range of pH in an adult is 7.35 to 7.45. These changes stimulate chemoreceptors in the aorta and carotid bodies to initiate respirations immediately after birth.

Fetal respiratory movements decrease greatly during labor. Fetal behavior persists as it did during pregnancy: 20 to 50 movements per hour, with periods of quiet and active sleep states and wakefulness. Fetal movements decrease after membranes rupture, but other behaviors continue.

Maternal Adaptation

A thorough understanding of maternal adaptations to pregnancy (discussed in Chapter 8) assists the nurse to anticipate and meet the woman's needs during labor. Further changes occur as the woman progresses through the stages of labor. Various body systems adapt to the process of labor, exhibiting both objective and subjective symptoms.

CARDIOVASCULAR CHANGES. The nurse can expect some changes in the woman's cardiovascular system during labor. During each contraction, 400 ml of blood is emptied from the uterus into the maternal vascular system. This increases *cardiac output* by about 10% to 15% in the first stage and by about 30% to 50% in the second stage.

The nurse can anticipate changes in *blood pressure*. Several factors alter blood pressure in the mother. Blood flow, reduced in the uterine artery by contractions, is redirected to peripheral vessels. Peripheral resistance occurs, blood pressure rises, and the *pulse rate* slows. During the first stage of labor, uterine contractions increase systolic readings by about 10 mm Hg. Therefore, assessing blood pressure between contractions provides more accurate data. During the second stage, contractions may increase systolic pressures by 30 mm Hg and diastolic readings by 25 mm Hg. However, both systolic and diastolic pressures remain somewhat elevated even between contractions. The woman already at risk for hypertension (Chapter 28) is then placed at increased risk for complications such as cerebral hemorrhage.

The woman must be discouraged from using the **Valsalva maneuver** (holding one's breath and tightening abdominal muscles) for pushing during the second stage. This activity increases intrathoracic pressure, reduces venous return, and increases venous pressure. The cardiac output and blood pressure increase and pulse slows temporarily. During the Valsalva maneuver, fetal hypoxia may occur. The process is reversed when the woman takes a breath.

As discussed previously and on p. 363, the woman's position affects blood pressure. Supine hypotension occurs when the ascending vena cava and descending aorta are compressed. The mother is at greater risk for supine hypotension if the uterus is particularly large because of multifetal pregnancy, hydramnios, obesity, or dehydration and hypovolemia. In addition, anxiety and pain, as well as some medications, can cause hypotension. Analgesics and anesthetics are discussed in Chapter 16.

White blood cells (WBCs) increase, often to ≥25,000/mm^3. Although the mechanism leading to this increase in WBCs is unknown, it may be secondary to physical or emotional stress or to tissue trauma. Labor is strenuous. Physical exercise alone can increase WBC count.

Some peripheral vascular changes occur, perhaps in response to cervical dilatation or to compression of maternal vessels by the fetus passing through the birth canal. Malar flush (reddened cheeks), hot or cold feet, and hemorrhoids may result.

RESPIRATORY CHANGES. Respiratory system adaptations also are seen. Increased physical activity with increased oxygen consumption is reflected in an increase in the respiratory rate. *Hyperventilation* may cause respiratory alkalosis (an increase in pH), hypoxia, and hypocapnia (decrease in carbon dioxide). In the unmedicated woman in the second stage, oxygen consumption almost doubles. Anxiety also increases oxygen consumption.

RENAL CHANGES. Several renal system adaptations occur. Diaphoresis (perspiration), increased insensible water loss through respirations, and occasionally the lack of food (NPO status) without adequate hydration leads to thirst and possible elevation in temperature. In the second trimester, the urinary bladder becomes an abdominal organ. When filling, it is palpable above the symphysis pubis. During labor spontaneous voiding may be difficult for various reasons: tissue edema caused by pressure from the presenting part, discomfort, sedation, and embarrassment. Proteinuria of 1+ is within normal limits inasmuch as the finding can occur in response to the breakdown of muscle tissue from the physical work of labor.

INTEGUMENTARY CHANGES. The integumentary system adaptations are evident especially in the great distensibility in the area of the vaginal introitus (opening). The degree of distensibility varies with the individual. Despite this ability to stretch, even in the absence of episiotomy or lacerations, minute tears in the skin around the vaginal introitus do occur.

MUSCULOSKELETAL CHANGES. The musculoskeletal system is stressed during labor. Diaphoresis, fatigue, proteinuria (1+), and perhaps an increased temperature accompany the marked increase in muscle activity. Backache and joint ache (unrelated to fetal position) occur as a result of increased joint laxity at term. The labor process itself and the woman's pointing her toes can cause leg cramps.

NEUROLOGIC CHANGES. The neurologic system reflects the stress and discomfort of labor. Sensorial changes occur as the woman moves through phases of the first stage of labor and as she moves from one stage to the next. Initially she may be euphoric. Euphoria gives way to increased seriousness, then to amnesia between contractions during the second stage, and finally to elation or fatigue after giving birth. Endogenous endorphins (morphinelike chemical produced naturally by the body) raise the pain threshold and produce sedation. In addition, physiologic anesthesia of perineal tissues, caused by pressure of the presenting part, decreases perception of pain. (For further discussion of discomfort during labor and its management, see Chapter 15.)

GASTROINTESTINAL CHANGES. Labor affects the woman's gastrointestinal system. Dry lips and mouth may result from mouth breathing, dehydration, and emotional response to labor. During labor, gastrointestinal motility and absorption are decreased and stomach emptying time is delayed. Nausea and vomiting of undigested food eaten after onset of labor are common. Nausea and belching also occur as a reflex response to full cervical dilatation. The mother may state that diarrhea accompanied the onset of labor, or the nurse may palpate the presence of hard or impacted stool in the rectum.

ENDOCRINE CHANGES. The endocrine system is active during labor. The onset of labor may be attributed to decreasing levels of progesterone and increasing levels of estrogen, prostaglandins, and oxytocin. Metabolism increases, and blood glucose levels may decrease with the work of labor.

■ SUMMARY

A firm grasp of the theory of essential factors and processes in labor and maternal and fetal adaptations provides a foundation for implementing the nursing process with women in labor. The anatomic structure of the maternal pelvis and the fetal skull affects the labor process. However, maternal and fetal physiology can be assisted by maternal position during labor. The effect of involuntary uterine contractions can be increased by voluntary bearing-down efforts in the second stage of labor. Maternal and fetal anatomy and physiology are uniquely suited to the process of labor and birth.

REFERENCES

Friedman EA: *Labor: clinical evaluation and management,* ed 2, New York, 1978, Appleton-Century-Crofts.

Friedman EA, Sachtleben MR: Station of the fetal presenting part, *Am J Obstet Gynecol* 93:522, 1965.

McKay S: Squatting: an alternate position for the second stage of labor, *MCN* 9:181, May/June, 1984.

Willson JR et al: *Obstetrics and gynecology,* ed 9, St Louis, 1991, Mosby–Year Book.

BIBLIOGRAPHY

Chez RA: Why it's important to help patients prepare for pregnancy, *Contemp OB/GYN* 33:9, 64, July 1989.

Cunningham FG, MacDonald PC, Gant NR: *Williams obstetrics,* ed 18, Norwalk, Conn, 1989, Appleton & Lange.

Curry J: Pregnancy health fair, *Can Nurse,* p 26, June 1988.

Friedman E: Normal and dysfunctional labor. In Cohen WR, Acker D, Friedman E, editors: *Management of labor,* Rockville, Md, 1989, Aspen.

Gaston-Johansson F, Fridh G, Turner-Norvell K: Progression of labor pain in primiparas and multiparas, *Nurs Res* 37:87, March/April 1988.

Liu YC: The effects of the upright position during childbirth, *Image J Nurs Sch* 21:14, 1989.

Malasanos L et al: *Health assessment,* ed 4, St Louis, 1990, Mosby–Year Book.

Rosen MG: Preconception care: why it is necessary, *Female Patient* 15:73, May 1990.

Scott JR et al: *Danforth's obstetrics and gynecology,* ed 6, Philadelphia, 1990, JB Lippincott.

chapter 14 review

Key Concepts

- Five essential factors affect the process of labor and delivery.
- Because of its size and relative rigidity, the fetal head has a major effect on the birth process.
- The diameters at the plane of the pelvic inlet, midpelvis, and outlet, plus the axis of the birth canal, determine whether vaginal delivery is possible and the manner by which the fetus may pass down the birth canal.
- The forces acting to expel the fetus and placenta are derived from involuntary uterine contractions during the first stage of labor, which are augmented by voluntary bearing-down efforts during the second stage.
- The mother's position affects her anatomic and physiologic adaptations to labor.
- The cardinal movements of the mechanism of labor are engagement, descent, flexion, internal rotation, extension, restitution and, external rotation, and expulsion of the baby.
- Many factors, including changes in the maternal uterus, cervix, and pituitary gland, are involved in the initiation of labor.
- An understanding of maternal adaptations to pregnancy is fundamental to anticipating and meeting the parturient's needs.
- A healthy fetus with an adequate uterofetoplacental circulation will respond in fairly predictable ways to stresses.

Key Terms

- attitude (p.358)
- bearing-down effort (p.362)
- biparietal diameter (p.358)
- bloody show p.364)
- breech presentation (p.358)
- bregma (p.357)
- cardinal movements of labor (p.365)
- cephalic presentation (p.358)
- descent (p.365)
- diagonal conjugate (p.354)
- dilatation (p.362)
- effacement (p.362)
- engagement (p.359)
- expulsion (p.365)
- Ferguson's reflex (p.363)
- fetal position (p.358)
- fontanelle (p.355)
- four stages of labor (p.364)
- gynecoid pelvis (p.353)
- labor (p.363)
- lie (p.358)
- lightening (p.364)
- maternal position (p.362)
- molding (p.357)
- onset of labor (p.364)
- partograms (p.365)
- passageway (p.352)
- passenger (p.355)
- position (p.358)
- powers (p.360)
- presentation (p.357)
- presenting part (p.358)
- prodromal labor (p.364)
- restitution (p.365)
- station (p.359)
- suboccipitobregmatic diameter (p.358)
- Valsalva maneuver (p.368)
- vertex (p.358)

Critical Thinking Exercises

You are assigned to a nullipara who is in early labor. She is lying in bed on her back and says, "I sure hope the baby doesn't take all day to come."

1. Discuss how the nurse can find out what the woman believes about the labor process.
2. Formulate a plan of care for the woman that incorporates the theory of the labor process.
3. What evaluation criteria would be appropriate?

Topic for Nursing Research

- What is the effect of maternal position on the length of the second stage of labor?

chapter 15

Pharmacologic Management of Discomfort

Irene M. Bobak

LEARNING OBJECTIVES

- Define the key terms listed.
- Discuss the types of analgesia and anesthesia used during labor.
- Compare the types of pharmacologic control of discomfort by stage of labor and method of delivery.
- Discuss the use of naloxone (Narcan) and naltrexone (Trexan).
- Relate each step of the nursing process to the pharmacologic management of labor discomfort.
- Describe the nursing responsibilities with women receiving analgesia or anesthesia during labor.
- Identify topics for nursing research related to management of discomfort during labor and birth.

Pregnant women commonly worry about pain during labor and childbirth and how they will react to and deal with that pain. There are many interventions to relieve the discomfort of labor. The interventions selected will depend on the situation and the preference of both the woman and her health care professionals. Nonpharmacologic nursing care of women in labor is discussed in Chapters 17 through 19. This chapter discusses pharmacologic intervention throughout all stages of labor. Discomfort during labor is discussed first; the causes, perception, and expression. Various methods of analgesia and anesthesia commonly used during childbirth are then presented. This information provides the basis for understanding the nurse's role in pharmacologic management of discomfort during labor.

■ DISCOMFORT DURING LABOR

Neurologic Origins

The discomfort experienced during labor has two origins (Cheek, Gutsche, 1987). During the *first stage of labor,* uterine contractions cause (1) cervical dilatation and effacement and (2) uterine ischemia (decreased blood flow and therefore local oxygen deficit) from contraction of the arteries to the myometrium.

The discomfort from cervical changes and uterine ischemia is **visceral pain.** It is located over the lower portion of the abdomen and radiates to the lumbar area of the back and down the thighs. Usually the woman experiences discomfort only during contractions and is free of pain between contractions.

During the *second stage of labor,* the stage of expulsion of the baby, the woman experiences perineal or **somatic pain.** Perineal discomfort results from stretching of perineal tissues to allow passage of the fetus and traction on the peritoneum and uterocervical supports during contractions. Discomfort also can be produced by expulsive forces or from pressure by the presenting part on the bladder, bowel, or other sensitive pelvic structures.

Pain may be *local,* with cramplike pain and a tearing or bursting sensation because of distention and laceration of the cervix, vagina, or perineal tissues. This discomfort is commonly perceived as an intense burning sensation as tissue stretches. Pain also may be **referred,** with the discomfort felt in the back, flanks, or thighs. Emotional tension from anxiety and fear may increase pain and perception of pain during labor (see Dick-Read method, p. 335).

Pain impulses during the first stage of labor are transmitted through the spinal nerve segment of T11-12 (Fig. 15-2) and accessory lower thoracic and upper lumbar sympathetic nerves. These nerves originate in the uterine body and cervix. Pain impulses during the second stage of labor are carried through S1-4 and the parasympathetic system from perineal tissues. Pain experienced during the *third stage* of labor, as well as so-called afterpains, is uterine, similar to that experienced early in the first stage of labor. Areas of discomfort are illustrated in Fig. 15-1.

Expression of Pain

Pain results in both psychic responses and reflex physical actions. The quality of physical pain has been described as prickling, burning, aching, throbbing, sharp, nauseating, or cramping. Pain in childbirth gives rise to symptoms that are identifiable. Increased activity of the sympathetic nervous system may occur in response to pain resulting in changes in blood pressure, pulse, respiration, and skin color. Pallor and diaphoresis may be seen (Potter, Perry, 1991). Bouts of nausea and vomiting and excessive perspiration also are commonplace. Certain **affective expressions** of suffering are often seen. Affective changes include increasing anxiety with lessened perceptual field, writhing, crying, groaning, gesturing (hand clenching and wringing), and excessive muscular excitability throughout the body. Childbirth pain is of a limited duration (at most 2 to 3 days).

Perception of Pain

Although the pain threshold is remarkably similar in all persons regardless of sexual, social, ethnic, or cultural differences, these differences play a definite role in the individual's **perception of pain.** The effects of factors such as culture, use of counterstimuli, or distraction in coping with pain are not fully understood. The meaning of pain and the verbal and nonverbal expressions given to pain are apparently learned from interactions within the primary social group. Pain is personalized for each individual. As pain is experienced, people develop various coping mechanisms to deal with it. Pain, or the possibility of pain, can induce fear in which anxiety borders on panic. Fatigue and sleep deprivation magnify pain. Parity may affect perception of labor pain (Gaston-Johansson et al, 1988).

At times, pain stimuli that are particularly intense can be ignored. Certain nerve cell groupings within the spinal cord, brain stem, and cerebral cortex may have the ability to modulate the pain impulse through a blocking mechanism. This **gate-control theory** is helpful in understanding the approaches used in parent education for childbirth programs or the use of hypnosis in labor. According to this theory, local physical stimulation, such as massage or stroking of the woman in labor, close the synaptic gates to pain stimuli. It is thought to work by closing down a hypothetic "gate" in the spinal cord, thus blocking pain signals from reaching the brain. Perception of pain stimuli is diminished. Also, when the laboring woman performs neuromuscular and motor skills, activity within the spinal cord itself further modifies the transmission of pain. Cognitive activities of concentration on breathing and relaxation require selective and directed cortical activity, which activates and closes the gating mechanism as well. The gate-control theory emphasizes the need for a supportive setting for birth (see discussion of parent education classes, p. 334). In such an environment the laboring woman can relax and allow the various higher mental activities to be implemented.

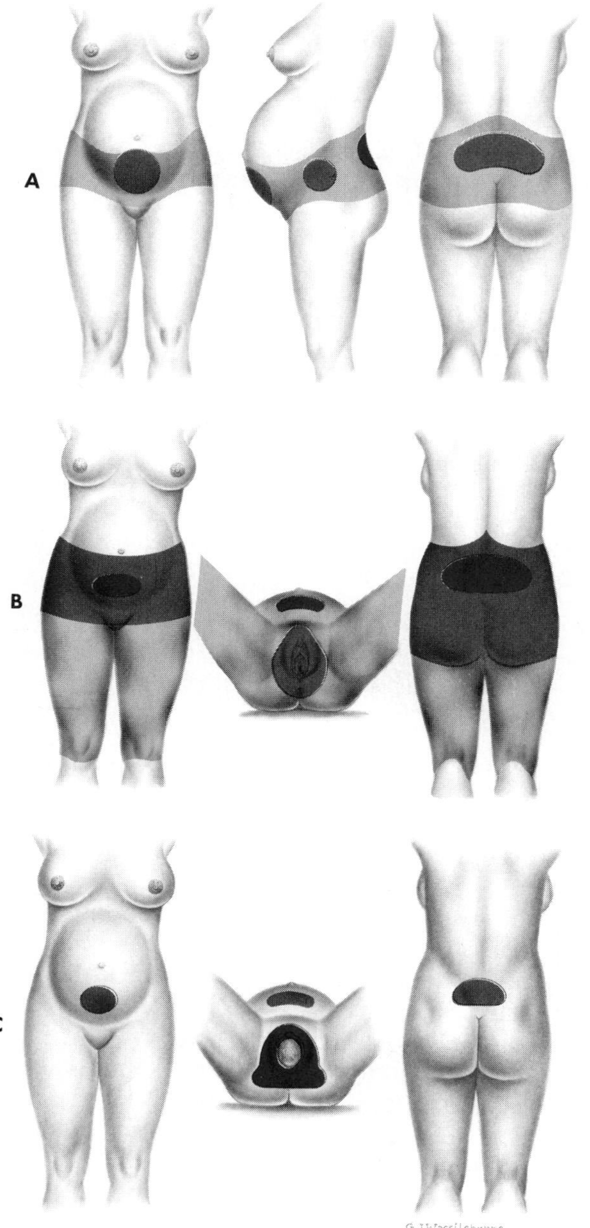

Fig. 15-1 Discomfort during labor. A, Distribution of labor pain during first stage. B, Distribution of labor pain during later phase of first stage and early phase of second stage. C, Distribution of labor pain during later phase of second stage and actual birth. (Gray shading indicates areas of mild discomfort: light colored shading indicates areas of moderate discomfort: dark colored areas indicate intense discomfort.)

At other times, maternal fatigue, fetal size or position, or other factors may require the use of medications in addition to comfort measures. Labor pain may result in physiologic responses that can decrease uterine contractility and lengthen the labor. Maternal pain is as severe as the woman describes it. Therefore nurses need to understand that each woman experiences and perceives pain in her own unique way. Concerns and anxieties can occur during later phases of labor and overcome the skills learned in parent education classes (see Research Highlight, p. 376).

Use of Sedatives

Sedatives such as barbiturates relieve anxiety and induce sleep only in prodromal or early latent labor and in the absence of pain. If the woman has pain, sedatives given without an analgesic may increase apprehension and cause the mother to become hyperactive and disoriented (Scott et al, 1990). Barbiturates should not be used late in the first stage or early in the second stage of labor if birth is expected within 1 or 2 hours, because the newborn may exhibit severe central nervous system (CNS) depression. Undesirable side effects include respiratory and vasomotor depression of both mother and newborn. Because of these disadvantages, barbiturates are seldom used (Scott et al, 1990). Sedatives do not cause amnesia but may confuse or distort recollection.

Barbiturates may be short-acting (1 hour), for example, secobarbital (Seconal); intermediate (2 hours), for example, pentobarbital (Nembutal); or of long duration (3 hours), for example, phenobarbital (Luminal). Each of these drugs can be given orally or by intramuscular injection.

■ ANALGESIA AND ANESTHESIA

The use of analgesia and anesthesia was not generally accepted as part of obstetric management until

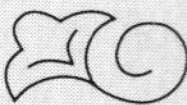 **Research Highlight** 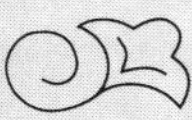

Perinatal Predictors of Pain and Distress During Labor

RESEARCH ABSTRACT

The purpose of the study was to determine whether women's attitudes and beliefs could predict pain and distress in labor and whether the relationships were specific to the phase of the first stage of labor. The sample consisted of 115 first-time mothers at low risk, who were recruited from clients of practitioners and participants in a hospital parent education program. Antenatal care was assumed to have been similar for all participants because the study was conducted in Canada where health care is available to all. During the third trimester, perinatal concerns were assessed with the Perinatal Self-Evaluation Inventory (PSEI). Practice and confidence in parent education techniques for childbirth were also assessed. Tape-recorded interviews were conducted during the three phases of the first stage of labor. Pain was measured by the Present Pain Intensity Scale. Coping and distress were assessed by asking women what was going on in their minds during contractions. Other physical and obstetric variables were obtained through a chart review. A positive correlation was found between women's confidence in their use of relaxation techniques and less pain and better coping during the latent, but not during the active or transition phases, of the first stage of labor. In the sample studies, high scores on the PSEI predicted distress during the latent phase. Two scales predicted pain and distress in active and transitional labor.

IMPLICATIONS FOR PRACTICE

Some responses of women to the latent phase of labor can be predicted with valid and reliable tools. However, concerns and anxieties of women appear during the active and transitional phases of labor and can overcome the skills learned in childbirth (parent education) classes. Nurses must listen to concerns expressed by women in the last trimester of pregnancy and then use their presence and their nursing skills to assist women through labor.

RELATED RESEARCH QUESTIONS

1. Does the presence of a trained labor coach reduce pain and distress in active and transitional phases of the first stage of labor?
2. What variables are associated with pain and distress in the three phases of the first stage of labor?
3. Is there a relation between pain and distress and administration of analgesics?
4. Is there a relation between pain and distress in labor and neonatal outcome?

REFERENCE

Wuitchik M, Hesson K, Bakal DA: Perinatal predictors of pain and distress during labor, *Birth* 17(4):186, 1990.

Queen Victoria used chloroform during the birth of her son in 1853. Since then much study has gone into the development of pharmacologic control of discomfort during the birth period. The goal of researchers is to develop methods that will provide adequate pain relief to women without adding to maternal or fetal risk or affecting the progress of labor.

Nursing management of obstetric analgesia and anesthesia combines the nurse's expertise in maternity care with a knowledge and understanding of anatomy and physiology, as well as of medications and their desired and undesired side effects and methods of administration.

Anesthesia encompasses analgesia, amnesia, relaxation, and reflex activity. It is the abolition of pain perception by interrupting the nerve impulses going to the brain. Loss of sensation may be partial or complete, sometimes with the loss of consciousness.

The term **analgesia** is best reserved to describe only those states in which there is alleviation of the sensation of pain or the raising of one's threshold for pain perception. With analgesia there is no loss of consciousness.

Analgesia can be induced by positive conditioning (e.g., Lamaze method, imagery, relaxation) and analgesic drugs. A basic understanding of the normal course of labor and delivery and physical and psychologic preparation by the pregnant woman may reduce pain during childbirth. Suggestion and reassurance are beneficial; good antenatal care is extremely important. Participation in parent education classes such as those proposed by Dick-Read (1959) or psychoprophylaxis by Lamaze (1972) or Bradley (1974) should do much to alleviate distress (for discussion of these methods, see Chapter 13).

The type of analgesic or anesthetic to be used is chosen in part by the stage of labor and by the method of birth (see boxes, p. 377).

Systemic Analgesia

Systemic analgesia remains the major method of analgesia for the woman in labor when personnel trained in epidural analgesia are not available or when epidural analgesia is contraindicated (Scott et al, 1990). Systemic analgesics cross the blood-brain barrier to provide central analgesic effects. They also cross the placental barrier. Effects on the fetus depend on the maternal dosage, the pharmacokinetics (degree of protein binding, lipid solubility, molecular weight, and metabolism) of the specific drug, and the route and timing of administration. Intravenous (IV) administration is often preferred over intramuscular (IM) administration because the onset of the drug effect is faster and more reliable. Classes of analgesic drugs used include narcotic drugs, narcotic agonist-antagonist compounds, and tranquilizers such as analgesic-potentiating drugs (**ataractics**).

NARCOTIC ANALGESIC COMPOUNDS. **Narcotic analgesics**—for example, meperidine (Demerol) and fentanyl (Sublimaze)—are especially effective for the relief of severe, persistent, or recurrent pain. Narcotic analgesics have no amnesic effect. Meperidine overcomes inhibitory factors in labor and may even relax the cervix (see Quick Reference medication cards).

Meperidine is the most commonly used narcotic for women in labor (Scott et al, 1990). After IV injection, onset is rapid (30 seconds), and maximum effect is reached in 5 to 10 minutes. Peak effect after IM injection of meperidine is reached in 40 to 50 minutes. The duration of effect of either IV or IM injection is 2 to 4 hours. After IM or IV administration of meperidine, birth ideally should occur within 1 hour or after 4 hours to minimize neonatal depression. Meperidine may cause tachycardia and therefore is administered with caution to women with cardiac disease.

Fentanyl is a potent, short-acting narcotic analgesic. After IV injection, onset of the drug effect occurs within 1 to 2 minutes and lasts about 30 to 60 minutes. Onset of the drug effect after IM injection occurs in 7 to 15 minutes, reaches its peak effect in 20 to 30 minutes, and lasts for 1 to 2 hours. Additive CNS and respiratory depression occurs if fentanyl is given with alcohol, antihistamines, antidepressants, and other sedative/hypnotics.

Fentanyl in combination with droperidol (Innovar) is used to produce tranquilization with analgesia. The effect of droperidol is longer lasting that that of fentanyl. Therefore, if additional analgesia is needed, fentanyl may be given alone to prevent accumulation of droperidol.

Pharmacologic Control of Discomfort by Stage of Labor

FIRST STAGE

- Sedatives*
  - Systemic analgesia*
  - Narcotic analgesic compounds
  - Mixed narcotic agonist-antagonist compounds, analgesic-potentiators
- Nerve block analgesia/anesthesia
  - Lumbar epidural analgesia
  - Paracervical block

SECOND STAGE

- Nerve block analgesia/anesthesia
  - Local infiltration anesthesia
  - Pudendal block
  - Subarachnoid (spinal) anesthesia
  - Epidural block
  - Epidural and spinal narcotics
- Inhalation analgesia/anesthesia
  - Self-administered
  - Nitrous oxide–oxygen
  - General anesthesia

*Administered by labor nurse.

Pharmacologic Control of Discomfort by Method of Birth

VAGINAL BIRTH

- Local infiltration
- Pudendal block
- Lumbar epidural block
  - Analgesia
  - Anesthesia
- Subarachnoid block
  - Analgesia
  - Anesthesia
- Inhalation analgesia

ABDOMINAL BIRTH

- Subarachnoid block
  - Spinal
  - Saddle block (low spinal)
- Lumbar epidural block
  - Anesthesia
- Inhalation
  - General anesthesia

MIXED NARCOTIC AGONIST-ANTAGONIST COMPOUNDS. Mixed narcotic **agonist-antagonist compounds** such as butorphanol (Stadol) and nalbuphine (Nubain), in the doses used during labor, provide analgesia without causing respiratory depression of the mother or neonate. An agonist is an agent that does something; an antagonist is an agent that blocks something from happening. Mixed narcotic agonist-antagonist compounds may be administered by IM or IV injection. Butorphanol (1 to 3 mg IM; 0.5 to 2 mg IV) or nalbuphine (0.2 mg/kg SC/IM; 0.1 to 0.2 mg/kg IV) may be given during the first stage of labor. If the woman has a preexisting narcotic dependency, the antagonist effect of these compounds will cause her to immediately exhibit symptoms of narcotic withdrawal.

ANALGESIC-POTENTIATORS (ATARACTICS). Phenothiazines, so-called tranquilizer drugs, have the property of augmenting most of the desirable, but few of the undesirable, effects of analgesics or general anesthetics. These drugs do not relieve pain but decrease anxiety and apprehension, as well as potentiate narcotic effects. Potentiation refers to the effect of a combination of two drugs resulting in action greater than the total effect of each used separately. Therefore, with the addition of an ataractic, narcotic dosages can be reduced. Analgesic potentiators include compounds such as promethazine (Phenergan), propiomazine (Largon), hydroxyzine (Vistaril), and promazine (Sparine).

In addition to potentiating the effects of the analgesic, the ataractic (tranquilizer) also acts as an antinauseant and antiemetic. The combination can be administered safely until the end of the first stage of labor. Usual dosages include the following: promethazine 25 to 50 mg IM or 15 to 25 mg IV; promazine 50 mg IM or 5 to 10 mg IV; hydroxyzine 25 to 50 mg IM. Because hydroxyzine is given only by IM injection, onset of effect is slower and less predictable. Fetal or neonatal problems rarely develop with these doses.

NARCOTIC ANTAGONISTS. Narcotics can cause excessive CNS depression in the mother or newborn. **Narcotic antagonists** such as naloxone (Narcan) or the newer narcotic antagonist, naltrexone (Trexan), promptly reverse the narcotic effects. In addition, the antagonist also counters the effect of stress-induced levels of endorphins. **Endorphins** are secreted by the pituitary gland and act on the central and peripheral nervous systems to reduce pain. Beta-endorphin is the most potent of the endorphins; it is a powerful analgesic in humans.

A narcotic antagonist is especially valuable if labor is more rapid than expected and birth is expected when the narcotic is at its peak effect. The antagonist may be given intravenously through the woman's IV line, or it can be administered intramuscularly into her gluteal muscle. Narcotic antagonists will counteract maternal and neonatal narcotic effects. The mother needs to be forewarned that administration of an antagonist will cause pain to return. Narcotic antagonists must be administered cautiously to a substance-dependent woman because withdrawal symptoms may occur.

A narcotic antagonist can be given to the newborn via the umbilical vein or into the neonate's thigh (see Fig. 21-10) (see Quick Reference medication card). **Neonatal narcosis** can be exhibited by respiratory depression, hypotonia, lethargy, and a delay in temperature regulation. Alterations of neurologic and behavioral responses may be evident for 72 hours after birth. Meperidine may be present in the neonate's urine for up to 3 weeks. Some depression of attention and social responsiveness can be evident for up to 6 weeks (Briggs et al, 1986).

Nerve Block Analgesia and Anesthesia

A variety of compounds are used in obstetrics to produce **regional analgesia** (minimal pain relief and motor block) and anesthesia (pain relief and motor block). Most of these drugs are related chemically to cocaine and carry the suffix *-caine*. This helps identify a local anesthetic.

The principal pharmacologic effect of local anesthetics is the temporary interruption of the conduction of nerve impulses, notably pain. Examples of common agents given in 0.5% to 1% solutions include lidocaine (Xylocaine), bupivacaine* (Marcaine), chloroprocaine* (Nesacaine), tetracaine (Pontocaine), and mepivacaine (Carbocaine).

Rarely, individuals are sensitive (allergic) to one or more local anesthetics. Sensitivity may be determined by testing with minute amounts of the drug to be used. Initially, the CNS is stimulated when excessive amounts of a regional anesthetic are injected. Stimulation may be followed by depression, hypotension, and other serious adverse effects. Atropine, antihistaminic drugs, oxygen, and supportive measures should bring relief.

As analgesia is established, a sympathetic block-

*On the basis of Apgar score assessment, blood gas analysis, drug concentration, and evaluation of newborn neurobehavioral response, bupivacaine and chloroprocaine offered some advantages over the other drugs: the neonates scored higher when these anesthetics were used than when the other agents were used (Lundberg, 1983).

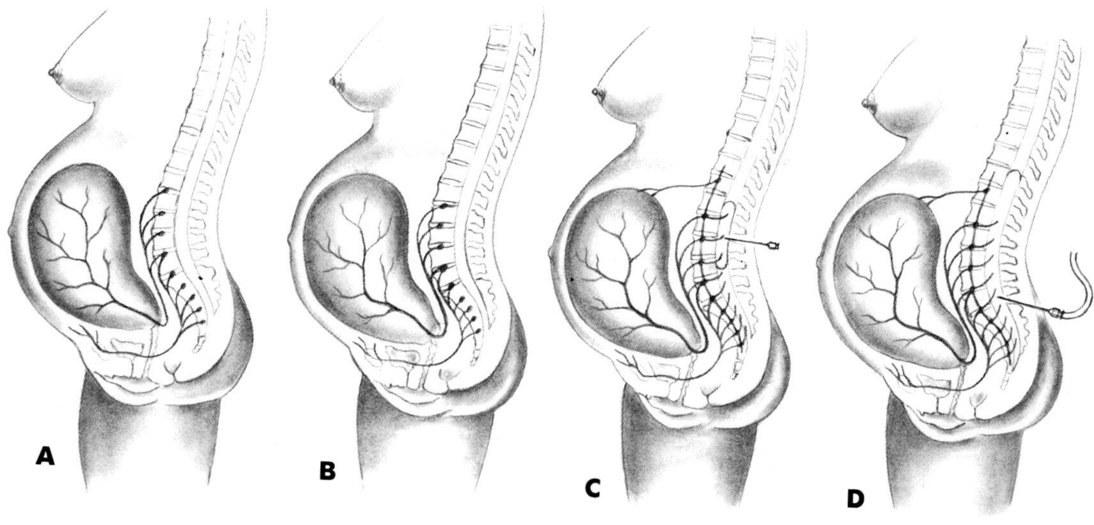

Fig. 15-2 Pain pathways and sites of pharmacologic nerve blocks. **A**, Pudendal block; suitable during second and third stages of labor and for repair of episiotomy. **B**, Paracervical (uterosacral) block: suitable during first stage of labor. **C**, Lumbar sympathetic block (one type of subarachnoid block): given as shown, suitable during first stage of labor (not usually method of choice; epidural is preferable). **D**, Epidural block: suitable during all stages of labor and for repair of episiotomy.

age occurs, causing vasodilation and pooling of blood in the lower extremities. Maternal hypotension also may occur. A fall of 20% to 30% in maternal blood pressure below the preblock average is regarded as hypotension and should be corrected promptly (Cheek, Gutsche, 1987). *Therefore, adequate hydration for blood volume expansion is a prerequisite.* Hydration is achieved with non–dextrose-containing balanced salt solution (e.g., Ringer's lactate or Plasma-Lyte A). *The mother receives IV hydration with 500 to 1000 ml solution within 20 minutes before the block. Facilities for cardiopulmonary resuscitation, including oxygen and suction, must be immediately available.* If maternal and fetal resuscitation is needed, left uterine displacement *must* be maintained to optimize venous return and therefore perfusion of the uterus (for discussion of aortocaval compression and supine hypotension, see pp. 275 and 368).

LOCAL INFILTRATION ANESTHESIA. **Local infiltration anesthesia** of perineal tissues is commonly used when an episiotomy is to be done and when time or the fetal head position does not permit a pudendal block to be administered (Scott et al, 1990). Rapid anesthesia is produced by injecting an average of 10 to 20 ml of local anesthetic with 1% lidocaine or 2% chloroprocaine into the skin and then subcutaneously into the region to be anesthetized. *Epinephrine* often is added to the solution to intensify the anesthesia in a limited region and to prevent excessive bleeding and systemic effects by constricting local blood vessels (Clark et al, 1990). Repeated injection will prolong the anesthesia as long as needed.

PUDENDAL BLOCK. **Pudendal block** is useful for the second stage of labor, for episiotomy, and for delivery. Although it does not relieve pain from uterine contractions, a pudendal block does relieve pain in the clitoris, labia majora and minora, and the perineum. Pudendal nerve block is administered 10 to 20 minutes before perineal anesthesia is needed. Once the presenting part descends through the cervix, vaginal and soon perineal distention occur. Vaginal and perineal pain can be eliminated by a pudendal anesthetic block (Fig. 15-2, *A*). The pudendal nerve traverses the sacrosciatic notch just medial to the tip of the ischial spine on each side. Injection of an anesthetic solution at or near these points will anesthetize the pudendal nerves peripherally (Fig. 15-3). The transvaginal approach usually is used because it is less painful for the woman, has a higher success rate, and tends to cause fewer fetal complications (Scott et al, 1990). Pudendal block does not change maternal hemodynamic or respiratory functions, vital signs, or fetal heart rate (FHR). The bearing-down reflex is lessened or lost completely.

If all branches of the pudendal nerve are anesthetized, analgesia is sufficient for a spontaneous vaginal birth or for an outlet (low) forceps-assisted birth. However, the degree of analgesia achieved with a pudendal nerve block is not adequate to allow midforceps delivery, uterine exploration, or manual removal of the placenta (Scott et al, 1990).

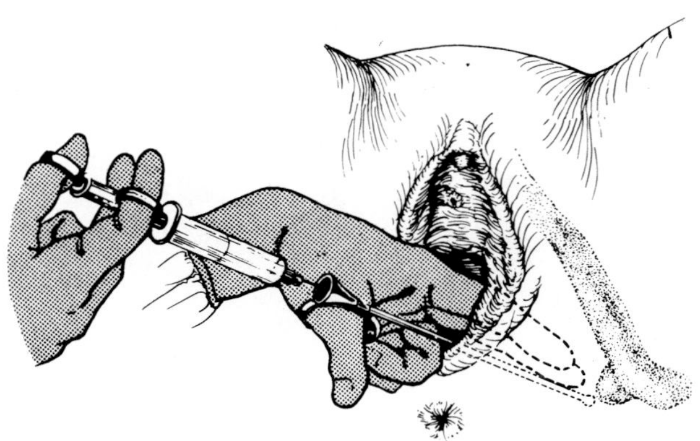

Fig 15-3 Pudendal block. Use of needle guide ("Iowa trumpet") and Luer-Lok syringe to inject medication.
Modified from Benson RC: *Handbook of obstetrics and gynecology,* ed 7, Los Altos, Calif, 1980, Lange Medical Publications.

SUBARACHNOID (SPINAL) ANESTHESIA. In **subarachnoid (spinal) block** anesthesia, local anesthetic is injected through the third, fourth, or fifth lumbar interspace into the subarachnoid space (Figs. 15-5), where the medication mixes with cerebrospinal fluid (see Fig. 15-2, *C*). This single-injection technique is useful for delivery, but not for labor. For vaginal delivery, the anesthetic solution is administered during the second stage of labor when delivery is imminent (e.g., fetal head is on the perineum).

The **low spinal (saddle) block** injection is made with the woman in a sitting position, her legs over the side of the delivery table and her feet supported on a stool. The nurse stands in front of her. The woman rests her chin on her chest, arches her back "like a rainbow," and leans on the nurse for support. The nurse comforts and coaches her. This posture is thought to widen the intervertebral space for ease in inserting the spinal needle and to allow the heavy anesthetic solution to gravitate downward. The injection is made between contractions to avoid an unexpected high block (medication rises above T10 with the potential of affecting the movement of the diaphragm and muscles of respiration). Once the anesthetic has been injected, the woman remains upright for a period of 30 seconds to 2 minutes (as directed by the anesthesiologist) to permit downward diffu-

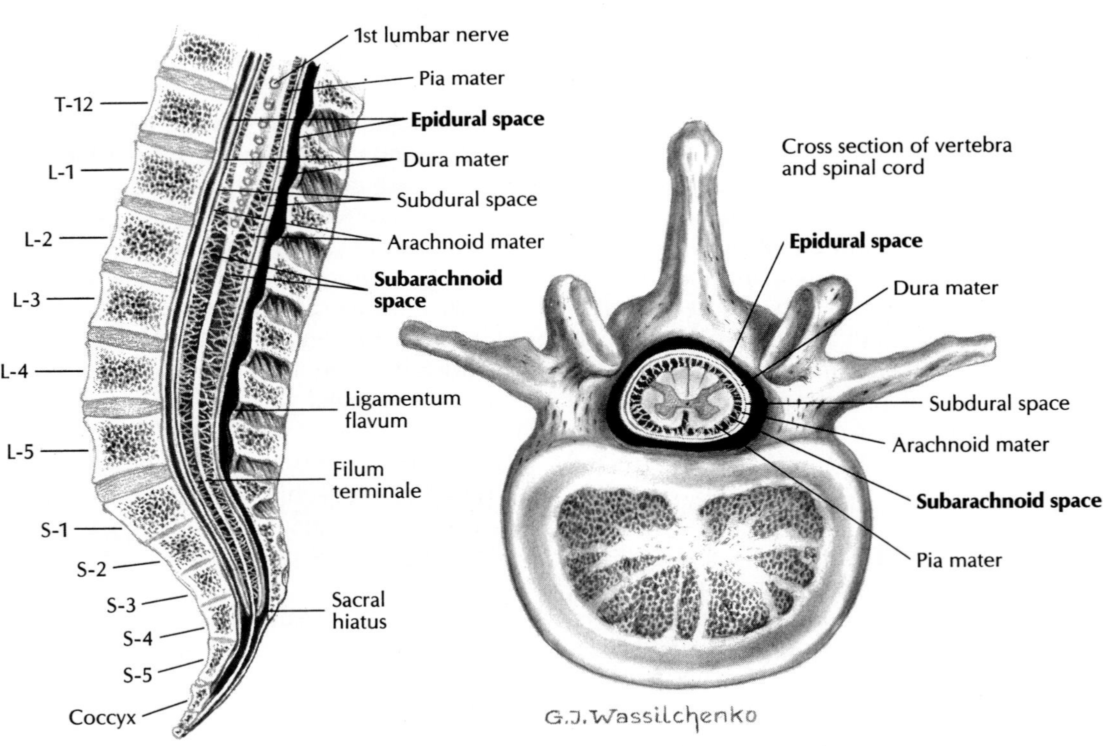

Fig. 15-4 Membranes and spaces of spinal cord; levels of sacral, lumbar, and thoracic nerves.

sion. Then the woman is assisted to a supine position. She must remain supine with the head elevated slightly. Onset of anesthesia usually occurs within 1 to 2 minutes after injection. Duration of anesthesia is 1 to 3 hours, depending on the anesthetic used.

Marked hypotension, decreased cardiac output and placental perfusion, and respiratory inadequacy tend to occur during any spinal anesthesia. Therefore the woman receives hydration with IV fluids before injection of anesthetic to decrease the potential for sympathetic blockade hypotension. After injection, maternal blood pressure, pulse, respirations, and FHR must be checked and recorded every 5 to 10 minutes. If signs of serious maternal hypotension or fetal distress develop, emergency care must be given (see box, p. 391). For further discussion of fetal distress and appropriate interventions, see Chapter 16.

Because the mother is not able to sense her contractions, she must be instructed when to bear down. If the birth occurs in a delivery room (rather than a labor-delivery-recovery room) the mother will need assistance in the transfer to recovery bed after delivery of the placenta.

Advantages of spinal anesthesia include ease of administration, maintenance of normotension and absence of fetal hypoxia. Maternal consciousness is maintained, excellent muscular relaxation is achieved; and blood loss is not excessive. Maternal alertness enables the woman to participate in the birth process. Usually no other anesthetic agents (e.g., inhalation drugs) are required. If stirrups are used for delivery, care must be taken to position them properly (for discussion of the use of stirrups, see Chapter 18). Spinal anesthesia may be the

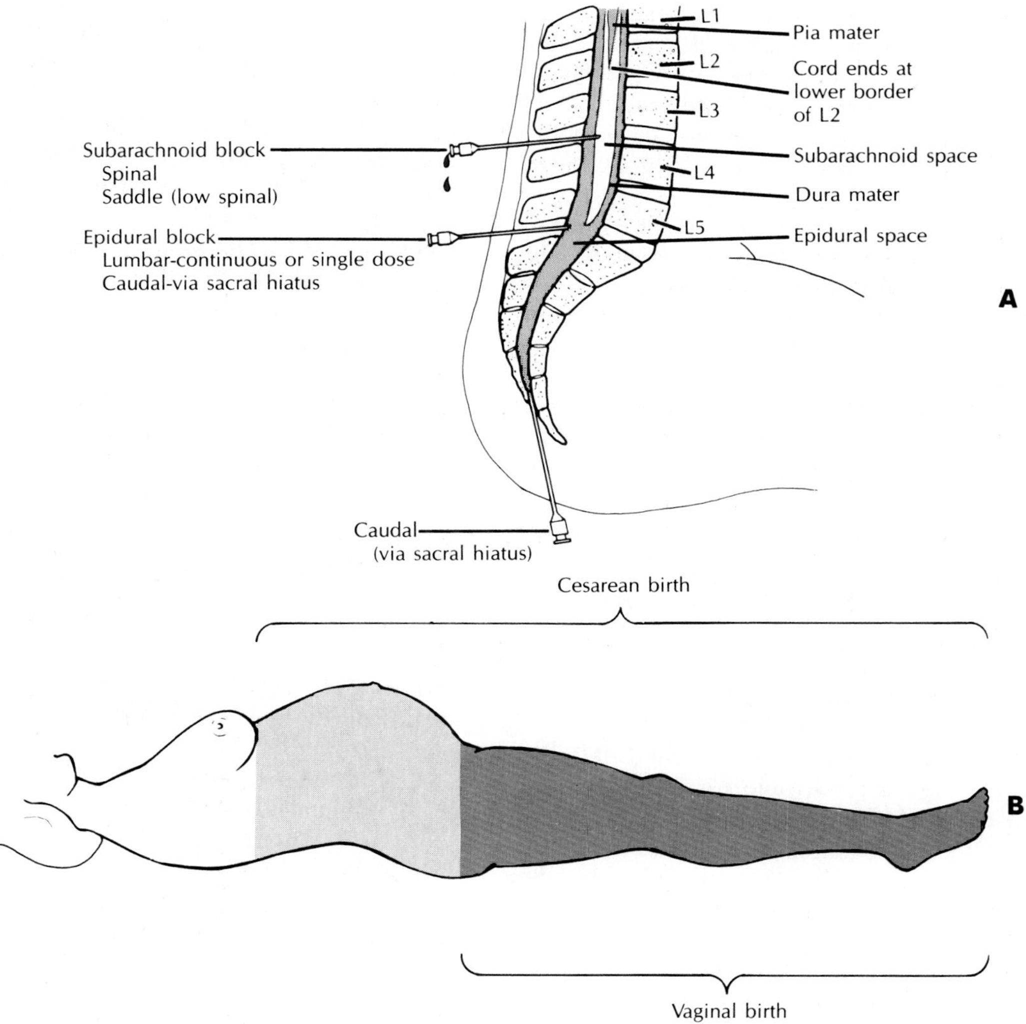

Fig. 15-5 A, Regional block analgesia and anesthesia in obstetrics. B, Level of anesthesia necessary for cesarean birth and for vaginal birth.
Courtesy Ross Laboratories, Columbus, Ohio.

method of choice for women with severe respiratory problems or with liver, kidney, or metabolic disease because it decreases the stress of labor and birth on these systems.

Disadvantages of spinal anesthesia include drug reactions (e.g., allergy), rare chemical myelitis or infection, hypotension, and respiratory paralysis. CPR may be needed. When spinal anesthesia is given, the need for operative delivery (episiotomy, low forceps extraction) tends to increase because of the elimination of voluntary expulsive efforts. After birth, the incidence of bladder and uterine atony, as well as postspinal headache, is higher.

HEADACHE AFTER SPINAL (LUMBAR) PUNCTURE. Leakage of cerebrospinal fluid from the site of puncture of the **meninges** (membranous coverings of the spinal cord) is thought to be the major causative factor in post–lumbar puncture (**postspinal headache**). Headache may be postural and occur only in the head-up or standing position. Presumably, the diminished volume of cerebrospinal fluid creates traction on pain-sensitive CNS structures with postural changes. Headache and auditory and visual problems may persist for days or weeks.

However, the likelihood of headache after lumbar puncture can be reduced if the anesthesiologist uses a small-gauge spinal needle and avoids multiple punctures of the meninges. A Spratt needle, for example, has a rounded tip with a hole on the side so that nerve fibers are not split as the tip is introduced. Positioning the woman flat in bed (with only a small, flat pillow for her head) for at least 8 hours has been recommended to prevent headache after spinal anesthesia, but there is no definitive evidence that this procedure is effective. Positioning the woman on her abdomen had been thought to decrease the loss of fluid through the puncture site. Vigorous hydration has been claimed to be of value, but there is no compelling evidence to support its use (Cunningham et al, 1989).

Initial treatment for headache after lumbar puncture usually includes analgesics, bed rest, caffeine, and increased fluid intake (i.e., 150 ml/hr IV) (Scott et al, 1990). An autologous **epidural blood patch** (a patch repairing a tear or a hole in the dura mater around the spinal cord) has proved helpful and may be considered if the headache does not resolve spontaneously (Scott et al, 1990). To create a patch, a few milliliters of the woman's own (autologous) blood without anticoagulant is injected epidurally at the site of the spinal tap (Fig. 15-6), forming a clot that covers the hole and prevents further fluid loss. Saline similarly injected in larger volumes also has been claimed to provide relief. Abdominal support with a girdle or abdominal binder has been helpful and is worth trying. For some women the headache may be remarkably improved by the third day and absent by the fifth day (Cunningham et al, 1989).

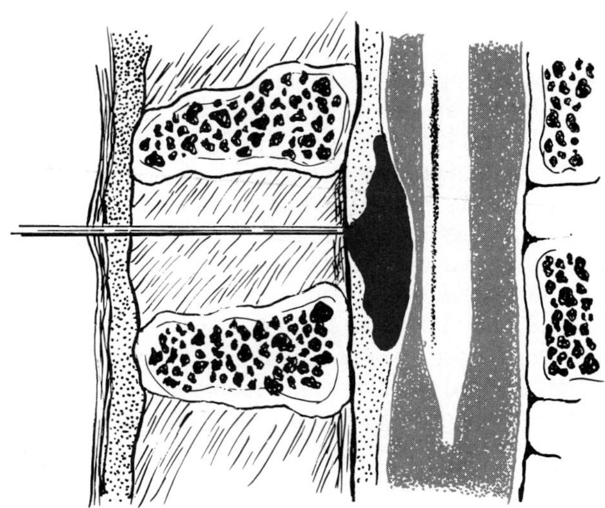

Fig. 15-6 Blood patch therapy for postspinal headache.

EPIDURAL BLOCK. Relief from the pain of uterine contractions and delivery (vaginal and abdominal) can be accomplished by injecting a suitable local anesthetic into the epidural (peridural) space (see Figs. 15-4 and 15-5). The portal of entry into this space for obstetric analgesia and anesthesia is through either a lumbar intervertebral space or caudally through the sacral hiatus and sacral canal.

The caudal space is the lowest extent of the epidural, or peridural, space (see Figs. 15-4 and 15-5). Emerging from the dural sac a few inches higher, a rich network of sacral nerves passes downward through the caudal space. A suitable anesthetic solution filling the caudal canal may eliminate the sensation of pain carried via the sacral nerves and thus produce anesthesia suitable for vaginal delivery. Higher levels with continuous caudal technique provide both analgesia in the first and second stages of labor and anesthesia for delivery. Because **caudal epidural block** is rarely used today, specifics regarding this method are not presented here. See medical texts in bibliography for this information.

Complete **lumbar epidural block** for the discomfort of labor and vaginal delivery requires a block from T10 to S5. For abdominal delivery, a block is essential from at least T8 to S1. The diffusion of epidural anesthesia depends on the location of the catheter tip, the dose and volume of anesthetic agent used, and the woman's position (e.g., horizontal or head-up position) (Cunningham et al, 1989).

For introduction of lumbar epidural anesthesia, the woman is positioned as for a spinal injection (i.e., sitting) (see p. 379) or in a modified Sims' position

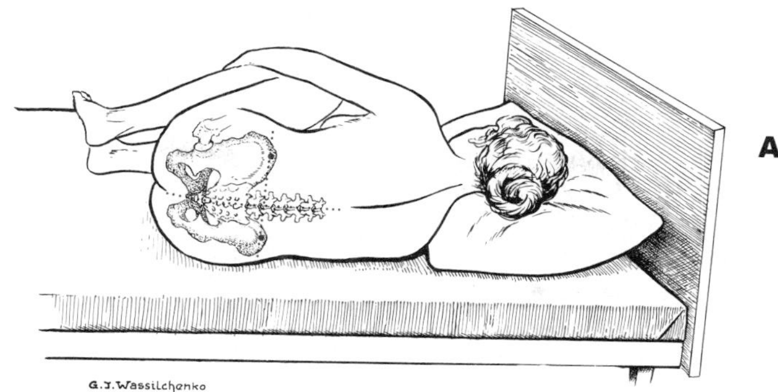

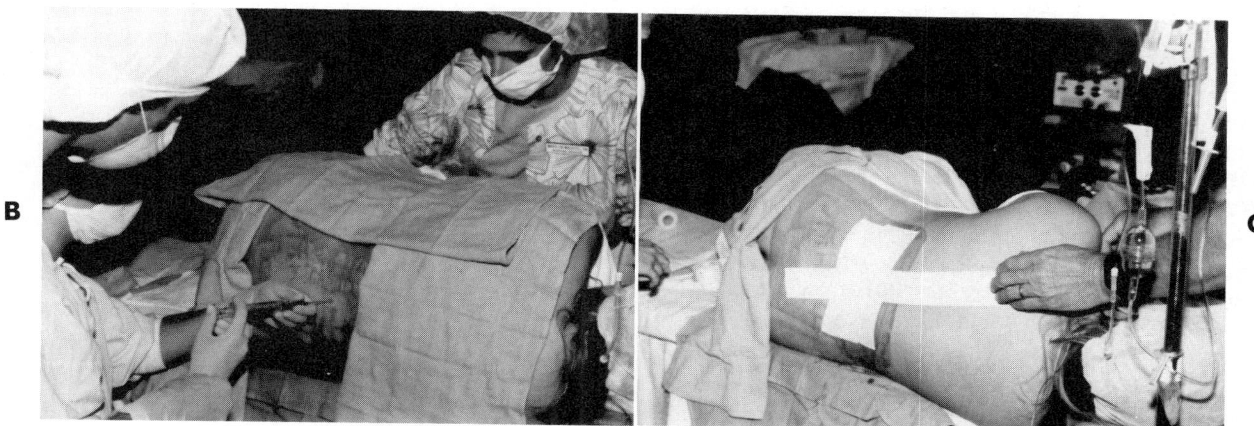

Fig. 15-7 **A,** Lateral decubitus position for epidural and subarachnoid block and anatomic landmarks to locate needle insertion site. **B,** Epidural anesthesia. Skin has been prepared with antiseptic solution (povidone-iodine) (Betadine). Area is draped with sterile towels. Nurse continues to support woman. **C,** Catheter is taped to woman's back; port segment is taped near her shoulder.
B and C courtesy Stanford University Hospital, Stanford, Calif.

(Fig. 15-7). For modified lateral Sims' position, the woman is placed on her left side, shoulders parallel, legs slightly flexed, and back arched.

The woman is positioned preferably on her left side to avoid weight of the uterus on the ascending vena cava and descending aorta, which can impair venous return and decrease placental perfusion. Oxygen is available should hypotension occur despite maintenance of IV fluid and displacement of maternal uterus to the left. The anesthesiologist may need to inject ephedrine (a vasopressor used to increase maternal blood pressure) and to accelerate IV fluid infusion (see Emergency Box, p. 391).

The FHR and progress in labor must be monitored carefully. The laboring woman will not be aware of changes in strength of uterine contractions or descent of the presenting part. Occasionally depression of contractions may result, necessitating augmentation of labor with oxytocin (for further discussion, see Chapter 35).

A single injection or continuous infusion (via pump) through an indwelling plastic catheter results in excellent analgesia-anesthesia (Fig. 15-2, *D*). The *advantages* of a continuous block are numerous: the mother remains alert and cooperative, airway reflexes remain intact, and only partial motor paralysis develops. In addition, good relaxation is achieved, and blood loss is not excessive. Fetal distress is rare but may occur with rapid absorption or marked maternal hypotension. Dose, volume, and type of anesthetic can be modified to allow the mother to push, to produce perineal anesthesia, and to permit forceps or even abdominal birth if required (Cunningham et al, 1989).

Some *disadvantages* to a continuous block exist. Anesthesiologists must have special training and experience to provide continuous blocks. Because a considerable amount of the drug must be used, reactions or rapid absorption of the anesthetic agent may result in maternal hypotension, convulsions, or paresthesia. The incidence of operative delivery (e.g., episiotomy, use of forceps) may be increased if the woman cannot bear down (push) effectively. If birth occurs on a delivery table instead of a labor-delivery-recovery room bed, the woman will need assistance to move to the recovery bed. Occasionally, accidental high-spinal anesthesia (and later, postspinal headache) may follow inadvertent perforation of the dural membrane when lumbar epidural anesthesia is administered.

The anesthetic selected may not be effective for some women, and a second form of anesthesia may be required. Establishment of effective pain relief with maximum safety takes time. The potential for pain relief during labor and for birth may not be realized in cases of rapid labor. Therefore epidural anesthesia for multiparous women in active labor is likely to prove not worth the bother, risk, and expense (Cunningham et al, 1989).

Complications also can occur. Severe respiratory and cardiac impairment resulting from inadvertent penetration of the epidural needle into the subarachnoid space is a rare complication with single injection or continuous epidural block. Diaphragmatic paralysis, breathing difficulty, and severe anxiety (from lack of oxygen) result.

Epidural catheter migration is another rare complication (Nicholson, 1990). Maternal response to *intravascular migration* of an epidural catheter is the return of pain. However, neither seizure nor cardiovascular collapse occurs (Cheek, Gutsche, 1987). Because the return of pain is a clear and unique signal of possible migration, another dose should not be added until migration is ruled out (O'Grady, Youngstrom, 1990).* *Migration of the epidural catheter into the subarachnoid space* is possible but highly unlikely. Excessive spinal block anesthesia could develop with subarachnoid migration. However, the progression of pronounced lower-limb motor block and very slow rise in level of sensory block allow for early diagnosis and treatment of subarachnoid migration of the epidural catheter (Cheek, Gutsche, 1987). Hourly observations of lower-limb movement would detect the migration of the catheter long before excessive spinal block develops (O'Grady, Youngstrom, 1990).

EPIDURAL AND SPINAL NARCOTICS. There is a high concentration of narcotic receptors along the pain pathway in the spinal cord, in the brain stem, and in the thalamus. Because these receptors are highly sensitive to narcotics, a small quantity of narcotic produces marked analgesia lasting for several hours. Medication is injected through a catheter placed in the epidural or subarachnoid space, which blocks pain transmission. Administration of epidural or spinal narcotics during labor has several advantages. These agents do not cause maternal hypotension or affect vital signs. The woman feels contractions but not pain. Her ability to bear down during the second stage of labor is preserved because the pushing reflex is not lost and motor power remains intact.

Fentanyl may be used alone. Its effects last up to 90 minutes. When added to the local anesthetic at the time of epidural administration, fentanyl extends the duration of anesthesia. There are no cardiovascular effects. However, fentanyl does not provide adequate analgesia for second-stage labor pain, episiotomy, or birth (Cunningham et al, 1989).

The most common indication for epidurally or spinally administered narcotics is for relief of postoperative pain. For example, women who give birth by the abdominal route receive Innovar or morphine through the catheter 1 hour after surgery. The catheter may then be removed, and the women are pain free for 24 hours. Occasionally the catheter is left in place in case another dose is needed.

Epidurally administered morphine allows the woman to be up with surprising ease and to care for her baby. Early ambulation and freedom from pain also facilitate bladder emptying. To women who have had a previous cesarean birth with the usual postoperative pain, the effects of this approach seem miraculous, and the nurse generally is amazed at the mother's ease in ambulation and relative freedom from pain. However, nurses must observe caution because the mother may not understand why she may experience pain after the narcotic effect wears off.

The side effects of morphine administered by the epidural or spinal route include nausea, vomiting, pruritus (itching), urinary retention, and delayed respiratory depression. Antiemetics, antipruritics, and narcotic antagonists are used to relieve these symptoms. For example, naloxone or naltrexone promethazine, or metoclopramide (Reglan) may be administered. Hospital protocols should provide specific instructions for treatment of these side effects. Some obstetricians believe that the risks of epidural or spinal injection are not sufficient to warrant its routine use. Respiratory depression is a serious concern; the woman's respiratory rate should be assessed and documented every 2 hours for 24 hours.

CONTRAINDICATIONS TO SUBARACHNOID AND EPIDURAL BLOCKS. Some contraindications to epidural analgesia apply equally to caudal and subarachnoid blocks (Scott et al, 1990):

1. *Client refusal.*

*In some hospitals, nurses are learning to "top off" (add another dose of medication) to indwelling catheters.

2. *Antepartum hemorrhage.* Acute hypovolemia leads to increased sympathetic tone to maintain the blood pressure. Any anesthetic technique that blocks the sympathetic fibers can lead to significant hypotension that can endanger the mother and baby.
3. *Anticoagulant therapy or bleeding disorder.* If a woman is receiving anticoagulant therapy or has a bleeding disorder, injury to a blood vessel may result in a hematoma. The hematoma may compress the cauda equina or the spinal cord and lead to serious CNS sequelae.
4. *Infection at the injection site.* Infection can be spread through the peridural or subarachnoid spaces if the needle traverses an infected area.
5. *Tumor at the injection site.* A tumor at the injection site is an unusual but definite contraindication.
6. *Allergy to anesthetic drug.*
7. *History of spinal injury or surgery.* The later occurrence of a spinal disorder could not be attributed to an epidural or subarachnoid block.

Relative contraindications to intraspinal blocks include CNS disorders, extensive back surgery, morbid obesity or anatomic abnormality in which landmarks cannot be identified, and current or prior disease of the CNS (Scott et al, 1990).

DRUG EFFECTS ON NEONATE. Debate persists concerning the effects of epidural anesthesia on the neonate's neurobehavioral responses. Studies of associations between neurobehavioral outcome and epidural anesthesia are far from consistent (Avard, Nimrod, 1985). Hodgkinson et al (1977) reported a beneficial effect whereas others have reported that neonates did not score as well on neurobehavioral tests (Rosenblatt et al, 1981). Others reported no difference (Abboud et al, 1982; Marx, 1984). However, the findings suggest a mild transient effect on neonatal behavior.

PARACERVICAL (UTEROSACRAL) BLOCK. **Paracervical block** is given to relieve pain from cervical dilatation and distention of the lower uterine segment in the first stage of labor during the active (acceleration) phase. (For a discussion of the acceleration phase, see Friedman curve, Fig. 17-7 and Table 17-3.) For paracervical anesthesia, a dilute local anesthetic drug (e.g., 5 mL of 1% procaine) is injected just beneath the mucosa adjacent to the outer rim of the cervix (9 and 3 o'clock positions) after the cervix is more than 5 cm dilated. A needle guide (e.g., the "Iowa trumpet") is useful but not indispensable for transvaginal administration (Fig. 15-8). Relief from discomfort is noticed within approximately 5 minutes. Excellent pain relief lasts for at least 1 hour.

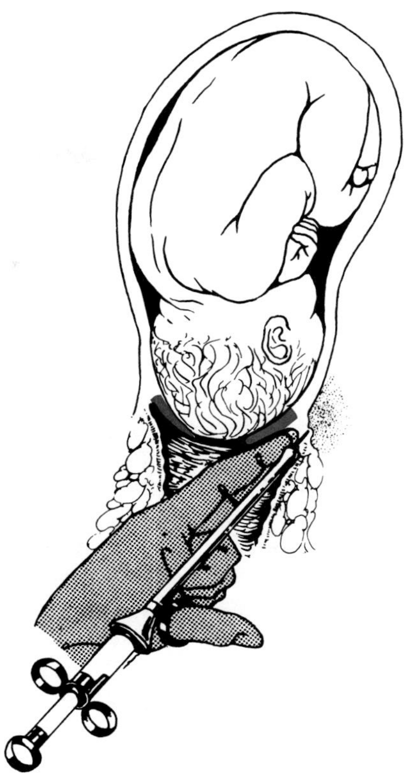

Fig. 15-8 Paracervical block. Note the position of the hand and fingers in relation to the cervix and fetal head and the shallow depth of the needle insertion. Note also that no undue pressure is applied at the vaginal fornix by the fingers or needle guide.
From Benson RC: *Handbook of obstetrics and gynecology,* ed 7, Los Altos, Calif, 1980, Lange Medical Publications.

Anesthesia extends from the lower uterine segment and cervix to the upper third of the vagina (see Fig. 15-2 *B*); there is no perineal anesthesia. Although there may be a transient depression of contractions, there is little or no effect on the labor. Repeat injections may be given until the cervix is dilated to 8 cm, whereupon another method, such as pudendal block, may be necessary.

Paracervical block anesthesia may cause fetal intoxication because of rapid absorption of the drug. When the anesthetic is injected into the tissues lateral to the cervix, it is picked up by the maternal circulation, which quickly involves the uterus and placenta. When overdosage occurs, the fetus may exhibit bradycardia because of the quinidine-like effect of the anesthetic on the myocardium or, as research indicates, because of a reduction in uterine blood flow. In addition, CNS medullary depression may develop, and the neonate may show vascular collapse and apnea at delivery. Hematomas can develop at the site of injection if a uterine vessel is damaged.

Because of these potential complications, paracervical block may not be the method of choice for labor but remains an option for anesthesia during abortion or other gynecologic procedures.

Inhalation Analgesia and Anesthesia

Self-administration of inhalation gases may be helpful, especially during the second stage of labor. The mother breathes subanesthetic concentrations of inhalation anesthetic such as methoxyflurane (Penthrane). If these agents are given properly, the woman remains conscious but has profound pain relief. The route is usually self-administered from a capsule and face mask strapped to the wrist. The physician sets the desired concentration, and the woman inhales the drug during contractions. The goal of this method is for the woman to remain conscious while profound analgesia, as well as some amnesia for painful events, is achieved. The nurse must stay with the woman and never administer the drug for her because overdose is a risk. The nurse also must monitor vital signs every 30 minutes and FHR every 15 minutes. The woman should remain conscious and not become delirious or excited. The nurse alerts the physician and removes the analgesic from the woman's hand if the mother has cardiac arrhythmia or loses consciousness or if FHR abnormalities occur. These inhalation analgesics are rarely used in the United States today.

Other inhalation agents include halothane (Fluothane) and nitrous oxide. Halothane inhalation relaxes the uterus quickly and facilitates intrauterine manipulation, version (see Chapter 35), and extraction. The desired effect is general loss of sensitivity to touch, pain, and other stimulation.

A combination of 50% nitrous oxide (laughing gas) and 50% oxygen may be given for analgesic effect late in the first stage and with contractions during the period of expulsion in the second stage. Nitrous oxide may be self-administered. Administered in low concentrations, nitrous oxide relieves the mother's pain but still allows her to bear down with her contractions during the second stage of labor. Care is needed to prevent maternal and neonatal respiratory depression when nitrous oxide is used as an analgesic/anesthetic.

GENERAL ANESTHESIA. General anesthesia rarely is indicated for uncomplicated vaginal birth. It may be necessary if there is a contraindication (including client refusal) to nerve block analgesia/anesthesia or if fetal indications necessitate a rapid (STAT) birth (vaginal or abdominal). The woman is not awake with this method, and there is danger of respiratory depression and vomiting followed by aspiration. For women with hypovolemia general anesthesia is safer than nerve block analgesia or anesthesia. It does not depress the newborn unless the mother is anesthetized deeply. Thiopental (Pentothal) is commonly used for general anesthesia. Administered intravenously (4 mg/kg of body weight), thiopental produces rapid induction of anesthesia and does not depress the fetus (Scott et al, 1990).

If general anesthesia is being considered, the nurse gives the woman nothing by mouth and sees that an IV infusion is established. If time allows, the nurse administers a nonparticulate oral antacid such as sodium citrate (30 mL) to increase gastric pH, which neutralizes acid contents of the stomach. If there is sufficient time, some physicians also order a histamine blocker such as cimetidine to decrease production of gastric acid and metoclopramide to increase gastric emptying (Scott et al, 1990). Before induction, a wedge should be placed under the woman's right hip to displace the uterus to the left. Uterine displacement prevents aortocaval compression, which interferes with placental perfusion. Sometimes the nurse is asked to assist with cricoid pressure during intubation. Priorities for recovery room care include maintaining an open airway and cardiopulmonary functions and preventing postpartum hemorrhage. Routine postpartum care is organized to facilitate parent-child attachment as soon as possible and to answer the mother's questions. When appropriate, the nurse assesses the mother's readiness to see the baby and her response to the anesthesia and to the event that necessitated general anesthesia (e.g., cesarean birth when vaginal birth was anticipated).

COMBINATION ANESTHESIA FOR CESAREAN BIRTH. Light general anesthesia is considered by many to be ideal for cesarean birth. A combination of thiopental, nitrous oxide–oxygen, and succinylcholine is used. The woman is given 100% oxygen for 3 minutes, followed by almost simultaneous rapid administration of thiopental and succinylcholine. During intubation, **cricoid pressure** is maintained, often by the nurse, to prevent aspiration of vomitus (Fig. 15-9). When the woman is drowsy, a nitrous oxide–oxygen mixture is given. Excellent tolerance of this combination is widely reported.

Anesthesia in the Obese Woman

Obesity affects 6% to 10% of pregnant women. Obesity is defined as an excess of body fat causing weight to be greater than 20% over ideal weight. Weight more than twice the ideal body weight is defined as morbid obesity. A study of anesthesia-related

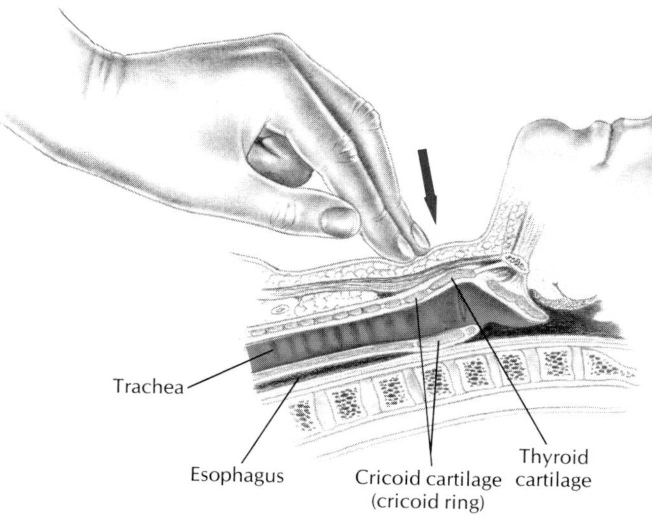

Fig. 15-9 Technique of applying pressure on cricoid cartilage to occlude esophagus prevents pulmonary aspiration of gastric contents during anesthesia induction.

maternal mortality in Michigan between 1972 and 1989 found that obesity was a risk factor in 80% of maternal mortalities (Endler, 1988).

Maternal physiologic changes are the result of hormonal influences and mechanical effects. In obesity, the weight of fat tissue and the added metabolic demands also affect maternal physiology (Endler, 1990). Blood volume and cardiac output increase during pregnancy (see Chapter 8) and obesity, expanding in proportion to the amount of fat tissue mass. During labor and vaginal birth, and in the immediate postpartum period, blood values and cardiac output reach levels 80% higher than prelabor values. The enlarged uterus and abdominal fat mass increase the possibility of aortocaval compression.

The respiratory system is also stressed (Endler, 1990). The obese laboring woman is in a precarious state of pulmonary function. Therefore oxygenation must be carefully monitored through birth and the immediate postpartum period. Monitoring by pulse oximeter has been suggested.

All pregnant women experience delayed gastric emptying time, decreased tone in the cardiac sphincter, and hyperacidity. In addition, the obese woman is more likely to have a hiatal hernia and a marked increase in intragastric pressure and volume. Therefore these women are at great risk for regurgitation and aspiration (Endler, 1990).

Management during labor should focus on efforts to minimize oxygen consumption and maximize pulmonary function. Epidural analgesia during the first stage of labor decreases demands on metabolic and respiratory systems and improves oxygenation. It also slows the rise in catecholamine levels caused by pain, and this rise leads to increased cardiac output.

Intravenous narcotics may be used during the first stage of labor. However, the dosage of drugs and their effects must be monitored carefully because obese women are extremely sensitive to the respiratory depressant effects of narcotics (Endler, 1990). Epidural block during the second stage of labor provides complete pain relief and supports cardiovascular function.

If cesarean birth is necessary, epidural block is preferred over general anesthesia. Problems associated with general anesthesia include potential difficulties during intubation, hypertensive effect of laryngoscopy and intubation, and danger of aspiration and pulmonary complications. Subarachnoid block may be used if there is insufficient time for an epidural block. Uterine displacement to prevent aortocaval compression is more difficult to achieve in the obese woman. If the woman is extremely obese, elevation of the right hip on a wedge may not be sufficient to avoid compression. It may be necessary to physically lift the abdominal fat pad off the abdomen until the peritoneal cavity has been entered (Endler, 1990).

■ THE NURSING PROCESS

The choice of pain relief depends on a combination of factors, including the woman's special needs and wishes, the availability of the desired method of analgesia or anesthesia, the physician's or certified nurse midwife's preference and expertise, and the phase and stage of labor. The nurse is responsible for continuous maternal and fetal assessment and for establishing mutual goals with the woman (and her family), planning and implementing nursing care, and evaluating the effects of care based on a plan of nursing care that includes nursing diagnoses.

ASSESSMENT

The assessment of the laboring woman, her fetus, and her labor is a joint effort of the nurse and the primary health care providers who then consult with the woman. The needs of each woman are different. Many factors enter into the nursing assessment to determine choice of analgesia and anesthesia.

History

The woman's prenatal record is read for relevant information. In addition to identifying data, the woman's parity, estimated date of delivery, complications and medications during pregnancy, and obstetric history are noted. History of allergies is noted and displayed prominently. History of smoking and neurologic, respiratory, cardiovascular, and spinal disorders are noted.

Interview

Interview data establish the time and type of food taken at the woman's last meal, existing medical respiratory conditions (cold, allergy), and unusual reactions (e.g., allergy) to medications, cleansing agents, or tape. The woman is asked whether she attended parent education for childbirth classes. Her preparation and preferences for management of discomfort are noted. Her knowledge of choices for management of discomfort is assessed. The woman's perception of discomfort and her expressed need for medication add to the data base. The events since the woman's last contact with the primary health care provider are reviewed (e.g., infections, diarrhea, change in fetal behavior). If verbal and physical signs suggest substance abuse, the nurse inquires about the type of drug used, time of last use, and method of administration (for further discussion of substance dependence, see Chapter 33).

The woman is asked about the onset of labor and status of membranes, or the reason for this admission is determined—for example, induction of labor or cesarean birth.

Physical Examination

The character and status of this labor and fetal response are assessed (see Chapters 14 and 17). The nurse notes the degree of hydration by assessing intake and output, moisture of mucous membranes, and skin turgor. Bladder distention is noted. Evidence of skin infection near sites of possible needle insertion is recorded and reported. Signs of apprehension such as fist clenching and restlessness are noted.

If the woman is in labor, maternal and fetal vital signs; uterine contractions; and cervical effacement and dilatation, station, and anticipated time until delivery are all considered. Length of labor and degree of fatigue are important considerations.

Laboratory Tests

Laboratory tests are reviewed for anemia (hemoglobin and hematocrit), coagulopathy (bleeding disorder), and infection (white blood cell count and differential). The prenatal record is reviewed for laboratory tests (e.g., blood, urine, amniotic fluid) related to disorders such as diabetes mellitus, cardiac disease, thyroid disease, infection, and concurrent disorders such as preeclampsia or substance abuse. Antenatal diagnostic studies (ultrasound, nonstress test, contraction stress test, amniocentesis, and biophysical profile) (see Chapter 27) and their findings are noted.

The choice of analgesia and anesthesia varies by phase and stage of labor (see box, p. 376).

Signs of Potential Problems. Any medication can cause an **allergic reaction** that may be minor or as severe as anaphylaxis. Minor reactions can be characterized by development of a rash, rhinitis, fever, asthma, and pruritus. Management of the less acute allergic response is not an emergency. The nurse should monitor the vital signs, respiratory status, cardiovascular status, platelet count, and white blood cell count. The woman is observed for side effects of drug therapy, especially drowsiness; the fluid intake and output are monitored to determine urinary retention; and frequency of bowel movements is monitored to assess constipation (Clark et al, 1990).

Severe reactions may occur suddenly and produce shock. The most dramatic form of anaphylaxis is sudden severe bronchospasm, vasospasm, severe hypotension, and death. Signs of anaphylaxis are largely caused by contraction of smooth muscles and may begin with irritability, extreme weakness, nausea, and vomiting. The reaction then proceeds to dyspnea, cyanosis, convulsions, and cardiac arrest. The acute allergic reaction, anaphylaxis, requires immediate diagnosis and treatment, usually with 1:1000 epinephrine injected subcutaneously or intramuscularly, followed by parenteral antihistamines. Supportive care addresses symptoms and is based on rapid assessment of the cardiovascular and respiratory response. Cardiopulmonary resuscitation (CPR) may be necessary. The nurse must also be alert to fetal well-being; FHR decelerations are noted and reported to the physician.

NURSING DIAGNOSES

Nursing diagnoses vary from individual to individual. Examples of nursing diagnoses relevant to pharmacologic control of discomfort during the labor and birth period include the following:

- High risk for altered tissue perfusion related to
  —Effects of analgesia or anesthesia
  —Maternal position

- Situational low self-esteem related to
  —Negative perception of the woman's (or her family's) behavior
- Pain related to
  —Processes of labor and birth
- Anxiety or fear related to knowledge deficit of
  —Procedure for nerve block analgesia
  —Expected sensation during nerve block analgesia
  —Mother's role during nerve block analgesia
  —Options for analgesia and anesthesia
- High risk for maternal injury related to
  —Effects of analgesia and anesthesia on sensation and motor control
- High risk for injury to fetus related to
  —Maternal hypotension
  —Maternal position (aortocaval compression)

PLANNING

A plan of care for each woman is developed that relates to her specific needs and nursing care. The plan involves the mother and family and incorporates their priorities and preferences. The nurse, in collaboration with the primary health care provider and laboring woman, selects those aspects of care relevant to the individual woman, as well as her family.

The goals for nursing care related to pharmacologic control of discomfort include the following considerations:

1. *Maternal* The mother will achieve adequate pain relief without adding to maternal risk (e.g., through appropriate medication, dosage, and timing and route of administration).
2. *Fetal and neonatal* The fetus will maintain well-being, and the neonate will adjust to extrauterine life.
3. *Family/significant others* The family/significant others will know their needs and rights in relation to the use of analgesia or anesthesia.

IMPLEMENTATION

The woman's *perception* of her behavior during labor is of utmost importance. If she planned a nonmedicated birth but then needs and accepts medication, her self-esteem may falter. Verbal and nonverbal acceptance of her behavior is given (as necessary) and reinforced by the nurse's visit the day after birth, if possible. Explanations about fetal response to maternal discomfort, the effects of maternal fatigue, and the medication itself are supportive measures. Support may be needed by family and other support persons if plans for a nonmedicated birth are altered.

Excessive stress (as yet undefined in perinatal medicine) causes increased maternal catecholamine production. Catecholamines have been linked to dysfunctional labor and fetal and neonatal distress and illness (Simkin, 1986 a, b). Parents may feel reassured somewhat by hearing that medication is sometimes indicated for the baby's benefit.

Informed Consent

The primary health care provider and anesthesia care provider are responsible for informing women of the alternative methods of pharmacologic pain relief available in the hospital setting. The description of anesthetic techniques is essential to informed consent, even if the woman has received information about analgesia and anesthesia earlier in her pregnancy. This interview should take place just before or early in labor so the woman has time to consider alternatives. Nurses play a part in the informed consent by clarifying and describing the procedures or by acting as a client's advocate and asking the primary health care provider for further explanations. The procedure and its advantages and disadvantages must be thoroughly explained (for a discussion of preparation for the procedure, see discussion that follows; for informed consent, see Chapter 4). The woman must be informed that the anesthetic is not always effective and that there are potential side effects for both mother and fetus.

Timing of Administration

Orders often are written to dispense or administer medications on the basis of the nurse's clinical judgment. These orders require clinical knowledge and expertise. It is often the nurse who alerts the primary health care provider that the woman is in need of pharmacologic relief for discomfort. The boxes on p. 377 list pharmacologic control by stage of labor and method of birth. A review of the origins of discomfort (see p. 374) provides the basis for understanding the laboring woman's changing needs during labor.

Preparation for Procedures

The nurse reviews or validates the woman's choices for relief from discomfort and clarifies the information for the mother as necessary. The woman needs an explanation of the procedure and what will be asked of her (e.g., to maintain flexed position during insertion of epidural). The woman benefits from knowing how the medication is to be given, the degree of discomfort to expect from administration of the medication, sensations she can expect, skin preparation, time requirement for administration, and interval before medication "takes hold." The nurse explains the need for emptying her bladder before analgesic or anesthetic is given and for keeping the bladder empty. If an indwelling epidural catheter is threaded and the woman feels a momentary twinge down her leg, hip, or back, she is assured that it is not a sign of injury.

For paracervical and pudendal blocks a long needle is used (see Fig. 15-8). The sight of this needle may be frightening. The woman can be reassured that only the tip of the needle will be inserted.

Administration of Medication

INTRAVENOUS ROUTE. The preferred route of administration of such medications as meperidine or fentanyl is through IV tubing. The infusion of IV solution is stopped while the medication is injected into the port nearest the client. The medication is given slowly in small doses at the *beginning* of three to five consecutive contractions (Petree, 1983). Because uterine blood vessels are constricted during contractions, the medication stays within the maternal vascular system for several seconds before the uterine blood vessels reopen. The IV infusion is restarted slowly to prevent giving a bolus of medication. This method of injection minimizes the amount of drug crossing the placenta to the fetus. With decreased placental transfer, the mother's degree of pain relief is maximized. The IV route has the following results:

Pain relief is obtained with small doses of the drug.
Onset of pain relief is more predictable.
Duration of effect is more predictable.

INTRAMUSCULAR ROUTE. IM injections of analgesics, although still used, are no longer the preferred route of administration for the laboring woman. Identified disadvantages of the IM route include the following:

Onset of pain relief is delayed.
Higher doses of medication are required.
Medication is released from the muscle tissue at an unpredictable rate and is available for transfer across the placenta to the fetus.

IM injections are given in the upper portion of the arm if regional anesthesia is planned later in labor. This is the preferred site because the autonomic blockage from the regional (e.g., epidural) anesthesia increases blood flow to the gluteal region and accelerates absorption of the drug. The maternal plasma level of the drug necessary to bring pain relief usually is reached 45 minutes after IM injection, followed by a decline in plasma levels. The maternal drug levels (after IM injections) are unequal because of uneven distribution (maternal uptake) and metabolism. The advantage of using the IM route is quick administration.

NERVE BLOCKS. An IV line is established before nerve blocks such as paracervical, epidural, and subarachnoid spinal and general anesthesia are introduced. Lactated Ringer's or Plasma-Lyte A and normal saline solutions are the preferred solutions. Infusion solutions without dextrose are preferred, especially when the solution needs to be infused rapidly (e.g., in the presence of severe dehydration or to maintain blood pressure). Solutions that contain dextrose raise maternal and fetal blood glucose levels rapidly. The fetus responds to high blood glucose levels by increasing insulin production; fetal or neonatal hypoglycemia may result. In addition, dextrose changes osmotic pressure so that fluid is excreted from the kidneys more rapidly.

The woman needs assistance in assuming and maintaining the correct position for epidural and spinal anesthesia (see pp. 379 and 382).

SAFETY AND GENERAL CARE. After IV or IM injection or nerve block, the woman is protected by raised side rails and a call bell within easy reach when the nurse is not in attendance. These women must be protected from prolonged pressure on an anesthetized part (e.g., lying on one side with weight on one leg; tight bedclothes on feet). If stirrups are used, the nurse pads them, adjusts both stirrups at the same level and angle, places both of the woman's legs into them simultaneously to avoid pressure to the popliteal angle, and applies restraints without restricting circulation.

The nurse monitors and records the woman's response to medication: level of pain relief, level of apprehension, return of sensations and perception of pain, and allergic or untoward reactions (e.g., hypotension, respiratory depression). Emergency care for maternal hypotension with decreased placental perfusion is outlined in the box on p. 391. The nurse continues to monitor maternal vital signs, blood pressure, strength and frequency of uterine contractions, changes in the cervix and station of the presenting part, presence of the bearing-down reflex, bladder filling, and state of hydration. Ascertaining fetal response after administration of analgesia or anesthesia is vital. The woman is asked if she (or the family) has any questions. The nurse assesses the woman's and her family's understanding of the need for ensuring her safety (e.g., keeping side rails up, calling for assistance as needed).

The time between the administration of a narcotic and the baby's birth is noted. The woman's record

EMERGENCY

Maternal Hypotension with Decreased Placental Perfusion

SIGNS/SYMPTOMS

Maternal hypotension (20% drop from preblock level or less than 100 mm Hg systolic)
Fetal bradycardia
Decreased beat-to-beat FHR variability (see Chapter 16)

INTERVENTIONS

Turn woman to left lateral position or place pillow or wedge under right hip (see Fig. 17.10) to deflect uterus.
Maintain IV infusion at rate specified, or increase prn per hospital protocol.
Administer oxygen by face mask at 10-12 L/min.
Elevate the woman's legs.
Notify the physician/midwife/anesthesiologist/nurse anesthetist.
Administer IV vasopressor (e.g., ephedrine).
Remain with woman; continue to monitor maternal BP and FHR q5 min until stable or per primary health care provider's order.

during childbirth serves as a documented means of communication among all members of the health care team. Documentation of the events is mandatory to meet legal requirements. Precise records also serve as a reservoir for research study.

EVALUATION

Evaluation is a continuous process. The nurse can be relatively assured that care was effective if the goals for care (p. 389) are met: the mother has adequate pain relief without increased risk; the unborn and neonate maintain well-being; and the family/significant others know their needs and rights in relation to analgesia and anesthesia.

A sample Case Study and Care Plan follow.

SUMMARY

Nursing management of obstetric analgesia and anesthesia combines the nurse's expertise in obstetrics and the labor process with knowledge and understanding of techniques, drugs, and their potential complications. Comprehensive care addresses the physiologic requirements of the woman and the effects on the unborn and newborn baby. The key is to provide the childbearing family with a choice in pain relief. It is then the duty of caring professionals to ensure safety in that choice by using their knowledge of drugs and techniques.

REFERENCES

Abboud TK et al: Maternal, fetal and neonatal responses after epidural anesthesia with bupivacaine, 2-chloroprocaine or lidocaine, *Anesth Analg* 61:638, 1982.

Avard DM, Nimrod CM: Risks and benefits of obstetric epidural analgesia: a review, *Birth* 12:215, Winter 1985.

Bradley RA: *Husband-coached childbirth,* New York, 1974, Harper & Row.

Briggs GC, Freeman RK, Yaffe SJ: *Drugs in pregnancy and lactation,* ed 2, Baltimore, 1986, Williams & Wilkins.

Cheek TG, Gutsche BB: Epidural analgesia for labor and vaginal delivery, *Clin Obstet Gyn* 30:515, 1987.

Clark JB, Queener SF, Karb VB: *Pharmacological basis of nursing practice,* ed 3, St Louis, 1990, Mosby–Year Book.

Cunningham FG, MacDonald PC, Gant NF: *Williams obstetrics,* ed 18, Norwalk, Conn, 1989, Appleton & Lange.

Dick-Read G: *Childbirth without fear,* ed 2, New York, 1959, Harper & Row.

Endler GC: The risk of anesthesia in obese parturients, *J Perinat* 10:175, June 1990.

Endler GC, et al: Anesthesia-related maternal mortality in Michigan, 1972-1984, *Am J Obstet Gynecol* 159:187, 1988.

Gaston-Johansson F, Fridh G, Turner-Norvell K: Progression of labor pain in primiparas and multiparas, *Nurs Res* 37:87, 1988.

Hodgkinson R et al: Neonatal neurobehavioral tests following vaginal delivery under ketamine, thiopental, and extradural anesthesia, *Anesth Analg* 56:548, 1977.

Lamaze F: *Painless childbirth,* New York, 1972, Pocket Books.

Lundberg GD, editor: Anesthetics and neonatal response, *JAMA* 250:2133, 1983.

Marx GF: Pain relief during labor—more than comfort, *J Calif Perinat Assn* 4:36, Winter 1984.

CASE STUDY

Lumbar Epidural Block During Labor

Rose N. is a 24-year-old married woman with one child and is in her second pregnancy. Obstetric history includes a spontaneous vaginal birth of a healthy male weighing 8 pounds 2 ounces after a 10-hour unmedicated labor. Rose's contractions began yesterday after supper 12 hours ago. She describes more discomfort than she had with her first labor. This morning at 7 AM, assessment of Rose N. revealed that she was in active labor. Her vital signs, blood pressure, labor pattern, and FHR were stable and within normal limits. She has been unable to sleep during the night. She felt she could no longer cope with the contractions and requested an epidural block. After Rose emptied her bladder, an IV infusion of lactated Ringer's solution was initiated and 100 ml were infused. An epidural block was started 30 minutes ago. At this time Rose states she is comfortable. Rose is apologetic about wanting an epidural block; her husband comments that they had hoped she would not need any medication.

ASSESSMENT

Rose's vital signs, blood pressure, labor pattern, and FHR remain stable and within normal limits. Her bladder is not palpable (distended) at this time. She is resting quietly. Her husband is at her side, holding her hand, and resting his head on his wife's pillow. The electronic fetal monitor is recording uterine contractions and FHR.

NURSING DIAGNOSIS

Epidural block causes vasodilation and pooling of blood in the pelvis and legs. Even though Rose's blood volume was expanded with 1000 ml of lactated Ringer's solution and she is still receiving an IV infusion, the nurse identifies the following nursing diagnosis: high risk for maternal and fetal injury related to maternal hypotension secondary to effects of epidural block.

PLANNING

Planning for Rose focuses on prevention of potential problems related to the epidural block. Rose and the nurse identified mutual *goals:* safe passage for herself and the baby and control of discomfort. The *expected outcome* is the avoidance of hypotension, the most common side effect of an effective epidural block. Hypotension is defined as a decrease in maternal blood pressure of 20% or more below the preblock average, or a systolic pressure under 100 mg Hg.

IMPLEMENTATION

Interventions are chosen based on knowledge of the effects of an epidural block on maternal and fetal physiology and on the primary health care provider's orders. According to hospital protocol, the nurse continues to monitor the following: maternal pulse, respirations, blood pressure, and degree of comfort; contractions; labor progress, IV infusion rate; bladder filling; and fetal well-being as evidenced by FHR and activity level. Rose is positioned on her left side, and her call button is within easy reach. Oxygen supply, face mask, and tubing are readily available. The electronic fetal monitor is functioning properly, and the alarm button is set. As appropriate, the nurse answers questions from and addresses concerns of Rose and her husband.

EVALUATION

Evaluation of effectiveness of nursing interventions is based on the degree to which the goals and expected outcomes are achieved. For example, the degree to which Rose's discomfort is controlled and she and her baby experience a safe and healthy labor and birth are evaluated. If hypotension occurs, the degree to which it is diagnosed and managed is evaluated. Optimal outcome is evaluated by the absence of adverse sequelae for the mother or fetus/neonate.

Nicholson C: Nursing considerations for the parturient who has received epidural narcotics during labor or delivery, *J Perinat Neonat Nurs* 4:14, July 1990.

O'Grady JP, Youngstrom P: Must epidurals always imply instrumental delivery? *Contemp OB/GYN* 35:19, Aug 1990.

Petree B: *A nursing perspective of obstetrical analgesia/anesthesia,* NAACOG update series, 1:lesson 12, 1983.

Potter PA, Perry AG: *Basic nursing:* theory and practice, ed 2, St Louis, 1991, Mosby–Year Book.

Rosenblatt DB et al: The influence of maternal analgesia on neonatal behavior. II. Epidural bupivacaine, *Br J Obstet Gynaecol* 88:407, 1981.

Scott JR et al: *Danforth's obstetrics and gynecology,* ed 6, Philadelphia, 1990, JB Lippincott Co.

Simkin P: Stress, pain, and catecholamines in labor. I. A review, *Birth* 13(4):227, 1986a.

Simkin P: Stress, pain, and catecholamines in labor. II. A pilot survey of new mothers, *Birth* 13(4):234, 1986b.

BIBLIOGRAPHY

Bucknell S, Sikorski K: Putting patient-controlled analgesia to the test, *MCN* 14:37, Jan/Feb 1989.

Chestnut DH et al: Continuous epidural infusion of bupivicaine-fentanyl during the second stage of labor, *Anesthesiology* 71:A841, 1989.

Dewan DM: Anesthesia for preterm delivery, breech presentation, and multiple gestation, *Clin Obstet Gynecol* 30:566, Sept 1987.

Dunajcik L: Controlling the dangers of epidural analgesia, *RN*, p 40, Jan 1988.

Faut-Callahan M, Paice J: Postoperative pain control for the parturient, *J Perinat Neonat Nurs* 4:27, July 1990.

Care Plan — Lumbar Epidural Block During Labor

GOALS	IMPLEMENTATION	RATIONALE	EVALUATION
Nursing diagnosis: High risk for maternal and fetal injury related to maternal hypotension secondary to effects of epidural block			
Rose will not experience hypotension: pulse and BP remain WNL. FHR remains WNL.	Position Rose in left lateral position. Maintain IV infusion. Monitor maternal pulse and BP. Monitor FHR. Be prepared to implement interventions for maternal hypotension (see Emergency Box, p. 391).	Avoids aortocaval compression; supports placental perfusion. Expands blood volume; increases cardiac output. Allows early identification of maternal hypotension and its effect on the fetus. Corrects maternal hypotension and placental perfusion.	Rose does not experience hypotension: Her BP and pulse stay WNL. FHR remains WNL—no bradycardia or change in beat-to-beat variabil ity.
Nursing diagnosis: Altered pattern of urinary elimination during labor related to effects of epidural block			
Rose's bladder does not become distended.	Palpate bladder superior to symphysis pubis and observe frequently for distention.	Rose received 1000 ml IV fluid before epidural block; IV is still infusing. Urinary retention is a side effect of epidural block: Rose may be unaware of the need to void. Rose may be unable to void spontaneously.	When Rose's bladder begins to fill, Rose is able to void spontaneously,
	Encourage frequent voiding. Catheterize if necessary.	Bladder distention may Impede progress of fetus down birth canal. Increase the possibility of trauma to the bladder, especially during birth. Result in decreased bladder tone after giving birth.	Rose's bladder does not become distended.
Nursing diagnosis: Situational low self-esteem related to negative perception of behavior (asking for and accepting an epidural block)			
Rose and her husband maintain self-esteem.	Explain effect of pain on labor. Discuss pros/cons of medicated labor.	Increases their understanding of benefits of pain reduction in labor. Parents experience a heightened sensitivity to other's opinions during labor.	Rose and her husband state they feel good about their decision.

Henrikson ML, Wild LK: A nursing process approach to epidural anesthesia, *JOGNN* 17:316, 1988.

Kangas-Saarela T et al: The effect of lumbar epidural analgesia on the neurobehavioral responses of newborn infants, *Acta Anaesthesiol Scand* 33:320, 1989.

Litwack K: Managing postanesthetic emergencies, *Nursing 91*, 21:49, Sept 1991.

Naulty JS, Smith R, Ross R: Effect of changes in labor analgesic practice on labor outcome, *Anesthesiology* 69:A660, 1988.

Nicholson C, Ridolfo E: Avoiding the pitfalls of epidural anesthesia in obstetrics, *J Am Assoc Nurse Anesth* 57(3):220, 1989.

Roberts SL, Chestnut DH: Anesthesia for the obstetric patient with cardiac disease, *Clin Obstet Gyn* 30:601, 1987.

Stampone D: The history of obstetric anesthesia, *J Perinat Neonat Nurs* 4:1, July 1990.

Youngstrom P et al: Continuous epidural infusion of low-dose bupivacaine-fentanyl for labor analgesia, *Anesthesiology* 69: A686, 1988.

Wright WC: Continuous epidural block for ob anesthesia, *Contemp OB/GYN* 36:89, Nov 1991.

Bibliography—Nursing Research

Perez-Woods MR et al: Pain control after cesarean birth: efficacy of patient-controlled analgesia vs traditional therapy (IM morphine), *J Perinat* 11:174, June 1991.

chapter 15 review

Key Concepts

- The type of analgesic or anesthetic to be used is chosen in part by the stage of labor and the method of delivery.
- Narcotic effects can be potentiated with ataractics.
- Naloxone or naltrexone are narcotic antagonists that can reverse narcotic effects, including/especially respiratory depression.
- Pharmacologic control of discomfort during labor requires collaboration among the nurse or primary health care provider, anesthesiologist, and laboring woman.
- The nurse must understand medications, their expected effects, potential side effects, and methods of administration.
- Placement of an IV line and maternal hydration are essential during regional nerve blocks.
- Maternal analgesia/anesthesia potentially affects neonatal neurobehavioral response.
- The use of narcotic agonist-antagonist compounds in women with preexisting narcotic dependency may cause symptoms of narcotic withdrawal.

Key Terms

- affective expressions (p. 374)
- agonist-antagonist compounds (p. 378)
- allergic reaction (p. 388)
- analgesia (p. 376)
- anesthesia (p. 376)
- ataractics (p. 377)
- caudal epidural block (p. 382)
- endorphins (p. 378)
- epidural blood patch (p. 382)
- cricoid pressure (p. 386)
- gate-control theory (p. 374)
- local infiltration anesthesia (p. 379)
- low spinal (saddle) block (p. 380)
- lumbar epidural block (p. 382)
- meninges (p. 382)
- narcotic analgesics (p. 377)
- narcotic antagonist (p. 378)
- neonatal narcosis (p. 378)
- paracervical block (p. 385)
- perception of pain (p. 374)
- post-spinal headache (p. 382)
- pudendal block (p. 379)
- referred pain (p. 374)
- regional analgesia (p. 378)
- somatic pain (p. 374)
- subarachnoid (spinal) block (p. 380)
- systemic analgesia (p. 377)
- visceral pain (p. 374)

Critical Thinking Exercises

1. You are assigned to a woman in labor who feels strongly that medications are to be avoided, but she is now experiencing pain and wants relief. You are convinced that discomfort should be avoided if possible.
   A. Examine assumptions that both the nurse and the woman may have about pain relief.
   B. Analyze arguments for and against use of pharmacologic agents for control of discomfort.
   C. Formulate a plan of care for pain relief in this situation, and justify your choice of interventions.
2. Talk to a woman who has experienced childbirth previously. Ask her to describe her reactions to pain, the atmosphere of the childbirth setting, and the attitudes of the health care providers.
   A. Analyze how the atmosphere and the attitudes might have influenced the woman's perception of pain.
   B. Examine the childbirth setting in which you are now assigned.
      1) What is the atmosphere of the setting, and what are the attitudes of the health care providers regarding pain?
      2) Evaluate the impact of these factors on the setting.

Topics for Nursing Research

- What are clients' preferred methods of pain relief compared with those of clinicians or caregivers?
- Are self-administered medication methods appropriate for labor and birth?
- What self-administered medication methods are appropriate for labor and birth?
- What effects do analgesia/anesthesia have on neonatal behavior?

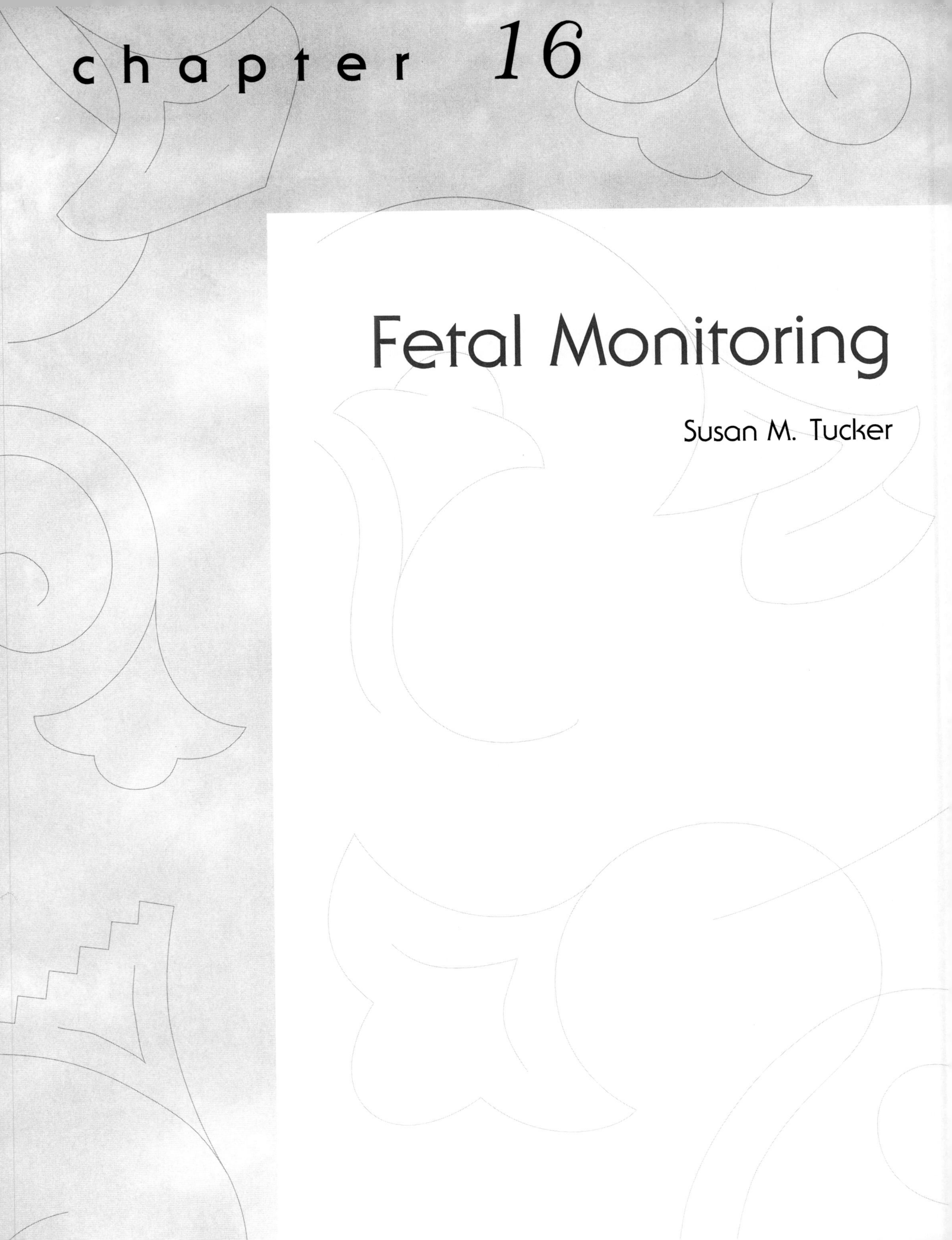

chapter 16

Fetal Monitoring

Susan M. Tucker

LEARNING OBJECTIVES

- Define the key terms listed.
- Identify typical signs of fetal distress.
- Discuss fetal heart rate (FHR) monitoring by periodic auscultation and electronic methods.
- Explain baseline FHR and evaluate periodic changes.
- Describe preventive measures to maintain FHR patterns within normal limits.
- Discuss intrauterine resuscitation.
- Differentiate between nursing interventions for specific FHR patterns: tachycardia and bradycardia; increased and decreased variability; and late and variable decelerations.
- Review guidelines for client care during electronic monitoring.
- Review application of monitor.
- Review documentation for monitoring during labor.
- Identify topics for nursing research related to fetal monitoring.

The psychologic climate surrounding pregnancy and childbirth has changed dramatically. "Have 11 and bury 7" is an old adage referring to couples' expectations that few pregnancies would result in newborn infants who would survive. Today each pregnancy is expected to go to term gestation and result in a perfect child; poor outcome for the product of pregnancy has become less acceptable (Cherry, Merkatz, 1991). Childbirth often is delayed, which, in many cases, reduces the woman's reproductive time and allows her to achieve only one or two pregnancies. Consequently each pregnancy and child is highly valued. In addition, the fetus has evolved as a person. These factors have promoted the development, refinement, and use of many diagnostic procedures such as electronic fetal monitoring. Technologic innovations in perinatal care over the past two decades have increased the understanding of fetal physiology and anatomy (Schifrin, Clements, 1990). In turn, greater understanding of maternal and fetal physiology and anatomy has been a driving force in fine-tuning technologic advances. Consumers are well aware of and expect to benefit personally from medical technology.

Since the 1970s, considerable expertise has evolved in assessing cardiovascular status as reflected by continuous electronic fetal monitoring (Scott et al, 1990). The evaluation of fetal heart rate (FHR) remains highly complex because of the number of factors that must be considered. Thus a consensus definition of fetal "distress" based on objective findings does not exist.

In this chapter, basic information about electronic fetal monitoring during labor is emphasized. Other methods of fetal surveillance (e.g., biophysical profile) are discussed in Chapter 27. Nurses caring for women in labor need to be knowledgeable about the methods of monitoring and the implications of various findings. Nursing responsibilities may include explaining procedures to the woman and family and responding to their questions and concerns. Nurses also may assist in various monitoring techniques. They must be alert for signs of fetal distress and be prepared to implement appropriate nursing interventions.

BASIS FOR MONITORING

Fetal Stress

Because labor represents a period of stress for the fetus, continuous monitoring of fetal health is instituted as part of the nursing care during labor. The fetal oxygen supply must be maintained during labor to prevent complicating conditions after birth. Fetal stress can result in fetal/neonatal compromise. The fetal oxygen supply can be reduced in a number of ways:

1. Reduction of blood flow through the maternal vessels as a result of maternal hypertension or hypotension (systolic blood pressure of 100 mm Hg in brachial artery is necessary for placental perfusion)
2. Reduction of the oxygen content of the maternal blood as a result of hemorrhage or severe anemia
3. Alterations in fetal circulation, occurring with compression of the cord, placental separation, or **head compression** (head compression causes increased intracranial pressure and vagal nerve stimulation with slowing of the heart rate)
4. Reduction in blood flow to the intervillous space in the placenta secondary to decrease in intervals during which the uterus is relaxed and an increase in resting uterine tonus (undesirable side effect of exogenous oxytocin) (Fanaroff, Martin, 1992).

Fetal well-being during labor can be measured by the *response of the FHR to uterine contractions*. In general, a reassuring FHR pattern is characterized by an FHR between 120 and 160 beats/min with normal baseline variability, the absence of nonreassuring periodic changes, and accelerations of FHR with fetal movement.

A normal uterine activity pattern in labor is characterized by contractions every 2 to 5 minutes, duration of contractions less than 90 seconds, intensity of contractions less than 100 mm Hg pressure, a period of 30 seconds or more from the end of one contraction to the beginning of the next contraction, and an average intrauterine pressure of 15 mm Hg or less between contractions.

Fetal Distress

Fetal distress is a compromise in fetal well-being. It can be an acute or chronic condition, depending on antepartum and intrapartum events, with the possibility of an acute insult superimposed on a condition of chronic fetal distress.

The goal of intrapartum FHR monitoring is the early detection of mild fetal hypoxia and the prevention of severe fetal hypoxia. The nurse must be thinking continually in terms of whether the FHR pattern is reassuring and whether fetal oxygenation is good. Distinctions can be made among reassuring patterns, nonreassuring or warning FHR patterns generally indicative of mild fetal hypoxia, and worrisome or ominous patterns that indicate severe fetal hypoxia. Reassuring FHR patterns include those that follow:

1. Baseline FHR in the normal range of 120 to 160 beats/min with no periodic changes and average baseline variability.
2. Early decelerations
3. Mild variable decelerations
4. Accelerations

Nonreassuring (warning) FHR patterns are given in the following list:

1. Progressive increase or decrease in baseline heart rate
2. Tachycardia of 160 beats/min or above
3. Progressive decrease in baseline variability

Potentially ominous FHR patterns are given in the following list:

1. Severe variable decelerations (FHR less than 70 beats/min lasting longer than 30 to 60 seconds, with rising baseline, decreasing variability, and/or slow return to baseline)
2. Late decelerations of any magnitude—especially those that are repetitive and uncorrectable, with a decreasing variability or rising baseline
3. Absence of variability
4. Prolonged deceleration
5. Severe bradycardia

■MONITORING TECHNIQUES

Periodic Auscultation

Periodic auscultation of the fetal heart may reveal tachycardia, bradycardia, or arrhythmia that may occur during a brief examination (Fig. 16-1). The Organization for Obstetric, Gynecologic, and Neonatal Nurses (NAACOG, 1990) has developed guidelines for auscultation of FHR during labor:

	Low-risk client	High-risk client
First stage:		
Latent phase	q60min	q30min
Active phase	q30min	q15min
Second stage	q15min	q5min

Meeting this standard for care may place considerable strain on nurses and other personnel. The frequency of auscultation requires a staffing ratio of one nurse per client. Nurses may become frustrated and anxious in trying to meet this standard of periodic auscultation (Fields, Boehm, 1989).

Auscultation is performed during a uterine contraction and for a period of 30 seconds immediately

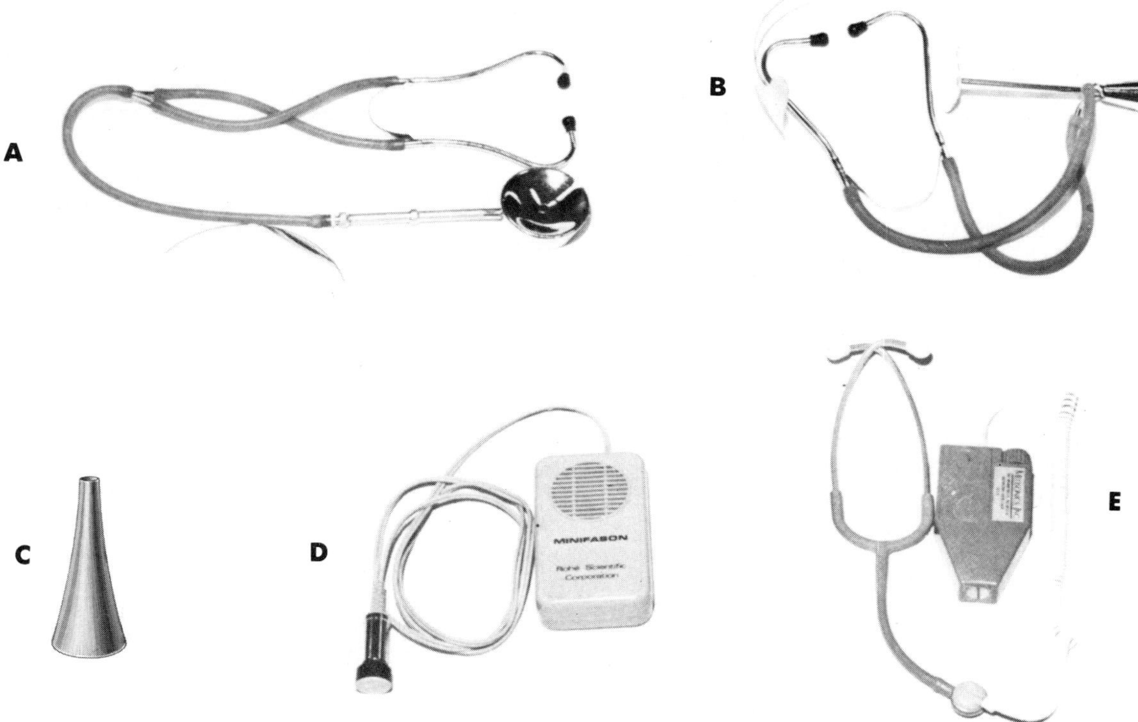

Fig. 16-1 A Leff scope. B, DeLee-Hillis scope. C, Pinard's stethoscope. D, Ultrasound fetoscope; amplifies sound to those in immediate area. E, Ultrasound stethoscope; amplifies mechanical movement of fetal heart to listener by means of ear pieces.

A, B, D, and E from Ingalls AJ, Salerno MC: *Maternal and child health nursing,* ed 7, St Louis, 1991, Mosby–Year Book.

after the end of the contraction. The most important sign of fetal distress, beat-to-beat variability of the FHR, cannot be assessed by periodic auscultation (Parer, 1984). Nonreassuring and potentially ominous FHR patterns may not occur during the periods of auscultation and may pass unrecognized by the examiner (AAP and ACOG, 1988; ACOG, 1989; Freeman et al, 1991). An improved method that is more likely to aid in diagnosing fetal compromise in the high-risk pregnancy is the counting of FHR during sequential contractions and for a full 3 minutes thereafter. Persistent, postcontraction bradycardia (e.g., FHR of 100 beats/min or a persistent drop of 30 beats/min or more below baseline) or gross irregularity can indicate fetal distress.

The woman can become anxious if the examiner cannot readily count the FHR. For the inexperienced listener it often takes time to locate the heartbeat and find the area of maximum intensity. The mother can be told that the nurse is "finding the spot where the sounds are loudest." If it has taken considerable time to locate them, the examiner can reassure the mother by offering her an opportunity to hear them too. If the examiner cannot locate the FHR, an experienced nurse should be asked for assistance.

Electronic Monitoring

There are two modes of electronic monitoring. The external mode employs the use of external transducers placed on the maternal abdomen to assess heart rate and uterine activity. Some monitors have the capability of monitoring twin gestations. The internal mode uses a spiral electrode applied to the fetal presenting part to assess the fetal electrocardiogram (ECG) and an **intrauterine catheter** to assess uterine activity and pressure. A brief description contrasting the external and internal modes of **electronic fetal monitoring** (EFM) is provided in Table 16-1.

EXTERNAL MONITORING. Separate transducers monitor the FHR and uterine contractions (Fig. 16-2). The *ultrasound transducer* acts through the reflection of high-frequency sound waves from a moving interface, in this case the fetal heart and valves. Therefore short-term variability and beat-to-beat changes in the FHR cannot be assessed accurately by this method. It also is difficult to reproduce a continuous and precise record of the FHR because of artifacts introduced by fetal and maternal movement. The FHR tracing is printed on a strip chart. Once the *area of*

TABLE 16-1 External and Internal Modes of Monitoring

External Mode	Internal Mode
FETAL HEART RATE (FHR)	
Ultrasound transducer: High-frequency sound waves reflect mechanical action of the fetal heart. Used during the antepartum and intrapartum period. *Phonotransducer:* Microphone amplifies sound, reflects excessive noise when woman is in labor. Used infrequently for antepartum monitoring. *Abdominal electrodes:* Fetal ECG is obtained when electrodes are properly positioned. Used infrequently for antepartum monitoring because of ease and reliability of ultrasound transducer.	*Spiral electrode:* Electrode converts fetal ECG as obtained from the presenting part to FHR via a cardiotachometer. This method can be used only when membranes are ruptured and cervix sufficiently dilated during the intrapartum period. Electrode penetrates fetal presenting part 1.5 mm and must be securely positioned to ensure a good signal.
UTERINE ACTIVITY	
Tocotransducer: This instrument monitors frequency and duration of contractions by means of pressure-sensing device applied to the maternal abdomen. Used during both the antepartum and intrapartum periods.	*Intrauterine catheter:* This instrument monitors frequency, duration, and *intensity of contractions*. Catheter is compressed during contractions, placing pressure on a strain gauge converting the pressure into millimeters of mercury on the uterine activity panel of the strip chart. It can be used when membranes are ruptured and cervix is sufficiently dilated during the intrapartum period.

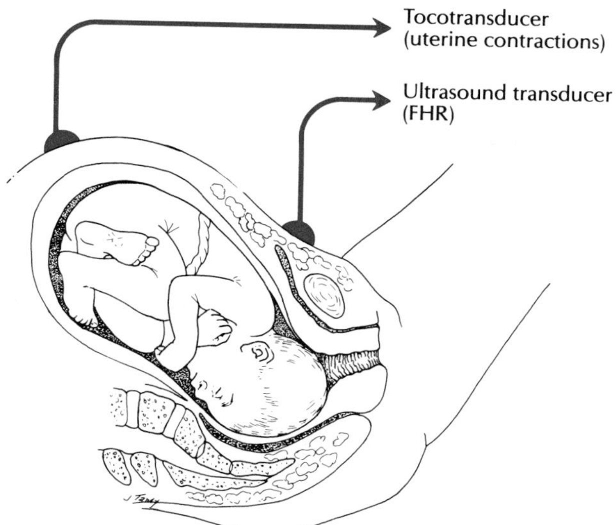

Fig. 16-2 Diagrammatic representation of external noninvasive fetal monitoring with tocotransducer and ultrasound transducer, with ultrasound transducer placed below umbilicus and tocotransducer placed on uterine fundus.

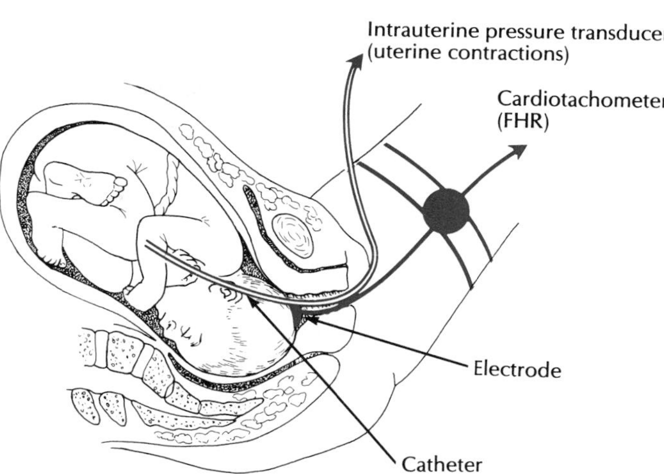

Fig. 16-3 Diagrammatic representation of internal invasive fetal monitoring with intrauterine catheter and spiral electrode in place (membranes ruptured and cervix dilated).

maximum intensity of FHR has been located, conductive gel is applied to the surface of the ultrasound transducer, and the transducer is then positioned over this area.

The **tocotransducer** (tocodynamometer) measures **uterine activity** transabdominally. A pressure-sensitive surface on the side next to the abdomen is depressed by uterine contractions or fetal movement. The device is placed over the fundus above the umbilicus. The tocotransducer can measure and record the frequency, regularity, and duration of uterine contractions but not their intensity. This method is especially valuable during the first stage of labor in women with intact membranes or for use in antepartum testing.

INTERNAL MONITORING. The technique of continuous internal monitoring provides an accurate appraisal of fetal well-being during labor (Fig. 16-3). For this type of monitoring the membranes must be ruptured, the cervix sufficiently dilated, and the presenting part low enough for placement of the electrode. A small fetal scalp electrode attached to the presenting part yields a continuous FHR on the fetal monitor strip. A pressure-sensitive catheter is introduced into the uterine cavity. As the catheter is compressed, pressure is placed on the strain gauge or pressure transducer, which is then converted into a pressure reading in millimeters of mercury. The normal pressure reading range during a contraction is 50 to 75 mm Hg. The intrauterine pressure catheter can measure frequency, duration, and intensity of uterine contractions. The display of FHR and uterine activity on the chart paper differs for the two modes of electronic monitoring (Fig. 16-4). *Note that each small square represents 10 seconds; each larger box of 6 squares equals 1 minute.*

Fetal Heart Rate Patterns

BASELINE FETAL HEART RATE. The intrinsic rhythmicity of the fetal heart and the fetal autonomic nervous system control the FHR. An increase in sympathetic response results in acceleration of the FHR. An augmentation in parasympathetic response produces a slowing of the FHR. The push-pull relationship between the two divisions of the autonomic nervous system serves to balance the fetal heart rate. (This process is described in the discussion of variability in this section.)

Baseline fetal heart rate (FHR) is the average rate when the woman is not in labor or is between contractions. At term this average is about 140 beats/min, a decrease from 160 beats/min early in pregnancy. The normal range at term is 120 to 160 beats/min.

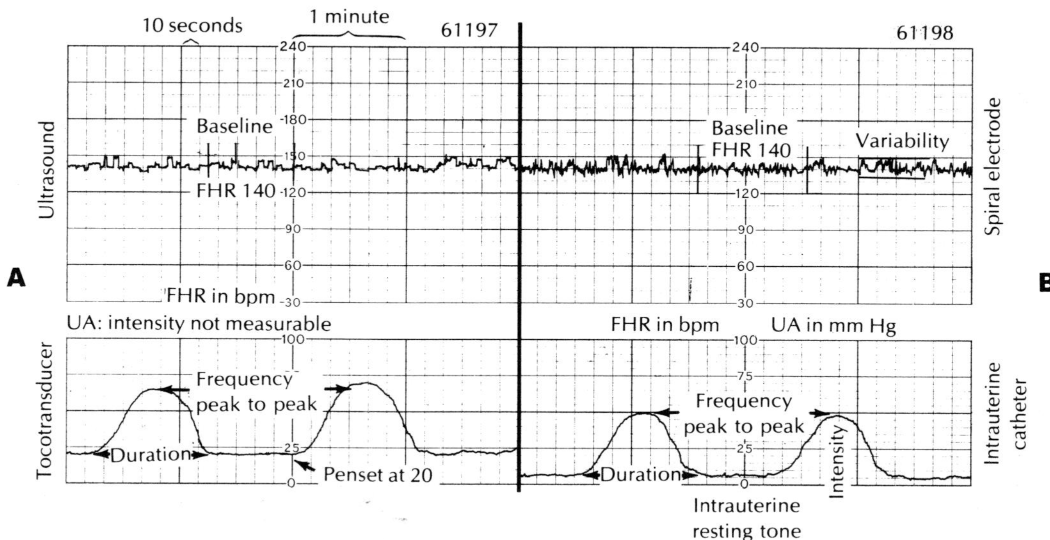

Fig. 16-4 Display of FHR and uterine activity on chart paper. **A,** External mode with ultrasound and tocotransducer as signal source. **B,** Internal mode with spiral electrode and intrauterine catheter as signal source. From Tucker SM: *Pocket guide to fetal monitoring* ed 2, St Louis, 1992, Mosby–Year Book.

TABLE 16-2 Tachycardia and Bradycardia

	Tachycardia	Bradycardia
Definition	FHR above 160 beats/min lasting longer than 10 min,	FHR below 120 beats/min lasting longer than 10 min
Cause	Early fetal hypoxia Maternal fever Parasympatholytic drugs (atropine, hydroxyzine) Beta-sympathomimetic drugs (ritodrine, isoxsuprine) Amnionitis Maternal hyperthyroidism Fetal anemia Fetal heart failure Fetal cardiac arrhythmias	Late fetal hypoxia Beta-adrenergic blocking drugs (propranolol; anesthetics for epidural, spinal, caudal, and pudendal blocks) Maternal hypotension Prolonged umbilical cord compression Fetal congenital heart block
Clinical significance	Persistent tachycardia in absence of periodic changes does not appear serious in terms of neonatal outcome (especially true if tachycardia is associated with maternal fever); tachycardia is an ominous sign when associated with late decelerations, severe variable decelerations, or absence of variability	Bradycardia with good variability and absence of periodic changes is not a sign of fetal distress if FHR remains above 80 beats/min; bradycardia caused by hypoxia is an ominous sign when associated with loss of variability and late decelerations
Nursing intervention	Dependent on cause; reduce maternal fever with antipyretics as ordered and cooling measures; oxygen* at 10-12 L/min may be of some value; carry out physician's orders based on alleviating cause	Dependent on cause; intervention not warranted in fetus with heart block diagnosed by ECG; oxygen at 10-12 L/min may be of some value; carry out physician's orders based on alleviating cause

*Some hospital protocols specify oxygen rates of 7-8 L/min

Tachycardia is a baseline FHR above 160 beats/min or an increase of more than 30 beats/min from the previous baseline for longer than 10 minutes. It can be considered an early sign of fetal hypoxia. Causes include maternal or fetal infection, such as sometimes occurs with prolonged rupture of membranes with amnionitis; maternal hyperthyroidism, or fetal anemia; and response to drugs such as atropine, hydroxyzine (Vistaril), or ritodrine.

Bradycardia is a baseline FHR below 120 beats/min or a decrease of more than 30 beats/min from the previous baseline for longer than 10 minutes. (Bradycardia should be distinguished from prolonged deceleration patterns, which are *periodic changes* that are described later in this chapter.) It can be considered a later sign of fetal hypoxia and is also known to occur before fetal death. Bradycardia can result from placental transfer of drugs such as anesthetics, prolonged compression of the umbilical cord, maternal hypothermia, and maternal hypotension. Maternal **supine hypotensive syndrome,** caused by uterine pressure (the weight of the gravid uterus) on the vena cava, decreases the return of blood flow to the maternal heart, which then reduces maternal cardiac output and blood pressure (Page, Young, 1986; Blackburn, Loper, 1992). These responses in the mother subsequently result in a decrease in the FHR and fetal bradycardia. Table 16-2 compares tachycardia with bradycardia.

Variability of the FHR can be described as the normal irregularity of the cardiac rhythm. It is characterized by a continuous balancing interaction of the parasympathetic (cardiodeceleration) and sympathetic (cardioacceleration) divisions of the autonomic nervous system. This "push-pull" effect results in an irregular FHR, which is an indicator of fetal health. Variability is described as being short-term or long-term. Short-term variability is the change in FHR from one beat to the next. That is, even though a fetal heart may beat 140 times over the course of a minute, there are moments in that minute when the heart rate is 134 or 146. This normal irregularity or unevenness from one heart beat to the next is termed *short-term variability*. *Long-term variability* appears as rhythmic cycles (or waves) from the baseline, and there are generally 3 to 5 cycles per minute. All monitors can present evidence of long-term variability whether the woman is monitored internally or externally. Only the internal signal source from a **spiral electrode** can accurately assess short-term variability (Fig. 16-5). However, monitors with autocorrelation can closely approximate short-term variability when the external signal source, the **ultrasound transducer,** is used.

Absence of variability, or a **smooth (flat) baseline,**

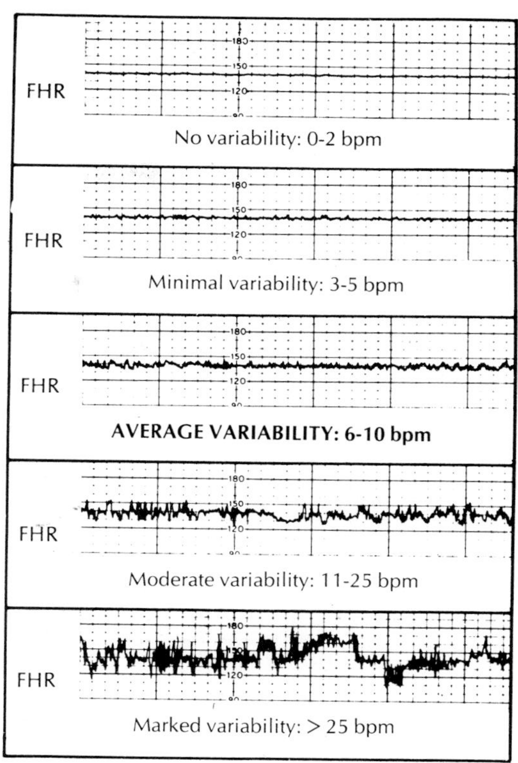

Fig. 16-5 Fetal heart rate variability. Short- and long-term variability tend to increase and decrease together. From Tucker SM: *Pocket guide to fetal monitoring,* ed 2, St Louis, 1992, Mosby–Year Book.

is considered nonreassuring and a sign of potential fetal distress. Decreased variability can result from fetal hypoxia and acidosis, as well as from certain drugs that depress the central nervous system (CNS), including analgesics, narcotics (meperidine [Demerol]), barbiturates (secobarbital [Seconal] and pentobarbital [Nembutal]), tranquilizers (diazepam [Valium]), ataractics (promethazine [Phenergan]), and general anesthetics. In addition, a temporary decrease in variability can occur when the fetus is in a sleep state. These sleep states do not usually last longer than 30 minutes before average variability resumes. Table 16-3 contrasts key differences between increased and decreased variability.

PERIODIC CHANGES IN FETAL HEART RATE. *Periodic changes* in the FHR are referred to as accelerations or decelerations, and the latter are described as early, late, or variable depending on their characteristics of timing, shape, and repetitiveness in relation to uterine contractions. **Accelerations** (caused by dominance of the *sympathetic* response) usually are encountered with breech presentations (Fig. 16-6, *A*). Pressure applied to the infant's buttocks results in

TABLE 16-3 Increased and Decreased Variability

	Increased Variability	Decreased Variability
Cause	Early mild hypoxia Fetal stimulation by the following: Uterine palpation Uterine contractions Fetal activity Maternal activity	Hypoxia/acidosis CNS depressants Analgesics/narcotics Barbiturates Tranquilizers Ataractics Parasympatholytics (atropine) General anesthetics Prematurity Fetal sleep cycles Congenital abnormalities Fetal cardiac arrhythmias
Clinical significance	Significance of marked variability not known; increased variability from a previous average variability, earliest FHR sign of mild hypoxia	Benign when associated with periodic fetal sleep states, which last 20 to 30 min; if caused by drugs, variability usually increases as drugs are excreted Decreased variability considered ominous if caused by hypoxia/asphyxia; occurring with late decelerations, decreased variability associated with fetal acidosis and low Apgar scores
Nursing intervention	Observe FHR tracing carefully for any sign of fetal distress, including decreasing variability and late decelerations; if using external mode of monitoring, consider using internal mode (spiral electrode)	Dependent on cause; intervention not warranted if associated with fetal sleep states or temporarily associated with CNS depressants; consider application of internal mode (spiral electrode) with physician; assist physician with fetal blood sampling for pH if ordered; prepare for birth if so indicated by physician

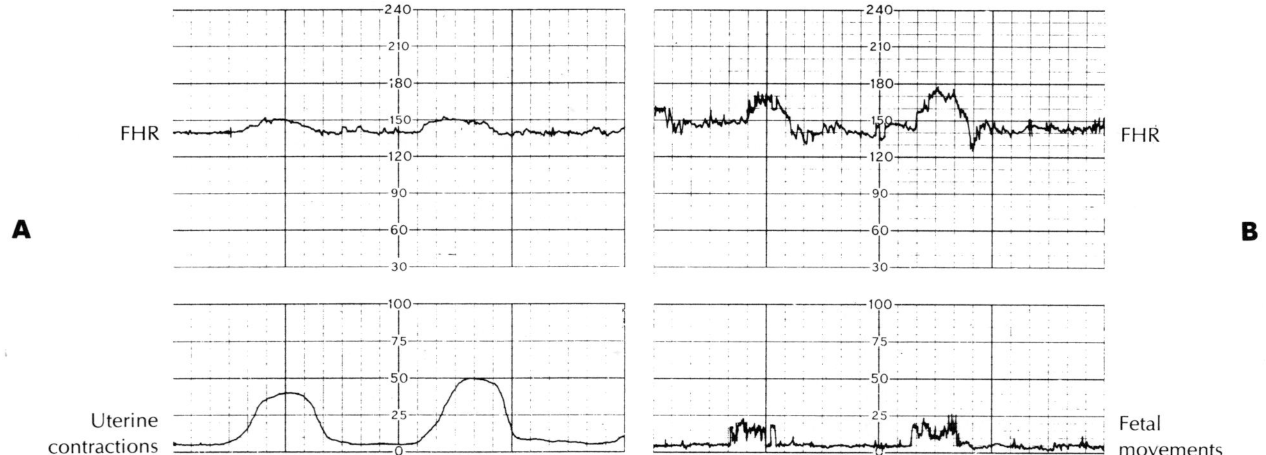

Fig. 16-6 **A**, Acceleration of FHR with uterine contractions. **B**, Acceleration of FHR with fetal movement. From Tucker SM: *Pocket guide to fetal monitoring*, ed 2, St Louis, 1992, Mosby–Year Book.

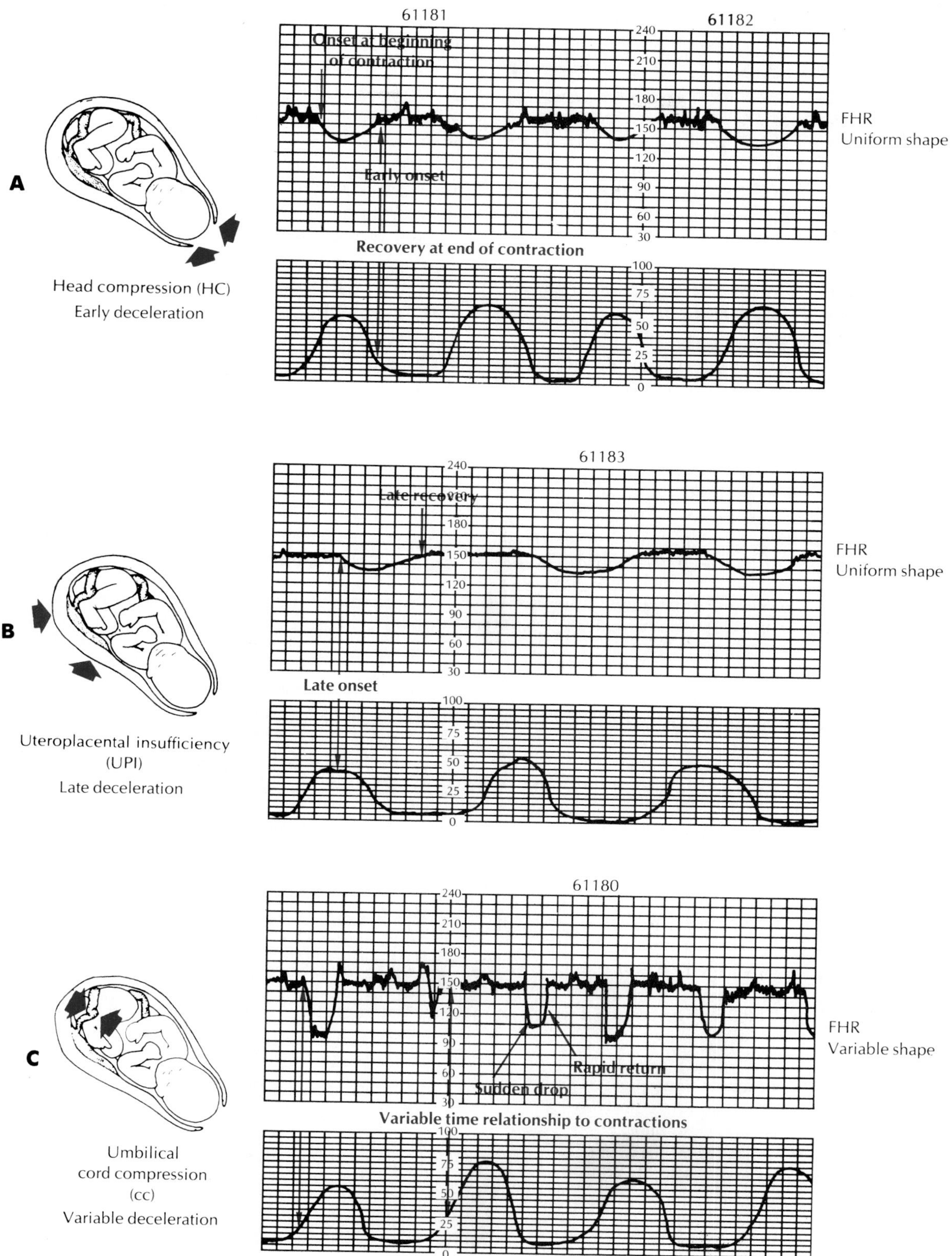

Fig. 16-7 A, Early decelerations caused by head compression. B, Late deceleration caused by uteroplacental insufficiency. C, Variable deceleration caused by cord compression.

accelerations, whereas pressure applied to the head results in decelerations. Accelerations may occur, however, during the second stage of labor in cephalic presentations. Accelerations (Fig. 16-6, *B*) of the FHR occurring during fetal movement are indications of fetal well-being (nonstress test, Chapter 27).

Decelerations (caused by dominance of *parasympathetic* response) may be benign or nonreassuring. The three types of decelerations that are encountered during labor are early, late, and variable. FHR decelerations are described by their relation to the onset and end of a contraction and by their shape.

Early deceleration (slowing of heart rate) in response to compression of the fetal head is normal and usually does not indicate fetal distress (Fig. 16-7, *A*). The deceleration is characterized by a uniform shape and an early onset corresponding to the rise in intrauterine pressure as the uterus contracts. It is not a common occurrence. When present, it usually occurs during the first stage of labor when the cervix is dilated 4 to 7 cm. Early deceleration sometimes is seen during the second stage when the woman is pushing. Early decelerations as a response to fetal head compression can occur during vaginal examinations, as a result of fundal pressure, during placement of the internal mode for fetal monitoring, and during uterine contractions.

Early decelerations are considered to be a benign pattern; therefore interventions are not necessary. The value of identifying early decelerations is to be able to distinguish them from late or variable decelerations, which can be nonreassuring, and for which interventions are appropriate. Table 16-4 contrasts accelerations of FHR with early decelerations.

Late decelerations are caused by **uteroplacental insufficiency** and appear as a smooth, curvilinear, uniform heart rate pattern that mirrors the pattern of intrauterine pressure during a contraction. However, the deceleration necessarily begins *after* the contraction has been established and consistently *persists into the interval after the contraction is over* (Fig. 16-7, *B*). Late deceleration patterns when persistent or recurrent usually indicate fetal hypoxia because of insufficient placental perfusion. Persistent and repetitive late decelerations are associated with fetal hypoxia and acidosis. They should be considered an ominous sign when they are uncorrectable, especially if they are associated with decreased variability

TABLE 16-4 Acceleration and Early Deceleration

	Acceleration	Early Deceleration
Description	Transitory increase of FHR above baseline (see Fig. 16-6)	Transitory decrease of FHR below baseline concurrent with uterine contractions (see Fig. 16-7, *A*)
Shape	May resemble shape of uterine contraction	Uniform shape; mirror image of uterine contraction
Onset	Variable; often precedes or occurs simultaneously with uterine contraction	Early in contraction phase before peak of contraction
Recovery	Variable	By end of contraction as uterine pressure returns to its resting tone
Amplitude	Usually 15 beats/min above baseline	Usually proportional to amplitude of contraction; rarely decelerates below 100 beats/min
Baseline	Usually associated with average baseline variability	Usually associated with average baseline variability
Occurrence	Variable; may be repetitive with each contraction	Repetitious (occurs with each contraction); usually between 4 and 7 cm dilatation and in second stage of labor.
Cause	Spontaneous fetal movement Vaginal examination Breech presentation Occiput posterior position Uterine contractions Fundal pressure Abdominal palpation	Head compression resulting from following: Uterine contractions Vaginal examination Fundal pressure Placement of internal mode of monitoring
Clinical significance	Acceleration with fetal movement signifies fetal well-being representing fetal alertness or arousal states	Reassuring pattern not associated with fetal hypoxia, acidosis, or low Apgar scores
Nursing intervention	None required	None required

and tachycardia. Late decelerations caused by maternal supine hypotensive syndrome are usually correctable when the woman turns to her side to displace the weight of the gravid uterus off the vena cava. This allows a better return of maternal blood flow to the heart, which increases cardiac output and blood pressure.

Late decelerations caused by uteroplacental insufficiency can result from uterine hyperstimulation with oxytocin, pregnancy-induced hypertension (PIH), preeclampsia, post-dating pregnancy (gestation past 42 weeks), amnionitis, small-for-gestational-age (SGA) fetus, maternal diabetes, placenta previa, abruptio placentae, conduction anesthetics (producing maternal hypotension), maternal cardiac disease, and maternal anemia.

Variable decelerations are those occurring any time during the uterine contracting phase and are caused by **umbilical cord compression.** Table 16-5 contrasts late deceleration with variable deceleration. The appearance of variable deceleration patterns is different from the early and late decelerations, which mirror the uterine contraction. In contrast, variable decelerations often are a U or a V shape characterized by a rapid descent and ascent to and from the nadir (or depth) of the deceleration (Fig. 16-7, *C*).

Variable decelerations may be related to partial, brief compression of the cord. If encountered in the first stage of labor, they usually can be eliminated by changing the mother's position, such as from one side to the other. Administration of oxygen by face mask to the mother is sometimes of value. Variable decelerations most commonly are encountered during the second stage of labor as a result of umbilical cord compression during fetal descent. Variable decelerations are associated with neonatal depression only when cord compression is severe or prolonged (i.e., tight nuchal cord, short cord, knot in cord, prolapsed cord). Variable decelerations occur in about half of all labors and usually are a temporary and correctable phenomenon with maternal position change. A nonreassuring sign is severe variable deceleration. In severe variable deceleration, the FHR is below 70 beats/min and lasts longer than 30 to 60 seconds. It is accompanied by any of the following: a rising baseline FHR, decreasing variability, or slow return of FHR to baseline. The return to baseline may occur with an "overshoot"; that is, the FHR goes above the baseline and then returns immediately to baseline.

Some physicians consider treatment with **amnioinfusion** for laboring women who have oligohydramnios (insufficient amniotic fluid). In this procedure normal saline (at 37°C) is infused rapidly via the intrauterine catheter into the uterine cavity in an attempt to add fluid around the umbilical cord and thus prevent its compression during contractions (Fanaroff, Martin, 1992).

PROLONGED DECELERATIONS. Prolonged decelerations are difficult to classify in as much as they can occur in many situations.

Generally the benign causes are pelvic examination, application of the spiral electrode, rapid fetal descent, and sustained maternal Valsalva's maneuver (pp. 368 and 411).

Other prolonged decelerations are caused by progressive severe variable decelerations, sudden umbilical cord prolapse, hypotension produced by spinal or epidural anesthesia, paracervical anesthesia, a tetanic contraction, and maternal hypoxia, which may occur during a seizure. When the duration of the deceleration is longer than 2 to 3 minutes, a loss of variability with rebound tachycardia usually occurs. Occasionally, a period of late decelerations follows. These responses normally clear spontaneously. However, when a prolonged deceleration is seen late in the course of severe variable decelerations or during a prolonged series of late decelerations, the prolonged deceleration may occur just before fetal death.

PATTERN RECOGNITION. Many factors must be evaluated to determine if an FHR pattern is reassuring or nonreassuring. This includes an assessment and evaluation of baseline rate, variability, accelerations, and decelerations, as well as consideration of the frequency and strength of uterine contractions. These factors must be evaluated on the basis of other obstetric information, including parity, maternal and obstetric complications, progress in labor, and analgesia or anesthesia. The estimated time interval until delivery also must be considered. Intervention and interruption of labor are therefore based on clinical judgment of a complex, integrated process.

The nurse's ability to interpret patterns and a comparison of nurses' and obstetricians' responses were studied (see Research Highlight, p. 410).

Fetal Blood Sampling: Acid-Base Monitoring

It is thought that fetal acidosis occurs as a result of hypoxia. As a part of the intrapartum fetal monitoring process, it may be useful to determine the fetal capillary pH, although the exact role of this procedure remains controversial (ACOG, 1989). Because blood gas values can vary so rapidly with transient circulatory changes, the use of fetal blood sampling during the intrapartum period is not routinely warranted. Some of the factors causing this variability include maternal acidosis or alkalosis, caput succedaneum,

TABLE 16-5 Late Deceleration versus Variable Deceleration

	Late Deceleration	Variable Deceleration
Description	Transitory decrease in FHR below baseline rate in contracting phase (see Fig. 16-7,*B*)	Abrupt transitory decrease in FHR that is variable in duration, intensity, and timing related to onset of contractions (Fig. 16-7,*C*)
Shape	Uniform; mirror image of uterine contraction	Variable; characterized by sudden drop in FHR in V or U shape
Onset	Late in contraction phase; after peak of contraction; low point of deceleration occurs well after peak of contraction	Variable times in contracting phase; often preceded by transitory acceleration
Recovery	Well after end of contraction	Return to baseline is rapid, sometimes with transitory acceleration or acceleration immediately preceding and following deceleration; slow return to baseline with severe variable decelerations
Deceleration	Usually proportional to amplitude of contraction; rarely decelerates below 100 beats/min	*Mild:* decelerates to any level, less than 30 sec with abrupt return to baseline *Moderate:* decelerates above 80 beats/min, any duration with abrupt return to baseline *Severe:* decelerates below 70 beats/min for more than 30 sec, with slow return to baseline
Baseline	Often associated with loss of variability and increasing baseline rate	Mild variables usually associated with average baseline variability; moderate and severe variables often associated with decreasing variability and increasing baseline rate
Occurrence	Occurs with each contraction; proportional to strength and duration of contractions	Variable; commonly observed late in labor with fetal descent and pushing
Cause	Uteroplacental insufficiency caused by the following: Uterine hyperactivity or hypertonicity Maternal supine hypotension Epidural or spinal anesthesia Placenta previa Abruptio placentae Hypertensive disorders Postmaturity Intrauterine growth retardation (IUGR) Diabetes mellitus Amnionitis	Umbilical cord compression caused by the following: Maternal position with cord between fetus and maternal pelvis Cord around fetal neck, arm, leg, or other body part Short cord Knot in cord Prolapsed cord
Clinical significance	Nonreassuring, worrisome pattern associated with fetal hypoxia, acidosis, and low Apgar scores; considered ominous if persistent and uncorrected, especially when associated with fetal tachycardia and loss of variability	Variable decelerations occur in about 50% of all labors and usually are transient, correctable, and not associated with low Apgar scores; mild variable decelerations reassuring; decelerations progressing from moderate to severe are associated with fetal acidosis, hypoxia, and low Apgar scores; severe variable decelerations with good baseline variability just before delivery usually well tolerated

TABLE 16-5 Late Deceleration versus Variable Deceleration—cont'd

	Late Deceleration	Variable Deceleration
Nursing intervention	Change maternal position Correct maternal hypotension Elevate legs Increase rate of maintenance IV Discontinue oxytocin if infusing Administer oxygen* at 10 to 12 L/min with tight face mask Assist with fetal blood sampling if ordered Assist physician with termination of labor if pattern cannot be corrected	Change maternal position; if decelerations do not yet meet criteria for mild variable deceleration, proceed with following measures: Discontinue oxytocin if infusing Administer oxygen* at 10-12 L/min with tight face mask Assist with vaginal or speculum examination, fetal blood sampling If cord is prolapsed, examiner will elevate fetal presenting part with cord between gloved fingers until cesarean birth is accomplished Assist with amnioinfusion if ordered Assist with birth

*Some hospital protocols specify 7-8 L/min

stage of labor, and time relationship of scalp sampling to uterine contraction.

The procedure is performed by a physician who obtains the sample from the fetal scalp transcervically after rupture of membranes. The scalp is swabbed with a disinfecting solution before the puncture is made. The sample is collected and sent to the laboratory for analysis.

MECONIUM-STAINED AMNIOTIC FLUID. The passage of meconium from the fetal bowel before birth may indicate fetal distress. Peristalsis of the bowel increases during hypoxia, and the contents are likely to be expelled. Although the presence of **meconium-stained amniotic fluid** is not always an indication of fetal difficulty, its presence requires immediate notification of the physician.

■ NURSING PROCESS

Implementing the nursing process with clients who require fetal monitoring during labor is possible even for a beginning student of nursing. Care of women in normal labor is the same as that of the woman undergoing fetal monitoring: assessment of maternal blood pressure and FHR, maternal position, care of emotional and knowledge needs, and recognition of meconium-stained amniotic fluid. Nursing students and new graduates will need additional education and experience for the application of internal electrodes and FHR pattern recognition.

ASSESSMENT

Prenatal records and current labor events must be assessed to determine the degree of risk for fetal compromise. Fetal membranes must be ruptured before internal monitoring is possible. Maternal mobility and positioning needs are assessed. Maternal and family's knowledge needs of FHR monitoring are determined.

The FHR pattern is assessed for baseline values, tachycardia, and bradycardia; variability (increased or decreased); and periodic changes (acceleration or deceleration). Decelerations are described as early, late, or variable. A checklist assists the nurse (see box, p. 411).

The need for fetal blood sampling–acid-base monitoring is determined. The character of amniotic fluid is assessed for evidence of meconium passage and infection and for amount.

NURSING DIAGNOSES

Assessment findings are reviewed and nursing diagnoses formulated. Several nursing diagnoses are possible, including the following:

- Decreased maternal cardiac output related to
  —Supine hypotension secondary to maternal position
- Ineffective individual coping related to
  —Lack of knowledge of fetal monitoring during labor

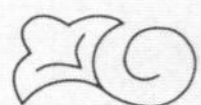 **Research Highlight** 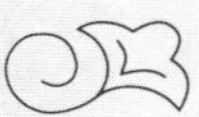

Interpretation of Nonstress Tests by Nurses

RESEARCH ABSTRACT

The purposes of this study were (1) to determine nurses' ability to interpret nonstress test (NST) results and factors associated with accurate interpretation and (2) to compare the patterns of responses of nurses to the responses of obstetricians who viewed the same NST results. A sample of 1000 members of the Organization for Obstetric, Gynecologic, and Neonatal Nurses (NAACOG), whose identified specialty was labor and birth or antepartum care, was selected to participate. The physician comparison group interpreted the strips for another study. The nurses were mailed a packet with a 16-item demographic (vital statistics) questionnaire, five NST strips, and a stamped, self-addressed envelope; 412 nurses (41%) returned the questionnaire. The nurses who returned the questionnaire had an average of 11.5 years of nursing experience, and 56% were staff nurses.

Each of the strips was evaluated on three scales with either two, three, or five choices. The two-choice options were "reactive" and "nonreactive," the three choice option added "equivocal," and the five-choice option included interpretation of fetal well-being on a Likert scale from "most healthy" to "most ill." Between 84% and 98% of the nurses agreed on a response on the two-point option; this response was designated as correct. There was no relation between the accuracy of response and the nurse's education, years of experience, years of NST experience, or self-evaluation of ability.

Correct responses on the three-point scale were generally predictable from the responses on the two-point scale. Many of those responding incorrectly changed their responses to "equivocal" when this option was available. On the five-point scale, the majority of nurses associated a healthy fetus with a reactive test result. In terms of correct labeling and interpretation of findings, the performance of the nurses as a group was equivalent to that of the physicians as a group. In using the two-point option, the nurses differed from the physician comparison group in the interpretation of one strip. On the three-point option, findings by the nurses and physicians were similar on all but one strip. On three strips, nurses and physicians indicated similar results on the five-point scale. On two strips, the nurses rated the fetus as less healthy than did the physicians.

IMPLICATIONS FOR PRACTICE

Nurses perform NSTs often. It is essential that they perform their functions accurately. The researchers found intraobserver (within subject) reliability (consistent results) in the majority of study participants. The discrepancies noted in evaluations on the two-, three-, and five-point scales are consistent with the observed lack of agreements among clinicians in interpretation of fetal heart monitoring data. The greatest clinical risk is the labeling of a test reactive when it is not. A system of checks needs to be in place so that such errors are minimized. Periodic audits of NST tracings are appropriate and would allow identification of persons who consistently err in one direction. Regular periodic joint review of tracings by physicians and nurses would increase standardization.

RELATED RESEARCH QUESTIONS

1. What factors are associated with inconsistent interpretation of NST tracings?
2. Will education increase the consistency of interpretation of NST tracings?
3. Which scale (two-, three-, or five-point) is most valid for evaluation of NST results?
4. What is the relation between a nonreactive NST and fetal outcome?

REFERENCE

Chez BF et al: Interpretations of nonstress tests by obstetric nurses, *JOGNN* 19:227, May/June 1990.

—Restriction of mobility or movement during EFM
- Impaired fetal gas exchange related to
  —Umbilical cord compression
  —Placental insufficiency
  —Nonrecognition of nonreassuring or ominous FHR pattern
  —Missed diagnosis because of poor tracing resulting from malposition of transducers
- High risk for fetal injury related to
  —Unrecognized hypoxia or anoxia
  —Infection secondary to internal monitoring or blood sampling
- Pain related to
  —Use of belts to position transducers
  —Maternal position
  —Application of internal electrode or obtaining blood sample

An example of the use of assessment findings in formulating nursing diagnoses is given in the case study and nursing plan of care pp. 416 and 417.

PLANNING

Interventions are derived from current knowledge of fetal monitoring during labor and standards for care. The woman's/family's concerns and questions are considered in planning.

Goals for the Fetus

1. The fetus will not suffer any hypoxic or anoxic episodes.
2. Should fetal distress occur, the distress is identified promptly and therapy instituted.

Goals for the Mother and Family

1. The mother and family will understand the need for monitoring.
2. The mother and family will assist the mother to avoid situations that compromise maternal/fetal circulation.
3. The mother and family will achieve the type of birth experience that is both physically safe for mother/fetus/neonate and emotionally satisfying.

IMPLEMENTATION

It is the responsibility of the nurse providing care to women in labor to assess FHR patterns, perform independent nursing interventions, document observations and actions according to the established standard of care, and report nonreassuring patterns to the primary care provider (e.g., physician, certified nurse midwife).*

Preventive Measures

DISCOURAGING VALSALVA'S MANEUVER. Valsalva's maneuver refers to closed-glottis (holding one's breath) pushing (see additional discussion on p. 368). Its use during the pushing process (bearing down) may adversely affect maternal hemodynamics and fetal status (Korner et al, 1976; Caldeyro-Barcia, 1979; Roberts, 1980; Barnett, Humenick, 1982; Yeates, Roberts, 1984; Liu, 1989). Prolonged Valsalva's pushing lasting more than 5 to 6 seconds can decrease maternal blood pressure and placental blood flow, alter maternal and fetal oxygenation, decrease

*Standards for competency have been established by the Organization for Obstetric, Gynecologic, and Neonatal Nurses (NAACOG, 1989; NAACOG, 1990).

Fetal Heart Rate Assessment Checklist

Client's name__________ Date/time__________

1. What is the baseline fetal heart rate (FHR)?
   ______ Beats per minute (bpm)
   Check one of the following as observed on the monitor strip:
   ______ Average baseline FHR (120 to 160 bpm)
   ______ Tachycardia (> 120 bpm or > 30 bpm from normal /previous baseline)
   ______ Bradycardia (<120 bpm or <30 bpm from normal/previous baseline)
2. What is the baseline variability?
   ______ Average short-term variability (6 to 10 bpm)
   ______ Average long-term variability (3 to 5 cycles per minute)
   ______ Minimal variability
   ______ Absence of variability
   ______ Marked variability
3. Are there any periodic changes in FHR?
   ______ Accelerations with fetal movement
   ______ Repetitive accelerations with each contraction
   ______ Early decelerations (head compression)
   ______ Late decelerations (uteroplacental insufficiency)
   ______ Variable decelerations (cord compression)
   ______ Mild
   ______ Moderate
   ______ Severe
4. What does the uterine activity panel show?
   ______ Frequency (peak to peak)
   ______ Duration (beginning to end)
   ______ Intensity (in mm Hg only with intrauterine catheter)
   ______ Resting time at least 30 seconds
   ______ Resting tone (<15 mm Hg pressure)

COMMENTS:__________

PANEL NUMBER	WHAT CAN BE OR SHOULD HAVE BEEN DONE

From Tucker SM: *Pocket Guide to fetal monitoring,* St Louis, 1992, Mosby–Year Book.

fetal pH and Po_2, increase fetal Pco_2, increase the incidence of FHR pattern changes, and delay recovery of FHR rate with fetal hypoxia (Caldeyro-Barcia, 1979; Caldeyro-Barcia et al, 1981; Barnett, Humenick, 1982; McKay, Roberts, 1985; Blackburn, Loper, 1992). Open-glottis (vocalization) pushing is not associated with changes in maternal blood pressure or increased fetal pH (Barnett, Humenick 1982). Therefore nurses should encourage the woman to keep her mouth and glottis open and to vocalize (e.g., grunt) while pushing. ***Nurses should not direct the woman to "be quiet, keep your mouth closed, and push."***

MATERNAL POSITION. Maternal hypotension and fetal hypoxia may develop more rapidly with supine position or epidural anesthesia (Page, Young, 1986; Blackburn, Loper, 1992; Fanaroff, Martin, 1992).

During the first stage of labor, the supine position compromises effective uterine activity, prolongs labor, and increases the use of drugs (e.g., oxytocin) to augment labor (Roberts, 1989). Oxytocin decreases the intervals during which the uterus is relaxed, and normal intervillous space perfusion occurs. Oxytocin also insidiously increases uterine resting tonus above the normal range of 10 to 15 mm Hg (Fanaroff, Martin, 1992). Therefore nursing care that supports a more efficient, shorter labor (e.g., maternal position changes) should be implemented.

During the second stage of labor, the laboring woman's involuntary pushing efforts with minimal straining is encouraged. In addition to maintaining maternal and fetal hemodynamics, this pushing pattern is associated with a shorter second stage of labor. A semirecumbent position and spontaneous short bursts of pushing in response to involuntary bearing-down urges are most conducive to favorable outcomes (Roberts, 1980; Cherry, Merkatz, 1991; Blackburn, Loper, 1992).

The nurse must coach the woman to avoid hyperventilatory breathing. Hyperventilation will result in hypoventilation between contractions. The attendant fall in Po_2 could be harmful to the fetus (Fanaroff, Martin, 1992).

Intrauterine Resuscitation

Intrauterine resuscitation refers to those interventions for fetal distress directed primarily toward improving uterine and intervillous space blood flow and secondarily toward increasing maternal oxygenation (Fanaroff, Martin, 1992). Preventive interventions have been described: avoiding the supine position and encouraging maternal position changes; encouraging spontaneous short bursts of pushing in response to involuntary bearing-down urges; and open-mouth, open-glottis with vocalizing during pushing.

Compression of the umbilical cord vessels results in variable decelerations. Amnioinfusion helps relieve pressure on the (nonprolapsed) umbilical cord. If maternal hypotension is caused by acute hemorrhage, rapid infusion of blood volume expanders may be ordered. Until the infusion is established, the nurse can elevate the woman's legs. Blood pooled in the legs, especially with sympathetic blockade (e.g., epidural anesthesia), will then drain quickly into the central venous circulation and augment the effective intravascular volume (Fanaroff, Martin, 1992).

Oxytocin always should be infused as a "piggyback" connection near the indwelling needle (ACOG, 1989). If FHR patterns change for any reason, oxytocin stimulation of uterine muscle activity needs to be stopped. The intravenous (IV) line from the piggyback (containing oxytocin) is clamped off and the primary infusion line is opened.

Nurses need to prioritize interventions to maximize intrauterine resuscitation. The first priority is to open the maternal/fetal vascular systems; the second priority, to increase blood volume; and the third priority, to optimize oxygenation of the circulating blood volume. For example, to relieve acute FHR deceleration, the nurse can do the following:

- Turn woman to side-lying position
- Increase maternal blood volume by increasing rate of primary IV infusion or raise woman's legs
- Provide oxygen by face mask

Some interventions are specific to the FHR pattern seen. Nursing interventions for tachycardia and bradycardia are given in Table 16-2 and those for increased or decreased variability, in Table 16-3. Nursing interventions specific for FHR acceleration or early deceleration are not required (Table 16-4). Late and variable FHR decelerations require aggressive intervention (Table 16-5). Review nursing interventions relevant to umbilical cord prolapse (see Chapter 17). The decision for medical intervention or termination of labor, achieved by expeditious vaginal or cesarean birth, is made by the physician.

Working with the Monitor

APPLICATION OF EXTERNAL ELECTRONIC FETAL MONITOR. The equipment is easily applied by the nurse but may need to be repositioned as the mother or fetus changes position. The woman is asked to assume a semisitting or left-lateral position. (Fig. 16-8). The nurse explains the procedure to the client and family and performs the following steps:

- Turns on monitor; taps transducer before use to ensure sound transmission

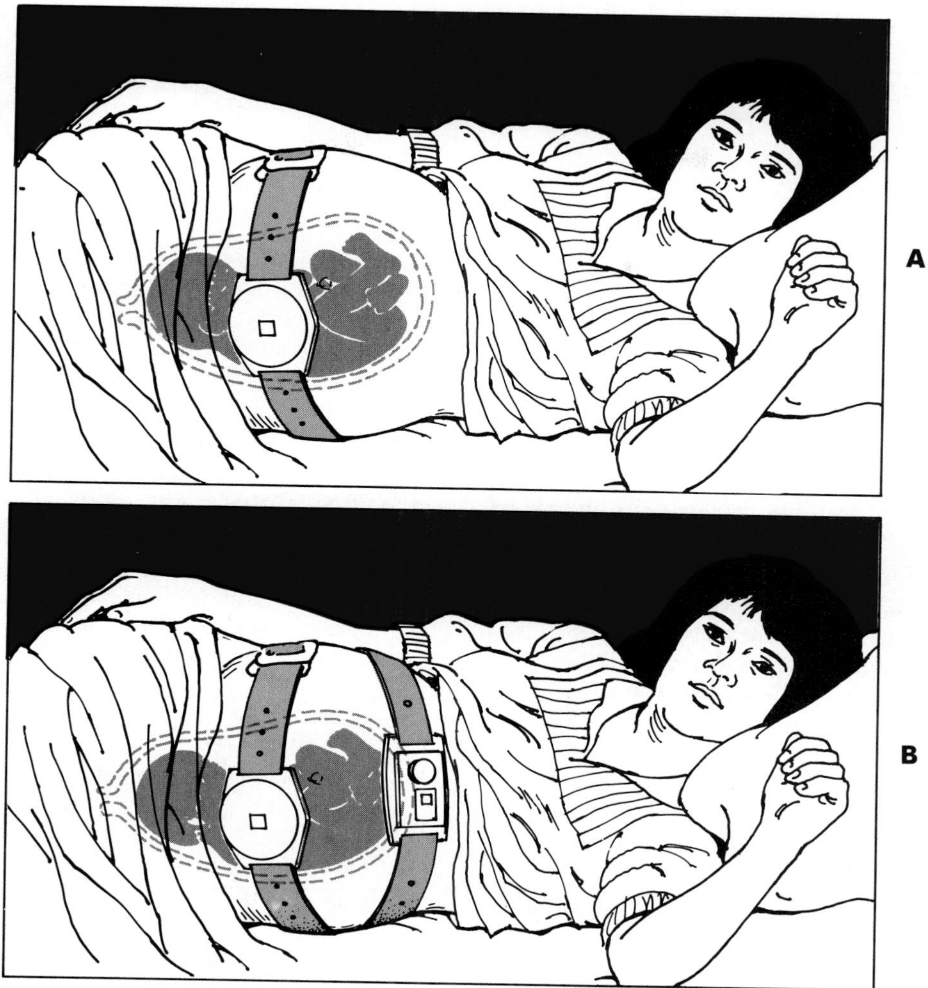

Fig. 16-8 Application of external electronic fetal monitoring. **A,** Ultrasound transducer in place over the fetal heart. **B,** Tocotransducer in place over the uterine fundus.

- Places both belts under the woman's back at about waist level
- Applies a thin coat of transmission gel to the face of the diaphragm
- Performs the first and second Leopold's maneuvers to locate the fetal back (for further discussion of Leopold's maneuvers, see Chapter 17 and Fig. 17-8)
- Positions the ultrasound transducer in place over the fetal heart (Fig. 16-8, *A*), and tightens the belt
- Obtains a tracing to ensure that the transducer is picking up the FHR
- Positions the tocotransducer over the uterine fundus where it contracts; it can be in the midline or slightly to one side
- Tightens the belt (Fig. 16-8, *B*)
- Checks placement by putting one hand on the fundus and palpating for a contraction
- Adjusts the pen-set knob so that the baseline reads between 5 and 15 mm Hg on the monitor strip

In addition to knowing how to apply the monitor and interpret tracings, the nurse functions as a trouble-shooter. A checklist for fetal monitoring equipment is presented in the box on p. 414.

CARE OF MOTHER UNDERGOING FETAL MONITORING. For quick reference, summary guidelines for the care of the woman undergoing electronic monitoring during labor are listed in the box on p. 415.

DOCUMENTATION. Clear and complete documentation is provided on the woman's monitoring strip be-

Checklist for Fetal Monitoring Equipment

PREPARATION OF MONITOR

1. Is the paper inserted correctly?
2. Are transducer cables plugged into the appropriate outlet of the monitor?

ULTRASOUND TRANSDUCER

1. Has ultrasound transmission gel been applied to the crystals?
2. Was the FHR tested and noted on the chart paper?
3. Does a signal light flash with each heart beat?
4. Is the strap secure and snug?

TOCOTRANSDUCER

1. Is the tocotransducer firmly strapped where the least maternal tissue is in evidence?
2. Has it been applied without gel or paste?
3. Was the pen-set knob adjusted between 20 and 25 mm marks and noted on chart paper?
4. Was this setting done between contractions?
5. Is the strap secure and snug?

SPIRAL ELECTRODE

1. Are the wires attached firmly to the posts on the leg plate?
2. Is the spiral electrode attached to the presenting part of the fetus?
3. Is the inner surface of the leg plate covered with electrode paste if necessary?
4. Is the leg plate properly secured to the woman's thigh?

INTERNAL CATHETER/STRAIN GAUGE*

1. Is the length line on the catheter visible at the introitus?
2. Is it noted on the chart paper that a calibration was done?
3. Was the uterine activity (UA) tested?

Modified from Tucker SM: Pocket guide to fetal monitoring, St Louis, 1992, Mosby–Year Book.
*New internal catheters are solid, without syringes or stopcocks.

fore the initiation of monitoring. This documentation is continued and updated as monitoring progresses. Observations and interventions are noted on the monitor strip to provide a comprehensive document that depicts the course of labor and the woman's care. Many of the aspects that should be documented on the monitor strip are listed in the box on this page.

The chart is labeled with the following information: woman's name, identification number, date, expected date of delivery (EDD); high-risk conditions such as preeclampsia, diabetes; membranes intact or ruptured; cervical dilatation and station of presenting part; and the time monitor was attached and the mode used (see Table 27-4) as well as a notation that the monitor paper has been reviewed and evaluated on a periodic basis.

Documentation: Monitor Strip

OBSERVATIONS

Maternal vital signs
Maternal position/repositioning
Vaginal examinations and findings
Medications; anesthesia
Voidings; emesis
Pushing/bearing down
Fetal movement
Baseline FHR, periodic changes

ADJUSTMENTS

Relocation of transducers
Flushing or adjustment of catheter
Replacement of electrode
Replacement of catheter
Time lapse when changing recording paper

INTERVENTIONS

Position change
Parenteral fluids
Discontinuance of oxytocin
Oxygen administration
Physician notification and response

EVALUATION

Evaluation is a continuous process. The nurse can assume that care was effective when the goals for care have been met. That is, the fetus will not suffer any hypoxic or anoxic episode, and should fetal distress occur, the distress is identified promptly and therapy instituted. In addition, the mother and family will understand the need for monitoring, will assist the mother to avoid situations that compromise maternal/fetal circulation, and will achieve the type of birth experience that is both physically safe for mother/fetus/neonate and emotionally satisfying. (See pp. 416 for a case study and nursing plan of care for the woman who is being monitored during labor.)

Care of Mother Undergoing Fetal Monitoring

The following guidelines relate to client teaching and functioning of the monitor:

Explain that fetal status can be continuously assessed by FHR even during contractions.

Explain that lower activity on strip chart shows uterine activity; upper panel shows FHR.

Reassure woman and significant other that prepared childbirth techniques can be implemented without difficulty.

Explain that during external monitoring effleurage can be performed on sides of abdomen or upper portion of thighs.

Relate that breathing patterns based on timing and intensity of contractions can be enhanced by observation of uterine activity panel of strip chart for onset of contractions.

Note peak of contraction; knowing that contraction will not get stronger and is half over usually is helpful.

Note diminishing intensity.

Coordinate with appropriate breathing and relaxation techniques.

Reassure woman/significant other that use of internal mode of monitoring does not restrict her movement although she is confined to bed.*

Explain that use of external mode of monitoring usually requires woman's cooperation in positioning and movement.

Reassure woman and significant other that use of monitor does not imply fetal jeopardy.

Reassure her that the equipment is removed periodically to permit washing of the applicator sites and giving of back rubs.

EXTERNAL MONITORING

Ultrasound transducer

Monitors FHR with high-frequency sound waves

Tap transducer before use to ensure sound transmission.

Apply ultrasound transmission gel to maternal abdomen; clean abdomen and transducer and reapply gel q2h and prn.

Massage reddened skin areas gently and reposition belt or adhesive device q2h and prn.

Auscultate FHR with stethoscope or fetoscope if in doubt as to validity of tracing.

Position and reposition transducer prn to ensure clear, interpretable FHR data.

Tocotransducer

Monitors uterine activity via a pressure-sensing device placed on the maternal abdomen

Position and reposition qh and prn on the fundus where least maternal tissue is in evidence.

Maintain abdominal strap snugly.

Adjust pen-set *between* contractions to print between 20 and 25 mm Hg on strip chart.

Palpate fundus q30min to 60min to gauge strength of contraction; only frequency and duration of contractions can be assessed with tocotransducer.

Do not assess woman's need for analgesic based on uterine activity displayed on strip chart.

Massage reddened areas gently under transducer and belt qh and prn.

INTERNAL MONITORING (FIG.16-3)

Spiral electrode

Obtains fetal ECG from presenting part and converts it into FHR

Ensure that color-coded wires are appropriately attached to push post on leg plate.

Apply electrode paste to leg plate q2h and prn.

Observe FHR panel of strip chart for long- and short-term variability.

Turn electrode counterclockwise to remove; never pull straight out from presenting part.

Administer perineal care after voiding during labor.

Intrauterine catheter

Catheter (may be fluid-filled) that internally monitors intrauterine pressure

Flush open system catheter with sterile water before insertion and prn.

Ensure that the length line on catheter is visible at introitus.

For open system catheters:

Turn stopcock off to woman, then with pressure valve of strain gauge released, flush strain gauge, remove syringe, and set stylus to 0 line of chart paper; test further according to manufacturer's instructions q3h to 4h and prn.

For closed system catheters set baseline rate between uterine contractions when uterus is relaxed.

Check proper functioning by tapping catheter, asking woman to cough, or applying fundal pressure; observe appropriate inflection on strip chart.

Maintain catheter taped to woman's leg to prevent dislodgement.

Modified from Tucker SM et al: *Patient care standards*, ed 5, St Louis, 1992, Mosby–Year Book.

*Portable telemetry monitors allow observation of the FHR and uterine contraction patterns by means of centrally located electronic display stations. These portable units permit ambulation during electronic monitoring.

■ SUMMARY

Nursing care of the woman in labor may include fetal and maternal monitoring. The nurse's knowledge and competence in this area can have a significant impact on the woman's labor experience.

Normal FHR patterns correlate with high Apgar scores and low neonatal morbidity. An abnormal pattern is equated with fetal hypoxia, low Apgar scores, and high neonatal morbidity in many but by no means in all cases. Because FHR patterns that suggest hypoxia may occur in the absence of fetal distress, intermittent and continuous FHR assessments are screening rather than diagnostic devices. More investigation and clarification of the factors and findings involved will be necessary to perfect the interpretation of fetal monitoring.

Although the use of monitoring can be reassuring to many parents, to some it is a source of anxiety. Therefore the nurse must be particularly sensitive to and respond appropriately to the emotional, knowledge, and comfort needs of the woman in labor as well as her family, during fetal monitoring.

Nursing responsibilities in implementing intrapartum FHR monitoring have been developed by NAACOG (see Appendix C).

CASE STUDY

Electronic Fetal Monitoring During Labor

Lana Resnik, 26 years old, in her first pregnancy, is in labor at full-term gestation. Her cervix is 100% effaced and 1 to 2 cm dilated. Intermittent external EFM has been ordered.

ASSESSMENT

All maternal and fetal assessment findings are within normal limits. The fetus is at term gestation and of normal size with a good FHR. Lana is to ambulate during labor. She is a candidate for intermittent electronic monitoring. Intermittent electronic monitoring includes an initial auscultation to detect possible arrhythmia and a 20-minute FHR and uterine activity tracing by means of external devices.

Lana assumes a supine position in bed. She asks why the physician ordered EFM when everything is so normal and he knows she cannot stay still in bed for long.

NURSING DIAGNOSES

Several nursing diagnoses are possible. One takes priority at this time: Decreased maternal cardiac output related to supine hypotension secondary to maternal position.

PLANNING

Whenever possible, the nurse plans care jointly with the client. One *goal* is mutually determined: The fetus will show no sign of distress. The nurse sets an additional *expected outcome:* Lana will increase her knowledge about position and blood flow and EFM.

IMPLEMENTATION

The nurse's first intervention is to prevent supine hypotension. Lana is asked to assume a semi-Fowler's or side-lying position. The nurse explains the anatomy and physiology of uterine compression of the ascending vena cava and descending aorta.

EVALUATION

Lana readily assumes the side-lying position. She states she understands why semi-Fowler's or side-lying position is beneficial to the fetus. Fetal bradycardia does not occur.

CARE PLAN Electronic Fetal Monitoring During Labor

GOALS	IMPLEMENTATION	RATIONALE	EVALUATION
Nursing diagnosis: Decreased maternal cardiac output related to supine hypotension secondary to maternal position			
Fetus will show no signs of distress. Lana will increase her knowledge of position and blood flow.	Ask Lana to assume a semi-Fowler's and side-lying position. Explain rationale for the requested position.	These positions allow the heavy uterus to be displaced off the ascending vena cava and descending aorta, thus preventing a decrease in cardiac output and drop in BP. Maternal hypotension results in fetal bradycardia.	Lana readily assumes the side-lying position. Her BP remains stable. No fetal bradycardia occurs.
Nursing diagnosis: High risk for impaired fetal gas exchange, undiagnosed, related to inaccurate tracing secondary to wrong placement of transducers			
Nurse applies transducers correctly and gets an accurate tracing.	Follow guidelines for initiating external monitoring. Complete checklist for fetal monitoring equipment.	Provides a back-up for memory when initiating monitor while explaining/teaching or intrusion of other external stimuli.	Nurse applies/initiates monitor correctly. Fetal heart rate and uterine activity tracings are accurate.
Fetus experiences no distress.	Auscultate FHR to cross-check information on tracing and to detect possible arrhythmia.	Double-checks accuracy of the machine. Reassures parent(s) (and nurse).	Monitor correctly displays FHR and uterine activity. The 20-min tracing showed the FHR pattern and long-term variability to be normal and periodic changes to be absent.
Nursing diagnosis: Pain related to use of belts to position transducers and perceived need to lie still			
Lana will not experience discomfort.	Ask Lana to empty her bladder. Explain reasons for emptying bladder and application of transducers.	Full bladder may cause discomfort as well as interfere with signal. Knowledge helps allay anxiety and gives client a sense of control.	Lana emptied her bladder and stated she had no discomfort. Lana stated she understood rationale.
	Use correct method to apply transducers and initiate monitoring. Ask Lana about comfort. Remind her that she has some room to move about; provide massage on back and effleurage on side of abdomen and thighs, prn.	Correctly applied, belts are usually not uncomfortable. Shows respect for her feelings and shows her she has some control over procedure; involves her in her care.	Lana experienced no discomfort.

chapter 16 review

Key Concepts

- Fetal well-being during labor is measured by the response of the FHR to uterine contractions.
- FHR characteristics include the baseline FHR and periodic changes in FHR.
- Monitoring techniques of fetal well-being include FHR assessment and watching for presence of meconium-stained amniotic fluid.
- It is the responsibility of the labor and delivery room nurse to assess FHR patterns, perform independent nursing interventions, and report nonreassuring patterns to the physician.
- NAACOG has established nursing standards for EFM.
- The emotional, informational, and comfort needs of the woman and her family must be addressed when the mother and her fetus are being monitored.

Key Terms

- accelerations (p. 403)
- amnioinfusion (p. 407)
- baseline fetal heart rate (p. 401)
- bradycardia (p. 403)
- decelerations (p. 406)
- electronic fetal monitoring (EFM) (p. 400)
- fetal distress (p. 398)
- head compression (p. 398)
- intrauterine catheter (p. 400)
- intrauterine resuscitation (p. 412)
- meconium-stained amniotic fluid (p. 409)
- prolonged decelerations (p. 407)
- smooth (flat) baseline (p. 403)
- spiral electrode (p. 403)
- supine hypotensive syndrome (p. 403)
- tachycardia (p. 403)
- tocotransducer (p. 401)
- ultrasound transducer (p. 403)
- umbilical cord compression (p. 407)
- uterine activity (p. 401)
- uteroplacental insufficiency (p. 406)
- Valsalva's maneuver (p. 411)
- variability (p. 403)

Critical Thinking Exercises

1. You are assigned to a woman who is in the first stage of labor. She is upset and unknowledgeable about the uses of the fetal monitor. You are using the monitor in an actual labor situation for the first time.
   A. Examine the significance of the woman's emotional state as well as what you might be feeling.
   B. Identify nursing diagnoses based on your analysis of the situation.
   C. Develop a plan of care, including interventions that would be reassuring and supportive, and justify your choices.
2. Review three sample or actual fetal monitor strips.
   A. Determine:
      (1) Fetal heart rate: baseline, variability,
      (2) Periodic changes, if any,
      (3) Contraction interval, duration, intensity, and resting tone.
   B. Corroborate your findings in clinical conference.
   C. Describe appropriate nursing actions for each of these periodic changes:
      (1) Accelerations
      (2) Early decelerations
      (3) Late decelerations
      (4) Variable decelerations

Topics for Nursing Research

- What factors affect the nurse's decision to use internal or external fetal monitoring?
- How do the Leff scope, DeLee-Hillis scope, and Pinard's stethoscope compare in accuracy and ease of use?
- How do the nonelectronic methods noted in the preceding topic compare in accuracy and ease of use with the ultrasound fetoscope and stethoscope?
- Is there a significant difference between FHR with directed (coached) pushing (in the second stage) and spontaneous pushing?
- Compare the FHR when the woman is in left-lateral versus right-lateral position.
- Compare continuous electronic monitoring and periodic auscultation, with one nurse supervising the electronic monitor and a second nurse taking periodic readings on the same woman.

REFERENCES

American Academy of Pediatrics/American College of Obstetricians and Gynecologists: *Guidelines for perinatal care,* Elk Grove Village, Ill, 1988, AAP/ACOG.

American College of Obstetricians and Gynecologists: *Guidelines for oxytocin induction,* Washington, DC, 1989, The College.

American College of Obstetricians and Gynecologists: *Intrapartum fetal heart rate monitoring* (ACOG Technical Bull No 132), Washington, DC, 1989, The College.

Blackburn ST, Loper DL: *Maternal, fetal and neonatal physiology: a clinical perspective,* Philadelphia, 1992, WB Saunders Co.

Caldeyro-Barcia R et al: The bearing down efforts and their effect on fetal heart rate, oxygenation and acid-base balance, *J Perinat Med* 9(6):3, 1981.

Caldeyro-Barcia R: The influence of maternal bearing-down efforts during second stage on fetal well being, *Birth Family J,* 6 17, Spring 1979.

Cherry SH, Merkatz IR: *Complications of pregnancy: medical, surgical, gynecologic, psychosocial, and perinatal,* Baltimore, 1991, Williams & Wilkins.

Fanaroff AA, Martin RJ: *Neonatal-perinatal medicine: diseases of the fetus and infant,* ed 5, St Louis, 1992, Mosby–Year Book.

Fields LM, Boehm FH: Changing issues in FHR monitoring, *Contemp OB/GYN* 33 (special issue), 145, 1989.

Freeman RK, Garite TJ, Nageotte MP: *Fetal heart rate monitoring,* Baltimore, 1991, Williams & Wilkins.

Korner PI, Tonkin AM, Uther JB: Reflex and mechanical circulatory effects of graded Valsalva maneuvers in normal man, *J Appl Physiol* 40:434, 1976.

McKay S, Roberts J: Second stage labor: what is normal? *JOGNN* 14:101, 1985.

NAACOG: *Nursing responsibilities in implementing intrapartum fetal heart rate monitoring* (Statement), Washington, DC 1989, NAACOG.

NAACOG: *Fetal heart rate auscultation* (OGN nursing practice resource), Washington, DC 1990, NAACOG.

Page L, Young K: Uterine activity in the second stage of labour and the effect of epidural analgesia, *Br J Obstet Gynaecol* 93:1017, 1986.

Parer JT: Fetal heart rate. In Creasy RK, Resnik R, editors: *Maternal/fetal medicine: principles and practice,* Philadelphia, 1984, WB Saunders.

Roberts JE: Alternative positions for childbirth. II. Second stage of labor, *J Nurse Midwife* 25:13, 1980.

Roberts JE: (1989). Maternal positioning during the first stage of labour. In Chalmers I, Enkin M, Keirse MJNC, editors: *Effective care in pregnancy and childbirth* Oxford, 1989, Oxford University Press.

Schifrin BS, Clements D: Why fetal monitoring remains a good idea, *Contemp OB/GYN* 35:70, 1990.

Scott JR et al: *Danforth's obstetrics and gynecology,* ed 6, Philadelphia, 1990, JB Lippincott Co.

Tucker SM: *Pocket guide to fetal monitoring,* ed 2, St Louis, 1992, Mosby–Year Book.

Tucker SM et al: *Patient care standards,* ed 5, St Louis, 1992, Mosby–Year Book.

References—Nursing Research

Barnett M, Humenick S: Infant outcomes in relation to second stage labor pushing, *Birth* 9:221, 1982.

Chez B et al: Interpretations of nonstress tests by obstetric nurses, *JOGNN* 19:227, May/June 1990.

Liu YC: The effects of the upright position during childbirth, *Image J Nurs Sch* 21:14, Spring 1989.

Yeates DA, Roberts JE: A comparison of two bearing down techniques during the second stage of labor, *J Nurse Midwife* 29(1):3, 1984.

BIBLIOGRAPHY

Afriat CI: *Electronic fetal monitoring,* Rockville, 1989, Aspen Publishers.

American College of Obstetricians and Gynecologists: *Standard for obstetric-gynecologic services,* ed 7, Washington, DC, 1989, ACOG.

Challis JRG: Characteristics of parturition. In Creasy RK, Resnik R editors: *Maternal-fetal medicine: principles and practice,* Philadelphia, 1989, WB Saunders.

Cohen WR, Acker DB, Friedman EA: *Management of labor* ed 2, Rockville, MD, 1989, Aspen Publishers.

Cunningham FG, MacDonald PC, Gant NF: *Williams' obstetrics,* ed 18, Norwalk, Conn, 1989, Appleton & Lange.

Devoe LD: Computerized analysis of fetal heart rate, *Female Patient* 15:41, April 1990.

Eganhouse DJ: Electronic fetal monitoring: education and quality assurance *JOGNN* 20:16, Jan/Feb 1991.

Fields LM: Electronic fetal monitoring: practices and protocols for the intrapartum patient, *J Perinat Neonat Nurs* 1:5, Jan 1987.

Freedman RM, Baltimore R: Fatal *Streptococcus viridans* septicemia and meningitis: relationship to fetal scalp electrode monitoring, *J Perinat* 10:272, Sept 1990.

Galvan B, Van Mullem C, Brockhuizen F: Using amnio-infusion for the relief of repetitive variable decelerations during labor, *JOGNN* 19:222, May/June 1989.

Garite TJ: FHR and contraction channels point to uterine rupture, *Contemp OB/GYN* 35:14, May 1990.

Garite TJ, Ray D: Intrauterine resuscitation with tocolysis, *Contemp OB/GYN* 31:24, March 1988.

Gilbert ES, Harmon JS: *Manual of high-risk pregnancy and delivery: nursing perspectives,* ed 2, St Louis, 1993, Mosby–Year Book.

Huszar G: Physiology of the myometrium. In Creasy RK, Resnik R, editors: *Maternal-fetal medicine: principles and practice,* 1989, Philadelphia, WB Saunders.

Kinnick VG: A national survey about fetal monitoring skills acquired by nursing students in baccalaureate programs, *JOGNN* 18:57, Jan/Feb 1989.

Knorr LJ: Relieving fetal distress with amnioinfusion, *MCN* 14:346, Sept/Oct 1989.

Perlow JH, Garite TJ: Update on EFM systems, *Contemp OB/GYN* 36(Technology):44, April 1991.

Pheigaru JL: Keeping staff up on electronic fetal monitoring, *MCN* 13:334, Sept/Oct 1988.

Pillai M, James D: The development of fetal heart rate patterns during normal pregnancy, *Obstet Gynecol* 76, 812, 1990.

Queenan J et al: Today's high C/S rate: can we reduce it? (Symposium), *Contemp OB/GYN* 32:154, Jan 1988.

Roussis P, Troiano NH, Shah DM: Fetal Assessment. I. Nonstress and contraction stress testing, *Female Patient* 15:33, Nov 1990.

Sarno AP, Phelan JP: Intrauterine resuscitation of the fetus, *Contemp OB/GYN* 32:143, Jan 1988.

Snydal SH: Responses of laboring women to fetal heart rate monitoring: a critical review of the literature, *J Nurse Midwife* 33:208, Sept/Oct 1988.

Strong TH, Phelan JP: Amnioinfusion for intrapartum management, *Contemp OB/GYN* 36:15, May 1991.

Thorp J, McNitt D, Leppert P: Effects of epidural analgesia: some questions and answers, *Birth* 17(3):157, 1990.

Legal Aspects

AIG Consultants, Inc: Fetal monitoring as a malpractice prevention tool, *Viewpoint: Risk Management Advisory for Healthcare Professionals* 2, Jan 1989.

Hankins GDV: Apgar scores: are they enough? *Contemp OB/GYN* (Ob-Gyn Law Special Issue) 36:13, Feb 1991.

Niswander KR: EFM and brain damage in term and postterm infants, *Contemp OB/GYN* (Ob-Gyn Law Special Issue) 36:39, Feb 1991.

Phelan JP: Was it intrapartum fetal distress? *Contemp OB/GYN* (OB-Gyn Law Special Issue) 36:26, Feb 1991.

Symposium: Confronting medical liability, *Contemp OB/GYN* (OB-Gyn Law Special Issue) 36:70, Feb 1991.

Twin Gestation

American College of Obstetricians and Gynecologists: *Multiple gestation* (Technical Bull No 131), Washington, DC, 1989, The College.

Eganhouse DJ: Fetal monitoring of twins, *JOGNN* 21:17, Jan/Feb 1992.

Jones JM, Sbarra AJ, Cetrulo CL: Antepartum management of twin gestation, *Clin Obstet Gynecol* 33:32, 1990.

Sherer DM et al: The occurrence of simultaneous fetal heart rate accelerations in twins during nonstress testing, *Obstet Gynecol* 76:817, 1990.

Sherer DM et al: Fetal vibratory acoustic stimulation in twin gestations with simultaneous fetal heart rate monitoring, *Am J Obstet Gynecol* 164:1104, 1991.

Nursing Research

Galvan B, Van Mullem C, Broekhuizen F: Using amnioinfusion for the relief of repetitive variable decelerations during labor, *JOGNN* 18:222, May/June 1989.

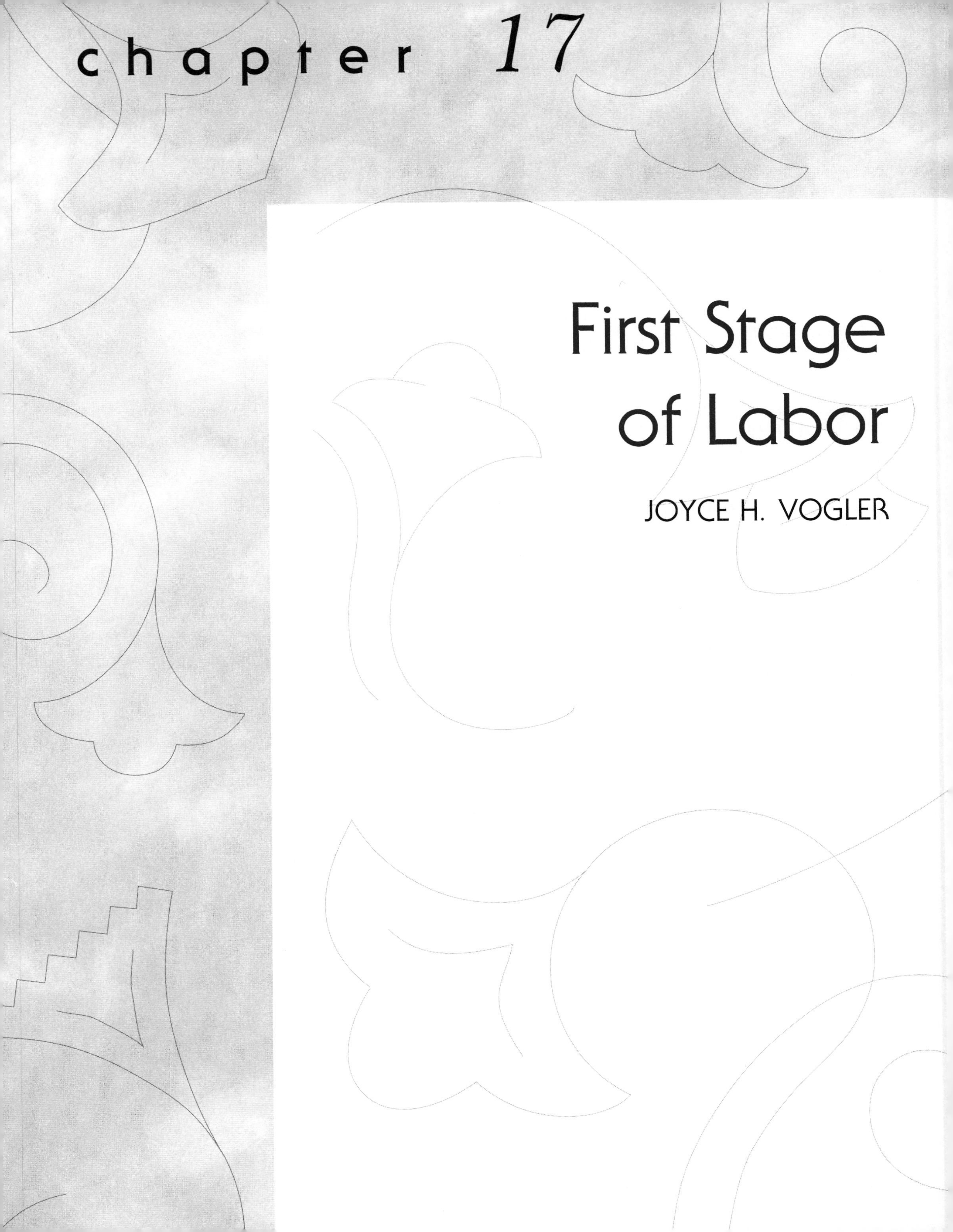

chapter 17

First Stage of Labor

JOYCE H. VOGLER

LEARNING OBJECTIVES

- Define the key terms listed at the end of the chapter.
- Review the factors involved in the initial assessment of the woman in labor.
- Summarize the subsequent assessment of progress during the first stage of labor.
- Identify nursing diagnoses, and develop an appropriate plan of care throughout the first stage of labor.
- Evaluate the role of the woman's supportive persons/family members during the first stage of labor.
- Summarize the nurse's role in supporting the woman and her supportive persons/family during the first stage of labor.
- Discuss assessment of the fetus during the first stage of labor.
- Outline those aspects of preparation for delivery that are appropriately done during the first stage of labor.
- Identify topics for nursing research related to the first stage of labor.

The first stage of labor begins a journey for the childbearing woman and her significant others that, in a matter of a relatively short time, will culminate in the birth of a baby whose arrival has been anticipated for months, sometimes years. Some pregnant women have prepared themselves to recognize the symptoms of the onset of labor and have certain expectations of what labor will be like. Nursing care is focused on supporting the laboring woman and her family through the journey to ensure the best possible outcome for all involved (Fig. 17-1). As they become more informed consumers of health care, many childbearing families are taking a more active role in developing a birth plan to outline their desires regarding the coming birth experience. Those desires may include experiencing the miracle of their baby's birth in nontraditional delivery settings, such as labor, delivery, recovery, postpartum (LDRP) rooms, that use more family-centered alternative approaches (Machol, 1988).

The **first stage of labor** begins with the onset of regular uterine contractions and ends with full dilatation of the cervix. The woman will either telephone or come to the perinatal unit. She will report one or more of the following:

1. History of contractions of sufficient strength, frequency, and duration to convince her that she is in labor
2. Vaginal discharge of mucus, often accompanied by some **bloody show**
3. Fluid discharge from the vagina (spontaneous rupture of membranes)

The first stage of labor consists of three phases; the **latent or early phase** (up to 3 cm of dilatation), the **active phase** (4 to 7 cm), and the **transitional phase** (7 to 10 cm). Most first-time mothers seek entry to the hospital in the latent phase because they have no basis for comparison and are unsure of the "right" time to come in (Bonovich, 1990). Multiparous women usually do not come to the hospital until they are in the active phase; sometimes they barely make it in time for delivery. Even though no two labors are identical, women who have given birth before appear less anxious about the process unless they have had a previous negative experience.

Comprehensive knowledge of the essential factors that trigger labor, the anatomic and physiologic adaptations, assessment of fetal and maternal well-being in labor, and recognition and treatment of problems are needed to provide quality physical nursing care to both mother and fetus during labor. The nurse who has or knows where to acquire this knowledge can provide the childbearing family with a quality of care that meets the high standards of nursing care (see Chapter 4).

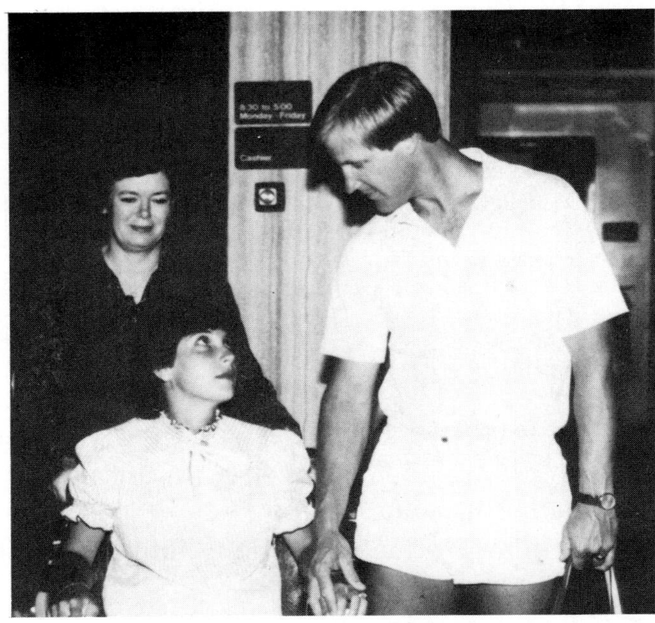

Fig. 17-1 Woman in labor, seated in wheelchair and accompanied by family members, being admitted by a nurse.

■ THE NURSING PROCESS

It is important for the nurse to be skilled in the nursing process as it relates to caring for women and their families in all stages of labor. Thus careful first-stage management is necessary to promote the best possible birth outcome.

ASSESSMENT

Assessment begins at the first contact with the woman, whether by telephone or in person. Many women will call the hospital first to receive validation that it is all right for them to come in. It is important for the nurse to respond in a pleasant manner to foster a caring attitude and encourage the client to verbalize her questions and concerns. If at all possible, the nurse needs to have the woman's prenatal record in hand when speaking to her or admitting her for evaluation of labor. Records usually are filed on the perinatal unit under the name of the physician or certified nurse midwife (the **primary care practitioner**).

Certain factors are assessed initially to determine if the woman is in **true labor** and should come to the hospital or be admitted (Cunningham, et al, 1989). (See Client Teaching box, p. 425) If there is any doubt about admission for the client who telephones,

TEACHING **Distinguishing True Labor from False Labor**

TRUE LABOR
Contractions

- Occur regularly, becoming stronger, lasting longer, occurring closer together
- Increase in intensity with walking
- Are felt in lower back, radiating to lower portion of abdomen
- Continue despite use of comfort measures

Cervix

- Shows progressive change (softening, effacement, and dilatation signaled by the appearance of bloody show)
- Moves to an increasingly anterior position; cannot be determined without vaginal examination

Fetus

- Presenting part becomes engaged in the pelvis, often referred to as the fetus "dropping" (lightening). This results in increased ease of breathing; at the same time the bladder is compressed from the downward pressure exerted by the presenting part.

FALSE LABOR
Contractions

- Occur irregularly or become regular only temporarily
- Often stop with walking or position change
- Are felt in the back or abdomen above the navel
- Often can be stopped with use of comfort measures

Cervix

- May be soft but there is no significant change in effacement or dilatation or evidence of bloody show
- Is often in a posterior position; cannot be detected without vaginal examination

Fetus

- Presenting part is not engaged in the pelvis

Telephone Interview with Woman in Latent Phase of Labor

The perinatal nurse performs the following steps of the nursing process.

ASSESSMENT

- Gathers data regarding client status, deciding whether the woman will come in to the hospital or be encouraged to continue her labor at home until contractions increase in duration and frequency

PLANNING AND IMPLEMENTATION

- Assures the woman that she is welcome to call the perinatal unit at any time to discuss her labor status
- Answers questions the woman and her family may have regarding labor or provides instruction as needed (e.g., which entrance of the hospital to come in)
- Suggests a variety of positions that maximally enhance uteroplacental and renal blood flow (e.g., left side-lying)
- Instructs the woman to come in immediately if membranes rupture

EVALUATION

- Evaluates whether instructions and information have been understood by asking for verbalization of understanding

the nurse either refers the woman to call her primary care practitioner or advises her to come to the hospital (see box above, right). The manner in which the nurse communicates with the woman during this first contact can set the tone for a positive experience in the hospital. Before the first meeting with the woman in labor, the nurse reviews the prenatal record.

When the woman arrives at the perinatal unit, assessment is top priority. The nurse will perform a detailed systems assessment, using the techniques of interview, physical assessment, and laboratory findings to determine the woman's status. The initial assessment consists of gathering information in a variety of ways to fully evaluate the woman's labor status and fill out the necessary hospital forms. Thus the nurse provides the primary care practitioner with the best possible evaluation of the woman's status.

Admission Forms

The admission forms can provide a guideline for important assessment information when a woman in labor is being evaluated or admitted. As previously mentioned, additional sources include (1) the prenatal record, (2) initial interview, (3) physical examination to determine baseline physiologic parameters, (4) laboratory results, (5) psychosocial and cultural factors, and (6) the clinical evaluation in progress. It is preferable to have a form that integrates admission and labor data as shown in Fig. 17-2.

ADMISSION LABOR RECORD

DATE:
GR T P L AB
ALLERGIES:
PHYSICIAN:
PEDIATRICIAN:
LMP: EDC: GEST:
CONTR: $\overline{q}$ FOR hrs.
BOW ☐intact ☐SR@
FLUID APPEAR.:

☐EVALUATION
☐ADMISSION: SONO/TOCO ON
☐ORIENTED TO UNIT ROUTINES CALL LIGHT, TELEPHONE, TV

Last Solid Food @
Curr. Meds. ☐ Vit. ☐Fe ☐Other:
Probs. this pregnancy:

*See Nurses Notes	Time												
VITAL SIGNS	BP												
	Pulse												
	Resp												
	Temp												
M = Mild MOD = Moderate S = Strong	FREQUENCY												
	DURATION												
	INTENSITY												
Fetal Heart (Enter baseline rate) LTV + = Long term variability present = 6-10 beats amplitude, 3-6 cycle changes/min. STV + = Beat to beat changes of 2-3 bpm; roughness of tracing line. AC=Accelerations present. P=Periodic													
Medications Pit=Pitocin Dem=Demerol Terb=Terbutaline Sta=Stadol Phen=Phenergan Vist=Vistaril													
Procedures/Activities													
I & O IV = Intravenous PO = Oral V = Void C = Cath E = Emesis													
Dilation and Effacement													
Station and Position													
RN Initial													

Ht: Reflexes: Clon:
Wt: Gain: Edema:
Hgb: Hct:
Type + Rh: Date
Rubella Titer: Done
Serology:
OTHER:

Classes Taken ☐No ☐Yes
☐Breast ☐Bottle

Protheses ☐No ☐Yes
If yes, specify ____________

Anesthesia Desired ☐Epidural
☐Local ☐None ☐Other:

URINE	PROT	GLU	KET	PH
Neg				
Pos				

LABOR

	From	To	Total time
Stage I			h m
Stage II			h m
Stage III			h m
TOTAL		hrs.	min.

Nurses Signature:

INIT:	
INIT:	
INIT:	

NURSES NOTES: ____________

ADDRESSOGRAPH

 OB 2791

Fig. 17-2 Admission labor record.
From Vogler/Perinatal Healthcare Consultants, 1990, Kailua, HI.

Prenatal Record

The prenatal record needs to be reviewed by the admitting nurse to assist in assessment of the woman's individual risks and needs. If the woman has not had any prenatal care, certain baseline information needs to be obtained. If the woman is experiencing discomfort, the nurse attempts to ask questions between contractions when the woman is better able to concentrate.

It is important to know the woman's *age* so that the plan of care can be individualized to her age-group. For example, a 14-year-old and a 40-year-old have different but specific needs, and their age places them at risk for different problems. *Height and weight* relationships are particularly important because most women are encouraged by their primary care practitioners to gain up to 30 pounds. For some women this places them at a higher risk for cephalopelvic disproportion (CPD) (see Chapter 35) and possible cesarean birth. This is especially true for women who were petite before pregnancy and have gained 35 or more pounds. Other factors for consideration are *general health,* any current *medical conditions or allergies, respiratory status,* the type and time of the last solid food taken, previous *surgeries.*

Past and present *obstetric and pregnancy history* are carefully noted on a perinatal risk assessment form (see Fig. 17-11) or on the admission form. Important *obstetric history* includes the following: pregnancies (gravidity), births over the age of viability (about 24 weeks' gestation), preterm labors and births, spontaneous abortions, and number of living children. Other *obstetric problems* to consider are history of the following: vaginal bleeding, pregnancy-induced hypertension, anemia, gestational diabetes, infections (bacterial or sexually transmitted), and immunodeficiencies.

If this is not the woman's first labor and delivery experience, it is important to note the characteristics of her previous labors and deliveries. Their duration, the type of anesthesia used, and the kind of delivery (spontaneous vaginal, forceps, vacuum- or cesarean-assisted birth) are important historic factors. After assessing past deliveries, the nurse must collect data related to the condition of the babies (their weight, Apgar scores, and general health at and following birth). For example, Mrs. Smith gained 31 pounds with her last pregnancy. Her baby was delivered by vacuum assistance after 2 hours of pushing, and Mrs. Smith had an extensive episiotomy. During this pregnancy, Mrs. Smith, who is at 38 weeks' gestation, has gained 43 pounds. With the information derived from the prenatal record, the nurse is better able to anticipate the delivery needs of this mother/baby couple. (It would not be surprising for this baby to need a vacuum- or cesarean-assisted delivery in light of the previous delivery history.)

It is important to confirm that the expected date of delivery (EDD) is as accurate as possible. EDD is confirmed during the second trimester (see Chapter 12). Other data in the prenatal record include patterns of maternal weight gain, physiologic measurements such as blood pressure, baseline fetal heart rate, and laboratory test results. These tests include blood type and Rh factor, complete or partial blood count (CBC or hemoglobin and hematocrit), rubella titer, serologic findings (VDRL or rapid plasma reagin [RPR]), hepatitis B surface antigen (HB_{sAG}), and urinalysis. Additional tests are for tuberculosis screen with purified protein derivative (PPD), human immunodeficiency virus (HIV), sickle cell trait, or other genetic screening.

Interview

Any information not found in the prenatal record is requested on admission. Pertinent data include birth plan, choice of infant feeding method, anesthesia desired, and pediatrician. A client profile is obtained; this profile indicates the woman's preparation for childbirth, supportive persons desired and available, and ethnic or cultural expectations or needs.

The woman's chief complaint or reason for coming to the hospital is determined. The chief complaint may be that her **bag of waters (BOW)** has broken, with or without contractions. In this case she is in for an **obstetric check.** The obstetric check is reserved for women who are unsure about onset of labor. This designation allows time on the unit for diagnosis of labor without official admission, which minimizes or avoids cost to the client.

The woman may have been scheduled for induction of labor (see Chapter 35). Induction of labor and other complications of labor, such as premature rupture of membranes, require special alterations in the nursing care plan. However, even in those instances much of the nursing care remains the same.

The onset of labor may be difficult to determine even for the experienced mother. The woman is asked to recall the events of the previous days. She is assessed for the prodromal signs of labor (see Chapter 14) and for the onset of regular contractions. She is asked to describe the following:

1. Frequency and duration of contractions.
2. Location and character of discomfort from contractions (i.e., back pain, suprapubic discomfort).
3. Persistence of contractions despite changes in maternal position, when walking or lying down.

4. Presence and character of vaginal discharge or show.
5. Status of amniotic membranes, such as gush or seepage of fluid. If there is a discharge that may be amniotic fluid, she is asked the date and time the fluid was first noted. In many instances a sterile speculum examination confirms that the membranes are ruptured (p. 442).

These questions also help the nurse assess the degree of progress by determining the character of the contractions and the nature of the vaginal discharge. *Bloody show* is distinguished from bleeding in that it is pink in color and feels sticky because of its mucoid nature. It is scant to begin with and increases with effacement and dilatation of the cervix. A woman may report a scant brownish discharge that may be attributed to cervical trauma as a result of vaginal examination or coitus within the last 48 hours.

In case general anesthesia may be required at a moment's notice, it is important to know about the woman's respiratory status. The nurse asks if the woman has a "cold" or related symptoms, "stuffy nose," sore throat, or cough. Allergies are rechecked, including allergies to drugs routinely used, such as meperidine (Demerol) or lidocaine (Xylocaine). Some allergic responses cause swelling of mucous membranes of the respiratory system. Because vomiting and subsequent aspiration into the respiratory tract can complicate an otherwise normal labor, the nurse records the type and time of the woman's last solid food.

This initial interview helps confirm the approximate time of onset of true labor and provides information on the woman's current clinical condition.

False labor may be experienced from the thirty-eighth week of pregnancy onward. It can be disheartening for the woman and her partner to find that the contractions she is having are not true labor contractions and that she must return home to await the onset of true labor (for a comparison of true and **false labor**, see box, p. 425).

The first-time mother, because of eagerness to complete labor, may come to the hospital early in the first stage. If she lives near the hospital, she may be asked to return home to wait for further progress either in frequency and strength of contractions or in amount of show. She is encouraged to walk about but is asked to restrict ingestion to clear fluids (those that one can see through). Clear fluids are advised because digestion slows significantly during labor and any food taken is liable to be vomited during transition or second stage. Examples of clear liquids are tea with sugar and juices such as apple or cranberry. Liquids should be sipped slowly and continuously during early labor to avoid nausea and to provide the woman with a source of nutrition inasmuch as labor burns extra calories.

It can be disheartening for the woman and her partner to find out that the contractions that feel strong and regular to her are not true labor contractions because they are not causing cervical dilatation. However, the woman who lives at a considerable distance from the hospital may be admitted in early labor.

Psychosocial Factors

The woman's general appearance and behavior (and that of her partner) provide valuable clues to the type of supportive care she will need. Factors to assess include the following:

Verbal interactions. Does the woman ask questions? Can she ask for what she needs? Does her partner do all the talking? Does she talk to her support person(s)? Does she talk freely with the nurse or respond only to questions?

Body language. Is she relaxed or tense? What is her anxiety level? How does she react to being touched by the nurse? Support person? Does she change position or lie rigidly still? Does she avoid eye contact? Where does her partner sit? Does she look tired? How much rest has she had during the last day?

Perceptual ability. Does she understand what the nurse says? Is there a language barrier? Does her anxiety level require repeated explanations? Can she repeat what she has been told or demonstrate understanding?

Discomfort level. To what degree does the woman relate what she is experiencing? How does she react to a contraction? Are there any nonverbal pain messages seen? Does she complain to the nurse? her partner? Can she ask for comfort measures?

Maternal Stress

The way women and their partners/significant others approach labor is related to the manner in which they have been socialized to the childbearing process. Their reactions provide a summary of their life experiences regarding childbirth—physical, social, and cultural. Societal teaching through media and literature instructs women that childbirth is a "wonderful" experience, which may include a few "pains" but ends in the glorious arrival of a perfect little baby. This idealized picture may create a feeling of guilt when the woman finds the process less than joyous, especially when the pregnancy is unplanned or is the product of a shaky or terminated relationship. Often women have heard horror stories or have seen friends or relatives going through labors that appear anything but easy. Mothers often will base their expectations of the present labor and delivery on their previous experience.

Usually women in labor have a variety of concerns that they will voice if asked but will rarely volunteer. It is therefore important for the nurse to ask the woman what she expects and thus clear up misinformation or suggest that the woman ask her primary care practitioner about an issue. Common concerns of women in labor are: Will my baby be all right? Will I be able to stand labor? Will my labor be long? How will I act? Will I need medication? Will it work for me? Will my partner/someone be there to support me? Do I have to have an IV, an enema, etc.?

The nurse's responsibility to the woman in the hospital is to answer her questions or find out the answers, to provide support to her and her family/significant others, to take care of her in a partnership with those persons the woman wants as her support team, and to be her advocate. It is imperative that the nurse tell the woman that she is not expected to act in any particular way and that the process will yield the birth of her baby, which is the only expectation she should have. The nurse needs to communicate with the woman regarding their individual perceptions of the nurse's role to promote the attachment or bonding that will become increasingly important to the woman as labor progresses.

The woman's level of anxiety may rise when she does not understand what is being said. The nurse need only observe the facial expression and body language of the woman who has just been examined vaginally when the physician, within the woman's hearing, tells the nurse, "She's a primigravida, EDD 2 weeks from now. She's 50% effaced but I can barely get a fingertip in there. She had bloody show but she'll have to drop the head some yet. If her membranes don't rupture by themselves, I'll pop them myself. The contractions are weak now; they'll have to get a lot harder to get the job done. Do a miniprep on her."

The woman who is unfamiliar with these terms could understandedly panic (Bentz, 1980). Many of the terms—bloody show, drop the head, membranes rupture—sound violent and could conjure up thoughts of injury or pain. If the woman perceives her "weak" contractions as painful, she may become tense anticipating the more intense uterine contractions that are needed "to get the job done."

Women prepare themselves for labor in a variety of ways. Some go to parent education classes, some read books and talk to friends and relatives, and some prepare elaborate birth plans of their wishes for their labor and delivery. The longer the list of "should be's," the greater the likelihood that expectations will not be met. The nurse tries to focus on the intent of the birth plan, not necessarily on every detail, and reassures the woman that every effort will be made to support her wishes. For example, a woman may desire to have her baby placed directly on her abdomen after birth, before the cord is clamped. The nurse can facilitate aspects of the birth plan by showing it to the physician or midwife and reminding the woman to ask her practitioner for what she wants in advance. It is the nurse's responsibility to include the desires of the client in formulating a plan of care.

Cultural Factors

It is important to note the woman's ethnic/cultural background to anticipate nursing interventions that may need to be added or deleted from the individualized plan of care. (See also Chapter 3.) If a special request is contrary to observed protocol, the woman will be encouraged to ask her primary care practitioner to write an order for the special request. For example, in some cultures it is traditional to take the placenta home; in others the woman is given only certain nourishments during labor.

Women are culturally taught the "right" way to behave in labor. These behaviors can range from total silence to moaning or screaming. If the woman primarily follows her mother's expectations, she may perceive the need to "behave" more strongly than if her coach is the father of the baby. She will perceive herself as failing or succeeding on the basis of her ability to adhere to these "standards" of behavior. A woman who moans with contractions may not be in as much physical pain as a woman who is silent but winces during contractions (see Table 17-1).

The Non–English-Speaking Woman in Labor

A woman's level of anxiety in labor will rise when she does not understand what is happening to her or what is being said. This can and does happen to English-speaking women (Bentz, 1980), causing some level of stress. The toll on non–English-speaking women is significantly more dramatic because they often feel a complete loss of control over their situation. They can panic and withdraw or become physically abusive to anyone who tries to do something they perceive might harm them or their babies. Sometimes they bring with them a support person who is able to communicate in English. However, this arrangement is not always an improvement because the "translator" friend may misrepresent what

TABLE 17-1 Sociocultural Basis of Pain Experience

	Woman in Labor	Nurse
Perception of meaning	Origin: Cultural concept of and personal experience with pain; for example: Pain in childbirth is inevitable, something to be borne Pain in childbirth can be avoided completely Pain in childbirth is punishment for sin Pain in childbirth can be controlled	Origin: Cultural concept of and personal experience with pain; in addition, nurse becomes accustomed to working with certain "expected" pain trajectories. For example, in obstetrics, pain is expected to increase as labor progresses, be intermittent in character, and have end point; relief can be derived from drugs once labor is well established and fetus or newborn can cope with amount and elimination of drug; relief can also come from woman's knowledge and attitude and support from family or friends
Coping mechanisms	Woman may do the following: Be traditionally vocal or nonvocal; crying out or groaning or both may be part of ritual of her response to pain Use counterstimulation to minimize pain; for example, rubbing, applying heat, or counterpressure Have learned to use relaxation, distraction, autosuggestion as pain-countering techniques Resist any use of "needles" as modes of administering pain relief	Nurse may do the following: Have learned to use self effectively; for example, tone of voice, closeness in space, touch, as media for message of interest and caring Use avoidance, belittling, or other distancing actions as protective device for self Use pharmacologic resources at hand judiciously Be skilled in use of comfort measures Assume accountability for control and management of pain
Expectations of others	Nurse may be seen as someone who will accept woman's statement of pain and act as her advocate Medical personnel may be expected to relieve woman of all pain sensations Nurse may be expected to be interested, gentle, kindly, and accepting of behavior exhibited	Nurse may accept only certain verbal or nonverbal behaviors as responses to pain Nurse may expect couple that is prepared for childbirth to refuse medication and to wish to "do everything on their own" Nurse may find it difficult to accept woman's definition of pain; that is, woman may wish to experience and participate in controlling pain or may not be able to accept any pain as reasonable

the nurse or others are saying and raise the woman's stress level even more.

If there is a list of employee translators, one may be contacted for help. If no one in the hospital is able to translate, a bilingual employee can be called and a telephone translation can take place. A set of cards with graphics that illustrate common situations the nurse will need to communicate to non–English-speaking clients can be generated to assist in the process. Even if the nurse is able to verbally communicate only marginally with the woman, in most cases it is meaningful to the woman that the nurse is making an effort to communicate with her. This attempt may initiate a nonverbal bond between the nurse and the woman/support persons.

Paternal Stress

The woman's support person is referred to as her partner and significant other because the identity of this person as the baby's father cannot be taken for granted. This section is addressed to the "father" of the baby, but can be applied to other support persons. It is important for the nurse to assess the father's behavior. Is he hesitant to stay by the woman's bedside? Does he watch television, sleep, read, or talk on the telephone instead of paying attention to the woman? Does he touch the woman? What is the character of the touch as observed by the nurse? Does he appear anxious, aggressive, or hostile to the woman or nurse? Does he look hungry, worried, confused?

TABLE 17-2 Minimum Assessment of Progress of First Stage of Labor

	Cervical Dilatation		
	0-5cm	6-7cm	8-10cm
Vital signs*	q4hr	q4h	q4h
Blood pressure (BP)	q60min	q30min	q30min
Contractions	q30min-1hr	q15min	q5-10min
Fetal heart rate (FHR)	q15min†	q15min†	q5min†
Show	q60min	q30min	q10-15min
Behavior, appearance, energy level	q30min	q15min	q5min

Vaginal examination‡ to be done only for following reasons:

1. To confirm diagnosis when symptoms indicate change (e.g., strength, duration, or frequency of contractions; increase in amount of bloody show; membranes rupture; or woman feels pressure on her rectum)
2. To determine whether dilatation and descent are sufficient for administration of analgesic or anesthetic
3. To reassess progress if labor takes longer than expected
4. To determine station of presenting part

*If membranes have ruptured, check temperature every 2 hours.
†For a period of 30 seconds immediately after a uterine contraction (Zuspan, Quilligan, 1982).
‡In presence of vaginal bleeding, physician performs vaginal examination, usually under double setup, or ultrasonography.

These fathers are viewed as providers of support to their woman partners. Often the support they are able to give is in direct relationship to the support they feel from the nurse, primary care practitioner, and others with whom they come in contact in the hospital environment.

Physical Examination

The initial examination confirms the onset of true labor. The findings serve as a baseline for assessing the woman's progress from that point in time. Knowledge of pregnancy, careful initial assessment, and follow-up of progress are necessary during labor. The initial physical examination includes general systems assessment, auscultation of fetal heart rate (FHR), assessment of uterine contractions, cervical effacement and dilatation, descent, tests for rupture of membranes, and Leopold's maneuvers. Clients often focus on contractions as the clearest indicator of how far advanced their labor is. However, the nurse considers the vaginal examination more conclusive, especially in first-time mothers, in estimating the woman's phase of labor. In addition, the presence of ruptured membranes has a significant effect on the woman's plan of care. The most vital aspect of assessment is that of fetal status. It is important to view as many related pieces of information as possible before planning and implementing care.

Complete and accurate assessment on admission provides the basis for ongoing care. Minimum assessment guidelines and normal limits of maternal progress during the first stage of labor are presented in Tables 17-2 and 17-3.

The assessment procedures that follow can be used as a basis for teaching women and their families. The purpose, equipment needed, and nursing actions and rationale of each procedure can be shared with the woman. All procedures are preceded by thorough hand washing. The procedures and findings are explained to the woman whenever possible. Universal precautions and precautions for invasive procedures are taken as needed (see Chapter 29). Findings and the time the procedure is performed are carefully noted and initialed on the chart. Hand washing is also important *after* the examinations. Accurate charting is done as soon as possible after interaction with a client.

Assessment is continuous throughout labor. The routine for assessment of progress and of the continued well-being of the mother and fetus is usually set on a minimum level by hospital policy (Table 17-2). Any unusual findings would prompt more frequent performance of assessment procedures.

The signs of progress in labor are well defined (Table 17-3). The character of the woman's uterine contractions, her behavior, and her appearance correlate with the phase of labor she is experiencing. The woman's culture, fatigue, and other factors may affect how she deals with labor.

TABLE 17-3 Maternal Progress in First Stage of Labor Within Normal Limits

Criterion	Phases Marked by Cervical Dilatation* 0-3 cm	4-7 cm	8-10 cm Transition
DURATION	About 8-10 hr	About 3 hr	About 1-2 hr
CONTRACTIONS			
Magnitude (strength)	Mild	Moderate	Strong to expulsive
Rhythm	Irregular	More regular	Regular
Frequency	5-30 min apart	3-5 min apart	2-3 min apart
Duration	10-30 sec	30-45 sec	45-60 (few to 90) sec
DESCENT			
Station of presenting part	Nulliparous: 0 Multiparous: 0 to −2 cm	About +1 to +2 cm About +1 to +2 cm	+2 to +3 cm +2 to +3 cm
SHOW			
Color	Brownish discharge, **mucous plug** or pale, pink mucus	Pink to bloody mucus	Bloody mucus
Amount	Scant	Scant to moderate	Copious
BEHAVIOR AND APPEARANCE	Excited; thoughts center on self, labor, and baby; may be talkative or mute, calm or tense; some apprehension; pain controlled fairly well; alert, follows directions readily; open to instructions	Becoming more serious, doubtful of control of pain, more apprehensive; desires companionship and encouragement; attention more inner directed; fatigue evidenced; malar flush; has some difficulty following directions	Pain described as severe; backache common; feelings of frustration, fear of loss of control, and irritability surface; vague in communications; amnesia between contractions; writhing with contractions; nausea and vomiting, especially if hyperventilating; hyperesthesia; circumoral pallor, perspiration on forehead and upper lips; shaking tremor of thighs; feeling of need to defecate, pressure on anus

*The pace of progress in cervical dilatation (according to Friedman and Sachtleben, 1965) varies as follows: from 0-2 cm (latent phase), progress is slow; from 2-4 cm (phase of acceleration), pace quickens; from 4-9 cm (phase of maximum acceleration), pace is most rapid; and from 9-10 cm (phase of deceleration), pace slows again (Figs. 17-6 and 17-7).
In the first-time mother, effacement is often complete before dilatation begins; in subsequent pregnancies, it occurs simultaneously with dilatation.

The woman's response to labor also may be reflected in vital signs and blood pressure (BP). Fear, anxiety, and fatigue can cause alterations in the baseline findings. Continued fetal well-being is monitored through assessment of the FHR and of the character of the amniotic fluid discharge.

Careful assessment provides the cues for selection and implementation of nursing actions. *The nurse assumes much of the responsibility for making the assessment of progress. It is the nurse's responsibility to keep the physician or midwife informed about progress and any deviations from normal findings.*

GENERAL SYSTEMS ASSESSMENT. A brief systems assessment needs to be performed by the nurse, including heart, lungs, and skin; presence of edema of the legs, face, hands or sacrum; and deep tendon reflexes and clonus. (See Chapter 28 for discussion of hypertensive states in pregnancy and Chapter 11 for review of physical examination.)

Vital signs and BP are assessed on admission of the client to the hospital. Findings are assessed for normality and are used for comparison with future values. If the BP is elevated, it should first be determined whether the correct size of BP cuff has been

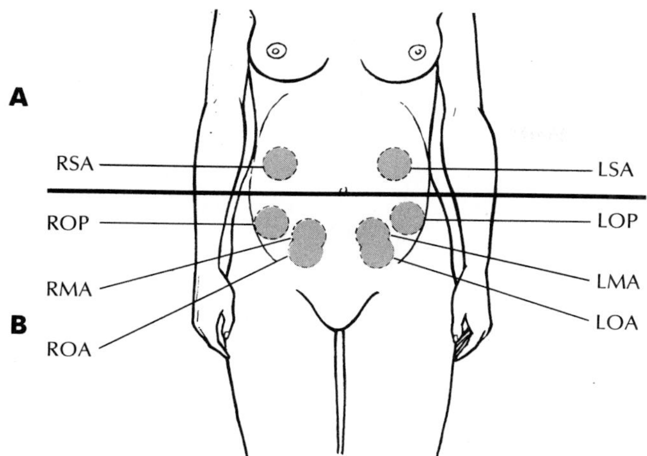

Fig. 17-3 Areas of maximum intensity of FHR for differing positions: *RSA,* right sacrum anterior; *ROP,* right occipitoposterior; *RMA,* right mentum anterior; *ROA,* right occipitoanterior; *LSA,* left sacrum anterior; *LOP,* left occipitoposterior; *LMA,* left mentum anterior; and *LOA,* left occipitoanterior. **A,** Presentation is *breech* if FHR is heard *above* umbilicus. **B,** Presentation is *vertex* if FHR is heard *below* umbilicus.

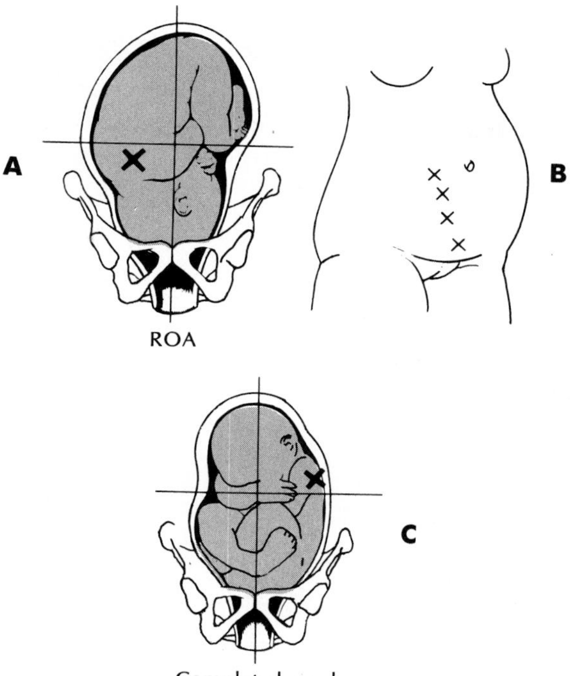

Lie: vertical
Presentation: breech (sacrum and feet presenting)
Reference point: sacrum (with feet)
Attitude: general flexion

Fig. 17-4 Area of the FHR. **A,** With fetus in ROA position. **B,** Changes in area of MI as fetus undergoes internal rotation from ROA to OA for delivery. **C,** With fetus in LSP (left sacrum posterior) position.
A and C courtesy Ross Laboratories, Columbus, Ohio.

used, and BP should then be reassessed 30 minutes later to obtain a true reading after the woman has relaxed. The woman also should be encouraged to lie on her left side and not in a supine position to avoid supine hypotension and fetal distress (see Fig. 17-9). Her temperature is monitored for signs of infection.

AUSCULTATION OF FETAL HEART RATE. It is important for the nurse to understand the relationship of location of points of maximum intensity (PMIs) of FHR to fetal presentation, lie, and position. Assessment of high risk for delivery complications may be diagnosed by variations in these factors. The PMI of the FHR is the location on the maternal abdomen where the FHR is heard the loudest. This is usually a place that is directly over the fetal back. The PMI is also an aid in determining the fetal position (Fig. 17-3). In a vertex presentation the FHR is heard *below* the mother's umbilicus in either the right or left lower quadrant of the abdomen. In a breech presentation, the FHR is heard *above* the mother's umbilicus (Fig. 17-3, *A,* and 17-4, *C*). As fetal descent and internal rotation occur, the FHR is heard lower and closer to the midline of the maternal abdomen. The PMI of the fetus in the right occipitoanterior (ROA) position is seen to move to the midline just over the symphysis pubis (Fig. 17-4, *A* and *B*). Just before delivery the fetal position is occipitoanterior (OA), and the fetal back is directly above the symphysis pubis. Fig. 17-3 presents diagrams of PMI for different presentations and positions. (See Chapter 16 for discussion of fetal monitoring, variability, periodic changes, appropriate designations for the woman's chart and the fetal monitor strip, and interventions required in response to fetal distress.) Table 17-2 notes the recommended assessment of fetal status during labor. *In addition, the FHR must be assessed immediately after rupture of membranes or after any change in contraction pattern.*

ASSESSMENT OF UTERINE CONTRACTIONS, CERVICAL DILATATION, AND DESCENT. A general characteristic of effective labor is regular uterine activity. Uterine activity is not directly related to labor progress. However, **uterine contractions** are considered the primary powers that involuntarily act to expel the fetus and the placenta from the uterus. (See

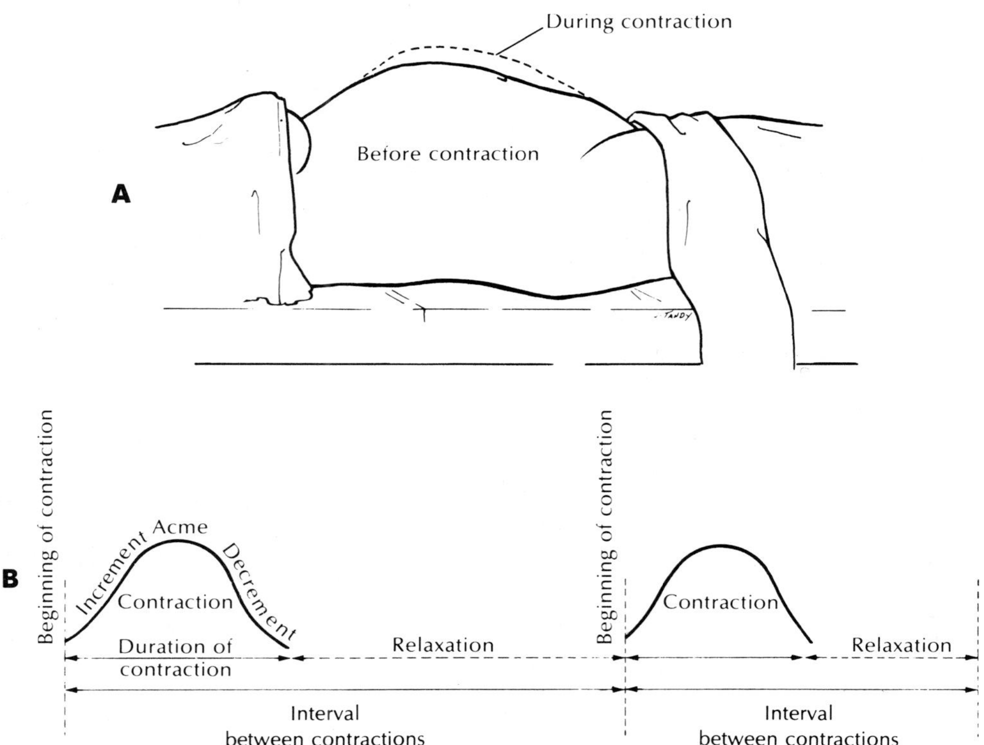

Fig. 17-5 Assessment of uterine contractions. **A,** Abdominal contour before and during uterine contraction. **B,** Wavelike pattern of contractile activity.

Chapter 14 for discussion of the physiology of involuntary uterine contractions.) Several methods are used for evaluation of uterine contractions: the woman's subjective description, palpation and timing of the contraction by a clinician, and electronic monitoring devices (see Chapter 16).

Each contraction exhibits a wavelike pattern; it begins with a slow **increment** (the "building up" of a contraction from its onset), gradually reaches an **acme** (the peak), and then diminishes rather rapidly (**decrement,** the "letting down" of the contraction). This is followed by an interval of rest (intrauterine pressure is 8 to 15 mm Hg), which is broken when the next contraction begins. (Fig. 17-5 diagrams a typical uterine contraction.)

The following characteristics describe a uterine contraction:

Frequency—how many contractions occur in a given period of time

Interval —the period of time from the beginning of one contraction to the beginning of the next

Intensity—the strength of a contraction at its peak

Duration—the period of time that elapses between the onset and the end of a contraction

Resting tone—the tension in the uterine muscle between contractions

The most common ways to measure uterine contractions are by palpation or by external or internal electronic monitor. Palpation is used in the early and active phases of the first stage of labor, when the woman often is still ambulatory. At the time when FHR is routinely assessed, contractions also are assessed. When the woman is admitted, a 20- to 30-minute baseline monitoring of uterine contractions and the FHR usually is done (Scott, et al, 1990). Table 17-2 indicates continued minimum assessment times in labor and description of what progress to expect as labor advances.

Palpation is a less precise method of determining the intensity of uterine contractions. The following terms are used to describe what is felt on palpation:

Mild—slightly tense fundus that is easy to indent with fingertips

Moderate—firm fundus that is difficult to indent with fingertips

Strong—rigid, boardlike fundus that is almost impossible to indent

Women in labor tend to describe the pain of contractions in terms of their sensations in the lower

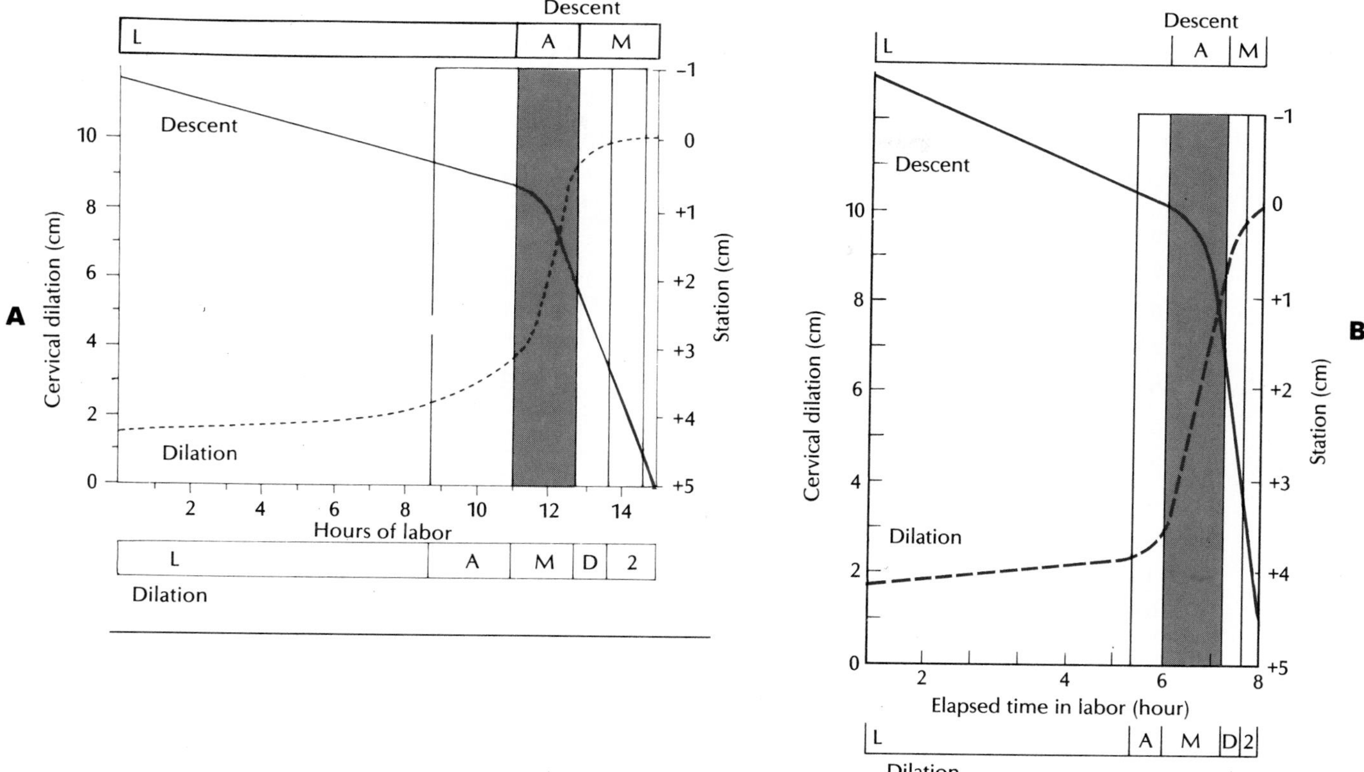

Fig. 17-6 Partogram showing relationship between dilatation and descent of presenting part. **A**, Nulliparous labor. **B**, Multiparous labor.
B modified from Friedman EA, Sachtleben MR: Station of the presenting part, *Am J Obstet Gynecol* 93:522, 1965.

uterine segment or in the back, which may be unrelated to the firmness of the uterine fundus. Thus their report of the strength of their contractions can be less reliable than that assessed by a clinician.

Electronic monitoring is the most reliable method of assessment of uterine contractions (see Chapter 16 for further discussion).

The nurse's responsibility in monitoring uterine contractions is to ascertain that they are powerful and frequent enough to accomplish the work of expulsion of the fetus and the placenta. If the characteristics of contractions are on either side of what is considered "acceptable" by standards, the nurse reports findings to the primary care practitioner.

When uterine activity is discussed, it must be related to its effect on cervical effacement and dilatation and on the degree of descent of the presenting part. The effect on the fetus also must be considered, as discussed in Chapter 16. Labor progress is effectively verified by the use of graphic charts (**partograms**) on which cervical dilatation and station (descent) are plotted. This assists in early identification of deviations from normal labor patterns. Figs. 17-6 and 17-7 show the normal pattern of cervical dilatation and descent for both nulliparous labor and multiparous labor. At each assessment, the nurse is responsible for recording the findings of labor progress on the partogram and for notifying the primary care provider should an abnormal pattern emerge.

CERVICAL EFFACEMENT. Effacement precedes cervical dilatation in the first pregnancy and often accompanies dilatation in subsequent pregnancies. The process of effacement plays a role in dilatation. As the cervix is retracted upward, it becomes a part of the lower uterine segment. The "taking up" of the cervix reduces the length of the cervix from about 2 cm to a few millimeters when it is 100% effaced. This upward pull on fibers of the lower uterus and downward push on the fetus presses the presenting part onto the cervix (see Figs. 14-16 and 14-17). As uterine contraction and retraction continue, the cervical os dilates (opens) progressively. Effacement does not appear on the partogram.

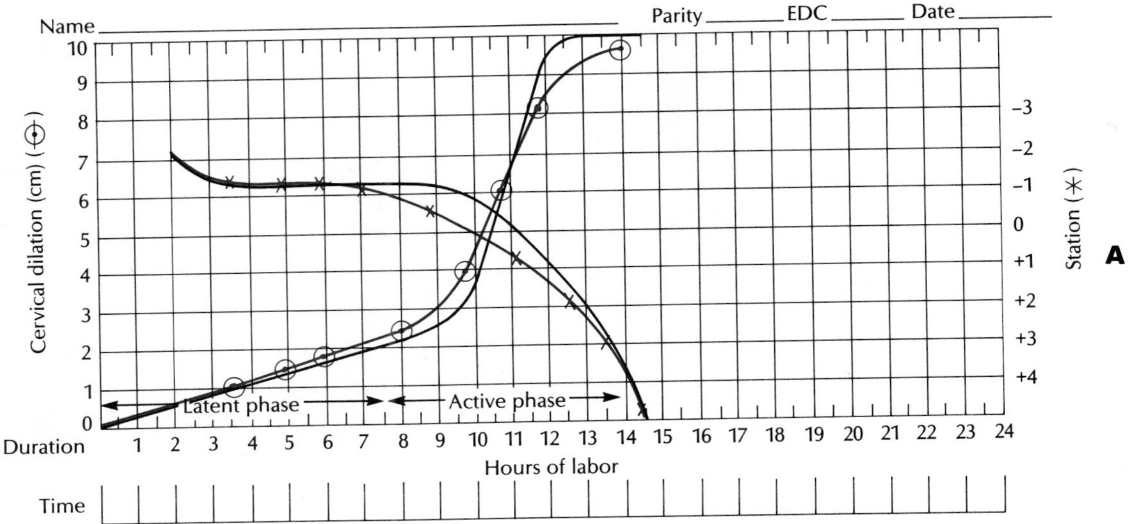

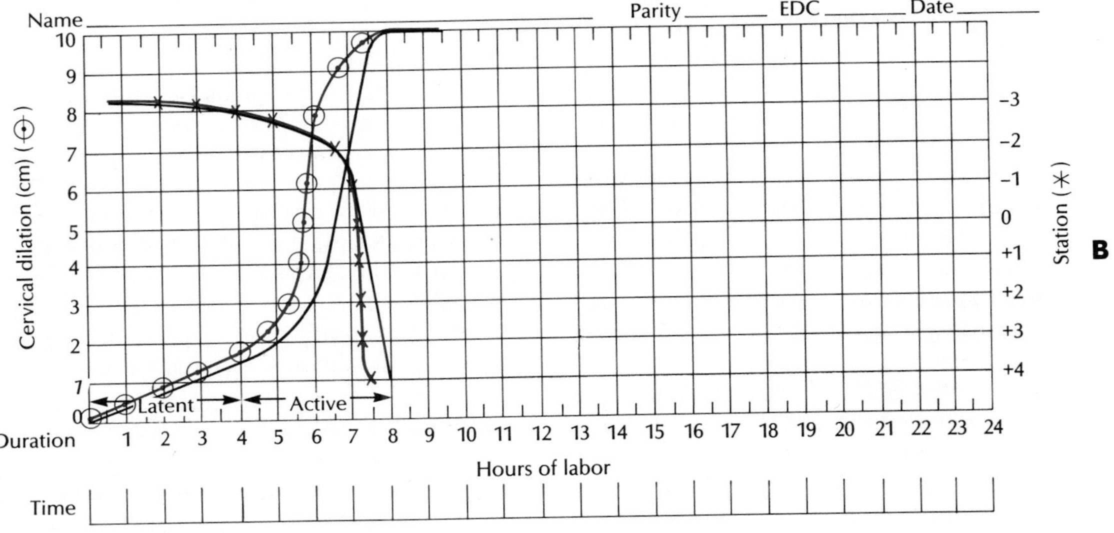

Fig. 17-7 Partogram for assessment of patterns of cervical dilatation and descent. Individual woman's labor patterns *(colored)* superimposed on prepared labor graph *(black)* for comparison. **A**, Nulliparous labor. **B**, Multiparous labor.

CERVICAL DILATATION. **Cervical dilatation** is the most conclusive sign that the power of the uterine contractions is effective and labor is progressing. In a nullipara the cervix softens and thins out before it dilates. Thus, if a cervix is long and closed, there is very little chance that delivery will occur within a few hours. Once a cervix has completely dilated (10 cm) in a previous delivery, as in a multiparous woman, it rarely will feel as closed as that of a nulliparous woman. Thus it is easier to predict length of the latent and active phases of labor for a woman with no delivery history than for one with a delivery history. The cervix will "remember" how to dilate (tissues are more elastic), and this event varies with individual women and their body's response to labor. The position of the cervix often will be posterior in early labor, particularly in nulliparous women. The cervix will move anteriorly as labor progresses and the presenting part descends, placing pressure on the cervical rim.

On the partogram the phases of cervical dilatation are identified by the letters *L, A, M,* and *D*. A number, for example, "2," refers to the stage of labor. The latent phase (L) of the first stage of labor is that time between the onset of labor and onset of acceleration. The active phase begins with the acceleration phase (A) and spans the time between the onset of the upward curve of cervical dilatation and full dilatation of the cervix. Friedman (1978) divides the active phase into three parts: (1) *acceleration phase* (A), (2) phase of *maximum slope* (M), and (3) *deceleration phase* (D). The dotted line in Fig. 17-6 denotes cervical dilatation. The rate of cervical dilatation is indicated by the symbol "O" in Fig. 17-7. A line drawn through the symbols depicts the slope of the curve.

DESCENT. Located over the graph are the letters *L, A,* and *M*. The L refers to the latent phase of minimum descent. Active descent (A) generally begins when the cervical dilatation curve reaches its phase of maximum slope. The rate of descent reaches its maximum at the beginning of the deceleration phase of cervical dilatation. Maximum descent (M) continues in a linear manner until the perineum is reached (Cunningham et al, 1989). In Fig. 17-6 the solid line shows the rate of descent. In Fig. 17-7, station is indicated with an *X*. A line drawn through the X's reveals the pattern of descent.

STATION. Station refers to the relationship of the lowermost portion of the presenting part to the mother's ischial spines. In early labor the presenting part often is above the level of the ischial spines; as labor progresses, the presenting part descends. If membranes are ruptured, station is usually lower if the presenting part has accommodated into the pelvic inlet. If membranes are intact, the presenting part may be floating or engaged in the inlet. If the vertex is at 0 station or below, most often engagement (p. 359) of the head has occurred; that is, the biparietal diameter of the head has passed through the pelvic inlet. *If the head is unusually molded or if there is an extensive formation of caput, or both, engagement might not have taken place even though the vertex is at 0 station or even lower* (Cunningham et al, 1989). (See Chapter 14 for discussion of presentation, attitude, lie, position, engagement, and cervical effacement and dilatation.)

LEOPOLD'S MANEUVERS (ABDOMINAL PALPATION). After the woman is in bed, the nurse asks her to lie flat on her back momentarily so that the nurse can perform Leopold's maneuvers (Procedure on p. 439 and Fig. 17-8). These maneuvers provide information about (1) the number of fetuses, (2) the identity of presenting part, the fetal lie, and attitude, (3) the degree of descent into the pelvis, and (4) the location of the PMI of FHR in relation to the woman's abdomen.

The next nursing action is to attach external monitor cables to the woman's abdomen to monitor contractions (see Fig. 16-8, *B*)and FHR (see Fig. 16-8, *A*). A baseline set of vital signs, including temperature, is taken, as well as a quick assessment of general physical condition, lung status, edema, rashes, respiratory conditions, and anything else noted that seems important.

VAGINAL EXAMINATION. A vaginal examination is performed by the nurse, who makes the following assessments:

Membranes—intact? bulging? ruptured? Color and character of amniotic fluid?

Cervix—soft? percentage of effacement, centimeters dilated?

Fetus—presenting part engaged? what is it?

Station—where is lowermost portion of presenting part in relation to the ischial spines? What is the position of the fetal occiput?

Labor is initiated by **spontaneous rupture of membranes (SROM)** in almost 25% of pregnant women. The lag period, rarely exceeding 24 hours, precedes the onset of labor. The length of uterine contractions is directly related to the duration of pregnancy.

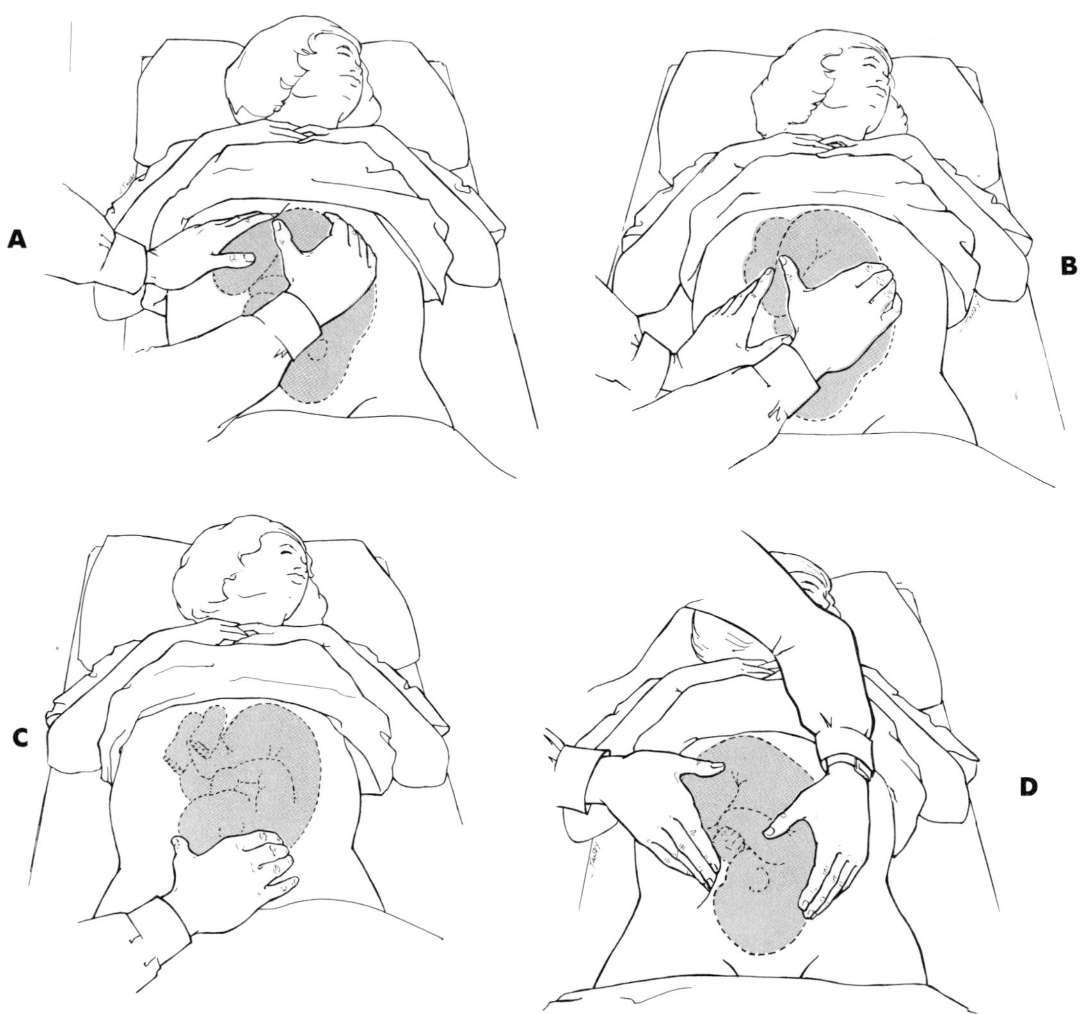

Fig. 17-8 Leopold's maneuvers.

Procedure: Leopold's Maneuvers and Determination of the Points of Maximum Intensity of the Fetal Heart Rate

Wash hands.

Ask woman to empty bladder.

Position woman supine with one pillow under her head and with her knees slightly flexed.

Place small rolled towel under woman's right hip to displace uterus to left off major blood vessels (avoids supine hypotensive syndrome, Fig. 17-9).

If right-handed, stand on woman's right, facing her:

1. Identify fetal part that occupies the fundus. The head feels round, firm, freely movable, and palpable by ballottement; the breech feels less regular and softer (identifies fetal lie [vertical or horizontal] and presentation [vertex or breech]) (Fig. 17-8,*A*).
2. Using palmar surface of one hand, locate and palpate the smooth convex contour of the fetal back and the irregularities that identify the small parts (feet, hands, elbows) (assists in identifying fetal presentation) (Fig. 17-8,*B*).
3. With the right hand, determine which fetal part is presenting over the inlet to the true pelvis. Gently grasp the lower pole of the uterus between the thumb and fingers, pressing in slightly (Fig. 17-8,*C*). If the head is presenting and not engaged, determine the attitude of the head.
4. Turn to face the woman's feet. Using two hands, outline the fetal head (Fig. 17-8,*D*) with palmar surface of fingertips.

When presenting part has descended deeply, only a small portion of it may be outlined.

Palpation of cephalic prominence assists in identifying attitude of head.

If the cephalic prominence is found on the same side as the small parts, the head must be flexed, and the vertex is presenting (Fig. 17-8,*D*). If the cephalic prominence is on the same side as the back, the presenting head is extended (Fig. 14-4,*C*).

Determination of PMI of FHR:

Wash hands.

Perform Leopold's maneuvers.

Auscultate FHR (Figs. 17-3, 17-4, and 12-2).

Apply monitor prn (Chapter 16).

Wash hands.

Chart fetal presentation, position, and lie; whether presenting part is flexed or extended, engaged or free floating.

Use hospital's protocol for charting (e.g., "Vtx, LOA, floating").

Chart PMI of FHR using a two-line figure to indicate the four quadrants of the maternal abdomen, right upper quadrant (RUQ), left upper quadrant (LUQ), left lower quadrant (LLQ), and right lower quadrant (RLQ):

RUQ	LUQ
RLQ	LLQ

The umbilicus is the point where the lines cross. The PMI for the fetus in vertex presentation, in general flexion with the back on the mother's right side, commonly is found in the mother's right lower quadrant and is recorded with an "x" or with the FHR as follows:

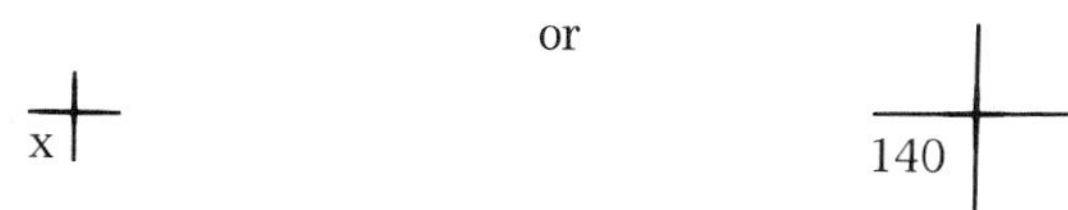

Fig. 17-9 Supine hypotension. Note relationship of gravid uterus to ascending vena cava in standing posture (**A**) and in supine posture (**B**). **C**, Compression of aorta and inferior vena cava with woman in supine position. **D**, Relieved by use of a wedge pillow placed under woman's right side.

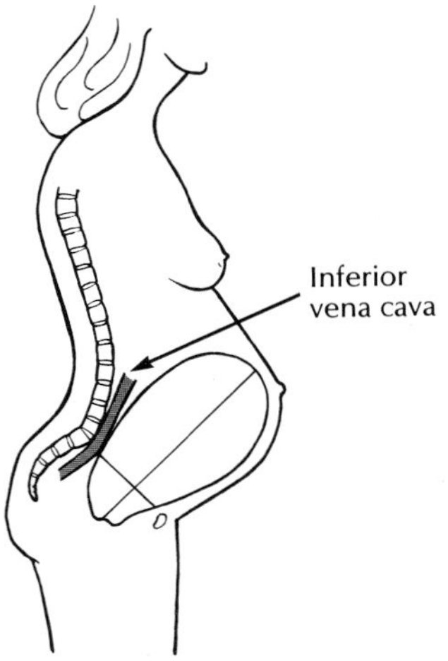

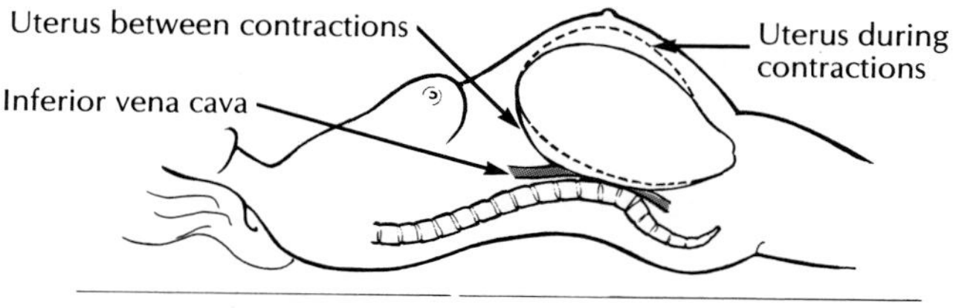

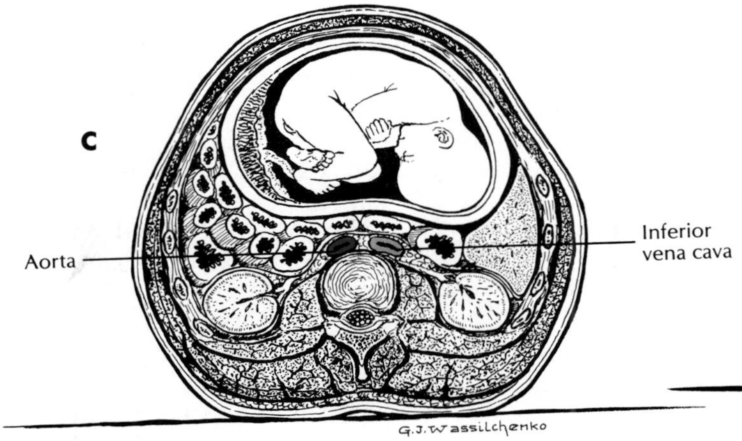

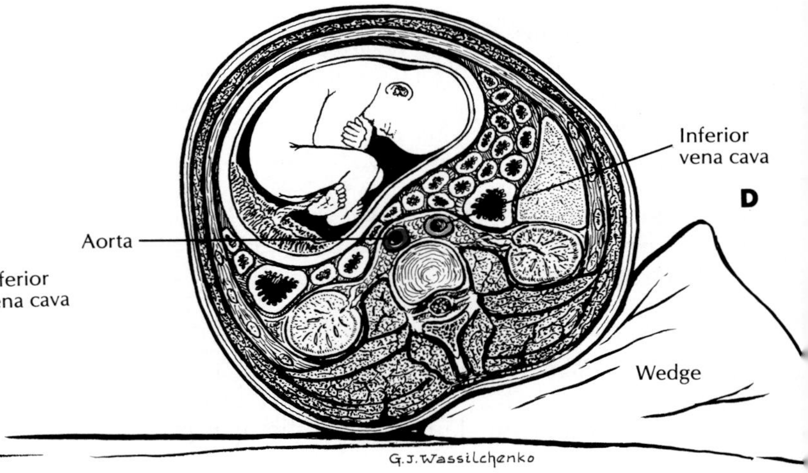

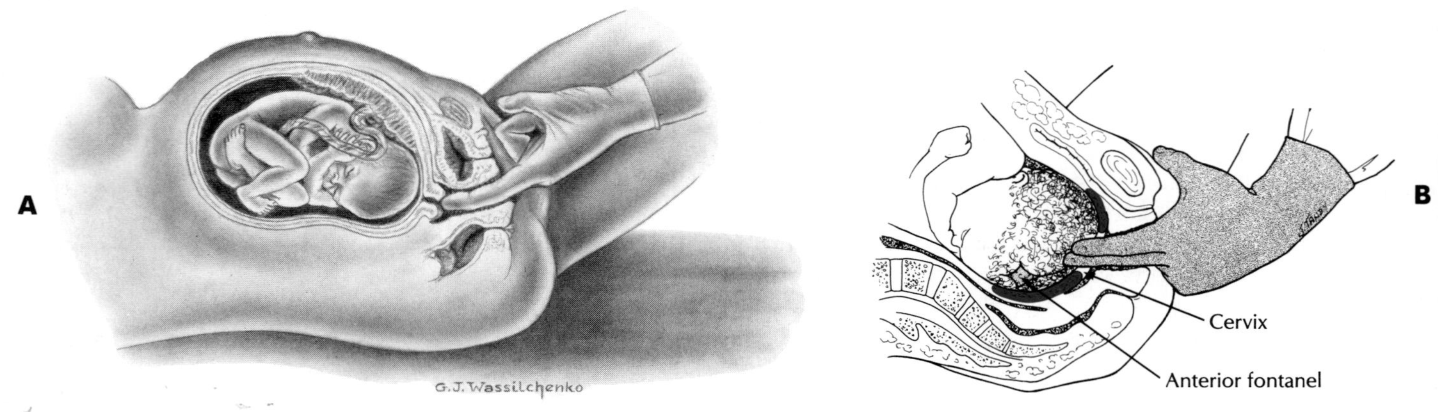

Fig. 17-10 Vaginal examination. **A**, Undilated, uneffaced cervix; membranes intact. **B**, Palpation of sagittal suture line. Cervix effaced and partially dilated.

The following steps are included in the vaginal examination:

1. The nurse assembles all the equipment needed, including single sterile glove, antiseptic solution or soluble gel, and a light source.
2. The woman is prepared through explanation of procedure and draping her to prevent chill and protect privacy.
3. The nurse begins with hand washing and applies sterile glove using aseptic technique. The nurse explains to the woman while gently inserting first and middle fingers into the vagina.
4. The woman is assessed for the following (Fig. 17-10):
   a. Dilatation and effacement of cervix
   b. Presenting part, position, station, and if vertex, any molding of the head
   c. Status of membranes, intact or ruptured
   d. Presence of stool in rectum
5. The woman is helped to a comfortable position, and the nurse reports and records all these data.

Laboratory and Diagnostic Tests

The nurse can anticipate the need for urinalysis and tests for blood values and rupture of membranes.

URINE SPECIMEN. A urine specimen is obtained to gather data about the pregnant woman's health. It is a convenient and simple procedure that can provide information about her hydration status (specific gravity, color, amount), nutritional status (ketones), or possible complications, for example, pregnancy-induced hypertension (protein). The results can be obtained quickly and will help the nurse determine appropriate interventions.

BLOOD TESTS. Blood tests vary with hospital protocol and client history. An example of minimum assessment is a hematocrit determination, in which the specimen is processed by use of a centrifuge on the perinatal unit. This can be accomplished with blood from a finger stick or the hub of a catheter used to start an intravenous (IV) line. More comprehensive blood assessments include hemoglobin and hematocrit values and a complete blood cell count (CBC).

If the woman's blood type has not been verified, blood will be drawn to establish type and Rh factor. If blood typing was previously done, the primary care practitioner may choose to repeat the test. If obvious signs of immunocompromise are present, other diagnostic blood tests may be ordered by the primary care practitioner.

RUPTURE OF MEMBRANES. Membranes (the bag of waters) can rupture spontaneously any time in labor. It is the nurse's responsibility to monitor FHR for several minutes immediately after **rupture of membranes (ROM),** to ascertain fetal well-being, and to document findings. Tests for assessing ROM are discussed in the procedure on p. 442. **Artificial rupture of membranes** (AROM) sometimes is done to augment or induce labor or to place internal monitors because fetal status is difficult to maintain by external means. Assessment of amniotic fluid includes the following routine measures.

AMNIOTIC FLUID

Color. Amniotic fluid normally is pale and straw colored, and may contain flecks of vernix caseosa. If it is greenish-brown, the fetus has probably undergone a hypoxic episode,* which has caused relaxation of the anal sphincter and the passage of byproducts of fetal ingestion in utero called *meconium.* Although it is thought that meconium-stained amniotic fluid is an ominous finding in labor, it is not always associated with fetal hypoxia and must be viewed in the context of the total clinical picture of labor (Scott, et al, 1990). Yellow-stained amniotic fluid may indicate fetal hypoxia that occurred 36 hours or more before ROM, fetal hemolytic disease (Rh or ABO incompatibility), or intrauterine infection. Meconium-stained amniotic fluid may be a normal finding in a breech presentation, resulting from pressure on the fetal rectum during descent.

Although meconium most often is associated with fetal hypoxia and asphyxia, it is not always a sign of fetal distress. The nurse's responsibility is to report it promptly to the primary care practitioner and to record findings in the labor record and on the monitor strip. After this finding, continuous electronic monitoring usually is employed for the duration of labor. The presence of meconium-stained amniotic fluid alerts the nurse to observe fetal status more closely. After birth, the newborn may be at high risk for alteration in respiratory status. Amniotic fluid that is port-wine colored may indicate premature separation of the placenta (abruptio) (see Chapter 30).

Character. Amniotic fluid normally has a watery consistency and lacks a strong odor. If fluid is thick or has an unpleasant odor, infection is suspected.

Amount. A normal range for the amount of amniotic fluid is 500 to 1200 mL. Most of the amniotic fluid originates from the maternal blood stream with additions of fetal urination.

Hydramnios (>2000 mL) often is associated with congenital anomalies of the fetus, resulting from the

*Also may be seen in response to maternal marijuana use (see Chapter 33).

Procedure: Tests for Rupture of Membranes

NITRAZINE TEST FOR pH

Explain procedure to woman/couple.

Procedure

Use **Nitrazine test** paper, a dye 1-1–impregnated test paper for pH. (Differentiates amniotic fluid, which is slightly alkaline, from urine and purulent material [pus], which are acidic.)

Wearing a sterile glove lubricated with water, place a piece of test paper at the cervical os

OR

Use a sterile, cotton-tipped applicator to dip deep into vagina to pick up fluid; touch applicator to test paper.

Read results:

Membranes probably intact: identifies vaginal and most body fluids that are acidic

Yellow	pH 5.0
Olive yellow	pH 5.5
Olive green	pH 6.0

Membranes probably ruptured: identifies amniotic fluid that is alkaline.

Blue-green	pH 6.5
Blue-gray	pH 7.0
Deep blue	pH 7.5

Realize that false test results are possible because of presence of bloody show, insufficient amniotic fluid, or semen.

Remove gloves and wash hands.

Chart results: positive or negative

TEST FOR FERNING OR FERN PATTERN
(usually performed by physician)

Explain procedure to client/couple.

Wash hands, apply gloves, obtain specimen of fluid (usually with sterile speculum examination).

Spread a drop of fluid from vagina on a clean glass slide with a sterile, cotton-tipped applicator.

Allow fluid to dry.

Assess slide under microscope: observe for appearance of ferning (a frondlike crystalline pattern) (do not confuse with cervical mucus test, when high levels of estrogen are responsible for the ferning).

Observe for absence of ferning (alerts staff to possibility that specimen was inadequate or that specimen was urine, vaginal discharge, or blood.)

Remove gloves and wash hands.

Chart results: either a positive or negative fern test finding

TEST FOR LANUGO HAIRS OR FETAL SQUAMOUS CELLS (usually performed by physician)

Explain procedure to client/couple.

Wash hands and apply gloves.

Aspirate fluid from posterior vaginal vault with sterile aspiration syringe.

Place on clean glass slide.

Observe under microscope for presence of fetal lanugo hairs or fetal squamous cells.

Stain with Nile blue stain to identify fetal cells because some squamous cells that contain lipids stain yellow; other squamous cells and hairs stain blue.

Assess findings.

Remove gloves and wash hands.

Chart results: Nile blue stain shows some squamous cells and some blue squamous cells and hair.

inability of the fetus to drink the fluid or for fluid to be trapped in the fetal body (see Chapter 38). Oligohydramnios (<500 mL) is an abnormally small amount of amniotic fluid and can be associated with incomplete formation or absence of the kidneys or obstruction of the urethra. If the fetus is unable to secrete and excrete urine, the volume of amniotic fluid is decreased. Fetal surgery can now correct some obstructive conditions.

Infection. When membranes rupture, microorganisms from the vagina can ascend into the amniotic sac. Amnionitis and placentitis may develop. Even when membranes are intact, microorganisms may ascend and directly cause premature ROM. There is a controversy regarding whether prophylactic antibiotic therapy will protect against infection known as chorioamnionitis, which involves both the maternal and fetal sides of the membrane. Maternal temperature and vaginal discharge are assessed frequently (every 1 to 2 hours) for early identification of a developing infection after ROM.

Signs of Potential Problems

Assessment findings serve as a baseline for evaluation of the woman's progress during the first stage of labor. Although some complications of labor are anticipated, others appear only in the clinical course of labor. Knowledge of pregnancy, careful initial assessment, and follow-up of progress are necessary during normal labor, as well as during a labor in which complications arise (see Fig. 17-11, and box, at right).

Nursing Diagnoses

Nursing diagnoses provide direction to types of nursing actions needed to implement a plan of care. When establishing nursing diagnoses, the nurse analyzes the significance of findings collected during assessment.

Initial Assessment

- Impaired verbal communication related to
  —Foreign language barrier
- Anxiety related to
  —Knowledge deficit regarding physical examination procedures
  —Lack of previous experiences or preparation-for-parenthood classes
- High risk for injury related to
  —Lack of prenatal testing of blood and urine

Subsequent Assessments

- Pain related to
  —Intense contractions
- Fluid volume deficit related to
  —Decreased fluid intake
- Impaired physical mobility related to
  —Station of fetal presenting part
  —Status of fetal membranes
  —Fetal monitoring
- Altered patterns of urinary elimination related to
  —Reduced fluid intake
  —IV fluids
  —Bed rest
  —Lack of privacy
  —Analgesia
  —Anesthesia

Assessment of Stress During Labor

- Impaired gas exchange, fetal, related to
  —Maternal position
  —Hyperventilation
- Spiritual distress, maternal, related to
  —Inability to meet self-expectations
- Ineffective family coping: compromised, related to
  —Knowledge deficit of comfort measures that can be used for the laboring woman

Planning

During this important step, *goals* are set in client-centered terms, and the goals are prioritized. Nursing actions are selected, with the client where appropriate, to meet the goals. Planning with the client is essential for the implementation of goals. Throughout the first stage of labor the woman will:

1. Demonstrate normal progression of labor
2. Express satisfaction with the assistance of her support person and nursing staff
3. Verbalize her desires for participation in labor and participate as tolerated throughout labor
4. Continue normal progression of labor while the FHR remains within normal range without signs of distress
5. Maintain adequate hydration status through oral or intravenous intake
6. Void every 2 hours to prevent bladder distention
7. Encourage participation of support person by verbalizing discomfort and indicating measures that help reduce discomfort and promote relaxation

Warning Signs—Labor Complications

Intrauterine pressure >75 mm Hg (by IUPC)
Contractions consistently lasting ≥90 sec
Contractions consistently occurring ≤2 min
Fetal bradycardia, tachycardia, or persistent decreased variability
Irregular FHR; suspected fetal arrhythmias
Absence of fetal heart beat
Appearance of fluid from the vagina that is meconium stained or bloody
Prolapsed umbilical cord
Arrest in progress of cervical dilatation/effacement and/or descent of the fetus
Maternal temperature ≥100.4° F (38° C)
Foul-smelling vaginal discharge
Persistent bright or dark-red vaginal bleeding

IUPC, Intrauterine pressure catheter (see Chapter 16).

Implementation

Standards of Care

Standards of care guide the nurse in preparing for and implementing procedures with the expectant mother (see Chapter 4). Protocols for care include the following:

1. Check the primary care practitioner's orders.
2. Assess the primary care practitioner's orders for appropriateness and correctness; for example, enema, and when not to carry out the procedure.

ADMISSION/RISK ASSESSMENT

NAME:					PHYSICIAN:	PEDIATRICIAN:
G	T	P	L	AB	EDC:	WKS GEST:

PREGNANCY RISK ON ADMISSION / DEVELOPING FACTORS DURING LABOR

1+ IMPORTANCE = 1 PT. EACH

Pregnancy risk on admission

- ☐ No prenatal care
- ☐ Parity >6
- ☐ Wt. <100 or >200 lb
- ☐ Nullip <18 or >35 yrs
- ☐ Multip >40 yrs
- ☐ Hx of >3 abortions
- ☐ Smokes >½ pack/day
- ☐ Anemia, <11 g Hgb
- ☐ Wight gain <15 lb
- ☐ Active pulmonary problem
- ☐ Active endocrine problem
- ☐ Unwed mother
- ☐ Rh neg, unsensitized
- ☐ Hx infertility
- ☐ Hx ABO imcompatibility
- ☐ Hx mitral valve prolapse
- ☐ Hx drug/alcohol abuse
- ☐ Hx stillbirth, neonatal death or major anomaly
- ☐ Other ______
- ☐ Other ______

Subtotal ______ X 1=

Developing factors during labor

- ☐ Maternal fever >100.4° F (0)
- ☐ 1+/2+ meconium in amniotic fluid
- ☐ Prolonged active phase
- ☐ Protracted active phase
- ☐ Precipitous labor
- ☐ Mild variable deceleration— decrease of <30 bpm lasting <60 sec.
- ☐ Other ______
- ☐ Other ______

Subtotal ______ X 1=

3+ IMPORTANCE = 3 PTS. EACH

Pregnancy risk on admission

- ☐ Diabetes, Class A
- ☐ Multiple gestation
- ☐ Suspected IUGR
- ☐ Maternal infection
- ☐ TORCH
- ☐ Hx drug/alcohol abuse this pregnancy
- ☐ Hx placenta previa or abruptio
- ☐ 36-38 wks of gestation
- ☐ Poly or oligo hydramnios
- ☐ Previous uterine incision
- ☐ Preeclampsia, mild to mod.
- ☐ Other ______
- ☐ Other ______
- ☐ Breech presentation
- ☐ Known fetal anomalies
- ☐ Hypertension, chronic
- ☐ Active liver disease
- ☐ Active renal disease
- ☐ Anemia <8 g Hgb
- ☐ Gest. >42 wks

Subtotal ______ X 3=

Developing factors during labor

- ☐ Intermittent late decelerations
- ☐ Mod. variable decelerations decrease of 30-45 bpm lasting 60-90 sec
- ☐ Rom >24 hr, maternal temp <100.0° F
- ☐ Labor >20 hrs of reg. contractions
- ☐ Thick (3+) meconium
- ☐ Painless maternal bleeding
- ☐ Secondary arrest of labor
- ☐ Failure to descend
- ☐ Baseline FHR <120 or >160
- ☐ Rise of baseline >30 bpm for >30 min, Maternal temp 99.0-100.0° F
- ☐ Suspected cord insult
- Other ______
- Other ______

Subtotal ______ X 3=

5+ IMPORTANCE = 5 PTS. EACH

Pregnancy risk on admission

- ☐ Diabetes Class B or R
- ☐ Symptomatic heart disease
- ☐ Rh sensitization
- ☐ Gestation <36 wks
- ☐ Maternal hypertension >160/100
- ☐ Bleeding during 3rd trimester
- ☐ Preeclampsia, severe (or eclampsia)
- ☐ Other ______
- Other ______

Subtotal ______ X 5=

Developing factors during labor

- ☐ Tetanic contractions
- ☐ Painful maternal bleeding
- ☐ Prolonged bradycardia >2 min
- ☐ Profound variable decelerations, dec. of >45 bpm for >90 sec
- ☐ Persistent late decelerations >3 consecutive
- ☐ Rom >24 hr maternal temp >100° F
- ☐ Rise of baseline >30 bpm for >1 hr
- ☐ Overt prolapsed cord
- ☐ Loss of baseline variability
- ☐ Fetal acidosis—pH <7.20
- Other ______
- Other ______

Subtotal ______ X 5=

Admission Risk Total | **Developing Factors Total**

ADDRESSOGRAPH

OB 1491

Admitting Rn Sig./Time ______

Labor Rn Sig./Time ______

TOTAL RISK SCORE

Fig. 17-11 Admission/risk assessment.
From Vogler/Perinatal Healthcare Consultants, 1990, Kailua, HI.

3. Check labels on IV solutions, drugs, and other materials used for nursing care.
4. Check expiration date on any packs of supplies used for ordered procedures.
5. Ensure that information on the woman's identification band is correct (also check that identification band is accurate; e.g., if she has allergies, the band is the appropriate color).
6. Employ an empathic approach when giving care:
   - Use words the woman can understand when explaining procedures
   - Establish a rapport with the woman and her support person(s)
   - Be kind, caring, and competent when performing necessary procedures
   - Be aware that pain and discomfort are as the woman describes
   - Repeat instructions as necessary and ensure that they are understood by the woman
   - Carry out appropriate comfort measures, for example, mouth care and back care, and ensure that support person is coping
   - Always wash hands before beginning and after completion of nursing care
7. Complete procedures, for example, label specimens and record procedures on chart regarding maternal and fetal well-being.

Admission to Labor Unit

First impressions are vivid. The woman and her partner are welcomed by name and introduced to staff members who will be involved in the woman's care. The nurse then determines whether the woman wishes her partner to stay throughout assessment and other admission procedures. The partner is included in the assessment and admission process through orientation and explanation. Family members not participating in this process are directed to the appropriate waiting area. The woman is asked to undress and get into bed. Her personal belongings are put away safely. For legal reasons, most hospitals have a checklist or other method of recording the woman's belongings that becomes part of her permanent record. If the woman prefers to wear some items of her own (such as knee socks), these are noted on her chart.

It is the nurse's responsibility to orient the woman and her partner to the unit and room. This includes use of the call light, telephone system, personal storage areas in the bedside and overbed tables, and lighting in the room. The woman with an electronic monitor is told how to notify the nurse of her wish to use the bathroom or to ambulate. If possible the nurse will undo the monitor belts or provide some alternative. An admissions bracelet will be placed on the woman, as well as an allergy bracelet (usually colored) if relevant. The woman should be reassured by the nurse that she is in competent, caring hands, can ask questions related to her care and status at any time during labor, and answers will be provided.

If the woman has not already done so, she signs the necessary papers giving permission for care for herself and her newborn. Her identification bracelet is secured. Legally a permit for care must be signed before the woman receives any medication or any procedures are instituted.

The nurse inquires if the woman came by car and ensures that the vehicle is properly parked. Some women, especially those who arrive in labor unexpectedly, welcome the offer of a telephone to notify their families. In some instances the nurse may have to make the calls for the woman.

The nurse should minimize the woman's anxiety by explaining terms commonly used during labor. During the review of the prenatal record, the nurse can add short definitions for technical terms and abbreviations. The woman's interest and response guide the nurse in choosing the depth and breadth of the explanations.

Physical Nursing Care during Labor

Physical nursing care of the woman in labor is an essential function. Physical needs, nursing actions, and rationale for care are presented in Table 17-4.

GENERAL HYGIENE. Women in labor should be offered showers or Jacuzzi baths if they are available to enhance a feeling of well-being and to minimize contraction discomfort. They should be encouraged to wash their hands after voiding and to perform self-hygiene activities. Their linen should be changed if wet or blood stained, and linen savers (Chux) should be used and changed as needed.

FLUID INTAKE

ORAL. The laboring woman is offered clear liquids during the active phase of labor and small amounts of ice chips thereafter. If conduction anesthesia (epidural) is employed, the woman usually is given nothing by mouth (NPO) or offered only small amounts of ice chips. This caution minimizes potential anesthesia complications and their sequelae (e.g., primarily aspiration of gastric contents and resultant compromise in oxygen perfusion, which may endanger the lives of the maternal/fetal couple).

Gastric motility is slowed or stopped during the process of labor. If the woman eats or drinks anything of substance, it is likely she will vomit during

TABLE 17-4 Physical Nursing Care During Labor

Need	Nursing Actions	Rationale
GENERAL HYGIENE		
Showers/bed baths	Assess for progress in labor.	Determines appropriateness for the activity
	Supervise showers closely if woman is in true labor.	Prevents injury from fall; labor may accelerate
	Suggest allowing warm water to strike lower back.	Aids relaxation; increases comfort
Vulva	Mini-prep if ordered.	Facilitates cutting and repair of episiotomy
Oral hygiene	Offer toothbrush, mouthwash, or wash the teeth with an ice-cold wet washcloth every hour.	Refreshes mouth; improves morale; helps counteract dry, thirsty feeling
Hair	Brush, braid per woman's wishes.	Improves morale
Hand washing	Offer washcloths before and after voiding and prn.	Maintains cleanliness; improves morale and comfort
Face	Offer cool washcloth.	Improves morale; relief from diaphoresis
Gowns/linens	Change prn; fluff pillows.	Improves morale and comfort, probably through the **Hawthorne effect (p. 452)**
FLUID INTAKE		
Oral	Per physician's orders, offer clear fluids, small amounts of ice chips, hard candy, or lollipops.	Meets standard of care; provides hydration; provides calories; absorbs quickly and is less likely to be vomited; provides positive emotional experience
IV	Establish and maintain IV.	Maintains hydration.
Nothing by mouth (NPO)	Inform family of NPO and rationale.	A precautionary measure if anesthesia is a possibility; deters vomiting and its possible sequelae
	Provide mouth care.	Promotes comfort
ELIMINATION		
Voiding	Encourage voiding at least every 2 hours.	A full bladder may impede descent of presenting part; overdistention may cause bladder atony and injury and postnatal voiding difficulty
Ambulatory	Allow ambulation to bathroom per physician's orders, *if:*	Reinforces normal process of urination
	The presenting part is engaged	Precautionary measure against prolapse of umbilical cord
	The membranes are not ruptured	Precautionary measure against injury
	The woman is not medicated.	
Bed rest	Offer bedpan.	Prevents hazards of bladder distention and ambulation
	Turn on the tap water to run; pour warm water over the vulva; and give positive suggestion.	Encourages voiding
	Provide privacy.	Shows respect for woman
	Put up side rails on bed.	Prevents injury from fall.
	Place call bell within reach.	
	Offer washcloth for hands.	Maintains cleanliness and comfort.
	Wash vulvar area.	Maintains standard of care.

TABLE 17-4 Physical Nursing Care During Labor—cont'd

Need	Nursing Actions	Rationale
ELIMINATION—CONT'D		
Catheterization	Catheterize per primary care practitioner's order per hospital protocols.	Prevents hazards of bladder distention
	Insert catheter between contractions.	Minimizes discomfort
	Avoid force if obstacle to insertion is noted.	"Obstacle" may be caused by compression of urethra by presenting part
	If presenting part is low, introduce two fingers of free hand into introitus to apply upward pressure on presenting part while other hand inserts the catheter.	Minimizes potential for injury and subsequent infection to urethra
Bowel elimination	After careful assessment *experienced* nurse ambulates woman to bathroom or offers bedpan.	Avoids misinterpretation of rectal pressure from the presenting part as the need to defecate

transition to the second stage of labor. It is important to instruct the woman to take small sips of clear liquids or water to prevent vomiting and its potential sequelae of tracheal irritation and aspiration of fluid into the lungs.

INTRAVENOUS. Fluids are administered to the laboring woman to maintain hydration; usually an electrolyte solution without glucose is adequate and avoids excess glucose in the blood stream. Excessive maternal glucose results in fetal hyperglycemia and fetal hyperinsulinism. After birth, the neonate's high levels of insulin will deplete the glucose stores, and hypoglycemia will result.

If the woman is in labor for a number of hours without calories, her urine may start to show ketone bodies (acetones from incomplete fatty acid metabolism). This is more common for women who have begun their labor early in the morning after a night without caloric intake. The primary care practitioner sometimes will order a small amount of IV solution with dextrose to provide the glucose needed to assist in fatty acid metabolism. Often after a dextrose infusion the woman's urine output will increase and her pulse will decrease.

ELIMINATION

VOIDING. Voiding must be encouraged by the nurse every 2 hours especially if the bladder is palpable or is visibly distended. A distended bladder may impede descent of the presenting part and cause decreased bladder tone or atony after birth. This could result in tissue injury, difficulty in voiding, or in completely emptying the bladder. If the woman wants to ambulate to the bathroom, it is the nurse's responsibility to assist her unless the primary practitioner has ordered bed rest or if in the nurse's judgment, ambulation would compromise the status of the laboring woman or her fetus, or both. If the electronic monitor cords will reach, the electronic monitor does not have to be turned off while the woman uses the bathroom. The laboring woman is able to retain control over very few aspects of her care in labor. The nurse acts as an advocate by respecting the woman's desire to void in the bathroom instead of in a bedpan.

CATHETERIZATION. If the woman is unable to void and her bladder is obviously distended and palpable, she may require catheterization. Most hospitals have protocols that rely on the nurse's judgment concerning the need for catheterization. Usually catheterization results in the woman's feeling less generalized discomfort. If there appears to be an obstacle to advancing the catheter, the nurse can insert two fingers into the vagina and try to move the presenting part away from obstructing the urethra. If the catheter still cannot be advanced, the nurse stops the procedure and notifies the primary care practitioner.

BOWEL EVACUATION. Most women do not have bowel movements during labor because of decreased intestinal motility. Stool that has formed in the large intestine often is moved downward toward the anorectal area by pressure of the fetal presenting part as it descends. This stool often is excreted during second stage pushing and delivery. If the presenting part is deep in the pelvis, even in the absence of stool in the anorectal area, the woman may feel rectal pressure and think she needs to defecate. The

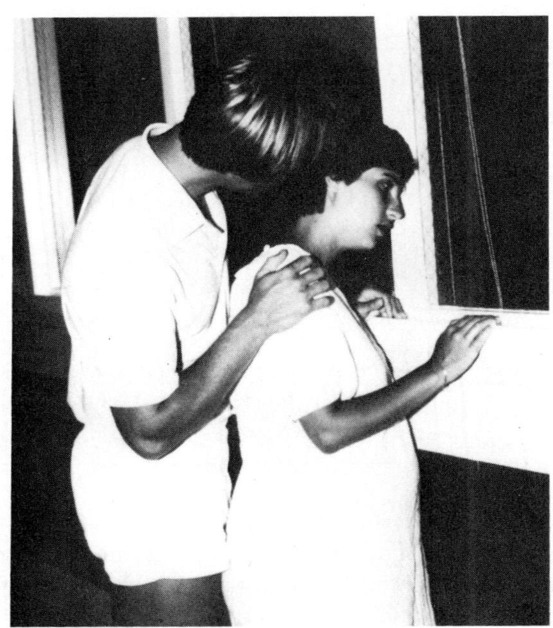

Fig. 17-12 Woman walking with husband.
Courtesy Marjorie Pyle, RNC, Lifecircle, Costa Mesa, Calif.

nurse should perform a vaginal examination to assess cervical dilatation and station. In a multiparous woman, verbalization of the urge to defecate often means birth will quickly follow.

AMBULATION AND POSITIONING. Ambulation ad lib may be encouraged if the fetal presenting part is engaged after ROM, if membranes are intact, and if the woman has not received medication for pain (Fig. 17-12). Ambulation may be contraindicated because of maternal and/or fetal status. (See Table 17-2 for minimum assessment of labor progress.)

When the woman is in bed, she is encouraged to lie on her left side to promote optimal uteroplacental and renal blood flow. If the woman wants to lie supine, the nurse may place a pillow under one side as a wedge to achieve the same result. Sitting is not contraindicated unless it adversely affects fetal status, which can be observed by visualization of the fetal monitor record. If the fetus is in the occiput posterior position, it may be helpful to encourage the woman to squat during contractions. This position increases pelvic diameter, allowing rotation of the head to a more anterior position.

Much research is being directed toward a better understanding of the physiologic and psychic effects of maternal position in labor (see Research Highlight, p. 449). It is important to appreciate that clini-

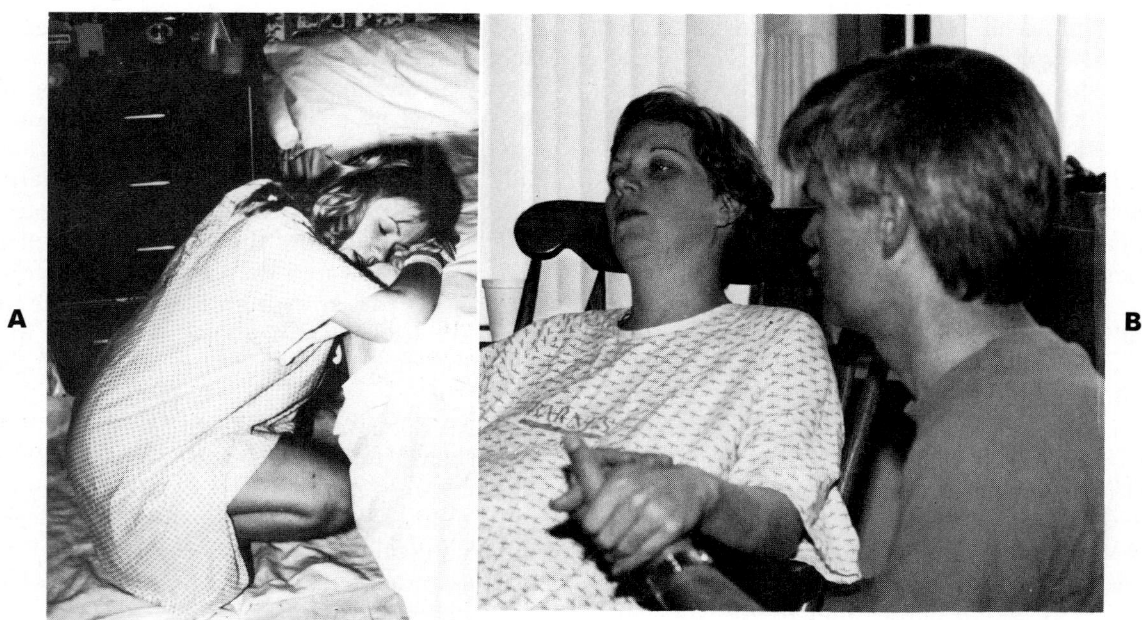

Fig. 17-13 Maternal positions for labor. **A,** Squatting. **B,** Woman using focusing and breathing with coaching from husband in rocking chair.
A, Courtesy Marjorie Pyle, RNC, Lifecircle, Costa Mesa, Calif. **B,** Courtesy Kathy Hanold, RN, MS, Birth place, Barnes Hospital at Washington University, Medical Center, St Louis, Mo.

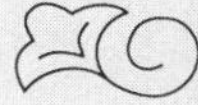 **Research Highlight** 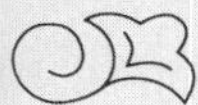

Maternal Position, Labor, and Comfort

RESEARCH ABSTRACT

The purpose of this study was to determine whether women who were in upright positions during the maximum slope of labor would have a shorter labor and be more comfortable than women who labored in a recumbent position. A convenience (one available to the researcher) sample of 40 nulliparous women in labor participated in the study. The women were randomly assigned to an upright or a recumbent position group. Women in the upright position could stand, walk, sit, squat, or kneel. Women in the recumbent position could be in lateral, supine, or prone positions.

Two data collection instruments developed by the researchers were used. One instrument was used to record information on demographics (such as age and education), the experience of childbirth pain, and the length of maximum slope of labor. The second instrument was the maternal comfort assessment tool, which estimates the level of maternal comfort. Vital signs, frequency, duration and intensity of contractions, medications, and monitoring equipment used also were recorded. The researchers found that women in the upright position had a shorter maximum slope of labor by an average of 90.25 minutes. Contractions of this group were more efficient, and cervical dilatation occurred more rapidly. Younger women had a shorter maximum slope than did older women; African-American women had a shorter maximum slope than did caucasian women. There was no difference in mean comfort scores between the two groups. The women in the upright position received less medication for discomfort. Women in the recumbent position were monitored with external monitoring more often. Apgar scores did not differ between groups.

IMPLICATIONS FOR PRACTICE

Women can safely labor in the upright position. Nurses can continue to advocate ambulation for healthy laboring women. They can educate women about the beneficial effects of the upright position.

RELATED RESEARCH QUESTIONS

1. Does an education program for pregnant women increase the number of women willing to labor in the upright position?
2. Does comfort score vary by age or race?
3. Is there a relation between length of labor and Apgar score?
4. Is there a relation between length of labor and neonatal behavioral assessment scores?

REFERENCE

Andrews CM, Chrzanowski M: Maternal position, labor, and comfort, *Appl Nurs Res* 3:7, Jan/Feb 1990.

cal entities such as fetal presentations or mechanisms of labor may be helped or hindered by maternal posture (Fig. 17-13) (Liu, 1989; McKay, Roberts, 1989; Andrews, Chrzanowski, 1990).

Emergency Interventions

Emergency conditions can arise with startling speed and require immediate nursing intervention. In this section the following conditions are addressed: prolapsed umbilical cord, fetal distress, inadequate uterine relaxation, and bleeding. Prolapsed umbilical cord is discussed in some detail. (Only indications for immediate intervention are presented in a box on p. 450; fetal distress [see Chapter 16], inadequate uterine relaxation [see Chapter 35], and bleeding [see Chapter 30] are discussed at length in the chapters indicated.) Infection does not require the same swift, emergency response. It is presented here to alert the nurse to this condition, which is potentially harmful to the fetus and mother.

PROLAPSED UMBILICAL CORD. **Prolapse of the umbilical cord** occurs when the cord lies below the presenting part of the fetus. Umbilical cord prolapse may be occult (hidden, not visible) at any time during labor whether or not membranes are ruptured (Fig. 17-14, *A* and *B*). It is most common to see frank (visible) prolapse directly after ROM, when gravity washes the cord in front of the presenting part (Fig. 17-14, *C* and *D*). This occurs in one of 400 deliveries. Contributing factors are a long cord (>100 cm or 40 inches), malpresentation (breech), transverse lie, or unengaged presenting part.

When the presenting part does not fit into the lower uterine segment, as in polyhydramnios or when the membranes rupture, a sudden gush of amniotic fluid may cause the cord to be displaced down-

EMERGENCY

Interventions for Emergencies

SIGNS	INTERVENTIONS
Fetal Distress	
Fetal bradycardia (FHR <120 bpm for >2 min) (except if FHR is 110-120 with average variability) Fetal tachycardia (if term, FHR is >160 bpm for >2 min) Irregular FHR, abnormal sinus rhythm with internal monitor Persistent decrease in FHR variability Absence of FHR	Change maternal position to side-lying (left preferred). Increase IV fluids, if infusing. Administer oxygen at 10-12 L/min by tight face mask. Start an IV if one is not in place.
Inadequate Uterine Relaxation	
Intrauterine pressure >75 mm Hg (by IUPC) Contractions consistently lasting >90 sec Contraction interval <2 min	Discontinue oxytocin (Pitocin) if infusing. Position woman on left side. Increase infusion rate of IV fluids. Administer oxygen at 10-12 L/min by tight face mask. If no IV is in place, start IV now. Palpate and evaluate contractions. Give tocolytics (terbutaline, ritodrine) as ordered.
Vaginal Bleeding	
Vaginal bleeding (bright red, dark red, or in an amount in excess of that expected during normal cervical dilation) Continuous vaginal bleeding with FHR changes Pain: may or may not be present	Notify primary care practitioner. Anticipate emergency (crash) cesarean delivery.
Infection	
Foul-smelling amniotic fluid Maternal temperature >100.4° F (38° C) (0) in presence of adequate hydration (straw-colored urine) Fetal tachycardia >160 beats/min for >2 min	Notify primary care practitioner. Institute cooling measures for laboring woman. Start IV hydration. Send catheterized urine specimen to the laboratory for urinalysis and amniotic fluid sample for culture.

ward. Similarly the cord may prolapse during AROM if the presenting part is high. A small fetus also may not fit into the lower uterine segment; as a result, cord prolapse is more likely to occur.

Other predisposing factors in cord prolapse that are associated with a high presenting part are multiparity, cephalopelvic disproportion, and placenta previa. Prolapse of the cord is difficult to diagnose; however, an alert nurse or physician may make the diagnosis on vaginal examination after a sudden gush of fluid (see warning signs: rupture of membranes). Prompt recognition is important because fetal hypoxia from prolonged cord compression (occlusion of blood flow to and from the fetus for more than 5 minutes) usually results in central nervous system (CNS) damage or demise of the fetus (see box on p. 452). Pressure on the cord is relieved by direct pressure on the presenting part applied by the examiner's fingers while the mother assumes a **modified Sims' position** (Fig. 17-15, *C*) or is placed in Trendelenburg's position* until preparation can be made for emergency cesarean delivery. If the cervix is fully dilated, rapid forceps or vacuum extraction–assisted delivery can be performed. Prompt delivery in the most appropriate manner is imperative for the safety of the mother and fetus.

At the first opportunity, the nurse explains to the woman what is taking place, what umbilical cord

*A position in which the mother's head is lowered to allow for gravity to relieve pressure from the presenting part on the cord.

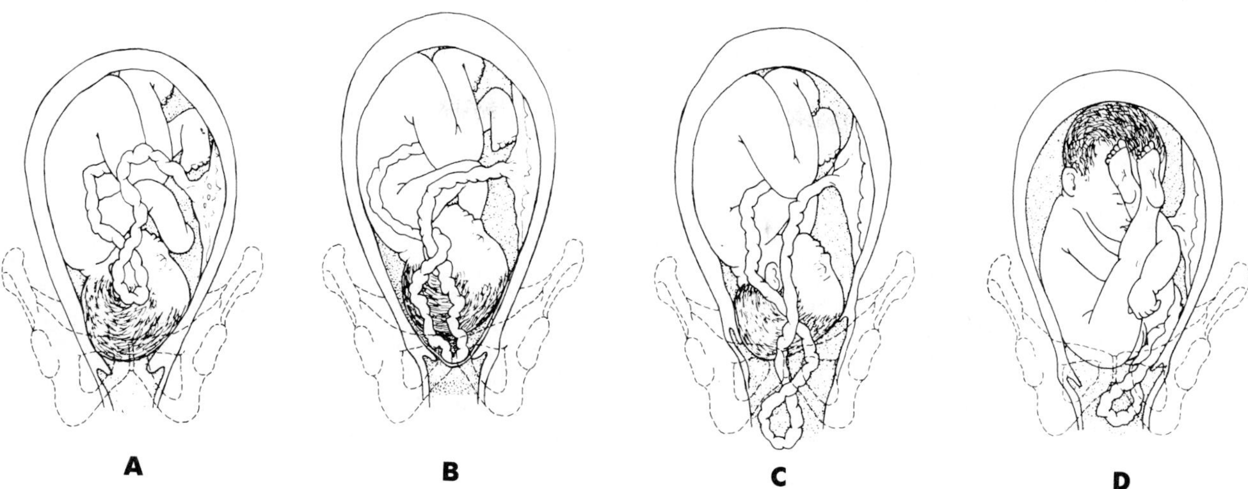

Fig. 17-14 Prolapse of umbilical cord. Note pressure of presenting part on umbilical cord, which endangers fetal circulation. **A**, Occult (hidden) prolapse of cord. **B**, Complete prolapse of cord. Note membranes are intact. **C**, Cord presenting in front of fetal head and may be seen within vagina. **D**, Frank breech presentation with prolapsed cord.

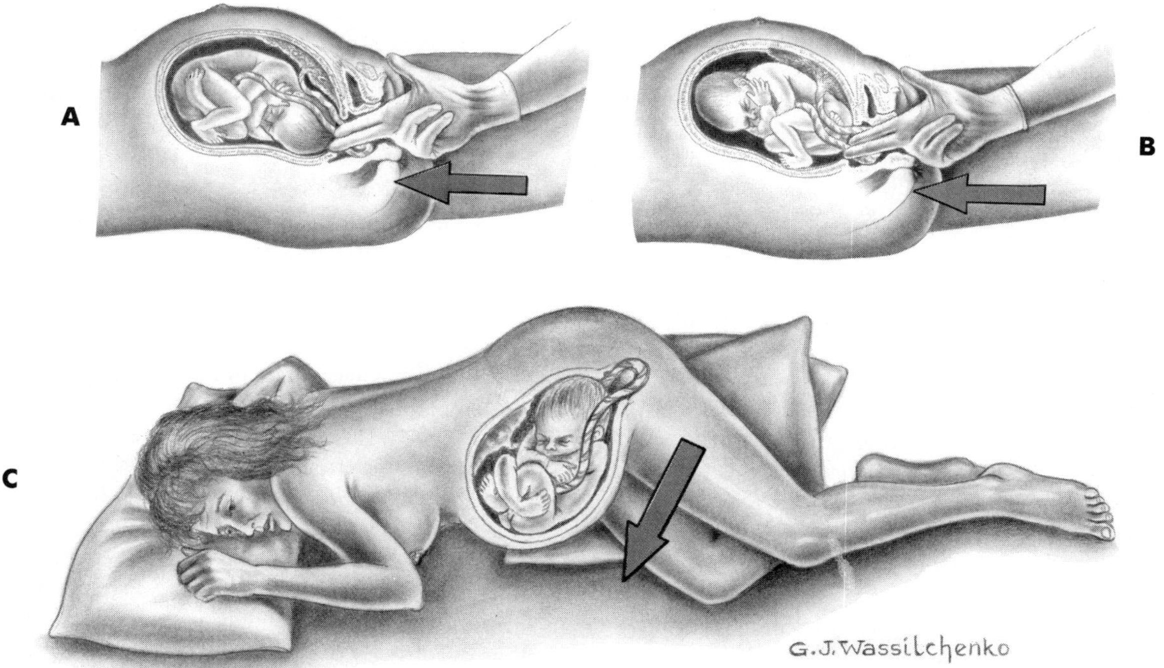

Fig. 17-15 *Arrows* indicate direction of pressure against presenting part to relieve compression of prolapsed umbilical cord. Pressure exerted by examiner's fingers in vertex presentation (**A**) and in breech position (**B**). **C**, Gravity relieves pressure with woman in modified Sims' position with hips elevated as high as possible with pillows.

EMERGENCY

Prolapse of Cord

SIGNS/SYMPTOMS

- Premature rupture of membranes
- Presenting part not engaged
- Polyhydramnios
- Fetal distress or abnormal FHR pattern
- Protruding cord from vagina (Fig. 17-14, *C*)

INTERVENTIONS

Call for assistance.

Glove the examining hand quickly and insert two fingers into the vagina to the cervix. With one finger on either side of the cord or both fingers to one side, exert upward pressure against the presenting part to relieve compression of the cord (Fig. 17-15, *A* and *B*). Apply a rolled towel under the woman's right hip.

Place woman into extreme Trendelenburg's or modified Sims' position (Fig. 17-15, *C*).

Notify physician immediately.

If cord is protruding from vagina, wrap loosely in a sterile towel wet with warm sterile normal saline.

Administer oxygen to the woman by mask, 10 to 12 L/min, until delivery is accomplished.

Start IV fluids or increase existing drip rate.

prolapse is, and how it is being managed. After vaginal or cesarean delivery, the mother and fetus are assessed for trauma or untoward effects. After cesarean delivery, the nurse performs postoperative assessment, monitors postanesthesia recovery, and charts the incident and results of treatment. The pediatrician usually is present at the birth and examines the infant.

Support Measures

By explaining unfamiliar terms to the woman and preparing her for sensations and procedures that will follow, the nurse can alleviate anxiety. By encouraging the woman or couple to ask questions and by providing honest, understandable answers, the nurse can play a significant role in achieving a satisfying birth experience.

Important components of the nursing care of the woman in labor relate to (1) helping the woman participate to the extent she wishes in the delivery of her infant, (2) meeting the woman's goals for herself, (3) helping the woman conserve her energy, and (4) helping control the woman's discomfort.

The nurse acts as an advocate for the woman and her family. Couples who have attended parenthood education programs using the psychoprophylactic approach will know something about the labor process, coaching techniques, and comfort measures (see Chapter 13). However, the staff's role is to be supportive and keep the couple informed of progress. Even if the expectant parents have not attended classes, the various techniques may be taught to a degree during the early phase of labor. The nurse will be expected to do more of the coaching and give supportive care.

The nurse serves as a coach to the woman in the absence of other support persons or as an adjunctive coach to the support persons present. The nurse must have a thorough knowledge of breathing and relaxation techniques to assist the woman and her partner in coping with labor. The nurse needs to provide comfort measures, such as warmth to the lower back in the case of back labor, a cool cloth to the forehead (Fig. 17-16), and room temperature controlled for the laboring woman's comfort. The **Hawthorn effect** is the "phenomenon that occurs when a person in pain begins to feel more comfortable as the nurse talks soothingly, fluffs a pillow, and promises to stay nearby. Positive support, especially by one in authority, enhances the ability to cope with stress" (Jimenez, 1983). (See Chapter 13 for complete discussion of methods of parent education and their use by the nurse during the woman's labor.)

Comfort measures vary with the situation. The nurse can draw on the couple's repertoire of comfort measures learned during the pregnancy. The comfort measures discussed here include maintaining a comfortable, supportive atmosphere in the labor and delivery area; using touch therapeutically; providing nonpharmacologic management of discomfort; and administering analgesics when necessary; but, most of all, just *being there*.

Labor rooms need to be light and airy. However, the bright overhead lights are turned off when not needed. The area should be large enough to accommodate the woman's partner in a comfortable chair, as well as the monitoring equipment and hospital personnel. In some hospitals, couples are urged to bring extra pillows to help make the hospital surrounding more homelike.

TOUCH. Most women respond positively to therapeutic touch in labor (Weaver, 1990). They appreciate gentle handling by staff members. Back rubs may be offered if the woman is experiencing back labor. A support person may be taught to provide **counterpressure** against the mother's sacrum (Fig. 17-17) over the occiput of the fetal head in a posterior position. Pain is caused from pressure of the occiput on spinal nerves, and pressure lifts the occiput off these nerves to provide some relief of pain. Once counterpressure is initiated, the woman usually requests that her partner continue the activity for each following contraction. The partner will need relief after a period of time because counterpressure is hard work.

The woman's awareness of the soothing qualities of touch changes as labor progresses. Many women develop hyperesthesia (increased sensitivity, especially in the skin) as labor progresses. They may tell their coach to "leave me alone," or they may say, "Don't touch me." The partner who is unprepared for this normal response may feel rejected and may react by withdrawing active support. The nurse can point out that this response on the part of the woman is a positive indication that the first stage is ending and that the transition stage is approaching. The woman's aggressive behavior is accepted; negative comments toward the woman are unwarranted and inappropriate (see Table 17-5).

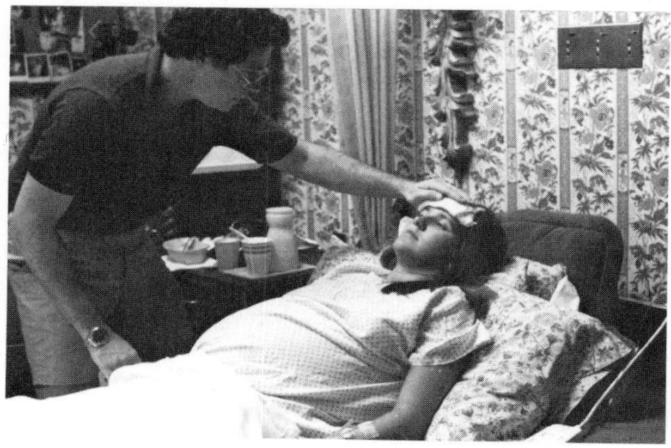

Fig. 17-16 Father providing comfort with a cool cloth to forehead.

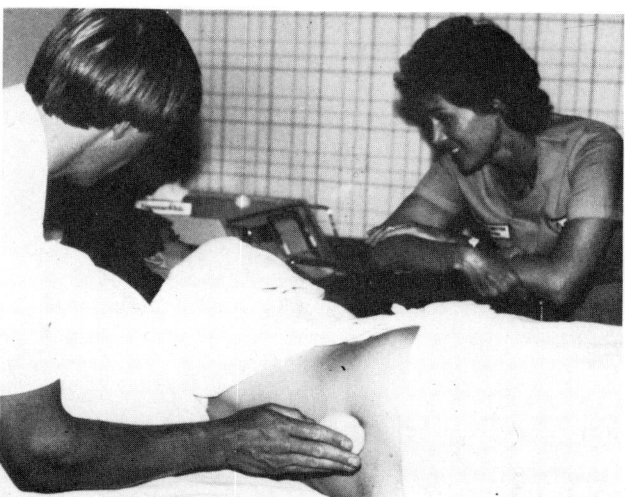

Fig. 17-17 Father applies sacral pressure with a tennis ball while nurse provides verbal encouragement.

NONPHARMACOLOGIC MANAGEMENT OF DISCOMFORT. The alleviation of pain is important. Commonly it is not the amount of pain the woman experiences, but *whether she meets her goals for herself in coping with the pain* that influences her perception of the birth experience as "good" or "bad." The observant nurse looks for cues to identify the woman's desired level of control in the management of pain and its relief.

The origins of discomfort during labor, the signs of pain, pain threshold, gate-control theory of pain, and pharmacologic control of discomfort are discussed in Chapter 15. The pain associated with parturition was accepted as a necessary part of childbirth until the discovery of the first anesthetics, nitrous oxide and ethyl ether. Since then much research has gone into the development of methods of pain control that bring effective relief for the mother without harm to the child. The perfect solution is yet to be found; therefore at times the safety of the child must take precedence over the comfort of the mother.

Nonpharmacologic methods for relief of discomfort are taught in many different types of prenatal preparation classes. Whether or not a woman or couple has attended these classes or read various books and magazines on the subject, the nurse can teach techniques to relieve discomfort during labor. The following section presents some nonpharmacologic methods of managing discomfort during labor.

TABLE 17-5 Woman's Expected Responses and Support Person's Actions During Labor

Woman	Support Person
DILATATION OF CERVIX 0-3 CM (contractions 10-30 sec long, 5-30 min apart, mild to moderate)	
Mood: alert, happy, excited, mild anxiety Settles into labor room; selects focal point Rests or sleeps if possible Uses breathing techniques Uses effleurage, focusing and relaxation techniques	Provides encouragement, feedback for relaxation, companionship Assists with contractions Uses focusing techniques Concentration on breathing technique Uses comfort measures Position most comfortable for woman Keeps woman aware of progress, explains procedures and routines Gives praise Offers ataractics as ordered (see Chapter 15)
DILATATION OF CERVIX 4-7 CM (contractions 30-40 sec long, 3-5 min apart, moderate to strong)	
Mood: seriously labor oriented, concentration and energy needed for contractions, alert, more demanding Continuous relaxation, focusing techniques Uses breathing techniques	Acts as buffer, limits assessment techniques to between contractions Assists with contractions May need to encourage woman to help her maintain breathing techniques Uses comfort measures Positions woman on side Encourages voluntary relaxation of muscles of back, buttocks, thighs, and perineum; effleurage Uses counterpressure to sacrococcygeal area Encourages and praises Keeps woman aware of progress Offers analgesics and anesthetics as ordered Checks bladder, encourages to void Gives mouth care, ice chips
DILATATION OF CERVIX 8-10 CM (TRANSITION) (contractions 45-60-90 sec long, 2-3 min apart, strong)	
Mood: irritable, intense concentration, symptoms of transition Continues relaxation, needs greater concentration to do this Breathing techniques Uses 4:1 breathing pattern if possible Uses panting to overcome response to urge to push	Stays with woman, provides constant support Assists with contractions Probably will need to remind, reassure, and encourage to reestablish breathing pattern and concentration If sedated or drowsy, woman needs warning to begin breathing pattern before contraction becomes too intense If woman begins to push, institutes panting respirations Uses comfort measures Accepts woman's inability to comply with instructions Accepts irritable response to helping, such as counterpressure Supports woman who has nausea and vomiting, gives mouth care as needed, gives reassurance regarding signs of end point of first stage Uses countertension techniques (effleurage and voluntary relaxation) Keeps woman aware of progress, tells woman when time to push

FOCUSING AND FEEDBACK RELAXATION. Some women bring a favorite device for use in focusing attention. Others choose some fixed object in the labor room. As the contraction begins, they may focus on this object to reduce their perception of pain. This technique, coupled with feedback relaxation, helps the woman work with her contractions rather than against them. The coach monitors this process, giving the woman cues as to when to begin the breathing techniques. A common feedback mechanism is for the woman and her coach to verbalize the word "relax" at the onset of each contraction and throughout it as needed. After the degree of relaxation has been assessed, relaxation techniques practiced in the prenatal period can be reviewed. The coach also keeps the woman from being disturbed by routine examinations for progress and checking of FHR. These procedures are postponed until the contraction is completed.

BREATHING TECHNIQUES. Different approaches to childbirth preparation stress varying techniques for using breathing as a "tool" to help the woman maintain control through contractions. *In the first stage,* breathing techniques can promote relaxation of abdominal muscles and thereby increase the size of the abdominal cavity. This lessens friction and discomfort between the uterus and the abdominal wall. Because the muscles of the genital area also become more relaxed, they do not interfere with descent. *In the second stage,* breathing is used to increase abdominal pressure and thereby assist in expelling the fetus. It also is used to relax the pudendal muscles to prevent precipitate expulsion of the fetal head.

For those couples who have prepared for labor by practicing such techniques, occasional reminders may be all that is necessary. For those who have had no preparation, instruction in simple breathing and relaxation can be given early in labor and often is surprisingly successful. Motivation is high, and learning readiness is enhanced by the reality of labor.

There are varied approaches to **breathing techniques** during contractions (see Chapter 13). The nurse needs to ascertain what if any information the laboring couple has before providing them with instruction. Generally, slow abdominal breathing, approximately half the woman's normal breathing rate, is initiated when the woman can no longer walk or talk through contractions (see "slow-paced breathing" in box on p. 456). As contractions increase in frequency and intensity, the woman may need to change to chest breathing, which is more shallow and approximately twice her normal rate of breathing (see "modified-paced breathing" in box on p. 456).

The most difficult time to maintain control during contractions comes when the cervical dilatation reaches 8 to 10 cm. This period is also called the **transition period.** Even for the woman who has prepared for labor, concentration on breathing techniques is difficult to maintain. The type used may be the 4:1 pattern: breath, breath, breath, breath, puff (as though blowing out a candle). This ratio may increase to 6:1 or 8:1. These patterns begin with the routine cleansing breath and end with a deep breath exhaled to "blow the contraction away." An undesirable side effect of this type of breathing may be **hyperventilation.** The woman must be aware of the accompanying symptoms of the resultant **respiratory alkalosis:** lightheadedness, dizziness, tingling of fingers, or circumoral numbness. Alkalosis may be overcome by having the woman breathe into a paper bag that is tightly held around the mouth and nose. This enables her to rebreathe carbon dioxide and replace the bicarbonate ion. She can breathe into her cupped hands if no bag is available.

As the fetal head reaches the pelvic floor, the woman will experience the urge to push and will automatically begin to exert downward pressure by contracting her abdominal muscles. Descent cannot continue until the cervix is fully dilated and the presenting part is free to move down the birth canal. *Pushing before full dilatation* is reached compresses the cervix between the fetal head and the pubic bone. This compression *may result in fetal distress or in cervical edema.* It may even slow the dilatation process. The woman can control the urge to push by taking panting breaths or by slowly exhaling through pursed lips. This is good practice for the type of breathing to be used as the fetal head is slowly delivered.

EFFLEURAGE AND SACRAL PRESSURE. Effleurage and sacral pressure, or massage, are two methods that have brought relief to many women during the first stage of labor. The gate-control theory may supply the reason for the effectiveness of these measures (see Chapter 15). **Effleurage,** which is a light stroking of the abdomen in rhythm with breathing during contractions, is used to distract the woman from contraction pain. The woman or her partner can perform effleurage on any area of her body. Many times the monitor belts make it difficult to perform effleurage on the abdomen; thus a thigh or the chest may be used.

JET HYDROTHERAPY. Jet hydrotherapy (whirlpool baths) is another nonpharmacologic method to use for increasing comfort and relaxation during labor (and after birth; see Chapter 25) (Aderhold, Perry, 1991; Rosenthal, 1991). Many new

Breathing Techniques

CLEANSING BREATH

Relaxed breath in through nose and out mouth. Used at the beginning and end of each contraction

SLOW-PACED BREATHING (APPROXIMATELY 6-8 BREATHS PER MINUTE)

Not less than half normal breathing rate (No. breaths/min divided by 2)

IN-2-3-4 / OUT-2-3-4 / IN-2-3-4 / OUT-2-3-4. . .

MODIFIED-PACED BREATHING (APPROXIMATELY 32-40 BREATHS PER MINUTE)

Not more than twice normal breathing rate (No. breaths /min × 2)

IN-OUT / IN-OUT / IN-OUT / IN-OUT / . . .

For more flexibility and variety, the woman may combine the slow and modified breathing by using the slow breathing for beginnings and ends of contractions and modified breathing for more intense peaks. This technique conserves energy and lessens fatigue.

PATTERNED-PACED BREATHING (SAME RATE AS MODIFIED)

Enhances concentration

a. 3:1 Patterned breathing
   IN-OUT / IN-OUT / IN-OUT / IN-BLOW
   (repeat through contraction)
b. 4:1 Patterned breathing
   IN-OUT / IN-OUT / IN-OUT / IN-OUT / IN-BLOW
   (repeat through contraction)

You may do any pattern desired, although ratios of 5:1 or higher tend to be very tiring. Some people like to do patterned breathing to a tune (Yankee Doodle, Old McDonald), to a repeated phrase (I think I can, I think I can), or in a pyramid pattern such as 1:1, 2:1, 3:1, 4:1, 5:1—5:1, 4:1, 3:1, 2:1, 1:1.

c. *Coach call:* May be used when woman needs more distraction and concentration (i.e., during transition). The woman's coach signals the breathing ratio with his/her fingers or by verbal cues, changing the ratio after each "IN-BLOW."
   Example:

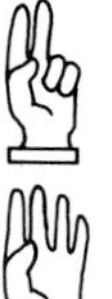

IN-OUT / IN-OUT / IN-BLOW

IN-OUT / IN-OUT / IN-OUT / IN-OUT / IN-BLOW

IN-OUT / IN-BLOW

From Shapiro HR et al: *The Lamaze ready reference guide for labor and birth,* ed2, Washington, DC, 1989, Chapter ASPO/Lamaze.

birthing units are installing baths with air jets. The buoyancy of the warm water, with or without air jets, provides support for tense muscles. Relaxing and soothing muscles have immediate benefits during labor and also reduce aftereffects of tense muscles during the immediate postpartum period (Fig. 17-18).

Several immediate benefits are seen (Aderhold, Perry, 1991). Relief from discomfort and general body relaxation reduce the woman's anxiety. Less anxiety decreases adrenalin production, which in turn allows an increase in levels of oxytocin (to stimulate labor) and endorphins (to reduce pain perception). In addition, the bubbles and gentle lapping of the water stimulate the nipples (hyperstimulation of uterine contractions has not occurred [Aderhold, Perry, 1991]). Cervical dilatation of 2 to 3 cm in 30 minutes often is noted. Blood pressure readings decrease and diuresis occurs. If the woman is experiencing "back labor" secondary to occiput posterior or transverse presentation, she is encouraged to assume the hands and knees or the side-lying position in the tub. Because this position decreases pain and increases relaxation and the production of oxytocin, the fetus can rotate to the occiput anterior position spontaneously.

Jet hydrotherapy must be ordered by the primary care practitioner. The mother's vital signs must be within normal limits, her cervix needs to be dilated 4 to 5 cm, and she must be in the active phase of the first stage of labor. If she is in the latent phase, her contractions may slow down. Fetal well-being must be established. Her membranes may be intact or ruptured. If ruptured, the fluid must be clear or only lightly stained with meconium (Aderhold, Perry, 1991). Heavy meconium staining necessitates an internal electrode, in which case jet hydrotherapy

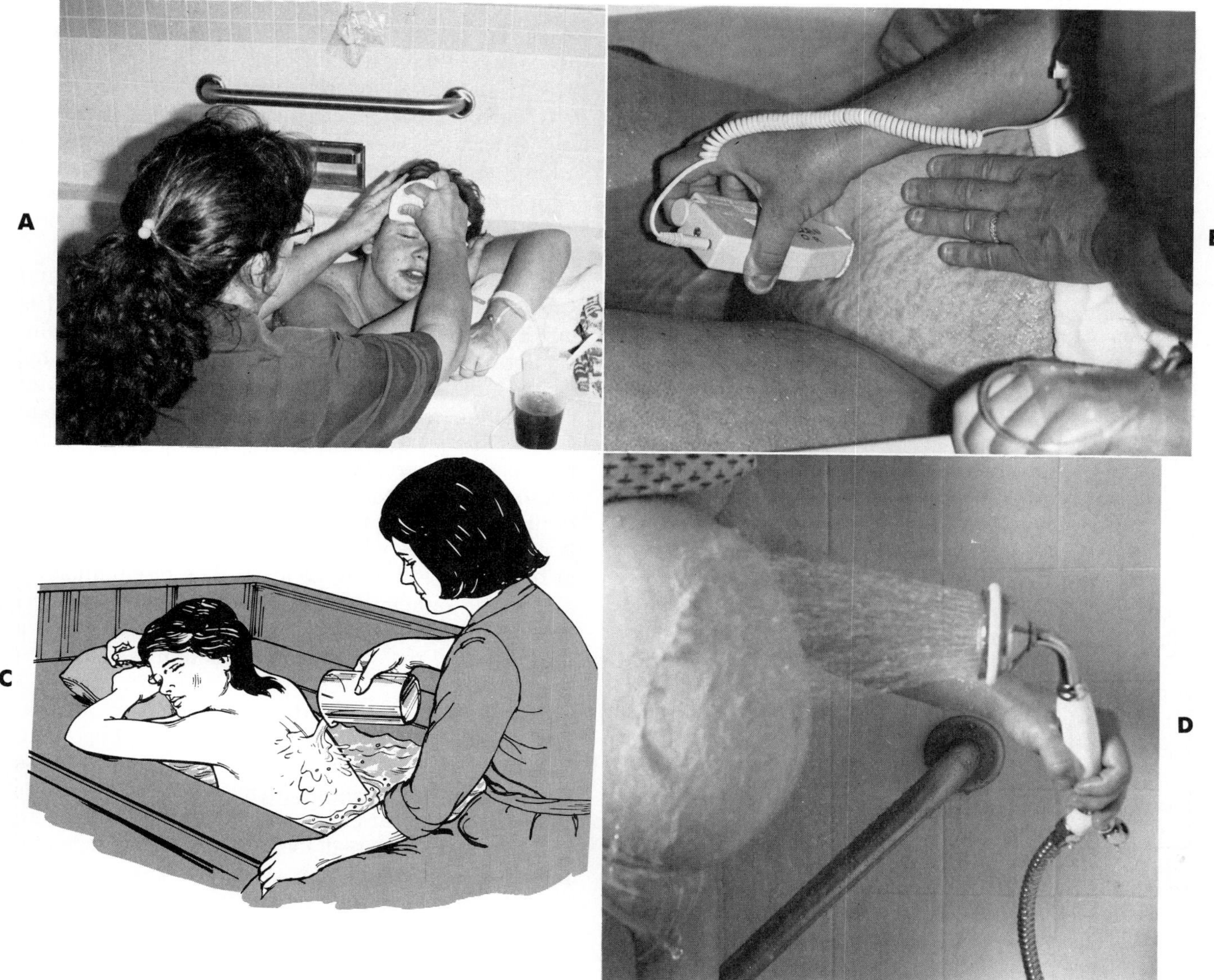

Fig. 17-18 Jet hydrotherapy during labor. **A**, Nurse provides comfort measures and ensures adequate hydration (note glass of clear fluid). **B**, Nurse assesses the FHR. **C**, Woman experiencing back labor, relaxing while nurse pours warm water over her back. **D**, Use of shower as one alternative to jet hydrotherapy during labor.
A, **B**, Courtesy Kathy Aderhold, CNM, Presbyterian/St. Luke's Medical Center, Denver, Colo. **D**, Courtesy Kathy Hanold, RN, MS, Birth Place, Barnes Hospital at Washington University, Medical Center, St. Louis, Mo.

would be contraindicated. Hydrotherapy also is available to the woman who has an IV or an IV heparin lock in place.

Jet hydrotherapy is an option if the women's cervix has been primed with PGE_2 gel (see discussion of induction of labor, Chapter 35). After application of the gel, the fetus is monitored for 2 hours before hydrotherapy is considered. Contraindications to jet hydrotherapy include stimulation of labor with oxytocin, the presence of thick meconium, or the use of internal electrodes for electronic fetal monitoring.

During the bath, if the woman's temperature and FHR increase, the water is cooled down or she is asked to step out of the bath to cool down. The bath water is kept between 96° to 98° F (35.6° to 36.7° C). The mother's temperature may remain slightly elevated for a short time after the bath. Fluids and ice chips and a cool face cloth are offered during the bath (Fig. 17-18, *A*). Maternal vital signs and labor and FHR are reassessed after the bath.

The tub must be kept meticulously clean. In one facility, it is cleaned after each use as follows (Aderhold, Perry, 1991). The tub is emptied and refilled to cover the jets; 1 cup bleach (Clorox) is added, and the jets are turned on for several minutes. The tub is drained again, cleaned with a nonabrasive cleanser, and rinsed. The tub is cultured each week. No infection has been reported to date.

TRANSCUTANEOUS ELECTRICAL NERVE STIMULATION. **Transcutaneous electrical nerve stimulation (TENS)** may be effective because of the "placebo effect"; that is, confidence in TENS may stimulate the release of endogenous opiates (enkephalins) in the woman's body and thus alleviate the discomfort (Scott et al, 1990).

Two pairs of electrodes are taped on either side of the thoracic and sacral spine. Continuous mild electrical currents are applied from a battery-operated device. During a contraction the woman increases the stimulation by turning control knobs on the device. Women describe the sensation as a tingling or buzzing and pain relief as good or very good. The use of TENS poses no risk to the mother or fetus. TENS is credited with reducing or eliminating the need for analgesia and with increasing the woman's perception of control over the experience.

The nurse assists the mother who is using TENS by explaining the device and its use, by carefully placing and securing the electrodes, and by closely evaluating its effectiveness.

■ ■ ■

Various other nonpharmacologic methods for control of discomfort are practiced. Many are learned in parent education classes (see Chapter 13). These include hypnosis, acupuncture, gate-control techniques, and relaxation techniques. Several relaxation techniques can be used for labor (and other life stresses): progressive relaxation, paced breathing, biofeedback, therapeutic touch, imagery, and music (see Research Highlight, p. 459). Aromatherapy—use of herbal teas or vapors—is employed by some to good effect (Valnet, 1990).

The Father/Partner during Labor

The father of the baby usually is the woman's partner who supports her in labor. He often is able to provide comfort measures and touch that the laboring woman needs. When the woman becomes focused on her pain, sometimes the father can persuade her to try nonpharmacologic variations of comfort measures. He usually is able to interpret the woman's needs and desires to staff members. He may be totally focused and involved with the woman, or he may be more passive because of cultural norms or fear. The nurse should assess his level of comfort in asking questions and in being present and involved during the second stage labor and birth. In this way the nurse can determine what level of support to provide to the couple during this time.

The father will be exposed to many sights and smells he may never before have experienced. It is important to tell him what to expect and to make him comfortable about leaving the room to gather his composure should something shock him. First, of course, provision should be made for someone else to support his partner during his absence. Staff members need to verbalize that the father's presence is helpful and to encourage his involvement in the care of his partner to the extent of his comfort level. This is especially true when his partner has just snapped at him and told him to go away. The nurse must reassure the father that this is normal behavior for a woman in transition and that if he reenters after a few minutes, the woman will ask him why he was gone so long.

Participation in the birth is ego building. The father *can* be of assistance; his presence *is* important. It is commonly observed that a caring person can be worth his or her weight in meperidine (Demerol). Recently a 16-year-old unwed mother in labor with her first child thrashed about, moaning and screaming with each contraction. A nurse remained at her bedside, coaching and comforting to no avail. The unwed adolescent father arrived and was immediately escorted into her room. The young woman continued her labor calmly and without medication through delivery.

When the father is active and supportive, the mother turns to him. The physician remains the medical-surgical expert, without taking on the father or husband-surrogate role as well. The couple's future relationship and their relationship with their child may be positively influenced. Mutuality is fostered when the mother can turn to the father and say, "I could never have done it without you. You were my pillar of strength."

Supporting the father, as well as the mother, in labor elevates the nurse's role. It is another step forward from merely providing custodial care to enacting a therapeutic role. Support of the father reflects the nurse's orientation and commitment to the person, the family, and the community. Therapeutic nursing actions convey to the father several important concepts.

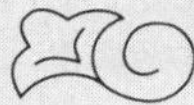 **Research Highlight** 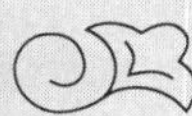

Effects of Music and Imagery on Analogued Labor Pain

RESEARCH ABSTRACT

Two studies were conducted. One examined the effects of music on pain and blood pressure, heart rate and respiratory rate. The second determined whether imagery combined with music was effective. The sample was recruited from undergraduate classes and consisted of 50 nulliparous women between the ages of 18 and 30 years. Subjects were randomly assigned to one of five groups: self-selected music, rock music, easy-listening music, placebo attention, or no treatment control. A pain stimulator was applied to the first phalanx of the left index finger. The stimulator is reported to produce pain that simulates pain of labor. Subjects listened to a recording through headphones. No significant effects were found, although the mean scores were in the predicted direction.

Sample size and selection were the same for the second study. Subjects were randomly assigned to one of five groups: music and self-generated imagery, self-generated imagery without music, music and guided imagery, guided imagery without music, and nontreatment control. They received 30 minutes of training in imagery 1 week before the laboratory experience. During application of the pain stimulus, subjects were asked to use music to assist in generating appropriate imagery. Significant differences in heart rate and in systolic and diastolic blood pressure were noted. The self-report of pain did not differ across groups although there may be a clinically meaningful difference. Music alone was not effective. However, when music was combined with imagery, subjects reported less subjective pain.

IMPLICATIONS FOR PRACTICE

Music can be used in early labor to assist in relaxing the woman. Music combined with imagery may be more effective later. Nurses should encourage women to use whatever means are available and safe to distract attention from and reduce the perception of labor pain.

RELATED RESEARCH QUESTIONS

1. What are the effects of music on pain in labor?
2. What are the effects of imagery on pain in labor?
3. Is imagery an effective adjunct to music in reducing perceptions of pain in labor?
4. Is listening to a preferred type of music more effective in reducing pain in labor than listening to music that is not preferred?

REFERENCE

Geden EA et al: Effects of music and imagery on physiologic and self-report of analogued labor pain, *Nurs Res* 38:37, Jan/Feb 1989.

First, he is of value as a person. He is not a comic-strip character, inept and bungling or idle, nervous, and inconsequential. Second, he can learn to be a partner in the mother's care. Finally, childbearing is a partnership.

The nurse can support the father/partner in the following ways:

1. Regardless of the degree of involvement desired, orient him to the maternity unit, including the woman's labor room and what he can do there (sleep, telephone), rest room, cafeteria, waiting room, nursery, visiting hours, and names and functions of personnel present.
2. Respect his or their decisions as to his degree of involvement, whether the decision is active participation in the delivery room or just being kept informed. When appropriate, provide data on which he or they can base decisions; offer freedom of choice as opposed to coercion one way or another. This is *their* experience and *their* baby.
3. Indicate to him when his presence has been helpful and continue to reinforce this throughout labor.
4. Offer to teach him comfort measures to the degree he wants to know them. Reassure him that he is not assuming the responsibility for observation and management of his partner's labor, but supporting her as she progresses.
5. Communicate with him frequently regarding her progress and his needs. Keep him informed of procedures to be performed, what to expect from procedures, and what is expected of him.
6. Prepare him for changes in her behavior and physical appearance.
7. Remind him to eat; offer snacks and fluids if possible.

8. Relieve him as necessary; offer blankets if he is to sleep in a chair by the bedside. Acknowledge the stress of the situation on each partner and identify normal responses. The nonjudgmental attitude of staff members helps the father and mother accept their own and the other parents' behavior.
9. Attempt to modify or eliminate unsettling stimuli (such as extra noise, extra light, chatter).

A well-informed father/partner can make a significant contribution to the health and well-being of the mother and child, their family interrelationship, and his self-esteem (Queenan, 1990). It has been found that a significantly lower percentage of women suffered postdelivery emotional upsets when their partners received support and assistance from parent education classes, physicians, midwives, and nurses throughout the childbearing cycle.

CULTURE AND FATHER PARTICIPATION. Many hospitals encourage the father's presence during labor and delivery. If he is not able to be there, another significant person may be present. In some cultures the father may be available, but his presence with the mother may not be appropriate and he may resist involvement at this time. His behavior could be misunderstood by the nursing staff as lack of concern, caring, or interest. Griffith (1982) identifies the importance of the affectional bond between a Mexican woman and her mother and sisters or other female relatives in regard to home-related activities such as childbearing. This is also true for many other groups, and the presence of another woman or women is highly desired. Among some cultures, if childbearing occurs in the hospital, at least one woman must be present for assistance. Cultures in which a woman's assistance during childbearing is preferred include Southeast Asians (Hollingsworth et al, 1980), African Americans (Carrington, 1978; Johnson, Snow, 1978), and Native Americans (Farris, 1978; Horn, 1982).

According to Pillsbury (1978), the Chinese husband is not allowed in the delivery room, lest he become polluted by the woman's blood. A nurse from a different culture might think it odd that a Chinese husband does not seem to give any emotional support to his wife during labor and delivery. However, Chinese women have significant others who can provide emotional support—mothers, in-laws, cousins, other members of the extended family, or close friends.

In India all attendants at birth are women; men are totally excluded (Flint, 1982). On the other hand, in Guatemala, a husband may assist his wife and the midwife during delivery (Cosminsky, 1982). During the labor process of the Navajo in the Southwestern United States, people passing by the hogan (home) are encouraged to enter and provide support for the mother (Newton, 1972). Because of the wide variation in the choice of the preferred person or persons, it is critical for the nurse to determine from the woman and her family what persons are wanted during labor and delivery.

Support of the Grandparents

Especially in situations in which the grandparents take the place of the husband as a labor coach, it is important to support them and treat them with respect. They may have a way to deal with pain relief that is based on their experience. They need to be given a chance to help if their actions will not compromise the status of the mother or the fetus, e.g., ingestion of herbal teas in labor. The nurse acts as a role model for parents by treating grandparents with dignity and respect, by acknowledging the value of their contributions to parental support, and by recognizing the difficulty parents have in witnessing their child's discomfort or crisis, regardless of the child's age.

Of particular value is the availability of another person or persons to relieve the father or coach. This may be necessary to assist the woman in labor with walking, especially if IV poles are to be pushed, as well as to help the woman when she needs two tasks performed simultaneously.

Whenever possible the nurse offers the grandparent emotional support. This can be done by providing liquid refreshment even if unsolicited and by initiating discussion with open-ended questions or statements, such as "It is sometimes hard to watch a daughter in labor. . . . "

These nursing actions are therapeutic for the entire family unit. According to Barnard (1978), "Rather than compete with family members, we can use them, provide support to them, and teach them. The family's influence will far outlast our contact with the client. If we can improve this social unit's ability to care, we will have a powerful health care system indeed." Support for the mother of a laboring woman—mothering *her* mother—is an important place to begin (Stephany, 1983).

Siblings during Labor

Preparation for acceptance of the new child helps with the attachment process. Parents, brothers and sisters, and other extended family members benefit from *cognitive rehearsal* for the new addition to the family. Preparation for and participation during pregnancy and labor may help the older children accept this change. The older child or children become *ac-*

tive participants who are important to the family (Bliss, 1980). Rehearsal for the event before labor is essential. Preparation for the entire family includes the additional support person who is to be responsible for the older children during the entire childbirth process.

The age and developmental level of children influence their responses. The child younger than 2 years of age shows little interest in pregnancy and labor; for the older child the experience may reduce fears and misconceptions. Preparation is adjusted to the age and developmental level of the child. Most parents have a "feel" for the maturational level and ability to cope of their children. Preparation includes description of anticipated sights and sounds. The children must learn that their mother will be working hard. She will not be able to talk to them during contractions. She may groan and pant at times. Labor is uncomfortable, but their mother's body is made for the job. The sights, sounds, smells, and behavior of participants will be similar to those for which fathers are prepared. Films are available for preparing older preschool and school-age children for participating in the birth experience (see Appendix H).

Leonard et al (1979) observed the behavior of children present during labor, delivery, and the postpartum period. In general the preschool-age children tended to interact eagerly with their parents during early labor. They were seen to withdraw from the happenings as labor progressed. None of the children seemed to become acutely distressed during the experience. However, children need to feel free to ask questions and express personal feelings (Daniels, 1983).

Preparation for Giving Birth

The first stage of labor ends with the complete dilatation of the cervix. For multiparous women, birth usually occurs within minutes of complete dilatation, perhaps only one push later. Nulliparous women usually push for 1 to 2 hours before delivery. If the woman has epidural anesthesia, pushing may be prolonged beyond 2 hours. The nurse will begin preparation for delivery when a multiparous woman is 6 to 7 cm dilated, because progression through the last few centimeters of dilation can occur any time from a few minutes to hours. Factors that are thought to influence the process are fetal position (e.g., occiput posterior) and size in relation to previous babies.

To prepare for delivery in any setting, the delivery table or case cart is usually set up during the transition phase for nulliparous women and during the active phase for multiparous women. (See Chapter 18 for description of a table set-up.) A radiant warmer is turned on when crowning begins to occur in the nulliparous woman and when the multiparous woman is 8 to 9 cm dilated. If a traditional delivery room is used, only a multiparous woman will be transferred during the first stage of labor. Transfer of the nulliparous woman will take place when the presenting part begins to distend the perineum between contractions during the second stage of labor (see Fig. 18-1 and Plates 1 to 3).

All nursing care and the woman's or couple's responses must be recorded to ensure continuity of care, ensure appropriate assessment of the woman's progress, and document the nursing and other care given. According to courts of law, nursing and medical care that is not documented on the client's record may not have been given.

The following are suggestions for preparation for delivery. These items may vary among different facilities so that the protocols from each facility's procedure manual should be consulted.

1. Scrubbing facilities, scrub brushes, cuticle sticks, cleaning agent, and masks with shield or protective glasses/goggles are available.
2. The following tasks have been done:
   a. Sterile gowns and gloves for physician or nurse-midwife, sterile drapes and towels for draping the woman, and sterile instruments and other supplies (such as bulb syringes, sutures, and anesthetic solutions) are arranged for convenience in use on sterile table.
   b. Sterile basin and water for hand washing during delivery process are readied for use.
   c. Supplies for cleansing vulva are available (sterile basin, sterile water, and cleaning solution).
   d. Delivery area is warmed and free of drafts.
   e. Infant identification materials have been readied.
   f. Infant receiving blankets and heated crib are readied. Material for prophylactic care of infant's eyes is available (see p. 494).
3. Equipment is in working order: delivery table (bed or chair), overhead lights, and mirror.
4. Emergency equipment, anesthesia, laryngoscope, and supplies are available and in working order if needed for emergency situations such as control of maternal hemorrhage or fetal respiratory distress.
5. Additional supplies (anesthetics, oxytocics for injection, and obstetric forceps) are available.
6. Woman's record is up-to-date and ready for use in delivery area. In areas such as the labor unit, recordings are made as symptoms are noted, assessments are made, and care is given. It is imperative to have recordings complete at all times.

A

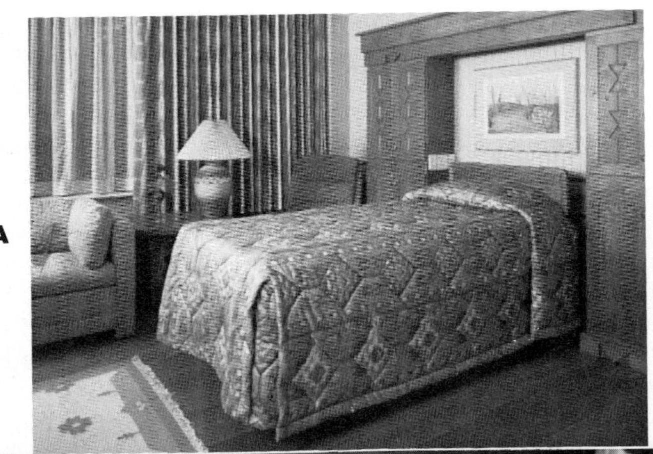

B

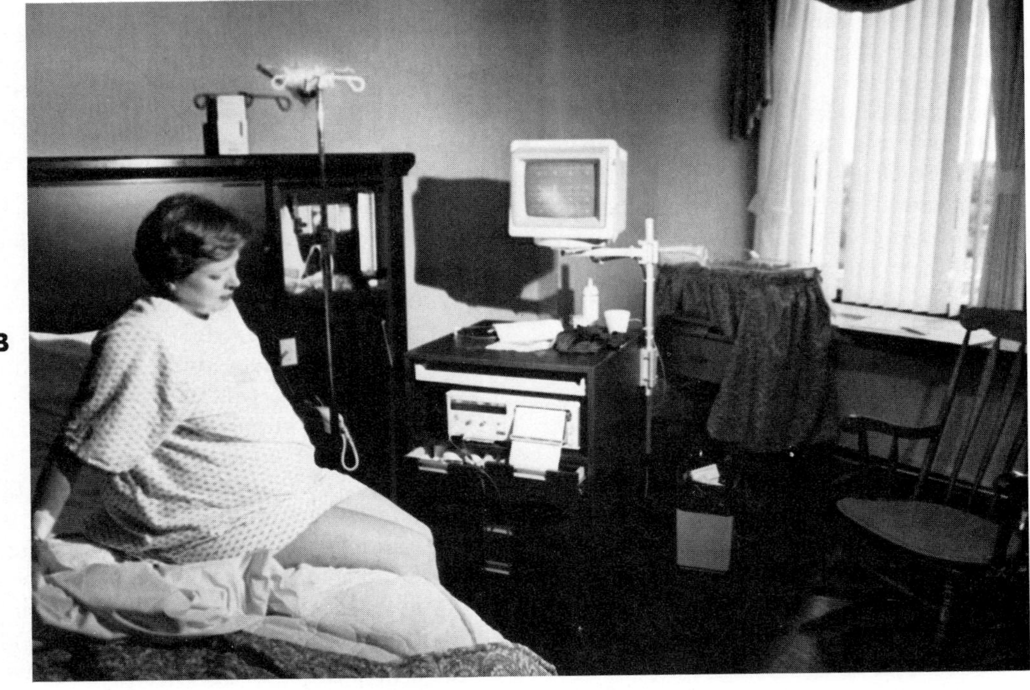

Fig. 17-19 Examples of a labor, delivery, recovery, postpartum (LDRP) room.
A, courtesy Vogler/Perinatal Healthcare Consultants, Kailua, HI. *B*, courtesy Kathy Hanold, RN, MS, Birth Place, Barnes Hospital at Washington University Medical Center, St. Louis, Mo.

Transfer to the delivery room*

Nulliparous woman	When the presenting part begins to distend the perineum
Multiparous woman	When the cervix is 8 to 9 cm dilated

The nurse estimates the time of delivery and will notify the primary care practitioner when there appears to be an hour or more of labor left. Even the most experienced nurse can mistake the time left before delivery. Thus every nurse who attends a woman in labor must be prepared to perform an emergency delivery if needed (see p. 483).

Significant changes have occurred in the location where birth takes place. Almost half of the hospitals that offer maternity care in the United States have, or are developing, birth settings that offer alternatives to what is known as "traditional" delivery rooms. The most common of these is the labor, delivery, recovery, postpartum (LDRP) room where the woman stays during her entire hospitalization. This avoids the confusion of multiple transfers of the woman from the labor room to delivery room to recovery room. Another option is the labor, delivery, and recovery (LDR) room, in which the woman stays dur-

*Transfer is unnecessary in LDR and LDRP rooms.

ing her labor and immediate postpartum recovery period (1 to 2 hours) and then is transferred to a "postpartum" room. Here she stays for the duration of her hospitalization (Fig. 17-19).

EVALUATION

Evaluation of progress and outcomes is a continuous activity during the first stage of labor. Each interaction with the mother-to-be and her family must be carefully evaluated by the nurse; the degree to which formulated goals for care are being met must be critically appraised. That is, effective care is reflected by the following results:

- The woman demonstrates normal labor progress while the FHR remains within normal range without signs of distress.
- She expresses satisfaction with the assistance of her support person and nursing staff.
- She verbalizes her desire for participation in her care during labor and participates as tolerated throughout labor.
- She maintains adequate hydration and empties her bladder as needed.
- She indicates to her support person or nurse those measures that help to reduce her discomfort and promote relaxation.

If the evaluation process identifies that results fall short of achieving any goal, further assessment, planning, and implementation are imperative to attain the correct nursing care for the woman and her family.

■ SUMMARY

In the first stage of labor the woman and her support persons begin preparation for the actual delivery of the baby that has been long awaited. The woman experiences some degree of stress as her system responds to the effects of physical changes that prepare her to give birth. Despite all the preparation she may have had during pregnancy to guide her through the labor experience, she will likely not be totally prepared for her individual experience. It is important for the nurse to assess what additional support the woman and her support persons require during the time labor is in progress and to provide interventions that will ease some of the stress felt by all parties involved. Nurses serve as an active client system advocate during labor. They provide information to members of the family system to assist their involvement in the process to the extent the laboring woman prefers. Nurses include the woman in care-planning decisions to achieve the goal of a labor experience that is as positive as possible.

CASE STUDY

Active Labor: First Stage

Paula Jones is a 24-year-old married woman with one child. At week 39 of gestation, she is in the process of being admitted to the perinatal unit.

ASSESSMENT

Paula states that she is very uncomfortable with contractions and is feeling anxious about her labor. She reports that she has not eaten or felt like taking any fluids all day before admission, and she has voided only once today. Physical examination reveals the following findings: cervical dilatation 5 cm, effacement 60%, station, −2, membranes intact; uterine contractions: regular every 4 to 5 minutes, moderate in intensity, lasting 40 to 60 seconds; temperature is 99.3° F (37.4° C). Otherwise, maternal vital signs, FHR, and fetal activity are within normal limits.

Examination of Paula's urine reveals clear amber color, ketones 2+, pH 5.0.

NURSING DIAGNOSIS

Assessment findings support several nursing diagnoses. The nursing diagnosis that takes priority is fluid volume deficit relating to inadequate fluid intake.

PLANNING

The nurse and Paula mutually agree on the following goal: Paula's fluid balance will be restored. The nurse sets the following expected outcomes: Within 3 hours Paula's urine will be within normal limits for color and pH, with an absence of ketones; her temperature will be 98.6° F (37° C).

IMPLEMENTATION

Paula's primary care practitioner has ordered an IV infusion of lactated Ringer's solution, 150 mL/hr, and clear liquid diet as tolerated. The nurse will start an IV infusion per hospital protocol, offer clear fluids of Paula's choice, and continue to monitor temperature every 2 hours while elevated and to monitor urinary output for amount, color, and ketones for each voiding until normal findings are obtained.

EVALUATION

Within 3 hours Paula has had 240 mL of clear fluids and 450 mL of IV fluids. She has voided 300 mL clear, straw-colored urine with a pH of 6.0 and 1+ ketone. Her temperature is now 98.6° F (37° C).

CARE PLAN Active Labor

GOALS	IMPLEMENTATION	RATIONALE	EVALUATION
Nursing diagnosis: Fluid volume deficit related to inadequate fluid intake			
Paula's fluid balance will be restored, as evidenced by adequate output of straw-colored urine, pH 6.0, absent ketones and by temperature of 9.6° F (37° C).	Start and maintain an IV infusion at 150 mL/hr. Provide ice chips or sips of clear fluids, as ordered. Monitor amount of urinary output; urine pH, ketones, color; temperature.	Hydration is essential for adequate blood supply to mother and fetus and to kidneys; and to maintain temperature of 98.6° F (37° C).	In 3 hours: Paula voided 300 mL straw-colored urine, pH 6.0, trace ketones. Paula's temperature is 98.6° F (37° C).
Nursing diagnosis: Pain related to increasing frequency and intensity of uterine contractions			
Paula reports increased comfort.	Assess Paula's verbal and nonverbal communication. Promote the use of focused breathing techniques	Reduction of perception of pain increases woman's ability to cope with labor. Focused breathing distracts.	Paula reports increased comfort. Paula is able to use relaxation techniques.
	Offer massage and other therapeutic touch techniques (p. 338) Involve her in decision-making regarding which comfort measures she prefers. Explain all procedures in simple language. Provide her with choice regarding administration of ordered medications.	Improves morale and comfort (Hawthorne effect).	
	Inform her regarding progress in labor.	Knowledge provides basis for decision-making.	

REFERENCES

Aderhold KJ, Perry L: Jet hydrotherapy for labor and postpartum pain relief, *MCN* 16:97, March/April 1991.

Barnard R: The family and you, *MCN* 3:83, 1978.

Bentz JM: Missed meanings in nurse/patient communications, *MCN* 5:55, Jan/Feb 1980.

Bliss J: New baby in the family, *Can Nurse* 76:42, 1980.

Carrington BW: The Afro-American. In Clark AI, editor: *Culture/childbearing/health professionals,* Philadelphia, 1978, FA Davis Co.

Cosminsky S: Knowledge and body concepts of Guatemalan midwives. In Kay MA, editor: *Anthropology of human birth,* Philadelphia, 1982, FA Davis Co.

Cunningham FG, MacDonald PC, Gant NF: *Williams obstetrics,* ed 18, Norwalk, Conn, 1989, Appleton & Lange.

Daniels MB: The birth experience for the sibling: description and evaluation of a program, *J Nurs Midwife* 28:15, Sept/Oct 1983.

Farris L: The American Indian. In Clark AL, editor: *Culture/childbearing/health professionals,* Philadelphia, 1978, FA Davis Co.

Flint M: Lockmi: an Indian midwife. In Kay MA, editor: *Anthropology of human birth,* Philadelphia, 1982, FA Davis Co.

Friedman EA, Sachtleben MR: Station of the presenting part, *Am J Obstet Gynecol* 93:522, 1965.

Friedman EA: *Labor: clinical evaluation and management,* ed 2, New York, 1978, Appleton-Century-Crofts.

Griffith S: Childbearing and the concept of children, *JOGNN* 11:181, 1982.

Hollingsworth AO et al: The refugees and childbearing: what to expect, *RN* 43:45, 1980.

Horn BM: Northwest coast Indians: the Muckleshoot. In Kay MA, editor: *Anthropology of human birth,* Philadelphia, 1982, FA Davis Co.

Jimenez SL: Application of the body's natural pain relief mechanisms to reduce discomfort in labor and delivery, *NAACOG Update Series,* lesson 1, vol 1, 1983.

Johnson SM, Snow LF: The profile of some unplanned pregnancies. In Bauwens EE, editor: *The anthropology of health,* St Louis, 1978, Mosby–Year Book.

Leonard CH et al: Preliminary observations on the behavior of children present at the birth of a sibling, *Pediatrics* 64:949, 1979.

Machol L: LDR: new factor in the OB equation, *Contemp OB/GYN* 31:176, Feb 1988.
McKay S, Roberts J: Maternal position during labor and birth: what have we learned? *IJCE, ICEA Rev* 13:19, Aug 1989.
Newton N: *Childbearing in broad perspective: pregnancy, birth and the newborn baby,* Boston, 1972, Delacorte Press.
Pillsbury BLK: "Doing the month": confinement and convalescence of Chinese women after birth, *Soc Sci Med* 12:11, 1978.
Queenan JT: Partners in the delivery room: a natural evolution, *Contemp OB/GYN* 35:8, Aug 1990.
Rosenthal MJ: Warm-water immersion in labor and birth, *Female Patient* 16:35, Aug 1991.
Scott JR et al: Danforth's obstetrics and gynecology, ed 6, Philadelphia, 1990, JB Lippincott Co.
Stephany T: Supporting the mother of a patient in labor, *JOGNN* 12:345, Sept/Oct 1983.
Valnet J: *The practice of aromatherapy,* Rochester, Vt, 1990, Healing Arts Press.
Zuspan FP, Quilligan EJ, editors: *Practical manual of obstetric care,* St Louis, 1982, Mosby–Year Book.

References Nursing Research

Andrews CM, Chrzanowski M: Maternal position, labor, and comfort, *Appl Nurs Res* 3:7, Jan/Feb 1990.
Bonovich L: Recognizing the onset of labor, *JOGNN* 19:141, March/April 1990.
Liu YC: Effects of the upright position during childbirth, *Image J Nurs Sch* 21:14, Spring 1989.
Weaver DR: Nurses' views on the meaning of touch in obstetrical nursing practice, *JOGNN* 19:157, March/April 1990.

BIBLIOGRAPHY

American Academy of Pediatrics, American College of Obstetricians and Gynecologists. In Frigoletto FD, Little GA, editors: *Guidelines for perinatal care.* ed 2, White Plains, NY, 1988, March of Dimes Birth Defects Foundation.
Benyon CL: Striving to better, oft we mar what's well—management of normal labour, *Midwives Chronicle* 101(1208):280, 1988.
Brown ST, Campbell D, Kurtz A: Characteristics of labor pain at two stages of cervical dilation, *Pain* 38:289, Sept 1989.
Chez RA, Katz Z: Umbilical cord prolapse, *Contemp OB/GYN* 34:83, Aug 1989.
Church LK: Water birth: one birthing center's observation, *J Nurse Midwife* 34:165, July/Aug 1989.
Clapp JF: The course of labor after endurance exercise during pregnancy, *Am J Obstet Gynecol* 163(6 PTI):1799, 1990.
Fraser WD et al: A randomized controlled trial of early amniotomy, *Br J Obstet Gynaecol* 98:84, 1991.
Gerlach C, Schmid M: Second skill educational development of personnel for a single-room maternity care system, *JOGNN* 17:388, Nov/Dec 1988.
Heminki E: Content of prenatal care in the United States: a historic perspective, Med Care 26:199, 1988.
Jordan PL: Laboring for relevance: expectant and new fatherhood, *Nurs Res* 39, Jan/Feb 1990.
Katz Z et al: Management of labor with umbilical cord prolapse, *Obstet Gynecol* 72:278, 1988.
Kitzinger S: *The complete book of pregnancy and childbirth,* rev ed, New York, 1989, Knopf.
Korbert LJ: Are universal precautions changing the "nurture" of obstetric nursing? *AJN* 89:1609, Dec 1989.
Malestic SL: Fathers need help during labor, too, *RN,* p 1990, July 1990.
Malinowski JS et al: *Nursing care during the labor process,* ed 3, Philadelphia, 1989, FA Davis.
McKay S: Consumer-provider relationships. In Nichols FH, Humenick SS, editors: *Childbirth education: practice, research, and theory,* Philadelphia, 1988, WB Saunders.
McKay S, Mahan C: Modifying the stomach contents of laboring women: why and how; success and risks, *Birth* 15:213, 1988.
Milner I: Water baths for pain relief in labour, *Nurs Times* 84:39, Jan 1988.
Morse JM, Park C: Differences in cultural expectations of the perceived expectations of parturition. In Michaelson, editor: *Childbirth in America: anthropological perspectives,* South Hadley, Mass, 1988, Bergin & Garvey.
Rooks JP: Value of a screening fetal heart rate tracing in the latent phase of labor, *J Reprod Med* 35:1990, 1990.
Rooks JP et al: Outcomes of care in birth centers. The National Birth Center Study, *N Engl J Med* 321:1804, 1989.
Strong TH et al: Prophylactic intrapartum amnioinfusion: a randomized clinical trial, *Am J Obstet Gynecol* 162:1370, 1990.
Stroud R, Cochrane S: Managing without drugs—physiological management of the third stage of labour, *Nurs Times* 86(48):70, 1990.
Sturrock WA, Johnson JA: The relationship between childbirth education classes and obstetric outcome, *Birth* 17:82, June 1990.
Swinnerton T: Alternative remedies during labor, *Nurs Times* 87:64, Sept 1991.
Thomson M: Unexplained differences in first stage labor duration in primipara at North American and European hospitals, *Birth* 15:205, Dec 1988.
Wuitchik M et al: Perinatal predictors of pain and distress during labor, *Birth* 17:186, Dec 1990.

Bibliography Nursing Research

Berry LM: Realistic expectations of the labor coach, *JOGNN* 17:354, Sept/Oct 1988.
Boylan PC, Parisi VM: Effect of active management on latent phase labor, *Am J Perinatol* 7:363, Oct 1990.
Fridh G et al: Factors associated with more intense labor pain, *Res Nurs Health* 11:117, 1988.
Gaston-Johansson F et al: Progression of labor pain in primiparas and multiparas, *Nurs Res* 37:86, 1988.
Mackey MC, Lock SE: Women's expectations of the labor and delivery nurse, *JOGNN* 18:505, Nov/Dec 1989.
Wilkie DJ et al: Use of the McGill pain questionnaire to measure pain: a meta-analysis, *Nurs Res* 39:36, 1990.

chapter 17 review

Key Concepts

- The onset of labor may be difficult to determine even for the woman who has given birth before.
- Although some complications of labor are anticipated, others appear only in the clinical course of labor.
- The nurse assumes much of the responsibility for making the assessment of progress and keeping the physician or certified nurse-midwife informed about that progress and any deviations from normal findings.
- Although meconium-stained fluid may be noted with fetal asphyxia, its presence is not always diagnostic of prospective fetal distress.
- Regardless of the actual labor and delivery experience, the woman's or couple's perception of the birth experience is most positive if events and performances are consistent with expectations.
- The woman's level of anxiety may rise when she does not understand what is being said to her and about her labor because of the medical terminology used or because of a language barrier.
- Prolapsed umbilical cord occurs in about 1 in 400 deliveries and requires prompt recognition and therapy to prevent fetal hypoxia.
- Coaching, support, and comfort measures assist the woman to use her energy constructively in relaxing and working with the contractions.
- Pushing before full cervical dilatation is reached compresses the cervix and may result in fetal distress or cervical edema.
- The nurse who is aware of sociocultural aspects of helping and coping acts as a protective agent for the woman in labor.
- The quality of the nurse-client relationship is a factor in the woman's ability to cope with the discomfort of the labor process.

Key Terms

- acme [of contraction] (p. 434)
- active phase [of labor] (p. 424)
- artificial rupture of membranes (AROM) (p. 441)
- bag of waters (BOW) (p. 427)
- bloody show (p. 424)
- breathing techniques (p. 455)
- counterpressure (p. 453)
- decrement [of contraction] (p. 434)
- duration [of uterine contractions] (p. 434)
- effleurage (p. 455)
- false labor (p. 425)
- first stage labor (p. 424)
- frequency [of uterine contraction] (p. 434)
- Hawthorn effect (p. 452)
- hyperventilation (p. 455)
- increment [of contraction] (p. 434)
- intensity [of uterine contraction] (p. 434)
- interval [of uterine contraction] (p. 434)
- jet hydrotherapy (p. 455)
- latent, or early, phase [of labor] (p. 424)
- modified Sims' position (p. 450)
- mucous plug (p. 432)
- Nitrazine test (p. 442)
- obstetric check (p. 427)
- partogram (p. 435)
- primary care practitioner (p. 424)

- prolapsed umbilical cord (p. 449)
- resting tone (p. 434)
- rupture of membranes (ROM) (p. 441)
- spontaneous rupture of membranes (SROM) (p. 437)
- transitional phase [of labor] (p. 424)
- transcutaneous electrical nerve stimulation (TENS) (p. 458)
- true labor (p. 424)
- uterine contractions (p. 433)

Critical Thinking Exercises

1. Compare the cervical dilatation and station of the fetal presenting part of a multiparous woman and a nulliparous woman during the first stage of labor.
   A. Examine how findings differ, whether they follow the normal labor curve, and how you account for any deviations.
   B. Identify nursing diagnoses and prepare a plan of care for each woman. Justify differences and similarities in the plans.

2. You are assigned to a laboring woman and her family who are culturally different from you.
   A. Compare their perceptions and beliefs about labor to your own.
   B. Analyze how these factors might affect the behavior of the woman, her family, and the nurse during the first stage of labor.
   C. How would you incorporate this knowledge into your plan of care?

Topics for Nursing Research

- Is there a difference in the length of the first stage of labor when a woman is allowed to ambulate as she pleases during her labor?
- Do women who consume an average of 100 mL/hr of fluids during the first stage of labor have lower temperatures at the beginning of the second stage of labor than women who neither receive IV hydration nor consume fluids regularly?
- Is there a difference in the timing of SROM in women who ambulate during the first stage of labor and those who do not?
- Is there a difference in the length of the first stage of labor for women who are allowed to shower or sit in a Jacuzzi than for women who do not bathe during labor?

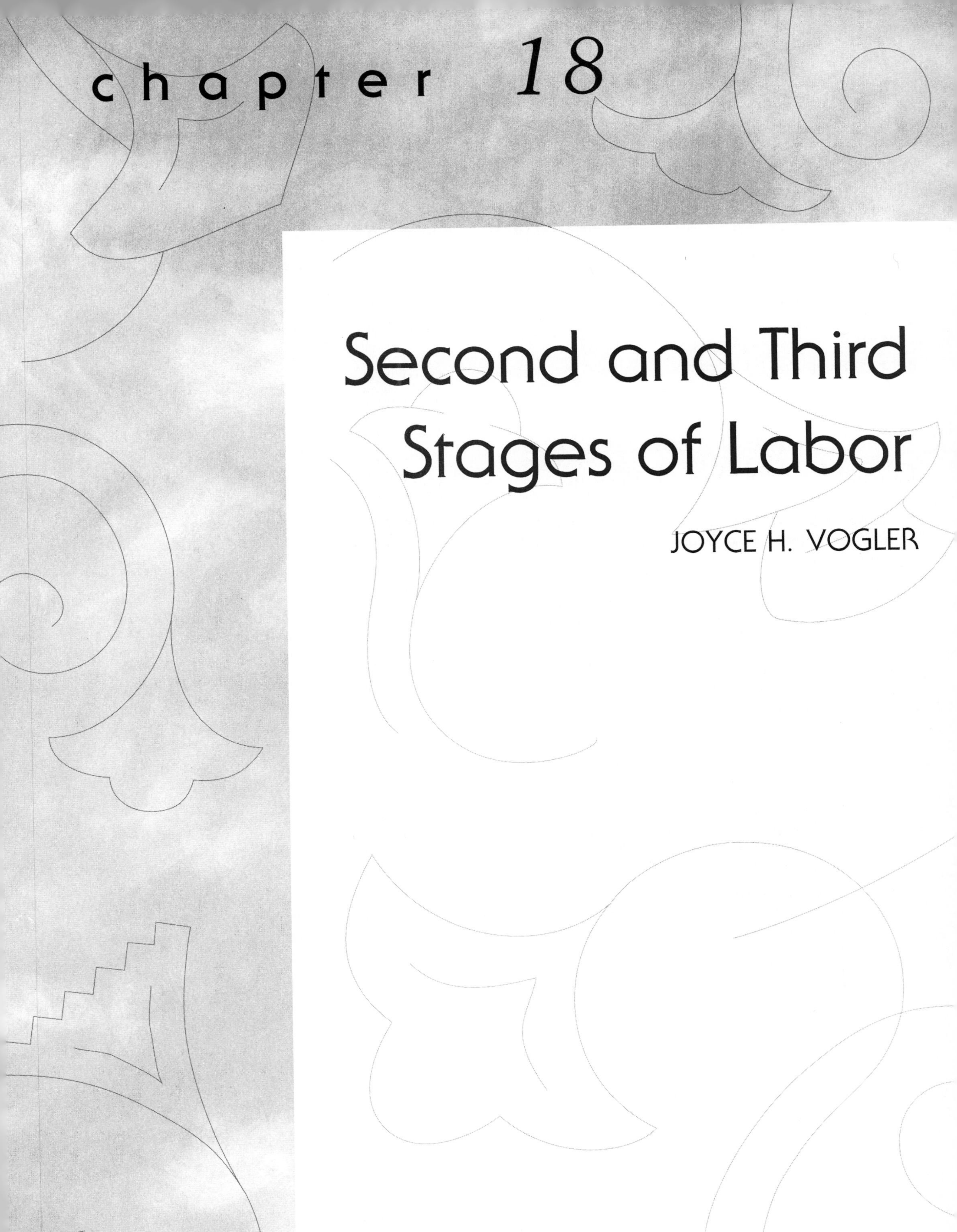

chapter 18

Second and Third Stages of Labor

JOYCE H. VOGLER

LEARNING OBJECTIVES

- Define the key terms listed.
- Describe assessment of the mother during the second stage of labor.
- Summarize the nurse's role with the mother and her family during the second stage of labor.
- Discuss assessment of the mother during the third stage of labor.
- Review the nurse's role with the new mother and her family during the third stage of labor.
- Discuss assessment of the neonate during the third stage of labor.
- Summarize the nurse's role with the neonate during the third stage of the mother's labor.
- Describe in detail and state in logical order the process of emergency childbirth.
- Outline the nurse's role in the care of the new mother who experienced an episiotomy or a laceration.
- Develop a complete nursing care plan for a woman and her family through the second and third stages of labor.
- Identify topics for nursing research related to the second and third stages of labor.

The journey through labor continues into the **second stage** and reaches its culmination at the end of the second stage when the process of new parenthood begins as the infant is born. The **third stage** is the period from the infant's birth until delivery of the placenta. This chapter covers the second and third stages of labor, outlining nursing care and responsibilities for women delivering in both traditional and alternative settings. During the third stage, nursing care shifts to support of the newborn's transition to extrauterine life, as well as monitoring the physical and psychosocial condition of the mother. The primary care practitioner may be involved with reestablishing skin integrity of the mother's perineum.

SECOND STAGE OF LABOR

The second stage of labor is the stage of expulsion of the fetus. It extends from full cervical dilatation (10 cm) through the birth of the baby. The three phases of the second stage are **latency/resting, descent,** and **final transition.** There is a rhythmic nature to the second stage of labor (Carr, 1983). The rhythm and movement emerge for the woman encouraged to listen to her body as she progresses through this stage. A woman normally will respond by changing body positions, pushing when she has an urge to push (Fig. 18-1), and vocalizing as she bears down. If a woman is confined to bed in a recumbent position, this rhythmic urge to push is lost. The rhythm also is lost if she is moved to another room and placed on a delivery table in the lithotomy position, as has been the custom in North America for the past 30 years. In most societies labor and delivery occur in the same room. In most non-Western societies women use a variety of positions for labor, such as kneeling, sitting, standing, or squatting. In Western society an active birth movement is developing in which women are asking for freedom of choice in relation to the position selected for both labor and birth.

"In the majority of cases, labor and delivery are physiologic processes, and do not, in the true sense, require 'management' " (Scott et al, 1990). In response to the question of whether the obstetrician should interfere with the process of labor during the second stage, Warrington (1842) replied, "He should let it alone if he has ascertained the position is correct."

ASSESSMENT

The only certain objective sign that the second stage of labor has begun occurs when, on vaginal examination, the examiner cannot feel the cervix (Myles, 1985). Other signs that suggest the onset of the second stage include the following:*

1. Sudden appearance of sweat on upper lip
2. An episode of vomiting
3. An increased bloody show
4. Shaking of extremities

*If the woman has an epidural block, she may not exhibit signs of being in the second stage.

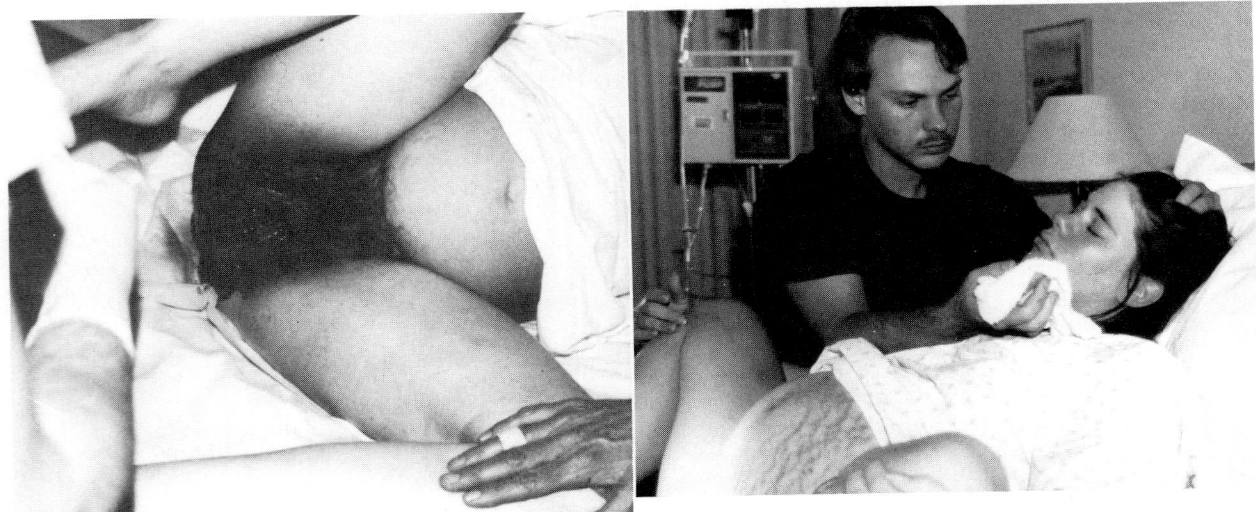

Fig. 18-1 **A,** Pushing, side-lying position, perineal bulging. **B,** Pushing, semi-sitting. Husband wiping woman's face with cool cloth between contractions.
Courtesy Marjorie Pyle, RNC, Lifecircle, Costa Mesa, Calif.

5. Increased restlessness; verbalization that "I can't go on"
6. Involuntary bearing-down efforts

These signs commonly appear at the time the cervix reaches full dilatation (Myles, 1985; Scott et al, 1990). Other indicators for assessing progress during each phase of the second stage can be found in Table 18-1.

Assessment is continuous during the second stage of labor. The specific type and timing of assessments are determined by hospital protocol.

In the second stage *each* contraction is monitored for frequency, strength, duration, intensity, and fetal response. Descent of the presenting part is confirmed by vaginal examination until the presenting part can be seen at the introitus. The degree of bladder filling is assessed because a full bladder can impede descent of the head and affect uterine contractions.

Maternal pulse and blood pressure are checked every 5 to 15 minutes. The blood pressure is obtained between contractions. The presence of amnesia between contractions may be noted. The partner's or father's response is assessed.

If the fetal heart rate (FHR) is monitored intermittently with a fetoscope, it is checked after every contraction or every 5 minutes. If continuous FHR monitoring is used (see Chapter 16), the nurse checks the tracings on the monitor with each contraction (AAP/ACOG, 1988). Observation of adequate variability is important in the presence of decelerations. Good variability indicates good fetal reserve. (See Chapter 16 for further discussion of variability.)

TABLE 18-1 Maternal Progress in Second Stage of Labor

Criterion	Latent/Resting (10-20 min)	Descent	Final/Transition
Contractions Magnitude (intensity) Frequency Duration	Period of physiologic lull for all criteria Period of peace and rest (Carr, 1983; Mahan, McKay, 1984)	Significant increase 2½ min 90 sec	Overwhelmingly strong Expulsive 2½ min 90 sec
Descent		Increases and **Ferguson's reflex*** activated	Rapid
Show: color and amount		Significant increase in dark-red bloody show	Fetal head visible at introitus; bloody show accompanies birth of head
Spontaneous bearing-down efforts	Slight to absent except with peaks of strongest contractions (Carr, 1983)	Increased urgency to bear down	Greatly increased
Vocalization		Grunting sounds or expiratory vocalization (Carr, 1983; Mahan, McKay, 1984)	Grunting sounds and expiratory vocalizations continue
Maternal behavior (Carr, 1983)	Experiences sense of relief that transition to second stage is finished Feels fatigued and sleepy Feels a sense of accomplishment and optimism, because the "worst is over" Feels in control	Senses increased urgency Alters respiratory pattern: has short 4 to 5 sec breath holds with regular breaths in between, 5-7 times per contraction Makes grunting sounds or expiratory vocalizations	Expresses sense of extreme pain Expresses feelings of powerlessness Shows decreased ability to listen or concentrate on anything but giving birth Describes **ring of fire†** Often shows excitement immediately after head emerges

**Ferguson's reflex,* Pressure of presenting part on stretch receptors of pelvic floor stimulates release of oxytocin from posterior pituitary, resulting in more intense uterine contractions.
†*Ring of fire,* Burning sensation of acute pain as vagina stretches and fetal head crowns.

Mild, brief bradycardia and decelerations can occur in 90% or more of women during the second stage of labor (Mahan, McKay, 1984). If recovery of the FHR from the deceleration is prompt after the contraction and expulsive forces cease, these episodes are not of major concern (Cunningham et al, 1989).

Protocols include assessment of show and amniotic fluid. Show is checked for evidence of excessive bleeding. Amniotic fluid is checked for meconium staining, odor, and amount (see p. 441). Amniotic fluid normally is odorless, but an odor can be detected when intrauterine infection (amnionitis) is present. Vaginal examinations are avoided or the number restricted whenever possible.

Duration of Second Stage

Considerable controversy exists over the precise duration of the second stage and the time limits that should be regarded as normal. Friedman's curves for nulliparous and multiparous women are commonly used to assess the progress of the second stage. A second stage of more than 2 hours in a first pregnancy and 1½ hours in subsequent pregnancies is considered abnormal and must be reported to a physician. Other factors that must be considered are the FHR pattern, the descent of the presenting part, the quality of the uterine contractions, and the fetal scalp blood pH (Mahan, McKay, 1984). On the basis of Friedman's data the range and average duration of the second stage of labor vary with parity:*

Parity	Range (min)	Average (min)
First pregnancy	25-75	57
Subsequent pregnancy	13-17	14.4

The nurse should be aware of the warning signs during labor (see Chapter 17, p. 443).

Yeates and Roberts (1984) compared the duration of the second stage when women engage in coached pushing or are allowed to push spontaneously when they feel the urge. Their findings are based on a small sample but suggest that spontaneous pushing may be the most effective aid in the descent and rotation of the newborn.

SIGNS OF POTENTIAL PROBLEMS. Prolonged second stage (see discussion above) is reported to the primary care practitioner. Signs and symptoms of impending birth (Table 18-1) may appear unexpectedly, requiring immediate action by the nurse.

*Duration of second stage may be prolonged for the woman who has had an epidural block, which causes loss of the bearing-down reflex.

NURSING DIAGNOSES

Nursing diagnoses lend direction to the nursing action needed to implement care. Before establishing diagnoses, the nurse analyzes the significance of the findings collected during assessment. Following are some nursing diagnoses indicating potential areas for concern during the second stage:

- High risk for injury to mother and fetus related to
  —Persistent use of Valsalva's maneuver
- Situational low self-esteem related to
  —Knowledge deficit of normal, beneficial effects of vocalization during bearing-down efforts
  —Inability to carry out birth plan for birth without medication
- Ineffective individual coping related to
  —Coaching that contradicts woman's physiologic urge to push
- Pain related to
  —Bearing-down efforts and distention of the perineum
- Anxiety related to
  —Inability to control defecation with bearing-down efforts
- Anxiety related to knowledge deficit regarding
  —Inexperience with reasons for perineal sensation
- High risk for injury to mother related to
  —Inappropriate positioning of mother's legs in stirrups
- Situational low self-esteem of father related to
  —Inability to support mother during final stage of labor

PLANNING

In both the second and third stages of labor, planning must be completed with speed and accuracy. Goals must be set and prioritized and may change as the second stage progresses. Nurses' ability and adaptability in relation to planning care will depend on their experience, which will influence their competence. A nursing plan of care for a woman in the second stage of labor is provided on p. 486.

Goals for the woman in second stage of labor may include that the woman will:

1. Actively participate in the labor process
2. Sustain no injury during the labor process (nor will the fetus)
3. Obtain comfort and support from family members of choice

IMPLEMENTATION

The nurse implements plans to monitor constantly the events of the second stage and mechanism of delivery, maternal physiologic and emotional responses to the second stage, the partner's response to the second stage, and fetal response to the stress of the second stage.

The nurse continues to provide comfort measures for the mother such as positioning, mouth care, maintaining clean, dry bedding, and avoiding extraneous noise, conversation, or other distractions (e.g., laughing, talking of attending personnel in or outside the labor area). The woman is encouraged to indicate other support measures she would like.

If the mother is to be transferred to another area for delivery, the nurse makes the transfer early enough to avoid rushing the client. The delivery area also is readied for the birth.

Prebirth Considerations

MATERNAL POSITION. The woman may want to assume various positions such as squatting (Supported Squatting, 1989; Gardosi et al, 1989; Andrews, Chrzanowski, 1990; McKay, Roberts, 1990). For this position a firm surface is required, and the woman will need side support. In a birthing bed a squat bar is available to assist (Fig. 18-2). Another position is the side-lying position with the upper part of the leg held by the nurse or coach or placed on a pillow. Some women prefer Fowler's position (can be attained with the support of a wedged pillow or with the father/partner supporting the woman). Others prefer the hands-and-knees or standing position when bearing down. When a woman is in the standing position, with weight being borne on both femoral heads, the pressure in the acetabulum will increase the transverse diameter of the pelvic outlet by up to 1 cm. This can be helpful if descent of the head is delayed as a result of failure of the occiput to rotate from the lateral (transverse diameter of pelvis) to the anterior position (Liu, 1989). The woman also may want to sit on the toilet to push because many women are concerned about stool incontinence during this stage. These women must be closely monitored and removed from the toilet before delivery becomes imminent.

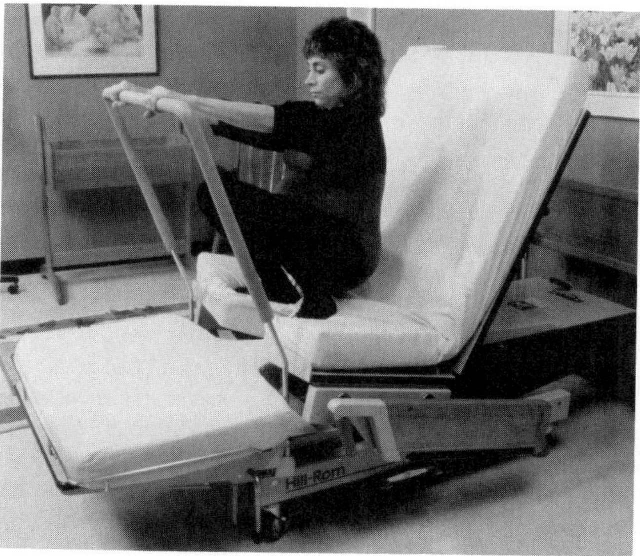

Fig. 18-2 Birth bed for a labor, delivery, recovery room (LDR) or labor, delivery, recovery, and postpartum room (LDRP).
Courtesy Borning Corp., Spokane, Wash.

BEARING-DOWN EFFORTS. As the fetal head reaches the pelvic floor, most women experience the urge to push. Automatically the woman will begin to exert downward pressure by contracting her abdominal muscles while relaxing her pelvic floor. This **bearing down** is an involuntary reflex response to the pressure of the presenting part on stretch receptors of pelvic musculature. A strong expiratory grunt may accompany the push (McKay, Roberts, 1990). When coaching women to push, the nurse encourages them to push as *they* feel like pushing rather than giving a prolonged push on command. The nurse monitors the woman's breathing so that the woman does not hold her breath more than 5 seconds at a time. Prolonged breath-holding may trigger **Valsalva's maneuver,** which results from the woman's closing the glottis, thereby increasing intrathoracic and cardiovascular pressure (Metzer, Therrien, 1990) (Fig. 18-3). In addition, holding the breath for more than 5 seconds diminishes the perfusion of oxygen across the placenta and results in fetal hypoxia. The nurse reminds the woman to take deep breaths to refill her lungs after each contraction.

To ensure slow birth of the fetal head, the nurse encourages the woman to control the urge to push. The urge to push is controlled by coaching the woman to take panting breaths or to exhale slowly through pursed lips as the baby's head crowns. The woman needs simple, clear directions from *one* coach.

Amnesia between contractions often is pronounced in the second stage, and the woman may have to be roused to cooperate in the bearing-down process. Parents who have attended parent education classes may have devised a set of verbal cues for the laboring woman to follow. It is helpful if they print

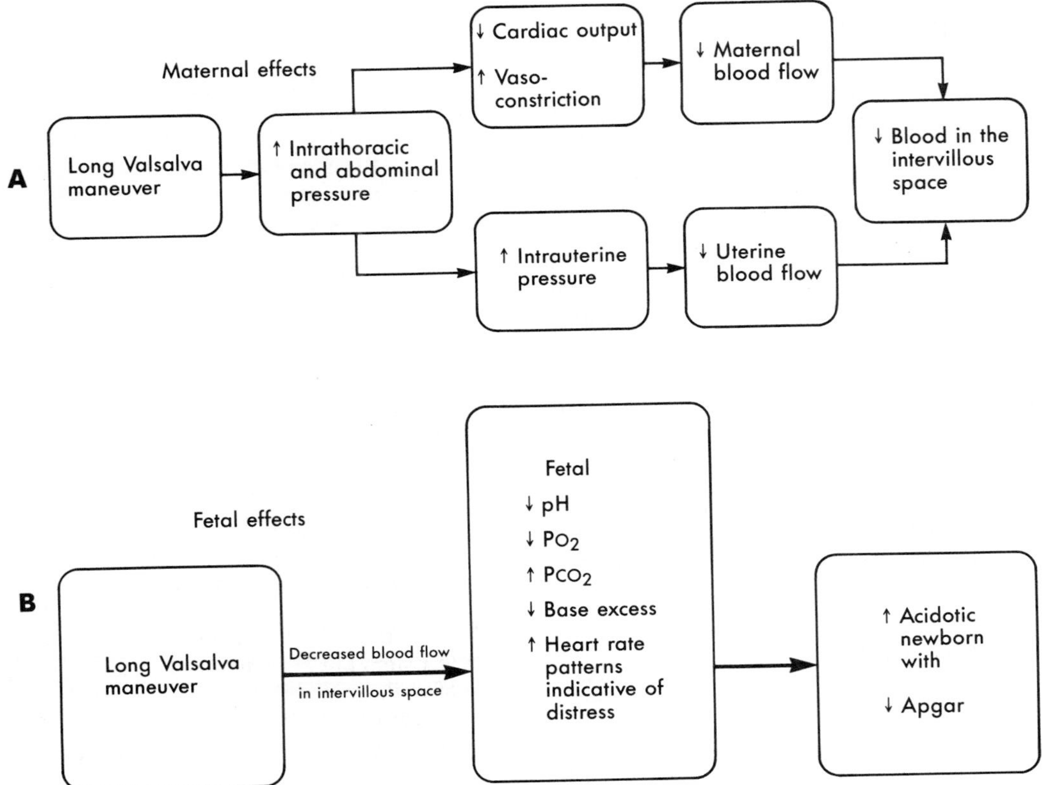

Fig. 18-3 Long Valsalva's push; possible effects to mother (A) and to fetus (B).
From Barnett M, Humenick S: Infant outcome in relation to second stage labor pushing method, *Birth* 9:221, Winter 1982.

these on a card that can be attached to the head of the bed so that the nurse can better substitute as coach if the partner has to leave.

FETAL HEART RATE. FHR must be checked as noted previously. If the rate begins to drop or if there is a loss of variability, prompt treatment must be initiated. The woman can be turned on her left side to reduce the pressure of the uterus against the ascending vena cava and descending aorta (see Fig. 17-9), and oxygen can be administered by mask at 10 to 12 L/min. This is often all that is required to restore the normal rate. If the FHR does not return to normal immediately, the physician should be quickly notified because medical intervention to hasten the birth may be indicated.

SUPPORT OF THE FATHER/COACH. During the second stage the woman needs continuous support and coaching. Because the coaching process can be physically and emotionally tiring for the father/coach (Jordan, 1990; Malestic, 1990; Queenan, 1990), the nurse can offer nourishment, fluids, and short breaks. The support person who is to attend the delivery in a delivery room is given instructions as to donning a cover gown, mask, hat, and shoe covers. Other information includes specifying support measures for the laboring woman and pointing out areas of the room in which the partner can move freely. If delivery occurs in a labor, delivery, recovery room (LDR) or a labor, delivery, recovery, postpartum room (LDRP), the partner usually can remain in street clothes (some come prepared to coach for pushing and panting) (Table 18-2).

BIRTHING BEDS AND CHAIRS. There is no single position for childbirth. Labor is a dynamic, interactive process among the mother's uterus, pelvis, and voluntary muscles. Angles between the baby and mother's pelvis constantly change as the infant turns and flexes down the birth canal. If able to, a mother will constantly change position in labor. The birthing bed (Fig. 18-4, p. 476) changes shape according to the mother's needs. The woman can squat, kneel, recline, or sit, choosing the position most comfortable for her (Kurokawa, Zilkoski, 1985). At the same time,

TABLE 18-2 Expected Responses and Support Person's Actions during Second Stage of Labor

Woman's Responses	Nurse/Support Person's Actions
LATENT/RESTING PHASE	
Experiences a short period (10-20 min) of peace and rest	Encourages woman to listen to her body (Carr, 1983) Continues support measures If descent phase does not begin after 20 min, suggests upright position to encourage progression of descent
DESCENT PHASE	
Senses increased urgency to bear down as Ferguson's reflex is elicited Notes increase in intensity of uterine contractions Demonstrates change in respiratory pattern (e.g., 5-sec breath-holds, 5-7 per contraction) Makes grunting sounds or expiratory vocalizations (see Research Highlight, p. 476).	Endorses respiratory pattern (short breath-holds with glottis closed) Stresses normality and benefits of grunting sounds and expiratory vocalizations Encourages pushing *with* urge to push Encourages/suggests maternal movement and position changes (upright, if descent is not occurring) If descent is occurring, encourages woman to listen to her body regarding movement and position change Discourages long breath-holding If transfer to a delivery room cannot be avoided, nurse transfers her early to avoid rushing or offers her option of walking to delivery room if permitted If descent is too fast, places woman in lateral recumbent position to slow descent (Carr, 1983)
FINAL/TRANSITIONAL PHASE	
Behaves in manner similar to transition during first stage (8-10 cm) Experiences a sense of severe pain and powerlessness (Carr, 1983) Shows decreased ability to listen Concentrates on delivery of baby until head is born Experiences contractions as overwhelming in intensity Reports "ring of fire" as head crowns Maintains respiratory pattern of 3 to 5, 5-sec breath-holds per contraction followed by forced expiration Eases head out with short expirations Responds with excitement and relief after head is born	Encourages slow, gentle pushing (Carr, 1983) Explains that "blowing away the contraction" facilitates a slower birth of the head Provides mirror or guides woman to see/touch emerging fetal head (best to extend over 2 to 3 contractions) to help her understand the perineal sensations Coaches relaxation of mouth, throat, and neck to relax pelvic floor Applies warm compresses to perineum to aid relaxation

there is excellent exposure for examination, electrode placement, fetal scalp sampling, and delivery. With the birthing bed the mother has full control of both seat and back functions and can adjust her position for maximum comfort. The mother and fetus can maintain a close personal contact and a new degree of involvement in the birth process if they desire. The bed can be positioned for administering anesthesia and can be used for transport to surgery in the event of a cesarean birth.

Birthing chairs also may be used and may provide women with a better physiologic position during childbirth, although some women feel restricted by a chair. Potentially there is both a physiologic and psychologic advantage to the upright position. The mother can see the birth as it occurs and also maintain *en face* contact with the attendant (Balaskis, 1983). Most chairs are designed so that if an emergency occurs, the chair can be adjusted to the horizontal or the Trendelenburg position. However, some evidence is offered for a higher incidence of postpartum hemorrhage when a chair is used. Coltrell and Shannahan (1986) also found that the pressure of the rim of the chair caused an increased risk of perineal edema, which may obstruct venous return from the perineal region.

In some hospitals oversize beanbag chairs are being used for both labor and delivery. These chairs mold around and support the mother in whatever position she selects. These chairs are of particular value

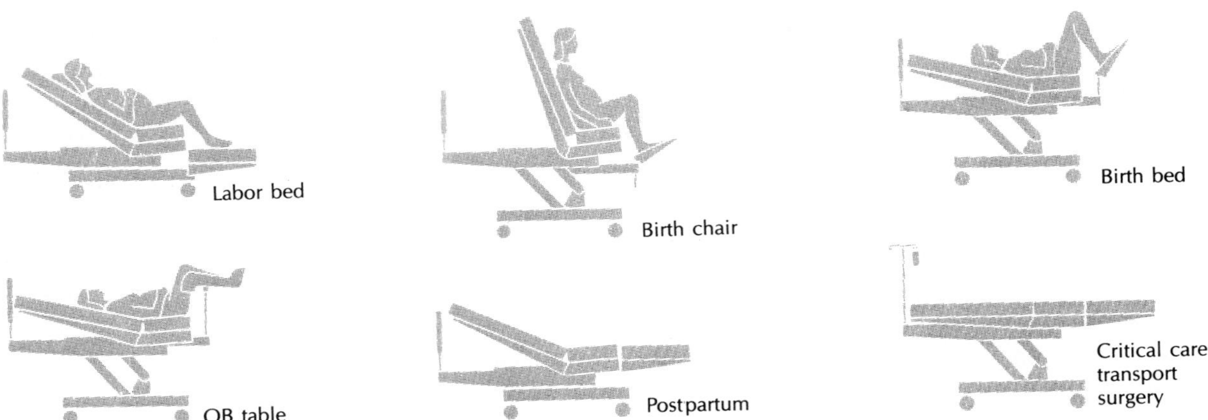

Fig. 18-4 Versatility of today's birthing bed makes it practical in a variety of settings.
Courtesy Hill-Rom.

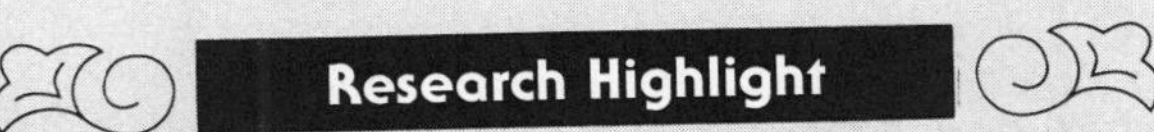

Meaning of Maternal Sounds during Second-Stage Labor

RESEARCH ABSTRACT

The purpose of this study was to examine the auditory perceptual skills used by caregivers in response to the behavioral cues of women in labor. Sixteen caregivers were interviewed: five certified nurse-midwives, four student nurse-midwives, five registered nurses, one obstetrics technician, and one lay midwife. All those interviewed were experienced labor attendants. Ten postpartum mothers also were interviewed about their responses to the experience. The caregivers listened to and watched videotapes of the second stage of labor in deliveries in which they had participated. They were interviewed about their perceptions of the experience. The 10 postpartum mothers viewed the videotapes and were interviewed about their responses to the videotapes. The researchers found that both caregivers and mothers clearly differentiated sounds of second-stage labor. Sounds and their significance were categorized as work/effort: adaptive/effective; coping: adaptive/self-comforting/soothing; childlike: emotions predominate/nonadaptive; out-of-control: emotions predominate/nonadaptive; and epidural anesthesia: body/mind split. Typical sounds of the categories were (1) work/effort—grunts, "uhhh," (2) coping—sighs, moans, (3) childlike—whimper, whine, (4) out of control—holler, yell, and (5) epidural anesthesia—quiet, normal conversation.

IMPLICATIONS FOR PRACTICE

Experienced caregivers can use the sounds of second-stage labor to judge progress. Open-glottis pushing allows for maternal grunting and making of other noises. There is some evidence that open-glottis pushing is more effective and safer for the mother and her fetus. When mothers are cautioned to refrain from making noise (vocalizing) when they push, valuable cues are lost to caregivers.

RELATED RESEARCH QUESTIONS

1. Will an education program focusing on sounds in labor increase the proportion of adaptive sounds?
2. Will the presence of a labor coach change the type of sounds made by a woman in labor?
3. Is there a relation between the type of sounds made in labor and length of labor?
4. Is there a relation between types of sounds made in labor and the perception of pain?

REFERENCE

McKay S, Roberts J.: Obstetrics by ear: maternal and caregiver perceptions of the meaning of maternal sounds during second stage labor, *J Nurse Midwife* 35:266, Sept/Oct 1990.

for mothers who seek active involvement in the birth process. Birthing stools also can be used (see Research Highlight, below).

Preparation for Birth in a Delivery Room

If the woman is to be transferred to a delivery area for completion of the birth process, the nurse uses the guidelines for transfer to the delivery room given on p. 479.

TIMING OF TRANSFER TO DELIVERY ROOM. Labor and delivery in the same room is becoming more common. Some hospitals, however, lack birthing rooms, and transfer during second stage is required. If birth is to occur in the delivery room, it is best to transfer the woman early enough to avoid a last-minute rush. For nulliparous women transfer can take place when the presenting part begins to distend the perineum. For multiparous women transfer should take place in the first stage, when the cervix is dilated 8 to 9 cm (Table 18-3, p. 479).

See also Table 18-2 for expected maternal behaviors during the descent phase of the second stage of labor.

If *any* laboring woman states, "The baby is coming!" the baby *is* coming, and it is too late for the transfer. The baby is coming *now,* and the nurse

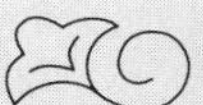 **Research Highlight** 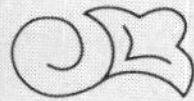

Birthing Stool or Semirecumbent Position for Second-Stage Labor

RESEARCH ABSTRACT

This study compared the effects of using a birthing stool or a semirecumbent position for vaginal delivery. At the end of the first stage of labor, 294 women with no fetal distress were randomly assigned to be encouraged to assume one of two birth positions: sitting on the birthing stool (experimental group) or lying in a semirecumbent position (control group). Two hours after delivery the women filled out a questionnaire describing their position, experience in this position, and preference for position in a future birth. The fathers completed a separate questionnaire about their experience, their satisfaction with their role, and whether they felt involved. Twenty-two midwives completed questionnaires about obstetric outcomes, birth position, partner's place, and their own posture during delivery. One half of the women actually delivered in the encouraged position. There were no differences in background characteristics between the two groups. There was no difference between groups in length of second stage of labor, but the estimated blood loss and the number of women with postpartum hemorrhage were greater in the experimental group. Length of active pushing was longer and use of oxytocin more frequent in the control group. There were more labial tears and vulvar edema in the experimental group. Women in the experimental group reported less pain and had a more positive delivery experience than did women in the control group. There were no group differences in Apgar scores of infants. Fathers in the experimental group felt more involved, supportive, and satisfied with their experience than did fathers in the control group. Some (14%) of the midwives described their posture during delivery as awkward.

IMPLICATIONS FOR PRACTICE

Alternative positions for delivery need continued investigation. Women who used the birthing stool, as well as their partners, reported satisfaction with the experience. However, half the women encouraged to use this position chose not to deliver on the birthing stool. Wishes of women must be respected, and efforts to decrease pain and distress in labor must continue. Health care providers must carefully document effects of alternative interventions.

RELATED RESEARCH QUESTIONS

1. Does blood loss differ in women who deliver in a squatting position as compared with women who use a birthing stool for delivery?
2. Does blood loss differ in women who deliver in a squatting position as compared with women who deliver in a semirecumbent position?
3. Is blood loss reduced by changing from a vertical to horizontal position immediately after delivery?
4. What is the effect of early ambulation on blood loss after delivery?

REFERENCE

Waldenstrom U, Gottvall K: A randomized trial of birthing stool or conventional semirecumbent position for second-stage labor, *Birth* 18(1):5, 1991.

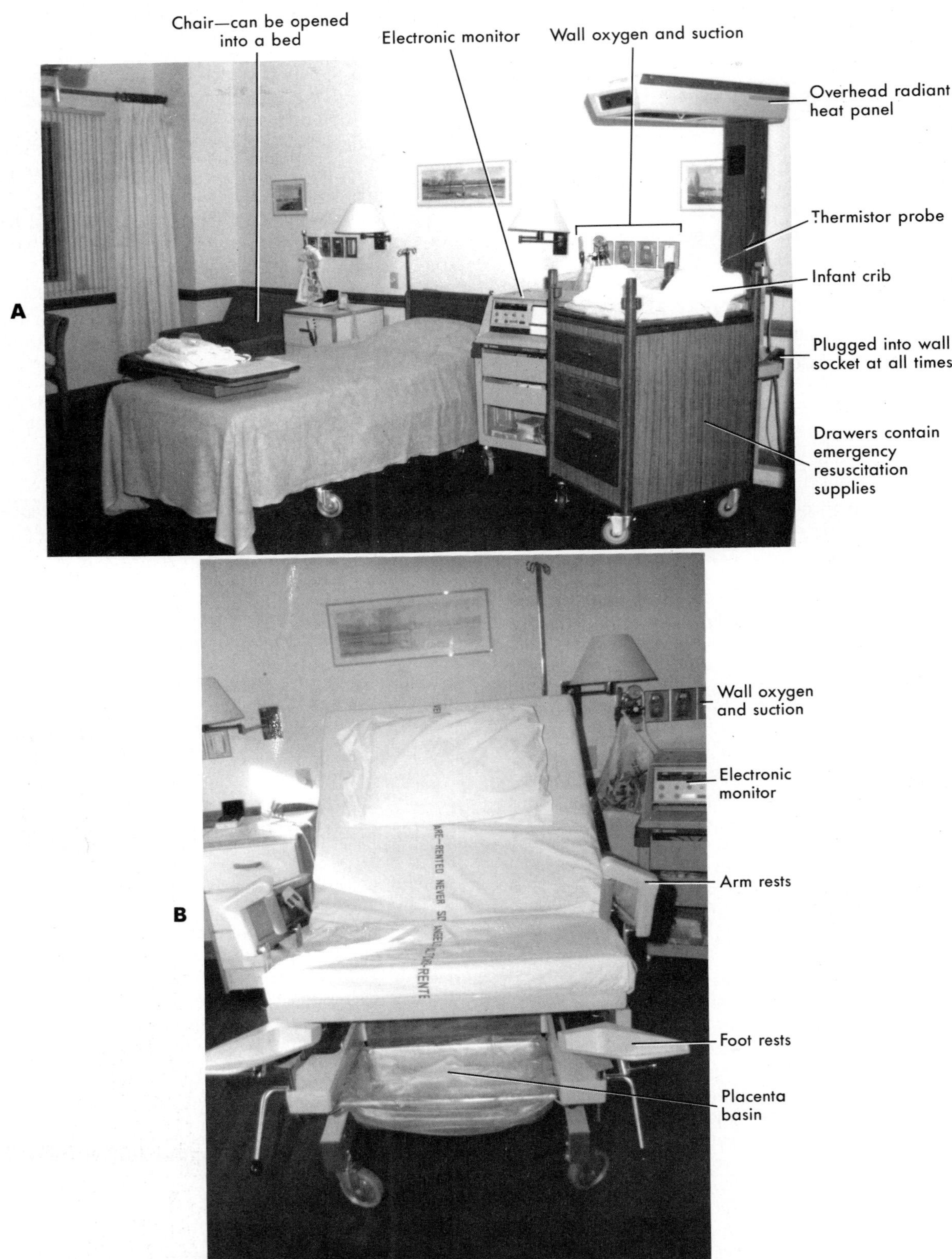

Fig. 18-5 Delivery room.

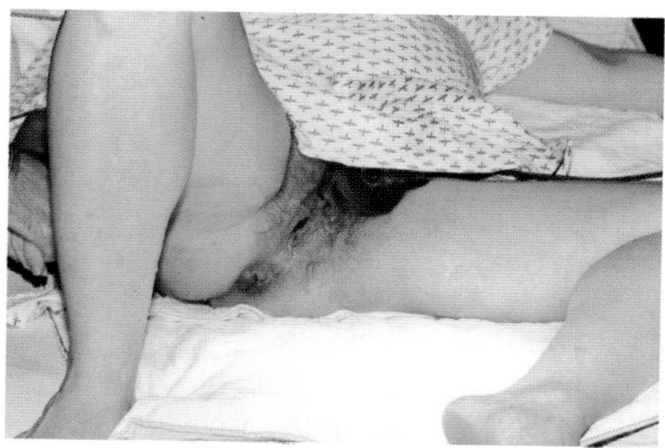

Plate 1 Anteroposterior slit. Vertex visible during contraction. Note fetal monitor.

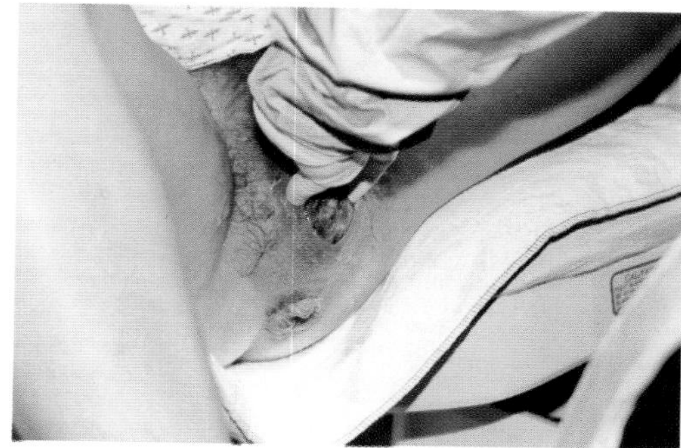

Plate 2 Oval opening. Vertex presenting.

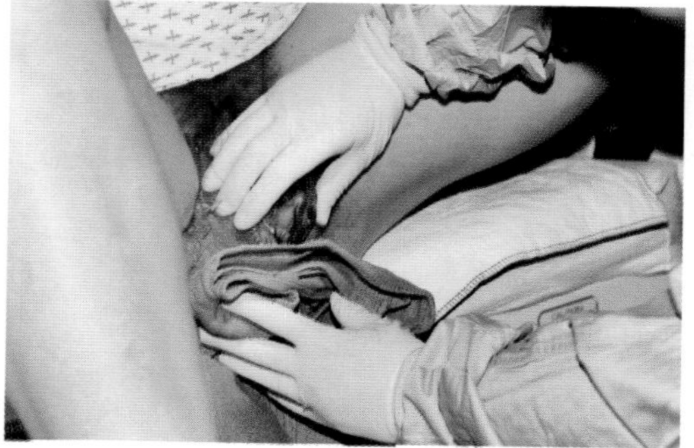

Plate 3 Circular shape. Midwife using Ritgen maneuver.

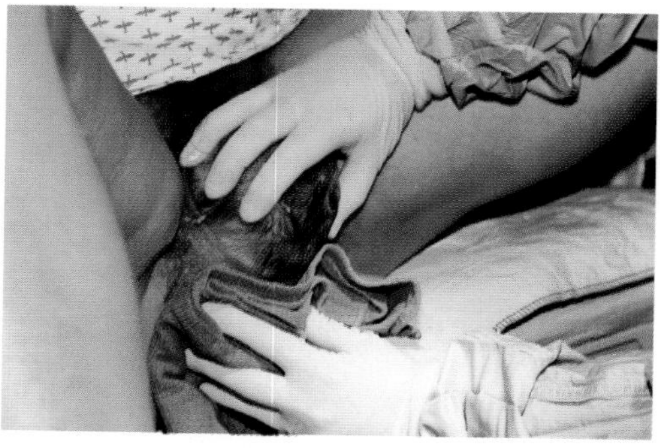

Plate 4 Crowning. Midwife continues with Ritgen maneuver as head is born by extension.

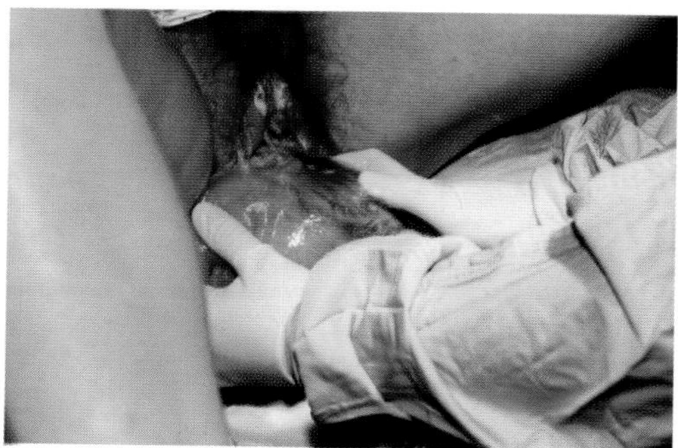

Plate 5 After checking for nuchal cord, midwife supports head during external rotation and restitution.

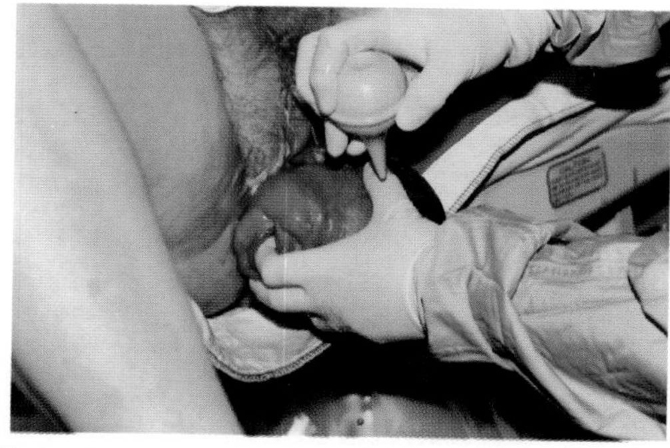

Plate 6 Use of bulb syringe to suction mucus.

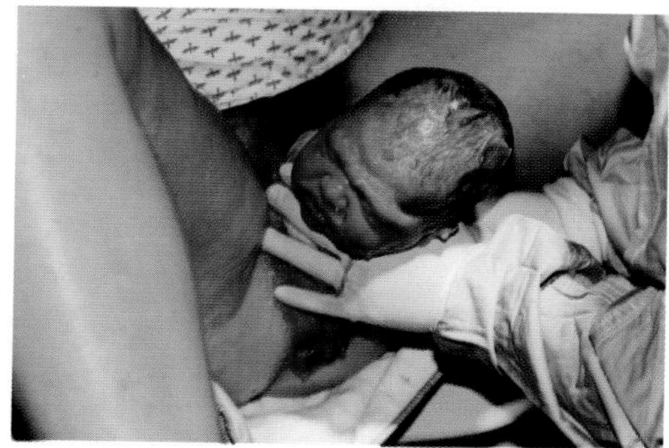

Plate 7 Birth of posterior shoulder.

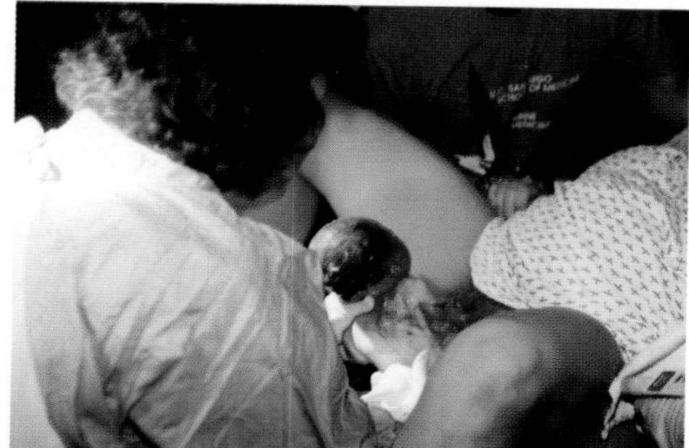

Plate 8 Birth by slow expulsion of fetus/newborn.

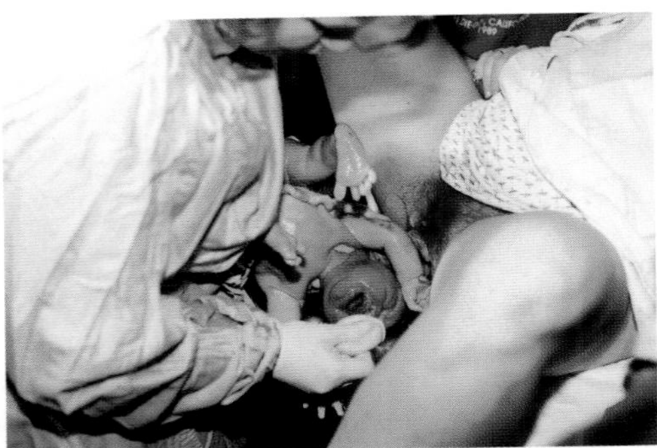

Plate 9 Second stage is complete. Newborn is supported in the head-down position while nasal and oral mucus is removed with a bulb syringe. Note that newborn is not completely pink yet.

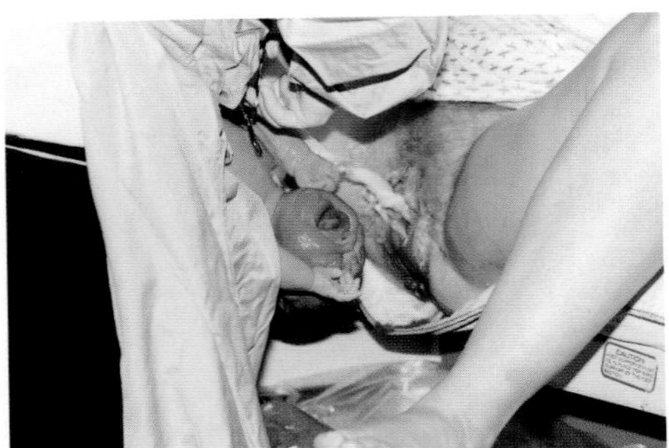

Plate 10 Cutting of the umbilical cord.

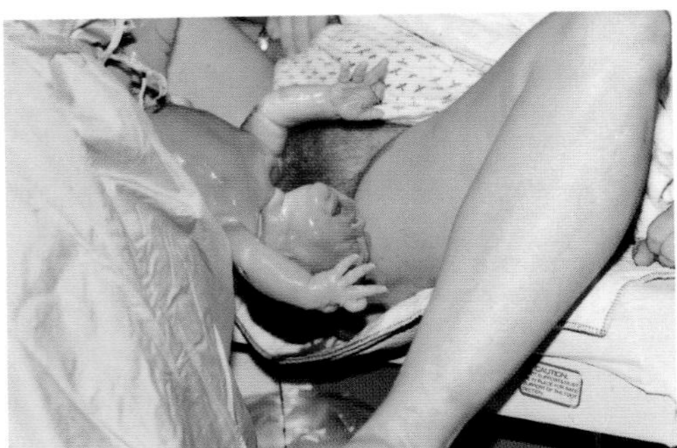

Plate 11 Newborn is now completely pink. Note increased vaginal bleeding as the placenta separates.

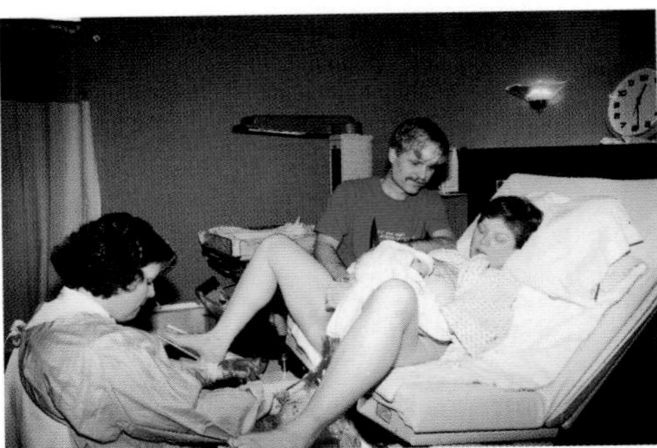

Plate 12 Newborn suckling at breast while midwife begins to deliver placenta. Note the intensity of the parents' gaze and their attentiveness to the newborn.

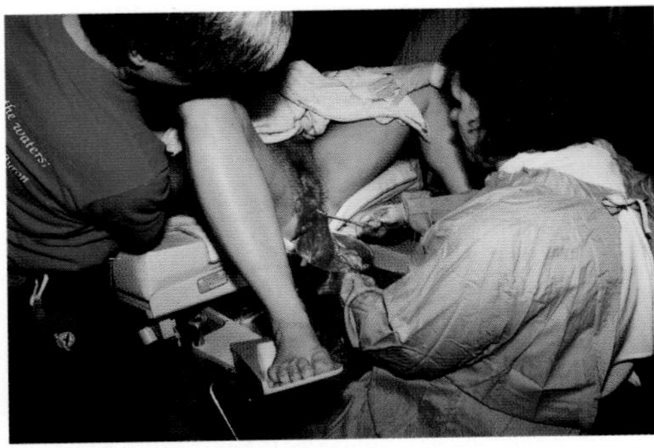

Plate 13 Delivery of placenta is complete, marking the end of the third stage of labor.

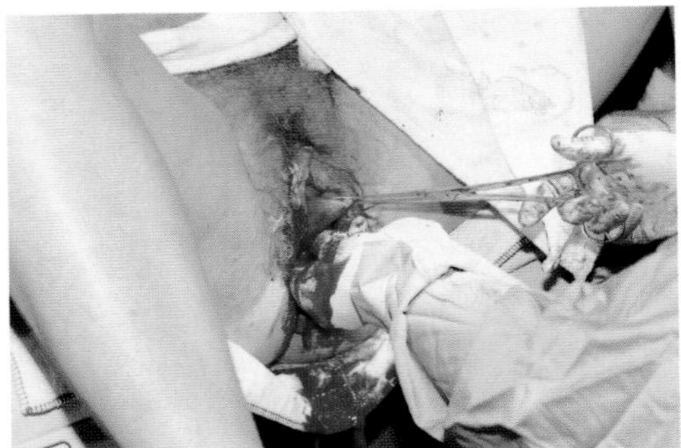

Plate 14 Assessment of the cervix for birth trauma.

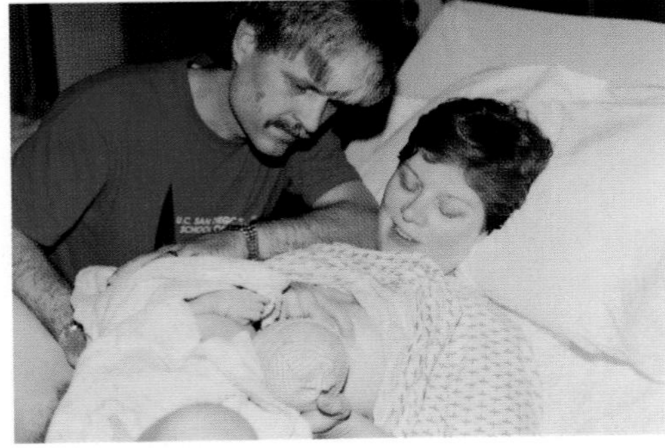

Plate 15 Parents are engrossed in their newborn, who is actively suckling at the breast.

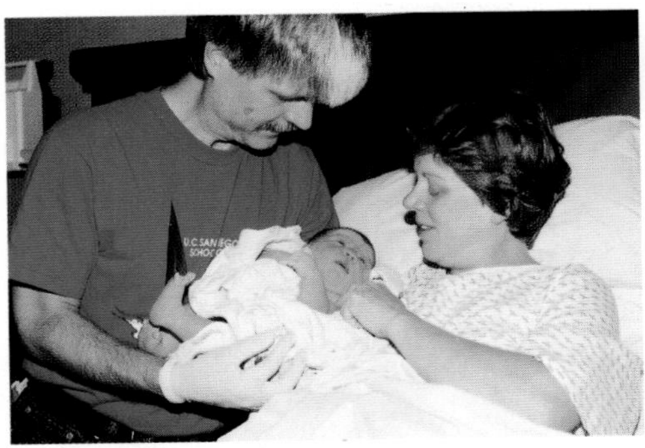

Plate 16 Father taking newborn to hold (newborn's cap fell off briefly).

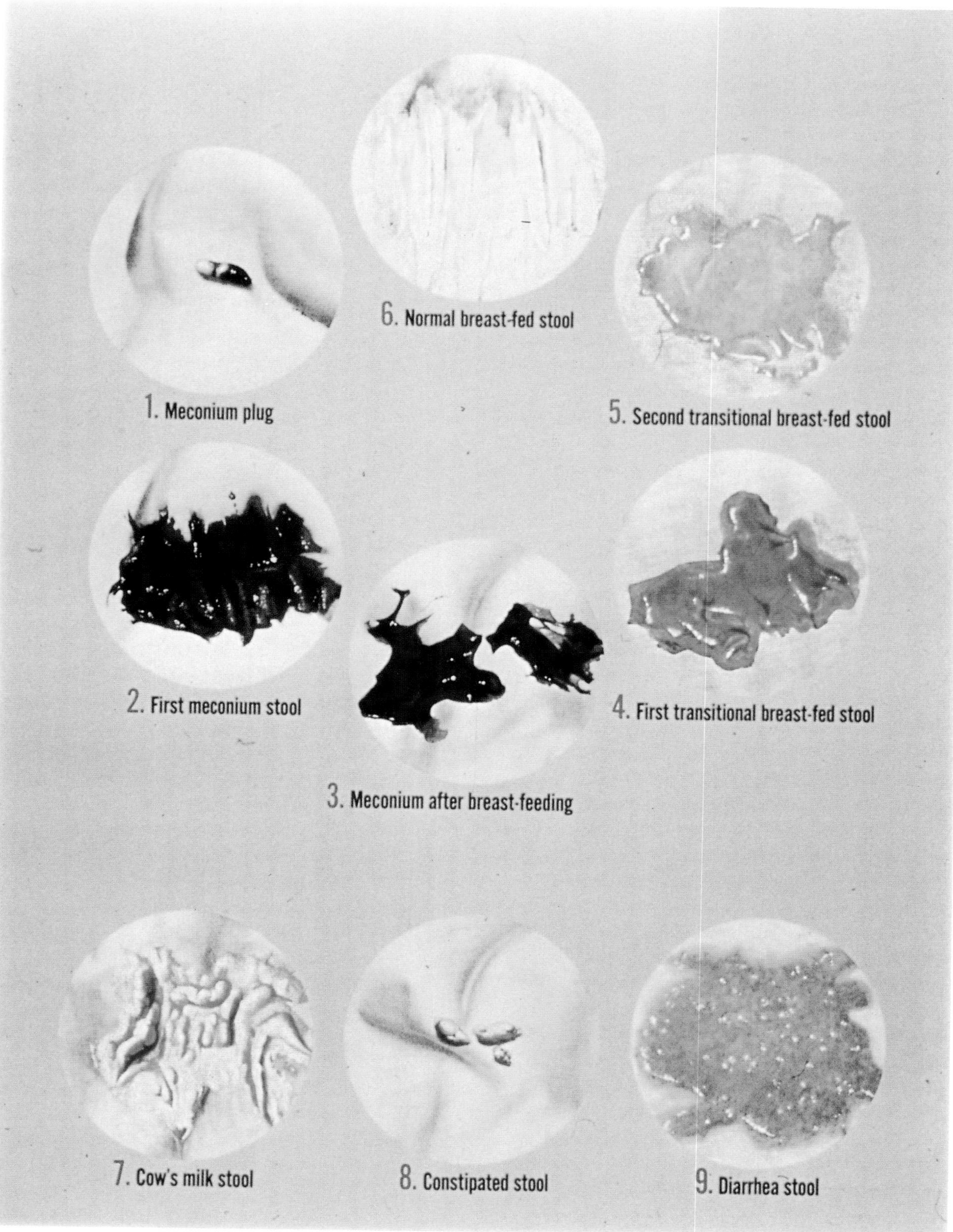

Plate 17 Normal stool cycle.
Reprinted with permission of Ross Laboratories, Columbus, OH 93126.

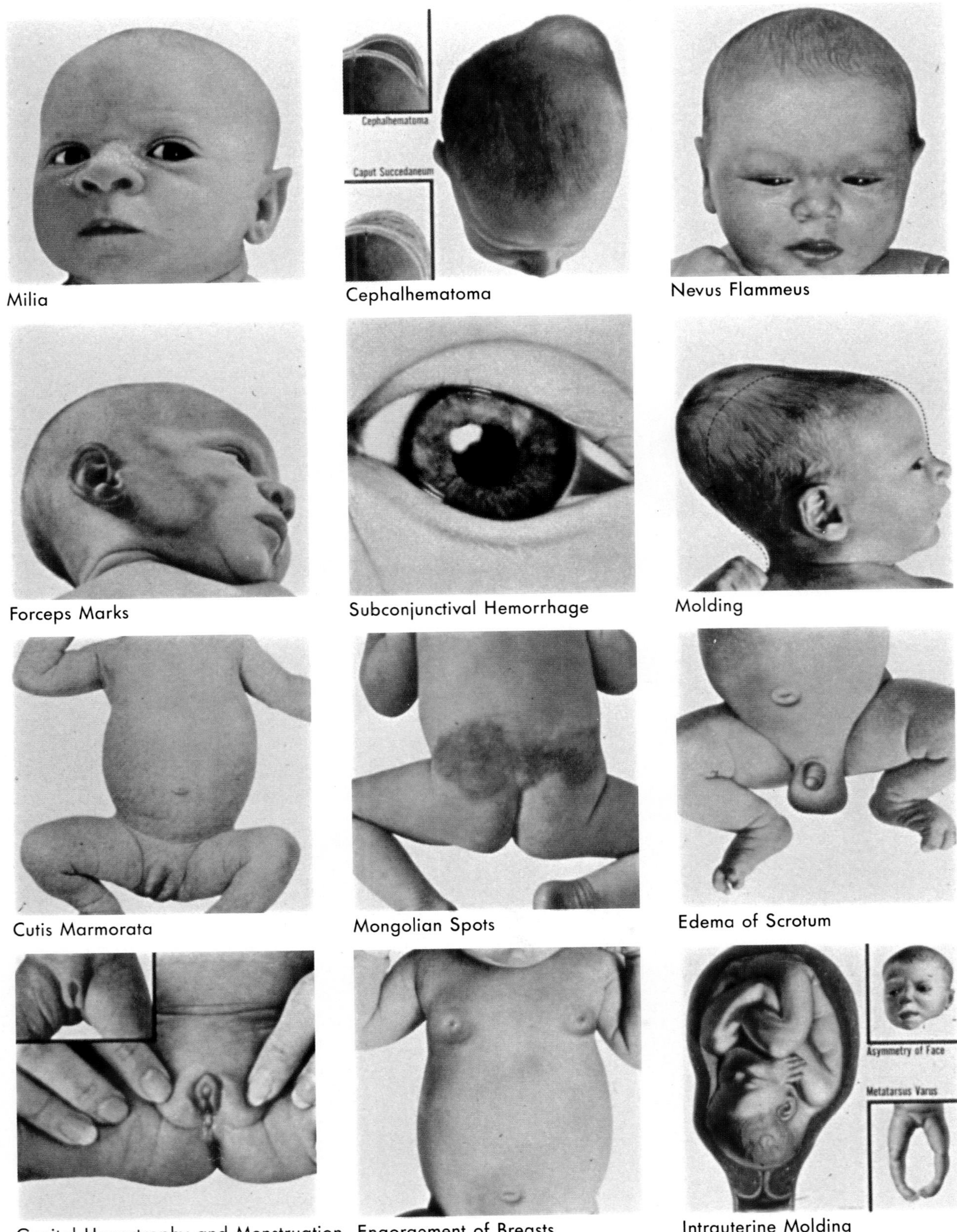

Plate 18 Common variations in the neonate.
Reprinted with permission of Ross Laboratories, Columbus, OH 93126.

TABLE 18-3 Transfer to Delivery Room

Parity	Stage	Characteristic
Nulliparous women	Second	When the presenting part begins to distend the perineum
Multiparous women	First	When the cervix is dilated to 8 to 9 cm

should prepare to assist her if the primary care practitioner is not yet present (see Emergency Childbirth, p. 483).

Recording of all vital signs and of labor progress must be done concurrently with care. The course of labor and maternal-fetal response may change without warning. It is of legal importance that all charting be accurate and complete. Charting is done in the labor record as well as on the monitor strip (for description of documentation on monitor strip, see Chapter 16, p. 415).

DELIVERY ROOM BIRTH TABLE. Delivery rooms are designed specifically to facilitate care during delivery (Fig. 18-5). The delivery table has many features: the entire table can be raised or lowered, and the head or foot may be raised or lowered. A wedge pillow or bolster can be inserted under the top of the mattress to raise it slightly, or the head of the table can be raised to prevent supine hypotension and to facilitate pushing. The table is equipped with stirrups for supporting the legs and handle grips to aid in bearing down. If stirrups are used, the bed can be "broken"; that is, the lower half of the bed can be lowered and rolled back to fit under the top half.

SUPPLIES, INSTRUMENTS, AND EQUIPMENT. The delivery table is prepared and instruments are arranged on the instrument table (Fig. 18-6). Standard procedures are followed for gloving, identifying and opening sterile packages, adding sterile supplies to the instrument table, and unwrapping and handing sterile instruments to the physician or nurse-midwife. The crib and equipment are readied for the support and stabilization of the infant (Fig. 18-5, *A*).

Birth in a Delivery Room or Birthing Room

The woman will need assistance to move from the labor bed to the delivery table. If this is done between contractions, the mother can help, but because of her awkwardness, she cannot be rushed.

The position assumed for birth may be **Sims' position** (if this is the case, the attendant will need to support the upper part of the leg), dorsal position, or lithotomy position.

The **lithotomy position** has been the position most commonly used for delivery in Western cultures although this is changing slowly. The lithotomy position makes it more convenient for the physician to deal with any complications that arise (Fig. 18-4). The buttocks are brought to the edge of the table, and the legs are placed in stirrups. Care must be taken to pad the stirrups, raise and place both legs simultaneously, and adjust the shanks of the stirrups so that the calves of the legs are supported. There should be no pressure on the popliteal space. If the stirrups are uneven in height, strained ligaments can develop in the woman's back as she bears down. This strain causes considerable discomfort in the postdelivery period. The lower portion of the table may be

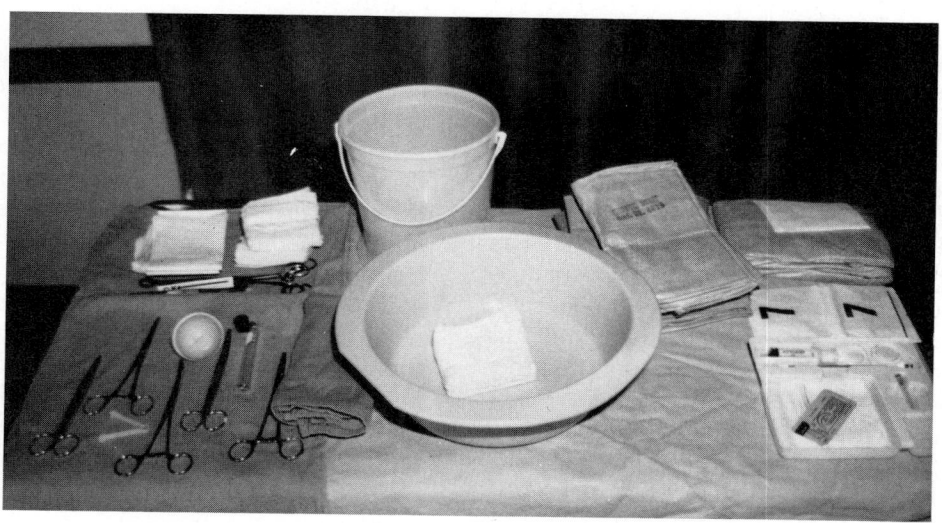

Fig. 18-6 Instrument table.

dropped down and rolled back under the table.

Once the woman is positioned for birth, the vulva is washed thoroughly with soap and water or sprayed with disinfectant to prevent bacterial contamination. A **mini-prep** may be performed at this time, shaving the area between the vagina and anus. Studies have shown that the presence of pubic hair does not increase the incidence of postpartum infection; thus shaving is not routinely done.

The physician or certified nurse-midwife dons cap and mask with shield or protective glasses/goggles, scrubs hands, and puts on the sterile gown (with waterproof front and sleeves) and gloves (see Universal Precautions, Chapter 29). The woman may then be draped with sterile towels and sheets. The partner helps the mother remember not to touch the sterile drapes.

The circulating nurse will continue to coach and encourage the woman. Once her legs are in the stirrups, the handle grips can be used to exert counterpressure. The nurse will check FHR for 30 seconds after every contraction or with continual electronic monitoring and notify the primary care practitioner as to the rate and regularity. The equipment for taking the blood pressure should be readied for instant use if signs of shock develop. However, the readings are distorted (increased) by the increase in thoracic and abdominal pressures as the woman pushes. A reading will be taken after delivery before transferring the woman to the recovery room. An oxytocic medication such as Pitocin may be prepared for administration after delivery. Observations and procedures are recorded on the chart.

Partners are encouraged to be present at the birth of their infants if this is in keeping with their cultural expectations. The psychologic closeness of the family unit is maintained, and the partner can continue the supportive care given in labor. The partner needs as much opportunity as does the mother to initiate the attachment process with the baby. Studies indicate, however, that it is the continuous long-term contact between father and child that acts to cement the bonds and that there is no immediate "magic moment" of bonding.

In some facilities, the partner is gowned in a clean scrub outfit and wears a cap and a mask. These supplies need to be provided in ample time for the person to don them before the birth. If the couple has decided that the partner is not to be present, their decision should be respected.

Contact with parents is maintained by touch, verbal comforting, instructions as to reasons for care, and sharing in parents' joy at birth of their child. The nurse notes and records the time of birth (i.e., when infant is born completely).

In many hospitals women have the opportunity to give birth without having to move to a birthing room or change beds (Machol, 1988). These settings can vary from a labor room of 60 to 80 square feet to a room the size of an operating room (300 to 350 square feet). The size of the setting dictates to a large degree who can attend the birth and what alternatives to traditional delivery room care can be offered. Women remain in these birthing rooms throughout labor, birth, recovery, and perhaps the postpartum period. A back table or case cart is set up with the items described in Chapter 17, p. 461, and Fig. 18-6. Position for delivery varies from that of lithotomy with legs in stirrups or feet resting on foot rests or squat bar to that of side-lying with legs propped up on a squat bar, which is part of the bed. The foot of the bed can be removed. This is done when the practitioner who is assisting at the birth specifies the need for better perineal access to perform episiotomy, for birth of a large baby, or for access to the emerging head to facilitate suctioning with a DeLee apparatus. Otherwise the foot of the bed is left in place and lowered slightly to form a ledge providing access for birth and a place to set the newborn infant. The primary care practitioner observes universal precautions and places drapes under the woman's buttocks.

Mechanism of Birth: Vertex Presentation

Most of the time the birth remains in the hands of the obstetrician or certified nurse-midwife. The time may come, however, when the nurse must assist the woman to give birth (p. 483). The nurse's knowledge of the birth process provides a basis for client preparation before and during delivery.

The nurse reviews with the woman or couple the cardinal movements of labor (see Chapter 14). Once the cervix is fully dilated, descent occurs. The vertex advances with each contraction and recedes slightly as the contraction wanes; descent is constant, and late in the second stage the head reaches the pelvic floor. *Bulging of the perineum* occurs during the **descent phase,** when the fetal presenting part is distending the perineum but is not yet visible at the introitus. The occiput generally rotates anteriorly, and with voluntary bearing-down efforts, the head appears at the introitus (Fig. 18-7 and Plates 1 to 3). Although more and more head may be seen with each push, **crowning** occurs when the head's widest part (the biparietal diameter) distends the vulva just before birth (Plate 4). Immediately before delivery, the perineal musculature becomes greatly distended. If an **episiotomy** is necessary, it is done at this time to minimize soft tissue damage (p. 496). The head is

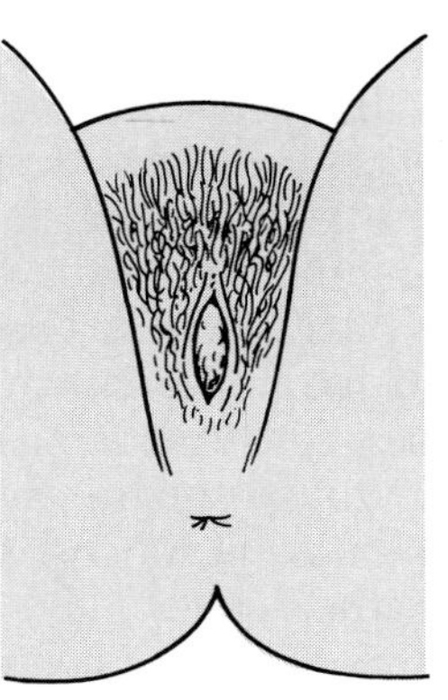
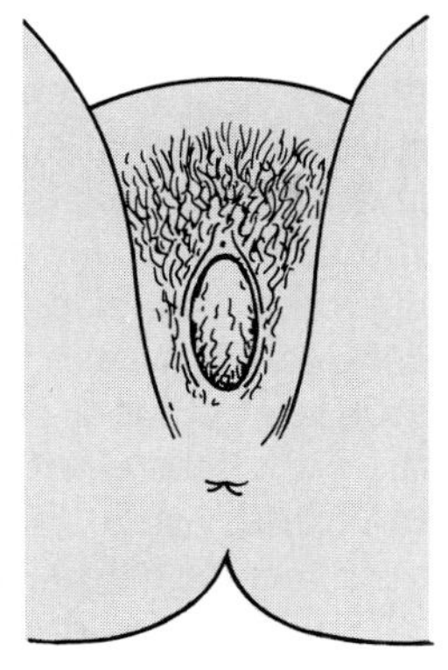
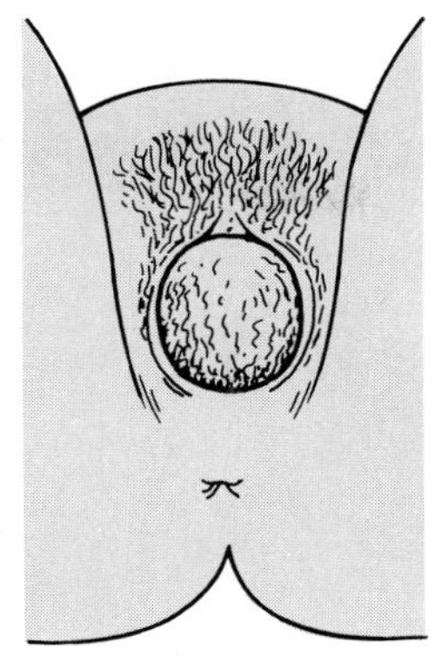
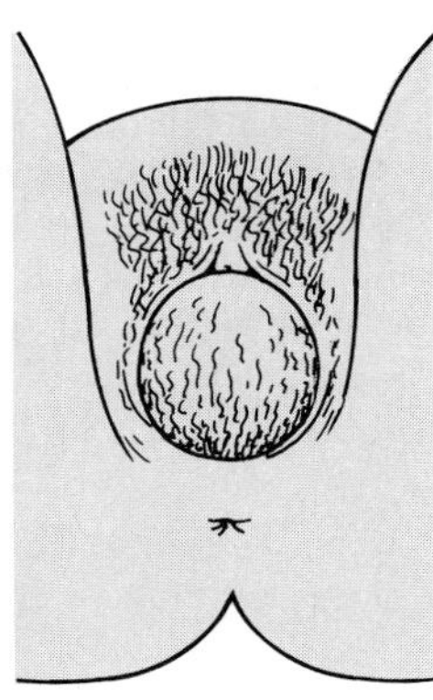

Fig. 18-7 Beginning birth with vertex presenting. **A**, Anteroposterior slit. **B**, Oval opening. **C**, Circular shape. **D**, Crowning.

born by extension and after birth restitutes with the shoulders (Plate 5). Interiorly the shoulders rotate into the anteroposterior diameter of the pelvis; external rotation of the head is observed. The body is born by lateral flexion.

The three phases of a spontaneous birth of the fetus in a vertex presentation are (1) birth of the head, (2) birth of the shoulders, and (3) birth of the body and extremities.

BIRTH OF HEAD. The vertex first appears, followed by the forehead, face, chin, and neck. The speed of the birth of the head must be controlled, or sudden birth of the head may cause severe **lacerations** through the anal sphincter or even into the rectum (p. 497). The physician or certified nurse-midwife controls the birth of the head by (1) applying pressure against the rectum, drawing it downward to aid in flexing the head as the back of the neck catches under the symphysis pubis; (2) then applying upward pressure from the coccygeal region (modified **Ritgen maneuver**) (Fig. 18-8 and Plates 3 and 4) to extend the head during the actual birth, thereby protecting the musculature of the perineum; and (3) assisting the mother with voluntary control of the bearing-down efforts by coaching her to pant. In addition to protecting the maternal tissues, gradual birth is imperative to prevent fetal intracranial injury.

The membranes may not be ruptured before delivery. During birth of the head these membranes look like a hood covering the head. This hood of intact amniotic membranes covering the head during birth is known as a **caul.** In Scotland a child born with a caul is thought to be gifted with "second sight."

The umbilical cord often encircles the neck (**nuchal cord**) but rarely so tightly as to cause hy-

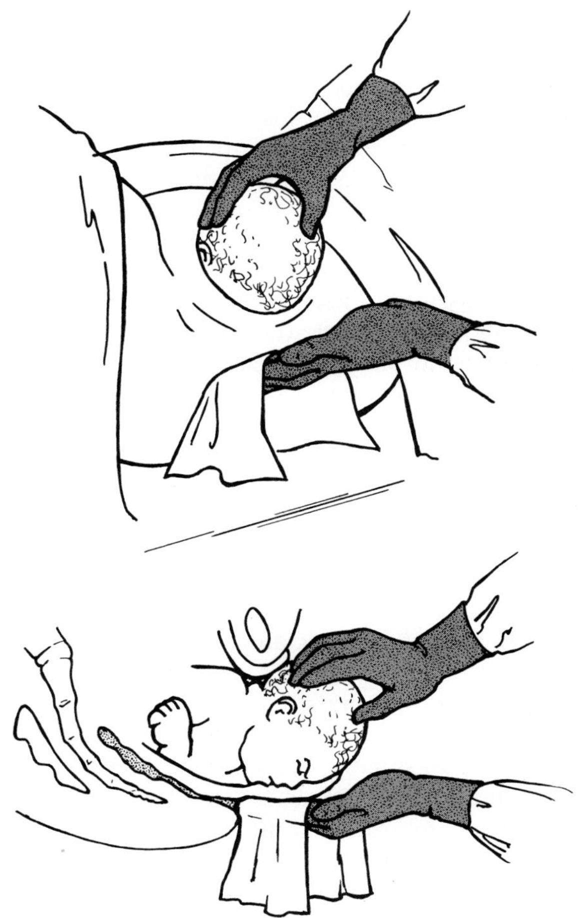

Fig. 18-8 Birth of head by modified Ritgen maneuver. Note control to prevent too-rapid birth of head.

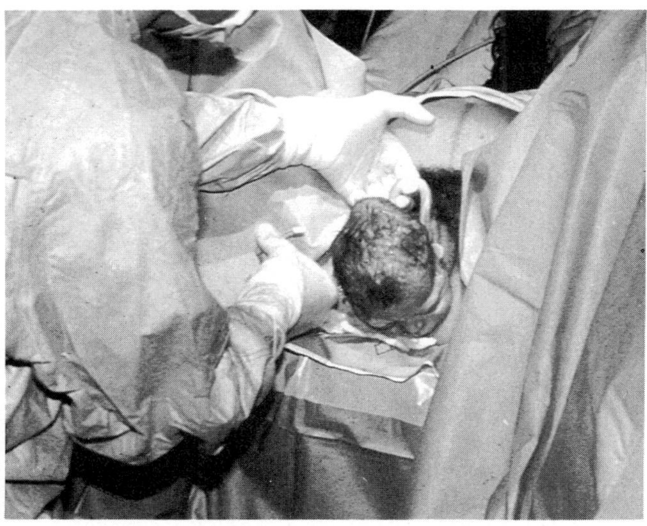

Fig. 18-9 Loosening nuchal cord (umbilical cord around neck).
Courtesy Marjorie Pyle, RNC, Lifecircle, Costa Mesa, Calif.

poxia. The cord should be slipped gently over the head (Fig. 18-9). If the loop is tight or if there is a second loop, the cord is clamped twice, severed between the clamps, and unwound from around the neck before the delivery is continued. Mucus, blood, or meconium in the nasal or oral passages may prevent the newborn from breathing. Moist gauze sponges are used to wipe the nose and mouth. A bulb syringe is inserted into the mouth and oropharynx first to aspirate contents (Plate 6). Next, the nares are cleared while the head is being supported (see discussion of suctioning the neonate, Chapter 21).

If, during labor, meconium has been present in the amniotic fluid, a DeLee suction apparatus is placed on the sterile field and wall suction is prepared. Thus, when the primary care practitioner is preparing for birth of the head, the old DeLee device is connected to the suction tubing. Birth is a time when nurses and physicians are exposed to a great deal of blood and fluid, and observation of universal precautions in hospitals reinforces the recommendation that the birth attendant wear a mask equipped with an eye shield. In addition, the practitioner should refrain from using the old DeLee device and oral suction to withdraw fluid from the infant. Instead, wall suction or oral suction using the new DeLee device is recommended (see Fig. 21-4). Perinatal infections most often are transmitted through contact with body fluids. Thus it is important for any health care worker to wear gloves when coming in contact with body fluids from the woman giving birth or when touching her baby.

BIRTH OF SHOULDERS. Before the shoulders can be born, they must engage in the pelvic inlet. Internal rotation of the shoulders, accompanied by restitution and external rotation of the head, occurs, and the shoulders now lie in the anteroposterior diameter of the inlet (see also Fig. 14-19, *E* and *F*). The shoulders can now pass through the pelvic cavity. While awaiting rotation, the primary care practitioner wipes the baby's face with sterile gauze squares and uses the bulb syringe to clear the nose of mucus in readiness for the baby's first breath.

The head is drawn downward and backward by the primary care practitioner to help the anterior shoulder impinge beneath the arch of the symphysis and slide beneath the pubic arch. Normally the anterior shoulder is delivered with this slight downward traction toward the perineum. The posterior shoulder distends the perineum, and to prevent perineal trauma, the head is lifted toward the symphysis pubis, the shoulder being delivered over the perineum (Myles, 1985) (Plate 7).

USE OF FUNDAL PRESSURE. The increased use of alternative positions for pushing has decreased the use of fundal pressure. Alternative positioning assists in fetal descent. In some cases in which regional or conduction anesthesia (epidural) is used, fundal pressure may be needed because of decreased maternal expulsive power. If fundal pressure is needed, a *skilled* nurse, in collaboration with the primary care practitioner, performs the procedure. Fundal pressure may be used when there is slight shoulder dystocia (see p. 1048 and Research Highlight, p. 483).

BIRTH OF BODY AND EXTREMITIES. Expulsion is controlled so that it occurs slowly. Lateral flexion is continued, the weight of the baby is supported by the primary care practitioner's lower hand (Plates 8 and 9), again to prevent perineal trauma. Slight rotation of the body to the right or left may be used to facilitate the birth. The time of birth is considered the precise time when the entire body is out of the mother. This must be recorded on the record.

The cord may be clamped at this time, and the primary care practitioner may ask if the woman's partner desires to cut the cord (Plate 10). If so, the practitioner will provide a clean pair of scissors and give instructions to cut the cord 1 inch above the clamp.

Siblings during the Second Stage

A young child may become frightened by the intensity of the second stage. Sights such as rupture of the membranes and sounds such as their mother's moans, screams, and grunts can be unsettling (Quinlan, 1983). It is not uncommon for a woman to say

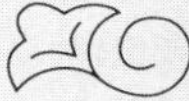
Research Highlight
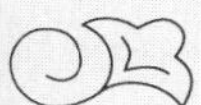

Use of Fundal Pressure during Delivery

RESEARCH ABSTRACT

The purpose of this study was to determine whether the use of fundal pressure during second-stage labor is accepted as part of nursing practice. Fundal pressure most often is used when there is shoulder dystocia. Nurses usually have no training in how to apply fundal pressure, and requests to apply fundal pressure usually occur under urgent conditions. A nationwide survey was mailed to 250 hospitals with obstetric services, randomly selected from all birthing centers and obstetric facilities in the nation. Seventy-four responses were received (30% response rate). Eighty-four percent of the respondents used fundal pressure. In some instances nurses applied the pressure; in other instances only physicians were responsible for fundal pressure. Few complications were noted: one respondent reported uterine rupture and nine respondents reported vaginal or cervical lacerations. Recording fundal pressure varied: 52% did not document the use of fundal pressure, 11% recorded it in the progress notes, 18% in the nursing notes, 9% in both medical and nursing notes, and 5% did not respond to the question. Nurses received no formal education in how to apply fundal pressure. No standard technique for the application of fundal pressure is available, and no current legal, professional, or regulatory standards for such application exist.

IMPLICATIONS FOR PRACTICE

Nurses with little or no knowledge or experience in application of fundal pressure may be requested to apply fundal pressure in emergency situations. Obstetric services should consider conducting an educational program on techniques of applying fundal pressure for nurses working in the labor suite. Some standardization of technique would be appropriate for individual units. Records should be kept of occurrences in which the primary care practitioner believed that fundal pressure was necessary, the technique used, length of time application occurred, and outcome of the delivery. With careful record keeping, standards can be developed and safety of women in labor enhanced.

RELATED RESEARCH QUESTIONS

1. What are indications for fundal pressure?
2. Does the use of fundal pressure vary by institution: public, private, teaching?
3. What is the incidence of complications from application of fundal pressure that resulted in a charge of medical or nursing negligence?
4. What is the response of the mother to fundal pressure during delivery?

REFERENCE

Kline-Kaye V, Miller-Slade D: The use of fundal pressure during the second stage of labor, *JOGGN* 19:511, Nov/Dec 1990.

things during the second stage and birth that she would not say otherwise and that might scare her child, such as "I can't take any more, take this baby out of me" or "This pain is killing me, I'm going to die." The child present during birth needs someone to be close and to give explanations simply and calmly. The child may want to be held.

Hospitals are more supportive of siblings' participation in the birth experience than in previous years. Organized sibling preparation classes now provide orientation to the birth environment, which is required for a sibling to attend the birth. Age limits, which vary, usually are set. However, most hospitals will not allow children younger than 3 years to attend the birth. Many hospitals deal with sibling attendance on an individual basis, taking into consideration the child's age, maturity, and preparation. Long-term effects on young children witnessing birth are not yet known.

An alternative to sibling presence at birth is for a trusted person to remain with the sibling in the waiting area until after the birth. At that time the child can be brought into the room and see the baby being held by the mother, who has become her "normal" self again.

Emergency Childbirth

Even under the best of circumstances there probably will come a time when the perinatal nurse will be required to deliver an infant without any medical assistance. Consider the multiparous woman who arrives at the community hospital fully dilated during the middle of the night. Because it is impossible to prevent an impending birth, the perinatal nurse needs to be able to function independently and also needs to be skilled in safely delivering a vertex fetus.

VERTEX PRESENTATION. The following measures are necessary for the emergency birth of a fetus in the vertex position:

1. The woman will usually assume the position most suitable for her. If she is in a bed and there is time, elevate the head of the bed about 45 degrees. This position, in addition to facilitating perfusion of the uterus, allows you to maintain eye-to-eye contact with the woman. Occasionally the woman will assume the crawling position, on hands and knees. Some women will stand and lean over a bed or their support person's shoulder. Others will assume a side-lying position.
2. Reassure the woman verbally with eye-to-eye contact and a calm, relaxed manner. If there is someone else available (e.g., the partner), that person could help support her in position, assist with coaching, and compliment her on her efforts.
3. Wash your hands with soap and water or wash-and-dry pledgets if possible.
4. Place under woman's buttocks whatever clean material is available. *Do not* "break" the table if no physician is available.
5. Avoid touching the vaginal area to decrease the possibility of infection. (If there is time, scrub your hands and fingernails for 5 minutes before touching the woman.) If hands are clean or sterile gloves are available, massage or support perineum as needed. Use Universal Precautions for body fluids at all times (see Chapter 29).
6. The perineum thins and distends. As the head begins to crown, the birth attendant should do the following:
   a. Tear the amniotic membrane (**caul**) if it is still intact.
   b. Instruct the woman to pant or pant-blow, thus avoiding the urge to push.
   c. Place the flat side of the hand on the exposed fetal head and apply *gentle* pressure toward the vagina to prevent the head from "popping out." The mother may participate by placing her hand under yours on the emerging head.
   NOTE: Rapid delivery of the fetal head must be prevented because it is followed by a rapid change of pressure within the molded fetal skull, which may result in dural or subdural tears, and it may cause vaginal or perineal lacerations.
7. Instruct the mother to pant or pant-blow as you check for an umbilical cord. If the cord is around the neck, try to slip it up over the baby's head or pull *gently* to get some slack so that it can slip down over the shoulders.
8. Support the fetal head as restitution (external rotation) occurs (Plate 5). After restitution, with one hand on each side of the baby's head, exert *gentle* pressure downward so that the anterior shoulder emerges under the symphysis pubis and acts as a fulcrum; then as *gentle* pressure is exerted in the opposite direction, the posterior shoulder, which has passed over the sacrum and coccyx, is delivered.
9. Be alert! Hold the baby securely because the rest of the body may emerge quickly. The baby will be slippery!
10. Cradle the baby's head and back in one hand and the buttocks in the other, keeping the head down to drain away the mucus (Plate 9). Use a bulb syringe to remove mucus if one is available.
    NOTE: Do not hold the baby upside down by the ankles because to do so (a) hyperextends the spine, which has been flexed since conception, (b) increases intracranial pressure and the danger of capillary rupture, (c) may cause direct tissue trauma to the ankles, and (d) increases the possibility of dropping a wet, slippery baby.
11. Dry the baby rapidly (to prevent rapid heat loss), keeping the baby at the same level as the mother's uterus.
    NOTE: Keep the baby at the same level to prevent gravity flow of baby's blood to or from the placenta and the resultant hypovolemia or hypervolemia. Also, do not "milk" the cord: hypervolemia can cause respiratory distress initially or hyperbilirubinemia subsequently (see Chapter 38). Also, if isoimmunization has occurred, the baby may receive an additional inoculation of harmful antibodies (e.g., anti-Rh positive or anti-A or anti-B antibodies).
12. As soon as the infant is crying, place the baby on mother's abdomen, cover baby (remember to keep head warm too) with her clothing, and have her cuddle baby. Compliment her (them) on a job well done and on the baby if appropriate. (If something appears to be the matter with the baby, do not lie!) She may wish to expose the part of the baby that will be touching her skin for skin-to-skin contact.
    NOTE: Soon after the **Wharton's jelly** in the cord is exposed to cool air and shrinks and the infant cries, the umbilical vessels stop pulsating and the blood flow ceases. The baby's presence on the mother's abdomen stimulates the release of oxytocin from her posterior pituitary and thus stimulates uterine contractions, which aid in placental separation.
13. *Wait* for the placenta to separate; *do not* tug on the cord.
    NOTE: Injudicious traction may tear the cord,

separate the placenta, or invert the uterus. Signs of **placental separation** include a slight gush of dark blood from the introitus, lengthening of the cord, and change in uterine contour from discoid to globular shape.

14. Instruct the mother to push to deliver the separated placenta. Gently ease out the placental membranes, using an up-and-down motion until membranes are removed. If delivery is occurring outside the hospital setting, to minimize complications, do not cut the cord without proper clamps or ties and a sterile cutting tool, and inspect the placenta for intactness. Place the baby on the placenta and wrap the two together for additional warmth.
    NOTE: There is no hurry to cut the cord. The infant will not lose blood through the placenta because the cord circulation ceases (clots) within minutes of birth. If a cord tie is needed, use the technique described in Fig. 18-10.
15. Check the firmness of the uterus. Gently massage the uterus and demonstrate to the mother how she can massage her own uterus properly.
16. Clean the area under the mother's buttocks.
17. Prevent or minimize hemorrhage.
    a. Hemorrhage from uterine atony
        (1) *Gently* massage fundus to stimulate uterine musculature to contract.
        NOTE: Overstimulation may fatigue the myometrium and cause atony.
        (2) Put the baby to the breast as soon as possible (Plate 12). Sucking or nuzzling and licking the breast stimulate the release of oxytocin from the posterior pituitary.
        NOTE: If the baby does not nurse, manually stimulate the mother's breasts.
        (3) If medical assistance is delayed, do not allow the mother's bladder to become distended.
        (4) Expel any clots from her uterus.
        NOTE: The fundus should be firm to prevent accidental inversion during this procedure. While holding the bottom of the uterus just above the symphysis pubis, apply gentle pressure on the firm fundus downward toward the vagina.
    b. Hemorrhage from perineal lacerations
        (1) Apply a clean pad to the perineum.
        (2) Instruct the mother to press her thighs together.
18. Comfort or reassure the mother and her family or friends. Keep her and the baby warm. Give her fluids if available and tolerated.
19. If this is a multifetal birth, identify the infants in order of birth (using letters A, B . . .).

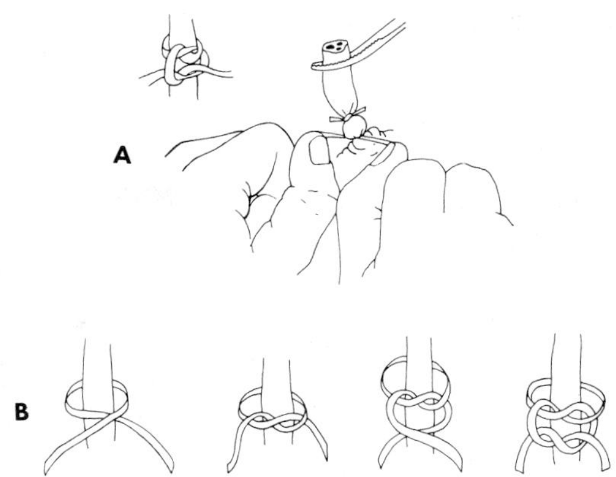

Fig. 18-10 Technique of tying off umbilical cord by use of soft flat tape to prevent cutting through cord as it is drawn tight (**A**), and square knot to prevent slippage (**B**).

20. Make notations on the birth.
    a. Fetal presentation and position.
    b. Presence of cord around neck (nuchal cord) or other parts and number of times cord encircles part.
    c. Color, character, and amount of amniotic fluid, if rupture of membranes (ROM) occurs immediately before birth.
    d. Time of delivery.
    e. Estimated time of Apgar score, resuscitation efforts, and ultimate condition of baby.
    f. Sex of baby.
    g. Time of placental expulsion, its appearance, and completeness.
    h. Maternal condition: affect, amount of bleeding, and status of uterine tonicity.
    i. Any unusual occurrences during the birth (i.e., maternal or paternal response, verbalizations, or gestures to birth or newborn).

LATERAL SIMS' POSITION FOR EMERGENCY CHILDBIRTH. A lateral Sims' posture may be the position of choice for birth when (1) the birth is progressing rapidly and there is insufficient time for slow distention of the perineum; (2) the fetal head seems too large to pass through the introitus without laceration, and episiotomy is not possible; or (3) the apparent size of the fetus is consistent with possible shoulder dystocia.

In the lateral Sims' position, less stress is placed on the perineum and better visualization of the perineum is possible. In the event of shoulder dystocia, lateral Sims' posture increases the space needed for delivery.

EMERGENCY CHILDBIRTH OF PRETERM INFANT. The actual process of birthing the preterm infant does not vary from that of the term infant. However, the care of the infant after birth requires some modification as follows:

1. Warmth is essential.
2. Minimize handling, maintain a clear airway, and feed and change the infant.
3. Nutrition may be a problem if a medical facility is not available. Although the infant may be unable to nurse at the breast, slow feeding is important, using a medicine dropper, for example.
4. Gently stimulate the preterm infant to breathe. When the infant "forgets" to breathe, rubbing the back or the soles of the feet usually is effective.
5. Transport the infant to a medical facility equipped to handle preterm infants as early as possible (see Chapter 37).

EVALUATION

Evaluation of outcomes is an ongoing activity. During each encounter with the woman and her family during the second stage of labor the nurse evaluates the degree to which goals for care are being met. For example, the woman has actively participated in the labor process, neither she nor her fetus has sustained any injury during the labor process, and she has been able to obtain comfort and support from family members of choice. If the evaluation shows that results fall short of achieving any goal, further assessment, planning, and implementation are warranted. (See case study and nursing plan of care for the woman in the descent phase of the second stage of labor.)

■ THIRD STAGE OF LABOR

The third stage of labor extends from the birth of the baby until the delivery of the placenta. The goal in the management of the third stage of labor is the prompt separation and expulsion of the placenta, achieved in the easiest, safest manner.

The placenta is attached to the decidual layer of the thin endometrium of the basal plate by numerous, randomized, fibrous anchor villi—much like a postage stamp is attached to a sheet of postage stamps. After the fetus is delivered, in the presence of strong uterine contractions, the placental site is markedly reduced in size. This reduced size causes the anchor villi to break and the placenta to separate from its attachments. Normally the first few strong

CASE STUDY

Descent Phase—Second Stage

Paula Jones is a 24-year-old, married woman with one child, who is at 39 weeks' gestation. She was admitted to the perinatal unit in active labor, with membranes intact, 6 hours earlier.

ASSESSMENT

Paula reports that the contractions are strong and that during them she is breathing quickly in and out through her mouth. Between contractions she states, "My water bag just broke." She feels a slight urge to push. She states she is worried that she will release stool when she gives birth and that she feels embarrassed. Paula's last vaginal examination 10 minutes ago showed she was completely dilated at +1 station with some molding. All other physical parameters are within normal limits.

NURSING DIAGNOSES

Assessment findings support several nursing diagnoses. The nursing diagnosis that takes priority is: High risk for injury to mother or newborn related to rapid delivery secondary to second-stage ROM.

PLANNING

The nurse decides on the following *goals*, which she communicates to Paula: Fetal well-being will remain within normal limits, Paula's progress toward and during the birth of her baby will be within normal limits, her primary care practitioner will arrive in time to deliver her baby, and Paula will understand the reasons for any procedures performed by the nurse.

IMPLEMENTATION

The nurse immediately assesses the FHR for a reassuring pattern, and the color, character, and amount of amniotic fluid. Because the primary care practitioner has not arrived yet, the nurse instructs Paula not to push unless the urge is unbearable but instead to blow or puff lightly until the peak of the contraction has passed. Paula is encouraged to lie on her left side with her head elevated only slightly.

EVALUATION

Paula's amniotic fluid is clear and watery and appears moderate in quantity. The FHR baseline for the 10 minutes after ROM is 140, with average long-term variability. Some FHR decelerations are present after the onset of contraction, lasting for 30 seconds, with abrupt return to baseline. Paula is following the nurse's directions regarding positioning and puffing with the peak of her contractions. There is no bulging of the perineum present. Paula's primary care practitioner arrives.

CARE PLAN Descent Phase—Second Stage of Labor

GOALS	IMPLEMENTATION	RATIONALE	EVALUATION
Nursing diagnosis: Impaired gas exchange (mother and fetus) related to respiratory alkalosis (hyperventilation)			
1. Paula resumes normal breathing pattern with no signs of alkalosis.	Provide a paper bag for Paula to breathe into, or she may breathe into her cupped hands if bag is unavailable.	Increases CO_2 levels and corrects respiratory alkalosis.	Paula ceases to hyperventilate and symptoms are relieved.
2. The fetus' FHR stays WNL.	Explain what is happening and how rebreathing her own air is therapeutic.	Information provides reassurance.	The fetus' FHR remains WNL.
	Assist coach to help her with verbal control of respirations. Coach her to breathe without hyperventilating. Identify stress (e.g., anxiety, knowledge deficit, or discomfort) that may underlie her hyperventilation; relieve the identified stress.	Provides opportunity for the coach to work with Paula to promote improved gas exchange and effective patterns.	Paula's concurrent stress is relieved.
	Assess FHR q5min.	Supports ACOG standards (1988) and promotes early identification of fetal compromise.	
Nursing diagnosis: High risk for injury to mother or newborn related to rapid delivery secondary to SROM			
1. Fetal well-being is maintained.	Assess FHR and progress of labor.	Precipitous labor increases the risk of fetal head trauma from inadequate time for molding to birth canal.	The fetus' status remains WNL.
2. Paula's amniotic fluid and progress of labor are WNL. 3. Infection does not develop 4. Paula's primary care practitioner is present for birth.	Assess the color or the fluid—normally straw-colored. Assess character of the fluid—normally looks like water and has a characteristic odor. Assess amount of fluid lost: an excessive amount (polyhydramnios) or abnormally small amount (oligohydramnios) signal congenital anomalies.	Meconium-stained amniotic fluid, greenish in color, may indicate fetal distress resulting from hypoxia. Polyhydramnios is associated with fetal disorders such as anencephaly, GI and renal disorders, maternal diabetes mellitus.	Paula's progress of labor continues WNL.
	Monitor pushing (bearing down) efforts as head emerges, instructing Paula to pant or blow during the process.	Prevents lacerations of perineal tissues by allowing them to stretch. Record findings and notify primary care practitioner.	Paula understands reasons for procedure.

GI, Gastrointestinal; *SROM*, spontaneous rupture of membranes; *WNL*, within normal limits.

Continued.

CARE PLAN Descent Phase—Second Stage of Labor—cont'd

GOALS	IMPLEMENTATION	RATIONALE	EVALUATION
Nursing diagnosis: Disturbance in self-concept related to loss of control of bodily function (i.e., stooling)			
1. Paula's perception of her birth experience will be positive.	Advise Paula that it is not uncommon for women to have a bowel movement during birth.	GI motility is decreased in labor, and expulsive efforts, coupled with descent of the presenting part, force out stool present in the anal canal.	Paula ceases to mention anything about stooling during birth.
2. Paula will cease to dwell on the possibility of passing stool during delivery. 3. Paula will accept having a bowel movement at the time of birth as normal.	If Paula begins to have a bowel movement while pushing, remove the fecal material as quickly and unobtrusively as possible, while giving Paula positive feedback on her pushing efforts.	If the nurse does not react negatively, Paula's attention will be diverted from her bowel movement to her pushing efforts.	Paula is giving her undivided attention to pushing.

contractions 5 to 7 minutes after the birth of the baby shear the placenta from the basal plate. A placenta will not be easily freed from a flaccid (relaxed) uterus because the placental site is not reduced in size.

ASSESSMENT

Placental separation is indicated by the following signs (Fig. 18-11 and Plates 11 to 13):

1. A firmly contracting fundus
2. A change in the uterus from a discoid to a globular ovoid shape, as the placenta moves to the lower segment
3. A sudden gush of dark blood from the introitus
4. Apparent lengthening of the umbilical cord as the placenta gets closer to the introitus
5. A vaginal fullness (the placenta) noted on vaginal or rectal examination, or fetal membranes seen at the introitus

Whether the placenta appears by its shiny fetal surface (Schultze mechanism) or whether it turns to show first its dark roughened maternal surface (Duncan mechanism) is of no clinical importance. After the placenta with its membranes emerges, it is examined for intactness to be certain that no portion of it remains in the uterine cavity (i.e., no retained fragments of the placenta or membranes) (Fig. 18-12).

Maternal Physical Status

Physiologic changes after birth are profound. The cardiac output is increased rapidly as maternal circulation to the placenta ceases and the pooled blood from the lower extremities is mobilized. The pulse rate slows in response to the change in cardiac output. During the first 7 to 10 days after delivery, pulse rates tend to remain slightly slower than before pregnancy.

Soon after the birth, the woman's blood pressure usually returns to prepregnancy levels. Several factors contribute to an elevated blood pressure: the excitement of the second stage, certain medications, and the time of day (blood pressure is highest during the late afternoon). Analgesics and anesthetics may lead to hypotension in the hour after birth.

SIGNS OF POTENTIAL PROBLEMS. Even as the primary care practitioner is completing delivery of the placenta, the nurse observes the mother for signs of an altered level of consciousness (LOC) or alteration in respirations. Because of the rapid cardiovascular changes (e.g., the increased intracranial pressure during pushing and the rapid increase in cardiac output), this period represents the risk of *rupture of a preexisting cerebral aneurysm* and of pulmonary emboli. The risk of pulmonary **amniotic fluid emboli**

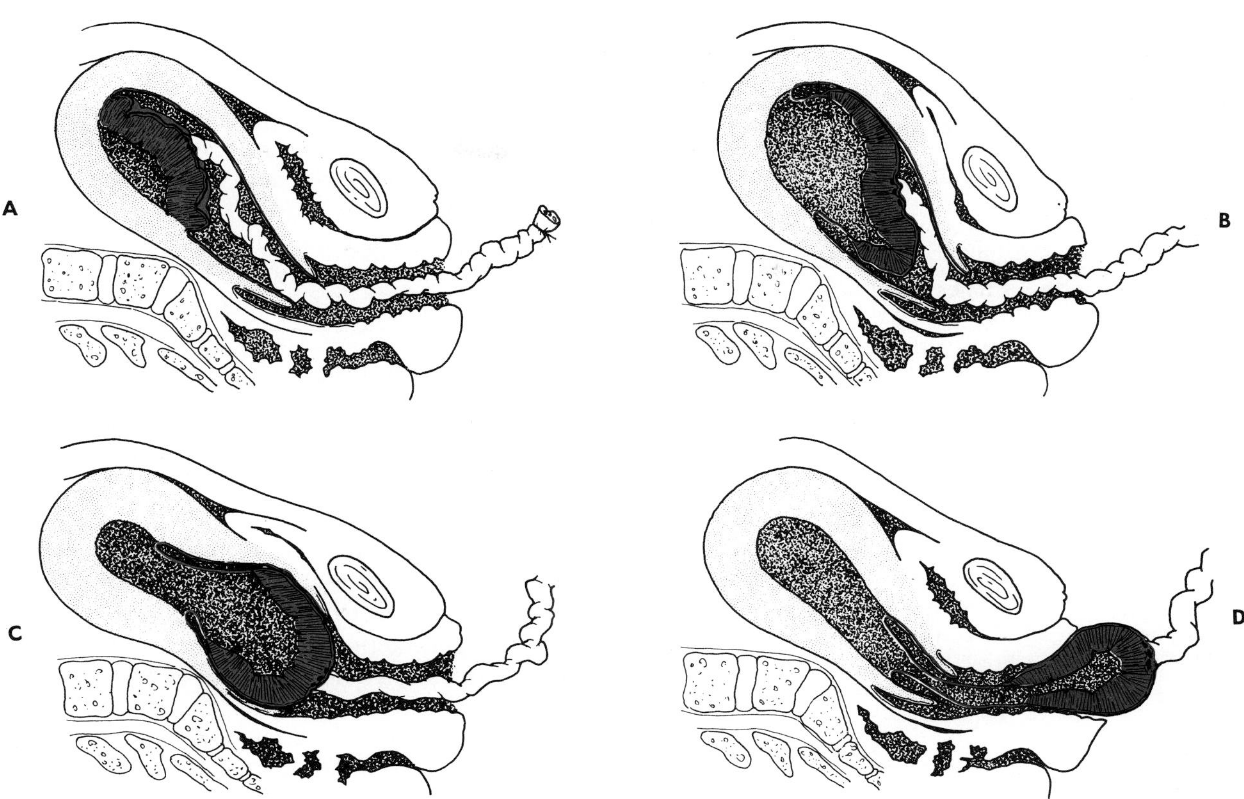

Fig. 18-11 Third stage of labor. **A,** Placenta begins the separation process in central portion with retroplacental bleeding. Uterus changes from discoid to globular shape. **B,** Placenta completes separation and enters lower uterine segment. Uterus is globular in shape. **C,** Placenta enters vagina, cord is seen to lengthen, and there may be increase in bleeding. **D,** Expression (birth) of placenta and completion of third stage.

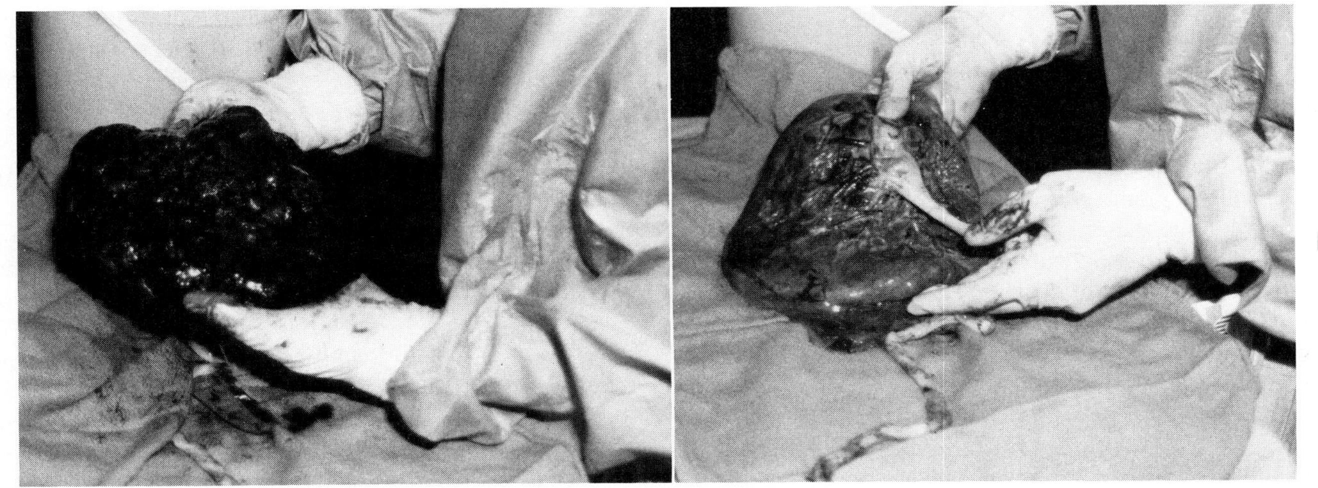

Fig. 18-12 Examination of the placenta. **A,** Maternal surface. **B,** Fetal surface.
Courtesy Marjorie Pyle, RNC, Lifecircle, Costa Mesa, Calif.

Warning Signs: Parent-Newborn Relationships Immediately After Birth

1. Passive reaction, either verbal or nonverbal (parents do not touch, hold, or examine baby or talk in affectionate terms or tones about baby)
2. Hostile reaction, either verbal or nonverbal (parents make inappropriate verbalization, glances, or disparaging remarks about physical characteristics of child)
3. Disappointment over sex of baby
4. No eye contact with baby
5. Nonsupportive interaction between parents (if interaction seems dubious, talk to nurse and primary care practitioner involved with delivery for further information)

Modified by permission from Gray JD et al: Prediction and prevention of child abuse, *Semin Perinatal* 3:95, Jan 1979.

arises from another source as well. As the placenta separates, there is a possiblity of amniotic fluid entering the maternal circulation if the uterine musculature does not contract rapidly and well. The incidence of these possible complications is small; however, the alert nurse can contribute to their immediate recognition and the prompt initiation of therapy.

Some warning signs in parent-child relationships that are apparent immediately after birth are listed in the box, above.

NURSING DIAGNOSES

Before establishing nursing diagnoses, the nurse correlates the events of the third stage and the mother's physical and emotional responses to the third stage of labor. The following are examples of nursing diagnoses:

- Ineffective individual (mother) coping related to
  —Lack of preparation for sensations that occur during third stage of labor
- Anxiety related to
  —Knowledge deficit regarding delivery of the placenta

PLANNING

Planning for this stage focuses on the woman's rapid physiologic changes and timely intact birth of the placenta. At the same time the emotional environment of the family is maintained.

Goals for the third stage of labor may include the following:

1. The mother's placenta is expelled and blood loss is less than 500 mL.
2. The mother is prepared for the sensations she will experience.
3. Mother and family initiate the processes of bonding and attachment.

IMPLEMENTATION

To assist the mother in the delivery of the placenta, the nurse or physician instructs the woman to push when signs of separation have occurred. If an oxytocic medication is ordered, the nurse administers the medication in the dosage and by the route indicated by the primary care practitioner. If possible, the placenta should be expelled by maternal effort during a uterine contraction, but assistance such as *alternate compression* and *elevation of the fundus,* plus *minimum,* controlled traction on the umbilical cord may be employed to facilitate delivery of the placenta and membranes. When the third stage is complete and lacerations are repaired or an episiotomy is performed (p. 496), the vulvar area is gently cleansed with sterile water by the physician or nurse-midwife. The nurse or practitioner performs the following:

1. Applies a sterile perineal pad
2. Removes the drapes if used, or places dry linen under the buttocks
3. Repositions the delivery table or bed
4. Lowers the mother's legs simultaneously from the stirrups if she is in lithotomy position
5. Assists the woman onto her bed if she is to be transferred from the birthing area to the recovery area; the nurse should request assistance to move the woman from a delivery table onto a bed if the woman has had anesthesia and does not have full use of her lower extremities
6. Provides the woman with a clean gown and covers her with a warmed blanket
7. Raises the side rails of the bed during the transfer (in some hospitals, the mother is given the baby to hold during the transfer; in some hospitals, the father/partner or significant other carries the baby; in other hospitals, the nurse carries the baby either to the nursery or to the recovery area for the duration of the mother's recovery period)

If the woman labors, gives birth, and recovers in the same bed and room, she is refreshed as already described. After the woman is transferred or discharged, the birthing area is cleaned as necessary.

The Family during the Third Stage

Most parents enjoy being able to handle, hold, explore, and examine the baby immediately after birth. Both parents can assist with the thorough drying of the infant. The infant may be wrapped in a receiving blanket and placed on the mother's abdomen. If skin-to-skin contact is desired, the unwrapped infant may be placed on the mother's abdomen and then covered with a warm blanket.

Holding the newborn next to her skin helps maintain the baby's body heat and provides skin contact; care must be taken to keep the head warm as well. Caps are sometimes used to cover the newborn's head (Plate 15). It is the nurse's responsibility to make sure the infant is kept warm and is in no danger of slipping from the parent's grasp.

Many women wish to begin to breast-feed their newborns at this time to take advantage of the infant's alert state (first period of reactivity) and to stimulate the production of oxytocin that promotes contraction (Plates 12 and 15) of the uterus. Others wish to wait until the newborn, parents, and older siblings are together in the recovery room.

While the primary care practitioner carries out the postbirth vaginal examination (Plate 14) and, if necessary, performs the episiotomy, the mother usually feels discomfort. Therefore while the process is being completed, the newborn's physical condition can be assessed; the baby can be weighed and measured, wrapped in warm blankets, and then given to the partner to hold (Plate 16).

Parent-Newborn Relationships

The mother's reaction to the sight of her newborn may range from excited outbursts of laughing, talking, and even crying to apparent apathy. A polite smile and nod may acknowledge the comments of nurses and physicians. Occasionally the reaction is one of anger or indifference; the mother turns away from the baby, concentrates on her own pain, and sometimes makes hostile comments. These varying reactions can arise from pleasure, exhaustion, or deep disappointment. Whatever the reaction and cause may be, the mother needs continuing acceptance and support from all staff. Notation regarding the parents' reaction to the newborn can be made in the recovery record. How do parents *look*? What do they *say*? What do they *do*?

Siblings, who may have appeared only remotely interested in the final phases of the second stage, tend to experience renewed interest and excitement and can be encouraged to hold the new family member (Fig. 18-13).

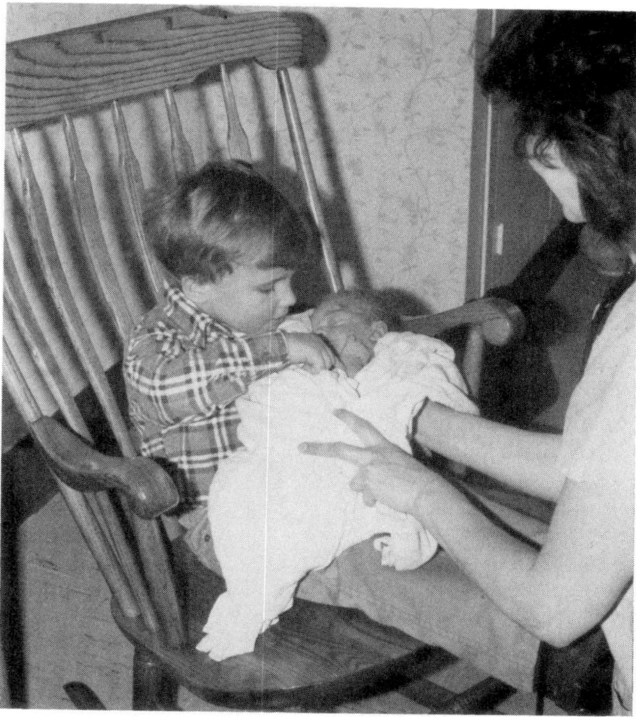

Fig. 18-13 Nurse helps big brother become acquainted with new baby sister.

Parents are responsive to praise of their newborn. Many require reassurance that the dusky appearance of their baby's extremities immediately after birth is normal until circulation is well established (Plate 9). The reason for the molding of the newborn's head must be reviewed with parents. Information about hospital routine can be communicated. Hospital staff members, by their interest and concern, can do much to make this a satisfying experience for parents, family, and significant others.

EVALUATION

Evaluation of outcomes is an ongoing activity. During each encounter with the new mother during the third stage of labor, the nurse evaluates the degree to which goals for care are being met. For example, the mother's placenta is expelled and blood loss is less than 500 mL, the mother was prepared for the sensations she would experience and was not concerned when they occurred, and the mother and father/partner and family initiated the process of bonding and attachment. If the evaluation shows that results fall short of achieving any goal, further assessment, planning, and implementation are warranted.

DELIVERY/RECOVERY RECORD

[ ] SVD [ ] VACUUM [ ] FORCEPS outlet low mid [ ] ROTATIONS ____________
[ ] Cesarean [ ] low cervical/transverse [ ] classical [ ] primary [ ] repeat X
Indications for Operative Delivery: ____________ CATH IN DR ____ cc @ ____________
Pres: [ ] Vtx [ ] Breech [ ] Other ____________ Rom ________ hrs.[ ] Mec. ________ [ ] Elevated maternal temp ______ F @ ______
Episiotomy: [ ] midline [ ] mediolateral [ ] episoproctotomy [ ] lacerations (type + grade) ____________ [ ] Repaired
Type & Rh _____ EBL [ ] Aver. [ ] _____ cc [ ] Transfusion _____ (amt.) [ ] Type: ____
Anesthesia: [ ] local [ ] pudendal [ ] epidural [ ] spinal [ ] general
Physician: ____________ Anesthesia: ____________
Assistant: ____________ Pediatrician: ____________
Nurse(s): ____________ Others: ____________

MEDICATIONS IV# ________

In Labor	In Delivery
☐Demerol _____ mg IV/IM @ ___	☐Pitocin ____ units @ ______
☐ _________ mg IV/IM @ ___	☐IV in ____ cc/ IM ☐
☐Stadol _____ mg IV/IM @ ___	☐ _______ mg IV/IM @ _____
☐ _________ mg IV/IM @ ___	☐ _______ mg IV/IM @ _____

INFANT

DATE: ________ TIME: ________ SEX: [ ] male [ ] female [ ] alive [ ] stillborn [ ] multiple _____
WEIGHT: _____ lbs. _____ oz. ____ _____ gm Electrode [ ] removed intact [ ] Cord blood to lab
CORD: [ ] 3 vessels [ ] nuchal X ____ [ ] abnormalities ____________ MR# ________
[ ] Voided [ ] Meconium [ ] Resuscitated ____________ I.D. band# ________

APGAR	0	1	2	1′	5′
Heart rate	Absent	<100	>100		
Resp Effort	Absent	Slow Irreg.	Good Cry		
Reflex Irrit	None	Grimace	Cry		
Tone	Limp	Some Flexion	Active Motion		
Color	Blue	Blue Extreme.	Pink		
Scored By: ________					

KEY:
V=Void
S=Stool E=Emesis
LOCHIA:
Sm=Small
Mod=Moderate
Lg=Large
PERINEUM:
Cl=Clear
RI=Repair intact
Sw=Swollen
I=Ice applied
UTERUS:
FF=Fundus firm
B=Boggy
MF=Massaged firm
@ U=at umbilicus
1/u = 1 finger above
u/1 = 1 finger below the umbilicus

NEWBORN **POST-DELIVERY ASSESSMENT** MATERNAL

NEWBORN									MATERNAL
Time									Time
Temp									Temp
Pulse									Pulse
Resp.									Resp.
Br. Fd.									I & O
RN Initial									BP
Latch-on good = L+ Nutritive Sucking = N+									Uterus
Comments:									Perineum
									Lochia
RN Init/Signature									Meds Dose Route
RN Init/Signature									R.N. Initital

RESUSCITATION
[ ] bulb syringe
[ ] gastric aspir./amt ______ cc
color ____________
Intubated X ____________
[ ] Cords Clear [ ] Mec below
[ ] Suctioned amt. ______ cc
color ____________
[ ] Free-flow Oxygen ______ %
[ ] mask [ ] tube for _____ min.
[ ] Pos. pressure ventilation:
_____ ETT [ ] bag & mask.
Resus. by ____________

NEWBORN ASSESSMENT RECORD

Admission date and time: ____________ Admission weight: ________ lbs. ______ oz. ______ gms.
Length _____ in. _____ cm. Vital Signs _____ temp ☐ Axillary ☐ Rectal
Head _____ in. _____ cm. ______ BP _____ pulse (AP) _____ resp.
Chest _____ in. _____ cm. BLD. GLUC. ______ @ _____ by ________
Abd. _____ in. _____ cm. ☐ Chemstrip ☐ Accucheck ☐ D-stix
Admission R.N. Sign/Init. ____________
Other comments: ____________

Admission Meds
Vit. K in L/R anterior thigh @ _____ by _____
Eye prophylaxis OU @ _____ by _____
Agent: ☐ Silver Nitrate* ☐ Other
☐Erythromycin/Ilotycin

INITIAL SYSTEMS ASSESSMENT

RN Init = item observed * = see nurses notes or comments

CNS: [ ] moves extremities, muscle tone good
[ ] reflexes present/strong
suck, root, Moro, step, grasps
[ ] symmetrical features, movements
CARD: [ ] ant. font. soft/flat
[ ] pulses strong/equal bilat.
[ ] heart ausc, strong/reg.
[ ] ∅ murmur ausc.
SKIN: Color: [ ] pink [ ] acrocyanosis
[ ] ∅ lesions, abrasions, rash
Peeling [ ] yes [ ] no
[ ] birthmarks ____________

RESP: [ ] lungs ausc. clear bilat.
[ ] ∅ upper airway congestion
[ ] resp. rate <60/min
[ ] chest expansion symmetrical
GU: [ ] ∅ bleeding/discharge
Male: [ ] testes descended bilat.
GI: [ ] abd. soft/∅ dist
[ ] bowel sounds active

ENT: [ ] eyes clear
[ ] mouth clear
[ ] palates intact
[ ] nares patent

Birth Inj./Variation
[ ] caput/molding
[ ] vacuum "cap"
[ ] forceps marks
[ ] other ____________

RN Init.	Signature

Comments/Transition Vital Signs: ____________

ADDRESSOGRAPH

 OB4791

* Silver nitrate has been banned in Canada; its use is declining in the United States.

Fig. 18-14 An example of delivery/recovery record.
Courtesy Joyce Vogler.

The Newborn

Care immediately after the birth focuses on assessing and stabilizing the newborn. The nurse has primary responsibility for the infant during this period, because the physician will be involved with delivery of the placenta and care of the mother. The nurse must be alert for any signs of distress and initiate appropriate interventions.

ASSESSMENT

Before birth, the nurse evaluates the maternal history, including labor, to identify potential problems for the neonate and alerts the nursery. Although an extensive examination will be performed later, a brief physical examination of the newborn is completed immediately after birth (Fig. 18-14).

The **Apgar score** permits a rapid and semiquantitative assessment based on five signs that indicate the physiologic state of the neonate (Fig. 18-14): ***heart rate,*** based on auscultation with stethoscope; ***respiration,*** based on observed movement of chest wall; ***muscle tone,*** based on degree of flexion and movement of the extremities; ***reflex ability,*** based on response to gentle slaps on the soles of the feet; and ***color*** (pallid, cyanotic, or pink). The 5-minute score correlates with neonatal mortality and morbidity. In addition, the nurse makes the following assessments and records findings:

1. Assesses respirations and neonate's ability to keep airway clear
2. Estimates infant's health status using Apgar rating at 1 and 5 minutes of age
3. Examines the cord for anomalies and verifies the presence of two arteries and one vein (Fig. 18-15), checks cord clamp is in place (Figs. 18-16 and 18-17)
4. Collects cord blood from placenta for analysis (Rh factor, blood grouping, and hematocrit)*
5. Assesses weight, length, head circumference, and gestational age
6. Notes passage of meconium or urine
7. Performs brief physical examination and assessment of neonate such as the following (see Chapter 20 for more in-depth discussion and techniques):

*Some hospitals do not send cord blood to the laboratory unless the mother has Rh negativity or blood type O or has had no prenatal care.

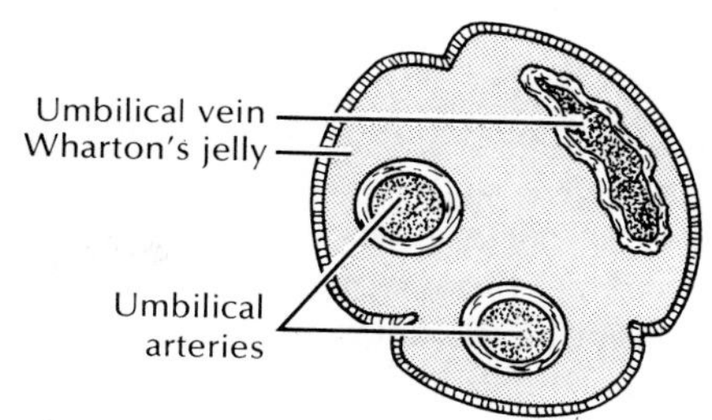

Fig. 18-15 Cross section of umbilical cord. Note collapsed appearance of thin-walled umbilical vein and contour of thicker, muscular-walled arteries.

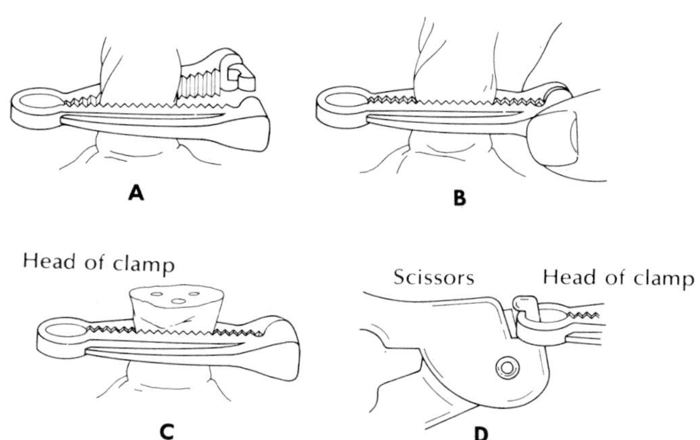

Fig. 18-16 Hollister cord clamp. **A,** Position clamp close to umbilicus. **B,** Secure cord. **C,** Cut cord. **D,** Remove clamp, using special scissors after cord dries (about 24 hours).

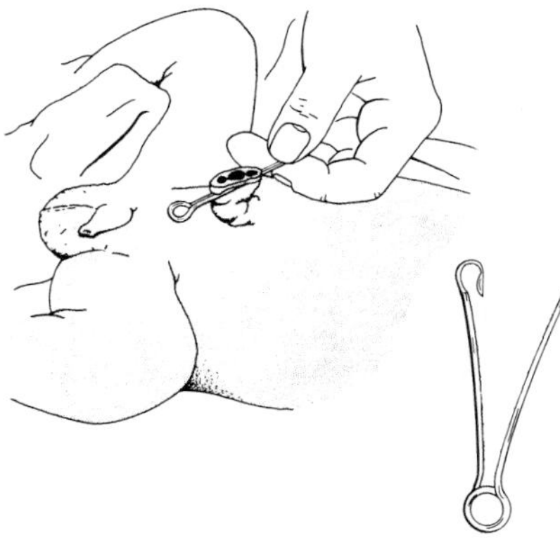

Fig. 18-17 Hesseltine cord clamp.

a. *External:* notes skin color, staining, peeling, or wasting (dysmaturity); considers length of nails and development of creases on soles of feet; checks for presence or absence of breast tissue; assesses nasal patency by closing one nostril at a time while observing the infant's respirations and color; notes meconium staining of cord, skin, fingernails, or amniotic fluid (may indicate fetal hypoxia; offensive odor may indicate intrauterine infection)
b. *Chest:* palpates for site of the point of maximum impulse (PMI) and auscultates for rate and quality of heart tones and murmurs; compares and notes character of respirations and presence of rales or rhonchi by holding stethoscope in each axilla
c. *Abdomen:* verifies presence of a domed abdomen and absence of anomalies; assesses umbilical cord (see Chapter 20)
d. *Neurologic:* checks muscle tone and reflex reaction and appraises Moro's reflex; palpates large (anterior) fontanelle for fullness or bulge; notes by palpation the presence and sizes of the sutures and fontanelles
e. *Other observations:* notes gross structure malformations obvious at birth (described in general terms and recorded on delivery record)

8. Assesses parents' response to newborn and to each other; assessment of the parent-child relationship is discussed under the nursing care of the mother during the fourth stage of labor (see p. 513)

SIGNS OF POTENTIAL PROBLEMS. The newborn with a low Apgar score requires immediate resuscitation (see Chapter 36). Gestational age (premature and dysmature) and birth-weight (small- and large-for-gestational age) problems are discussed in Chapter 37. Findings suggestive of developmental and/or acquired problems are presented in depth in Chapter 38 and 39, respectively. Loss and grief are covered in Chapter 40.

NURSING DIAGNOSES

Nursing diagnoses lend direction to the nursing actions needed to implement a plan of care. Before establishing nursing diagnoses, the nurse analyzes the significance of findings collected during assessment. Following are examples of nursing diagnoses:

- Ineffective airway clearance related to
  —Airway obstruction with mucus and amniotic fluid
- Ineffective thermoregulation related to
  —Environmental factors
  —Amniotic fluid moisture
- Altered health maintenance related to
  —Congenital disorders

PLANNING

During this important step, goals are set in client-centered terms. The goals are prioritized. Nursing actions are selected to meet the goals. *Goals* for the newborn during the recovery period include the following:

1. The newborn's airway remains clear.
2. The newborn's temperature remains within normal limits.
3. The newborn does not experience injury.
4. The parent—newborn's bonding process is facilitated.

IMPLEMENTATION

Events move rapidly during this time period. Assessment must be followed quickly by appropriate implementation. The primary care practitioner may be concentrating on the progress of the third stage for the mother. The nurse assumes responsibility and accountability for accurate assessment of and timely intervention for the newborn.

GENERAL CARE. Initiation and maintenance of respiration are top priorities. Abnormal breathing must be recognized and treated (see warning signs box, p 593, and emergency box, pp. 591 and 593).

Nursing actions that usually apply to this period include a variety of activities. Among them are actions related to the care of the airway, cord clamping, attachment and warmth, Apgar score, eye prophylaxis, measurement of weight and length, and identification. A summary of these nursing actions and the rationale for each are given in Table 18-4.

EYE PROPHYLAXIS. Instillation of a prophylactic agent in the eyes of all neonates is mandatory in the United States (Fig. 18-18). It is a precaution against ophthalmia neonatorum. **Ophthalmia neonatorum** refers to inflammation of the eyes from gonorrheal or chlamydial infection contracted by the newborn's passage through the mother's infected birth canal. In some Canadian institutions the parents may sign a form refusing **eye prophylaxis.** In the United States, if the family objects to this treatment, the primary

TABLE 18-4 Nursing Care of the Neonate

Intervention	Rationale
AIRWAY	
Hold baby with head lowered (10 to 15 degrees).	Uses gravity to help remove fluids.
Suction oral pharynx with small bulb syringe as soon as head is born.	Expedites drainage and prevents aspiration of amniotic fluid, mucus, and blood (maternal).
Suction nares next.	Prevents inspiration after stimulation of nares before mouth is clear.
Avoid deep suctioning with catheter, if possible.	May cause bradycardia or laryngospasm, or both.
Avoid suspending neonate by ankles.	Results in hyperextension of baby whose entire development occurred in flexed position.
CORD CLAMPING	
Immediately after birth, neonate is kept at about the same level as uterus, until cord clamp is applied or until cord has stopped pulsating.	If neonate is held above level of uterus, gravity drains blood to placenta.
Without "stripping" it, cord is clamped close to umbilicus approximately 30 sec after birth if neonate appears normal and mature.	Ordinarily it is unwise to strip cord before clamping and cutting because postdelivery red blood cell destruction will be increased and hyperbilirubinemia may ensue; in addition, polycythemia (increased number of red blood cells) increases blood viscosity, leading to cardiopulmonary problems.
Cord is clamped 8 to 10 cm from umbilicus if there is a possibility for exchange transfusion.	Permits access to umbilical vessels.
Assess cord for two arteries and one vein (Fig. 18-15).	Absence of one artery indicates need for further assessment.
ATTACHMENT AND WARMTH	
Unless immediate intervention is required, dry infant and place on mother's abdomen, covering both; or wrap infant in warm blanket first.	Facilitates attachment. Assures and relaxes mother.
Caution parents to keep neonate's head covered.	Prevents cold stress.
Permit mother to breast-feed as desired.	Facilitates uterine contractions and expulsion of placenta.
APGAR SCORE	
Appraise neonate at 1 min and again at 5 mins, using Apgar scoring method (see p. 493 and Fig. 18-14).	Permits rapid and semiquantitative assessment of physiologic state; 5-min score correlates with neonatal mortality and morbidity.
EYE PROPHYLAXIS	
Instill medication per agency policy (Fig. 18-18).	Meets legal requirements.
NEWBORN WEIGHT AND LENGTH	
Weigh and measure the neonate; this may be delayed until the fourth stage.	Parents usually are anxious to know and want to share data with relatives and friends.
IDENTIFICATION	
Identify the neonate by one of a number of techniques *before mother or baby leaves the delivery area.*	Although rare, an occasional mix-up in the identity of neonates occurs; identification and care to check both mother's and infant's ID numbers prevent unnecessary anxiety and legal complications.

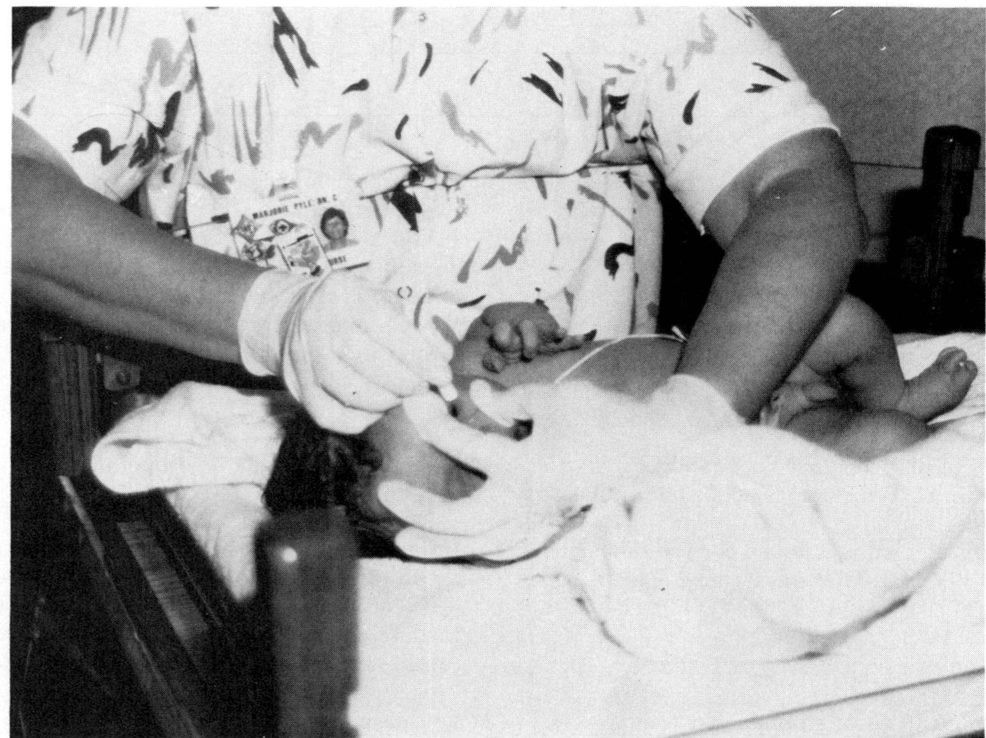

Fig. 18-18 Instillation of ophthalmic erythromycin drops into conjunctival sac. Note that nurse is wearing gloves.
Courtesy Marjorie Pyle, RNC, Lifecircle, Costa Mesa, Calif.

care practitioner will request that the parents sign an informed consent, and their refusal will be noted in the neonate's record. The agent used for prophylaxis varies according to hospital protocols. Usual agents include forms of erythromycin and tetracycline. Canadian hospitals have not recommended the use of silver nitrate since 1986. Its use in the United States is declining because silver nitrate does not protect against chlamydial infection and can cause chemical conjunctivitis. In some institutions instillation of eye prophylaxis is delayed until an hour or so after birth. This facilitates eye contact and enhances attachment and bonding. The Centers for Disease Control specify that a delay of up to 2 hours is safe.

EVALUATION

Evaluation of nursing care and outcomes is an ongoing activity in the care of both mother and baby. During the third stage of labor, the nurse evaluates the degree to which goals for care are being met. That is, the newborn's airway remains clear, temperature remains within normal limits, the infant does not experience an injury, and the parent/newborn bonding process is facilitated. If the evaluation shows that results fall short of achieving any goal, further assessment, planning, and implementation are warranted.

■ INTERRUPTION IN SKIN INTEGRITY RELATED TO CHILDBIRTH

EPISIOTOMY. An episiotomy is an incision made in the perineum to enlarge the vaginal outlet. Episiotomies are performed more commonly in the United States and Canada than in Europe. The use of the side-lying position for delivery is used routinely in Europe whereas the position with legs in stirrups is more commonly used in the United States and Canada. With the side-lying position there is less tension on the perineum and a gradual stretching of the perineum is possible. As a result the indications for use of episiotomies are less.

The proponents of use of the episiotomy maintain it serves the following purposes:

1. Prevents tearing of the perineum. The clean and properly placed incision heals more properly than does a ragged tear. Some conditions

that predispose a woman to perineal tearing and are therefore indications for episiotomy are a large infant, rapid labor in which there is not sufficient time for stretching of the perineum to take place, a narrow subpubic arch with a constricted outlet, and malpresentations of the fetus (e.g., the face).

2. May minimize prolonged and severe stretching of the muscles supporting the bladder or rectum, which may later lead to stress incontinence or to vaginal prolapse.
3. Reduces duration of the second stage, which may be important for maternal reasons (e.g., a hypertensive state) or fetal reasons (e.g., persistent bradycardia).
4. Enlarges the vagina in case manipulation is needed to deliver an infant, for example, in a breech presentation or for application of forceps.

Those opposed to the *routine* use of episiotomies maintain the following:

1. The perineum can be prepared for delivery through use of the Kegel exercises and massage in the prenatal period. Use of Kegel exercises in the postpartum period improves and restores the tone of the perineal muscles.
2. Lacerations may occur even with the use of an episiotomy.
3. Pain and discomfort from episiotomies can interfere with mother-infant interactions and the reestablishment of parental sexual intercourse.
4. Episiotomies *are indicated* (a) if the well-being of the mother or fetus is in jeopardy, to shorten the second stage of labor, (b) if the infant is preterm and cerebral hemorrhage is a possibility because of capillary fragility, (c) if the infant is large (greater than 4000 g [9 lb]), or (d) in most forceps and breech deliveries (Pernoll, Benson, 1987).

The type of episiotomy is designated by site and direction of the incision (Fig. 18-19).

Midline episiotomy is most commonly used. It is effective, easily repaired, and generally the least painful. Occasionally there may be an extension through the rectal sphincter (third-degree laceration) or even into the anal canal (fourth-degree laceration). Fortunately primary healing and a good repair usually will be followed by good sphincter tone.

Mediolateral episiotomy is employed in operative delivery when posterior extension is likely. Although a fourth-degree laceration may thus be avoided, a third-degree laceration may occur. Moreover, as compared with a midline episiotomy, blood loss is greater and the repair more difficult and painful. Repair of left mediolateral episiotomy is shown in Fig. 18-20.

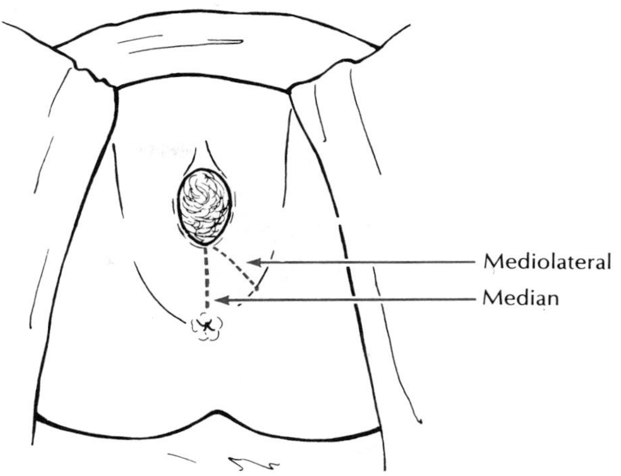

Fig. 18-19 Types of episiotomies.

LACERATIONS. Most acute injuries and lacerations of the perineum, vagina, uterus, and their support tissues occur during childbirth, and their management is an obstetric problem. Some injuries to the supporting tissues, whether they were acute or nonacute and whether they were repaired or not, may become gynecologic problems later in life (for further discussion, see Chapter 41).

The soft tissues of the birth canal and adjacent structures suffer some damage during every delivery. Damage usually is more pronounced in nulliparous women because the tissues are firmer and more resistant than in multiparous women. Perineal skin and vaginal mucosa may appear intact, obscuring numerous small lacerations in underlying muscle and its fascia. Damage to pelvic supports usually is readily apparent and thus is repaired after delivery.

The individual woman's tendency to sustain lacerations varies; that is, the soft tissue in some women may be less capable of distention. Heredity may be a factor. For example, the tissue of very light-skinned women, especially those with reddish hair, is not as readily distensible as that of a darker-skinned woman. Women whose tissues show a tendency to lacerate also may have varicose veins (see Fig. 12-3) and diastasis recti abdominis (see Fig. 8-13). In addition, healing may occur less efficiently in these women.

Immediate repair promotes healing and limits residual damage, as well as decreases the possibility of infection. Immediately after every delivery the cervix, vagina, and perineum are inspected. During the early postdelivery days, the nurse and primary care practitioner carefully inspect the perineum and evaluate lochia and symptoms to identify any previously missed damage (see Chapters 23 and 25).

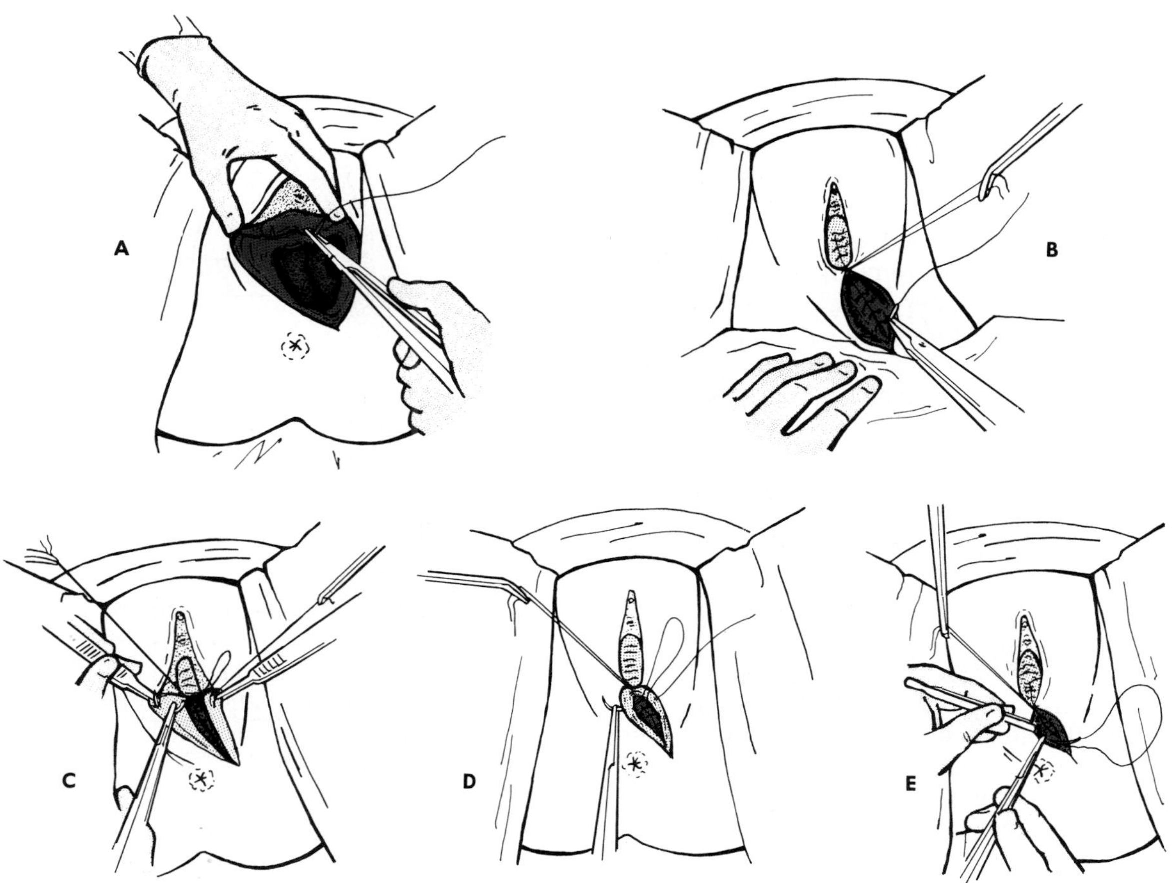

Fig. 18-20 Repair of left mediolateral episiotomy. **A** and **B,** Repair of levator muscle and its severed fascia. Attendant approximates cut edges of vaginal orifice, using forceps to exert traction on suture of bulbocavernosus muscles. **C,** Repair of cut ends. **D,** Repair of muscle and fascial components of urogenital diaphragm. **E,** Closure of skin edges. Sutures are placed just under dermis so that no sutures are visible when skin edges are approximated.

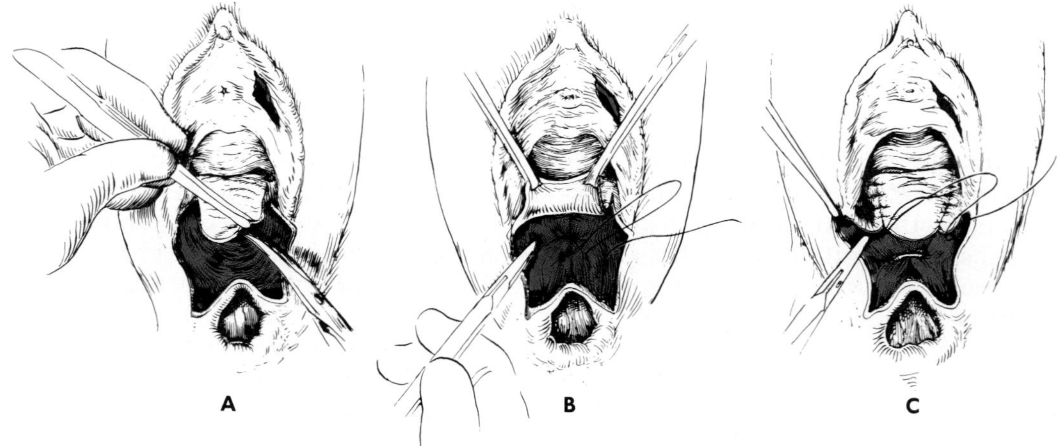

Fig. 18-21 Perineal lacerations. **A,** Bilateral sulcus tears, periurethral tear, and separation of anal sphincter. **B,** Exposure and approximation of levator ani structures. **C,** Approximation of torn bulbocavernosus muscle.
From Willson JR: *Atlas of obstetric technic,* ed 2, St Louis, 1969, Mosby–Year Book.

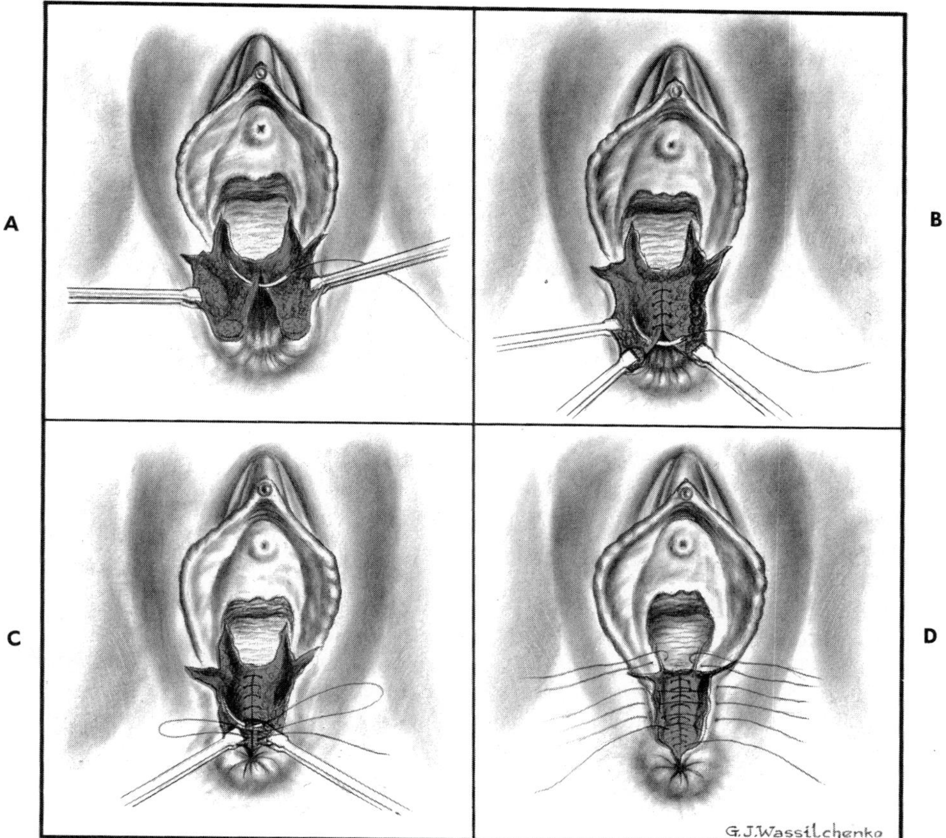

Fig. 18-22 Repair of fourth-degree laceration. **A,** Repair of rectal mucosa, with inverted sutures buried in muscles of rectal wall. **B,** Sutures of levator muscles to be buried; ends of sphincter drawn forward—first step of sphincter suture. **C,** Second step of sphincter suture—beginning figure-of-eight sutures. **D,** Sphincter suture completed and ready for tying. Remainder of perineal repair in usual manner.

PERINEAL LACERATIONS. Perineal lacerations usually occur as the fetal head is being born. The extent of the laceration is defined on the basis of depth:

1. *First degree.* Laceration extends through the skin and structures superficial to muscles.
2. *Second degree.* Laceration extends through muscles of perineal body.
3. *Third degree.* Laceration continues through anal sphincter muscle.
4. *Fourth degree.* Laceration also involves the anterior rectal wall.

Lacerations in the lower portion of the vagina occur along one or both lateral walls (sulci), rather than up the midline. The fascia of the elevator ani muscle is injured in all but the most superficial perineal tears. Perineal injury often is accompanied by small lacerations in the medial surfaces of the labia minora below the pubic rami and to the sides of the urethra and clitoris. Lacerations in this greatly vascular area often result in profuse bleeding.

Immediate repair with absorbable suture (Fig. 18-21) is indicated. Third- and fourth-degree lacerations require special attention so that the woman retains fecal continence. (Postdelivery nursing care is discussed in Chapters 23 and 25.) The woman's comfort is increased and healing is promoted by measures taken to ensure soft stools for a few days. Antimicrobial therapy may be used in some cases.

When the levator ani (including the iliococcygeus and pubococcygeus muscles, which form the sling-like support of pelvic viscera) is not involved, simple perineal injuries usually heal without permanent disability regardless of whether they were repaired. However, the *vaginal introitus may gape* if torn or severed (episiotomy) ends of superficial perineal muscles (e.g., bulbocavernosus) are not well approximated during repair.

The ends of the torn or severed anal sphincter muscles must be repaired adequately to avoid *fecal incontinence* (Fig. 18-22). It is easier to repair a new perineal injury to prevent sequelae than it is to correct long-term damage.

VAGINAL LACERATIONS. Vaginal lacerations often accompany perineal lacerations. Vaginal lacerations tend to extend up the lateral walls (sulci) and, if deep enough, to involve the levator ani. Additional injury may occur high in the vaginal vault near the level of the ischial spines. Vaginal vault lacerations may be circular and may result from forceps rotation, especially in the presence of cephalopelvic disproportion CPD (see Chapter 35).

A cervical or vaginal laceration extending into the broad ligament should *not* be repaired vaginally. Laparotomy with evacuation of the resultant hematoma and hemostatic repair or hysterectomy will be required (Pernoll, Benson, 1987).

The location of lacerations and the rapid and profuse bleeding make it difficult to expose and repair these types of tears. Late sequelae and management depend on the injury and the results of subsequent repair of injuries to the levator ani (see Chapter 41).

CERVICAL INJURIES. The greatest percentage of cervical injuries are obstetric in origin and occur when the cervix is being retracted over the advancing fetal head. Obstetrically acquired *cervical lacerations* usually occur at the lateral angles of the external os; most are shallow and bleeding is minimal (Fig. 18-23). More extensive lacerations may extend to the vaginal vault or beyond the vault into the lower uterine segment; serious bleeding may occur. Extensive lacerations may follow hasty attempts to enlarge the cervical opening artificially or to deliver the fetus before full cervical dilatation is achieved.

Anterior lip incarceration can occur. Occasionally the cervix is injured if the anterior lip is trapped between the fetal head and the pubic bone, an event that occurs most often when there is some degree of cephalopelvic disproportion (see Chapter 35). Because the trapped (incarcerated) cervix cannot be retracted upward around the descending head, the lower uterine segment above it thins excessively and may rupture. The anterior lip becomes edematous, bruised and almost black in color, and diffused with blood. The condition is exacerbated by women pushing before full dilatation of the cervix (p. 455). Unless the anterior lip is freed by pushing the head upward and easing the cervix over the head, the entire cervix may be torn loose; this condition is called *anular amputation*.

UTERINE RUPTURE. The most serious of childbirth injuries, rupture of the uterus, occurs approximately once in 1500 to 2000 births. Although the uterus may rupture during pregnancy, the uter-

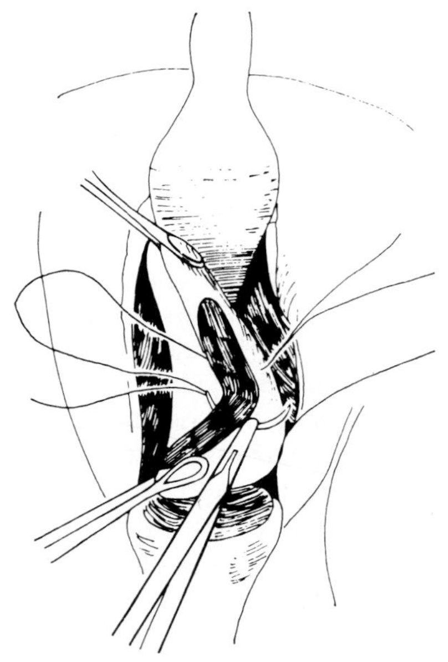

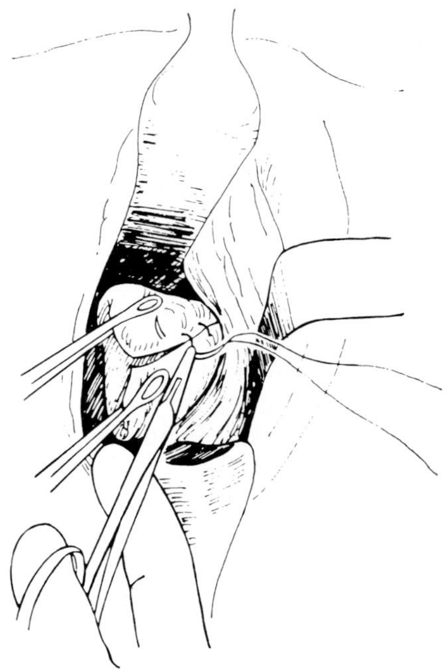

Fig. 18-23 Exposure and repair of cervical laceration. Interrupted sutures are placed through entire thickness of cervix.
From Willson JR, et al: *Obstetrics and gynecology,* ed 9, St Louis, 1991, Mosby–Year Book.

ine wall usually gives way during the stresses of labor. Hysterectomy may be indicated if the uterus is severely damaged. Uterine rupture is discussed in Chapter 30.

■ SUMMARY

Nursing care during the second and third stages of labor considers all members of the childbearing family. The new mother has now completed what in most instances is an exhilarating and rewarding experience. The perinatal nurse is in an ideal position to encourage and promote early family participation and attachment and to focus on the individual health care needs of each member of the childbearing family. The perinatal nurse uses specialized skills to provide safe, quality nursing care during the second and third stages of labor.

REFERENCES

American Academy of Pediatrics, American College of Obstetricians and Gyncologists. In Frigoletto FD, Little GA, editors: *Guidelines for perinatal care,* ed 2, White Plains, NY, 1988, March of Dimes Birth Defects Foundation.

Balaskis J: *Active birth,* London, 1983, Unicorn.

Carr KG: Management of the second stage of labor, *NAACOG Update Series,* lesson 9, vol 1, 1983.

Coltrell BH, Shannahan MD: Effect of the birth chair duration of second stage labor an maternal outcome, *Nurs Res* 35:364, 1986.

Cunningham FG, MacDonald PC, Gant NF: *Williams obstetrics,* ed 18, Norwalk, Conn, 1989, Appleton & Lange.

Gray JD et al: Prediction and prevention of child abuse, *Semin Perinatol* 3:95 Jan 1979.

Kurokawa J, Zilkoski MW: Adapting hospital obstetrics to birth in the squatting position, *Birth* 12:87, Summer 1985.

Machol L: LDR: new factor in the OB equation, *Contemp OB/GYN* 31:176, Feb 1988.

Mahan CS, McKay S: Are we overmanaging second stage labor? *Contemp OB/GYN* 24:37, Dec 1984.

Malestic SL: Fathers need help during labor, too, *RN* Vol. 53 1990, July 1990.

McKay S, Roberts J: Maternal position during labor and birth: what have we learned? *IJCE, ICEA Rev* 13:19, Aug 1989.

Myles M: *Textbook for midwives,* ed 10, Edinburgh, 1985, Churchill Livingstone.

Pernoll ML, Benson RC: Current obstetric and gynecologic diagnosis and treatment, ed 6, Los Altos, Calif, 1987, Appleton & Lange.

Queenan JT: Partners in the delivery room: a natural evolution, *Contemp OB/GYN* 35:8, Aug 1990.

Quinlan P: Genevieve's birth at Pithiviers, *Birth* 10:187, Fall 1983.

Scott JR et al: Danforth's obstetrics and gynecology, ed 6, Philadelphia, 1990, JB Lippincott Co.

Supported squatting enhances the second stage of labor, *AJN* 89:1266, Oct 1989.

Warrington J: *The obstetric catechism,* Philadelphia, 1842, Crolius & Clading.

References—Nursing Research

Andrews CM, Chrzanowski M: Maternal position, labor, and comfort, *Appl Nurs Res* 3:7, Jan/Feb 1990.

Coltrell BH, Shannahan MD: Effect of the birth chair on duration of second stage labor and maternal outcome, *Nurs Res* 35:364, 1986.

Gardosi J, Sylvester SB, Lynch C: Alternative positions in the second stage of labour; a randomized controlled trial, *Br J Obstet Gynaecol* 96:1290, 1989.

Jordan PL: Laboring for relevance: expectant and new fatherhood, *Nurs Res* 39, Jan/Feb 1990.

Liu YC: Effects of the upright position during childbirth, *Image* 21:1, 1989.

McKay S, Roberts J: Obstetrics by ear. Maternal and caregiver perceptions of the meaning of maternal sounds during second stage labor, *J Nurse Midwife* 35:266, Sept/Oct 1990.

Metzer BL, Therrien B: Effect of position on cardiovascular response during the Valsalva maneuver, *Nurs Res* 39:198, July/Aug 1990.

Yeates J, Roberts J: A comparison of 2 bearing down techniques during the second stage of labor, *J Nurse* 29:3, 1984.

BIBLIOGRAPHY

Brown A: After birth—management of the third stage of labour, *Nurs Times* 85:52, Sept 1989.

Manyonda IT, Shaw DE: The effect of delayed pushing in the second stage of labor with continuous epidural analgesia, *Acta Obstet Gynecol Scand* 69:291, 1990.

Moon JM, Smith CV, Rayburn WF: Perinatal outcome after a prolonged second stage of labor, *J Reprod Med* 35:229, 1990.

Piquard F et al: The validity of fetal heart rate monitoring during the second stage of labor, *Obstet Gynecol* 72:746, 1988.

Roberts JE: Managing fetal bradycardia during second stage of labor, *MCN* 14:394, Nov/Dec 1989.

Rooks JP et al: Outcomes of care in birth centers. The National Birth Center Study, *N Engl J Med* 321:1804, 1989.

Strong TH et al: Prophylactic intrapartum amnioinfusion: a randomized clinical trial, *Am J Obstet Gynecol* 162:1370, 1990.

Stroud R, Cochrane S: Midwives' managing without drugs, *Nurs Times* 86:70, Nov 28, 1990.

Swinnerton T: Alternative remedies during labor, *Nurs Times* 87(9):64, 1991.

Wuitchik M et al: Perinatal predictors of pain and distress during labor, *Birth* 17:186, Winter 1990.

Bibliography—Nursing Research

Begley CM: A comparison of "active" and "physiological" management of the third stage of labour, *Midwifery* 6:3, March 1990.

Harding JE, Elbourne DR, Prendiville WJ: Views of mothers and midwives participating in the Bristol randomized, controlled trial of active management of the third stage of labor, *Birth* 16:1, Spring 1989.

Mackey MC, Lock SE: Women's expectations of the labor and delivery nurse, *JOGNN* 18:505, Nov/Dec 1989.

McKay S, Barrows T, Roberts J: Women's views of second-stage labor as assessed by interviews and videotapes, *Birth* 17:192, Winter 1990.

Weaver DR: Nurses' views on the meaning of touch in obstetrical nursing practice, *JOGNN* 19:157, March/April 1990.

chapter 18 review

Key Concepts

- When allowed to respond to the rhythmic nature of the second stage of labor, the woman normally will change body positions, push when she has an urge, and vocalize as she bears down.
- The only certain objective sign that the second stage has begun is that, on vaginal examination, the cervix cannot be palpated.
- If any laboring woman states, "The baby is coming!" the baby *is* coming, and it is too late for transfer to a delivery room.
- During the second stage, the woman needs continuous monitoring, support, and coaching.
- Five signs indicate that placental separation has occurred and the placenta is ready to be expelled; before placental separation, excessive traction can result in immediate or delayed injury to the mother.
- Most parents/families enjoy being able to handle, hold, explore, and examine the baby immediately after the birth.
- Nurses must be alert to the appearance of warning signs in parent-child relationships during the postdelivery period.
- As the neonate makes the transition from intrauterine to extrauterine life, initiation and maintenance of respiration and prevention of cold stress are top priorities.
- In a situation such as emergency childbirth out of the hospital, in the absence of injectable oxytocin, the neonate's sucking or nuzzling and licking the breast stimulate the release of natural oxytocin from the mother's posterior pituitary.
- Episiotomies and lacerations may be seen even with "normal" childbirth, and their appropriate and prompt repair is essential.

Key Terms

- amniotic fluid emboli (p. 488)
- Apgar score (p. 493)
- bearing down (p. 473)
- caul (p. 481)
- crowning (p. 480)
- descent phase (p. 475, 480)
- episiotomy (p. 480, 496)
- eye prophylaxis (p. 494)
- Ferguson's reflex (p. 471)
- final/transition phase (p. 470, 475)
- lacerations (p. 481, 497)
- latency/resting phase (p. 470, 475)
- lithotomy position (p. 479)
- mini-prep (p. 480)
- nuchal cord (p. 481)
- ophthalmia neonatorum (p. 494)
- placental separation (p. 488)
- ring of fire (p. 471)
- Ritgen maneuvers (p. 481)
- second stage (p. 470)
- Sims' position (p. 479)
- third stage (p. 470)
- Valsalva's maneuver (p. 473)
- vocalization (p. 471)
- Wharton's jelly (p. 484)

Critical Thinking Exercises

You are assigned to a woman and her family during the second and third stages of labor.

1. Develop assumptions about the behaviors observed among the family members.
2. Examine your response to and feelings about the birth. Identify your positive or negative feelings, and explore their causes.
3. Examine the birth setting and the procedures performed during these stages, and assess their potential effect on parent-infant attachment.
4. Observe parent-infant interactions.
   A. Identify behaviors that make you uncomfortable.
   B. Explore the cause of those behaviors.
   C. What impact could these feelings have on your ability to facilitate parent-infant interactions?

Topics for Nursing Research

- Is there a difference in the length of the second stage if women push when they have the urge to push and in the manner they wish to push as compared with that of women who push as directed by a coach?
- Are there effects on siblings who witness their mother's labor and birth?
- Is there a "profile" of siblings (e.g., age, level of maturation) who could benefit from—or who could be traumatized by—witnessing their mother's labor and birth?

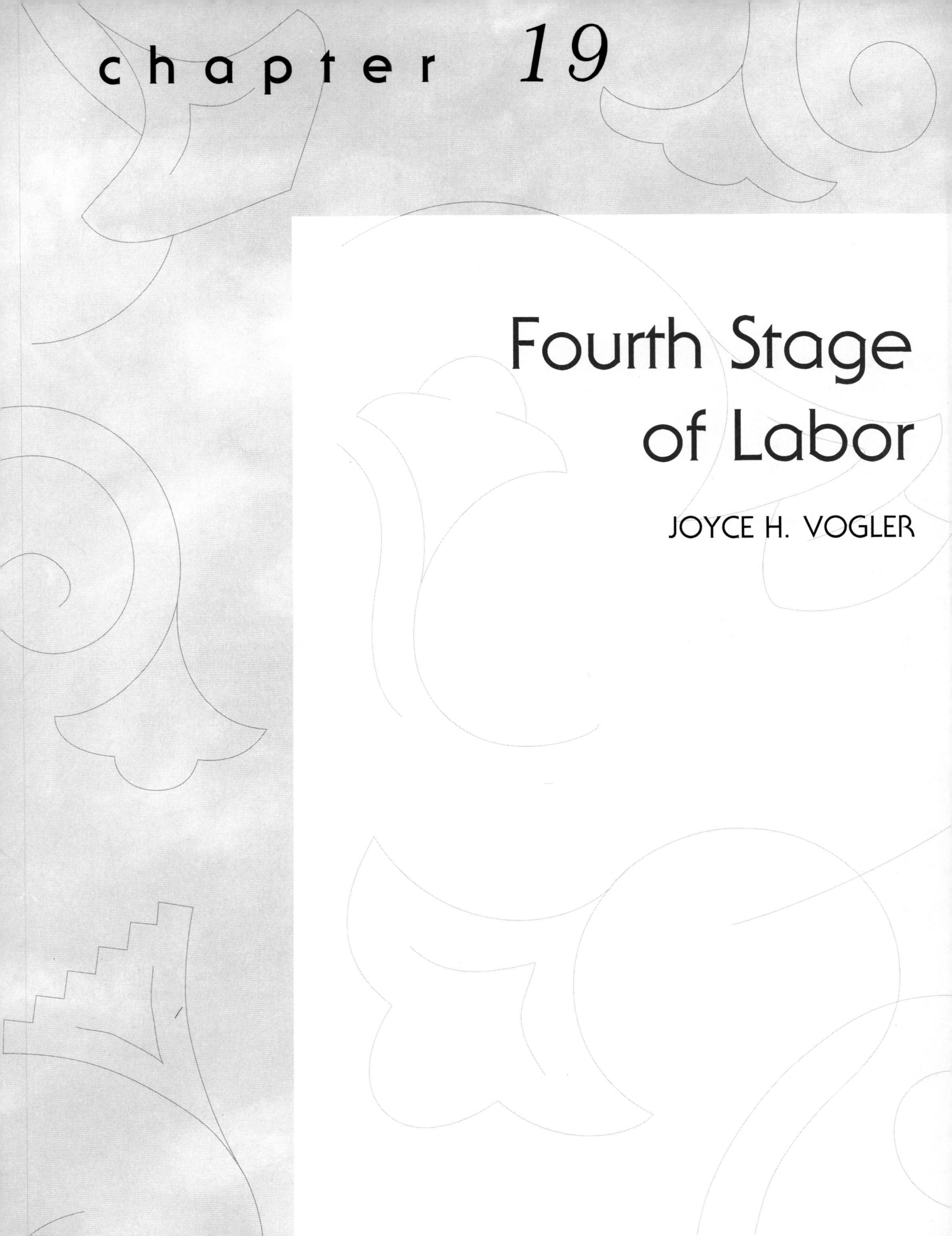

chapter 19

Fourth Stage of Labor

JOYCE H. VOGLER

LEARNING OBJECTIVES

- Define the key terms listed.
- Review the immediate care of the mother after the birth.
- Identify priorities of maternal care immediately after the birth.
- Discuss the maternal fluid balance and nutritional needs.
- List measures to prevent hemorrhage.
- Formulate measures to prevent bladder distention.
- Develop measures to support parental emotional needs.
- Explain measures to facilitate parent-infant interaction.
- Summarize measures to promote comfort and support emotional needs.
- Outline the nurse's role in the care of the new mother with an episiotomy or a laceration.
- Review transfer of mother and newborn to postdelivery area.
- Identify topics for nursing research related to the fourth stage of labor.

The **fourth stage of labor,** the stage of recovery, is a critical period for the mother and newborn. They not only are recovering from the physical process of birth but also are initiating new relationships.

During the first 2 hours after the birth, maternal organs are undergoing their initial readjustment to the nonpregnant state, and body systems begin to stabilize. For several hours the newborn continues the transition from intrauterine to extrauterine existence. Many parents are choosing early discharge from the hospital; others must leave because of diagnosis-related group (DRG) and insurance requirements. The health care team must be reasonably assured that there is no potential for disruption in these normal processes for the mother or newborn. The nurse's skills can make a critical difference during the fourth stage. Some terms important in this stage follow:

involution Process that results in the healing of the birth canal and the return of the uterus and all systems to or almost to the prepregnant state. Generally, changes reflect reversals of the anatomic and physiologic adaptations to pregnancy.

lochia Uterine discharge after delivery

atonic uterus A lack of tone in the uterine muscle caused by interference with the ability of the muscle to contract and retract

■ NURSING PROCESS

It is important for the nurse to be skilled in the nursing process as it relates to the mother/newborn/family during the fourth stage of labor. Careful management of this stage is necessary to promote the best possible outcome for all.

ASSESSMENT

If the nurse has not previously cared for the new mother, assessment begins with review of the prenatal and labor records (see Fig. 18-14). In many institutions the labor nurse now follows the woman through the initial 1 to 2 hours after the birth. Of primary importance are conditions that could predispose the mother to hemorrhage (such as precipitous labor, large baby, grand multiparity, or induced labor), which is a potential danger during the fourth stage of labor.

Selected data from the prenatal and intrapartal records may include the following information:

Item	Examples
Relevant information from prenatal record	Blood type, Rh factor, medical conditions, prenatal care
Length of labor and type of delivery; unusual events (e.g., nuchal cord)	Spontaneous vaginal, after short unmedicated labor; Cesarean: elective, or after long labor
Gravidity and parity, age of mother	Primiparous woman, grand multiparous woman, adolescent, after age 35
Baby's condition at birth, sex and weight, events since birth*	Healthy or unhealthy, average for gestational age, weight >9 lb 8 oz
Parents' response to labor and birth.	Happy; disappointed in sex of baby; need for cesarean

General Systems Assessment

To help the nurse provide comprehensive care, a worksheet outlining a schedule for assessments is suggested for this 2-hour postdelivery period. During the first hour in the recovery room, physical assessment of the mother occurs frequently. All factors except temperature are assessed every 15 minutes for 1 hour. After the fourth 15-minute assessment, if all parameters have stabilized within the normal range, assessment is repeated twice more at 30-minute intervals. A physical assessment of the mother during the fourth stage of labor is performed by the recovery nurse.

The findings for the first recovery hour can be charted on a delivery/recovery record (see Fig. 18-14) or in a postpartum record.

NOTE: Hand washing precedes assessment. Latex gloves are worn while the perineum is inspected or when contact with mucous membranes, nonintact skin, blood, or other body fluids is possible.

VITAL SIGNS. *Blood pressure* readings provide a data base for diagnosis of potential complications such as hemorrhage (see Chapter 30) and hypertensive states (see Chapter 28). It usually stabilizes at prelabor values during the first hour. An appropriate-sized cuff must be used. The *pulse* is counted and assessed for rate, amplitude (indicating volume), rhythm and symmetry, and regularity. Readings provide a data base for diagnosis of complications (e.g., hemorrhage). The pulse usually stabilizes at prelabor levels during the first hour. **Bradycardia** (50 to 70 beats/min) may occur in some women as a result of cardiovascular changes that occur immediately after

*Neonatal adjustment to extrauterine existence and recovery of the neonate are discussed in detail in Chapter 20 and Unit 4.

giving birth. At the moment of birth, intraabdominal pressure is drastically reduced, pressure on veins is removed, the vessels in the abdominal organs engorge with blood (splanchnic engorgement), and blood flow to the heart is increased. When blood flow to the heart is increased, reflex bradycardia may result (Guyton, 1987).

UTERUS. *Uterine tone, fundal position, and height* are assessed frequently during this time. An empty bladder makes assessment easier and findings more accurate. The woman is positioned with her head slightly elevated and her knees flexed to relieve tension on abdomen and to facilitate palpation. The nurse begins palpation just below the umbilicus by cupping the hand and pressing firmly into the abdomen. If the fundus is firm (and the bladder is empty), with the uterus in the midline, the nurse measures its position relative to the woman's umbilicus. With the fingers flat on the abdomen, the nurse measures the number of fingerbreadths that fit between the umbilicus and the top of the fundus. Most authors identify a normal fundal height to be below the umbilicus, but variations exist. The position of the contracted fundus immediately after expulsion of the placenta has been described in the following ways:

- Immediately after delivery the globular uterus is an abdominal organ extending halfway up to the umbilicus; after several hours, it ascends to about the level of the umbilicus (Scott et al, 1990, p. 189).
- Immediately after expulsion of the placenta, the fundus is about midway between the umbilicus and symphysis, or slightly higher; during the next two days it remains approximately the same size and then begins to shrink (Cunningham et al, 1989, p. 245).
- The fundus is two-thirds to three-fourths up from the symphysis pubis; it rises to level of umbilicus within a few hours and remains at approximately the level of the umbilicus or 1 fingerbreadth below for a day or two (Varney, 1991, p. 476).
- After the uterus regains its tone, the superior surface can be felt below the umbilicus (Willson et al, 1991, p. 541).

If the fundus is *not* firm, the nurse must stimulate the uterine muscle ("living ligature"; see Fig. 6-10) to regain tone and to expel any clots before measuring the distance from the umbilicus. The uterus is massaged *gently* only until it is firm; overstimulation causes uterine muscle fatigue and results in atonia (relaxation).

The uterus can contract only if it is free of **intrauterine clots.** Care must be taken to avoid inversion of the uterus during expulsion of clots. To expel clots the nurse keeps the hands placed as in Fig. 19-1 to support the uterus from below with one hand. With the upper hand, the nurse applies firm pressure downward toward the vagina while observing the perineum for the number and size of expelled clots. As the nurse performs these assessments, the woman is taught the rationale for the assessment and how to maintain uterine tone herself by self-massage.

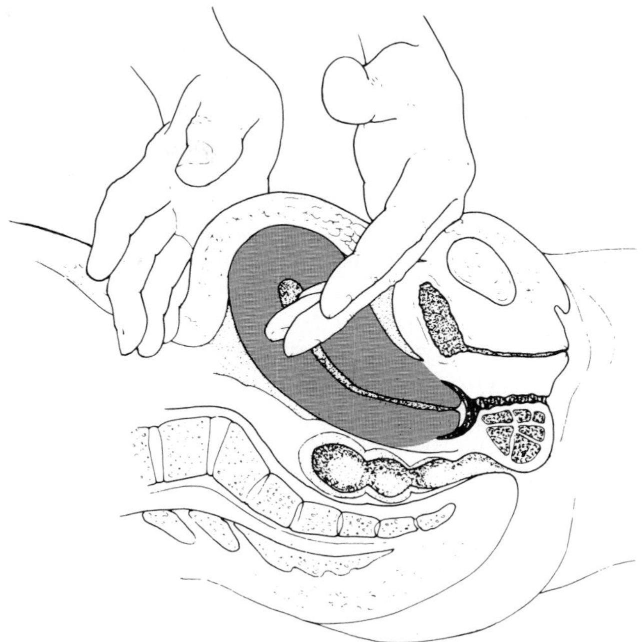

Fig. 19-1 Palpating fundus of uterus during first hour after delivery. Note that upper hand is cupped over fundus; lower hand dips in above symphysis pubis and supports uterus while it is massaged gently.

BLADDER. **Bladder distention** is assessed by noting the location and firmness of the uterine fundus and by observation and palpation of the bladder (located just above the symphysis pubis). If the bladder is distended, it appears as a suprapubic rounded bulge that is dull to percussion and fluctuates like a water-filled balloon. When the bladder is distended, the uterus may be boggy, well above the umbilicus, and usually to the woman's right side (dextrorotated). The degree to which normal bladder function has returned is assessed by asking the new mother to void and measuring the volume. Small frequent voidings occur when there is urinary retention. Catheterization may be necessary to prevent bladder distention and subsequent bladder atony. Overdistention causes maternal discomfort and results in uterine atony and hemorrhage. The distending bladder pushes the uterus higher into the abdominal cavity, interfering with its ability to contract. Signs of an empty bladder include a firm fundus in the midline and a nonpalpable bladder.

LOCHIA. The amount and character of lochia are assessed by observation of peripads, the woman's perineum, and the linens under the woman's buttocks. The number and size of clots, if present, are noted. Findings provide a data base to assist the nurse to differentiate between lochia of normal involution and discharge signaling complications such as infection (see Chapter 29) or hemorrhage (see Chapter 30). At this time, the *lochia rubra* is *moderate* in amount and may contain some small clots. The odor should be "fleshy," much like that of menstrual flow. The nurse observes the perineum for the source of bleeding; lochia does not come out of the vagina in a continuous trickle or in spurts. An episiotomy or laceration may be the source of the bleeding.

PERINEUM. The nurse asks the woman, or assists her, to turn on to her side, flex her thigh against her hip, and *gently* lifts the upper buttock to assess the perineum. Good lighting is essential for adequate observation. After vaginal birth, mild edema or labial swelling and slight bruising may be seen. If the woman has had an episiotomy or a laceration, the nurse needs to assess for redness, edema, ecchymosis, discharge, and approximation of the wound edges (**REEDA**). During inspection, the nurse notes the degree of discomfort the new mother is experiencing. A painful perineum, bruising, and swelling may indicate a hematoma in the area (see p. 509). The primary care practitioner needs to be informed of these findings to perform a more thorough evaluation.

TEMPERATURE. The woman's temperature is assessed at 1 hour and then per hospital protocol. Temperature usually stabilizes within normal range during the first hour. A slight elevation during this period may be related to dehydration or fatigue.

COMFORT. The woman is assessed for discomfort, the type and location. The amount and type of analgesia or anesthesia she received during labor and birth will affect her perception of discomfort. Perineal discomfort and fatigue frequently are reported.

Assessment and support for parents' psychologic needs are noted on p. 513. Assessment for psychosocial adaptations is discussed extensively in Chapters 10 and 24.

SIGNS OF POTENTIAL PROBLEMS. Because hemorrhage is a significant potential complication, it is discussed extensively in this chapter and in Chapters 25 and 30. The nurse must always be on the alert for other potential complications: postspinal headache (Chapter 15), hypertensive states (Chapter 28), infections (Chapter 29), endocrine disorders (Chapter 31), psychosocial disorders (Chapter 33), and loss and grief (Chapter 40). A box on p. 490 lists warning signs of dysfunctional parent-neonate relationships.

NURSING DIAGNOSES

Nursing diagnoses lend direction to the type of nursing action needed to implement a plan of care. Before establishing nursing diagnoses, the nurse analyzes the significance of findings collected during assessment. Examples of nursing diagnoses include the following:

- High risk for fluid volume deficit (hemorrhage) related to
  —Uterine atony after childbirth
- Urinary retention related to
  —Effects of labor and delivery on urinary tract sensation
- Pain related to
  —Interruption in skin integrity secondary to the process of childbirth
- High risk for injury related to
  —Early ambulation
- High risk for altered parenting related to
  —Postpartum pain or fatigue
  —Disappointment in sex or appearance of newborn
- Altered family processes related to
  —Addition of new member
- Ineffective breast-feeding related to
  —Lack of experience

PLANNING

During the planning step, *goals* are set in client-centered terms. The goals are prioritized. Nursing actions are selected, with the client where appropriate, to meet the goals. Goals for the fourth stage of labor may include that the woman will:

1. Saturate no more than one pad per hour
2. Void within 6 to 8 hours after delivery
3. Verbalize acceptance of labor process after expressing concerns
4. Begin the bonding/attachment process with infant and family
5. Verbalize increased comfort after initiation of comfort measures

IMPLEMENTATION

During the fourth stage of labor, the nurse must organize care to include observation of vital signs, provision of comfort measures, education of the mother, and care of the infant. Nursing concerns include prevention of hemorrhage, prevention of urinary bladder distention, maintenance of comfort, maintenance of cleanliness, maintenance of fluid balance and nutrition, support of parental emotional needs, and promotion of maternal and infant care education.

During the fourth stage of labor, the nurse uses every opportunity to teach the new mother. Regardless of parity, new mothers can benefit from explanations for the various nursing actions during the immediate puerperium (Mercer, 1979). Teaching is correlated with goals, assessment findings, nursing actions, and evaluation.

Prevention of Hemorrhage

Assessments are designed for early identification of events that may lead to **hemorrhage.** Postpartum hemorrhage is considered to be the loss of 500 ml of blood or more (for further discussion, see Chapter 30). The mother's temperature, pulse, and blood pressure (BP) are assessed and recorded and should be within normal limits. The pulse rate will generally be between 60 and 70 beats/min. If the pulse rate is more than 90 beat/min, investigation and continued supervision are necessary. The temperature may be below normal because of loss of body heat. On occasion it may be higher than 37.2° C (99° F) because of dehydration or long labor. After a difficult labor, systolic BP less than 110 mm Hg, accompanied by a pulse over 100 beats/min, usually is the result of hemorrhage or shock.

The uterus must be palpated at frequent intervals to ascertain that it is not filling with blood (Fig. 19-1). The pad must be checked frequently to ensure that blood is not excessive (Fig. 19-2). Lochia may be described as scant, light, moderate, or heavy (profuse). Normally, the fundus is firm or may be returned to a state of firmness with intermittent gentle massage. As noted earlier, **atony** *(relaxation) of the uterine musculature* may occur. As the relaxed uterus distends with blood and clots, blood vessels in the placental site are not clamped off and bleeding results. The uterus is unable to function as the "living ligature" that promotes sustained uterine contraction.

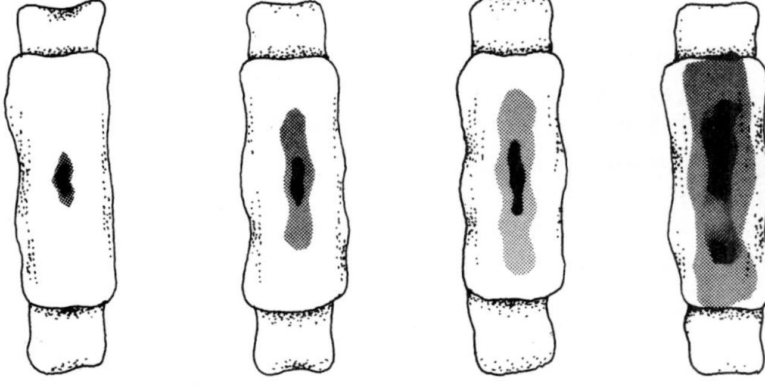

Fig. 19-2 Peripad-saturation volumes.

NOTE: To express clots it is necessary to express gently the accumulated blood and clots before the uterus will contract again. First, make certain the fundus is firm, then support the base of the uterus with one hand while pressing gently on the uterus in the direction of the vagina with the other hand. If atony is not controlled by this treatment, medical intervention must be instituted (see Chapter 25).

As the effect of the oxytocic medication administered after delivery wears off, the amount of lochia will increase because the myometrium relaxes somewhat. The nurse *always checks* under the mother's buttocks, as well as on the perineal pad. Bleeding may flow between the buttocks onto the linens under the mother while the amount on the perineal pad is slight. A perineal pad that is soaked through from tail to tail contains approximately 68 to 80 mL of blood (Luegenbiehl et al, 1990). Higgins (1982) found that most nurses overestimate blood loss but were consistent in their observations. When hemorrhage is suspected, the nurse should save all peripads and underpads for the primary care practitioner to assess. If a pad is found to be soaked through in 15 minutes, or if blood is seen pooled under the buttocks, continuous observation of blood loss, vital signs, and maternal color and behavior is essential.

Another potential source of hemorrhage is the development of a **hematoma** under the vaginal mucosa or in the connective tissue of the vulva. This may occur as a result of injury to a blood vessel during the delivery or in repairing the laceration/episiotomy. The bleeding may be slow but continuous as the blood oozes from the vessel and distends the surrounding tissue. In many cases this distention of the tissue may not be visualized by the nurse. The initial complaint by the woman is that of severe and intense pressure and/or pain in the perineal or rectal area. The nurse should carefully inspect the perineum, monitor vital signs, and report all findings to the primary care practitioner immediately, with emphasis placed on the woman's complaint and the location of pain.

A vulvar hematoma may be visualized as the swelling increases. It usually is unilateral and becomes purplish. A vaginal hematoma is usually found only through manual examination. A soft mass may be palpated through a vaginal or rectal examination. The blood loss with this type of hematoma may be excessive. A loss of 500 mL or more is not unusual.

The hematoma continues to be evaluated, and if it

remains small, treatment is unnecessary because the hematoma will reabsorb. However, many times it is necessary for the nurse to prepare the woman for surgical incision and evacuation of the hematoma. The procedure is performed with general anesthesia or regional anesthesia in the area from which the clots are removed and ligation of the blood vessel is necessary. Nursing care after the procedure includes careful monitoring of the perineum and blood loss, maintenance of intravenous (IV) fluids, monitoring of vital signs and laboratory work, preparing for a possible blood transfusion, and administering prescribed antibiotics as prophylaxis against infection (see Chapter 25 for additional information).

If bleeding is in the form of a continuous trickle or is seen to come in spurts, lacerations of the vagina or cervix or the presence of an unligated vessel in the episiotomy are suspected. The woman most likely will be returned to the delivery area to permit visualization of the site and surgical correction.

HYPOVOLEMIC SHOCK. Hypovolemic shock as a result of hemorrhage may occur in an otherwise normal fourth stage of labor. Prompt identification, diagnosis, and intervention usually result in rapid stabilization of the woman's BP, pulse, and other signs. This occurs if adequate circulating blood volume to assist the body to compensate for the loss is available or is infused intravenously. If compensatory mechanisms become ineffective, shock may ensue. The woman will experience symptoms that include lightheadedness, pallor, air hunger, and cool clammy skin. These are caused by sympathetic nervous system stimulation and hypoxia of both brain and tissue cells.

Beta-adrenergic receptors are stimulated and the circulatory system attempts to compensate for tissue hypoxia and metabolic acidosis. The BP falls, and in response the pulse will increase. Measures such as uterine massage and IV administration of oxytocin are implemented to prevent further blood loss. If the woman feels faint, aromatic ammonia* is used as a respiratory stimulant to increase intake of oxygen. It is important for the nurse to stay with and reassure the woman and family to decrease their anxiety. The nurse then documents all nursing and medical interventions that have been employed and their results. The emergency procedure box below provides a quick reference for danger signs and symptoms and interventions for hypovolemic shock.

Prevention of Bladder Distention

Palpation to determine the amount of *bladder distention* should accompany palpation of the fundus. The full bladder forces the uterus upward and to the right of the midline. Such a position interferes with the contractility of the uterine muscles, and hemorrhage results. In addition to the possibility of causing

*CAUTION: Do not use aromatic ammonia for women with history of cardiac disease.

EMERGENCY

Hypovolemic Shock

SIGNS/SYMPTOMS

Persistent significant bleeding—perineal pad soaked within 15 minutes; *may not be accompanied by a change in vital signs or maternal color or behavior.*
Mother states she feels light-headed, "funny," "sick to my stomach," or sees "stars"
Mother begins to act anxious or exhibits air hunger
Woman's color turns ashen or grayish
Temperature of skin feels cool and clammy
Increasing pulse rate
Falling BP
Intense perineal pain (possible hematoma)

INTERVENTIONS

Call for help immediately—summon help to *you.*
Tilt woman onto her side and raise her legs *high.* Increase flow of IV drip.
If uterus is atonic, massage gently and expel clots to allow uterus to contract; compress uterus manually, as needed, using two hands. Add oxytocic to IV drip, as ordered.
Break ampule of aromatic ammonia, a respiratory stimulant; give oxygen by face mask or nasal prongs at 8 to 10 L/min.
Reassure woman (couple). *Do not leave* the woman.
Prepare for possible incision and evacuation of hematoma.
Chart incident and medical and nursing interventions employed. Chart results of treatments.

uterine relaxation, distention of the urinary bladder can result in atony of the bladder wall. Atony leads to **urinary retention,** which provides a favorable environment for infection.

A nurse encourages the woman to void naturally, employing one or more of the following methods: placing a bedpan under the mother, giving her water to drink if the physician has ordered oral fluids, turning on the water faucet, pouring warm water over the perineum, helping her walk to the bathroom (if ordered), and providing privacy. If after these measures the woman cannot void, most physicians write an order for catheterization.

Spirits of peppermint are sometimes used to aid the woman to void naturally. "Spirits" are concentrated alcohol solutions of volatile substances; they are also known as essences. Spirits of peppermint give off vapors. These vapors have an external, local relaxing effect on the sphincter muscle of the urinary meatus. Use of peppermint spirits may make it unnecessary to catheterize. The nurse places a bedpan under the woman and pours a few drops of peppermint spirits *into the bedpan.* The vapors rise to flow over the vulvar area, the urinary meatus relaxes, and urine is released. Nothing touches the woman except the vapors; the woman feels no sensation, only notices the aroma of peppermint. Most hospitals do not require a physician's order for the technique.

Maintenance of Safety

The mother is settled comfortably in bed. A woman who has just given birth may need to remain in bed for a period of time to allow her body systems to adjust to fluid volume changes. The nurse caring for the woman will decide the appropriate time for the first ambulation. The nurse takes several things into consideration when making this decision: baseline BP, the amount of blood loss, type and amount of analgesic or anesthetic medications administered during labor and birth, the level of pain evident in the woman's movements, and the woman's desire to ambulate. The rapid decrease in intraabdominal pressure after birth results in a dilation of blood vessels supplying the intestines, which is known as **splanchnic engorgement,** causing blood to pool in the viscera. This contributes to **orthostatic hypotension,** which tends to occur when a woman who has recently given birth stands up; consequently she may faint or feel light-headed.

It is imperative to keep within the nurse's reach aromatic ammonia ampules, which can be easily broken, to revive the woman who is ambulating for the first time. The nurse must caution the woman to use her call bell to summon help before she attempts to get out of bed. The nurse will assess her color, pulse, and level of consciousness (LOC) in response to conversation and then assist her in ambulating to the bathroom. Once the woman has reached the bathroom, the nurse should remain outside the door and inquire as to her well-being every minute or so. If there is no answer, the nurse enters the bathroom to assess the woman's condition. A wheelchair should be handy in the room or just outside in case the woman feels too weak to walk back to bed. She is encouraged to rest after the ambulation, so that she can regain her strength.

The woman who has received conduction anesthesia (epidural block) is kept in bed until she is able to fully move and feel sensation in her legs and her BP and pulse are within normal limits. Ambulation can occur within the first 2 hours, depending on whether the last dose was administered just before birth. If the woman had local anesthesia and some intravenously or intramuscularly administered analgesic shortly before birth, the nurse will need to assess her ability to communicate, her LOC, and her vital signs for stability (within normal limits) before allowing the woman to get out of bed. Other types of anesthesia consist of saddle block, spinal block, and paracervical block (see Chapter 15 for discussion of methods and postspinal headache). The nurse will check that the woman is wearing slippers before she ambulates.

The woman who has received analgesics needs to be watched until she is fully recovered from the medication (i.e., vital signs are stable within her normal range, and she is fully awake).

Maintenance of Comfort

Uterine contractions may result in **discomfort** known as **afterpains.** The volume within the uterus is decreased after delivery. The force of the myometrial contractions is considerable; the intrauterine pressure is much greater than that during labor, reaching 150 mm Hg or more.

During the first 2 hours after delivery, uterine contractions are regular and strong, especially in multiparous women. The nurse adds to the woman's comfort by performing the following measures:

1. Explaining the normal physiology of afterpains
2. Helping the mother keep her urinary bladder empty
3. Placing a warmed blanket on the mother's abdomen
4. Administering analgesics ordered by the physician
5. Encouraging relaxation and breathing exercises

As the bladder fills, it presses against the uterus, causing it to relax. The uterus attempts to stay firm by increasing the force of contractions, thereby increasing the discomfort of afterpains. Gentle massage of the fundus increases uterine contractions, thereby intensifying afterpains. To help the new mother cope with the discomforts of assessment measures, the nurse explains what is being done and why and then encourages the woman to perform the procedure.

The episiotomy site or hemorrhoids often contribute to a new mother's discomfort. Immediately after the birth, cold therapy such as ice packs are applied to the perineum directly over the episiotomy to minimize edema formation. Edema adds to perineal discomfort. After the first 2 hours, ice packs have little effect on minimizing edema; they are used to increase comfort by numbing the area. Chemical ice packs attached to sanitary pads are used if available, but they are expensive.

Disposable ice packs are easily made from rubber examining gloves filled with ice chips and covered with something clean such as a disposable wash cloth or one of the disposable towels in the perineal prep kit. The primary care practitioner may order any one of several antiseptic or anesthetic ointments or sprays to ease discomfort in the perineal area. A side-lying position relieves direct pressure on the area.

If the woman has had a saddle block or other regional anesthetic, the nurse's description of sensations to expect as the anesthetic wears off can be reassuring. Women describe the sensation as tingling or prickly, much like that experienced after one has been sitting cross-legged for a long time and the legs have "gone to sleep."

Some women experience intense **postpartum tremors** that resemble the shivering of a chill. The chilling may be related to the sudden release of pressure on pelvic nerves. According to another theory, chilling may be symptomatic of a fetus-to-mother transfusion that sometimes occurs during placental separation. The feeling of a chill may be a reaction to epinephrine (adrenaline) production during delivery. The nurse can help the woman relax or feel comforted by providing her with warm blankets and an explanation that the tremors are commonly seen after delivery and are not related to infection. Some women experience the tremors without any feeling of chill; these women also should be covered with a blanket, preferably warm if tolerated. The tremors usually are self-limiting and last only a short while. The warm blanket also provides a means of "mothering the mother." This helps restore her energy so she can move from a focus on herself to a focus on her baby as she moves from "taking-in" to "taking-hold" (see chapter 24).

If the nurse administers analgesics, the sedating effect of these analgesics necessitates such protective care as raising side rails, placing call bell within reach, and cautioning about remaining in bed. The woman must be warned about any expected dizziness or drowsiness resulting from the medications.

Maintenance of Cleanliness

Perineal Care increases the mother's comfort and safety (prevention of infection). A clean perineal pad is placed in position, buttocks dried, and any wet linen removed so the woman will be warm and comfortable. The nurse dons clean gloves before touching the mother's linens, soiled perineal pad, or perineal area. The nurse instructs the mother first to wash her hands, then cleanse the vulvar area from front to back, using a separate tissue for each wipe, and end by rewashing her hands. A woman who has had a repair to her perineum may be encouraged not to use tissue to wipe her vulva after voiding but to use the hospital's available perineal cleansing alternatives. A plastic "peri-bottle," which can be filled with warm tap water that is squeezed out to cleanse the perineal area, may be used. Also available is an electrical apparatus that runs warm water through a plastic wand containing a soap cartridge (see Fig. 25-1). The woman holds the wand under her perineum and experiences a type of sitz bath. Clean pads usually are left in the bathroom, and the woman is instructed to change her pad each time she uses the bathroom.

The nurse's attention to the mother's needs demonstrates a sense of caring. The woman feels more comfortable even if the same amount of discomfort is still present (Hawthorne effect [p. 452]).

Maintenance of Fluid Balance and Nutrition

Restriction of food and fluid intake and the loss of fluids (blood, perspiration, or emesis) during labor cause many women to express a sudden desire to eat and drink soon after they give birth. The type of nourishment the nurse offers depends on several factors, including type of anesthesia used and the amount of blood loss after the birth. If local or pudendal anesthesia was used in preparation for episiotomy or for perineal repair and if lochia flow is small to moderate, the woman usually can have sips of a drink of her choice (Fig. 19-3), followed by a regular diet. She is cautioned to drink *small* amounts of fluid initially. Rapid drinking, especially of large amounts, can lead to nausea and possibly vomiting.

If the woman had another type of anesthesia, the

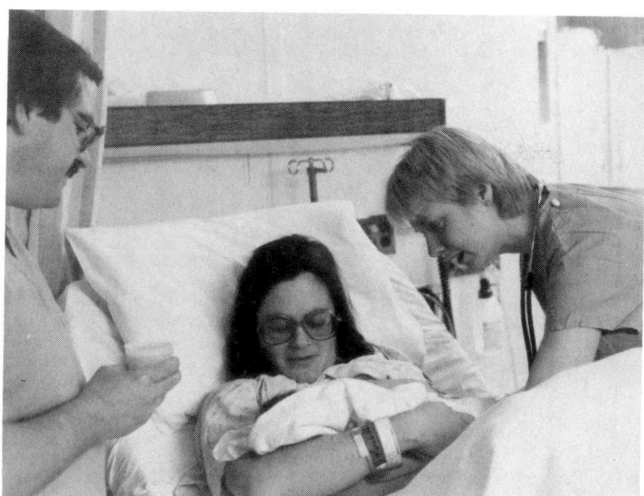

Fig. 19-3 Father offers his partner orange juice while she breast-feeds their baby. Nurse is explaining technique of breast-feeding.
Courtesy Stanford University Medical Center, Stanford, Calif.

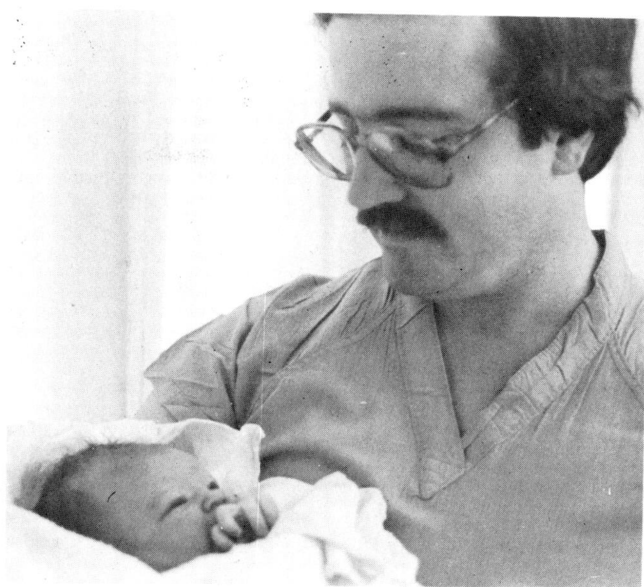

Fig. 19-4 A proud father's pensive moment with his son.
Courtesy Stanford University Medical Center, Stanford, Calif.

anesthesiologist will decide when the effect of the anesthesia is worn off significantly and the woman can resume oral intake. Heavy bleeding may signal retained placental fragments (see Chapter 30), which may require the administration of general anesthesia to remove the placental fragments and stop the bleeding. Thus the woman with heavy bleeding usually will be given nothing by mouth (NPO) until the bleeding is under control. The IV line will be maintained, and its contents often are switched to a solution that contains dextrose to provide some calories until oral feedings resume. The nurse monitors the IV line and notes in the woman's chart the type, amount, and tolerance of any oral intake. (See Chapter 30 for pharmacologic control of postpartum hemorrhage, e.g., Hemabate sterile solution.)

Support of Parental Psychosocial Needs

It is acceptable for the nurse to share openly in the excitement and emotion of birth. The nurse assists the parents by accepting any expressions of disappointment about the child's sex or appearance and reassures them that these feelings are normal. The nurse may reassure the mother that her behavior during labor was acceptable if the mother appears worried about this. The new mother may need to talk about her labor and may endeavor to fill in gaps ("missing pieces") that she cannot remember, particularly if the delivery was hurried (Affonso, 1977).

Psychologic states of new mothers range from euphoria and a feeling of well-being to a sleepy state marked by an unawareness of surroundings. As noted earlier, first reactions of new mothers and fathers to their newborns vary widely. These reactions give the perinatal team cues to use in individualizing plans of care. Women who have experienced long, difficult labors or who are in pain are commonly too exhausted to extend interest to the child. The nurse can offer to take the baby to the nursery until the mother is rested. The father/coach/partner may be invited to accompany the nurse to the nursery at this stage (Fig. 19-4). After sufficient rest a mother's attitude can be surprisingly different. The child unwanted for diverse reasons may continue to be rejected or be viewed with only mild interest. The attitude of the father is often reflected in the mother. His pleasure arouses a responsive pleasure, or his disappointment arouses corresponding disappointment.

Ethnic or cultural origins dictate behaviors that are deemed appropriate for special occasions. Some parents may not be able to express their delight openly; others wish to welcome the newcomer noisily (see Chapter 3 for discussion of culture and ethnicity).

The single or teenage mother may express mixed emotions at the birth of the baby. The nurse can help her express her emotions, involve any significant other/family/friends, or refer her to a social worker (see Chapter 34 for discussion of adolescent parenthood).

Some mothers, particularly with their firstborn, are surprised and disturbed by the passivity or disin-

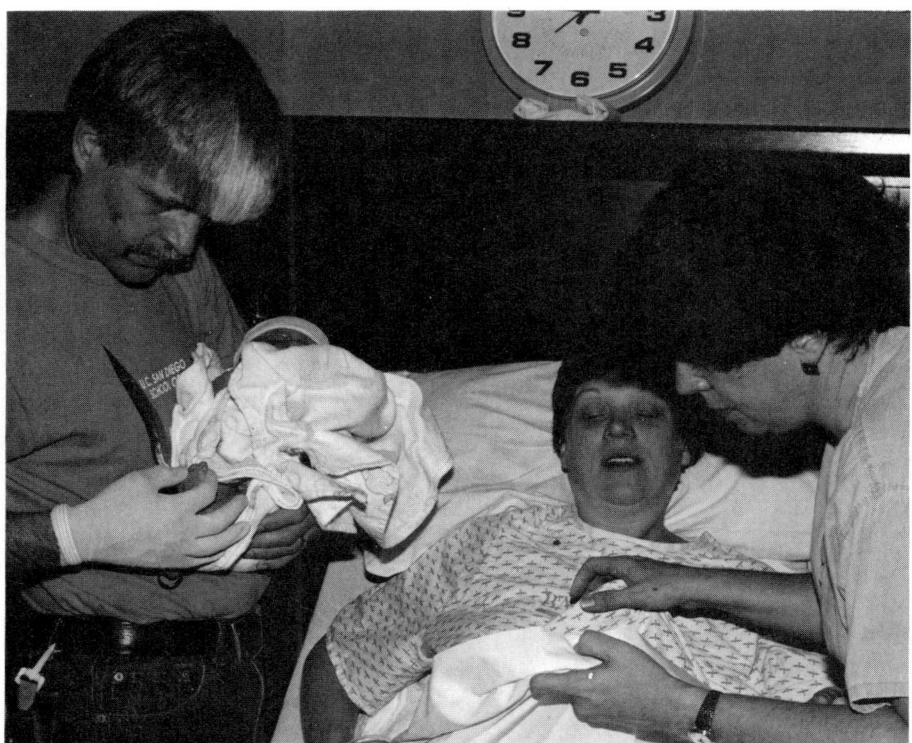

Fig. 19-5 Father engrossed in examining newborn as nurse prepares for mother's fourth-stage care.
Courtesy Kathy Hanold, RN, MS, Birth Place, Barnes Hospital at Washington University Medical Center, St. Louis, Mo.

terest they experience on seeing their long-awaited infant. The nurse can reassure the mother of the normality of these feelings. The idealized "mother love" does not necessarily appear right after delivery. The gradual growth of such love comes to some as they assume the care of and responsibility for their child.

Some interventions can facilitate parent-child acquaintance and beginning bonding or attachment. The father/partner can be encouraged to hold the baby in the birth room or the recovery area (Fig. 19-5) (see Research Highlight, p. 515). In a warm, quiet, dimly lighted environment, an infant responds by opening the eyes. Parents are encouraged to hold the infant ***en face.*** In the en face position, parents and newborns gaze into each other's eyes. Newborns focus best at about 20.3 cm (8 in) distance. Body odor can be noticed (mothers have remarked that each child smells different). Skin contact between mother and baby should be encouraged during this time. Neonatal temperatures remain stable if mother and newborn are placed chest-to-chest and covered by a blanket. The mother is encouraged to explore her baby and put her baby to the breast if she plans to breast-feed. Immediately after birth the baby has a strong desire to suck; thus this early feed is most encouraging for the mother and bonding is promoted.

Transfer from the Recovery Area

During the recovery period of 1 to 2 hours, the recovery nurse (who often functions as the delivery nurse) will complete any required paperwork while performing the frequent postpartum assessments. After the initial recovery period has passed (per hospital protocol), the woman may be transferred to a postpartum room in the same or another nursing unit. In labor, delivery, recovery, postpartum room (LDRP) settings the nurse who has provided care during the recovery period usually will continue caring for the woman. In the labor, delivery, recovery room (LDR) or traditional setting the woman is transferred to a "postpartum" area where she is cared for by the postpartum nursing staff. In some settings, nurses are responsible for both members of the mother-baby couple. Research has shown this type of care to enhance continuity and increase job satisfaction of nurses while also being cost-effective for the hospital (Phillips, 1988).

In preparing the transfer report, the recovery

nurse needs information from the admission record, the delivery record, and the recovery record. Information that needs to be communicated includes identity of the primary care practitioner, gravidity and parity, age, anesthesia used, duration of labor and rupture of membranes, type of delivery and repair, blood type, the state of rubella immunity, VDRL and hepatitis serology test results, the IV infusion of any fluids, physiologic status since delivery; description of fundus, lochia, bladder, perineum, and hemorrhoids; sex and weight of infant, time of birth, pediatrician, chosen method of feeding, any abnormalities noted; and assessment of initial parental-infant interaction (Table 19-1).

This information also must be documented for the nursing staff in the newborn nursery. In addition, specific information should be provided regarding the infant's Apgar scores, weight, voiding, and feeding since the birth. Nursing interventions that have been completed (e.g., eye prophylaxis, vitamin K injection) also should be recorded (Table 19-2).

EVALUATION

Evaluation of progress and outcomes is a continuous activity through the fourth stage of labor. Physiologic recovery from pregnancy and labor, as well as development of parent-infant attachment and new family interrelationships, is evaluated by the nurse. The degree to which formulated goals of care are being met must be critically appraised in terms of the following factors:

- The new mother does not saturate more than one perineal pad per hour.
- She voids if her bladder is filling during the fourth stage.
- She verbalized acceptance of the labor process after expressing concerns.
- She (and other family members, if present) begin the bonding/attachment process.
- She verbalizes increased comfort after initiation of comfort measures.

If the evaluation process identifies that results fall short of achieving any goal, further assessment, planning, and implementation are imperative to attain the correct nursing care for the woman and her family.

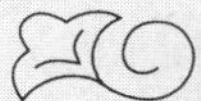 **Research Highlight** 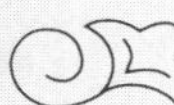

Postpartum Interaction of Fathers, Infants, and Mothers

RESEARCH ABSTRACT

The aim of this study was to describe behaviors of first-time fathers with their infants immediately after the birth. The subjects were 24 first-time fathers and their partners. Data were collected by videotaping the birth just before, during, and after delivery. The Paternal Behavior Observation form was used to measure the frequency of nonverbal paternal behavior noted on the video films. The four categories of behavior assessed were proximity, gaze, touch, and movement. Gaze and proximity were the most frequently exhibited paternal behavior. The most frequent type of proximity behavior was "distant behavior"; next was "embrace." Most of the time, fathers gazed at their infants; they looked at the mothers less. Movement and proximity increased slightly over time. Touch remained constant at a low frequency.

IMPLICATIONS FOR PRACTICE

Most fathers remained in the area designated for them in the birth room; this restriction may have interfered with their ability to interact more with their infants. The traditional birth room setting may interfere with the father's desire to move about or interact more with his partner or the infant. Nurses can more directly include the father by ensuring that he has an opportunity to hold the baby in the birth room and by specifying permissible movement within the birth room environment.

RELATED RESEARCH QUESTIONS

1. Does paternal interaction behavior vary with gender of the infant?
2. Is the paternal interaction behavior of first-time fathers different from that of second-time fathers?
3. Does an education program increase the amount and type of paternal behavioral interaction?
4. Is there a relation between paternal interaction behavior in the delivery room and later father-infant interaction?

REFERENCE

Tomlinson PS, Rothenberg MA, Carver LD: Behavioral interaction of fathers with infants and mothers in the immediate postpartum period, *J Nurse Midwife* 36:232, July/Aug 1991.

TABLE 19-1 Recovery Nurse's Report to Postpartum Nurse

Item	Example
Type of labor and delivery; unusual observations, if any, of the placenta	Spontaneous or assisted (forceps) vaginal delivery; vertex presentation
Gravidity and parity, age	GI, PI, 22 years old
Anesthesia and analgesia used	None; epidural, low spinal, local
Condition of perineum	Episiotomy; repair of lacerations
Events since delivery	Vital signs, BP, fundus, lochia, intake and output, medications (dosage, time of administration, and results), response to newborn, observation of family interactions, including siblings, if present
Condition and sex of newborn; other information	Apgar at 1 and 5 min; time of birth; eye prophylaxis given; weight; whether breast- or bottle-feeding; if breast-feeding, whether newborn was at breast; name of pediatrician
Relevant information from prenatal record	Need for rubella vaccination
Miscellaneous information	
IV drip	If IV drip is infusing, rate of infusion, medications added (e.g., Pitocin), whether to keep open or discontinue after completion of bag that is hung
Social factors	If woman is giving baby up for adoption, whether she wants to see baby, breast-feed, allow visitors, or other preferences she may have

TABLE 19-2 Recovery Nurse's Report on Newborn

Item	Example
Type of labor and delivery; unusual events (e.g., cord around neck)	Spontaneous or assisted (forceps, vacuum extractor) vaginal birth in vertex presentation
Gravidity and parity, age of mother	GI, PI, 22 years old
Analgesia and anesthesia	None; epidural, low spinal, or local
Condition at birth	Apgar scores at 1 and 5 min
Sex and weight	Male; 3400 g (7 lb 8 oz)
Events since birth*	Nursed at breast; took nipple well Voided ×1; meconium ×1 Eye prophylaxis Vitamin K injection Held by siblings who are happy (or have other response to newborn)
Relevant information from prenatal record	Unremarkable pregnancy

*Neonatal adjustment to extrauterine existence and recovery of the neonate are discussed in detail in Chapter 20 .

■ SUMMARY

The childbearing family has many special needs and concerns throughout the labor process. Nursing care begins with the initial assessment during the admission procedure, and a plan of care is begun that is modified and updated throughout the labor process. Nurses must utilize their expertise in caring for the physical needs of the woman and in providing for a safe delivery of the infant. They must recognize complications and intervene appropriately.

The nurse is also sensitive to the cultural preferences of the woman and family and modifies the plan of care accordingly. All family members are integral parts of the birthing team, and they require support in their support of the laboring woman.

Throughout the fourth stage of labor, the nurse continues to modify the plan of care and prepare the woman for the tasks of the postpartum period as well as for care of the infant. This is accomplished through education and physical and emotional support of both the woman and her family. The plan of care continues during the postpartum period and beyond if continued support is required.

CASE STUDY

Fourth Stage of Labor

Paula is a 24-year-old married woman, G2P2, who gave birth to her second baby boy a half hour ago. Both she and her husband Jeff were hoping for a girl. After birth, the baby boy was placed skin-to-skin on Paula's chest where he remains. Her certified nurse-midwife has just repaired a midline episiotomy.

ASSESSMENT

Paula verbalizes she is experiencing (uterine) cramps that she does not remember having after her first baby, as well as pain in her perineal area. She states she is glad that the baby is healthy even though she had wanted a girl. Jeff stands at Paula's bedside watching his new son. Paula's fundus is firm at one fingerbreadth above the umbilicus (1/U) with a moderate amount of lochia rubra on her perineal pad.

NURSING DIAGNOSIS

Because this is the immediate postbirth period, the nurse's assessments and interventions center on the priority of care during this time: the prevention of hemorrhage. The following nursing diagnosis is identified: High risk for fluid volume deficit related to hemorrhage secondary to uterine atony or perineal trauma or repair.

PLANNING

In most instances, it is possible to consult with the client regarding the goals for care. In this instance, the nurse takes the initiative to establish the primary *goal:* Paula will not experience hemorrhage during the fourth stage of labor. In addition, the nurse identifies the *goal:* Paula will learn how to do self-massage and observe for amount and character of bleeding. The nurse's *expected outcome* is that hemorrhaging will not occur during the fourth stage and that Paula's knowledge about self-care will prevent hemorrhage during the following postpartum days.

IMPLEMENTATION

Every 15 minutes for the first hour the nurse monitors the following factors to assess for excessive bleeding and impending hypovolemic shock: BP, pulse, respirations, uterine tone and height of fundus, character and amount of lochia or clots, status of perineum (condition of episiotomy; laceration; formation of hematoma), skin color, and LOC.

If the uterus is firm in the midline and below the umbilicus, no further action (other than teaching the mother) is taken. If the fundus is relaxed, the nurse gently massages it until firm, expresses any clots, and notes the amount and character of lochia expressed. If the uterus does not remain contracted and the woman's bladder is empty, an oxytocic medication and an IV infusion may be ordered. If the uterus is relaxing as a result of a filling urinary bladder, the woman is asked to void or is catheterized as needed.

If the fundus is remaining firm and bright-red bleeding continues, the woman needs to be assessed for cervical, vaginal, or perineal trauma (see Chapter 30), and the primary care practitioner is notified.

EVALUATION

Paula's fundus is firm at one fingerbreadth above the umbilicus, and her vaginal bleeding covers half of one peripad in the first postpartum hour. Her BP and pulse are within normal limits of the baseline identified on her prenatal chart. Her bladder is not palpable.

CARE PLAN Fourth Stage of Labor

GOALS	IMPLEMENTATION	RATIONALE	EVALUATION
Nursing diagnosis: High risk for hemorrhage related to immediate postpartum uterine changes and childbirth			
1. Paula maintains normal physiologic status, as evidenced by bleeding within normal limits and stable vital signs.	Monitor BP, pulse, skin color, and uterine tone q15min for the first hour and q30min for the next hour. Assess uterine position and lochial flow; massage fundus as needed. Assess bladder for distention.	It is important to identify changes in vital signs and uterine tone early to identify postpartum hemorrhage. If the fundus is not felt in the midline near the level of the umbilicus, it may indicate bladder distention. A distended bladder can push the uterus out of place and promote uterine atony. Massage of fundus stimulates the uterine muscle to contract.	Paula's vital signs are within normal limits. Her uterine fundus is 1/U. Lochia is moderate rubra. Paula's lochial flow saturated one peripad in the first hour. Bladder is not palpable.
Nursing diagnosis: Pain related to interruption in skin integrity secondary to midline episiotomy and afterpains			
1. Paula verbalizes reduction of pain. 2. Paula displays relaxed posture and facial expression.	Encourage Paula to change positions at intervals and to avoid sitting up for extended periods. Provide Paula with a pillow to sit on when sitting in a chair.	Pressure from remaining in one position may result in increased pain. Allows for increased comfort.	Paula changes position from right to left side at intervals and refrains from sitting except when eating. Paula sits on pillow when using chair, displays relaxed posture and facial expression.
3. Paula asks for analgesics when needed and reports relief of pain within 30 min.	Administer analgesics as ordered. Check with Paula and document relief of pain in nurse's notes.	Analgesics act on higher brain centers to reduce the perception of pain.	Paula takes analgesics when needed, q3-4h. Paula states pain is relieved within 30 min of taking medication.
4. Paula verbalizes understanding of rationale for afterpains and asks questions as they arise.	Inform Paula of rationale for afterpains, and massage uterus gently if needed. Ask Paula if she has any questions. Provide and educate Paula in use of various topical aids for episiotomy pain.	An informed client is less anxious about the postpartum period if she knows what to expect and why. Use of topical aids promotes immediate comfort in the perineal area.	Paula verbalizes understanding of rationale for afterpains and asks questions as they arise. Paula understands use of topical aids prn.
Nursing diagnosis: Alteration in family process related to addition of new member			
1. Paula will hold and touch newborn within 10 min of birth.	Dry the newborn and present him to his parents as soon as his condition is assessed as stable. Wrap the baby and hand him to his father to hold.	Close physical contact soon after birth facilitates bonding/attachment and capitalizes on the newborn's first period of reactivity when he is particularly receptive.	The baby's initial assessment is within normal limits. While Paula's perineum is being repaired, Jeff holds his son.

CARE PLAN Fourth Stage of Labor—cont'd

GOALS	IMPLEMENTATION	RATIONALE	EVALUATION
2. Baby will look into his parents' eyes, grasp one of their fingers, and snuggle into their arms.	Point out baby's positive features and ask questions such as, "Who does he look like . . . ?"	Touch helps to facilitate paternal attachment/bonding with newborn.	The baby makes eye contact with Jeff. While holding the baby's hand, Jeff feels his son grasp his finger and snuggle into his arms.
3. Paula and Jeff will express pleasure at seeing their newborn.	Encourage parents to hold their son, and invite them to be present during the initial care and assessment.		
4. Paula will be able to breast-feed during recovery.	Assist Paula to comfortably position herself to promote baby's sucking.	Comfortable positioning and correct latch-on are essential in promoting a positive initial breast-feeding experience for Paula and her baby.	Paula and Jeff smile at son, stroke him, and talk to him while he is breast-feeding.

REFERENCES

Affonso D: Missing pieces: a study of postpartum feelings, *Birth Fam J* 4:159, Winter 1977.

Cunningham FG, MacDonald PC, Gant NF: *Williams obstetrics*, ed 18, Norwalk, Conn, 1989, Appleton & Lange.

Guyton AC: *Textbook of medical physiology, ed 7, Philadelphia, 1987, WB Saunders.*

Luegenbiehl DL et al: Standardized assessment of blood loss, *MCN* 15:241, July/Aug 1990.

Mercer RT: "She's a multip . . . she knows the ropes," *MCN* 4:30, Sept/Oct 1979.

Phillips C: *Survey of mother-baby staffing patterns in U.S. Correspondence*, 1988.

Scott JR et al: *Danforth's obstetrics and gynecology*, ed 6, Philadelphia, 1990, JB Lippincott Co.

Varney H: *Nurse-midwifery*, ed 3, Boston, 1991, Blackwell Scientific.

Willson JR et al: *Obstetrics and gynecology*, ed 9, St Louis, 1991, Mosby–Year Book.

References—Nursing Research

Higgins PG: Measuring nurses' accuracy of estimating blood loss, *J Adv Nurs* 7:175, 1982.

BIBLIOGRAPHY

Ament LA: Maternal tasks of the puerperium reidentified, *JOGNN* 19:330, July/Aug 1990.

Gjerdingen DK, Froberg DG, Fontaine P: A causal model describing the relationship of women's postpartum health to social support, length of leave, and complications of childbirth, *Women Health* 16(2):71, 1990.

Korbert LJ: Are universal precautions changing the "nurture" of obstetric nursing? *AJN* 89:1609, Dec 1989.

Machol L: LDR: new factor in the OB equation, *Contemp OB/GYN* 31:176, Feb 1988.

Mackey MC, Lock SE: Women's expectations of the labor and delivery nurse, *JOGNN* 18:505, Nov/Dec 1989.

Morse JM et al: Initiating breast feeding: a world survey of the timing of postpartum breastfeeding, *Int J Nurs Stud* 27(3):303, 1990.

Oleen MA, Mariano JP: Controlling refractory atonic postpartum hemorrhage with Hemabate sterile solution, *Am J Obstet Gynecol* 162:205, 1990.

Rhode MA, Barger MK: Perineal care. Then and now, *J Nurs Midwife* 35:220, July/Aug 1990.

St. George L, Crandon AJ: Immediate postpartum complications, *Aust N Z J Obstet Gynecol* 30:52, Jan 1990.

Smith MP: Postnatal concerns of mothers: an update, *Midwifery* 5:182, Dec 1989.

Sturrock WA, Johnson JA: The relationship between childbirth education classes and obstetric outcome, *Birth* 17:82, June 1990.

Bibliography—Nursing Research

Jordon PL: Laboring for relevance: expectant and new fatherhood, *Nurs Res* 39, Jan/Feb 1990.

chapter 19 review

Key Concepts

- The fourth stage of labor, the stage of recovery, is a critical period for the mother and newborn.
- A primary nursing concern during this period is the prevention of hemorrhage.
- Other physical nursing concerns include the prevention of urinary bladder distention and the maintenance of comfort, cleanliness, fluid balance, and nutrition.
- Safety for the mother is an issue until she is fully recovered from analgesia or anesthesia, splanchnic engorgement, and fatigue.
- The mother needs to fill in the "missing pieces" to begin to integrate the experience of labor and delivery.
- The nurse can facilitate mother-infant attachment by meeting the new mother's physical, support, and teaching needs.
- Meeting the family's ethnic and cultural expectations for care is an important component of the nursing care plan.
- Regardless of parity, marital status, or age, new mothers can benefit from explanations of the various nursing actions during the immediate puerperium.

Key Terms

- afterpains (p. 511)
- atonic uterus (p. 506)
- bladder distention (p. 507)
- bradycardia (p. 506)
- discomfort (p. 511)
- en face (p. 514)
- fourth stage of labor (p. 506)
- hematoma (p. 509)
- hemorrhage (p. 509)
- hypovolemic shock (p. 510)
- intrauterine clots (p. 507)
- involution (p. 506)
- lochia (p. 506)
- orthostatic hypotension (p. 511)
- perineal care (p. 512)
- postpartum tremors (p. 512)
- REEDA (p. 508)
- splanchnic engorgement (p. 511)
- urinary retention (p. 511)

Critical Thinking Exercises

1. The nurse has just received a postpartum mother and her husband in the recovery area. They are expressing disappointment over the sex of their child, and the father is hinting that it is his wife's fault.
   A. Identify the assumptions of the father.
   B. Analyze the significance of these assumptions for the family and the nurse.
   C. Formulate a plan of care that provides the family with information about sex determination.

2. Provide care for a woman in the fourth stage of labor. Meet with other members of your clinical group to examine your experiences.
   A. Discuss your nursing assessments, diagnoses, plans, and evaluations for each woman. Justify your actions.
   B. Compare physiologic and psychologic aspects of the fourth stage of labor for each woman. Examine the reasons for any differences.

Topics for Nursing Research

- Is there a difference in the amount of vaginal bleeding during the fourth stage of labor in women who deliver in a side-lying position versus those who deliver in lithotomy?
- Do women who have had local anesthesia for birth and ambulate within 1 hour of delivery request analgesics less than do women who first ambulate more than 1 hour after they give birth?
- Is there a difference in the number of episiotomies performed by physicians in women who have spent their last hour of labor in a squatting position versus those who have remained in bed?
- Is there a difference in maternal perception of the neonate in mothers who are allowed to touch their babies before the cord is cut and those who must wait until after the cord is cut?

unit 4

Normal Newborn

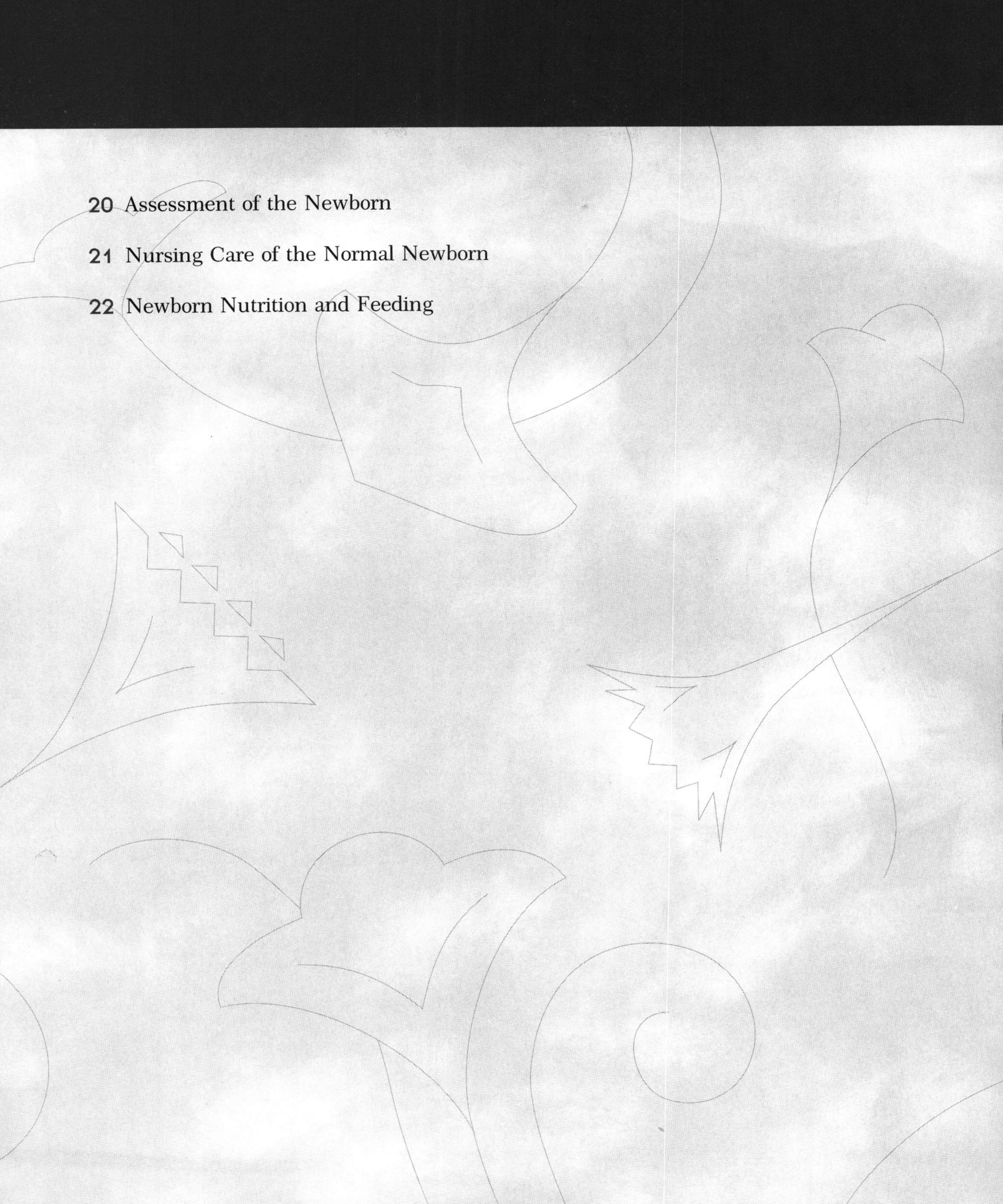

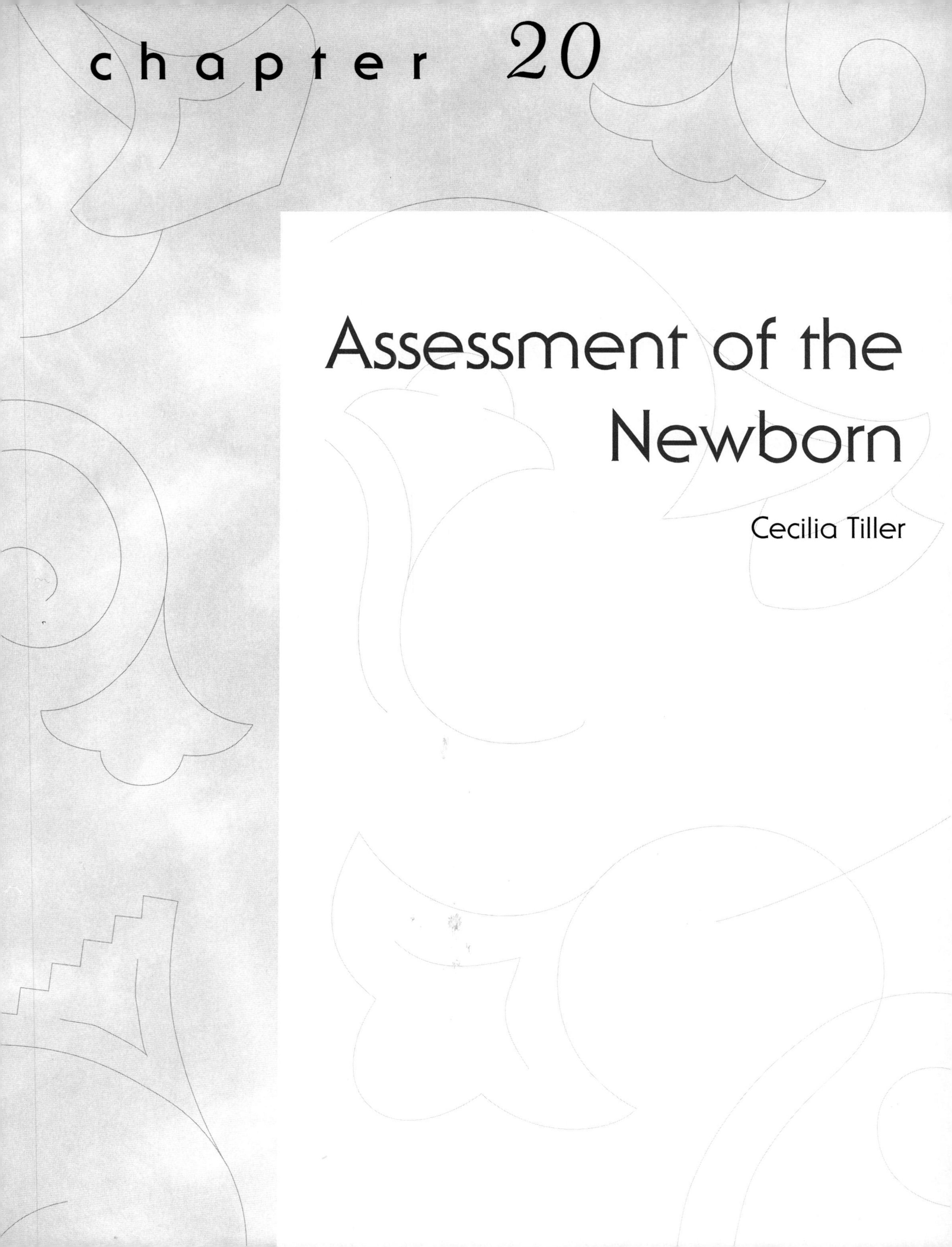

chapter 20

Assessment of the Newborn

Cecilia Tiller

LEARNING OBJECTIVES

- Define key terms listed.
- Describe the biologic system changes of the neonate's transition to extrauterine life.
- Compare neonatal systems to adult systems.
- Identify the sensory and perceptual functioning of the neonate.
- Provide anticipatory guidance to parents.
- Describe assessment of a newborn.
- Identify topics for nursing research related to assessment of the newborn.

The neonatal period includes the time from birth through the twenty-eighth day of life. During this time the neonate must make many adjustments to extrauterine life. Many of these developmental tasks occur shortly after birth. *Biologic tasks* are those that involve (1) establishing and maintaining respirations, (2) circulatory changes, (3) regulation of temperature, (4) ingesting, retaining, and digesting nutrients, (5) elimination of waste, and (6) regulation of weight. *Behavioral tasks* include (1) establishing a regulated behavioral tempo independent of the mother, which involves self-regulation of arousal, self-monitoring of changes in state, and patterning of sleep, (2) processing, storing, and organizing multiple stimuli, and (3) establishing a relationship with caregivers and the environment. The infant at *term gestation* (infant born between 38 and 42 weeks of gestation) normally makes these adjustments with little or no difficulty.

A classic study (Desmond et al, 1966), which still applies today, found that infants pass through phases of instability during the first 6 to 8 hours after birth. These phases collectively are termed the **transition period** between intrauterine and extrauterine existence (Fig. 20-1). To be able to detect disorders in adaptation soon after birth, each nurse must be aware of normal features of the transition period. During labor, the fetus is exposed to a host of sensory input; at birth a new set of stimuli influence neonatal adaptation to the extrauterine environment. Labor and immediate neonatal events stimulate a sympathetic response that is reflected in changes in heart rate, color, respiration, motor activity, gastrointestinal function, and temperature of the infant (Fanaroff, Martin, 1992). Behavioral characteristics also change during this transitional period (see p. 569).

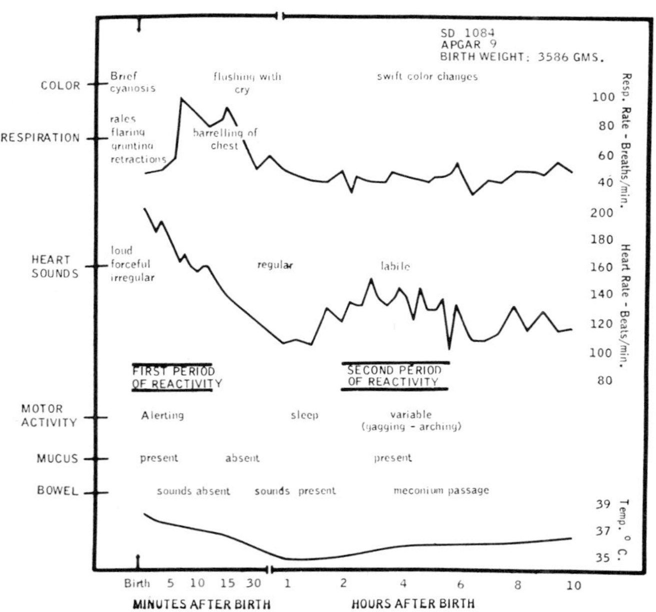

Fig. 20-1 Normal transition period.
From Desmond M, Rudolph A, Phitakspharaiwan P: The transitional care nursery, *Pediatr Clin North Am* 13:651, 1966.

The first phase lasts up to 30 minutes after birth and is called the *first period of reactivity*. The *second period of reactivity* occurs roughly between the fourth and eighth hours after birth. This sequence occurs in all newborns, regardless of gestational age or type of birth (vaginal or cesarean). There will be variations, however, in the length of time the periods last, depending on amount and kind of stress experienced by the fetus.

During the late stages of labor, the fetus's heart rate normally fluctuates with a certain degree of variability around a baseline of 120 to 140 beat/min. After birth, the newborn's heart rate increases rapidly to the range of 160 to 180 beats/min for 10 to 15 minutes, with a gradual fall by 30 minutes to a baseline rate of between 100 to 120 beats/min. During the first 15 minutes of life, respirations are irregular with rates between 60 and 80 breaths per minute. During this period, rales are also present on auscultation; audible grunting, nasal flaring, and retractions of the chest may be noted. In addition, there may be brief periods of apnea. Coincident with these changes in heart rate and respiratory rate, the infant is alert. The infant's behavior is marked by spontaneous startle reactions, tremors, crying, and movements of the head from side to side. This characteristic exploratory behavior is accompanied by a decrease in body temperature and a generalized increase in motor activity, with increase in muscle tone (Fanaroff, Martin, 1992). Gastrointestinal manifestations of this first period of reactivity include the onset of bowel sounds, passage of meconium, and production of saliva. The duration of this first period of reactivity, although varying between 15 and 30 minutes in healthy term infants, is prolonged in term infants who have had an abnormal labor or birth and in sick infants and normal preterm infants (Fanaroff, Martin, 1992).

After the first period of reactivity, the newborn either sleeps or has a marked decrease in motor activity. The heart rate falls to between 100 and 120 beats/min, respiratory rates slow and become irregular, and the newborn becomes relatively unresponsive. This period of unresponsiveness, frequently accompanied by sleep, lasts from 60 to 100 minutes and is followed by a second period of reactivity.

The second period of reactivity lasts from 10 minutes to several hours. Periods of tachycardia and tachypnea occur, associated with increased muscle tone, skin color, and mucus production. Meconium frequently is passed during this time.

BIOLOGIC CHARACTERISTICS

With the cutting of the umbilical cord the infant must undergo rapid and complex changes. Many biologic adaptations occur that make it possible for the infant to adapt to extrauterine life. All systems within the infant change their functions or become established during the neonatal period.

Respiratory System

The most critical adjustment a newborn must make at birth is the establishment of respirations. At term the lungs hold approximately 20 ml fluid/kg (Blackburn, Loper, 1992). Air must be substituted for fluid that filled the respiratory tract to the alveoli. During the course of normal vaginal delivery, some fluid is squeezed or drained from the newborn's trachea and lungs. With the first breath of air, the newborn begins a sequence of cardiopulmonary changes. These changes include (1) converting from fetal to neonatal circulation, (2) emptying the lungs of fluid, and (3) establishing the characteristics of pulmonary function (Nelson, 1987). During the first hour of life, large amounts of fluid continue to be removed by the pulmonary lymphatics. Removal of fluid is also a result of the pressure gradient from alveoli to interstitial tissue to blood capillary. Reduced vascular resistance accommodates this flow of lung fluid; however, it is the diminished intravascular pressure that is ultimately responsible.

Abnormal respiration and failure to completely expand the lungs retard the egress of fetal lung fluid from alveoli and interstices into the pulmonary circulation. Retention of fluid in turn alters pulmonary function. The infant must breathe strongly enough to expand the lungs completely, and the lungs must remain expanded. **Initial breathing** is probably the result of a reflex triggered by pressure changes, chilling, noise, light, and other sensations related to the birth process. In addition the chemoreceptors in the aorta and carotid bodies initiate neurologic reflexes when arterial oxygen pressure (PO_2) falls from 80 to 15 mm Hg, arterial carbon dioxide pressure (PCO_2) rises from 40 to 70 mm Hg, and arterial pH falls below 7.35. When these changes are extreme, respiratory depression can occur. In most cases an exaggerated respiratory reaction follows within 1 minute of birth, and the infant takes a first gasping breath and cries.

With the first breath considerable negative intrathoracic pressure develops in the infant. Air is drawn in, and about half of this remains as residual pulmonary volume. Normally only a few breaths are required to expand the lungs; subsequently the pressure will be lower than at the onset of respiration.

After respirations are established, **respiratory patterns** are shallow and irregular, ranging from 30 to 60 breaths per minute, with short periods of apnea (less than 15 seconds). Apnea (periodic breathing) is characteristic of the newborn. It occurs most often during the active (rapid eye movement [REM]) sleep cycle and decreases in frequency and duration with age. However, any apneic period should be evaluated. Tactile or other sensory stimulation increases the infant's respiratory rate. It is best to observe the respirations while the infant is at rest. Respirations should be counted for a full minute. Crackles (rales) may be present during the first few hours while lung fluid is still present. Auscultation of the chest of an infant reveals loud, clear breath sounds that seem very near because little chest tissue intervenes.

Infants are **preferential nose breathers.** The reflex response to nasal obstruction is opening the mouth to maintain an airway. This response is not present in most babies until 3 weeks after birth but may occur earlier in certain ethnic groups. The infant's tongue is relatively large (macroglossia), whereas the glottis and trachea are small. All lumina of the infant are narrower and more easily collapsed. Respiratory tract secretions of the infant are more abundant than those of the adult. Nasal blockage resulting in cyanosis and asphyxia may occur rapidly. The mucous membranes of the infant are delicate and therefore more susceptible to trauma. The ciliated columnar epithelium just below the vocal cords is especially prone to edema. The alveoli of the infant are sensitive to changes in pressures, and the capillary network of the infant is not well developed. Capillaries are friable (easily damaged) and have minimal vasoconstrictive and dilative abilities. The infant's bony rib cage and respiratory muscles are not well developed.

The infant's chest circumference is approximately 30 to 33 cm (12 to 13 in) at birth. The ribs of the infant articulate with the spine at a horizontal rather than a downward slope; consequently the rib cage cannot expand as readily as does the adult's with inspiration. Neonatal respiratory function is largely a matter of diaphragmatic contractions. The negative intrathoracic pressure is created by the descent of the diaphragm, much as negative pressure is created in the barrel of a syringe when medication is drawn up by retracting the plunger. The infant's chest and abdomen should rise simultaneously with inspiration (Fig. 20-2, *A*).

The alveoli of the infant's lungs are lined with surfactant. Lung expansion augments surfactant secretion. Surfactant functions (1) to lower surface tension therefore requiring less pressure to keep the al-

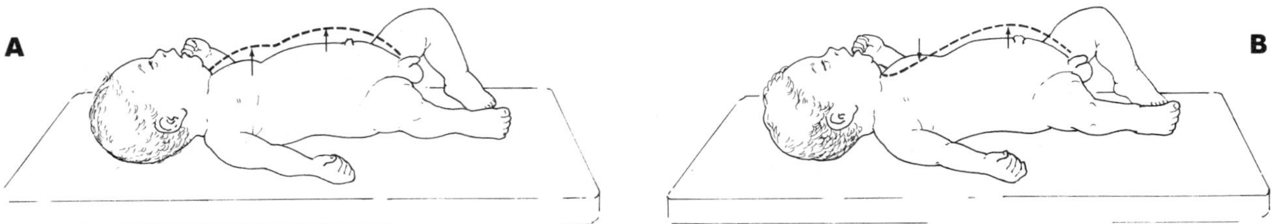

Fig. 20-2 **A,** Normal respiration. Chest and abdomen rise with inspiration. **B,** Seesaw respiration. Chest wall retracts and abdomen rises with inspiration.
Courtesy Mead Johnson & Co, Evansville, Ind.

veolus open and (2) to maintain alveolar stability by changing surface tension as the size of the alveolus changes. The surfactant system develops as the infant develops in utero (for further discussion, see Chapter 7). Fetal pulmonary maturity can be determined by examining amniotic fluid for lecithin/sphingomyelin ratio (L/S) and other phospholipid levels. Phosphatidylglycerol appears at 35 to 36 weeks; its presence is a more predictable index of lung maturity (see discussion in Chapter 31).

The concentration of lecithin and sphingomyelin increases with gestational age (for further discussion, see Chapter 7). Mature fetal lungs have an L/S ratio greater than 2:1. The infant born before the L/S ratio is 2:1 will have varying degrees of respiratory distress.

SIGNS OF RISK FOR RESPIRATORY PROBLEMS. Most term infants breathe spontaneously and continue to have normal respirations. However, infants can manifest other problems through **respiratory distress.** Signs of respiratory distress include nasal flaring, retractions (indrawing of tissue between ribs, below rib cage, or above sternum and clavicles), or grunting with expirations. Any increased use of the intercostal muscles may be a sign of distress. Seesaw respirations are not normal and should be reported immediately (Fig. 20-2, *B*). A respiratory rate less than 30 or greater than 60 breaths per minute, with the infant at rest, need to be reported immediately to the pediatrician. The respiratory rate of the infant is influenced by the analgesics or anesthetics the mother received during labor and birth. Apneic episodes also can be related to rapid warming or cooling of the infant, whereas tachypnea may result from aspiration or a diaphragmatic hernia. Apneic periods longer than 15 seconds must be reported to the pediatrician for evaluation. A normal-appearing infant bears close observation because changes in the respiratory system can occur very rapidly (for further discussion, see Chapter 37).

Cardiovascular System

While respiratory changes are occurring, the cardiovascular system also is making many changes (Fig. 20-3). **Fetal circulation** ceases and extrauterine circulation begins. (Review fetal circulation in Chapter 7.) The infant's first breath inflates the lungs, thereby reducing pulmonary vascular resistance to the pulmonary blood flow. As a result there is a drop in pulmonary artery pressure. This sequence is the major mechanism by which pressure in the *right atrium declines*. The increased pulmonary blood flow returned to the left side of the heart increases the pressure in the *left atrium*. This change in pressures causes a functional closure of the shunt between the atria, the **foramen ovale.** Temporary reversal of flow through the foramen ovale may occur with crying and lead to mild cyanosis during the first few days of life.

Within the first 12 hours of extrauterine life, the shunt between the pulmonary artery and the aorta, the **ductus arteriosus,** constricts in response to a decrease in circulating prostaglandin E_2 and the establishment of a high oxygen level in the arterial blood. Anatomic closure takes more time; approximately 80% are closed by the end of the third month (Blackburn, Loper, 1992). After anatomic closure, it becomes a ligament. With the clamping and severing of the cord, the two umbilical arteries and one umbilical vein and the ductus venosus close immediately and are converted into ligaments. The umbilical arteries also occlude and become ligaments. The changes in blood flow at birth have the effect of transforming the circulatory system. Before birth the two ventricles act in parallel (simultaneously), with shunts (foramen ovale and ductus arteriosus) adjusting any unequal outputs. After birth the two ventricles act in series (one following the other), which requires that the outputs of the right and left sides of the heart be equal (Fanaroff, Martin, 1992). Table 20-1 summarizes the cardiovascular changes at birth.

A relative hypoxia is present at birth. Within 10

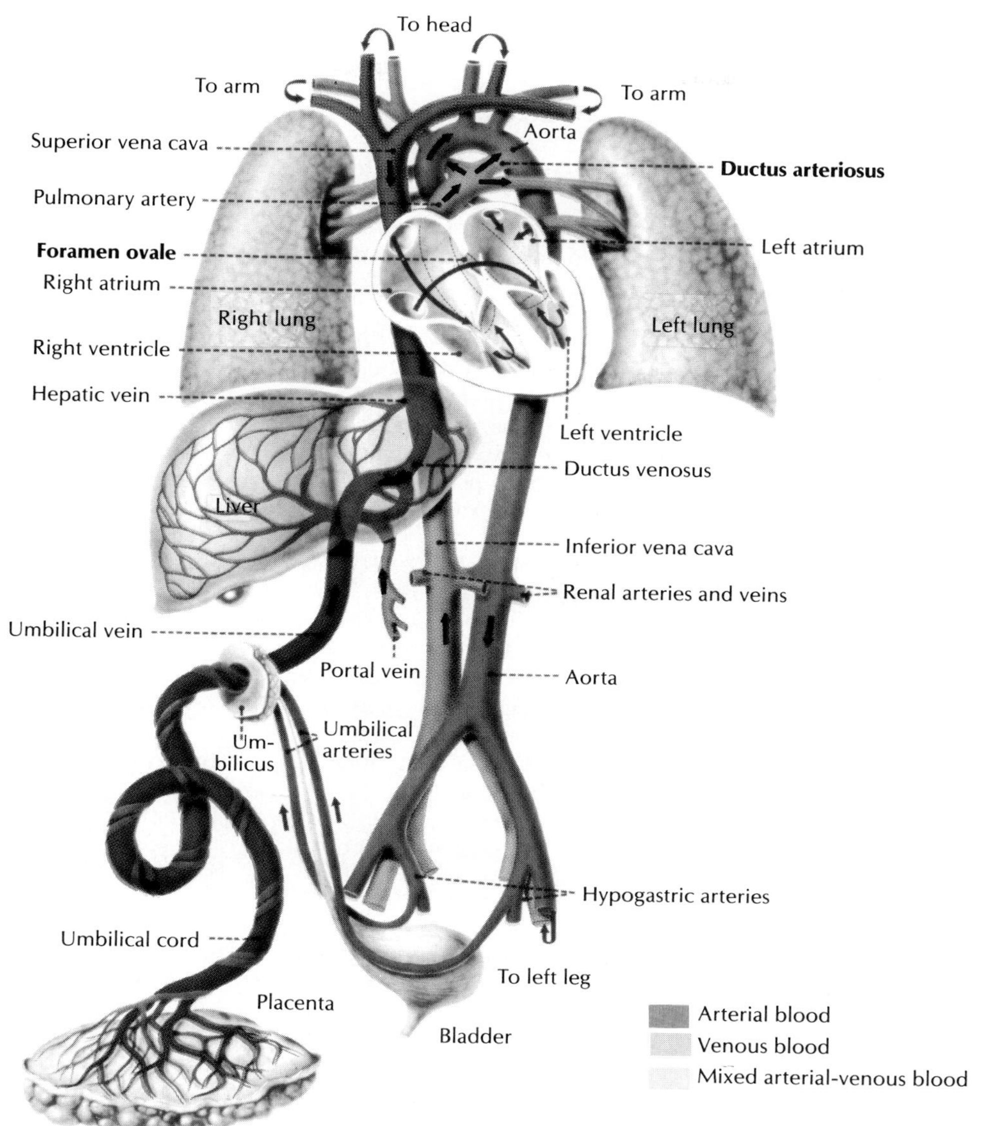

Fig. 20-3 Fetal circulation. *Before birth.* Arterialized blood from the placenta flows into the fetus through the umbilical vein and passes rapidly through the liver into the inferior vena cava; from there it flows through the foramen ovale into the left atrium, soon to appear in the aorta and arteries of the head. A portion by-passes the liver through the ductus venosus. Venous blood from the lower extremities and head passes predominantly into the right atrium, the right ventricle, and then into the descending pulmonary artery and ductus arteriosus. *Thus the foramen ovale and the ductus arteriosus act as bypass channels,* allowing a large part of the combined cardiac output to perfuse body tissues without flowing through the lungs. *After birth.* The foramen ovale closes; the ductus arteriosus closes and becomes a ligament; the ductus venosus closes and becomes a ligament; and the umbilical vein and arteries close and become ligaments.
Courtesy Ross Laboratories, Columbus, Ohio.

TABLE 20-1 Cardiovascular Changes at Birth

Prenatal Status	Postbirth Status	Associated Factors
PRIMARY CHANGES		
Pulmonary circulation: high pulmonary vascular resistance; increased pressure in right ventricle and pulmonary arteries	Low pulmonary vascular resistance; decreased pressure in right atrium, ventricle, and pulmonary arteries	Expansion of collapsed fetal lung with air
Systemic circulation: low pressures in left atrium, ventricle, and aorta	High systemic vascular resistance; increased pressure in left atrium, ventricle, and aorta	Loss of placental blood flow
SECONDARY CHANGES		
Umbilical arteries: patent; carry blood from hypogastric arteries to placenta	Functionally closed at birth; obliteration by fibrous proliferation may take 2-3 months; distal portions become lateral vesicoumbilical ligaments; proximal portions remain open as superior vesicle arteries	Closure precedes that of umbilical vein; probably accomplished by smooth muscle contraction in response to thermal and mechanical stimuli and alteration in oxygen tension; mechanically severed with cord at birth
Umbilical vein: patent; carries blood from placenta to ductus venosus and liver	Closed; after obliteration it becomes *ligamentum teres hepatis*	Closure shortly after umbilical arteries; hence blood from placenta may enter neonate for short period after birth; mechanically severed with cord at birth
Ductus venosus: patent; connects umbilical vein to inferior vena cava	Closed, after obliteration it becomes *ligamentum venosum*	Loss of blood flow from umbilical vein
Ductus arteriosus: patent; shunts blood from pulmonary artery to descending aorta	Functionally closed almost immediately after birth; anatomic obliteration of lumen by fibrous proliferation requires 1-3 months; becomes *ligamentum arteriosum*	High systemic resistance increases aortic pressure; low pulmonary resistance reduces pulmonary arterial pressure Increased oxygen content of blood in ductus arteriosus creates vasospasm of its muscular wall
Foramen ovale: forms a valve opening that allows blood to flow directly to left atrium (shunts blood from right to left atrium)	Functionally closes at birth; constant apposition gradually leads to fusion and permanent closure within a few months or years in majority of persons	Increased pressures in left atrium together with decreased pressure in right atrium cause closure of valve over foramen

Modified from Whaley LF, Wong DL: *Nursing care of infants and children,* ed 4, St Louis, 1991, Mosby–Year Book.

minutes the infant's arterial oxygen pressure (Pao_2) rises to about 10 mm Hg. At 1 hour of age, it reaches 62 mm Hg. Pao_2 stabilizes between 75 and 85 mm Hg during the next 2 days (Blackburn, Loper, 1992).

HEART RATE AND SOUNDS. The heart rate averages 140 beats/min at birth, with variations noted during sleeping and waking states. Shortly after the first cry the infant's heart rate may accelerate to 175 to 180 beats/min. The range of the heart rate in the full-term infant is 70 to 90 beats/min during deep sleep and 120 to 150 beats/min while awake. It is not unusual to find a heart rate of 180 beats/min when the infant cries. A heart rate that is either high (>150) or low (<120) should be reevaluated within an hour or when the activity of the infant changes.

Immediately after birth the heart rate can be palpated by grasping the base of the umbilical cord. By term the infant's heart lies midway between the crown of the head and the buttocks, and the axis is more transverse than that of the adult (Fig. 20-4) (Guyton, 1987). The apical impulse (point of maximal impulse [PMI]) in the newborn is at the fourth intercostal space and to the left of the midclavicular line. The PMI is often visible.

Apical pulse rates should be obtained on all in-

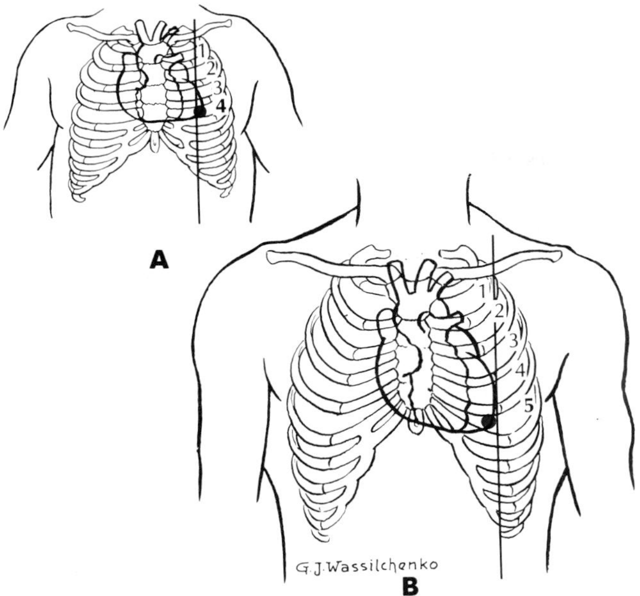

Fig. 20-4 Differences in location of apical pulse in newborn from that of adult. **A,** Neonate. **B,** Adult.
From Whaley LF, Wong DL: *Nursing care of infants and children,* ed 4, St Louis, 1991, Mosby–Year Book.

fants. Auscultation should be for a full minute, preferably when the infant is asleep. Sinus arrhythmia (irregular heart rate) may be considered a physiologic phenomenon in infancy and an indication of good heart function. It is not uncommon to detect irregular heart rates in normal newborns.

Heart sounds during the neonatal period are of higher pitch, shorter duration, and greater intensity than during adult life. The first sound is typically louder and duller than the second sound, which is sharp in quality. Most heart murmurs heard during the neonatal period have no pathologic significance, and more than half disappear by 6 months.

BLOOD PRESSURE. Blood pressure (BP) tends to be highest immediately after birth and lowest about 3 hours later. BP in infants varies from day to day. A drop in systolic BP (about 15 mm Hg) the first hour after birth is common. Values from several hours after delivery through the neonatal period average a systolic pressure of 60 to 80 mm Hg and a diastolic pressure of 40 to 50 mm Hg. Crying and movement result in changes in BP, especially systolic. BP is also sensitive to the changes in blood volume that occur with the adaptations in circulation. The measurement of BP is best accomplished with a Doppler device and while the infant is at rest. It is very important to use the correct-sized BP cuff when taking an infant's BP. When arm pressure measurement is followed by leg pressure measurement, different-sized cuffs may be needed because arms and legs rarely are the same size.

BLOOD VOLUME. Blood volume in the newborn ranges from 80 to 110 ml/kg during the first several days and doubles by the end of the first year. The newborn has approximately 10% greater blood volume and nearly 20% greater red blood cell (RBC) mass than does the adult. However, the plasma volume of the newborn's blood compared with that of the adult by kilogram of body weight, is about 20% less. The preterm infant will have a greater blood volume than the term newborn. This occurs because the preterm infant has a greater plasma volume, not a greater RBC mass.

A number of differences in the circulatory dynamics of the newborn result from early or delayed clamping of the cord. Holding the newborn below the level of the placenta and delaying clamping for several minutes after birth result in an expansion of blood volume from the so-called placental transfusion, an increase of 40% to 60%. This in turn causes an increase in heart size, higher systolic BP, and an increased respiratory rate. Pulmonary crackles (rales) and transient cyanosis also are seen after delayed clamping. To date the value of early or late clamping of the cord has not been determined. Although the increased blood volume may stress the heart and pulmonary vasculature, a decreased incidence of neonatal respiratory distress has been reported in infants for whom cord clamping was delayed. Furthermore, breakdown of the additional RBCs increases the storage supply of iron; 80 ml of placental blood yields 50 mg of iron (Cunningham et al, 1989). However, breakdown of excess RBCs may contribute to hyperbilirubinemia (Fanaroff, Martin, 1992).

HEMATOPOIETIC SYSTEM. The hematopoietic system of the newborn exhibits certain variations from that of the adult. There are differences in RBCs and leukocytes and relatively few differences in platelets.

RED BLOOD CELLS AND HEMOGLOBIN. Because the fetal circulation is less efficient at oxygen exchange than are the lungs, the fetus needs additional RBCs for transport of oxygen in utero. Therefore, at birth the average values of RBCs and hemoglobin are higher than those values in the adult. Cord blood of the term newborn may have a hemoglobin concentration from 14 to 29 g/dL, with a mean of 17 g/dL. The hematocrit ranges from 43% to 63% (mean 55%). RBC count is correspondingly elevated, ranging from between 5.7 to 5.8/mm.^{3} These values fall and reach the average levels of 11 to 17 g/dL and 4.2 to 5.2/mm,^{3} respectively, by the end of the first month. The blood values may be affected by delayed clamping of the cord, which results in a rise in hemoglobin, RBCs, and hematocrit. The source of the sample is another significant factor because capillary blood will give higher values than does venous blood. The time after birth when the blood sample was obtained is significant inasmuch as the slight rise in RBCs after birth is followed by a substantial drop. At birth the infant's blood contains about 80% fetal hemoglobin, but because of the shorter life span of the cells containing fetal hemoglobin, the percentage falls to 55% by 5 weeks and 5% by 20 weeks. Fortunately iron stores generally are sufficient to sustain normal RBC production for 6 months, and thus the slight brief anemia is not serious.

LEUKOCYTES. Leukocytosis, with the white blood cell (WBC) count approximately 18,000/mm^3 (range: 10,000 to 30,000/mm,^{3}) is normal at birth. The number, largely polymorphs, increases to about 23,000 to 24,000/mm^3 during the first day after birth. A resting level of 11,500/mm^3 normally is maintained during the neonatal period. Serious infection is not well tolerated by the newborn, and marked increase in the WBC count is unlikely even in critical sepsis (infection). In most instances sepsis is accompanied by a decline in white cells, particularly in neutrophils. The activity of the bone marrow is accurately reflected by the number of circulating cells—both erythrocytes and leukocytes. The early high WBC count of the newborn decreases rapidly (see Appendix F). A relative leukopenia found in African-American children and adults is apparent by 1 year of age and is caused primarily by a decreased number of neutrophils. By 6 years of age the peripheral blood picture is approximately the same as that of an adult.

PLATELETS. Platelet count ranges between 150,000/mm^3 and 350,000/mm^3 and is essentially the same in newborns as in adults. One exception is the infant of a mother who has taken acetylsalicylic acid (ASA, or aspirin) or chlorpromazine (Thorazine). Both interfere with the release of adenosine diphosphate (ADP). Factors II, VII, IX, and X, found in the liver, are decreased during the first few days of life because the newborn is unable to synthesize vitamin K (pp. 535 and 539). However, bleeding tendencies in the newborn are rare, and unless there has been a marked **vitamin K deficiency,** clotting is sufficient to prevent hemorrhage. The administration of Aquamephyton (vitamin K), 0.5 to 1 mg IM, at birth enhances clotting and serves to help prevent bleeding (see Fig. 21-10).

BLOOD GROUPS. The infant's group is genetically determined and is established early in fetal life. However, during the neonatal period there is a gradual increase in the strength of the agglutinogens present in the RBC membrane. Samples of cord blood may be drawn after birth, especially if the mother's blood type is O or Rh negative. The cord blood samples usually are sent to the laboratory for identification of the infant's blood type and Rh determination.

SIGNS OF RISK FOR CARDIOVASCULAR PROBLEMS. Awareness of normal vital signs is necessary for the nurse to detect any abnormalities. It is important to closely monitor the infant's vital signs for early detection of impending problems. Persistent tachycardia ($\geq$170 beats/min) could be an indication of respiratory distress syndrome (RDS) whereas persistent bradycardia ($\leq$120 beats/min) could be a sign of a congenital heart block (see Chapter 38). Any prolonged cyanosis other than in the hands or feet could indicate respiratory or cardiac problems, or both (see Chapter 38). A difference between upper and lower extremity BP may indicate early signs of coarctation of the aorta (see Chapter 38). It is also important to know the mother's and the infant's blood group so that measures can be taken to prevent ABO or Rh factor problems (see Chapter 38).

Thermogenic System

Heat regulation ranks next to establishment of respirations and circulation as a most critical component to an infant's survival. Temperature regulation is the maintenance of thermal balance between heat loss and heat production. Newborns are homeothermic, which means they attempt to stabilize their internal body temperature within a narrow range. Hypothermia from excessive heat loss is a prevalent and dangerous problem in neonates. The newborn infant's ability to produce heat often approaches the capacity of the adult. However, the tendency toward rapid heat loss in a cold environment is increased in the newborn and often is hazardous to well-being.

THERMOGENESIS. **Thermogenesis** refers to the production of heat (*thermo,* heat; *genesis,* origin). The shivering mechanism of thermogenesis (heat production) rarely is functioning in the newborn. Nonshivering thermogenesis is accomplished primarily by the metabolism of **brown fat** and secondarily by increased metabolic activity in the brain, heart, and liver. Nonshivering thermogenesis is a complex process that increases the metabolic rate and rate of oxygen consumption. Brown fat (adipose tissue) begins to appear during weeks 17 to 20 of gestation. At term brown fat accounts for 2% to 6% of the total body weight of the newborn. It is located in superficial deposits in the interscapular region (below the nape of the neck) and axillas and posterior to the sternum, as well as in deep deposits at the thoracic inlet, surrounding the kidneys and adrenals, along the vertebral column, and in the perineal area. Brown fat is unique to the newborn (Blackburn, Loper, 1992; Fanaroff, Martin, 1992). Brown fat has a richer vascular and nerve supply than does ordinary fat. Heat produced by intense lipid metabolic activity in brown fat can warm the neonate by increasing heat production as much as 100%. Reserves of brown fat, usually present for several weeks after birth, are rapidly depleted with cold stress. The less mature the infant, the less reserve of this essential fat is available at birth.

HEAT LOSS. Heat loss in the newborn occurs in four ways:

1. *Convection:* the flow of heat from the body surface to cooler ambient air. For this reason nursery ambient temperatures are kept at 24° C (75° F), and newborns are wrapped to protect them from the cold.
2. *Radiation:* the loss of heat from the body surface to cooler solid surfaces not in direct contact but in relative proximity to each other. Nursery cribs and examining tables are placed away from outside windows.
3. *Evaporation:* the loss of heat that occurs when a liquid is converted to a vapor. In the newborn, heat loss by evaporation occurs as a result of vaporization of moisture from the skin. The process is invisible and is knows as *insensible water loss* (IWL). This heat loss can be intensified by failure to dry the newborn directly after birth or by bathing and drying the infant too slowly.
4. *Conduction:* the loss of heat from the body surface to cooler surfaces in direct contact. The newborn, when admitted to the nursery, is placed in a warmed cot to minimize heat loss. Loss of heat must be controlled to protect the infant. As already noted, control of such modes of heat loss is the basis of caregiving policies and techniques.

TEMPERATURE REGULATION. Anatomic and physiologic differences among the newborn, child, and adult are notable. The newborn's thermal insulation is less than an adult's. Blood vessels are closer to the surface of the skin. Changes in environmental temperature alter the temperature of the blood, thereby influencing temperature-regulation centers in the hypothalamus. The newborn has a larger body surface to body weight (mass) ratio than do children and adults. The flexed position of the newborn helps to guard against heat loss because it diminishes the amount of skin surface exposed to the environment. Infants also can reduce loss of internal heat to body surfaces by vasoconstricting peripheral vessels. The neonate's sweat glands have little function until the fourth week of age or later. When exposed to high temperatures, the newborn is unable to sweat.

SIGNS OF RISK FOR THERMOGENIC PROBLEMS. Changes in environmental temperature have the potential to disturb the core body temperature. This may cause serious consequences in the newborn. Brown fat metabolism is activated in response to changes in environmental temperature that are perceived by the thermal sensors in the newborn's skin, even when the core temperature of the newborn is unchanged. The newborn does not have the capabilities of the adult to change body posture to decrease the amount of skin surface exposed (e.g., flexion of extremities) in response to cold. When exposed to cold, the newborn may cry, become restless, and increase muscular activity in an effort to generate heat. However, crying increases the work load and energy is expended. Newborns also may increase their respiratory rate in an attempt to stimulate muscular activity.

Cold stress imposes metabolic and physiologic problems in all infants, regardless of gestational age and condition. The respiratory rate is increased as a response to the increased need for oxygen when the oxygen consumption increases significantly in cold stress. Oxygen consumption and energy in the cold-stressed infant are diverted from maintaining normal brain cell and cardiac function and growth to thermogenesis for survival (see Chapter 37). If the infant cannot maintain an adequate oxygen tension, vasoconstriction follows and jeopardizes pulmonary perfusion. As a consequence, arterial blood gas levels of Po_2 are decreased, and the blood pH drops. These changes aggravate existing RDS, also known as hyaline membrane disease (see Chapter 37). Moreover, decreased pulmonary perfusion and oxygen tension may maintain or reopen the right-to left shunt across the patent ductus arteriosus.

The basal metabolic rate will be increased with cold stress. If cold stress is protracted, anaerobic glycolysis occurs, resulting in increased production of acids. Metabolic acidosis develops, and if there is a defect in respiratory function, respiratory acidosis also develops. Excessive fatty acids displace the bilirubin from the albumin-binding sites. The increased level of circulating unbound bilirubin that results increases the risk of kernicterus (defined, p. 1150) even at serum bilirubin levels of 10 mg/dL or less.

Hyperthermia develops more rapidly in the newborn than in the adult because of the larger surface volume. Although newborn infants have six times as many sweat glands per unit area as adults, these glands do not function to allow the infant to sweat. Serious overheating of the newborn can cause cerebral damage from dehydration, heat stroke, and even death.

Renal System

By the fourth month of fetal life the kidneys are formed. In utero, urine is formed in the kidneys and excreted into the amniotic fluid. Small amounts of urine usually are present in the bladder at birth.

At term gestation the kidneys occupy a large portion of the posterior abdominal wall. The bladder lies close to the anterior abdominal wall and is partially an abdominal, as well as a pelvic, organ. In the newborn almost all palpable masses in the abdomen are renal in origin.

Kidney function comparable to that of the adult is not approached until the second year of life. The newborn has a minimal range of chemical balance and safety. Diarrhea, infection, or improper feeding can lead rapidly to acidosis and fluid imbalances—dehydration or edema. Renal immaturity also limits the neonate's ability to excrete drugs.

About 17% of newborns void at delivery, 92% by 24 hours, and 99% within 48 hours (Fanaroff, Martin, 1992). An infant who has not voided after 24 hours should be assessed for adequacy of fluid intake, bladder distention, restlessness, and symptoms of pain. At 40 weeks' gestation the bladder volume capacity is approximately 40 mL. The frequency of voiding varies from two to six times during the first and second days of life and from five to 25 times during the subsequent 24 hours. Generally, term infants void 15 to 60 mL of urine per kilogram per day (Blackburn, Loper, 1992; Fanaroff, Martin, 1992). In addition to excretion of urine, infants lose additional water through insensible fluid loss (water evaporated from the skin [70%] and respiratory tract [35%]) and stool. Stool water loss is estimated at 5 to 10 mL/kg/day.

Full-term infants are unable to concentrate urine; therefore the specific gravity may range from 1.005 to 1.015. The ability to fully concentrate urine is attained by about 3 months of age. After the first voiding, the infant's urine may appear cloudy (because of mucus content) and have a much higher specific gravity. This decreases as fluid intake increases. Normal urine during early infancy is usually straw-colored and almost odorless. Sometimes pink-tinged stains (brick dust) appear on the diaper. These stains are caused by uric crystals and are normal. Blood may be found on a diaper of female infants. The *pseudomenstruation* is caused by the withdrawal of maternal hormones. Male infants may have some bloody spotting from a circumcision. If there is no apparent cause of bleeding, the physician should be notified.

Loss of fluid through urine, feces, lungs, increased metabolic rate, and limited fluid intake results in a 5% to 15% loss of the birth weight. This usually occurs over the first 3 to 5 days of life. If the mother is breast-feeding and her milk supply has not come in yet (usually happens on the third or fourth day after birth), the neonate is protected from dehydration by its increased extracellular fluid volume. The neonate should regain the birth weight within 10 days.

Because renal thresholds are low in the infant, bicarbonate concentration and buffering capacity are decreased. This may lead to acidosis and electrolyte imbalance.

FLUID AND ELECTROLYTE BALANCE. Differences exist between the newborn and adult physiologic response. First, the distribution of extracellular and intracellular fluid differs. About 40% of the body weight of the newborn is extracellular fluid, whereas in the adult it is 20%. The rate of exchange of extracellular fluid also is different. The newborn daily takes in and excretes 600 to 700 mL of water, which is 20% of the total body fluid, or 50% of the extracellular fluid. In contrast, the adult exchanges 2000 mL of water, which is 5% of the total body fluid and 14% of the extracellular fluid. The glomerular filtration rate (GFR) is about 30% to 50% of that of the adult. This results in a decreased ability to remove nitrogenous and other waste products from the blood. However, the newborn's ingested protein is almost totally metabolized for growth.

The sodium reabsorption is decreased as a result of a lowered sodium potassium–activated adenosine triphosphatase (ATPase) activity. The decreased ability to excrete excessive sodium results in hypotonic urine compared with plasma. The composition of body fluids shows variations. There is a higher concentration of sodium, phosphates, chloride, and organic acids and a lower concentration of bicarbonate ions. These findings mean that the newborn is in a compensated acidotic state and in a state of potential manifest edema. The infant has a higher renal threshold for glucose.

The newborn can dilute urine down to 50 milliosmols (mOsm). An osmol is a measure of total number of particles. One gram molecular weight (mole) of nondiffusible and nonionizable substance is equal to 1 osmol. Capacity to dilute urine exceeds capacity to concentrate it. There is some limitation in the ability to increase urinary volume. The newborn can concentrate urine to 600 to 700 mOsm compared with the adult's capacity of 1400 mOsm. The inability to concentrate urine is not absolute, but in terms of adult function, it is somewhat limited. Comparative laboratory values for newborns and adults appear in Appendix F.

SIGNS OF RISK FOR RENAL SYSTEM PROBLEMS. The renal system has a wide range of functions, and dysfunction can result from a multitude of physiologic abnormalities. Any infant who has not voided within a 24 hour period must be assessed further. The pediatrician must be notified and further evaluation conducted. Gross anomalies, hypospadias, or exstrophy of the bladder (see Chapter 38) can be easily identified at birth. Some kidney anomalies also can be detected by ultrasound during pregnancy (see Chapter 38).

Gastrointestinal System

The infant's gastrointestinal system is not mature at birth. The gastrointestinal tract reaches adult maturity levels in 2 to 3 years. The full-term newborn is capable of swallowing, digesting, metabolizing, absorbing proteins and simple carbohydrates, and emulsifying fats. With the exception of pancreatic amylase, the characteristic enzymes and digestive juices are present even in low-birth-weight neonates.

In the adequately hydrated infant the mucous membrane of the mouth is moist and pink. The hard and soft palates are intact.

Drooling of mucus is common in the first few hours after birth. Retention cysts, small whitish areas (Epstein's pearls), may be found on the gum margins and at the juncture of the hard and soft palate. The cheeks are full because of well-developed sucking pads. These, like the labial tubercles (sucking calluses) on the upper lip, disappear when the sucking period is over.

Even though in utero sucking motions have been recorded by ultrasound, these motions are not coordinated in any infant born who is less than 1500 g or less than 32 weeks' gestation. Sucking behavior is influenced by neuromuscular maturity, maternal medications received in labor and delivery, and the type of initial feeding.

A special mechanism present in normal newborns coordinates the breathing, sucking, and swallowing reflexes necessary for oral feeding. Sucking in the newborn takes place in small bursts of three or four sucks at a time. In the term newborn, longer and more efficient sucking attempts occur a few hours after birth. The infant is unable to move food from the lips to the pharynx; therefore it is necessary to place the nipple (breast or bottle) well inside the baby's mouth (see Chapter 22). Peristaltic activity in the esophagus is uncoordinated in the first few days of life. It quickly becomes a coordinated pattern in normal infants, and they swallow easily.

Teeth begin developing in utero with enamel formation continuing until about age 10. Tooth development is influenced by neonatal/infant illnesses, medications, and illnesses of, or medications taken by, the mother during pregnancy. The fluoride level in the water supply also influences tooth development. Occasionally an infant may be born with one tooth or even two teeth.

Bacteria are not present in the infant's gastrointestinal tract at birth. Soon after birth, oral and anal orifices permit entrance of bacteria and air. Generally the highest bacterial concentration is found in the lower portion of the intestine, particularly in the large intestine. Normal colonic bacteria are established within the first week after birth. The normal intestinal flora help synthesize vitamin K, folic acid, and biotin. Bowel sounds usually can be heard 1 hour after birth.

The capacity of the stomach varies from 30 to 90 mL depending on the size of the infant. Emptying time for the stomach is highly variable. Several factors, such as time and volume of feedings, type and temperature of food, and psychic stress, may affect the emptying time. The stomach empties intermittently, starting within a few minutes of the beginning of a feeding and completing between 2 to 4 hours after feeding. The cardiac sphincter and nervous control of the stomach are immature; thus some regurgitation may occur. Regurgitation during the first day or two of life can be decreased by avoiding overfeeding and by burping the infant.

DIGESTION. The infant's gastric acidity at birth normally equals the adult level but is reduced within a week and may remain reduced for 2 to 3 months. The reduction in gastric acidity may lead to "colic." Infants with colic usually remain awake, crying in apparent distress between two feedings, often the same ones every day. Nothing seems to appease them. Infant massage may help. They appear to "grow out" of this behavior by age 3 months.

Further digestion and absorption of nutrients occur in the small intestine. This complex process is made possible by pancreatic secretions, secretions from the liver through the common bile duct, and secretions from the duodenal portion of the small intestine.

The infant's ability to digest carbohydrates, fats, and proteins is regulated by the presence of certain enzymes. Most of these are functional at birth. One exception is *amylase*, produced by the salivary glands after about 3 months and by the pancreas at about 6 months of age. This enzyme is necessary to convert starch into maltose. The other exception is *lipase,* also secreted by the pancreas; it is necessary for the digestion of fat. Thus the normal term newborn is capable of digesting simple carbohydrates and proteins but has a limited ability to digest fats (for further discussion, see Chapter 22).

STOOLS. **Newborn stools** consist of meconium and are followed by transitional stools. At birth the lower intestine is filled with meconium. *Meconium* is formed during fetal life from the amniotic fluid and its constituents, intestinal secretions (including bilirubin) and cells shed from the mucosa. Meconium is greenish black and viscous and contains occult blood (Plate 17). The first meconium passed is sterile, but within hours all meconium passed contains bacteria. About 69% of normal term infants pass meconium within 12 hours of life; 94% by 24 hours; and 99.8% in 48 hours (Blackburn, Loper, 1992).

The number of stools varies during the first week, being most numerous between the third and sixth days. Newborns fed early pass stools sooner (Boyer, Vidyasagar, 1987). *Transitional stools* (thin, slimy, and brown to green because of the continued presence of meconium) are passed from the third to the sixth day (Plate 17). The stools of the breast-fed infant are loose, golden yellow in color, and nonirritating to the infant's skin (Plate 17). It is normal for the breast-fed infant to have a bowel movement as often as each feeding or as infrequently as once in 3 to 4 days. Even in the latter case, the stools remain loose and unformed. The stools of the formula-fed infant are formed but soft, pale yellow, and have a typical stool odor. They tend to be irritating to the infant's skin (Plate 17). The number of stools decreases in the first 2 weeks from five or six each day (after every feeding) to one or two per day.

During feeding, distention of the stomach muscles causes a corresponding relaxation and contraction of the muscles of the colon, stimulating peristalsis. As a result of this **gastrocolic reflex,** infants often have bowel movements during or just after a feeding. Breast-fed infants are more likely to stool during a feeding than are formula-fed infants.

The infant develops an elimination pattern by the second week of life. With the addition of solid food the baby's stool gradually assumes the characteristics of an adult's stool.

FEEDING BEHAVIORS. Variations occur among infants regarding interest in food, symptoms of hunger, and amount ingested at any one time. The amount that the infant takes at any one formula feeding depends on the size of the infant, the hunger level, and the alertness of the infant. When an infant is put to breast, some feed immediately, whereas others require a learning period of up to 48 hours before breast-feeding can be said to be effective. Random hand-to-mouth movement and sucking of fingers have been seen in utero. These actions are well developed at birth and are intensified with hunger, which enhances feeding (see Chapter 22).

SIGNS OF RISK FOR GASTROINTESTINAL PROBLEMS. It is important to note the time, color, and character of the infant's first stool. A lack of passage of stool could indicate an inborn error of metabolism (e.g., cystic fibrosis) or congenital disorder (e.g., Hirschsprung disease or an imperforate anus) (for further discussion of congenital anomalies, see Chapter 38). An active rectal "wink" reflex (contraction of anal sphincter muscle in response to touch) usually is a good sign of anal patency. Some infants do not digest specific formulas well. If an infant is allergic to or unable to digest the formula, the stools may become very soft with a high water content that is seen as a distinct water ring around the stool on the diaper. Forceful ejection of stool and a water ring around the stool are signs of diarrhea (Plate 17). Care must be taken to avoid misinterpreting transitional stools for diarrhea stools. The loss of fluid in diarrhea can rapidly lead to fluid and electrolyte imbalance.. Passage of meconium from the vagina or urinary meatus is a possible sign of a fistulous tract to the rectum. Other deviations from normal findings that require further investigation involve the umbilical cord, as in the following examples:

- A single artery is sometimes associated with internal anomalies.
- Redness surrounding the cord stump may indicate infection.
- Bleeding may be a sign of hemorrhagic disorder.
- Oozing of urine results from persistence of the urachus (normal in fetal life).
- Oomphalocele is herniation of abdominal contents into the cord.
- Gastroschisis is a congenital fissure of the abdominal cavity.

Abdominal distention at birth usually indicates a serious disorder, such as ruptured viscus or tumors. Distention that occurs later may be the result of something simple such as overfeeding or may signal gastrointestinal disorders. A scaphoid (sunken) abdomen with bowel sounds heard in the chest and signs of respiratory distress indicates diaphragmatic hernia. The amount of regurgitation ("spitting up") after feedings needs to be recorded. Color change, gagging, and projectile (very forceful) vomiting occur in association with esophageal or tracheoesophageal anomalies (for further discussion of congenital anomalies, see Chapter 38).

Hepatic System

The liver and gallbladder are formed by the fourth week of gestation. In the newborn, the liver can be palpated about 1 cm below the right costal margin because it is enlarged and occupies about 40% of the abdominal cavity. The infant's liver plays an important role in iron storage, carbohydrate metabolism, conjugation of bilirubin, and coagulation.

IRON STORAGE. The fetal liver (which serves as the site for production of hemoglobin after birth) begins storing iron in utero. The infant's iron store is proportional to total body hemoglobin content and length of gestation. At birth the term neonate has approximately 270 mg of iron (depending on the neonate's gestational age and birth weight) of which about 140 to 170 mg is hemoglobin (Cunningham et al, 1989). If the mother had adequate iron intake during pregnancy, the infant will have an iron store that will last until the fifth month of life.

CARBOHYDRATE METABOLISM. The infant's carbohydrate reserves are low. Glucose is a main source of energy during the first 4 to 6 hours of life. Blood glucose levels fall rapidly and then stabilize at about 50 to 60 mg/dL. By the time the infant is 3 days old, blood glucose levels should be around 60 to 70 mg/dL. The infant's liver may not be mature enough to form glucose from protein; therefore newborns are susceptible to hypoglycemia. If the infant appears to be jittery, a blood glucose determination should be obtained to rule out hypoglycemia.

CONJUGATION OF BILIRUBIN. The fetal liver begins to metabolize bilirubin at 12 weeks' gestational age but loses this ability at 36 weeks. The fetus does not conjugate bilirubin so that it can cross the placenta and be excreted.

Bilirubin is a yellow pigment that results from the breakdown of hemoglobin and myoglobin in muscle cells (Valmin, 1989). The hemoglobin is phagocytosed by the reticuloendothelial cells, converted to bilirubin, and released in an unconjugated form. Unconjugated bilirubin, termed *indirect bilirubin,* is relatively insoluble and is almost entirely bound to circulating albumin, a plasma protein. The unbound bilirubin can leave the vascular system and permeate other extravascular tissues (e.g., the skin, sclera, oral mucous membranes). The resultant yellow coloring is termed *jaundice*.

In the liver the unbound bilirubin is conjugated with glucuronide in the presence of the enzyme glucuronosyl transferase. The conjugated form of bilirubin is excreted from liver cells as a constituent of bile. It is termed *direct bilirubin* and is soluble. Along with other components of bile, direct bilirubin is excreted into the biliary tract system that carries the bile into the duodenum. Bilirubin is converted to urobilinogen and stercobilin within the duodenum through the action of the bacterial flora. Urobilinogen is excreted in urine and feces; stercobilin is excreted in the feces (Fig. 20-5). Total serum bilirubin is the sum of conjugated (direct) and unconjugated (indirect) bilirubin.

Adequate serum albumin–binding sites are also available unless the infant experiences asphyxia neonatorum, cold stress, or hypoglycemia. Maternal prebirth ingestion of drugs such as sulfa drugs and aspirin can reduce the amount of serum albumin–binding sites in the newborn. Although the neonate has the functional capacity to convert bilirubin, physiologic hyperbilirubinemia occurs in most infants.

PHYSIOLOGIC HYPERBILIRUBINEMIA. **Physiologic jaundice** or neonatal hyperbilirubinemia is a normal

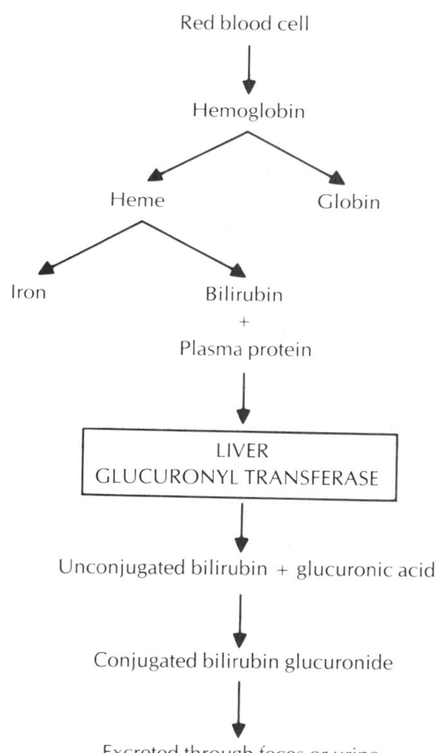

Fig. 20-5 Formation and excretion of bilirubin.
From Whaley LF, Wong DL: Nursing care of infants and children, ed 4, St Louis, 1991, Mosby–Year Book.

occurrence in 50% of full-term and 80% of preterm newborns. Korones (1986) noted that neonatal jaundice occurs for the following reasons:

1. The newborn has a higher rate of bilirubin production. The number of fetal RBCs per kilogram of weight is greater than the adult's. Fetal RBCs have a shorter survival time, 40 to 90 days compared with 120 days in the adult.
2. There is considerable reabsorption of bilirubin from the neonatal small intestine.

Although neonatal jaundice is considered benign, bilirubin may accumulate to hazardous levels and become pathologic (see Chapter 38). Physiologic jaundice fulfills the following specific criteria (Korones, 1986):

1. The infant is otherwise well.
2. In term infants, jaundice first appears after 24 hours and disappears by the end of the seventh day.
3. In preterm infants, jaundice is first evident after 48 hours and disappears by the ninth or tenth day.
4. Serum unconjugated bilirubin concentration does not exceed 12 mg/100 mL, either in term or preterm infants.
5. Hyperbilirubinemia is almost exclusively of the unconjugated variety, and conjugated (direct) bilirubin should not exceed 1 to 1.5 mg/100 mL.
6. Daily increments of bilirubin concentration should not surpass 5 mg/100 mL.

Bilirubin levels in excess of 12 mg/100 mL may indicate either an exaggeration of the physiologic handicap or the presence of disease. *At any serum bilirubin level, the appearance of jaundice during the first day of life or persistence beyond the ages previously noted usually indicates a pathologic process.*

Jaundice is noticeable first in the head and then progresses gradually toward the abdomen and extremities because of the neonate's circulatory pattern (cephalocaudal developmental progression). The appearance of jaundice in the various body locations give a rough estimate of the circulating levels of unbound bilirubin. For example, when jaundice appears over the nose, the circulating level of unbound bilirubin is approximately 3 mg; levels at which other body areas appear jaundiced are as follows:

Approximate level of hyperbilirubinemia by cephalocaudal distribution

Nose:	3 mg/dL	Abdomen:	10 mg/dL
Face:	5 mg/dL	Legs:	12 mg/dL
Chest:	7 mg/dL	Palms:	20 mg/dL

Several nursery practices may influence the appearance and degree of physiologic hyperbilirubinemia. *Early feeding* tends to keep the serum bilirubin level low by stimulating intestinal activity (the gastrocolic reflex) and the passage of meconium and stool.

Cold stress of the newborn may result in acidosis and raise the level of free fatty acids. In the presence of acidosis, albumin binding of bilirubin is weakened and bilirubin is freed. *Kernicterus*, the most serious complication of neonatal hyperbilirubinemia, is caused by the precipitation of bilirubin in neuronal cells, resulting in their destruction (see Chapter 38). Cerebral palsy, epilepsy, and mental retardation are expected in survivors.

There is an increase in the number of mothers and infants being discharged from the hospital between 2 and 48 hours after birth and others who have elected to give birth at home. As a result the professional attendant may not be available to assess levels of jaundice. *Therefore, all parents need instructions in how to assess jaundice and to whom to report the findings* (see Chapter 38).

BREAST MILK JAUNDICE. **Breast milk jaundice** has been defined as progressive indirect hyperbilirubinemia beyond the first week of life. Jaundice from ingestion of breast milk occurs in 0.5% to 2% of full-term neonates (Wilkerson, 1988). It is thought that an enzyme present in the milk of some women inhibits the enzyme glucuronyl transferase, which is necessary for the conjugation of bilirubin. Although breast milk jaundice is a form of physiologic jaundice, it occurs after the mature milk comes in, usually about the fifth or sixth day of life in a thriving infant whose mother is lactating well. This type of jaundice usually persists longer—up to 6 weeks. Unconjugated bilirubin rises beyond physiologic limits (15 to 20 mg/dL) by the seventh day. The levels subside by 5 to 10 mg if breast-feeding is discontinued for 12 to 24 hours; then usually 3 to 5 days pass before the previous high level is again reached. Mothers are encouraged to maintain their milk supply during this test period by pumping or manually expressing the milk. Mothers need reassurance that nothing is wrong with their milk (Brovten et al, 1985; Locklin, 1987).

BREAST-FEEDING JAUNDICE. **Breast-feeding jaundice** usually becomes apparent about the third day of life. There is no other apparent clinical cause. Dehydration, lack of fluid, and weight loss are not causes (Lascari, 1986; Lawrence, 1989). Recent research has documented that the number of breast-feedings during the first 3 days of life is related to bilirubin levels and has a significant relationship. The greater the number of feedings, the lower the bilirubin level

(Lascari, 1986; Lawrence, 1989). The number of feedings per day should be eight or more. The mother is encouraged to feed around the clock. Colostrum (a precursor to milk) is a natural laxative that helps promote passage of meconium. Consequently early, frequent nursing will enhance meconium excretion and decrease bilirubin levels (Lawrence, 1989).

COAGULATION. The liver has an important role in blood coagulation. Coagulation factors, which are synthesized in the liver, are activated by vitamin K. The lack of intestinal bacteria needed to synthesize vitamin K results in transient blood coagulation deficiency between the second and fifth days of life. The levels slowly rise to reach adult levels by 9 months of age. An injection of Aquamephyton (vitamin K) on the day of birth helps prevent clotting problems. Any bleeding problems noted in an infant should be reported immediately and clotting studies ordered.

SIGNS OF RISK FOR HEPATIC SYSTEM PROBLEMS. Some problems such as kernicterus and hypoglycemia have been discussed. It is necessary to assess the infant's hemoglobin levels for anemia. Because infants have a potential for coagulation deficiency, a male child needs to be observed closely for signs of hemorrhage after circumcision. Hemorrhage could be due to a clotting defect, indicating a serious problem such as hemophilia (see Chapters 38 and 39).

Immune System

The cells that supply the infant's immunity are developed early in fetal life; however, they are not activated for several months. For the first 3 months of life, the infant is protected by passive immunity received from the mother. Natural barriers such as the acidity of the stomach or the production of pepsin and trypsin, which maintain sterility of the small intestine, are not fully developed until 3 to 4 weeks (Medici, 1983). The membrane-protective IgA is missing from the respiratory and urinary tracts, and unless the newborn is breast-fed, it is absent from the gastrointestinal tract as well. The infant begins to synthesize IgG, and about 40% of adult levels are reached by 1 year of age. Significant amounts of IgM are produced at birth, and adult levels are reached by 9 months of age. The production of IgA, IgD, and IgE is much more gradual, and maximum levels are not attained until early childhood. The infant who is breast-fed receives passive immunity through the colostrum and the breast milk. The protection provided varies with the age and maturity of the infant, as well as the mother's own immune system (Lawrence, 1989).

SIGNS OF RISK FOR IMMUNE SYSTEM PROBLEMS. All newborns and especially preterm newborns are at high risk for infection during the first several months of life. During this period, infection represents one of the leading causes of morbidity and mortality. The newborn is unable to limit the invading pathogen to the portal of entry because of a generalized hypofunction of the inflammatory and immune mechanisms. Any unusual discharges from the infant's eyes, nose, mouth, or other orifice must be investigated. If a rash does appear, it must be closely evaluated because there are many normal newborn rashes not associated with any infection. When an infant is septic, the usual response will be respiratory distress (see Chapter 39). Infants need to be protected from infections by the use of good hand-washing techniques.

Integumentary System

All the skin structures are present at birth but are immature. The epidermis and dermis are loosely bound and are very thin. Vernix caseosa is also *fused with* the epidermis and serves as a protective covering. The infant's skin is very sensitive and can be easily damaged. The term infant has an erythematous (very red) skin for a few hours after birth, after which it fades to its normal color. The skin often appears blotchy or mottled, especially over the extremities. The hands and feet appear slightly cyanotic. This bluish discoloration, *acrocyanosis,* is caused by vasomotor instability, capillary stasis, and a high hemoglobin level. This is normal and appears intermittently over the first 7 to 10 days, especially with exposure to cold.

The healthy term newborn is plump. Subcutaneous fat accumulated during the last trimester acts to insulate the neonate. The preterm infant has difficulty maintaining an even body temperature because of the lack of brown fat. The newborn's skin may be slightly tight, suggesting fluid retention. Fine *lanugo* hair may be noted over the face, shoulders, and back. Actual edema of the face and *ecchymosis* (bruising) may be noted as a result of face presentation or forceps delivery.

CAPUT SUCCEDANEUM. **Caput succedaneum** is a generalized, easily identifiable edematous area of the scalp, most commonly found on the occiput area (Fig. 20-6, *A*). The sustained pressure of the presenting vertex against the cervix results in compression of local vessels, thus slowing venous return. The slower venous return causes an increase in tissue fluids within the skin of the scalp, and an edematous swelling develops. This boggy edematous swelling,

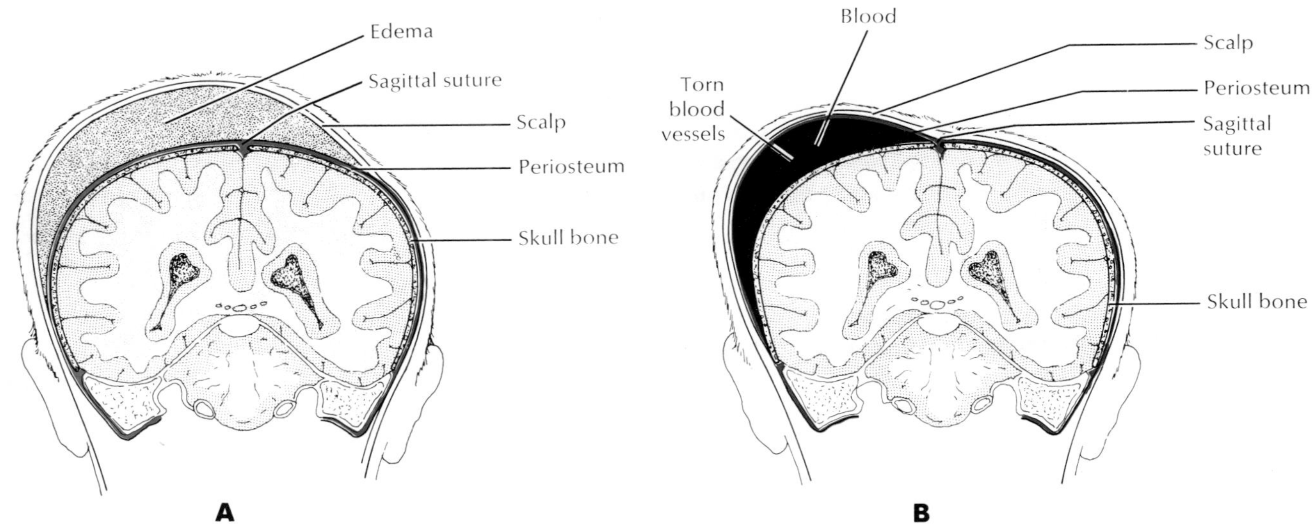

Fig. 20-6 Differences between caput succedaneum and cephalhematoma. **A,** Caput succedaneum: edema of scalp noted at birth; crosses suture lines. **B,** Cephalhematoma: bleeding between periosteum and skull bone appearing within first 2 days; does not cross suture lines.

present at birth, extends across suture lines of the fetal skull and disappears spontaneously within 3 to 4 days. Excessive pressure to the presenting vertex as it passes over the bony maternal pelvis may cause a cephalhematoma to develop. Often, caput succedaneum and cephalhematoma occur simultaneously.

CEPHALHEMATOMA. **Cephalhematoma** is a collection of blood between a skull bone and its periosteum. Therefore a cephalhematoma never crosses a cranial suture line (Fig. 20-6, *B*). Bleeding may occur with spontaneous delivery from pressure against the maternal bony pelvis. Low forceps delivery, as well as difficult forceps rotation and extraction, also may cause bleeding. This soft, fluctuating, irreducible fullness does not pulsate or bulge when the infant cries. It appears several hours after birth or the day after delivery. It may not become apparent until a caput succedaneum is absorbed (Fig 20-6, *A*). A cephalhematoma usually is largest on the second or third day, by which time the bleeding stops. The fullness of cephalhematoma spontaneously resolves in 3 to 6 weeks. It is not aspirated because infection may develop if the skin is punctured.

As the hematoma resolves, the hemolysis of RBCs occurs. Hyperbilirubinemia (jaundice) may result after the newborn is home. Therefore the parents are instructed to observe the newborn for jaundice and may be asked to bring the infant in to be rechecked before the usual 4-week visit.

DESQUAMATION. Desquamation (peeling) of the skin of the term infant does not occur until a few days after birth. Its presence at birth is an indication of postmaturity. Parents should be instructed to avoid harsh drying soap and refrain from overuse of lotions on the infant's skin. Humidifying the air sometimes helps this condition.

SWEAT AND OIL GLANDS. Sweat glands are present at birth but do not function effectively because they do not respond to increases in ambient or body temperature. There is some fetal sebaceous (oil) gland hyperplasia and secretion of sebum as a result of the hormonal influences of pregnancy. *Vernix caseosa,* a cheeselike substance, is a product of the sebaceous glands. Removal of the vernix is followed by desquamation of the epidermis in most infants (Fanaroff, Martin, 1992). Distended sebaceous glands, noticeable on the newborn face, are known as *milia* (small white pimples). Although sebaceous glands are well developed at birth, they are only minimally active during childhood. They become more active as androgen production increases before puberty (Plate 18).

MONGOLIAN SPOTS. **Mongolian spots,** bluish-black areas of pigmentation, may appear over any part of the exterior surface of the body, including the extremities. They are more commonly noted on the back and buttocks (Plate 18). These pigmented areas most frequently are noted in babies whose ethnic origins are the Mediterranean shores, Latin America, Asia, or a number of other areas in the world. They

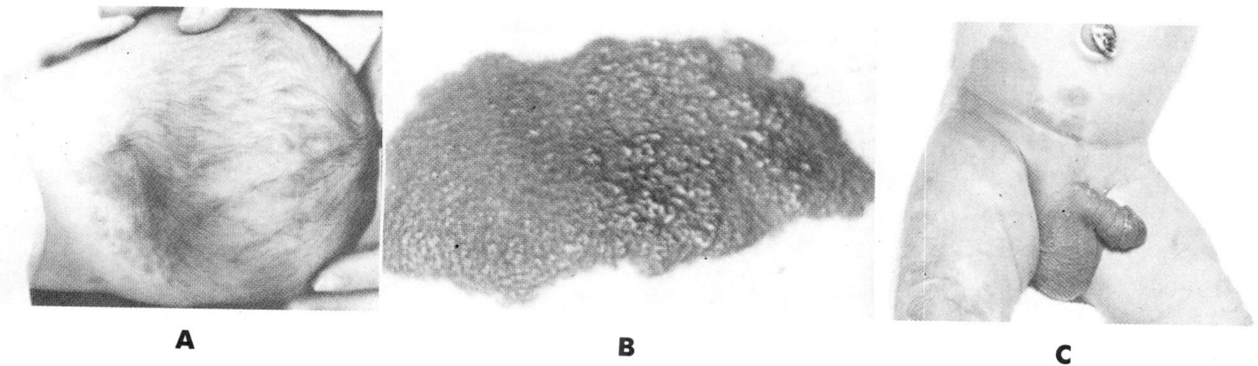

Fig. 20-7 **A**, Telangiectatic nevus (stork bite). **B**, Strawberry mark, or nevus vasculosus. **C**, Port-wine stain, or nevus flammeus.
Courtesy Mead Johnson & Co, Evansville, Ind.

are more common in dark-skinned individuals regardless of race. They fade gradually over a period of months or years.

NEVI. Known as stork bites, *telangiectatic nevi* are pink and easily blanched (Fig. 20-7, *A*). They appear on the upper eyelids, nose, upper lip, lower occiput bone, and nape of the neck. They have no clinical significance and fade between the first and second year.

The *strawberry mark,* or nevus vasculosus, is the second most common type of capillary hemangioma (Fig. 20-7, *B*). It consists of dilated, newly formed capillaries occupying the entire dermal and subdermal layers, with associated connective tissue hypertrophy. The typical lesion is a raised, sharply demarcated, and bright or dark-red, rough-surfaced swelling that resembles a strawberry. Lesions usually are single but may be multiple, with 75% occurring on the head. These lesions can remain until the child is of school age or sometimes even longer.

A *port-wine stain,* or nevus flammeus (Fig. 20-7, *C*), usually is observed at birth and is composed of a plexus of newly formed capillaries in the papillary layer of the corium. It is red to purple, varies in size, shape, and location, and is not elevated. True port-wine stains do not blanch on pressure and do not disappear. They most frequently are found on the face.

ERYTHEMA TOXICUM. A transient rash, *erythema toxicum,* also is called erythema neonatorum, "newborn rash" or "fleabite" dermatitis. It has lesions in different stages, erythematous macules, papules, or small vesicles. The lesions may appear suddenly anywhere on the body. The rash is thought to be an inflammatory response. Eosinophils, which help decrease inflammation, are found in the vesicles. The rash is seen only in term neonates (36 or more weeks' gestational age) during the first 3 weeks of age (Medici, 1983). Although the appearance is alarming, it has no clinical significance and requires no treatment.

SIGNS OF RISK FOR INTEGUMENTARY PROBLEMS. Close observation of the newborn's skin color can lead to early detection of potential problems. Any pallor, plethora (deep purplish color from increased circulating RBCs), cyanosis, or jaundice should be noted and described. The skin should be examined for signs of birth injuries, such as forceps marks (Plate 18) or lesions related to fetal monitoring. Ecchymoses (bruises) may be present. When bruises are present, the infant's bilirubin levels may be elevated. Petechiae may be present if increased pressure was applied to an area. Petechiae scattered over the infant's body, should be reported to the pediatrician because their presence may indicate underlying problems such as low platelet count or infection. Unilateral or bilateral periauricular papillomas (skin tags) occur fairly frequently. They usually are a familial trait and of no consequence. However, they may be helpful in identifying potential urinary tract abnormalities (see Chapter 38).

Reproductive System

FEMALE. At birth the ovaries contain thousands of primitive germ cells. These represent the full complement of potential ova because no oogonia form after birth in term infants. The ovarian cortex, which is made up primarily of primordial follicles, forms a thicker portion of the ovary in the female newborn than in the adult. The number of ova decreases from birth to maturity by approximately 90%.

The infant's uterus, enlarged during pregnancy because of maternal estrogen, undergoes involution in the first weeks of life and decreases in size and weight. Hyperestrogenism of pregnancy, followed by a drop after delivery, may result in a mucoid vaginal discharge and even some slight bloody spotting (pseudomenstruation) (See Plate 18). If this occurs, it will disappear in 2 to 4 weeks. Vaginal tags are common findings and have no clinical significance. External genitals usually are edematous, with increased pigmentation (Fig. 20-8, *A*).

The preterm girl of 30 to 36 weeks' gestation usually has a prominent clitoris that extends from the labia minora and majora. The labia majora are small and widely separated. At 36 to 40 weeks' gestation, the labia majora are larger and almost cover the clitoris. In term neonates, labia majora and minora obscure the vestibule and cover the clitoris. Vernix caseosa may be present in large amounts between the labia (Jones et al, 1984).

If the female was delivered in the breech position, the labia may be very edematous. It is not uncommon for bruising to appear because of the trauma of the breech delivery. These two problems usually self-correct within a few days and no further treatment is needed.

MALE. The testes descend into the scrotum by birth in 90% of newborn boys. Although this percentage drops with preterm birth, by 1 year of age the incidence of undescended testes in all boys is less than 1%. Spermatogenesis does not occur until puberty (see Chapter 6).

Adhesions of the foreskin (prepuce) are almost universally present in newborn boys. During prenatal development the tissue of the prepuce is continuous with the epidermis that covers the glans. Gradually the preputial space between the prepuce and glans forms. The complete separation of the two tissue areas generally is not complete at birth. For this reason the prepuce of the newborn usually is not fully retractable. Smegma, a white cheesy substance, commonly is found under the foreskin. Small white, firm lesions called epithelial pearls may be seen at the tip of the prepuce. In the preterm boy of less than 28 weeks' gestation, the testes remain within the abdominal cavity and the scrotum appears high and close to the body. By 28 to 36 weeks' gestation, the testes can be palpated in the inguinal canal and a few rugae appear on the scrotum. At 36 to 40 weeks' gestation, the testes are palpable in the upper scrotum and rugae appear on the anterior portion. After 40 weeks the testes can be palpated in the scrotum and rugae cover the scrotal sac. The postterm neonate has deep rugae and a pendulous scrotum. The scrotum usually is more deeply pigmented than the rest of the skin (Fig. 20-8, *B*). This pigmentation is a response to maternal estrogen. Hydroceles, caused by an accumulation of fluid around the testes, are a common finding. They can easily be transilluminated with a light and usually will decrease in size without treatment.

If the male infant was delivered in a breech pre-

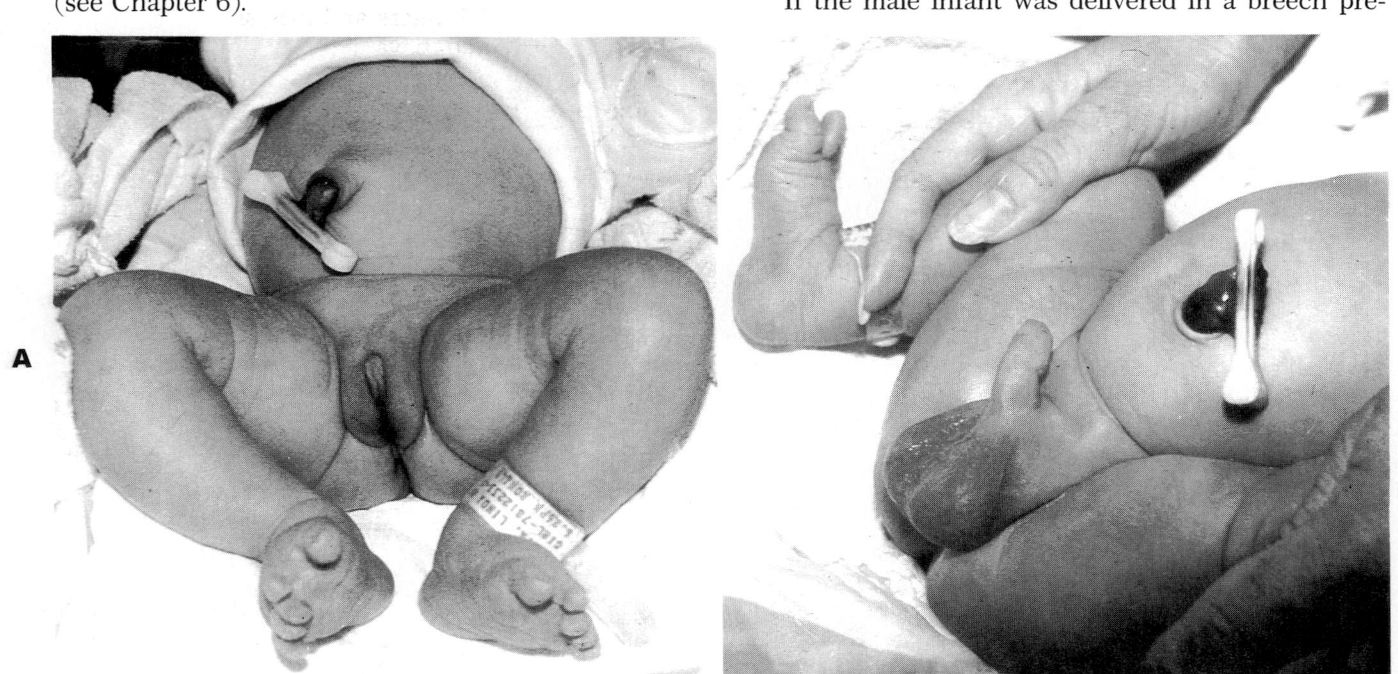

Fig. 20-8 **A,** Genitals in female term infant. Note mucoid vaginal discharge. **B,** Genitals in male infant. Uncircumcised penis. Rugae cover scrotum, indicating term gestation. Cord has been swabbed with ethylene blue to prevent infection.

sentation, the scrotum will appear very edematous (Plate 18). Often the scrotum is also very bruised from the trauma of the breech delivery. The swelling and discoloration will subside within a few days.

SWELLING OF BREAST TISSUE. Swelling of the breast tissue (Plate 18) in infants of both sexes is caused by the hyperestrogenism of pregnancy. In a few infants a thin discharge (witch's milk) can be seen. This finding has no clinical significance, requires no treatment, and will subside as the maternal hormones are eliminated from the infant's body. The nipples should be symmetric on the chest.

Breast tissue and areola size increase with gestation. The areola appears slightly elevated at 34 weeks' gestation. By 36 weeks a breast bud of 1 to 2 mm is visible and increases to 12 mm by 42 weeks. Increased breast tissue may indicate subcutaneous fat in larger babies. However, generally the more breast tissue, the greater is the gestational age (Jones et al, 1984).

SIGNS OF RISK FOR REPRODUCTIVE PROBLEMS. The infant must be closely inspected for ambiguous genitalia and other abnormalities. Normally in a female infant the urethral opening is located behind the clitoris. Any deviation from this may mistakenly suggest that the clitoris is a small penis, which can occur in conditions such as adrenal hyperplasia. Nearly all females are born with hymenal tags. Absence of such could indicate vaginal agenesis. Fecal discharge from the vagina indicates a rectovaginal fistula. Any of these findings need to be reported for further evaluation.

The male infant's scrotum always should be palpated for testes. Inguinal hernias may be present and become more obvious when the infant cries. If the urinary meatus is not at the tip of the glans penis, hypospadias or epispadias may be present. These problems usually are associated with other anomalies (see Chapter 38).

Skeletal System

The infant's skeletal system undergoes rapid development during the first year of life. At birth there are larger amounts of cartilage than ossified bone. Because of **cephalocaudal** (head-to-toe) **development**, the newborn looks somewhat out of proportion.

The head at term is one fourth of the total body length. The arms are slightly longer than the legs. In the newborn the legs are one third of the total body length but only 15% of the total body weight. In the adult the legs comprise one half of the total body height and 30% of total body weight. As growth proceeds, the midpoint in head-to-toe measurements gradually descends from a level even with the umbilicus at birth to the level of the symphysis pubis at maturity.

The face appears small in relation to the skull. The skull is large and heavy in comparison. Cranial size and shape can be distorted by molding. Molding is the shaping of the fetal head by overlapping of the cranial bones to facilitate movement through the birth canal during labor (Fig. 20-9, *B* and *C*). This shaping gives the infant's head a cone appearance (Fig. 20-9, *A* and Plate 18). The bones in the vertebral column of the newborn form two primary curvatures, one in the thoracic region and one in the sacral region (Fig. 20-10, *A*). Both are forward, concave curvatures. As the infant gains control of the head, at approximately 3 months of age, a secondary curvature appears in the cervical region (Fig. 20-10, *B*).

In some newborn infants there is a significant separation of the knees when the ankles are held together, resulting in an appearance of bowlegs (Fig. 20-11, *A*). If the infant's presentation was breech, the knees many be extended and the infant will continue to maintain the in utero position for several weeks. What sometimes appears as a gross anomaly may simply be a result of in utero positioning. These conditions are self-limiting. The newborn is also very flat footed because there is no clearly apparent arch to the foot (Fig. 20-11, *B*).

The infant's extremities should be symmetric and of equal length. Fingers and toes should be equal in count and should have nails present. Extra digits (polydactyly) sometimes are found on hands or feet. Fingers or toes may be fused (syndactyly). Creases can be found on the palms of the hands. The simian line, a single palmar crease, often is found in Down syndrome (see Fig. 7-3). The soles of the feet should be inspected for number of creases. Preterm newborns have little if any creases. The more creases present, the greater is the gestational age.

The infant's hips should be inspected for symmetry. Skin folds should be equal and symmetric. Hip integrity is assessed by using the Ortolani's maneuver (Fig. 20-12). The index and middle fingers of each hand are placed over the greater trochanters of the hips at the same time. Downward pressure is exerted on the hips while the neonate's knees are flexed. The hips are flexed at least 70 degrees and then abducted. The motion should be smooth without any unusual clicks felt. Presence of a click, unequal movement, or extra skin folds is considered a positive response, indicating that the hip is dislocated, and the physician should be notified.

The newborn's spine appears straight and can be

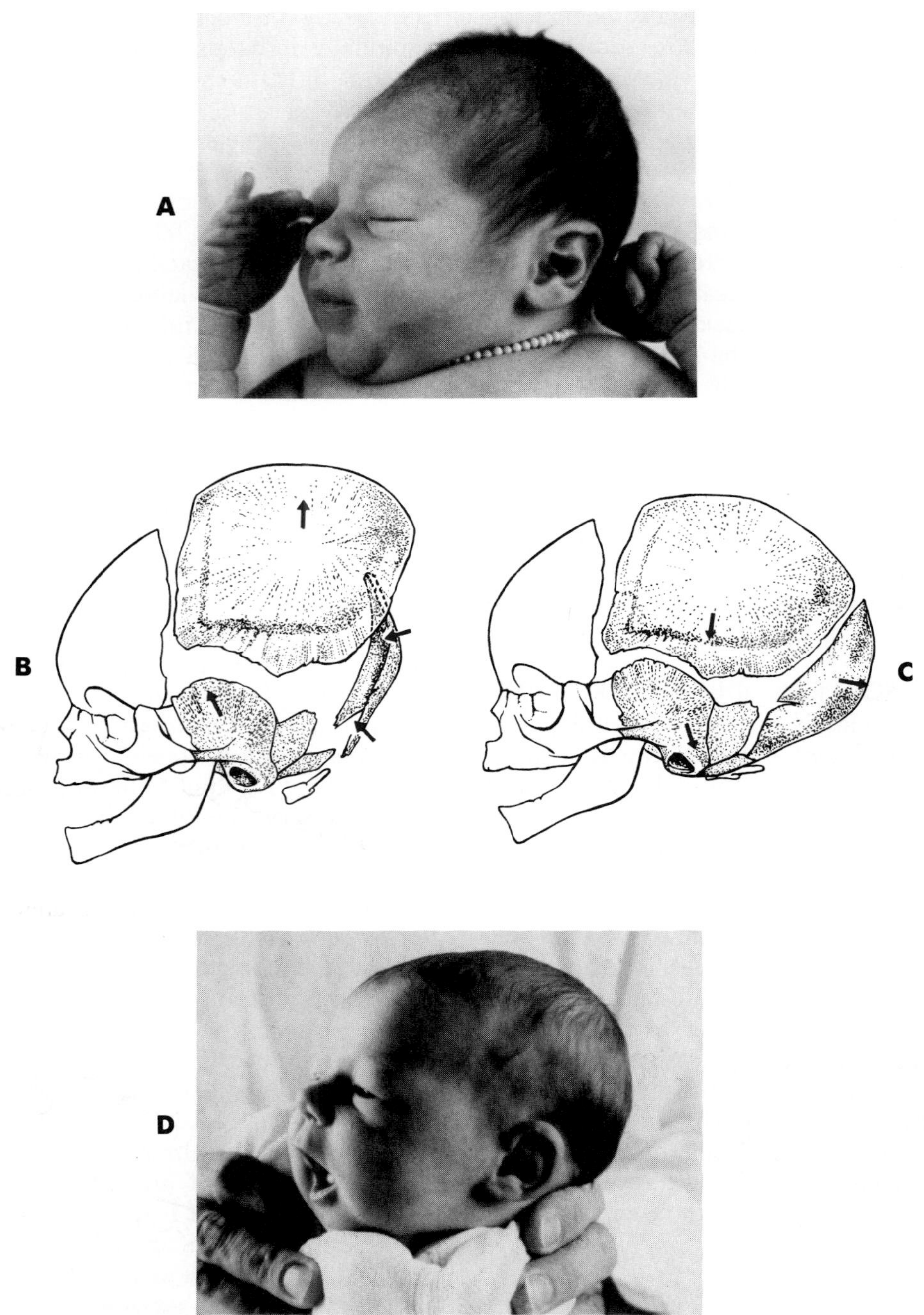

Fig. 20-9 **A,** Molding after vaginal birth. **B,** Movement of cranial bones during molding. **C,** Return of cranial bones to alignment. **D,** Absence of molding.

easily flexed. The newborn can lift its head and turn it from side to side when prone. The vertebrae should appear straight and flat. The base of the spine should be free from a dimple. If a dimple is noted, further inspection is required to determine if a sinus is present. A pilonidal dimple, especially with a sinus along with a nevus pilosus (hairy nevus), is significant because it is associated with spina bifida.

SIGNS OF RISK FOR SKELETAL PROBLEMS. Skeletal deformities may be congenital problems or drug induced. Clubfoot (talipes equinovarus), a deformity in which the foot turns inward and is fixed in a plantar flexion position, as well as any absence of limb or digit should be recorded and reported. Additional digits or webbing of digits also must be recorded and reported (see Chapters 38 and 39).

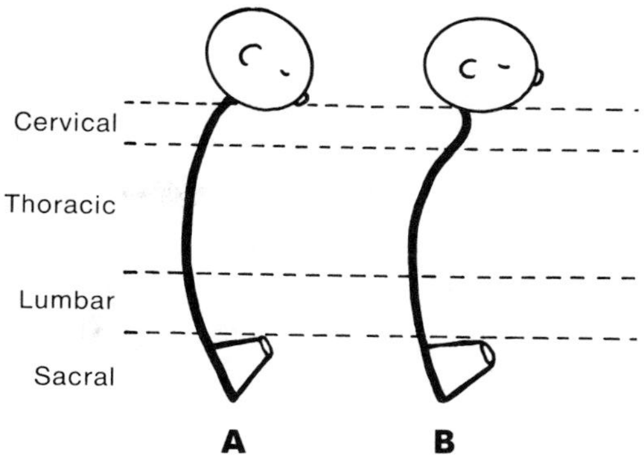

Fig. 20-10 Development of spinal curvatures. **A,** Newborn infant. **B,** Cervical secondary curvature.
From Whaley LF, Wong DL: *Nursing care of infants and children,* ed 4, St Louis, 1991, Mosby–Year Book.

Cervical
Thoracic
Lumbar
Sacral
A B

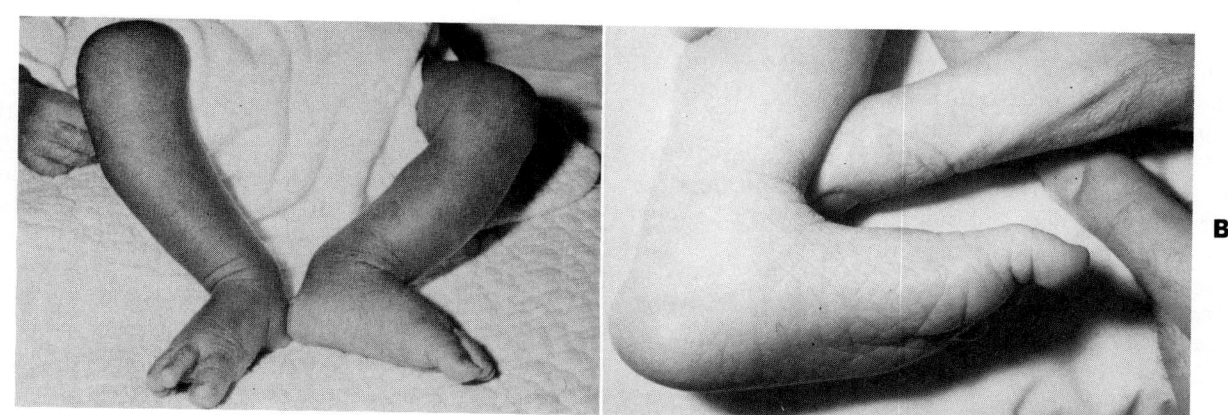

Fig. 20-11 Extremities. **A,** Bowed appearance of legs. **B,** Normal absence of arch in newborn.

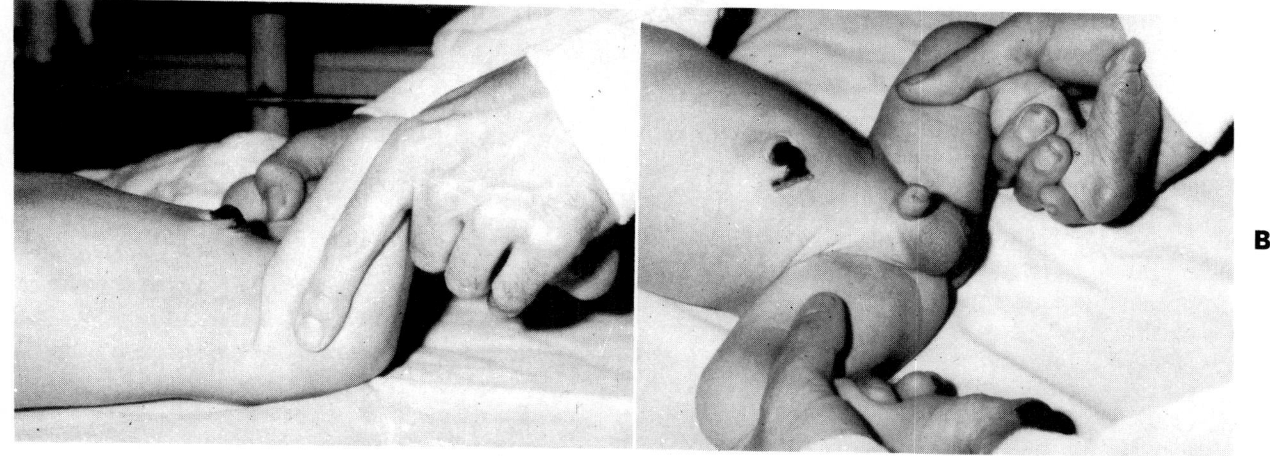

Fig. 20-12 Method of assessing for hip dysplasia using Ortolani's maneuver. **A,** Examiner's middle fingers are placed over greater trochanter and thumbs over inner thigh opposite lesser trochanter. **B,** Gentle pressure is exerted to further flex thigh on hip, and thighs are rotated outward. If hip dysplasia is present, head of femur can be felt to slip forward in acetabulum and slip back when pressure is released and legs returned to their original position. A click is sometimes heard (Ortolani's sign).

Neuromuscular System

Unlike the skeletal system, the muscular system is almost completely developed at birth. Until the late 1950s the human newborn was considered to be immature, disorganized, and able to function only at a brain-stem level. Neurobehavioral assessment of the neonate was, therefore, based mainly on evaluation of muscle tone and primitive reflexes. Recent studies have recognized the term newborn to be a vital, responsive, and reactive being. The newborn shows remarkable sensory development and an amazing ability for self-organization and social interaction (Fanaroff, Martin, 1992).

Postdelivery growth of the brain follows a predictable pattern: rapid during infancy and early childhood, more gradual during the remainder of the first decade, and minimal during adolescence. The cerebellum ends its growth spurt, which began at about 30 gestational weeks, by the end of the first year. This is perhaps why it is vulnerable to nutritional or other trauma in early infancy (see discussion of newborn nutrition, Chapter 22, and kernicterus, Chapter 38).

The brain requires glucose as a source of energy and a relatively large supply of oxygen for adequate metabolism. Oxygen requirements range from 5 to 8 mL/100 g. Such requirements signal a need for careful assessment of the infant's oxygen therapy. The necessity for glucose requires an awareness of those neonates who may have hypoglycemic episodes.

Spontaneous motor activity may be seen in transient tremors of the mouth and chin, especially during crying episodes, and of extremities, notably the arms and hands. The transient tremors are normal and can be observed in nearly every newborn. These tremors should not be present when the infant is quiet and should not persist beyond 1 month. Persistent tremors or tremors involving the total body may indicate pathologic conditions. Marked tonicity, clonicity, and twitching of facial muscles are signs of convulsions. There is a need for the physician to differentiate among normal tremors, tremors of hypoglycemia, and central nervous system (CNS) disorders so that corrective care can be instituted as necessary (Parker et al, 1990).

Neuromuscular control in the newborn, although still very limited, can be noted. If newborns are placed face down on a firm surface, they will turn their heads to the side to maintain an airway. They attempt to hold their heads in line with their bodies if they are raised by their arms. Various reflexes serve to promote their safety and adequate food intake.

NEWBORN REFLEXES. The normal infant has many primitive reflexes. The times at which these **newborn reflexes** appear and disappear reflect the maturity and intactness of the developing nervous system. The infant is dependent upon these reflexes for survival. Absences of reflexes may indicate CNS damage. Persistence of reflexes beyond the time they should disappear also may indicate CNS problems.

The most common reflexes found in the normal neonate are as follows.

MORO'S REFLEX. Moro's reflex is one of the most important to elicit in the neonate, because it reflects neurologic status (Fig. 20-13). This is also known as the startle reflex. The neonate responds to any sudden, intense stimulation, such as a loud noise, by extending the arms and legs and then drawing them inward; crying may occur at the same time. The reflex may be elicited by striking a flat surface adjacent to where the neonate is lying supine. The neonate should abduct and extend the arms symmetrically. The fingers will fan out, with the thumb and forefinger forming a C. The arms then adduct in an embracing movement and return to their relaxed position. The legs also may follow in a similar motion. The Moro reflex should be present at birth and usually disappears by 3 to 4 months of age. Persistence of the reflex beyond 6 months of age is abnormal and should be further investigated.

PALMAR AND PLANTAR GRASP REFLEXES. When an object is placed in the palm of the neonate, the grasp reflex causes the fingers to tighten around it (Fig. 20-14). A similar response can be elicited when the sole of the foot is stroked near the toes, causing the toes to flex. When a finger is placed in the neonate's palm, the neonate will firmly grasp the finger. The grasp is so strong that the neonate can be slowly lifted from a prone position to a slight sitting position. The palmar grasp usually lasts 3 to 4 months. The plantar grasp can be stimulated by placing a finger at the base of the neonate's toes. The toes will curl downward in response (Fig. 20-14, *B*). This reflex decreases by 8 months of age but may still be present at 1 year of age.

TONIC NECK REFLEX. The tonic neck reflex or fencing reflex is observed with the neonate in the supine position (Fig. 20-15). When the neonate's head is turned to the right or left, the infant extends the arm on the side toward which the head is turned and flexes the opposite arm. This gives the neonate the appearance of a "fencer." This reflex may not be seen in the early days of the neonate's life; however, once it appears it can be observed until the third or fourth month of age. Many children continue to assume this posture during sleep and maintain the posture until 2 or 3 years of age. Persistence of this reflex in an alert infant beyond 4 months of age may indicate cerebral palsy.

SUCKING AND ROOTING REFLEXES. The

A

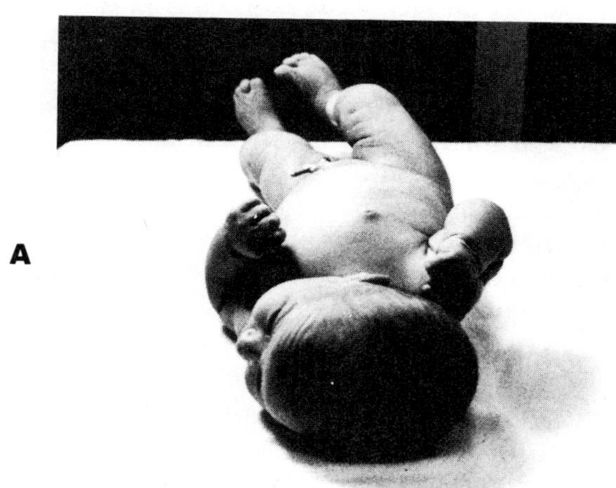

Fig. 20-13 A, Position of rest. B, Moro's reflex consists predominantly of abduction and extension of arms. C, Interesting subtlety of Moro's response in newborn infants is C position of fingers.
Courtesy Mead Johnson & Co, Evansville, Ind.

B

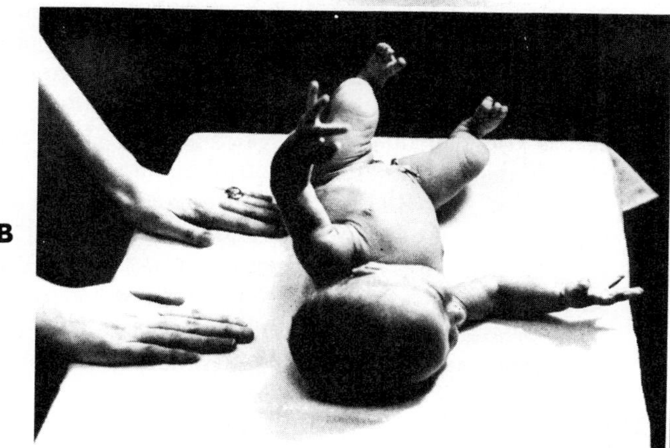

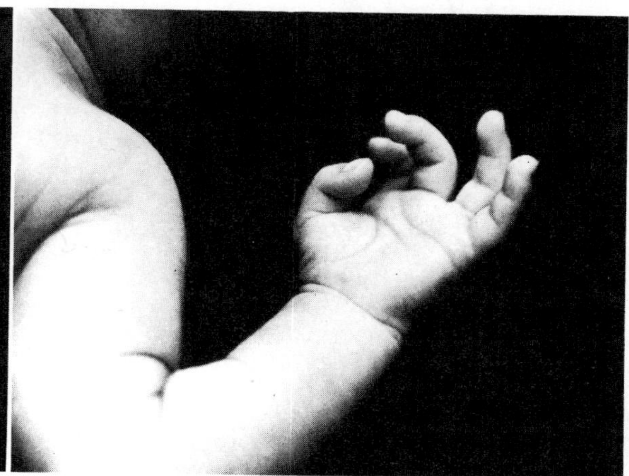

C

A

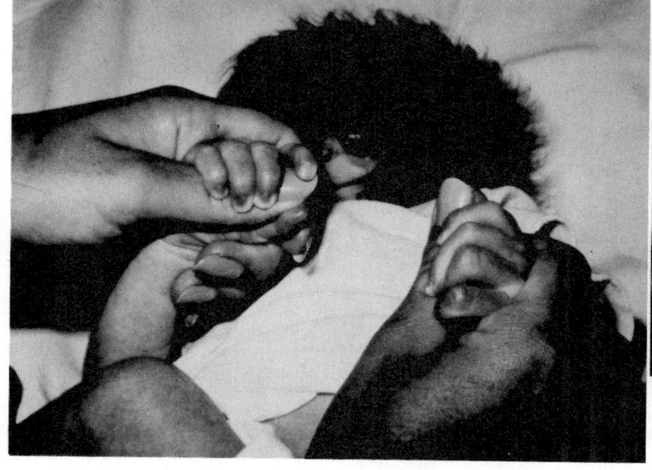

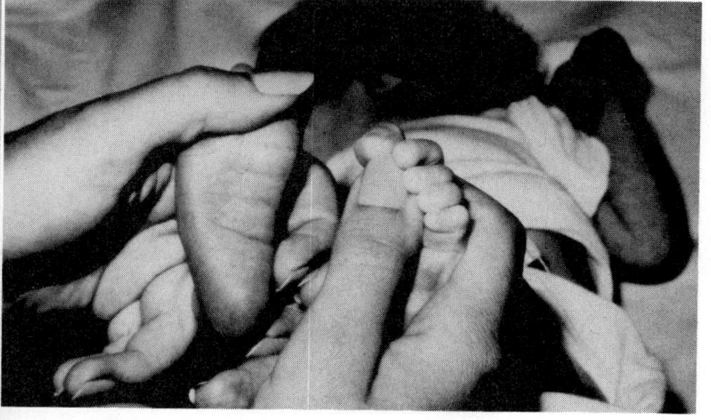

B

Fig. 20-14 A, Palmar (hand) grasp. B, Plantar grasp.
Courtesy Joan Edelstein and Ralph Levy, San Jose, Calif.

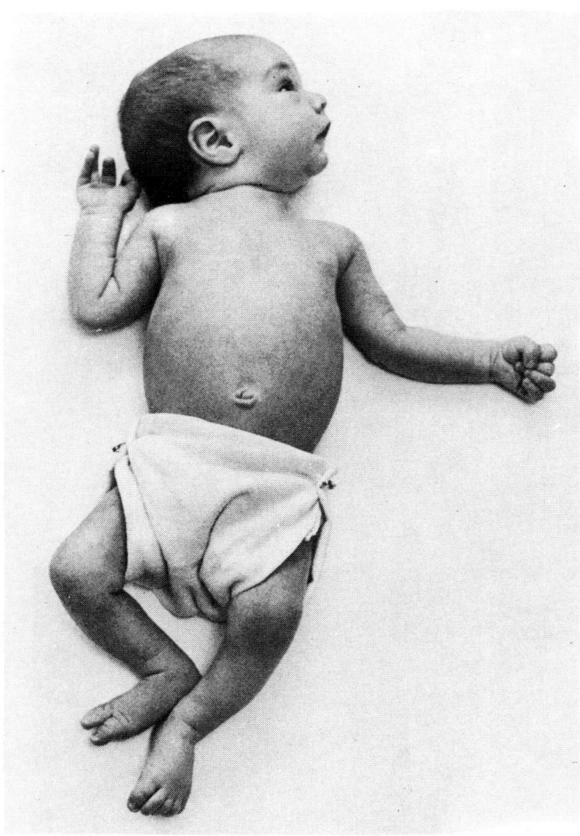

Fig. 20-15 Classic pose in spontaneous tonic neck reflex.
Courtesy Mead Johnson & Co, Evansville, Ind.

sucking reflex is the vigorous sucking of the finger or nipple when introduced into the mouth (Fig. 20-16, *A*). The rooting reflex is closely related to the sucking reflex and can be seen as movement of the neonate's head, mouth, and tongue toward a touch at the corner of the mouth or on the cheek (Fig. 20-16, *B*). If the neonate's cheek or corner of mouth is lightly stroked, the infant will turn in the direction of the stroking, open its mouth and begin to suck. These reflexes usually disappear by 7 months of age. Absence of these responses in a term infant would imply developmental delay or abnormality.

SWALLOWING REFLEX. The swallowing reflex is the appropriate swallowing of liquid introduced into the mouth. This reflex can easily be observed during a feeding. Fluids should be easily swallowed, without gagging, coughing, or vomiting. Swallowing may be poorly developed in a preterm infant or in a term infant with a neurologic defect.

BABINSKI'S REFLEX. Babinski's reflex, or hyperextension of the toes, occurs when the lateral aspect of the sole is stroked from the heel upward and across the ball of the foot (Fig. 20-17). This reflex usually disappears after 1 year of age.

STEPPING REFLEX. The neonate can make stepping motions that are sometimes called dancing (Fig. 20-18). When the neonate is held in an upright position and the feet are allowed to touch a flat surface, alternate stepping movements that simulate walking are observed. This reflex sometimes is diffi-

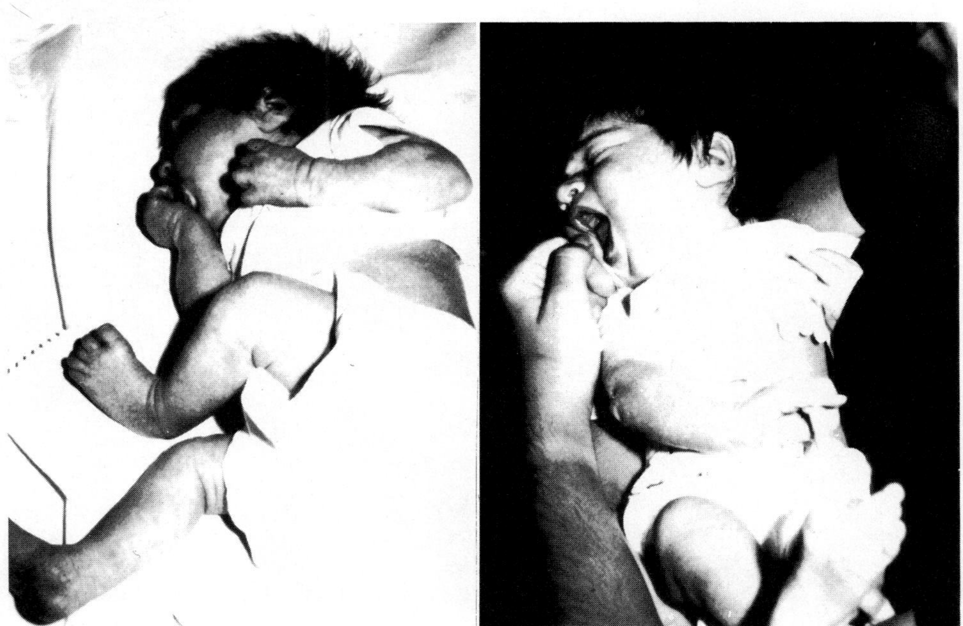

Fig. 20-16 **A,** Sucking. Also note hand-to-mouth facility with prolonged sucking. **B,** Rooting reflex is apparent when corner of newborn's mouth is touched. Bottom lip lowers on same side; tongue moves toward stimulation.
Courtesy Joan Edelstein and Ralph Levy. San Jose, Calif.

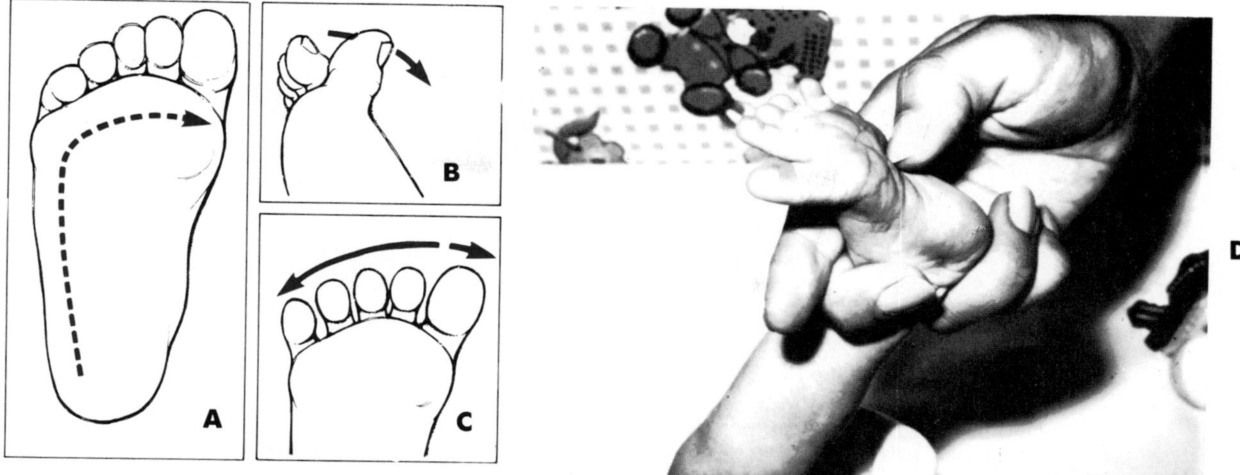

Fig. 20-17 Babinski's reflex. **A,** Direction of stroke. **B,** Dorsiflexion of big toe. **C,** Fanning of toes. **D,** Babinski's reflex in newborn.
From Whaley LF, Wong DL: *Nursing care of infants and children,* ed 4, St Louis, 1991, Mosby–Year Book.

cult to elicit because not all neonates cooperate. However, with persistence, the reflex usually can be observed. Stepping generally disappears by 4 months of age.

TRUNK INCURVATION REFLEX. When the neonate is prone, stroking the spine causes the pelvis to turn to the stimulated side (Fig. 20-19). This is called trunk incurvation or Galant's reflex. If the back is firmly stroked about 5 cm (2 in) from the spine in a downward motion, the neonate responds by curving the body to the side stroked. The opposite side also should be checked. This response diminishes by 2 to 3 months of life.

CROSSED EXTENSION REFLEX. With the infant in a supine position, the examiner extends one leg and stimulates the sole of the foot with a finger flick or other object (Fig. 20-20). The neonate will swiftly flex and extend the opposite leg as though trying to push the stimulus away from the other foot.

TRACTION REFLEX. Traction reflex (pull-to-sit or head lag) is normally seen in a newborn (Fig. 20-21). When the neonate is pulled up by the wrists from a supine position, the head will lag and fall back. As the newborn continues to be pulled, the head will be lifted and be held upright before it falls forward onto the chest. The amount of head lag depends on the maturity and muscle tone of the newborn.

ARM RECOIL. When both arms are extended by pulling them down by the wrist, the neonate quickly flexes the elbows when the arms are released. This is a normal reaction and should be observed equally in both arms.

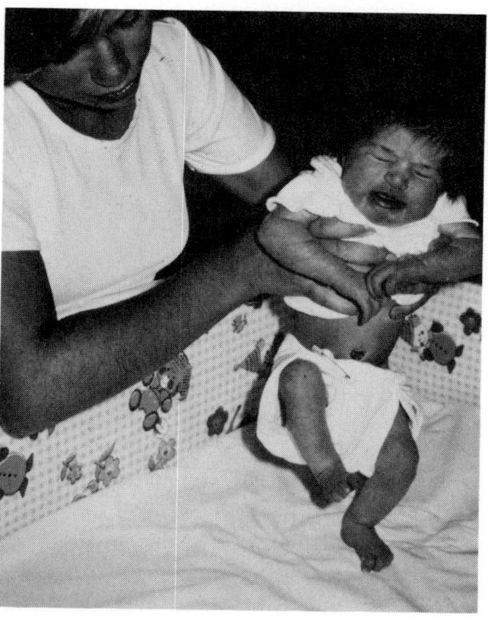

Fig. 20-18 Automatic walking reflex is phase of neuromuscular maturity from which infant normally graduates after 3 to 5 weeks. If infant is held so that the sole of the foot touches table, reciprocal flexion and extension of leg occur, simulating walking.
Courtesy Joan Edelstein and Ralph Levy, San Jose, Calif.

BAUER'S REFLEX. Bauer's reflex (crawling) will be seen in a term neonate (Fig. 20-22). With the neonate in a prone position, the examiner places pressure on the soles of the feet. The neonate should respond by making crawling movements. This usually disappears by 6 weeks of age.

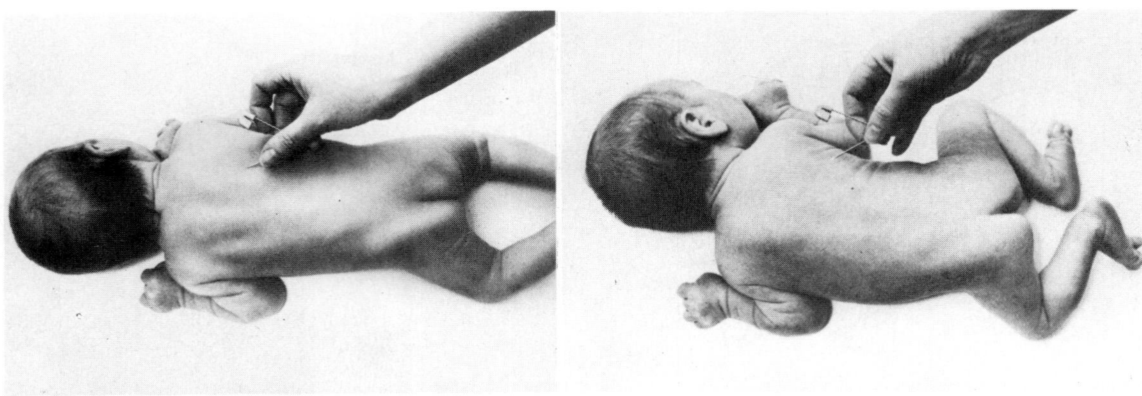

Fig. 20-19 Trunk incurvation reflex. In prone position, infant responds to linear skin stimulus (pin or finger) along paravertebral area by flexing trunk and swinging pelvis toward stimulus. With transverse lesions of cord, there will be no response below that level. Complete absence of response suggests general depression or nervous system abnormality. Response may vary but should be obtainable in all infants, including premature ones. If not seen in the first few days, it usually is apparent by 5 to 6 days.
Courtesy Mead Johnson & Co, Evansville, Ind.

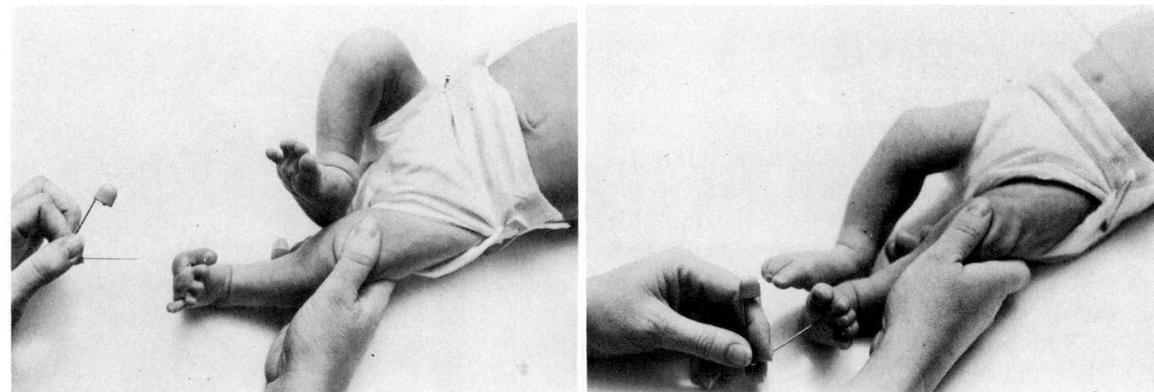

Fig. 20-20 Crossed extension reflex. With child in supine position, examiner extends one of infant's legs and presses knee down. Stimulation of sole of foot of fixated limb should cause *free* leg to flex, adduct, and extend as if attempting to push away stimulating agent. This reflex should be present during newborn period. Absence of response suggests a spinal cord lesion; weak response suggests peripheral nerve damage.
Courtesy Mead Johnson & Co, Evansville, Ind.

DOLL'S EYE REFLEX. With the neonate supine, the examiner slowly turns the newborn's head to the left or right. The infant's eyes remain stationary. This reflex usually disappears a few weeks to 2 months of age.

SIGNS OF RISK FOR NEUROMUSCULAR PROBLEMS. Any absence of a newborn reflex could indicate major neurologic problems. Birth trauma may cause nerve damage that results in facial asymmetry and paralysis. CNS depression, because of maternal medications received during labor and delivery, also will influence neuromuscular functioning. Observation of the neonate for any abnormalities must be made and documented. A thorough physical examination of the newborn assists to detect any potential complications.

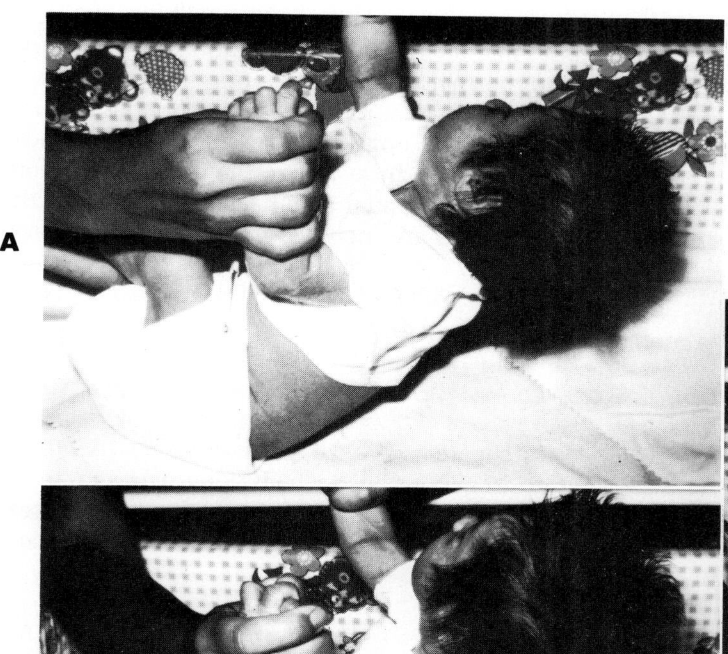

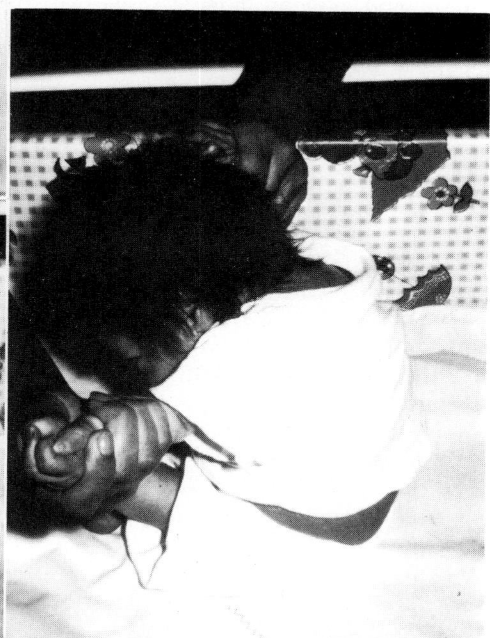

Fig. 20-21 Pull-to-sit (or traction reflex). A, Head falls backward. **B**, Infant attempts to right head. **C**, Infant unable to maintain head up.
Courtesy Joan Edelstein and Ralph Levy, San Jose, Calif.

Physical Assessment

The assessment of the newborn should progress from head-to-toe, with each system being evaluated. Findings provide a data base for implementing the nursing process with newborns and providing anticipatory guidance for the parents. The immediate assessment of the newborn is carried out in the delivery room. The Apgar score (see Chapter 18), determined at 1 and 5 minutes, provides a source that must be considered in the context of data from the total assessment. Some authors question the usefulness of the Apgar score (Editorial, 1989a; Editorial, 1989b), and the scores may vary on the basis of the reliability of the raters (see Research Highlights. p. . .).

A complete physical assessment is done within 12 hours of birth. It may be performed in the nursery, labor and delivery room, or recovery room. This assessment includes appearance, behavior, cardiorespiratory function, skin, vital signs, and maternal-infant

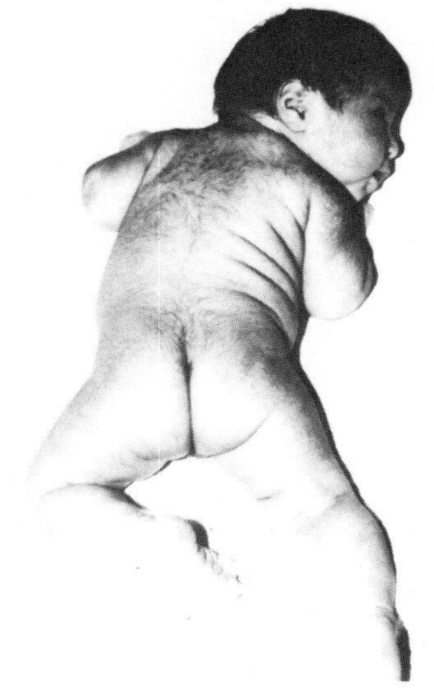

Fig. 20-22 Crawling.
Courtesy Marjorie Pyle, RNC, Lifecircle, Costa Mesa, Calif.

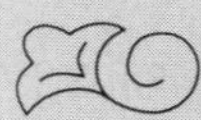 **Research Highlight** 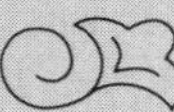

Interrater Reliability of the Apgar Score

RESEARCH ABSTRACT

This study examined the interrater reliability (agreement between raters) of the Apgar score in both term and preterm infants. Fifty-two infants were included in the study; 11 were preterm and 41 were born at term. The investigator assigned them Apgar scores and then compared these scores with those recorded in the mothers' charts.

Percentage agreement at 1 and 5 minutes for each of the five indicators of the Apgar was calculated. For preterm infants, the agreement of 1-minute scores ranged from a high of 82% for tone and respiratory rate to a low of 55% for heart rate. At 5 minutes the agreement was highest for heart rate (100%) and lowest for reflex irritability (36%). There was a 69% agreement for the total score at both 1 and 5 minutes. The percentage agreement for the term infants was highest for heart rate (98%) and lowest for reflex irritability (82%). At 5 minutes, percentage agreement for heart rate, tone, and reflex irritability was 98%; for color and respiratory rate, percentage agreement was 95%. The percentage agreement for the total score was 87% at 1 minute and 97% at 5 minutes. For preterm infants, the interrater reliability estimates were very low. The poor results may be due to recall errors in recording; that is, the Apgar scores, which were recorded after resuscitative efforts were completed, were based on the recorders' memory of the infant's condition at 1 and 5 minutes.

IMPLICATIONS FOR PRACTICE

Apgar scores are used as indicators of condition and need for resuscitation. It is important for the scorer to have adequate training in use of the Apgar instrument before assuming responsibility for assigning the score. Periodic review and interrater checks may be necessary to improve reliability. Efforts should be directed to assigning the score at 1 and 5 minutes so that recall errors are minimized.

RELATED RESEARCH QUESTIONS

1. Will use of a timing device improve the interrater reliability of the Apgar score?
2. What factors are associated with discrepancies among observers in assignment of Apgar scores?
3. Does the interrater reliability of the Apgar score vary with gestational age?
4. Does interrater reliability of the Apgar score vary with specialization of the scorer (nurse, obstetrician, anesthesiologist, neonatologist)?

REFERENCE

Livingston J: Interrater reliability of the Apgar score in term and premature infants, *App Nurs Res* 3(4):164, 1990.

interactions. The nurse performs a complete physical assessment, including descriptions of any variations from normal, as well as abnormal findings. Table 20-2 on p. 559 summarizes newborn assessment. After the birth, ongoing assessments of the newborn are made and an evaluation is performed before discharge. After initial stabilization is effected, the following steps are included in a newborn assessment.

GENERAL APPEARANCE. The neonate's maturity level can be gauged by assessment of general appearance. Features to assess in the general survey include posture, head size, lanugo, vernix caseosa, cry, and state of alertness. The normal resting position of the neonate is one of general flexion. The head is large in proportion to body length, averaging about one fourth of the total. The umbilicus is the center of the newborn's body. The neck is short and the abdomen is prominent.

VITAL SIGNS. Temperature, heart rate, and respiratory rate are always obtained. BP may not be routinely assessed unless there is a potential for cardiac problems.

In the past a rectal temperature was obtained after the birth to establish patency of the rectum. Today it is generally accepted that passage of meconium is sufficient validation of a patent anus. Bliss-Holtz (1989) found that axillary temperatures are a safe, accurate substitute for rectal temperatures. Comparing rectal, axillary, and inguinal temperatures, the researcher found the greatest discrepancy (0.8° F) between rectal and inguinal temperatures. Rectal and axillary temperatures differed by only 0.2° F.

Therefore temperature should be measured by the axillary route. The use of electronic thermometers has expedited the performance of this task and provides a reading within 1 minute. If a standard mercury thermometer is used, it should be held in place for 3 minutes. Taking an infant's temperature may cause the baby to cry and struggle against the placement of the thermometer in the axilla. Tympanic thermometers may be used after the newborn's ear canals are free of vernix. Before taking the temperature, the examiner may want to count the heart and respiratory rates while the infant is quiet and at rest.

The normal axillary temperature averages between 97.6° to 98.6° F (36.5° and 37° C) with a range from 97° to 99° F (36.1° to 37.2° C). The temperature should be stabilized by 10 hours of age. An axillary temperature above the range reflects hyperthermia or fever; below the range, poor peripheral perfusion or prematurity (Coen et al, 1988b).

External heat or cooling sources may affect the neonate's temperature. Many neonates take on the temperature of the environment. For example, a neonate who is exposed to direct sunlight may experience a rapid increase in core and skin temperatures, which will cause the infant to become restless and irritable. Consequently, room temperature must be kept constant to prevent overheating or excessive cooling of the neonate (Judd, 1985).

The respiratory rate varies with the state of alertness after birth. The respiratory rate will vary between 30 to 60 breaths per minute. If the newborn is very active or crying, respiratory rates often are greater than 60/min. Respirations are abdominal in nature and can easily be counted by observing the rise and fall of the abdomen. Neonatal respirations are shallow, irregular, and may include short periods of apnea from 5 to 15 seconds in length. Therefore it is important to count the respirations for a full minute to obtain an accurate count.

In the first few hours after birth, the heart rate fluctuates from 120 to 180 beats/min; it may be altered by activity or crying. The neonate's heart rate may range from as low as 70 to 90 beats/min in deep sleep to as high as 180 beats/min while crying. Because of these variations, it is very important to count the heart rate for a full minute. Apical pulse rates are always taken.

Coen et al (1988b) reported that both heart and respiratory rates are affected by age. Full-term neonates usually have a decreased respiratory rate with a mean of 38.5/min at 4 week of age compared with a mean of 45.1/min at birth. Heart rate increases from a mean of 116.3/min at birth to 141.3/min at 15 days, and then decreases to 136.2/min at 4 weeks of age. A racial difference in the heart rate of African-American and white neonates of the same gestational age and socioeconomic class has been identified, with the African-American neonates averaging 8 beats/min higher.

If BP is taken, a Doppler device (electronic monitoring) facilitates this procedure. Neonatal BP usually is highest immediately after birth and falls to a minimum within 3 hours after birth. It then begins to rise steadily and reaches a plateau between 4 to 6 days after birth. This measurement usually is equal to that of the immediate postdelivery BP. Average BP for a term neonate is 67/41 mm Hg. This reading varies with the neonate's activity.

BP is measured in both arms and legs to detect any discrepancy between the two sides or between the upper and lower parts of the body. A discrepancy of 10 mm Hg or more between the arms and legs may signal a cardiac defect, such as coarctation of the aorta. Weak or absent femoral pulses also may indicate coarctation of the aorta, hip dysplasia, or thrombophlebitis. To palpate femoral pulses, the thighs are flexed on the hips, the fingers are placed along the inguinal ligament about midway between the symphysis pubis and the iliac crest, and pulses are palpated bilaterally at the same time. Femoral pulses should be equal and strong in the absence of a disorder.

BASELINE MEASUREMENTS OF PHYSICAL GROWTH. Baseline measurements must be taken and recorded to help assess the progress of the neonate. Measurements are used to determine the neonate's growth patterns. These may be recorded on growth charts. The following measurements are made every time the neonate is assessed (Deter et al, 1990).

WEIGHT. The parents are always curious about the infant's measurements, and often the first question asked is "How much does the baby weigh?" The newborn usually is weighed shortly after birth. This may be done in the labor and delivery area or on admission to a nursery. Care must be taken to make sure the scales are balanced. The totally unclothed neonate is placed in the center of the scale. The nurse should place one hand over the neonate to prevent the infant from falling off the scales (Fig. 20-23). It is not uncommon for the newborn to jerk and have tremors or even cry when placed on the scales. It is common practice to weigh the infant at the same time every day of the hospital stay.

Birth weight of a term infant averages from 2500 to 4000 g (5 lb 8 oz to 8 lb 13 oz). Neonates lose about 10% of their birth weight or less after birth. This is due to the excretion of fluids through the lungs, urinary bladder, bowels, and small amount of intake during the first few days of life. They begin to regain their birth weight by 10 to 14 days of age.

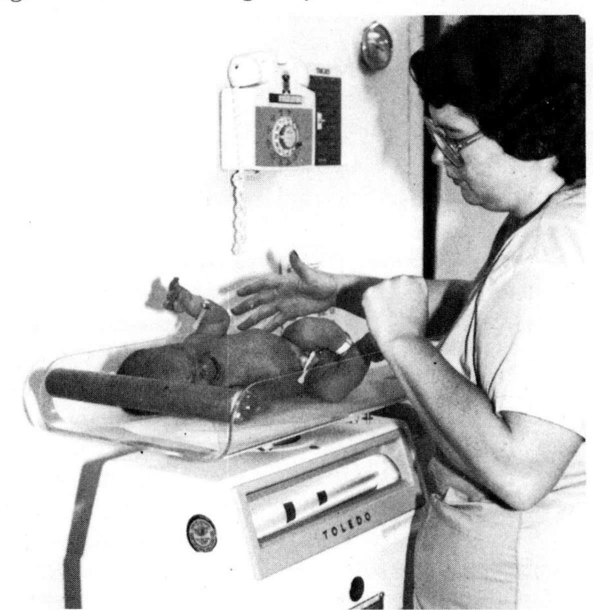

Fig. 20-23 Weighing infant. Note hand is held over infant as safety measure. Scale is covered to provide warmth and protection against cross infection.

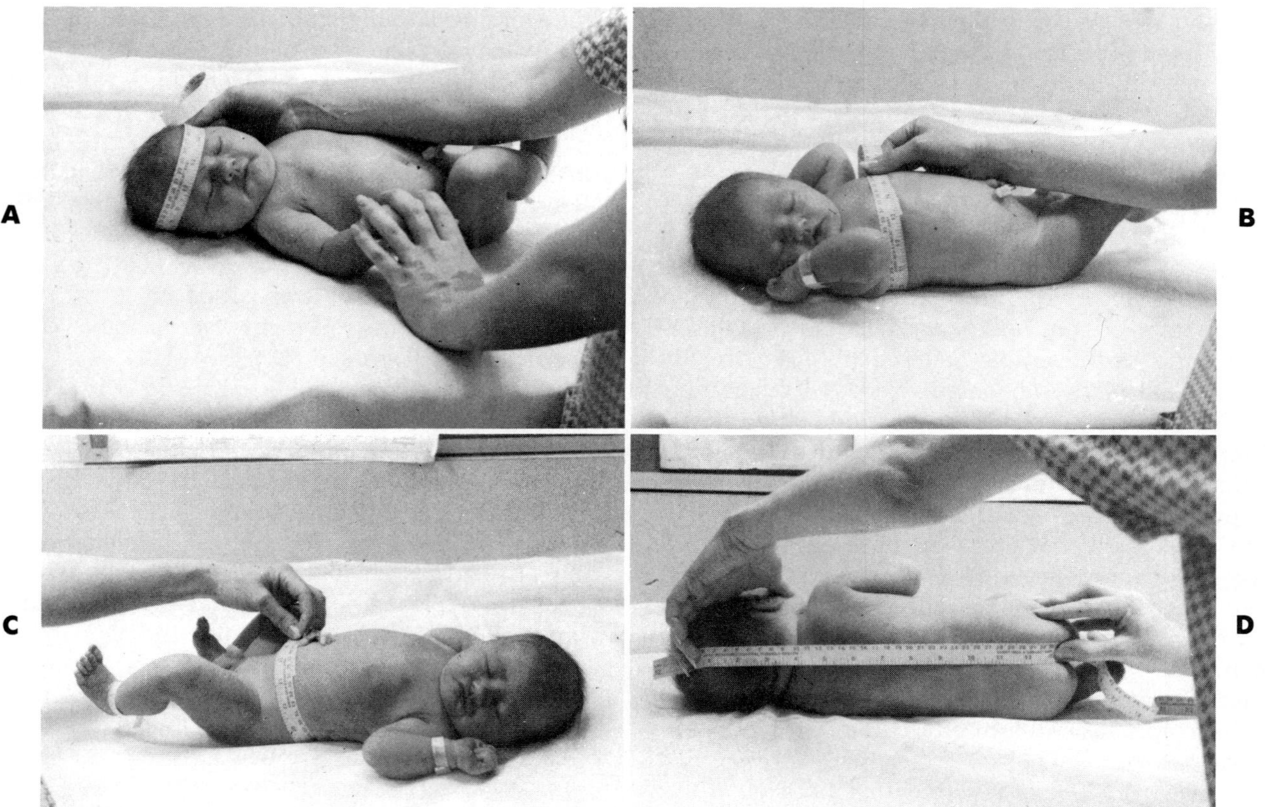

Fig. 20-24 Measurements. **A**, Circumference of head. **B**, Circumference of chest. **C**, Abdominal circumference. **D**, Length, crown to rump. To determine total length, length of legs is included.

CIRCUMFERENCES AND LENGTH. The term neonate's head circumference is 32 to 35 cm (12½ to 13¾ in). The head is measured at the widest part, which is the occipitofrontal diameter (Fig. 20-24, A). The tape measure is placed around the head at the infant's eyebrows. It is a good idea to remeasure the head again within 48 hours because molding may misshape the head and make the measurement inaccurate.

The chest circumference usually measures about 2 cm less than head circumference. Frequently it is the same as the head but should not exceed it. The tape is placed around the infant's chest at the nipple line (Fig. 20-24, *B*).

Abdominal circumference is measured by placing the tape around the abdomen just below the umbilicus (Fig. 20-24, *C*). Measurements will vary with the size of the infant. The abdomen should be cylindric in shape and protrude slightly. Abdominal measurements are not always taken but should be measured when there is suspicion of abdominal distention. Abdominal measurements are approximately the same as chest measurements.

In the term neonate, head-to-heel length averages 45 to 55 cm (18 to 22 in). The length may be difficult to obtain because of the flexed posture of the newborn (Fig. 20-24, *D*). The examiner places the newborn on a flat surface and extends the leg until the knee is flat against the surface. Placing the head against a perpendicular surface and extending the leg may assist with this measurement. Some nurses make a pen mark on the surface of the examining table, especially if it is covered with a disposable covering, at the top of the infant's head, extend the leg, and make another mark at the infant's heel. The distance between the two marks is then accurately measured.

SKIN TEXTURE, COLOR, AND OPACITY. Certain physical features vary with gestational age and usually reflect neonatal maturity (for extensive discussion, see Chapter 37). The preterm neonate has thin, translucent, ruddy skin with easily seen veins and venules (especially over the abdomen). As term approaches, the skin thickens and becomes pinker; also the number of large vessels visible over the abdomen decreases. The postterm neonate typically has thick, parchmentlike skin, with peeling and cracking; few if any blood vessels appear over the abdomen (NAACOG, 1991).

Observations should be made for color and color changes during activity, familial and racial features, rashes, milia, anomalies or deformities, birth marks, jaundice, petechiae, forceps marks, tone, and hydration status. Any of these characteristics should be noted and recorded.

Color varies with racial background, pigmentation, and physiologic changes. **Acrocyanosis** is characterized by bluish discoloration of the hands and feet. It is a normal condition caused by vasomotor instability and poor peripheral circulation. To distinguish between true cyanosis and acrocyanosis, the examiner vigorously rubs the sole of the foot. If the sole turns pink, the discoloration is due to acrocyanosis. It will not turn pink with true cyanosis. In addition, acrocyanosis should disappear when the infant is crying.

The newborn's skin often appears mottled (Plate 18), which is a response to temperature changes. Harlequin color changes may be seen. This occurs when one side of the body develops a deep red color. Harlequin color is a response to a normal vasomotor disturbance causing the blood vessels on one side of the body to constrict while those on the other side dilate. Even though this is not an uncommon occurrence, it should be recorded and reported.

The skin is inspected for any signs of lesions or birthmarks. Location, size, color, characteristics, and distribution should be noted and recorded. The examiner inspects the scalp for any sign of lesion from an internal scalp electrode. Forcep marks also should be recorded. *Lanugo* —soft, downy hair—appears at approximately 20 weeks' gestation. From 21 to 33 weeks it covers the entire body. It begins to vanish from the face at 34 weeks and by 38 weeks may appear only on the shoulders. Lanugo rarely appears after 42 weeks' gestation.

HEAD AND NECK. The cranial bones commonly slide over each other during labor and delivery, causing head molding (see Fig. 20-9). In the first few hours after birth, the conical, elongated, asymmetric shape of the molded head may complicate measurements of head circumference. The examiner palpates the suture lines to determine how much the bony edges overlap. Assessment of the anterior and posterior fontanelles may reveal a third fontanelle along the sagittal suture. In most cases, this represents a normal variation (see Fig. 14-1).

The fontanelles are palpated and measured. The anterior fontanelle is located at the junction of the sagittal and coronal sutures and is diamond-shaped. The fontanelle usually feels soft, and it may pulsate. The posterior fontanelle is a triangular depression located at the junction of the lambdoidal and sagittal sutures.

The fontanelles vary in size, with the anterior fontanelle being 3 to 4 cm long and 2 to 3 cm wide. The posterior fontanelle is smaller, between 0.5 and 1.0 cm. African-American neonates usually have larger anterior and posterior fontanelles than do white neonates.

If the anterior fontanelle is very large, it may indicate hypothyroidism. A tense or bulging fontanelle may indicate increased intracranial pressure. A normal fontanelle may appear slightly depressed; however, one that is severely depressed indicates dehydration.

The scalp also should be palpated for signs of caput succedaneum or cephalhematoma. Any occurrence should be documented. Their presence may cause the head to appear misshapen.

Hair distribution, texture, and color are other important aspects of the head examination. The amount and color will vary and depend on genetic factors. Unusual hair distribution may represent a minor abnormality and should be noted.

The examiner inspects the neonate's face for symmetry of features. Facial asymmetry may occur from prenatal pressure (Plate 18), and the lopsided appearance disappears spontaneously in time. The mouth should appear at the midline, and its size should be appropriate for the face. The lips should be sensitive to the touch; gentle stroking should trigger the sucking reflex. The chin normally is slightly receding. The term neonate has fat pads in both cheeks. The examiner touches the tongue lightly to check for the normal reaction—a forward tongue thrust. The oral cavity should never be inspected just after a feeding because the gag reflex could be stimulated, causing vomiting and subsequent aspiration. The examiner inserts the smallest finger into the infant's mouth, allowing assessment of the hard and soft palates. This also stimulates the suck reflex, and intensity of the reflex can be evaluated. The neonate has moist oral mucous membranes but does not drool constantly.

Eyebrows should be present. The eyes are examined for placement on the face; the eyelids should be of equal size, freely movable, and open adequately. Both eyeballs should be present, of equal size and shape (round), and firm (Fig. 20-25). Shortly after birth, the eyelids commonly appear edematous from birth trauma or irritation caused by erythromycin instillation. In the white neonate, the sclerae should be clear and white; in other neonates, they may appear slightly yellow. The conjunctivae should be clear and may be somewhat bluish in color. The iris color should be distributed evenly (Coen et al, 1988b). Occasionally, subconjunctival hemorrhage, a result of pressure while traversing the birth canal during labor and birth, may be seen (Plate 18). Most neonates do not have tears; occasionally, however, tears are seen.

If the neonate's eyes are closed during the head-to-toe assessment, the examiner delays the eye inspection until the ophthalmic examination (which should be conducted last because it upsets the neonate). The pupils are examined with use of a penlight or flashlight and dim room lights. If this examination must be conducted in an incubator or nursery, the neonate's eyes should be shielded.

The retina should be transparent and intact and the pupils round and centered in the iris. When exposed to light in a darkened room, the pupils should constrict equally bilaterally. If all pupil findings are normal, they are documented as PERRLA (pupils equal, round, reactive to light, accommodation). To assess for the red reflex, the examiner places the penlight or ophthalmoscope directly in front of the pupil and turns on the light. The pupils should appear red bilaterally (Cohen, Byrne, 1989).

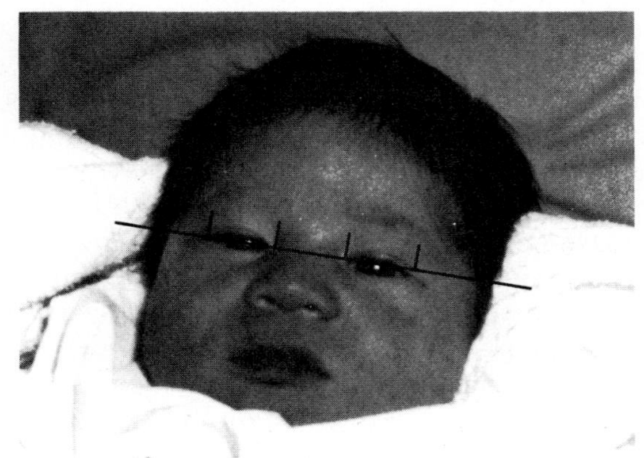

Fig. 20-25 Eyes. Pseudostrabismus. Inner epicanthal folds cause eyes to appear malaligned; however, corneal light reflexes fall perfectly symmetric. Eyes are symmetric in size and shape and are well placed.

Movement of the eyeballs is noted. The neonate can focus momentarily and may follow to midline. Eye movements are characterized by being random and uneven. Occasionally the eyes may appear crossed, a condition known as strabismus. In the neonate, however, transient strabismus (pseudostrabismus) and nystagmus may be seen until the third or fourth month; it persists until the eye muscles develop sufficiently to act in a coordinated fashion (Fig. 20-25). When the neonate's head is rotated from side to side, the eyes do not follow in response to head movements. This doll's-eye phenomenon persists for about 10 days.

The ears are inspected for symmetric shape and size. The top of the ear should align with the inner and outer canthi of the eyes (Fig. 20-26). Skin tags, pinpoint holes, and sinus tracts along the helix or preauricular surface may represent minor abnormalities. The neonate's hearing also should be checked. A loud noise should elicit the startle reflex or crying. The ear appears flat and shapeless until 23 weeks' gestation when incurvation of the pinna (the external part of the ear) begins. At 36 weeks' gestation, the upper two thirds of the pinna are incurved and the pinna recoils instantly. In the term neonate the pinna has well-defined incurvation. Old blood and vernix may be present in the ear canal for several days, and therefore the tympanic membrane may not be visible.

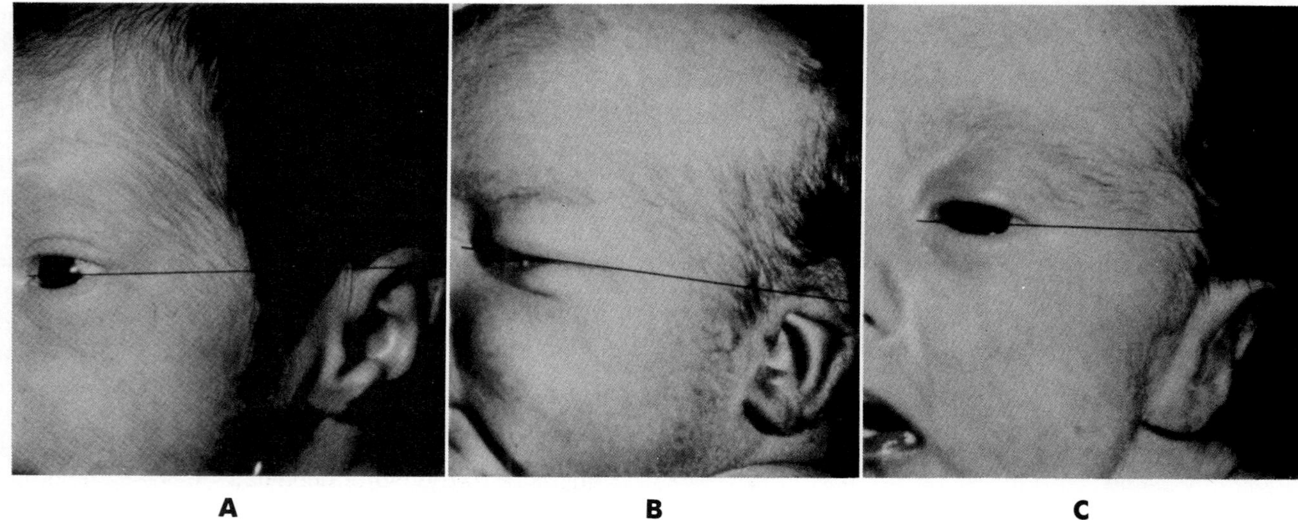

Fig. 20-26 Placement of ear insertion on head in relation to line drawn from inner to outer canthus of eye. **A**, Normal position. **B**, Abnormally angled ear. **C**, True low-set ear.
Courtesy Mead Johnson & Co, Evansville, Ind.

Because the neonate cannot coordinate tongue movements well, the tongue often falls backward, occluding the oral airway. Consequently, the neonate is a preferential nose breather who depends on patent nares (nostrils). To assess the nares for patency, the examiner occludes them one at a time and holds the infant's mouth closed. The neonate should be able to breathe through the open naris. To check for the sneeze reflex, the examiner occludes both nares for 1 to 2 seconds, which should trigger sneezing (Coen et al, 1988a). The neonate's nose also is examined for size, shape, mucous membrane integrity, and discharge. The placement of the nose should be midline on the face. The mucous membranes will appear pink and moist with no copious drainage.

The mouth should be inspected and palpated. Symmetry of the lips and lip movement, as well as the internal structure of the mouth, should be noted. Lips appear pink and moist. Some neonates are born with precocious teeth. If they are loose, they may be pulled to prevent aspiration. The hard and soft palates are inspected for cleft palate. The shape of the palate is examined. The uvula should be midline.

The tongue should be freely movable and symmetric in shape and movement. Occasionally a neonate may have a shortened frenulum ("tongue-tie"). If the tongue can extend to the alveolar ridge, usually no intervention is needed. If the frenulum is too short, it may need to be clipped to assist in sucking.

Small white epithelial cysts—Epstein's pearls—on the hard palate and on the gums sometimes are seen. Sucking pads can be palpated inside the cheeks. The examiner places a finger inside the neonate's mouth to elicit the sucking reflex and strokes the neonate's cheek to check the rooting reflex.

The posterior pharynx is easiest to see when the neonate is crying. Saliva usually is scant because the salivary glands are immature. The presence of excessive saliva in a neonate should alert the nurse to the possibility of tracheoesophageal fistula or esophageal atresia. The infant should not have an odor. Meconium staining sometimes can cause a foul odor. If an odor is detected, a sepsis work-up may be needed.

The neck should appear symmetric and without webbing; it also should be flexible enough to allow the head to move freely and equally to each side. The examiner palpates the front of the neck at the midline for the thyroid gland, as well as for the lymph nodes, which normally are not palpable (Coen et al, 1988b).

The cardiovascular status is assessed by palpating the carotid pulses one side at a time. They should be equal and strong bilaterally. Palpation requires caution. Massage of the carotid artery may stimulate pressure receptors, causing reflex bradycardia (Coen et al, 1988b).

When palpating the clavicles, the examiner moves the fingers slowly over the anterior clavicular surface. If a mass or lump is detected, one tries to move the neonate's arm gently while palpating with the other hand. A grating sensation and uneven movement of two juxtaposed bone fragments indicate a fracture, which could result from delivery trauma (Coen et al, 1988b).

THORAX. The thoracic cavity should be cylindric and symmetric. In the small-for-gestational-age (SGA) or preterm neonate, decreased chest circumference is to be expected. Normally, chest wall excursion is bilaterally equal.

The ribs should be flexible and symmetric, with no palpable masses. The xiphoid process may be palpable at the bottom of the sternum. In a thin neonate, it may be visible.

BREAST SIZE. The examiner assesses breast tissue through observation and palpation. To measure breast tissue, the nipple is palpated gently between the second and third fingers. The thumb and index finger are not used because surrounding skin may be measured inadvertently this way.

Breast tissue and areola size increase with gestation. Increased breast tissue may indicate subcutaneous fat accumulation from accelerated intrauterine growth (such as occurs in the large-for-gestational-age [LGA] neonate). In contrast, the SGA or postterm neonate may have decreased breast tissue from inadequate fetal growth or lost fetal weight. The nipples are inspected for spacing and number. Supernumerary nipples may appear as darkened spots just below or beside natural nipples. Any discharge is noted and documented.

ABDOMEN. The abdomen should have a symmetric, slightly rounded contour. Peristaltic waves normally are not visible; however, the abdomen should move visibly during breathing. The umbilical cord remnant should appear bluish-white, contain two arteries and one vein, and be free of urine leakage, a sign of a fistula from the bladder to the cord (persistent urachus) (Judd, 1985).

The umbilical cord begins to dry several hours after birth, and it shrivels and blackens by the second or third day of life. The umbilicus should be inspected frequently for signs of infection (foul odor, redness, purulent drainage), granuloma (small red, raw-appearing polyp where the umbilical cord separates), bleeding, and discharge. The cord normally falls off by 2 weeks after birth. By the time the neonate is 1 month old, the umbilicus should be healed.

Auscultation of the abdomen is performed before palpation and percussion. The examiner listens for peristaltic sounds in all four quadrants. The sounds usually are present within 1 to 2 hours after birth.

Palpation of the abdomen begins with gentle pressure and gradually deeper pressure as the neonate relaxes. To promote relaxation and comfort during palpation, the neonate's legs are flexed in the fetal position. If the neonate has an asymmetric abdomen, which suggests an internal mass, great caution must be used during the assessment. Palpation of a Wilms' tumor may cause the tumor to seed to other areas. In the preterm neonate, palpation may reveal a wide separation along the rectus abdominis muscles. This condition, termed *diastasis recti abdominis,* results from abdominal muscle immaturity.

The liver normally lies at the right costal margin. Its sharp edge should be palpated no more than 1 cm below the right costal margin; it can be felt during inspiration. The spleen, on the opposite side of the abdomen, is approximately 1 cm below the left costal margin.

The posterior position of the kidneys makes them less accessible to palpation. If they cannot be palpated with one hand, bimanual palpation is used. In this technique, the examiner places one hand behind the neonate's back while palpating the abdomen with the fingertips of the other hand. The kidney should be felt between the hands (Coen et al, 1988b).

Unless the bladder is distended, it should not be visible. The bladder may be percussed just above the symphysis pubis. The presence of urine will produce a tympanic sound. The time of the first voiding should be noted.

The abdomen is percussed just after the neonate voids to prevent misleading findings. Percussion should reveal tympany below the left costal margin, reflecting a gastric bubble. Most other abdominal areas also should be tympanic. However, dullness should be percussed over the liver, spleen, and bladder. Percussion delineates the borders of these organs to detect enlargement, indicated by increased areas of dullness. Decreased areas of dullness suggest fluid or air where solid tissue is expected (Coen et al, 1988b).

BACK AND ANUS. To assess the back, the examiner positions the neonate prone and inspects for spinal alignment, enlargement, and masses. The back should be straight. The sacrum is examined for dimpling or a tuft of hair and observed for bulges. The vertebral column is palpated for enlargement and signs of pain (Judd, 1985).

The perineum should be smooth, without dimpling or extra orifices. The anus should be midline and patent. The examiner assesses the anal sphincter by lightly stroking the anus with a cotton-tipped applicator and observing anal constriction—a reaction called the anal wink (Judd, 1985). Passage of meconium should be noted. This indicates patency of the rectum.

GENITALIA. In the male neonate, the genitalia should be assessed for testicular descent, scrotal size, and number of rugae (skin folds). A hydrocele, caused by an accumulation of fluid around the testes, may be found. Hydroceles are a common finding and usually decrease without intervention.

The female genitalia should be assessed for signs of gestational maturity. The degree to which the labia majora and minora have come together and reduced the visual prominence of the labia minora and clitoris reflects the stage of the infant's maturity (Coen et al, 1988a). Any discharge or abnormalities should be recorded and reported.

EXTREMITIES. The extremities are inspected for length, symmetry relative to each other and to the body as a whole, equality, muscle tone, and range of motion. Normally, the term neonate has a full range of motion, which can be tested either actively or passively. The preterm neonate has limited flexion, especially of the arms. The hands and feet are inspected for number of digits, palmar and plantar creases, and such abnormalities as webbing (Judd, 1985).

Movement of the arms should be assessed. Trauma to the brachial plexus during a difficult delivery may result in brachial palsy. The most common type of palsy involves the fifth and sixth cervical nerve roots (Duchenne-Erb paralysis). In this condition, the affected arm is held in a position of tight adduction and internal rotation at the shoulder. The grasp reflex on the affected side may be intact; however, the Moro reflex will be absent on that side. With treatment most neonates have complete recovery.

To assess leg length both legs are extended simultaneously. They should be equal, with symmetric skin folds. The legs are inspected in both the prone and supine positions. Hip integrity is assessed by using the Ortolani movement as described earlier in this chapter.

Plantar (sole) creases should be assessed immediately after birth because the drying effect of environmental exposure causes additional creases to form. The preterm neonate of 34 to 35 weeks' gestation has one or two anterior creases at 36 to 38 weeks' gestation; creases cover the anterior two thirds of the sole. In the term neonate, creases appear over both the sole and the heel. In the postterm neonate, deeper creases line the entire sole (Coen et al, 1988b).

■ ■ ■

Table 20-2 summarizes the physical assessment of the newborn.

Text continued on p. 569.

TABLE 20-2 Physical Assessment of Newborn

Area Assessed and Appraisal Procedure	Normal Findings	Deviations from Normal Range: Possible Problems (Etiology)
POSTURE		
Inspect newborn before disturbing for assessment Refer to maternal chart for fetal presentation, position, and type of birth (vaginal, surgical), since newborn readily assumes prenatal position	Vertex; arms, legs in moderate flexion; fists are clenched Newborn resists having extremities extended for examination or measurement and may cry when this is attempted Crying ceases when allowed to reassume curled-up fetal position Normal spontaneous movement is bilaterally asynchronous (legs move in bicycle fashion) but equally extensive in all extremities	Hypotonia, relaxed posture while awake (prematurity or hypoxia in utero, maternal medications) Hypertonia (drug dependence, CNS disorder) Opisthotonos (CNS disturbance) Limitation of motion in any of extremities (see Extremities, below)
VITAL SIGNS		
Heart rate and pulses		
Thorax (chest Inspection Palpation Auscultation Apex: mitral valve Second interspace, left of sternum: pulmonic valve	Pulsations visible in left midclavicular line; fifth intercostal space Apical pulse; fourth intercostal space 120-140 bpm Quality: *first sound* (closure of mitral and tricuspid valves) and *second sound* (closure of aortic and pulmonic valves) should be sharp and clear	Tachycardia: persistent; ≥170 (RDS) Bradycardia: persistent; ≤120 (congenital heart block) Murmurs (may be functional) Arrhythmias: irregular rate
Second interspace, right of sternum: aortic valve Junction of xiphoid process and sternum: tricuspid valve		Sounds Distant (pneumomediastinum) Poor quality Extra Heard on right side of chest: dextrocardia; often accompanied by reversal of intestines
Femoral pulse palpation: flex thighs on hips; place fingers along inguinal ligament about midway between symphysis pubis and iliac crest; feel bilaterally simultaneously	Femoral pulses should be equal and strong	Weak or absent femoral pulses (hip dysplasia, coarctation of aorta, thrombophlebitis)
TEMPERATURE		
Axillary: method of choice until 6 years of age Rectal: before passage of meconium, check for patent anus; insert thermometer with great caution, gently; hold in place for 90 sec, keeping legs immobilized Electronic: thermistor probe (avoid taping over bony area)	Axillary: 37° C (98.6° F) Rectal: may be misleading—even in cold stress may remain unchanged until metabolic activity can no longer maintain core temperature Temperature stabilization by 8-10 hours of age Shivering mechanism underdeveloped	Subnormal (prematurity, infection, low environmental temperature, inadequate clothing, dehydration) Increased (infection, high environmental temperature, excessive clothing, proximity to heating unit or in direct sunshine, drug addiction, diarrhea and dehydration)

Continued.

TABLE 20-2 Physical Assessment of Newborn—cont'd

Area Assessed and Appraisal Procedure	Normal Findings	Deviations from Normal Range: Possible Problems (Etiology)
		Temperature not stabilized by 10 hours after birth (if mother received magnesium sulfate, newborn is less able to conserve heat by vasoconstriction; maternal analgesics may reduce thermal stability in newborn)
Respiratory rate and effort		
Observe respiration when infant is at rest Count respirations for full minute Apnea monitor Listen for sounds audible without stethoscope Observe respiratory effort	40/min Tend to be shallow, and when infant is awake, irregular in rate, rhythm, and depth No sounds should be audible on inspiration or expiration Breath sounds: bronchial; loud, clear, near	Apneic episodes: ≥15 sec (preterm or premature infant: "periodic breathing," rapid warming or cooling of infant) Bradypnea: ≤25/min (maternal narcosis from analgesics or anesthetics, birth trauma) Tachypnea: ≥60/min (RDS, aspiration syndrome, diaphragmatic hernia) Sounds Rales, rhonchi, wheezes (fluid in lungs) Expiratory grunt (narrowing of bronchi) Distress evidenced by nasal flaring, retractions, chin tug, labored breathing (RDS, fluid in lungs)
Blood pressure (BP) (usually assessed only if a problem is suspected) Electronic monitor BP cuff: BP cuff width affects readings; use cuff 2.5 cm (1 in) wide and palpate radial pulse	75/42 (approximately) At birth Systolic: 60-80 mm Hg Diastolic: 40-50 mm Hg At 10 days Systolic: 95-100 mm Hg Diastolic: slight increase	Difference between upper and lower extremity pressures (coarctation of aorta) Hypotension (sepsis, hypovolemia) Hypertension (coarctation of aorta)
WEIGHT*		
Put protective liner cloth or paper in place and adjust scale to 0 Weigh at same time each day Protect newborn from heat loss	Female 3400 g (7 lb 8 oz) Male 3500 g (7 lb 11 oz) Regain birth weight within first 2 weeks	Weight ≤2500 g (prematurity, small for gestational age, rubella syndrome) Weight ≥4000 g (large for gestational age, maternal diabetes, heredity: normal for these parents) Weight loss over 10% (dehydration)
LENGTH*		
Measure recumbent length from top of head to heel; difficult to measure in full-term infant because of presence of molding, incomplete extension of knees	50 cm (20 in)	<45 or >55 cm (chromosomal aberration, heredity: normal for these parents)

*NOTE: Weight, length, and head circumference should all be close to same percentile for any child.

TABLE 20-2 Physical Assessment of Newborn—cont'd

Area Assessed and Appraisal Procedure	Normal Findings	Deviations from Normal Range: Possible Problems (Etiology)
HEAD CIRCUMFERENCE*		
Measure head at greatest diameter: occipitofrontal circumference May need to remeasure on second or third day after resolution of molding and caput succedaneum	33-35.5 cm (13-14 in) Circumferences of head and chest may be about the same for first 1 or 2 days after birth	Small head ≤32 cm: microcephaly (rubella, toxoplasmosis, cytomegalic inclusion disease) Hydrocephaly: sutures widely separated, circumference ≥4 cm more than chest Increased intracranial pressure (hemorrhage, space-occupying lesion)
CHEST CIRCUMFERENCE		
Measure at nipple line	2 cm (¾ in) less than head circumference; averages between 30-33 cm (12-13 in)	≤30 cm (prematurity) Postmaturity (some small-for-gestational age [SGA] and some large-for-gestational age [LGA])
ABDOMINAL CIRCUMFERENCE		
Measure below umbilicus (not usually measured unless specific indication)	Abdomen enlarges after feeding because of lax abdominal muscles Same size as chest	Enlarging abdomen between feedings (Abdominal mass or blockage in intestinal tract)
INTEGUMENT		
Color		
Inspection and palpation Inspect naked newborn in well-lit, warm area without drafts; natural daylight provides best lighting Inspect newborn when quiet and when active	Varies with ethnic origin; skin pigmentation begins to deepen right after birth in basal layer of epidermis Generally pink Acrocyanosis, especially if chilled	Dark red (prematurity) Pallor (cardiovascular problem, CNS damage, blood dyscrasia, blood loss, twin transfusion, nosocomial infection) Cyanosis (hypothermia, infection, hypoglycemia, cardiopulmonary diseases, cardiac, neurologic, or respiratory malformations) Petechiae over any other area (clotting factor deficiency, infection) Ecchymoses in any other area (hemorrhagic disease, traumatic birth)
Check for jaundice	None at birth	Jaundice within first 24 hr (Rh isioimmunization) Gray (hypotension, poor perfusion)
Birthmarks		
Inspect and palpate for location, size, distribution, characteristics, color	Transient hyperpigmentation Areolae Genitals Linea nigra	Hemangiomas Nevus flammeus: port-wine stain Nevus vasculosus: strawberry mark Cavernous hemangiomas

Continued.

TABLE 20-2 Physical Assessment of Newborn—cont'd

Area Assessed and Appraisal Procedure	Normal Findings	Deviations from Normal Range: Possible Problems (Etiology)
Condition		
Inspect and palpate for intactness, smoothness, texture, edema	No skin edema Opacity: few large blood vessels seen indistinctly over abdomen	Edema on hands, feet; pitting over tibia Texture thin, smooth, or of medium thickness; rash or superficial peeling seen Numerous vessels easily seen over abdomen (prematurity) Texture thick, parchment-like; cracking, peeling (postmaturity) Skin tags; webbing Papules, pustules, vesicles, ulcers, maceration (impetigo, candidiasis, herpes, diaper rash)
Hydration and consistency		
Weigh infant routinely Inspection and palpation Gently pinch skin between thumb and forefinger over abdomen and inner thigh to check for turgor Check subcutaneous fat deposits (adipose pads) over cheeks, buttocks	Dehydration: best indicator is loss of weight After pinch is released, skin returns to original state immediately	Loose, wrinkled skin (prematurity, postmaturity, dehydration: fold of skin persists after release of pinch) Tense, tight, shiny skin (edema, extreme cold, shock, infection) Lack of subcutaneous fat, clavicle or ribs prominent (prematurity, malnutrition)
Check voiding	Voids within 24 hrs of delivery Voids 6-10 times per day	
Vernix caseosa		
Observe amount		Absent or minimal (postmaturity) Excessive (prematurity)
Observe its color and odor before bath or wiping If not readily apparent over total body, check in folds of axilla and groin	Whitish, cheesy, odorless	Yellow color (possible fetal anoxia 36 hours or more before birth, Rh or ABO incompatibility) Green color (possible in utero release of meconium or presence of bilirubin) Odor (possible intrauterine infection)
Lanugo		
Inspect for this fine, downy hair: amount, distribution	Over shoulders, pinnas of ears, forehead	Absent (postmaturity) Excessive (prematurity, especially if lanugo is abundant and long and thick over back)
HEAD		
Palpate skin Inspect shape and size	See Integument Makes up one fourth of body length	Cephalhematoma Molding Severe molding (birth trauma)

TABLE 20-2 Physical Assessment of Newborn—cont'd

Area Assessed and Appraisal Procedure	Normal Findings	Deviations from Normal Range: Possible Problems (Etiology)
	Molding	Lack of molding (prematurity, breech presentation, cesarean birth)
Palpate, inspect, measure fontanelles	Anterior fontanelles 5 cm diamond; increases as molding resolves Posterior fontanelle triangle; smaller than anterior	Fontanelles Full, bulging (tumor, hemorrhage, infection) Large, flat, soft (malnutrition, hydrocephaly, retarded bone age, hypothyroidism) Depressed (dehydration) Large mastoid and sphenoid fontanelles (hydrocephaly)
Palpate sutures	Sutures palpable and not joined	Sutures Widely spaced (hydrocephaly) Premature synostosis closure
Inspect pattern, distribution, amount of hair; feel texture	Silky, single strands, lies flat; growth pattern is toward face and neck	Fine, wooly (prematurity) Unusual swirls, patterns, hairline or coarse, brittle (endocrine or genetic disorder)
EYES		
Placement on face	Eyes and space between eyes each ⅓ the distance from outer-to-outer canthus	
Symmetry in size, shape	Symmetric in size, shape	
Eyelids: size, movement, blink	Blink reflex Epicanthal folds: normal racial characteristic	Epicanthal folds when present with other signs (chromosomal disorders such as Down syndrome, cri du chat syndrome)
Discharge	None No tears	
Eyeballs: presence, size, shape	Both present and of equal size; both round, firm	Agenesis or absence of one or both eyeballs Small eyeball size (rubella syndrome) Lens opacity or absence of red reflex (congenital cataracts, possibly from rubella) Lesions: coloboma, absence of part of iris (congenital) Pink color of iris (albinism) Jaundiced sclera (hyperbilirubinemia) Discharge: purulent (infection)
Pupils	Present, equal in size, react to light	Pupils: unequal, constricted, dilated, fixed (intracranial pressure, medications, tumors)
Eyeball movement	Random, jerky, uneven, can focus momentarily, can follow to midline	Persistent strabismus Doll's eyes (increased intracranial pressure) Sunset (increased intracranial pressure)
Eyebrows: amount, pattern	Distinct (not connected in midline)	

Continued.

TABLE 20-2 Physical Assessment of Newborn—cont'd

Area Assessed and Appraisal Procedure	Normal Findings	Deviations from Normal Range: Possible Problems (Etiology)
NOSE		
Observe shape, placement, patency, configuration of bridge of nose	Midline Apparent lack of bridge, flat, broad Some mucus but no drainage Obligatory nose breathers Sneezes to clear nose	Copious drainage, with or without regular periods of cyanosis at rest and return of pink color with crying (choanal atresia, congenital syphilis) Malformed (congenital syphilis, chromosomal disorder) Flaring of nares (respiratory distress)
EARS		
Observe size, placement on head, amount of cartilage, open auditory canal	Correct placement: line drawn through inner and outer canthi of eye should come to top notch of ear (at junction with scalp) Well-formed, firm cartilage	Agenesis Lack of cartilage (prematurity) Low placement (chromosomal disorder, mental retardation, kidney disorder) Preauricular tags Size: may have overly prominent or protruding ears
Hearing	Responds to voice and other sounds	Deaf: no response to sound
FACE		
Observe overall appearance of face	Infant looks "normal"; features are well placed, proportionate to face, symmetric	Infant looks "odd" or "funny" Usually accompanied by other features, such as low-set ears and other structural disorders (hereditary, chromosomal aberration)
MOUTH		
Inspection and palpation Placement on face Lips: color, configuration, movement	Symmetry of lip movement	Gross anomalies in placement, size, shape (cleft lip and/or palate, gums) Cyanosis; circumoral pallor (respiratory distress, hypothermia) Asymmetry in movement of lips (seventh cranial nerve paralysis)
Gums	Pink gums	
Tongue: attachment, mobility, movement, size	Tongue does not protrude, is freely movable; symmetric in shape, movement	Macroglossia (prematurity, chromosomal disorder) Excessive saliva (esophageal atresia, tracheoesophageal fistula)
Cheeks	Sucking pads inside cheeks	
Palate (soft, hard)		Micrognathia (Pierre Robin or other syndrome)
Arch	Soft and hard palates intact	Teeth: predeciduous or deciduous (hereditary)
Uvula	Uvula in midline	Thrush: white plaques on cheeks or tongue that bleed if touched (*Candida albicans*)
Saliva: amount, character		
Chin	Distinct chin	

TABLE 20-2 Physical Assessment of Newborn—cont'd

Area Assessed and Appraisal Procedure	Normal Findings	Deviations from Normal Range: Possible Problems (Etiology)
Reflexes Rooting Sucking Extrusion	Reflexes present	
NECK		
Inspection and palpation Length Movement of head Sternocleidomastoid muscles; position of head Trachea: position; thyroid gland Reflex response	Short, thick, surrounded by skinfolds; no webbing Head held in midline, i.e., sternocleidomastoid muscles are equal; no masses Freedom of movement from side to side and flexion and extension; cannot move chin past shoulder Thyroid not palpable	Webbing Restricted movement; head held at angle (torticollis [wryneck], opisthotonos) Masses (enlarged thyroid) Distended veins (cardiopulmonary disorder) Skin tags Absence of head control (prematurity; Down syndrome)
CHEST		
Inspection and palpation Shape Clavicles Ribs Nipples: size, placement, number Breast tissue Respiratory movements Amount of cartilage in rib cage Auscultation Heart tones and rate and breath sounds (see Vital signs, above)	Almost circular; barrel shaped Symmetric chest movements; chest and abdominal movements synchronized during respirations Breast nodule: approximately 6 mm in term infant Nipples prominent, well formed; symmetrically placed	Bulging of chest (pneumothorax, pneumomediastinum) Malformation (funnel chest—pectus excavatum) Fracture of clavicle (trauma) Nipples Supernumerary, along nipple line (congenital) Malpositioned or widely spaced (congenital) Lack of breast tissue (prematurity) Poor development of rib cage and musculature (prematurity) Sounds: bowel sounds (see Abdomen, below) Retractions with or without respiratory distress (prematurity, RDS)
ABDOMEN		
Inspect, palpate, and smell umbilical cord	Two arteries, one vein (AVA) Whitish gray Definite demarcation between cord and skin; no intestinal structures within cord Dry around base; drying Odorless Cord clamp in place for 24 hr	One artery (internal anomalies) Bleeding or oozing around cord (hemorrhagic disease) Redness or drainage around cord (infection, possible persistence of urachus) Hernia: herniation of abdominal contents into area of cord (e.g., omphalocele); defect covered with thin, friable membrane, may be extensive (congenital) Gastroschisis: congenital fissure of abdominal cavity Meconium stained (intrauterine distress)

Continued.

TABLE 20-2 Physical Assessment of Newborn—cont'd

Area Assessed and Appraisal Procedure	Normal Findings	Deviations from Normal Range: Possible Problems (Etiology)
Inspect size of abdomen and palpate contour	Rounded, prominent, dome shaped because abdominal musculature is not fully developed Liver may be palpable 1-2 cm below right costal margin No other masses palpable No distention	Distention at birth (ruptured viscus, genitourinary masses or malformations: hydronephrosis; teratomas, abdominal tumors) Mild (aerophagia, over-feeding, high gastrointestinal tract obstruction) Marked (lower gastrointestinal tract obstruction, imperforate anus) Intermittent or transient (aerophagia, overfeeding) Partial intestinal obstruction (stenosis of bowel) Annular pancreas (congenital) Malrotation of bowel or adhesions (congenital) Sepsis (infection)
Auscultate bowel sounds, and note number, amount, and character of stools, and behavior—crying, fussiness—before or during elimination	Sounds present within 1-2 hours after birth Meconium stool passes within 24-48 hours after birth	Scaphoid, with bowel sounds in chest and respiratory distress (diaphragmatic hernia)
Color		
Movement with respirations	Respirations primarily diaphragmatic; abdominal and chest movements synchronous	Decreased abdominal breathing (intrathoracic disease, diaphragmatic hernia)
GENITALS		
Girl		
Inspection and palpation		
General appearance	Female genitals	Ambiguous genitals—enlarged clitoris with urinary meatus on tip; fused labia (chromosomal disorder; maternal drug ingestion)
Clitoris	Usually edematous	
Labia majora	Usually edematous; cover labia minora in term newborns	
Labia minora	May protrude over labia majora	Stenosed meatus (congenital) Labia majora widely separated and labia minora prominent (prematurity)
Discharge	Smegma	
Vagina	Orifice open Mucoid discharge Hymenal/vaginal tag present	Absence of vaginal orifice or imperforate hymen (congenital) Fecal discharge (fistula)
Urinary meatus	Beneath clitoris; hard to see—watch for voiding	
Boy		
Inspection and palpation		
General appearance	Male genitals	Ambiguous genitals (congenital)
Veins Urinary meatus seen as slit	Meatus at tip of penis	Urinary meatus not on tip of glans penis (hypospadias, epispadias)

TABLE 20-2 Physical Assessment of Newborn—cont'd

Area Assessed and Appraisal Procedure	Normal Findings	Deviations from Normal Range: Possible Problems (Etiology)
Prepuce	Prepuce (foreskin) covers glans penis and is not retractable	
Scrotum Rugae (wrinkles)	Large, edematous, pendulous in term infant; covered with rugae	Scrotum smooth and testes undescended (prematurity, cryptorchidism) Hydrocele Inguinal hernia (congenital) Round meatal opening (congenital)
Testes	Palpable on each side	Undescended (prematurity)
Urination	Voiding within 24-48 hr, stream adequate, amount adequate	
Reflexes Erection Cremasteric	Erection may occur spontaneously and when genitals are touched Testes are retracted, especially when newborn is chilled	
EXTREMITIES		
General		
Inspection and palpation Degree of flexion Range of motion Symmetry of motion Muscle tone	Assumes position maintained in utero Attitude of general flexion Full range of motion, spontaneous movements	Limited motion (malformations) Poor muscle tone (prematurity, maternal medications, CNS, anomalies)
Clavicles	Intact	Positive scarf sign Crepitus/fracture (trauma)
Arms Inspection and palpation Color Intactness Appropriate placement Number of fingers Palpate humerus	Longer than legs in newborn period Contours and movement are symmetric 5 on each hand Fist often clenched with thumb under fingers	Asymmetry of movement (fracture/crepitus, brachial nerve trauma, malformations) Asymmetry of contour (malformations, fracture) Amelia or phocomelia (teratogens) Webbing of fingers: syndactyly Absence or excess of fingers Palmar creases Simian line seen with short, incurved little fingers (Down syndrome)
Joints Shoulder Elbow Wrist Fingers Reflex: grasp	Full range of motion; symmetric contour Brachial pulses palpable and equal	Strong, rigid flexion, persistent fists; fists held in front of mouth constantly (CNS disorder) Increased tonicity, clonicity, prolonged tremors (CNS disorder)
Legs Inspection and palpation Color Intactness Length—in relation to arms and body and to each other Major gluteal folds Number of toes	Appear bowed since lateral muscles more developed than medial muscles Major gluteal folds even	Amelia, phocomelia (chromosomal defect, teratogenic effect) Webbing, syndactyly (chromosomal defect) Absence or excess of digits (chromosomal defect, familial trait) Femoral fracture (difficult breech delivery)

Continued.

TABLE 20-2 Physical Assessment of Newborn—cont'd

Area Assessed and Appraisal Procedure	Normal Findings	Deviations from Normal Range: Possible Problems (Etiology)
Femur Head of femur as legs are flexed on hips and abducted; placement in acetabulum; femoral pulses	Femur should be intact No click should be heard; femoral head should not override acetabulum Soles well lined (or wrinkled) over two thirds of foot in term infants	Congenital hip dysplasia/dislocation Absent femoral pulses Soles of feet Few lines: (prematurity) Covered with lines (postmaturity)
Inspection and palpation Joints Hip Knee Ankle Toes Reflexes	Plantar fat pad gives flat-footed effect	Congenital clubfoot Hypermobility of joints (Down syndrome) Yellowed nail beds (meconium staining) Temperature of one leg differs from that of the other (circulatory deficiency, CNS disorder) Asymmetric movement (trauma, CNS disorder)
BACK		
Anatomy		
Inspection and palpation Spine Shoulders Scapulae Iliac crests Base of spine—pilonidal area	Spine straight and easily flexed Infant can raise and support head momentarily when prone Shoulders, scapulae, and iliac crests should line up in same plane	Limitation of movement (fusion or deformity of vertebra) Pigmented nevus with tuft of hair when located anywhere along the spine is often associated with spina bifida occulta Spina bifida cystica (meningocele, myelomeningocele)
Reflexes (spinal related) Test reflexes		
ANUS		
Inspection and palpation Placement Number Patency Test for sphincter response (active "wink" reflex) Observe for following: Abdominal distention Passage of meconium Passage of fecal drainage from surrounding orifices	One anus with good sphincter tone Passage of meconium within 24 hr after birth Good "wink" reflex of anal sphincter	Low obstruction: anal membrane (congenital) High obstruction: anal or rectal atresia (congenital) Drainage of fecal material from vagina in female or urinary meatus in male (rectal fistula)
STOOLS	Meconium followed by transitional and soft yellow stools	

NEUROLOGIC ASSESSMENT. The physical assessment includes a neurologic assessment of the newborn's reflexes (p. 546). This provides useful information about the infant's nervous system and state of neurologic maturation. Many of the reflex behaviors are important for survival, for example, sucking and rooting. Other reflexes act as safety mechanisms, for instance, gagging, coughing, and sneezing. The assessment needs to be carried out as early as possible because abnormal signs present in the early neonatal period may disappear. They may reappear months or years later as abnormal functions.

■ BEHAVIORAL CHARACTERISTICS

The healthy infant must achieve behavioral as well as biologic tasks to develop normally. Behavioral characteristics form the basis of the social capabilities of the infant. Through the first half of this century the focus of developmental research was on how the infant was affected by the environment. Infants were considered to be born with neither personality nor ability to interact.

Today it is recognized that newborns are well equipped to begin social interactions with their parents. The behavioral characteristics of the newborn represent a second phase in human development. The first phase, fetal phase, indicates that the individual personalities and behavioral characteristics of infants play a major role in the ultimate relationship between infants and their parents.

Brazelton (1984) and others brought the behavioral states of the newborn into prominence. The behavioral assessment scale developed by Brazelton (1984) (known as the ***Brazelton Neonatal Behavioral Assessment Scale [BNBAS]***) and the Mother's Assessment of the Behavior of her Infant (MABI) developed by Field et al (1978) provide a psychologic assessment of a newborn's capabilities. These capabilities are relevant to later personality development. It was the authors' contention that the behavioral responses of infants indicate cortical control, responsiveness, and eventual ability to manage the environment. They emphasized the importance of infant-parent interaction. Infants' responses can either consolidate relationships or alienate the persons in their immediate environment. By their actions infants encourage or discourage attachment and care-taking activities. The development of parent-child love does not occur without feedback. The absence of feedback because of separation or incorrectly interpreted feedback can impair the growth of parental love (see Chapter 24).

One of the first tasks parents must accomplish is to become aware of the unique behavioral response of their child. Brazelton (1984) demonstrated that normal babies differ from the moment of birth in such things as activity (active, average, quiet), feeding patterns, sleeping patterns, and responsiveness. He suggested that the parents' reactions to their infants were determined in part by these differences.

Behavioral characteristics, like physical characteristics, change during the transition period (p. 526). Knowledge of these phases and the parents' presence during the infant's reactive phases help promote attachment and successful feeding.

The newborn is in a state of quiet alertness during the first period of reactivity. The eyes are open and alert. The newborn can focus attention on the parents' faces and attend to voices, especially the voice of the mother. This phase lasts about 15 minutes and is followed by a phase of active alertness. In the active alertness period, the neonate has frequent bursts of movement and may cry. The neonate demonstrates a strong suck reflex and may appear hungry. This is a good time to initiate breast-feeding.

The first period of reactivity facilitates attachment. Parents should have time to hold and talk to their newborn. Eye-to-eye contact can be fostered by delaying eye treatment so the baby can interact with the parents.

After this first 30 minutes the newborn becomes drowsy and falls asleep. The newborn appears relaxed and is unresponsive and difficult to awaken during this period. This period of inactivity may last from 2 to 4 hours.

After the rest period the neonate enters the second period of reactivity. Once again the newborn is awake and alert and demonstrates states of quiet alertness, active alertness, and crying. This period may last 4 to 6 hours in a normal newborn. Feeding may be initiated if it was not begun during the first period of reactivity. The neonate sucks, roots, and swallows during this second period of reactivity and becomes interested in feeding.

Sleep-Wake Cycles

Infant variations in *state of consciousness* are called the **sleep-wake cycles** (Fig. 20-27) (Brazelton, 1984). These cycles form a continuum, with deep sleep, narcosis, or lethargy at one end and extreme irritability at the other end. There are two sleep states, deep sleep and light sleep, and four wake states, drowsiness, quiet alert, active alert, and crying. The ability of infants to control or modify their responses varies as they move from a particular sleep or wake state to another. Their reactions to external and internal stimuli reflect their potential for organization of behavior.

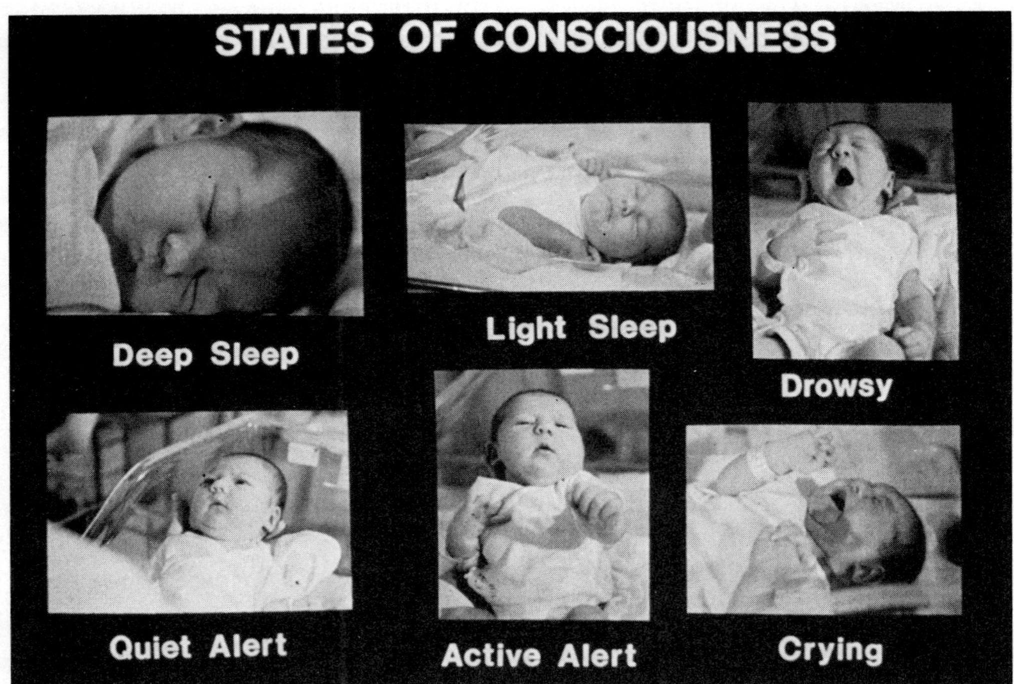

Fig. 20-27 Summary of sleep-wake states of newborn. States of consciousness: deep sleep, light sleep, drowsy, quiet alert, active alert, crying.
Courtesy March of Dimes Birth Defects Foundation.

As listed in Table 20-3 each state has its distinguishing characteristics and **state-related behaviors.** The quiet alert state is also termed *the optimum state of arousal.* During this state infants may be observed smiling, vocalizing, or moving in synchrony (occurring simultaneously). Even during the first day of life, smiling is evident in a surprising number of infants (Bamford et al, 1990). The newborns seem to watch their parents' faces carefully and respond to other persons talking to them. Many infants begin a type of vocalizing by the time they are 2 weeks of age, making cooing, small, throaty noises while feeding.

The infant employs purposeful behavior to maintain the optimum arousal state: (1) active withdrawal by increasing physical distance, (2) a rejecting motion of pushing away with hands and feet, (3) decreasing sensitivity by falling asleep or breaking eye contact by turning head, or (4) use of signaling behaviors, such as fussing or crying (Brazelton, 1984). Use of such behaviors permits infants to quiet themselves and reinstate readiness to interact again.

The first 6 weeks of life involves a steady decrease in the proportion of active REM sleep to total sleep. A steady increase in the proportion of quiet sleep to total sleep time also occurs. There is a 25% increase in wakefulness over the first 3 or 4 weeks. For the first few weeks the wakeful periods seem dictated by hunger, but soon thereafter a need for socializing appears to function as well. The newborn sleeps a total of about 17 hours a day, with the periods of wakefulness gradually increasing. By the fourth week of life, some infants are staying awake from one feeding session to the next. It is not until 4 to 5 years of age that children achieve the adult pattern of sleeping.

Other Factors Influencing Newborn's Behavior

Several other variables, in addition to sleep-wake state, affect the newborn's responses. Several factors are discussed here.

GESTATIONAL AGE. The gestational age of the infant (see Chapters 22 and 37) and level of CNS maturity will affect observed behavior. An infant with an immature CNS will have an entire body response to a pinprick of the foot. The mature infant will withdraw the foot. CNS immaturity also will be reflected in reflex development and sleep-wake cycles.

TIME. Length of time to recuperate from labor and birth will affect the behavior of infants as they attempt to become initially organized. Time since the last feeding and time of day may influence infants' responses.

TABLE 20-3 Behavioral States and State Behavior

	Characteristics of State				
State	Body Activity	Eye Movements	Facial Movements	Breathing Pattern	Level of Response
SLEEP STATES					
Deep sleep	Nearly still, except for occasional startle or twitch	None	Without facial movements, except for occasional sucking movement at regular intervals	Smooth and regular	Threshold to stimuli is very high so that only very intense and disturbing stimuli will arouse infants
Light sleep	Some body movements	Rapid eye movements (REMs), fluttering of eyes beneath closed eyelids	May smile and make brief fussy or crying sounds	Irregular	More responsive to internal and external stimuli; when these stimuli occur, infants may remain in light sleep, return to deep sleep, or arouse to drowsy
AWAKE STATES					
Drowsy	Activity level variable, with mild startles interspersed from time to time; movements usually smooth	Eyes open and close occasionally, are heavy-lidded with dull, glazed appearance	May have some facial movements; often there are none, and face appears still	Irregular	Infants react to sensory stimuli although responses are delayed; state change after stimulation commonly noted
Quiet alert	Minimum	Brightening and widening of eyes	Faces have bright, shining, sparkling looks	Regular	Infants attend most to environment, focusing attention on any stimuli that are present; optimum state of arousal
Active alert	Much body activity; may have periods of fussiness	Eyes open with less brightening	Much facial movement; faces not as bright as quiet alert state	Irregular	Increasingly sensitive to disturbing stimuli (hunger, fatigue, noise, excessive handling)
Crying	Increased motor activity, with color changes	Eyes may be tightly closed or open	Grimaces	More irregular	Extreme response to unpleasant external or internal stimuli

From Barnard KE et al: Behavioral states and state behaviors. In *Early parent-infant relationships,* copyright 1978 by the March of Dimes Birth Defects Foundation, White Plains, NY, Reprinted by permission.

STIMULI. Environmental events and stimuli will affect the behavioral responses of infants. Nurses in intensive care nurseries observe that infants respond to loud noises, bright lights, monitor alarms, and tension in the unit. It has been well documented that infants of mothers who are tense have more muscle activity and their heart rates change according to those of their mothers during feeding. In addition, the newborn responds differently to animate and inanimate stimulation.

MEDICATION. There is controversy concerning the effects on infant behavior of maternal medication (analgesia, anesthesia) during labor. Some researchers have noted that infants of mothers who were given medications may continue to demonstrate poor state organization beyond the fifth day. Others maintain that the effect can be beneficial or that there is no effect (see Chapter 15).

ETHNICITY. Some of the most interesting research findings have been the ethnic differences in infant behavior (Freedman, 1979; Chitty, Winter 1989). Freedman and Freedman (1969) found that Chinese-American infants had more self-quieting activities, fewer state changes, and more rapid responses to consoling activities than did white American infants. A study of Navajo newborns paralleled the stereotype of the stoic impassive Native American (Freedman, 1979). Among Navajo babies, crying was rare and limb movements were reduced, and calming was almost immediate after tests for the Moro reflex. In Freedman's study (1979), Japanese newborns were more sensitive and irritable than either the Chinese or Navajo newborns. Mexican mothers use tactile stimulation more often than vocalizations to quiet their newborns (Garcia-Coll, 1990). These studies suggest that neonatal behavior represents a behavioral phenotype, which expresses a complex relation among genetic endowment, intrauterine environment, and maternal obstetrical history.

Sensory Behaviors

From birth, infants possess **sensory capabilities** that indicate a state of readiness for social interaction. Infants are able to use behavioral responses effectively in establishing their first dialogues. These responses, coupled with the newborn's "baby appearance" (the face is proportioned so that the forehead and eyes are larger than the lower portion of the face) and their smallness and helplessness, rouse feelings of wanting to hold, protect, and interact with them.

VISION. At birth the eye is structurally incomplete and the muscles are immature. The pupils react to light, blink reflex is easily stimulated, and the corneal reflex is activated by light touch. Tear glands usually do not begin to function until the infant is 2 to 4 weeks of age.

However, tears have been seen in some newborns' eyes. The clearest visual distance is 17 to 20 cm (7 to 8 in), which is about the distance the infant's face is from the mother's face as she breast-feeds or cuddles. Infants are sensitive to light. They will frown if a bright light is flashed in their eyes and will turn toward a soft red light. If the room is darkened, they will open their eyes widely and look about. This is noticeable when the delivery area is darkened after birth. By 2 months of age they can detect color, but under 5 days of age they seem more attracted by black-and-white patterns (Luddington-Hoe, 1983).

Response to movement is noticeable. If a bright object is shown to newborns (even at 15 minutes of age), they will follow it visually, and some will even turn their heads to do so. Because human eyes are bright, shiny objects, newborns will track their parents' eyes. Parents will comment on how exciting this behavior is.

Visual acuity is surprising. Even at 2 weeks of age infants can distinguish patterns with stripes 3 mm (1/8 in) apart. By 6 months their vision is as acute as that of an adult (Luddington-Hoe, 1983). They prefer to look at patterns rather than plain surfaces, even if the latter are brightly colored. They also prefer more complex patterns to simple ones. They prefer novelty (changes in pattern) by 2 months of age. This is significant because it means that the infant of a few weeks of age is capable of responding actively to an enriched environment.

From birth onward, infants are able to fix their eyes and gaze intently at objects. They gaze at their parents' faces and respond to changes in them with apparent imitative effect. This ability permits parents and children to gaze into each other's eyes, and a subtle communication pattern is thereby set up. The development of eye-to-eye contact in very important for parent-infant attachment. Children of blind parents and parents who have blind children must circumvent this obstacle in the formation of a relationship (see Chapter 24).

HEARING. As soon as the amniotic fluid drains from the ear, the infant's hearing is similar to an adult's. This may occur as early as 1 minute of age. Loud sounds of about 90 decibels cause the infant to respond with a startle reflex. The newborn responds to low-frequency sounds, such as a heartbeat or a lullaby, by decreasing motor activity or crying. The response to a high-frequency sound elicits an alerting reaction (Barr, 1990).

Studies have indicated that the infant responds readily to the mother's voice (Brazelton, 1984; Redshaw et al, 1985; Curnock, 1989). This may be a response to having heard or felt sound waves from the mother's voice while the infant was in utero.

All these studies indicate a selective listening to the maternal voice sounds and rhythms during intrauterine life that prepares newborns for recognition and interaction with their primary caregivers—their mothers. Newborns are accustomed in the uterus to hearing the regular rhythm of the mother's heartbeat. As a result they respond by relaxing and ceasing to fuss and cry if a regular heartbeat simulator is placed in their cribs.

The acute sensitivity to the human voice has been tested experientially. In observations of the responses of quiet, alert newborns to computer-simulated cries and the cries of human newborns, more restlessness and crying occurred in response to the genuine cry. Newborns less than 35 hours old typically began to cry when subjected to the cry of other newborns but quieted at the sound of their own cry (Barr, 1990).

The internal and middle portions of the ear are large at birth, but the external canal is small. The mastoid process and the bony parts of the external canal have not developed. Therefore the tympanic membrane and facial nerve are very close to the surface and can be easily damaged.

TOUCH. The infant is responsive to touch on all parts of its body. The face, especially the mouth, the hands, and the soles of the feet appear to be the most sensitive. Reflexes can be elicited by stroking the infant. The newborn's responses to touch suggest this sensory system is well prepared to receive and process tactile messages. Touch and motion have been reported as being essential to normal growth and development (Gunzenhauser, 1990). However, each infant is unique, and variations can be seen in newborns' responses to touch.

The new mother uses touch as one of the first interaction behaviors: fingertip touch, soft stroking of the face, and gentle massage of the back. Because touch between strangers is avoided in some cultures, it would seem that this automatic maternal touching behavior evidences an already intimate relationship. Birth trauma or stress and depressant drugs taken by the mother decrease the infant's sensitivity to touch or painful stimuli.

TASTE. The newborn has a well-developed taste system, and different solutions elicit different facial expressions. A tasteless solution produces no response whereas a sweet solution causes eager sucking. A sour solution results in puckering of the lips, and a bitter solution causes anger. Newborns have been reported to prefer glucose water over sterile water (Pete, 1989). These studies demonstrate not only the newborn's response to various tastes but also the strength of the taste response and its independence from cortical levels of the nervous system.

It is generally accepted that young infants are particularly oriented toward the *use of their mouths,* both for meeting their nutritional needs for rapid growth and for releasing tension through sucking. The early development of circumoral sensation and muscle activity, as well as taste, would seem to be preparation for survival in the extrauterine environment.

SMELL. The newborn's sense of smell has been reported to be well developed at birth. Newborns appear to react similarly to adults when exposed to strong or pleasant odors. Breast-fed infants are able to smell breast milk and can differentiate their mothers from other lactating women (Lawrence, 1989). These maternal odors are believed to influence bonding and adequate feeding.

The significance of smell in maternal identification of offspring and vice versa in the animal world is well documented. Maternal identification of the human newborn by smell has not been studied extensively. Stainton (1985) noted that mothers reported that from the time of birth their infants had a unique smell.

Response to Environmental Stimuli

Infants respond to the environment in a number of ways. Classic studies have identified individual variations in the primary reaction pattern of newborns and described them as *temperament* (Thomas, 1961, 1970). Their style of behavioral response to stimuli is guided by the temperament that affects the newborn's sensory threshold, ability to habituate, and response to maternal behaviors.

TEMPERAMENT. The behavioral styles of infants and children "show distinct individuality in temperament in the first weeks of life, independently of their parents' handling or personality style." In addition, "the original characteristics of temperament tend to persist in most children over the years" (Chess, 1969; Chess, Thomas, 1977).

Chess's classic work (1969) led to the development of nine categories of primary reactivity to evaluate **behavioral style:**

1. Activity level—the diurnal proportion of active to inactive periods
2. Rhythmicity—the regularity and predictability of bodily function and sleep-wake cycle
3. Approach or withdrawal—the response to a new stimulus
4. Adaptability—the speed and ease with which current behavior is modified in response to environmental changes
5. Intensity of reaction—the energy in a response regardless of its quality or direction
6. Threshold of responsiveness—the intensity of stimuli required to evoke a response
7. Quality of mood—the proportion of happy behavior to unhappy behavior

8. Distractibility—the efficacy of external stimuli in changing the direction of ongoing behavior
9. Attention span and persistence—duration one activity is pursued and effect of distraction

These nine categories were then grouped into three major patterns of behavioral style or temperament:

1. The easy child who demonstrates regularity in bodily functions, readily adapts to change, has a predominantly positive mood and a moderate sensory threshold, and approaches new situations or objects with a moderate response.
2. The slow-to-warm-up child who has a low activity level, withdraws on first exposure to new stimuli, is slow to adapt and low in intensity of response, and is somewhat negative in mood
3. The difficult child who is irregular in bodily functions, intense in reactions, generally negative in mood, resistant to change or new stimuli, and often cries loudly for long periods

The human newborn possesses sensory receptors capable of responding selectively to various stimuli present in the internal and external environment. The infant also possesses individual characteristics that define her or him as a unique personality. The range of these responses may impress the parent with the newborn's formidable neurologic capacity.

HABITUATION. **Habituation** is a protective mechanism. It allows the infant to become accustomed to environmental stimuli. Habituation is a psychologic and physiologic phenomenon whereby the response to a constant or repetitive stimuli is decreased. In the term newborn this can be demonstrated in several ways. Shining a bright light into a newborn's eyes will cause a startle or squinting the first two to three times. The third or fourth flash will elicit a diminished response and by the fifth or sixth flash, the infant ceases to respond (Brazelton, 1984). The same response pattern holds true for the sounds of a rattle or a pinprick to a heel. A newborn presented with new stimuli will become wide-eyed and alter its gaze for a time but eventually will show a diminished interest.

The ability to habituate also allows the newborn to select stimuli that promote continued learning about the social world, thus avoiding overload. The intrauterine experiences seem to have programmed the newborn to be especially responsive to human voices, soft lights, soft sounds, and sweet tastes.

The newborn quickly learns the sounds in a newborn nursery and in the home and is able to sleep in their midst. The selective responses of the newborn indicate cerebral organization capable of remembering and making choices. The ability to habituate depends on state of consciousness, hunger, fatigue, and temperament. These factors also affect consolability, cuddliness, irritability, and crying.

CONSOLABILITY. Korner (1971) reported studies that describe variations in the ability of newborns to console themselves or to be consoled. In the crying state, most newborns will initiate one of several ways to reduce their distress. Hand-to-mouth movements are common, with or without sucking, as well as alerting to voices, noises, or visual stimuli.

CUDDLINESS. Cuddliness is especially important to parents because they gauge their ability to care for the child by the child's responses to their actions. The degree to which newborns will mold into the contours of the person holding them varies. Barr (1990) tested the effect of body contact and vestibular stimulation in both soothing babies and creating alertness. The vestibular stimulation of being picked up and moved had the greater effect.

IRRITABILITY. Some newborns cry longer and harder than others do. For some the sensory threshold seems low. They are readily upset by unusual noises, hunger, wetness, or new experiences, and they respond intensely. Others with a high sensory threshold require a great deal more stimulation and variation to reach the active, alert state (Barr, 1990).

CRYING. Crying in an infant may signal hunger, pain, desire for attention, or fussiness. Some mothers state that they eventually are able to distinguish the reasons for crying. This is a means of communication.

Barr (1990) reported five characteristics of crying. First, there is a progressive increase in crying that peaks in the second month, then gradually decreases. Second, there is a diurnal rhythm, with more crying occurring in the evening hours. Third, there is considerable variation among different babies. Fourth, there also appears to be individual day-to-day variation, and fifth, the crying does not seem to differ with the caretaker.

■ SUMMARY

During the period of infancy the infant within the "protective envelope of nurturing adults" (Brazelton, 1984) can learn complex coping mechanisms and control systems. These in turn help the infant to be alert, to pay attention, and to master rules of communication. The newborn and adult learn about each other and about themselves. Thus, a feeling of mutuality and identification with the "other" are accomplished. The nurse uses knowledge of the biologic and behavioral characteristics of the newborn as a basis for the care of the infant and the teaching and counseling of the parents.

REFERENCES

Bamford, FN et al: Sleep in the first year of life, *Dev Med Child Neurol* 32:718, 1990.

Barr RG: The normal crying curve: what do we really know? *Dev Med Child Neurol* 32:356, 1990.

Blackburn ST, Loper DL: *Maternal, fetal and neonatal physiology: a clinical perspective,* Philadelphia, 1992, WB Saunders.

Brazelton TB: *Neonatal behavioral assessment scale,* ed 2, Philadelphia, 1984, JB Lippincott Co.

Brovten D et al: Breastmilk jaundice, *JOGNN* 14:220, May/June 1985.

Chess S: Individuality and baby care, *Dev Med Child Neurol* 11:749, 1969.

Chess S, Thomas A: Temperament and the parent-child interaction, *Pediatr Ann* 6(9):26, 1977.

Chitty LS, Winter RM: Perinatal mortality in different ethnic groups, *Arch Dis Child* 64:1036, 1989.

Coen RW et al: The detailed newborn examination, *Patient Care* 22:93, Dec 1988b.

Coen RW et al: A fast, efficient newborn exam, *Patient Care* 22:192, Nov 1988a.

Cohen KW, Byrne SM: The role of the nurse in assisting with eye examinations on premature infants, *Neonatal Network* 8(2):31, 1989.

Cunningham FG, MacDonald PC, Gant NF: Williams obstetrics, ed, 18 Norwalk, Conn, 1989, Appleton & Lange.

Curnock DA: The senses of the newborn: tests for hearing and vision have improved, *BMJ* 299:1478, 1989.

Desmond MM, Rudolph A, Phitakspharaiwan P: The transitional care nursery, *Pediatr Clin North Am* 13:651, 1966.

Deter RL, Harrist RB, Hill RM: Neonatal growth assessment score: a new approach to the detection of intrauterine growth retardation in the newborn, *Am J Obstet Gynecol* 162:1030, 1990.

Editorial: The Apgar score . . . revisited, *J Perinat* 9:338, Sept 1989a.

Editorial: Is the Apgar score outmoded? *J Perinat* 9:338, Sept. 1989b.

Fanaroff AA, Martin RJ: *Neonatal-perinatal medicine: diseases of the fetus and infant,* ed 5, St Louis, 1992, Mosby–Year Book.

Field R et al: Mothers' assessments of the behavior of their infants, *Infant Behav Dev* 1:156, 1978.

Freedman DG: Ethnic differences in babies, *Hum Nature,* p 36, Jan 1979.

Freedman DG, Freedman N: Behavioral differences between Chinese-American and European-American newborns, *Nature* 224:1227, 1969.

Garcia Coll CT: Developmental outcome of minority infants: a process-oriented look into our beginnings, *Child Dev* 61:270, 1990.

Gunzenhauser N, editor: *Advances in touch: new implications in human development,* Skillman, JN, 1990, Johnson & Johnson Consumer Products.

Guyton A: *Textbook of medical physiology,* Philadelphia, 1985, WB Saunders Co.

BIBLIOGRAPHY

Feeg VD: New legislative efforts to improve child health and decrease infant mortality, *Pediatr Nurs* 15(2):145, 1989.

Giger JN, Davidhizar RE: *Transcultural nursing: assessment and intervention,* St Louis, 1991, Mosby–Year Book.

Jones MB: A physiologic approach to identifying neonates at risk for kernicterus, *JOGNN* 19:313, July/Aug 1990.

Malasanos L, Barkauskas V, Stoltenberg-Allen K: *Health assessment,* ed 4, St Louis, 1990, Mosby–Year Book.

NAACOG: *Neonatal skin care* (OGN Nursing Practice Resource), Jan 1992.

Seidel HM et al: *Mosby's guide to physical examination,* St Louis, 1991, Mosby–Year Book.

Jones DA, Lepley MK, Baker BA: *Health assessment across the life span,* St Louis, 1984, Mosby–Year Book.

Judd JM: Assessing the newborn from head to toe, *Nursing* p 34, Dec 1985.

Korner AF: Individual differences at birth: implications for early experiences and later development, *Am J Orthospychiatry* 41:608, 1971.

Korones SB: *High-risk newborn infants: the basis for intensive nursing care,* ed 4, St Louis, 1986, Mosby–Year Book.

Lascari AD: "Early" breast-feeding jaundice: clinical significance, *J Pediatr* 108:156, 1986.

Lawrence RA: Breastfeeding: a guide for the medical profession, ed 3, St Louis, 1989, Mosby–Year Book.

Locklin M: Assessing jaundice in full-term newborns, *Pediatr Nurs* 13:15, Jan 1987.

Luddington-Hoe SM: What can newborns really see? *Am J Nurs* 83:1286, 1983.

Medici MA: The fight against infection: neonatal defense mechanisms, *J Calif Perinat Assoc* 3(2):25, 1983.

Nelson NM: The onset of respirations. In Avery G, editor: *Neonatology: pathophysiology and management of the newborn,* ed 3, Philadelphia, 1987, JB Lippincott.

Physical assessment of the neonate (OGN Nursing Practice Resource), Aug 1991, NAACOG

Parker S et al: Jitteriness in full-term neonates: prevalence and correlates, *Pediatrics* 85:17, 1990.

Pete J: Newborn infant's preference for sterile water versus five-percent glucose and water, *J Pediat Nurs* 4:263, 1989.

Redshaw ME, Rivers RPA, Rosenblatt DB: *Born too early: special care for preterm baby,* New York, 1985, Oxford University Press.

Schaffer HH, Emerson P: Patterns of response to physical contact in early human development, *J Child Psychol Psychiatry* 5:1, 1964.

Stainton C: *Origins of attachment, culture, and cue sensitivity,* doctoral dissertation, San Francisco, 1985, University of California.

Thomas A et al: Individuality in responses of children to similar environmental situations, *Am J Psychiatry* 117:798, 1961.

Thomas A et al: The origin of personality, *Sci Am* 223:102, 1970.

Valmin HB: Jaundice in the newborn, *BMJ* 299:1272, 1989.

Wilkerson N: A comprehensive look at hyperbilirubinemia, *Matern Child Nurs J* 13:360, 1988.

References—Nursing Research

Bliss-Holtz J: Comparison of rectal, axillary, and inguinal temperatures in full-term newborn infants, *Nur Res* 38:85, 1989.

Boyer DB, Vidyasagar D: Serum indirect bilirubin levels and meconium passage in early fed normal newborns, *Nurs Res* 36:174, 1987.

Bibliography—Nursing Research

Greer PS: Head coverings for neonates under radiant heat warmers, *JOGNN* 17:265, July/Aug 1988.

Jones MA: Identifying signs that nurses interpret as indicating pain in newborns, *Pediat Nurs* 15:76, Jan 1989.

Keefe MR et al: Development of a system for monitoring infant state behavior, *Nurs Res* 38:344, 1989.

Kunnel MT et al: Comparisons of rectal, femoral, axillary, and skin-to-mattress temperatures in stable neonates, *Nurs Res* 37:162, 1988.

Medoff-Cooper B, Weininger S, Zukowsky K: Neonatal sucking as a clinical assessment tool: preliminary findings, *Nurs Res* 38:162, 1989.

Zahr LK, Khoury M, Nugent K: Neonatal behavior of prenatally stressed Lebanese infants, *Image* 20(4):200, 1988.

chapter 20 review

Key Concepts

- By term the infant's various anatomic and physiologic systems have reached a level of development and functioning that permits a physical existence apart from the mother and sensory capabilities that indicate a state of readiness for social interaction.
- Several significant differences between the newborn's respiratory, renal, and thermogenetic systems and those of the adult affect nursing care.
- At any serum bilirubin level, the appearance of jaundice during the first day of life or persistence of jaundice usually indicates a pathologic process.
- Chilling of a newborn, even a healthy term newborn, may result in acidosis and raise the level of free fatty acids.
- Many reflex behaviors are important for the newborn's survival.
- The individual personalities and behavioral characteristics of infants play a major role in the ultimate relationship between infants and their parents.
- Behavioral responses of infants indicate cortical control, responsiveness, and eventual ability to manage their environment.
- The development of parent-child love does not occur without feedback.
- Sleep-wake cycles and other factors influence the newborn's behavior.
- Each newborn has a predisposed capacity to handle the multitude of stimuli in the external world.

Key Terms

- acrocyanosis (p. 539)
- behavioral style (p. 573)
- Brazelton Neonatal Behavioral Assessment Scale (BNBAS) (p. 569)
- breast-feeding jaundice(p. 538)
- breast-milk jaundice (p. 538)
- brown fat (p. 532)
- caput succedaneum (p. 539)
- cephalhematoma (p. 540)
- cephalocaudal development (p. 553)
- cold stress (p. 533)
- ductus arteriosus (p. 528)
- fetal circulation (p. 528)
- foramen ovale (p. 528)
- gastrocolic reflex (p. 536)
- habituation (p. 574)
- initial breathing (p. 527)
- mongolian spots (p. 540)
- newborn reflexes (p. 546)
- newborn stools (p. 536)
- physiologic jaundice (p. 537)
- preferential nose breather (p. 527)
- respiratory distress (p. 528)
- respiratory patterns (p. 527)
- sensory capabilities (p. 572)
- sleep-wake cycles (p. 569)
- state-related behaviors (p. 570)
- thermogenesis (p. 532)
- transition period (p. 526)
- vitamin K deficiency (p. 532)

Critical Thinking Exercises

1. Observe and record findings of a normal newborn immediately after birth and in follow-up periods for several days thereafter. Include both physiologic and behavioral data; compare data, and identify questions for further research.
2. Prepare teaching materials that could be used for a new-parent class on changes and challenges to one of the newborn's body systems. Justify selections.
3. Research theories of newborn behavior and sensory abilities before 20 years ago and over the last 10 years. Discuss changes in attitude and expectations toward the newborn and how these might affect treatment and care of the newborn. Discuss how this new information can be used to update grandparents (or older pregnant women).
4. Use research on newborn's sensory abilities and social responses to design a nursery for the new baby (in the home) that incorporates these findings with a list of suggestions of parent-child interactions appropriate to the findings. Justify your design and suggestions.

Topics for Nursing Research

- Compare the ages at which bottle-fed and breast-fed infants sleep through the night.
- Compare leaning techniques of drying the umbilical cord: Q-tip and alcohol versus alcohol prep pad.
- Compare jitterness in newborns who are small for gestational age (SGA), appropriate for gestational age (AGA) and large for gestational age (LGA).
- Study different states of consciousness in infants whose mothers received different types of anesthesia during delivery.
- Compare various cultures in terms of methods of attachment with the newborn.

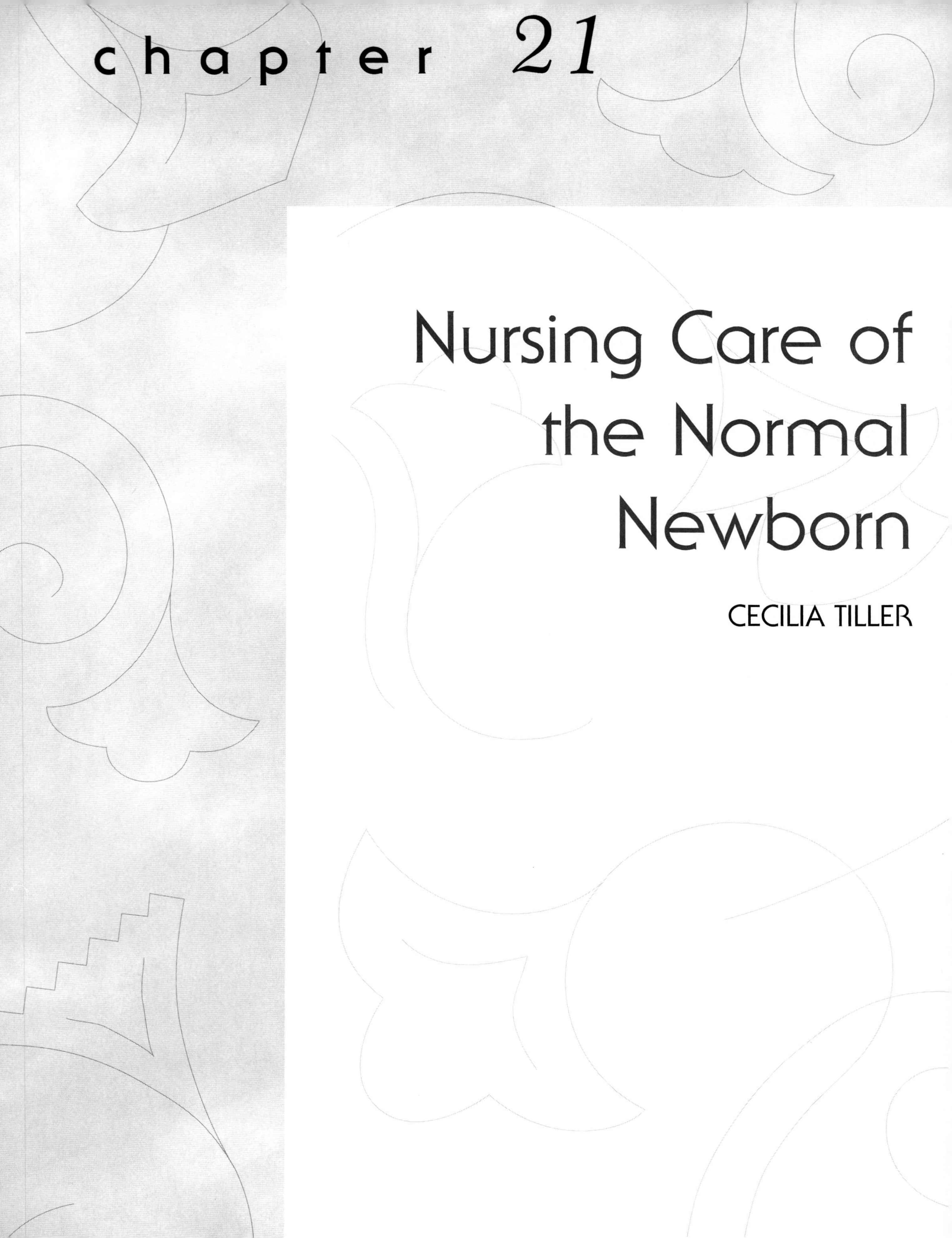

chapter 21

Nursing Care of the Normal Newborn

CECILIA TILLER

LEARNING OBJECTIVES

- Define key terms.
- Gather appropriate health history information from the prenatal and intrapartal periods.
- Identify the sequence to follow in assessment of the newborn.
- Explain what is meant by a safe environment.
- Discuss methods to maintain the newborn's temperature.
- Compare methods of maintaining an adequate oxygen supply.
- Outline in detail the emergency procedure for cardiopulmonary resuscitation and relieving airway obstruction.
- Describe precautions in administering an intramuscular injection to a newborn.
- Discuss phototherapy and guidelines for teaching parents.
- Explain circumcision purposes and methods, postoperative care, and parent teaching.
- Review procedures for heel stick, collection of urine specimen, assisting with venipuncture, and restraining the newborn.
- Review anticipatory guidance for parents.
- Identify topics for nursing research related to nursing care of the normal newborn.

The preceding chapter presented the numerous biologic changes the neonate undergoes during the transition to extrauterine life. The first 24 hours of life are critical because respiratory distress and circulatory failure can occur rapidly and with little warning.

Although most infants make the necessary biopsychosocial adjustment to extrauterine existence without undue difficulty, their well-being depends on the care they receive from others. The nursing care described in this chapter is based on careful assessment of biologic and behavioral responses and formulation of nursing diagnoses. It includes planning and implementing appropriate nursing actions and evaluating their effectiveness. (See p. 612 for an example of a nursing plan of care.)

ASSESSMENT

Routine assessment of the infant is a continuous process. An Apgar score (see Chapter 18), assigned to the infant after birth, provides an indication of the infant's stability. Knowledge of the mother's prenatal history, duration and events of labor, and maternal analgesia and anesthesia helps alert the nurse to any potential problems.

An initial assessment of the newborn is performed at birth. The first thorough examination should be done within 24 hours, following the guidelines presented in Chapter 20. A head-to-toe assessment is conducted, and each system is evaluated.

Whenever any care is given to a newborn, observations and recordings of the infant's progress are made. During each 8-hour shift the following assessments are made, compared with the norm, and recorded:

- Temperature
- Respiratory rate, rhythm, and effort
- Breath sounds
- Heart rate and rhythm
- Skin color
- Activity level and muscle tone
- Feeding and elimination behavior
- Fontanelles
- Parent/child interactions

Admission to the Nursery

The admission to the nursery may be delayed or may never actually occur. Depending on the routine of the hospital, the infant frequently remains in the labor area and is transferred to the postpartum unit with the mother. Many hospitals have adopted variations of the **single-room maternity care (SRMC)** for postpartum care (Phillips, 1988). One nurse provides care for the mother and newborn. SRMC allows the infant to remain with the parents after the birth. Many procedures, such as weight and measurement, eye medication, intramuscular (IM) administration of vitamin K, and physical assessment, may be carried out in the labor and birth unit. Nurses who work in an SRMC unit; labor, delivery, recovery room (LDR); or labor, delivery, recovery, postpartum room (LDRP) must be educated to provide obstetric, neonatal, and postpartum nursing care (Gerlach, Schmid, 1988). Regardless of the physical organization for care, most hospitals have a small holding nursery, which is available for procedures or on request of the mother who wishes her infant to be placed there. This set-up promotes parent-infant bonding while still allowing the new parents some time to be alone.

Even with modifications in nursery placement, the routine procedures and admission process are still necessary. All these procedures can be carried out in any LDR, LDRP, SRMC, or separate nursery setting. (See Chapter 18 for immediate care of the newborn.)

The first assessment of the newborn occurs at birth with use of the Apgar scoring system that judges heart rate, respiratory rate, muscle tone, reflex irritability, and skin color (see Chapter 18). The assessment for gestational age should be done within the first 2 hours of birth and the complete physical assessment within 24 hours. Initial assessment is done within 2 hours because drying of the infant's skin may increase creases, especially in the sole of the foot, and may make the infant appear more mature than he or she really is.

After verifying the infant's identification with the transfer nurse from the delivery unit, the nursery nurse places the baby in a warm environment and begins the admission assessment. This includes obtaining pertinent information from the mother's prenatal record and the record of events during the mother's labor and the newborn's birth. Often a form (see individual hospital forms or Fig. 21-1) is used to record findings. This form shows at a glance, significant data from the antenatal period through nursery admission. (An example of newborn nursery routine orders is shown in the box on p. 582.)

Extensive Physical Examination

Reviewing the maternal history and the prenatal and intrapartal records provides a background for any potential problems. Knowing the type of analgesia and anesthesia the mother received in labor also alerts the nurse to any potential problems or helps explain the infant's current status. During the initial physical assessment the infant's gestational age should be evaluated (see Chapter 37).

Neonatal Health History

Date ________ Infant ________
Date of delivery ________ Sex ________
Time of delivery ________ Age (in hours) now ________

Prenatal data
Maternal age ________ Blood type and Rh ________
Indirect Coombs' ________ EDB via dates ________

Previous obstetric history
Parity (explain all items) ________
Previous pregnancies:
Date ________ Gestational age ________ Sex________ Weight ________ Delivery ________ Complications ________

Complications of this pregnancy
Preeclampsia ________ Hypertension ________
Diabetes (class) ________ Bleeding ________
Viral/bacterial infection ________
Environmental teratogens ________
Drug use ________
Over-the-counter ________ Alcohol ________
Prescription ________ Cocaine ________
Heroin ________ Methadone ________
Other ________

Results of fetal testing
AFP assay ________
Ultrasound ________ Amniocentesis ________
NST ________ BPS ________

Intrapartum data
Onset of contractions ________
Rupture of membranes (ROM) ________ When? ________
Bloody ________ Meconium stained ________ Foul smell ________
Abnormalities of maternal vital signs ________
Medications during labor ________
Anesthesia/analgesia ________ Time last administered ________
Fetal monitoring (external/internal) ________
Fetal distress ________ Fetal pH ________
Length of stages of labor: 1st ________ 2nd ________ 3rd ________

Delivery
Time ________ Route ________
Reason for operative delivery ________

Resuscitation
Apgar score: 1 minute ________ 5 minute ________
Suction ________ Whiffs of O_2 ________
Positive pressure ________ via mask/endotracheal tube ________
Length ________
Time of first spontaneous breath ________
Medications ________

Other
Voided in delivery room ________ Stool ________
Breastfed ________ Bonding time ________
Observations of bonding behavior ________

In nursery
Time of transfer to nursery if applicable ________
First temperature ________ Placed in warmer/Isolette ________
Eye prophylaxis ________
Vitamin K ________ Time ________ Location ________

Fig. 21-1 Neonatal health history.
From Dickason EJ, Schultz MO, Silverman BL: *Maternal-infant nursing care,* St Louis, 1990, Mosby–Year Book.

Routine Admission Orders

Vital signs: on admission and q30min × 2, q1h × 2, then q8h
Weight, length, and head and chest circumference on admission; then weigh daily
Erythromycin ophthalmic ointment 5 mg/g 1 line each eye (ou)
Vitamin K 1 mg IM
Hematocrit by warm heel stick within 3 to 8 hr of age; call physician if <50 or >65
Dextrostix prn; notify physician if <45 mg%; offer early D_5W po
Feedings: sterile water × 1 by nurse within first 4 hr of life; if tolerated, begin breast-feeding or formula q3h to q4h on demand
Rooming in as desired and infant's condition permits
Newborn screen for *phenylketonuria* (PKU), *thyroxine* (T_4), and *galactosemia* on day of discharge

A second, more thorough, physical examination is performed within 24 hours after delivery, when the newborn's temperature is stabilized. The *goal* of this examination is to compile a complete record of the newborn that will provide a data base for subsequent assessment and care. The parents' presence during this extensive examination permits prompt discussion of parental concerns and actively involves the parents in the health care of their child from birth. Also, *parental interactions with the child* can be observed. This aids in early diagnosis of concerns in parent-child relationships and learning needs.

The area used for the examination should be well lighted, warm, and free from drafts. The child is undressed as needed and placed on a firm, flat surface. The infant may need to be picked up and cuddled at times for reassurance. The examination is carried out in a systematic manner. It begins with a general evaluation of such characteristics as appearance, maturity, nutritional status, activity, and state of well-being. This general evaluation is followed by more specific observations. (See Chapter 20.)

Data are recorded as descriptive notes or are summarized on standard forms. Identifying data are entered first: addressograph, birth date, weight, length, chest and head circumferences, race, sex, mother's and infant's blood type and Rh factor, Coombs' test results, and time of examination.

The *general appearance* (posture, maturity, activity, tone, cry, color, edema) and *sleep-wake state* are assessed before disturbing the infant. These observations aid in the interpretations of the findings. Each examiner has a preferred pattern for assessment. Blood pressure (BP) is not assessed routinely. *Heart and respiratory rates* are easiest to assess when the newborn is quiet (Margolius et al, 1991). Respirations are counted by observing the chest wall, noting whether the sternum retracts, the nares flare, and the chin lags on inspiration. The examiner notes whether the infant is a normal nose breather (i.e., sleeps with mouth closed, does not have to interrupt feedings to breathe), assesses breath sounds, and notes abnormal sounds—grunting or wheezing—during inspiration or expiration.

The examiner notes the efficiency of the gagging, sneezing, and swallowing reflexes related to maintaining a clear airway.

The examiner watches for bouts of rapid and irregular respirations, gagging, and regurgitation of mucus during "reactivity" periods after birth and after 4 to 6 hours of life (see p. 526).

The infant's *color* is assessed for cyanosis. A pink color over the head and trunk and mucous membranes indicates adequate oxygenation. Feet and hands may remain slightly cyanotic for 48 hours, especially when they are cold.

On admission and each time the *skin* is exposed while giving care, the infant's skin is assessed for rashes, excoriations (e.g., from fingernails), color (e.g., petechiae, ecchymosis, jaundice, mottling), wounds (e.g., from internal fetal monitoring, forceps, scalpel during cesarean birth, circumcision, cord, heel sticks, injections), vernix caseosa, and lanugo. The axillary *temperature* is measured. Taking the temperature rectally ordinarily is contraindicated. Rectal temperatures may be taken to assess patency of the anus. Waiting for the first stool to appear, however, is the preferable means of assessing anal patency.

The baby's *head* is assessed for skin, hair pattern and distribution, molding, fontanelles and sutures, size, shape, symmetry, eyes, nose, mouth, ears, and facies. The neck is inspected and palpated. *Chest assessment* includes measuring the chest circumference and noting the shape of the thorax, the breasts and nipples, and chest movement with respirations. The rate and rhythm of the heart and presence or absence of murmurs are noted. Lung fields are auscultated. The shape of the *abdomen* and the condition of the umbilical cord are assessed. Abdominal circumference may be measured. Bowel sounds and record of stooling behavior are noted. The newborn's *genitals, urinary meatus,* and *anus* are assessed carefully. The *skeletal system* also is inspected.

Neonatal *reflexes* are assessed. The responses reveal the status of the neuromuscular and skeletal systems. State-related behaviors are assessed, and implications for caregiving are suggested in Table 21-1.

TABLE 21-1 Infant State-Related Behavior Chart

Behavior/Description of Behavior	Infant State Consideration	Implications for Caregiving
ALERTNESS		
Widening and brightening of the eyes. Infants focus attention on stimuli, whether visual, auditory, or objects to be sucked.	From drowsy or active alert to quiet alert.	Infant state and timing are important. When trying to alert infants, try to: 1. Unwrap infant (arms out at least). 2. Place infant in upright position. 3. Talk to infant, putting variation in your pitch and tempo. 4. Show your face to infant. 5. Elicit the rooting, sucking, or grasp reflexes.
VISUAL RESPONSE		
Newborns have pupillary responses to differences in brightness. Infants can focus on objects or faces about 7-8 inches away. Newborns have preferences for more complex patterns, human faces, and moving objects.	Quiet alert.	Newborn's visual alertness provides opportunities for eye-to-eye contact with caregivers, an important source of beginning caregiver-infant interaction.
AUDITORY RESPONSE		
Reaction to a variety of sounds, especially in the human voice range. Infants can hear sounds and locate the general direction of the sound, if the source is constant.	Drowsy, quiet alert, active alert.	Enhances communication between infants and caregivers. Crying infants can often be consoled by voice.
IRRITABILITY		
How easily infants are upset by loud noises, handling by caregivers, temperature changes, removal of blankets or clothes, etc.	From deep sleep, light sleep, drowsy, quiet alert, or active alert to fussing or crying.	Irritable infants need more frequent consoling and more subdued external environments. Parents can be helped to cope with more irritable infants.
READABILITY		
The cues infants give through motor behavior and activity, looking, listening, and behavior patterns.	All states.	Parents need to learn that newborns' behaviors are part of their individual temperaments and not reflections on their parenting abilities. By observing and understanding an infant's characteristic pattern, parents can respond more appropriately.
SMILE		
Ranging from a faint grimace to a full-fledged smile. Reflexive.	Drowsy, active alert, quiet alert, light sleep.	Initial smile in the neonatal period is the forerunner of the social smile at 3-4 weeks of age. Important for caregivers to respond to it.

Modified from Barnard KE et al: Infant state-related behavior chart. In *Early parent-infant relationships*, copyright 1978 by the March of Dimes Birth Defects Foundation, White Plains, NY. Reprinted by permission.

Continued.

TABLE 21-1 Infant State-Related Behavior Chart—cont'd

Behavior/Description of Behavior	Infant State Consideration	Implications for Caregiving
HABITUATION The ability to lessen one's response to repeated stimuli. This is seen where the Moro response is repeatedly elicited. If a noise is continually repeated, infants will usually cease to respond.	Deep sleep, light sleep, also seen in drowsy.	Because of this ability families can carry out normal activities without disturbing infants. Infants who have more difficulty with this will probably not sleep well in active environments.
CUDDLINESS Infant's response to being held. Infants nestle and work themselves into the contours of caregivers' bodies.	Primarily in awake states.	Cuddliness is usually rewarding behavior for the caregivers. If infants do not nestle and mold, show the caregivers how to position infants to maximize this response.
CONSOLABILITY Measured when infants have been crying for at least 15 seconds. The ability of infants to bring themselves or to be brought by others to a lower state.	From crying to active alert, quiet alert, drowsy, or sleep states.	Crying is the infant behavior that presents the greatest challenge to caregivers. Parents' success or failure in consoling their infants has a significant impact on their feelings of competence as parents.
SELF-CONSOLING Maneuvers used by infants to console themselves and move to a lower state: ■ Hand-to-mouth movement. ■ Sucking on fingers, fist, or tongue. ■ Paying attention to voices or faces. ■ Changes in position.	From crying to active alert, quiet alert, drowsy, or sleep states.	If caregivers are aware of these behaviors, they may allow infants the opportunity to gain control of themselves. This does not imply that newborns should be left to cry. Once newborns are crying and do not initiate self-consoling activities, they may need attention from caregivers.
CONSOLING BY CAREGIVERS After crying for longer than 15 seconds, the caregivers may try to: ■ Show face to infant. ■ Talk to infant in a steady, soft voice. ■ Hold both infant's arms close to body. ■ Swaddle infant. ■ Pick up infant. ■ Rock infant. ■ Give a pacifier or feed.	From crying to active alert, quiet alert, drowsy, or sleep states.	Often parental initial reaction is to pick up infants or feed them when they cry. Parents could be taught to try other soothing maneuvers.
MOTOR BEHAVIOR AND ACTIVITY Spontaneous movements of extremities and body when stimulated vs. when left alone. Smooth, rhythmical movements vs. jerky ones.	Quiet alert, active alert.	Smooth, nonjerky movements with periods of inactivity seem most natural. Some parents see jerky movements and startles as negative response to their caregiving and are frightened.

Signs of Potential Problems. Behavioral patterns, sensory capabilities, and signs of potential problems are described in Table 21-2. Knowledge of normal physical and behaviorial characteristics and signs of potential problems (see Chapter 20) is essential for the nurse. Gestational age assessments can identify the preterm, postterm, or postmature infant or one who is small or large for age (see Chapter 37). General assessment may reveal developmental problems such as jaundice or congenital anomalies (see Chapter 38). Assessment findings may suggest acquired problems such as birth injuries and sequelae to a pregnancy complicated by diabetes, infection, or substance abuse (see Chapter 39).

NURSING DIAGNOSES

Analysis of the significance of findings collected during assessment leads to the establishment of nursing diagnoses. Possible nursing diagnoses for the *newborn* are as follows:

- Ineffective breathing pattern related to
  —Obstructed airway
- Impaired gas exchange related to
  —Hypothermia (cold stress)
- High risk for ineffective thermoregulation related to
  —Heat loss to environment
- High risk for infection related to
  —Environmental factors
- High risk for pain related to
  —Circumcision

Possible nursing diagnoses *for the parent or parents* are as follows:

- Family coping, potential for growth related to
  —Knowledge of newborn's social capabilities
  —Knowledge of newborn's dependency needs
  —Knowledge of biologic characteristics of the newborn
- Situational low self-esteem related to
  —Misinterpretation of newborn's responses

The nursing plan of care on p. 612 provides examples of formulating nursing diagnoses from specific assessment findings.

PLANNING

Plans for care of the newborn reflect the rapid growth and development during the neonatal period. Changes in biologic and behavioral states are measured in minutes and hours since birth. The neonatal period extends through the first 28 days after birth. By that time the rate of changes has slowed enough so that the child's appearance and needs can be referred to in terms of weeks and months.

The focus of care changes between birth and 28 days. During the first 2 hours of life (HOL) the main focus is on the infant's physiologic adaptation. By the end of the neonatal period the infant's socialization needs assume equal importance with physiologic needs.

The care given the neonate during the *first* 2 HOL is part of the care given parents and newborns in the fourth stage of labor (see Chapter 19). Care related to *nutritional needs* of infants, including techniques of feeding, is presented in Chapter 22. *Parent-child interactions* are discussed in detail in Chapters 24 and 25.

The information in this chapter pertains to the maintenance of vital functions, the daily care of infants, and the forms of general therapy carried out routinely in newborn nurseries. Parental education before discharge from the hospital and at the well-baby visit is outlined.

Goals

The expected outcomes for newborn care relate to the infant and to the caregiver. The *goals for the infant* include the following:

- The infant will make the transition from intrauterine to extrauterine life.
- The infant will maintain effective breathing patterns.
- The infant will experience minimal pain related to circumcision.
- The infant will maintain effective thermoregulation.
- The infant will remain free from infection.

Goals for the parents include the following:

- The parent(s) will attain knowledge, skill, and confidence relevant to child-care activities.
- Parents will state understanding of biologic and behavioral characteristics of the newborn.
- Parent(s) will demonstrate behavior/life-style changes to reduce potential for development of problems.
- The parent(s) will have opportunities to intensify relationships with their newborn.

IMPLEMENTATION

Neonatal care includes techniques for health maintenance, detection of disability, and institution of remedial measures. These techniques can be used for teaching purposes. Careful and concise recording of client responses or laboratory results contributes to the continuous supervision vital to mother, newborn, and family.

TABLE 21-2 Infant Behavioral Patterns and Sensory Capabilities

Item	Normal Parameters	Deviations From Normal/Probable Conditions
BEHAVIORAL PATTERNS		
Feeding	Cortical control and responsiveness	Central nervous system (CNS) disorders
	Variations in interest, hunger; usually feeds well within 24 hr of birth	Lethargic, tires easily or may perspire while attempting to feed; poor suck, poor coordination with swallow, cyanosis, choking
Social	Cry is lusty, strong; soon indicative of hunger, pain, attention seeking	Weak or absent; high pitched
	Smiling, focusing evident within first week	Absence; no focusing on person holding her or him; unconsolable
	Responds by quietness and increased alertness to cuddling, voice	
Sleep-wakefulness	Transitional period with two periods of reactivity: at birth and 6-8 hr later (see Chapter 20)	Lethargy; drowsiness
	Stabilization with wakeful periods about every 3-4 hr	Disorganized pattern
Elimination	Develops own pattern within first 2 weeks:	See pp. 536 and 568
	Stooling, see p. 536	
	Urination (see Renal System, p. 534)	Diminished number: dehydration
	First few days: 3-4 times daily	
	End of first week: 5-6 times daily	
	Later: 6-10 times daily with adequate hydration	
Reflex response	Brain-stem development and musculoskeletal intactness	Present in anencephalic newborns also
	See Reflexes (p. 546)	Absence; hyperreactive; incomplete; asynchronous
SENSORY CAPABILITIES		
Vision	Limited accommodation with clearest vision within 18-20 cm (7-8 in)	Absence of these responses may be caused by absence of or diminished acuity or by sensory deprivation.
	Detects color by 2 months but attracted by black-white pattern at 5 days or less	
	Focuses and follows by 15 min of age	
	Prefers patterns to plain surfaces	
	Prefers changes in patterns by 2 mo	
	At birth, can gaze intently	
Hearing	By 2 min of age, moves eyes in direction of sound	Absence of response: deafness
	Responds to high pitch by "freezing," followed by agitation; to low pitch (crooning) by relaxation	
	Can hear beginning in last trimester of fetal life	
Touch	Sensitivity to pain may be diminished (because of β-endorphins present prenatally)	Unable to be comforted; possible drug dependence
	Soothed by massaging, warmth, weightlessness (as in warm water bath)	
Smell	By days 2-7 can distinguish between own mother's used breast pads and those of another woman	
Taste	By 3 days of age, can distinguish between sucrose and glucose and grimaces in response to drop of lemon juice on tongue	
Motor	Coordinates body movement to parent's voice and body movement; imitates parent's actions by 2 wk of age	Absence

A nurse working with infants has a responsibility to assess the health of the newborn and provide appropriate care. An eight-point check system (Ragan, Weinfield, 1989) has been developed to assist with assessing the newborn. The memory device, *v*ery *a*ctive *c*hildren *n*eed *e*xcellent *c*omforting *c*are *a*lways for the acronym VACNECCA (*v*ital signs, *a*ctivity, *c*olor, *n*utrition, *e*limination, *c*ord, *c*ircumcision, and *a*ttachment), facilitates a quick and thorough assessment. Such assessments should occur on every shift. The nurse's ease in handling and caring for the infant encourages new parents and serves as a role model. To anticipate and answer new parents' questions, the nurse needs to fully understand newborn care.

Protective Environment

The provision of a **protective environment** is basic to the care of the newborn. The construction, maintenance, and operation of nurseries in accredited hospitals are monitored by national professional organizations such as the American Academy of Pediatrics and local or state governing bodies. Prescribed standards cover areas such as the following:

1. *Environmental factors:* provision of adequate lighting, elimination of potential fire hazards, safety of electric appliances, adequate ventilation, controlled temperature (warm and free of drafts) and humidity (lower than 50%)
2. *Measures to control infection:* adequate floor space to permit positioning bassinets at least 60 cm (24 in) apart, hand-washing facilities, techniques for safe formula preparation and storage, and cleaning and sterilizing of equipment and supplies

In addition, hospital personnel develop their own policies and procedures directed toward protecting the newborns under their care, such as those that follow.

1. Nursery personnel are restricted to those directly involved in the care of mothers and infants, thereby reducing the opportunities for the introduction of pathogenic organisms. Personnel are instructed to use good hand-washing techniques: "The most important single measure in the prevention of neonatal infection is handwashing between each infant handling" (Larson, 1987).
2. In light of the acquired immunodeficiency syndrome (AIDS) issue the Centers for Disease Control (CDC) in Atlanta recommended the following practice (NAACOG, 1986a): *health care workers must wear gloves when touching mucous membranes or nonintact skin of all patients.* In addition, masks, eye coverings, and gowns must be used when indicated. Health care personnel must *wear gloves and gowns when handling the infant until blood and amniotic fluid have been removed from the infant's skin, when drawing blood (e.g., heel stick), and when caring for a fresh wound (e.g. circumcision).*
3. Persons coming from "outside" are expected to wash their hands before coming in contact with infants or equipment, for example, nurses, physicians, parents, brothers and sisters, department supervisors, electricians, and housekeepers.
4. Individuals with infectious conditions are excluded from contact or must take special precautions when working with newborns. This includes persons with upper respiratory tract infections, gastrointestinal tract infections, and infectious skin conditions. Most agencies have now coupled this day-to-day self-screening of personnel with yearly health examinations.
5. Health care workers should wear gowns and gloves when caring for people with herpes. Good hand-washing techniques are required at all times. Visitors usually are not restricted.

Cover gowns do not need to be worn in providing care for healthy newborns (see Research Highlight, p. 588).

Maintenance of Vital Functions

BODY TEMPERATURE. During all procedures heat loss must be avoided or minimized for the newborn. This can be accomplished by placing the newborn under overhead radiant heat or using another source of heat (e.g., an incubator). Cold stress is detrimental to the newborn (see Chapter 20). It increases the need for oxygen and can upset the acid-base balance. The infant may react by increasing its respiratory rate and may become cyanotic. An axillary temperature should be taken every hour until the newborn's temperature stabilizes. Initial temperatures as low as 96.8° F (36° C) are not uncommon. By the twelfth hour, the temperature should stabilize within the normal range.

The nurse can help stabilize the newborn's body temperature in several ways. One is to check the temperature in the nursery. (The ambient temperature of the nursery unit should be 75° F [24° C].) A second is to keep the newborn dry and wrapped in warmed blankets immediately after birth, taking care to keep the head well covered while the parent is holding the newborn. (The newborn's body temperature should be checked at least every hour until it is stabilized. This also helps prevent hyperthermia.)

During the first 1 to 2 hours after birth, the nurse places the thoroughly dried, unclothed baby under a radiant heat panel until the body temperature is stabilized. In an incubator with a servocontrol mechanism the infant's skin temperature is used as the point of control. The control panel usually is maintained between 96.8° and 98.6° F (36° and 37° C). This setting should maintain the infant's skin temperature around 97.6° F (36.5° C). A **thermistor probe** (automatic sensor) is taped to the right upper quadrant of the abdomen immediately below the right intercostal margin, never over a bone. This will ensure detection of minor changes resulting from peripheral vasconstriction, dilatation, or increased metabolism long before a change in deep (core) body temperature develops. The other end of the probe cord is attached to the control panel. The sensor needs to be checked periodically to make sure it is securely attached to the infant's skin. The core temperature of the newborn is checked by axilla every hour with a thermometer.

Other examinations and activities are performed with the newborn under a heat panel. The initial bath is postponed until the newborn's skin temperature reaches 97.6° F (36.5° C) and is maintained for at least for 1 hour. To minimize the heat loss, an overhead radiant heat source is used during a newborn assessment. To prevent overheating, the infant should remain unclothed while under an overhead heat panel or in an incubator with a servocontrol mechanism.

WARMING INFANT WITH HYPOTHERMIA. Even a normal full-term baby in good health can become hypothermic. Birth in a car on the way to the hospital, a cold delivery room, or inadequate drying and wrapping immediately after birth may cause the infant's temperature to fall below the normal range (**hypothermia**). Warming the hypothermic baby is accomplished with care. Rapid warming or cooling may cause apneic spells and acidosis in an infant. Therefore the warming process is monitored to progress slowly over a period of 2 to 4 hours.

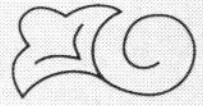 **Research Highlight** 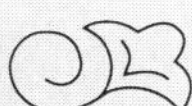

Wearing Cover Gowns to Care for Healthy Newborns

RESEARCH ABSTRACT

The wearing of cover gowns by nurses and visitors while handling newborn infants is a routine practice in many health care settings. The purpose of this study was to determine whether the rate of colonization with *Staphylococcus aureus* in the neonatal nares or umbilicus on the third day of life or day of discharge was increased when cover gowns were not worn. The 222 infants in the experimental group were cared for without cover gowns; the 230 infants in the control group were cared for with cover gowns. The researchers found that 20% of the experimental group and 21% of the control group had positive culture results. Two infants in each group had symptoms of *S. aureus* infection. Infants with positive culture results had mothers with longer labors, more vaginal examinations, and included more male infants who had been circumcised. The researchers concluded that routine use of cover gowns is unnecessary.

IMPLICATIONS FOR PRACTICE

Wearing cover gowns as a means to control infections may give nurses and others a false sense of security. This study supports the view that nurses and visitors who are healthy and use good hand-washing technique do not present a hazard to a newborn. Discarding routine use of cover gowns results in a significant cost saving for the nursery.

RELATED RESEARCH QUESTIONS

1. Does type of cord care make a difference in colonization rate?
2. Does type of preparation for circumcision make a difference in colonization rate?
3. Does type of postcircumcision care make a difference in colonization rate?
4. Do visitors and nurses routinely use good hand-washing technique before handling a newborn?

REFERENCE

Rush J et al: A randomized controlled trial of a nursery ritual: wearing cover gowns to care for healthy newborns, Birth 17(1):25, 1990.

ADEQUATE OXYGEN SUPPLY. Establishing a patent airway is a primary objective during delivery and remains a primary nursing goal. Four conditions are essential for maintenance of an adequate oxygen supply:

- A clear airway, fundamental to adequate ventilation
- Respiratory efforts, necessary to ensure continued ventilation
- A functioning cardiopulmonary system, essential to maintain oxygen
- Heat support, necessary because exposure to cold stress increases oxygen needs

MAINTENANCE OF CLEAR AIRWAY. Generally the normal full-term infant born vaginally has little difficulty clearing the air passages. Most secretions are drained by gravity, propelled to the oropharynx by the cough reflex, to be drained or swallowed. The infant is maintained in a side-lying position with a rolled blanket at the back to facilitate drainage (Fig. 21-2). If excessive mucus is present, the foot of the crib is elevated and the oropharynx is suctioned with a bulb syringe (Fig. 21-3) or a DeLee mucous-trap catheter (Fig. 21-4). The nurse's knowledge and skill in suctioning may be critical in helping both normal and distressed infants to establish or maintain adequate respirations. "Milking" the trachea is ineffective, it may injure cartilage and often will delay effective suctioning.

SUCTIONING OF UPPER AIRWAY. If the infant has excess mucus in the respiratory tract, the nurse may need to aspirate the mouth and nasal passages with a bulb syringe. The infant who is coughing and choking on the secretions should be supported with its head downward. The infant should never be suspended by the ankles. The mouth is suctioned first. This prevents the infant from inhaling pharyngeal secretions by gasping as the nares are touched. The bulb is compressed and inserted into one side of the mouth. The center of the infant's mouth is avoided because this could stimulate the gag reflex. The nasal passages are suctioned one nostril at a time. When the infant's cry does not sound as though it were through mucus or a bubble, suctioning can be stopped. The bulb syringe should always

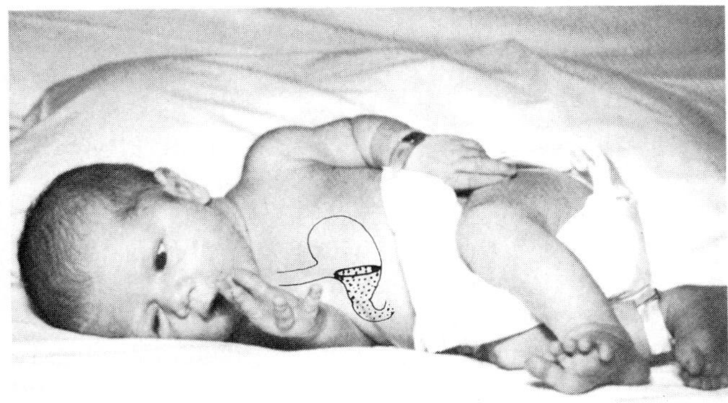

Fig. 21-2 Infant is turned to right side and supported in this position to facilitate drainage from mouth and to promote emptying of stomach contents into the small intestine.

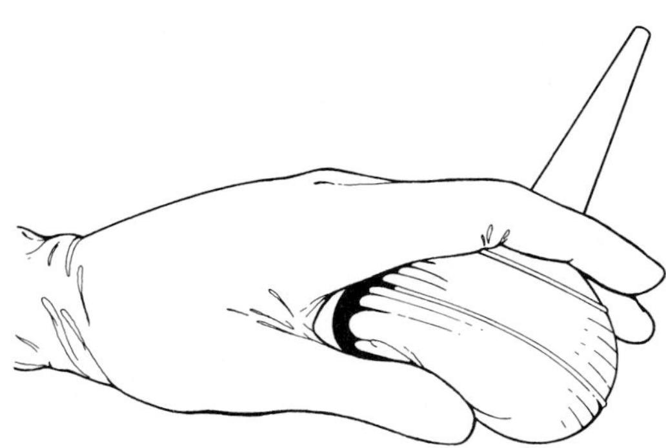

Fig. 21-3 Bulb syringe. Bulb must be compressed before insertion.
From Smith DP et al: *Comprehensive child and family nursing*, St Louis, 1991, Mosby–Year Book.

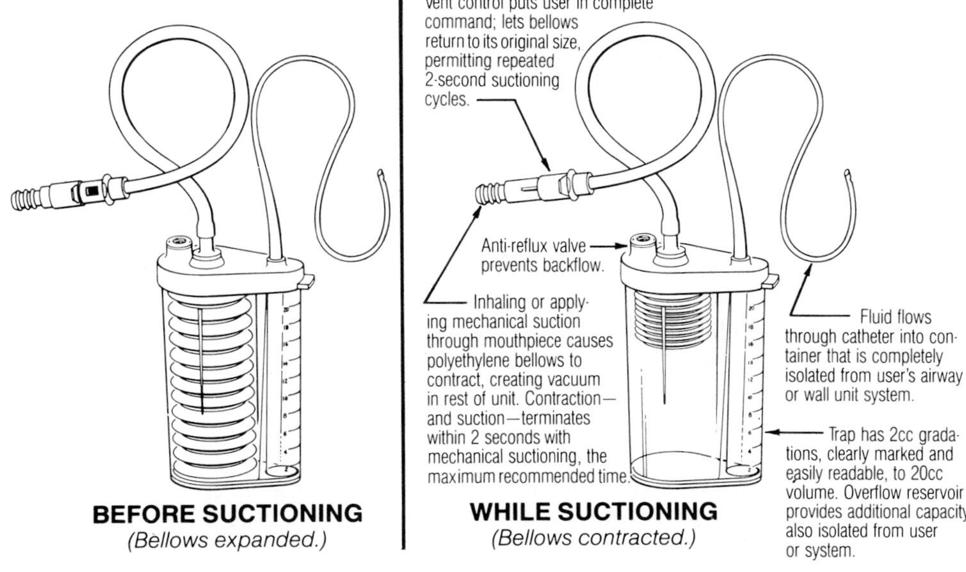
Vent control puts user in complete command; lets bellows return to its original size, permitting repeated 2-second suctioning cycles.
Anti-reflux valve prevents backflow.
Inhaling or applying mechanical suction through mouthpiece causes polyethylene bellows to contract, creating vacuum in rest of unit. Contraction—and suction—terminates within 2 seconds with mechanical suctioning, the maximum recommended time.
Fluid flows through catheter into container that is completely isolated from user's airway or wall unit system.
Trap has 2cc gradations, clearly marked and easily readable, to 20cc volume. Overflow reservoir provides additional capacity, also isolated from user or system.
BEFORE SUCTIONING
(Bellows expanded.)
WHILE SUCTIONING
(Bellows contracted.)

Fig. 21-4 (Isolated) DeLee suction method with catheter and mucus trap.
Courtesy Busse Hospital Disposables, PO Box 011067, Hauppauge, NY 11788-0920.

be kept in the infant's crib. The parents should be given demonstrations on how to use the bulb syringe. They should be asked to perform a return demonstration.

A DeLee mucous-trap suction apparatus may be needed to remove secretions. The catheter tip should be lubricated with sterile water before it is inserted through the nares. A 120 mL (4 oz) bottle of sterile water for feeding is convenient, already in a sterile container, and decreases risk of contamination possible with large stock bottles. The suction apparatus is placed in the user's mouth, and gentle suction is applied as the tube is rotated and removed from the infant's nose. The procedure also can be performed by inserting the tube through the infant's mouth along the base of the tongue. To prevent tissue trauma, forcing the catheter should be avoided. Correct placement is determined by the stimulation of the infant's gagging reflex, which indicates entrance into the esophagus, or coughing, which indicates entrance into the trachea. Suctioning should be discontinued when the cry is clear. The amount of mucus obtained may be sent to the laboratory for examination and cultures if necessary.

The DeLee mucous-trap suction apparatus is used most commonly in labor and delivery. Many health care facilities have discontinued use of the regular DeLee device because of AIDS precautions and the possibility of the users' drawing mucus from the infant into their own mouth. The isolated DeLee suction method (Busse bac/shield) provides safe oral or mechanical suctioning of neonates while preventing the transmission of bacteria, viruses, and other infectious material from the newborn to the user (Fig. 21-4).

USE OF A NASOPHARYNGEAL CATHETER WITH MECHANICAL SUCTION APPARATUS. Deeper suctioning may be necessary to remove excessive or tenacious mucus from the infant's nasopharynx. The same procedure is followed for deep suctioning as just described with the DeLee device. Proper tube insertion and suctioning 5 seconds or less per tube insertion will help prevent laryngospasms and oxygen depletion. If wall suction is used, the pressure should be adjusted to less than 100 mm Hg. The catheter is lubricated in sterile water (see above). After the catheter is properly placed, suction is created by placing one's thumb over the control as the catheter is carefully rotated and gently withdrawn. This procedure may need to be repeated until the infant's cry sounds clear and air entry into lungs is heard by stethoscope. Allow time between suctioning for adequate ventilation with 100% oxygen as needed.

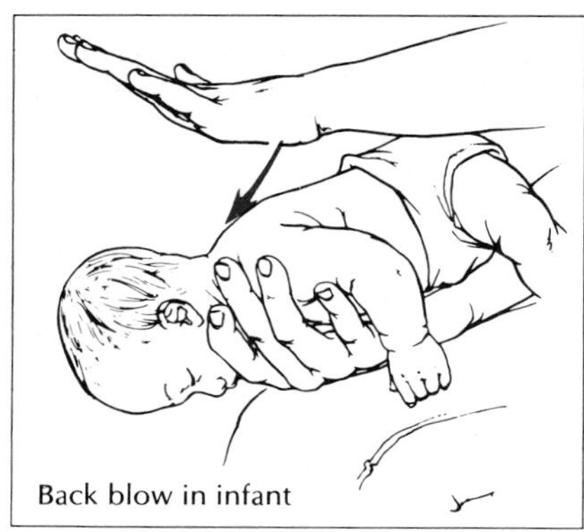

Fig. 21-5 Back blow in infant for clearing airway obstruction.
From Guidelines for Cardiopulmonary Resuscitation (CPR) and Emergency Cardiac Care (ECC): *JAMA* 268(16):2171, 1992.

RELIEVING AIRWAY OBSTRUCTION. A choking infant needs immediate attention. The infant is placed face down over the rescuer's arm with the head lower than the trunk and the head supported. Additional support can be achieved if the rescuer supports her or his own arm firmly against her or his thigh (American Academy of Pediatrics, 1986). Four quick, sharp back blows are delivered between the infant's shoulder blades with the heel of the rescuer's hand (Fig. 21-5). After delivery of the back blows, the rescuer's free hand is placed flat on the infant's back so that the infant is "sandwiched" between the two hands, making certain the neck and chin are well supported. While the rescuer maintains support with the infant's head lower than the trunk, the infant is turned and placed supine on the rescuer's thigh, where four chest thrusts are applied in rapid succession in the same manner as external chest compressions described for **cardiopulmonary resuscitation (CPR)** (see emergency procedures, pp. 591 and 593).

Often, simply repositioning the infant and suctioning the mouth and nose with the bulb syringe corrects the situation. The nurse listens to respirations and lung sounds with a stethoscope to determine the presence of rales, rhonchi, and wheezes. The infant is positioned with head down to facilitate gravity drainage. If the lungs are clear, the bulb syringe is used to clear the mouth and nose. If the bulb syringe does not provide relief, a DeLee mucous-trap suction apparatus may be needed to remove mucus obstructing the nasopharynx and oropharynx. If available, mechanical suction can be used.

All personnel working with infants must have current infant CPR certification. Many institutions offer infant CPR courses to new parents (Donaher-Wag-

EMERGENCY

Cardiopulmonary Resuscitation (CPR)

Wash hands before and after touching infant and equipment. Glove.

RESUSCITATION (Fig. 21-6)

Observe color; tap, or gently shake shoulders.
Yell for help; if alone, perform CPR for 1 min before calling for help again.
Turn infant to back, supporting head and neck.
Place on firm, flat surface.
Clear airway, prn (see below).
Tilt head back gently to "sniffing" or neutral position; use head-tilt/chin-lift maneuver (Fig. 21-6).
Do not hyperextend neck.
Assess for evidence of breathing:
Observe for chest movement.
Listen for exhaled air.
Feel for exhaled air flow.
Breathe for infant (Fig. 21-6):
Take a breath.
Open mouth wide and place over mouth and nose of infant to create seal. (See emergency procedure, p. 593).
NOTE: Repeat the word *ho* as you gently puff volume of air *in your* cheeks into infant. *Do not* force air.
Infant's chest should rise slightly with each puff; keep fingers on chest wall to sense air entry.
Give two slow breaths (1 to 1.5 sec/breath), pausing to inhale between breaths.
Check pulse of brachial artery (Fig. 21-6) while maintaining head tilt.
If pulse is present, initiate rescue breathing. Continue until spontaneous breathing resumes at rate of every 3 sec or 20 times/min.
If pulse is not present, initiate chest compressions and coordinate with breathing.
NOTE: When two people are present, breathing and compressions are shared.
Provide compressions/breathing:
Pause at end of every fifth compression to allow chest to fall by passive recoil.
Maintain 5:1 ratio for 1 or 2 rescuers.
Reassess after 20 cycles, and every few minutes thereafter.
Chest compressions:
Maintain head tilt. With other hand, position fingers for chest compressions.
Place index finger of hand farthest from infant's head just under imaginary line drawn between nipples (Fig. 21-6). Move index finger to a position one fingerbreadth below this intersection.
Using 2 or 3 fingers, compress sternum to depth of ½ or ¾ inch.
Release pressure without moving fingers from the position.
Repeat at a rate of at least 100 times/min; 5 compressions in 3 sec or less.
Perform 20 cycles of 5 compressions and 1 ventilation. (If possible, compressions are accompanied by positive-pressure ventilation at a rate of 40 to 60/min.) Use this memory device: one-two-three-four-five-pause-head tilt-chin lift-ventilate-continue compressions. After cycles, check the brachial pulse to determine presence of pulse.
Discontinue compressions if the infant's spontaneous heart rate reaches or exceeds 80 beats/min.

RELIEVING AIRWAY OBSTRUCTION

Use no blind finger sweeps.
Initiate back blows and chest thrusts (Fig. 21-5).
HAZARD: To avoid the risk of injury to abdominal organs, the Heimlich maneuver (abdominal thrusts) should not be used for infants of 1 year of age or younger.
Position child prone over forearm with head down and with infant's jaw firmly supported.
Rest supporting arm on thigh.
Deliver up to five back blows forcefully between infant's shoulder blades with heel of free hand.
Place free hand on infant's back to sandwich the baby between both hands: one hand supports the neck, jaw, and chest; the other supports the back.
Turn infant over and place head down, supporting head and neck. Provide up to five quick downward chest thrusts to same location as chest compressions.
Open the airway with a head-tilt/chin-lift maneuver and attempt to ventilate.
Repeat the sequence until it is effective.
Alternative position: Place infant face down on your lap with head lower than trunk and head firmly supported. Apply back blows, turn infant, and apply chest thrusts as above.
Continue emergency procedures until signs of recovery occur, as indicated by palpable peripheral pulses, return of pupils to normal size and responsiveness, and the disappearance of mottling and cyanosis.
Record time and duration of procedure and effects of intervention.
Teach procedure to parents or other caregivers.

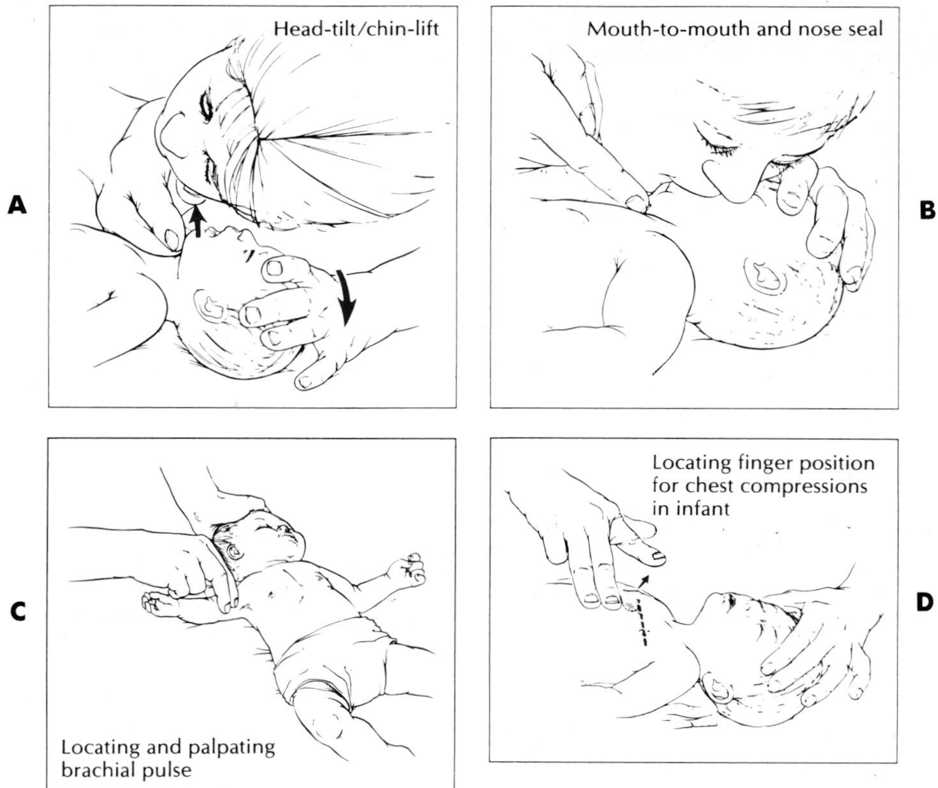

Fig. 21-6 Procedures for cardiopulmonary resuscitation.
From Guidelines for Cardiopulmonary Resuscitation (CPR) and Emergency Cardiac Care (ECC): *JAMA* 286(16):2171, 1992.

ner, Braun, 1992). Cardiac and respiratory arrest can occur in infants. Careful monitoring is necessary so that rapid treatment can be instituted (see emergency box p. 591).

If an abnormal or difficult breathing pattern is observed in an infant (see warning signs, p. 593), steps must be taken to relieve the problem. If respirations cease, mouth-to-mouth resuscitation should be started (see emergency procedure, p. 593). When respiration are reestablished and fairly regular, start oxygen therapy.

Hygienic Care and Safety

Caregiving activities for the newborn are shared by the nurse and the parents. The nurse acts as teacher and support person. As soon as the mother feels physically able, she is encouraged to participate in her child's care. The mother's need for knowledge and the factors that may hinder her learning are determined through questioning and observation. The parent is alerted to the newborn's state-related behaviors and implications for caregiving (Table 21-1) and the newborn's behavioral patterns and sensory capabilities (Table 21-2). The content taught and teaching aids used should reflect the mother's level of understanding. Films and tapes can be valuable timesavers in teaching. Most hospitals provide parents with written instructions for infant care. The care given the child is supervised, and the parents are encouraged to ask questions. The nursing plan of care (p. 612) can serve as a guide for teaching parents.

POSITIONING AND HOLDING. After feeding, positioning the infant on the right side promotes gastric emptying into the small intestine (Fig. 21-2). Placing the infant in the crib in a side-lying position also permits drainage of mucus from the mouth and applies no pressure to the cord or the sensitive circumcised penis. The infant's position is changed from side to side to help develop even contours of the head and to ease pressure on the other parts of the body.

Anatomically the infant's shape—barrel chest and flat, curveless spine—makes it easy for the child to roll and startle. A folded or rolled blanket against the spine will prevent rolling to the supine position and will promote a feeling of security. Care must be taken

EMERGENCY

Mouth-to-Mouth and Mouth-to-Nose Resuscitation

Wash hands before and after touching infant and equipment. Apply gloves.
Clear airway of any mucus or debris.
Position infant in "sniffing" position by putting rolled towel under head to move it slightly forward from neck, or leave infant on flat surface.
Insert plastic airway if available.
Place your mouth over infant's nose and mouth to create seal.
Repeat the word *ho* as you gently *puff* volume of air *in your cheeks* into infant. Do *not* force air.
Repeat puffs at rate of 30/min.
Infant's chest should rise slightly with each puff; keep fingers on chest wall to sense air entry.
Allow chest to fall by passive recoil.
If available, place tubing of oxygen in your mouth as you inhale quickly between puffs.
Consider airway obstruction. Prepare for laryngoscopy and endotracheal intubation aspiration.
Record procedure.

to prevent the infant from rolling off flat, unguarded surfaces. The parent or nurse who must turn away from the infant even for a moment keeps one hand securely on the infant.

The infant is held securely with support for the head because newborns are unable to maintain an erect head posture for more than a few moments. Fig. 21-7 illustrates various positions for holding an infant with adequate support. Too much stimulation is avoided after feeding and before a sleep period.

UMBILICAL CORD CARE. The care of the umbilical cord is the same as that for any surgical wound. The goals of care are prevention and early identification of hemorrhage or infection. If bleeding from the blood vessels of the cord is noted, the nurse checks the clamp (or tie) and applies a second clamp next to the first one. If bleeding is not stopped immediately, the nurse calls for physician assistance at once.

Hospital protocol directs the time and technique for routine cord care. The nurse cleanses the cord and skin area around the base of the cord with the prescribed preparation (e.g., erythromycin solution, triple-blue dye, or alcohol) and checks daily for signs of infection. The cord clamp is removed after 24 to 48 hours when the cord is almost dry (see Fig. 18-16, *D*).

WARNING SIGNS—Abnormal Newborn Breathing

1. Bradypnea: respirations ≤ 25/min
2. Tachypnea: respirations ≥ 60/min
3. Abnormal breath sounds: crackles (rales), rhonchi, wheezes, expiratory grunt
4. **Respiratory distress:** nasal flaring, retractions, chin tug, labored breathing

RASHES

DIAPER RASH. Treatment of diaper rash involves exposing the rash to warmth and air. Immediately washing and drying the wet and soiled area and changing the diaper after voiding or defecating prevents and helps treat diaper rash. The warmth can be achieved with a 25-watt bulb placed 45 cm (18 in) from the affected area. Parents must be cautioned to prevent the lamp from falling on the baby.

The most severe type of diaper rash occurs when the area becomes infected, indurated (hardened), and tender. Medical advice should be sought and a prescribed medication applied.

OTHER RASHES. A rash on the face may result from the infant's scratching **(excoriation)** or from rubbing the face against the sheets, particularly if regurgitated stomach contents are not washed off promptly. Newborn rash, or erythema toxicum, is a common finding (see Chapter 20).

CLOTHING. Parents commonly ask how warmly they should dress their infant. A simple rule of thumb is to dress the child as they dress themselves, adding or subtracting clothes and wraps for the child as necessary. A shirt or diaper may be sufficient clothing for the young infant. A bonnet is needed to protect the scalp and to minimize heat loss if it is cool or to protect against sunburn and to shade the eyes if it is sunny and hot. Wrapping the infant snugly in a blanket maintains body temperature and promotes a feeling of security. Overdressing in warm temperatures can cause discomfort and prickly heat. Underdressing in cold weather also can cause discomfort; cheeks, fingers, and toes can easily become frostbitten.

CARE OF THE INFANT'S LINENS. Care of the infant's clothes and bedding is directed toward minimizing cross infection and removing residues from soap, feces, or urine that may irritate the infant's skin. In the

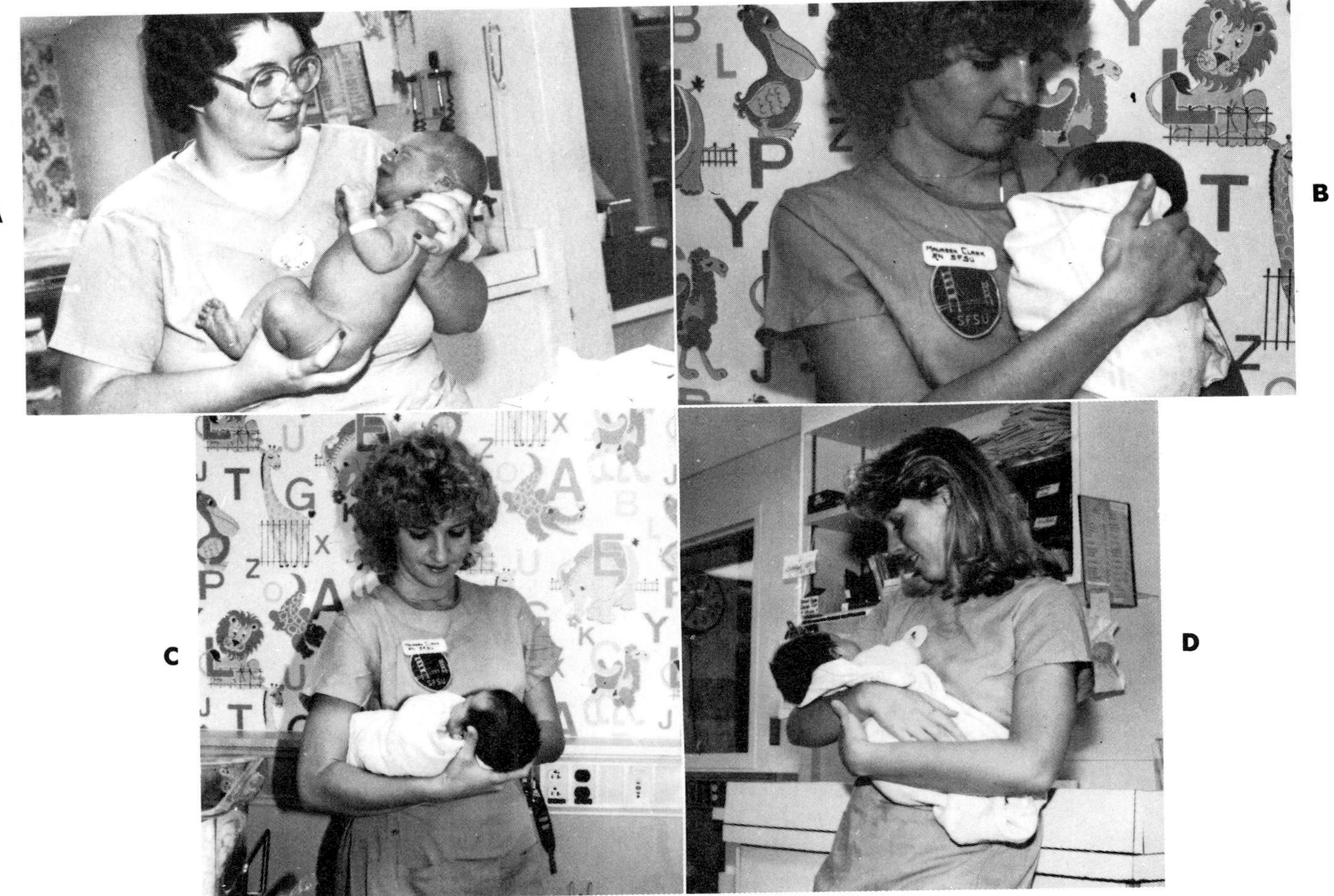

Fig. 21-7 Holding baby securely with support for head. A, Holding infant while moving infant from one place to another. Baby is undressed to show posture. B, Holding baby upright in"burping" position. C, "Football" hold. D, Cradling hold.

hospital, clothing and bedding may be washed separately from other linens and autoclaved. Some hospitals use disposable shirts and diapers. At home the baby's clothes should be washed separately with a mild detergent or soap and hot water. A double rinse usually removes traces of the potentially irritating cleansing agent or acid residue from the urine or stool. If it is possible to do so, drying the clothing and bedding in the sun neutralizes residues. Parents who must use coin-operated machines to wash and dry clothes may find it expensive or impossible to wash and rinse the baby's clothes well.

Bedding requires frequent changing. The plastic-coated, firm mattress must be washed daily and the crib or bassinet damp dusted. The infant's toilet articles may be kept separate and convenient for use in a box or basket.

BATHING. Bathing serves a number of purposes. It provides opportunities for (1) a complete cleansing of the infant, (2) observing the infant's condition, (3) promoting comfort, and (4) parent-child-family socializing (see client teaching box, p. 596). The initial bath is postponed until the infant's skin temperature stabilizes at 36.5° C (97.6° F) or core temperature stabilizes at 37° C (98.6° F) for 2 hours. Until the initial bath is completed, personnel must wear gloves when handling the newborn. In some hospitals the infant is given the initial bath with mild soap to remove blood and amniotic fluid. Cleansing of the genitals as necessary is deemed sufficient for the first 3 to 4 days. Bathing with warm water is sufficient for the first week. Then a mild soap may be used (NAACOG, 1985b). A newborn may not need a bath everyday. Creases under the neck and arms and in the diaper area need more attention. If a documented staphylococcal skin infection outbreak occurs in a nursery, the newborn is bathed with dilute hexachlorophene detergent (pHisoHex) (less than 3%), followed by thorough rinsing of the skin. As pHisoHex is a potential neurotoxin, particularly for infants who weigh less than 2000 g, it is no longer used in many nurseries (see boxes on pp. 596 and 597 for teaching sponge bathing and tub bathing). The nurse does not need to wear gloves during the bath demonstration (Fig. 21-8, p. 598).

Questions have arisen about some routine practices: use of soap, oils, powder, lotion, and sponging. Nursing research can provide needed answers. One of the most important considerations in skin cleansing is a preservation of the skin's **acid mantle,** which is formed from the uppermost horny layer of the epidermis, sweat, superficial fat, metabolic products, and external substances such as amniotic fluid, microorganisms, and cosmetics. At birth, the skin pH is less acidic than that of older infants and adults. Within 4 days, the pH of the newborn's skin surface falls to within the bacteriostatic range (pH < 5) (NAACOG, 1992). Consequently, only plain warm water should be used for the bath (NAACOG, 1985b). Alkaline soaps such as Ivory, oils, powder, and lotions are not used because they alter the acid mantle, thus providing a medium for bacterial growth. The sponging technique generally is used. However, bathing the newborn by immersion has been found to cause less heat loss and less crying, but it should not be done until the umbilical cord falls off (about 10 days to 2 weeks).

Infant's Social Needs

The sensitivity of the caregiver to the social responses of the infant is basic to the development of a mutually satisfying parent-child relationship (see Chapter 24). Sensitivity increases over time as parents' awareness of their infant's social capabilities becomes more acute. (The newborn's social capabilities are discussed in Chapter 20 and Tables 21-1 and 21-2.)

PARENTAL AWARENESS. The mother's assessment of the behavior of her infant (MABI) determines how mothers perceive their infants (Field et al, 1978). It was found that mothers perceived their infants in much the same way as the professional examiner did. For example, mothers noted that postmature infants were not as adaptable or in tune rhythmically with parents. There was one notable exception: mothers were not as aware of the social capabilities of their infants as were the examiners.

Other questionnaires have been developed to study parent-infant relationships. The neonatal perception inventory developed by Broussard and Hartner (cited in Johnson, 1986), compared how a mother perceives her infant in relation to how she views an average baby. This tool can be used to screen for potential maladaptive mother-infant relationship. One way nurses can promote parental sensitivity is to share with the parents the process of the newborn assessment. Performing the newborn assessment in the parents' presence allows them to ask questions about their infant.

PLANNING TIMES FOR SOCIAL INTERACTIONS. The activities of daily care during the neonatal period offer the best time for infant and family interaction. While caring for their baby, parents can talk to the infant, play baby games, and caress and cuddle the child. Parents and infant can engage in arousal, imitation of facial expression, and smiling (Fig. 21-9, p. 599). Older children's contact with a newborn needs to be supervised for strength of hugs, exploring of eyes and nose, and attempts to feed the baby. Parents often keep baby books that record their infant's progress.

Therapeutic Interventions

INTRAMUSCULAR INJECTION. Certain techniques, such as administering vitamin K intramuscularly, are routine in newborn nurseries; however, this is sometimes done in the birth room. Newborn infants offer little, if any, resistance to injections. Although they squirm and may be difficult to hold in position if they are awake, they usually can be restrained without assistance from a second person if the nurse is skilled.

In most cases a 25-gauge ⅝-inch needle should be used. This allows the medication to reach the muscle. A 22-gauge needle may be necessary if thick medications such as some penicillins are to be given.

Selection of the site for injection is important. Injections must be placed in muscles large enough to accommodate the medication, yet major nerves and blood vessels must be avoided. The muscles of newborns may not tolerate a volume of more than 0.5 mL/IM injection. The preferred site for newborns is the vastus lateralis muscle (Fig. 21-10, p. 599), although the rectus femoris muscle also can be used. These two muscles, except for the femoral artery on the medial aspect of the thigh, are free of important nerves and blood vessels. The vastus lateralis muscle is the larger of the two and is well developed in the newborn. The posterior gluteal muscle is very small, poorly developed, and dangerously close to the sciatic nerve, which occupies a larger proportion of space in infants than in older children. Therefore it is not recommended as an injection site until the child has been walking for at least 1 year.

The neonate's leg should be stabilized. It may be necessary to ask someone to hold the leg while the injection is being given. The nurse cleanses the injection site with alcohol and then pinches up the infant's muscle with the thumb and first finger. The

TEACHING Sponge Bathing (Fig. 21-8)

Fitting baths into family's schedule

Give a bath at any time convenient to you but not immediately after a feeding period because the increased handling may cause regurgitation of the feeding.

Preventing heat loss

The temperature of the room should be (75° F) 24° C, and the bathing area should be free of drafts.

Control heat loss during the bath period to conserve the infant's energy. Bathing the infant quickly, exposing only a portion of the body at a time, and thorough drying are therefore parts of the bathing technique.

Preventing skin trauma

The fragile skin can be injured by too vigorous cleansing.

If stool or other debris has dried and caked on the skin, soak the area to remove it. Do not attempt to rub it off because abrasion may result. Gentleness, patting dry rather than rubbing, and use of a mild soap without perfumes or coloring are recommended. Chemicals in the coloring and perfume can cause rashes in sensitive skin.

Gathering supplies and clothing before starting

Clothing suitable for wearing indoors: diaper, shirt; stretch suit or nightgown optional

Unscented, mild soap

Baby lotion, not powder; baby powder can be inhaled by the infant

Pins, if needed for diaper, placed well out of baby's reach

Cotton balls

Towels for drying infant and a clean washcloth

Receiving blanket

Bathing the baby

Bring infant to bathing area when all supplies are ready.

Never leave the infant alone on bath table or in bath water, not even for a second! If you have to leave, take the infant with you or put back into crib.

Test temperature of the water. It should feel pleasantly warm to the inner wrist (about 98° to 99° F).

Do not hold infant under running water—water temperature may change and infant may be scalded or chilled rapidly.

Wash infant's head before unwrapping and undressing to prevent heat loss.

Cleanse the eyes from the canthus outward, using a *clean* washcloth. For the first 2 to 3 days a discharge may result from the reaction of the conjunctiva to the substance (erythromycin) used as a prophylactic measure against infection. Any discharge should be considered abnormal and reported to the physician. When removing eye discharge, avoid contamination of one eye with the discharge from the other by using a separate cotton swab and water source (running water from a tap is best) for each eye.

Wash the *scalp* daily with water and mild soap; rinse well and dry thoroughly. Scalp desquamation, called **cradle cap,** often can be prevented by removing any scales with a fine-toothed comb or brush after washing. If condition persists, the physician may prescribe an ointment to massage into the skin.

Creases under the chin and arms and in the groin may need daily cleansing. The crease under the chin may be exposed by elevating the infant's shoulders 5 cm (2 in) and letting the head drop back.

Cleanse *ears* and *nose* with twists made of moistened cotton. Do not use cotton-tipped swabs.

Undress baby and wash body and arms and legs. Pat dry gently. Baby may be tub bathed after the cord drops off and umbilicus and circumcised penis are completely healed.

Care of the cord

Use a cotton swab. Dip swab in solution the physician has ordered and cleanse around base of the cord, where it joins the skin. Notify your physician of any odor, discharge, or skin inflammation around the cord. The clamp is removed when the cord is dry (about 24-48 hours) (see Fig. 18-16, *D*). When you diaper the infant, the diaper should not cover the cord. A wet or soiled diaper will slow or prevent drying of the cord and foster infection. When the cord drops off in a week to 10 days, small drops of blood can be seen when the baby cries. This will heal itself. It is not dangerous.

Care of hands and feet

Wash and dry between the fingers and toes daily.

Do not cut fingernails and toenails immediately after birth. The nails have to grow out far enough from the skin so that the skin is not cut by mistake. Before the nails can be cut, if the baby scratches himself or herself, you can apply loosely fitted mitts over each hand. Do so as a last resort, however, because it interferes with the baby's ability for self-consolation. When the nails have grown, the *fingernails* and *toenails* can be

Continued.

TEACHING Sponge Bathing—cont'd

cut more readily with manicure scissors (preferably with rounded tips) when the infant is asleep. Nails are kept short.

Cleansing genitals

Cleanse the *genitals* of infants daily and after voiding and defecating. For girls, cleansing of the genitals may be done by separating the labia and gently washing from the pubic area to the anus. For uncircumcised boys, gently pull back (retract) the foreskin. Stop when resistance is felt. Wash the tip (glans) with soap and warm water and replace the foreskin. The foreskin must be returned to its original position to prevent constriction and swelling. In most newborns, the inner layer of the foreskin adheres to the glans. By the age of 3 years, in 90% of boys the foreskin can be retracted easily without pain or trauma. For others, the foreskin is not retractable until the teens. As soon as the foreskin is partly retractable, and the child is old enough, he can be taught self-care.

Dressing the infant

When dressing the child, do not pull shirts roughly over the face or catch fingers in shirt sleeves. Bunch up the shirt in both hands and expand the neck opening before placing the neck opening over the face; then slip the shirt over the rest of the head.

Diapering the infant may be done before and after feeding. It is not necessary to wake the infant for changing.

If cloth diapers are used, absorbency can be increased by bringing the bulk of the diaper in the front for a boy and in the back for a girl. This will help absorb urine so that skin is protected. The diaper between the infant's legs should not be bulky because it can cause outward displacement of the hips. A soaker pad can be placed under the infant as a protection for the blanket. The continued use of plastic or rubber pants may lead to diaper rash.

Store infant's towels, washcloths, and supplies apart from the family for 2 to 4 months to prevent infection.

TEACHING Tub Bathing

See guidelines for sponge bathing.

Place liner on bottom of tub to prevent infant from slipping.

Add 3 inches of comfortably warm water (98° to 99° F—pleasantly warm to the inner wrist).

Wash face and shampoo hair as for sponge bath. Undress baby.

Hold your baby safely. Have your fingers under your baby's armpit, with your thumb around the shoulder. Your other hand supports your baby's bottom and legs.

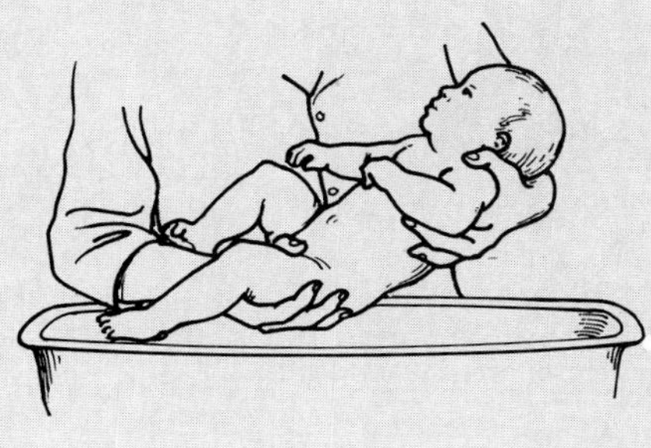

Wash the front of your baby.

Go from front to back between the legs. Rinse with the wet washcloth.

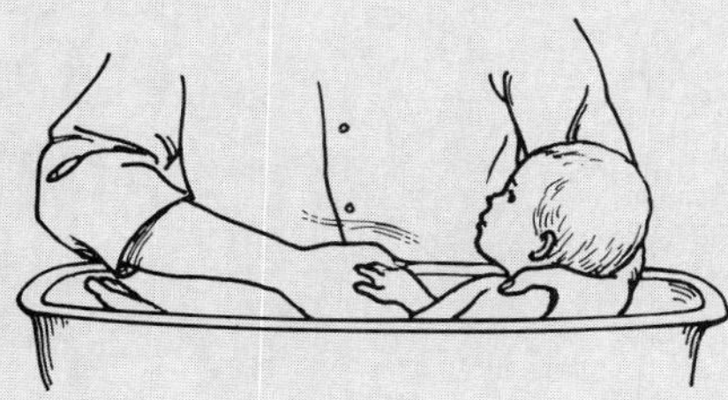

Wash the back of your baby with your free hand lathered with soap.

Rinse well with the wet washcloth.

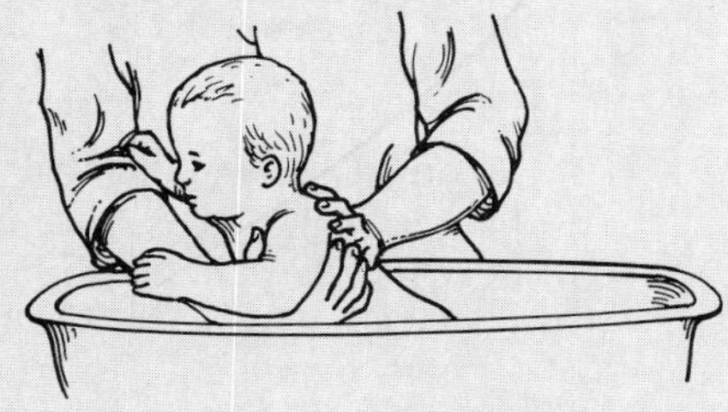

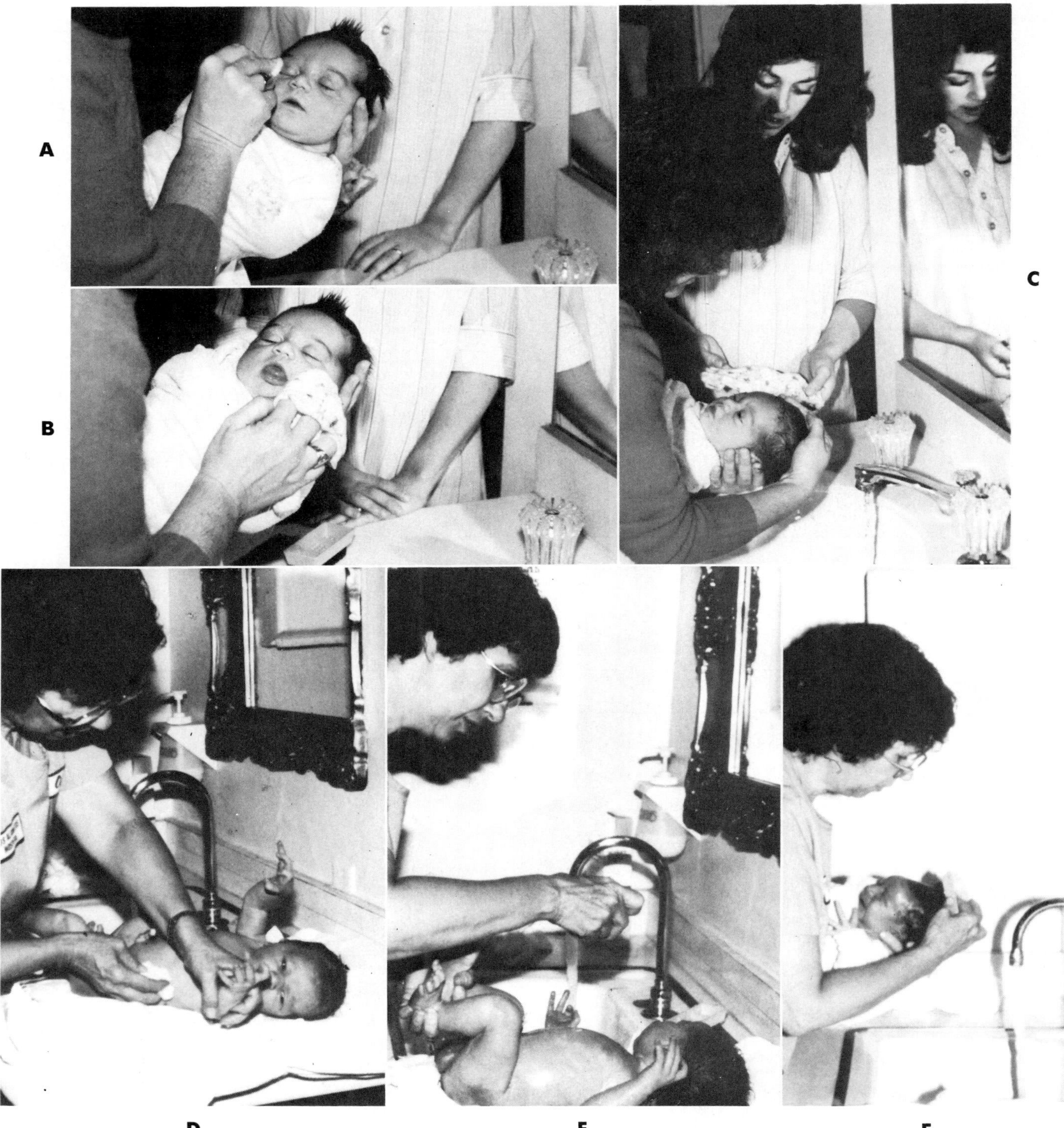

Fig. 21-8 Demonstration baby bath. **A**, Eyes. **B**, Face. **C**, Head and hair. **D**, Sponge-bathing baby. **E**, Rising baby. Do not rinse (or wash) under running water. **F**, Brushing hair. Mother in **A**, **B**, and **C** is being supervised. Note in **D** and **E** that nurse keeps one hand on baby at all times. (Gloves are used only until baby has first bath to remove blood and amniotic fluid.)

Courtesy Marjorie Pyle, RNC, Lifecircle, Costa Mesa, Calif.

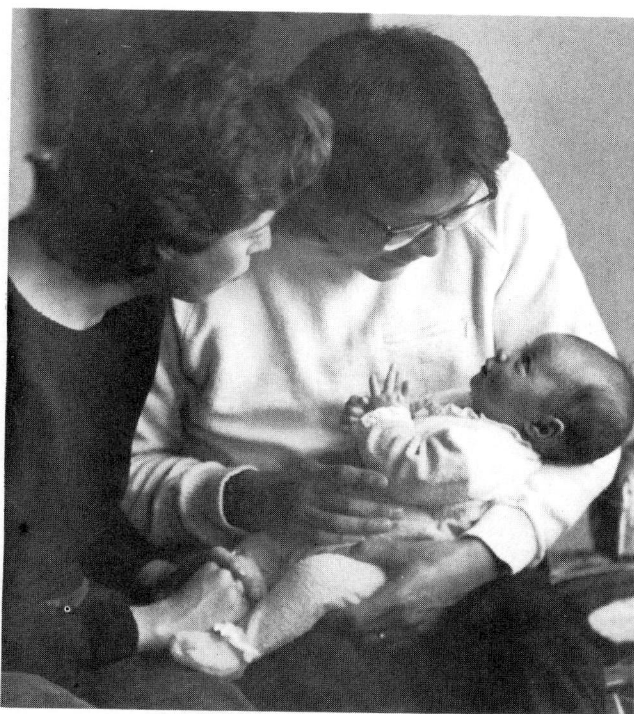

Fig. 21-9 Mother-father-baby interaction.
Courtesy Colleen Stainton.

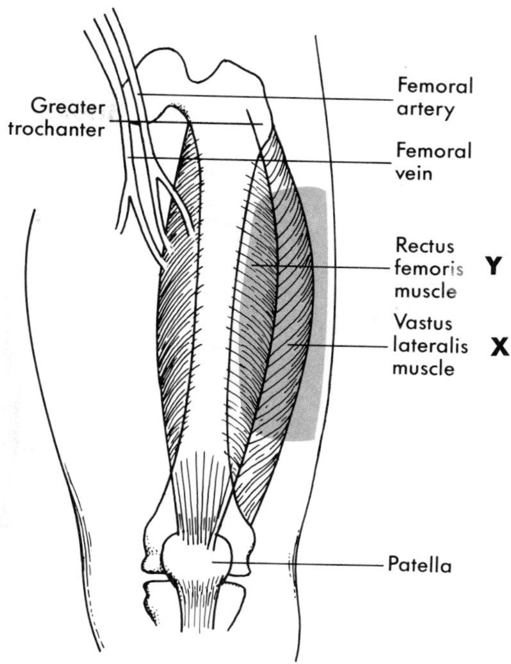

Fig. 21-10 Acceptable intramuscular injection site, lateral aspect of muscle mass in middle third of distance between greater trochanter and patella. *X*, Preferred injection site in vastus lateralis muscle; *Y*, alternate injection site in rectus femoris muscle.

needle is inserted into the vastus lateralis at a 90-degree angle. The muscle is released and the syringe is gently aspirated. If no blood is aspirated, the medication is injected. The needle is withdrawn quickly and the site massaged with an alcohol wipe. It is not uncommon for blood to ooze from the injection site. It is not necessary to cover the site with an adhesive bandage.

The nurse should always remember to comfort the infant after an injection. Then equipment should be properly discarded. It is important to record medication, amount, route, site of injection, and infant's tolerance of injection.

THERAPY FOR HYPERBILIRUBINEMIA. The best therapy for hyperbilirubinemia is prevention. Feeding of the newborn soon after birth stimulates the gastrocolic reflex and the passage of meconium. Because **bilirubin** is excreted in meconium, early feeding stimulates the bowels and may help prevent jaundice. The goal of hyperbilirubinemia treatment is to help the newborn's body reduce serum levels of unconjugated bilirubin. The term infant may have trouble conjugating the increased amount of bilirubin derived from disintegrating fetal red blood cells. Thus the serum levels of unconjugated bilirubin rise beyond normal limits (**hyperbilirubinemia**) (see Chapter 20). If untreated, the levels can continue to rise and the risk of kernicterus increases (see Chapter 38).

There are two principal methods for reducing serum bilirubin levels: exchange blood transfusion and phototherapy. Exchange transfusion is used to treat infants whose levels of bilirubin cannot be controlled by phototherapy (see Chapter 38).

PHOTOTHERAPY. Phototherapy causes reversible isomerization of unconjugated bilirubin in the skin (NAACOG, 1986b; Valman, 1989). During phototherapy infants form a substance called *lumirubin,* a water-soluble product. Lumirubin is formed slowly and excreted rapidly. Lumirubin is excreted both in the urine and feces. Because lumirubin is excreted efficiently by infants, increasing the formation of lumirubin improves the effectiveness of phototherapy in the treatment of neonatal jaundice.

Traditional phototherapy consists of a light source (e.g., four special blue and four daylight bulbs) that will most effectively accomplish the isomerization process. The light source is situated about 18 to 20 inches from the newborn in an incubator, who must wear eye patches. The fluorescent bulbs currently used (daylight, cool light, blue and special blue) have

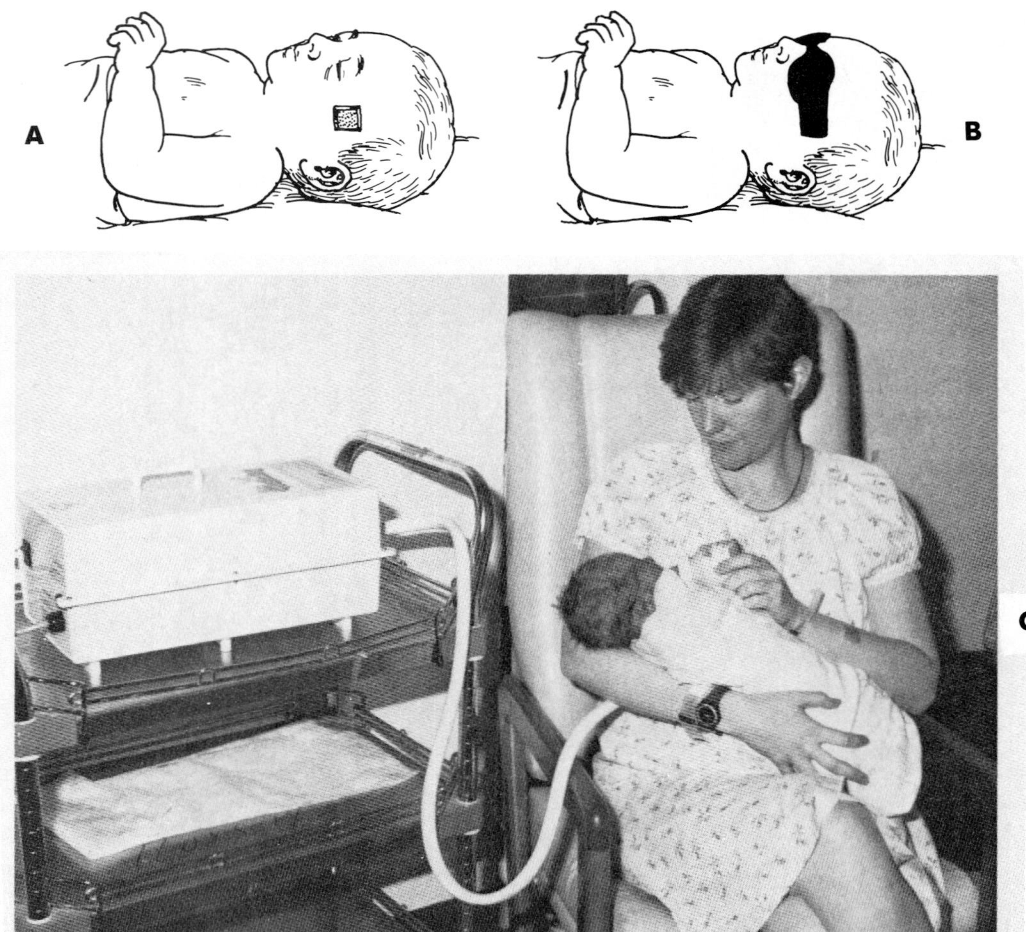

Fig. 21-11 Eye patches for newborn receiving phototherapy. **A,** Small Velcro patch stuck to both sides of head. **B,** Eye cover sticks to Velcro patch, which reduces movement of eye cover and facilitates removal for feedings. **C,** Fiberoptic phototherapy blanket permits baby to be fed, held, and changed without the need for eye patches.
C, Courtesy Rosefeld W, Twist P, Concepcion L: A new device for phototherapy treatment of jaundiced infants, *J Perinatology* (3):243, Sept 1990.

different distribution points on the light spectrum and different peaks of maximal emission. The generally accepted light range for maximum absorption by bilirubin is 400 to 500 nanometers. Blue or special blue lights are considered to be more specific and effective. Blue lights can make the detection of cyanosis in the infant difficult and may strain the nursery staff's eyes (NAACOG, 1986b). The side effects of phototherapy do not appear to produce any long-term effects (Tan, 1989). *Bronze baby syndrome* has occurred in some newborns receiving phototherapy. The serum, urine, and skin turn bronze (brown-black). The cause is unclear. Almost all newborns recover from bronze baby syndrome without sequelae.

In this procedure, the unclothed infant is placed approximately 18 to 20 inches under a bank of lights for several hours or days until the serum bilirubin level drops to an acceptable range. The decision to discontinue therapy is based on a definite downward trend in bilirubin values. After therapy has been terminated, the infant should be retested in several hours to ascertain whether rebound occurs (NAACOG, 1986b).

Several precautions need to be taken while the infant is under phototherapy. The infant's eyes must be protected by an opaque mask to prevent overexposure to the light. The eye shield should be the correct size to completely cover the eyes but not occlude the nares. Before the mask is applied, the infant's eyes should be closed gently to prevent excoriation of the corneas. The mask should be removed during infant feedings so that the eyes can be checked and the infant can receive visual contact with the parents (Fig. 21-11, *A* and *B*).

TEACHING Hyperbilirubinemia

Terms you will hear

Hyperbilirubinemia: higher levels of bilirubin than normal

Bilirubin: end product of RBCs when they mature and break down

Jaundice: yellow color of whites of eyes, skin, and mucous membranes caused by circulating bilirubin

Phototherapy: the use of fluorescent light to break down bilirubin in the skin into substances that can be excreted in the feces (stool) or urine

How jaundice happens

When RBCs break down, they release bilirubin. Bilirubin circulates in the blood. In the liver it is combined with another substance. In the combined form it goes via the blood to the kidneys and the intestines. It gives the yellow color to urine and the brown color to the stool.

Before birth the infant's RBCs were more numerous than the adult's. They also had a shorter life span, 70 to 90 days instead of 120 days. When the RBCs broke down, the baby's blood carried most of the bilirubin via the placenta to the mother's liver to be excreted.

After birth the infant's liver began to take care of all the bilirubin. Even though the baby's liver functions well, it cannot handle the whole load. Bilirubin seeps out of the blood and into the tissues, coloring them yellow. The blood level of bilirubin rises quickly up to the fifth day, and then goes down; the jaundice usually clears up by the end of the week.

If the baby is breast-feeding, a certain amount of the jaundice may be caused by the free fatty acids that interfere with the conjugation of bilirubin.

RBCs, Red blood cells.

The danger of excess bilirubin

Some babies seem to have extra bilirubin to excrete. The amount in the tissues becomes too great when the blood level reaches 12 mg/dL. There is a danger that the bilirubin at high levels will cause damage to the brain. Consequently your physician wants the baby to be placed under the Bililight for phototherapy. This will help the baby eliminate the extra bilirubin and prevent damage to the baby's brain.

Your baby's care

We place eye masks on the baby to keep the light out of the baby's eyes.

We keep the baby undressed so as much light as possible can reach the skin.

We use a paper diaper or the face mask as a small diaper (a "string bikini").

We will take your baby's temperature often so that the infant will not become too hot or too cold.

We will give the baby extra water to drink because infants have watery, green stools from the extra bilirubin being excreted.

We will be taking your baby out from under the lights for feedings and cuddling. We will let you know when to come for feedings and to hold your baby.

We will be taking blood tests to check the amount of bilirubin, and we will let you know the results.

After baby goes home

If you have any questions, ask us any time. We will give you our telephone number, and you can call at any hour. It is hard not being able to take your baby home with you.

Often a "string bikini" made from a disposable face mask is used. This allows optimum skin exposure, yet sufficient protection to the genitals and bedding. The metal strip must be removed from the mask to prevent its overheating and burning the infant. Lotions and ointments also should be avoided because they too can cause the infant to become burned.

Phototherapy may cause the infant to sleep for longer than the usual 4-hour periods. The infant should be kept on a regular feeding schedule. The number and consistency of stools should be monitored. Bilirubin breakdown increases gastric motility, which results in loose stools that can cause skin excoriation and breakdown. The infant's buttocks should be cleaned after each stool to help maintain skin integrity.

Because the infant is unclothed and the lights produce heat, the infant's temperature needs to be monitored. The lights also increase the rate of insensible water loss (NAACOG, 1992). Therefore fluid loss and dehydration also can occur. The infant should be turned every 2 hours to expose all body surfaces to the lights. Accurate charting for phototherapy is necessary.

A new device for phototherapy consisting of a fiberoptic panel attached to an illuminator was compared with traditional phototherapy (Rosenfeld et al, 1990). The researchers found no complications of therapy; the fiberoptic panel proved effective and safe. This new fiberoptic blanket, which wraps light around the newborn's torso, delivers continuous phototherapy. The newborn can remain in the mother's room in an open crib or in her arms during treatment without the need for eye patches (Fig. 21-11, *C*) (Murphy, Oellrich, 1990).

PARENT EDUCATION. Serum levels of bilirubin in the newborn continue to rise until the fifth day of life. Most parents leave the hospital by the third or fourth day and some as early as 2 hours after delivery. Therefore parents must be able to assess the newborn's degree of jaundice. They should have written instructions that include the contact person to whom they should report the infant's condition. Some hospitals have a nurse make a home visit to evaluate the infant's responses. (See the box on p. 601 for parental guidelines concerning hyperbilirubinemia.)

CIRCUMCISION

HISTORICAL PERSPECTIVE. Circumcision has been a rite in many cultures for centuries. It continues to be a religious ritual, for example, in the Jewish faith. Circumcision became a common practice in the United States in the early 1870s. From that time until the 1930s people thought masturbation was harmful and that removal of the foreskin would discourage it by making it less pleasurable. Circumcision also was credited with preventing or curing a number of conditions such as epilepsy, syphilis, asthma, mental illness, and tuberculosis. About 25% of the world's population circumcise their males sometime between birth and young adulthood.

Circumcision is the most commonly performed surgical procedure in the United States. In 1975 the American Academy of Pediatrics (AAP) released a report that supported not circumcising infants (Wiswell, 1990). Past studies indicated there was no connection between circumcision and penile or prostatic cancer and cervical cancer in the female partner.

The use of circumcision for all males to prevent phimosis is unwarranted. **Phimosis** is a *rare* condition that can interfere with or impede the flow of urine (if the foreskin opening is tiny) and can predispose the male to infection between the foreskin and glans.

CURRENT VIEWS. A study conducted at U.S. Army hospitals in 1985 demonstrated a greater than tenfold increase in urinary tract infections in uncircumcised male infants. Circumcision also has been associated with a decrease in the incidence of cancer of the penis among males in the United States. However, evidence regarding the relationship of circumcision to sexually transmitted diseases is conflicting as is evidence linking uncircumcised men to female cervical carcinoma (AAP, 1989). In early 1989 the AAP released a report delineating potential medical benefits and advantages of newborn circumcision (Wiswell, 1990). Controversy still exists, and the elective surgery is left up to the parents.

Circumcision is a matter of personal parental choice. The parents' decision to have their newborn circumcised usually is based on one or more of the following factors: hygiene, religious conviction, tradition, culture, or social norms. Some people do not like to touch their infant's genitals. For these parents, circumcision may be the wisest choice. Regardless of the reason for the decision, it should be made only after parents have the available facts and sufficient time to review their options.

Parents need to begin learning about circumcision during the prenatal period (NAACOG, 1985a). However, circumcision often is not discussed with the parents before labor. In many instances, it is during

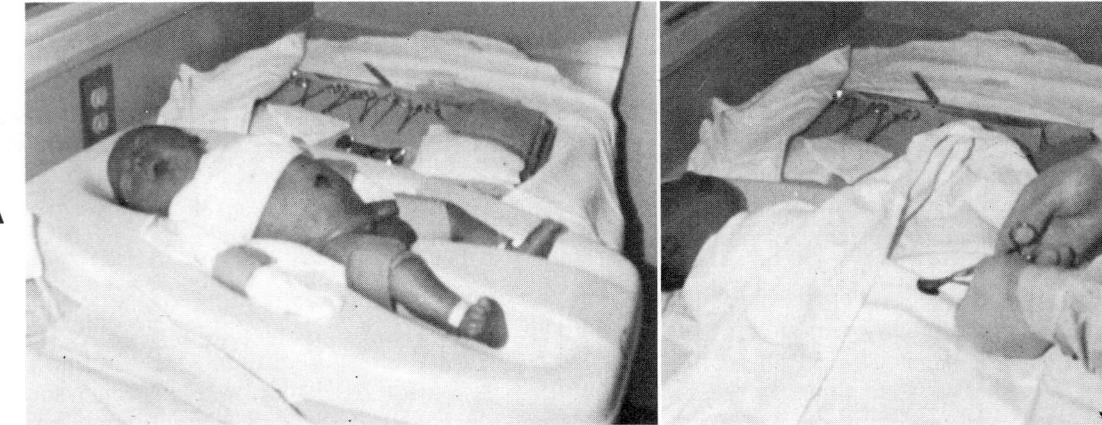

Fig. 21-12 A, Proper positioning of infant in Circumstraint. B, Physician performing circumcision. Baby is completely covered to prevent cold stress.

admission to the hospital or labor unit that the mother confronts the decision regarding circumcision. The stress of the intrapartal period makes this a difficult time for parental decision making, although consenting to their boy's circumcision is ultimately the parent's personal choice. The mother usually is asked to sign a circumcision permit form during this admission procedure. Some hospitals are requiring parents to sign a different form stating they do not wish their male infant to be circumcised if that is their desire.

PROCEDURE. In **circumcision** the prepuce (foreskin) of the glans is removed. The operation is performed in the hospital before the infant's discharge. The circumcision of a Jewish male is performed on the eighth day after birth and is done at home unless the infant is unwell. The procedure is no longer done immediately after birth because the amount of cold stress had proved detrimental to the infant. Clotting factors drop somewhat immediately after birth and return to prebirth levels by the end of the first week. Therefore performing the circumcision after the baby is a week old has a firmer physiologic basis.

For the circumcision procedure the infant is positioned on a plastic restraint form so that his movements are restricted (Fig. 21-12). The penis is cleansed with soap and water or Betadine. The infant is draped to provide warmth and a sterile field. The sterile equipment is readied for use.

Some procedures require no special equipment or appliances (Fig. 21-13). However, numerous instruments have been designed for circumcision. The Yellen clamp (Fig. 21-14) may make this an almost bloodless operation. The procedure takes only a few minutes. After it is completed, a small petrolatum gauze dressing may be applied for the first day to prevent a cloth diaper from adhering. If a Plastibell is used, the bell applies constant direct pressure to prevent hemorrhage. It also protects against infection, sticking to the diaper, and pain with urination. The bell is fitted over the glans. The suture is tied around the rim of the bell. Excess prepuce is cut away. The plastic rim remains in place for about a week until it

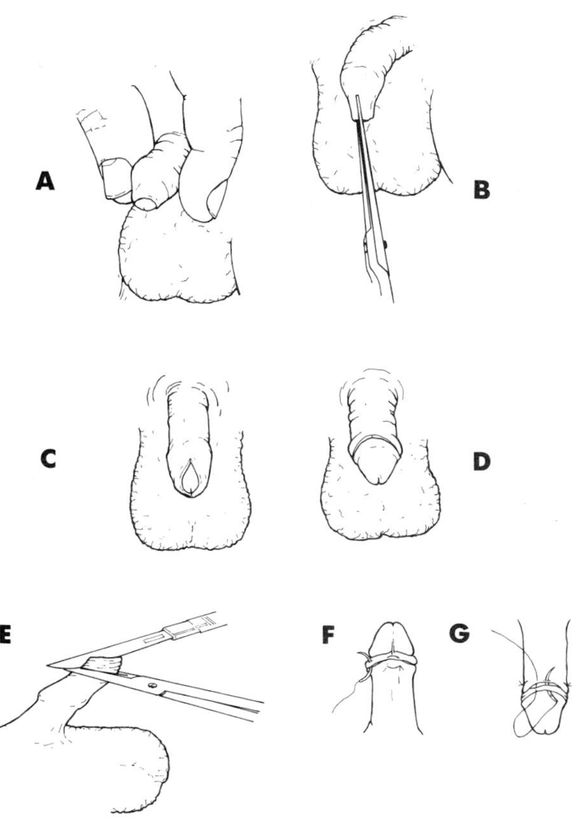

Fig. 21-13 Technique of circumcision. A to D, Prepuce is stripped and slit to facilitate its retraction behind glans penis. E, Prepuce is now clamped and excessive prepuce cut off. F and G, Suture material used is plain 00 or 000 catgut in very small needle, but some physicians prefer silk.

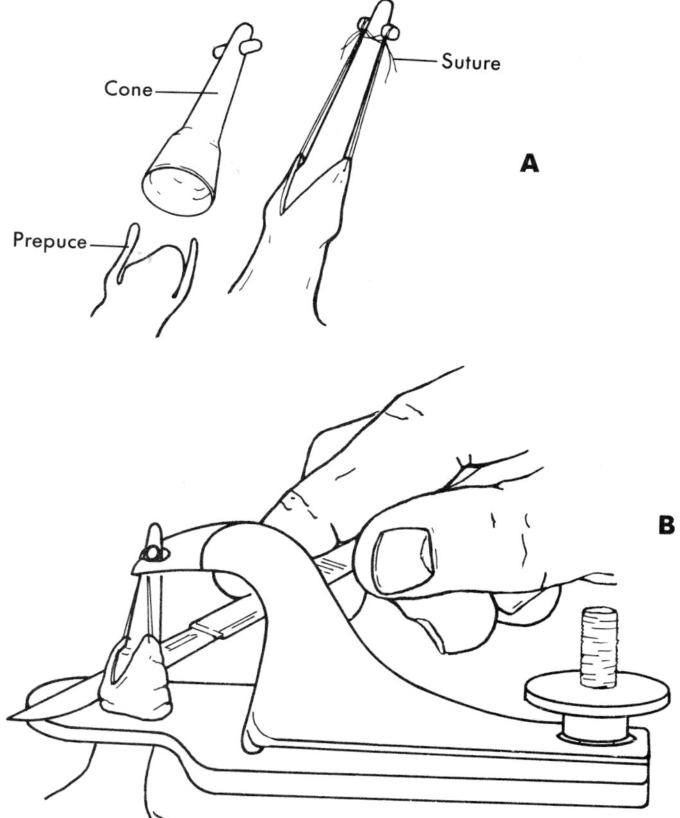

Fig. 21-14 Circumcision with Yellen clamp. A, Prepuce drawn over cone. B, Yellen clamp is applied, hemostasis occurs, then prepuce (over cone) is cut away.

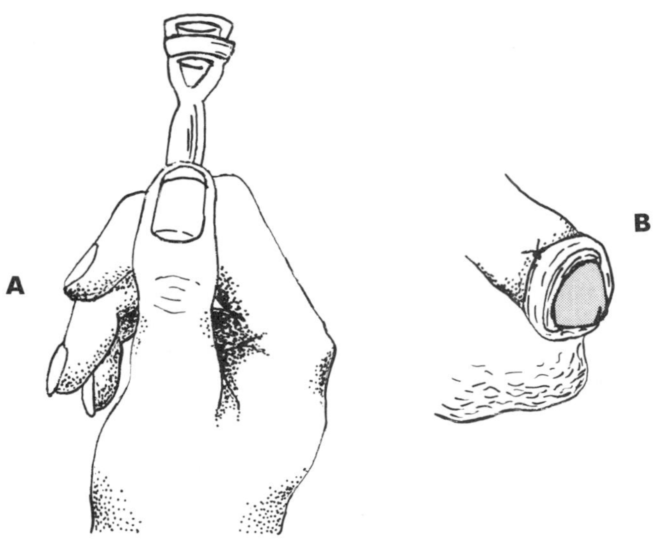

Fig. 21-15 Circumcision using the Plastibell.

falls off, after healing has taken place (Fig. 21-15). Petrolatum gauze is not needed when the bell is used.

DISCOMFORT. If the infant has undergone this surgery without anesthesia, he is comforted until he is quieted (Campos, 1989; Marchette et al, 1991). Then he is returned to his mother. These infants usually are fussy for about 2 to 3 hours and may refuse a feeding. It is not uncommon for the infant to have a loose, green stool after the circumcision.

In the Jewish ritual the newborn is given a few drops of wine to relax him in preparation for the surgery. Dorsal penile nerve blocks may reduce pain and stress during newborn circumcision. Reported use of local anesthesia for circumcision is limited and needs further study. Pain may not end when the operation is over because the wound requires as long as a week to heal.

CARE OF THE NEWLY CIRCUMCISED PENIS. The nurse observes the infant for bleeding and voiding. If bleeding is noted from the circumcision, the nurse applies gentle pressure to the site of bleeding with a folded sterile gauze pad, 4 × 4 inches, or sprinkles on powdered gel foam. If bleeding is not easily controlled, a blood vessel may need to be ligated. One nurse notifies the physician and prepares equipment (circumcision tray and suture) while the other nurse maintains pressure *intermittently* until the physician arrives. The penis is checked hourly for bleeding for 12 hours. If the parents take the baby home before the end of 12 hours, they have to be taught the preceding actions. Before the infant's discharge, the nurse checks to see that the parents have the physician's telephone number.

Nursing actions are planned and implemented to prevent infection. Prepackaged wipes should be avoided because they contain alcohol. The infant should not be placed on his abdomen until the circumcision heals. The nurse washes the penis gently with water to remove urine and feces and reapplies a fresh sterile petrolatum gauze around the glans after each diaper change. The glans penis, normally dark red in appearance during healing, becomes covered with a yellow exudate in 24 hours. This is part of the normal healing process, not an infective process. No attempt is made to remove the exudate, which persists for 2 to 3 days. Parents should be taught to fan-fold the diaper so that it does not press upon the circumcised area. They should be encouraged to change the diaper at least every 4 hours to prevent it from sticking to the penis.

RESTRAINING THE NEWBORN. Reasons for restraining an infant include (1) protecting the infant from injury, (2) facilitating examinations, and (3) limiting discomfort during tests, procedures, and specimen collections. When restraining an infant, one must keep in mind special considerations:

- Check the infant hourly, more frequently if indicated.
- Apply restraints and check them to prevent skin irritation and circulatory impairment.
- Maintain proper body alignment.
- Apply restraints without use of knots or pins if possible. If knots are necessary, make the kind that can be released quickly. Use pins with care to prevent puncture wounds and pressure areas—and to prevent the infant's swallowing one of them.
- If the infant is in an incubator, secure the infant to the mattress to protect the extremities, especially when the lid is raised or the mattress moved.

MUMMY TECHNIQUE. The mummy technique is used with the stronger, more vigorous newborn. It is used during examinations, treatments, or specimen collections that involve the head and neck.

Equipment includes a blanket and one or two large safety pins (Fig 21-16, *A*). The procedure is as follows:

1. Spread blanket on flat surface; a crib could suffice.
2. Fold over one corner (12 o'clock position).
3. Lay newborn on blanket so that neck is at fold.
4. Fold corner at 9 o'clock position over right shoulder; tuck this corner securely under infant's left side.
5. Bring corner at 6 o'clock position up over feet, and either tuck it under infant's left side or, if

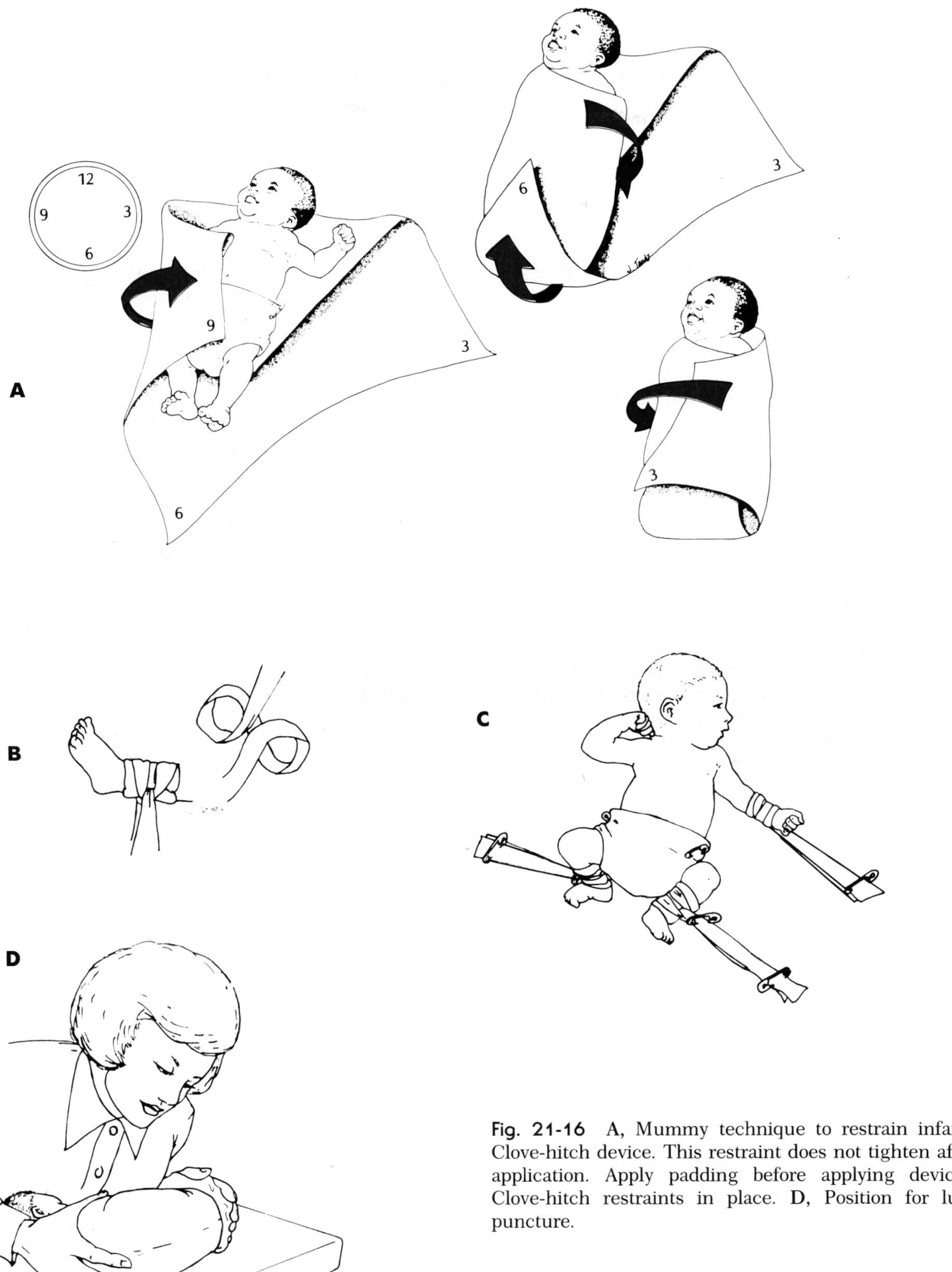

Fig. 21-16 A, Mummy technique to restrain infant. B, Clove-hitch device. This restraint does not tighten after its application. Apply padding before applying device. C, Clove-hitch restraints in place. D, Position for lumbar puncture.

long enough, fold it over blanket, crossing it under infant's chin.

6. Swing corner of 3 o'clock position snugly over infant, and fold under infant's right side. Pin this corner into place. When tucked tightly, it is not always necessary to use a pin.

EXTREMITY RESTRAINTS. This type of restraint is used to control movements of the infant's arms or legs. It is used during many procedures, such as intubating, gavage feedings, or intravenous (IV) infusion.

Equipment includes gauze strips or wide strips of soft material and cotton wadding. Pins are optional.

The procedure depends on which type of extremity restraint is used.

Following are examples:

1. *Pad extremity with cotton wadding.* Fold one end of gauze strip over extremity and pin. Pin other end to mattress.
2. *Clove-hitch restraint.* Arrange a long strip of material that is 5 cm (2 in) wide, as shown in Fig. 21-16, *B*. Loop device over extremity, which has been padded with cotton, and pin loose ends to mattress (Fig. 21-16, *C*). The clove-hitch does not tighten even if infant's movements tug on restraint.

TOWEL SUPPORT. Although the towel support is not a true restraint, it controls the infant's position and movement. The towel may be rolled and placed at the infant's back or sides or folded and placed under the neck or upper part of the back. A towel support has the following advantages:

1. It provides comfort and security by stabilizing the infant's position.
2. It maintains positioning to assist respiratory effort and gastrointestinal functions and to prevent skin breakdown.
3. It prevents the infant from rolling against the incubator wall, where the child may lose heat by convection.
4. It prevents the infant from falling out of the incubator when the lid is lifted.

RESTRAINT WITHOUT APPLIANCE. The nurse may restrain the infant by using the hands and body. Fig. 21-16, *D,* illustrates restraints of the infant in position for lumbar puncture.

COLLECTION OF SPECIMENS. Ongoing evaluation of a newborn requires obtaining blood and urine specimens. The following procedures are used for heel stick, collection of urine specimen, and assisting with venipuncture.

HEEL STICK. Most blood specimens are drawn by laboratory technicians. Nurses, however, may be required to perform heel sticks to obtain blood for glucose monitoring and to measure hematocrit levels. The same technique is needed to complete the phenylketonuria (PKU) form or to test for galactosemia and hypothyroidism.

Before the sample is taken, it is helpful to warm the heel. However, second- and third-degree thermal burns have been reported from inappropriate heel warming techniques: "Plastic wraps and plastic covered diapers prevent heat dissipation and can result in thermal burns" (NAACOG, 1992). A cloth soaked with warm water and wrapped loosely around the foot provides effective warming (Fig. 21-17). Application of heat for 5 to 10 minutes help dilate the vessels in the area. Nurses should wear gloves when collecting any specimen. The nurse cleanses the area with alcohol, restrains the infant's foot with the free hand, and punctures the selected site with a Bard-Parker No. 11 or Redi-Lance blade.

The most serious complication of infant heel stick is necrotizing osteochondritis from lancet penetration of the bone. To avoid this, the stick should be no deeper than 2.4 mm and should be made at the outer aspect of the heel (Whaley, Wong, 1991). To identify the appropriate puncture sites, the nurse draws an imaginary line from between the fourth and fifth toes that runs parallel to the lateral aspect of the heel, or a line running from the great toe that runs parallel to the medial aspect of the heel (Fig. 21-17, *B*). Repeated trauma to the walking surface of the heel can cause fibrosis and scarring that may lead to problems with walking (Reiner et al, 1990; Whaley, Wong, 1991).

After the specimen has been collected, pressure is applied with a dry gauze square. Reapplying alcohol will cause the site to continue to bleed. The site is covered with an adhesive bandage. The nurse ensures proper disposal of the equipment used, reviews the laboratory slip for correct identifications, and checks the specimen for adequate labeling and routing.

A heel stick can be traumatic for the infant and can cause pain. After several heel sticks infants have been observed to withdraw their foot when it is touched. Pain pathways are present and functional in the infant (Shapiro, 1989). To reassure the infant and promote feelings of safety, the neonate should be cuddled and comforted when the procedure is completed.

OBTAINING URINE SPECIMEN. Examination of urine is a valuable laboratory tool for infant assessment. The way in which the specimen is collected may influence the results. The urine sample should be fresh and examined within 1 hour of collection.

A variety of urine collection bags are available, including the Hollister U-Bag (Fig. 21-18). These bags

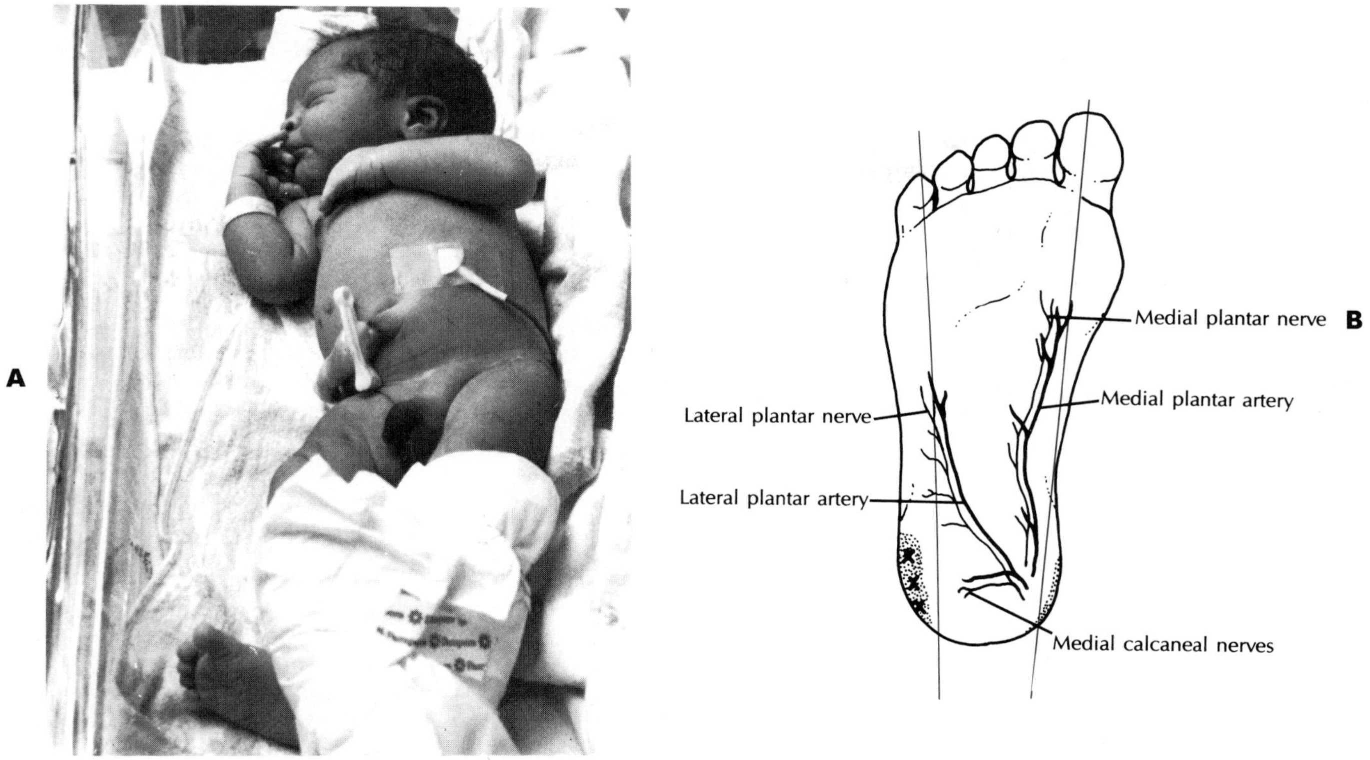

A

Medial plantar nerve B

Lateral plantar nerve

Medial plantar artery

Lateral plantar artery

Medial calcaneal nerves

Fig. 21-17 A, Newborn with foot wrapped for warmth to increase blood flow to extremity before heel stick. B, Puncture sites (x) on infant's foot for heel stick samples of capillary blood.

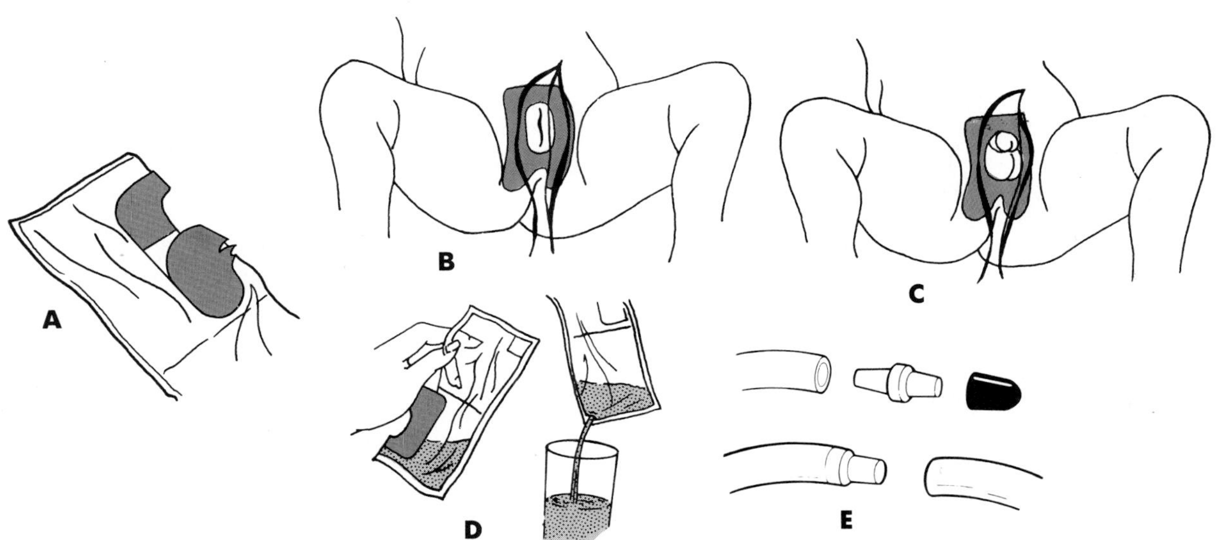

Fig. 21-18 A, Protective paper is being removed from the adhesive surface. B, Applied to girls. C, Applied to boys. D, Cut to drain urine. E, Collection tube.
Courtesy Hollister, Inc, Chicago, Ill.

are clear plastic, single-use bags with self-adhering material around the opening at the point of attachment.

To prepare the infant, the nurse removes the diaper and places the infant in a supine position. The genitalia, perineum, and surrounding skin are washed and thoroughly dried because the adhesive of the bag will not stick to moist, powdered, or oily skin surfaces. The protective paper is removed to expose the adhesive. (Fig. 21-18, *A*). For girls, the perineum, is stretched to flatten skin folds. Then the adhesive is pressed firmly to the skin all around the urinary meatus and vagina. (NOTE: Start with the narrow portion of butterfly-shaped adhesive patch.) *The nurse must be sure to start at the bridge of skin separating the rectum from the vagina and work upward* (Fig. 21-18, *B*). For boys, the penis and scrotum are tucked through the aperture of the collector before the nurse removes the protective paper from the adhesive. The bag is fitted over the penis, and the flaps are pressed firmly to the perineum, making sure the entire adhesive coating is firmly attached to the skin with no puckering of the adhesive (Fig. 21-18, *C*). This helps ensure a leak-proof seal and decreases the chance of contamination from stool. Cutting a slit in the diaper and pulling the bag through the slit also may help prevent leaking.

The diaper is carefully replaced, and the bag is checked frequently. When 1 to 2 mL of urine have been obtained, the bag is removed. The infant's skin is observed for signs of irritation. The specimen can be aspirated with a syringe or drained directly from the bag. For draining, the bag is held in the left hand and the bag is tilted to keep urine away from the tab. The tab is removed, and the urine is drained into a clean receptacle (Fig. 21-18, *D*).

Collection of a 24-hour specimen can be a challenge. The infant may need to be restrained. The 24-hour U-Bag is applied in the manner just described, and the drainage is directed into a receptacle. The collection tube can be shortened or capped (Fig. 21-18, *E*). The infant's skin is watched closely for signs of irritation and lack of a proper seal.

For some types of urine testing, urine can be aspirated directly from the diaper by means of a syringe without a needle. If the diaper has absorbent gelling material that traps urine, a small-gauge dressing or some cotton balls are placed inside the diaper and the urine is aspirated from them (Whaley, Wong, 1991).

ASSISTING WITH VENIPUNCTURE. Venous blood samples can be drawn from radial veins, jugular veins, or femoral veins or through heparin lock devices. The use of a heparin lock device is not very successful and may shorten the life of the device (Whaley, Wong, 1991). If an IV site is used to obtain a blood specimen, it also is important to consider the type of infusion fluid.

When venipuncture is required, positioning of the needle is extremely important. Although regular venipuncture needles usually are used, some personnel prefer scalp-vein needles. It is necessary to be very patient during the procedure because small veins yield slow blood return and the small needle must remain in place longer.

The mummy restraint frequently is used to help secure the infant. If the radial vein is used, the infant's arm is exposed and securely held in place.

For external jugular venipuncture: "Mummy" the infant as necessary. Lower the infant's head over rolled towel, edge of table, or your knee, and stabilize.

For femoral venipuncture: Position the infant in frog posture. Place hands over infant's knees. Avoid pressure of fingers over inner aspect of thigh.

These positions will ensure safety and exposure of the puncture sites.

If venipuncture or arterial puncture is performed for blood gas studies, crying, fear, and agitation will affect the values. Every effort needs to be taken to try to keep the infant quiet during the procedure. For blood gas studies the blood sample tubes are packed in ice to reduce blood cell metabolism and are taken immediately to the laboratory for analysis (Whaley, Wong, 1991).

For an hour after any venipuncture, the nurse should observe the child frequently for evidence of bleeding or hematoma at the puncture site. Determination of the infant's tolerance of the procedure should be made and recorded. The infant should be cuddled and comforted when the procedure is completed.

Discharge Planning

For the new parent, child care activities can cause much anxiety (see nursing plan of care, p. 612). Support from nursing staff members in the mother's beginning efforts can be an important factor in her seeking and accepting help in the future. Whether or not this is the couple's first baby, parents appreciate **anticipatory guidance** in the care of their child. The nurse should avoid covering all content at once because the parents can be overwhelmed and become anxious. To set priorities for teaching, the nurse follows parental cues. Normal growth and development and the changing needs of the infant (e.g., for stimulation, exercise, and social contacts), as well as the following topics, should be included during **discharge planning** with parents.

TEMPERATURE. The following topics are reviewed:

1. The causes of elevation in body temperature (such as exercise, cold stress with resultant vasoconstriction, minimum response to infection) and the body's response to extremes in environmental temperature
2. Symptoms to be reported, such as high or low temperatures, with accompanying fussiness, stuffy nose, lethargy, irritability, poor feeding, and crying
3. Ways to reduce body temperature, such as giving a cool tub bath, dressing the infant appropriately for the temperature of the air, and protecting the infant from long exposure to sunlight
4. Use of warm wraps in cold weather or extra blankets
5. How to take the baby's axillary temperature

RESPIRATIONS. The following points are reviewed:

1. Normal variations in rate and rhythm
2. Reflexes such as sneezing to clear the air passage
3. The need to protect the infant from the following:
   a. People with upper respiratory tract infections (an efficient mask can be made by wrapping toilet tissue around the head to cover the mouth and nose if the parent or another has a cold)
   b. Pollution from a smoke-filled environment
   c. Suffocation from loose bedding, drowning (bath water), entrapment under excessive bedding, anything tied around the infant's neck, poorly constructed playpens, bassinets, or cribs
   d. Aspiration pneumonia: A commonly aspirated substance is baby powder, which usually is a mixture of talc (hydrous magnesium silicate) and other silicates (Whaley, Wong, 1991). Although the use of talc has been discouraged, it is a common baby care product and can cause severe and often fatal aspiration pneumonia. A factor involved in talc aspiration is the similar appearance of baby powder containers and nursing bottles. Talc containers often become favorite playthings and are placed in the mouth (Mofenson et al, 1981). Improper use of powder by sprinkling it directly on the skin creates a cloud of talc dust that is easily inhaled. Parents are advised of the danger of baby powder and discouraged from using it. If they prefer to use a powder, a cornstarch preparation can be substituted. Whenever a powder is used, it should be placed in the caregiver's hand and then applied to the skin. The container is kept closed and immediately stored in a safe place, especially away from curious toddlers who often imitate caregiving activities and may accidentally shake it on the infant.
4. *Symptoms of the* **common cold:** nasal congestion, coughing, sneezing, difficulty in swallowing (sore throat), low-grade fever. Advise parents on measures to help the infant, for example:
   a. Feed smaller amounts but more frequently to avoid overtiring the infant.
   b. Hold the baby in an upright position to feed.
   c. Offer extra sterile water or nursing time.
   d. For sleeping, raise the infant's head and chest by raising the mattress 30 degrees (do not use pillow).
   e. Avoid drafts, and do not overdress the baby.
   f. Use only medications prescribed by a physician (do not use nose drops because aspiration may result in lung involvement).
   g. Cover the upper lip with a light film of petrolatum to minimize excoriation from nasal secretions.

ELIMINATION. A review includes the following reminders:

1. Changes to be expected in the color of the stool and the number of bowel evacuations, plus the odor of stools for breast- or bottle-fed infants (see Chapter 20)
2. The color of normal urine and the number of voidings to expect each day (see Chapter 20)

SAFETY. The following measures are reviewed:

1. Protecting the infant from trauma, for example, keeping objects such as pins and scissors closed and well out of baby's reach. When infant clothes are purchased, the type of closure used should be considered. A front button can easily be pulled off and swallowed. Even though a young infant may not search for buttons or other small objects at this time, practicing this good habit from the beginning prevents future injuries.
2. Preventing overheating or chilling.
3. Care in transporting infants, particularly in automobiles (Fig. 21-19). The use of approved car seats for infants is a law in 33 states.
4. Supervising brothers' and sisters' attention to the new baby.

PACIFIERS/THUMBSUCKING. Sucking is the infant's chief pleasure. It may not be satisfied by breast- or formula-feeding (Whaley, Wong, 1991). It is such a strong need that infants who are deprived of sucking, such as those with cleft lip repair, will suck on their tongue. Some newborns are born with sucking pads on their fingers that developed from in utero sucking

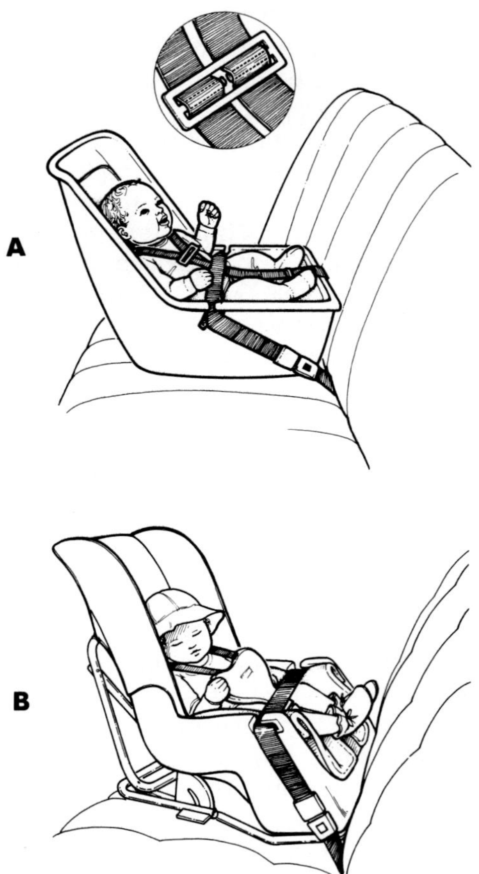

Fig. 21-19 Rearward-facing shell car seat. Infant is placed in car seat when going home from hospital.
From Whaley LF, Wong DL: *Nursing care of infants and children,* ed 4, St Louis, 1991, Mosby–Year Book.

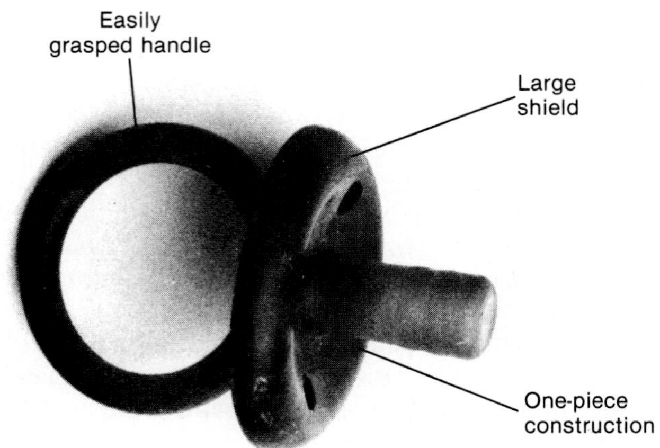

Fig. 21-20 Design of a safe pacifier.
From Whaley LF, Wong, DI: *Nursing care of infants and children,* ed 3, St Louis, 1987, Mosby–Year Book.

activity. Several benefits of nonnutritive sucking have been documented, such as increased weight gain in premature infants and decreased crying (Anderson, 1986).

Problems arise when parents are concerned about sucking of fingers, thumb, or pacifier and attempt to restrain this natural tendency. Before giving advice, nurses investigate the parents' feelings and base guidance on this information. For example, some parents may see no problem with the use of a finger but may find the use of a pacifier objectionable. In general, there is no need to restrain either unless thumbsucking persists past 4 years of age or past the time when the permanent teeth erupt. Parents are advised to work with their pediatrician and pediatric nurse practitioner about this topic.

To decrease dependence on nonnutritive sucking, sucking pleasure can be increased by prolonging feeding time. A small-holed, firm nipple causes stronger sucking and slower feeding. Also, the parent's excessive use of the pacifier to calm the child should be explored. It is not unusual for parents to place a pacifier in the infant's mouth as soon as crying begins, thus reinforcing a pattern of distress-relief (Whaley, Wong, 1991). If the child uses a pacifier, safety considerations in purchasing one must be stressed. A homemade or poorly designed pacifier can be dangerous because the entire object may be aspirated if it is small, or a portion may become lodged in the pharynx. Improvised pacifiers, such as those commonly made in hospitals from a padded nipple, also present dangers. The nipple may separate from the plastic collar and be aspirated (Millunchick, McArtor, 1986). In addition, parents may continue to offer this pacifier to the infant at home. Safe pacifiers should be of one-piece construction, have a shield or flange that is large enough to prevent entry into the mouth, and have a handle that can be grasped (Fig. 21-20).

IMMUNIZATIONS. The schedule for immunizations should be reviewed. The *ability* to protect against antigens by formation of antibodies *develops sequentially*. The fetus or infant must be developmentally capable of responding to antigens. This is the reason for planning sequential immunizations in infants. A form of passive immunity is present in colostrum and breast milk. It is specific for microbial agents present in the mother's own gastrointestinal tract. As fresh colonization occurs in the newborn, *these antibodies limit bacterial growth in the gastrointestinal tract and protect against overgrowth* (see also Chapter 6). This information helps health care professionals plan for the use of poliomyelitis vaccine in breast-fed infants. According to Korones (1986), for its effectiveness, oral polio vaccine depends on multiplication in the intestinal tract. The vaccine fails to immunize babies receiving maternal breast milk with high antibody titers to poliovirus, because vaccine virus is inactivated in the gut by secretory IgA from breast milk.

INFANT FOLLOW-UP CARE. Parents should plan for infant health follow-up care: at 2 to 4 weeks of age, then every 2 months until 6 to 7 months of age, then every 3 months until 18 months, at 2 years, at 3 years, at preschool age, and every 2 years thereafter.

The newborn's record provides a source of documented communication among all members of the health care team. The record contains accurate and complete recordings of the history, physical examination, laboratory test results, sequential observations, expected outcomes, interventions, and the newborn's responses. The record should be readily accessible to health care professionals caring for the infant and family. Documentation of the parents' health education, counseling, and responses to information is included. These data provide valuable information for the pediatrician and nurse for the infant's follow-up care and serve as a reservoir for data for future research.

EVALUATION

The nurse can be reasonably assured that care was effective to the degree that the goals for care have been met. For the infant this includes the following.

- Successful transition from intrauterine to extrauterine life
- Maintenance of effective breathing patterns and thermoregulation
- Minimal pain related to circumcision
- Freedom from infection

The mother/parent has achieved the following goals:

- Attained knowledge, skill, and confidence relevant to child care activities
- Can state understanding of biologic and behavioral characteristics of the newborn
- Has demonstrated behavioral/life-style changes to reduce potential for development of problems
- Has taken the opportunity to intensify relationships with the newborn

SUMMARY

The care the newborn receives in the first months of life is reflected in the normal growth and development of a healthy infant. The nurse in the roles of teacher and support person acts as an advocate for the vulnerable infant. The nurse's skills in caring for the newborn and teaching these skills to parents are of paramount importance. Nurses are present during the formative stages of parent-child interactions. From their unique perspective they can do much to help both parents and child.

CASE STUDY

Parent's Care of Newborn: Gagging, Circumcision Care, and Crying

Karen Sponselli, age 20, just gave birth to her first baby. Ernest was circumcised yesterday; Karen is going home this evening. When you walk into the room, you find Karen about to clean the circumcision with an alcohol wipe. Further questioning reveals that Karen has many questions about child care.

ASSESSMENT

Karen has completed 2 years of college and earned an AA degree in interior design. She states that school and her new job are "not nearly as hard as learning to care for a new baby." Karen states she has never been around babies and knows nothing of newborn care or how newborns are supposed to look and act. Ernest is a healthy boy, 8 pounds 4 ounces, born at full term 2 days ago. All health assessment findings are within normal limits. Ernest gags and spits up a small amount of formula. Karen states she does not know what to do "when he does that." Within the next few minutes, Ernest begins to move around and looks as if he may start to cry. Karen appears anxious, quickly picks him up, and says, "My husband and I don't know what to do when he cries."

NURSING DIAGNOSIS

Karen will need assistance and anticipatory guidance for all her concerns. However, the mother's need to learn what to do when Ernest gags takes priority. The following nursing diagnosis is chosen: High risk for ineffective airway clearance related to parent's knowledge deficit regarding suctioning and positioning the newborn.

PLANNING

Planning of interventions is derived from accepted methods of clearing the mouth and nose. The nurse and Karen mutually agree on the *goal:* Karen will learn how to use a bulb syringe and to place Ernest in a head-down position. The nurse sets the *expected outcome:* Newborn will maintain an open airway.

IMPLEMENTATION

The nurse demonstrates how (1) to hold Ernest face downward with head slightly lowered, (2) to aspirate his mouth and nose with bulb syringe, and (3) to position him on his side to facilitate drainage from mouth. After the demonstration, the nurse encourages Karen to practice with the bulb syringe and positioning. The nurse explains that gagging, coughing, and sneezing are normal and expected in babies to clear their airways. The nurse encourages Karen to comfort Ernest after a bout of gagging and regurgitation. The nurse refers Karen to new parents' classes.

EVALUATION

Assessment of the newborn indicated that interventions were successful: Ernest maintains a clear airway and remains free of respiratory distress. In addition, Karen's child-care skills and self-confidence increased: Karen verbalized understanding of instruction; demonstrated skill in helping Ernest keep a clear airway; expressed satisfaction with her new skill; and states she is ready to learn more. At the next visit, she tells the nurse that she will attend parents' classes at least once per week.

CARE PLAN Parent's Care of Newborn: Gagging, Circumcision Care, and Crying

GOALS	IMPLEMENTATION	RATIONALE	EVALUATION
Nursing diagnosis: High risk for ineffective airway clearance related to Karen's knowledge deficit regarding suctioning and positioning of Ernest			
Karen will learn how to use a bulb syringe and to place Ernest in a head-down position.	Hold Ernest face downward with head slightly lowered and aspirate mouth and nose with bulb syringe. Position Ernest on side to facilitate drainage from mouth.	Gravity assists drainage of fluid. Properly used bulb syringe effectively removes material from the mouth.	Ernest maintains clear airway. Ernest remains free of respiratory distress.
	Encourage practice with positioning and use of bulb syringe.	A return demonstration and practice increase skill and self-confidence.	Karen verbalizes understanding of instructions. Karen demonstrates skill in helping Ernest keep a clear airway.
	Tell Karen that gagging, coughing, and sneezing are normal and expected to clear airway. Encourage Karen to comfort Ernest after gagging and regurgitation.	Knowledge can be reassuring and provide a basis for decision making. Increased skill leads to increased self-confidence.	Karen expresses satisfaction and states she is ready to learn more.
	Refer Karen to new parents' classes.	Provides peer group support regarding concerns, similar experiences, and problem-solving.	Karen attends parents' classes.
Nursing diagnosis: High risk for injury to infant related to parent's knowledge deficit regarding circumcision care			
Ernest's circumcision will heal rapidly with no hemorrhage or infection and with a minimum of discomfort.	Demonstrate circumcision care: ■ Wash penis gently with water to remove urine or feces. ■ Apply a fresh sterile petrolatum gauze around the glans; fanfold diaper and apply loosely; change diaper at least q4h.	Role models appropriate care: ■ Cleansing ■ Preventing adherence to diaper, which increases chance of causing hemorrhage and delaying healing ■ Decreasing possibility of infection Adds looseness to decrease chance of sticking to diaper.	Karen correctly describes circumcision care, diaper application, positioning, use of pressure (in the event of hemorrhage).
	Position Ernest on his side (not abdomen) ■ Caution about use of alcohol. ■ Demonstrate, and ask for return demonstration for controlling possible hemorrhage. ■ Describe the yellow exudate that normally forms in 24 hr.	Prevents pressure on penis and promotes comfort. Alcohol delays healing and causes discomfort. Increases Karen's skill and self-confidence; teaches accepted therapy for hemorrhage. Provides anticipatory guidance about normal healing process; allays parental anxiety.	

Continued.

CARE PLAN Parent's Care of Newborn: Gagging, Circumcision Care, and Crying—cont'd

GOALS	IMPLEMENTATION	RATIONALE	EVALUATION
Nursing diagnosis: Family coping, potential for growth, related to anticipatory guidance regarding responses to son's crying			
Parents will learn how to cope effectively with Ernest's crying.	Alert parents to crying as a child's form of communication and that soon they will be able to differentiate the cries: hunger, pain, loneliness. Differentiate self-consoling behaviors from fussing/crying.	Provides reassurance that crying is not a sign of infant's rejection of them and that they will soon be able to interpret the different cries. Presents parents with concrete examples of interventions.	Karen states she understands about crying and methods to cope with it.
	Discuss methods of consoling infant (Table 21-1) who has been crying: ■ Show face to infant. ■ Talk to infant in a steady, soft voice. ■ Hold both infant's arms close to body. ■ Swaddle infant. ■ Pick up infant. ■ Rock infant. ■ Give a pacifier or feed.	Reassures parents that no one intervention works all the time. Anticipating a problem and considering a number of options increase one's self-confidence.	At next visit, Karen ■ States she/they are "getting better" in coping with Ernest's crying ■ Relates the techniques that work the best ■ Describes some successes in accurately interpreting Ernest's cries.

REFERENCES

AAP releases circumcision statement, *Pediatr Nurs* 15:203, Feb 1989.

American Academy of Pediatrics Committee on Accidents and Poison Prevention: Revised first aid for the choking child, *Pediatrics* 78:177, 1986.

Anderson G: Pacifiers: the positive side, *MCN* 11:122, March/April 1986.

Campos RG: Soothing pain-elicited distress in infants with swaddling and pacifiers, *Child Dev* 60:781, 1989.

Field R et al: Mother's assessments of the behavior of their infants, *Infant Behav Dev* 1:156, 1978.

Gerlach C, Schmid M: Second skill educational development of personnel for a single-room maternity care system, JOGNN 17:388, Nov/Dec 1988.

Guidelines for cardiopulmonary resuscitation and emergency cardiac care, JAMA 268(16):2171, 1992.

Johnson SH: *Nursing assessment and strategies for the family at risk: high-risk parenting,* ed 2, New York, 1986, JB Lippincott Co.

Korones SB: *High-risk newborn infants: the basis for intensive care,* ed 4, St Louis, 1986, Mosby–Year Book.

Larson E: Rituals in infection control: what works in the newborn nursery? *JOGNN* 16:411 Nov/Dec, 1987.

Millunchick E, McArtor R: Fatal aspiration of a makeshift pacifier, *Pediatrics* 77:369, 1986.

Mofenson HC et al: Baby powder—a hazard! *Pediatrics* 68:265, 1981.

NAACOG: Neonatal skin care, *OGN Nursing Practice Resource,* Jan 1992.

NAACOG: Nurses' role in neonatal circumcision, *OGN Nursing Practice Resource* 14:3, 1985a.

NAACOG: Neonatal skin care, *OGN Nursing Practice Resource* 12:3, March 1985b.

NAACOG: CDC reports caution about AIDS virus, *NAACOG Newsletter* 13, June 1986a.

NAACOG: Phototherapy and nursing care of the newborn with hyperbilirubinemia, *OGN Nursing Practice Resource* 15 July, 1986b.

Phillips CR: Single-room maternity care for maximum cost efficiency, *Perinat Neonat* 12:22, 1988.

Ragan J, Weinfield AM: VACNECCA: an eight-point check for neonatal assessment, *J Pract Nurs* p 39, June 1989.

Reiner CB, Meltes S, Hayes JR: Optimal sites and depths for skin puncture of infants and children as assessed from anatomical measurements, *Clin Chem* 36:547, 1990.

Rosenfeld W, Twist P, Concepcion L: A new device for phototherapy treatment of jaundiced infants, *J Perinat* 10:243, Sept 1990.

Shapiro C: Pain in the neonate: assessment and intervention, *Neonatal Network* 8:7, Jan 1989.

Tan KL: Efficacy of fluorescent daylight, blue, and green lamps in

the management of nonhemolytic hyperbilirubinemia, *J Pediatr* 114:132, 1989.
Valman HB: Jaundice in the newborn, *BMJ* 299:1272, 1989.
Whaley LF, Wong DL: *Nursing care of infants and children,* ed 4, St Louis, 1991, Mosby–Year Book.
Wiswell TE: Routine neonatal circumcision: a reappraisal, *Am Fam Physician* 41:859, 1990.

References—Nursing Research

Marchette L et al: Pain reduction interventions during neonatal circumcision, *Nurs Res* 40:241, July/Aug 1991.
Margolius FR, Sneed NV, Hollerbach AD: Accuracy of apical pulse rate measurements in young children, *Nurs Res* 40:378, Nov/Dec 1991.
Murphy MR, Oellrich RG:(1990). A new method of phototherapy: nursing perspectives, *J Perinat* 10:249, Sept 1990.

BIBLIOGRAPHY

Bamford FN et al: Sleep in the first year of life, *Dev Med Child Neurol* 32:718, 1990.
Barr RG: The normal crying curve: what do we really know? *Dev Med Child Neurol* 32:356, 1990.
Blackburn ST, Loper DL: *Maternal, fetal and neonatal physiology: clinical perspective,* Philadelphia, 1992, WB Saunders Co.
Brown LP et al: Transcutaneous bilirubinometer: intermeter reliability, *J Perinat* 10:167, June 1990.
Coen RW et al: The detailed newborn examination, *Patient Care* 22:93, Dec 1988b.
Coen RW et al: A fast, efficient newborn exam, *Patient Care* 22:192, Nov 1988a.
Cunningham FG, MacDonald PC, Gant NF: *Williams obstetrics,* ed 18, Norwalk, Conn 1989, Appleton & Lange.
Dobrusin R, Zaprudsky P: Circumcising neonates with the Mogen clamp, *Contemp OB/GYN* 36:79, June 1991.
Donaher-Wagner BM, Braun DH: Infant cardiopulmonary resuscitation for expectant and new parents, *MCN* 17:27, Jan/Feb 1992.
Fanaroff AA, Martin RJ: *Neonatal-perinatal medicine: diseases of the fetus and infant,* ed 5, St Louis, 1992, Mosby–Year Book.
Giger JN, Davidhizar RE: *Transcultural nursing: assessment and intervention,* St Louis, 1991, Mosby–Year Book.
Gunzenhauser N, editor: *Advances in touch: new implications in human development,* Skillman, JN, 1990, Johnson & Johnson Consumer Products.
Hulman S et al: Blood pressure patterns in the first three days of life, *J Perinat* 11:231, Sept 1991.
Jones MA: A physiologic approach to identifying neonates at risk for kernicterus, *JOGNN* 19:313, July/Aug 1990.
Keating SB, Kelman GB: *Home health care nursing: concepts and practice,* Philadelphia, 1988, JB Lippincott Co.
Leduc E: The healing touch, *MCN* 14:41, Jan/Feb 1989.
Long CA: Teaching parents infant CPR—lecture or audiovisual tape? *MCN* 17:30, Jan/Feb 1992.
Marchette L, Main R, Redick E: Pain reduction during neonatal circumcision, *Pediatr Nurs* 15:207, March/April 1989.
Nelson NM: The onset of respirations. In Avery G editor: *Neonatology: pathophysiology and management of the newborn,* ed 3, Philadelphia, 1987, JB Lippincott.
NAACOG: Physical assessment of the neonate, *OGN Nursing Practice Resource,* Aug 1991.
Savinetti-Rose B, Kempfer-Kline RE, Mabry CM:(1990). Home phototherapy with the fiberoptic blanket: the nurse's role in caring for newborns and their caregivers, *J Perinat* 10:435, Dec 1990.
Shibley B: Phototherapy at home. *NURSEweek,* p 12, Jan 7, 1991.
Stang HJ et al: Local anesthesia for neonatal circumcision: effects on distress and cortisol response, *JAMA* 259:1507, 1988.
Weiss GN: Local anesthesia for neonatal circumcision, *JAMA* 260:637, 1988.
Wilkerson NN: A comprehensive look at hyperbilirubinemia, *MCN J* 13(5):36, May 1988.
Wilkerson NN: Treating hyperbilirubinemia, *MCN* 14:32, Jan/Feb 1989.
Wilkerson NN, Barrows TL: Synchronizing care with mother-baby rhythms, *MCN* 13:264, July/Aug 1988.
Willens JC, Copel LC: Performing CPR on infants, *Nursing 89* 52:47, March 1989.

Bibliography—Nursing Research

Covington C, Cronenwett L, Loveland-Cherry C: Newborn behavioral performance in colic and noncolic infants, *Nurs Res* 40:292, Sept/Oct 1991.
Fuller BF: Acoustic discrimination of three types of infant cries, *Nurs Res* 40:158, May/June 1991.
Goodwin BA: Pediatric resuscitation, *Crit Care Nurs Q* 10(4):69, 1988.
Greer PS: Head coverings for neonates under radiant heat warmers, *JOGNN* 17:265, July/Aug 1988.
Jones MA: Identifying signs that nurses interpret as indicating pain in newborns, *Pediatr Nurs* 15:76, Jan 1989.
Keefe MR et al: Development of a system for monitoring infant state behavior, *Nurs Res* 38:344, Nov/Dec 1989.
Kunnel MT et al: Comparisons of rectal, femoral, axillary, and skin-to-mattress temperatures in stable neonates, *Nurs Res* 37:162, May/June 1988.
Lane AT, Rheder PA, Helm K: Evaluation of diapers containing absorbent gelling material with conventional disposable diapers in newborn infants, *Am J Dis Child* 144:315, 1990.
Medoff-Cooper B, Weininger S, Zukowsky K: Neonatal sucking as a clinical assessment tool: preliminary findings, *Nurs Res* 38:162, May/June 1989.
Reams PK, Deane DM: Bagged versus diaper urine specimens and laboratory values, *Neonatal Network* 6:17, June 1988.

chapter 21 review

Key Concepts

- Assessment of the newborn requires data from the prenatal, intranatal, and postnatal periods.
- Knowledge of the biologic and behavioral characteristics is essential for guiding assessment and interpreting data.
- Providing a protective environment is a key role for the nurse that includes such actions as careful identification procedures, restraining techniques, measures to prevent infection, and support of physiologic functions.
- Maintenance of adequate ventilation includes ensuring an adequate airway and body temperature.
- Each nurse must develop skill in CPR and relieving airway obstruction.
- Parent education is a major role for the nurse and includes involving parents in all phases of the nursing process.
- Circumcision is an elective surgical procedure.
- The newborn has social, as well as physical, needs.
- Whether or not this is the couple's first baby, parents appreciate anticipatory guidance in the care of their child.

Key Terms

- acid mantle (p. 595)
- anticipatory guidance (p. 608)
- bilirubin (p. 599, 601)
- cardiopulmonary resuscitation (CPR) (p. 590)
- circumcision (p. 603)
- common cold (p. 609)
- cradle cap (p. 596)
- discharge planning (p. 608)
- excoriation (p. 593)
- hyperbilirubinemia (p. 599, 601)
- hypothermia (p. 588)
- jaundice (p. 601)
- phimosis (p. 602)
- phototherapy (p. 599, 601)
- protective environment (p. 587)
- respiratory distress (p. 593)
- single-room maternity care (SRMC) (p. 580)
- thermistor probe (p. 588)

Critical Thinking Exercises

1. Select one emergency and one daily care procedure. Describe what supplies and equipment are needed and how you would perform the procedure yourself and/or teach it to new parents. Justify your decisions and actions.
2. Prepare and conduct one 20-minute class in infant care for parents. Before class, prepare a written teaching plan that includes assessment of clients' learning needs; a teaching-learning diagnosis; a plan with prioritized client-centered goals; content and teaching methods with rationale; and evaluative criteria. If possible, several students can present teaching plans to the group for debate, critique, and adjustment. Following the class, critique the total experience. What insights have you achieved?

Topics For Nursing Research

- Compare mother's ability to bathe infant after viewing videotape versus personal demonstration. Compare healing time of different types of circumcision (Plastibell, Gomco, Yellen clamp, Mogen clamp).
- Compare father's and mother's responses to reactivity periods.
- Compare similarities or differences, or both, between maternal and paternal attachment.
- Compare types of cord care employed until the cord dries and falls off.

chapter 22

Newborn Nutrition and Feeding

Cecilia Tiller
Mary Courtney Moore

LEARNING OBJECTIVES

- Define keyterms.
- Identify factors that affect parent and newborn readiness for feeding.
- Evaluate nutrient needs in relation to infant's growth and development.
- Identify how breast milk and infant formula differ in composition and nutritional value.
- Review the physiology of lactation.
- Formulate nursing diagnoses relative to the infant's nutritional status and the parents' needs and preferences.
- Examine breast-feeding in relation to advantages, care of breasts, diet and fluids, infant responses, secretion of drugs in milk, maintaining a job, and infant-related and maternal-related concerns.
- Discuss formula-feeding in relation to advantages, care of breasts, diet and fluids, infant responses, and formula preparation.
- Develop guidelines for teaching self-care for breast-feeding, formula-feeding, and formula preparation.
- Recognize the impact of nursing interventions on success of feeding.
- Teach the client positioning techniques that promote infant feeding.
- Explore cultural aspects of breast-feeding.
- Describe the nurse's role in identifying and reducing barriers to successful breast-feeding.
- Compare nutrition supplements recommended for the breast-fed and formula-fed infant.
- Identify topics for nursing research related to newborn nutrition and feeding.

Good nutrition in infancy not only fosters good health and optimal growth and development during the first few months of life but also establishes a basis for lasting good eating habits. Moreover, the feeding process is an important mechanism in the formation of a close, trusting relationship between the infant and primary caregiver(s), a key step in the infant's emotional development. Skillful health supervision of infants requires knowledge of their nutritional needs. This chapter focuses on nutritional needs for normal growth and development from birth to 3 months. Breast-feeding and formula-feeding are addressed.

INFANT DEVELOPMENT AND NUTRITIONAL NEEDS

Discussion of the child's **growth pattern** is often the starting point for effective communication with parents regarding proper nutrition for their child.

The full-term infant generally will double the birth weight by the age of 5 months and triple it in 1 year. Most newborn infants experience a 5% to 10% weight loss during the first few days of life. Full-term infants usually regain this weight within 10 days.

Length increases about 50% during the first year. Doubling of birth length does not occur until about 4 years of age. Head circumference also increases rapidly during the first year in conjunction with rapid growth of the brain.

At birth the term infant's body is composed of about 16% fat (by weight). Between 2 and 6 months of age, the increase in adipose tissue is more than twice as great as the increase in muscle mass; fat deposition occurs at a steady pace until about 9 months of age. Throughout infancy, girls add a greater percentage of weight as fat than boys do; this trend continues throughout the remaining developmental years.

To assist in the clinical evaluation of physical growth of children in the United States, growth "standards," or "norms," have been developed for height or length, body weight, and head circumference.

The rank of an individual child's measurements in relation to American children of the same sex and age can be determined by examining the percentiles of the National Center for Health Statistics (Hamill et al, 1979). Adjustments can be made for children from segments of the population that might differ on the basis of race, socioeconomic status, and geography. Measurements outside the extreme percentiles may indicate nutritional problems sufficiently severe to affect growth. Measurements within the control or intermediate percentiles indicate that growth is within normal limits by current standards.

Readiness for Feeding

At birth and for several months thereafter all the secretions of the infant's digestive tract contain enzymes especially suited to the digestion of human milk. The ability to handle foods other than milk depends on the physiologic development of the infant. The capacities for salivary, gastric, pancreatic, and intestinal digestion increase with age, indicating what may be a natural pattern for introduction of various solid foods (Table 22-1).

At birth the infant produces little salivary or pancreatic amylase and thus is poorly prepared to digest the complex carbohydrates found in solid foods. Lipase production by the pancreas is lower than in older children or adults. Human milk fat and the vegetable oils used in commercial formulas are fairly well digested, but significant malabsorption of butterfat and other fats occurs. During the first few months of life, rapid maturation occurs so that digestion of the starches found in cereals and vegetables is adequate by about 4 months of age. Therefore introduction of solid foods is practical after this age.

Kidney function of the full-term infant is not completely mature. Well-developed glomeruli satisfactorily filter the blood presented to the kidneys. The tubules, which are functionally less mature, are somewhat limited in their ability to reabsorb water and some solutes. Therefore it is important that the kidneys not be presented with excess solutes (renal solute load) to excrete. For this reason protein beyond that needed for growth and the extra sodium sometimes added to baby foods as sodium chloride (NaCl, or table salt) should be avoided.

The percentage of body water decreases from 75% at birth to 60% at 1 year of age. This reduction is almost entirely in extracellular water. The ability to retain body water through kidney function improves in the early months of life. To the infant this means that risk of dehydration decreases as renal concentrating capacity increases.

The development of feeding behavior depends on the maturation of the central nervous system (CNS). The **rooting, sucking,** and **swallowing reflexes** are present in the term newborn (see Chapter 20). The infant also has an **extrusion reflex** that automatically pushes food out of the mouth when it is placed on the tongue. Between 3 and 6 months of age the extrusion reflex becomes less pronounced.

Early emotional, psychologic, and social attachment of the parent to the infant may influence future aspects of the infant's personality. Feeding is the

TABLE 22-1 Digestion in Infancy: Birth to 6 Months

Location	Function of Enzyme or Other Factor	Comments/Implications for Feeding
Human milk	Lipase hydrolyzes triglycerides into free fatty acids and glycerol	Functions in the small bowel because it must be activated by bile salts. Helps to compensate for the low pancreatic lipase activity at birth.
Mouth	Some salivary amylase is available at birth for starch digestion.	Insufficient to compensate for low pancreatic amylase levels.
	Lingual lipase released by serous glands hydrolyzes triglycerides.	Activity continues in the stomach, making an important contribution to milk fat digestion in the infant.
Stomach	Hydrochloric acid (HCl) and pepsin denature protein and begin hydrolysis.	Protein digestion begins. HCl output is low at birth but reaches adult levels by 6 mo of age. Pepsin levels do not equal the adult's until 2 years.
	Gastric lipase hydrolyzes triglycerides.	Along with lingual lipase, serves as an important compensatory mechanism for low pancreatic lipase levels.
Pancreas/intestine	Trypsin, chymotrypsin, the carboxypeptidases, and elastase from the pancreas hydrolyze proteins into peptides and amino acids. Dipeptidases and tripeptidases in the intestinal brush border further digest the peptides.	Although pancreatic proteolytic enzyme release is lower than in the adult, the infant has the ability to digest at least 80% of the protein ingested during the first month.
	Bile salts emulsify dietary fats, increasing the surface area available to pancreatic lipase activity.	Bile salt and pancreatic lipase levels are low at birth, but the activity of other lipases enables the newborn to digest 90% to 95% of dietary fat.
	Pancreatic amylase hydrolyzes starches.	Activity in term neonates is approximately 10% that of the adults. Activity increases by the end of 6 mo, but maximal activity is not achieved until 2 yr of age. Starch digestion may be incomplete in the young infant.
	Disaccharidases (lactase, sucrase, maltase) in the intestinal brush border hydrolyze specific disaccharides (lactose, sucrose, and maltose, respectively) to their component monosaccharides, in which form they can be absorbed.	Levels of these disaccharidases are higher at birth than they are in adults. Thus the neonate is well prepared to digest the carbohydrate in human milk, as well as the carbohydrates commonly used in preparation of formulas.

Modified from Tsang RC, Nichols BL, editors: *Nutrition during infancy,* Philadelphia, 1988, Hanley & Belfus.

main means by which the newborn establishes a human relationship with the parent. Development of trust is built on the close relationship between parent and infant. If the infant's needs are satisfied through food and love, a sense of trust is developed between the child and the parent. Food becomes the means by which infants bring together their parents and their own world. The newborn communicates by vigorous and sustained crying to express hunger, thirst, pain, and discomfort.

Feeding practices from birth, whether by breast or formula, influence the infant's exposure to tactile stimulation. Tactile stimulation is essential to the infant's physical and emotional growth.

Nutrient Needs

ENERGY (Calories or kcal). The energy requirements of the infant may be considered in terms of three areas: (1) the basal energy requirement that sustains organ metabolic function, (2) the energy needed for physical activity and digestion of food, and (3) the energy needed for growth. During the first 4 months of life, 50% to 60% of the infant's energy is expended for basal metabolism, 25% to 40% for growth, and approximately 10% to 15% for activity and other needs.

The recommended daily dietary allowance (RDA) for energy for the first year is approximately 108 kcal/kg (49 kcal/lb) for the first 6 months and 98 kcal/kg (44.5 kcal/lb) for the second half of the year (Food and Nutrition Board, 1989). Both human milk and infant formulas supply approximately 67 kcal/dL (20 kcal/oz); thus 720 mL (24 oz) of human milk or formula will supply about 480 kcal, sufficient for an infant weighing approximately 4.2 kg (9¼ lb).

CARBOHYDRATE. There is no absolute requirement for carbohydrate. However, newborns have only small hepatic glycogen stores. Moreover, they may have limited ability for gluconeogenesis (formation of glucose from amino acids and other substrates) and ketogenesis (formation of ketone bodies from fat), which are mechanisms that provide alternative energy sources. Thus carbohydrate should provide at least 40% to 45% of the calories in the newborn's diet.

Lactose is the primary carbohydrate of milk. It also is the most abundant carbohydrate in the diet of infants to 6 months of age. Lactose provides calories in an easily available form. Its slow breakdown and absorption probably benefit calcium absorption. Commercial formulas may contain corn syrup solids or glucose polymers in addition to lactose. These carbohydrate sources are well utilized by the infant.

FAT. For infants to acquire adequate calories from the limited amount of milk or formula they are able to consume, at least 15% of the calories provided must come from fat (triglycerides). The fat must be easily digestible. Fat in human milk is easier to digest and absorb than that in cow milk. This is caused in part by the arrangement of fatty acids on the glycerol molecule. It also is related to the natural lipase activity present in human milk. Fecal loss of fat and therefore loss of energy may be excessive if whole or evaporated milk without added carbohydrate is fed to infants. Cow milk is used in preparing most commercial formulas, but the milk fat is removed, and a fat source such as corn oil, which is well digested and absorbed by the infant, is added.

In addition to the energy contributions made by fat, certain fats, the essential fatty acids (EFA), are required for growth and tissue maintenance. EFA are components of cell membranes and precursors of some hormones. Inadequate intake of EFA results in eczema and growth failure. Infants should not be fed skim or low-fat milk, since these products are lacking in EFA.

PROTEIN. The protein requirement is greater per unit of body weight in the newborn than at any other time of life. The RDA for protein during the first 6 months is 2.2 g/kg.

The *protein* content of human milk, lower than that of unmodified cow milk, is sufficient for the newborn. Human milk contains far more lactalbumin in relation to casein, and lactalbumin is more easily digested than casein. In addition, the *amino acid* composition of human milk is ideally suited to the newborn infant's metabolic capabilities. For example, phenylalanine and methionine levels are low and cystine and taurine levels are high. The protein in some commercial formulas is modified to increase the amount of lactalbumin, or "whey" protein, and to decrease the relative proportion of casein. The amino acid composition of these formulas more closely resembles that in human milk than unmodified cow milk.

FLUIDS. The fluid requirement for normal infants is about 105 mL (3.5 oz)/kg/24 hr. This usually is consumed from the breast or in properly prepared formulas. Infants receiving this amount of water have approximately 100 mL/24 hr available for secretion of urine.

Water intoxication resulting in hyponatremia, weakness, restlessness, nausea, vomiting, diarrhea, polyuria or oliguria, and convulsions can result from excessive feeding of water to infants (David et al, 1981).

MINERALS AND VITAMINS. Most of the recommended minerals and vitamins are present in appropriate amounts in human milk and formula feedings. In contrast, unmodified cow milk is much higher in mineral content than is human milk, which is one important reason why it is unsuitable for the feeding of infants. The minerals and vitamins most likely to be a problem in various types of infant feedings are discussed next.

Human milk is low in calcium in comparison with cow milk and formulas, but the ratio of calcium to phosphorus is 2:1, optimal for bone mineralization. As a result, breast-fed term infants receive ample calcium. Cow milk is very rich in calcium, but the calcium to phosphorus ratio is low. Because of the imbalance, hypocalcemia, tetany, and seizures frequently develop in young infants fed unmodified cow milk. The calcium to phosphorus ratio in commercial formulas is midway between human and cow milk.

Milk of all types is low in iron. However, iron from human milk is better absorbed (50%) than that from cow milk (10%), iron-fortified formula, or infant cere-

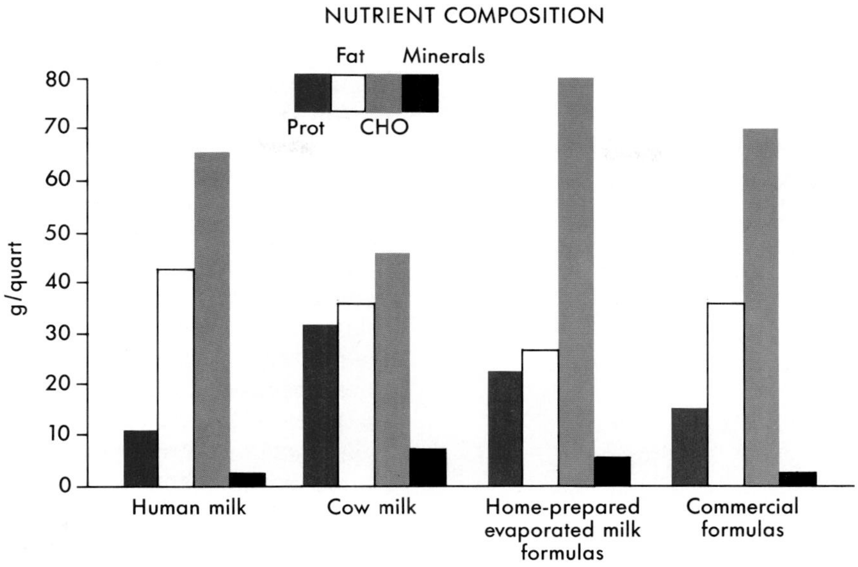

NUTRIENT COMPOSITION

Fat Minerals
Prot CHO
g/quart
0 10 20 30 40 50 60 70 80
Human milk
Cow milk
Home-prepared evaporated milk formulas
Commercial formulas

Fig. 22-1 Nutrient composition comparison of human milk/commercial formulas and cow milk/home-prepared evaporated milk formulas.
Modified from Dallman PR: Nutritional anemia of infancy. In Tsang RC, Nichols BL, editors: *Nutrition during infancy*, Philadelphia, 1988, Hanley & Belfus.

als (5%). Moreover, the fetus and the newborn infant deposit iron stores to draw upon for the first few months of life. Therefore the infant who is totally breast-fed normally maintains adequate hemoglobin levels for the first 6 months of life. After that time, iron-fortified infant cereals and other iron-containing foods are increasingly being included in the diet so that dietary intake usually is sufficient. Formula-fed infants (and infants who are initially breast-fed but then are weaned from the breast) should receive an iron-fortified formula until 12 months of age. Even though only a small percentage of the iron is absorbed from formulas, fortified formulas contain so much iron that the amount absorbed is sufficient.

Fluoride levels in human and cow milk and commercial formulas are low. This mineral is involved in tooth development, which is very active during early infancy. A reduction in dental caries is seen in children who receive adequate fluoride from birth. Thus a supplement is recommended for infants not receiving fluoridated water (p. 645).

Vitamin K levels in human milk are much lower than in cow milk or formulas. This vitamin, which is required for blood coagulation, can be produced by intestinal bacteria. However, the gut is sterile at birth, and time is required for intestinal flora to become established and produce vitamin K. Hemorrhagic disease of the newborn results from low vitamin K levels. Excessive bruising, petechiae, prolonged bleeding from blood-sampling sites or circumcisions, and intracranial hemorrhage may occur in affected infants.

Cow milk is low in vitamins C and E, but human milk and commercial formulas provide sufficient amounts. (See Fig. 22-1 for a graphic comparison of the nutrient composition of human milk and other infant feedings.)

Lactation

Lactation is under the control of numerous endocrine glands, particularly the pituitary hormones prolactin and oxytocin. It is influenced by the suckling process and by maternal emotions. The establishment and maintenance of lactation in the human are determined by at least three factors: (1) the anatomic structure of the mammary gland and the development of alveoli, ducts, and nipples, (2) the initiation and maintenance of **milk secretion,** and (3) **milk ejection,** or propulsion of milk from the alveoli to the nipple.

BREAST DEVELOPMENT. The female human breast, a large exocrine gland, is largely quiescent during most of the woman's life span. It is composed of about 18 segments embedded in fat and connective tissues and lavishly supplied with blood vessels, lymphatic vessels, and nerves. The *size of the breast* is largely related to the amount of fat present and *gives no indication of functional capacity*. The principal

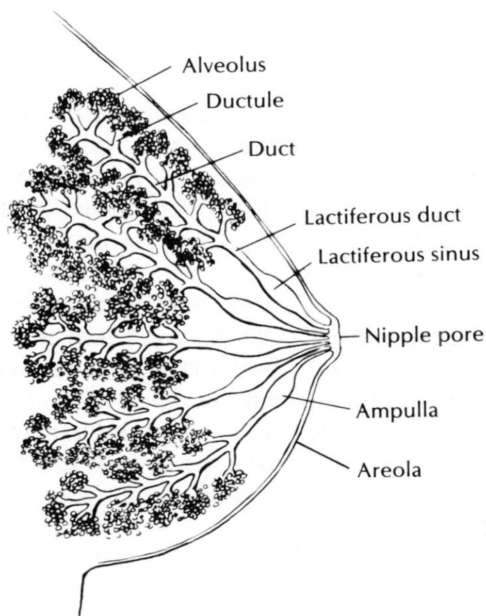

Fig. 22-2 Detailed structural features of human mammary gland.
From Worthington-Roberts BS, Williams SR: *Nutrition in pregnancy and lactation*, ed 4, St Louis, 1989, Mosby–Year Book.

feature of mammary growth in pregnancy is a great increase in ducts and alveoli under the influence of many hormones (see Chapter 8). Fig. 22-2 shows terminal glandular (alveolar) tissue of each lobule leading into the duct system. This eventually enlarges into lactiferous ducts and sinuses (ampullae). Lactiferous sinuses rest beneath the areola and converge at the nipple pore. Late in pregnancy there is maximum development of the lobuloalveolar system and presumably a sensitization of glandular tissue for action by prolactin. Colostrum is secreted in small amounts during the last 3 months of pregnancy.

STAGES OF LACTATION. *Lactation,* or more properly the process of breast-feeding, results from the interplay of hormones, instinctive reflexes, and learned behavior of the mother and newborn.

Lactogenesis (milk initiation) begins during the later part of pregnancy. Colostrum is secreted as a result of stimulation of the mammary alveolar cells by placental lactogen, a prolactin-like substance. It continues after birth as an automatic process.

The continuing secretion of milk is mainly related to (1) sufficient production of the anterior pituitary hormone prolactin and (2) maternal nutrition. Milk secretion occurs by a process of extrusion from the cells.

Movement of milk from alveoli, where it is secreted, to the mouth of the infant is an active process within the breast. This process is brought on by the let-down, or milk-ejection, reflex. The **let-down reflex** is primarily a response to an infant's sucking on the breast. The sucking stimulates the posterior pituitary gland to secrete oxytocin. Under the influence of oxytocin, the cells surrounding the alveoli contract, propelling the milk through the ductal system into the infant's mouth.

Colostrum, a yellow, premilk substance, is high in protein and contains antibodies. The production of colostrum gradually diminishes after childbirth, and the production of true milk begins. The bluish white true milk usually comes in between the third to fifth postpartum day. At the beginning of a feeding, the milk, known as *fore milk,* contains less fat and flows at a faster rate than at the end of the feeding. Toward the end of the feeding the hind milk is whiter and contains more fat calories. The higher fat content at the end of the feeding is believed to satisfy the infant and signal that the feeding should come to an end (Lawrence, 1989).

The last stage of human lactation is the ingestion of milk by the suckling baby. The full-term, healthy newborn baby possesses three instinctive reflexes needed for successful breast-feeding: the rooting, sucking, and swallowing reflexes (for a discussion of these reflexes, see Chapter 20).

MATERNAL BREAST-FEEDING REFLEXES. Three major maternal reflexes involved in breast-feeding are secretion of prolactin, nipple erection, and the let-down reflex (Fig. 22-3).

Prolactin can be considered the key lactogenic hormone in initiating and maintaining milk secretion. Its production by the anterior pituitary is mainly the result of the **prolactin reflex,** resulting from the infant's suckling at the breast. The sucking stimulus provided by the baby sends a message to the hypothalamus. The hypothalamus stimulates the *anterior* pituitary to release *prolactin,* the hormone that promotes milk production by the alveolar cells of the mammary gland. The amount of prolactin secreted, and hence the milk produced, is related to the amount of sucking stimulus, that is, the frequency, intensity, and duration with which the baby breast-feeds (Garza, Hopkinson 1988; Lawrence 1989, Worthington-Roberts, 1989).

Stimulation of the breast nipple by the infant's mouth leads to nipple erection. The stimulation makes the nipple more prominent. The **nipple erection reflex** assists in the propulsion of milk through the lactiferous sinuses to the nipple pores.

The ejection of milk from the alveoli and milk ducts occurs as a result of the milk-ejection, or **let-down, reflex.** The let-down reflex is regulated in part

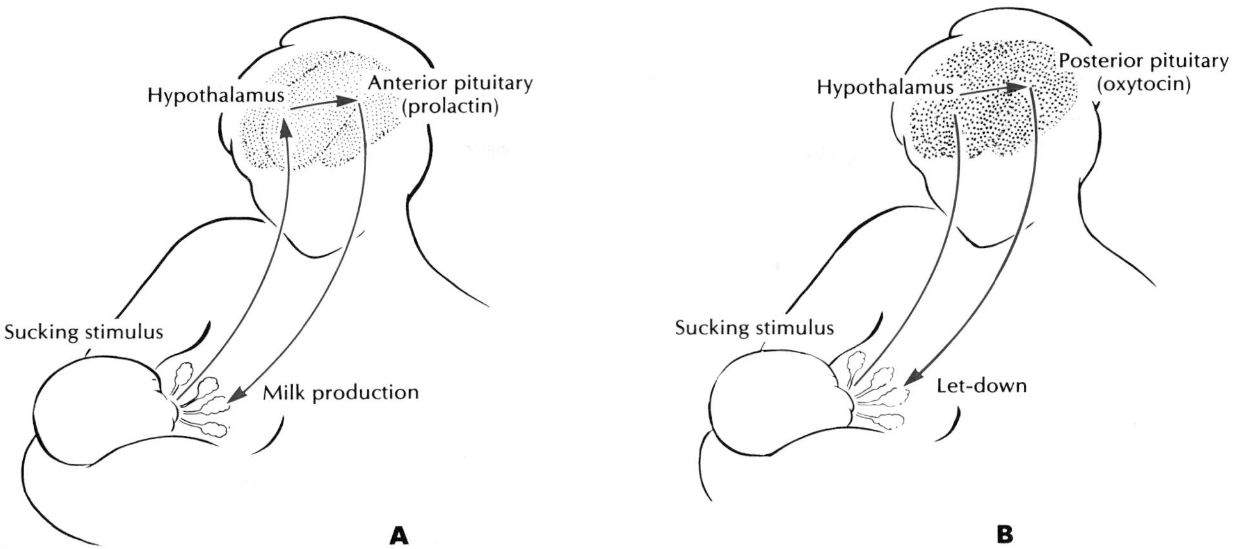

Fig. 22-3 Maternal breast-feeding reflexes. **A,** Milk production. **B,** Let-down.
From Worthington-Roberts BS, Williams SR: *Nutrition in pregnancy and lactation,* ed 4, St Louis, 1989, Mosby–Year Book.

by the CNS. The sucking stimulus arrives at the hypothalamus, which promotes release of *oxytocin* from the *posterior* pituitary. Oxytocin stimulates contraction of the myoepithelial cells around the alveoli in the mammary glands. Contraction of these musclelike cells causes milk to be propelled through the duct system and into the lactiferous sinuses, where it becomes available to the breast-feeding infant (Lawrence, 1989).

The let-down reflex appears to be sensitive to small differences in circulating oxytocin levels. Signs of successful let-down are easily recognized by the breast-feeding mother. The let-down reflex is characterized by a tingling sensation that progresses to a feeling of pulling or of being squeezed from the inside. Many women will experience the let-down reflex when simply thinking about their baby or hearing another baby cry. The let-down reflex appears to be somewhat consciously controlled. Common and significant signs of let-down include milk dripping from the breasts before the baby starts to suckle, milk dripping from the breast opposite to the one being used, and uterine cramping during feeding caused by the action of oxytocin on the uterus. Minor emotional and psychologic disturbances may influence the ease with which breast milk is released to the baby. The attitude of the mother toward breast-feeding (positive, doubtful, or negative) is a powerful factor in achieving successful lactation, influencing milk production, and facilitating the art of breast-feeding. Even minimal breast-feeding can be successful and rewarding for many women.

CULTURAL ASPECTS OF LACTATION. Cultural beliefs need to be considered in the case of a client whose background differs from that of the nurse's. In the Philippines, if the mother's milk does not flow regularly, a meal of chicken and green papaya boiled in coconut "milk" is suggested (Hart, 1965). According to Hart, the Filipino mother also is advised to eat a soup of boiled clams and ginger. Hart noted that Filipinos use hot applications of special medicinal preparations to stimulate lactation. Furthermore, the Filipino mother believes that raising either arm over her head while lying down will decrease, if not actually stop, lactation. Hart also noted the Filipino women's belief that heavy work will make their milk "hot." Korean mothers eat seaweed soup with rice to increase milk production (Chung, 1977). Currier (1978) reported that Spanish Americans believe that exposing mothers to cold diminishes the flow of milk. Yaqui women massage their breasts to drain them (Shutler, 1977).

Other differences can be observed in Finland, where no infant formula is manufactured. All women breast-feed (Carr, 1989). Countries such as Colombia, Brazil, Thailand, and New Guinea have reversed the recent decline in breast-feeding through vigorous breast-feeding promotion.

Filipinos, Mexican Americans, Vietnamese, and some Nigerians do not give colostrum to their infants. These mothers begin breast-feeding after their milk has come in. Some Korean women do not begin breast-feeding until 3 days after delivery whereas others begin breast-feeding immediately and offer the breast every time the infant cries (Choi, 1986). Mexican Americans tend to overfeed their babies because they believe that a fat baby is a healthy baby (Alexander, Blank, 1988). These mothers are more likely to offer a child a nonnutritive food as a substitute for acceptance, relieving boredom, resisting depression, and promoting relaxation.

In Kenya, mothers feed preterm neonates only by breast. They also begin breast-feeding preterm infants earlier than is the practice in most other countries. Kenyans never use gavage tubes. They feed preterm infants from small cups until they can suck (Armstrong, 1987). To provide proper assistance to a new mother from a different culture, the nurse should become aware of that culture's practices.

■ NURSING PROCESS

The nurse is one of the most important contributors to the health care team. Nurses can assist with nutrition assessment and provide education, support, and counseling.

ASSESSMENT

Feeding an infant involves the infant and the primary caregiving parent, usually the mother. Therefore both need to be assessed.

Assessment of the Infant

The infant is assessed for developmental **readiness for feeding,** nutritional needs, and success of the feeding program (Shrago, Bocar, 1990). Infant factors affecting readiness for feeding are assessed shortly after birth for the breast-fed and formula-fed infant. In addition, the suck is evaluated further by placing a finger in the baby's mouth, with the finger pad touching and stroking the palate. The examiner should be able to feel the tongue cushioning the joint of the finger and stroking the finger, while keeping the gum covered. The examiner should *not* feel an insecure or loose suction on the finger or a tapping of the gum on the finger alone, or a combination of both, with the tongue slipping back and forth across the gum (licking).

As the infant grows and matures, nutrition needs reflect the change. The infant who is obtaining the necessary nutrients and fluid will exhibit a steady increase in weight, good skin and muscle tone, vigorous feeding behavior, and satisfaction. The satisfied newborn sleeps, cries in moderation, and is interested in socializing.

Assessment of the Mother

The mother (couple) is assessed as follows:

1. Physical ability and psychologic readiness for feeding the newborn
2. Knowledge of the advantages of breast- and formula-feeding so that an informed choice of method can be made
3. Knowledge of the infant's nutrition needs and capabilities
4. Knowledge and skill in feeding methods
5. Knowledge of an adequate and safe diet during lactation

The techniques used to assess these areas include primarily interviews, discussion, and observation of skill in feeding methods.

SIGNS OF POTENTIAL PROBLEMS. The nurse must be alert for signs that the mother needs information about the newborn's reflexes (e.g., rooting, sucking, gagging, and extrusion), cues indicating readiness to feed, and feeding techniques (either breast or formula). Lack of knowledge can lead to mother-and-child frustration and maternal loss of self-esteem and can negatively affect the mother-child relationship. Mother-related problems and nursing actions are described in Table 22-2. The infant is assessed for readiness to feed, feeding skill, number and character of urine and stool, weight, and general behavior. Failure to thrive must be identified promptly (see Fig. 22-13). Gestational age and birth weight (see Chapter 37), developmental and acquired disorders (see Chapters 38 and 39) influence infant nutrition and feeding.

NURSING DIAGNOSES

When dietary data have been collected and analyzed, nursing diagnoses relative to the infant's nutrition status can be made. Examples include the following:

- High risk for ineffective breast-feeding related to
  - —Maternal anxiety or ambivalence
  - —Nonsupportive partner/family
- High risk for situational low self-esteem related to
  - —Difficulties encountered in breast-feeding secondary to knowledge deficit
- Effective family coping, potential for growth related to
  - —Knowledge of infant readiness to feed
  - —Skill in implementing chosen feeding method

A nursing plan of care on p. 648 presents examples of nursing diagnoses based on assessment findings.

PLANNING

While planning care, the nurse needs to consider many factors. These factors include the infant's and parent's readiness for feeding, the chosen feeding method, and relevant cultural influences. Community resources can be helpful, for example, the La Leche League, as well as teaching aids such as videotapes available in the hospital or clinic.

Goals

The goals or expected outcomes for the *infant* include the following:

1. The infant will receive the levels and types of nutrients to support the infant's body composition, activity, and growth.
2. The infant will have minimal physiologic stress associated with digestion, metabolism, and excretion of nutrients.
3. The infant will receive sufficient water to maintain adequate body water balance.

The *goals* for the *mother*/parent include the following:

1. The mother will receive knowledge that can be used for sound nutritional selection and feeding practices.
2. The mother will become skilled and confident in the feeding method of her choice.
3. The mother will develop closeness and pleasure with the child during feeding.

IMPLEMENTATION

General Considerations

PRENATAL PERIOD. A pregnant woman is encouraged to select a method of infant feeding before the birth. Information should be provided so that the woman can make a knowledgeable choice. Promotion of breast-feeding has been encouraged since 1981. However, breast-feeding rates among women, especially low-income women, has steadily declined (Barber-Madden, 1990). A basic lack of information regarding the benefits of breast-feeding appears to contribute to its decline.

Counseling should begin the first or second trimester of pregnancy when the mother is unrushed and has time to consider her choices. Women are encouraged to express their opinions and feelings so that they can be discussed and any misinformation be corrected. During the last months of pregnancy, counseling about the lactation process is made available to women who have decided to breast-feed. Fathers/partners are encouraged to participate in counseling sessions because their encouragement and emotional support contribute to successful lactation (see Research Highlight, p. 628). Many mothers have never seen a woman breast-feeding an infant; they therefore find it especially helpful to have a woman who has successfully breast-fed an infant available to answer questions and to provide reinforcement.

Over the past 10 years there has been an increase in the number of women who choose to breast-feed. This increase is more likely to be seen among middle-class and educated women. Reports indicate that low-income women participate in Special Supplement Food Programs for Women, Infants, and Children (WIC) and tend to bottle-feed instead of breast-feed (Barber-Madden, 1990). However, WIC has initiated successful programs to encourage mothers to breast-feed their babies.

To assist mothers in making a choice, a nurse must be knowledgeable about methods for infant feeding. Nurses can educate expectant mothers and provide support and guidance once a feeding method has been selected.

POSTNATAL PERIOD. With the birth of the infant, the parents' choice of feeding method is accepted and supported. Feeding is an emotionally charged area of infant care. Culturally the size and growth of an infant are equated with excellence and evidence of mothering/parenting ability. The infant who is a fussy eater can raise parental anxiety levels. The anxious parent appears to compound the problem, and a vicious cycle can develop. If relatives or friends can take over a feeding period or two, this help seems to break the cycle so that the mother can view the feeding session in a more relaxed manner rather than as a condemnation of her care. Mothers need positive feedback to develop a feeling of confidence in their own abilities. Often just listening and praising is the most effective intervention. Tension tends to lessen milk production. The first few days the mother is home with the baby often are filled with excitement and anxiety about mothering activities. Entertaining company or undertaking extended family commitments may have to be restricted. Many mothers need considerable assistance with infant feeding. Both group and individual teaching may be necessary.

INITIATING FEEDING. It is the practice in many hospitals to offer the newborn plain sterile water 1 to 4 hours after birth. Should it be aspirated, sterile water

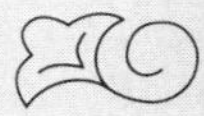 **Research Highlight** 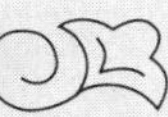

Insufficient Milk Supply Syndrome

RESEARCH ABSTRACT

Mothers often stop breast-feeding because they think they do not have enough milk. This study was conducted to determine what factors are associated with an inadequate supply of breast milk. The sample included 384 mothers with infants between 8 and 14 weeks of age; 190 mothers participated in the WIC (Women, Infant, and Children supplemental food) program and 194 did not. Data were collected using an author-developed breast-feeding questionnaire. Factors addressed in the questionnaire included maternal time constraints, maternal comfort factors, breast-feeding behaviors, maternal psychologic and physiologic factors, sociocultural factors, infant factors, and possible insufficient milk syndrome (IMS) factors. Of the subjects, 100 (26%) reported they did not have enough milk to satisfy their baby during the first 8 postpartum weeks. Mothers who had IMS knew less about breast-feeding, did not intend to breast-feed as long, and were less confident about breast-feeding. Lack of support from the mother-in-law was associated with IMS. Mothers with IMS reported more illness and poorer health while breast-feeding. Larger babies breast-fed longer. Introducing solid food was associated with IMS.

IMPLICATIONS FOR PRACTICE

Many factors are associated with IMS. Some factors were identifiable in pregnancy. Nurses can address these factors in childbirth preparation classes and reinforce the teaching in breast-feeding classes after childbirth. Support for successful breast-feeding is necessary. Whether the milk produced is insufficient or whether breast-feeding factors contribute to a decrease in quantity of milk is still unknown.

RELATED RESEARCH QUESTIONS

1. What is the incidence of IMS?
2. Does an educational intervention decrease the incidence of IMS?
3. Are ethnic and cultural factors related to the incidence of IMS?
4. Does quantity and quality of milk produced differ in mothers with IMS and mothers who do not have the syndrome?

REFERENCE

Hill PD, Aldag J: Potential indicators of insufficient milk supply syndrome, *Res Nurs Health* 14:11, Jan 1991.

is less irritating than glucose water. However, neither is colostrum irritating, and, if aspirated, it is readily absorbed by the respiratory system. The initial feeding allows the nurse to assess the newborn for any signs of tracheoesophageal fistula or atresia. If there are no complications with the mother or the infant and the mother wishes to breast-feed, the infant should be put to breast immediately after birth. As soon as the placenta separates, lactation is established (Lawrence, 1989). With encouragement and taking advantage of the infant's first period of reactivity, breast-feeding can be established early.

For the term, nonstressed newborn, early oral or parenteral feeding prevents dehydration, spares the available stores of glycogen, maintains blood glucose levels, and lessens initial weight loss. Serum bilirubin levels within normal limits often follow. Protein catabolism that would result in metabolic acidosis, hyperkalemia, or elevated levels of blood urea nitrogen is curtailed. Energy is conserved for growth, and the sucking response is stimulated.

Breast-Feeding

Milk from a healthy mother is the food of choice for a healthy infant. Breast-feeding offers many advantages: nutritional, immunologic, and psychologic. According to Worthington-Roberts (1989), breast feeding offers the following advantages:

1. The infant receives immunoglobulins to protect against some infections.
2. The infant usually has less diarrhea or constipation.
3. The type of protein ingested is less likely to cause allergic reactions.
4. The infant has fewer problems with overfeeding because the need to "empty the bottle" is eliminated.
5. Bottle washing, preparation of formula, and refrigeration are unnecessary.
6. Maternal organs return more quickly to their nonpregnant condition.
7. Breast-feeding promotes close mother-child contact.

Women who have had no contact with other mothers who breast-feed and who have had little or no contact with newborns require assistance to become proficient (Lawrence, 1989). The guidelines in the box on p. 629 outline a plan for helping an inexperienced mother with the first breast-feeding session with her baby.

IMMUNOLOGIC BENEFITS. There is evidence that the newborn infant acquires certain important elements of host resistance from breast milk while mat-

TEACHING Breast-Feeding

Here are some things to know before you start.

About Yourself

You can assume any comfortable position (Figs. 22-4 and 22-5). Let the breast fall forward without tension. Leave one hand free to guide the nipple into the child's mouth.

The nipple can be made more prominent by gently rolling it between your fingers. The areolar area will be put in the baby's mouth with the nipple. This prevents bruising the nipple.

Colostrum is the yellow fluid you can express from your breasts now. It is good for the baby. It contains some fat and protein and helps baby resist infections.

Milk may be expected to appear 48 to 96 hours after delivery. Before the milk comes in, the breasts feel soft to the touch. After the milk comes in, the breasts feel full and hard.

The Breast-Feeding Technique

Hold the baby so that the infant's cheek touches the breasts. The pressure against the outer angle of the lip begins the rooting reflex. The baby will turn toward the nipple. The baby can smell the colostrum and milk, which also will cause turning toward the nipple.

Put the baby to breast by guiding the nipple and areolar tissue into the infant's mouth and over the tongue. Compress the breast with thumb above and fingers below areola to permit infant to latch on effectively.

Expected Infant Responses and Maternal Sensations

At first the baby sucks in short bursts of three to five sucks followed by single swallows. In 1 to 2 days a sucking pattern evolves. This consists of 10 to 30 sucks followed by swallowing. The infant's lips and jaws exert pressure on the areola, and the tongue "cradles" the nipple so that the tip is not retracted. The pressure, combined with negative intraoral pressure, brings milk into the mouth (Fig. 22-6).

When the baby is sucking properly, there is no "clicking" noise. This clicking noise means the infant is sucking on her or his own tongue in the back of the throat, past the nipple. You should hear the rhythmic suck-swallow breathing pattern that indicates milk is flowing.

Some mothers can sense if the infant has drawn the areolar tissue into the mouth along with the nipple.

Breast-Feeding the Baby

Get the baby ready to put to breast by first making sure the infant is awake. If necessary, waken the baby by stroking the cheek, rubbing the feet, and talking to her or him. The nurse may help you position the baby so that the head is directly facing the breast and the nipple is not pulled to one side.

Now put the infant to breast by bringing the baby to the breast, not the breast to the baby. The baby's face, chest, genitals, and knees should all be facing your body. Touch the infant's upper lip with your nipple, and watch how the baby will turn toward you with an open mouth. Pull the baby as close to you as you can.

Feel how the baby's jaws fit behind the nipple and the nipple is deep in the infant's mouth.

If infant needs more breathing space, lift your breast, or make a "dimple" in your breast for breathing space (Fig. 22-5, *A* and *B*).

CAUTION: Making a "dimple" may be done too vigorously, which may dislodge the nipple.

You may need to hold your nipple throughout the entire feeding for a few weeks.

It is a good idea to use both breasts at each feeding. You need to empty both breasts because an empty breast signals the woman's body to produce more milk. Once the milk has come in, you can tell which breast to start with next time by feeling the weight. The heaviest one has the most milk, so start with that one. In the meantime, put a safety pin on your bra on the side that you finished, so you will know which side to start out with next time.

To remove the baby from the breast, place a finger in the corner of the baby's mouth until the suction is broken (Fig. 22-4, *D*). The breast can then be comfortably removed.

Before putting the baby to the other breast, burp the infant (Fig. 22-7). Some babies never burp; others do so frequently. Gently rub or pat the baby's back.

After feeding, place the baby on the right side. This allows air in the stomach to come up and not bring the milk with it (see Fig. 21-2).

uration of the infant's own immune system is taking place. Human milk contains high levels of immunoglobin A (IgA) and affords protection against several bacterial and viral diseases, especially those of the respiratory and gastrointestinal system (Whaley, Wong, 1991).

Immunoglobulins are believed to function directly in the infant's gastrointestinal tract by diminishing antigen contact with intestinal mucosa until the infant's own antibody responses are developed. **Lactoferrin,** which is secreted in human milk, is believed to play a role in controlling bacteria growth in the gastrointestinal tract. It works by competing with microorganisms that require iron for replication. The presence of these factors is believed to explain the reduced incidence of illness in breast-fed babies that has been reported not only in developing countries but also in the United States.

IgA probably protects against development of food allergies. In addition, human milk contains numerous other host defense factors, such as macrophages, granulocytes and T- and B-lymphocytes (Lawrence, 1989).

CARE OF BREASTS. Daily washing of the breasts with water is sufficient for cleanliness. If possible, it is helpful to expose the breasts to the air for 20 to 30 minutes. Expressed breast milk, vitamin E, or a lubricant may then be massaged gently into the nipple area. The lubricant should not clog pores or contain alcohol because its drying effects tend to encourage cracking of the tissue. Some infants object to either the taste or the smell of ointments and will refuse to suckle until the breast has been washed.

The brassiere needs to be well-fitted, with broad shoulder straps and the flaps over the breasts large enough to release the breast without discomfort. Milk leaking from the breasts, particularly just before the next feeding (milk-ejection reflex), can be uncomfortable and embarrassing. The brassiere can be padded with folded squares of soft cotton, a perineal pad cut in two, or commercially designed pads. Lining the brassiere cup with plastic material is not recommended because moisture tends to soften the nipple and predispose it to erosion.

A tingling sensation in the nipple area precedes leaking of the milk. Pressure with the heel of both hands over the nipple areas often will prevent the milk from forming so that leaking from the breast is prevented.

DIET AND FLUIDS. During lactation there is increased need for maternal energy, protein, minerals, and vitamins. This increase restores what the mother loses in secreting milk, it provides adequate nutrients for the nourishment of the infant, and it protects the mother's own stores. A well-balanced diet containing an extra 500 calories per day (per baby) is necessary for both mother and infant. Because this amount of calories is inadequate to compensate completely for the energy costs of producing milk, the mother will experience a gradual weight loss as fat stores deposited during pregnancy are expended.

The breast-feeding mother requires *extra fluids,* as much as 3 L/day. Fluids can be taken routinely before each feeding. Glasses of water, fruit juices, decaffeinated tea, and milk can be alternated. The mother can keep a pitcher of water close by when breast-feeding, because she often becomes thirsty. The use of beer or wine to aid lactation is *not* recommended (Blume et al, 1987). (See Chapter 9 for additional discussion about nutrition.)

BREAST-FEEDING POSITIONS AND TECHNIQUES. There are several positions for nursing a baby. The mother should find a position that is comfortable for her (Figs. 22-4 and 22-5, p. 632). The mother should lightly touch the baby's lips with her nipple. The baby will respond with a natural rooting reflex and turn toward the nipple and open his or her mouth. The nipple and as much of the areola as possible should be in the baby's mouth (Fig. 22-6, p. 632). If the baby's nose seems to be blocked by the breast, the mother should gently press the breast away from the nose with her finger (Fig. 22-5, *A* and *B*). When the mother is ready to change breasts, she should gently insert her finger into the corner of the baby's mouth between the gums to break the suction (Fig. 22-4, D). Pulling the baby away without breaking suction could be painful and lead to sore nipples. After burping the baby, the mother should offer the other breast. There are several positions for burping (bubbling) the baby (Fig. 22-7, p. 633). The next time the mother breast-feeds, she should offer the breast from which the infant last nursed. A safety pin on the brassiere may help remind the mother where to start the next time. She needs to remember to move the pin before starting to breast-feed.

Breast-feeding is more successful if the baby is awake and eager to nurse. Talking to, rubbing, patting, and unwrapping the baby will help the infant wake up. Washing the baby's face with a warm washcloth also may help. The baby should not have to turn the head or strain the neck to reach the nipple. The baby should be in a comfortable position to facilitate feeding.

Limiting time at the breast does not prevent sore nipples. When the baby is nursing correctly, there will not be pain or tissue damage. Getting the baby on and off the breast carefully, positioned correctly and sucking properly, will enhance feeding for both the mother and the baby. Some soreness is common, and mothers should be encouraged to continue breast-feeding. Often the soreness occurs only at the beginning of a feeding. When the milk lets down and lubricates the nipple, the soreness abates. The mother may need to try a different position to adjust the infant's sucking (Fig. 22-5). This often decreases soreness (Storr, 1988).

INFANT RESPONSES. Breast-fed babies may wish to feed more often than do formula-fed babies. If the baby wants to breast-feed, there is no reason not to do so. Breast-fed babies consume what they need and

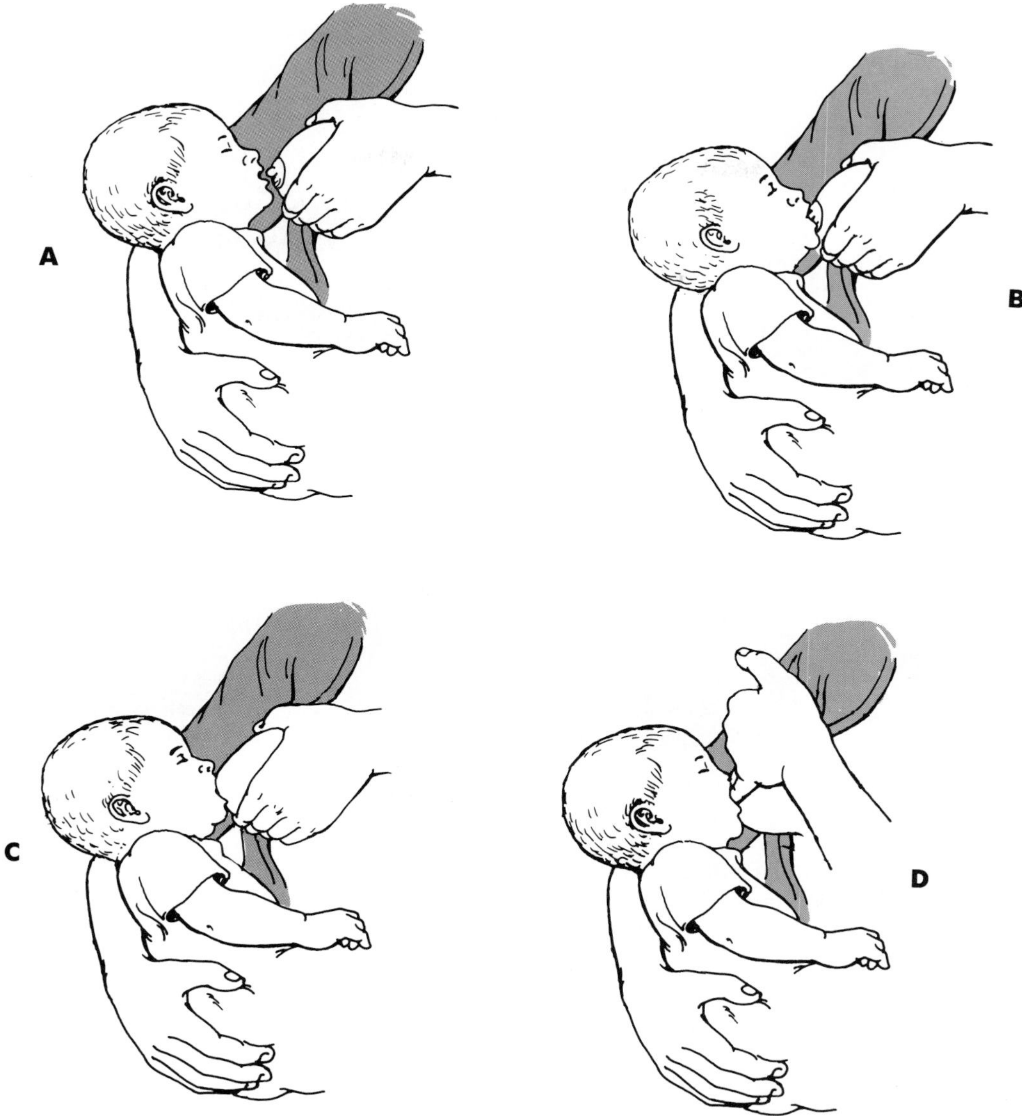

Fig. 22-4 Cradle hold. **A,** Mother touches corner of infant's mouth to elicit rooting reflex; infant responds by turning to breast and opening mouth. **B,** Infant begins to latch on. **C,** Infant latched on correctly. **D,** Mother uses finger to release suction at end of feeding.

no more. Breast-feeding whenever the baby is hungry is easy to do because the milk is always ready. Some babies may be hungry as frequently as every hour or two on some days, on other days only every 4 hours. *The more often the baby breast-feeds, the more milk the breasts produce. Thus whenever a woman's supply is low (e.g., during or after an illness), she should breast-feed more often*. If the woman has too much milk, the baby may need to breast-feed on only one side at a feeding for a while. This will reduce overall stimulation and reduce the milk supply.

Crying does not always mean that the baby is hungry (see Chapter 25). The baby may be physically uncomfortable or just want to be held, burped, or changed. The mother can be reassured that she is producing sufficient milk if the infant has 6 to 10 voidings of pale, straw-colored urine in 24 hours. In warm weather the baby may be thirsty. The mother can give the baby a bottle of water (preboiled in areas with poor sanitation or purchased, plain bottled water) (1 to 2 oz) or increase the number of breast-feedings.

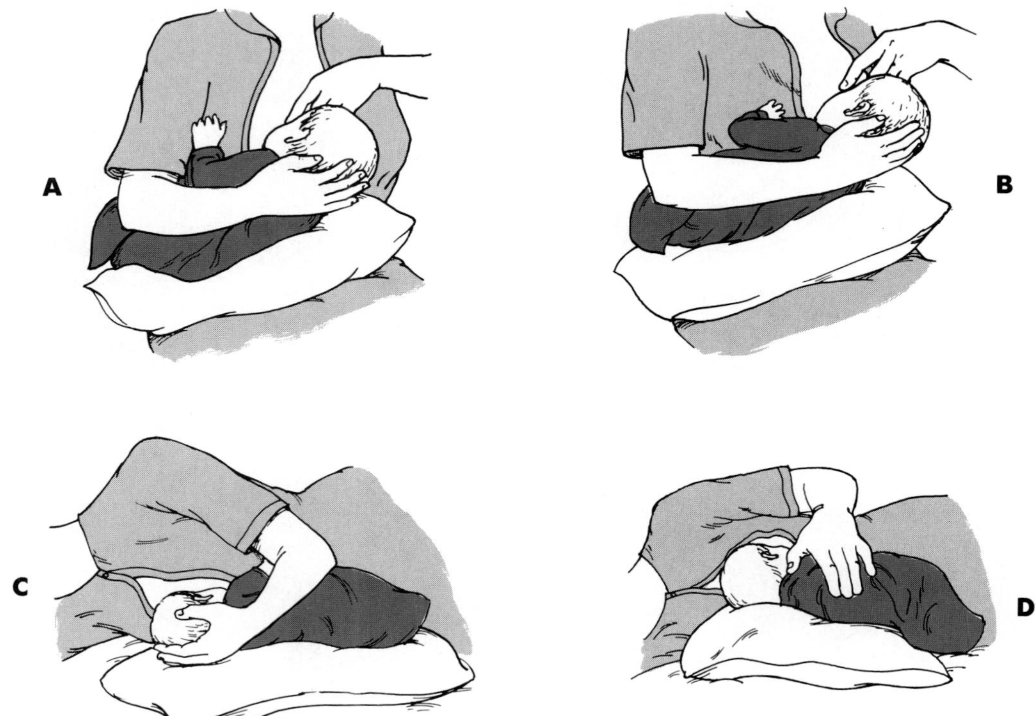

Fig. 22-5 Alternate positions for breast-feeding. **A**, Football hold (right breast). **B**, Transitional hold (left breast). **C**, and **D**, Side-lying. These positions often are used after cesarean birth to prevent pressure on abdominal incision.

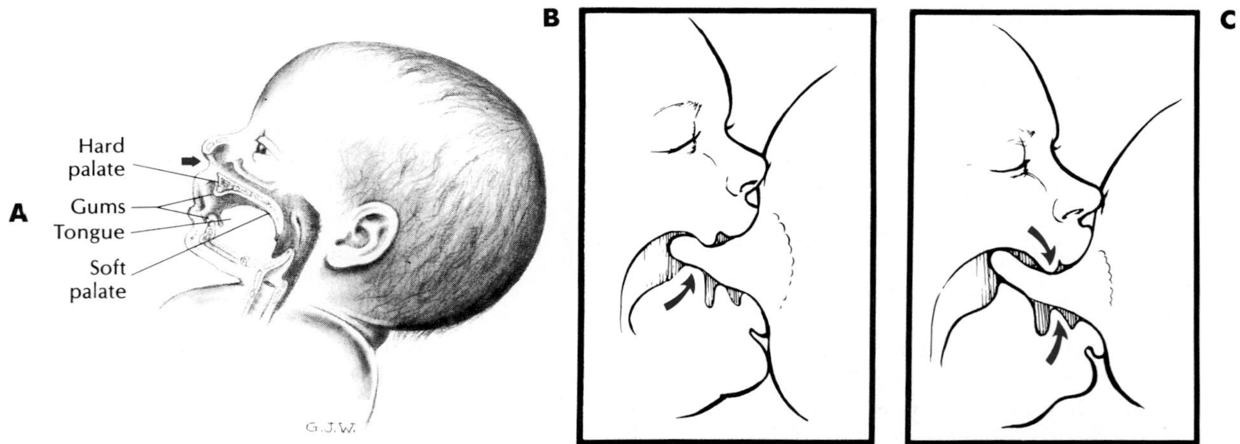

Fig. 22-6 Suckling process: **A**, Infant breathes through nose *(arrow)*. Tongue and palate meet, closing esophagus. **B**, Tongue thrusts up and forward to grasp nipple. **C**, Gums compress areola, and tongue moves backward creating, negative pressure for suction.
B and C from Riordan J: A *practical guide to breastfeeding,* St Louis, 1987, Mosby–Year Book.

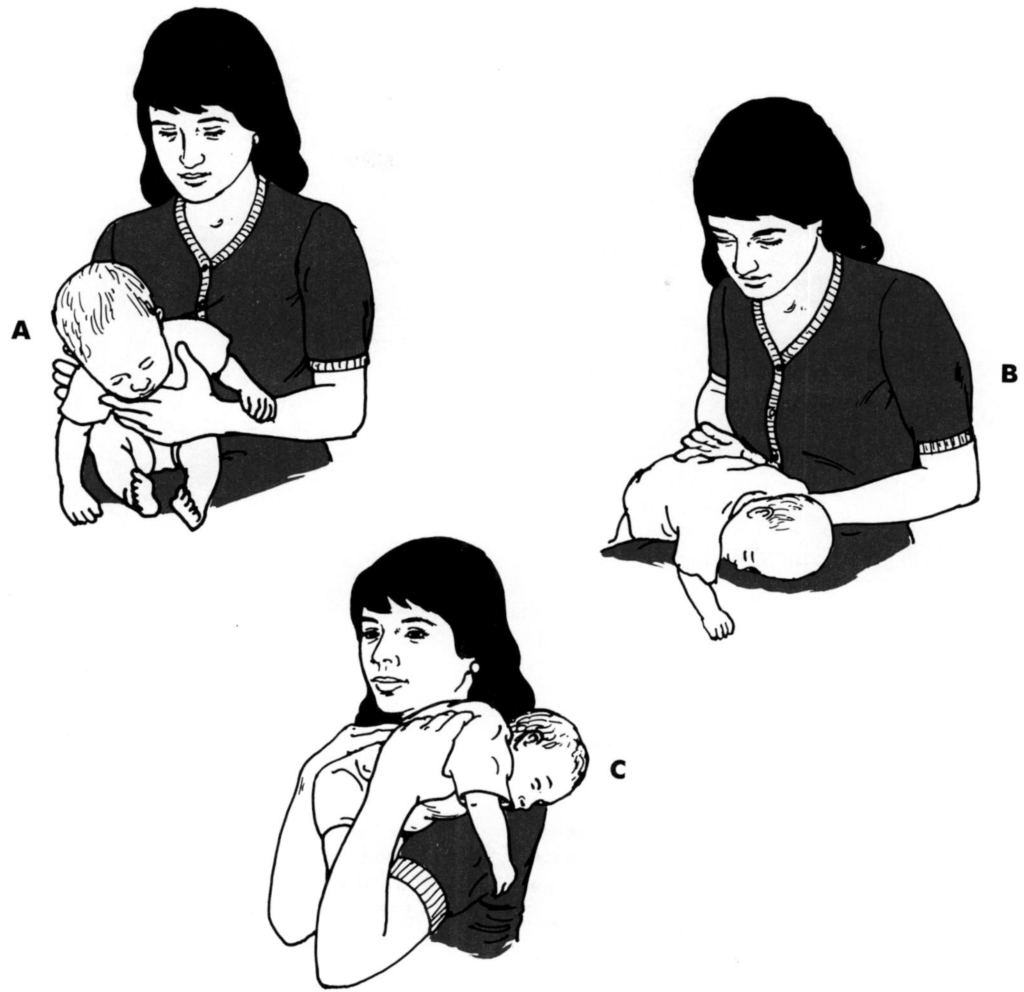

Fig. 22-7 Positions for burping (bubbling) infant. **A,** Upright. Note position of hand on jaw supporting head. **B,** Across the lap. **C,** Over the shoulder.

The *stools* of breast-fed babies are loose. Some infants have a bowel movement at each feeding, whereas others may go up to 5 days without one. Babies who are fed only breast milk do not become constipated, although they may strain considerably in passing the stool. The stool is not irritating to the skin.

BREAST-FEEDING TWINS. Breast-feeding twins takes planning and patience. If the mother elects the rooming-in regimen, the added care of two infants may prove too taxing to her strength. However, many mothers have stated that the early adjustment made going home easier. It is suggested that these mothers remain longer in the hospital unless there is help at home. It is important to establish a feeding schedule as soon as possible. The mother may use a modified **demand feeding** schedule. She can feed the first baby who wakes up, then wake up the second baby. She may decide to breast-feed them simultaneously (Fig. 22-8).

A record of the feeding times, which breast was used by which baby, and which side was used first is essential during the early weeks. If one twin feeds more readily than the other, an effort should be made to have that twin feed on alternate breasts to equalize stimulation. If feeding simultaneously, the mother should experiment with positions. Each baby may be supported on pillows and in the football hold. One may be held in the football hold and the other in the cradle hold. Obviously the mother with twins will need extra assistance from her family, extra nourishment (500 cal/day for each baby), and extra rest. She will need sufficient energy not only to care for and

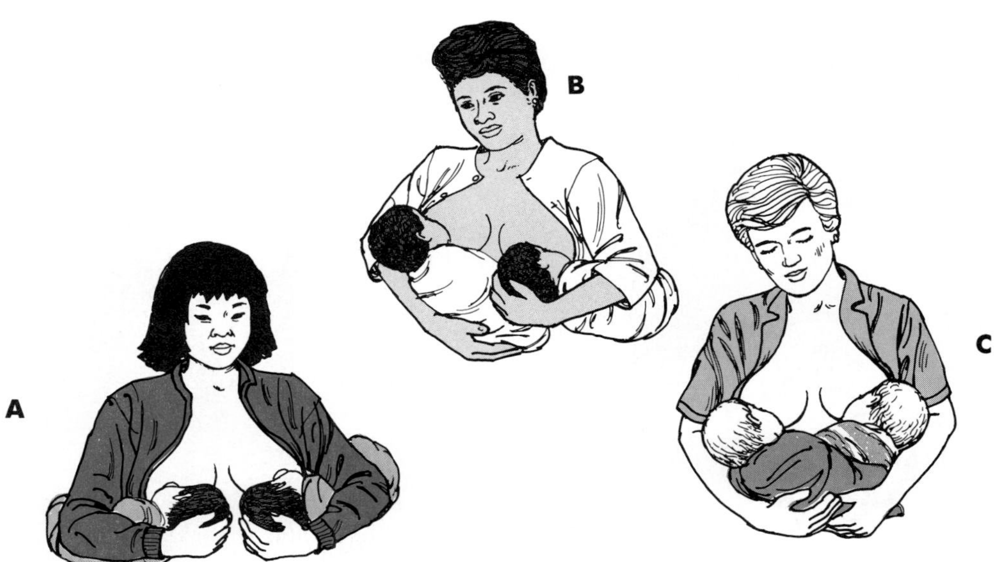

Fig. 22-8 Breast-feeding twins. **A,** Football hold. **B,** Combination cradle hold and modified cradle hold. **C,** Criss-crossed, double-cradle hold.

breast-feed each baby but also to provide the mothering each child needs.

EXPRESSING AND STORING BREAST MILK. During the early days of breast-feeding, engorgement may make the mother very uncomfortable. Expressing breast milk will provide her some relief. If a mother returns to work, it may be necessary for her to pump her breasts while away from the baby. Breast milk can be expressed by hand (manually) or with the aid of a breast pump. The process is facilitated if the mother is relaxed. The mother should be encouraged to drink liquids before and while expressing milk. Breast massage and stroking will help the let-down reflex occur before and in between expressing breast milk (see Table 22-2, p. 638 and Fig. 22-9).

To manually express milk the mother should place her hand on her breast at the edge of the areola (see Table 22-2 and Fig. 22-10). With the thumb above and the other fingers below the areola, the woman presses in toward the chest and squeezes the breast by rolling the thumb and fingers forward. These motions should be repeated in a rhythmic motion until the milk begins to flow. The fingers should not slip across the areola to the nipple. The mother should rotate her hand to reach all sections of each breast. She should return to the first breast and then the second breast, repeating until all milk is expressed.

Several types of breast pumps are available on the market today (Fig. 22-11). Some are easier to use than others, and they vary greatly in price. After the mother has selected a pump, she should moisten the inside of the breast cup with warm water. This assists to form a better seal. The mother should be instructed to lean over slightly and place the nipple and areola in the cup. The position of the cup should be changed throughout the pumping process. The cup is gently pressed toward the chest, and the pump is turned on. When the flow of milk decreases, the pump should be moved to the other breast. When the milk flow decreases in the second breast, the woman returns to the first breast.

The expressed milk may be fed to the baby in a bottle, or the milk can be stored and frozen. Plastic is preferable for storage because some of the beneficial substances in breast milk cling to the surface of glass. If breast milk is to be transported, it should be kept cold. Breast milk can be safely stored in a refrigerator 24 to 48 hours. If it is not to be used within 48 hours, it should be frozen immediately after being expressed. Breast milk may be frozen for 2 weeks. To thaw, the container should be shaken under lukewarm tap water. Thawed breast milk should be used right away. It should not be refrozen, and *a microwave oven should not be used to thaw or heat breast milk* (Worthington-Roberts, 1989). Microwaving causes "hot spots," which can cause thermal burns in the infant's mouth and throat.

BREAST-FEEDING BY DIABETIC WOMEN. Breast-feeding by diabetic women is encouraged not only for its psychologic benefits and its advantages for the infant but also for its antidiabetogenic effect. Breast-feeding decreases the insulin dosage for

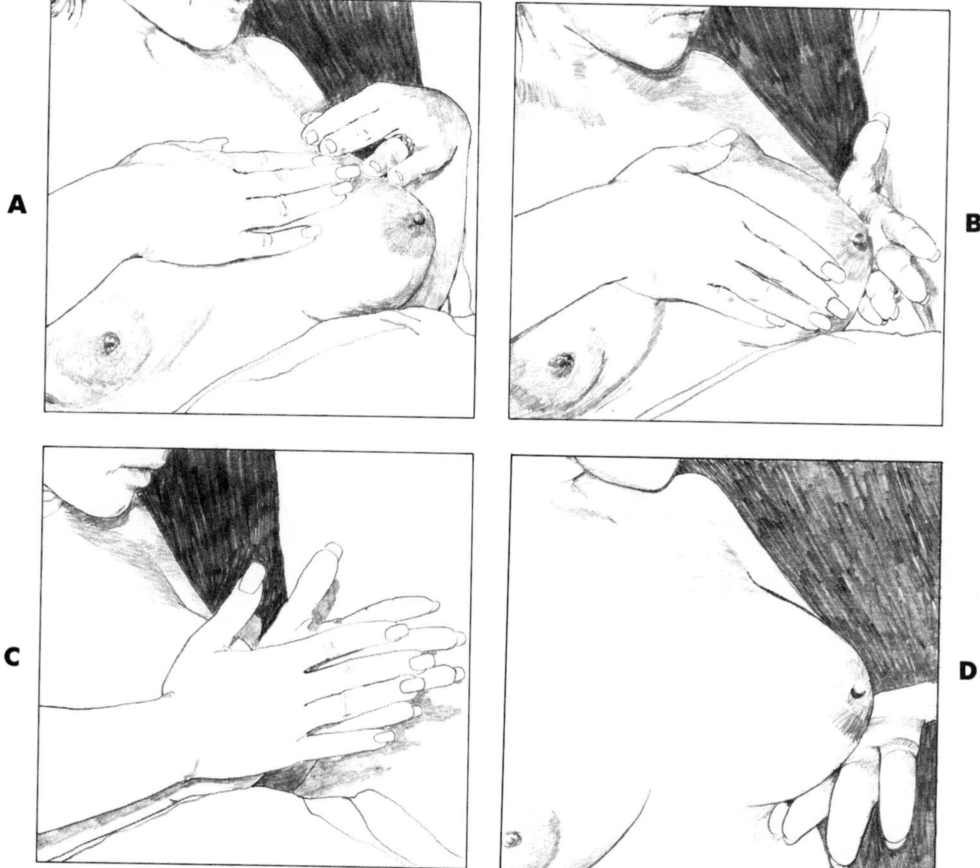

Fig. 22-9 Breast massage. **A,** Begin by placing one hand over the other above the breast. **B,** Gently, but firmly, exert pressure evenly with the thumbs across the top and fingers underneath the breast. **C,** Come together with the heel of the hand on each side and release at the areola, being careful not to touch the areola and nipple. **D,** Then gently lift the breast from beneath and drop lightly. Repeat four to five times with each breast.
Courtesy Marjorie Pyle, RNC, Lifecircle, Costa Mesa, Calif.

insulin-dependent women. The insulin dosage must be readjusted at the time of weaning (see Chapter 31).

CONTAMINANTS IN MATERNAL MILK. Nonnutrients enter human milk from the blood stream of the lactating mother. Such compounds include environmental pollutants, nicotine, methadone, marijuana, caffeine, and alcohol. The distribution of a compound across the membrane between plasma and milk is influenced by (1) its solubility in fat, (2) its degree of ionization, (3) its degree of protein binding, and (4) active vs. passive transport.

Substance abuse creates significant difficulties for the nursing infant. Regular use of *alcohol* is common in our society. However, during both pregnancy and lactation, even moderate drinking can cause problems for the unborn child or infant (Little et al, 1989). *Smoking* by the lactating woman can cause a decrease in her milk supply. Another reason not to smoke is the secondhand smoke in the baby's atmosphere. This smoke can aggravate or even trigger asthma symptoms, and babies of parents who smoke have a higher incidence of lung disease. *Caffeine* should be taken in moderation by the breast-feeding mother. Although only 1% of the mother's ingested caffeine passes to the milk, the baby's immature system cannot get rid of the caffeine as effectively as an adult can. Some babies are sensitive to even a small amount of caffeine. Caffeine is found in coffee, tea, chocolate, and some soft drinks. It is best to limit these drinks to no more than a total of 24 oz/day. If *cathartics* are taken, they may cause loose stools in the infant.

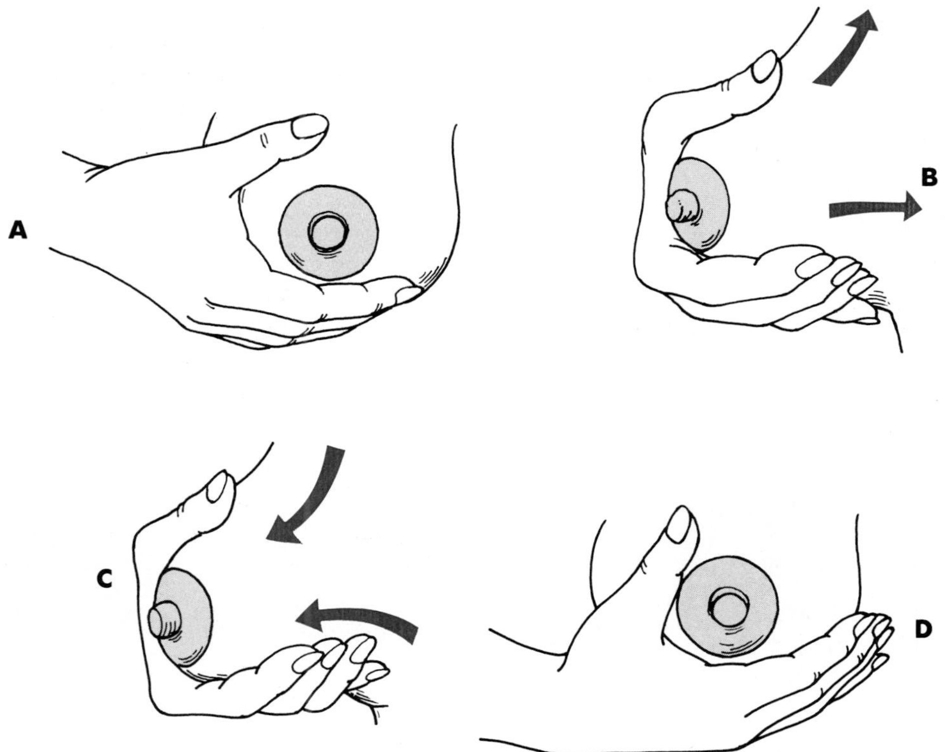

Fig. 22-10 Manual expression of human milk. A, Start with thumb above areola and other fingers below. B, Press in toward the chest. C, Squeeze milk from lactiferous sinuses by compressing the breast as the thumb and fingers slide forward. D, Rotate hand one-quarter turn around breast, and repeat steps in a rhythmic motion until the milk begins to flow. The fingers should not slip across the areola to the nipple.

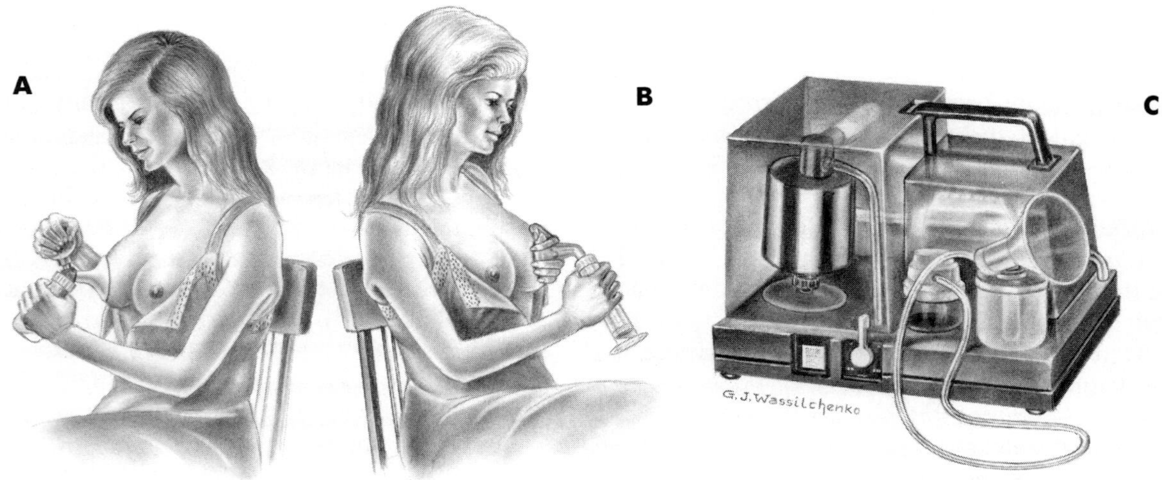

Fig. 22-11 Commonly used breast pumps. A, Swedish (rubber bulb) pump requires two hands. B, Syringe or cylinder pump requires two hands inasmuch as the cylinder must be moved back and forth. C, Electric pump. Only one hand is needed to operate this efficient and gentle pump.

EFFECT OF ORAL CONTRACEPTIVES. If *oral contraceptives* are taken sooner than 6 weeks after delivery, the amount of milk a woman produces may be diminished. Most women will not have difficulty producing an adequate amount of milk if they do not use oral contraceptives until after weaning the infant.

EFFECT OF MENSTRUATION. If menstruation occurs, the mother can continue to breast-feed. Although some babies may act fussy, the quality and quantity of the milk are not affected (Lawrence, 1989).

MATERNAL COMMITMENTS. On occasions when the mother needs to be away from the infant at feeding time, a bottle of breast milk, expressed earlier, can be substituted. If the mother returns to the workplace, she can continue to breast-feed (Morse, Bottorff, 1989). The length of time a woman breast-feeds her infant will depend on her own feelings and situation. Milk will continue to be produced as long as it taken from the breast.

CONCERNS. The inexperienced breast-feeding mother is likely to encounter major or minor problems in the course of adjusting to breast-feeding. Success or failure at breast-feeding effort may depend largely on the availability of help in the early weeks and the support of a clinician or friend who provides useful tips.

Some common concerns related to the infant may be experienced. If the infant does not open his or her mouth wide enough to grasp the nipple, the mother should depress the infant's lower jaw with one finger as she guides the nipple into the mouth. Sometimes the infant may latch on properly but will not suck. If this occurs, the mother can stimulate sucking motions by pressing upward under the baby's chin. Expression of colostrum results, and the infant is stimulated by the taste and begins sucking.

In the beginning, the infant may make frantic rooting, mouthing motions but will not grasp the nipple and eventually begins to cry and stiffen his or her body. The mother should stop trying to feed for a few minutes. If she comforts the infant and takes time to relax herself, the infant should calm down. Then she may begin again.

The infant may suck for a few minutes and then fall asleep. Methods to waken the baby should be attempted. Stimulation may include loosening the wraps, holding the baby upright, talking to the baby, or gently rubbing her or his back or the soles of the feet. A sleepy infant will not nurse satisfactorily. If it is impossible to wake the baby, it is better to postpone the feeding.

Usually an infant will suck vigorously at first and then may begin taking short, rapid sucks with frequent rest periods. This behavior indicates a slowing of the flow of milk. If the mother massages the breast toward the nipple, the flow of milk will resume. As soon as sucking resumes, the massage should be discontinued so that the infant will not be overwhelmed and choked by the milk flowing too rapidly.

Women may encounter other problems relating to breast-feeding (Graef et al, 1988). Individual counseling by a skilled clinician can greatly simplify the process of learning to cope with any problems. Table 22-2 presents mother-related problems in breast-feeding.

BREAST-FEEDING AND BIRTH CONTROL. Breast-feeding generally has been considered an ineffective method of birth control, although it has been found to delay the return of ovulation after childbirth. However, predicting the return of ovulation is difficult because ovulation may occur before menses resumes. Women who use breast-feeding as a contraceptive must be taught methods of determining ovulation. For example, basal body temperature, presence of cervical mucus, and the cervical position may be used to predict the onset of ovulation (Lethbridge, 1988). *Breast-feeding is not a method of birth control.* (For a discussion of birth control, see Chapter 42.)

SUPPORT SYSTEM/REFERRALS. Breast-feeding is very important to a new mother. It provides a closeness with the child and maternal fulfillment. A strong support system enhances the breast-feeding process. (See Research Highlight on cesarean birth and breast-feeding, p. 642).

New mothers may need some advice or encouragement when they begin breast-feeding. Being shown how to position the baby correctly will help prevent sore nipples. Childbirth educators, the perinatal nurse, or a member of the local La Leche League, a support group for breast-feeding mothers, can provide valuable information and suggestions for breast-feeding. The mother's commitment to breast-feeding and the support from partner, family, and friends greatly increases the chances of success. The father can be included by offering water or expressed milk to the baby during a mother's absence. Parents can be confident that their support of breast-feeding will give their new baby the best start in life. Prenatal breast-feeding education also can help the expectant mother prepare for breast-feeding (Wiles, 1984; Coreil, Murphy, 1988; Neifert et al, 1990; Emery et al, 1990).

TABLE 22-2 Mother-Related Problems in Breast-Feeding

Problem	Nursing Action
ENGORGED BREASTS If feeding has been on demand since birth, painful **engorgement** of the breasts is not likely to occur. However, because of the lag between the production of milk and the efficiency of the ejection reflexes, engorgement of the breasts may occur for up to 48 hours after the milk comes in. The mother often complains that the breast is tender and that the tenderness extends into the axilla. The breasts usually feel firm, tense, and warm as a result of the increased blood supply, and the skin may appear shiny and taut. The unyielding areolae makes it difficult for the infant to grasp the nipple. Breast-feeding can be uncomfortable to the mother and frustrating for both mother and infant.	1. Application of moist heat: apply wet cloths as hot as can be endured to the whole breast and, at the same time, express milk from the nipple. As the wet cloth cools, replace with another one. Shower and direct the hot water to the breasts. 2. **Breast massage** (Fig. 22-9): (a) Begin by placing one hand over the other above the breast. (b) Gently, but firmly, exert pressure evenly with the thumbs across the top and fingers underneath the breast. (c) Come together with the heel of the hand on each side and release at the areola, being careful not to touch the areola and nipple. (d) Then gently lift the breast from beneath and drop lightly. Repeat four to five times with each breast. 3. **Manual expression of milk** (Fig. 22-10): Place the thumb and forefinger on opposite sides of the breast just outside the areola, press downward into the rib cage, and then gently squeeze together and downward; the nipple should not be pulled outward. Repeat the procedure, moving the thumb and forefinger around the nipple until as much milk as desired has been expressed. If the milk is to be used later, *it should be expressed into a sterile plastic bottle and frozen.* Milk expression is not easy for some women at first, but persistence usually brings success if the mother takes the time.
SORE NIPPLES The nipples may become sore during the early days of breast-feeding. **Sore nipples** may be prevented or limited by using a correct position and avoiding undue breast engorgement. If soreness occurs, it usually is temporary until the nipples become accustomed to the baby's sucking (Storr, 1988). Some mothers report soreness for up to 3 months (Chapman et al, 1985).	1. Expose the nipples to air. 2. Use a heat lamp to dry the nipples after the feeding (40-watt bulb in a desk lamp, positioned 45 cm [18 in] from breast). 3. If soreness occurs, limit sucking time to 5 min on each breast, the time it takes to empty the breasts of milk. 4. Use a pacifier if the infant's sucking needs have not been met. 5. Use a nipple shield. 6. Discontinue breast-feeding for 48 hr. During this time the milk is expressed manually or with a breast pump, collected in a sterilized bottle, and given to the baby by bottle. Precautions for maintaining the milk in a safe condition must be followed. Bottles and nipples must be sterilized by immersing them in water and boiling for 10 minutes; any milk not immediately consumed must be refrigerated or frozen.
PLUGGED DUCTS Occasionally a milk duct will become plugged, creating a tender spot on the breast, which may appear lumpy and hot. **Plugged ducts** might result from inadequate emptying of the milk ducts or from wearing a brassiere that is too tight.	1. Offer the sore breast first so that it will be emptied more completely. 2. Nurse longer and more often; if the breast gets too full, the plugged duct becomes worse and infection may develop. 3. Change positions at every feeding so that the pressure of the feeding will be applied to different places on the breast.

TABLE 22-2 Mother-Related Problems in Breastfeeding—cont'd

Problem	Nursing Action
	4. Apply warm compresses to the breasts between feedings to reduce the risk of infection by keeping the ducts open.
INCREASED LOCHIAL FLOW The breast-feeding mother may note an increase in lochial flow once feeding begins. At times afterpains are intensified to such a degree that the mother becomes uncomfortable, and her tension interferes with feeding the infant.	Offer a mild analgesic for pain 40 min before the feeding period. The mother may be reassured that this discomfort is transitory and will be gone in about 2 days.
PERCEPTION OF INADEQUATE AMOUNT OF MILK Insufficient milk supply rarely is a problem for the well-nourished mother. Because sucking stimulates the flow of milk, feeding on demand for adequate duration should supply ample amounts of milk.	1. Increase frequency of feedings to increase supply. 2. Note frequency of infant urination; 6 to 10 voidings every 24 hr is adequate. 3. Weight gain of 1/2 oz/day indicates adequate intake. 4. Reassure mother if infant seems satisfied.
BREAST PUMPING For a number of reasons, mothers may wish to remove milk from their breasts and save it for a later feeding, take it to their hospitalized newborn, or donate it to a milk bank. Under such circumstances, milk can be expressed by hand, and for some women **pumping the breasts** by hand is satisfactory. For many women, however, a manual or electric breast pump provides a better stimulus for milk flow and a more efficient mode of milk collection.	Instruct the mother in the use of the breast pump (Fig. 22-11).
MATERNAL INFECTION If breast tenderness is accompanied by fever and a general flulike feeling, a breast infection probably is present (see Chapter 29).	Instruct the mother to notify her physician immediately.
SEXUAL SENSATIONS For some women the rhythmic uterine contractions occurring while breast-feeding are akin to those experienced during orgasm. These unexpected sexual sensations within the context of child care may be disturbing.	Reassure as to normality of such feelings.
RELACTATION AND LACTATION AFTER ADOPTING Occasionally a mother starts breast-feeding late or discontinues it but decides at a much later date that she would like to begin again. *After adopting an infant,* a small number of women decide to attempt lactation even though they have never done so before or, at best, have breast-fed a baby of their own. With much sucking stimulus, lactation can be induced but only with great perseverance and in most cases only if a woman has once carried a pregnancy well into the second trimester. Because the mammary glands complete their development for lactation during the first 6 months of pregnancy, a woman who has never been pregnant or never carried a pregnancy beyond the first trimester is a poor candidate for successful induction of lactation.	Instruct the mother to attempt relactation or induced lactation through providing the infant substantial opportunities to suck at the breast. With much sucking stimulus over several days' time, many patient and persistent women can initiate the lactation process late or once again. Their volume of milk production may be less than the infant demands, in which case a supplemental feeding after breast-feeding may be necessary. Alternatively, some women find the Lact-Aid Nursing Trainer to complement their own milk production (Fig. 22-12) (Edgehouse, Radzyminski, 1990). While sucking at the breast, the baby also obtains milk via suction through a small tube leading to a bag of fresh formula that is clipped to the mother's brassiere. As the infant sucks, the mother's milk supply is built up and the infant receives adequate nutrition through the Lact-Aid feeding device.

Continued.

TABLE 22-2 Mother-Related Problems in Breast-Feeding—cont'd

Problem	Nursing Action
FAILURE OF INFANT TO THRIVE Occasionally, an infant will experience **failure to thrive** (have an inadequate weight gain) while seeming to feed properly.	1. Assist in the explanation of potential problems (Fig. 22-13). 2. Encourage mother to turn to commercial infant formula for at least partial nutritional support of the infant if the cause of the problem cannot be identified or the defined problem cannot be corrected. 3. Refer the mother to a pediatrician if condition continues, or prn.

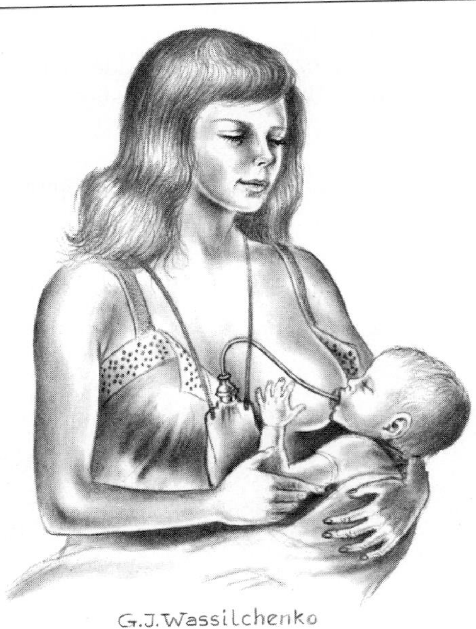

Fig. 22-12 Lact-Aid Nursing Trainer in use.

Formula-Feeding

Formula-feeding has proved a successful substitute for breast-feeding in certain instances, including the following:

1. The family decides against breast-feeding or the mother is unable to breast-feed because of disease or anomalies.
2. The mother's schedule does not permit her to breast-feed.
3. Special formula is required because of infant allergies or special dietary needs.
4. It provides supplementation for infants of mothers who occasionally choose to omit breast-feeding.
5. It complements human milk if the mother's milk production is inadequate (Tsang, Nichols, 1988).
6. The infant is adopted.

Formula feeding should be the choice if the mother has an active infection such as tuberculosis, syphilitic breast lesions, or acquired immunodeficiency syndrome (AIDS). Other medical reasons such as diabetes need to be evaluated. If a mother is taking medication for a specific disease, such as thyroid medication, the infant must be closely followed. It is best to refrain from taking medications if the mother is breast-feeding. The mother should consult the pediatrician in regard to any medication she may be taking (see Appendix E).

Physicians recommend formulas on the basis of the infant's nutrition needs, cost, need for refrigeration, convenience, and the mother's ability to prepare the formula accurately and safely.

FEEDING PROCESS AND CARE OF THE MOTHER AND INFANT. Inexperienced mothers who are formula-feeding their infants need the same teaching, counseling, and support as do the mothers who are breast-feeding. They need assistance with the feeding process and with problems they experience. Some mothers who elect formula-feeding express concern that the baby will suffer as a result of their decision. They need assurance that knowledge of their infant's nutrition needs and skill in use of formula-feeding can be an acceptable substitute for breast-feeding. Emphasis on the beneficial use of the feeding time for close contact with their infant can help relieve their tensions. (See guidelines for teaching for self-care to mothers who are formula-feeding, p. 643.)

FEEDING SKILLS. The formula-feeding mother needs teaching regarding feeding skills. During feedings, she should be encouraged to assume an *en face*

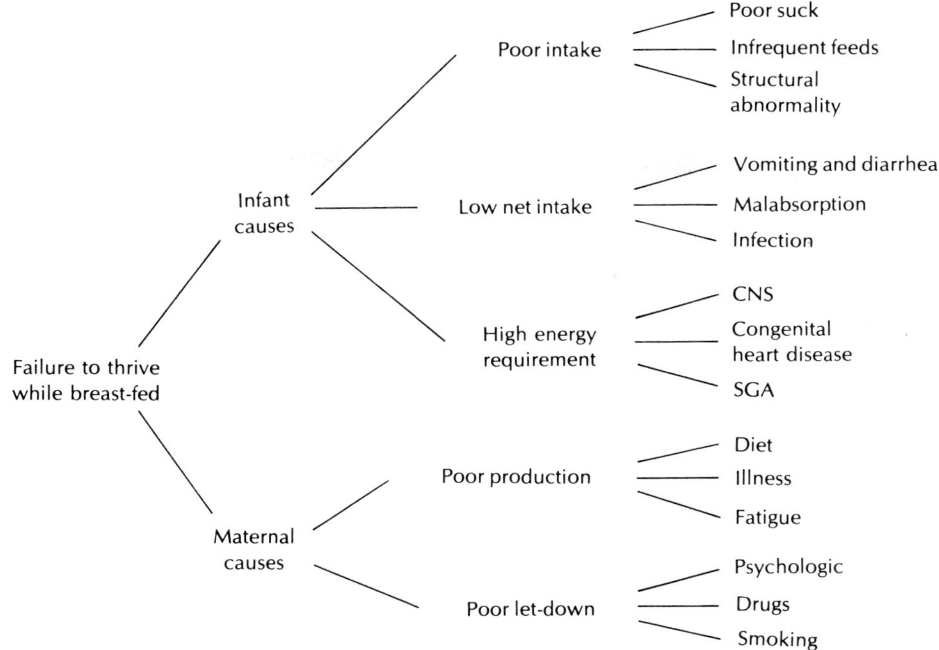

Fig. 22-13 Diagnostic flow chart for failure to thrive.
From Lawrence RA: Breastfeeding: a guide for the medical profession, ed 3, St Louis, 1989, Mosby–Year Book.

position with the infant (looking into each other's eyes) and to hold the infant closely and securely. Feedings provide a good time for her to talk, sing, or read to the infant or simply enjoy a time of peaceful relaxation with her baby.

A new bottle has been designed that allows only fluid, not air, to travel through the nipple. A bend at the top of the bottle forces air bubbles to the top, away from the nipple. The Degree bottle helps eliminate feeding-related disorders such as excessive spitting up and colic. Designed to promote correct, upright feeding posture, the Degree baby bottle has a soft, clear, no-drip, cross-cut silicone nipple and a leak-proof travel cap. The bubbleless bottle comes in 5-ounce and 8-ounce sizes.

A bottle should never be propped with a pillow or other inanimate object and left with the infant. This practice may result in choking, and it deprives the infant of important interaction during feeding. Moreover, propping the bottle has been implicated in causing **nursing bottle caries,** or decay of the first teeth resulting from continuous bathing of the teeth with carbohydrate-containing fluid as the infant sucks sporadically on the nipple.

The bottle should be held so that fluid fills the nipple and none of the air in the bottle is allowed to enter the nipple (Fig. 22-14). After the newborn period, the infant who falls asleep, turns aside the head, or ceases to suck usually is signaling that enough formula has been taken. The mother should be taught to look for these cues and avoid overfeeding, which could contribute to obesity (see box on p. 643).

CARE OF BREASTS. The breasts should be washed daily with clear water or a mild soap. A well-fitting brassiere provides needed support. During the early postpartum period, a tight binder, ice packs, and a mild analgesic may be necessary to relieve discomfort caused by pressure if the milk comes in. Nipple and breast stimulation should be avoided. When in the shower, women should stand so that the shower beats on their back and not on their breasts. An antilactogenic, bromocriptine (Parlodel), frequently is prescribed for non–breast-feeding mothers. The mother must be instructed to continue to take the bromocriptine for 14 to 21 days (for a discussion of Parlodel, see Chapter 25).

DIET AND FLUIDS. A formula-feeding mother needs a well-balanced diet to restore maternal energy, provide protein for healing, and provide minerals and vitamins. An adequate fluid intake is important to maintain renal function and bowel regularity.

INFANT RESPONSES. Because cow milk formula forms a larger curd, stomach emptying time is slower than with breast milk. Formula-fed babies eat

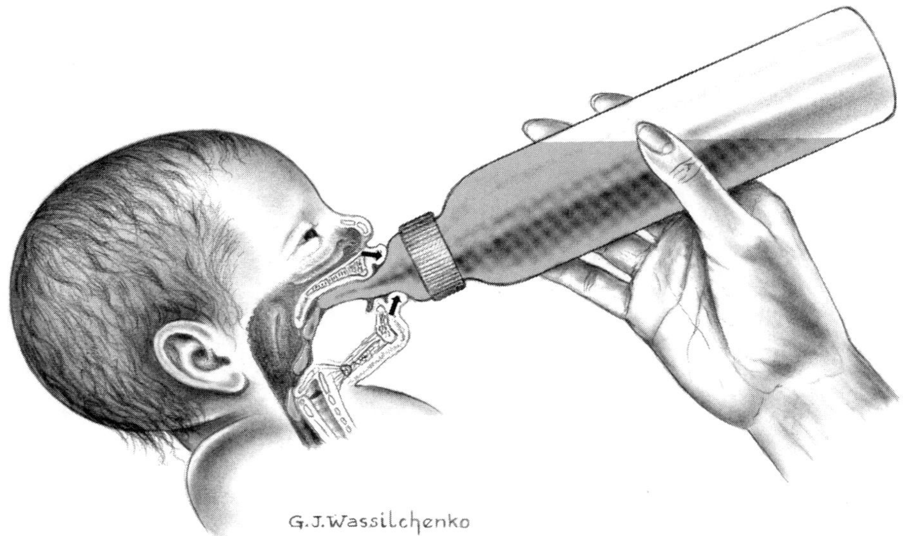

Fig. 22-14 Bottle-feeding. Bottle is held in hand like a pencil. Note milk covers nipple area so infant will not suck in air.

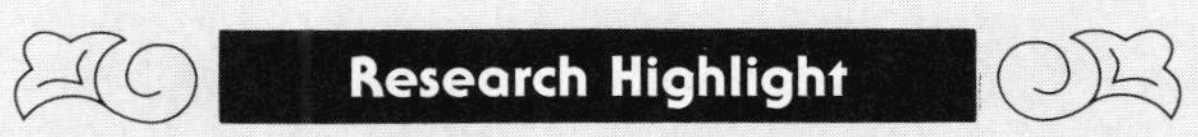

Cesarean Birth and Breast-Feeding Outcomes

RESEARCH ABSTRACT

The purpose of this study was to determine the effect of cesarean delivery on the time of the first breast-feeding as well as breast-feeding problems and duration. Subjects were 121 first-time mothers who were enrolled in a larger study. The subjects were randomly assigned to one of two groups: a planned formula-feeding group (who offered one bottle feeding per day) and a total breast-feeding group. A scale that measured attitudes toward breast-feeding was used to collect prenatal data. Other variables were collected by means of chart review and structured interviews 1 week after birth. Breast-feeding outcomes were assessed by telephone interviews through 6 months postpartum. In this sample the cesarean rate was 23%. Mothers giving birth by cesarean breast-fed later for the first time and reported less satisfaction with the birth experience than those who had vaginal births. There was no difference between groups in any other variables. There was no relation between the type of birth and duration of breast-feeding or in the amount of pain or fatigue attributed to breast-feeding.

IMPLICATIONS FOR PRACTICE

Breast-feeding support and not time of first breast-feeding was the important factor in breast-feeding success. Nurses must provide a supportive environment for breast-feeding at the time of childbirth and during the postpartum stay. They can assure mothers that cesarean birth need not prevent them from breast-feeding. Nurses can assist mothers to identify supportive individuals in their own networks and arrange for follow-up telephone calls or referrals to groups of breast-feeding mothers.

RELATED RESEARCH QUESTIONS

1. Does breast-feeding outcome differ between mothers who attend childbirth preparation classes and those who do not?
2. Will providing a support person during the early postpartum period change the breast-feeding outcome?
3. Is the time milk "comes in" related to breast-feeding success?
4. Is the time milk "comes in" related to satisfaction with breast-feeding success?

REFERENCE

Kearney MH, Cronenwett LR, Reinhardt R: Cesarean delivery and breastfeeding outcomes, *Birth* 17:97, Summer 1990.

every 3 to 5 hours. The physician provides instructions as to the amounts of formula to be fed the infant over 24 hours and when to increase the amounts to ensure meeting the growing infant's nutrition needs. Formula may be fed at room temperature or warmed until the milk feels warm when tested on the caregiver's inner arm. The infant may need extra water in warm weather.

Infants swallow more air when fed from a bottle and should be burped after every ½ to 1 ounce of formula. Unused formula should be discarded after a feeding. Bottles, nipples, water, and formula need not be sterilized unless the water is not safe.

The stools of formula-fed babies are firmer than those of breast-fed babies and have a characteristic odor. Infants may have one to two stools per day. The diaper should be changed and the skin thoroughly cleaned to prevent irritation to the skin.

INFANT FEEDING FORMULATIONS

COMMERCIAL FORMULAS. Commercial formulas are available in three forms: ready-to-feed, concentrate, and powder. All forms are equivalent in nutritional content, but there may be a considerable difference in price. Parents should be helped to weigh the considerations of convenience and cost carefully and to choose the form that best suits their needs. Powdered formulas are especially well-suited

TEACHING Formula-Feeding

Baby needs to be wide awake.

The hospital bottles of formula can be stored at room temperature. You may use this brand or the one your pediatrician recommends. They contain 4 oz of formula (120 mL). Your baby will probably drink 2 to 3 oz (60 to 90 mL) at a feeding for a few days and then increase. If you do not use all the formula, throw the remainder away because it spoils once opened.

You can keep track of how many ounces the baby drinks in 1 day by writing it down. When you take the baby for a check-up, your physician or nurse will ask you the amount of intake.

Your baby will probably be hungry every 2½ to 3 hours. If your baby fusses or cries in between feedings, check the diaper or the infant's need to be picked up and cuddled. As the baby gets older, thirst may occur. Check with the pediatrician concerning water supplementation.

Test the temperature of the formula by letting a few drops fall on the inside of your wrist. If the formula feels comfortably warm to you, it is the correct temperature. If the formula is refrigerated, warm it by placing the bottle in a pan of hot water. Check it often for correct temperature.

Test the size of the nipple hole by holding the bottle and nipple upside down. The formula should drip from the nipple. If it runs in a stream, the hole is too big. If it has to be shaken for the formula to come out, the hole is too small. To correct this, you can try a softer nipple or enlarge the hole in the nipple or both. To enlarge the hole, heat a needle stuck into a cork (used as a handle) and insert the hot needle into the nipple. New nipples may be softened by boiling for 5 minutes before using. If the nipple collapses, unscrew the bottle lid to let air in.

Some newborns need burping. They tend to swallow air when sucking. Burp the baby who has been crying before feeding, then after every ounce of formula. As the infant gets older and you get more experienced, you will know when to burp the baby.

To feed the baby, place the the nipple in the infant's mouth over the tongue. It should rest against the roof of the mouth. This stimulates the sucking reflex.

Hold the bottle like a pencil. Keep nipple filled with milk so the infant does not suck air.

Start out with the baby held away from you until the nipple is in the mouth. The baby who is too close will turn toward you and not the nipple; this is the rooting reflex.

After the baby starts feeding, you can hold the infant close.

Some newborns take longer to feed than others. Slow, patient feeding, keeping the baby awake and encouraging the infant to take more may be necessary.

The stools of a formula-fed newborn are soft but formed. They will be yellow with a characteristic odor. The baby probably will defecate either during the feeding or after. Change the diaper immediately because the composition of the stool is irritating to the skin.

SAFETY TIPS

Do not prop the bottle. The nipple may fall against the throat and block the air, or the baby could drown in the formula or aspirate any that was regurgitated.

Newborns should never be left alone while feeding until they are old enough to remove the bottle from their mouth.

Bottles taken to bed can lead to early dental problems in young children (nursing bottle caries, or baby bottle syndrome).

Practice how to hold the newborn, and use the bulb syringe in case the baby should choke.

After the baby is finished, place the infant in the crib on the right side so air can come up easily.

to the needs of families who travel or who are away from home frequently at feeding time, because they are lightweight, not bulky, and require no refrigeration. Ready-to-feed and concentrated formulas usually come in multiserving cans that must be refrigerated after opening. Some ready-to-feed formula is sold in disposable bottles, but ordinarily this is the most costly type of formula.

Cow milk is used as the basis of most formulas, although soy-based formulas and other specialized formulas are available for the infant who does not tolerate milk-based formulas. A comparison of human milk with commercial formulas is given in Fig. 22-1. The following list summarizes the modifications used in preparing milk-based commercial formulas:

1. Butterfat is removed and vegetable oils are added to ensure adequate fat absorption and to provide essential fatty acids.
2. Protein is heated to produce a softer, more flocculent curd that is more easily digested by the infant.
3. Protein and mineral concentrations are decreased to more nearly resemble those in human milk. Carbohydrate is then added to provide sufficient calories.

HOME-PREPARED FORMULAS. Some families may wish to make their own formula at home to reduce the expense of formula feeding. However, it is impossible for home-prepared formulas to resemble human milk as closely as do commercial products (Fig. 22-1). Because human milk is uniquely designed to meet the needs of the human infant, it is commonly used as the standard for judging all infant feedings. Thus mothers who do not breast-feed should be encouraged to use commercial formulas whenever possible. If finances are an overwhelming factor, the family usually is eligible for services through the WIC program, which will provide iron-fortified infant formula.

CAUTION: *Honey* sometimes is used as a sweetener for home-prepared infant foods or formula, and occasionally it is recommended for use on pacifiers to promote sucking in hypotonic babies. Use of honey for any of these purposes, however, is discouraged because some sources contain spores of *Clostridium botulinum* (Whaley, Wong, 1991). These spores are extremely resistant to heat and therefore are not destroyed in the processing of honey. If ingested by an infant, spores may germinate and lethal toxin may be released into the lumen of the bowel. Infant botulism may ultimately develop, and in some cases it is fatal.

FORMULA PREPARATION. Recent recommendations for labeling commercial infant formulas require that the directions for preparation and use of the formula include pictures and symbols for nonreading individuals. In addition, manufacturers are translating the directions into foreign languages, such as Spanish and Vietnamese, to prevent misunderstanding and errors in formula preparation. It is important to impress upon families that the proportions *must not be altered*—neither diluted to extend the amount of formula nor concentrated to provide more calories.

Although manufacturers of commercial formula include directions for preparing and administering their products, the nurse should review **formula preparation** with the mother. It is especially important that formula be diluted properly. The newborn's kidney is immature, and overly concentrated formula may provide protein and minerals that exceed the kidney's excretory ability. In contrast, if formula is too dilute (a practice sometimes followed to conserve formula and save money), the infant may be unable to consume an increased volume to compensate, and poor growth may result.

Sterilization of formula rarely is recommended now where families have access to a safe public water supply. Instead, formula is prepared with scrupulous cleanliness. Where water comes from a private well or a public supply of questionable safety, parents should be advised to boil for 15 minutes all water that is to be fed to the infant or used for formula preparation.

If sanitary conditions within the home appear unsafe, it may be necessary to teach the mother to sterilize the formula. The two traditional methods for sterilization are terminal heating and the aseptic method. In the terminal heating method, the formula is placed in the bottles, which are topped with the nipples and caps, and they are boiled together in a water bath for 25 minutes. In the aseptic method, the bottles, nipples, and any other necessary equipment such as a funnel are boiled separately, after which the formula is poured into the bottles. (The teaching box summarizes steps in formula preparation.)

UNMODIFIED COW MILK. Unmodified cow milk is unsuited to meeting the nutritional needs of the infant (Fig. 22-1). Specific concerns include its excessive amounts of calcium, phosphorus, and other minerals, imbalance of calcium and phosphorus, excessive protein content, poorly absorbed fat, and low iron concentration. In addition, for reasons that are not completely understood its use is apt to cause gastrointestinal blood loss in the infant (Zeigler et al, 1990). This blood loss, as well as the low levels of

TEACHING Formula Preparation

- Clean all necessary equipment (e.g., bottle, nipple, can opener), and wash hands carefully before preparing formula.
- Read formula label and dilute formula exactly as recommended by the manufacturer.
- Use tap water for preparation of concentrated or powdered formula, unless directed otherwise by physician or nurse.
- Opened cans of ready-to-feed or concentrated formula should be discarded after 24 hours.

TEACHING Fluoride Supplementation

- Administer fluoride drops daily as prescribed by the physician.
- Leave supplement in childproof container, and store it where children cannot reach it. (The drops have a pleasant taste. Long-term overdose causes mottling of teeth, and acute poisoning can cause symptoms ranging from vomiting and other gastrointestinal disturbances to death.)
- If infant begins to consume 240 mL or more of fluoridated water/day (either alone or in other feedings such as juices), consult the physician regarding discontinuing the supplement.

iron in the milk, increases the likelihood of iron deficiency anemia. Anemia in the infant may have serious and long-lasting consequences; some evidence suggests that infants who have anemia (corrected with iron therapy) have learning delays that may persist throughout the preschool years (Oski, 1990).

Thus the use of unmodified cow milk cannot be advocated before the end of the first year of life.

Some infants have an allergic reaction to the formula and may be switched to a soy milk formula (Tsang, Nichols, 1988). The soy protein used in infant formulas appears to equal and, in some cases, exceed the amount of protein in cow milk formula (Witherly, 1990). Some infants benefit from a change from one brand of formula to another.

Some infants cannot tolerate sucrose or glucose oligosaccharide formulas. Signs of intolerance are diarrhea and failure to thrive. If hypersensitivity to cow milk protein is suspected, a hydrolyzed casein formula is used. If carbohydrate intolerance is suspected, a modular formula is substituted (Tsang, Nichols, 1988).

Discharge Planning

If the mother elects early discharge anticipatory guidance can be given before the mother leaves the hospital, at the well-baby checkups, or during a home visit. The following information is helpful to the parent (Pyle, 1985).

FREQUENCY OF FEEDING. During the daytime, the mother awakens and feeds the infant so that the baby is not sleeping more than 3 hours at a time. At night, the infant is allowed to sleep and is fed only upon awakening. Night feedings should be businesslike so that the baby learns that nights are not play time. At the beginning, most mothers prefer to take the baby to bed to breast-feed or formula-feed. Mothers also find that baby will sleep better if laid across the upper portion of her abdomen, so that baby hears her heartbeat and has the warm body contact.

Ideally for the newborn, feeding schedules are determined by the infant's hunger. Feeding infants when they signal readiness is called *demand feeding*. *Scheduled feedings* are arranged at predetermined intervals to meet family routines. The newborn will feed every 1½ to 3 hours during the daytime and usually every 3 to 5 hours at night. Breast-fed infants need to feed *at least every 3 hours* during the daytime. "Good" babies who rarely cry, who sleep, and who awaken only to nurse every 4 to 6 hours usually do not have an adequate weight gain, and the mother may not maintain an adequate milk supply. Most babies will average 10 feedings during a 24-hour period. The following guide indicates the average intake by formula-fed infants:

Age	Quantity per feeding	Number of feedings 24 hr
Birth-3 wk	2-3 oz (60-90 mL)	6-10
3 wk-2 mo	5 oz (150 mL)	5-8
2-3 mo	5-7 oz (150-210 mL)	5-6

Mothers will notice spurts in the infant's appetite between 10 days and 2 weeks; 6 weeks and 9 weeks; and 3 months and 6 months. These appetite spurts correspond to growth spurts. The infant wants to breast-feed more frequently and for longer periods. For the breast-feeding baby, increasing the feedings results in a greater production of milk. The satisfied infant then tapers off her or his demands. For the formula-fed baby, the amount of formula offered can be increased by 2 to 4 oz (60 to 120 mL).

SUPPLEMENTAL FEEDINGS FOR BREAST-FED BABIES. *Supplemental feedings* should *not* be offered to breast-fed infants in the nursery because, if satiated, they will not suck vigorously at the breast. Lactation depends on emptying the breast at each feeding. If milk is allowed to accumulate in the ducts, breast engorgement and ischemia result, suppressing the activity of the acini (milk-secreting cells). Consequently milk production is reduced. In addition, the process of sucking from a bottle is different from breast-nipple compression. The relatively inflexible rubber nipple prevents the tongue from its usual rhythmic action. Infants learn to put the tongue against the nipple holes to slow down the more rapid flow of fluid. When infants use these same tongue movements during breast-feeding, they may push the human nipple out of the mouth and may not grasp the areola properly (Lawrence, 1989).

Usually by 3 to 4 weeks after birth, lactation is well established and a feeding schedule has been formed. Formula-fed infants ingest about 2 to 3 ounces of formula at each feeding and are fed about six times a day. Breast-fed infants may feed as frequently as 10 to 12 times daily. Larger infants are able to retain increased amounts because of greater stomach capacity; as a result they generally sleep through the night sooner than do smaller infants. After the milk supply is established, an occasional bottle will not affect lactation and breast-feeding.

In contrast to the occasional bottle-feeding, the regular use of solid foods before 4 to 6 months of age is more likely to result in an inadequate maternal milk supply and early cessation of breast-feeding (Grossman et al, 1990; Hill, Aldag, 1991).

MINERAL AND VITAMIN SUPPLEMENTATION. Shortly after birth, vitamin K is administered intramuscularly to prevent hemorrhagic disease of the newborn (see Chapter 21). Normally, vitamin K is synthesized by the intestinal flora. However, because the infant's intestine is sterile at birth and breast milk contains low levels of vitamin K, the supply is inadequate for at least the first 4 to 7 days.

The normal infant receiving breast milk from a well-nourished mother needs no specific vitamin and mineral supplements, with the exceptions of fluoride in a dose of 0.25 mg daily and iron by 6 months of age (when fetal iron stores are depleted) (see box, p. 645). Supplements of 400 IU of vitamin D daily may be indicated if the mother's vitamin D intake is inadequate or if the infant does not benefit from adequate ultraviolet light because of dark skin color or little exposure to light (American Academy of Pediatrics, 1980 a,b).

Milk from strict vegetarian mothers (those who include no animal products in their diet) may be too low in vitamin B_{12} to meet the infant's needs. These infants (and/or mothers) require a supplement (Specker et al, 1988). Like human milk, commercial iron-fortified formula supplies all the nutrients needed by the infant for the first 6 months. The only supplementation required is 0.25 mg of fluoride if the local water supply is not fluoridated or if the infant is given ready-to-feed formula, which eliminates the use of fluoridated tap water (American Academy of Pediatrics, Committee on Nutrition, 1986).

WEANING. Weaning the baby from the breast can be a smooth process if it is done gradually. If the mother eliminates feedings gradually over a period of several weeks, this creates less discomfort for both mother and infant and gradually decreases the amount of milk being produced.

One breast-feeding a day can be substituted with formula if the infant is younger than 1 year of age. Many mothers wean directly from the breast to a cup. The feeding eliminated is a matter of personal choice. Frequently the feeding before bedtime is the last feeding eliminated. The weaning process should continue until all breast-feeding is eliminated.

Sometimes situations require the mother to stop breast-feeding suddenly. If this happens, the mother may have engorgement. This discomfort can be diminished by wearing a snug brassiere and avoiding stimulation of the breast. Ice packs and a mild analgesic may help. The idea is to avoid milk expression, thereby reducing the milk supply.

INTRODUCING SOLID FOODS. The infant receives the right balance of nutrients from breast milk or formula during the first 4 to 6 months (Broussard, 1984). It is not true that the feeding of solids will help the baby sleep through the night. Introduction of solid foods before the infant is 4 to 6 months of age may result in overfeeding and decreased intake of breast milk or formula (Madgic, 1986). The infant cannot communicate feeling full as can an older child, who is able to turn her or his head away. The proper balance of carbohydrate, protein, and fat for an infant to grow properly is in breast milk or formula.

The infant's individual growth pattern should help determine the right time to start solids. The physician will advise when to introduce solid foods. The schedule for introducing solid foods and the types of foods to serve will be discussed during well-baby supervision visits with the pediatrician and pediatric nurse (American Academy of Pediatrics, 1980 b, 1983 a, b).

REFERRALS. Referral procedures provide an opportunity for individuals and groups to take advantage of services available from other sources. A properly coordinated health service delivery for infants and children that includes a registered dietitian can contribute to a sense of continuity and to consistency of care and advice. The mother is encouraged to contact the local association that assists with breast-feeding (see Appendix H).

The mother who is formula-feeding needs teaching and support as much as does the breast-feeding mother. It is important that she understands how to mix the formula and how to prepare the bottles. The mother should be encouraged to hold the baby while feeding and discouraged from propping the bottle. Above all, she should not be made to feel guilty or a less adequate mother for not electing to breast-feed.

Nurses are in an ideal position to provide the support the mother needs. If the mother experiences problems, she should feel free to contact the nursery or her pediatrician for assistance.

EVALUATION

Parental knowledge and infant well-being and the findings that represent normal response form the basis for selecting appropriate nursing actions and evaluating their effectiveness. The nurse can be reasonably assured that care was effective to the degree that the following goals for care have been met.

- The infant received the level and type of nutrients to support body composition, activity, and growth.
- The infant experienced minimal physiologic stress associated with digestion, metabolism, and excretion of nutrients.
- The infant received sufficient water to maintain adequate body water balance.

The following goals apply to the mother/parents.

- They received information that can be used for sound nutritional selection and feeding practicies.
- They became skilled and confident in the feeding method of choice.
- They developed closeness and pleasure with the child during feeding.

■ SUMMARY

Parental knowledge is a key factor in infant nutrition and feeding. Providing nutrition services to parents and their infants is a function of the health care team. Physicians, nurses, registered dietitians, social workers, and health educators are major contributors to the care. One of the most important contributors, the nurse, can assist with nutrition assessment and provide education, support, and counseling. Nurses can help interpret dietary prescriptions and make appropriate referrals of more complicated problems to nutrition personnel.

CASE STUDY

Maternal Self-Esteem, Breast Feeding, and Infant Nutrition

Mindy Jonus, a 32-year old first-time mother, called for a nurse to help her with breast-feeding. Jason (7 pounds 10 ounces) is 1 day old and is making frantic rooting and mouthing motions but appears unable to latch on. When you enter the room, the baby is crying lustily and is very stiff. Mindy is trying to push Jason's cheek to turn his head to face the breast. Mindy is near tears and equally frustrated. She cries out, "I just do not know what to do! I can't remember everything the nurse did for me last night. I feel like such a failure."

ASSESSMENT

Mindy states she and her husband have been looking forward to her breast-feeding. She has "read every book" she could find, but now she "can't remember what to do." She gave birth to Jason vaginally after a 12-hour unmedicated labor. All physical assessment and laboratory test findings for her and Jason are within normal limits. After Jason breast-feeds successfully, Mindy changes Jason's diaper and comments, "How will I know he's getting enough milk from me—that is, after my milk comes in?"

NURSING DIAGNOSIS

The assessment findings support several nursing diagnoses. Two problems require immediate attention: Mindy is anxious and has low self-esteem at this time, and Jason is hungry and frustrated. Mindy's needs take priority because the current situation could affect her self-perception as a mother and her attachment to Jason. One nursing diagnosis is chosen: Situational low self-esteem related to lack of experience with breast-feeding.

PLANNING

The nurse and Mindy mutually agree on a *goal:* reduction of her anxiety by learning how to comfort her son and relax before starting to breast-feed. The nurse sets an *expected outcome:* Mindy's self-esteem as a mother will be enhanced.

IMPLEMENTATION

Several nursing interventions are possible. For Mindy, the nurse chooses the following: suggests that Mindy wrap Jason up snugly, pick him up, "bubble," cuddle, and talk or sing to him to relax him; comments on Mindy's success in relaxing Jason; touches Mindy's neck and shoulders and asks her to consciously relax each muscle group touched; remarks that this is the first time for both her and her son to breast-feed, and each needs time to learn because knowing is not instinctive; states that the nurse will remain with her as *she* initiates and completes the feeding.

EVALUATION

The nurse can be assured that their goal was met when Jason quiets down in response to Mindy's actions. Mindy is gratified by her son's response and is able to relax.

CARE PLAN Maternal Self-Esteem, Breast-Feeding, and Infant Nutrition

GOALS	IMPLEMENTATION	RATIONALE	EVALUATION
Nursing diagnosis: Situational low self-esteem related to lack of experience with breast feeding			
1. Mindy's anxiety is relieved.	Suggest that she wrap Jason snugly, pick him up, "bubble," cuddle, and talk or sing to him to relax him.	A frantic, frustrated newborn is unable to initiate feeding; he may have a bubble causing abdominal discomfort.	Jason relaxes and stops frantic rooting, mouthing, and crying.
2. Mindy's self-esteem is maintained as she understands that she and Jason both need to learn to breast-feed.	Comment on her success in relaxing Jason.	Focuses mother on her accomplishment of a parental skill.	Mindy states her pleasure from seeing Jason respond to her.
	Touch her neck and shoulders to teach her to relax specific tense muscle groups (as she had learned to do in parent education classes for childbirth).	Reinforces self-care method to reduce muscle tension.	Mindy's posture and facial expression indicate relaxed muscles in neck and shoulders.
3. Mindy's self-esteem is enhanced as she learns and implements methods to console Jason.	Remark that this is the first time for both her and Jason to breast-feed, and each needs time to learn.	Reaffirms that breast-feeding is a learned behavior for both and learning takes time.	Mindy states she had never grasped the fact that breast-feeding needs to be learned by both of them.
4. Mindy feels supported.	State that you will remain with her as *she* initiates the feeding.	Offers supportive presence while Mindy *learns by doing*.	Mindy states she "would feel better having someone nearby" as she starts the feeding.
Nursing diagnosis: High risk for ineffective breast-feeding related to insufficient knowledge regarding newborn reflexes and breast-feeding techniques			
1. Mindy will learn about newborn reflexes, e.g., rooting.	Describe rooting reflex.	Provides knowledge so newborn reflexes can be used effectively.	Mindy states she understands content taught and demonstrated.
2. Mindy will learn breast-feeding techniques.	Ask Mindy to assume a comfortable position and let the breast fall forward without tension. Assist Mindy to position Jason so that his face, chest, and knees face her body. Coach Mindy to bring Jason to the breast, compress her breast with thumb above and fingers below areola, touch his cheek and outer angle of his lip, and guide her nipple and areolar tissue into his mouth and over his tongue.	Provide support as Mindy learns by doing.	Mindy completes breast-feeding at this time. Mindy is able to breast-feed successfully at the next feeding. Mindy states pleasure with her accomplishment and with breast-feeding.

Continued.

CARE PLAN Maternal Self-Esteem, Breast-Feeding, and Infant Nutrition—cont'd

GOALS	IMPLEMENTATION	RATIONALE	EVALUATION
	Describe, demonstrate, and watch Mindy do the following: ■ Make a breathing space by dimpling ■ Remove baby from breast ■ Bubble him ■ Try alternate positions ■ Care for breasts ■ Lay Jason on his right side, after feeding		
Nursing diagnosis: Potential for altered nutrition related to parent's lack of knowledge of infant's behaviors, elimination patterns, and growth (weight)			
1. Mindy will learn infant's behaviors and elimination patterns. 2. Jason will sleep after feedings. 3. Jason will void pale, straw-colored urine 6-10 times/day.	Discuss infant's: ■ Behavior indicating satiety (enough food), e.g., sleeps 3 hours ■ Stooling pattern ■ Voiding pattern ■ Immediate weight loss less than 10% of birth weight ■ Regaining birth weight within 10 days	Anticipatory guidance provides reassurance and serves as a basis for decision making. Knowledge helps to allay anxiety regarding the unknown and thereby assists in maintaining parent's self-confidence.	Mindy states she understands content. Jason loses less than 10% of his birth weight and has normal elimination patterns.
4. Jason will not lose more than 10% of his birth weight and will regain his birth weight within 10 days.	Discuss need to empty each breast at each feeding. While Mindy is changing Jason's diaper, encourage questions regarding Jason's elimination pattern. Encourage questions regarding Jason's behaviors, characteristics, and parameters of normal growth and development.	Emptying the breasts is the stimulus for lactation. Readiness for learning enhances retention of content. Reassures Mindy that all questions are legitimate and that answers are available for the asking.	At his next visit to the physician, nurse practitioner, or home health care nurse, Jason's growth is within normal parameters; he shows no signs of failure to thrive. Mindy indicates satisfaction with her mothering.

REFERENCES

American Academy of Pediatrics, Committee on Nutrition: Vitamin and mineral supplement needs in normal children in the United States, *Pediatrics* 66:1015, 1980a.

American Academy of Pediatrics, Committee on Nutrition: On the feeding of supplemental foods to infants, *Pediatrics* 65:1178, 1980b.

American Academy of Pediatrics, Committee on Nutrition: The use of whole cow's milk in infancy, *Pediatrics* 72:253, 1983a.

American Academy of Pediatrics, Committee on Nutrition: Toward a prudent diet for children, *Pediatrics* 71:78, 1983b.

American Academy of Pediatrics, Committee on Nutrition: Fluoride supplementation, *Pediatrics* 77:758, 1986.

Armstrong H: Breastfeeding and low birth weight babies: advances in Kenya, *J Human Lactation* 3:34, 1987.

Barber-Madden R: Design and implementation of a citywide breastfeeding promotion program: the New York City approach, *Fam Community Health* 12:71, April 1990.

Blume S et al: Beer and breast-feeding mom, *JAMA* 258:2126, 1987.

Broussard A: Anticipatory guidance: adding solids to the infant's diet, *JOGNN* 13:239, 1984.

Carr C: A four-week observation of maternity care in Finland, *JOGNN* 18:100, 1989.

Choi EC: Unique aspects of Korean-American mothers, *JOGNN* 15:394, 1986.

Chung HJ: Understanding the Oriental maternity patient, *Nurs Clin North Am* 12:67, 1977.

Currier RL: The hot-cold syndrome and symbolic balance in Mexican and Spanish-American folk medicine. In Martinez RA, editor: *Hispanic culture and health care: fact, fiction, folklore,* St Louis, 1978, Mosby–Year Book.

David R et al: Water intoxication in normal infants: role of antidiuretic hormone in pathogenesis, *Pediatrics* 68:349, 1981.

Edgehouse L, Radzyminski SG: A device for supplementing breast-feeding, *MCN* 15:34, Jan/Feb 1990.

Emery JL, Scholey S, Taylor EM: Decline in breastfeeding, *Arch Dis Child* 65:369, 1990.

Food and Nutrition Board: Recommended dietary allowances, Washington, DC, 1989, National Academy of Sciences.

Garza C, Hopkinson J: Physiology of lactation. In Tsang RC, Nichols BL, editors: *Nutrition during infancy,* St Louis, 1988, Mosby–Year Book.

Graef P et al: Postpartum concerns of breastfeeding mothers, *J Nurse Midwife* 33:62, March/April 1988.

Grossman LK et al: The effect of postpartum lactation counseling on the duration of breast-feeding in low-income women, *Am J Dis Child* 144:471, 1990.

Hamill PVV et al: Physical growth: National Center for Health Statistics percentiles, *Am J Clin Nutr* 32:607, 1979 (data from the Fels Research Institute, Wright State University School of Medicine, Yellow Springs, Ohio).

Hart DV: From pregnancy through birth in a Bisayan Filipino village. In Hart DV, Rajadhon PA, Coughlin RJ, editors: *Southeast Asian birth customs: three studies in reproduction,* New Haven, Conn, 1965, Human Relations Area Files.

Lawrence RA: *Breastfeeding: a guide for the medical professional,* ed 3, St Louis, 1989, Mosby–Year Book.

Lethbridge DJ: The use of breastfeeding as a contraceptive, *JOGNN* 18:31, 1989.

Little RE et al: Maternal alcohol use during breastfeeding and infant mental and motor development at one year, *N Engl J Med* 321:425, 1989.

Madgic D: *Nutrition notes for new mothers,* Stanford, Calif, 1986, Department of Dietetics, Stanford University Hospital.

Morse JM, Bottorff JL: Intending to breastfeed and work, *JOGNN* 18:493, 1989.

Neifert M et al: Factors influencing breastfeeding among adolescents, *J Adolesc Health Care* 9:209, 1990.

Oski FA: Whole cow milk feeding between 6 and 12 months of age? Go back to 1976, *Pediatr Rev* 12:187, 1990.

Shrago L, Bocar D: The infant's contribution to breastfeeding, *JOGNN* 19:209, 1990.

Shutler ME: Disease and curing in a Yaqui community. In Spicer EH, editor: *Ethnic medicine in the Southwest,* Tucson, Ariz, 1977, The University of Arizona Press.

Specker BL et al: Increased urinary methylmalonic acid excretion in breast-fed infants of vegetarian mothers and identification of an acceptable dietary source of vitamin B_{12} *Am J Clin Nutr* 47:89, 1988.

Storr GB: Prevention of nipple tenderness and breast engorgement in the post-partal period, *JOGNN* 17:203, 1988.

Tsang RC, Nichols BL: *Nutrition during infancy,* St Louis, 1988, Mosby–Year Book.

Whaley LE, Wong DL: *Nursing care of infants and children,* ed 4, St Louis, 1991, Mosby–Year Book.

Wiles LS: The effect of prenatal breastfeeding education on breastfeeding success and maternal perception of the infant, *JOGNN* 13:253, 1984.

Witherly SA: Soy formulas are not hypoallergenic, *Am J Clin Nutr* 51:705, 1990.

Worthington-Roberts B: Lactation and human milk: nutritional considerations. In Worthington-Roberts B, Williams SR, editors: *Nutrition in pregnancy and lactation,* ed 4, St Louis, 1989, Mosby–Year Book.

Zeigler EE et al: Cow milk feeding in infancy: further observations on blood loss from the gastrointestinal tract, *J Pediatr* 116:11, 1990.

References—Nursing Research

Alexander MA, Blank JJ: Factors related to obesity in Mexican-American preschool children, *Image* 20(2):79, 1988.

Chapman J et al: Concerns of breast-feeding mothers from birth to 4 months, *Nurs Res* 34:374, 1985.

Coreil J, Murphy, JE: Maternal commitment, lactation practices, and breastfeeding duration, *JOGNN* 17:273, 1988.

Hill PD, Aldag J: Potential indicators of insufficient milk supply syndrome, *Res Nurs Health* 14:11, 1991.

BIBLIOGRAPHY

Giger JN, Davidhizar RE: *Transcultural nursing: assessment and intervention,* St Louis, 1991, Mosby–Year Book.

McCoy R et al: Nursing management of breast feeding for preterm infants, *J Perinat Neonatal Nurs* 2:42, 1988.

Morse JM et al: Leaking: a problem of lactation, *J Nurse Midwife* 34:15, 1989.

Nice FJ: Can a breast-feeding mother take medication without harming her infant? *MCN* 14:27, 1989.

Uvnas-Moberg K: The gastrointestinal tract in growth and reproduction, *Sci Am,* p 78, July, 1989.

Walker M, Driscoll JW: Sore nipples: The new mother's nemesis, *MCN* 14:260, July/Aug 1989.

Bibliography—Nursing Research

Anderson E, Geden E: Nurses' knowledge of breastfeeding, *JOGNN* 20:58, 1991.

Hughes RB et al: Relationship between neonatal behavior responses and lactation outcomes, *Issues Comp Pediatr Nurs* 11:271, 1988.

Janke JR: Breastfeeding duration following cesarean and vaginal births, *J Nurse Midwife* 33:159, July/Aug 1988.

Kaufman KJ, Hall LA: Influence of the social network on choice and duration of breastfeeding in mothers of preterm infant, *Res Nurs Health* 12:149, 1989.

Kearney MH: Identifying psychosocial obstacles to breast-feeding success, *JOGNN* 17:98, 1988.

Kearney MH, Cronenwett LR, Barrett JA: Breastfeeding problems in the first week postpartum, *Nurs Res* 39:90, 1990.

Martone DJ et al: Initial differences in postpartum attachment behavior in breastfeeding and bottlefeeding mothers, *JOGNN* 17:212, 1988.

Matthews MK: Mothers' satisfaction with their neonates' breastfeeding behaviors, *JOGNN* 20:49, 1991.

Medoff-Cooper B: (1991). Changes in nutritive sucking patterns with increasing gestational age, *Nurs Res* 40:245, 1991.

Rentschler DD: Correlates of successful breastfeeding, 23:151, Fall 1991.

Serdula MK et al: Correlates of breast-feeding in a low-income population of whites, blacks, and Southeast Asians, *J Am Diet Assoc* 91:41, 1991.

Virden SF: The relationship between infant feeding method and maternal role adjustment, *J Nurse Midwife* 33:31, 1988.

Wood CS et al: Exclusively breast-fed infants: growth and caloric intake, *Pediatr Nurs* 14(2):117, 1988.

chapter 22 review

Key Concepts

- Healthy term babies are developmentally ready for feeding.
- Teaching and counseling concerning the feeding of infants are important aspects of the daily care plan for maternity clients.
- The mother/parent is presented with the benefits of both breast-feeding and formula-feeding as a basis for decision making.
- Feeding is an emotionally charged area of infant care.
- Most parents benefit from teaching related to chosen method of feeding.
- The attitude of the mother (and the partner) toward breast-feeding is a powerful factor in achieving successful lactation.
- The size of the breast gives no indication of its functional capacity.
- Limiting breast-feeding time does not prevent nipple soreness.
- The composition and characteristics of commercial formulas are based on those of mature human milk.
- Use of honey in home-prepared formulas can be fatal (botulism); parents should be warned.
- Neither skim nor low-fat milk is suitable for infant feeding. Infants fed whole cow milk are at risk for iron deficiency.

Key Terms

- breast massage (p. 638)
- colostrum (p. 624)
- demand feeding (p. 633, 645)
- engorgement (p. 638)
- extrusion reflex (p. 620)
- failure to thrive (p. 640)
- formula-feeding (p. 640)
- formula preparation (p. 644)
- growth pattern (p. 620)
- lactation (p. 623)
- lactoferrin (p. 629)
- lactogenesis (p. 624)
- let-down reflex (p. 624)
- manual expression of milk (p. 634, 638)
- milk ejection (p. 623)
- milk secretion (p. 623)
- nipple erection reflex (p. 624)
- nursing bottle caries (p. 641)
- plugged ducts (p. 638)
- prolactin reflex (p. 624)
- pumping the breasts (p. 639)
- readiness for feeding (p. 626)
- rooting reflex (p. 620)
- sore nipples (p. 638)
- sucking reflex (p. 620)
- supplemental feedings (p. 646)
- swallowing reflex (p. 620)
- weaning (p. 646)

Critical Thinking Exercises

1. A new mother calls you to assist her with breast-feeding. She is crying as she hands you the baby, saying, "I just can't do this."
   a. What additional information do you need?
   b. Based on assessment data, formulate nursing diagnoses. Plan and prioritize client-centered goals for the diagnosis that takes priority. Choose interventions, giving rationale and expected outcomes. Justify your decisions and actions.
2. Repeat Exercise 1 with a new mother who has chosen to formula-feed her infant.
3. You overhear two mothers talking. One says she plans to start feeding her infant solid foods as soon as possible so that the baby sleeps all night. The other mother states she wants to feed her baby natural foods only and that she plans to use honey as a natural sweetener. Role-play how you would approach this situation, what you plan to say, and how you will say it while showing respect for each woman. Justify your decisions and actions.

Topics for Nursing Research

- Compare growth charts of breast-fed infants to formula-fed infants.
- How much breast milk is needed to provide increased resistance to disease?
- Compare the ability to let-down and success with manual expression of breast milk.
- Compare mother/child attachment with satisfaction about chosen methods of feeding.
- If breast-feeding was discontinued, discover reasons bottle-feeding was initiated and breast-feeding stopped.
- Compare the current percentage of breast-fed versus formula-fed infants.
- Determine effective (and low cost) methods of providing support to breast-feeding mothers and helping them to develop their coping and problem-solving skills in an effort to encourage them to breast-feed longer.

unit 5

Normal Postpartum

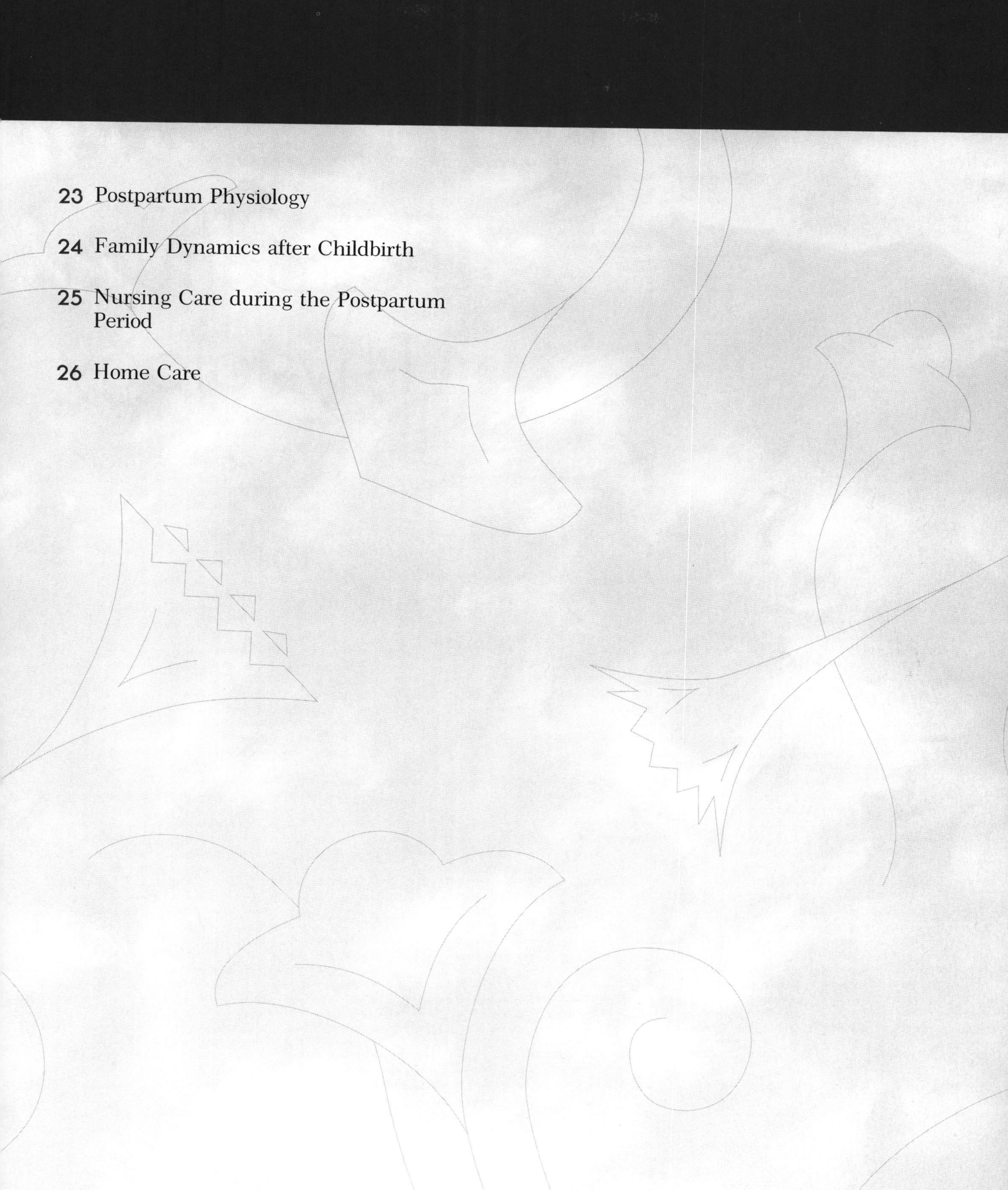

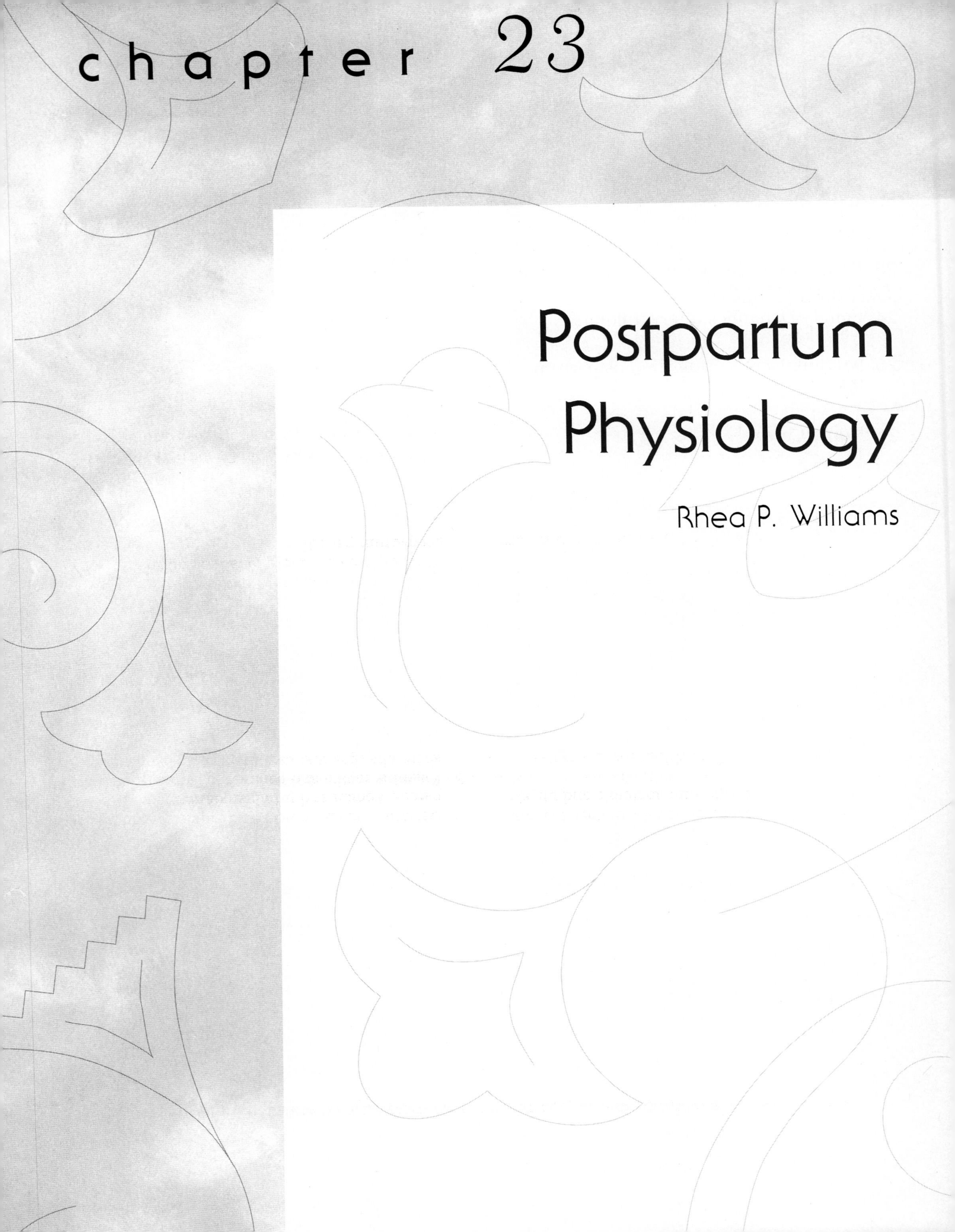

chapter 23

Postpartum Physiology

Rhea P. Williams

LEARNING OBJECTIVES

- Define the key terms listed.
- Describe normal maternal anatomy and physiology during the postpartum recovery and return to the nonpregnant state.
- Review characteristics and measurement of normal uterine involution and lochia.
- List expected values for vital signs and blood pressure, deviations from normal findings, and probable causes.
- Identify topics for nursing research related to maternal physiology during the immediate postpartum period.

The postpartum period (**puerperium**) is the 6-week interval between the birth of the newborn and the return of the reproductive organs to their normal nonpregnant state. This period through the first 3 months after birth is commonly referred to as the **fourth trimester** of pregnancy. The physiologic changes that occur during the puerperium are distinctive, although considered normal as the processes of pregnancy are reversed. Many factors, including energy level, degree of psychologic and physical comfort, health of the newborn, and care and encouragement given by the health professionals, contribute to the mother's well-being and response to her infant during this time. To provide care beneficial to the mother, her infant, and her family, the nurse must use a holistic approach. Knowledge must be synthesized from maternal anatomy and physiology of the recovery period, the newborn's physical and behavioral characteristics, infant care activities, and family response to the birth of the child. This chapter focuses on anatomic and physiologic changes during the postpartum period.

Knowledge of these changes serves as a rationale for ongoing postpartum care related to anatomy and physiology. Family dynamics during this period is the focus of Chapter 24. In Chapter 25, concepts from anatomic and physiologic recovery and family dynamics provide the bases for nursing process with new mothers and their families. Home care of new families is discussed in Chapter 26.

■ REPRODUCTIVE SYSTEM AND ASSOCIATED STRUCTURES

Uterine Corpus Changes

UTERINE INVOLUTION. The return of the uterus to its normal size and condition after childbirth is known as **involution.** At the end of the third stage of labor the uterus is in the midline, about 2 cm *below* the level of the umbilicus, with the fundus resting on the sacral promontory. At this time, uterine size approximates the size at 16 weeks of gestation (about the size of a grapefruit). The uterus is about 14 cm (5½ in) long, 12 cm (4¾ in) wide, and 10 cm (4 in) thick and weighs about 1000 g (2 lb).

Within 12 hours the fundus may be approximately 1 cm *above* the umbilicus (Fig. 23-1). From then on, involution progresses rapidly. With improved tone of the uterine supports, the fundus descends about 1 to 2 cm every 24 hours. By the sixth postpartum day the fundus normally will be half the distance from the symphysis pubis to the umbilicus. The uterus should not be palpable abdominally after the ninth postpartum day.

The uterus, which at full term weighs about 11 times its prepregnant weight, rapidly involutes to about 500 g (1 lb) 1 week after childbirth and 350 g (11 to 12 oz) 2 weeks after the birth. A week after childbirth the uterus lies in the true pelvis once again. At 6 weeks it weighs 50 to 60 g (Fig. 23-1).

The level of estrogen, which stimulated myometrial growth primarily by increase in cell size, and the level of progesterone, which was responsible for much of the increased uterine weight and collagen formation during gestation, drop rapidly after childbirth. Uterine involution within 4 to 6 weeks occurs principally by a decrease in the size of individual myometrial cells. However, the augmentation of connective tissue and elastin in the myometrium and blood vessels and the increase in the total uterine cell number are permanent. Thus uterine size is increased slightly after each pregnancy.

UTERINE CONTRACTIONS. The intensity of uterine contractions increases significantly immediately after childbirth, presumably in response to the greatly diminished intrauterine volume. During the first 1 to 2 postpartum hours, uterine activity decreases smoothly and progressively and stabilizes.

Uterine contractions contribute to hemostasis by compressing the intramural blood vessels (see Fig. 6-10).

In first-time mothers uterine tone is increased so that the fundus remains firm. Periodic relaxation and vigorous contraction are more common in subsequent pregnancies and may cause uncomfortable cramping called **afterpains** that persist throughout the early **puerperium.** Afterpains are more acute after births in which the uterus was overdistended (e.g., large baby, twins). Breast-feeding usually intensifies afterpains because oxytocin is released by the posterior pituitary gland in response to nipple stimulation. Increased intensity also may occur after administration of **oxytocic medication** (Table 25-3).

PLACENTAL SITE. Immediately after the placenta and membranes are expelled, vascular constriction and thromboses reduce the placental site to an irregular nodular and elevated area. **Exfoliation,** the sloughing off of necrotic tissue, occurs with the upward growth of the endometrium to prevent scar formation. This unique process is characteristic of normal wound healing. It enables the endometrium to resume its usual cycle of changes and to permit implantation and placentation in future pregnancies. Endometrial regeneration is completed by the end of the third postpartum week except at the placental site. Regeneration at the placental site usually is not complete until 6 weeks after childbirth.

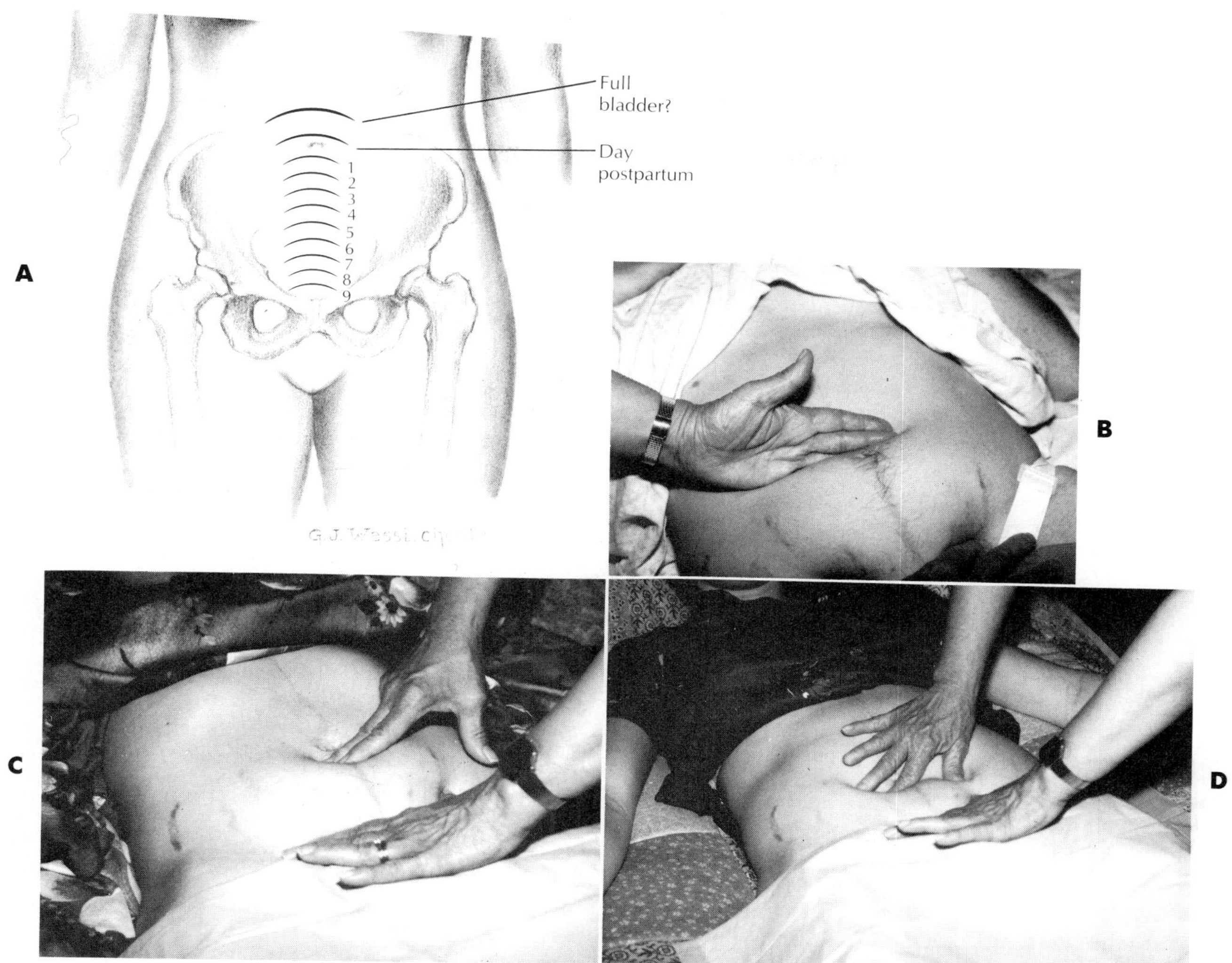

Fig. 23-1 Assessment of involution of uterus after childbirth. **A,** Normal progress, days 1 through 9. **B,** Size and position of uterus 2 hours after the birth. **C,** Two days after the birth. **D,** Four days after the birth.
B, C, and D, courtesy Marjorie Pyle. RNC, Lifecircle. Costa Mesa, Calif.

Failure of the placental site to heal completely is called *subinvolution* of the placental site (see Chapter 30). Women with this condition have persistent lochia and episodes of brisk, painless bleeding (Cunningham et al, 1989). Curettage usually is required.

LOCHIA. Postdelivery uterine discharge initially is bright red, changing to dark red or reddish brown; it may contain small clots. **Lochia** refers only to uterine discharge. The blood seen on the peripad or bed linens may be from a different source (Table 23-1). Regardless of the source of bleeding, if the peripad is soaked through in 15 minutes or less, the flow is considered excessive.

Lochia rubra consists mainly of blood, decidual and trophoblastic debris and bacteria (Cunningham et al, 1989). The flow pales, becoming pink or brown after 3 to 4 days (lochia serosa). **Lochia serosa** consists of old blood, serum, leukocytes, and tissue debris. About 10 days after childbirth the drainage becomes yellow to white (lochia alba). **Lochia alba** consists of numerous leukocytes, decidua, epithelial cells, mucus, serum, and bacteria. Lochia alba may continue until about 2 to 6 weeks after the birth.

The amount of lochia is described as scant, light, moderate, and heavy (Jacobson, 1985):

scant—blood only on tissue when wiped or less than 2.5 cm (1 in) on a peripad (see Fig. 19-2)
light—less than 10 cm (4 in) stain on a peripad
moderate —less than 15 cm (6 in) stain on peripad
heavy—saturated peripad within 1 hour

TABLE 23-1 Lochia and Nonlochia Bleeding

Lochia	Nonlochia Bleeding
Lochia usually trickles from the vaginal opening. The steady flow is greater as the uterus contracts.	If the bloody discharge spurts from the vagina, there may be cervical or vaginal tears in addition to the normal lochia.
A gush of lochia may result as the uterus is massaged. If it is dark in color, it has been pooled in the relaxed vagina and the amount soon lessens to a trickle of bright red lochia (in the early puerperium).	If the amount of bleeding continues to be excessive and bright red, a tear may be the source.

If the woman receives an oxytocic medication, regardless of the route of administration, the flow of lochia usually is decreased until the effects of the medication wear off. Flow of lochia usually increases with ambulation and breast-feeding. After lying in bed for a prolonged period, the woman may experience a gush of blood upon standing, which is not to be confused with hemorrhage.

Persistence of lochia rubra early in the postpartum period suggests continued bleeding as a result of retained fragments of the placenta (Cunningham et al, 1989). Recurrence of bleeding about 10 days after childbirth indicates bleeding from the placental site, which is healing. However, after 3 to 4 weeks bleeding may be caused by infection or subinvolution of the placental site. Continued lochia serosa or lochia alba may indicate endometritis, particularly if fever, pain, or tenderness is associated with the discharge. Lochia should smell like normal menstrual flow, sometimes described as "fleshy"; an offensive odor usually indicates infection. Lochia clots, whereas normal menstrual blood does not (see Chapter 6).

Cervix

The cervix up to the lower uterine segment remains edematous, thin, and fragile for several days after childbirth. The ectocervix (portion of the cervix that protrudes into the vagina) is soft, appears bruised, and has some small lacerations, optimum conditions for the development of infection. It remains easily distensible; two fingers may still be introduced for the first 4 to 6 days after the birth, but only the smallest curette may be introduced by the end of 2 weeks. By the eighteenth hour the cervix has shortened, has a firm consistency, and has regained its form. By the end of the first week, recovery is almost complete. The external os, however, does not regain its pre-pregnant appearance (Cunningham et al, 1989); it is no longer shaped like a circle but appears as a jagged slit often described as "fish mouth" (see Fig. 6-11). Production of cervical and other estrogen-influenced mucus and mucosal characteristics may be delayed in the lactating woman.

Vagina and Perineum

Postpartum estrogen deprivation is responsible for the thinness of the *vaginal mucosa* and the absence of rugae. The greatly distended, smooth-walled vagina gradually returns to its prepregnant size by 6 to 8 weeks after childbirth. Rugae reappear by about the fourth week, although they are never as prominent as they are in the nulliparous woman. Most rugae may be permanently flattened. The mucosa remains atrophic in the lactating woman at least until menstruation begins again. Thickening of the vaginal mucosa occurs with the return of ovarian function. Profuse vaginal discharge usually is not present at 4 to 6 weeks after childbirth unless there is an associated vaginitis. The hypoestrogenic condition of the vaginal epithelium is responsible for the decreased amount of vaginal mucus production and thinner vaginal mucosa. Local dryness and coital discomfort may persist until ovulation and menstruation resume.

Initially the vaginal *introitus* is erythematous and edematous, especially in the area of the episiotomy or laceration repair. Careful repair, prevention or early treatment of hematomas, and good hygiene during the first 2 weeks after childbirth usually result in an introitus barely distinguishable from that of a nulliparous woman. The torn hymen heals with the development of fibrosed nodules of mucosa called *hymenal caruncles*.

Most *episiotomies* are visible only if the woman is lying on her side and her buttock is raised. A good light source is essential for visualization of some episiotomies. The healing process of an episiotomy is the same as for any surgical incision. As suggested by Davidson (1974), it should be examined for redness, edema, ecchymosis, discharge and approximation, (REEDA). The incision edges should be well approximated without signs of infection. Some bruising may be present. Healing should occur within 2 to 3 weeks.

Hemorrhoids (anal varicosities) commonly are seen and are associated with symptoms such as itching, discomfort, and bright-red bleeding with defeca-

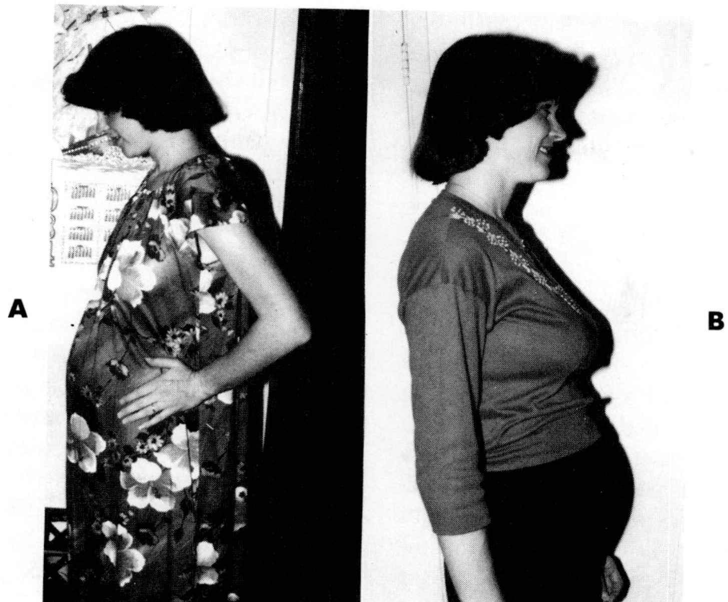

Fig. 23-2 Abdomen after childbirth. A, Two hours after childbirth. B, Eight days after childbirth.
Courtesy Marjorie Pyle, RNC, Lifecircle. Costa Mesa, Calif.

tion. These hemorrhoids usually decrease in size within weeks of childbirth.

Pelvic Muscular Support

Injury of the supporting structures of the uterus and vagina may occur during childbirth and may become gynecologic problems later in life. The term *relaxation* refers to the lengthening and weakening of the fascial supports of pelvic structures. These include the uterus, upper posterior vaginal wall, urethra, bladder, and rectum. Although relaxations can occur in any woman, most are direct but delayed sequelae to childbirth (see Chapter 41).

Abdominal Wall

When the woman stands up during the first days after childbirth, abdominal muscles cannot retain abdominal contents. The abdomen protrudes and gives her a still-pregnant appearance (Fig. 23-2). During the first 2 weeks after childbirth the abdominal wall is relaxed. About 6 weeks are required before the abdominal wall almost returns to its nonparous state. The skin regains most of its previous elasticity, but some striae persist. The return of muscle tone depends on previous tone, proper exercise, and amount of adipose tissue. On occasion, with or without overdistention because of a large fetus or multiple fetuses, the abdominal wall muscles separate, a condition termed ***diastasis recti abdominis*** (see Fig. 8-13). Peristence of this defect may be disturbing to the woman, but surgical correction rarely is necessary. With time, the defect becomes less apparent.

Breasts

The concentrations of hormones that stimulated breast development during pregnancy (estrogen, progesterone, human chorionic gonadotropin, prolactin, cortisol, and insulin) decrease promptly after childbirth. The time it takes for the return of these hormones to prepregnancy levels is determined in part by whether the mother breast-feeds her infant.

NON–BREAST-FEEDING MOTHERS. The breasts generally feel nodular (in nonpregnant women they feel granular). The nodularity is bilateral and diffuse.

If the woman chooses not to breast-feed and no antilactogenic medication is taken, prolactin levels drop rapidly. Colostrum secretion and excretion persist for the first few days after childbirth. Palpation of the breast on the second or third day, as milk production begins, reveals tissue tenseness. On the third or fourth postpartum day the breasts become *engorged*. They are distended (swollen), firm, tender, and warm to the touch (vasocongestion makes them feel warm). Milk can be expressed from the nipples. Axillary breast tissue (the tail of Spence) and any accessory breast or nipple tissue along the milk line may be involved. Breast distention is caused primarily by temporary congestion of veins and lymphatics rather than from an accumulation of milk. **Engorgement** resolves spontaneously, and discomfort decreases usually within 24 to 36 hours. If suckling is never begun (or is discontinued), lactation ceases within a few days to a week. Antilactogenic medications are discussed in Chapter 25.

BREAST-FEEDING MOTHERS. As lactation is established, a mass (lump) may be felt; however, a filled milk sac will shift position from day to day. Before lactation begins, the breasts feel soft and a yellowish fluid, **colostrum** can be expressed from the nipples. After lactation begins, the breasts feel warm to the touch and firm. Tenderness persists for about 48 hours. Bluish white milk (skim-milk appearance) can be expressed from the nipples. The nipples are examined for erectility as opposed to inversion and for cracks or fissures.

For a discussion of breast changes associated with lactation, see Chapter 22.

■ ENDOCRINE SYSTEM

Numerous changes occur in the endocrine system during the puerperium. These changes are summarized in Table 23-2.

Placental Hormones

Plasma levels of placental hormones fall rapidly after childbirth. *Human placental lactogen (hPL)* levels reach undetectable levels within 24 hours (see also discussions of growth hormone and carbohydrate metabolism). Levels of *human chorionic gonadotropin (hCG)* decline rapidly and remain low until ovulation occurs.

TABLE 23-2 Endocrine Changes in the Puerperium

Hormone	Change	Lowest Level
Human placental lactogen (hPL)	Decreases	<24 hr
Estrogen	Decreases	Day 7
Progesterone	Decreases	Day 7
Follicle-stimulating hormone (FSH)	Decreases	Day 10-12
Luteinizing hormone (LH)	Decreases	Day 10-12
Prolactin	Decreases	Day 14
Growth hormone	Stays low through day 3	
Thyroid	No change	
Corticosteroids	Decreases	Day 7
Plasma renin	Decreases	<2 hr
Angiotensin II	Decreases	<2 hr

Estrogen levels in plasma fall to 10% of the prenatal value within 3 hours after childbirth; the lowest levels occur about day 7. The significant decline in estrogen is accompanied by the onset of breast engorgement on about postpartum day 3. Plasma levels of estrogen do not increase to follicular levels until 19 to 21 days after the birth. In lactating women, return to normal estrogen levels is somewhat delayed.

Progesterone levels in plasma fall below luteal levels by the third postpartum day and cannot be detected in serum after the first postdelivery week. Progesterone production begins with the first ovulation.

Pituitary Hormones

Prolactin levels in blood rise progressively throughout pregnancy. After childbirth, in nonlactating women, prolactin levels decline, reaching the prepregnant range within 2 weeks. Initially, suckling and lactation are accompanied by dramatic increases in prolactin concentration. Serum prolactin levels are influenced by the number of times per day breast-feeding occurs. Normal basal values of prolactin are reached by 6 months if breast-feeding occurs only 1 to 3 times per day. High prolactin levels persist for more than a year if suckling occurs more than 6 times per day.

Levels of *follicle-stimulating hormone (FSH)* and *luteinizing hormone (LH)* are low in all women for 10 to 12 days after childbirth. FSH levels rise to follicular phase concentration by the third postpartum week, whereas LH levels remain low until after ovulation occurs.

Hypothalamic-Pituitary-Ovarian Function

Little is known about the physiology of the hypothalamus, the pituitary gland, and the ovaries during the puerperium after term gestation. The exact nature of the changing endocrine milieu is unclear at this time (Scott et al, 1990). However, considerable information is available on the time of appearance of the first ovulation and the reestablishment of menstruation for lactating and nonlactating women. For all women, the first menses *usually* follows an **anovulatory cycle** or a cycle associated with inadequate corpus luteum function (low LH and progesterone).

Among lactating women, 15% resume menstruation by 6 weeks, and 45% by 12 weeks. Among nonlactating women, 40% menstruate by 6 weeks, 65% by 12 weeks, and 90% by 24 weeks. For lactating women, 80% of first menstrual cycles are anovulatory; for nonlactating women 50% of first cycles are anovulatory (Scott et al, 1990).

Much of the variability in the reestablishment of menstruation and ovulation observed in lactating women may result from individual differences in the strength of the suckling stimulus. Partial weaning (formula supplementation) and breast-feeding less than six times per day also may play a role. This emphasizes the fact that *breast-feeding must not be used as a form of birth control.*

The first menstrual flow usually is heavier than normal. Within three to four cycles the amount of menstrual flow has returned to the woman's prepregnant volume.

Other Endocrine Changes

Growth hormone secretion remains depressed during late pregnancy and the early puerperium. The low level of growth hormone and the rapid decline in the hormones hPL, estrogens, and cortisol and in the placental enzyme, insulinase, *reduce the anti-insulin factors* in the early puerperium. Therefore new mothers have low fasting plasma glucose levels, and insulin requirements for insulin-dependent diabetic women usually fall after childbirth (see Chapter 31). Normal hormonal alterations render the early puerperium a transitional period for *carbohydrate metabolism* so that interpretation of glucose tolerance tests is difficult at this time.

Thyroid function is difficult to evaluate during the early puerperium because of the rapid fluctuation in many endocrine hormones. Postpartum hypothyroidism is suspected if the woman fails to lactate or if recovery from childbirth is delayed.

A progressive increase of plasma levels of *corticosteroids* during pregnancy and labor is followed by a decline to nonpregnant values by the end of the first week after childbirth. Within 2 hours after the birth, *plasma renin* and *angiotensin II* levels drop to within the normal range for the nonpregnant woman. This finding may indicate that the fetoplacental unit is one source of maternal plasma renin.

BASAL METABOLIC RATE. The basal metabolic rate remains elevated for 7 to 14 days after childbirth. Normal nonpregnant values for respiratory system function are given in Appendix D.

FATIGUE. Fatigue is customary during the first few days after childbirth. The underlying cause is unclear, but may be related to the rapid endocrine changes, the labor process (including energy expenditure and sleep loss), and sleep disturbances during the third trimester. The excitement of the actual birth and the disruption of the woman's normal sleep pattern also may contribute to fatigue during the early postpartal period.

■ CARDIOVASCULAR SYSTEM

Blood Volume

Changes in blood volume depend on several variable factors, for example, blood loss during childbirth, and mobilization and subsequent excretion of extravascular water (physiologic edema). Blood loss results in immediate but limited decrease in total blood volume. Thereafter, normal shifts in body water result in a slow decline in blood volume. By the third to fourth week after the birth the blood volume usually has regressed to prepregnancy values (Fig. 23-3).

Maternal Response to Normal Blood Loss

Pregnancy-induced hypervolemia (increase of at least 40% from 1 to 2 L near term) allows most women to tolerate a considerable blood loss during childbirth. Many women lose 300 to 400 mL of blood

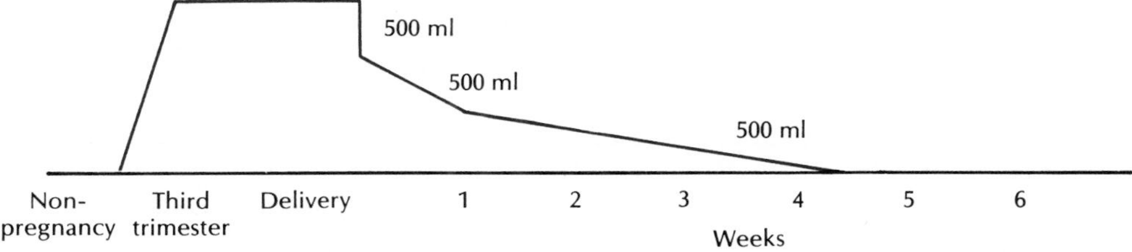

Fig. 23-3 Rate of loss of 1500 mL in blood volume during first postnatal month. Greatest change at delivery, then in week after childbirth.
From Wiggins JD: *Childbearing: physiology, experiences, needs*, St Louis, 1979, Mosby–Year Book.

TABLE 23-3 Vital Signs and Blood Pressure after Childbirth

Normal Findings	Deviations from Normal Findings and Probable Causes
TEMPERATURE	
During first 24 hrs, may rise to 100.4° F (38° C) as a result of dehydrating effects of labor. After 24 hrs the woman should be afebrile.	A diagnosis of puerperal sepis is suggested if a rise in maternal temperature to 100.4° F (38° C) is noted after the first 24 hrs after the birth and recurs or persists for 2 days. Other possibilities are mastitis, endometritis, urinary tract infections, and other systemic infections.
PULSE	
Bradycardia is a common finding for the first 6 to 8 days after childbirth. Bradycardia is a consequence of increased cardiac output and stroke volume. The pulse returns to prepregnancy levels by 3 mo after the birth. A pulse rate of between 50 and 70 beats/min may be considered normal.	A rapid pulse rate or one that is increasing may indicate hypovolemia secondary to hemorrhage.
RESPIRATIONS	
Respirations should fall to within the woman's normal prepregnancy range.	Hypoventilation and hypotension may follow an unusually high subarachnoid (spinal) block.
BLOOD PRESSURE	
Blood pressure is altered *slightly* if at all. Orthostatic hypotension, as indicated by feelings of faintness or dizziness immediately after standing up, can develop in the first 48 hrs as a result of the splanchic engorgement that may occur after the birth.	A low or falling blood pressure may reflect hypovolemia secondary to hemorrhage. However, it is a late sign, and other symptoms of hemorrhage usually alert the staff. An increased reading may result from excessive use of vasopressor drugs or oxytocic drugs. Since pregnancy-induced hypertension can persist into or occur first in the postpartum period, routine evaluation of blood pressure is needed. If a woman complains of headache, hypertension must be ruled out as a cause before analgesics are administered. If the blood pressure is elevated, the woman is confined to bed and the physician notified. (See also Chapter 28.)

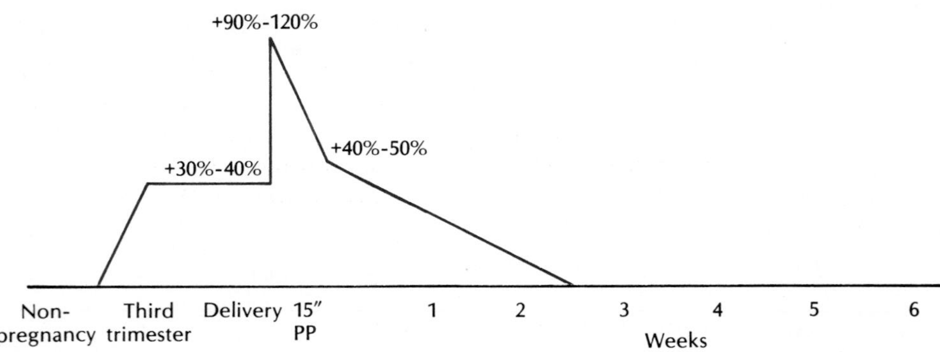

Fig. 23-4 Cardiac output. Work of heart increases during labor and decreases significantly immediately after birth of baby.
From Wiggins JD: *Childbearing: physiology, experience, needs*, St Louis, 1979, Mosby–Year Book.

during vaginal delivery of a single fetus and about twice this amount during cesarean delivery.

Readjustments in the maternal vasculature after childbirth are dramatic and rapid. The woman's response to blood loss during the early puerperium differs from that in a nonpregnant woman. Three postpartal physiologic changes protect the woman: (1) elimination of uteroplacental circulation reduces the size of the maternal vascular bed by 10% to 15%; (2) loss of placental endocrine function removes the stimulus for vasodilation; and (3) mobilization of extravascular water stored during pregnancy occurs. Thus hypovolemic shock usually does not occur with normal blood loss.

Cardiac Output

The cardiac output continues to increase during the first and second stages of labor. It peaks during the puerperium regardless of the type of delivery or use of conduction anesthesia (Fig. 23-4). Cardiac output remains elevated for up to 48 postpartum hours. This most likely is due to increased stroke volume from increased venous return; bradycardia is seen during this time (Cunningham et al, 1989). Cardiac output returns to prepregnancy levels within 2 or 3 weeks (Robson et al, 1987).

Vital Signs and Blood Pressure

Few alterations in vital signs and blood pressure are seen under normal circumstances (Table 23-3). Respiratory function returns to prepregnancy levels by 6 months after childbirth. After the uterus is emptied, the diaphragm descends, the normal cardiac axis is restored, and cardiologic features (point of maximal impulse and electrocardiogram) are normalized.

Blood Constituents

HEMATOCRIT AND HEMOGLOBIN. During the first 72 hours after childbirth, there is a greater loss in plasma volume than in blood cells. The decrease in plasma volume plus the increase in red blood cell (RBC) mass of pregnancy is associated with a rise in hematocrit and hemoglobin levels by the third to seventh day after the birth. There is no RBC destruction during the puerperium, but any gain will disappear gradually in accordance with the life span of the RBC. In uncomplicated cases the hematocrit and hemoglobin levels will have returned to the normal prepregnancy range by the fourth or fifth postpartal week.

WHITE BLOOD CELL COUNT. Normal leukocytosis of pregnancy averages about $12{,}000/mm^3$. During the first 10 to 12 days after childbirth, values between 20,000 to $25{,}000/mm^3$ are common. Neutrophils are the most numerous WBCs, with a consequent shift to the left. Leukocytosis, coupled with the normal increase in erythrocyte sedimentation rate, may confuse the interpretation of acute infections at this time.

COAGULATION FACTORS. An extensive activation of blood-clotting factors occurs after childbirth. This activation, together with immobility, trauma, or sepsis, encourages thromboembolism. Factors I, II, VIII, IX, and X decrease within a few days to prepregnancy levels. The elevated levels of fibrin split products are probably the result of their release from the placental site.

THROMBOSIS. The woman's legs are examined daily for signs of **thrombosis** (pain, warmth, and tenderness; swollen reddened vein that feels hard or solid to touch). There may be a positive Homans' sign (dorsiflexion of foot [see Fig. 13-2, *A*], which causes calf muscles to compress tibial veins and produce pain if thrombosis is present). It is important to remember that deep venous thrombosis may be silent, that is, not cause pain.

VARICOSITIES. Varicosties of the legs and around the anus (hemorrhoids) are common during pregnancy. Varices, even the less common vulvar varices, regress (empty) rapidly immediately after childbirth.

■ URINARY SYSTEM

Renal Function

The hormonal changes of pregnancy (high steroid levels) contribute to the increase in renal function. Conversely, the diminishing steroid levels after childbirth may partly explain the reduced renal function during the puerperium. Kidney function returns to normal within a month after the birth. About 2 to 8 weeks are required for the pregnancy-induced hypotonia and dilation of the ureters and renal pelves to return to the prepregnant state (Cunningham et al, 1989). In a small percentage of women, dilation of the urinary tract may persist for 3 months.

URINE CONSTITUENTS. The renal glycosuria induced by pregnancy disappears. *Lactosuria* may be expected in lactating women. The *blood urea nitrogen increases* during the puerperium as **autolysis**

(self-digestion; breakdown of excess protein in the uterine muscle cells) of the involuting uterus is accomplished. As a result of the **catalyic processes** of involuting, *mild proteinuria* (+1) is a normal finding for 1 to 2 days after childbirth in about 50% of women. *Acetonuria* may even occur in women with an uncomplicated birth or after a prolonged labor with dehydration.

REVERSAL OF WATER METABOLISM OF PREGNANCY. **Profuse diaphoresis,** especially at night (night sweats), is not unusual for 2 to 3 days after childbirth. Diaphoresis is a mechanism to reduce the retained fluids of pregnancy and usually is not a symptom of infection.

The renal plasma flow and glomerular filtration rate that increased by 25% to 50% during pregnancy remains elevated for at least the first postpartal week. Normally a marked **diuresis** begins within 12 hours after the birth. The volume of urinary output along with the water loss through perspiration accounts for a large portion of the weight loss during the early puerperium. This weight loss is approximately 5.5 kg (12 lb) after delivery of the fetus, placenta, and amniotic fluid and an additional 4 kg (9 lb) during the puerperium because of excretion of fluids and electrolytes accumulated during pregnancy. The mechanism that facilitates elimination of the excess tissue fluid accumulated during pregnancy is often referred to as the *reversal of the water metabolism of pregnancy*.

Urethra and Bladder

Trauma occurs to the urethra and bladder as the infant passes through the pelvis. The bladder wall is hyperemic and edematous, often with small areas of hemorrhage. Clean-catch or catheterized urine specimens after the birth often reveal hematuria from bladder trauma. Later in the puerperium, hematuria may be a sign of urinary tract infection. The urethra and urinary meatus may be edematous. Birth-induced trauma and the effects of analgesia, especially conduction anesthesia, cause relative insensitivity that depresses the urge to void. In addition, pelvic soreness caused by the forces of labor, vaginal lacerations, or the episiotomy reduces or alters the voiding reflex. This alteration, together with postpartum diuresis, may allow rapid filling of the bladder.

Distention of the bladder can readily occur as the water metabolism of pregnancy is reversed and fluids are mobilized in the elimination of end products of protein catabolism. Overdistention, incomplete emptying, and excessive residual urine can make the bladder more susceptible to infection as well as impede the resumption of normal voiding (Cunningham et al, 1989). If prolonged bladder overdistention occurs, further damage to the bladder wall (atony) may result. Bladder tone usually is restored within 5 to 7 days after childbirth, with adequate emptying of the bladder.

■ GASTROINTESTINAL SYSTEM

Appetite

The mother usually is hungry shortly after the birth and can tolerate a light diet. After full recovery from analgesia, anesthesia, and fatigue, most new mothers are hungry. Requests for double portions of food and frequent snacks are common. For a discussion of diet during lactation, see Chapters 9 and 22.

Motility

Typically decreased muscle tone and motility of the gastrointestinal tract persist for only a short time after childbirth. Excess analgesia and anesthesia could delay a return to normal tonicity and motility.

Bowel Evacuation

A spontaneous bowel evacuation may be delayed until 2 to 3 days after childbirth. This can be explained by decreased muscle tone (**adynamic ileus**) in the intestines during labor and the immediate puerperium, prelabor diarrhea or a predelivery enema, lack of food, dehydration, or perineal tenderness because of episiotomy, lacerations, or hemorrhoids. Regular bowel habits need to be reestablished after the birth once bowel tone returns.

■ NEUROLOGIC SYSTEM

Neurologic changes during the puerperium are those resulting from a reversal of maternal adaptations to pregnancy and those resulting from trauma during labor and childbirth.

Pregnancy-induced neurologic discomforts abate after the birth. Elimination of physiologic edema through the diuresis that follows the birth relieves *carpal tunnel syndrome* by easing the compression of the median nerve. The periodic numbness and tingling of fingers that afflict 5% of pregnant women usually disappear after the birth unless lifting and carrying the baby aggravate the condition. (For a discussion of nerve injury incurred during childbirth, see Chapter 32.) *Headache* requires careful assessment. Postpartum headaches may be caused by various conditions, including pregnancy-induced hypertension, stress, and leakage of cerebrospinal fluid into the extradural space during placement of the needle for spinal anesthesia. Duration of the headaches varies from 1 to 3 days to several weeks, depending on the cause and effectiveness of the treatment.

■ MUSCULOSKELETAL SYSTEM

Adaptations in the mother's musculoskeletal system are reversed in the puerperium. The adaptations include those that contribute to relaxation and subsequent hypermobility of the joints and in the change in the mother's center of gravity because of the enlarging uterus. *Stabilization of joints* is complete by 6 to 8 weeks after childbirth. However, although all other joints return to their normal prepregnancy position before restabilization, those in the parous woman's feet do not; the new mother may notice a permanent increase in shoe size.

■ INTEGUMENTARY SYSTEM

Chloasma of pregnancy usually disappears at the termination of pregnancy. *Hyperpigmentation* of the areolae and linea nigra may not regress completely after childbirth, and some women will have permanent darker pigmentation of these areas.

Vascular abnormalities such as spider angiomas (nevi), palmar erythema, and epulis generally regress in response to the rapid decline in estrogens after termination of pregnancy. For some woman, spider nevi persist indefinitely.

The abundance of fine *hair* seen during pregnancy usually disappears after the birth; however, any coarse or bristly hair that appears during pregnancy usually remains. *Fingernails* return to their prepregnant characteristics of consistency and strength.

Diaphoresis is the most noticeable change in the integumentary system (see reversal of water metabolism of pregnancy, p. 666).

■ IMMUNE SYSTEM

The mother's need for *rubella vaccination* or for prevention of Rh isoimmunization is determined.

For discussion of acquired immunodeficiency syndrome (AIDS) and other questions concerning immunology, see the section on immunology in Chapter 6.

■ SUMMARY

The perinatal nurse needs a thorough understanding of normal physiologic responses during the postpartum period. This serves as a basis or guide for providing quality nursing care. Knowledge of normal physiologic adaptations enables the nurse to make and interpret pertinent assessments and to recognize deviations so that the proper plan of care may be instituted. Proper application of this knowledge will contribute to the woman's overall sense of well-being and her adaptation to motherhood.

REFERENCES

Cunningham FG, MacDonald PC, Gant NF: *Williams obstetrics,* ed 18, Norwalk, Conn, 1989, Appleton & Lange.

Davidson N: Reeda: evaluating postpartum healing, *J Nurse Midwife* 19:6, 1974.

Jacobson H: A standard for assessing lochia volume, *MCN* 10:174, 1985.

Robson SC, Dunlop W, Hunter S: Haemodynamic changes during the early puerperium, *Br Med J* 294:1065, 1987.

Scott JR et al: *Danforth's obstetrics and gynecology,* ed 6, Philadelphia, 1990, JB Lippincott Co.

BIBLIOGRAPHY

Brewer MM et al: Postpartum change in maternal weight and body fat deposits in lactating vs. non-lactating women, *Am J Clin Nutr* 49:259, 1989.

Butters L et al: The influence of breast and bottlefeeding on blood pressure, *Midwifery* 4(3):130, 1988.

Drake ML et al: Physical and psychological symptoms experienced by Canadian women and their husbands during pregnancy and the postpartum, *J Adv Nurs* 13:436, 1988.

Gerlach C, Schmid M: Second skill educational development of personnel for a single-room maternity care system, *JOGNN* 17:388, 1988.

Giger JN, Davidhizar E: *Transcultural nursing: assessment and intervention,* St Louis, 1991, Mosby Year–Book.

Greene GW et al: Postpartum weight change: how much of the weight gained in pregnancy will be lost after delivery? *Obstet Gynecol* 71:701, 1988.

Parham ES: The association of pregnancy weight gain with the mother's postpartum weight. *J Am Diet Assoc,* 90:550, 1990.

Seidel HM et al: *Mosby's guide to physical examination,* ed 2, St Louis, 1991, Mosby–Year Book.

Tulman LJ: Recovery from childbirth—does the "postpartum period" last only 6 weeks? *NJ Nurse* 19:11, Jan 1989.

Bibliography—Nursing Research

Dougherty MC et al: The effect of exercise on the circumvaginal muscles in postpartum women, *J Nurse Midwife* 34:8, Jan/Feb 1989.

Mead-Bennett E: The relationship of primigravid sleep experience and select moods on the first postpartum day, *JOGNN* 19:146, 1990.

Tulman LJ, Fawcett J: Return of functional ability after childbirth, *Nurs Res* 37:77, 1988.

chapter 23 review

Key Concepts

- The uterus involutes rapidly after childbirth, returning to the true pelvis within 1 week.
- The rapid drop in estrogen and progesterone levels after expulsion of the placenta is responsible for many of the anatomic and physiologic changes in the puerperium.
- Changes in lochia and fundal height are important indicators of the progress of normal involution, as well as indications of potential problems.
- Breast-feeding is *not* a form of birth control.
- Bradycardia is a common finding for the first 6 to 8 days.
- Activation of blood clotting factors, immobility, and sepsis predispose the woman to thromboembolism.
- Marked diuresis, decreased bladder sensitivity, and overdistention of the bladder can lead to problems with urinary elimination.
- Postpartum physiologic changes allow the woman to tolerate considerable blood loss during childbirth.

Key Terms

- adynamic ileus (p. 666)
- afterpains (p. 658)
- anovulatory cycle (p. 662)
- autolysis (p. 666)
- bradycardia (p. 664)
- catabolism (p. 666)
- colostrum (p. 662)
- diaphoresis (p. 666)
- diastasis recti abdominis (p. 661)
- diuresis (p. 666)
- engorgement [breast] (p. 662)
- exfoliation (p. 658)
- fourth trimester (p. 658)
- involution (p. 658)
- lochia (p. 659)
- lochia alba (p. 659)
- lochia rubra (p. 659)
- lochia serosa (p. 659)
- oxytocic medication (p. 658)
- prolactin (p. 662)
- puerperium (p. 658)
- thromboembosis (p. 665)

Critical Thinking Exercise

Prepare a teaching plan for the new mother that will cover all aspects of postpartum anatomic and physiologic changes.

1. Correlate these changes with prenatal adaptations.
2. Describe the differences and similarities in multiparous women and primiparous women.
3. Examine myths and common misunderstandings about changes that can affect postpartum recovery.

Topics for Nursing Research

- How do nurses use knowledge of the physiologic changes during the postpartum period to develop a nursing plan of care?
- How does the amount and character of lochia vary in (a) women with vaginal and cesarean births and (b) in primiparous and multiparous women?
- What factors contribute to fatigue during the early postpartum period?

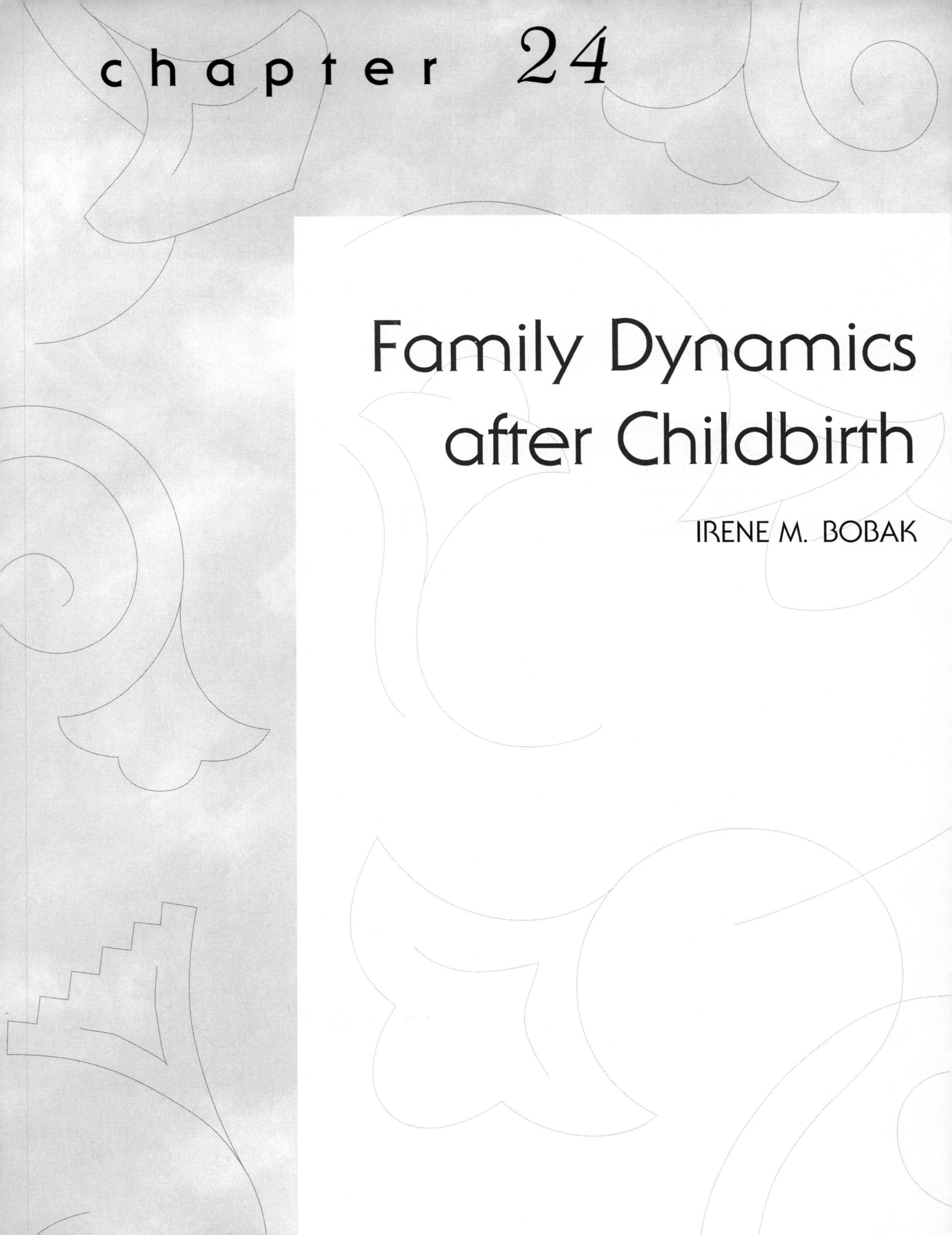

chapter 24

Family Dynamics after Childbirth

IRENE M. BOBAK

LEARNING OBJECTIVES

- Define the key terms listed.
- Describe the two components of the parenting process.
- Discuss five preconditions that influence attachment.
- List the sensual responses that strengthen attachment.
- Differentiate the three periods in parental role change after childbirth.
- List six parental tasks and responsibilities.
- Identify infant behaviors that facilitate and inhibit parental attachment.
- Identify behaviors of the three phases of maternal adjustment.
- Discuss maternal age over 35 as a factor influencing parental response.
- Explain paternal adjustment.
- List three ways to facilitate parent-infant adjustment.
- Explain effects of a parent's sensory impairment on the attachment process.
- List three activities that facilitate sibling attachment.
- Describe grandparent adjustment.
- Identify topics for nursing research related to family dynamics after the birth of an infant.

The birth of a child poses a fundamental challenge to the existing interactional structure of the family. Becoming a parent creates a period of instability. This change requires behaviors that promote the transition to parenthood. Parents must explore their relationship with the infant as well as redefine the relationship between themselves. If there are other children, parents must adjust their own life space to include another child. The older children, on the other hand, must adjust to the infant's claim on parental time and love (Walz, Rich, 1983). This chapter reviews the parenting process, including adjustments of parents, siblings, and grandparents.

PARENTING PROCESS

Biologic parenthood for both parents begins with the union of ovum and sperm. During the prenatal period the mother is the primary agent in providing an environment in which the unborn child may develop and grow. This close symbiotic union of mother and child ends with birth. Others may then assume partial or complete involvement in the infant's care. Whoever—whether biologic or substitute parent, woman or man—assumes the parental role enters into a crucial relationship with a child that will persist throughout the life of each. Men and women, of course, may exist without a child; thus, in essence, parenthood is optional. Regardless of whether parenthood is biologically based, it can contribute to the maturation of the couple. For children, parenthood is all important; their continued existence depends on the quality of care they receive.

The tasks, responsibilities, and attitudes that make up parenting care have been designated by Steele and Pollack (1968) as the **mothering function.** It is a process in which an adult (a mature, caring, capable, self-sufficient person) assumes the care of an infant (an immature, helpless, dependent person). Either parent may exhibit "motherliness." Motherliness is now recognized to be a non–gender-related ability. The ability to show gentleness, love, and understanding and to place another's welfare above one's own is not limited to women—it is a human characteristic.

Steele and Pollack (1968) also describe parenting as one process with two components. The first, being practical or mechanical in nature, involves cognitive and motor skills; the second, emotional in nature, involves cognitive and affective skills. Both components are essential to the infant's well-being and future development.

Cognitive-Motor Skills

The first component in the process of parenting includes child-care activities such as "feeding, holding, clothing, and cleaning the infant, protecting it from harm, and providing mobility for it" (Steele, Pollack, 1968). These task-oriented activities, or **cognitive-motor skills,** are not automatically supplied at the birth of one's child. The parents' abilities in these respects have been influenced by cultural and personal experiences. Many parents have to learn how to do these tasks, and this learning process can be difficult. However, almost all parents with the desire to learn and with the support of others become adept in caregiving activities.

Cognitive-Affective Skills

The psychologic component in child care, motherliness or fatherliness, appears to stem from the *parents'* earliest experiences with a loving, accepting mother figure. In this sense parents may be said to "inherit" the ability to show concern and tenderness and to pass on this ability to the next generation by repeating the kind of parent-child relationship they experienced. The **cognitive-affective skills** of parenting include an attitude of tenderness, awareness, and concern for the child's needs and desires. This component of parenting has a profound effect on the manner in which the practical aspects of child care are performed and on the emotional response of the child to the care. A positive parent-child relationship is mutually rewarding. This relationship is fundamental to a person's development of confidence in the expectations that others will be willing to help and that the person is worth helping.

Erikson's concept (1959, 1964) of "basic trust" is similar. He claims that development of a sense of trust determines the infant's responses to others throughout life. Persons who experienced a positive parent-child relationship tend to be social or outgoing and able to seek and accept assistance from others. In contrast, those deficient in a sense of trust tend to be alienated and isolated. They are most likely to have crises because of their inability to make use of situational supports in times of stress.

PARENTAL ACQUAINTANCE, BONDING, AND ATTACHMENT

Although much research has been directed toward unraveling the process by which a parent comes to love and accept a child and a child comes to love and

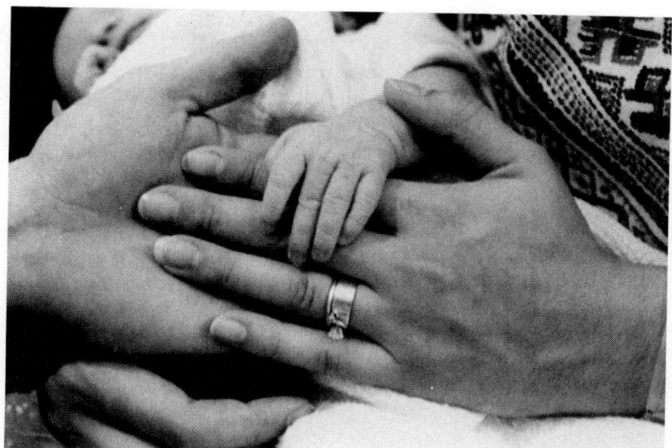

Fig. 24-1 Hands.
Courtesy St Luke's Hospital, Kansas City, Mo.

accept a parent (Fig. 24-1), we still do not know what motivates and commits them to decades of supportive and nurturing care of each other. This process often is referred to as attachment or bonding, terms that often are used interchangeably. Definitions differ somewhat. **Bonding,** as defined by Brazelton (1978), describes the initial mutual attraction between people, such as between parent and child at first meeting. **Attachment** occurs at critical periods, such as birth or adoption. It describes a feeling of affection or loyalty that binds one person to another; it is unique, specific, and enduring (Klaus, Kennell, 1976). The attachment process has been described as linear, beginning during pregnancy, intensifying during the early postbirth period, and being constant and consistent once established. It is critical to mental and physical health across the life span (Parkes, Stevenson-Hinde, 1982).

Mercer (1982) lists *five preconditions that influence attachment:*

1. A parent's emotional health (including the ability to trust another person)
2. A social support system encompassing mate, friends, and family
3. A competent level of communication and caregiving skills
4. Parental proximity to the infant
5. Parent-infant fit (including infant state, temperament, and sex)

If any of these preconditions are not present or are distorted, skilled intervention is necessary to ensure the attachment process.

According to Stainton (1983b), attachment is a mutual exchange of feelings based on attractiveness, responsiveness, and satisfaction. It is subject to changes in intensity as circumstances change over time. Attachment is developed and maintained by proximity and interaction. As with any developmental process, it is characterized by periods of progress and regression. Thus temporary or permanent withdrawal from attachment figures can occur.

Mercer (1982) notes that attachment is facilitated by **positive feedback:** "Positive feedback includes the social, verbal and nonverbal responses, either real or perceived, that indicate acceptance of one partner by the other." She notes that attachment occurs through "a mutually satisfying experience." The newborn infant grasps a finger or a strand of hair, becoming attached to the parent. A mother commented on her son's grasp reflex, "I put my finger in his hand, and he grabbed right on. It is just a reflex, I know, but it felt good anyway."

Various theories have attempted to explain the basis for attachment. Freudian psychoanalytic theory emphasizes the development of a bond between child and mother as a result of the mother's satisfying the infant's innate needs to socialize with another and the physical needs for survival. Social learning theory contributed the principles of reinforcement to the attachment process. As discomfort is reduced or removed by the mother (or other caregiver) and is substituted with pleasure, the mother becomes associated with the pleasurable feeling of being satisfied. She becomes important to the infant, is loved, and can therefore act as a reinforcing agent or event. The mother becomes a **significant other** in the infant's life.

Bowlby (1958) and others (Ainsworth, 1969, 1970; Ainsworth, Bell, 1970; Brazelton, 1963, 1973) have extended the concept of attachment to include **mutuality;** that is, the infant's behaviors and characteristics call forth a corresponding set of maternal behaviors and characteristics. The infant displays **signaling behaviors** such as crying, smiling, and cooing that initiate the contact and bring the mother near the child. These behaviors are followed by **executive behaviors** such as rooting, grasping, and postural adjustments that maintain the contact. The caregiver is attracted to an alert, responsive, cuddly infant and repelled by an irritable, apparently disinterested infant. Attachment occurs more readily with the infant whose temperament, social capabilities, appearance, and gender fit the parent's expectations. If the child does not meet these expectations, resolution of disappointment can delay the attachment process.

An important part of attachment is **acquaintance** (Klaus, Kennell, 1983). Parents use eye contact (Fig. 24-2), touching, talking, and exploring as they be-

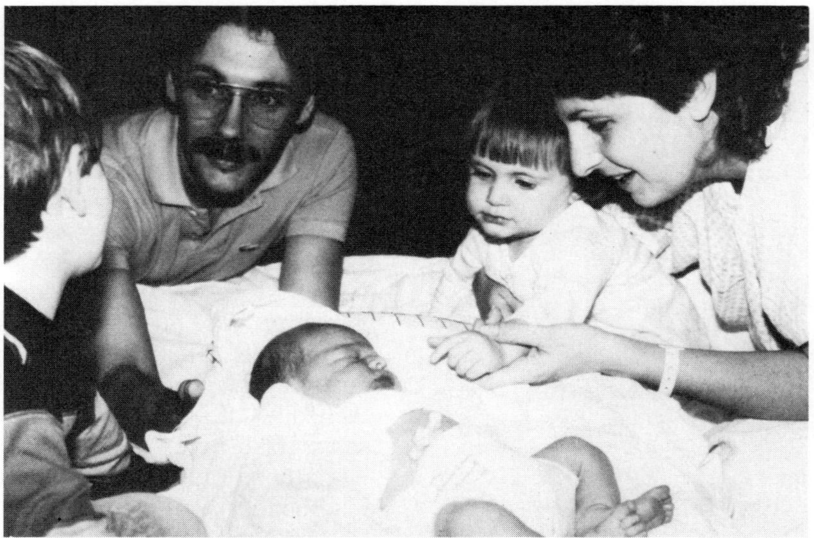

Fig. 24-2 Family members examine the new baby. They discuss her appearance and admire her.
Courtesy Marjorie Pyle, RNC, Lifecircle, Costa Mesa, Calif.

come acquainted during the immediate postbirth period. Adoptive parents undergo the same process when they first meet their new child. During this period, families engage in identification of the new baby, known as the **claiming process.** The child is first identified in terms of "likeness" to other family members, then in terms of "differences," and finally in terms of "uniqueness." The unique newcomer is thus *incorporated* into the family. Mothers and fathers scrutinize an infant carefully. They point out characteristics that the child shares with other family members and indicate recognition of a relationship between them. Mothers make comments such as the following that reveal the claiming process: "Russ held him close and said, 'He's the image of his father,' but I found one part like me—his toes are shaped like mine. Look, he's smiling; he likes his mother's jokes."

On the other hand, some mothers react negatively. They "claim" the infant in terms of the discomfort or pain the baby causes the mother. The mother interprets the infant's normal responses as being negative toward her. The mother reacts to her child with dislike or indifference. She does not hold the child close or touch the child to be comforting; for example, "The nurse put the baby into Marie's arms. She promptly laid him across her knees and glanced up at the television. 'Stay still 'til I finish watching—you've been enough trouble already.' "

Parental responses have direct implications for nursing. Nurses can establish an environment that enhances positive parent-child contacts. They can encourage parental awareness of infant responses and ability to communicate, provide support and encouragement as parents attempt to become competent and loving in their role, and enhance the attachment process.

COMMUNICATION BETWEEN PARENT AND CHILD

Attachment is strengthened through the use of sensual responses or abilities by both partners in the parent-child interaction. The sensual responses and abilities used in the communication between parent and child include the following.

TOUCH. Touch, or the tactile sense, is used extensively by parents and other caregivers as a means of becoming acquainted with the newborn. The fingertip, one of the most touch-sensitive areas of the body, is used to explore the infant's head, face, and body surfaces. The open palms and arms are used to handle the infant (Tulman, 1985). Many mothers reach out for their infants as soon as they are born and the cord is cut. They lift them to their breasts, enfold them in their arms, and cradle them. Once the child is close to them, they begin the exploration process with their fingertips. For some mothers and other caregivers (fathers, nursing and medical students) studies have depicted a predictable pattern of touch behavior (Rubin, 1963; Klaus, Kennell, 1982; Tulman, 1985). The caregiver begins with a **fingertip**

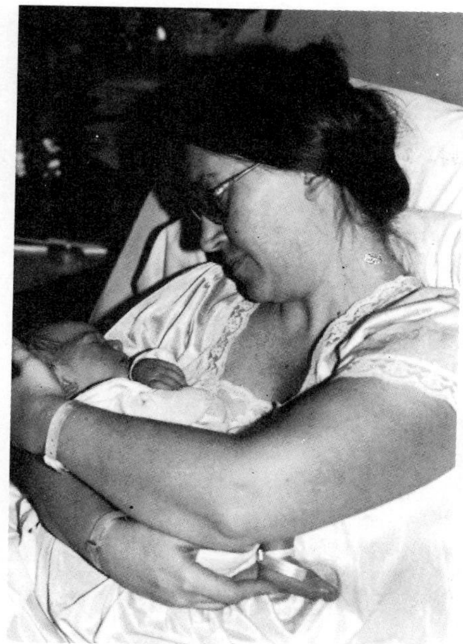

Fig. 24-3 Mother interacts with daughter through touching infant's head and feet.
Courtesy Judy Bamber, San Jose, Calif.

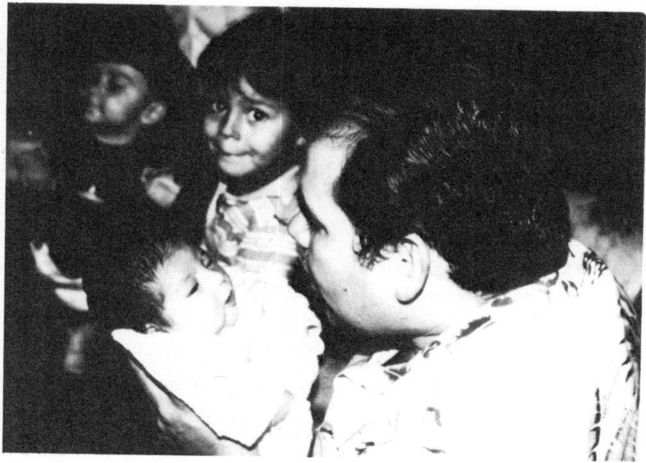

Fig. 24-4 Father and new baby make eye contact in *en face* position.
Courtesy Marjorie Pyle, RNC, Lifecircle, Costa Mesa, Calif.

exploration of the infant's head and extremities. Within a short time the caregiver uses the palm to caress the baby's trunk and eventually enfolds the infant in her or his arms. Gentle stroking motions are used to soothe and quiet the infant. Mothers pat or gently rub their infant's back after feedings. Infants pat the mother's breast as they nurse. Parents want to touch, pick up, and hold their infant (Fig. 24-3). They comment on the softness of the baby's skin and are aware of milia and rashes. Infant massage helps relax the baby and promotes attachment (see guidelines for teaching infant massage p. 722).

Parents and child seem to enjoy sharing each other's body warmth. Mothers will say, "I love her warm little body against mine."

Parents can be helped to recognize and respond to the similarities of their child's responses before and after birth. *The unborn comes "not as a stranger" but as one known to the parents and alert to the sound of their voices and their soothing actions.* Increasing sensitivity to the infant's like or dislike of types of touch brings parents closer to their babies. Stainton (1983b) reports the following instance:

> The unborn baby was perceived to be distressed at times and communicated this to the parents through excessive movement, especially kicking, indicating a need for, in their words, "calming down." One or both parents typically responded by rubbing the baby's body through the abdominal wall and all reported this resulted in a "settling" or "quieting." The majority stated the unborn baby liked to be rubbed. Mothers and fathers were observed rubbing or patting the abdomen.*

Prenatal strategies that have been used to promote intrauterine attachment include having the mother feel for fetal parts abdominally, massaging and rubbing the abdomen, and noting what maternal activities cause changes in fetal activity. Studies have found the fetus is more active when the mother engages in activities like jogging and will become quiet when the mother relaxes, for example, when she takes a warm shower (Davis, Akridge, 1987).

EYE-TO-EYE CONTACT. Interest in having eye contact is demonstrated again and again. Some mothers remark that once their babies have looked at them, they feel much closer to them (Klaus, Kennell, 1982). Others have also noted this response: "I was a mother and looked into his eyes so clear; fell into his eyes, and in love" (Lang, 1972). Parents spend much time getting their babies to open their eyes and look at them. In our culture eye contact appears to have a cementing effect on the development of a beginning and trusting relationship and is an important factor in human relationships at all ages.

As newborns become functionally able to sustain eye contact, parents and child spend much time gazing at one another, often in the *en face* position (Fig. 24-4). ***En face,*** "face-to-face," is a position in which the mother's face and the infant's face are approxi-

*Stainton MD: Maternal newborn attachment origins & processes. III. Interactions synchrony: the prelude to attachment, doctoral dissertation, San Francisco, 1983, University of California.

mately 8 inches apart and on the same plane. We need to implement medical and nursing practices that encourage this exchange. Instillation of protective eye drops can be withheld until the infant and parents have some time together. Lights can be dimmed so that the child's eyes will open. Newborns can be held close enough to see the parents' faces.

VOICE. The shared response of parents and infant to each other's voice also is remarkable. Parents wait tensely for the first cry. Once it has reassured them of the baby's health, they begin comforting behaviors. As the parents talk in high-pitched voices, the infant is alerted and turns toward them.

ODOR. Another behavior shared by parents and infant is response to each other's odor. Mothers comment on the smell of their babies when first born and have noted that each child has a unique odor. Infants learn rapidly to distinguish the odor of their own mother's breast milk (Stainton, 1985).

ENTRAINMENT. Newborns have been found to move in time with the structure of adult speech (Condon, Sander, 1974). They wave their arms, lift their heads, kick their legs, seemingly "dancing in tune" to their parent's voice. This means that the infant has developed *culturally determined rhythms* of speech long before using the spoken language in communicating. A *carryover* (**entrainment**) occurs once the child begins to talk. This shared rhythm also acts to give the parent positive feedback and to establish a positive setting for effective communication.

BIORHYTHMICITY. The unborn child can be said to be in tune with the mother's natural rhythms, such as heartbeats. After birth, a crying infant may be soothed by being held in a position in the mother's arms where her heartbeat can be heard or by hearing a recording of a heartbeat. One of the newborn's tasks is to establish a personal rhythm (**biorhythmicity**). Parents can help in this process by giving consistent loving care and by using their infant's alert state to develop responsive behavior and thereby increase social interactions and opportunities for learning. The more quickly parents become competent in child-care activities, the more quickly their psychologic energy can be directed toward observing the communication cues the infant gives them.

RECIPROCITY AND SYNCHRONY. **Reciprocity** is a type of body movement or behavior that provides the observer with cues. The observer/receiver interprets those cues and responds to them. Reciprocity often takes several weeks to develop with a new baby. For example: the newborn fusses and cries; the mother responds by picking up and cradling the child; the child becomes quiet and alert, establishes eye contact; the mother verbalizes, sings, and coos while the child maintains eye contact. The child then averts her or his eyes and yawns; the mother decreases active response. Should the parent continue to stimulate the infant, the child may become fussy.

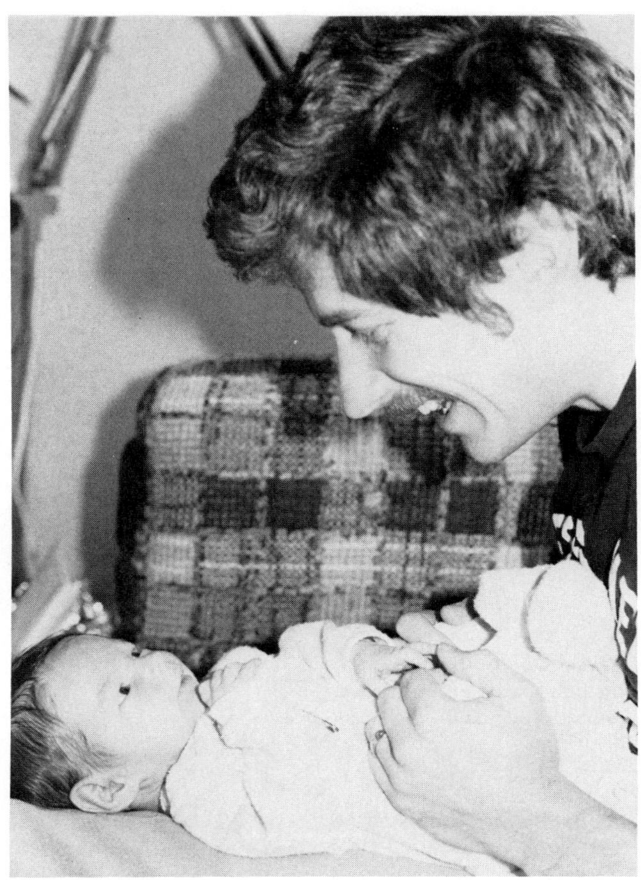

Fig. 24-5 Sharing a smile: example of synchrony. Courtesy Chris Cowing.

Synchrony refers to the "fit" between the infant's cues and the parent's response (Censullo et al, 1985). When parent and child experience a synchronous interaction, it is mutually rewarding (Fig. 24-5). It takes time for the parent to correctly interpret the infant's cues. For example, it takes some time for the infant to acquire a different cry for different reasons, such as boredom, loneliness, hunger, or discomfort. The parent may need assistance, along with trial and error interventions, before synchrony develops.

Early Contact

Research with mammals other than humans indicates that early contact between mother and offspring is important in developing future relationships. *To date, no scientific evidence has demonstrated that immediate contact after birth is essential for the human parent-child relationship.* According to Siegel (1982), carefully controlled replicated investigations appear to document the following finding:

> Early contact, irrespective of its supplementation by extended contact, favorably affects maternal affectional behavior during the first postpartum days. The results are consistent across low and middle socioeconomic status mother-infant pairs as well as in developed and less developed countries.

Siegel also noted that early contact has a positive effect on the duration of breast-feeding. However, long-range effects of early contact have yet to be documented (Lamb, 1982).

The physiologic benefits of early contact between mother and infant have been documented (Klaus, Kennell, 1982). For the mother, levels of oxytocin and prolactin rise; for the infant, sucking reflexes are employed early. The process of developing active immunity begins as the infant inhales flora from the mother's skin.

The first hours or days after birth may be a sensitive time for parent-infant interaction. Early close contact *may facilitate* the attachment process between parent and child. This is not to say a delay will inhibit this process (humans are too resilient for that), but additional psychologic energy may be needed to accomplish the same effect. For parents unable or unwilling to expend this energy the delay may affect the infant's future well-being.

In one of the first texts on newborn disorders, Budin (1907) noted that "mothers separated from their young soon lost all interest in those whom they were unable to nurse or cherish." Subsequent investigators have noted similar behaviors when interactions between parent and child meet interference. Bowlby's work (1958, 1969) emphasizes the attachment process between infant and mother and details the effects of loss of that attachment to the infant. Research in the area of child abuse documents the greater percentage of neglect, abuse, and failure to thrive among infants separated from parents for relatively long periods because of illness or preterm birth (Klaus, Kennell, 1982).

Parents who desire but are unable to have early contact with their newborn infant *can be reassured that such contact is not essential for optimum par-child interactions*. Otherwise, ***adopted infants*** would not form the usual affectional ties with their parents. Nor does the mode of infant-mother contact after birth (skin-to-skin versus wrapped) appear to have any important effect. Nurses need to counsel mothers to assure them that their emotional bond to their infant is not necessarily weaker because they missed early contact or because the contact was not skin to skin (Curry, 1979). Women who have experienced a long and difficult labor often are too exhausted to respond other than in a superficial way to the newborn. They may welcome the attention of others and be grateful that the infant is healthy, but their primary need centers on recovery from the physical and emotional aspects of pregnancy and childbirth. Infants born at risk as a result of either fetal or maternal disabilities usually are transferred to the intensive care nursery as quickly as possible. Concerns for their need for intensive medical and nursing care take priority over the need for close contact with the parents. Opportunities to be with the infant in the intensive care nursery, to touch or hold the baby if at all possible, and to receive reports of the infant's progress must be part of the nursing plan of care.

Extended Contact

Since the early 1970s, consumers have worked for childbirth practices that promote the family as the focus of care. The alternatives of home birth, birthing centers, and family-centered maternity care units reflect this desire by parents to share in the birth process and to have more contact with their infants.

One widely used method of family-centered care is the provision of rooming-in facilities for the mother and her baby. The infant is transferred to the area from the transitional nursery after satisfactory postbirth adjustment is ensured. The father is encouraged to visit and to participate in the care of the infant. Siblings and grandparents also are encouraged to visit and become acquainted with the infant. Some hospitals have established family birth units such as labor, delivery, recovery (LDR); labor, delivery, recovery, postpartum (LDRP) rooms and single room maternity care (SRMC). The mother is accompanied by the father during the birth of the infant, and all three may remain together until discharged. Medical and nursing personnel are available for any care necessary for the mother and child. Other hospitals arrange for the discharge of the mother and infant any time from 2 to 24 hours after the birth if the condition of the mother and that of the child warrants it. Follow-up care with nursing personnel from a health agency is part of this plan.

Mother-baby care is another form of family-centered care. Care for the mother and baby is provided by a primary nurse, fostering family unity (Fig. 24-6). Parents involved in this approach are likely to be more self-confident in care, and maternal attachment and role attainment is promoted (NAACOG, 1989).

Extended contact with the infant should be available for all parents, but especially for those at risk for parenting inadequacies, such as adolescents and low-

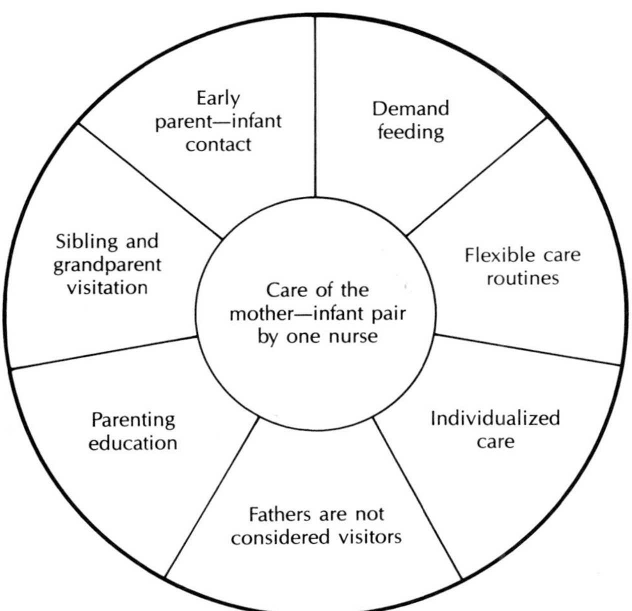

Fig. 24-6 The wheel of family-centered postpartum and newborn care.
Modified from Watter NE: *JOGNN* 6:480, 1985.

income women. Any activity that optimizes family-centered care is worthy of serious consideration by postpartum nurses.

■ PARENTAL ROLE AFTER CHILDBIRTH

For the biologic parent the parental role does not begin at birth but rather enlarges and intensifies. Care and nurturing of the child are not initiated in the postbirth period. Before birth the mother who carried out the dictates of health (e.g., diet, rest, exercise) for the "good of her baby," the father who supported and sheltered her, and the parents who became aware of and attached to their unborn child were already functioning in the parental role.

During the postbirth period, new tasks and responsibilities arise and old behaviors need to be modified or new ones added. Mothers' and fathers' responses to the parental role change over time and tend to follow a predictable course.

During the early period parents have to reorganize their relationship with the newborn infant. The child's needs for shelter, nourishment, protection, and socializing continue. What was accomplished through the biologic process of pregnancy now requires an array of caregiving activities. This period is characterized by intense learning and need for nurturing. The family structure and functioning as a system have been forever altered. The duration of this period varies with individuals but lasts about 4 weeks.

The next period represents a time of drawing together and uniting the family unit. This consolidation period involves negotiations as to roles (wife-husband, mother-father, parent-child, sibling-sibling). It involves a stabilizing of tasks, a coming to terms with commitments. Parents demonstrate growing competence in child-care activities and become sensitive to the meaning of their infant's behavior. This period lasts approximately 2 months and in conjunction with the early period forms what is now termed the ***fourth trimester.***

Parents and children grow in their roles until separated by death. The most outstanding feature of the lifelong process of parent-child interaction is change, consistent evolution over time. The people involved deal not only with the present but also with the future. They need support and care in the here and now and anticipatory guidance for coming changes.

Parental Tasks and Responsibilities

Parents need to reconcile the actual child with the fantasy and dream child. This means coming to terms with the infant's physical appearance, sex, innate temperament, and physical status. If the real child differs greatly from the fantasy child, parents may delay acceptance for a period. In some instances they may never accept the child. Mothers describe the differences between the real and the imagined child as follows (Stainton, 1983a):

> In the words of one mother, "I was surprised that she seemed to me to be a complete person with a personality of her own. I expected a blank tablet, a piece of clay for me to mold or a sponge for me to fill." Another, "I could not believe how determined and demanding he could be. I was going to control him and get him fitted into our life-style."

Some parents are startled by the appearance of the infant—size, color, molding of the head, or bowed appearance of the legs (see Chapter 20). Many fathers have commented that they thought the odd shape of the child's head (molding) meant the child would be mentally retarded.

Disappointment over the sex of the infant can take time to resolve. The mother or father may be able to give adequate physical parenting but may find it difficult to be sincerely involved with the infant until these feelings have been resolved. As one mother remarked:

> I really wanted a boy, I know it is silly and irrational, but when they said, "She's a lovely little girl," I was so disappointed and angry—yes, angry—I could hardly look at her. Oh, I looked after her okay, her feedings and baths and things, but I couldn't feel excited. To tell the truth, I

felt like a monster not liking my child. Then one day she was lying there and she turned her head and looked right at me. I felt a flooding of love for her come over me, and we looked at each other a long time. It's okay now. I wouldn't change her for all the boys in the world.

Nursing care plans need to include time for explanations about the child's appearance. Nurses need to provide opportunities for parents to discuss their lack of motherly feelings without fear of censure or ridicule. Often the expression of doubts and concerns provides relief and makes it easier for parents to accept help with such feelings.

Parents need to establish the newborn as a person separate from themselves, that is, as someone having many dependency needs and requiring much nurturing.

Parents need to become adept in the care of the infant. This includes caregiving activities, noting the communication cues given by the infant to indicate needs, and responding appropriately to the infant's needs.

Parents need to establish reasonable evaluative criteria to use in assessing the success or failure of the care given the infant. Parents are surprisingly sensitive to infant responses. One father told of his first attempt to give his child a kiss. At that moment the child turned her head. The father felt hurt, although he understood that the baby was totally unaware of her own movements. How the infant responds to the parental care and attention is interpreted by the parent as a comment on the quality of the care being given. These responses may include crying, weight gain or loss, or sleeping at a designated time. Continued responses that the parent views as negative can result in alienation of parent and child to the infant's detriment (Table 24-1).

Self-esteem grows with competence. Mothers of preterm infants have noted that the skillful handling of their infants by nurses made their own efforts appear inadequate. Mothers who have supplied breast milk for their infant comment that this makes them feel they are contributing in a unique way to the welfare of their child.

Criticism, real or imagined, of new parents' ability to provide adequate physical care, nutrition, or social stimulation for their infant can prove devastating. These "critics" may need constructive direction. Assistance, including advice by husbands, wives, mothers, mothers-in-law, and professional workers, can be seen as supportive. Conversely, it can be seen as an indication of how inept these persons have judged the new parents to be.

Parents must establish a place for the newborn within the family group. Whether the infant is the first born or last born, all family members must adjust their roles to accommodate the newcomer. An only child needs support to accept a rival to parental affections. An older child needs support when losing a favored position. The parents are expected to negotiate these changes.

TABLE 24-1 Infant Behaviors Affecting Parental Attachment

Facilitating Behaviors	Inhibiting Behaviors
Visually alert; eye-to-eye contact; tracking or following of parent's face	Sleepy; eyes closed most of the time; gaze aversion
Appealing facial appearance; randomness of body movements reflecting helplessness	Resemblance to person parent dislikes; hyperirritability or jerky body movements when touched
Smiles	Bland facial expression; infrequent smiles
Vocalization; crying only when hungry or wet	Crying for hours on end; colicky
Grasp reflex	Exaggerated motor reflex
Anticipatory approach behaviors for feedings; sucks well; feeds easily	Feeds poorly; regurgitates; vomits often
Enjoys being cuddled, held	Resists holding and cuddling by crying, stiffening body
Easily consolable	Inconsolable; unresponsive to parenting, caretaking tasks
Activity and regularity somewhat predictable	Unpredictable feeding and sleeping schedule
Attention span sufficient to focus on parents	Inability to attend to parent's face or offered stimulation
Differential crying, smiling, and vocalizing; recognizes and prefers parents	Shows no preference for parents over others
Approaches through locomotion	Unresponsive to parent's approaches
Clings to parent; puts arms around parent's neck	Seeks attention from any adult in room
Lifts arms to parents in greeting	Ignores parents

From Gerson E: *Infant behavior in the first year of life,* New York, 1973, Raven Press, Copyright © 1973. With permission.

Parents need to establish the primacy of their adult relationships to maintain the family as a group. Because this includes reorganizing many roles—for example, sexual roles, child-care roles, career roles, and community roles—time and energy must be provided for this vital task.

Maternal Adjustment

Three phases are evident as the mother adjusts to her version of the parental role. These phases of **maternal adjustment** are characterized by dependent behavior, dependent-independent behavior, and interdependent behavior.

DEPENDENT PHASE. During the first 1 to 2 days after childbirth, the mother's dependency needs predominate. To the extent that these needs are met by others, the mother is able to divert her psychologic energy to her child rather than to herself. She needs "mothering" to "mother." Rubin (1961) has aptly described these few days as the **taking-in phase:** a time when nurturing and protective care are required by the new mother.

For a few days after the birth, mature and apparently healthy women appear to suspend involvement in everyday responsibilities. They rely on others to respond to their needs for comfort, rest, nourishment, and closeness to their families and newborn.

The **dependent phase** is a time of great excitement, and most parents are extremely talkative. They need to verbalize their experience of pregnancy and birth. Focusing on, analyzing, and accepting these experiences help the parents move on to the next phase. Some parents are able to use staff members or other mothers as an "audience." Others are unable to do this and need the opportunity to be with family or friends.

Because anxiety and preoccupation with her new role often narrow a mother's perceptions, information may have to be repeated. The new mother may require reminders to rest, or conversely, to ambulate enough to promote recovery. Ward routine may not necessarily be an important priority to the new mother; she may take showers when examinations are scheduled and be involved in a telephone conversation rather than "being ready" for the baby. Regulations seem cumbersome, and sometimes mothers and their families have difficulty accepting rules that interfere with their needs to share reactions about their child.

Physical discomfort from an episiotomy, sore nipples, hemorrhoids, afterpains, and occasionally a sprained coccygeal joint can interfere with the mother's need for rest and relaxation. The selective use of comfort measures and medication depends on the nurse. Many women hesitate to ask for medication, believing that any pain they experience is normal and to be expected; few have a knowledge of the use of heat or cold to relieve local pain.

DEPENDENT-INDEPENDENT PHASE. If the mother has received adequate nurturing in the first few days, by the third day her desire for independent action reasserts itself. In the **dependent-independent phase,** the mother alternates between a need for extensive nurturing and acceptance by others and the desire "to take charge" once again. She responds enthusiastically to opportunities to learn and practice the care of the baby or, if she is an accomplished mother, to carry out or direct this care.

Regardless of the desire for the baby and the amount of prenatal preparation undertaken, the reality of parenthood must be experienced to be understood fully. One young mother expressed it as follows (Lang, 1972):

> But then in my second week, as my strength began to return, my energies began to focus on the overwhelming task of motherhood that stood before me. And I realized then that I faced that task alone. Not that my husband wouldn't stand by me, not that my friends would not share experiences with me, but I stood alone with the realization that only I could be the child's mother.

In the period of 6 to 8 weeks after childbirth the mastery of the tasks of parenthood are crucial. Realistic expectations promote the future functioning of the family as a unit.

Some women adjust with considerable difficulty to the isolation of infant care and resent the endless coping with home and child-care responsibilities. The mothers who appear to need additional supportive counseling include the following:

1. First-time mothers inexperienced in child care
2. Women whose careers had provided outside stimulation
3. Women who lack friends or family members with whom to share delights and concerns
4. Adolescent mothers

Depressive states are not uncommon during this phase. *Feelings of extreme vulnerability* may arise from a number of factors. Psychologically the mother may be overwhelmed by the actuality of parental responsibilities. She may feel deprived of the supportive care she received from family members and friends during her pregnancy. Some mothers regret the loss of the mother-unborn child relationship and mourn its passing. Still others experience a letdown feeling when labor and birth are complete. They had prepared themselves for an elemental experience, a walk "through the shadows," and now it is safely over.

Once immediate tasks and adjustments have been

undertaken and brought under control, a plateau is reached. At this time the life-long effects of the parents' new responsibilities come into focus. Some parents experience a feeling of being trapped and wonder what life is all about.

Occasionally the mother becomes increasingly fatigued during the last month of pregnancy, when sleep is interrupted by shortness of breath and urinary frequency. Leg cramps, or inability to lie in a comfortable position can disturb sleep. *Fatigue* after childbirth is compounded by around-the-clock demands of the new baby and can accentuate the feelings of depression. It has been suggested that a lowered level of circulating glucocorticoids or a condition of subclinical hypothyroidism may exist during the puerperium. This physiologic state could explain some minor degrees of **postpartum depression ("baby blues")**.

Depressive reactions are not necessarily expressed verbally. A depressive state can be recognized by such typical behavior as withdrawal, loss of interest in surroundings, and crying (p. 720).

It is hoped that toward the end of the dependent-independent phase the tasks and adjustments of daily routine will begin to follow a pattern. The baby begins to take an established position in the family. Many of the feeding problems, whether related to breast-feeding or bottle-feeding, have been largely resolved. The mother's physical energy and strength return; the **taking-hold phase** (Rubin, 1961) is ending. By the fifth week the infant has been examined by the physician and the mother also has been examined or has made arrangements for a checkup. It is time to move on to the next phase of adjustment.

INTERDEPENDENT PHASE. In this phase interdependent behavior reasserts itself, and the mother and her family move forward as a system with interacting members. The relationship of the partners, although altered by the introduction of a child, resumes many of its former characteristics. A primary need is to establish a life-style that includes, but in some respects excludes, the child. The couple must share interests and activities that are adult in scope.

Most couples begin intercourse by the third or fourth week after the child is born; some begin earlier, as soon as it can be accomplished without discomfort for the woman. Sexual intimacy increases the man-woman aspect of the family, and the adult pair shares a closeness denied to other family members. Many new fathers speak of the alienation experienced when they observe the intimate mother-child relationship, and some are frank in expressing feelings of jealousy toward the infant. The resumption of the marital relationship seems to bring the parents' relationship back into focus.

The **interdependent phase (letting-go phase)** is often stressful for the parental pair. Career patterns of men from their 20s through their 40s show intense activity centering around advancement in their profession or job. This often necessitates long hours away from the home or moving from one locale to another. Meanwhile the women are engrossed in home activities directed toward the care of the young children. Interests and needs differ, and there may be a gradual estrangement, which is ignored for the time being because of the individual needs of each. A special effort must be undertaken to strengthen the adult-adult relationship as a basis for the family unit.

Paternal Adjustment

During the last decade a growing interest in the relationship between the father and the child has become evident. It is now recognized that the mother-child relationship does not exist in a vacuum but within the context of the family system. Parents' attitudes toward the expectations of each other's parental behavior affect the behavior of each couple. In our culture the newborn has been found to have a powerful impact on the father. Fathers have demonstrated intense involvement with their babies (Fig. 24-7). Greenberg and Morris (1976) named the father's absorption, preoccupation, and interest in the

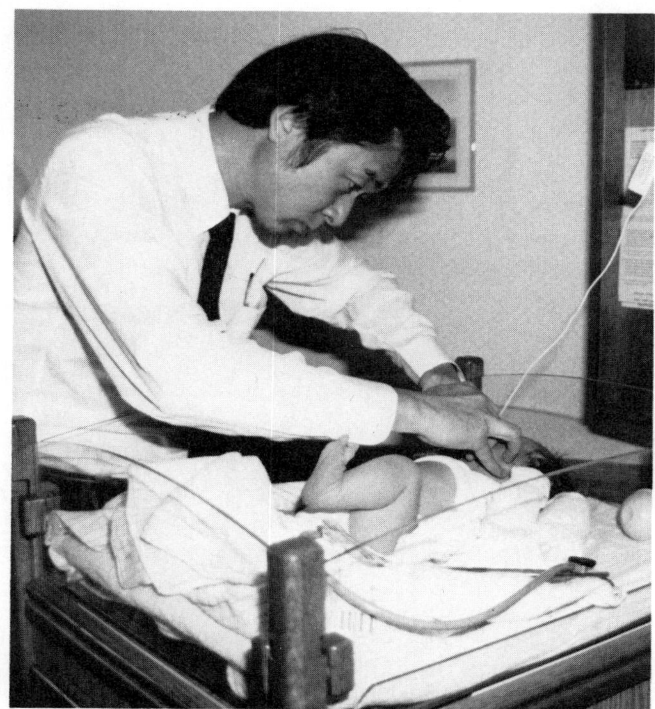

Fig. 24-7 Engrossment. Father looking at and touching his newborn.
Courtesy Marjorie Pyle, RNC, Lifecircle, Costa Mesa, Calif.

infant **engrossment.** These researchers described a number of characteristics of engrossment. Some of the sensual responses relating to touch and eye-to-eye contact are the same as discussed earlier. The father's keen awareness of features both unique and similar to himself is another characteristic related to the father's need to claim the infant. An outstanding response is one of *strong attraction* to the newborn. Much time is spent "communicating" with the infant and taking delight in the infant's response to the father. Fathers feel a sense of increased self-esteem, a sense of being "proud, bigger, more mature, and older" after seeing their baby for the first time. Studies have revealed distinct features in father-infant relationships. Fathers tend to take the lead in initiating play and other social situations. Mothers tend to take the lead in caregiving activities (Clarke-Stewart, 1978). The subtle, as well as the more open, differences in stimulation from two sources, mother and father, provide a wider social experience for the child. In addition, the child has improved chances of developing at least one good parenting relationship (Kunst-Wilson, Cronenwett, 1981).

Much has still to be learned about the relationships between fathers and their offspring. The mother's biologic relationship with the child provides a basis for predicting behaviors in the mother-child relationship. However, the knowledge that a man is the father of a child gives us no clues as to his relationships or behaviors with the child.

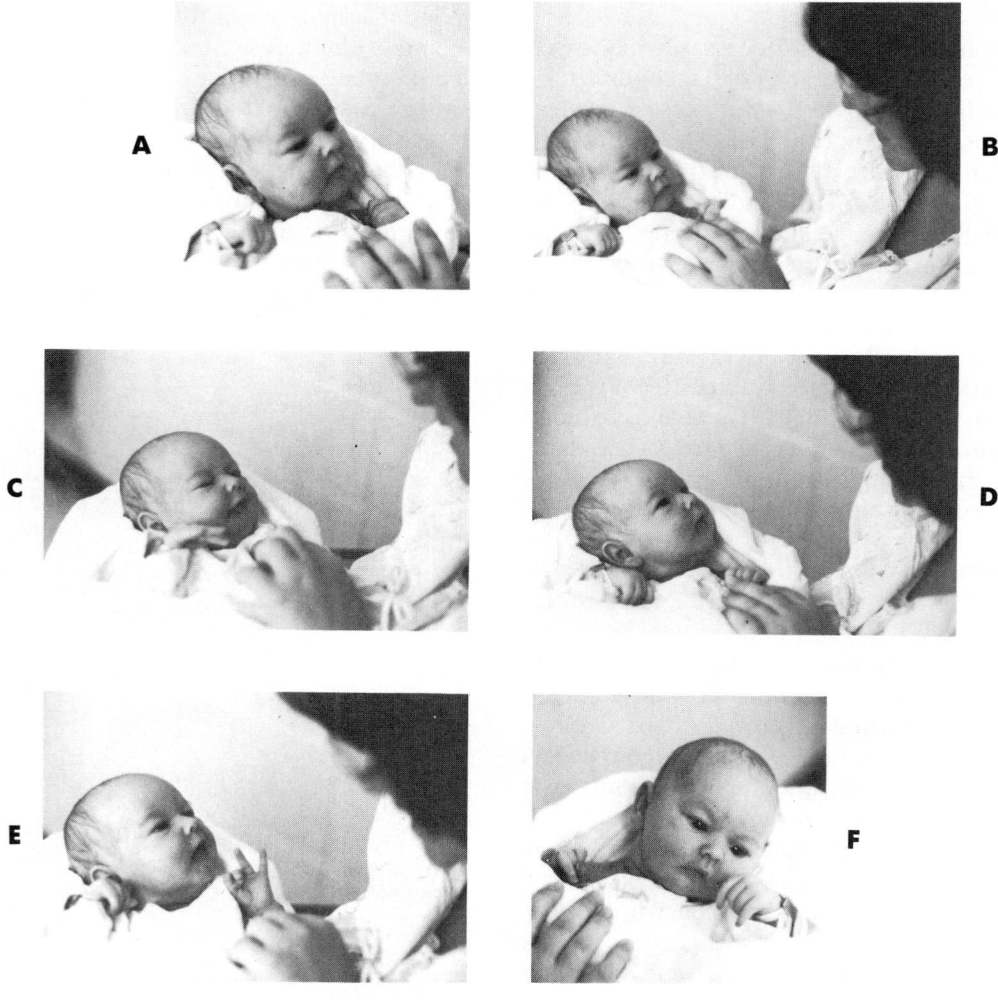

Fig. 24-8 Holding newborn in *en face* position, mother works to alert her daughter, 6 hours old. **A,** Infant is quiet and alert. **B,** Mother begins talking to daughter. Note frown of concentration. **C,** Infant responds, opens mouth, like her mother. **D,** Infant gazes at her mother. **E,** Infant waves hand, opens mouth. **F,** Infant glances away, resting. Hand relaxes.
Courtesy Colleen Stainton, RN, DNS, University of Calgary, Alberta, Canada.

As yet, no evidence exists as to how the father's individual style affects his actual experience with one particular child. Despite their active involvement in the perinatal period, fathers tend to gravitate toward more traditional roles as they become more involved in job-related activities and less in child-care activities. However, if the father does involve himself in caregiving, he responds much as the mother in talking to the infant (Field, 1978a).

Infant-Parent Adjustment

The **infant-parent interaction** is characterized by a "set of rhythms, behavioral repertoires, and responsivity or response styles" (Field, 1978a). These traits are unique to each partner. Interactions can be facilitated in any of three ways: (1) modulation of **rhythm,** (2) modification of **behavioral repertoires,** and (3) mutual **responsivity.**

RHYTHM. To modulate the rhythm, both parent and infant must be able to interact. Therefore the infant must be in the alert state, one of the most difficult of the sleep-wake states to maintain. The alert state occurs most often during a feeding or in face-to-face play. The parent must work hard to help the infant maintain the alert state long enough and often enough for interactions to take place. The ***en face*** position (parent positions face in same plane as that of newborn) is usually assumed (Fig. 24-8). Evidently mothers learn how to do this: multiparous mothers show particular sensitivity and responsiveness to their infant's feeding rhythms. The mother who is sensitive to feeding rhythms reserves stimulation for pauses in sucking activity. For example, the mother learns not to talk or smile excessively while the infant is sucking because the infant will stop feeding to interact with her (Field, 1978b). With maturity the infant can sustain longer interactions by modulating activity rhythms, that is, limb movement, sucking, gaze alternation, and **habituation** (Fig. 24-9). "In the interim, the adult learns to attend to these rhythms, modulate her or his own rhythms, and thereby facilitate a rhythmical turn-taking interaction" (Field, 1978a).

REPERTOIRES. Both contributors to the infant-parent interaction have a repertoire of behaviors they can use to facilitate interactions. Fathers and mothers engage in these behaviors depending on the amount of contact and caregiving of the infant. (Review reciprocity and synchrony, p. 676).

The *infant's repertoire* includes gaze, behaviors, vocalizing, and facial expressions. The infant is able to focus and follow the human face from birth. The infant also is able to use gaze alternation. These abilities are under voluntary control. "The infant appears to look away from the mother's face when under-or over-aroused to modulate his or her arousal level and process the stimulation he or she is receiving." (Field, 1978a). Brazelton et al (1974) suggest that one of the key responses for the parents to learn is *sensitivity to the infant's capacity for attention and inattention.* Developing this sensitivity is especially important in interacting with preterm infants (Sammons, Lewis, 1985). Field (1978b) states, "Mothers who are more active or 'overstimulating' and less sensitive or responsive to their infant's pauses or turning away during the conversation are less able to elicit or hold their infants' gaze."

Body gestures form a part of the infant's "early language." Babies greet parents with waving hands or with a reaching out of hands. They can raise an eyebrow or soften their expression to elicit loving attention. They can be stimulated to smile or laugh with game playing. To end an interaction they use pouting or crying, arching of the back, and general squirming.

The parents' repertoire includes various behaviors for interacting with their infant. One of these behaviors is constantly looking at the infant and noting the infant's behavior. New parents often remark that they are exhausted from looking at the baby and

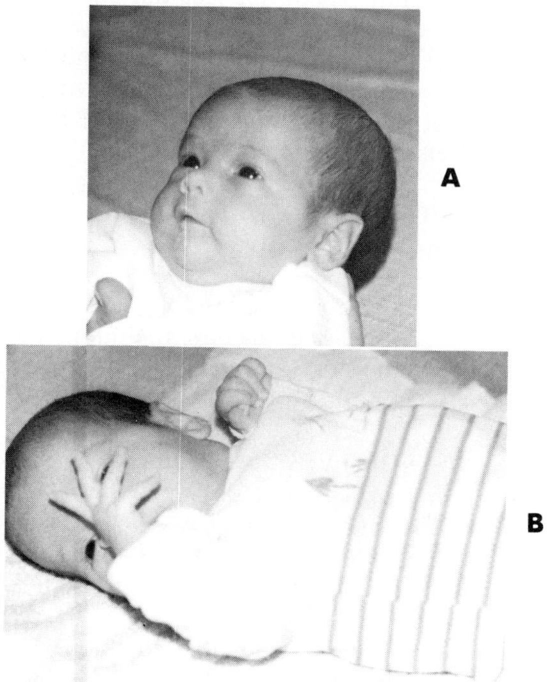

Fig. 24-9 **A,** Alerting. **B,** Habituating.
Courtesy Colleen Stainton, RN, DNS, University of Calgary, Alberta, Canada.

smiling. Adults also "infantilize" their speech to help the infant "listen." They do this by slowing the tempo, speaking loudly and rhythmically, and by emphasizing key words. They repeat phrases frequently. Infantilizing does not mean using "baby talk," which involves distortion of sounds.

Parents also will use facial expressions as a means of interaction. They may slow and exaggerate expressions such as surprise, happiness, and confusion to communicate them to the infant. Playing games, such as "peek-a-boo," is another means of interaction. Parents also can be observed imitating the infant's behaviors. If the baby smiles, so does the parent. If the baby frowns, the parent responds in kind.

RESPONSIVITY. Contingent responses are those that occur within a specific time and are similar in form to a stimulus behavior. They elicit a feeling in the person originating the behavior of having an influence on the interaction. In other words, they act as positive feedback. Adults view infant behaviors such as smiling, cooing, and sustained eye contact, usually in *en face* position, as contingent responses. That is, the adults are encouraged to continue the same game when the infant responds in such a way. These responses act as rewards to the initiator. When the adult imitates the infant, the infant appears to enjoy the responses. The infant in turn imitates behaviors of adults soon after birth. The parent shows progression in presenting behaviors for the baby to imitate; for example, in early interactions the parent will grimace rather than laugh, which is in keeping with the infant's developmental level. Such "turnabout" behaviors sustain interactions and promote harmony in the relationship.

Factors Influencing Parental Responses

How the parents respond to the birth of their child is influenced by various factors, including age, social networks, socioeconomic conditions, and personal aspirations for the future.

MATERNAL AGE OVER 35. Maternal age has a definite effect on pregnancy outcome. The mother and fetus are both at highest risk when the mother is an adolescent or is over 35 years old. Adolescent pregnancy, which is a significant issue in North America, is addressed in Chapter 34.

Issues and concerns related to the over-35 age-group have become increasingly more prominent in the last decade. There have always been women over 35 who have continued their childbearing either by choice or because of lack or failure of contraception during the perimenopausal years. Added to this group are women who have postponed pregnancy because of careers or other reasons, as well as women with infertility problems who have become pregnant because of technologic advances that have expanded alternatives for couples desiring children.

Studies have identified certain factors that can influence parental responses in this older group. *Fatigue and the need for more rest* seem to be the major concerns of older parents with newborns (Queenan, 1987; Winslow, 1987). Many of these mothers, being less resilient than younger women, may need to stay in the hospital longer, rather than be forced to an early discharge as some third party payers are requiring.

Measures designed to assist the mother in regaining strength and muscle tone (e.g., prenatal and postnatal exercises) are emphasized. Some older mothers may find that the care of the newborn infant exhausts their physical capabilities. Many women might benefit from referral to supportive resources in the community (Scott et al, 1986).

SOCIAL NETWORKS. First-time mothers may have different needs from women who have given birth before. The latter group may be more realistic in anticipating their physical limitations and can adjust to changes in roles and relationships more easily. First-time mothers may need more supportive care and follow-up for parenting, including referral to community resources. The families and friends of the parents and their newborn child form an important dimension of the parent's social network. Social networks provide a support system on which parents can rely for assistance (Crawford, 1985; Cronenwett, 1985 a, b). Positive emotional and affectional relationships appear critical to the enhancement of parenting skills and nurturance of children (Gottlieb, 1980; Schornkoff, 1984). Social networks promote the growth potential of children and the prevention of their maltreatment. Mercer (1982) and Crawford (1985) found that social networks provided support but also were a source of conflict. Grandparents or in-laws who assist with household responsibilities and who did not intrude into the parents' privacy or critically judge them were most appreciated. Sometimes a large network caused problems because it resulted in conflicting advice to the new parents.

SOCIOECONOMIC CONDITIONS. Parents whose economic condition is made worse with the birth of each child and who are unable to use an effective method of fertility management may find childbirth complicated by concern for their own health and a sense of helplessness. Mothers who are alone, deserted by husband, a partner, family, and friends, or who have serious financial problems may view the birth of the child with dread. The difficulties in which they find themselves may overcome any desire for mothering the infant (see Chapter 33).

Nursing measures designed to help persons in these circumstances involve social and economic community agencies as well as health agencies. Satisfactory outcomes of such problems often require long-term commitments from both the woman or couple and the community. Adequate situational supports need to be instituted in the prenatal period.

PERSONAL ASPIRATIONS. For some women parenthood interferes with or prevents their plans for personal freedom or advancement in their career. Resentment concerning their loss may not have been resolved during the prenatal period. If this resentment is not resolved, it will spill over into caregiving activities and may result in indifference and neglect. Conversely, it may result in excessive concern and the setting of impossibly high standards by the mother for her own behavior or the child's performance (Shainess, 1970).

Nursing intervention includes providing opportunities for parents to express their feelings freely to an objective listener; to discuss measures to permit personal growth of the parent, for example, by part-time employment, volunteer work, and use of agencies that provide baby-sitting care or mother substitutes during parents' vacations; and to learn about the care of the child.

PARENTAL SENSORY IMPAIRMENT

In the early dialogue between parent and child, all senses—sight, hearing, touch, taste, and smell—are used by both to initiate and sustain the *attachment process*. A parent who is deprived of one of the senses needs to develop an enriched use of the remaining sensory sources.

Blind Parent

Although parents who are blind need the presence as well as the support of another responsible person, they can become adept in some child-care activities, as the following report indicates:

> We had always planned to have a child. My family and Dick's both wanted us to have the happiness of children and were willing to help us with the baby care. First I bathed and changed a doll; then I practiced caring for my sister's baby. I would feel in all the creases with my finger to see if they were clean and dry. We used disposable diapers that do not need pins. My mother made baby clothes with fastenings of press cloth (Velcro) so I would not have to fiddle with buttons. I feel really confident now. I know I can't do everything for her, but I can do enough to feel like a "mother," and I know she will have all the love she needs.

One of the major difficulties blind parents experience is the skepticism, open or hidden, of the professional worker. Blind persons sense a reluctance on the part of others to acknowledge that they have a right to be parents. One blind mother-to-be noted that the best approach by the nurse is for the nurse to assess the mother's capabilities (Asrael, 1983). From that basis the nurse can make plans to assist the woman (i.e., the same as for a sighted mother). Another mother talked about the shyness, fear, or reluctance she sensed in nurses that resulted in her being left alone or being involved in awkward conversations.

Another mother expressed how sensitive the blind can become to other sensory output. She remarked that she could tell when her infant was facing her because she could feel his breath on her face.

Three mothers who are blind volunteered the following suggestions for providing care for the needs of women such as themselves during childbearing:

1. Clients who are blind need verbal teaching from health care providers because maternity information is not accessible to blind people.
2. Clients need an orientation to the hospital room that allows the client to move about the room independently. For example, "Go to the left of the bed and trail the wall until you feel the first door. That is the bathroom."
3. Clients need explanations of routines.
4. Clients need opportunities to feel devices (e.g., monitors, pelvic models) and to hear descriptions of the devices.
5. Clients need "a chance to ask questions!"
6. Clients need the opportunity to hold and touch their baby after childbirth.
7. Nurses need to demonstrate baby care by touch and to follow with, "Now let me see you do it."
8. Nurses need to give instructions such as "I'm going to give you the baby. The head is to your left side."

Eye-to-eye contact is considered important in our culture. With a parent who is blind, this critical factor in the parent-child attachment process is obviously missing. However, the blind parent, who may never have experienced this method of strengthening relationships, cannot be said to miss it. The infant will need other sensory input from the blind parent. Perhaps an infant looking into the eyes of a mother who is blind is not conscious that the eyes are unseeing. Other persons in the newborn's environment can participate in active eye-to-eye contact to supply this lack. Another problem may arise if the parent who is blind has an impassive facial expression. One observer noticed an infant making repeated attempts to engage in face play with his mother, who was blind. After repeated failure of his efforts, he abandoned the behavior with his mother and intensified it with his father. This problem might be overcome by the person's learning to accompany talking and cooing to the infant with head nodding and smiling.

Deaf Parent

The parent who has a hearing impairment faces another set of problems, particularly if the deafness dates from birth or early childhood. The mother and her partner are likely to have established an independent household. A number of devices that transform sound into light flashes are now marketed. The infant's room can be fitted with such a device to permit immediate detection of crying. Even if the parent is not speech trained, her or his vocalizing can serve as both stimulus and response to the infant's early vocalizing. Deaf parents can provide additional vocal training by use of records and television so that from birth onward the child is aware of the full range of the human voice. Sign language is acquired readily by the young child, and the first sign used is as varied as the first word.

Barnanowski (1983) described childbirth education classes for expectant deaf parents: "The students were attentive, asked questions, and readily participated in discussions. Their regular attendance indicated that they were interested in the classes."

Section 504 of the Rehabilitation Act of 1973 requires that hospitals and other institutions receiving funds from the U.S. Department of Health and Human Services use various communication techniques and resources with the deaf, including staff members or a certified interpreter who are proficient in sign language. The nurse who is bilingual has an advantage in providing care for clients.

■ SIBLING ADAPTATION

Introduction of the infant into a family with one or more children may pose problems for the parents. They are faced with the task of caring for a new child while not neglecting the others. Parents need to distribute their attention in a manner that they consider fair.

Older children have to assume new positions within the family hierarchy. The older child's goal is to maintain a leading position. The child who is next in birth order to the infant has to gain a superior position over the newcomer (Kreppner et al, 1982). As the infant develops and begins to assert herself or himself, the older child works towards dominance: "He or she takes away toys and other objects the younger child is grasping for, thereby demonstrating that he or she has control over the situation. The older child also intervenes more openly when parents are interacting with the younger child" (Kreppner et al, 1982). One 3-year-old child encouraged his mother to put the new baby "out with the garbage because we've seen enough of her."

Regression to an infantile level of behavior may be seen in some children. They may revert to bed-wetting, whining, or refusing to feed themselves. An older child who is still young wavers between thinking "I'm big now" and thinking "I'm still a baby, so look after me." Because the baby absorbs the time and attention of the important persons in the other children's lives, jealous reactions are to be expected once the initial excitement of having a new baby in the home is over.

Parents, especially mothers, spend much time and energy promoting sibling acceptance of a new baby. Sibling preparation classes for mothers make a difference in their ability to cope with sibling rivalry (see Research Highlight, p. 687). Older children are involved actively in preparation for the infant, and involvement intensifies after the birth of the child. Mother and father face a number of tasks related to **sibling rivalry** and adjustment. The tasks include the following:

1. Making the older child feel loved and wanted
2. Managing guilt arising from feelings that older children are being deprived of parental time and attention
3. Developing feelings of confidence in the ability to nurture more than one child
4. Adjusting time and space to accommodate the new baby
5. Monitoring behavior of older children toward the more vulnerable infant and diverting aggressive behavior.

The new parent can learn many innovative techniques by listening to other parents describe their efforts to ease the older siblings' acceptance of the new child (see sibling preparation, p. 258). Walz and Rich (1983) have described a number of creative parental interventions.

1. A mother took her first-born child on a tour of her hospital room and pointed out similarities to the birth of the first child. "This is the same room I was in with you, and I think the baby is in the same cot that you were in."
2. The newborn was described as a "special gift" for the older child.

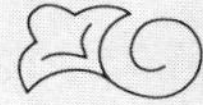 **Research Highlight** 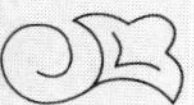

Adjustment of Siblings to Newborn

RESEARCH ABSTRACT

The study was conducted to determine whether sibling preparation classes made a difference in the behavior of the children and the perceptions of the mothers' ability to cope with the children. The sample consisted of 20 mothers pregnant with their second child and 20 mothers who had just given birth to their second child. The first group of mothers attended sibling preparation classes with their first-born children. They completed questionnaires after the class and at 1 month after childbirth. The second group of mothers were contacted in the hospital after childbirth and completed the questionnaires then and 1 month postpartum. There was a significant difference between the two groups. The group of women who had attended the class experienced fewer sibling rivalry behaviors. Mothers who had attended the class felt better prepared to cope with the behavior of their children. Parents used a variety of strategies in addition to the class to prepare the children for the birth of the baby.

IMPLICATIONS FOR PRACTICE

Preparation of siblings for childbirth is important. Consideration might be given to the routine addition to childbirth preparation classes of one session on sibling preparation. Nurses can provide counseling to expectant mothers and fathers so that they are better able to deal with behavioral changes of their first-born child and the sibling's interactions with the newborn.

RELATED RESEARCH QUESTIONS

1. Does age or sex of the sibling make a difference in behaviors exhibited after birth of a newborn?
2. Does birth order of parents affect sibling preparations and expressions of jealousy by the sibling?
3. Do expressions of jealousy of second- and third-born children differ from expressions of jealousy of first-born children?
4. What strategies are effective in preparing siblings for the birth of an infant?

REFERENCE

Fortier JC et al: Adjustment to a newborn: sibling preparation makes a difference, *JOGNN* 20:73, 1991.

3. The children were in the *first* group (grandparents, sister) to see the newborn.
4. Time was planned for both children. A mother remarked, "When I get home, I'll arrange my day so that I can have the baby's care done in the morning while Sam (first child) is at school. Maybe the baby will sleep part of the afternoon and I can spend some time with Sam."

Fathers were enlisted as the main support for mothers arranging time to include older children. "My husband will take care of Becca [first child] and I will have the baby, because he can do things with Becca she will enjoy. I will give the baby things my husband can't." Other fathers were expected to help with the care of the newborn to permit the mother to spend more time with the older child. Studies (Umphenour, 1980; Wranesh, 1982; Kowaba et al, 1985) have demonstrated that direct sibling contact does not place healthy newborns at risk for exposure to pathogenic organisms. Therefore separation of newborns and older siblings does not appear to be justified.

Acquaintance behaviors of siblings with the newborn have been described by Marecki et al (1985) and Anderberg (1988). The acquaintance process depends on the information given to the child before the baby is born and on the cognitive developmental level of the child. The initial behaviors of siblings with the newborn include looking at the infant and touching the head (Fig. 24-10).

The initial adjustment of older children to a newborn takes time. Children should be allowed to interact at their own pace rather than being forced. To expect a young child to accept and love a rival for the parents' affection assumes a too-mature response. Sibling love grows as does other love, that is, by being with another person and sharing experiences (Fig. 24-11).

■ GRANDPARENT ADAPTATION

The amount of involvement of grandparents in the care of the newborn depends on many factors, for ex-

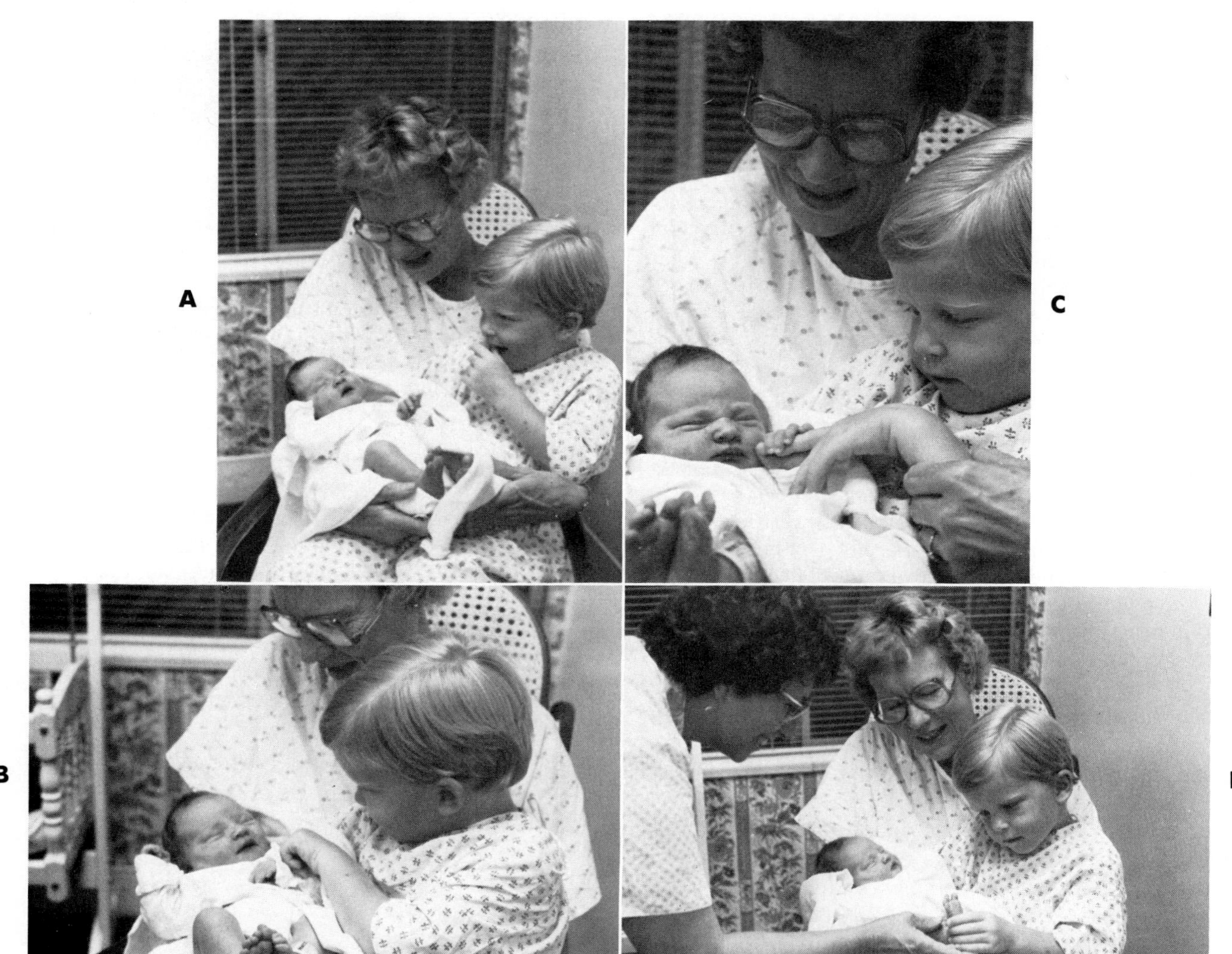

Fig. 24-10 First meeting. **A,** Boy with grandmother during first meeting with new sister. On first sight brother seems overwhelmed; sucks thumb for comfort and withdraws from contact. **B,** First tentative touch. **C,** testing with fingertip. **D,** Relationship more secure: it is now okay to hold with whole hand.
Courtesy Marjorie Pyle, RNC, Lifecircle, Costa Mesa, Calif.

ample, willingness of the grandparents to become involved, proximity of the grandparents, and ethnic and cultural expectations of the role grandparents play (Grosso et al, 1981).

The woman's mother is an important model for child-rearing practices (Rubin, 1975). She acts as a source of knowledge and as a support person (see Research Highlight, p. 689). Grandchildren are tangible evidence of continuity, of immortality. Often grandparents comment that the presence of grandchildren helps relieve loneliness and boredom (Fig. 24-10).

"There are many ways to encourage new parents to include the grandparents, enriching their child's life and benefiting from the extended family themselves" (Olson, 1981). As parents are assisted in working through differing opinions and unresolved conflicts (e.g., dependency, control) between themselves and their parents, they can move toward mastery of the developmental tasks of adulthood. Grandparental support can be a stabilizing influence for families undergoing developmental crises such as childbearing and new parenthood (Newell, 1984). Grandparents can foster the learning of parental skills and

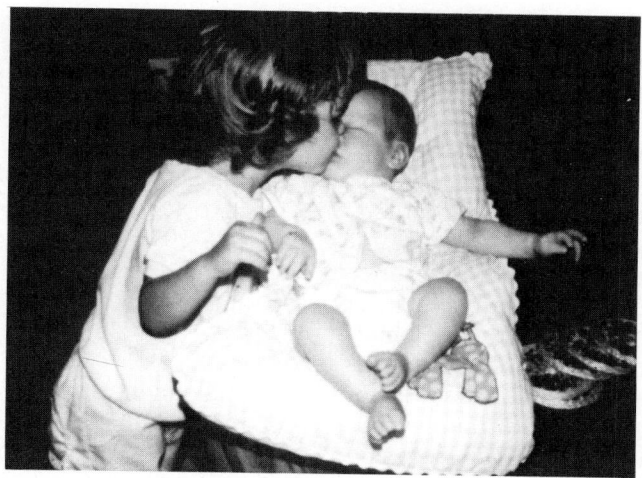

Fig. 24-11 Sister kisses her new brother. Family contacts are important for newborn and siblings.
Courtesy Marjorie Pyle, RNC, Lifecircle, Costa Mesa, Calif.

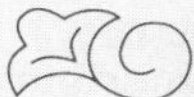 **Research Highlight** 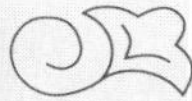

Grandparents as Supporters of Families with Infants

RESEARCH ABSTRACT

This study compared interaction patterns of grandparent-infant and parent-infant dyads (or couples). The extent to which grandparents act as social support agents for their children and grandchildren also was examined. Subjects were 30 white three-generation families with 7-month-old infants. Families were observed in the children's home with the parents and grandparents present. Each parent and grandparent was observed while playing with the infant individually for a period of 5 minutes. Observers coded behavior of adults and infants in a global behavioral category system using a 15-second sampling technique. A social support resource questionnaire was completed by the parents. Grandparents completed a questionnaire describing contact with their children and grandchild.

The Bayley scale of infant development was administered on a separate home visit. Results showed no differences between parents and grandparents in interactive behaviors. Grandparents were more gentle, and parents were more competent, confident, calm, and flexible. Mothers and grandmothers interacted in similar fashion as did fathers and grandfathers. Higher Bayley scores were related to higher levels of interactive behavior. Families with male infants had more contact, and grandparents reported more satisfaction with contact than did parents. Infants having more contact with grandparents had higher Bayley scores.

IMPLICATIONS FOR PRACTICE

Interaction with grandparents is important for support of their adult children and for infant development. Inclusion of grandparents by nurses in classroom and other teaching situations relating to the childbearing family should be encouraged. Classes on grandparenting can be initiated and included in childbirth education classes.

RELATED RESEARCH QUESTIONS

1. Does interaction with other adult relatives increase infant development scores?
2. Are interaction patterns of adult relatives similar to interaction pattern of grandparents?
3. What is the optimal level of intergenerational contact?
4. Is there a difference in interaction styles between maternal and paternal grandparents?

REFERENCE

Tinsley BJ, Parke RD: Grandparents as interactive and social support agents for families with young infants, *Int J Aging Human Dev* 25(4):259, 1987.

preserve tradition. One simple technique to help people span the generation gap is through a printed "letter to new parents" (written from the grandparents' perspective), which can be included in prenatal kits distributed in childbirth preparation classes and made available to all family members on the postpartum unit (Olson, 1981). Another way to help grandparents bridge the generation gap and understand their adult children's parenting concepts is to offer classes (Maloni et al, 1987). Included in these classes would be information about up-to-date childbearing practices, especially family-centered care; infant care, feeding, and safety (car seats); and exploration of roles grandparents play in the family unit. Both techniques can foster open discussion between the generations about feelings and needs of parents and grandparents.

Grandparents can do things that no one else can do. They can tell their grandchildren about their roots and stories about their parents. They contribute to a sense of family continuity and provide for maintenance of cultural traditions.

Grandparents who are free to love the grandchild "crazily, blindly, lavishly," and without reservation (LeShan, 1975) can have a significant positive influence on the child's life. Praise and encouragement from a significant person foster the development of a positive self-image and a sense of being worthy (see Fig. 22-10).

SUMMARY

The childbearing family faces a constant challenge of maintaining balance between the integration of new family members and changing established interaction patterns and problem-solving strategies. The family's ability to meet the challenge is critical for parents and children. Nursing actions designed to strengthen family bonds and to facilitate the mother's and father's attainment of parental roles serve an important social purpose.

REFERENCES

Ainsworth MD: Object relations, dependency, and attachment: a theoretical review of the infant-mother relationship, *Child Dev* 40:969, 1969.

Ainsworth MD: The development of infant-mother attachment. In Caldwell BM, Reccurti HN, editors: Review of child development research, vol 3, New York, 1970, Russell Sage Foundation.

Ainsworth MD, Bell SM: Attachment, exploration and separation: illustrated by the behavior of one-year-olds in a strange situation, *Child Dev* 41:49, 1970.

Anderberg GJ: Initial acquaintance and attachment behavior of siblings with the newborn, *JOGNN* 17:49, 1988.

Asrael W: Disabled women and childbearing: the nurse's role, *NAACOG Update Series* 1 (lesson 8), 1983.

Baranowski E: Childbirth education classes for expectant deaf parents, *MCN* 8:143, 1983.

Bowlby J: The nature of the child's tie to his mother, *Int J Psychoanal* 39:350, 1958.

Bowlby J: *Attachment and loss,* vol 1, *Attachment,* New York, 1969, Basic Books.

Brazelton TB: The early mother-infant adjustment, *Pediatrics* 32:931, 1963.

Brazelton TB: Effect of maternal expectations on early infant behavior, *Early Child Dev Care* 2:259, 1973.

Brazelton TB: The remarkable talents of the newborn, *Birth Fam J* 5:187, Winter 1978.

Brazelton TB et al: The origins of reciprocity: the early mother-infant interaction. In Lewis M, Rosenblum LA, editors: *The effect of the infant on its caregiver,* New York, 1974, John Wiley & Sons.

Budin P: *The nursling,* London, 1907, Caxton Publishing Co.

Clarke-Stewart K: And daddy makes three: the father's impact on mother and young child, *Child Dev* 49:466, 1978.

Condon W, Sander L: Neonate movement is synchronized with adult speech: interactional participation and language acquisition, *Science* 183:99, 1974.

Curry MS: Contact during first hour with the wrapped or naked newborn: effect on maternal attachment behaviors at 36 hours and three months, *Birth Fam J* 6:4, Winter 1979.

Erikson EH: Identity and the life cycle: selected papers. In *Psychological issues,* vol 1, no 1, New York, 1959, International Universities Press.

Erikson EH: *Childhood and society,* New York, 1964, WW Norton.

Field T: The three Rs of infant-adult interactions: rhythms, repertoires, and responsibility, *J Pediatr Psychol* 3:131, 1978a.

Field T: Visual and cardiac responses to animate and inanimate faces by young term and preterm infants, *Child Dev* 49, 1978b.

Gottlieb BH: The role of individual and social support in preventing child maltreatment. In Garbarino J, Stocking S, editors: *Protecting children from abuse/neglect,* San Francisco, 1980, Jossey-Bass.

Greenberg M, Morris N: Engrossment: the newborn's impact on the father, *Nurs Digest* 4:19, Jan/Feb 1976.

Grosso C et al: The Vietnamese American family . . . and grandma makes three, *MCN* 6:177, 1981.

Klaus MH, Kennell JH: Human maternal and parental behaviors. In Klaus MH, Kennell JH, editors: *Maternal-infant bonding,* St Louis, 1976, Mosby–Year Book.

Klaus MH, Kennell JH: *Bonding: the beginnings of parent-infant attachment,* St Louis, 1983, Mosby–Year Book.

Klaus MH, Kennell JH: *Parent-infant bonding,* ed 2, St Louis, 1982, Mosby–Year Book.

Kreppner K et al: Infants and family development from triads to tetrads, *Hum Dev* 25:373, 1982.

Lamb M: Early contact and maternal-infant bonding: one decade later, *Pediatrics* 70:325, 1982.

Lang R: *Birth book,* Ben Lomond, Calif, 1972, Genesis Press.

LeShan E: *The wonderful crisis of middle age,* New York, 1975, Warner Books.

Maloni JA, McIndoe JE, Rubenstein G: Expectant grandparents classes, *JOGNN* 16:26, 1987.

Marecki M et al: Early sibling attachment, *JOGNN* 14:418, 1985.

Mercer RT: Parent-infant attachment. In Sonstegard LJ et al: editors: *Women's health,* vol 2, *Childbearing,* New York, 1982, Grune & Stratton.

NAACOG, Committee on Practice: *Mother-baby care* NAACOG OGN Nursing Practice Resource, NAACOG. Washington, DC, 1989, NAACOG.

Newell NJ: Grandparents, the overlooked support system for new parents during the fourth trimester, *NAACOG Update Series* 1 (lesson 21), 1984.

Olson ML: Fitting grandparents into new families, *MCN* 6:419, 1981.

Parkes CM, Stevenson-Hinde J: *The place of attachment in human behavior,* New York, 1982, Basic Books.

Queenan JT, moderator: Managing pregnancy in patients over 35, *Contemp OB/GYN* 29(5):180, 1987.

Rubin R: Maternal behavior, *Nurs Outlook* 9:682, 1961.

Rubin R: Maternal touch at first contact with the newborn infant, *Nurs Outlook* 11:828, 1963.

Rubin R: Maternal tasks in pregnancy, *Matern Child Nurs J* 4:143, Fall 1975.

Sammons WA, Lewis JM: *Premature babies: a different beginning,* St Louis, 1985, Mosby–Year Book.

Schornkoff JP: Social support and the development of vulnerable children, *Am J Public Health* 74:310, 1980.

Scott L, Meredith A, Angwin J: *Time out for motherhood: a guide for today's working woman to the financial emotional and career aspects of having a baby,* Los Angeles, 1986, Jeremy P Tarcher.

Shainess N: Abortion is no man's business, *Psychology Today,* p 18, March 1970.

Siegel E: A critical examination of studies of parent-infant bonding. In Klaus M, Robertson M, editors: *Birth interaction and attachment,* Evansville, Ind, 1982, Johnson & Johnson Baby Products Co.

Stainton MC: A *comparison of prenatal and postnatal perceptions of their babies by parents.* Paper presented to the First International Congress on Pre-and Para-natal Psychology, Toronto, July 8, 1983a.

Stainton MC: *Maternal newborn attachment origins and processes.* III. *Interactional synchrony: the prelude to attachment,* doctoral dissertation, San Francisco, 1983b, University of California.

Stainton MC: Origins of attachment: Culture and cue sensitivity, *Dissertation Abstracts Int* 46:3786-B (University Microfilms No. 8600606), 1985.

Steele B, Pollock C: A psychiatric study of parents who abuse infants and small children. In Helfer RE, Kempe C, editors: *The battered child,* Chicago, 1968, University of Chicago Press.

Umphenour JH: Bacterial colonization in neonates with sibling visitation, *JOGNN* 9:73, 1980.

Walz B, Rich O: Maternal tasks of taking on a second child in the postpartum period, *Matern Child Nurs J* 12:3, Fall 1983.

Winslow W: First pregnancy after 35: what is the experience? *MCN* 12:92, 1987.

Wranesh BL: The effect of sibling visitation on bacterial colonization rate in neonates, *JOGNN* 11:211, 1982.

References—Nursing Research

Anderberg GJ: Initial acquaintance and attachment behavior of siblings with the newborn, *JOGGN* 17:49, 1988.

Censullo M, Lester B, Hoffmann J: Rhythmic patterning in mother-newborn interaction, *Nurs Res* 34:342, 1985.

Crawford J: A theoretical model of support network conflict experienced by new mothers, *Nurs Res* 34:100, 1985.

Cronenwett LR: Network structure, social support, and psychological outcomes of pregnancy, *Nurs Res* 34:93, 1985a.

Cronenwett LR: Parental network structured and perceived support after birth of first child, *Nurs Res* 34:347, 1985b.

Davis MI, Akridge KM: The effect of promoting intrauterine attachment in primiparas on postdelivery attachment, *JOGNN* 16:430, 1987.

Fortier JC et al: Adjustment to a newborn: sibling preparation makes a difference, *JOGNN* 20:73, 1991.

Kowba MD et al: Direct sibling contact and bacterial colonization in newborns, *JOGNN* 14:412, 1985.

Kunst-Wilson W, Cronenwett L: Nursing care for the emerging family: promoting paternal behavior, *Res Nurs Health* 4:201, 1981.

Solheim K, Spellacy C: Sibling visitation: effects on newborn infection rates, *JOGGN* 17:43, 1988.

Tulman L: Mothers and unrelated persons' initial handling of newborn infants, *Nurs Res* 34:205, 1985.

BIBLIOGRAPHY

Bradshaw MJ: *Nursing and the family in health and illness,* East Norwalk, Conn, 1988, Appleton & Lange.

Evans CJ: Description of a home follow-up program for childbearing families, *JOGNN* 20:113, 1991.

Friedman MM: *Family nursing: theory and assessment.* ed 2, East Norwalk, Conn, 1986, Appleton & Lange.

Gay JT, Edgil AE, Douglass AB: Reva Rubin revisited, *JOGNN* 17:394, 1988.

Giger JN, Davidhizar RE: *Transcultural nursing: assessment and intervention,* St Louis 1991, Mosby–Year Book.

Jacob T, Tennenbaum DL: *Family assessment: rationale, methods, and future directions,* New York, 1988, Plenum Press.

Martell LK: Postpartum depression as a family problem, *MCN* 15:90, 1990.

Norr KF, Roberts JE, Freese U: Early postpartum rooming-in and maternal attachment behaviors in a group of medically indigent primiparas, *J Nurse Midwife* 34:85, 1989.

Palkovitz R: Sources of father-infant bonding beliefs: implications for childbirth education, *Matern Child Nurs J* 17:101, 1988.

Wilkerson NN, Barrows TL: Synchronizing care with mother-baby rhythms, *MCN* 13:264, 1988.

Zwergel J, Ende ML: Maternal-infant early discharge: making one home visit count, *J Home Health Care Pract* 1(2):16, 1989.

Bibliography—Nursing Research

Dormire SL, Strauss SS, Clarke BA: Social support and adaptation to the parent role in first-time adolescent mothers, *JOGNN* 18:327, 1989.

Fortier JC: The relationship of vaginal and cesarean births to father-infant attachment, *JOGNN* 17:128, 1988.

Hall LA et al: Psychosocial predictors of maternal depressive symptoms, parenting attitudes, and child behavior in single-parent families, *Nurse Res* 40:214, 1991.

Martone DJ, Nash BR: Initial differences in postpartum attachment behavior in breastfeeding and bottle-feeding mothers, *JOGNN* 17:212, 1988.

Matthews MK: Mothers' satisfaction with their neonates' breastfeeding behaviors, *JOGNN* 20:49, 1991.

chapter 24 review

Key Concepts

- The birth of a child necessitates changes in the existing interactional structure of a family.
- Either parent may exhibit "motherliness."
- Attachment is the process by which parent and child come to love and accept each other.
- Attachment is strengthened through the use of sensual responses or abilities by both partners in the parent-child interaction.
- Early contact with the newborn is not essential for optimum parent-child interactions.
- For the biologic parent, the parental role does not begin at birth but rather enlarges and intensifies from the gestational period.
- In adjusting to the parental role, the mother moves from a dependent state to an interdependent state.
- Mothers may be overwhelmed by the actuality of parenting responsibilities and may exhibit signs of postpartum depression ("baby blues").
- A primary need of parents is to establish a life-style that includes, but in some respects excludes, the child.
- In Western culture the newborn has been found to have a powerful impact on the father.
- Modulation of rhythm, modification of behavioral repertoires, and mutual responsivity facilitate infant-parent adjustment.
- Many factors influence parental responses (e.g., their age, socioeconomic level, and their expectations of what their child will be like).
- Parents face a number of tasks related to sibling adjustment that require creative parental interventions.
- Grandparents can be a source of knowledge and support and can have a positive influence on the postpartal family.

Key Terms

- acquaintance (p. 673)
- attachment (p. 673)
- behavioral repertoires (p. 683)
- biorhythmicity (p. 676)
- bonding (p. 673)
- claiming process (p. 674)
- cognitive-affective skills (p. 672)
- cognitive-motor skills (p. 672)
- dependent phase (p. 680)
- dependent-independent phase (p. 680)
- en face (p. 675)
- engrossment (p. 682)
- entrainment (p. 676)
- executive behaviors (p. 673)
- fingertip exploration (p. 674)
- habituation (p. 683)
- infant-parent interaction (p. 683)
- interdependent phase (p. 681)
- letting-go phase (p. 681)
- maternal adjustment (p. 680)
- maternal age over 35 (p. 684)
- mothering function (p. 672)

- mutuality (p. 673)
- positive feedback (p. 673)
- postpartum depression ("baby blues") (p. 681)
- reciprocity (p. 676)
- responsivity (p. 683)
- rhythm (p. 683)
- sibling rivalry (p. 686)
- signaling behaviors (p. 673)
- significant other (p. 673)
- synchrony (p. 676)
- taking-hold phase (p. 681)
- taking-in phase (p. 680)

Critical Thinking Exercises

1. You are asked to participate in a group discussion on parenthood. Consider the following.
   a. Examine your feelings regarding parenthood and how these might affect your perceptions of parenting.
   b. Identify how experiences with your own parents might affect your parenting style.
   c. Discuss your feelings with the group and compare experiences.
   d. Identify possible interventions to facilitate parenting in the postpartum period.
2. You are providing postpartum care for a woman and her newborn. The woman's 2-year-old daughter comes for a visit and states that she "hates the baby."
   a. What are possible reasons for this reaction?
   b. How can you check them out? What assessments are needed to determine if sibling rivalry is a problem?
   c. Formulate a plan of care to counteract the problem and justify choices.

Topics for Nursing Research

- Is there a difference in reciprocity and synchrony depending on the age of the parent—for example, young adults (20 through 30 years of age); after age 35?
- Compare the mother's (parent's) consoling behaviors for the unborn fetus with that demonstrated after the infant's birth.
- Describe how parents with sensory impairment develop reciprocity and synchrony with the newborn.
- Identify and validate nursing diagnoses related to family dynamics after childbirth.

chapter 25

Nursing Care during the Postpartum Period

RHEA P. WILLIAMS

LEARNING OBJECTIVES

- Define the key terms listed.
- Review the components of the postpartum interview, physical examination, and laboratory tests.
- Outline the normal progression of puerperal changes and schedule of assessment from day 1 through day 3.
- Formulate examples of potential nursing diagnoses for physical and emotional care.
- Identify goals for postpartum physical and emotional care.
- Summarize general care for rest, ambulation and exercise, bed rest, immunizations, comfort, and safety.
- Compare parental responses to the birth of a child, focusing on adaptive and maladaptive behaviors of the mother, infant, and family.
- Explain mother's need to integrate the birth experience.
- Discuss anticipatory guidance for helping new parents during the transition to parenthood.
- Explore the cultural aspects of postpartum care, both physical and emotional.
- List physical warning signs during the postpartum period.
- Determine the nurse's responsibilities related to discharge.
- Identify topics for nursing research related to nursing care during the postpartum period.

The postpartum (puerperal) period offers nurses a challenging opportunity to assist women in their achievement of motherhood. The approach to care of women during the postpartum period has changed from one modeled on the concept of sickness to one that is wellness oriented. The nurse provides holistic care, focusing not only on the woman's physical recovery but also on her psychologic well-being and her ability to care for herself and her infant. Furthermore, the common practice of early discharge, often within 24 hours of giving birth, makes accurate and effective nursing care during this time extremely important.

Psychologic and physiologic factors interact to help the mother adjust to the aftermath of childbirth and return to a prepregnancy state. For example, unless the mother recovers physically—that is, she is free from hemorrhage, pain, fatigue, and other problems—her psychologic well-being will be in jeopardy. In turn, if she experiences low self-esteem or is doubtful of her maternal abilities, the chances of achieving her recovery goals—caring for herself, caring for and bonding with her infant—will be decreased. On the other hand, a mother's success in caring for herself and her baby can improve her physical and psychologic well-being. A breakdown or inability to achieve any one of these recovery and growth goals may contribute to breakdown in a second area. To achieve these goals, women are now active participants in their care, along with the nurse, physician, and family.

To assess possible abnormalities in the postpartum recovery process, nurses must be knowledgeable about physical (see Chapter 23) and psychologic changes in the mother, as well as emotional changes in the entire family (see Chapter 24). This chapter focuses on using the nursing process to meet both the mother's and the family's needs during this crucial time.

■ NURSING CARE OF PHYSICAL NEEDS

Care of the woman during the postpartum period begins with assessment, including both interview and physical examination. This is followed by the development and implementation of an individualized plan of care (see example p. 728). The nurse should be careful at every stage to determine the needs of the woman and the family to ensure that these needs are met, and to build the woman's confidence and ability to care for herself and her newborn.

ASSESSMENT

ADMISSION TO POSTPARTUM UNIT. In the fourth stage of labor (see Chapter 19) the mother's physiologic processes are stabilized and maternal-infant bonding is begun. Then the woman's care may continue in the labor, delivery, recovery, postpartum (LDRP) room, or she may be transferred to the more traditional postpartum unit. In the LDRP, ongoing assessments continue. On the woman's transfer to the postpartum unit, the admitting nurse is responsible for the initial assessment. This includes taking into account the report from the nurse in the labor (or recovery) unit, who provides a summary of the woman's prenatal and labor records. The nursing plan of care is based on this information and ongoing assessments of physical, psychologic, cultural, and learning needs by means of interview, physical examination, and review of laboratory test results.

INTERVIEW. The nurse-client interview is an important assessment technique to use with postpartum women. Early discharge from the hospital requires rapid assessment, and a properly focused interview provides the nurse with information necessary to begin the plan of care as soon as possible. During the interview the nurse can determine the mother's emotional status, energy level, degree and location of physical discomfort, hunger, and thirst. To some degree, the new mother's history and knowledge level concerning self-care and infant care also can be determined.

The interview process offers the nurse the opportunity to gather information about the woman as a unique and special individual within a cultural and family context. Thus significant family members should be included in the interview process if they are available and the woman so wishes. As appropriate, ethnic and cultural expectations are assessed regarding postpartum recovery patterns.

Learning Needs

A nurse's accurate assessment helps to identify those areas in which clients most need education. With shortened hospital stays, it may be unrealistic to teach everything the nurse thinks should be taught. Studies affirm that maternity clients can articulate their personal learning needs. Therefore, mothers should routinely be asked about their learning needs as part of the postpartum assessment. Martell et al (1990) comment that "mothers seem pleased that their individual needs were being considered, while nurses found that their teaching became more

TEACHING Information Priorities of New Mothers in a Short Stay Program

TOPICS
Signs and symptoms of infant illness
Maternal illness
Feeding and infant care
Comfort measures
Uterine massage
Involution
Rest
Breast care

From Martell et al: Information priorities of new mothers in a short stay program, *West J Nurs Res* 11:320, 1989.

TEACHING Mothers' Postpartum Teaching Priorities

TOPIC	PERCENT (VERY IMPORTANT)
Infant illness	68
Postpartum complications	67
Feeding baby	58
Stitches/episiotomy	56
Cord care	50
Temperature taking	50
Infant medications	50
Well-baby care	45
Infant bowel/urinary patterns	44
Infant safety	43
Infant skin care	42
Crying	42
Circumcision	41
Breast care	40
Constipation/hemorrhoids	39
Baby bath	38

From Davis JH, Brucker MC, MacMullen NJ: A study of mothers' postpartum teaching priorities, *Matern Child Nurs J* 17(1):41, Spring 1988.

efficient because they could focus on fewer concepts."

In addition, results of nursing research can assist nurses to identify important areas for educating new mothers. For example, Davis et al (1988) found that the topic of highest priority for all age and parity groups was postpartum complications, followed by episiotomy/stitches. Mothers also wanted education about infant illness, feeding baby, cord care, temperature taking, and infant medications (see box, above right). In another study (Martell et al, 1989) signs and symptoms of infant illness, feeding and infant care, comfort measures, uterine massage, involution, rest, and breast care were seen as priorities (see box, above).

Cultural Considerations

Many of the woman's responses during the postpartum period are strongly influenced by her cultural background. The nurse should be familiar with a variety of cultural patterns so that normal cultural practices are not confused with abnormal behaviors and maladaptation (see Table 10-1). This familiarity provides a starting point. The nurse also must determine the specific beliefs and values of the individual woman and her family. Only then can the nurse accurately differentiate normal from abnormal behavior and design a plan of care to meet the individual needs of each client.

The greatest conflict between Western and non-Western beliefs and practices in childbearing occurs in the postpartum period. If a woman gives birth in a hospital, she and her family are directly confronted with culture-related problems that are not as easily resolved as those encountered in the prenatal, labor, and birthing stages. Nurses must be aware that cultural prescriptions (those behaviors allowed or expected of new mothers) for women in many cultures include a period of seclusion lasting from 7 to 40 days, with a minimum of activity allowed for mothers. These practices are based on two beliefs: (1) that childbirth has upset the balance of the mother's body and (2) that the mother, infant, and those caring for them are in a **state of pollution** (impure).

Because the idea of postpartum imbalance tends to affect the physical treatment and behavior of the mother, relevant cultural beliefs will be further discussed in this section. The idea of a pollution state, however, relates more to the woman's psychosocial well-being and is discussed later in this chapter under nursing assessment of psychologic adjustment. In addition, each of these concepts is discussed in Chapter 3.

BALANCE OF HEAT AND COLD. Cultures that subscribe to the need for body balance believe that the body has lost a great deal of heat during the labor and birthing process and that the mother is therefore subject to a number of illnesses. Thus certain practices must be followed to restore the balance of heat and cold. Adherents of both humoral and yin and yang theories have **cultural prescriptions** and **proscriptions** (those behaviors that are prohibited, or taboo, for new mothers) for restoration of balance of heat and cold (Ahumada, 1991).

After birth, hot and cold restrictions prevail. The mother must remain on strict bed rest without a pillow. Hot or steam baths (but not showers) are permitted only after the second postpartum day. Physical warmth is essential; blankets may be added even on the warmest day. Liquids must be served without ice (Ahumada, 1991) (see also Chapter 10).

FOOD. Food is one way in which heat can be restored and cold diminished. The classic Chinese diet (Campbell, Chang, 1975) represents an effort to decrease yin forces, which are cold. Included are an abundance of hot foods. The quality of heat and cold cannot always be measured by actual temperature. The essence of cold might be retained in a food even if the food is heated. Pillsbury (1978) noted that some foods are considered cold because they are grown in the damp earth or in watery places. Green vegetables, fruits, meats, and fish are commonly considered cold foods. Asians rank rice, eggs, and chicken high on the heat scale and thus believe they should be eaten frequently. It is obvious that many, if not most, of the foods served on hospital trays, such as meats, vegetables, fruits, and fruit juices, are considered cold. These probably will not be eaten by many Asian, Southeast Asian, and Spanish-speaking women.

However, if a hot substance is added to boiled water, it may counteract the coldness. For example, the chicken soup is so powerful that the cold quality of the water with which it is made is counteracted. Ginger added to hot water that has been boiled may cause the same effect. It is obvious then that ice water, used frequently in hospitals, is forbidden.

Clark (1970) wrote that Mexican-American women are forbidden to eat "cold" foods such as hot chilies, pickles, any food prepared with vinegar (e.g., sour foods [Cassidy, 1982]), tomatoes, spinach, any pork product, and most fruits. Fruits such as bananas and grapefruit and other citrus fruits must be avoided because of their acidity and because they are believed to cause varicose veins in mothers. Although fruits and vegetables also are prohibited in the pregnant Vietnamese woman's diet, pork legs and knuckles are allowed because pork is believed to improve the secretion of milk. To prevent stomachaches, Filipino women avoid "cold" foods such as eels, oysters, squash, and uncooked fruits and vegetables. Filipino women also refrain from eating sour foods because they supposedly cause the mother's milk to curdle. "Tasty" foods with strong, rich flavor, such as peanuts, canned fish, and fatty meats, are avoided because they are believed to cause lactation to stop. The nurse also should understand that Filipino and Chinese women prefer to drink warm water instead of ice water (Campbell, Chang, 1975; Ahumada, 1991). According to Campbell and Chang, two possible reasons for this preference are (1) the belief that drinking ice water "shocks" the body and (2) the history of poor sanitation in the Philippines and China, which has made it a custom for people in those countries to boil drinking water.

Inasmuch as disagreement may occur among Latin Americans and Filipinos about the classifications of basic foods into hot and cold categories, *nurses should use clients as their major cultural informants*. With flexibility and creativity, the nurse can plan with clients and other health team members nutritious and culturally acceptable diets. To this end, the nurse can allow, as much as possible, family members to bring the mother foods that are not readily available in the hospital but are highly recommended in the woman's culture.

LACTATION. Many cultural beliefs and practices focus on improving the mother's production of milk. In the Philippines, if the mother's milk does not flow regularly, a meal of chicken and green papaya, boiled in coconut "milk" may be suggested. Chicken soup also is believed important in the production of a nursing mother's milk. The Filipino mother may be advised by her family to eat a soup of boiled clams and ginger. Filipinos use hot applications of special medicinal preparations to stimulate lactation. Furthermore, the Filipino mother may believe that raising either arm over her head while lying down will decrease, if not actually stop, lactation. Filipino women also may believe that heavy work will make their milk "hot." Korean mothers eat seaweed soup with rice to increase milk production (Chung, 1977). Currier (1978) reported that Spanish-Americans believe that exposing mothers to cold diminishes the flow of milk. Latino and Asian mothers may believe that they must refrain from breast-feeding until their milk is in (Lee, 1988; Lee, 1989 et al, Ahumada, 1991). Offering the breast to the infant before the milk comes in is thought to further deplete the mother of vital heat and fluids during this perilous time (Lee, 1989). Mexican-Americans may even view colostrum as dirty (Hahn, Muecke, 1987). A common practice among Hispanics is to give honey water to their infants. These parents need to be informed about the risk of botulism in honey (Ahumada, 1991).

ACTIVITIES OF DAILY LIVING. In addition to food, contact with air and wind is proscribed by Asians, Filipinos, Mexican-Americans, and southern African Americans (Snow, 1983). To counteract further imbalance, cold must be prevented from entering the body. Air is considered cold, whatever the temperature, and thus windows and doors must be kept closed. The Chinese belief that a woman's pores are open for 30 days after childbirth coincides with the period in which they believe the mother has an excess of cold (Campbell, Chang, 1975; Pillsbury, 1978). Air conditioners can be a source of fear for some women in the hospital. Fans are to be avoided. New mothers may keep themselves totally covered with blankets despite how hot the room may be. Some Chinese also believe that for the 30 days after birth, cold air can enter the body through the vagina (Campbell, Chang, 1975). This is consistent with the Chinese belief that during the postbirth period some balance of the yang, or "hot" air, should be returned by decreasing the yin energy forces, or "cold" air in the body. Similarly, many Spanish women believe that during the 40-day postbirth period, they should avoid exposing themselves to any condition that could cause bad air *(malaire)* to enter the vagina (Baca, 1973).

Water is considered cold at all times, even if it is heated. Therefore not bathing for a period of time is a widely held belief. Recognizing these beliefs, the nurse can encourage the mother to take frequent sponge baths and emphasize perineal care, breast care, and other measures for good hygiene and comfort. Some mothers will use all kinds of strategies to avoid the daily shower but will not directly refuse, complying by going to the shower room, turning on the water, and remaining in such a position that the water will not touch them. Pillsbury (1978) notes that Chinese women who have been westernized in so many ways often still adhere to the postpartum practice of avoiding water. They must not wash themselves, their dishes, or their clothes. To the Chinese and other Asians, contact with water, considered cold, causes wind to enter the body and will result in asthma, arthritis, and chronic aches and pains.

In some cultures women use abdominal binders during the pregnancy, as well as during the postbirth period. Some Mexican-Americans use binders during the first 40 days of the puerperium (Clark, 1970). It is believed by these persons that binders help organs in the stomach return to their normal positions, push the hips together, and firm up the stomach muscles. Binders are used in conjunction with massage to help the woman with the "slipped" uterus. In some regions in the Philippines, binders are worn by women both during pregnancy and after childbirth to prevent *buhî-buhî*. *Buhî-buhî* is a syndrome in which ascending gas, starting under the lowest left rib, produces symptoms ascribed to postbirth hemorrhage, such as tachycardia, vertigo, partial blindness, and impaired respiration. The use of the binder also is thought to prevent the postbirth expansion of the uterus. Another reason this practice is followed by Filipino women is the notion that the "cold" womb should be protected.

When making a cultural assessment, the nurse must remember that most of these cultural beliefs and customs reflect the traditional culture and are not universally practiced by all members of the cultural group. Variables such as degree of acculturation, socioeconomic status, amount of contact with older generations, and subculture influence the extent to which these customs are practiced. It is important that the nurse validate the cultural beliefs that are meaningful to the individual client. This can be accomplished only if the nurse creates an atmosphere that makes the woman comfortable in discussing her cultural preferences. The nurse must not interpret the client's cultural practices as placing the woman at high risk for alteration in parenting.

The woman's ability to speak and understand verbal and written English should be assessed. If the woman does not communicate in English and the nurse does not understand her language, the nursing process will be jeopardized. An interpreter should be used to ensure accurate communication.

PSYCHOSOCIAL FACTORS. During the first few hours after childbirth, as physical parameters are monitored, the nurse observes and interviews the mother and family for healthy attachment (bonding) behaviors. The family interactions continue to be monitored and documented every 4 to 8 hours throughout the hospital stay. Assessment of the mother's self-esteem, her body image, her expectations and her feelings about this birth are important aspects in exploring the woman's psychologic well-being.

Physical Examination

Postpartum assessment is based on expected maternal changes as discussed in Chapter 23. A head-to-toe assessment is performed when the client is admitted to the unit and at least daily throughout her hospital stay to determine any potential problems.

The length of the fourth stage and the time of transfer to the postpartum unit varies with each institution. Included in the daily assessments are vital signs; reproductive and genitourinary concerns; and cardiovascular and gastrointestinal function. Expected findings during the first 72 hours are summarized in Table 25-1.

The blood pressure, pulse, and respirations are assessed every 15 minutes for the first hour after birth (see Chapter 19,) every 30 minutes for the next 2 hours, and then every hour for the next 2 hours. Vital signs continue to be monitored every 4 hours for the

TABLE 25-1 Progression of Puerperal Changes: Days 1 through 3

Assessment	2-24 hr (Day 1)	25-48 hr (Day 2)	49-72 hr (Day 3)
Temperature	97.1° F (36.2° C) 100.4° F (38° C)	Within normal range	Within normal range
Pulse	Bradycardia: 50-70 beats/min	Bradycardia may persist or rate may return to within normal range	Bradycardia may persist or rate may return to within normal range
Blood pressure	Within normal range	Within normal range	Within normal range
Energy level	Euphoric, happy, excited, or fatigued; may show need for sleep	Often tired, slow moving	Anxious to go home; level within normal range but variable
Uterus	At umbilicus or just below; firm	1 cm or more below umbilicus; firm	2 cm or more below umbilicus; firm
Lochia	Rubra; moderate; few clots, if any; fleshy odor of normal menstrual flow	Rubra to serosa; moderate to scant; odor continues to be "fleshy" or absent	Rubra to serosa; scant; odor continues to be "fleshy" or absent
Perineum	Edematous; clean, healing, intact	Edema lessening; clean, healing	Edema lessening or absent; clean, healing
Legs	Pretibial or pedal edema; Homans' sign negative	Edema lessening; Homans' sign negative	Edema minimal or absent; Homans' sign negative
Breasts	Remain soft to palpation; colostrum can be expressed	Begin to feel firmer; occasionally feel lumpy	Increase in vascularity and initiation of swelling; feel firmer and warmer to touch; milk expected within 2-4 days after birth
Appetite	Excellent; may ask for double helpings, snacks	Usually remains excellent	Varies; appetite may have returned to normal range or may lessen (especially if client is constipated)
Elimination			
Voiding	Up to 3000 mL	Large amounts	Amount/24 hr is lessening
Defecation	None expected	None expected	Usually defecates; may need enema, etc.
Discomfort	Generalized aching; perineal area: episiotomy, hemorrhoids	Muscle aches; perineal area: episiotomy, hemorrhoids	Possible tension headache, perineal area: usually lessening; breasts, nipples

first 24 hours after birth and then once every 8 hours. When the mother is admitted to the recovery area, her temperature is assessed. The temperature is assessed 1 hour later, then every 4 hours for the first 24 hours, then every 8 hours unless problems develop.

Alteration in vital signs necessitates more frequent assessments, as well as additional assessments to determine the underlying cause of the alteration. For example, a slightly elevated temperature in the early puerperium might suggest dehydration. However, the nurse also would want to question the woman about other possible causes of elevated temperature, such as sore throat or painful urination. In addition, the nurse would monitor the temperature, inspect the perineum and breasts, auscultate the lungs, and inspect skin integrity (i.e., intravenous [IV] site). In the presence of a rapid pulse the nurse assesses for indications of anxiety in addition to signs of abnormal bleeding.

During the first hour after childbirth the fundus, lochia, bladder, and perineum are assessed every 15 minutes. The fundus is assessed for firmness, location, and position (Chapter 19). To avoid discomfort, the nurse's fingers should be warm while palpating the uterus through the abdomen. The woman's size may affect the initial ease with which the uterus is felt. The heavier the woman, the deeper the palpation that might be necessary (see Fig. 23-1). Encouraging the woman to take deep breaths and relax during the procedure will promote comfort. Palpation of a relaxed, **atonic (boggy) uterus** and an increase in the amount of lochia indicate uterine atony (see nursing plan of care, 728). Massage may be necessary to firm up a boggy uterus. At the same time the suprapubic area should be palpated for bladder fullness. The peripad is examined for color, amount, and any odor of the lochia. Clots also may be expelled during this time and should be carefully assessed for amount and documented. Also the linens under the buttocks should be checked for any pooling of blood.

Assessment of the perineum begins with a review of the woman's chart to determine if an episiotomy was performed or if a laceration occurred during the birth process. A good light source is essential for visualization of the incision. The nurse dons gloves, asks the woman to turn onto her side, and inspects the perineal area using the REEDA (see Chapter 23) guideline for *r*edness, *e*dema, *e*cchymosis, *d*rainage, and *a*pproximation. The anal area should be assessed for hemorrhoids. If they are present, this should also be noted. These assessments should be performed twice in the second hour, and then once in the third and fourth hours after the birth. Assessments continue for the next 24 hours, along with vital signs.

Whether the woman plans to breast-feed or bottle-feed her baby, the breasts should be assessed every 8 hours throughout the hospital stay for nipple soreness, fissures, redness, tenderness, or engorgement.

The woman's legs are inspected every 8 hours throughout the hospital stay for evidence of edema or thrombophlebitis. Each foot is flexed with the leg extended (see Fig. 13-2, *A*) to assess for pain in the calf area along with inspection for redness or swelling and palpation for increased warmth. Evidence of pain in the calf is a positive **Homans' sign.** Pulses may be absent in the presence of thrombophlebitis.

The woman should be asked daily if she has had a bowel movement. Stool softeners or laxatives may be part of the physician's regimen.

LABORATORY TESTS. Findings of these tests are reviewed to detect indications of abnormalities and to determine implications for nursing. Hemoglobin and hematocrit determinations may be obtained on the first postpartum day for assessment of blood loss during the birth. The white blood count is assessed as an indicator of infection. However, the leukocytosis of labor (25,000 to 30,000/mL) persists into the early postpartum period (Cunningham et al, 1989; Scott et al, 1990) without the presence of infection. The prenatal record will provide information about the woman's rubella and Rh status and the need for possible treatment. A clean-catch or catheterized urine specimen may be obtained and sent for routine urinalysis or culture and sensitivity testing.

SIGNS OF POTENTIAL PROBLEMS. Nurses must be on the alert for potential physiologic problems while assessing the "normal" new mother. Early identification of such problems allows for timely intervention (see box above).

Signs of Potential Physiologic Problems

Temperature	More than 100.4° F (38° C) after the first 24 h.
Pulse	Tachycardia, marked bradycardia
Blood pressure	Hypotension or hypertension
Energy level	Lethargy, extreme fatigue
Uterus	Deviated from the midline, boggy, remains above the umbilicus after 24 hours
Lochia	Heavy, foul odor
Perineum	Pronounced edema, not intact, signs of infection, marked discomfort
Legs	Homans' sign positive; painful, reddened area; warmth on posterior aspect of calf
Breasts	Redness, heat, pain, cracked and fissured nipples, inverted nipples, palpable mass
Appetite	Lack of appetite
Elimination	*Urine:* inability to void, urgency, frequency, dysuria; *bowel:* constipation, diarrhea
Rest	Inability to rest or sleep

Nursing Diagnoses

Although women experience similar problems during the postpartum period, certain factors act to make each woman's experience unique. The length and difficulty of the labor, whether the woman plans to bottle-feed or breast- feed, whether she had an episiotomy, and whether she has other children are some factors to consider. After analyzing the data from the assessment, the nurse establishes nursing diagnoses that will provide a guide for action. Examples of nursing diagnoses frequently established for the postpartum client include the following:

- High risk for infection related to
  - —Childbirth trauma to tissues
- Constipation or urinary retention related to
  - —Postpartum discomfort
  - —Childbirth trauma to tissues
- Sleep pattern disturbance related to
  - —Discomforts of postpartum period
  - —Long labor process
  - —Infant care and hospital routine

- Pain related to
  - —Involution of uterus
  - —Trauma to perineum
  - —Episiotomy
  - —Hemorrhoids
  - —Engorged breasts
- High risk for injury related to
  - —Postpartum hemorrhage
  - —Effects of anesthesia
- Fluid volume deficit related to
  - —Postpartum blood loss
- Situational low self-esteem related to
  - —Actual vs. expected birth experience
- Ineffective breast-feeding related to
  - —Maternal discomfort
  - —Infant positioning
  - —Normal physiologic response
- Altered parenting related to
  - —Lack of knowledge about infant care and feeding

Tribotti et al (1988) identified nursing diagnoses selected by mothers during the first 72 hours after birth. They found that on the average each mother selected nine diagnoses. Most client concerns focused on the physical discomforts and physiologic changes inherent in the immediate postpartum period. Parity, type of birth, and length of postpartum time influenced the diagnoses selected. (See Table 25-2 for the most frequently selected nursing diagnoses in this study; for an example of how to establish nursing diagnoses from assessment data, see the nursing plan of care, p. 728.)

TABLE 25-2 Nursing Diagnoses for the Postpartum Woman

Diagnosis	Percent of Women Who Selected Diagnosis
Alteration in comfort	87
Potential for growth	80
Fluid volume deficit/excess	69
Impaired mobility	66
Sleep pattern disturbances	66
Alteration in bowel elimination	56
Anxiety	45
Alteration in urinary elimination	40
Alteration in nutrition	38
Lack of knowledge	35

From Tribotti et al: Nursing diagnoses for the postpartum woman, *JOGNN* 17:410, 1988.

PLANNING

The nursing plan of care is individualized for the postpartum woman and her infant, even if the nursery retains the primary responsibility for the infant (for an example of a nursing plan of care, see p. 728). In many areas **couplet care** (mother and baby) (single room maternity care) is in practice. The nurse has been educated in both mother and infant care and functions as the primary nurse for both mother and infant even if the newborn is kept in the central nursery. This approach is a variation of rooming-in, in which the mother and child room together and mother and nurse share the care of the infant. The organization of care must take the newborn into consideration. The day actually revolves around the baby's feeding and care times. In couplet care, responsibility and accountability for infant care and client education rest with the primary nurse.

Once the nursing diagnoses are formulated, the nurse plans with the client what nursing measures would be appropriate and which are to be given priority. After a period of rest the mother is encouraged to assume increasing responsibility for her own self-care and her infant's care. The nurse is responsible for consistent assessment of actual and potential problems.

The nursing plan of care will include assessments to detect deviations from normal physical and psychosocial status, comfort measures to relieve discomfort or pain, and safety measures to prevent injury or infection. The nurse also will provide teaching and counseling measures designed to promote a mother's (and father's) feeling of competence in the care of herself and the newly born child. The nurse evaluates continuously and is ready to change the plan if indicated. The nurse's ability to adapt the care plan to specific medical and nursing diagnoses results in individualized client care. Caution is advised against total reliance on a standardized plan: the uniqueness of the individual may be overlooked.

Goals during the postpartum period are based on the nursing diagnoses identified for the individual client. They may include the following goals for the woman:

1. She will remain infection free.
2. She will demonstrate normal bowel and bladder patterns.
3. She will verbalize that she is able to obtain sufficient sleep.
4. She will verbalize that her comfort level is adequate; she will be free from injury.
5. She will demonstrate normal involution and lochia changes without hemorrhage.
6. She will express understanding and some degree of satisfaction with the birth experience.
7. She will demonstrate effective infant feeding techniques.

8. She will verbalize and demonstrate infant care skills.

IMPLEMENTATION

The nurse fulfills many roles in implementing the nursing care plan. These include providing physical care, teaching self- and infant care, and providing anticipatory guidance and counseling. Postpartum nurses provide a special type of care to new mothers—care that comes through nurturing. This nurturing (or "high-touch" care) fosters the woman's growth, development, and success with mothering. Postpartum nurses should use their skills to nurture while intervening most effectively on behalf of these women.

All nursing care given during the postpartum period is provided simultaneously with teaching. The rationale for each action can be provided, and questions are encouraged during each encounter with the new mother. The short span of time allotted the nurse to provide care necessitates that every opportunity for teaching be used. The puerperium period is characterized by a heightened interest in learning and readiness to change by the new mother and often by her family as well.

The first step in providing individualized care is to confirm the client's identity by checking her arm band. At the same time, the infant's identification number is matched with the corresponding band on the mother's wrist. The nurse demonstrates caring and respect by determining how the mother wishes to be addressed. This is especially important for women from certain cultures. Her preference is noted in her record and in her nursing plan of care.

The woman and her family are oriented to their surroundings. Familiarity with the unit, routines, resources, and personnel reduces one potential source of anxiety—the unknown. The mother is reassured through knowing whom and how she can call for assistance and what she can expect in the way of supplies and services. If the woman's usual daily routine before admission differs from the facility's routine, the nurse works with the woman to develop a mutually acceptable and workable routine.

Ethnic and cultural variations in care of the woman after childbirth can be discussed and plans for modifying nursing actions made (see pp. 697 to 699). An example of a cultural variation follows:

A Vietnamese woman who had been in the United States for 4 years requested rooming-in facilities after the birth. Instead of participating in the care of her infant, she refused to do so, remained in bed, wore a woolen cap, and appeared distressed and angry. One nurse decided to put newly learned concepts concerning cross-cultural nursing into effect. She began by praising the woman's ability to speak English and after eliciting a smile, remarked, "Every country has developed good ways to look after mothers and babies. Would you tell me about the care in Vietnam?" There was an immediate response. The woman explained that in her country women remained in bed for 10 days after the birth and the biggest danger to their health was getting a cold. The baby was kept in the room with the mother, but either a grandmother or nurse took complete charge of the care.

Evidently the woman was behaving in terms of cultural expectations, and the nurses were performing within theirs. This rather simple approach to resolving a nursing problem can be applied successfully to similar situations.

Prevention of Infection or Hemorrhage

In the case of mothers and newborns, special consideration must be given to the prevention of infection and hemorrhage. To guard against infection, facilities (unit kitchens, bathroom, and bed units) and supplies (linens) must be kept scrupulously clean. Frequent changes of draw sheet and a daily change of linen are recommended. Supervision of use of facilities to prevent cross infection among women is necessary (e.g., common sitz bath must be scrubbed after each woman's use, ventilation system is monitored). Personnel must be conscientious about their hand-washing techniques to prevent cross infection. Universal precautions must be practiced (see Chapter 29). Personnel with colds, coughs, or skin infections (e.g., a cold sore on the lips [herpes simplex virus, type 1]) must follow hospital protocol when in contact with women during the puerperium.

Setting priorities in nursing interventions is important in the prevention of hemorrhage. (See nursing plan of care, p. 728.) The first intervention is stimulation of uterine tone (**living ligature**) by gently massaging the fundus until firm. Clots may be expelled. While massaging the fundus, the nurse palpates for a full bladder. Frequent monitoring for a full bladder and uterine atony may be the only interventions needed at this time.

Education of the woman also is important to maintain uterine tone. Fundal massage can be a very uncomfortable procedure. Teaching the woman about the procedure enables her to maintain some control and decrease her anxiety. The teaching plan should include a demonstration of self-fundal palpation and massage, information regarding the importance of voiding at regular intervals, and possibly breast-feeding or nipple stimulation to release oxytocin. The woman and her family also may want to know why uterine atony occurs. The nurse must be able to ex-

TABLE 25-3 Pharmacologic Measures to Stimulate Uterine Tone

Intervention	Action, Uses during Puerperium	Onset of Effect, Duration, Usual Dose	Contraindications, Precautions	Caution
OXYTOCIN INJECTION				
USP (Pitocin, Syntocinon, Uteracon); oxytocic, synthetic posterior pituitary hormone	Stimulates phasic uterine muscle contraction, promotes milk-ejection (let-down) reflex, facilitates flow of milk during engorgement	IV injection, 10 U/mL; onset in 1 min IV infusion, 10-40 U/1000 mL 5% dextrose or physiologic electrolyte solution IM injection, 3-10 U; onset in 3-7 min; duration 30-60 min	Hypersensitivity; return of atony when effect wears off. May cause severe hypertension if client also is receiving ephedrine, methoxamine, or other vasopressors	Assess for return of atony; store in cool place.
ERGONOVINE				
USP, NF (Ergotrate Maleate); oxytocic, ergot alkaloid	Stimulates prolonged, nonphasic uterine contractions	Oral: 0.2-0.4 mg q6-12 h for 48 hr; onset in 6-15 min IM injection: 0.2 mg (1 mL) if nausea precludes oral preparation, onset "in a few minutes" Initial response: firm, tetanic contraction Subsequent response: alternating minor relaxations and contractions for 1½ hr; then vigorous rhythmic contractions for 3-4 hr after injection.	Severe hypertensive episodes may occur if given to hypertensive clients or those receiving vasconstrictors; hypersensitivity; nausea, vomiting; sudden change in BP or pulse	Assess for changes in BP, pulse; store in cool place.

plain the physiologic events that precipitate hemorrhage.

The uterus may remain atonic (boggy) even with massage and expulsion of clots. If this occurs, it is important that the nurse remain with the woman and summon help. Some hospitals may have standard protocols for postpartum hemorrhage. The protocol may specify IV therapy, medication (Table 25-3), and contacting the physician for possible surgical intervention. The primary nurse should keep the mother and family informed and assist them to remain calm. Efforts of the other health team members are coordinated by the primary nurse. **Oxytocic medications** (drugs that stimulate the smooth muscle of the uterus to contract) are presented in Table 25-3.

Evaluation of the woman's responses to intervention is an ongoing part of the nursing process. All responses to interventions should be carefully recorded. If goals are not met or new needs emerge, the woman's plan of care is modified accordingly.

Care of Episiotomy, Lacerations, and Hemorrhoids

A variety of interventions aid the healing process, maintain cleanliness, prevent infection, and enhance comfort. Teaching the woman to wipe from front to back (vagina to anus) is the first step in preventing contamination of the vaginal and genitourinary areas. In many hospitals a squeeze bottle filled with warm water or a Surgi-Gator or Hygienic is used after each voiding to cleanse the perineal area (see box on p. 707). The woman also is taught to change her peripad with each voiding and to avoid inserting anything (i.e., tampons) into the vagina. Educating the mother while assisting her will encourage coopera-

TABLE 25-3 Pharmacologic Measures to Stimulate Uterine Tone—cont'd

Intervention	Action, Uses during Puerperium	Onset of Effect, Duration, Usual Dose	Contraindications, Precautions	Caution
METHYLERGONOVINE				
NF (Methergine); oxytocic, ergot alkaloid and congener of lysergic acid (LSD)	Stimulates rapid, sustained tetanic uterine contractions; used in treatment of subinvolution; has only minimum vasoconstrictive effect	Oral: 0.2 mg tab, q6-8 h for maximum of 1 wk; onset in 5-10 min IM injection 0.2 mg (1 mL) q2-4 h; onset in 2-5 min IV infusion *(emergency only)*: 0.2 mg (1 mL) *slowly over 60 sec;* onset immediate	Nausea, vomiting; transient hypertension; dizziness, headache; tinnitus; diaphoresis; palpitations; temporary chest pains	Do not administer with Percodan—may result in hallucinations; assess BP; store in cold place, away from light.
CARBOPROST				
(Prostin/M15); oxytocic, prostaglandin	Stimulates rapid, sustained uterine contractions; used for treatment of uterine atony and uterine inversion	IM injection 1 ampule (250 μg), onset within minutes; intramyometrial injection (by physician only), ½-2 ampules (125-500 μg) diluted with 10 mL saline (injected transabdominally into anterior wall of uterus); onset within minutes	Severe hypertension (systolic >170 mm Hg or diastolic >100 mm Hg); avoid in clients with severe symptomatic asthma Diarrhea commonly seen with dosage above 1 ampule; there is usually a rise in systolic and diastolic BP; possible bronchoconstriction and wheezing	Monitor BP, appearance of adverse reactions; store in refrigerator.

NF, National Formulary; *USP*, United States Pharmacopeia.

tion and ensure that necessary measures are continued upon discharge.

Simple comfort measures include encouraging the woman to lie on her side or to use a pillow while sitting. Other interventions include application of an ice pack, topical applications, dry heat, cleansing with a squeeze bottle or Surgi-Gator (Fig. 25-2), and a cleansing shower or **sitz bath** Fig. 25-1. (The box on p. 707 details nursing actions for various interventions.) Many of these interventions also are effective for hemorrhoids, especially ice packs, sitz baths, and topical applications. Some women may report that their hemorrhoids are more bothersome than their episiotomy. The woman who has previously experienced hemorrhoids should be asked what measures have proved helpful for her. Whenever possible these measures should be continued.

The performance of Kegel exercises, especially af-

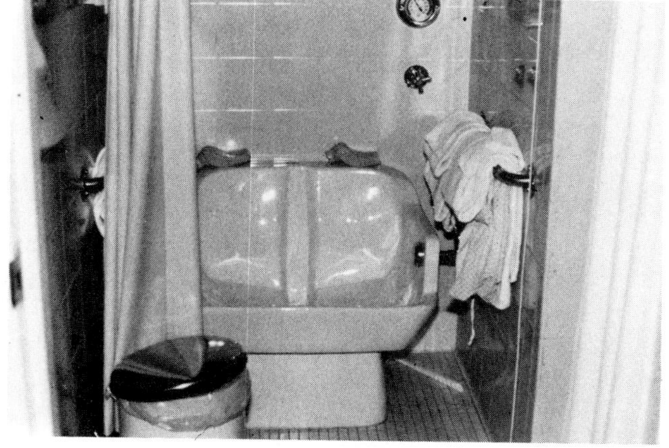

Fig. 25-1 Sitz bath.
Courtesy Marjorie Pyle, RNC, Lifecircle, Costa Mesa, Calif.

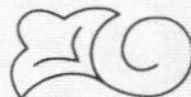 **Research Highlight** 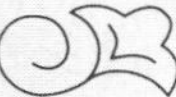

Pelvic Muscle Strength and Stress Urinary Incontinence

RESEARCH ABSTRACT

Pelvic muscle strength was measured in 20 nulliparous women between 32 and 36 weeks' gestation and at 6 weeks postpartum to identify stress urinary incontinence and relate these two factors to childbirth. The women were recruited from a midwifery and obstetric service at a university medical center. Pelvic muscle strength was obtained by a digital measure and use of two gloved fingers. A uroflometer graphed the ability to stop the flow of urine on a verbal command. The presence of stress urinary incontinence was measured with a standing stress test. In this test a woman with a full bladder stood with her feet 18 inches apart with the external urinary meatus exposed. She was asked to cough vigorously. Leakage of urine signified a positive reaction to the standing stress test. Women who had vaginal births exhibited a significant decrease in pelvic muscle strength from the antepartum to the postpartum period. The pelvic muscle strength of women who had cesarean births remained unchanged. Women who had strong pelvic muscles antepartally had high levels of pelvic muscle strength postpartally. The strength of the pelvic muscle was positively associated with the ability to interrupt the flow of urine.

IMPLICATIONS FOR PRACTICE

Vaginal childbirth results in relaxation of the pelvic muscles. The retention of muscle strength from the antepartum to postpartum period supports nursing interventions of teaching the importance of good nutrition and pelvic muscle exercises to strengthen muscle tone. Women experiencing urine loss should be strongly encouraged to follow a rigorous regimen of pelvic muscle exercise.

RELATED RESEARCH QUESTIONS

1. Do women of childbearing age routinely perform pelvic muscle exercises?
2. Do health care providers routinely teach pelvic muscle exercises?
3. Do adolescent women have knowledge about pelvic muscle exercises and the benefits of the exercises?
4. Does the pelvic muscle strength vary with the body weight of women?

REFERENCE

Sampselle CM: Changes in pelvic muscle strength and stress urinary incontinence associated with childbirth, *JOGNN* 19:371, 1990.

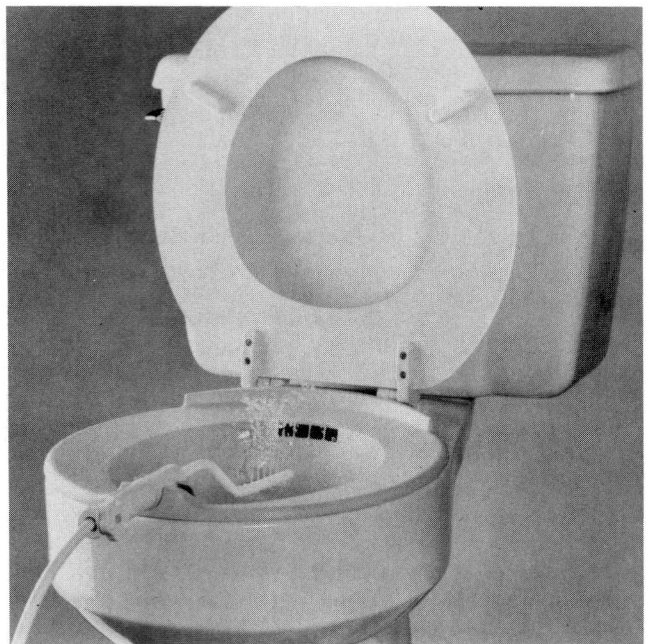

Fig. 25-2 Hygienic sitz bath (Surgi-Gator) for perineal care.
Courtesy Andermac, Inc, Yuba City, Calif.

ter vaginal birth, are discussed. Pelvic muscle exercises to strengthen muscle tone supports the nursing intervention: retention of muscle strength from antepartum to postpartum periods. Women who maintain muscle strength may benefit years later (see Research Highlight regarding stress urinary incontinence).

The nurse needs to evaluate the various options and along with the woman, determine the care method that is most effective for her. The client's cultural practices must be taken into account when using heat and cold therapy and teaching care of the perineum and Kegel exercises.

Comfort

Assessment for comfort should be ongoing. Mothers often report some discomfort during the puerperium. Alteration in comfort was the most frequently identified diagnosis by women in the study by Tribotti et al (1988) (see nursing plan of care, p. 728).

The woman's description of the type and severity of her pain is the nurse's best guide in choosing an appropriate intervention. One method used to quantify pain is to have the woman rate her pain on a 10-point scale, with 10 being the most severe pain she can imagine. To confirm the location and extent of discomfort the nurse inspects and palpates areas of pain, as appropriate, for redness, swelling, discharge,

Interventions for Episiotomy, Lacerations, and Hemorrhoids

ICE PACK

Apply a covered ice pack to perineum.

1. During first 2 hours to decreases edema formation and increase comfort
2. After the first 2 hours following the birth to provide anesthetic effect

SITZ BATH

Built-in type (Fig. 25-1):

Prepare bath by thoroughly scrubbing with cleaning agent and rinsing.

Pad with towel before filling.

Fill ⅓ to ½ full with water of correct temperature: 100.4°-105° F, or 113° F* (38°-40.6° C, or 45° C).

Encourage woman to use at least twice a day for 20 min.

Place call bell within easy reach.

Teach woman to enter bath by tightening gluteal muscles and keeping them tightened and then relaxing them after she is in the bath.

Place dry towels within reach.

Ensure privacy.

Check woman in 15 min; assess pulse as needed.

Disposable type:

Clamp tubing and fill bag with warm water.

Raise toilet seat, place bath in bowl with overflow opening directed toward back of toilet.

Place container above toilet bowl.

Attach tube into groove at front of bath.

Loosen tube clamp to regulate rate of flow; fill bath to about ½ full; continue as above for built-in sitz bath.

SQUEEZE BOTTLE

Demonstrate for and assist woman; explain rationale.

Fill bottle with tap water warmed to approximately 100° F (38° C) (comfortably warm on the wrist).

Instruct woman to position nozzle between her legs so that squirts of water reach perineum as she sits on toilet seat. Explain that it will take whole bottle of water over perineum.

Remind her to blot dry with toilet paper or clean wipes.

Remind her to avoid contamination from anal area.

Apply new clean pad.

SURGI-GATOR

Assemble Surgi-Gator (Fig. 25-2).

Instruct woman regarding use and rationale.

Follow package directions.

Instruct woman to sit on toilet with legs apart and to put nozzle so tip is just past the perineum, adjusting placement as needed.

Remind her to return her applicator to her bedside stand.

DRY HEAT

Inspect lamp for defects.

Cover lamp with towels.

Position lamp 50 cm (20 in) from perineum; use 3 times a day for 20-min periods.

Teach regarding use of 40-watt bulb at home.

Provide draping over woman.

If same lamp is being used by several women, clean it carefully between uses.

TOPICAL APPLICATIONS

Apply anesthetic cream or spray; use sparingly 3 to 4 times per day.

Offer witch hazel pads (Tucks) after voiding or defecating; woman pats perineum dry from front to back, then applies witch hazel pads.

CLEANSING

Wash perineum with mild soap and warm water at least once daily.

Cleanse from symphysis pubis to anal area.

Apply peripad from front to back, protecting inner surface of pad from contamination.

Wrap soiled pad and place in covered waste container.

Remind to change pad every time she voids or defecates or at least 4 times per day.

Wash hands before and after changing pads.

Assess amount and character of lochia with each pad change.

*Some authors propose cool sitz bath (Droegemueller, 1980; Ramler, Roberts, 1986).

and heat and observes for body tension, guarded movements, and facial tension. Blood pressure, pulse, and respiration may be elevated in response to acute pain. Diaphoresis may accompany severe pain. A lack of objective symptoms does not necessarily mean there is no pain because there also may be a cultural component to the expression of pain.

Nursing actions are chosen so that the pain sensation is eliminated or reduced to a tolerable level that allows the woman to perform self-care activities and begin infant care. Most physicians routinely order a variety of analgesics to be administered as needed, including both narcotic and nonnarcotic choices, with their dosage and time frequency ranges. Many women will want to participate in decisions about analgesia. Women should routinely be asked what pain control methods have been helpful to them in the past. Some women may prefer nonpharmacologic pain measures, such as ice packs, warm compresses, warm drinks, distraction, imagery, therapeutic touch, relaxation, and bonding with the infant, before taking analgesics.

Jet hydrotherapy (whirlpool baths), discussed in Chapter 17, can be used during the postpartum period as well. Total submersion in warm water soothes tired and tense muscles throughout the entire body, thus increasing relaxation and pain relief (Aderhold, Perry, 1991; Rosenthal, 1991). It also is similar to the sitz bath in that the warm bath cleanses damaged tissues and increases circulation. This facilitates healing and reduces pain. The same nursing measures used in labor are important here—prevention of dehydration and overheating (p. 455).

Severe pain, however, may interfere with active participation in choosing pain-relief measures. If an analgesic is to be given, the nurse must make a clinical judgment of the type, dosage, and frequency from the medication ordered. The client is informed of the prescribed analgesic and its common side effects. Breast-feeding mothers often have concerns about the effects of taking an analgesic on the infant. The nurse should inform the mother of any such effect.

A woman may prefer a different analgesic or pain control measure if she considers a side effect unacceptable. For example, a new mother planning to keep her infant at her bedside may not be comfortable with an analgesic that may make her drowsy. Pain is a frightening, lonely experience, and a woman should feel confident that her need for pain relief will be attended to. Therefore the nurse evaluates the effectiveness of the analgesic every 15 minutes until acceptable pain relief is achieved.

If evaluation reveals there is no improvement in reported pain in 30 minutes, to enhance the analgesic, the nurse institutes appropriate *nonpharmacologic pain measures* that were not previously instituted. Pain relief is enhanced by using more than one method or route.

If acceptable pain relief has not been achieved in 1 hour and there has not been a change in the initial assessment, the nurse may need to contact the physician for additional pain relief orders or directions. Unrelieved pain results in fatigue, anxiety, and worsening perception of pain. Once pain has become severe, a larger dose or stronger analgesia is required.

When acceptable analgesia has been achieved, the nurse evaluates with the woman her pain relief and her expectations and desire to participate in pain control. The nurse identifies any changes the mother desires in her regimen and adds changes to the care plan. *A woman's belief regarding what is helpful to achieve pain relief is vital to the success of any pain regimen.*

A "spinal" (postsubarachnoid) headache may begin up to 7 days after spinal puncture (see discussion in Chapter 15). It usually is a positional headache, worsening in the upright position and improving in the flat-lying position. The nurse must be prepared to provide reassurance and explanations and to administer analgesics, caffeine, or an IV infusion at 150 mL/hr. In addition, the nurse should be ready to prepare the woman for and to assist with the application of a blood patch (p. 382).

Rest, Ambulation, and Exercise

The excitement and exhilaration experienced after the birth of the infant make rest difficult (Tribotti et al, 1988). The new mother who is uncomfortable or anxious about her ability to care for her infant also may have difficulty sleeping. In the ensuing days the demands of the infant, along with the influence of the hospital environment and routines, contribute to alterations in her sleep pattern. In addition, patterns of medication administration and postpartum assessment are based on hospital routines rather than the mother's needs. This also contributes to sleep pattern disturbances. The Research Highlight on p. 709 discusses the results of a study of reported changes in sleep patterns during the postpartum period.

The need for rest during the postpartum period, however, is critical to the mother's sense of well-being and to her ability to participate in her own care as well as care of her infant. Mead-Bennet (1990) suggests that "sleep loss in the postpartum period may have implications for early mother and infant interactions." As a priority, immediate postpartum care should provide the new mother with the opportunity to rest (see nursing plan of care, p. 728).

Interventions must be planned to meet the client's individual needs for sleep and rest. Backrubs, other comfort measures, and medication for sleep for the first few nights may be necessary. Hospital and nursing routines also may be adjusted to meet individual needs. In addition, the nurse can assist the family to limit visitors and provide a comfortable chair or bed for the father.

Early ambulation has proved successful in reducing the incidence of thromboembolism and in pro-

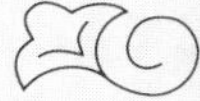 **Research Highlight** 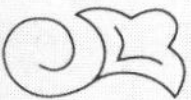

Sleep Patterns during Postpartum Hospitalization

RESEARCH ABSTRACT

Women have documented changes in sleep patterns during the perinatal cycle. The objective of this study was to describe one aspect of physiologic adaptation during the postpartum period by assessing sleep patterns during the first 2 days after childbirth. Data were collected from 34 normal women in two hospitals during the first 48 hours after the birth. Data collection methods included observation, self-report, and a review of records. Observations of body position, open or closed eyes, and respirations were made at 15-minute intervals between 11 PM and 7 AM by trained observers. Other information recorded was noise, light level, temperature, and activity of others in the environment. The first postpartum sleep for eight women was the night after childbirth; 13 others said they had less than 90 minutes' sleep during that time. Sixteen women reported they were awakened by nurses, five were awakened by visitors, four by the infant, and three awoke on their own. Subjects were judged as awake during a range of 5 to 30 of the 32 observations. Fourteen of the women felt rested and 19 felt tired or sleepy upon awakening. Women who had more sleep-cycle opportunities reported sleeping more soundly. The most common cause of awakening during the night was to feed the infant, to have vital signs assessed by the nurse, and to urinate. Environmental activities were noted on numerous occasions.

IMPLICATIONS FOR PRACTICE

This study documents sleep patterns of new mothers and the disruptive nature of a hospital environment on sleep. Women may have no opportunity for uninterrupted sleep in the first several hours after giving birth. The lack of sleep may interfere with early postpartum recovery. Nursing interventions should be timed to interfere as little as possible with sleep of new mothers. Environmental disruptions should be minimized.

RELATED RESEARCH QUESTIONS

1. What is the effect of modifying the environment on sleep in new mothers?
2. What nursing care activities can be clustered safely?
3. What is the effect of clustering nursing care activities on sleep in new mothers?
4. What is the minimum safe level of monitoring of new mothers in the postpartum period?

REFERENCE

Lentz MJ, Killien MC: Are you sleeping? Sleep patterns during postpartum hospitalization, *J Perinat Neonatal Nurs* 4(4):30, 1991.

moting women's more rapid recovery of strength. Exercise also promotes rest. Confinement to bed is not required for women who had general anesthesia, who had *epidural* or *caudal anesthesia,* or who had local anesthesia such as paracervical or pudendal block. Free movement is permitted once the anesthetic wears off unless an analgesic has been administered. After the first vital rest period is over (usually about 2 to 8 hours), the mother is encouraged to ambulate frequently. Postpartum exercises are begun as soon as the woman indicates readiness. Fig. 25-3 illustrates a number of exercises appropriate for the new mother.

Prevention of **thrombosis** (the formation or development of a blood clot) is part of the nursing care plan. If a woman is confined to bed longer than 8 hours (e.g., after spinal anesthesia or cesarean birth), exercise to promote circulation in the legs is indicated:

1. Alternate flexion and extension of feet
2. Rotate feet
3. Alternate flexion and extension of legs
4. Press back of knee to bed surface; relax

If the woman's history suggests that she is susceptible to **thromboembolism** (clot that becomes dislodged and is transported through the blood vessel), the physician may avoid use of estrogens to inhibit or suppress lactation. Women with varicosities are advised to wear support hose. The woman is encouraged to walk about actively for true ambulation and discouraged from sitting immobile in a chair. If a thrombus is suspected (as evidenced by a positive Homans' sign, warmth, redness, or tenderness in the suspected leg), the physician should be notified immediately; meanwhile the woman should be confined to bed, with the affected limb elevated on pillows.

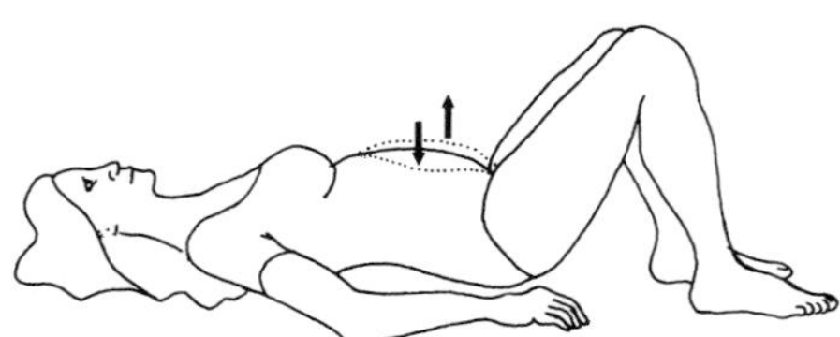

Abdominal Breathing. Lie on back with knees bent. Inhale deeply through the nose. Keep ribs as stationary as possible and allow abdomen to expand upwards. Exhale slowly but forcefully while contracting the abdominal muscles; hold for 3 to 5 seconds while exhaling.

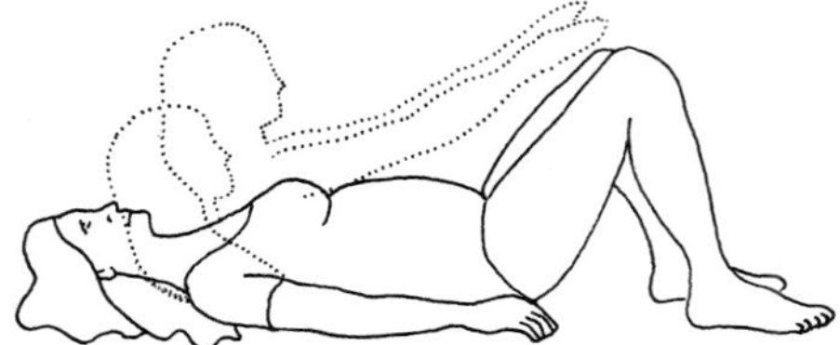

Reach for the Knees. Lie on back with knees bent. While inhaling deeply lower chin onto chest. While exhaling, raise head and shoulders slowly and smoothly and reach for knees with arms outstretched. The body should only rise as far as the back will naturally bend while waist remains on floor or bed (about 6 to 8 inches). Slowly and smoothly lower head and shoulders back to starting position. Relax.

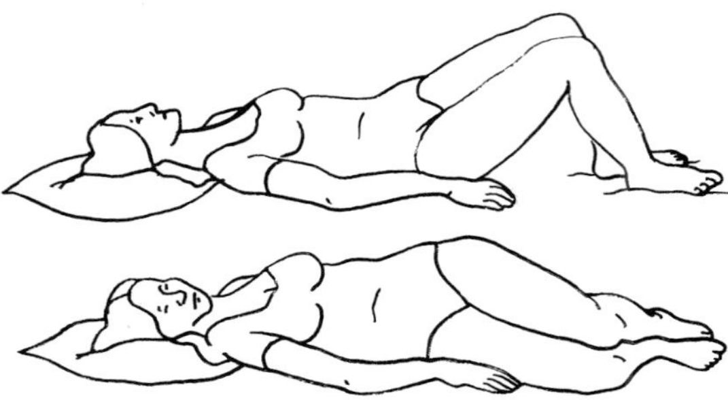

Double Knee Roll. Lie on back with knees bent. Keeping shoulders flat and feet stationary, slowly and smoothly roll knees over to the left to touch floor or bed. Maintaining a smooth motion, roll knees back over to the right until they touch floor or bed. Return to starting position and relax.

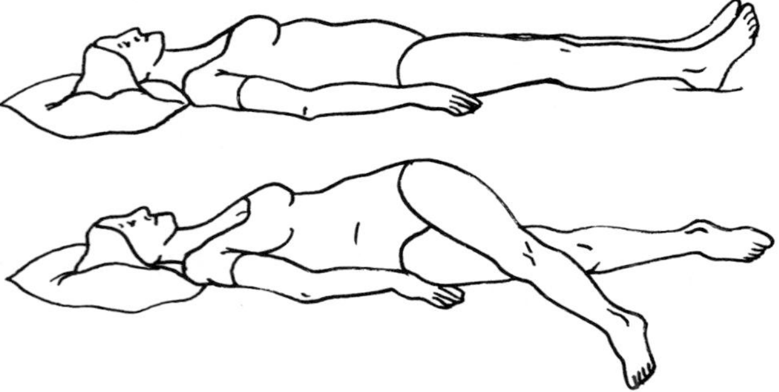

Leg Roll. Lie on back with legs straight. Keeping shoulders flat and legs straight, slowly and smoothly lift left leg and roll it over to touch the right side of floor or bed and return to starting position. Repeat, rolling right leg over to touch left side of floor or bed. Relax.

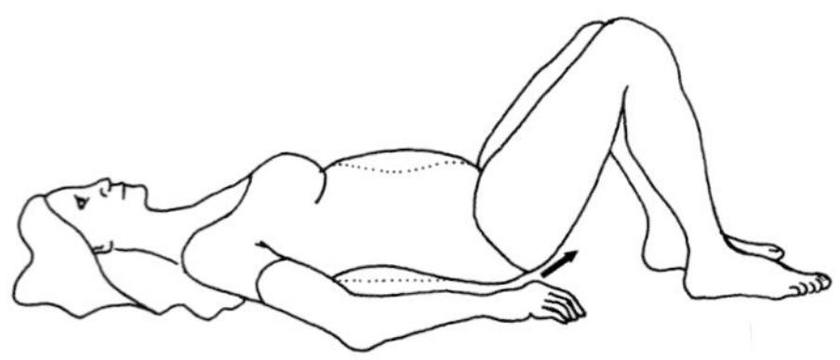

Combined Abdominal Breathing and Supine Pelvic Tilt (Pelvic Rock). Lie on back with knees bent. While inhaling deeply, roll pelvis back by flattening lower back on floor or bed. Exhale slowly but forcefully while contracting abdominal muscles and tightening buttocks. Hold for 3 to 5 seconds while exhaling. Relax.

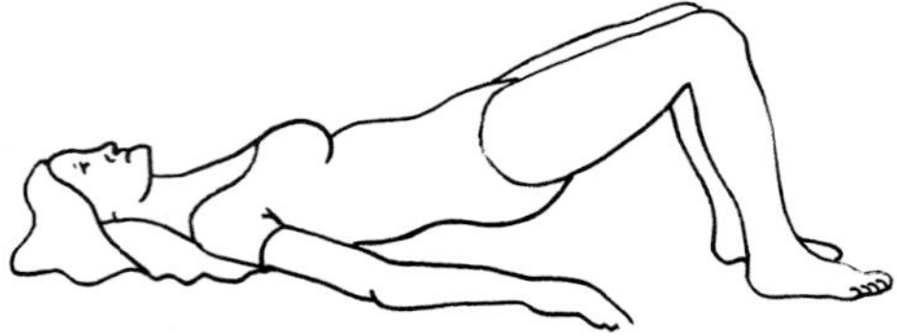

Buttocks Lift. Lie on back with arms at sides, knees bent and feet flat. Slowly raise buttocks and arch back. Return slowly to starting position.

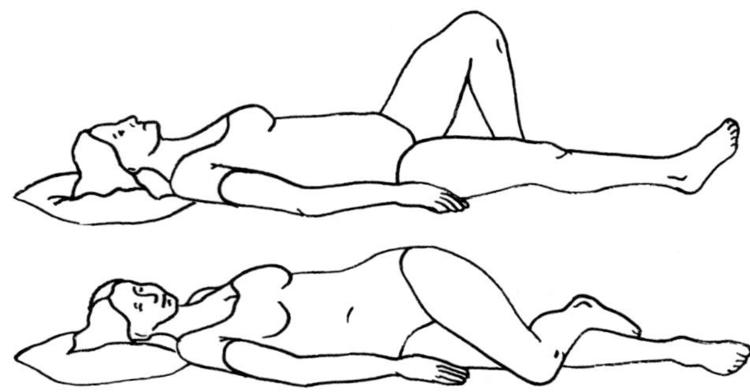

Single Knee Roll. Lie on back with with right leg straight and left leg bent at the knee. Keeping shoulders flat, slowly and smoothly roll left knee over to the right to touch floor or bed and then back to starting position. Reverse position of legs. Roll right knee over to the left to touch floor or bed and return to starting position. Relax.

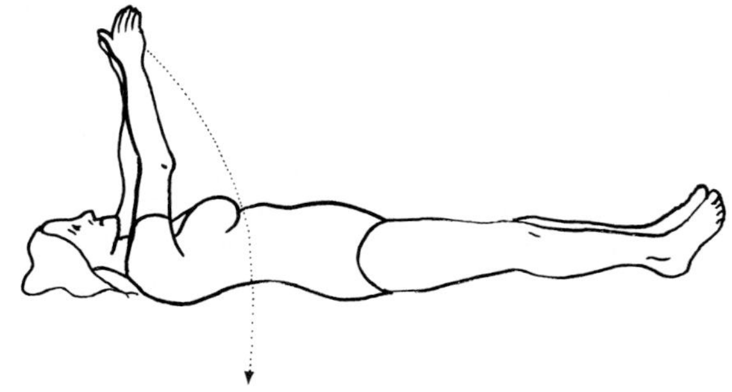

Arm Raises. Lie on back with arms extended at 90° angle from body. Raise arms so they are perpendicular and hands touch. Lower slowly.

Fig. 25-3 Postpartum exercise should begin as soon as possible. The woman should start with simple exercises and gradually progress to more strenuous ones.

Nutrition

After giving birth women usually are hungry and demonstrate interest in food in general. This presents an ideal opportunity for continued nutritional counseling (see discussion of nutrition in Chapter 9 for detailed information). The woman's weight, expectations of weight loss, usual food habits, cultural preferences, laboratory findings (hemoglobin and hematocrit levels), and knowledge about nutritional needs after pregnancy should be reassessed.

Nursing interventions might include teaching about nourishment needed to facilitate healing and increase energy. A regular diet high in protein, vitamin C, and dietary fiber, along with sufficient fluids and calories, generally is recommended for the postpartum woman to prevent constipation and promote well-being. Nutritional snacks usually are welcome. Prenatal vitamins and iron supplements often are continued. (Specific dietary needs of the nursing mother are discussed in Chapters 9 and 22.)

Cultural dietary preferences must be respected. Special arrangements for inclusion of ethnic items with meals may be made with the dietary department. The family should be permitted and encouraged to bring in any special ethnic foods the woman prefers.

Elimination

After giving birth the mother should void spontaneously within 6 to 8 hours. The first three voidings are measured to ensure adequate emptying of the bladder; a volume of at least 150 mL is expected for each voiding. Some women experience difficulty in emptying the bladder, possibly a result of diminished bladder tone, edema from trauma, or fear of discomfort. The suprapubic area should therefore be palpated for bladder fullness when fundal checks are done. In the presence of a full bladder the fundus may be displaced to the side or well above the umbilicus. The nurse also notes any increase in the amount of lochia. Other data may include unequal input and output. The woman may indicate that she has the urge to void but is unable to do so.

Nursing interventions focus on helping the woman spontaneously empty her bladder as soon as possible. The first priority is to assist the woman to the bathroom or onto a bedpan if she is unable to ambulate. Running water in the sink, placing the woman's hands in warm water, or pouring water from a squeeze bottle over the perineum may stimulate voiding. Other techniques include assisting the woman into the shower or sitz bath and encouraging her to void or placing oil of peppermint (wintergreen) in a bedpan under the woman. The vapors may relax the urinary meatus and trigger spontaneous voiding. Fluid intake should be encouraged. Cranberry juice often is recommended as a deterrent to urinary tract infection.

If these measures are unsuccessful, a sterile catheter may be inserted to drain the urine. Care must be taken not to drain too much urine at once. If the bladder appears to be overdistended, a Foley (retention) catheter should be inserted, 800 mL removed, and the tube clamped. Additional urine should be removed at intervals. Many hospitals have standard orders for this condition. In some institutions the physician must be informed.

The woman should be asked daily if she has had a bowel movement. Nursing interventions to promote normal bowel elimination include educating the client about measures to avoid constipation. These include ensuring adequate roughage and fluid intake and promoting exercise. Alerting the woman to side effects of medications such as narcotic analgesics (i.e., decreased gastrointestinal tract motility) may encourage her to implement measures to reduce the risk of constipation. Stool softeners or laxatives often are necessary during the early postpartum period.

Care of Breasts

The 2 hours after childbirth provide an excellent time to encourage the mother to breast-feed if she desires. The infant is in an alert state and ready to breast-feed. Breast-feeding at this time will aid in the contraction of the uterus and help prevent hemorrhage. This is an outstanding opportunity for the nurse to demonstrate and instruct the mother in breast-feeding. (Chapter 22 includes a thorough discussion of lactation and breast-feeding.) If the woman elects to breast-feed soon after giving birth, the nurse also can use that opportunity to assess the physical appearance of the woman's breasts.

Suppression of lactation (efforts to prevent or stop the development of breast milk) is implemented when the woman has decided not to breast-feed or in the case of neonatal death. These women should be instructed about nonpharmacologic suppression techniques, known as mechanical suppression. The first priority in mechanical suppression is wearing a snug support brassiere, one that fits tightly, or a breast binder for at least 72 hours after the birth. The woman should avoid any breast stimulation, including running warm water over the breasts, newborn suckling, or pumping of the breasts.

In some cases, pharmacologic therapy is prescribed by the physician. The most commonly prescribed medication for suppression of lactation is bromocriptine (Parlodel). This nonestrogen medication suppresses lactation by preventing the secretion of prolactin. The drug is taken twice a day for 14 days. There may be a rebound breast engorgement when the medication is discontinued. These symptoms usually are mild, and mechanical suppression may be helpful. Some physicians may prescribe estrogens (Tace or Deladumone) to suppress lactation. The nurse should follow the hospital protocols to obtain informed consent and provide and discuss literature included with the drug package regarding estrogen and its possible association with cancer. Women who receive these estrogen-containing antilactogenics have an increased incidence of thrombus formation and should be observed closely.

Should engorgement occur, the nurse assures the woman that it is temporary and that ice packs and analgesia will decrease the symptoms. The woman is instructed to maintain an adequate fluid intake and to avoid taking diuretics.

Immunizations

If the assessment data indicate the need, rubella vaccination and Rh_o (D) immune globulin are administered during the puerperium. (For a detailed discussion of the Rh factor and isoimmunization, see Chapter 38; for a general discussion of the immune system, see Chapter 6.)

For women who have not had rubella (10% to 20% of all women) or women who show serologic negativity (i.e., titer of 1:8 or less), **rubella vaccination** is recommended in the immediate post-birth period to prevent fetal anomalies in future pregnancies. Seroconversion occurs in approximately 90% of women vaccinated after the birth. The live attenuated rubella virus is not communicable; therefore breast-feeding mothers can be vaccinated. However, the live attenuated rubella vaccine is made from duck eggs. Women who have allergies to these eggs may develop a hypersensitivity reaction to the vaccine, for which they will need adrenalin. A transient arthralgia or rash is common in vaccinated women but is benign. Because the vaccine may be teratogenic, the client should sign an informed consent and should receive written information about the vaccine, its side effects and risks, and the necessity for practicing contraception to avoid pregnancy for a period of 2 to 3 months after vaccination.

Injection of **Rh_0(D) immune globulin** (solution of gamma globulin that contains Rh antibodies) within 72 hours of childbirth will prevent sensitization in the Rh-negative woman who has had a fetomaternal transfusion of Rh-positive fetal red blood cells (RBCs). The administration of 300 μg of Rh_0(D) immune globulin usually is sufficient to prevent maternal sensitization. Rh_0(D) immune globulin promotes lysis of fetal Rh-positive RBCs circulating in the maternal blood stream before the mother forms her own antibodies against them. If a large fetomaternal transfusion is suspected, the dose needed can be assessed by either the Betke-Kleihauer or the D^u test, which detects 20 mL or more of Rh-positive fetal blood in the maternal circulation. The Rh_0(D) immune globulin is administered after all known abortions (gestational age of 8 weeks or more) because the risk of sensitization after abortion is about half the risk after a full-term pregnancy.* *It is administered after the birth to any woman who meets the following three criteria:* (1) the mother must show Rh_0(D) negativity with no Rh antibodies (i.e., indirect Coombs' test result is negative), (2) the infant must show Rh_0(D) or D^u positivity, and (3) results of direct Coombs' test on the cord blood must be negative. If the woman meets these criteria, a 1:1000 dilution of Rh_0(D) immune globulin† is cross-matched to the mother's red cells to ensure compatibility. To ensure that the immune globulin is administered to the correct woman, the same precautions are followed for a blood transfusion. *If administered to a person with Rh positivity, immune globulin will act to promote lysis of the Rh-positive RBCs.* The dose is administered to the mother intramuscularly, *never* intravenously or to the infant.

EVALUATION

The nurse can be reasonably assured that care was effective when the goals for care have been met:

- The woman remains infection free.
- She demonstrates normal bowel and bladder patterns.
- She verbalizes that she has had sufficient sleep and adequate comfort levels.
- She is free from injury.
- She demonstrates normal involution.
- She expresses understanding and some degree of satisfaction with the birth experience.
- She verbalizes knowledge of and demonstrates mastery of infant care skills.

Any goals that have not been met should be reviewed with the client. New goals may be necessary or additional intervention strategies may be required, or both.

*For prenatal prophylaxis, see Chapters 13 and 38.
†A blood product. Certain religions proscribe use of blood or blood products.

■ NURSING CARE OF PSYCHOSOCIAL NEEDS

Psychologic care of the mother includes assessing parental responses and parent-infant interactions, particularly within the family and cultural context. A plan of care must be developed that will help ensure the woman's success in her parental role and ease her return to the home and, if relevant, the work environment. Meeting the emotional needs of a new mother will strongly promote her success as a mother. In providing emotional care, postpartum nurses play a key role in assisting women to make positive adaptations to parenting. The woman must be viewed and treated as a unique individual as well as a unique mother. Her self-esteem, self-concept, and body image are important determinants of psychologic well-being. Cultural expectations and the role of the family during the postpartum period also may have a strong influence on her emotional adaptation, as well as on the physical behaviors already discussed.

ASSESSMENT

When assessing the woman's psychologic state, nurses must be aware of a number of factors. For example, many women indicate a need to examine the birth experience itself in retrospect (Konrad, 1987). The mother's critical self-evaluation of her intrapartum behavior is one of the important psychologic tasks of the postpartum period. The nurse needs to identify, within a cultural context, the mother's perception of the fit between her prenatal expectation for her behavior and the intrapartum reality experienced. Other factors to be assessed include integration of the birth experience, parental responses to the birth of the child, parent-infant interactions, and the mother's self-image.

Parental Responses

Parental responses to the birth of a child include behaviors that are either adaptive or maladaptive. Both mother and father exhibit these behaviors, although to date most research has centered on the mother. Parents who are faced with the crisis of a severe life stress may not be able to provide supportive parenting for their child. Life stress reduces both psychologic well-being and physical health. These are two important factors in establishing and maintaining relationships with others. Another critical factor is a feeling of personal control.

Many new mothers will experience **parenting difficulties** (find it hard to adjust to the mothering role) until their skills become established. Once they feel confidence in their skills, the increase in self-esteem promotes a positive affective response to the child. However, some parents will exhibit **parenting disorders** (altered parenting) of varying degrees that place the child in jeopardy and at risk. Protocols for the physical screening of high-risk pregnant women and fetuses have been developed and confirmed. However, tools predicting high-risk parenting behaviors require more replication over larger population samples before they can be used with the same precision.

The quality of motherliness or fatherliness in parent's behavior prompts nurturing and protection as opposed to neglect or abuse of the child. Cues that indicate the presence or absence of this quality appear early in the postbirth period as parents react to the newborn child and continue the process of establishing a relationship (Table 25-4).

The parents' response is profoundly affected by their interpretation of the infant's behaviors. Feedback is an important component in any relationship. Mothers and fathers make value judgments about their infant's behavior and respond as though the baby had either "praised" or "criticized" them. Table 25-5 provides a listing of infant behaviors and their evaluation by parents as either adaptive (positive feedback) or maladaptive (negative feedback).

Adaptive behaviors stem from the parents' realistic perception and acceptance of their newborn's needs and her or his limited abilities, immature social responses, and helplessness (Steele, Pollock, 1968). Parental unity can be said to be satisfactory when parents can find pleasure in their infant and in the tasks done for and with the baby; when they understand their infant's emotional states and provide comfort; and when they read the infant's cues for new experience and can sense the infant's fatigue level.

Maladaptive behaviors are exhibited when parents respond inappropriately to the needs of their infant. They expect responses from the infant far in excess of the infant's ability to perform. They interpret inadequate responses as defiance or as negative judgment of parental capabilities. They obtain no pleasure from physical contact with their child. Such infants tend to be handled roughly. They are held in a manner that allows the head to dangle without support, and they are not cuddled. The parents see the child as unattractive. The child-caring tasks of bathing and changing are viewed with disgust or annoyance. There is a lack of discrimination in responding to the infant's signals relative to hunger, fatigue, need for soothing or stimulating speech, and need for

TABLE 25-4 Mothering Behaviors*

Adaptive Behaviors	Maladaptive Behaviors
FEEDING	
Offers appropriate amount and type of food to infant	Provides inadequate type or amount of food for infant
Holds infant in comfortable position during feeding	Does not hold infant, or holds in uncomfortable position during feeding
Burps baby during and after feeding	Does not burp infant
Prepares food appropriately	Prepares food inappropriately
Offers food at comfortable pace for infant	Offers food at pace too rapid or slow for infant's comfort
INFANT STIMULATION	
Provides appropriate verbal stimulation for infant during visit	Provides no, or only aggressive, verbal stimulation for infant during visit
Provides tactile stimulation for infant at times other than during feeding or moving infant away from danger	Does not provide tactile stimulation or only that of aggressive handling of infant
Provides age-appropriate toys	No evidence of age-appropriate toys
Interacts with infant in a way that provides for infant's satisfaction	Frustrates infant during interactions
INFANT REST	
Provides quiet or relaxed environment for infant's rest, including scheduled rest periods	Does not provide quiet environment or consistent schedule for rest periods
Ensures that infant's needs for food, warmth, and dryness are met before sleep	Does not attend to infant's needs for food, warmth, and dryness before sleep
PERCEPTION	
Demonstrates realistic perception of infant's condition in accordance with medical and nursing diagnoses	Shows unrealistic perception of infant's condition
Has realistic expectations for infant	Demonstrates unrealistic expectations of infant
Recognizes infant's unfolding skills or behavior	Has no awareness of infant's development
Shows realistic perception of own mothering behavior	Shows unrealistic perception of own mothering
INITIATIVE	
Shows initiative in attempts to manage infant's problems, including actively seeking information about infants	Shows no initiative in attempts to meet infant's needs or to manage problems; does not follow through with plans
RECREATION	
Provides positive outlets for own recreation or relaxation	Does not provide positive outlets for own recreation or relaxation
INTERACTION WITH OTHER CHILDREN	
Demonstrates positive interaction with other children in home	Demonstrates hostile-aggressive interaction with other children in home
MOTHERING ROLE	
Expresses satisfaction with mothering	Expresses dissatisfaction with mothering

Reprinted by permission from Mercer RT: In Sonstegard LJ et al, editors: *Women's health: childbearing,* vol 2, New York, 1982, Grune & Stratton, Inc.
*These describe paternal as well as maternal behaviors.

comforting body or eye contact. The parents of these infants often show excessive concern over the health of their child and cannot distinguish between the expected minor illnesses of childhood and serious disabilities. It appears difficult for them to accept their child as healthy and happy.

Culturally sensitive interventions intended to establish healthy early family relationships can be the unique contribution of nursing. Healthy family relationships promote the growth potential of the newborn and other family members. Caregivers need to be alert to parents who have positive family circum-

TABLE 25-5 Infant Behaviors

Adaptive Behaviors	Maladaptive Behaviors
SLEEPING	
Receives adequate sleep for normal growth—at least 17 hours each day without restless sleep patterns or prolonged crying at nap or bedtime after other needs have been met	Receives inadequate sleep for normal growth—less than 16 hours each day; shows restless sleep patterns or prolonged crying at nap or bedtime
FEEDING	
Actively seeks food offered Actively sucks and swallows food Demonstrates pleasurable relief after eating	Resists food offered Does not suck effectively Remains fussy after adequate amount of feeding—no pleasurable relief
RESPONSE TO ENVIRONMENT	
Demonstrates active response to environment by ignoring or reaching-out behavior	Seems apathetic to environment
VOCALIZING	
Demonstrates vocalizations when alert if developmentally ready	Makes infrequent or no vocalizations during visit although developmentally ready
SMILING	
Demonstrates smiling behavior if older than 2 months	Does not demonstrate smiling behavior during visit
CUDDLING	
Cuddles when held	Resists being held or stiffens when held

Reprinted by permission from Mercer RT: In Sonstegard LJ et al, editors: *Women's health: childbearing,* vol 2, New York, 1982, Grune & Stratton, Inc.

stances, as well as to those who exhibit warning signs during the postbirth period.

PARENT-INFANT INTERACTIONS. To assess parent and child relationships and competency in child care, the nurse observes parental attitudes toward themselves and their responsibilities. The nurse assesses the mother's perceptual acuity and the amount of physical and psychic energy she possesses. Cultural or ethnic variations in maternal and paternal roles also are noted. This information provides the context within which the parents will give care to their child. Competency in child care can be determined during feeding periods or when the mother or father is giving general care to the infant. In Fig. 25-4, a nursing student observes a new father's technique as he bathes his infant.

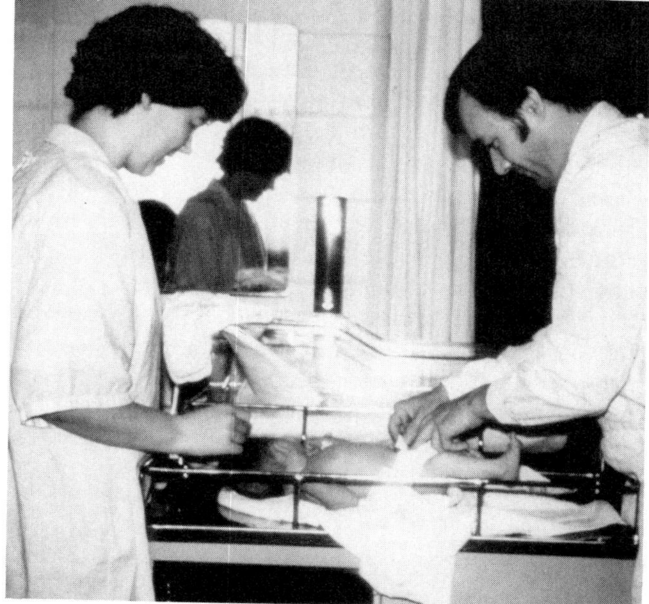

Fig. 25-4 Father bathes his infant with support of nursing student.
Courtesy Colleen Stainton, RN, DNS, University of Calgary, Alberta, Canada.

MATERNAL SELF-IMAGE. Other important psychosocial assessments that should be made by postpartum nurses relate to the woman's self-concept, her body image, and sexuality. How this new mother feels about herself and her body during the puerperium may affect her behavior and adaptation to parenting. The woman's self-concept and the view she holds of her body image also may affect her sexuality.

Feelings related to sexual adjustment after childbirth are often a cause of concern for new parents. Because many new mothers are reluctant to bring up the topic, postpartum nurses must include questions related to sexuality as an integral part of their assessment. This must be done with sensitivity because some cultural groups do not discuss these topics openly. The woman's knowledge and concerns about resumption of menstruation, sexual activity, and the use of contraceptives should be determined so that necessary teaching can take place (see boxes, pp. 726 and 727).

Cultural Considerations

In addition to the influence of cultural beliefs on a woman's physical behavior discussed earlier in this chapter, the mother's postpartum psychosocial adaptation may be affected. Some cultural beliefs may contradict the hospital practice of early ambulation after childbirth, early infant care responsibilities, and early discharge from the hospital.

Mexican-Americans may observe *la cuarentina* for 40 days after the baby's birth (Clark, 1970). For the Chinese mother, going out during the first month after birth will offend the gods because dirty birth blood remains throughout the month (Pillsbury, 1978). The Filipino mother (Stern et al, 1980) is commonly misunderstood as lazy and not caring when she refuses to do what is requested in the hospital and at home. Cambodian women may express concern about how they will manage after the baby is born because they do not have an extended family to assist during the required time of seclusion and limited activity. The fear of subsequent illness, especially arthritis, in later years is very real to them. Homemaker services are not available to them because according to the Western view, they are able-bodied and assistance cannot be justified. They believe they can counteract the bad effects of neglecting postpartum cultural proscriptions only by going through a subsequent pregnancy correctly. Their chances of "doing" future pregnancies "correctly" are remote, however. The cultural quandary for these women is clear.

The cultural knowledge of childbearing Cambodian women was studied (Kulin, 1988). A number of unique beliefs were identified: birthmarks are attributed to a mark made by soot in the person's previous life, and activities such as jumping could cause the umbilical cord to break. Herbal medicines are used prenatally to ensure a fast and short labor and to prevent the birth of a baby with vernix (Kulin, 1988). Vernix is believed to be sperm. Because sexual activity is prohibited after the sixth month of pregnancy, the presence of vernix would indicate to others the woman's transgression of this restriction.

Snow (1974) described the view of southern African Americans that blood is a pollutant that carries contaminants from the body. This group and others believe that an adequate lochia flow is essential and that going outside in the wind or air could thicken and halt the flow of blood, extending the time of pollution. Some Filipino mothers may remain bedfast for 2 weeks, after which time a special bath is taken to further remove the debris of pregnancy believed to be found in perspiration.

"Mother roasting" is an old Southeast Asian custom. In this practice the mother sits on a cane-bottom (or bamboo-slat) chair draped in a blanket from head to floor, while a bowl of glowing hot coals is placed under her. There she "roasts" until the coals are cold. This is repeated daily for 11 to 30 days. According to Stern et al (1980), "roasting" is practiced by Filipinos in the most remote provinces only. Its purpose is to hasten the healing process, much like perineal heat lamps and warm sitz baths used in recent times. At the end of the 30 to 40 days, the woman usually takes a cleansing bath. Then she resumes her normal activities in the community. Because she has been "cleansed," members of the community need not avoid contacts with a recently pregnant woman.

Some cultural groups have unique practices. For example, the women of Northern Thailand bind their wrists with string. The purpose of wrist binding is to prevent the loss of the soul, which may lead to wind disease, a specific complex of symptoms indicating a state of humoral imbalance characterized by weakness, nausea, and hypersensitivity to odors (Kundstadter, 1978). Northern Thai women giving birth will most likely have their wrists bound and would be extremely frightened and upset if the strings were removed.

It is important that nurses do not use their own cultural beliefs as a framework for care. They must assist women in carrying out their beliefs and practices as completely as possible and assist them with necessary adjustments when their expectations are not feasible. The nurse *never* assumes conformance to cultural practices by ethnic origin. Many young women who are first- or second-generation Americans follow their cultural traditions when their grandmother is present but request a shower and cold drink when the family leaves. The nurse uses discretion to assist the woman to integrate her cultural beliefs into her life-style.

Signs of Potential Problems: Psychosocial Needs

Inability or refusal to discuss labor and birth experience
Refusal to interact with or care for baby (e.g., does not name baby, does not want to hold or feed baby.)
Refusal to attend infant care (including breast-feeding) classes
Refusal to discuss contraception
Refers to self as ugly and useless
Excessive preoccupation with self (body image)
Marked depression
Lack of support system

Signs of Potential Problems

No assessment of psychosocial needs is complete without assessing for signs of potential problems. Not all potential psychosocial problems are easily identified. However, there are some signs that may indicate a need for further evaluation by a caregiver skilled in that area. Nor does the presence of one or more of these signs provide absolute proof that a problem actually exists. The box above presents some signs that may indicate a need for further assessment.

NURSING DIAGNOSES

After analyzing the data obtained from assessment, the nurse establishes nursing diagnoses that will act as guides to action. The following are examples of diagnoses that relate to postpartum clients:

- Altered family processes related to
  - —Unexpected birth of twins
- Impaired verbal communication related to
  - —Client's deafness
  - —Client's language not same as nurse's
- Altered parenting related to
  - —Long, difficult labor
  - —Unmet expectations of labor and the birth
- Knowledge/skill deficit related to
  - —Usual infant behaviors
  - —Holding, cuddling, interacting with infant
- Anxiety related to
  - —Newness of parenting role, sibling rivalry, or grandparental response
- High risk for situational low self-esteem related to
  - —Lack of knowledge of infant characteristics or of caregiving skills
  - —Grandparental responses
- Anxiety related to
  - —Insufficient knowledge of contraception and resumption of sexual activity

PLANNING

The postnatal period is a crucial one for the family. It contains the potential for crisis in family adjustment. Developing a plan of care that recognizes family strengths and provides support for family weaknesses does much to help family members take on new tasks and responsibilities.

Goals may include the following:

1. Family members express healthy self-esteem, self-concept.
2. Parents demonstrate a healthy parent-child relationship
3. They participate in the care of the infant with beginning confidence
4. They meet cultural and personal expectations of their childbirth experience
5. They verbalize a choice of contraception and understanding of sexuality after childbirth.

IMPLEMENTATION

Adaptation to the parental role is a complex process. The nurse's application of knowledge related to family dynamics after childbirth (see Chapter 24) and to psychosocial concepts in the care of new parents can help with this role transition. Psychosocial nursing care is primarily directed toward increasing the mother's mastery of the "art of motherhood," thereby increasing or sustaining her self-esteem. Nursing interventions encompass measures that encourage assertive, self-reliant behaviors in family members. Intervention strategies to promote emotional adaptation recognize the need to meet the mother's "taking-in" needs and supporting her "taking-hold" behaviors (for a discussion of these behaviors, see p. 680).

One of the new mother's first psychologic tasks is to integrate the birth experience.

Integration of the Birth Experience

The nurse who interviews a new mother about her birth experience in a thoughtful, sensitive manner has already intervened therapeutically. Inviting the new mother to review the events and describe how she felt helps her understand what happened and begin the integration process. The new mother usually initiates this portion of the interview with such statements as, "I'm sorry I . . ."; "You should have seen how I screamed . . ." "I just can't remember some things." Feelings of anger and resentment and vocalizing are understandable, temporary responses to an acute, stressful situation. The normality of these reactions can be validated by the nurse. However, statements such as "everyone does it" puts all women in the same category and may be perceived as a lack of regard for the individual (Konrad, 1987). Restating or rephrasing are useful communication techniques. These techniques help the woman fill in the whole picture for herself, reflect on her meaning behind her words, and identify connections between this experience and previous ones. The need for input regarding the birth experience is consistent with Rubin's "taking-in" phase (1961) seen in the early postpartum period (p. 680). Assisting the new mother with this postpartum psychologic task is a valuable function of the nurse. The nurse in the LDRP or SRMC setting is in an ideal position to help the new mother integrate the birth experience. In traditional settings with separate postpartum units, the labor and delivery nurse can be instrumental in this process by taking time for a follow-up visit to the new mother. The nurse can best help the mother put in perspective the events that occurred during the labor and birth process.

Other needs of the more passive taking-in phase—rest and food—should be met so that the woman can more readily move into the more independent "taking-hold" phase.

The time during which new mothers are allowed to meet their taking-in needs may contribute to their psychological adaptation to parenting. A study by Ament (1990) supports Rubin's concepts (1961) of taking-in and taking-hold (see Chapter 24). Women today were found to progress through the taking-in to the taking-hold stage much more rapidly than Rubin described, however. Ament suggests that, although the taking-in now only lasts about 24 hours, women are not ready to absorb the vast amount of information presented to them at that time because they are highly involved in taking-in phenomenon.

Because most mothers are discharged within 24 to 48 hours, teaching often takes place during a period when the mother may have difficulty absorbing a great deal of new information. Supporting the mother's attempts at taking-hold behaviors through anticipatory guidance is an important nursing intervention. Care during the early puerperium needs to reflect the mother's and father's psychologic readiness for learning new skills. Ament (1990) suggests that the presentation of only vital highlights may be more practical during the early puerperium. Parents should be encouraged to use follow-up programs—home or telephone visits when feasible (see Chapter 26).

Transition into the Parental Role

One of the main concepts to be stressed repeatedly is that parenthood is a learned role. As with any other learned role, it takes time to master, improves with experience, and evolves gradually and continually as the needs of the parents and child change.

Caplan (1957) noted that intervention during the early puerperium had a much greater influence on the attitudes of family members than it did at periods of stable emotional functioning. Therefore, care needs to reflect the mother's and father's psychologic readiness for learning new skills.

Parents have been found to be receptive to information regarding their infant's interactive capabilities during the early puerperium. During this time the parents' awareness of their own behavioral responses toward their infant can be reinforced. Parents' anxiety levels must be addressed, because anxiety can reduce their ability to learn.

Care of the newborn may be limited to feeding during the first few days. When the mother's strength returns, she also may wish to bathe and change the infant. Demonstrations and discussions of these techniques with the parents and supervision of their efforts are incorporated into the nursing care. Through the loving and attentive manner nurses exhibit while providing physical care, they act as role models. As one nurse described it:

> I found the mother crying and distraught as she wrapped and unwrapped her baby. She said, "I don't seem to be able to do anything right." I took the baby from her and talked to him. "What are you doing to your mother? You've got her all upset!" The baby alerted to my voice and looked at me. Then I said to the mother, "Now, you talk to him." She said, "You're a big lovely boy, don't cry so much." The baby hearing her voice promptly turned his head from me to look at her. I said, "You see, he knows his mother's voice and prefers it to mine." The mother was surprised and seemed very pleased and excited. We then reviewed how to wrap a baby snugly.

Recognition and praise of her successes increase the mother's feeling of competence and control in her ability to mother. Feelings of self-esteem in the mother are increased through positive feedback. Fig. 25-5 shows a feedback circle in which the left side presents an example of a positive mother-infant interaction based on the sequence outlined on the right side.

Researchers in their studies of mother-infant in-

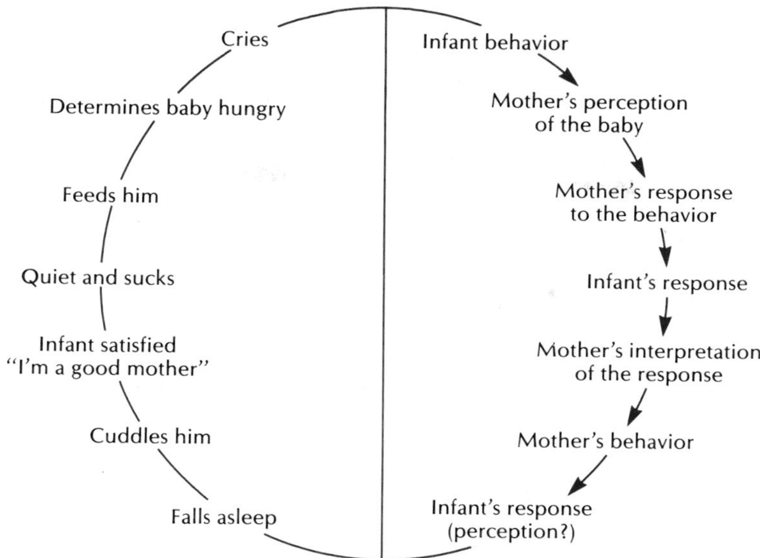

Fig. 25-5 Maternal-infant feedback mechanisms.
From Stainton MC: *Assessment and support of healthy parent-child relationships.* Proceedings of POGP: Pediatrics, Obstetrics and Gynaecology Workshop for Nurses, Saskatoon, 1977, University of Saskatchewan.

teractions have used various techniques to promote the mother's awareness of the behavioral and social capabilities of their newborns. In one of Field's early studies (1977) mothers were asked to imitate their babies rather than attempt to keep their babies' attention. By doing this the mothers decreased their activities and increased responsiveness to infant behavior. By advising mothers to repeat phrases and to be silent during gaze aversion, Field noted mothers were increasingly sensitive to their infants' behavioral cues and responsive to their signals. (see discussion of synchrony p. 676). Anderson (1981) combined providing information to the mother about neonatal behavior with a demonstration of the infant's behavior as a means of enhancing the quality of mother-infant interaction. Riesch and Munns (1985) provided an audiotape with accompanying text for the mothers to listen to privately. They reported the following:

> Mothers who received the intervention to inform them of the neonate's social capabilities and of the maternal behaviors to enhance and support their infants reported significantly more of their own behavior than did mothers who did not receive the treatment. Awareness of one's own behavior undoubtedly was a significant factor in the mother's reporting of her own behavior that her infant noticed.

The new mother is concerned about how she will perform her new role; she needs to meet her own expectations and those of others in the performance of her maternal role (Humenick, Bugen, 1987). The mother's expectations may or may not be realistic. Unrealistic expectations may serve as a detriment to a mother's accomplishments. Informing the mother of the responses she can initiate in order to enhance or support her particular infant may relieve some of her role uncertainty, thus allowing her to interact freely with her infant.

Because of the sheltered environment provided after childbirth, women may misjudge the actual amount of physical and psychic energy they possess. They may expect to resume tasks too soon and then feel discouraged when they are not able to do so. Their still-pregnant look prompts well-meaning people to ask them when they expect their baby (Fig. 25-6). These remarks can add to the mother's feelings of discouragement. In addition, the baby's behavior does not always meet expectations. Sore nipples, worry about adequate milk supply, or even lack of sensations anticipated with breast-feeding can lead to a mother's disappointment. Some babies cry more than expected or do not seem satisfied with their feedings. Many babies have fussy periods that do not respond to any ministrations:

> But my husband, too, was disconcerted at first, for the intense, unending plaintive cries of our firstborn reached to the very depths of our hearts. And we both had really believed that, somehow, a baby born naturally at home and never separated from his mother would not be so fretful. However, it becomes apparent that all babies cry.*

Mothers also are faced with the need to help siblings adjust to the new sister or brother. **Sibling rivalry** (competition between brothers and sisters) may

*Lang R: *Birth book,* Ben Lomond, Calif, 1972, Genesis Press.

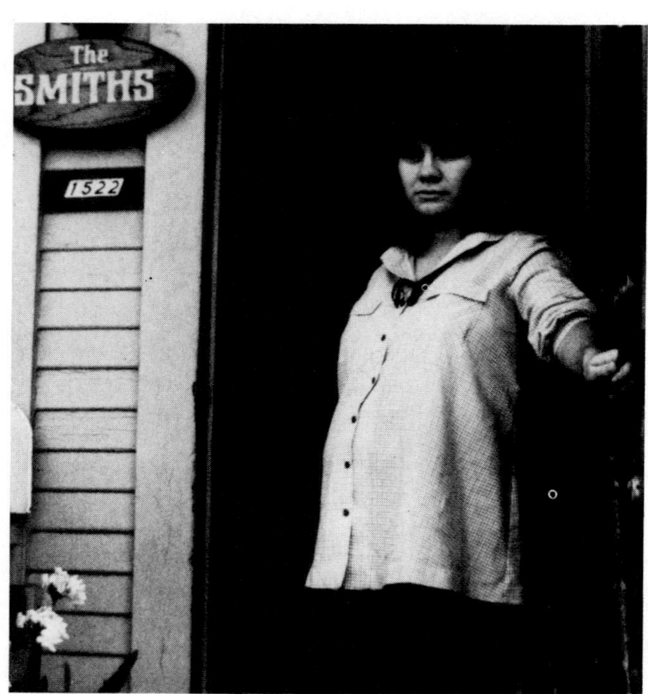

Fig. 25-6 Lack of abdominal muscle tone shortly after childbirth gives mother still-pregnant appearance.
Courtesy Marjorie Pyle, RNC, Lifecircle, Costa Mesa, Calif.

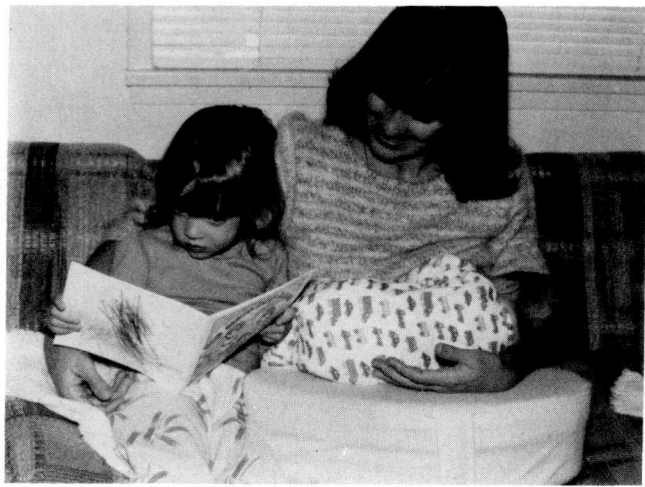

Fig. 25-7 Mother shares feeding time of newborn with older sibling. Baby is supported on an adjustable pad (Keiki Designs).
Courtesy Marjorie Pyle, RNC, Lifecircle, Costa Mesa, Calif.

require parental time and attention to be handled successfully (Fig. 25-7). Even if the children have participated in planning for the new baby, they may be unable to accept the reality of diminished parental attention. Their behavior may reflect their feelings of frustration.

Forewarning about the possibility of such happenings even in the best-regulated homes permits the parents to judge themselves less harshly. They are better prepared to seek assistance, change routine, or accept the happening as a passing phase.

Family Adjustment and Crisis Prevention

Nursing care of the postpartum mother must include interaction with the family. The entire family (mother, father, siblings, and grandparents) needs to be aware of the difficulties, as well as the joys, brought by a new family member. Knowledge of the potential pitfalls can help family members prevent crisis situations from developing. Postpartum nurses have an excellent opportunity to instruct mothers and their families about the transition into the parental role. They should discuss the problems families commonly encounter, as well as potential coping mechanisms and support systems.

POSTPARTUM DEPRESSION. **Depressive states,** often called **the baby blues,** may occur after childbirth and should not be dismissed lightly (Hansen, 1990; Martell, 1990). Symptoms begin 2 or 3 days after the birth and usually disappear within a week or two. The woman experiences a letdown feeling accompanied by irritability. She may cry easily, lose her appetite, have trouble sleeping, and feel anxious. Mothers of preterm infants have been found to initially experience higher levels of anxiety and depression (Gennaro, 1988). Severe depressive psychosis occurs rarely (see Chapter 33).

The nurse can best assist the woman and family by assuring them that this depression is both normal and temporary. Recognizing the state, helping the woman verbalize her feelings, and providing support and understanding are important nursing actions. The nurse can explain to the woman and family that the depression may be caused by hormonal changes, emotional reaction to the role transition, discomfort, or fatigue. Setting up tasks the woman can accomplish easily and successfully are interventions that can help counteract the feelings of depression. It also is important to encourage adequate rest and nutrition. Because the woman will likely experience symptoms after discharge, the nurse should always include the woman's partner in all interventions to support the woman and to express concerns.

INFANT CRYING. Babies cry because they are hungry or wet, too hot or too cold, because they are ill, or simply because they want attention. And, if the baby is crying just to be held, who is to say that this is not a legitimate reason to cry? The way babies cry seems to contain the message they want to convey. Parents soon recognize the difference between cries. When parents want to respond to their baby's cry, they need to be encouraged not to be put off by friends or relatives who say they are spoiling the child. *A tiny infant cannot be spoiled.* Bell and Ainsworth (1972) found that "mothers who ignore and delay in responding to the crying of an infant when he is tiny have babies who cry more frequently and persistently later on." A baby's cry requires an investigation to identify the specific need.

Nurses, and often knowledgeable grandparents, have a special role in helping parents and baby synchronize (Darbyshire, 1985). Reciprocal signalling and responding is an important part of parenting (Lamb, 1981) (see discussion of reciprocity. p. 676). Attachment is greatly enhanced for the mother/parent who is able to detect and respond to the baby's distress signals and who can comfort and console the baby effectively (Darbyshire, 1985). Conversely, the effect on a mother/parent faced with a crying, fussing, irritable, and unconsolable baby can be devastating for all concerned (Kirkland, 1985; Mortimer and Kevill, 1985).

Life with a crying baby can create a crisis situation. Eventually, parents are "ground down," worrying that something is wrong, facing guilt and loss of self-esteem about their inability to comfort a crying baby. Physical and emotional fatigue compound the crisis.

Parents benefit from concrete suggestions. Knowing that "all parents go through this" is not helpful. If the crying signal is not yet set, several possibilities are explored and tested—hunger, cold, wet diaper. Pain is suspected if there are areas of redness or diaper rash. Loneliness, the need to make contact, may be the sole cause. First the cold, hunger, wet diaper, and pain are treated. Then other comforting techniques are used—carrying and rocking, sounds, nonnutritive sucking, swaddling, and **infant massage** (see box, p. 722).

People who care for newborns soon become aware that rocking a crying baby vertically and intermittently promotes a "bright-alert" state, whereas continuous horizontal rocking induces the baby to sleep (Byrne Horowitz, 1981). Studies also have shown that the ideal rate to rock a baby is around 60 to 90 rocks a minute (Pederson, 1975.)

The sound of a human voice or soft music can be an effective means to soothe a baby. The old practice of swaddling (wrapping snugly) has been found to pacify some infants. Nonnutritive sucking on a pacifier is another effective method. (See Chapter 21 for the use of safe pacifiers.) Infant massage has benefits for both parent and child.

SIBLINGS AND GRANDPARENTS. Preparation of siblings and parents for the reactions of siblings begins before childbirth. Preparation of siblings and grandparents is discussed in Chapter 13.

Classes for grandparents-to-be are designed to help the givers and receivers of advice understand one another (see Chapter 13) and update the grandparents to contemporary thinking. Examples of contemporary child-rearing theories with which grandparents may be unfamiliar are that one cannot spoil a newborn, breast-feeding is superior to formula-feeding, and bright colors are better than pastels for the baby's room because they are more stimulating. Safer infant car seats and disposable diapers are advances that most grandparents readily appreciate.

Few people move gracefully or fearlessly into new identities. Nurses support the grandparents who are the role models and support network for the new parents. Nurses also help new parents bridge the generation gap by keeping communication open. On occasion, the nurse suggests the "scripts" parents need to develop to achieve the kind of loving relationship they would like to have. Many hospitals distribute pamphlets to grandparents concerning the topic of helping the new parents "without interfering." Several publications on the topic are available at local bookstores.

MULTIFETAL BIRTH. The mother with a multifetal pregnancy (e.g., twins) requires the same physical care as any other new mother. She is more at risk for postbirth hemorrhage because of excessive uterine distention. Therefore she must be carefully assessed.

Psychologically, however, even the most willing of mothers can find their coping-mechanisms overwhelmed by both the idea and the reality of caring for two or more newborns. Mother-child attachment takes longer because the mother attaches first to one newborn and then to the other. Nurses must help parents organize simplified and flexible plans of care. The almost constant attention required until the infants' schedule of care can be synchronized may prove exhausting. If possible, help is obtained, particularly to guarantee sufficient rest for the mother. The added expense also can be burdensome to a young family. One mother expressed anger at the surprise birth of twins. The explanation of such errors did not placate her. She needed time to vent these feelings before she could be helped with changing her anticipated plan for care. Some communities have support groups for parents of twins, and these can be a great resource for new parents. Another resource that may

TEACHING Infant Massage

"When from the wearying ware of life
I seek release,
I look into my baby's face,
And there find peace."
—Martha F. Crow

Benefits to you, the parent:
Helps you recognize infant's cues
Soothes baby and reduces effects of stress caused by potentially overwhelming new environment
Provides baby with regular nurturing attention
Deepens attachment between parent and child
Provides fun and feels good.

Appropriate materials:
Assemble 2-3 pillows, 2 towels, a change of diapers and clothes
Purchase cold-pressed vegetable oil: almond, apricot kernel, sunflower, safflower, or coconut oil; powder.
CAUTION: Do not use mineral oil (leaches vitamins D, E, and K from skin) and scented oils or any product if baby has developed rashes from it.

To provide conducive environment:
Choose place that is warm, quiet, dimly lit, out of mainstream of activity.
Choose time when parent and baby are in good mood; use relaxation methods first if needed before starting.

To avoid injury to baby:
Handle infant gently; avoid jerking, pulling.
Place infant on lap or sit on floor with infant between legs.
Avoid creating cloud of powder near infant's face.

Head

Do not use oil on head and face.
Caution parents against jabbing or poking.
Demonstrate technique, using gentle pressure as thumbs are moved outward.
Smile at baby.

- Do gentle head "tapping" around base of neck and skull.†
- Once eyes are closed, place thumbs together over bridge of nose and move thumbs outward, gently over eyes; repeat over bridge of nose and outward over checks; repeat over lips and move thumbs outward in a "smile."
- With two fingers of each hand starting at forehead, make small circles around face at hairline and under chin.
- Gently massage each ear between thumb and forefinger; do one ear at a time.

Chest

Apply 1-2 tablespoons vegetable oil over hands.

- Do "open book" over infant's stomach. Starting with both hands flat over chest, make heart-shaped pattern down sides and over groin three or four times.
  Use this pattern:

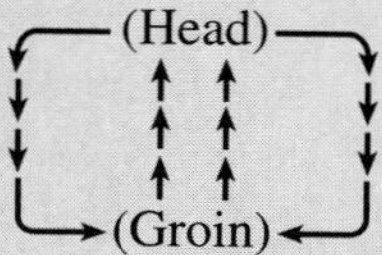

- Place hands together over abdomen, press in gently, and push outward to sides; hold baby under buttocks while thumbs are on abdomen.
- Do "butterfly." Place one hand on infant's shoulder, pull downward to opposite groin; repeat with other hand.
  Repeat each technique three or four times.

To avoid stressing baby:
Watch for infant's cues to end massage; fussing, squirming, turning away.
Talk to infant, sing, hum, smile.
Limit massage to 20 minutes.

To perform massage:
Read Schneider or LeBoyer reference, and follow pictures, because not all the techniques can appear here.*

To perform techniques:
Greet infant: "Hi, I love you."

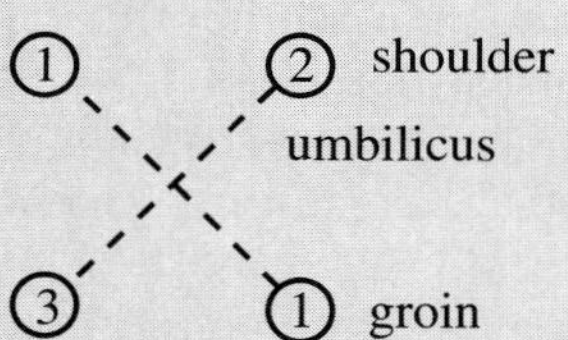

Stomach

- Do waterwheel: with outside edge of one hand, start at umbilicus and move hand downward to groin; alternate hands like a water wheel.

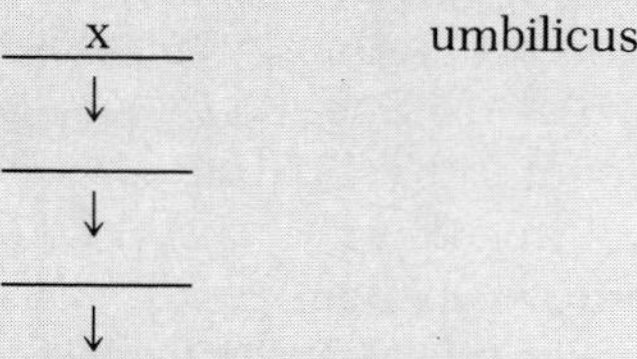

This technique is good for helping the baby with gas.

*Leboyer F: *Loving hands,* New York, 1981, Alfred A. Knopf; Schneider V: *Infant massage: handbook for loving parents,* New York, 1982, Bantam Books.
†Each bullet starts a new technique.

TEACHING Infant Massage—cont'd

- Place thumbs together in center of abdomen, then pull out to sides.
- Perform "I love you" using this pattern

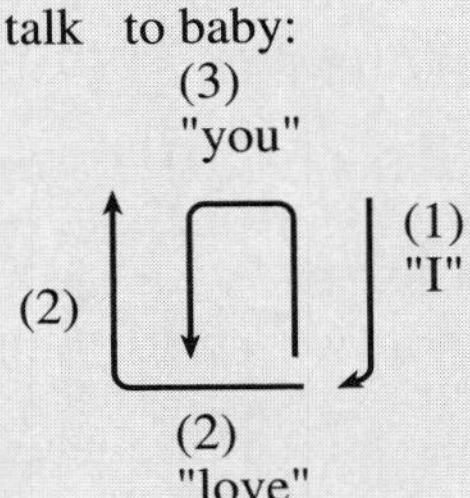

- Perform "walking": tap with fingers of both hands simultaneously, over infant's abdomen.

Arms

- Perform "Indian (Swedish) milking": hold one hand at wrist, encircle wrist with other hand and "milk" downward.
  Repeat with other arm.
- Perform rolling: between palms of both hands, roll infant's arm back and forth; repeat with other arm.

Hands

- Make little circles in palms of each hand; then gently pull on each finger.

Legs and Feet

- Push on bottom of foot with both thumbs, making small circles; pull on each toe; roll leg between both hands; press on dorsal surface of foot to gently plantarflex foot.

Back

Carefully turn infant back onto abdomen.

- Perform "butterfly" technique making an "X" over baby's back down to the buttocks, starting at the shoulders. Use one hand at a time.
- Make small circles over baby's back with fingers of both hands simultaneously; start at shoulders and move down to buttocks.
- Perform "milking" with one hand, starting at shoulders, moving to feet. Use other hand to support infant.

Ending

- "Comb" infant's back with fingers of both hands simultaneously, starting at shoulders, moving to feet. Gradually lighten pressure so that last "combing" is barely touching skin.

Variations

Teach older child who can perform massage on doll with mother.

Learn technique during prenatal period by practicing on maternal abdomen.

be available is a list of community agencies or retail operations that provide services to parents of twins; this may be useful in easing the added financial burden.

Most parents are anxious to know if their children are identical or fraternal. Gross examination of the placenta at birth cannot prove whether twins are identical. Therefore it is best to tell parents that the distinction cannot be made at this time.

If the infants are born prematurely or are small-for-gestational age, their prolonged hospital stay can cause parental separation anxiety. If this is the case, the mother may be encouraged to visit or care for the infant in the hospital. She can use this waiting time to recover as much physical strength as possible. It provides time for the family to prepare for the infants' homecoming. Introduction of multiple siblings into a family also can result in intense rivalry. All children compete for the mother's attention. Substitute mothering by interested relatives can do much to ease the strain.

Coping Mechanisms and Support Systems

Family commitments involve having both time and energy for individual family members—mother, father, and children. In addition to learning the techniques for care of themselves and their babies, parents have found other suggestions helpful in coping with readjusting their lives. A list of these suggestions can be given to new parents, but discussion of specific ways of handling them also is necessary (see box, p. 724). These suggestions may need to be tailored to the cultural needs and expectations of the family.

The North American culture emphasizes the instinctual aspects of motherhood. As a result, many parents hesitate to seek help from nurses, physicians, family, and friends. Long-term support by nurses or physicians is a positive factor in the ultimate adjustment of the family. Besides providing emotional sup-

TEACHING Coping Mechanisms

- *Set priorities for tasks.* Many tasks can be left for a later period or done by others. Be firm about not taking on extra tasks for family, friends, or community. Try not to schedule a move to a new location soon after giving birth.
- *Do not become overly concerned with appearances*—tidiness in the home is not as important as time spent with the family. Taking up the role of "super housekeeper" can be postponed until other adjustments are made.

  Sometimes new mothers become overburdened with visits from relatives eager "to take over the baby." Husbands or partners can help redirect these well-meaning people toward helping with the housework and cooking. This leaves the parent free to interact with the child.
- *Get plenty of rest and sleep;* rearrange schedules if necessary. Because naps may not be possible if there are other children in the family, going to bed early is recommended; let friends know when to visit.
- *Do not undertake the care of another incapacitated relative* at this point; such responsibilities should be undertaken by other family members.
- *Arrange for some time away from the baby;* enlist the help of friends, family, or others for baby-sitting. Relaxation for parents is necessary. Baby-sitting, if at all possible, must be planned and a regular schedule developed. This includes time off during the day so that you can get away from the home and its responsibilities. In some localities, churches or other agencies have developed programs attuned to the needs of mothers. The young children are cared for while the mothers take part in activities with other mothers. This helps them establish relationships with others who also are involved in the care of young children. A mutual sharing of successes and failures in this regard helps a new mother maintain a feeling of equilibrium.

  At the very least you need to plan to get out of the house at least once each day. Access to a car and being able to drive are assets. Taking the baby out for a walk or shopping helps break up the daily routine.
- *Make plans regarding fertility management* before intercourse is resumed and the possibility of pregnancy arises.
- *Be open in your communication with others.* Share incidents of delight or of worry with others. Be open in your requests for support. Discussions with other mothers are helpful.
- *Learn what health facilities are available,* for example, well-baby centers, immunization clinics, mother-infant classes (e.g., exercise, massage) and how to get in touch with the physician or nurse. If you have questions, remember that the hospital is open all day and night and you can call the emergency or maternity department at any time.
- *Prepare for returning to work.* Most women are physically able to return to work by the end of the sixth week. If plans for child care were not in place before the birth, adjustments for child care must be made. Ideally a substitute parent would be one who could come to the home and provide love, as well as care, for the child. Some parents are fortunate enough to have grandparents or other relatives willing and able to fill such a role. Others must take the child to another person's home or a day-care center early in the morning and pick the child up at night. The care provided by day-care centers is needed by some children whose mothers must work to help support them or who are the sole support of the child. For families who require this type of service, assistance in locating such help can be obtained from the local health department and parent referrals. Unfortunately there are not enough quality places available for all children requiring day-care.
- *Include the father/partner in caregiving activities.* Research shows that most fathers/partners participate in infant care to the extent that the mother allows (Stainton, 1985).

port, families and friends can assist with housework, baby-sitting with older children, and eventually, the new baby. Being able to verbalize experiences with others who are interested and experienced also tends to reassure the new mother. A mother, in discussing visits by the family to see the new baby, commented as follows:

> I want the family to come. You people praise him so and think he is the most wonderful baby. All my friends have their own babies and are too busy trying to get compliments for them to give us any. All babies need aunties and grandmothers!

Providing information about the availability of health facilities and telling the family how to get in touch with the nurse or physician relieves new parents of feeling total responsibility for the health of the new baby.

Home visits by nurses can be used to relieve stress and help parents anticipate and prepare for other

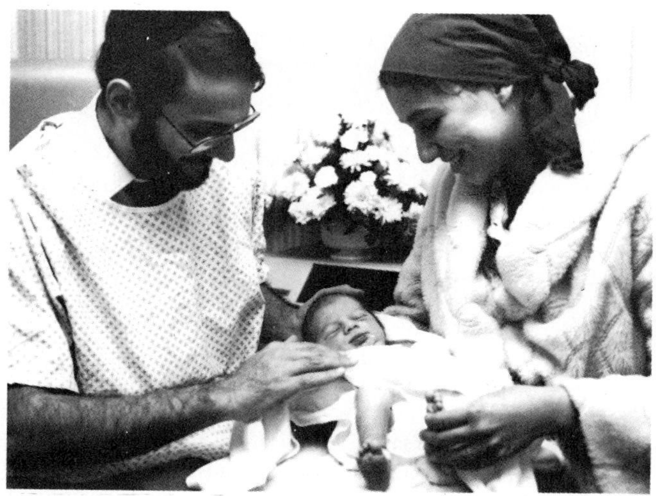

Fig. 25-8 Parents admire their new baby.

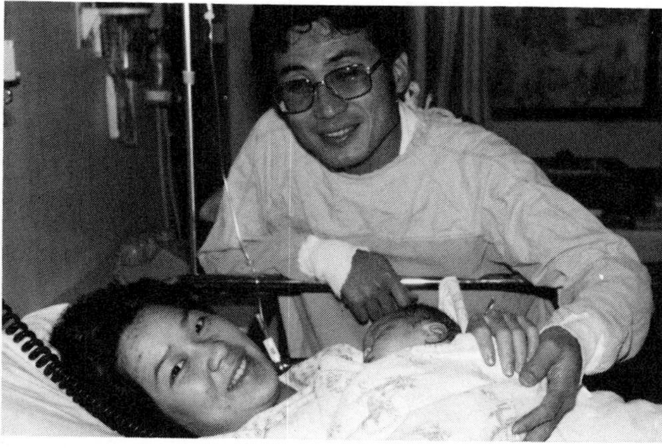

Fig. 25-9 New parents after the cesarean birth of their daughter.

possible stresses (see Chapter 26). Hospital stays are short; the parents leave the hospital in the "honeymoon" phase of transition. The realities of recovery and the parenting role become evident quickly, especially for those without assistance in the home. Rubin (1961) defines this as *letting go*. Parental expectations of each other, even if discussed thoroughly prenatally, usually do not go as expected by either partner (Humenick, Bugen, 1987). Parents need to be encouraged to communicate openly with each other regarding their stresses. Some anticipatory guidance before discharge and during the home visit may enable new parents to negotiate constructively any conflicts they may experience in their new roles and to have more realistic expectations of each other and the baby and baby care. Visits may be spaced to take into account potential stress time, such as 2 or 3 days after coming home from the hospital and the third and sixth weeks at home (see Chapter 26).

Nursing Strategies to Meet Changing Parental Needs

The infant, parents, and family must pass through three distinct periods as the parents learn more about the infant, themselves, and their relationship to the family. These three periods are known as the early, consolidation, and growth periods.

EARLY PERIOD. The nurse encourages infant contact during the early period by timing the contact with the newborn's normal wake/sleep cycles. The parents are encouraged to care for and examine the infant as the nurse describes any normal variations. The couples in Figs. 25-8 and 25-9 are obviously pleased with their new babies. The parents are given a demonstration of infant care, beginning with the use of a bulb syringe. Videotapes and written materials may supplement actual demonstrations. The family is introduced to the infant, with reassurance provided to the siblings as appropriate for their age.

CONSOLIDATION PERIOD. This is the time when the infant, parents, and family are working together to incorporate the new person into the family. Parents should be praised for their successes in caring for the infant. They need to discuss their role as parents and their response to the complexities of the role. Support people, such as social service workers, may be contacted to provide additional support if the family expresses a need. The nurse should discuss typical sibling reactions and explore with the parents methods of coping with difficult family situations.

GROWTH PERIOD. This period may not begin until weeks after the birth, when the family can absorb more information regarding growth and development of the infant and family. The parents are taught normal physical and psychosocial growth and development patterns. This may include concrete information about adding solids to the infant's diet or the type of toy appropriate to stimulate the baby. The parents are encouraged to discuss any problems in child care (e.g., feeding problems) and how they react to the infant. Parents may be referred to telephone crisis centers or social service agencies if problems are identified. The nurse also will discuss with the parents and families their reactions, including sibling reaction or demands placed on other family members. The parents in Fig. 25-10 share their at-

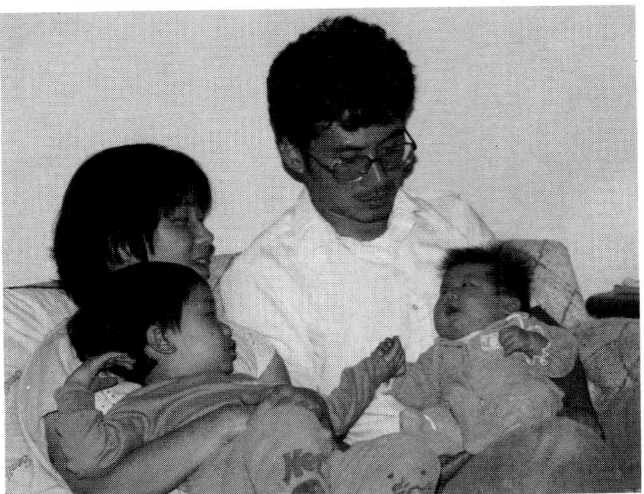

Fig. 25-10 Healthy family relationships promote the growth potential of the newborn and other family members.

tention with the new baby and her older brother. Anticipatory guidance also includes helping new parents explore coping mechanisms during the transition to parenthood.

■ DISCHARGE FROM HOSPITAL

Bridging the gap between hospital and home care requires sensitive and knowledgeable nursing care. Discharge planning and extended postpartum care are discussed in detail in Chapter 26. Criteria for early discharge are presented in Table 26-1. Before a client leaves the hospital, her readiness for learning should be determined. A teaching plan is developed that may include the following: resumption of sexual intercourse, postbirth contraception, postpartum home visits, telephone follow-up, warm lines/help lines, and support groups (see Chapter 26).

Some parents are interested in hearing about resumption of sexual intercourse (see box at right) and postbirth contraception (see box, p. 727). The nurse can offer parents the opportunity to discuss these topics.

Just before the time of discharge the nurse reviews the client's chart (audits the chart) to see that laboratory reports, medications, signatures, and so on are in order. Some hospitals have a checklist to follow before the client's discharge. The nurse verifies that medications, if ordered, have arrived on the unit, that

TEACHING Resumption of Sexual Intercourse

You can safely resume sexual intercourse by the third or fourth postbirth week if bleeding has stopped and the episiotomy has healed. For the first 6 weeks to 6 months the vagina does not lubricate well because steroid depletion inhibits the vasocongestive response to sexual tension.

Your physiologic reactions to sexual stimulation for the first 3 postbirth months are marked by a reduction in both rapidity and intensity of response. Vasocongestion of the labia majora and minora is delayed well into the plateau phase. The walls of the vagina are thin and pink, a condition similar to senile vaginitis. This results from the hormonal starvation of the involutional period. Finally, the size of the orgasmic platform and strength of the orgasmic contractions are reduced.

A water-soluble gel, cocoa butter, or a contraceptive cream or jelly might be recommended for lubrication. If some vaginal tenderness is present, your partner can be instructed to insert one or more clean, lubricated fingers into the vagina and rotate them within the vagina to help relax it and to identify possible areas of discomfort. A coital position in which the woman has control of the depth of the penile penetration also is useful. The side-by-side or female-superior position often is recommended.

The presence of the baby influences postbirth lovemaking. Parents hear every sound made by the baby; conversely they may be concerned that the baby hears every sound they make. In either case any phase of the sexual response cycle may be interrupted by hearing the baby cry or move, leaving one partner or both frustrated and unsatisfied. The amount of psychologic energy expended by the parents in child care activities may lead to fatigue. Newborns require a great deal of attention and time, not to mention what is necessary to take care of twins or triplets, and older children as well.

Some women have reported sexual stimulation to plateau and orgasmic levels when nursing their babies. Although nursing mothers have a longer delay in ovarian steroid production, they often are interested in returning to sexual activity before nonnursing mothers. Nursing mothers also report higher levels of postbirth eroticism.

You should be instructed to perform the Kegel exercises to strengthen your pubococcygeal muscle. This muscle is the major sphincter of the pelvis. It is associated with bowel and bladder function and with vaginal perception and response during intercourse.

TEACHING Postbirth Contraception

Women *may* not ovulate while they successfully breast-feed their infants because ovarian functions *usually* are suppressed by a high level of serum prolactin. Therefore breast-feeding is *not* a contraceptive method.

Follicle formation usually is suspended, and ovulation usually does not occur.

Women who do not breast-feed frequently or on demand (e.g., every 3 to 4 hours) or who *supplement the infant's feeding* do not maintain an effectively high level of serum prolactin. If these women do not employ contraceptives, they may conceive again, sometimes without having a menstrual period after the previous pregnancy.

If the mother is not breast-feeding, she may resume use of oral contraceptives (after the birth) under the physician's direction. If she is breast-feeding, barrier contraception, such as a diaphragm, condom, gel, or foam, should be employed until the first postbirth examination, at which time the desired method can be instituted (see Chapter 42).

any valuables kept secured during the client's stay have been returned to her and that she has signed a receipt for them, and that the infant is ready to be discharged.

The nurse is careful not to administer any medication that would make the mother sleepy if she is the one who will be holding the baby on the way out of the hospital. In most instances, the woman is seated in a wheelchair and usually is given the baby to hold. Some families leave unescorted and ambulatory, depending on hospital protocol. The woman's possessions are gathered and taken out with her and her family; usually they are placed on some type of cart or carried by family members. *The woman's and the baby's identification bands are carefully checked.* As the client and the baby are assisted into the car, the nurse should make sure that there is a car seat in which to secure the baby.

CAUTION: Whether or not the woman and her family have chosen early discharge, the nurse and the physician are held responsible if the woman is discharged before her condition has stabilized within normal limits. If complications occur, the medical and nursing staff could be sued for "abandonment."

EVALUATION

Evaluation is a continuous process. Parental, infant, and family relationships are consistently assessed as indicators of healthy family adjustments after the birth of a child. The nurse can be reasonably assured that care was effective to the extent that the goals for care have been met; that is, the parents express a healthy self-esteem, demonstrate a healthy parent-child relationship, participate in the care of the newborn, reconcile their childbirth experience with their cultural and personal expectations, and verbalize their choice of contraception and understanding of sexuality after childbirth.

A case study (p. 728) and nursing plan of care (p. 729) detail three common concerns of new mothers: hemorrhage, perineal discomfort, and getting sufficient rest. The case study and nursing plan of care provide examples of how a nurse can integrate content from Chapters 23 through 25.

■ SUMMARY

The normal postpartum period is a time of rapid change. Physiologic and psychosocial change takes place in the woman, the newborn, and their family. The nurse who makes pertinent assessments, plans and implements client-centered care, and evaluates the effectiveness of the care plays an important role in the health of the child-bearing family.

CASE STUDY

Spontaneous Vaginal Birth

Mary Williams, a 24-year-old first-time mother experienced a spontaneous vaginal birth with a midline episiotomy after 15 hours of labor and epidural anesthesia. She plans to breast-feed her healthy daughter, who weighs 9 pounds 2 ounces. She is admitted to the postpartum unit after 2 hours in the recovery room.

ASSESSMENT

The recovery nurse's report to the postpartum nurse includes the following information. Mary had a period of heavy vaginal bleeding after the birth; however, her fundus is now firm, and the lochia is moderate rubra. Her vital signs are temperature 99° F, BP 110/70 mm Hg, pulse 80 beats/min, respirations 18/min. An IV infusion of 5% dextrose and ½ normal saline with Pitocin is infusing at 20 drops per minute. Although fatigued and hungry, Mary and her husband, who was with her throughout the labor and birth, verbalize their excitement about the birth of their daughter.

Three hours after admission to the postpartum unit Mary complains of perineal pain and increased fatigue. She asks "Why is there so much bleeding?" Her vital signs are now BP 110/70 mm Hg, pulse 80 beats/min, respirations 20/min. Mary's uterus was found to be one finger-breadth above and to the right of the umbilicus and boggy. Her lochia had increased, with one peripad saturated in less than 1 hour. Several small clots also were expelled.

NURSING DIAGNOSIS

On the basis of the assessment the nurse identifies the nursing diagnosis: High risk for fluid volume deficit related to uterine atony.

PLANNING

A plan of care is developed with Mary's input. The mutually agreed upon *goal* for Mary is that the uterine bleeding will be controlled and will progress at expected levels while ensuring her rest and comfort levels. The nurse sets the following *expected outcomes*: no hemorrhage as evidenced by vital signs within normal limits, fundus firm and midline, lochia moderate, and client resting comfortably.

IMPLEMENTATION

Nursing actions are derived from medical management, physician's orders, and nursing diagnoses. Specific interventions will include assessment of vital signs, uterine tone, lochia flow, and bladder fullness. Uterine massage is performed, and Mary is encouraged to empty her bladder as indicated. The nurse will monitor prescribed IV therapy of oxytocic medication. When Mary's fatigue and pain are controlled, self-care activities, including fundal massage, are taught and encouraged.

EVALUATION

The expected outcomes were used to evaluate the effectiveness of these interventions. Mary experienced no further episodes of increased bleeding. Within 30 minutes her fundus was firm in midline at the level of the umbilicus. The lochia was rubra and moderate. Her vital signs were BP 110/70 mm Hg, pulse 70 beats/min, respirations 18/min.

On the basis of these findings the goal set for Mary was met (See the related plan of care.)

CARE PLAN Spontaneous Vaginal Birth

GOAL	IMPLEMENTATION	RATIONALE	EVALUATION
Nursing Diagnosis: High risk for fluid volume deficit related to uterine atony			
Mary's fundus will remain firm, lochia moderate without evidence of hemorrhage.	Assess tone and response to gentle massage.	Massage promotes contraction of uterus. Continued assessment determines need for further interventions.	Mary's fundus firm at midline, lochia rubra and moderate in amount.
	Check IV flow of oxytocin (Pitocin).	Pitocin stimulates uterine contraction; adequate infusion maintains level of oxytocin.	Mary's vital signs are normal and stable.
	Express clots.	Empties uterus and promotes contractions.	Mary demonstrates ability to assess and massage uterus.
	Assess bladder for fullness and encourage voiding.	Full bladder interferes with uterine contraction.	
	Assess amount and character of lochia.	Indicates amount of blood loss.	
	Assess vital signs.	Further indication of amount of blood loss.	
	Teach Mary how to assess and massage fundus.	Involvement in own self-care maintains sense of control.	
Nursing Diagnosis: Perineal pain related to episiotomy and hemorrhoids			
Mary will state decreasing level of pain in the perineal area.	Explain and demonstrate:	Knowledge promotes selfcare.	Mary states stitches and hemorrhoids feel more comfortable.
	Use of hot or cold procedures to perineal area	Decreases pain: heat increases circulation; cold decreases edema.	
Mary will state and demonstrate understanding of proper perineal self-care techniques.	Perineal hygiene: proper wiping, proper changing, and placement of peripad	Prevents contamination and infection that could cause pain.	Mary performs self-perineal care using proper technique at appropriate time.
	Side-lying position and sitting technique through tensing of gluteal muscles	Decreases pressure on area.	
	Use of analgesics	Reduces pain perception.	
Nursing Diagnosis: Sleep pattern disturbances related to excitement, interrupted sleep, and discomfort			
Mary will state ability to sleep restfully and to feel rested while awake.	Individualize nursing routine to fit Mary's schedule.	Promotes individual sleep pattern.	Mary states, "I slept well during night and at nap time."
	Keep noise level in hall and at nursing station to minimum; close Mary's door while resting.	Reduces distracting external stimuli.	
	Arrange uninterrupted nap while baby sleeps.		Mary states, "I feel rested and refreshed."
	Advise Mary to limit visitors and telephone calls.		
	Discuss with Mary techniques used by her in the past to promote rest, for example, warm drink, reading, TV at bedtime.	Provides feeling of control. Promotes relaxation.	
	Provide specific comfort measures if experiencing pain: back rub, analgesics.	Reduces pain and tension. Promotes relaxation and rest.	

REFERENCES

Aderhold KJ, Perry L: Jet hydrotherapy for labor and postpartum pain relief, *MCN* 16:97, 1991.

Ahumada LS: Multicultural perinatal health care, *Matern Child Health Educ Resources* 6, Spring 1991 (Center for Health Educaiton Resources).

Baca J: Some health beliefs of the Spanish-speaking. In Reinhardt AM, Quinn MD, editors: *Family-centered community nursing*, St Louis, 1973, Mosby–Year Book.

Bell RQ, Ainsworth MDS: Infant crying and maternal responsiveness. *Child Dev* 43:1171, 1972.

Byrne JM, Horowitz FS: Rocking as a soothing intervention: the influence of direction and type of movement, *Infant Behav Dev* 4:207, 1981.

Campbell T, Chang B: Health care of the Chinese in America. In Spradley BW, editor: *Contemporary community nursing*, Boston, 1975, Little, Brown & Co.

Caplan G: Psychological aspects of maternity care, *Am J Public Health* 47:25, 1957.

Cassidy CM: Subcultural prenatal diets of Americans. In *Alternative dietary practices and nutritional abuses in pregnancy: proceedings of a workshop*, Washington, DC, 1982, National Academy Press.

Chung HJ: Understanding the Oriental maternity patient, *Nurs Clin North Am* 12:67, 1977.

Clark M: *Health in the Mexican-American culture: a community study*, Berkeley, Calif, 1970, University of California Press.

Cunningham FG, MacDonald PC, Gant NF: *Williams Obstetrics*, ed 18, Norwalk, Conn., 1989, Appleton & Lange.

Currier RL: The hot-cold syndrome and symbolic balance in Mexican and Spanish-American folk medicine. In Martinez RA, editor: *Hispanic culture and health care: fact, fiction, folklore*, St Louis, 1978, Mosby–Year Book.

Darbyshire P: Comfort for the crying child, *Nurs Times*, p 59, Sept 11, 1985.

Droegemueller W: Cold sitz bath for relief of postpartum perineal pain, *Clin Obstet Gynecol* 23:1039, 1980.

Field TM: Effects of early separation, interactive deficits, and experimental manipulation on infant-mother face-to-face interaction, *Child Dev* 48:763, 1977.

Hahn RA, Muecke MA: The anthropology of birth in five U.S. ethnic populations: implications for obstetrical practice, *Curr Probl Obstet Gynecol Fertil* 138, April 1987.

Hansen CH: Baby blues: identification and intervention, *NAACOG'S Clin Issues Perinatal Women's Health Nurs* 1(3):359, 1990.

Humenick SS, Bugen LA: Parenting roles: expectation versus reality, *MCN* 12:36, 1987.

Increasing culturally relevant practice with Hispanic clients, *NPA Bulletin*, 3:23, Nov/Dec 1988.

Kirkland J: *Crying and babies: helping families cope*, Kent, UK, 1985, Croom Helm.

Konrad CJ: Helping mothers integrate the birth experience, *MCN* 12:268, 1987.

Kulin J: Childbearing Cambodian refugee women, *Can Nurse*, p 46, June 1988.

Kundstadter P: Do cultural differences make any difference? Choice points in medical systems available in northwestern Thailand. In Kleinman A et al, editors: *Culture and healing in Asian societies*, Cambridge, Mass, 1978, Schenkman Books.

Lamb ME: The development of social expectations in the first year of life. In Lamb M, Sherrod L, editors: *Infant social cognition*, Hillside, N.J. 1981, Lawrence Erlbaum Associates.

Lee RV: Understanding Southeast Asian mothers-to-be, *Childbirth Educ* 8(3):32, 1989.

Lee RV et al: Southeast Asian folklore about pregnancy and parturition, *Obstet Gynecol* 71:243, 1988.

Martell LK: Postpartum depression as a family problem, *MCN* 15:90, 1990.

Mortimer P, Kevill F: Infant care: frustration and despair, *Nurs Times* (Community Outlook), p. 19, May 1985.

Pederson DR: The soothing effects of rocking as determined by the direction and frequency of movement, *Can J Behav Sci* 7:237, 1975.

Pillsbury BLK: "Doing the month": confinement and convalescence of Chinese women after childbirth, *Soc Sci Med* 12:11, 1978.

Rosenthal MJ: Warm-water immersion in labor and birth, *Female Patient* 16:35, Aug 1991.

Rubin R: Puerperal change, *Nurs Outlook* 9:753, 1961.

Scott JR et al: Danforth's obstetrics and gynecology, ed 6, Philadelphia, 1990, JB Lippincott Co.

Snow LF: Folk medical beliefs and their implications for care of patients, *Ann Intern Med* 81:82, 1974.

Snow LF: Traditional health beliefs and practices among lower class black Americans, *West J Med* 139:820, 1983.

Steele B, Pollock C: A psychiatric study of parents who abuse infants and small children. In Helfer RE, Kempe C, editors: *The battered child*, Chicago, 1968, University of Chicago Press.

Stern PN et al: Culturally induced stress during childbearing: the Filipino-American experience, *Issues Health Care Women* 2(3-4):67, 1980.

References—Nursing Research

Ament L: Maternal tasks of the puerperium reidentified, *JOGNN* 19:330, 1990.

Anderson CJ: Enhancing reciprocity between mother and neonate, *Nurs Res* 30:89, 1981.

Davis JH, Brucker MC, MacMullen NJ: A study of mothers' postpartum teaching priorities, *Matern Child Nurs J* 17(Spring):41, 1988.

Gennaro S: Postpartal anxiety and depression in mothers of term and preterm infants, *Nurs Res* 37:82, 1988.

Martell LK et al: Information priorities of new mothers in a short stay program, *West J Nurs Res* 11:320, 1989.

Mead-Bennett E: The relationship of primigravid sleep experience and select moods on the first postpartum day, *JOGNN* 19:146, 1990.

Ramler D, Roberts J: A comparison of cold and warm sitz baths for relief of postpartum perineal pain, *JOGNN* 15:471, 1986.

Riesch S, Munns S: Promoting awareness: the mother and her baby, *Nurs Res* 33:271, 1985.

Stainton MC: Maternal newborn attachment origins and processes. III. Interactional synchrony: the prelude to attachment, doctoral dissertation, San Francisco, 1985, University of California.

Tribotti S et al: Nursing diagnoses for the postpartum woman, *JOGNN* 17:410, 1988.

BIBLIOGRAPHY

Auerbach KG, Jacobi AM: Postpartum depression in the breast-feeding mother, *NAACOG's Clin Issues Perinatal Women's Health Nurs* 1(3):375, 1990.

Berchtold N, Burrough M: Reaching out: depression after delivery support group network, *NAACOG's Clin Issues Perinatal Women's Health Nurs* 1(3):385, 1990.

Boyer KB: Prediction of postpartum depression, *NAACOG's Clin Issues Perinatal Women's Health Nurs* 1(3):359, 1990.

Busch P, Perrin K: Postpartum depression: assessing risk, restoring balance, *RN*, 46, Aug 1989.

Casiano ME: Outpatient medical management of postpartum psychiatric disorders, *NAACOG's Clin Issues Perinatal Women's Health Nurs* 1(3):395, 1990.

Comitz S, Comitz G, Semprevivo DM: Postpartum psychosis: a family's perspective, *NAACOG's Clin Issues Perinatal Women's Health Nurs* 1(3):410, 1990.

Degenhart-Leskosky SM: Health education needs of adolescent and nonadolescent mothers, *JOGNN* 18:238, 1989.

Gerlach C, Schmid M: Second skill educational development of personnel for a single-room maternity care system, *JOGNN* 17:388, 1988.

Gjerdingen, DK, Froberg DG, Fontaine P: A causal model describing the relationship of women's postpartum health to social support, length of leave, and complications of childbirth, *Women Health* 16(2):71, 1990.

Hansen CH: Baby blues: identification and intervention, *NAACOG's Clin Issues Perinatal Women's Health Nurs* 1(3):369, 1990.

Johnstone HA, Marcinak JF: Candidiasis in the breast-feeding mother and infant, *JOGNN* 19:171, 1990.

Keefe MR: The impact of infant rooming-in on maternal sleep at night, *JOGNN* 17:122, 1988.

Kumar R: An overview of postpartum psychiatric disorders, *NAACOG's Clin Issues Perinatal Women's Health Nurs* 1(3):351, 1990.

Malasanos L, Barkauskas V, Stoltenberg-Allen K: *Health assessment*, ed 4, St Louis, 1990, Mosby–Year Book.

Mercer R: Facilitating parent-infant interaction, *NURSEweek*, p 10, Jan 13, 1992.

Morse JM et al: Initiating breastfeeding: a world survey of the timing of postpartum breastfeeding, *Int J Nurs Studies* 27(3):303, 1990.

NAACOG: Nurses offer home health-care alternatives, *NAACOG Newsletter* 15:4, May 1988.

Norr KF et al: Early discharge with home follow-up: impact on low income mother and infants, *JOGNN* 18:133, 1989.

Oleen MA, Mariano JP: Controlling refractory atonic postpartum hemorrhage with Hemabate sterile solution, *Am J Obstet Gynecol* 162:205, 1990.

Redman BK: *The process of parent education*, ed 6, St Louis, 1988, Mosby–Year Book.

Rhode MA, Barger MK: Perineal care. Then and now, *J Nurs Midwife* 35:220, July/Aug 1990.

Seidel HM et al: *Mosby's guide to physical examination*, ed 2, St Louis, 1991, Mosby–Year Book.

Semprevivo DM: A select psychiatric mother and baby unit in Britain: implications for care in the United States, *NAACOG's Clin Issues Perinatal and Women's Health Nurs* 1(3):402, 1990.

Smith MP: Postnatal concerns of mothers; an update. *Midwifery*, 5:182, Dec 1989.

Starn J, Niederhauser V: A MCN model for nursing diagnosis to focus intervention, *MCN* 15:180, 1990.

St. George L, Crandon AJ: Immediate postpartum complications, *Aust NZJ Obstet Gynaecol* 30:52, 1990.

Storr GB: Prevention of nipple tenderness and breast engorgement in the postpartal period, *JOGNN* 17:203, 1988.

Tucker SM et al: *Patient care standards, nursing process, diagnosis, and outcome*, ed 4, St Louis, 1988, Mosby–Year Book.

Waxler-Morrison N, Anderson J, Richardson E, editors: *Crosscultural nursing*, Vancouver, 1990, University of British Columbia Press.

Weaver DR: Nurses' views on the meaning of touch in obstetrical nursing practice, *JOGNN* 19:157, 1990.

Bibliography—Nursing Research

Alder E, Bancroft J: The relationship between breastfeeding persistence, sexuality and mood in postpartum women, *Psychol Med* 18:389, 1988.

Blackburn S et al: Patients' and nurses' perceptions of patient problems during the immediate postpartum period. *Appl Nurs Res* 1(3):141, 1988.

Brouse AJ: Easing the transition to the maternal role, *J Adv Nurs* 13:167, 1988.

Fawcett J, Yorke R: Spouses' physical and psychological symptoms during pregnancy and the postpartum, *Nurs Res* 35:144, 1986.

Keefe MR: The impact of infant rooming-in on maternal sleep at night, *JOGNN* 17:122, 1988.

LaFoy J: Postepisiotomy pain: warm versus cold sitz bath. *JOGNN* 18:399, 1989.

Laizner AM, Jeans ME: Identification of predictor variable of a postpartum emotional reaction, *Health Care Women Int* 11(2):191, 1990.

Morales-Mann ET: Comparative analysis of the perceptions of patients and nurses about the importance of nursing activities in a postpartum unit, *J Adv Nurs* 14:478, 1989.

Norr KF, Roberts JE, Freese U: Early postpartum rooming-in and maternal attachment behaviors in a group of medically indigent primiparas, *J Nurse Midwife* 34(2):85, 1989.

Tulman L, Fawcett J: Return of functional ability after childbirth, *Nurs Res* 37:77, 1988.

Tulman L, et al: Changes in functional status after childbirth, *Nurs Res* 39:70, 1990.

Webster J: Lactation suppression: a pilot study, *Aust J Adv Nurs* 4:36, Jan 1986.

chapter 25 review

Key Concepts

- Postpartum care is modeled on the concept of health.
- The nursing care plan includes assessments to detect deviations from normal, comfort measures to relieve discomfort or pain, and safety measures to prevent injury or infection.
- The nurse provides teaching and counseling measures designed to promote a mother's (and father's) feeling of competence and control in the care of herself and newly born child.
- The nurse's clinical expertise is required to implement many therapeutic measures for physical care, including care of the boggy uterus, the full urinary bladder, the need for pharmacologic relief of discomfort, care after episiotomy or laceration repair, care of hemorrhoids, and suppression of lactation.
- Nurses have a role in helping clients establish healthy early family relationships.
- The parents' response is profoundly affected by their interpretation of the infant's response.
- Crisis prevention is an important function of the nurse and includes anticipatory guidance for postpartum depression, the infant's crying, sibling responses, and interactions with the grandparents.
- Mothers (and fathers) often misjudge the actual amount of physical and emotional energy required for the role transition to parenthood.
- The behaviors of the mother, the infant, the partner, and others may not always meet expectations.
- Nursing interventions to promote emotional adaptation recognizes the need to meet the mother's "taking-in" needs and supporting her "taking-hold" behaviors.
- The greatest conflict between Western and non-Western beliefs and practices in childbearing occurs in the postpartum period.
- Cultural beliefs and practices affect the client's response to the puerperium.

Key Terms

- adaptive behaviors (p. 713)
- atonic (boggy) uterus (p. 700)
- couplet care (p. 702)
- cultural proscriptions (p. 697)
- depressive states ("the baby blues") (p. 720)
- Homans' sign (p. 701, 709)
- infant massage (p. 721, 722)
- living ligature (p. 703)
- maladaptive behaviors (p. 713)
- oxytocic medications (p. 704)
- parenting difficulties (p. 713)
- parenting disorders (p. 713)
- Rh_0(D) immune globulin (p. 712)
- rubella vaccination (p. 712)
- sibling rivalry (p. 719)
- sitz bath (p. 705, 707)
- state of pollution (p. 697)
- suppression of lactation (p. 711)
- thromboembolism (p. 709)
- thrombosis (p. 709)

Critical Thinking Exercises

1. You are assigned to care for an Asian mother on the postpartum unit. She does not want to get out of bed, and you think it is related to her cultural practices. Nursing staff members tell you to make her follow the physician's order for activity, that is, to get out of bed as needed and to perform self-care activities.
   a. Identify the issues that are in conflict in this situation.
   b. Analyze arguments pro and con for integrating the woman's cultural practices into a plan of care.
   c. Formulate a plan of care based on your analysis.
2. In the newborn nursery, select a baby that you "really like" and the one that you "can't stand."
   a. Identify those characteristics of the newborn that influence your response to the babies.
   b. Reflect on what you would do if *your* baby had the characteristics of the one you "can't stand."
   c. Devise strategies for intervention for the mother (or father) whose baby does not meet her (or his) expectations.

Topics for Nursing Research

- Applications of warm/hot vs. cool/cold for perineal discomfort
- Culturally sensitive teaching priorities checklist and teaching plan for short-stay postpartum care
- Cost effectiveness of postpartum nurses participating in postdischarge (home-based), postpartum nursing care; for example, telephone follow-up, postpartum group teaching
- Strategies to help older siblings cope with addition of new family member
- Strategies to help grandparents cope with grandparent vs. parent role

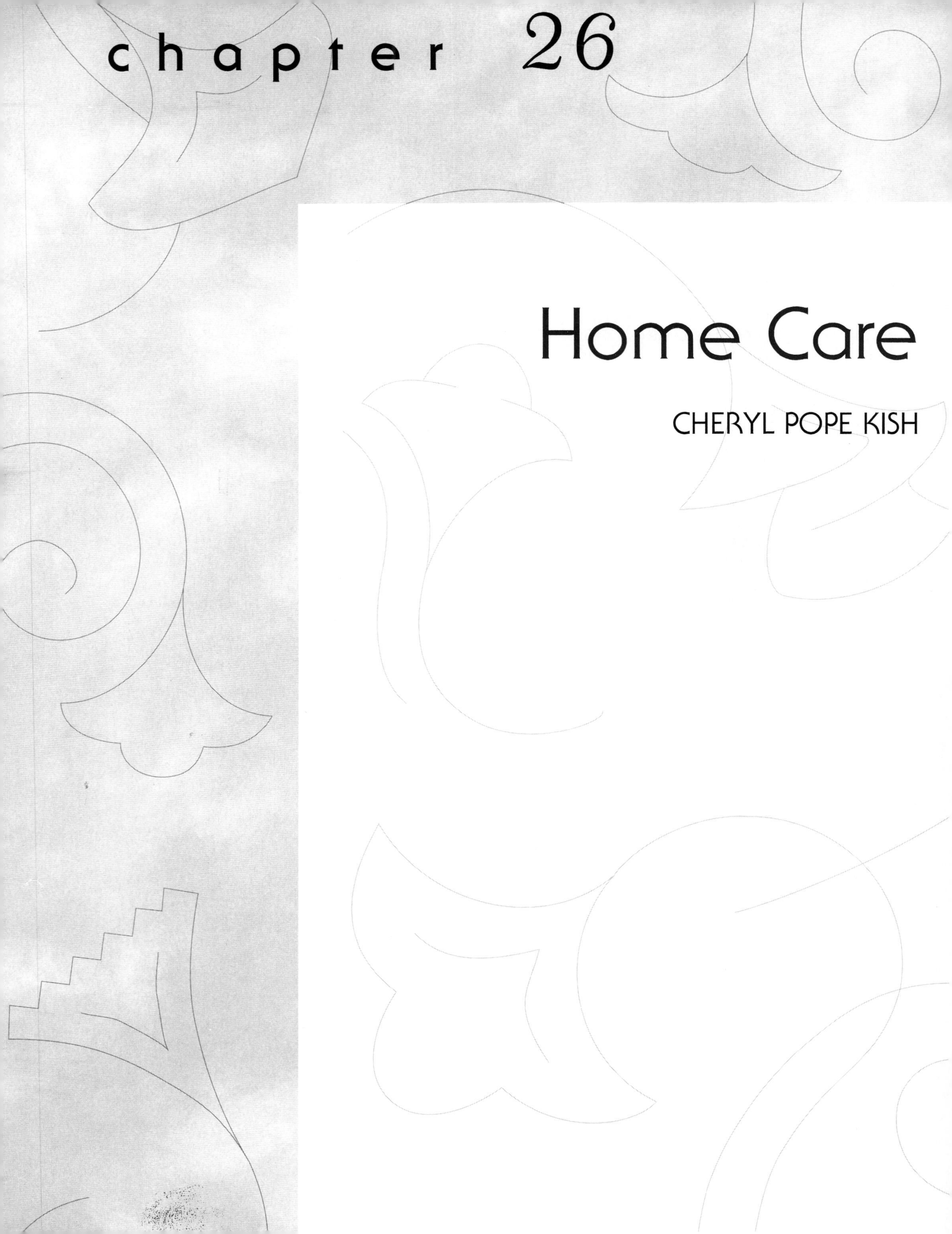

chapter 26

Home Care

CHERYL POPE KISH

LEARNING OBJECTIVES

- Define the key terms listed.
- Identify common selection criteria for safe early postpartum discharge.
- List the potential advantages and disadvantages of early postpartum discharge, including those justified by research findings.
- Summarize the nurse's role in these postpartum follow-up strategies: early discharge preparatory classes, home visits, telephone follow-up, warm lines, support groups, and perinatal coaching.
- Suggest ways in which the professional nurse may be involved in planning, implementation, and evaluation of postpartum home care strategies.
- Identify topics for nursing research related to home care.

Early postpartum discharge is a trend affecting increasing numbers of maternity clients and the nurses who provide their care. Early postpartum discharge refers to a postbirth hospital stay of 48 hours or less and is generally based on criteria that indicate low-risk status (see box at right). To gain perspective on how maternity hospital stays have changed over time, one can draw a quick comparison between 1950 and 1990. In 1950 the traditional postpartum stay after a vaginal birth was 6 days; in 1990 the mother who has had a vaginal birth is likely to remain in the hospital for 2 days or less. There is speculation that by 1995, the postpartum stay will shrink to 24 hours or less (Nichols, Humenick, 1988). Today medicaid will pay only for 24 hours.

The nurse in contemporary maternity practice is well advised to examine the circumstances contributing to early postpartum discharge and the implications of shorter stays for the well-being of clients/families and for maternity practice. The first issue is best addressed by examining the role of the current health care environment in early discharge.

Criteria for Early Discharge

MOTHER

Uncomplicated pregnancy, labor, birth, and postpartum course
No evidence of premature rupture of membranes
Stable blood pressure; temperature < 100.4° F (38° C)
Ability to ambulate
Ability to void without difficulty
Intact perineum without third- or fourth-degree perineal laceration
Hemoglobin > 10 g
No significant vaginal bleeding

INFANT

Term infant (38-41 wk) with birth weight of 2500-4500 g*
Normal findings on physical assessment performed by physician*
Normal laboratory data, including negative Coombs' test result and hematocrit 40%-65%*
Stable vital signs*
Temperature stability*
Successful feeding (normal sucking and swallowing)*
Apgar score > 7 at 1 and 5 min
Normal voiding and stooling
PKU and thyroid screening tests completed; repeat of PKU test scheduled for 2 wk*

GENERAL

Attendance at classes that include maternal and infant care, with an emphasis on problems of the first week at home*
Presence of a support person in the home to assist with care*
Presence of a strategy for follow-up*
Uncomplicated pregnancy, labor, birth, and postpartum course for mother and baby*
Demonstration of skill by mother in feeding, providing skin and cord care, measuring temperature with a thermometer, assessing infant well-being and signs of illness, and providing emergency care*

PKU, Phenylketonuria.
*Recommendations of American Academy of Pediatrics: Criteria for early infant discharge and follow-up evaluation, *Pediatrics* 65:651, 1980.

■ THE HEALTH CARE ENVIRONMENT THAT SUPPORTS EARLY DISCHARGE

Escalation of health care costs has contributed to cost-containment efforts on the part of both care providers and agencies that fund care. One such measure, prospective payment, enables the fee structures to be determined in advance of treatment, rather than retrospectively or after-the-fact. Prospective payment systems impose cost-containment measures and provide incentives to providers who decrease costs. A prospective payment system, the diagnosis-related group (DRG), was initiated by the federal government in 1983 to enable containment of Medicare costs so that the system might remain solvent. The DRG fee structure specifies that providers may recover only the preset (prospective) fee associated with a particular diagnosis, regardless of the actual cost incurred in delivering such care. Hospitals that contain costs are allowed to keep the overage in payment. In the event that actual costs incurred are greater than those allowable by diagnosis, hospitals absorb the loss.

Success of prospective payment systems, including the DRG model for cost containment, have encouraged other health care financiers (private insurers, the health maintenance organization [HMO], and the preferred provider organization [PPO]) to enact similar measures. Prospective payment systems have resulted in other major changes in health care: fewer unnecessary hospitalizations, more diagnostic tests and minor procedures performed in out-of-hospital settings, increasing acuity of in-hospital health problems, and early discharge.

An appreciation of the potential effects of those

changes, especially early discharge, and the existence of an intensely competitive health care market have led to the development of innovative services to bridge hospital and home. The maternity nurse can play a vital role in developing and implementing home care options. To do so effectively involves first recognizing the advantages and disadvantages of early discharge, including those with research support.

Potential Advantages of Short-Stay Maternity Care

Proponents of early postpartum discharge cite the following advantages of the practice:

- Reinforce the concept of childbirth as a normal physiologic event
- Allow shorter separations between mothers and other children
- Extend a couple's sense of control and participation beyond the birth itself
- Capitalize on the security of the home environment during the stressors of early parenting
- Decrease unnecessary exposure to the pathogens in the hospital environment (Harrison, 1990)
- Allow beds on the maternity service to be used more effectively (i.e., quick turnover in clients or for someone with a complication)
- Take advantage of increasing numbers of nonmedicated births
- Allow more time for mother/father/partner/infant and other family members to bond (Fig. 26-1)
- Create less disruption in the daily life of the family

Potential Disadvantages of Short-Stay Maternity Care

The day that a couple brings the newborn home for the first time is generally joyous and memorable. It also can be profoundly unsettling. Although some new parents anticipate early discharge eagerly, others feel unprepared for the reality they face. The woman with another child or children, feeling unrested, may be concerned about going home to their demands. Not uncommonly, the first-time mother will report astonishment at her level of discomfort. As one young mother explained, "I thought when labor was over, there would be no more pain. Why didn't someone warn me about stitches and sore nipples?" Another, while packing to go home, shared these feelings, "Almost from the minute I was brought from the delivery room, I have been bombarded with facts about baby care. There's so much to learn, everything is jumbled in my brain. What if I don't remember something or do it backwards and hurt my

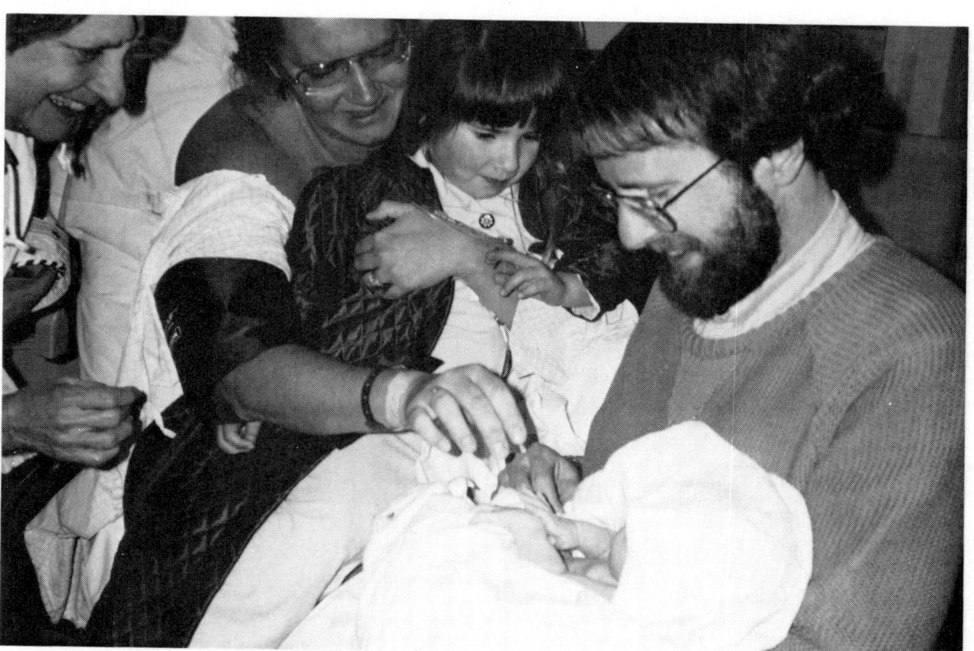

Fig. 26-1 Bonding and attachment begun early after birth is fostered in the postpartum period. Grandmother, parents, and older sibling meet the newborn.
Courtesy Nancy Mason, MD.

baby? The ink isn't dry on the birth records and I'm about to be wheeled out the door."

During the immediate days and weeks of the fourth trimester, the parents will be experiencing a major life transition: recovering from the events surrounding birth, adjusting to the demands of a newborn, parenting, applying the knowledge and skill from their postdischarge instructions, shifting priorities, and realigning some roles while assuming new ones. When there are other children, an additional challenge occurs: helping them to adjust to sharing home and parents with the newborn. The stress inherent in such profound transitions contributes tremendous crisis potential to the early postpartum experience. Table 26-1 differentiates between those clients discharged early who are at high risk for crisis and those who are at low risk.

Opponents of early postpartum discharge cite these predominant concerns: the risk of undetected complications and the vulnerability and crisis potential that exists for both clients and families. Goer (1990) cites recommendations of the American College of Obstetrics and Gynecologists (ACOG) for a 96-hour recovery time after a cesarean birth and 48 hours after vaginal birth: "ACOG also recommends 96 hours following uncomplicated abdominal hysterectomy—and hysterectomy [clients] won't be taking home a new baby."

The protest against early discharge becomes magnified in the conventional health care arena, in which there is a 4- to 6-week interval between discharge and the first scheduled visit to a physician for follow-up. To some extent, without some innovative approach, families are on their own, attempting a major life transition without benefit of health care resources. Postpartum nurses have been expected to be responsive to the changes in practice dictated by cost containment. In a small pilot survey, Lukacs (1991) found postpartum nurses frustrated, feeling harried, and occasionally ineffective in meeting the needs of the short-stay client. Although they were concerned about providing quality care in the abbreviated time frame, nurses in the study planned to remain in the setting. Continued attention must be given to the ways in which nurses and nursing are affected by this short-stay model of practice.

TABLE 26-1 Postpartum Clients and Risk of Crisis Related to Early Discharge

Perception of Event	Coping Skills	Support
CRISIS UNLIKELY		
Perception of uneventful, healthy pregnancy	Effective coping/problem/solving skills evident	Presence of supportive, helpful partner
Positive labor and birth experience that met expectations		Helper in home for 1-2 weeks
Elective or desired early discharge; feels "ready" for homecoming		Readily available resources (funds, persons, agencies)
HIGH RISK FOR CRISIS		
Perception that includes unresolved negative feelings about pregnancy	Ineffective coping skills or failure coping as a result of feeling overwhelmed, by lack of preparation or lack of control	Partner or other support person physically or emotionally unavailable
Traumatic birth experience; expectations unmet; sense of failure or loss of control		Lack of help at home
Physically or emotionally uncomfortable postpartum course		
Concerns/worries about parenting ability, skills, maternal recovery, finances, family relations		Limited financial resources
Unresolved feelings of loss		
Nonelective or undesired early discharge; feels unprepared for homecoming		

Modified from Aguilera DC: *Crisis intervention: theory and methodology,* ed 6, St Louis, 1990, Mosby–Year Book.

Are the concerns about early postpartum discharge supported by research findings? When the early discharge option is supplemented by extensive preparatory and postpartum follow-up strategies, it appears to be a safe and cost-effective alternative to traditional care (Jansson, 1985; Norr, Nacion, 1987). Norr and Nacion (1987), who conducted an extensive review of program outcomes with early postpartum discharge between 1960 and 1986, found on average less than 2% maternal readmission and approximately 4% infant readmission. The most common indications for maternal readmission to the hospital were endometritis and late postpartum hemorrhage. For the infants the most likely problem necessitating readmission was hyperbilirubinemia. Any of these problems could have occurred equally in those experiencing a longer postpartum stay.

Most research studies in the area of early postpartum discharge are based on groups of relatively advantaged clients or those for whom early discharge was an elective choice. Additional research is necessary to determine if equally favorable outcomes can be associated with those for whom early discharge is nonelective, even unsettling, or for those from disadvantaged groups (Norr, Nacion, 1987).

Favorable outcomes are not ensured when preparation for early discharge and postpartum home follow-up are not components of the shorter-stay alternative. The potential exists for the early postpartum discharge program to be compromised by the very normality of its clients. For example, educating for early discharge may cease to be a priority on understaffed, hectic units where there are numerous clients with complications demanding the nurses' time and attention. Further, in the face of the large number of short-stay cases, nurses must guard against complacency in assessment of these low-risk clients. Complacency can contribute to undetected complications: "Perhaps the most serious potential danger is that once the safety of early discharge is well established, cost containment pressures may lead to decreases in the follow-up care and careful client selection that now make early discharge a high quality care alternative" (Norr, Nacion, 1986).

The Future of Early Postpartum Discharge

As evaluative studies and research continue to show favorable client and economic outcomes of early postpartum discharge, the approach will likely become more common. Caseloads will tend to be increased as selection criteria are relaxed, so that those at minor risk will experience shorter postpartum hospitalization. In addition, common problems such as maternal infection and infant hyperbilirubinemia, identified after discharge, may be treated in the home (Norr, Nacion, 1986).

Existing home care follow-up programs are likely to extend their services to greater numbers of clients, including those from lower socioeconomic groups and those who stay longer than 24 hours in the hospital setting (Evans, 1991). Programs will offer increased outreach services, allowing those at greater geographic distances to take advantage of the short-stay option. As more maternity nurses extend their practice into client homes, the subspecialty of postpartum home care will emerge. More nurse-entrepreneurs will initiate private agencies, such as St. Louis' Healthy Homecomings, to serve the needs of short-stay clients.

■ NURSING CARE AND EARLY POSTPARTUM DISCHARGE: BRIDGING HOSPITAL AND HOME

The hospital-based maternity nurse assumes an invaluable role as caregiver, teacher, and client/family advocate in settings with early postpartum discharge options. In collaboration with the obstetrician and pediatrician, the nurse is instrumental in determining the readiness of mother and infant for early discharge. On the basis of careful assessment, the nurse plans an approach for meeting the needs of mother and infant during the brief hospitalization and provides anticipatory guidance, teaching, and/or referral to help to ensure the couplet's continued well-being at home.

Critical Path

One innovation to achieve these ends during the shortened hospital stay is the use of **critical path case management** for delivery of nursing care (Zander, 1989). Critical paths are defined as shortened case management plans (Gillerman, Beckham, 1991). The schedule of care and the goals for physical recovery remain the same as those described in Chapter 25. The critical path clearly delineates what teaching/discharge planning should occur within specified times. Nurses have an average of only 24 hours to prepare the postpartum mother for discharge. Therefore each nurse on each shift is expected to complete the prescribed interventions.

For example, the mother-baby care path standard after vaginal birth may include the following schedule—as long as uneventful maternal or newborn recovery continues. Starting by the third hour on the postpartum unit until the end of the first 8-hour shift, the woman is assisted with ambulation; is taught about self-perineal care (including medication), hand washing, involution, bleeding (lochia); and is given booklets and introduced to available video tapes. When the baby is with her, she learns about supporting the infant's head and extremities and proper positioning for feeding and burping. If she is breast-feeding, she also learns about rooting, latching on, and release of the nipple.

By the end of the second 8-hour shift, the woman is taught about diet, activity/rest, elimination, and medication. When her baby is with her, she is taught about bonding/attachment, usual parent concerns, normal newborn characteristics, diaper changes, cord care, frequency/timing of feedings, use of water feedings, pacifiers, and suckling patterns.

By the end of the third 8-hour shift, the woman needs a review of danger signs for which to call her health care provider. If she will need a consultation —for example, with a lactation specialist—this call is made before discharge. She is taught about safety: baby positioning, car seat, the need for baby to be attended at all times, and no bottle propping or use of microwave oven to heat baby's bottle. Sibling rivalry is discussed. Teaching is reinforced, questions are answered. The mother is asked for return demonstrations/explanations, for example, newborn characteristics, including crying, sneezing, diaper changes, feeding, circumcision care, and recognition of jaundice. As the woman is preparing to go home, she is reminded again of the person to call should a question arise and of the follow-up appointments.

During any one shift, the nurse may have one client who, immediately after the birth, needs frequent postpartum checks; others who are completing their first, second, or third shifts; and a mother who is preparing for discharge home. With clearly delineated interventions for each, nurses can provide more efficient care without worry about duplication or gaps. The critical path provides clear direction to coordinating care, teaching essential information, preparing the clients for discharge, and supporting the parent toward independence (Gillerman, Beckham, 1991).

The critical plan needs to be adapted to a client's special needs, e.g., English as a second language or inability to read; impaired mental capacity such as retardation; substance abuse; very young chronologic age; or physical problems such as extreme fatigue, infection, or anemia. The critical plan is a standard. Any deviation is noticed quickly and must be acted on. Therefore the critical plan can enhance and secure quality care. It is one appropriate vehicle for high-technology nursing and developing professional independence. It provides one method to effect the transition from hospital to home care.

Postpartum Follow-Up Services

For clients discharged early, there is an obvious need for bridging hospital and home, especially early in the course of the fourth trimester when rapid physiologic and psychosocial transitions are occurring. Maternity nurses, wishing to offer continuity of care, have extended their practice arena outside the hospital, offering a variety of postpartum follow-up services:

- Early-discharge preparatory classes
- Telephone follow-up
- Home visit follow-up
- Warm lines/help lines
- Parent-support groups
- Perinatal coaching

Although home care packages for postpartum follow-up may be offered by hospitals, maternity centers, public health agencies, private physicians, or independent entrepreneurs, it is the nurse who is a constant presence in each of these approaches.

ASSESSMENT

Systematic nursing assessment of the postpartum client and her newborn assumes special significance when early discharge is anticipated. Nursing assessment data may be used to help establish that criteria have been met for early discharge, thereby safeguarding mother and infant. A careful assessment enables the nurse to note normality of findings and to recognize and promptly report any complications. Further, these assessment findings represent baseline data for continued assessment in the home.

The postpartum assessment focuses on the mother's physiologic and psychologic status, her level of comfort, any relevant knowledge deficit and readiness to learn, the bonding behaviors evident, and adjustment to the transitions required for mothering. The focus of the newborn assessment is physiologic adjustment to an extrauterine environment, normality of physical and behavioral findings, and ability of the parents to meet the infant's needs.

NURSING DIAGNOSIS

As each client and family anticipates postpartum discharge, they will have unique responses. After a careful analysis of data obtained from the assessment, the nurse establishes data-based nursing diagnoses that will guide nursing actions. The following nursing diagnoses may be relevant for a client or family experiencing early postpartum discharge:

- Altered health maintenance related to
  —Insufficient knowledge of signs of complications
- Anxiety related to
  —Perceived lack of readiness for early discharge
- Ineffective breast-feeding related to
  —Inadequate knowledge or insufficient support
- Ineffective family coping related to
  —Disorganization and role changes of early discharge and parenting
- Fatigue related to
  —Lack of opportunities to rest during brief hospitalization
- High risk for altered parenting related to
  —Lack of knowledge/skill and unrealistic expectations

PLANNING

A plan of care is formulated that relates specifically to the needs of the client and her family. To the extent possible, the nurse involves them all in the planning and incorporates their priorities and preferences for any actions planned. *Goals* are set in client-centered terms and prioritized in collaboration with the client and family. Expected outcomes appropriate for clients/families experiencing early postpartum discharge include the following:

1. The postpartum client experiences uncomplicated physiologic recovery.
2. The woman experiences uncomplicated psychologic adjustment to parenting.
3. The postpartum client verbalizes an accurate knowledge base and/or demonstrates appropriate care of self and infant.
4. The woman lists available resources for home care and support and the manner in which these may be accessed.
5. The new parents demonstrate positive interactions with each other, the newborn, and other family members.
6. The postpartum client has attended preparatory classes for early discharge and is scheduled for follow-up at home.

IMPLEMENTATION

Nurses assume both caregiving and teaching roles in preparing the client and her family for early discharge. They know what home care follow-up alternatives are available to their postpartum clients and make appropriate referrals. Nurses who are providers of postpartum home care extend continuity of care to the postdischarge setting in a variety of ways: supportive counseling, teaching, and referral, which are based on continued additions to the data base.

The specific roles assumed by nurses in home care follow-up programs are summarized in detail later in the chapter.

EVALUATION

Evaluation of client outcomes is a continuous process. To be effective, evaluation is based on client-centered expected outcomes identified during the planning stage of nursing care. The nurse can be reasonably assured that care was effective if the following goals have been achieved:

- The postpartum client has experienced uncomplicated physiologic recovery and psychologic adjustment to parenting.
- She verbalizes an accurate knowledge base and/or demonstrates appropriate self-care and infant care.
- She lists available resources for home care and support and the manner in which these may be obtained.
- The new parents demonstrate positive interactions with each other, the newborn, and other family members.
- The postpartum client has attended preparatory classes for early discharge and has scheduled a follow-up visit.

If the nurse determines that client goals are being achieved, implementation of the nursing actions continues as planned. When evaluation data suggest that expected outcomes have not been attained, the plan is revised.

EARLY DISCHARGE PREPARATORY INSTRUCTION

To ensure the client's safety and well-being, a basic criterion for client selection in short-stay maternity programs is educational preparation before discharge. Either formal classes or one-on-one instruction, both supplemented with written material, may be provided at various times throughout the pregnancy. The necessary instructions may be given initially or expanded during the short hospital stay. Attempting to provide essential teaching only within the time constraints of a short-stay setting presents a special challenge for nurses who are trying to teach more in less time, often with fewer staff members. In addition, the nurse who is doing the teaching may be carrying a caseload that also includes women with complications. Postpartum teaching is further complicated because the learner is tired and uncomfortable from the demands of labor and distracted by visitors and her desire to spend time with the baby and her family: "The attention span of short-stay mothers may be affected by sensory overload, postdelivery fatigue, and sleep deprivation" (Martell et al, 1989).

The nurse recognizes that the adult's *readiness to learn* is associated with an acknowledgement that a problem exists or with recognition of a gap or deficit in knowledge or skill. The postpartum client may not identify knowledge deficit as a priority concern (Blackburn et al, 1988; Tribotti et al, 1988) (see Research Highlight). The inexperienced mother may not realize her limitations or know what questions to ask until she is at home with the dependent newborn. The multiparous woman, not yet appreciating how unique each child is, may not realize that her existing knowledge base is insufficient. For example, one mother of an especially fussy newborn son reported that she had not learned quieting behaviors when caring for her first baby, a quiet, easily comforted daughter. Although the mother of daughters may be willing to acknowledge a need to learn how to care for the genitalia of a male newborn, she may be hesitant to reveal a knowledge deficit in other basic skills, believing it might put her previous mothering ability in question.

A **teaching plan** is essential to avoid duplication of content and to ensure that all essential information is given. A teaching plan also offers consistency of the information being provided. Few things are more frustrating than hearing conflicting information, especially when the learner is pressed for time or is feeling stressed. Written and audiovisual materials can be used effectively to reinforce the verbal instructions.

Teaching plans should be based on systematic assessment of the client's learning needs, rather than on the nurse's perceptions of what constitutes essential information. Blackburn et al (1988) and Tribotti et al (1988) indicate that differences often exist between what nurses believe clients should know and what clients want to know. However, focusing on the informational needs common to new mothers can assist the nurse in collaborating with the client in planning instruction. Mothers in short-stay perinatal programs have identified as priorities health threats to themselves and their babies, feeding, and infant care (Davis et al, 1988; Martell et al, 1989). Of concern to multiparous women are family relationships (Hiser, 1987).

Once home, the postpartum woman is likely to turn to the infant's father or another support person as a source of information. For that reason it is imperative to include the woman's partner or support person in the instruction whenever possible. Grandparents also may be invited because they frequently are caregivers for the new family during early days at home (Fig. 26-2).

When postpartum follow-up is planned, especially home visits, not all the essential teaching must be

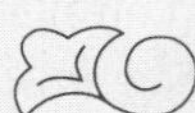 **Research Highlight** 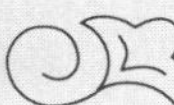

Early Postpartum Transition

RESEARCH ABSTRACT

Adaptation to motherhood requires major changes. The purpose of this study was to explore the relationship between selected variables and transition to parenthood. The selected variables were parity, age, education, infant feeding plan, support and stress during labor, and the birthing experience. The sample consisted of 108 vaginally delivered women who returned completed questionnaires. Parity was a significant variable in preparation for birthing and in evaluation of parenting. Breast-feeding mothers perceived more support during labor and birth. Preparation for birthing was a significant factor in how well labor and birth went. Postpartum learning experience influenced how well prepared mothers were to care for the infant and themselves. Better educated and first-time mothers had lower evaluations of their parenting skills and their ability to care for their infant and themselves.

IMPLICATIONS FOR PRACTICE

Nurses need to provide education and support during labor and birth and the postpartum period regardless of the parity or education of the mother. Supports for breast-feeding are necessary. Because perceptions of infant care and self-care capabilities may change after discharge, follow-up care is important.

RELATED RESEARCH QUESTIONS

1. What are the effects of parity, age, education, and childbirth preparation on self-care and infant-care capabilities 1 month postpartum?
2. What are the effects of the childbirth experience and perceived support in labor and birth on postpartum adaptation 1 month postpartum?
3. What are the effects of feeding plans and support for breast-feeding on breast-feeding success?
4. Do individual qualities or childbirth factors that affect self-care and infant-care capabilities differ between multiparous and primiparous mothers?

REFERENCE

Pridham KF et al: Early postpartum transition: progress in maternal identity and role attainment, *Res Nurs Health* 14:21, Jan 1991.

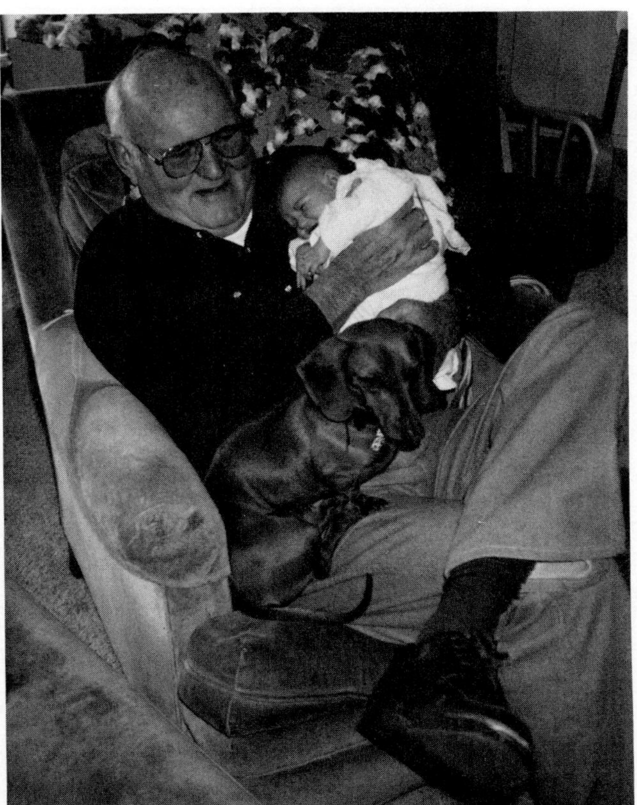

Fig. 26-2 Grandfather tends to newborn while assisting family dog with "sibling" rivalry.
Courtesy Nancy Mason, MD.

provided during the hospital stay. Some information, even if considered somewhat essential, can be temporarily delayed to the next nurse-client contact. The nurse can help the family to anticipate what their most pressing informational needs will be between discharge and the initial follow-up contact. Together, nurse and clients can plan to meet those prioritized needs. For example, the mother and nurse may reach a mutual decision to delay the total bath demonstration until the first home visit, focusing in-hospital teaching on cleaning the diaper area. Subsequently, the mother will learn to bathe her infant in the home, where she can work with the items she will use on a daily basis. Learning is facilitated because she is not forced to adapt to agency routine, supplies, or equipment; instead, she works within the security of her home with items familiar to her (Evans, 1991).

The nurse is, of course, compelled to provide emergency information and to help clients gain knowledge or skills they will need between discharge and the initial postdischarge contact (see warning signs above). All couples need to be helped to anticipate the reality of homecoming with a new infant and the stressors of the first hours and days of transition. Table 26-2 shows a checklist devoted to self-assessment of learning needs of women anticipating early postpartum discharge. Other topics include breast-feeding, formula feeding, and infant care.

Warning Signs—Postpartum (Physical)

1. Fever, with or without chills
2. Foul-smelling or irritating vaginal discharge
3. Excessive lochia or vaginal discharge
4. Recurrence of bright red vaginal bleeding after the lochia has changed to rust color
5. A swollen area on the leg that is painful, red, or hot to the touch
6. Localized swelling or a painful, hot area on the breast
7. A burning sensation during urination or an inability to urinate
8. Pelvic or perineal pain

Instructions for the First Hours or Days at Home

New parents often romanticize homecoming with their newborn to the extent that they are inadequately prepared for the reality. One new mother explains, "By the time we drove an hour through traffic, my stitches were hurting and all I wanted was a warm sitz bath and some private time with Bill and the baby, in that order. Instead, a carload of visitors pulled into the driveway as we were unbuckling the baby from his car seat. I thought I would surely cry."

All couples, especially those anticipating early discharge, must be helped to anticipate what the transition from hospital to home will be like so that reality shock will not negate their joy or cause undue stress. Anticipatory guidance should focus on the immediacy of homecoming: the trip itself, providing essential infant care, ensuring rest and comfort for the mother, dealing with visitors, and enlisting help. Sometimes the most simple nursing strategies provide enormous support.

The Trip Home

With guidance from the nurse, the couple anticipates the actual journey home. The nurse reinforces the use of an infant car seat that meets appropriate safety standards and helps the parents consider how they will respond if the baby becomes fussy during the trip. Some new mothers prefer to ride home sit-

TABLE 26-2 Self-Assessment of Learning Needs: Early Postpartum Discharge Unit

As a client anticipating early postpartum discharge, your time in the hospital will be limited. To help the nursing staff make sound use of that time to meet your learning needs, please complete this checklist by placing a check (✔) in the column that best describes your priority for learning the information listed. Use the following key:

Cr, Critical to know before discharge
HV, Prefer to learn during home visit
PI, Printed sheet or brochure will be adequate
OK, Knowledge in area is adequate or not desired

Topic	Learning Priority				Documentation of Teaching/Date/Nurse	Client Outcome
	CR	HV	PI	OK		
Self-care of vaginal flow						
Care of stitches						
Afterpains						
Diet						
Postbirth exercises						
Warning signs						
Resuming sex/birth control						

ting in the back seat beside the infant in the car seat. A fluffy pillow on the seat can provide comfort for a painful perineum, especially during a long trip. Before discharge the nurse may wish to administer whatever mild analgesic has been ordered for postpartum pain relief. The nurse first determines that the mother has had at least one previous dose of the medication without untoward effect.

Before the discharge a family member may wish to take all unnecessary items and any flowers or gifts home and to have any prescriptions filled. This minimizes the time necessary for unloading the car or shopping, thereby increasing the availability of that person as a support after the trip home.

Dealing with Activities of Daily Life

Even the small details of daily life may become stressful, given the demands of a newborn or the discomfort or fatigue associated with birth and a busy homecoming day, or both. The nurse may intervene by suggesting that even if the plan is to use cloth diapers, the parents may wish to purchase one box of disposables for those first hours at home. The nurse, offering preparatory instructions during the pregnancy, may encourage the woman to freeze extra casseroles or leftovers to be ready for use for the first few meals at home. Even a take-out meal can be planned if necessary to decrease one additional parental responsibility or concern during the initial hours at home.

Planning for discharge soon after an infant feeding ensures that the couple will have adequate time to get home and relatively settled before the next feeding (Fig. 26-3). Offering a sample carton of premixed bottles for the formula-fed infant prevents an immediate need for rushed preparation of formula. *Offering the samples to nursing mothers is inappropriate because it may be confused as discouragement of breast-feeding.*

Dealing with Visitors

A newborn in the family or neighborhood often seems to draw visitors like a magnet. Although the new parents may be unsettled by the trip home, they may serve as unwilling hosts to avoid strained relationships with friends and family. The nurse can help the parents in advance to explore ways in which they can assert their needs in such situations. They also may want to work out some signal for alerting the partner that the new mother is becoming tired or uncomfortable and needs to have the partner invite the visitors into another part of the house.

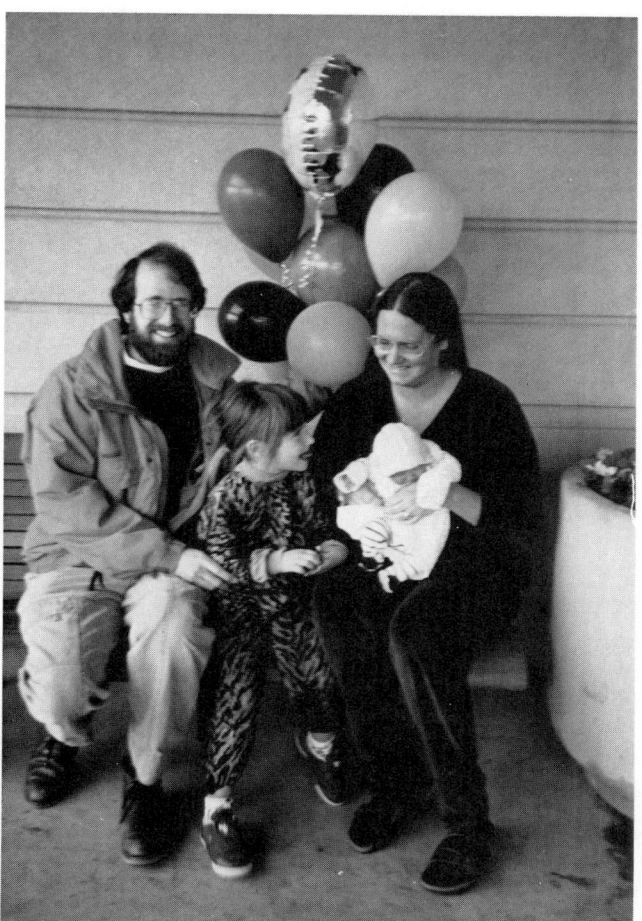

Fig. 26-3 A happy homecoming requires some preplanning.
Courtesy Nancy Mason, MD.

Dealing with Self-Imposed and Infant-Imposed Demands

New parents often report surprise at the amount of fatigue they experience initially with a new infant in their lives. Schedules must be readjusted and priorities realigned to accommodate infant care and interruptions in sleep. It is not uncommon for the new mother to find it difficult even to schedule time for her own shower. One first-time mother expressed amazement when her husband returned home from work and she realized that she had not found time to change out of her nightgown and robe. A father expressed his fatigue in this way, "It never ceases to amaze me that an 8-pound baby girl can wear down a 200-pound father and a 136-pound mother."

The woman needs to be cautioned not to overexert herself and to set priorities so that she can rest whenever possible. The nurse might help her to explore the daily routines and ways she can best obtain rest intervals. She may need help in considering her workload more realistically, asserting her need for help or support, or limiting unnecessary tasks. The new mothers should be introduced to the woman Edwards (1974) introduced as **fantasy Mom** —a composite of the ideal mother she envisions in her mind's eye, who may have enviable but totally unrealistic accomplishments to her credit. For example, a typical fantasy Mom or supermother has an immaculate house, gourmet meals with home-baked bread, and freshly made brownies; she is perfectly groomed in a size 6, black, sexy negligee; she mothers a cherubic baby; and she is always available for an uninterrupted intimate relationship. The woman who strives for this perfection may become unduly fatigued and experience unnecessary guilt and depression.

By encouraging the woman to list all the perfect qualities she expects of herself because of her image of the ideal mother, the nurse may enable the mother to experience less guilt. The nurse can help the new mother examine those ideal behaviors and choose to concentrate on the ones she considers most important. Together, client and nurse can explore ways of adapting to a lack of perfection, perhaps modifying those behaviors she cannot willingly let go, and asserting her need for help and support (Edwards, 1974). The nurse can use this opportunity to clarify misconceptions, provide reinforcement of strengths and positive behaviors, and refer the client to appropriate resources, such as postpartum support groups or warm lines.

■ POSTPARTUM CARE

Home Visits

Many early discharge programs are using **postpartum home visits** as an additional measure for postpartum follow-up. Home visits may be a service of the hospital, the private physician, a public health department, or a private agency providing home care to maternity clients. Regardless of their source, home visits are planned collaboratively with the family and are scheduled on the basis of identified need. A visit may occur as early as 24 hours after discharge; rarely would an initial visit be delayed beyond the third day at home. Additional visits are planned throughout the course of the first week, as needed. A decision to extend the contract for home visits beyond that time will be made on the basis of the family's needs.

During the home visit the nurse conducts a systematic assessment of mother and newborn to determine physiologic adjustment and to identify any ex-

Outcome Criteria

PHYSIOLOGIC RECOVERY, INVOLUTION, AND HEALING IN MOTHER

- Lists signs of problems that should be reported to primary care provider immediately
- Verbalizes understanding of normal findings
- Confirms decreasing discomfort, controlled by prescribed comfort measures
- Confirms patterns reflecting adequate rest

Breasts

- Supported by well-fitted brassiere
- Nontender; no signs of inflammation
- Intact nipples without cracks, fissures, or undue soreness

  If breast-feeding
- Describes or demonstrates technique for placing baby on and removing baby from breast, positioning to decrease stress of nipple area

  If not breast-feeding:
- No engorgement
- Taking lactation suppressants correctly (if prescribed) and knows warning signs to report
- Discusses importance of not stimulating breasts

Uterus

- Fundus firm, descending below umbilicus approximately 1 cm/day

Bowels/bladder

- Resumption of usual pattern of bowel elimination
- Hemorrhoids (if present) decreasing in size; not causing undue discomfort
- Resumption of usual pattern of urinary elimination; no burning or difficulty in initiating stream

Lochia

- Reveals normally progressing involution—rubra, serosa, alba in decreasing amounts—normal fleshy odor, no clots

Incision: perineal or abdominal

- Episiotomy (if present) well-approximated without undue redness, edema, ecchymosis, discharge, or tenderness
- Cesarean incision (if present) clean, dry, well-approximated; skin staples, sutures, or Steri-strips intact (if still present); evidence of normal healing process

Legs

- Nontender, with negative Homans' sign bilaterally

PHYSIOLOGIC ADAPTATION OF INFANT

Temperature

97.7°-98.6° F (36.5-37° C) axillary route

Heart rate

120-160 beats/min, strong, regular, normal variations with activity

Respiration

30-50 breaths/min, normal breath sounds, irregular rhythm; no retractions, or grunting; normal variations with activity

Skin

Warm, good turgor; no rashes

Head

Symmetric, with flat fontanelles; molding or caput decreasing; no hematoma

Abdomen

Soft, nondistended; audible bowel sounds

Color

Consistent with racial background; no evidence of jaundice

Activity

Alert with good muscle tone; moving all extremities normally

Umbilical cord

Normal atrophy noted, dry base without redness; not malodorous

Circumcision

Bell in place (if appropriate); clean and healing; no evidence of oozing; urinary stream normal

Elimination

Wetting a minimum of 6-10 diapers/day; stools consistent with feeding method in color, number, and consistency

Sleep pattern

Sleeps well

Feeding

- Sucking well without excessive spitting
- Burping well

Outcome Criteria—cont'd

- Length of breast-feeding (if done) consistent with recommendations
- Amount of formula per feeding (if done) consistent with recommendations

EFFECTIVE ADJUSTMENT TO PARENTING

- Parents interact with newborn in a loving and nurturing way.
- Parenting behaviors reflect appreciation of sensory and behavioral capacities of infant.
- Parents respond to cues provided by infant.
- Parents verbalize increasing confidence and competence in physical care of infant feeding, diapering, dressing, hygiene, sensory stimulation.
- Parents identify deviations from normal in the infant that should be brought to the immediate attention of the primary caregiver.
- Parents relate not only stressful or challenging factors in life style change but also positive or joyous ones.
- Parents describe or demonstrate emergency procedures and verbalize ways for accessing emergency help.
- Parents interact in a supportive manner.
- Parents collaborate effectively with each other in caring for newborn and other children.
- Parents relate effectively to newborn's grandparents and siblings.

isting complications. The assessment also focuses on the mother's emotional adjustment, including the presence of balancing factors (perception, coping, and support) that prevent crisis, and her knowledge of self-and infant care (see also discussions in Chapter 25). Ideally, the father is present during a home visit so that the couple's adjustment to parenting can be considered. If not, the mother's perception of their adjustment can be noted. The visit also affords the nurse an opportunity to observe interaction among those family members present within the familiarity and security of their home setting where they are in control. Observing new parents, the newborn, and other family members in this natural setting enables the nurse to elicit data about their life circumstances not accessible in any other way (Clemen-Stone et al, 1991). The box on p. 746 indicates criteria for evaluating the visit's outcome.

Although the primary nursing interventions during a home visit involve supportive counseling, anticipatory guidance, teaching, or referral, on occasion physical care might be given. For example, on order from the physician, the nurse may remove sutures or staples from the mother's abdominal incision, change a dressing, or initiate home phototherapy for the infant (Fig. 26-4). On occasion, it may be necessary for the nurse to collect blood or urine specimens for laboratory study. For example, a clean-catch urine specimen might be needed for a mother with suspected urinary tract infection; infant blood might be collected to follow up hyperbilirubinemia in the newborn. Throughout procedures of this kind, careful techniques are used to prevent the spread of pathogens.

Careful records that document assessment findings and all interventions, including counseling and teaching, are imperative. Not only does such documentation serve as a legal record of the visit; it also justifies appropriate reimbursement. Fig. 26-5 shows an example of a document for recording a postpartum home visit.

Although a nurse's purpose in visiting is different from that of a guest in the home, visiting nurses extend the same courtesy they would show to friends they might visit. For example, the nurse will call ahead to verify that the time scheduled for the visit is still convenient. (Not only is this common courtesy; it occasionally saves an unnecessary, sometimes costly trip.) Nurses will show respect for the privacy and personal property of family members. For example, the woman is given the choice of where the interview and physical examination will be conducted to best safeguard her privacy. The nurse will seek permission before using the family's hand washing facilities, placing equipment in a particular place, or using the family telephone to call the physician.

A home visit progresses more effectively if it is preplanned and well organized. The nurse reviews the hospital's discharge summary, teaching plan, and any other records, including physician's orders, that will serve to structure the interview and physical assessment and that will provide a sense of continuity in care. After the visit is so planned, the nurse collects necessary equipment, supplies, and instructional materials and ensures that they are clean and in working order before placing them securely in the bag. In addition to a name tag, the nurse who is not known to the family places other identification in the

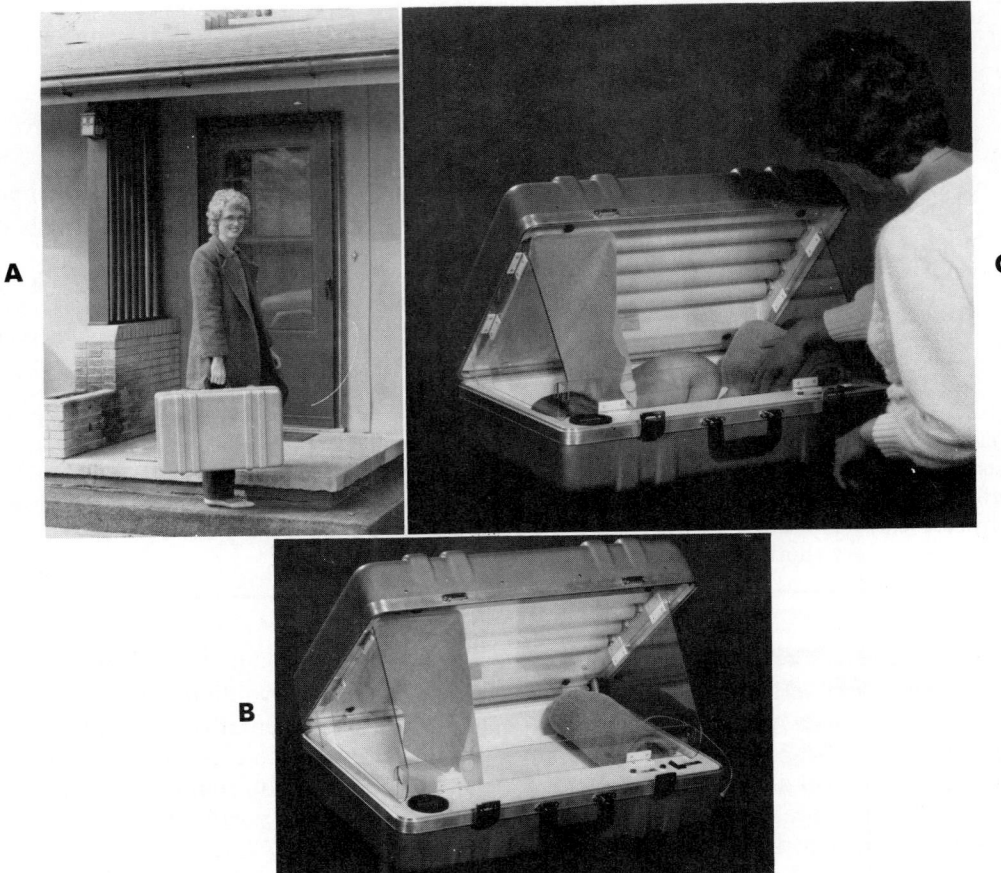

Fig. 26-4 Portable phototherapy for home use. **A**, Nurse brings portable unit to the home. **B**, Assembled unit. **C**, Infant under phototherapy with face shielded from the light. Courtesy PEP Inc., Park Rapids, Minn. (see appendix H for address).

bag for use in securing access to the home.

Before the visit, the nurse obtains directions to the family's home and secures a map, if necessary. If public transportation will be used, it is necessary to become familiar with the route and to obtain the necessary fare or tokens. Before using a personal or agency automobile, the nurse ensures that it has been adequately serviced and fueled for the trip. In case of emergency, the agency should always have a copy of the nurse's daily itinerary and the nurse should have emergency telephone numbers and appropriate coins for toll calls and emergency transportation. The box on p. 752 summarizes the protocol for a postpartum home visit.

The visiting nurse will need to enter unsafe areas on occasion. Taking necessary safety precautions and avoiding dangerous visits is imperative. A confident, nonvulnerable manner is appropriate. For visits in particularly dangerous settings, nurses may wish to visit in pairs. Nurses also may wish to report to the agency by telephone at specified intervals. The same precautions and common sense that guide a lone woman's behavior in any potentially hazardous setting should be used on home visits. For example, the

Text continued on p. 753.

MATERNAL ASSESSMENT

HEALTH PERCEPTION – HEALTH MANAGEMENT
_____ Reports overall health status as positive.
_____ Free from signs/symptoms of infection.
_____ Lochia is scant; reddish-brown or serosanguineous; no clots or foul odor.
_____ Exhibits behaviors compliant with plan of care.
_____ Verbalizes plan for medical follow-up.
Comments:

NUTRITION – METABOLIC
_____ Usual food intake is adequate for healing/lactation.
_____ Usual fluid intake is adequate for healing/lactation.
Comments:

ELIMINATION
_____ Reports an acceptable, regular pattern of bowel movements.
_____ Reports a normal pattern of urinary elimination.
Comments:

ACTIVITY – EXERCISE
_____ Activity level and exercise activities are appropriate.
Comments:

COGNITIVE – PERCEPTUAL
_____ Communicates effectively.
_____ Verbalizes relief from or a minimal amount of pain.
_____ No behavioral characteristics/physical responses to pain are observed.
_____ Verbalizes comfort with current knowledge level related to self and newborn care.
_____ Expresses correct knowledge related to self and newborn care.
_____ Demonstrates cognitive ability to problem solve and/or to make appropriate decisions for self and newborn.
Comments:

SLEEP – REST
_____ Recognizes need for sleep and/or rest.
_____ Reports napping and/or retiring early.
_____ Reports feeling rested.
_____ No behavioral characteristics related to fatigue are observed.
Comments:

SELF-PERCEPTION – SELF-CONCEPT
_____ Experiencing a low to normal level of anxiety.
_____ Exhibits a positive self-image, body image, and sense of personal identity.
Comments:

ROLE – RELATIONSHIP
_____ Verbalizes and/or demonstrates signs of newborn attachment.
_____ Mother/father/siblings show signs of adaptation to new roles.
_+/–_ If relevant, exhibits appropriate grief response.
Comments:

SEXUALITY – REPRODUCTIVE
_____ Verbalizes a positive adaptation to restrictions and/or changes in sexual relations.
Comments:

COPING – STRESS TOLERANCE
_____ Verbalizes experiencing an appropriate amount of stress and a smooth transition to changes.
_____ Verbalizes use of positive coping mechanisms.
_____ Verbalizes assistance and/or support from another person.
_____ Verbalizes family (or family verbalizes) experiencing an appropriate amount of stress and a smooth transition to changes.
_____ Verbalizes family (or family verbalizes) use of positive coping mechanisms.
Comments:

VALUE – BELIEF
_+/–_ If relevant, shows signs of spiritual well-being.
Comments:

NEWBORN ASSESSMENT

HEALTH PERCEPTION – HEALTH MANAGEMENT
_____ Overall health status reported as positive.
_____ Free from all signs/symptoms of infection.
_____ Free from signs/symptoms of increasing jaundice.
_____ Free from presence of rash or skin irritation.
_____ Environment free from obvious threats to newborn's safety.
_____ Caregiver exhibits behaviors compliant with plan of care for newborn.
_____ Caregiver verbalizes plan for medical follow-up of newborn.
Comments:

NUTRITIONAL – METABOLIC
_____ Weight gain is appropriate (Weight: _____ Date: _____).
_____ Observable signs of adequate infant intake.
_____ Caregiver verbalizes satisfaction with feeding process.
Comments:

ELIMINATION
_____ Stool is yellow-brown, soft and passed easily.
_____ Voids at least six times in 24 hours.
Comments:

SWEDISH HOSPITAL MEDICAL CENTER
MATERNAL-NEWBORN HOME SERVICES
SEATTLE, WASHINGTON 98104

NB-1207 Rev. 6/91 FC/SHMC SN-5846

Fig. 26-5 Document for recording a postpartum home visit, and example of a standard of care.
Copyright jointly held by Swedish Hospital Medical Center and Cynthia J. Evans, RN, MN, Coordinator, Maternal-Newborn Home Services, Seattle, Wash. (see Appendix H for address).

Continued.

CONTACT RECORD

TELEPHONE / HOME VISIT				CALLS RECEIVED		
DATE / TIME	NURSING NOTES	STANDARDS OF CARE	SIGNATURE	DATE / TIME	STANDARDS OF CARE	SIGNATURE
	No answer – 1st attempt					
	No answer – 2nd attempt					
	No answer – 3rd attempt					
	No answer – 4th attempt					
	Message left to call MNHS					
	Message left to call MNHS					
	Telephone Assessment Protocol completed					
	Home Visit Assessment Protocol completed					

STANDARDS OF CARE INDEX

A = Anxiety
B = Breastfeeding, Ineffective
b = Breastfeeding, Interruption
C = Constipation
c = Constipation, Newborn
F = Coping, Family
O = Coping, Individual
D = Diarrhea
d = Diarrhea, Newborn
G = Grieving
I = Infection
i = Infection, Newborn
V = Involution
Y = Injury
j = Jaundice
K = Knowledge Deficit
N = Nutrition
n = Nutrition, Newborn
P = Pain
R = Parenting
X = Sexuality
t = Skin Integrity
S = Sleep
U = Urinary
u = Urinary, Newborn

NURSING NOTES

DATE / TIME	

Fig. 26-5, cont'd

SLEEP PATTERN DISTURBANCE – STANDARD OF CARE

INITIATED: DATE / TIME ____________________

RN ____________________

RESOLVED: DATE / TIME ____________________

RN ____________________

RELATED TO:
1. Frequent night feedings.
2. Infant waking periods at night.
3. Inability to take naps/rest due to:
   a. other children.
   b. outside responsibility.
   c. limited help.
   d. difficulty sleeping.
4. Knowledge deficit of need for rest.
5. Pain/discomfort.
6. Anxiety/emotional state.
7. Inactivity.
8. Pregnancy.
9. Other:

CHARACTERIZED BY:
1. Verbal complaints of not feeling rested.
2. Verbal complaints of interrupted sleep.
3. Verbal complaints of difficulty falling asleep.
4. Observation of physical characteristics related to fatigue.
5. Other:

OUTCOME STANDARDS

DATE / RN

____________ 1. Recognizes need for sleep/rest.
____________ 2. Reports feeling rested.
____________ 3. Verbalizes retiring early and/or naps during the day.
____________ 4. Nurse does not observe any of the behavioral characteristics related to fatigue.

INTERVENTIONS

DATE / RN

____________ 1. Stress importance of rest.
____________ 2. Recommend resting if unable to sleep.
____________ 3. Provide positive reinforcement for any attempts at resting/sleeping.
____________ 4. Teach relaxation techniques.
____________ 5. Recommend restricting or lessening outside activities.
____________ 6. Remind of importance of vitamin/iron and balanced diet.
____________ 7. Teach techniques to minimize night time interruptions.
____________ 8. Encourage having someone else attend to household chores.
____________ 9. Recommend priority setting; do only highest priority items or basic tasks.
____________ 10. Recommend napping during infant's longest nap period.
____________ 11. Recommend lying down when infant first goes down.
____________ 12. Recommend unplugging telephone when napping.
____________ 13. If bottle feeding, suggest having someone else feed infant at night.
____________ 14. Encourage separating daytime rest from night time sleep.
____________ 15. Provide comfort measures and aids.
____________ 16. Other:

EVALUATION

DATE / RN

____________ 1. Receptive to interventions.
____________ 2. Other:

ADDRESSOGRAPH

SWEDISH HOSPITAL MEDICAL CENTER
MATERNAL-NEWBORN HOME SERVICES
Seattle, Washington 98104

NB-1323 6/91 FC/SHMC

Fig. 26-5, cont'd

Protocol for Postpartum Home Visit

PREVISIT INTERVENTIONS

1. Contact family to arrange details for home visit:
   a. Identify self, credentials, and agency role.
   b. Review purpose of home-visit follow-up.
   c. Schedule convenient time for visit.
   d. Confirm address and route to family home.
2. Review and clarify appropriate data.
   a. All available assessment data for mother and infant (i.e., referral forms, hospital discharge summaries, family identified learning needs).
   b. Review records of any previous nursing contacts.
   c. Contact other professional caregivers, as necessary to clarify data (i.e. obstetrician, nurse-midwife, pediatrician, referring nurse).
3. Identify community resources and teaching materials appropriate to meet needs already identified.
4. Plan the visit, and prepare bag with equipment, supplies, and materials necessary for assessments of mother and infant, actual care anticipated for mother and infant, and client teaching.

IN-HOME INTERVENTIONS: ESTABLISHING A RELATIONSHIP

1. Reintroduce self and establish purpose of postpartum follow-up visit for mother, infant, and family; offer family opportunity to clarify their expectations of contact.
2. Spend brief time socially interacting with family to become acquainted and establish trusting relationship.

IN-HOME INTERVENTIONS: WORKING WITH FAMILY

1. Conduct systematic assessment of mother and newborn to determine physiologic adjustment and any existing complications.
2. Throughout visit, collect data to assess the emotional adjustment of individual family members to newborn and life-style changes. Note evidence of family-newborn bonding and sibling rivalry; note relationships among mother, father, children, and grandparents.
3. Determine adequacy of support system.
   a. To what extent does someone help with cooking, cleaning, and other home-management tasks?
   b. To what extent is help being provided in caring for the newborn and any other children?
   c. Are support persons encouraging the new mother to care for herself and get adequate rest?
   d. Who is providing helpful information? Emotional support?
4. Throughout the visit, observe home environment for adequacy of resources:
   a. Space: privacy, safe play of children, sleeping
   b. Overall cleanliness and state of repair
   c. Number of steps new mother must climb
   d. Adequacy of cooking arrangements
   e. Adequacy of refrigeration and other food storage areas
   f. Adequacy of bathing, toileting, and laundry facilities
   g. Arrangements in home for newborn: sleeping, bathing, formula preparation (if needed), layette items and diapers
5. Throughout the visit, observe home environment for overall state of repair and existence of safety hazards:
   a. Storage of medications, household cleaners, and other substances hazardous to children
   b. Presence of peeling paint on furniture, walls, or pipes
   c. Factors that contribute to falls, such as dim lighting, broken steps, scatter rugs
   d. Presence of vermin
   e. Use of crib or playpen that fails to meet safety guidelines
   f. Existence of emergency plan in case of fire; fire alarm or extinguisher
6. Provide care to mother and/or newborn as prescribed by their respective primary care provider or in accord with agency protocol
7. Provide client teaching on basis of previously identified needs
8. Refer family to appropriate community agencies or resources, such as warm lines and support groups
9. Ascertain that client knows potential problems to watch for and whom to call if they occur
10. Ensure that used disposable items have been handled appropriately and that reusable items are cleaned and repacked appropriately in the nurse's bag.

IN-HOME INTERVENTIONS: ENDING THE VISIT*

1. Summarize the activities and main points of the visit.
2. Clarify future expectations, including schedule of next visit.
3. Review teaching plan, and provide major points in writing.
4. Provide information about reaching the nurse or agency if needed before the next scheduled visit.

*If this is the nurse's final planned encounter with the client/family, it is important to recognize that both the client and nurse may have feelings evoked by ending a meaningful relationship and by saying goodbye. Such feelings as anger, denial, and sadness are normal in this situation. Freely expressing these feelings at the end of the relationship is encouraged. Often clients are encouraged to do so if the nurse shares such feelings first.

Protocol for Postpartum Home Visit—cont'd

POSTVISIT INTERVENTIONS

1. Document the visit thoroughly, using the necessary agency forms to serve as a legal record of the visit and to allow third-party reimbursement, as possible.
2. Initiate the plan of care on which the next encounter with the client/family will be based.
3. Communicate appropriately (by telephone, letter, progress notes, or referral form) with primary care provider, other health professionals, or referral agencies in behalf of client/family.

nurse should park near the home or in a well-lighted public area with an unobstructed route to the home's entrance. Automobile keys spread between the fingers with sharp ends outward not only allows quick access to an automobile but also can be used as a weapon if necessary. The automobile should always be locked and any valuables stored out of sight. The nurse should not accept rides with strangers, enter vacant buildings, walk near groups of strangers in doorways or alleys, enter a yard with an unrestrained dog, or carry valuables. Neither should unfamiliar shortcuts be used. If nurses are concerned about entering a home or other building, they are best advised not to enter without an escort (Humphrey, 1986). If the nurse has an intuitive feeling that the house is unsafe, it is wise to leave immediately.

ADVANTAGES AND LIMITATIONS. A home visit has the obvious advantage of allowing the visitor to observe and interact with family members in their most natural and secure environment. Because they are at home, they are no longer anticipating how an infant will affect their lives; they are experiencing it. For that reason family members may have questions or concerns about areas that had not been anticipated before discharge. The use of open-ended questions by the nurse may serve to elicit those kinds of issues. For example, "What is it like being home?" "What has happened that you least expected?" "What has been your greatest joy in bringing the baby home?" "Now that you are at home, what needs do you have?"

The nurse is able to assess the adequacy of resources in the home, as well as evidence of safety in both the home and immediate surroundings. Both kinds of data are helpful in planning health teaching. Teaching that was not possible during the short hospital stay can be continued on a priority basis. For example, nurse and mother may explore what must be learned to get through the hours until the next visit. Learning about infant care is facilitated because the exact items to be used on a daily basis are available for demonstration and return demonstration; the mother is not required to adapt what she has learned to her own setting.

Nurses may find that the in-hospital care they provide is enhanced as a result of what they have learned during practice in client homes. Further, they may experience more job satisfaction as a result of extending the setting of their practice (Evans, 1991).

Although telephone follow-up must, of necessity, address the mother's perceptions of her status and that of the newborn and family, home visit allows direct assessment. It is therefore more likely to facilitate identification of complicated physical or psychologic adjustment.

There are several limitations in home visits as a postpartum follow-up strategy: (1) the cost of visiting families separated by great geographic distances, (2) the availability of the number of nurses with expertise in caring for maternity clients and newborns in the home, and (3) concerns about safety in accessing families in certain areas.

Telephone Follow-Up

As part of their early discharge package, many providers are implementing one or more **postpartum telephone follow-up** calls to their clients for assessment, provision of health teaching, identification of complications to effect timely intervention, and referrals. Telephone follow-up may be part of the services offered by the hospital, private physician, or a private agency and may be used separately or in combination with other strategies for extending postpartum care.

The nature of the telephone follow-up calls should be explained to the family before discharge from the hospital. A mutually agreeable time is scheduled for the initial call. The ideal time for a telephone call varies according to family needs and provider philosophy and protocol. In some cases the initial call might be placed within the first few hours after early discharge to ascertain that the homecoming has not been a problem. Donaldson, in her classic work on postpartum telephone follow-up (1977), suggests that an ideal time for the follow-up call is 3 to 7 days after discharge, and she provides a scientific rationale in support of that schedule. By that time the reality of the transition home has been realized and couples have begun to explore their concerns and options. Calls made earlier than 3 days may not allow adequate time for the "honeymoon" phase of homecoming to disappear; therefore the client's perception of the situation may not be realistic.

The number of calls and the time intervals between calls also vary and may be based on the family's assessed need and the other strategies being provided. For example, *Healthy Homecomings*, a private agency providing obstetric and gynecologic home recovery care in St. Louis, alternates daily telephone calls with scheduled home visits (Seibold, personal communication, 1991).

All therapeutic dialogue between nurse and client, including that by telephone, is purposive and goal-directed. This is not a social call even though there may be limited small talk in reestablishing rapport between nurse and client. During the telephone follow-up the nurse will ask questions with the following goals:

- To determine evidence of the mother's physiologic recovery, comfort, and rest
- To determine evidence of psychologic well-being in the mother, including the presence of crisis-preventing balancing factors
- To determine selected evidence of physiologic adaptation in the newborn
- To establish the perceived level of parental adjustment to parenthood and the stresses inherent in the early fourth trimester
- To identify learning needs of the family
- To determine the extent to which a relationship is being formed between the newborn, siblings, parents, and grandparents (Fig. 26-6)
- To explore the areas creating special concerns or challenges, as well as placing unsettling demands on family members

In opening the conversation, the nurse should provide reintroduction to family members and reinforce the reason for the telephone call. The nurse should ascertain if the call has been made at a convenient time; otherwise, the effectiveness of the call is questionable. For example, a mother who has just settled a fussy baby and is attempting to relax herself will not be well served by a follow-up call at this time. Further, common courtesy dictates that nurses determine if the call will create an unwelcome interruption for whatever reason. If so, a more suitable time should be mutually set.

The particulars of a follow-up call are planned on the basis of the discharge summary or records from the postpartum hospital stay. The use of discharge notes to guide the assessment ensures that an area of particular concern will not be overlooked. It also prompts the nurse to follow-up on the basis of the woman's history. An additional advantage is in the personalization and sense of warmth and regard it communicates. For example, rather than asking how other children are reacting to the new baby, the nurse can ask specifically, "How is Leslie responding to his new brother?" or "Is your Mom still with you, or has she gone back to South Carolina?" The latter question shows more interest than "Who is helping you at home?"

The nurse allows the conversation to develop as naturally as possible so that the client will not feel rushed or interrupted as rapport is established. This will be particularly important if the telephoner is not the nurse who cared for the family in the health care facility. A natural progression has the additional advantage of providing cues, such as the topic the mother chooses to address first, which often indicates her area of greatest concern. Open-ended questions facilitate the telephone interaction most effectively, for example: "How are things going since you left the hospital?" "You mentioned frequent headaches since you got home. Tell me more about those." Or "How are you and Peter collaborating on the baby's care?" Because specific assessment data about the mother, infant, and family are necessary, the nurse eventually will guide the assessment to these areas so that the aforementioned goals for the call can be met.

An effective postpartum telephone follow-up should assess the well-being of mother and infant and the transitions each family member is making to the new life-style and changes in the family constellation. To determine the crisis potential in the family, the nurse is careful to address each of the balancing factors. Consider, for example, the nurse making a return call to check on the status of a new mother who has been experiencing sore nipples. At an earlier call, the nurse had reinforced teaching about varying the infant's position on the breast to minimize stress to the nipple and had referred the mother to La Leche League. Today the nurse moves quickly to an assessment of the balancing factors, starting with "How have things been going since we spoke last?" Depending on the answer, the nurse may address a second factor by asking, "What have you been able to try?" After hearing the answer, the nurse might follow-up by asking, "And how is that working?" The nurse would determine if the mother has called La Leche and how productive this inter-

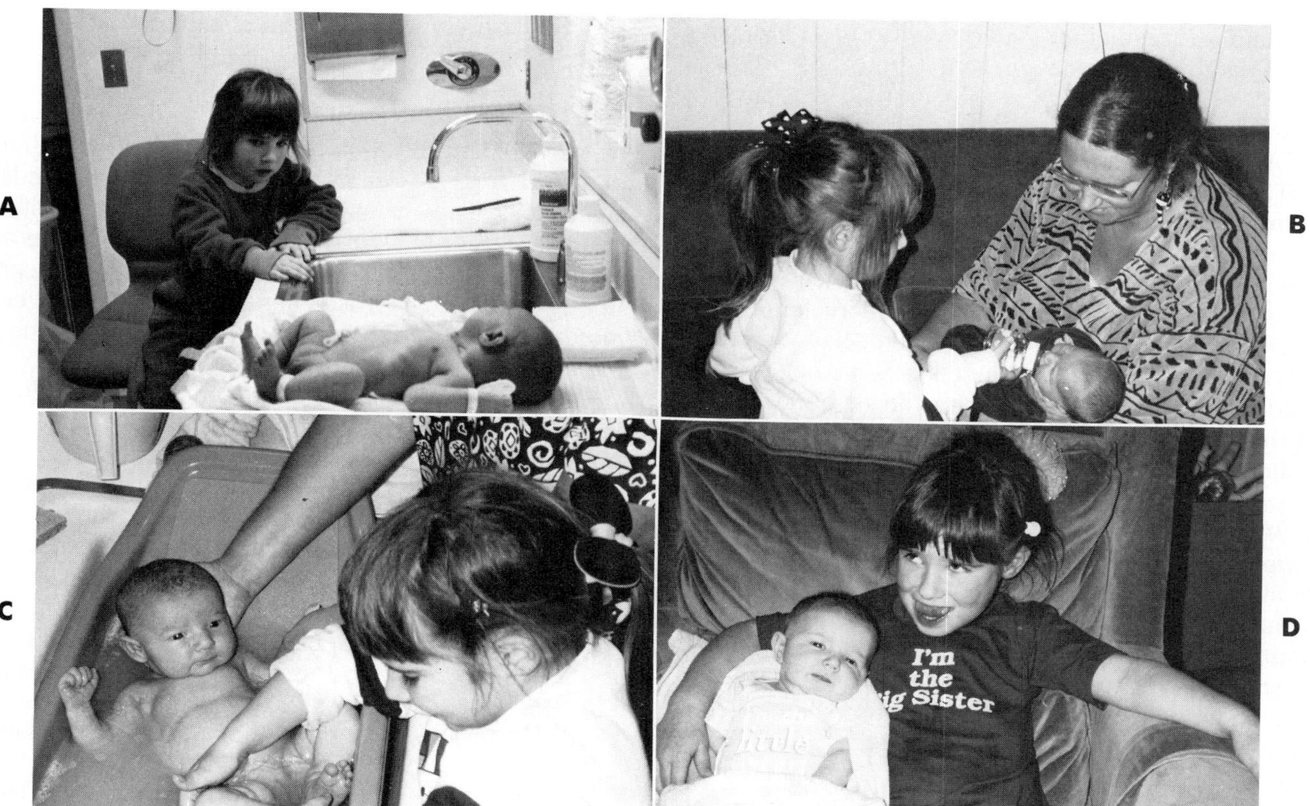

Fig. 26-6 Progress in sibling bonding and attachment. **A,** Watching during her new sister's first bath before discharge. **B,** Sibling feeds new sister under mother's watchful eye. **C,** Sibling gives her 2-week old sister a bath; both seem to be enjoying this time together. **D,** Sibling bonding and attachment between big sister and 1-month old little sister.
Courtesy Nancy Mason, MD.

vention has been. Additional teaching or referral, possibly to the primary caregiver, may be necessary at this time.

The primary interventions available to providers extending care by telephone include client advocacy, provision of teaching, reassurance/positive feedback, corrective feedback, supportive counseling, anticipatory guidance, and referral. Interventions are selected on the basis of a careful assessment and are provided in collaboration with the family.

Both the assessment data elicited and interventions employed during the postpartum follow-up call are recorded. Documentation serves both legal and reimbursement purposes.

ADVANTAGES AND LIMITATIONS. Telephone follow-up affords contact with the postpartum family during the vulnerable time interval in which support and intervention may be particularly effective. Most clients can be reached by telephone; according to Donaldson's research (1988), 92% of homes are accessible by telephone. Calls are most cost effective than are home visits but are limited by the indirect nature of the assessment. If the mother's perception of her well-being (or that of the newborn or family) is inaccurate or falsely reported, problems may be missed and intervention will not be supported by relevant data. This disadvantage can be overcome by combining both strategies: telephone calls and home visits.

On average, the call itself lasts 19 minutes (Rhode, Groejes-Finke, 1980). Preplanning and documentation time can easily expand the time commitment to 30 minutes per call. Consequently, there is a potential limit to the numbers of calls that can be handled each day. The effectiveness of telephone calls to postpartum women also is limited by the telephone skills and listening ability of the caller and by the comfort the mother experiences in providing personal data to the faceless caller.

Warm Lines/Help Lines

The **warm line** represents another type of telephone link between the new family and concerned caregivers or experienced parent volunteers. Warm line services sometimes are best understood in contrast to "hot lines," which may be more familiar to new parents. For example, they might have seen advertisements of hot lines in their area that provide emergency help to prevent suicide or child abuse. Perhaps they have heard of the White House hotline that links the president with other countries at times of crisis.

In contrast, *a warm line is a helpline,* or consultation service, not a crisis line. The warm line is appropriately used for less extreme concerns that may seem urgent at the time the call is placed but are not actual emergencies. Calls to warm lines commonly relate to infant feeding, prolonged crying, or sibling rivalry. One new mother called because she noticed a drop of blood on her daughter's diaper. With an explanation of the reason for the blood and that its presence was normal, she was appropriately reassured. Another mother called to talk about how it felt when her 4-year-old son screamed out, "I hate you and I hate that baby." Warm line services may extend beyond the fourth trimester. Even parents with adolescent children may profit from the helping relationship of a warm line.

Individuals who answer warm line calls need to be good listeners, who are empathic and able to use techniques such as open questions, restating, and reflecting to encourage the caller to communicate. The caller is given an unhurried opportunity to share feelings or concerns. It is her story, and she is allowed to tell it in her own way. Questions often are used to clarify what the caller is saying.

The caller is assessed for evidence of impending crisis: What is the situation or concern? What has already been tried in order to cope? What resources are available? Advice is not given; rather callers are helped to explore options available to them. Referrals may be made to support groups or to community agencies. When medical problems are identified, referrals are made to the appropriate physician.

Rauen (1985), who refers to the "telephone as stethoscope," maintains that communication can be blocked when the caregiver "talks too much, makes judgmental remarks, conveys differences, takes sides, dwells on personal experiences or assumes that the first problem mentioned is the real problem." Warm line calls always end with the caregiver summarizing the call—what concerns were identified and what resolutions have been explored. Also, the caller is invited to call again if the need arises.

ADVANTAGES AND LIMITATIONS. Individuals may be less hesitant to call an established warm line than to disturb a physician, especially at night, weekends, or holidays. The primary advantage of the warm line is quick access to a good listener, whether nurse or trained volunteer, 24 hours a day, 365 days a year. Because it is an advertised helpline, couples may feel more comfortable and less intimidated about making the call.

Inasmuch as the warm line offers round-the-clock service, there are potential difficulties in staffing; when a limited staff necessitates an answering recorder or message service, the resource is less effective. Having to leave a message negates the advantage of immediate access. Although some individuals welcome the anonymity of a faceless listener, they may be less willing to record a message.

The cost of the warm line is minimal if volunteers are used; the only costs are the telephone service itself and advertisement. The financial commitment obviously increases when any of the staff members are salaried.

For some nurses the inability to evaluate the effectiveness of their interventions is frustrating. There are generally no provisions for follow-up with the caller to determine the extent to which the problem has been resolved, if at all.

Support Groups

Humans are inherently social beings, involved on a daily basis in some kind of group—groups of family members, classmates, co-workers, and friends. Often, education, work, worship, and leisure time take place in groups. Thus it seems reasonable that at times of difficult transitions, people might turn to groups for support. Nurses are generally familiar with the benefits of support groups for such diverse groups as the newly divorced or widowed, those with recently diagnosed acquired immunodeficiency syndrome (AIDS) or cancer, and those undergoing mastectomy, colostomy, or heart attack.

A special group experience is sometimes sought by the woman adjusting to motherhood. On occasion, postpartum women who have met earlier in prenatal clinics or on the hospital unit may begin to associate for mutual support. Members of Lamaze classes who attend a postpartum reunion may decide to extend their relationship during the fourth trimester. Realizing the value of group support, nurses may wish to make postpartum support groups available as a strategy for bridging hospital and home.

A **postpartum support group** is a collection of individuals living the postpartum experience who are (1) striving to satisfy a personal need by belonging to a group, (2) interacting with respect to mutual goals, common interests or concerns, and (3) experiencing the reward of an interdependent relationship. They perceive themselves to be members of a group; others recognize them as a group. Group behavior is governed by rules and norms that are collectively chosen; for example, "We will protect each other's confidences" and "Husbands are invited to group meetings only when members agree unanimously to invite them."

An observer of a postpartum support group would be able to distinguish between content and process within the group's exchanges. Group content refers to what is discussed, for example, dealing with infant colic or concern over "still looking pregnant." Group process involves what actions, interactions, and reactions are occurring within the group. For example, who sits by whom, who does or does not talk, what interconnections form, and who takes on leadership roles are all elements of group process.

In a classic reference that examined group dynamics, Yalom (1975) identified several therapeutic advantages of group membership. Several of these factors have relevance for a postpartum support group: instillation of hope, cohesiveness, universality, catharsis, imparting concrete information, and imitating behavior.

During successful experiences, the instillation of hope provided within the group helps members believe that things can be different, perhaps better. Seeing others and themselves benefit from the group experience keeps members coming back. As they are accepted within the group and feel valued by other group members, individuals feel a bond with the group, and cohesiveness develops. Cohesion in a group also tends to reinforce the value of group membership.

Recognizing the universality of their feelings—that others feel the same way and that they are not alone or unique by virtue of their feelings or concerns—decreases anxiety and reassures members of their normality. It is comforting and offers a sense of catharsis to feel free to share feelings with others. For many women, it is a welcome relief to unburden deeply held emotions such as guilt, anger, or grief in a supportive setting where others, because of their shared emotions, are likely to be nonjudgmental.

Often in a postpartum support group, an experienced mother can impart concrete information that can be valuable to other group members. For example, one new mother shared her nurse-midwife's advice about placing warm, newly brewed tea bags on sore nipples for the comfort and healing value of warmth and the tannic acid. Another shared the use she had made of her husband's socks with the foot cut out. Sliding the sock over her left arm provided enough traction to keep the wet, soapy baby from slipping off the supporting arm while she gave the infant his bath. An inexperienced mother may find herself imitating the behavior of someone in the group whom she perceives as particularly capable. She may imitate someone's way of positioning a baby or find herself folding her daughter's diapers differently after watching someone else's technique.

Finally, sharing oneself in a group, whether in expressing feelings or expertise, has the therapeutic value of altruism. When the woman believes that she has helped someone else, it increases her sense of esteem and self-worth. In addition to its therapeutic benefit, this factor, as well as those discussed, encourage ongoing group membership.

In addition to organizing and marketing the group, the nurse may serve in a participant-observer role in a postpartum support group. This role would involve observing how the group is functioning and facilitating effective group process. In addition, the nurse might participate in the group as a resource person or content expert. The box below lists criteria by which the nurse would assess whether a postpartum support group is functioning effectively. A nurse who wishes to serve as a leader of a postpartum support group will be well served to enroll in a course in group dynamics, to study the literature on group dynamics, or to work initially with an experienced

Postpartum Support Groups: Signs of Effective Functioning

- Efforts are made to make each member feel welcome, included, supported, and trusted.
- Goals are identified and/or modified so that group goals and individual goals are congruent or compatible.
- Communication is open. Expression of ideas and feelings is welcomed, even when they are not those held by others in the group.
- Being oneself is encouraged in a nonjudgmental atmosphere.
- Group members participate in group work and group leadership tasks.
- Decisions are effectively made, and problems are solved with group input.
- Conflict and controversy are allowed and seen as positive events in the group's life.
- Personal growth and self-actualization are encouraged.

group leader. In planning a support group, the nurse may wish to consult experts in conducting needs assessment and marketing surveys.

ADVANTAGES AND LIMITATIONS. Yalom's classic list of therapeutic benefits to be gained from group membership lends support to the potential value of postpartum support groups. Although numerous studies focus on the advantages of support groups for psychologic health and well-being, few relate exclusively to the postpartum period. Cronenwett (1980) confirmed the value in sharing feelings that are universally experienced in a postpartum support group. She also found that the presence of infants and husbands in such groups adversely affected both attendance and expression of genuine feelings. Further, she noted that mothers may not participate in a support group until the baby is 1 month old. Such delayed participation in a group could well negate any immediate benefit in the fourth-trimester transition.

It may prove difficult to initiate a postpartum support group at an ideal time to meet the needs of families in transition. Although they may believe that group membership would be of value, new mothers may initially be too overwhelmed to consider seeking out such a group, much less attend consistently. Some of the questions that must be considered by the nurse who hopes to organize and market a postpartum support group include the following:

- Will women of all ages and experiences be invited to the same group?
- Will fathers and newborns be invited or excluded?
- How can the group be marketed to benefit the new mother in the early postpartum period?
- How can ongoing commitment to the group be encouraged, given the obvious demands of this life stage?
- How can the group best be advertised?
- How can the nurse prepare most effectively for a leadership role?

Perinatal Coaching

As the name suggests, **perinatal coaching** occurs in the period surrounding birth and employs behaviors expected of an effective athletic coach: modeling, directing, instructing, overseeing practice, and providing cues and prompts while a learner attempts a particular skill. In this case the learners are first-time parents and the skill being coached is two-way communication between them and their newborn infant. This primary prevention model was first described by Helfer (1979) as a way of preventing child abuse and neglect by facilitating a positive parent-child relationship. Perinatal coaching offers short-term support and basic information about the newborn's amazing capacity to respond, as well as skill learning and practice in a nonthreatening environment. Parents experience less stress and more enjoyment in interaction with their newborn as result of perinatal coaching (Bristor et al, 1984).

Interacting with a newborn involves an ability to **"speak sensory"**—to use the sensory system to communicate special messages. Helfer (1987) refers to the sensory messages that occur "when a child is picked up, cuddled, looked at with warmth and loving eyes, talked to, sung to, touched, soothed, and rocked." Such messages reach beyond the capacity of words to communicate what words sometimes cannot. The ability to speak sensory does not occur naturally because new parents typically do not fully appreciate the amazing ability of the newborn to interact with them.

Perinatal coaching can become an integral component of existing maternity care, performed by nurses or managed by nurses using experienced parents as trained volunteers. The latter approach ensures a self-perpetuating system: those who learn can subsequently volunteer for the coach's role. Perinatal coaches are trained in a 6- to 8-hour program that employs materials available from Gerber products.* Materials introducing the concept of perinatal coaching are available at no cost. Actual training materials, including *The Perinatal Coaching Picture Book,* may be purchased. Audiovisual materials that support training of both coaches and parents are available for rental or purchase.

Once trained, the perinatal coach will spend four 1- to 1½-hour sessions with the first-time parents, often initiating the relationship and describing the program in the final weeks of the woman's pregnancy. The box on p. 759 shows a plan of typical coaching sessions. At least one follow-up session is scheduled during the mother's postpartum stay; at least one home visit is made. The four sessions provide multiple opportunities for repetition and for reinforcing learning by both positive and corrective feedback, all of which enhance skill learning. Further, continued direct contact with a skillful coach offers ongoing support during the difficult transitions of the early fourth trimester. The home visit enables the perinatal coach to assess the progression of parent-infant attachment in the security of the familiar environment. It also provides an additional opportunity to determine a need for referral.

Although new parents involved in perinatal coach-

*Gerber Products Co, Medical Marketing Services, 445 State St, Fremont, MI 49412, 616-920-2000.

ing programs tend to evaluate the experience favorably, there is little empiric support for the program. A study by Bristor et al (1984) found that coached mothers looked at, talked to, and played with their infants more during routine care activities than did their noncoached peers. Their findings, however, were limited by a small (n = 42), nonrepresentative sample. Other studies are needed to consider the outcome of perinatal coaching programs for diverse groups of clients, including teens and those with poor parental role models.

ADVANTAGES AND LIMITATIONS. Advantages of perinatal coaching include the obvious benefit of parent education and the addition of another means of social support during the transition to parenthood. It is limited by the need for trained volunteers, by the time commitment involved, and by the lack of research support.

THE ROLE OF NURSING IN HOME CARE SERVICES

Nurses may wish to serve in expanded roles in postpartum care by helping to design, implement, and evaluate home care for new parents. In this effort, the nursing process will be completed in a different way. All prospective clients will be evaluated in terms of the phases of process, assessment, planning, implementation, and evaluation. Further, the process will occur on a larger scale.

ASSESSMENT

A comprehensive needs assessment ideally precedes any attempt to extend postpartum care through some form of home care follow-up. A marketing survey will determine what services, if any, are available, what level of support is evident, and the current and projected needs for such services (Postpartum follow-up, 1986). Consideration of the following marketing areas can be advantageous in developing postpartum home care follow-up:

- Survey of postpartum clients and what they identify as their needs
- Assessment of the availability of services that are in place or can be extended.
- Identification of competitive programs in the area
- Assessment of the level of support/sanction from providers of maternity care
- Review of obstetric statistics reflecting the number of births, including the percentages of both

The Perinatal Coaching Strategy: An Overview

Session No. 1: 1-1½–hour session with a one-on-one or small group format held in prenatal setting

Interventions

Establish rapport with individuals.

Provide overview of perinatal coaching, and offer opportunity to participate in the program.

Provide basic information about infants' sensory capabilities, wake/sleep states, reflexes, other newborn characteristics and ways of responding.

Introduce content from *The Perinatal Coaching Picture Book* and leave copy with each mother for subsequent review/reinforcement of content.

Session No. 2: 1-1½–hour private session with mother and father held in postpartum setting

Interventions

With the infant present, demonstrate and model touching, holding, looking at, rocking, talking to, and quieting behaviors.

Assist parents to identify infant's unique responses to the behaviors.

Observe as couples return the demonstration of learned skills.

Encourage couples to practice learned skills before next scheduled session.

Session No. 3: 1-1½–hour private session with mother and father held in the hospital setting or during the early days at home.

Interventions

With the infant present, observe as mother and father apply what they have learned to "speak sensory" with their newborn.

Provide reassurance by reinforcement of correctly performed skills.

Provide supportive corrective feedback of incorrectly performed skills; reteach/remodel as necessary.

Encourage continued practice.

Session No. 4: 1-1½–hour session with mother, father, and newborn in their home environment 1 to 2 weeks after discharge.

Interventions

Repeat strategies of session No. 3 as necessary.

Summarize and offer continued availability as social support person accessible by telephone.

Refer for additional types of assistance as necessary.

Modified from Helfer RE, Wilson AL: The parent-infant relationship: promoting a positive beginning through perinatal coaching, *Pediatr Clin North Am* 29:249, 1982.

vaginal and cesarean births, and the average length of hospital stay
- Review of projections about the future nature of obstetric services in the area
- Identification of existing agencies and support groups to which appropriate referrals may be made
- Existence of reimbursement sources for cost containment
- Review of literature and research findings on stressors of the fourth trimester and needs of new parents

A few key questions asked of in-hospital postpartum clients may provide invaluable data for customizing follow-up programs. For example: As you anticipate going home with your newborn, what needs do you have? What services do you wish were available to meet those needs? For what do you feel most prepared? Least prepared? What worries or concerns, if any, do you have?

A survey of postpartum clients who have experienced early discharge can elicit their retrospective views on their needs. For example: What has it been like for you to come home with a newborn? Can you speculate about what services would have been of value to you during those early days and weeks of transition? Answers to questions such as these from representative individuals and families provide a key to the scope of services needed. For example, the expressed needs of first-time parents may be very different from those of third-time parents; the teen-aged father and the thirty-year-old father may be stressed by totally unlike factors. The needs of different ethnic or socioeconomic groups also should be represented in the survey.

PLANNING

An analysis of assessment data provides planners with a profile of prospective clients and their needs, an overview of the setting in which their follow-up service will be implemented, and a determination of the degree of available support, sanction, and cooperation. Given those data, planners consider how other communities are meeting home care needs of postpartum clients and their families. There are numerous details to consider during the planning stage, not the least of which are soliciting funds; reviewing relevant standards, regulations and laws; finding a facility; hiring staff members or enlisting volunteers; developing protocols and forms for documentation; and marketing the service. Details may range in scope from naming the service to selecting carpet color. At every stage the assessment data provide a basis for decision making.

Ultimately, plans for postpartum home care programs must address three critical areas: access, cost, and quality terms of developing criteria that will meet the needs identified in the assessment. The following goals, for example, focus attention on the critical areas.

1. The program will be available, within a thirty-mile radius of the agency, to all postpartum clients who request the service, without regard to age, color, creed, national origin, or socioeconomic status.
2. The cost of basic home care service is $250.00. Documentation of professional contact will be provided to justify reimbursement.
3. All home care protocols will be based on standards of quality care developed by the Organization for Obstetric, Gynecologic, & Neonatal Care (NAACOG). To ensure quality programs, input will be solicited from both client evaluations and readmission statistics.

IMPLEMENTATION

The nurse may provide care, teaching, and referral directly or may serve as a coordinator or manager of care provided by other staff members or volunteers. To ensure quality care based on appropriate standards, the nurse's role in program implementation also may include education for staff members or volunteers.

EVALUATION

It is important that the program design be created on the basis of a thorough needs assessment. Equally important is developing a system of evaluating outcome effectiveness. Ideally, the effectiveness of postpartum follow-up services or home care strategies is evaluated in three dimensions: access, cost, and quality. Findings from such evaluation are used to make decisions about maintaining, expanding, or revising existing services.

An outcome evaluation is based on the specific objectives of the service. For example, evaluation of warm line service might include questions about the nature of calls placed, effectiveness of telephone counseling provided, and the timeliness with which return calls were made. In its outcome evaluation, a program employing homemakers might address such issues as cleanliness of the home and the quality of any meals prepared by the homemaker.

The outcome evaluation may elicit both verbal and written comments from clients and may be either formative or summative in nature. *Formative evaluation* is conducted while the clients are receiving the service and time is available to alter the plan of care as indicated. *Summative evaluation* occurs after the follow-up care has ended and summarizes what the experience was like for the client. Survey data obtained after the experience—that is, summative evaluation—may be more honest because anonymity is possible. Both formative and summative evaluation data are used in decision making about continuation, revision, or expansion of the program or of particular strategies offered.

Evaluation of Access

In evaluating access to the postpartum follow-up program, the evaluator will wish to collect demographic data showing what types of individuals are utilizing the program's services and what types of clients are not. These data will allow the program to market its services in a more representative way to access new client populations. If it becomes obvious that a particular group is underserved by the program, specific attention can be given to determining why certain clients are not using the services of the program. The results can guide an appropriate revision of the services.

The evaluation instrument will ask how respondents learned of the services provided by the program. Did they hear a television or radio advertisement? Were they referred by a professional caregiver? Did a newspaper advertisement appeal to them? Did they learn about the service through the program brochure? Perhaps the program was recommended by a satisfied previous client. If so, who was that individual? Taking the time to call or write to a client to thank them for recommending the agency is time and effort well spent.

An evaluation of access also will consider what specific services the client used. For example, in a program that offered a variety of services, did the family use only one service or several? Would the family be inclined to use the program again? Would they recommend it to others? If not, what problems prevent that recommendation?

Evaluation of Cost

A cost comparison can be made of the cost of early discharge supplemented by the particular home care follow-up program versus the cost of a prolonged hospital stay. A cost-benefit ratio must be established to evaluate whether the client has benefited from the service to the extent that additional physician visits or hospitalization have been prevented. Was a complication recognized and treated in a more timely manner than would have occurred without the follow-up program?

In evaluating cost, the agency providing the program will wish to determine whether part or all of the cost of services is being borne by clients. Is reimbursement available from private insurance, an HMO, or PPO? To what extent are charges being reimbursed? Is the agency providing necessary documentation for reimbursement? Is paperwork provided in a timely manner, and does it reflect actual services rendered? Might Medicaid funding be available to allow eligible clients to receive services provided by the program?

An internal audit will enable the agency manager to determine if the program is operating in the most cost-efficient manner possible. Comparing the actual costs of the agency's services with those being offered by similar agencies may provide helpful data for financial planning.

Evaluation of Quality

An analysis of a program's quality addresses areas of evaluation in addition to access and cost. For example, a program that consistently fails to meet the needs of a particular group or one that charges unreasonable fees or fails to provide documentation for timely reimbursement may be perceived as ineffective or of poor quality. A declining number of clients is equated with questionable quality as surely as client recommendations reflect satisfaction with the level of care provided.

Ensuring the quality of the program involves eliciting data that address clients' perceptions of the care they received and the extent to which they believe they benefited from the care. To that end, the evaluation may consist of questions that can be answered by a yes or no, a 0 to 10-scale on which effectiveness of care may be ranked, or an open-ended questionnaire. Some evaluation tools combine one or more formats. Regardless of format, the language is geared to the reader's level.

The following types of questions may be considered for inclusion in the evaluation:

- Was the early-discharge class informative? Did it prepare you thoroughly for the first hours or days at home?
- Did educational materials reinforce or expand verbal instructions?

- Were the physical examinations of the mother and baby comprehensive? Were any problems identified? Did the nurse explain her findings in an understandable way?
- Was the nurse responsive to your needs and concerns?
- Did the nurse look and behave professionally?
- Was it a comfort to you to have telephone or home visits? Did you feel more secure because of the 24-hour warm line?
- Did the nurse's care enhance your ability to care for yourself or your infant?
- How was your family's transition to parenting a newborn facilitated by the program?
- What suggestions do you have for improving the program's services?

An evaluation of quality requires data about the extent to which a particular client or family used a particular service. For example, how many calls did they place to the warm line? What types of information or support were sought? How many calls or visits did the nurse make? Was the schedule effective? Did clients feel better prepared as a result of perinatal coaching, early discharge classes, or written instructions?

Documentation of calls or visits serves to support the available data concerning the nature and quality of services. The records, which may be evaluated themselves, offer an explanation of the appropriateness of assessment, intervention, and referral.

To fully evaluate the quality of services provided and the effectiveness of a particular strategy or strategies, a comprehensive evaluation must examine readmission statistics. How many mothers and newborns are developing problems significant enough to require additional physician visits or hospital readmissions? What is the nature of such problems? Might they have been more quickly recognized and treated if the early discharge had not been an option? Would the problems have been missed or become more serious had follow-up care not been available? Is there a correlation between a particular strategy and the need for readmission? For example, do clients who are being visited at home by a follow-up nurse have fewer complications? Which clients are more likely to require readmission? Which follow-up strategy is most likely to be associated with readmission? The answers to these kinds of questions provide reliable evidence about the quality of a particular postpartum follow-up program.

■ SUMMARY

The trend for early postpartum discharge continues, creating a challenge for the nursing profession: to prepare families for the vulnerabilities of the fourth trimester in less time and with fewer staff members. Without systematically planned strategies to bridge hospital and home, a gap in postpartum health care, 4 to 6 weeks in duration, is possible. To an extent, families are on their own as they attempt to adjust to a major life transition without health care resources.

A variety of strategies—early discharge classes, telephone follow-up, home visits, warm lines, parent support groups, and perinatal coaching—may be used individually or collectively to extend postpartum care outside the hospital walls. Nurses have an invaluable role in each of these strategies. Their involvement has the potential to negate the hazards of early discharge and to facilitate healthy adjustment to the stressors of childbearing and early parenting.

CASE STUDY

Client Experiencing Early Postpartum Discharge: Nursing Process by Telephone

Ann Klaric is a 27-year-old postpartum client who was discharged from a short-stay unit 48 hours after the birth of her first child, a son named Jason. At midnight on her day of discharge, Ann called the warm line with medically related questions. She was referred to a hospital-based maternity clinical nurse specialist.

ASSESSMENT

The telephone interview revealed that Ann expelled "a large blood clot" when she last voided 10 minutes earlier. This is the first blood clot she has experienced since the birth, and even though she is now bleeding much less, Ann has obviously been alarmed by the experience. She says, "I'm so keyed up that I don't think I can relax enough to rest. Plus, I'm afraid to go to sleep—what if I start to hemorrhage and don't wake up?"

Ann's husband, Tom, is asleep in another room. A city bus driver, he must report for his next route in a few hours, while his sister stays with Ann and the baby. Because Tom has slept so erratically during the last 2 days, Ann decided to speak with the nurse before awakening him unnecessarily. The newborn also is sleeping.

Prompted by the nurse's assessment, Ann describes the expelled clot as "golf-ball size," dark red, and smooth; she did not notice any tissue fragments. The mild cramping she experienced earlier has ceased. In response to the nurse's specific inquiries, Ann describes her physical activity since leaving the hospital at 7 PM as follows. She unpacked, breast-fed and provided other care for the baby, prepared a snack for her and her husband, and washed a load of clothes.

Later, after resolution of her more urgent problems, Ann says, "While I have you on the line, let me ask you another question. I've noticed that my bra is becoming tighter. Can that affect my breasts and cause me not to have enough milk for the baby? I wish I knew more about breast-feeding."

NURSING DIAGNOSIS

On the basis of the subjective data elicited during the telephone interview, the nurse identifies three nursing diagnoses. The diagnosis that takes priority is: Fluid volume deficit related to postpartum bleeding secondary to overactivity during the first hours at home.

PLANNING

Ann is involved in developing her plan of care after she and the nurse explore several options. They agree on mutual *goals* for Ann: that she will experience decreased uterine bleeding over the next 2 hours with decreased activity and that her concerns about the bleeding will be resolved. Moreover, the nurse is hopeful that gaining confidence in her skill at handling this perceived emergency will enable Ann to cope with future emergencies more effectively. *Expected outcomes* set by the nurse include decreasing Ann's activity in an attempt to decrease uterine bleeding. Ann agrees to reassess the amount of bleeding at the end of 2 hours and to call the nurse with a condition report. At that time a decision will be made regarding further intervention.

IMPLEMENTATION

Nursing actions, which are derived from the nursing diagnoses, may be based on agency protocol or specific standards of care. For the initial diagnosis the nurse will assess the nature of the uterine bleeding on the basis of Ann's perception and determine if a 2-hour interval of bed rest will significantly decrease the amount of bleeding. Ann is encouraged to reassess her bleeding and to telephone the nurse at the end of the 2 hours of bed rest or earlier, if heavy bleeding recurs.

EVALUATION

The expected outcomes were used to evaluate the effectiveness of nursing interventions. As mutually agreed upon, after relaxing in bed for 2 hours, Ann reassessed the amount of uterine bleeding. She reported to the nurse that there was a 4-inch dark red stain on her perineal pad; no additional clots were seen. She agreed to call back in case the bleeding recurred. While sharing her feelings during the initial care and listening to the accurate information provided by the nurse, Ann was reassured that the blood clot was associated with overactivity. She stated that she felt better and much calmer as a result. Further, she seemed confident in her ability to cope.

CARE PLAN Telephone Follow-Up after Early Postpartum Discharge*

GOAL/EXPECTED OUTCOME	IMPLEMENTATION	RATIONALE	EVALUATION
Nursing diagnosis: Fluid volume deficit related to postpartum bleeding secondary to overactivity during first hours at home			
Ann will decrease her activity level, and bleeding will have decreased in amount when she calls the nurse in 2 hours.	Assess amount of blood loss on basis of perineal pad count, Ann's description of blood clot expelled, and history of bleeding since discharge from hospital.	Accurate assessment of actual/potential hemorrhage and contributing factors enables planning appropriate interventions.	
	Identify Ann's activity level since discharge as a possible contributing factor in increased bleeding. Encourage decreased activity (bed rest) for next 2 hours followed by reassessment. Suggest that applying a clean perineal pad before bed rest will facilitate more accurate data about the effects of decreased activity.	Decreasing activity level and avoiding heavy lifting generally is associated with decreased uterine bleeding.	After 2 hours in bed, Ann reports that bleeding has decreased in amount.
	Review telephone number of nurse, and encourage Ann to call back in 2 hours to report on condition. Advise Ann to call earlier if heavy bleeding recurs (>1 pad/hr).	Offering the client an opportunity to provide self-care to the extent possible increases self-confidence in decision making and in ability to cope with future emergency.	
Nursing diagnosis: Anxiety related to concerns about possibility of postpartum hemorrhage			
Ann will report diminished anxiety, and her concerns about excessive bleeding will be resolved.	Listen carefully with an attitude of warm regard and empathy to establish a trusting relationship. Assist Ann to acknowledge and express her feelings and concerns. Clarify misconceptions, and provide accurate information about uterine bleeding and overactivity.	An atmosphere of trust is basic to sharing private feelings, anxiety, and concerns not only with this care provider but also in future health care encounters.	
	Suggest that Ann lie down for 2 hours and use familiar Lamaze techniques. Provide positive reinforcement for Ann's decision making/coping as demonstrated by her calling for help. Assure Ann that nurse is immediately accessible by telephone, if needed, and that her call in 2 hours with a status report is welcomed and anticipated.	Relaxation techniques and knowledge that a concerned caregiver is immediately available will decrease anxiety and enhance the client's feelings of emotional comfort.	By the end of the telephone call, Ann reports that she is more relaxed and reassured about her condition.

CARE PLAN Telephone Follow-Up after Early Postpartum Discharge*—cont'd

GOAL/EXPECTED OUTCOME	IMPLEMENTATION	RATIONALE	EVALUATION
Nursing diagnosis: Health maintenance altered related to knowledge deficit regarding breast-feeding			
Ann will verbalize understanding of the process of production of breast milk and will evaluate her nursing bra according to criteria provided by nurse.	Assess learning needs. Prioritize learning needs to plan timely teaching that capitalizes on readiness to learn. Answer Ann's questions first. Provide opportunity for follow-up to meet other learning needs at more opportune time. Provide telephone number of contact person to answer questions and validate information or arrange home visit.	Prioritizing instructions in such a way that the client's most urgent need for information is met early reduces anxiety and enhances learning.* Ensuring readiness to learn, eliminating environmental barriers, and being responsive to client's needs and preferences are essential components in providing instruction for health maintenance.	Ann acknowledges understanding of the concept of supply and demand in breast-milk production and determines that her nursing bra is providing nonconstrictive support according to the following criteria: ■ Nonbinding ■ No underwires ■ Seams stitched toward underarm (to prevent obstruction of milk ducts) ■ 1-2 cup sizes larger than prepregnancy ■ Nonelastic straps ■ Comfortable and easy to fasten ■ Support to place nipples at midline
Ann will identify her preference for follow-up to enable additional learning, as needed.			Ann requests a home visit to learn more about breast-feeding.

*Only Ann's most pressing concern and request for information was addressed during this telephone encounter because of the late hour (midnight) and her need to rest. Follow-up to meet Ann's other learning needs is essential.

REFERENCES

Bristor MW et al: Effects of perinatal coaching on mother-infant interaction, *Am J Dis Child* 138:254, 1984.

Clemen-Stone S, Eigsti DG, McGuire SL: *Comprehensive family and community health nursing,* ed 3, St Louis, 1991, Mosby–Year Book.

Donaldson NE: Fourth trimester follow-up, *Am J Nurs* 77:1176, 1977.

Edwards M: The crisis of the fourth trimester, *Birth Fam J* 1:19, Jan 1974.

Evans CL: Description of a home follow-up program for childbearing families, *JOGNN* 20:113, 1991.

Gillerman H, Beckham MH: The postpartum early discharge dilemma: an innovative solution, *J Perinat Neonatal Nurs* 5:9, Jan 1991.

Goer H: The incredible shrinking postpartum stay, *Bay Area Baby,* 25, Fall/Winter 1990.

Harrison LL: Patient education in early postpartum discharge programs, *MCN* 15:39, 1990.

Helfer RE: Perinatal coaching guide. In *Pediatric basics,* No 26, Fremont, Mich, 1979, Gerber Products Co.

Helfer RE: The perinatal period, a window of opportunity for enhancing parent-infant communication: an approach to prevention, *Child Abuse Neglect* 11:565, 1987.

Helfer RE, Wilson AL: The parent-infant relationship: promoting a positive beginning through perinatal coaching, *Pediatr Clin North Am* 29:249, 1982.

Humphrey CJ: *Home care nursing handbook,* Norwalk, Conn, 1986, Appleton-Century-Crofts.

Jansson P: Early postpartum discharge, *Am J Nurs* 85:547, 1985.

Lukacs A: Issues surrounding early postpartum discharge: effects on the caregiver, *J Perinat Neonatal Nurs* 5:33, Jan 1991.

NAACOG: Postpartum follow-up: A nursing practice guide, *OGN Nursing Practice Resource R25,* Oct 1986.

Nichols FH, Humenick SS: *Childbirth education: practice, research, and theory,* Philadelphia, 1988, WB Saunders Co.

Norr KF, Nacion KW: Early postpartum discharge, *NAACOG Nursing Update Series* 4:2, Oct 1986.

Norr KF, Nacion KW: Outcomes of postpartum early discharge, 1960-1986: a comparative review, *Birth* 14:135, Fall 1987.

Rauen KC: The telephone as stethoscope, *MCN* 10:122, 1985.

Rhode MA, Groenjes-Finke JM: Evaluation of nurse initiated telephone calls to postpartum women, *Issues Health Care Women,* 2:23, Feb 1980.

Yalom I: *Inpatient group psychotherapy,* New York, 1975, Basic Books.

Zander K: Second generation critical paths, Definition: *Center for Nursing Care Management* 4(4):00, 1989.

References—Nursing Research

Blackburn S et al: Patients' and nurses' perception of patient problems during the immediate postpartum period, *Appl Nurs Res* 1:141, March 1988.

Cronenwett LR: Elements and outcomes of a postpartum support group program, *Res Nurs Health* 3:33, 1980.

Davis JH et al: A study of mothers' postpartum teaching priorities, *Matern Child Nurs J* 17:41, Spring 1988.

Donaldson NE: Effect of telephone postpartum follow-up: a clinical trial, *Diss Abstr Int* 49:2567B (University Microfilms No DA8809495), 1988.

Hiser PL: Concerns of multiparas during the second postpartum week, *JOGNN* 16:195, 1987.

Martell LK et al: Information priorities of new mothers in a short-stay program, *West J Nurs Res* 11:320, 1989.

Tribotti S et al: Nursing diagnoses for the postpartum woman, *JOGNN* 17:410, 1988.

BIBLIOGRAPHY

Ament LA: Maternal tasks of the puerperium reidentified, *JOGNN* 19:330, 1990.

Arnold LS, Blakewell-Sacho S: Models of perinatal home follow-up, *J Perinat Neonatal Nurs* 5:18, Jan 1991.

Auerbach KS, Jacobi AM: Postpartum depression in the breastfeeding mother, *NAACOG's Clin Issues* 12:375, May/June 1990.

Avery MD et al: An early postpartum hospital discharge program, *JOGNN* 11:233, 1982.

Bristor MW et al: Perinatal coaching: program development, *Clin Perinatol* 12:367, 1985.

Brooten D et al: Early discharge and specialist transitional care, *Image* 20:65, 1988.

Brouse AJ: Easing the transition to the maternal role, *J Adv Nurs* 13:167, 1988.

Cunningham FG, MacDonald PC, Gant NF: *Williams obstetrics,* ed 18, Norwalk, Conn, 1989, Appleton & Lange.

Davis J, Brucker M, MacMullen N: A study of mothers' postpartum teaching priorities, *Matern Child Nurs* 17:41, 1988.

Donaldson NE: A review of nursing intervention research on maternal adaptation in the first 8 weeks postpartum, *J Perinat Neonatal Nurs* 4(4):1, 1991.

Drummond RC et al: Mother care—cost effective program in maternal-infant care, *Home Health Nurse* 2:41, May 1984.

Elmer E, Maloni JA: Parent support through telephone consultation, *Matern Child Nurs J* 17:13, Jan 1988.

Gillerman H, Beckham MH: The postpartum early discharge dilemma: an innovative solution, *J Perinat Neonatal Nurs* 5:9, Jan 1991.

Gjerdingen DK, Froberg DG, Fontaine P: A causal model describing the relationship of women's postpartum health to social support, length of leave, and complications of childbirth, *Women Health* 16:71, Feb 1990.

Gosha J, Brucker MC: A self-help group for new mothers: an evaluation, *MCN* 11:20, 1986.

Hampson SJ: Nursing interventions for the first three postpartum months, *JOGNN* 18:116, 1989.

Luegenbiehl DL et al: Standardized assessment of blood loss, *MCN* 15:241, 1990.

Marrelli TM: *Handbook of home health standards and documentation: guidelines for reimbursement,* St Louis, 1988, Mosby–Year Book.

Martell LK: Postpartum depression as a family problem, *MCN* 15:90, 1990.

Morse JM et al: Initiating breast feeding: a world survey of the timing of postpartum breastfeeding, *Int J Nurs Stud* 27:303, 1990.

NAACOG: Physical assessment of the neonate, *OGN Nursing Practice Resource,* Washington, DC, 1991, NAACOG.

NAACOG: Postpartum nursing care: vaginal delivery, *OGN Nursing Practice Resource,* Washington, DC, 1991, NAACOG.

Norr KF Nacion K: Outcomes of postpartum early discharge, 1960-1986, a comparative review, *Birth* 14:135, Fall 1987.

Pelletier, Blovin A<; Case study: case management: Success in a community hospital, *Definition: center for Nursing Care Management* 5(3), 1990.

Rhode MA, Barger MK: Perineal care. Then and now, *J Nurs Midwife* 35:220, July/Aug 1990.

St. George L, Crandon AJ: Immediate postpartum complications. *Aust NZ J Obstet Gynaecol* 30:52, 1990.

Smith MP: Postnatal concerns of mothers: an update, *Midwifery* 5:182, Dec 1989.

Stanhope M, Lancaster J: *Community health nursing: process and practice for promoting health,* ed 2, St Louis, 1988, Mosby–Year Book.

Stern TE: An early discharge program: an entrepreneurial nursing practice becomes a hospital-affiliated agency, *J Perinat Neonatal Nurs* 5:1, Jan 1991.

Worthington-Roberts BS, Williams SR: *Nutrition in pregnancy and lactation,* ed 4, St Louis, 1989, Mosby–Year Book.

Zwergel J, Ende ML: Maternal-infant early discharge: making one home visit count, *J Home Health Care Pract* 1(2):16, 1989.

Bibliography—Nursing Research

Brooten D et al: A randomized clinical trial of early hospital discharge and home follow-up of very-low-birth-weight infants, *N Engl J Med* 315:934, 1986.

Donaldson NE: A review of nursing intervention research on maternal adaptation in the first 8 weeks postpartum, *J Perinat Neonatal Nurs* 4(4):1, 1991.

Elmer E, Maloni JA: Parent support through telephone consultation, *Matern Child Nurs J,* 17:13, 1988.

Golas GA, Parks P: Effects of early postpartum teaching on primiparas' knowledge of infant behavior and degree of confidence, *Res Nurs Health* 9:209, 1986.

chapter 26 review

Key Concepts

- The trend for early postpartum discharge will continue as a result of cost-containment measures, increasing technologic advances, and consumer demand.
- The short-stay option in perinatal care is safer when selection criteria are used and when home care follow-up is available.
- Early discharge classes, postpartum telephone follow-up, home visits, warm lines, support groups, and perinatal coaching used individually or in combination are effective means of preventing crisis and facilitating physiologic and psychologic adjustments in the postpartum period.
- Postpartum follow-up programs are most effective when planned on the basis of needs assessment and when revision is based on an evaluation of access, cost, and quality.

Key Terms

- critical path case management (p. 739)
- early postpartum discharge (p. 736)
- fantasy Mom (p. 745)
- perinatal coaching (p. 758)
- postpartum home visits (p. 745)
- postpartum telephone follow-up (p. 753)
- postpartum support groups (p. 756)
- speak sensory (p. 758)
- teaching plan (p. 742)
- warm lines (p. 756)

Critical Thinking Exercises

You are making a home visit to a new mother on her third postpartum day. She has two other children, ages 2 and 4. Assessment reveals the following findings:

1. Skin problems show that the infant is not being bathed properly.
2. Interactions of siblings with the newborn show that they have not accepted the necessity for correct hand washing and attitudes toward the newborn.
3. The mother shows a lack of knowledge concerning the newborn's jaundice.
4. The mother quotes family members regarding proper care of the umbilicus; the infant is wearing a flannel belly band that overlaps the diaper.

For each of the identified problems:

1. Formulate a nursing diagnosis.
2. Prioritize nursing diagnoses.
3. Plan and prioritize client-centered goals and expected outcomes.
4. Choose interventions and indicate rationale.
5. Indicate how you would know your interventions were effective.
6. Verify and justify your claims, beliefs, conclusions, decisions, and actions.

Topics for Nursing Research

- What is the relationship between postpartum home care follow-up strategies and hospital readmission for postpartum or newborn complications?
- Is a particular home care strategy (home visit, telephone follow-up, support group, perinatal counseling, or warm line) associated with easier transition to parenthood? With lower costs?
- How do postpartum outcomes compare when a single home-care strategy is used versus a combination?
- What is the level of satisfaction among nurses in traditional perinatal settings compared with perinatal nurses in postpartum follow-up care programs?
- What is the relationship between specific content areas in early-discharge classes and the level of anxiety in new mothers 12 hours after discharge?
- What are the anticipated needs of new mothers in the first 12 hours after homecoming?
- How do the postpartum mother's anticipated needs for homecoming compare with those of the perinatal nurse?

unit 6

Complications of Childbearing

27 Assessment for Risk Factors and Environmental Hazards

28 Hypertensive Disorders in Pregnancy

29 Maternal Infections

30 Maternal Hemorrhagic Disorders

31 Endocrine and Metabolic Disorders in Pregnancy

32 Medical-Surgical Problems and Trauma

33 Psychosocial Problems

34 Adolescent Sexuality, Pregnancy, and Parenthood

35 Labor and Birth at Risk

chapter 27

Assessment for Risk Factors and Environmental Hazards

SUSAN MATTSON
IRENE M. BOBAK

LEARNING OBJECTIVES

- Define key terms listed.
- Explore the scope of high-risk pregnancy.
- Discuss regionalization of health care services.
- List risk factors identified through history, physical examination, and diagnostic techniques.
- Understand diagnostic techniques and implications of findings.
- Explain diagnostic techniques to clients and their families.
- Identify topics for nursing research related to assessment for risk factors.

Of the approximately 3 million births that occur in the United States each year, 500,000 will be categorized as high risk because of maternal or fetal complications. Because the fetus in any given pregnancy is now at greater risk than the mother, the concept of "at risk" is applied to both maternal and fetal outcomes. The perinatal period is unique in that outcome depends on the early recognition and management of problems. Assessment of the existence of risks, together with appropriate and timely intervention, can help prevent disabling conditions both during the neonatal period and in future stages (Aumann, Baird, 1986). The united efforts of all medical and nursing personnel are required to care for these high-risk clients. In this chapter the high-risk client and the factors associated with diagnosis of high risk are identified. Diagnostic techniques used to monitor the maternal-fetal unit are emphasized.

DEFINITION AND SCOPE OF THE PROBLEM

A high-risk pregnancy is one in which the life or health of the mother or infant is jeopardized by a disorder coincidental with or unique to pregnancy. For the mother the high-risk status arbitrarily extends through the puerperium (30 days after childbirth). Post-birth maternal complications usually are resolved within a month of birth, but perinatal morbidity may continue for months or years.

There has been a significant decrease in maternal mortality and morbidity as a result of advances in the management of disorders that have adversely affected pregnant women. However, there has been a less significant decline in perinatal mortality and morbidity. In 1985 (the latest date for which figures are available), 66% of all pregnancies ended in a live birth, 28% in induced abortions, and 14% in fetal loss (spontaneous abortion or stillbirth). This has changed little since 1976. The aim of obstetric care is to concentrate resources on improving perinatal outcomes.

Of the approximately 6 million pregnancies that occur in the United States each year, about 3.5 million reach viability (22 to 24 weeks of gestation), but of these at least 30,000 fetuses fail to survive. About the same number of newborns die during the first month of life. Another 30,000 babies have severe but perhaps correctable congenital anomalies. Pregnancy and childbirth complications may be at least partly responsible for mental retardation in approximately 90,000 individuals. In addition, these complications have partially handicapped more than 150,000 persons, who have difficulty coping in our complex society (Pernoll et al, 1986).

When viewed in this perspective, high-risk pregnancy presents one of the most critical problems of modern medical and nursing care. A new social emphasis on the quality of life has developed. Family planning has reduced family size and the number of unwanted pregnancies. Technologic advances permit pregnancies in previously infertile couples. With these trends the wanted child has become increasingly important. As a consequence, emphasis is on the safe birth of normal infants who can develop to their maximum potential. Advances along many scientific fronts have provided the technology to achieve a level of perinatal health care far beyond that previously available.

Although pregnancy often is referred to as a maturational crisis, the diagnosis of high risk imposes another crisis, a situational crisis (e.g., the pregnancy terminates before the anticipated date; gestational diabetes mellitus with its potential complications develops; a neonate is born who does not meet cultural, societal, or familial norms and expectations). Understanding of the high-risk client will allow the nurse to provide individualized therapeutic nursing care (see Research Highlight, p. 775).

Maternal Health Problems

Different parts of the world have different leading causes of maternal death attributable to pregnancy. In general, three major causes have persisted for the last 35 years: hypertensive disorders, infection, and hemorrhage.

In 1988, 330 women were reported to have died of maternal causes (those attributable to complications of pregnancy, childbirth, and the puerperium). The maternal mortality rate for that year was 8.4 deaths per 100,000 live births. Data available indicate that the rate for 1989 (6.5) declined to approximately the 1987 level (National Center for Health Statistics, 1990).

In the United States, maternal mortality for white women is still less than for all other women. In 1988 African-American women were 3.3 times as likely as Caucasian women to die of causes associated with pregnancy, childbirth, and the puerperium. Further, African-American women have 40% more hospitalizations during pregnancy than do white women (National Center for Health Statistics, 1990).

Although the number of maternal deaths overall is small, maternal mortality remains a significant problem because a high proportion of deaths are preventable, mainly through improving the access to and utilization of prenatal care services. Nurses can be instrumental in educating the public about the importance of obtaining early and regular care during pregnancy.

Fetal and Neonatal Health Problems

Fetal and neonatal health problems are described under certain categories: fetal death (demise), neonatal death, perinatal death, perinatal death rate, and infant mortality. Definitions for these terms are found in Chapter 1. The incidence of each cause of infant mortality is expressed as the number of deaths per 100,000 live births. The infant mortality rate includes neonatal deaths. In 1988 more than 3.9 million babies were born in the United States. Of these, 38,910 died before their first birthday; 63% of these deaths occurred during the neonatal period (the first month of life). African-American infants died at twice the rate of Caucasian infants.

As demonstrated in Table 27-1, the majority of the 10 leading causes of death during infancy continue to occur during the perinatal period. Although a number of perinatal problems have benefited from improved treatment, congenital anomalies continue to be the leading cause of infant mortality. Increased rates of survival during the neonatal period have resulted largely from the improvement in perinatal services, including the technology of neonatal intensive care units, high-quality prenatal care, and the use of obstetric technology.

As can be seen in Table 27-1, the leading causes of death in the neonatal period are congenital anomalies, disorders relating to short gestation and low birth weight, respiratory distress syndrome, and the effects of maternal complications. The four leading causes of death in the post–neonatal period are sudden infant death syndrome (SIDS), congenital anomalies, injuries, and infections (National Center for Health Statistics, 1990). African-American women are twice as likely as white women to experience prematurity, low birth weight, and infant and fetal death (Kessel et al, 1988).

A significant decline of the infant mortality rate, as well as the elimination of racial and ethnic differences in pregnancy outcomes, requires a national, state, and local commitment to that goal. Reducing infant mortality rates requires the removal of financial, educational, social, and logistic barriers to care so that health services are received by those who need them.

Regionalization of Health Care Services

Significant evidence indicates that mortality decreases when high risk is identified and intensive care applied. In addition, follow-up studies have

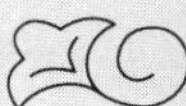 **Research Highlight** 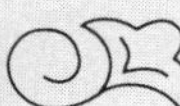

Stress and Social Support in High-Risk Pregnancy

RESEARCH ABSTRACT

This study examined the relationship among stress, social support, and risk in pregnancy. Participants were 19 high-risk and 20 low-risk women, between 26 and 38 weeks' gestation, who were receiving outpatient prenatal care. Data were collected with use of Brown's Support Behavior Inventory and the State Anxiety Inventory and by measuring urine catecholamine levels to assess physiologic stress. Most participants were African American (85%); all had a partner; all but four had other children. No significant differences were found between groups in anxiety, norepinephrine levels, or support scores. The high-risk group had significantly higher levels of epinephrine. In the high-risk group, women with lower norepinephrine levels were more satisfied with their partner's social support. In the low-risk group, women who were satisfied with their partner had lower anxiety scores. Younger women had higher anxiety scores and more partner satisfaction.

IMPLICATIONS FOR PRACTICE

High-risk pregnancy creates physiologic stress. Nurses can work with women to help them identify sources of stress and means to deal with the stress. Partner support is important, and nurses can counsel families on ways in which the partner can be of assistance. Stress-reduction techniques may be of value to pregnant women regardless of risk status.

RELATED RESEARCH QUESTIONS

1. Are anxiety levels during high-risk pregnancy affected by the time at which the high-risk status was identified?
2. Does an education program directed at partners of high-risk women increase supportive behaviors of the partner and lower anxiety and catecholamine levels in the women?
3. Is there a relation between anxiety of a woman experiencing a high-risk pregnancy and anxiety of her partner?
4. What factors affect stress and coping in high-risk pregnancy?

REFERENCE

Kemp VH, Hatmaker DD: Stress and social support in high-risk pregnancy, *Res Nurs Health* 12:331, 1989.

TABLE 27-1 Deaths Under 1 Year and Infant Mortality Rates for the 10 Leading Causes of Infant Death: United States, 1988*

Rank order†	Cause of death (Ninth Revision International Classification of Diseases, 1975)	No.	Rate
	All causes	38,910	995.3
1	Congenital anomalies	8,141	208.2
2	Sudden infant death syndrome	5,476	140.1
3	Disorders relating to short gestation and unspecified low birth weight	3,268	83.6
4	Respiratory distress syndrome	3,181	81.4
5	Newborn affected by maternal complications of pregnancy	1,411	36.1
6	Accidents and adverse effects	936	23.9
7	Newborn affected by complications of placenta, cord, and membranes	907	23.2
8	Infections specific to the perinatal period	878	22.5
9	Intrauterine hypoxia and birth asphyxia	777	19.9
10	Pneumonia and influenza	641	16.4
	All other causes	13,294	340.0

From National Center for Health Statistics: Advance report of final mortality statistics, 1988, *Monthly Vital Statistics Report* 39 (7) (suppl), Nov 28, 1990.
*Rates per 100,000 live births.
†Rank based on no. of deaths.

shown that serious residual handicaps (physical and mental) of surviving infants have been dramatically reduced.

It is neither feasible nor reasonable for each hospital to develop and maintain the full spectrum of medical and nursing specialists, laboratory capabilities, and equipment necessary to care optimally for all clients. As a consequence, **regionalization of health care** has come into being; that is, facilities are organized to provide different levels of care within a given area.

Ideally, a regionalized system includes primary care and three levels of facilities within the designated area. Level I facilities have three main functions: (1) the management of normal pregnancy, labor, and childbirth, (2) the earliest possible identification of high-risk pregnancy and high-risk neonates, and (3) the provision of stabilization care in the event of unanticipated obstetric or neonatal emergencies.

Level II facilities provide care for a specified type of maternal and neonatal complications, as well as offer a full range of maternity and neonatal care in uncomplicated cases. Staff members are specially educated and prepared for those particular complications, and appropriate equipment is available.

Level III facilities, the *regional centers,* have the capacity to manage the most complex disorders, both maternal and neonatal. Often mothers are transported to these centers *before* the birth of the baby to optimize the outcome. In addition, the regional centers provide outreach educational services for medical and nursing staff within the region.

■ ■ ■

The idea that certain events that occur during the prenatal and intranatal periods can have an adverse effect on the infant in later life is not a new one. Serious biologic handicaps, health problems, obstetric disorders, and social deprivation may compromise the mother and the infant in subtle or more obvious ways. Identification of the high-risk client is critical to minimize maternal and neonatal mortality or morbidity, or both. Ample evidence indicates that known risk factors can be used to identify high-risk clients early in the prenatal course as well as intrapartally. Approximately 20% of pregnant women can be identified prenatally to be at risk, accounting for 55% of poor pregnancy outcomes (American College of Obstetricians & Gynecologists [ACOG], 1988).

Commonly it is the alert nurse, conversant and familiar with deviations from normal, who notes and reports potential or actual high-risk factors (see Tables 27-2 and 27-3 and boxes, p. 782 and p. 783). The interrelationship of risk factors that influence pregnancy outcomes are summarized in Fig. 27-1.

The major goal of **antepartum testing** is the detection of potential fetal compromise. Ideally, the technique used will identify the compromise before intrauterine asphyxia of the fetus so that the health

Text continued on p. 783.

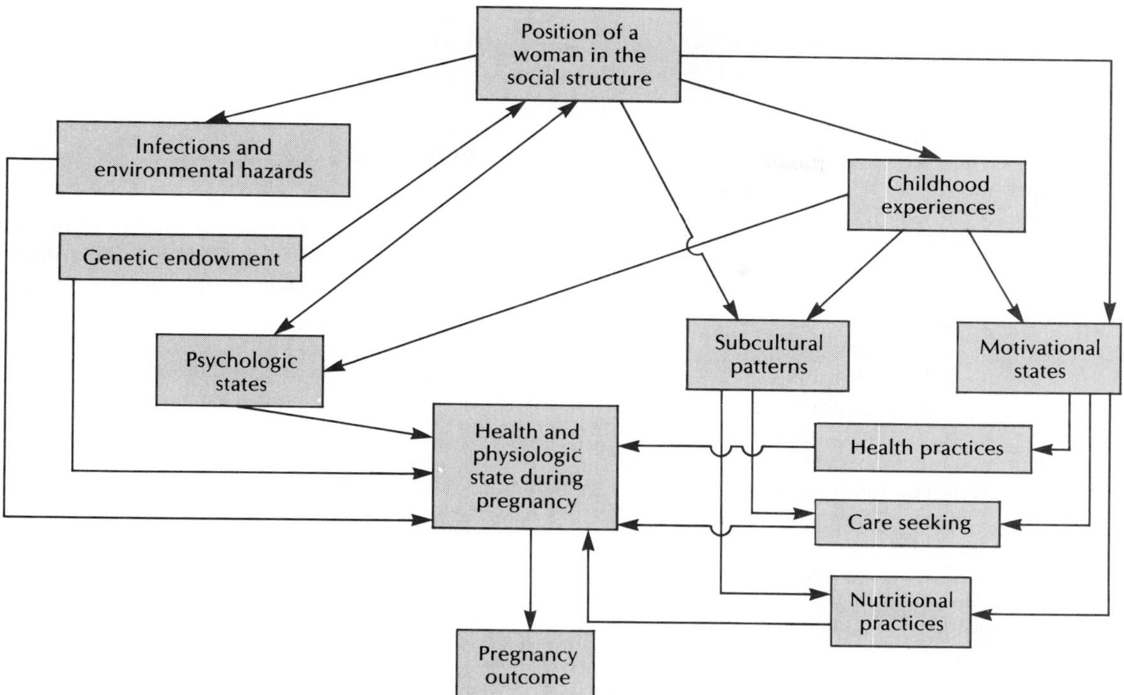

Fig. 27-1 Summary of risk factors that may affect pregnancy outcome.
From Fogel CI, Woods DF: *Health care of women*, St Louis, 1981, Mosby–Year Book.

TABLE 27-2 Factors that Place the Pregnancy and Fetus/Neonate at High Risk by Trimester and during Labor

Category	Factors that Result in Risk	Category	Factors that Result in Risk
FIRST TRIMESTER		Psychologic	Psychologic shock
Anatomic	Maternal		Drugs
	Ectopic pregnancy	Therapeutic	Elective abortion (aspiration, saline solution, prostaglandin) before this pregnancy
	Uterine abnormality		Drug therapy
	Retroversion of uterus		X-ray therapy
Physiologic	Fetal	Infection	Viral infection
	Gross chromosomal defect	Genetic	Sporadic mutation
	Hydatidiform mole		Inherited characteristics
	Multifetal pregnancy		Sex-linked disease
	Poor trophoblast invasiveness	Environmental	Poverty
	Folate deficiency		Drugs, tobacco, alcohol
	Endocrine deficiency		Inadequate nutrition
	Hyperemesis gravidarum		
	Defective sperm		

Modified from Fogel CI, Woods NF: *Health care of women: a nursing perspective,* St Louis, 1981, Mosby–Year Book.
HIV, Human immunodeficiency virus; *TORCH*, toxoplasmosis, rubella, cytomegalovirus, and herpes simplex.

Continued.

TABLE 27-2 Factors that Place the Pregnancy and Fetus/Neonate at High Risk by Trimester and during Labor—cont'd

Category	Factors that Result in Risk
SECOND TRIMESTER	
Anatomic	Maternal Uterine abnormality Incompetent cervical os Fetal Gross abnormality Acute hydramnios Multifetal pregnancy Poor implantation
Maternal complications	Rh incompatibility Cyanotic heart disease Hypertension Renal disease Urinary tract infections Accidents Anoxia of hypertensive disease or epilepsy
Infections	Polio, syphilis, hepatitis, TORCH, HIV
Genetic	Amniocentesis
Environmental	Poverty Drugs, tobacco, alcohol Inadequate nutrition
THIRD TRIMESTER	
Anatomic	Malpresentation Cord complications Placenta previa*
Maternal complications	Hypertensive disease* Rh incompatibilities Diabetes Thyrotoxicosis
Infections	Viral infection* Pneumonia
Nutritional	Protein lack Iron deficiencies Abruptio placentae*
Therapeutic to mother	Antibacterial drugs Tetracycline Antithyroid drugs Corticosteroids Anticonvulsants Anticoagulants
Fetal complications	Premature rupture of membranes Preterm labor; postmaturity Hydramnios or oligohydramnios Multifetal gestation
Environmental	Poverty Drugs, tobacco, alcohol Inadequate nutrition
LABOR	
Anatomic	Fetal head compression Malpresentation Umbilical cord prolapse Breech presentation Placenta previa; abruptio placentae Rigid soft tissues Multifetal gestation Placental or umbilical cord compression Excessive or inadequate fetal size
Physiologic	Dehydration Ketosis Fetal acidosis (pH 7.25 or less in the first stage of labor) Meconium staining of amniotic fluid Fetal bradycardia or tachycardia (>30 min) Abnormal nonstress test or oxytocin challenge test results Immature fetal lungs Severe preeclampsia-eclampsia
Maternal complications, iatrogenic	Sedative depression Hypotension; anesthesia; supine position Oxytocin (Pitocin) augmentation or induction of labor Prolonged labor; precipitous labor (<3 hr) Operative birth; cesarean, forceps, vacuum extraction
Uterine and placental	Uterine hypotonicity, hypertonicity, inertia Placental insufficiency

*Associated with intrauterine growth retardation (IUGR).

TABLE 27-3 Psychosocial Perinatal Warning Indicators for Families at High Risk for Abnormal Parenting Practices*

Pregnancy	Labor and birth	Postpartum
PARENTS' PHYSICAL AND PSYCHOLOGIC WELL-BEING		
Pregnancy is perceived as very difficult or burdensome Mother feels her health will suffer from childbearing or child rearing Mother intellectually subnormal Mother shows great depression over pregnancy Mother persists in feeling frightened and alone, especially before birth; careful explanations do not dissipate the fear Excessive visits for health care or expresses multiple psychosomatic complaints Evidence of emotional instability or mental illness History of drug or alcohol abuse Child wanted to fill unmet need in parents' lives Evidence of low self-esteem ("I'm no good"), particularly in parenting ability Mother aged under 20 years Previous pregnancy terminating in spontaneous abortion, fetal or neonatal death, or birth of a damaged child History of previous child's death or removal from home because of abuse or neglect	Mother experiencing excessive discomfort, fatigue, drug effects, or physical complications immediately after birth Mother or father perceive labor or birth as traumatic or unsatisfactory Obvious lack of supportive interaction between couple Hostile interaction between couple	Mother does not see attention focused on infant as something positive for herself Mother bothered by infant's crying; makes her feel helpless, hopeless, or unloved Mother relinquishes control to physicians and nurses for meeting needs of infant Evidence of low self-esteem ("I'm no good"), especially in parenting ability Parents express excessive feelings of failure concerning performance during labor or birth Parents express resentment or anger toward infant over childbirth experience Express excessive doubt about ability to care for infant
CHARACTERISTICS OF CHILD	Preterm Physically or mentally defective Immature or defective reflex behaviors Unresponsive Condition necessitates separation from parents "Wrong" sex Looks or behavior perceived in negative way by parents	As in column 2 Perceived by parent as being different or "not normal" despite normal findings Sex of infant remains unacceptable to parent Denies or exaggerates handicapped infant's capabilities Difficult feeder Unresponsive, e.g., sleepy baby Irritable or difficult to console Hyperreflexive infant Rigid or noncuddly infant

Modified from Ledger KE, Williams DL: *Parents at risk: an instructional program for perinatal assessment and preventive intervention,* Victoria, BC, Canada, 1981, Ministry of Health and Queen Alexandra Solarium for Crippled Children Society.

*It must be noted that it is not merely the presence or number of warning indicators that signify a high-risk situation. It is the unique combination of these indicators and their degree of expression in each individual family situation that is of importance. Factors such as culture, educational level, age of parents, receptiveness to change *must* be taken into consideration.

Continued.

TABLE 27-3 Psychosocial Perinatal Warning Indicators for Families at High Risk for Abnormal Parenting Practices—cont'd

Pregnancy	Labor and birth	Postpartum
PARENT-CHILD ATTACHMENT		
Pregnancy unplanned or unwanted Parents considered abortion or relinquishment Denial of pregnancy, e.g., unwilling to gain weight, refusal to talk about pregnancy In advanced pregnancy, mother dresses and acts as though she is not pregnant Absent or disturbed response to quickening Mother perceives fetal movement as abusive or aggressive actions Mother reports an experience she fears will damage baby (e.g., a "scare," accident) Undue concern about infant's sex or performance Absence of any fantasies about what baby will be like or predominantly negative fantasies Mother attributes negative characteristics to fetus Apparent lack of concern for physical well-being of unborn fetus, as evidenced by refusal to make health and life-style changes (e.g., poor nutrition, excessive use of drugs and alcohol) Absence of "nesting" behavior in the third trimester (e.g., preparation of clothing, equipment, space for infant)	Mother looks distressed, disappointed Does not talk to infant in affectionate terms Makes negative or hostile remarks to infant Expresses disappointment with sex of infant Mother makes inappropriate verbalizations, glances, or disparaging remarks about or toward infant Avoids eye contact and direct *en face* position Mother does not hold, touch, or examine infant Mother handles infant in rough manner	Does not comfort crying infant and does not heed physical needs Appears apathetic toward or disinterested in infant Expresses excessive doubt about ability to care for infant Remains disappointed over sex of infant Frequently voices negative feelings about or toward infant Repelled by messiness and diaper changing Negative identification of infant by name or association with someone disliked No feelings of attachment or bonding toward infant after 1 mo Mother does not appear to enjoy playing with infant
PARENTING KNOWLEDGE, BELIEFS, AND EXPECTATIONS		
Perceive own upbringing as abusive or neglectful Experienced harsh physical punishment during childhood Express belief that physical force is necessary in rearing and disciplining children Express a strong desire to parent in manner different from that of own parents Express inaccurate knowledge of infant care and development Express rigid or unrealistic expectations for infant's physical characteristics, behavior, development		As in column 1 Unaware of infant's characteristics and ability See infant as demanding or manipulative Inadequate preparation for child rearing Express expectations developmentally far beyond infant's capabilities Express fear of "spoiling" the infant

Continued.

TABLE 27-3 Psychosocial Perinatal Warning Indicators for Families at High Risk for Abnormal Parenting Practices—cont'd

Pregnancy	Labor and birth	Postpartum
SUPPORT SYSTEMS		
No spouse, mate, or significant other Express dissatisfaction with spouse or mate relationship Chronic marital discord, especially if focus of conflict is around child-bearing or child rearing Chronic conflict with or alienation from one's own mother or other female relatives History of loss of mother's own mother before her own puberty Mate or family's reaction to pregnancy is negative or nonsupportive Lack or loss of support systems, e.g., no supportive friends or relatives nearby Show evidence of social isolation, i.e., no telephone, outside interests, use of community resources	Mother expresses hostility toward father, who "put her through all this" As in column 1	As in column 1
FAMILY CIRCUMSTANCES		
Parent seems unaware or denies impact of new baby on relationship with mate, own time, other siblings Express concern that this child is going to be "one too many" Inadequate housing for family's needs Children too closely spaced Recent death or loss of loved one Have recently moved Financial, health, social, or interpersonal problems in the family Parents describe stresses of chaotic nature (e.g., physical fights, heavy drinking, arguments among immediate family members, abandonment by mate) Parents exhibit few skills for dealing with stress Express inability to cope with present life circumstances Dissatisfied with career or career change	As in column 1	As in column 1

Categories of High-Risk Pregnancy

Maternal age and parity factors

1. Age 16 years or under
2. Nullipara 35 years or over
3. Multipara 40 years or over
4. Interval of 8 years or more since last pregnancy
5. High parity (5 or more)
6. Pregnancy occurring 3 mo or less after last birth

Nonmarital pregnancy

Pregnancy-induced Hypertension, Hypertension, Kidney Disease

1. Preeclampsia with hospitalization before labor
2. Eclampsia
3. Kidney disease—e.g., pyelonephritis, nephritis, nephrosis
4. Chronic hypertension, severe (160/100 mm Hg or over)
5. Blood pressure 140/90 mm Hg or above on two readings 30 min apart

Anemia and Hemorrhage

1. Hematocrit 30% or below in pregnancy
2. Hemorrhage (previous pregnancy)—severe, requiring transfusion
3. Hemorrhage (present pregnancy)
4. Anemia (hemoglobin below 10 g) for which treatment other than oral iron preparations is required (hemolytic, macrocytic)
5. Sickle cell trait or disease
6. History of bleeding or clotting disorder at any time

Fetal Factors

1. Two or more previous preterm births (twins = one parity)
2. Two or more consecutive spontaneous abortions (miscarriages)
3. One or more stillbirths at term
4. One or more gross anomalies
5. Rh incompatibility or ABO immunization problems
6. History of previous birth defects—cerebral palsy, brain damage, mental retardation, metabolic disorders such as PKU
7. History of large infants (4032 g [9 lb])

Paternal age (?) and other factors (?)

Dystocia (history of or anticipated)

1. Contracted pelvis or CPD
2. Multifetal pregnancy in current pregnancy
3. Two or more breech births
4. Previous operative births, e.g., cesarean or midforceps birth
5. History of prolonged labor (more than 18 hr for nulliparous woman; more than 12 hours for multiparous woman
6. Previously diagnosed genital tract anomalies (incompetent cervix, cervical or uterine malformation, solitary ovary or tube) or problem (ovarian mass, endometriosis
7. Short stature (1.5 m [60 in] or less)

History of or concurrent conditions

1. Diabetes mellitus; gestational diabetes
2. Hyperemesis gravidarum
3. Thyroid disease (hypothyroidism or hyperthyroidism)
4. Malnutrition or extreme obesity (20% over ideal weight for height; 15% under ideal weight for height)
5. Organic heart disease
6. Syphilis and TORCH infections: toxoplasmosis, rubella in first 10 weeks of *this* pregnancy, CMV, and herpes simplex; HIV
7. Tuberculosis or other serious pulmonary pathologic condition (e.g., emphysema, asthma)
8. Malignant or premalignant tumors (including hydatidiform mole)
9. Alcoholism, drug addiction
10. Psychiatric disease or epilepsy (documented)
11. Mental retardation

Previous history

1. Late registration
2. Poor clinic attendance
3. Home situation making clinic attendance and hospitalization difficult
4. Mothers, including minors, without family resources (including desertions, adoptions, injuries, separations, family withdrawals, sole support)

CMV, Cytomegalovirus; *CPD*, cephalopelvic disproportion; *PKU*, phenylketonuria. Modified from Fogel CI, Woods NF: *Health care of women: a nursing perspective*, St Louis, 1981, Mosby–Year Book.

Factors that Place the Postpartum Woman and Neonate at High Risk

THE MOTHER

Hemorrhage
Infection
Abnormal vital signs
Traumatic labor or birth
Psychosocial factors

THE INFANT (FOR ADMISSION TO NICU)

High-risk category

Infants continuing or developing signs of RDS or other respiratory distress
Asphyxiated infants (Apgar score <6 at 5 min); resuscitation required at birth
Preterm infants; dysmature infants
Infants with cyanosis or suspected cardiovascular disease; persistent cyanosis
Infants with major congenital malformations requiring surgery; chromosomal anomalies
Infants with convulsions, sepsis, hemorrhagic diathesis, or shock
Meconium aspiration syndrome
CNS depression for > 24 hr.
Hypoglycemia
Hypocalcemia
Hyperbilirubinemia

Moderate risk

Dysmaturity
Prematurity (weight between 2000 and 2500 g)
Apgar score of < 5 at 1 min
Feeding problems
Multifetal birth
Transient tachypnea
Hypomagnesemia or hypermagnesemia
Hypoparathyroidism
Failure to gain weight
Jitteriness or hyperactivity
Cardiac anomalies not requiring immediate catheterization
Heart murmur
Anemia
CNS depression for <24 hr

CNS, Central nervous system; *NICU*, Neonatal intensive care unit; *RDS*, respiratory distress syndrome.

care provider can take measures to prevent or minimize adverse perinatal outcomes. Unfortunately, no single test can provide this information. The results of such tests must be interpreted in light of the complete clinical picture. The remainder of the chapter describes those available diagnostic techniques and their use in detecting fetuses at risk.

■ BIOPHYSICAL ASSESSMENT

Ultrasonography

Sound is a waveform of energy that causes small particles in a medium to oscillate. The frequency of sound, which refers to the number of peaks or waves that traverse a given point per unit of time, is expressed in hertz (Hz). Sound with a frequency of one cycle, or one peak per second, would have a frequency of 1 Hz. When directional beams of sound strike an object, an echo is returned. The time delay between the emission of the sound and the return of the echo is noted, as well as the direction from which the echo comes. From these data the object's distance and location can be calculated.

First introduced in the 1960s, diagnostic ultrasound has developed rapidly to enjoy a principal position in antepartum fetal surveillance. **Ultrasound** is sound having a frequency higher than that of normal human hearing, that is, greater than 20,000 Hz. Diagnostic ultrasound instruments operate in a range of frequency varying from 2 to 10 million Hz (or 2 to 10 megahertz [MHz]), still well below that used by sonar and radar.

The biophysical principles of diagnostic ultrasound are beyond the scope of this text, but several excellent resources are available (see Bibliography at the end of this chapter).

OPERATIONAL MODES. Table 27-4 presents a summary of modalities, imaging, and principal uses of diagnostic ultrasound. Static image scanners are useful for gynecologic as well as obstetric diagnoses. Dynamic image scanners provide direct visualization of indicators of fetal viability—fetal cardiac and body movement.

INDICATIONS FOR USE. Major indications for the use of obstetric sonography by trimester appear in Table 27-5. During the *first trimester* ultrasound examination is performed to obtain the following information: (1) number, size, and location of gestational sacs (Fig. 27-2), (2) presence or absence of fetal cardiac and body movement, (3) presence or absence of uterine abnormalities (e.g. bicornuate uterus or fi-

TABLE 27-4 Diagnostic Ultrasound: Operational Modes*

Modality	Product	Principal Use
Pulsed wave		
A Mode	Static image	Diagnostic evaluation of brain
B Mode (gray scale)*	Static image	Images of abdominal and pelvic structures
M Mode	Dynamic imaging	Monitoring of heart and measuring of heart wall displacement
Real time*	Static image and dynamic imaging	Provides dynamic imaging and static images
Continuous wave		
Doppler mode*	Ranging mode	Fetal heart monitoring

Pulsed wave, Sound emitted at intervals; *continuous wave,* sound emitted continuously; *A mode,* one-dimensional image that appears as spikes on a horizontal base; distance between spikes can be measured (e.g., biparietal diameter [BPD]; *B mode (gray scale),* rough, two-dimensional image of various tissue densities for visualizing tissue texture and contour; *M mode,* time-related tracings showing straight lines for motionless structures and wiggly lines for structural motion (e.g., atrial septal defects and patent ductus arteriosus); *static,* stationary; *dynamic,* moving; *Doppler mode,* detection of change in frequency (wavelength) of structures rather than in amplitude motion (e.g., blood flow in umbilical cord and placenta, closure of fetal cardiac valves) *real time,* dynamic imaging (limb and respiratory movements), as well as static images (BPD, placental location);
*Used extensively in obstetrics and gynecology

TABLE 27-5 Major Indications for Obstetric Sonography

First Trimester	Second Trimester	Third Trimester
Confirm pregnancy	Establish or confirm dates*	If no fetal heart tones:
Confirm viability	If no fetal heart tones:	Clarify dates/size discrepancy
Rule out ectopic pregnancy	Clarify dates/size discrepancy	Large for dates—rule out:
Confirm gestational age†	Large for dates—rule out:	Macrosomia (diabetes mellitus)
Birth control use	Poor estimate of dates	Multifetal gestation
Irregular menses	Molar pregnancy	Polyhydramnios
No dates	Multifetal gestation	Congenital anomalies
Postpartum pregnancy	Leiomyomata	Poor estimate of dates‡
Previous complicated pregnancy	Polyhydramnios	Small for dates—rule out:
Cesarean birth	Congenital anomalies	Fetal growth retardation
Rh incompatibility	Small for dates—rule out:	Oligohydramnios
Diabetes mellitus	Poor estimate of dates	Congenital anomalies
Fetal growth retardation	Fetal growth retardation	Poor estimate of dates‡
Clarify dates/sizes discrepancy	Congenital anomalies	Determine fetal position—rule out:
Large for dates—rule out:	Oligohydramnios	Breech
Leiomyomata	If history of bleeding—rule out total placenta previa	Transverse lie
Bicornuate uterus	If Rh incompatibility—rule out fetal hydrops	If history of bleeding—rule out:
Adnexal mass		Placenta previa
Multifetal gestation		Abruptio placentae
Poor dates		Determine fetal lung maturity
Molar pregnancy*§		Amniocentesis for lecithin/sphingomyelin ratio
Small for dates—rule out;		Placental maturity (grade 0-3)
Poor dates		If Rh incompatibility—rule out fetal hydrops
Missed abortion		
Blighted ovum		

Modified from Athey PA, Hadlock, FP: *Ultrasound in obstetrics and gynecology,* ed 2, St Louis, 1985, Mosby–Year Book.
*Accuracy ± 1 to 1½ weeks.
†Accuracy ± 3 days
‡Accuracy only ± 3 weeks
§Hydatidiform mole.

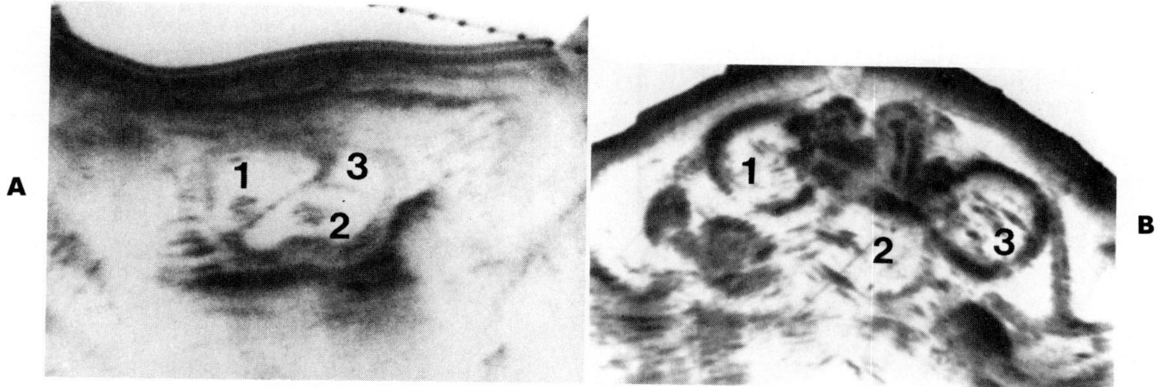

Fig. 27-2 **A,** Transverse static image scan demonstrates three well-formed gestational sacs. **B,** Subsequent static image scan demonstrates three well-defined fetal heads in this woman carrying triplets.
From Athey PA, Hadlock FP: *Ultrasound in obstetrics and gynecology*, ed 2, St Louis, 1985, Mosby–Year Book.

broids) or adnexal masses (e.g. ovarian cysts or ectopic pregnancy), (4) pregnancy dating (i.e., crown-rump length), and (5) coexistence and location of an intrauterine device (IUD).

During the *second* and *third trimesters*, the following information is sought: (1) fetal viability, number, position, gestational age, growth pattern, and anomalies, (2) amniotic fluid volume, (3) placental location and maturity, (4) uterine fibroids and anomalies, and (5) adnexal masses.

FINDINGS. In general, the use of ultrasound has hastened diagnoses so that appropriate therapy can be instituted early in the pregnancy. Early therapy may decrease the severity and duration of morbidity, both physical and emotional, of the family. Early diagnosis of a fetal anomaly, for instance, makes possible choices such as (1) intrauterine surgery or other therapy for the fetus, (2) discontinuation of the pregnancy, and (3) preparation of the family for the care of a child with a disorder.

FETAL VIABILITY. Fetal heart activity can be demonstrated as early as 6 to 7 weeks by real-time echo scanners and at 10 to 12 weeks by Doppler mode. By 9 to 10 weeks, gestational trophoblastic disease can be diagnosed (Fig. 27-3). Confirmation of fetal death can be detected by lack of heart motion, the presence of fetal scalp edema, and maceration and overlap of the cranial bones.

GESTATIONAL AGE. Several indicators have been established for the need of gestational dating: (1) uncertain dates for the last normal menstrual period, (2) recent discontinuation of oral contraceptives, (3) bleeding episode during the first trimester, (4) uterine size that does not agree with dates, and (5) other high-risk conditions.

During the first 18 weeks of gestation, the use of ultrasound permits an extremely accurate assessment of gestational age because most normal fetuses grow at the same rate. However, the accuracy of assessment is inversely related to fetal age inasmuch as fetuses do not grow at a constant rate. Rather they move from an exponential rate at conception toward a linear rate in later pregnancy. Thus the distribution of physical measures for a population of fetuses at the same age broadens as age advances. With advanced age the accuracy of gestational age estimates by means of ultrasound increases, however, as more variables are measured (Manning, 1989).

Four methods of fetal age estimation are used: (1) determination of gestational sac dimensions (about 8 weeks), (2) measurement of crown-rump length (between 7 and 14 weeks), (3) measurement of the **biparietal diameter (BPD)** (about 12 weeks), and (4) measurement of femur length (after 12 weeks). Fetal BPD at 36 weeks should be approximately 8.7 cm. Term pregnancy and fetal maturity can be diagnosed with some confidence if the biparietal cephalometric measurement by ultrasound is greater than 9.8 cm (Fig. 27-4 and Table 27-6), especially when combined with appropriate femur length measurement.

In later gestations the accuracy of fetal age determination is enhanced by serial measurements. Two, preferably three, composite measurements are recommended, at least 2 weeks apart, and plotted against standard fetal growth curves. When applied between 24 and 32 weeks' gestation, this method yields an estimate error of 10 days more or less (Manning, 1989).

FETAL GROWTH. Fetal growth is a result of interaction between intrinsic growth potential and environmental factors that may enhance or inhibit that

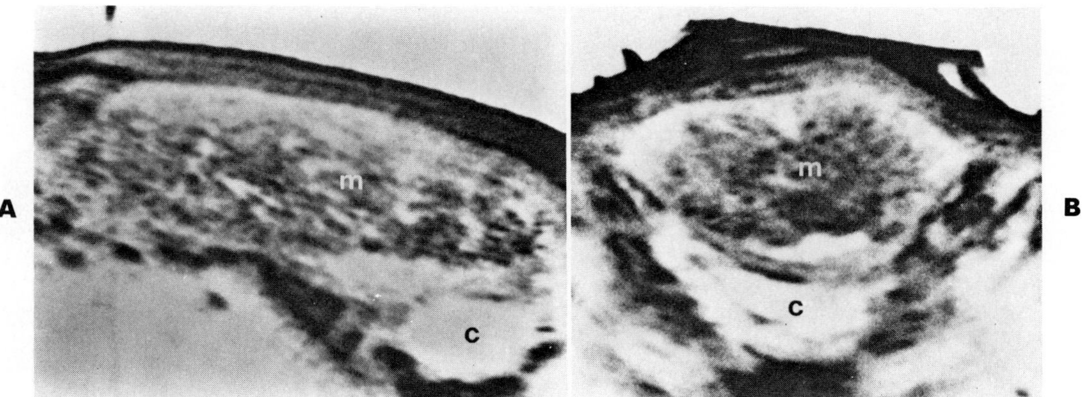

Fig. 27-3 Longitudinal (**A**) and transverse (**B**) scans of molar pregnancy *(m)*. Note typical vesicular (grapelike) pattern. Also demonstrated are multiloculated lutein ovarian cysts *(c)* in cul-de-sac.
From Athey PA, Hadlock FP: *Ultrasound in obstetrics and gynecology,* ed 2, St Louis, 1985, Mosby–Year Book.

growth. Conditions that serve as indicators for ultrasound assessment of fetal growth include (1) poor maternal weight gain or pattern of weight gain, (2) previous **intrauterine growth retardation (IUGR),** (3) chronic infections, (4) ingestion of drugs, (5) maternal diabetes mellitus, (6) pregnancy-induced or other hypertension, (6) multifetal pregnancy, and (7) other medical or surgical complications.

Serial evaluations of BPD and limb length can differentiate between wrong dates and true IUGR. IUGR may be symmetric (the fetus is small in all parameters) or asymmetric (head and body growth vary). Symmetric IUGR, which implies a chronic or long-standing insult, may be caused by low genetic growth potential, intrauterine infection, maternal undernutrition or heavy smoking, or chromosomal aberration. Asymmetric growth reflects an acute, or late-occurring deprivation, such as placental insufficiency resulting from hypertension, renal disease, or cardiovascular disease. Reduced fetal growth is still among the most frequent complications associated with stillbirth (Morrison, Olsen, 1985). Macrosomic infants (those weighing >4000 g) are at increased risk for birth trauma; macrosomic fetuses associated with maternal glucose intolerance are at increased risk of intrauterine death as well (Fig. 27-5) (Manning, 1989).

TABLE 27-6 Correlation of Fetal Weight and Biparietal Diameter

BPD (cm)	Estimated Fetal Weight
8.2	2290 g (5 lb 1 oz)
8.5	2500 g (5 lb 8 oz)
8.8	2730 g (6 lb 0 oz)
9.4	3180 g (7 lb 0 oz)
10.0	3630 g (8 lb 0 oz)
10.6	4070 g (9 lb 0 oz)

ADJUNCT TO AMNIOCENTESIS. The safety of amniocentesis is increased when the physician knows the exact position of the fetus, placenta, and pockets of amniotic fluid. The use of ultrasound scanning has greatly reduced previous risks associated with amniocentesis, such as a fetomaternal hemorrhage from a pierced placenta.

FETAL ANATOMY. Depending on the gestational age, the following structures may be identified: head (including ventricles and blood vessels), neck, spine, heart, stomach, small bowel, liver, kidneys, bladder, and limbs. Ultrasonography permits the confirmation of normal anatomy or the detection of major fetal malformations. The recognition of an anomaly may influence the location and method of birth so that neonatal outcomes may be optimal. Beyond 36 weeks of gestation, more than 85% of all major anomalies can be detected by ultrasound. As a general rule the earlier in gestation a lesion is detected, the worse the prognostic significance (Manning, 1989).

The number of fetuses and their presentation also may be assessed. This knowledge often will govern therapy and mode of birth.

PLACENTAL POSITION AND FUNCTION. The pattern of uterine and placental growth and the fullness of the maternal bladder influence the apparent location of the placenta. During the first trimester, differentiation between the endometrium and the small placenta is difficult. By 14 to 16 weeks the pla-

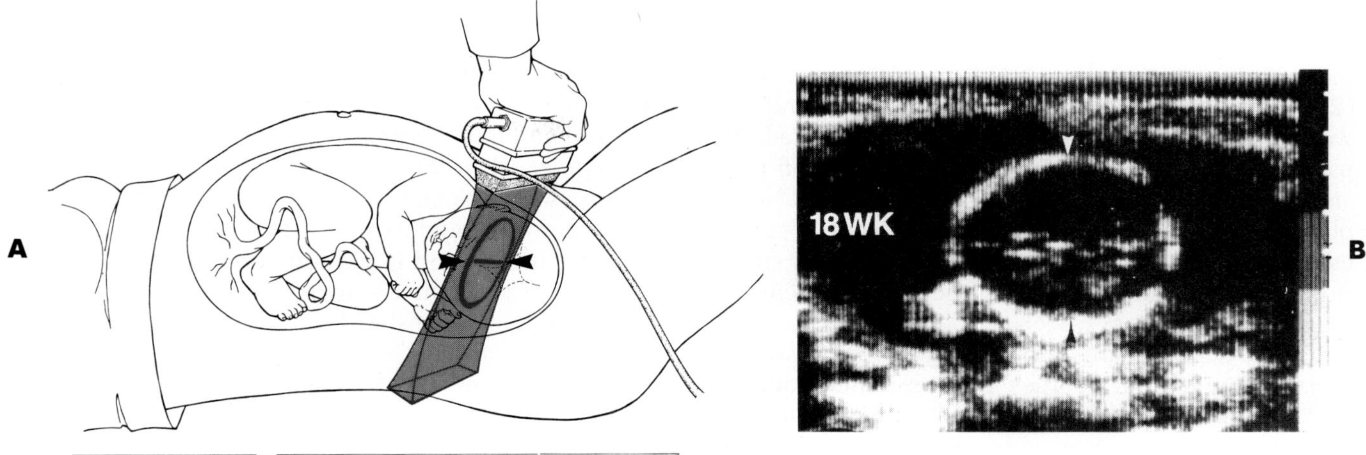

Fig. 27-4 **A,** Biparietal *(arrow)* cephalometry by ultrasound. **B,** Linear-array, real-time image demonstrates fetal BPD *(arrow)* at 18 weeks.
B from Athey PA, Hadlock FP: *Ultrasound in obstetrics and gynecology,* ed 2, St Louis, 1985, Mosby–Year Book.

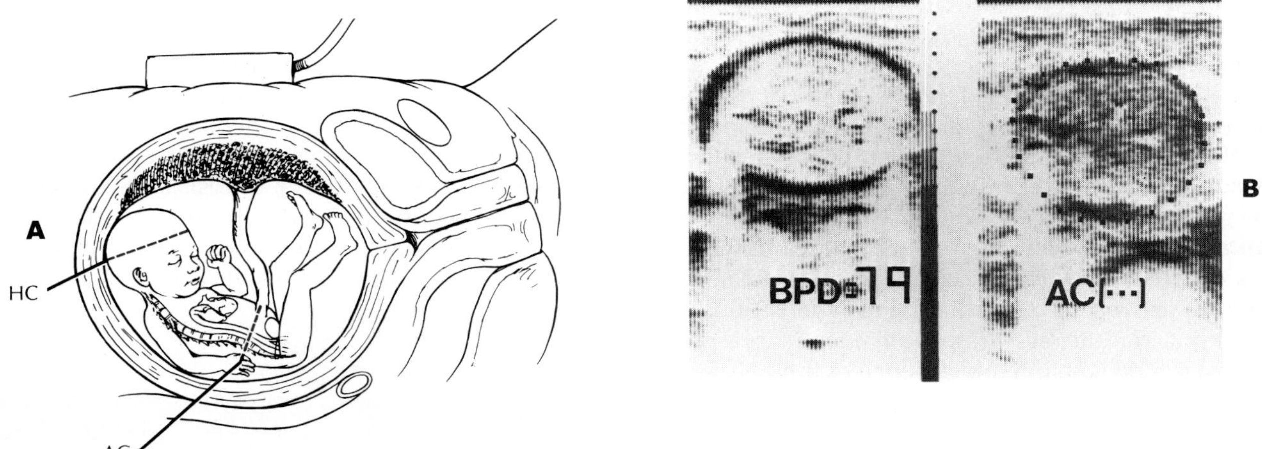

Fig. 27-5 **A,** Schematic presentation of appropriate planes of sections *(dotted lines)* for BPD, head circumference *(HC),* and abdominal circumference *(AC).* **B,** Real-time ultrasound image demonstrates typical head and body images that correspond to planes in **A.** Using these two images, one can determine BPD (7.9 cm), HC (30 cm), AC (28 cm), and estimated fetal weight *(EFW)* (1840 g) in this normal 32-week fetus.
From Athey PA, Hadlock FP: *Ultrasound in obstetrics and gynecology,* ed 2, St Louis, 1985, Mosby–Year Book.

centa can be clearly defined, but if it is seen to be low lying, its relationship to the internal cervical os sometimes can be altered dramatically by changing the degree of fullness of the maternal bladder. In approximately 15% to 20% of all pregnancies in which ultrasound scanning is performed in the second trimester, the placenta seems to be overlying the os; at term the incidence of placenta previa is only 0.5%. The diagnosis of *placenta previa* can seldom be confirmed until 27 weeks, mainly because of the elongation of the lower uterine segment as pregnancy advances.

Third-trimester grading of placental maturation can be accomplished by means of ultrasound scanning. It has been recognized that throughout gestation the placenta undergoes detectable maturational changes; a relationship has been noted between advancing placental grade and fetal pulmonary maturity. Placentas are graded on a scale of 0 to 3 (with 3 being the most mature) that is based on the identification and distribution of calcium deposits within the fetal component (Manning, 1989). Ultrasound examination can identify changes in the chorionic plate, placental substance, and basal layer of the placenta that correspond to the following grades: (1) grade 0 placentas are seen in the first and second trimesters; (2) grade I placentas appear between 30 and 32 weeks and may even persist until term; (3) grade II placentas are observed at around 36 weeks and persist until term in 45% of pregnancies; (4) grade III placentas are seen at 38 weeks and reflect the greatest maturation; however, this occurs in only a small number of placentas (Scherwen et al, 1991; Schruefer, Warsof, in press).

These deposits are also significant in *postterm pregnancies* in that as they increase, the available surface area that can be adequately bathed by maternal blood decreases. At exactly what point this results in fetal wastage and hypoxia cannot be pinpointed precisely; however, effects usually are observable by 42 weeks and progress thereafter (Gilbert, Harmon, 1992).

FETAL WELL-BEING. Among the many physiologic measurements that can be performed with ultrasound scanning are the following: heart motion, fetal breathing movements, fetal urine production, fetal limb and head movements, and analysis of vascular waveforms from the fetal circulation. Assessment of these parameters yields a fairly reliable picture of fetal well-being, singly or in cohort fashion. The significance of these findings is discussed in the following sections.

Amniotic Fluid Volume. Abnormalities of amniotic fluid volume, whether excessive or diminished, frequently are associated with fetal disorders. Subjective criteria for the assessment of *oligohydramnios* (decreased fluid) include the absence of fluid pockets throughout the uterine cavity and the impression of crowding of fetal small parts. Objective determination of decreased volume is made when the largest pocket of fluid measured in two perpendicular planes is less than 1 cm. In the case of *polyhydramnios* (increased fluid), subjective criteria include multiple large pockets, the impression of a floating fetus, and free movement of fetal limbs. The diagnosis may be made when the largest pocket of fluid exceeds 8 cm in two perpendicular planes (Gabbe, 1986; Manning, 1989).

The total volume can be evaluated by a method developed by Rutherford et al (1987) whereby the depths (in centimeters) of amniotic fluid in all four quadrants surrounding the maternal umbilicus are totaled, resulting in an *amniotic fluid index* (AFI). An AFI of less than 5 cm is considered to indicate oligohydramnios, 5 to 8 cm is considered borderline, and a measurement greater than 8 cm reflects polyhydramnios.

Oligohydramnios has been associated with congenital anomalies (such as renal agenesis), growth retardation, and fetal distress in labor. Polyhydramnios has been found with neural tube defects, obstruction of the fetal gastrointestinal tract, multiple fetuses, and fetal hydrops (Gabbe, 1986).

Doppler Blood Flow Analysis. One of the major advances in perinatal medicine is the ability to study blood flow noninvasively in the fetus and placenta. **Doppler ultrasound** is a helpful adjunct in the management of pregnancies at risk because of hypertension, IUGR, diabetes mellitus, multifetal gestation, and preterm labor.

When a sound wave is reflected from a moving target, there is a change in frequency of the reflected wave relative to the transmitted wave. This is called the Doppler effect. An ultrasound beam scattered by a group of red blood cells (RBCs) is an example of this effect. The velocity of the RBCs can be determined by measuring the change in the frequency in the sound wave reflected off them (Trudinger, 1989).

Doppler-shifted frequencies can be displayed as velocity versus time. The shape of these waveforms can be analyzed to give information about blood flow and resistance in a given circulation (Schulman, 1990). Velocity waveforms from umbilical and uterine arteries, reported in systolic/diastolic (S/D) ratios, can first be detected at 15 weeks of pregnancy. Because of progressive decline in resistance in both the umbilical and uterine artery circulation, decreasing measurement values occur as pregnancy advances. Most fetuses will achieve an S/D ratio of 3 or less by 30 weeks (Fig. 27-6).

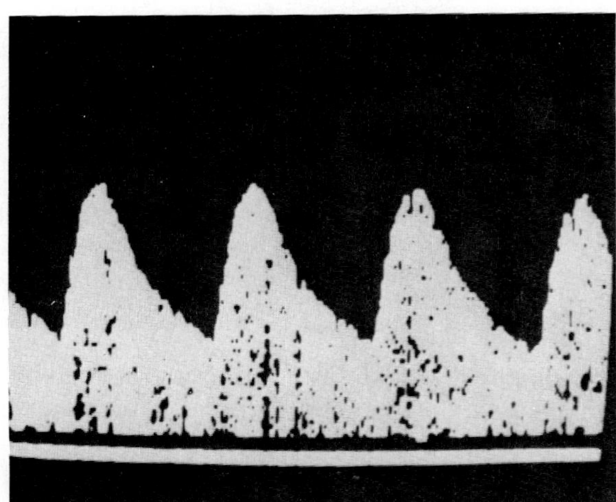

Fig. 27-6 Normal umbilical artery velocity wave forms, and measurements from systole and end-diastole.
From Schulman H: Doppler, ultrasound. In Eden R, Boehm R, editors: *Assessment and care of the fetus: physiological, clinical and medicolegal principles,* Norwalk Conn, 1990, Appleton & Lange, p. 399.

Persistent elevation of S/D ratios after 30 weeks is associated with IUGR, usually resulting from *uteroplacental insufficiency*. Abnormal velocity study results also are seen with certain chromosome abnormalities (trisomy 13 and 18) in the fetus and lupus erythematosus in the mother (Schulman, 1990). Nicotine from maternal smoking also has been reported to increase the S/D ratio (Fig. 27-7) (Trudinger, 1989).

Biophysical Profile. The advent of real-time ultrasound now permits detailed assessment of the physical and physiologic characteristics of the developing fetus to such an extent that it is possible to examine the fetus in detail and to catalogue normal and abnormal biophysical responses to stimuli. The **biophysical profile (BPP)** is a noninvasive dynamic assessment of a fetus and its environment, employing ultrasonography and external fetal monitoring. It was introduced in 1980 by Manning and colleagues (1980).

Fetal BPP scoring is a method of fetal risk surveillance based on the composite assessment of both acute and chronic markers of fetal disease. It also yields fetal morphologic data. The procedure may be viewed as undertaking a physical examination of the fetus, including determination of vital signs. The fetus responds to central hypoxia by alterations in movement, muscle tone, breathing, and heart rate patterns. The implication has major importance: the presence of normal fetal biophysical activities shows that the central nervous system is fully functional and therefore not hypoxemic (Manning, Harman, 1990). The absence of the following three distinct biophysical variables (Table 27-7)is significant:

1. **Fetal breathing movements (FBM)** —Defined by initial inward movement of the thorax with descent of the diaphragm and abdominal contents, followed by a return to the original position.
2. Fetal movements (FM)—Defined as single or clusters of activity involving the limbs and fetal body; isolated hand and arm movements represent normality.
3. Fetal tone (FT)—The definition has been refined to at least one episode of opening of the hand with finger and thumb extension with a return to closed fist formation. In the absence of any hand movement, tone is still recorded as normal if the hand remains in the fist formation for the entire 30-minute observation.

Scoring also includes two other findings:

- Qualitative amniotic fluid volume—Normal is a finding of at least one pocket that measures at least 1 cm in two perpendicular planes.
- Nonstress test—Often performed before the BPP as a screening procedure.

Table 27-7 includes scoring and management factors. Although some clinicians advocate the use of a 3-point scoring system (0-1-2), the 0 or 2 points assigned to these factors remain the more generally applied system.

The BPP provides an accurate estimate of the risk

A

B

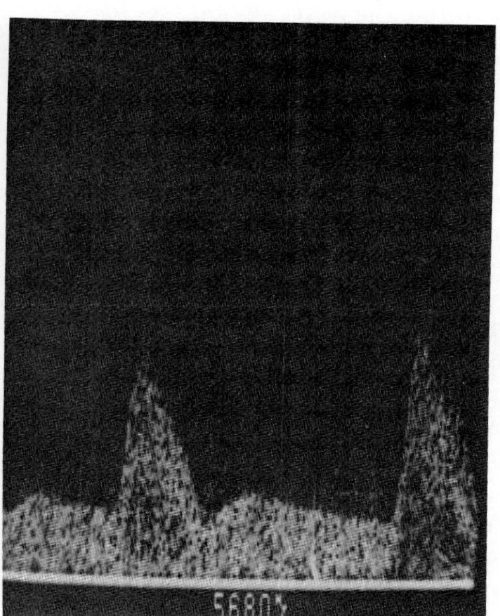

Fig. 27-7 Normal and abnormal uteroplacental vessels at 34 weeks. *Left,* Normal S/D of 2.1. *Right,* S/D = 3.4. The difference is 1.3.

From Schulman H: Doppler, ultrasound. In Eden R, Boehm R, editors: *Assessment and care of the fetus: physiological, clinical and medicolegal principles,* Norwalk Conn, 1990, Appleton & Lange, p. 399.

TABLE 27-7 Biophysical Profile Scoring: Technique and Interpretation

Biophysical Variable	Normal (Score = 2)	Abnormal (Score = 0)
Fetal breathing movements (FBM)	At least one episode of FBM of at least 30-sec duration in 30-min observation	Absent FBM or no episode of >30 sec in 30 min
Gross body movement	At least three discrete body or limb movements in 30 min (episodes of active continuous movement considered as single movement)	Two or fewer episodes of body or limb movements in 30 min
Fetal tone	At least one episode of active extension with return to flexion of fetal limb(s) or trunk. Opening and closing of hand considered normal tone	Either slow extension with return to partial flexion or movement of limb in full extension, absent fetal movement
Reactive FHR	At least two episodes of FHR acceleration of >15 beats/min and of at least 15-sec duration associated with fetal movement in 30 min	Less than two episodes of acceleration of FHR or acceleration of >15 beats/min in 30 min
Qualitative AFV	At least one pocket of AF that measures at least 1 cm in two perpendicular planes,	Either no AF pockets or a pocket <1 cm in two perpendicular planes

From Manning F, Harman C: The fetal biophysical profile. In Eden R, Boehm F, editors: *Assessments and care of the fetus: physiological, clinical and medicolegal principles,* Norwalk, Conn, 1990, Appleton & Lange. Used with permission.
FBM, Fetal breathing movement; *FHR,* fetal heart rate; *AFV,* amniotic fluid volume; *AF,* amniotic fluid.

of fetal death in the immediate future. Data support the BPP as an early predictor of an acidotic fetus in the face of a nonreactive nonstress test result and absent FBM. In addition, when an abnormal score and oligohydramnios are encountered, labor induction is warranted (Manning, Harman, 1990). The BPP also has proved effective as an early predictor of fetal infection in women whose membranes rupture prematurely (at less than 37 weeks' gestation). The change in biophysical activities precedes the clinical signs of infection and indicates the necessity for immediate birth (Gaffney et al, 1990). When risk is low, as with a normal score, intervention is indicated only for obstetric or maternal factors.

NURSING ROLE. Although a growing number of nurses perform ultrasound scans and BPPs in certain centers, most nurses are involved mainly in counseling and educating women about the procedure. Accurate information regarding the procedure is imperative to allay the mother's anxiety. Although ultrasound scanning has become a widely used diagnostic tool, recommendations for the procedure are based on expectations of a fetal problem and therefore may cause concern. The nurse should provide ample opportunity to answer the woman's questions and reassure her that the procedure is safe.

Early in pregnancy the woman usually is directed to come for the examination with a full bladder because it supports the uterus in position for the imaging. She is then positioned comfortably with small pillows under her head and knees. The display panel should be positioned so that the woman can observe the images on the screen if she so desires; some women may *not* want to watch (Fig. 27-8).

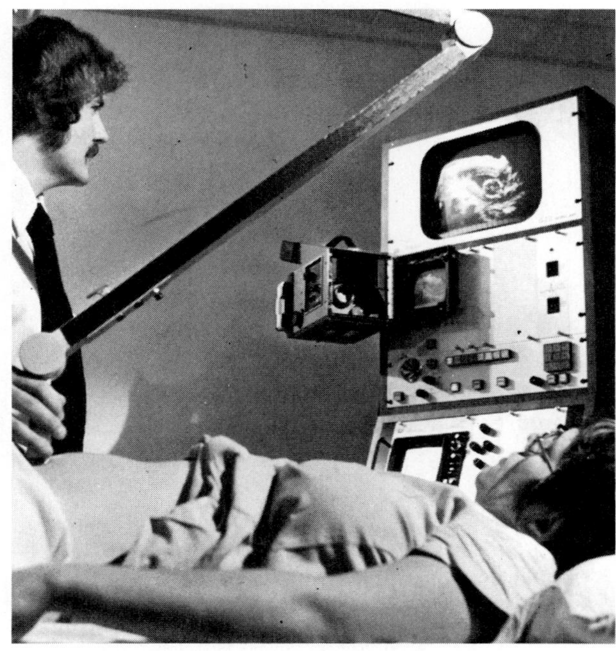

Fig. 27-8 Ultrasound examination.
Courtesy March of Dimes Birth Defects Foundation.

SAFETY OF DIAGNOSTIC ULTRASOUND. Although there is no conclusive evidence that humans have been harmed by diagnostic ultrasound during the 25 years it has been used, a hypothetical risk cannot be ignored. However, no biologic damage has been measured at ultrasonic intensity of less than 100 mW/cm^2, even for extended exposure times. Diagnostic ultrasonic beams all have intensities less than 10 mW/cm^2 and are applied for relatively short times. Diagnostic units also employ pulsed ultrasound with a usual duty cycle of 1/1000, which during 24 hours of continuous sampling produces only 86 seconds of ultrasonic exposure (Manning, 1989). Thus the total ultrasound exposure for a fetus will depend on the number of ultrasonic examinations performed, the type of equipment used, and the amount of energy received, which depends on the duration of the procedure. It has been recommended that the length of ultrasound study and the type of equipment used be recorded. Although the possibility exists that some biologic effects may be identified in the future, current data indicate that the benefits to the client of prudent use of diagnostic ultrasound far outweigh the possible risk (Gabbe, 1986).

Magnetic Resonance Imaging

Magnetic resonance imaging (MRI) is a noninvasive tool that can be used for obstetric and gynecologic diagnosis. Like computerized tomography (CT), MRI provides excellent pictures of soft tissue. Unlike CT, ionizing radiation is not used; thus vascular structures within the body can be seen and evaluated without the need to inject an iodinated contrast medium, which eliminates any known biologic risk. Like sonography, MRI is noninvasive and can provide images in multiple planes; yet interference from skeletal, fatty, or gas-filled structures is not a problem. Also, imaging of deep pelvic structures does not depend on a full bladder.

MRI can evaluate (1) fetal structure—CNS, thorax, abdomen, genitourinary tract, musculoskeletal system, and overall growth, (2) placenta—position, density, and evaluation of gestational trophoblastic disease, (3) amniotic fluid quantity, (4) maternal structures—uterus, cervix, adnexa, and pelvis, (5) biochemical status (pH, adenosine triphosphate [ATP] content) of tissues and organs, and (6) soft tissue, metabolic, or functional malformations.

The woman is placed on a table in a supine position and slid into the bore of the main magnet that is similar in appearance to a CT scanner. Depending on the reason for the study, the entire procedure may take anywhere from 20 to 60 minutes, during which time the woman must be perfectly still except for short respites. Because of the long time needed to produce magnetic resonance images, it is likely that the fetus will move, which will obscure anatomic details. The only way to ensure that the fetus will not move is to administer a sedative to the mother, but this approach should be reserved for selected cases in which visualization of fetal detail is critical (Weinreb, Brown, 1990). Although the procedure appears to have many advantages, its total safety has not been accurately determined. Thus broad usage should not be encouraged until results of further study are known (Mattison, Angtuaco, 1988).

Fetoscopy, Amnioscopy and Roentgenography

Direct fetoscopic visualization is possible by means of a tiny telescope-like instrument with the caliber of a large hypodermic needle. The fetoscope is introduced into the uterus through the abdominal wall with the woman under local anesthesia. This method is not used extensively because there is a risk of causing preterm labor. The fetoscope is used most often to obtain fetal blood samples for diagnosing serious hereditary blood disorders (e.g., sickle cell anemia). However, newer techniques to obtain fetal blood cells have largely supplanted this technique.

Fetal hypoxia often results in meconium passage by the mature fetus. Transcervical visualization of greenish amniotic fluid through the intact membranes (amnioscopy) will confirm the presence of meconium. Unfortunately, because the cervix must be more than 1 cm dilated and special equipment is needed, this technique is used only rarely.

A special x-ray technique, termed *amniography* or *fetography,* allows visualization of gross structural abnormalities during the third trimester. There has been little experience with its use in early pregnancy.

The procedure involves the instillation of a radio contrast medium into the amniotic fluid. The medium adheres to fetal skin to produce a clear fetal silhouette on the x-ray film. Before the development of diagnostic ultrasound, amniography was used to visualize suspected fetal malformations and localize the fetal gastrointestinal (GI) tract before an intrauterine transfusion. Fetal swallowing of the dye resulted in visualization of the GI tract. Both procedures, which expose the fetus to the dangers of ionizing radiation, have largely been replaced by ultrasound (Gabbe, 1986).

Daily Fetal Movement Count

Maternal assessment of fetal activity is a simple yet valuable method for monitoring the fetal condition. **Daily fetal movement count (DFMC)** can be done at home, is noninvasive, is simple to understand, and does not interfere with most daily routines. In general, the presence of fetal movements is a reassuring sign of fetal health. It has been well-documented in the literature that decrease in or absence of fetal movements was noted by most women who experienced stillbirth (Calhoun, 1990).

Maternal awareness of fetal movements is reported to be at least 90% accurate as demonstrated by simultaneous observation of the fetus by real-time ultrasound. It also is important to note that no mothers reported *more* movements than were documented. Several protocols are used for counting. Except for very low daily fetal movements or a trend toward decreased motion, the clinical value of the absolute number of fetal movements has not been established. The only exception is if fetal movements cease entirely for 12 hours (the fetal alarm signal). Generally, less than three FM within 1 hour warrants further evaluation through nonstress or contraction stress testing, BPP, or a combination. Gabbe (1986) reported most success using a combination of the fetal alarm signal and less than 10 movements during a 12-hour period.

■ BIOCHEMICAL ASSESSMENT

Biochemical assessment involves the study of biologic components such as genes or exfoliated cells and of chemical components such as the lecithin/sphingomyelin ratio and bilirubin level. Specific procedures are used to obtain the specimens needed for study: amniocentesis, percutaneous umbilical blood sampling, chorionic villi sampling, and maternal assays.

Amniocentesis

Amniocentesis is performed to obtain amniotic fluid, which contains fetal cells. Under direct ultrasound visualization, a needle is inserted transabdominally into the uterus. Amniotic fluid is withdrawn into a syringe and various **amniotic fluid assessments** performed. Amniocentesis is possible after week 14 of pregnancy, when the uterus becomes an abdominal organ and sufficient amniotic fluid is available for this procedure (Table 27-8 and Fig. 27-9).

Overall complications are less than 1% for both mother and fetus and include the following:

Maternal: hemorrhage, fetomaternal hemorrhage with possible maternal Rh isoimmunization, infection, labor, abruptio placentae, inadvertent damage to the intestines or bladder, amniotic fluid embolism

TABLE 27-8 Typical Amniotic Fluid Increase during Pregnancy

Weeks of Gestation	Amniotic Fluid Volume (mL)
12	50
14	100
16	175
18	250
20	325

From Queenan JT: *Contemp OB/GYN* 15:61, Feb 1980.

Fetal: death, hemorrhage, infection (amnionitis), direct injury from the needle, abortion or preterm labor, leakage of amniotic fluid.

Many of the complications have been minimized or eliminated by performing the procedure with use of ultrasound examination.

Indications for the procedure include prenatal diagnosis of genetic disorders, assessment of pulmonary maturity, and diagnosis of fetal hemolytic disease. Amniotic fluid may be analyzed for investigation of a number of factors.

GENETIC PROBLEMS. Prenatal assessment of genetic disorders is indicated in women of advanced age, those with a previous child with a chromosome abnormality, or a family history of chromosome anomalies. Inherited errors of metabolism also may be detected (such as Tay-Sachs disease, hemophilia, and thalassemia) and other disorders for which marker genes are known.

Cells are cultured for *karyotyping* of chromosomes (see Chapter 7). Chromosome aberrations appear in 1% to 2% of fetuses of women between 35 and 38 years of age, in 2% of women between 39 and 44 years of age, and in 10% of women older than 45 years of age. Fetal cells also are assessed for *sex chromatin* inasmuch as sex determination is important if a sex-linked disorder (occurring almost always in a male fetus) is suspected.

Biochemical analysis of enzymes produced from a cell culture can detect inborn errors of metabolism. Assessment of **alpha-fetoprotein (AFP)** levels is done as a follow-up for elevated levels of maternal serum AFP. Elevated levels in the amniotic fluid help confirm the diagnosis of a open neural tube defect such as spina bifida or anencephaly, or an open abdominal wall defect such as omphalocele. Elevated levels result from the increased leakage of cerebrospinal fluid into the amniotic fluid through the open defect. AFP values are normally high in fetal circulation but low in amniotic fluid. The amount of AFP should decrease to 18.5 μg/mL at 15 weeks and to 0.26 μg/mL at term.

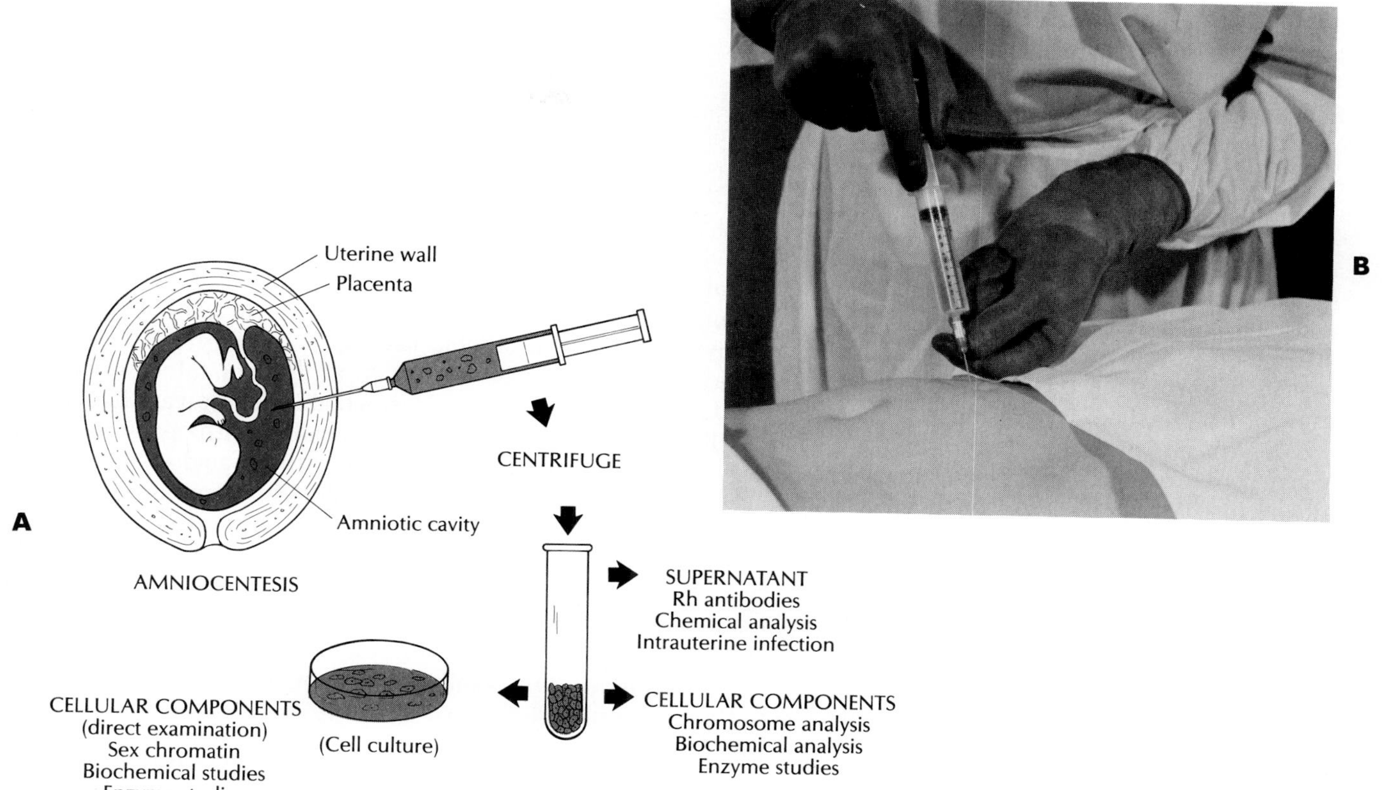

Fig. 27-9 A, Amniocentesis and laboratory utilization of amniotic fluid aspirant. B, Transabdominal amniocentesis.

A, from Whaley LF: *Understanding inherited disorders*, St Louis, 1974, Mosby–Year Book; B, courtesy of March of Dimes Birth Defects Foundation.

Levels also may be elevated in a normal multifetal pregnancy and with intestinal atresia, presumably caused by lack of fetal swallowing. A concurrent test for the presence of acetylcholinesterase virtually always indicates a fetal defect (Burton, 1988). Follow-up with ultrasound examination is recommended in these instances.

FETAL MATURITY. Greater accuracy in estimating fetal maturity is now possible through examination of amniotic fluid or its exfoliated cellular contents. Term pregnancy and fetal maturity can be demonstrated by the following laboratory studies.

PHOSPHOLIPIDS. A **lecithin/sphingomyelin (L/S) ratio** greater than 2:1 indicates adequate lung maturity for extrauterine life in most cases (see Chapter 7). This is generally achieved by 36 weeks of gestational age. A quick means of determining an approximate L/S ratio is the rapid surfactant test, also known as the **shake test** or bubble test. Equal parts of fresh amniotic fluid and normal saline solution are added to two parts 95% ethyl alcohol. The mixture is shaken vigorously for 30 seconds. If bubbles are still present at the meniscus 15 minutes after shaking, the fetal lung is judged to be mature.

The presence of *phosphatidylglycerol* (PG), another phospholipid, also reflects fetal lung maturity. In the presence of PG, the incidence of respiratory distress syndrome (RDS) is virtually 0%. The turbidity of the specimen itself is believed to depend on the total amniotic fluid phospholipid concentration. Optical density (OD) 650 greater than 0.15 correlates extremely well with the absence of RDS (Sonek et al, 1990).

BILIRUBIN. A Δ OD of bilirubinoid pigments of 450 nm <0.01 indicates a gestational age of greater than 38 weeks inasmuch as bilirubin disappears after 36 weeks.

CREATININE. When the creatinine (estimate of renal maturity) value is greater than 2 mg/dL, the gestational age is greater than 36 weeks in the absence of maternal renal disease and dehydration or of fetal anomaly.

LIPID CELLS. After fetal lipid-containing exfoliated cells are stained with Nile blue sulfate, a finding of more than 20% orange-staining cells indicates a gestational age of greater than 35 weeks; the fetus probably weighs 2500 g.

FETAL HEMOLYTIC DISEASE. Identification and follow-up of fetal hemolytic disease in cases of isoimmunization is another indication for amniocentesis. The procedure usually is not done until the mother's antibody titer reaches 1:8 and is rising.

APT TEST. This test is used to differentiate maternal and fetal blood when vaginal bleeding occurs during pregnancy or labor. It may be performed quickly by the following method: Add 0.5 mL bloody fluid to 4.5 mL distilled water and shake. Add 1 mL 0.25N sodium hydroxide. Fetal and cord blood will remain pink for 1 to 2 minutes. Maternal blood turns brown in 30 seconds. For further confirmation, a Kleihauer-Betke examination can be done in the laboratory.

MECONIUM. The presence of meconium in the amniotic fluid may be determined, usually by visual inspection of the sample.

ANTENATAL PERIOD. Before early labor, the presence of meconium is not usually associated with poor fetal outcome. The finding cannot be used to distinguish an acute and subsequently corrected fetal stress from either a chronic ongoing one or simply the physiologic passage of meconium. Because there has been some association between meconium in amniotic fluid in the third trimester and hypertensive conditions and postmaturity, the fetus should undergo further antepartum evaluation if the birth is not imminent (Brady, Goldman, 1986).

INTRAPARTAL PERIOD. Intrapartal **meconium stained amniotic fluid** is an indication for more careful evaluation, such as through electronic fetal monitoring (EFM) and fetal scalp blood sampling. The presence of meconium should not be used as the sole indication for intervention (Depp, 1990). When membranes are ruptured and the fetal head can be touched, fetal well-being can be assessed by *fetal scalp stimulation*. Those fetuses whose heart rates respond with a brisk acceleration usually have a scalp blood pH >7.23, which suggests fetal well-being (Harvey, 1987).

There are three possible reasons for the passage of meconium during the intrapartal period: (1) it is a normal physiologic function that occurs with maturity (meconium passage is infrequent before weeks 23 to 24, with an increased incidence after 38 weeks); (2) it is the result of hypoxia-induced peristalsis and sphincter relaxation; and (3) it may be a sequela to umbilical cord compression–induced vagal stimulation in mature fetuses.

The following criteria have been proposed for evaluating meconium-stained amniotic fluid during the intrapartal period (Depp, 1990):

1. *Consistency:* "old and thin" vs. "new and thick." A new and thick consistency is more likely to be the result of fetal stress.
2. *Timing.* Thick, fresh meconium passed for the first time in late labor, associated with nonremediable severe variable or late FHR decelerations, is an ominous sign. However, the presence of meconium alone is not necessarily a sign of fetal distress.
3. *Presence of other indicators.* Meconium passage and nonremediable severe variable or late decelerations (especially with poor baseline variability), with or without acidosis confirmed by scalp-blood sampling, are ominous signs.

In the presence of meconium, the birth team should anticipate the need for careful suctioning of the nasopharynx at time of the birth, ideally before the first breath is taken. Suctioning at this time is effective in reducing the incidence and severity of meconium aspiration in the neonate (Brady, Goldman, 1986).

Percutaneous Umbilical Blood Sampling

Direct access to the fetal circulation during the second and third trimesters is now possible through **percutaneous umbilical blood sampling (PUBS)**, or *cordocentesis*. It is the most widely used method for fetal blood sampling and transfusion (Nicolaides et al, 1990). PUBS involves the insertion of a needle directly into a fetal umbilical vessel under ultrasound guidance. Ideally, the umbilical cord is punctured 1 to 2 cm from its placental insertion (Fig. 27-10). At this point the cord is well anchored and will not move, and the risk of maternal blood contamination (from the placenta) is slight (Ludomirski, Weiner, 1988). Generally, 1 to 4 mL of blood are removed during the puncture and immediately tested by the Kleihauer-Betke procedure to ensure fetal blood.

In a study of more than 1600 pregnant women from 14 major North American centers, only a 1.6% mean fetal loss rate resulted from this procedure (Nicolaides et al, 1990). The three main complications reported are blood leakage from the puncture site, fetal bradycardia, and chorioamnionitis; none of the procedures were followed by premature rupture of the membranes (PROM) (Ludomirski, Weiner, 1988).

Indications for use include prenatal diagnosis of inherited blood disorders or karyotyping of malformed fetuses, detection of fetal infection, determination of the acid-base status of IUGR fetuses, and assessment and treatment of isoimmunization and thrombocytopenia in pregnant women (see Research Highlight, p. 796).

Inasmuch as a fetal blood specimen will yield a karyotype in 2 to 3 days, PUBS may be the procedure of choice when time limitations do not permit amniotic fluid cultures to be used.

In fetuses at risk for isoimmune hemolytic anemia, PUBS now permits precise identification of fetal blood type and RBC count and may avoid further interventions. If the fetus is antigen positive for maternal antibodies, a direct blood test can confirm the degree of anemia resulting from hemolysis. PUBS is now the procedure of choice for intrauterine transfusion for severely anemic fetuses; it can be done 4 to 5 weeks earlier than through the intraperitoneal route (Ludomirski, Weiner, 1988).

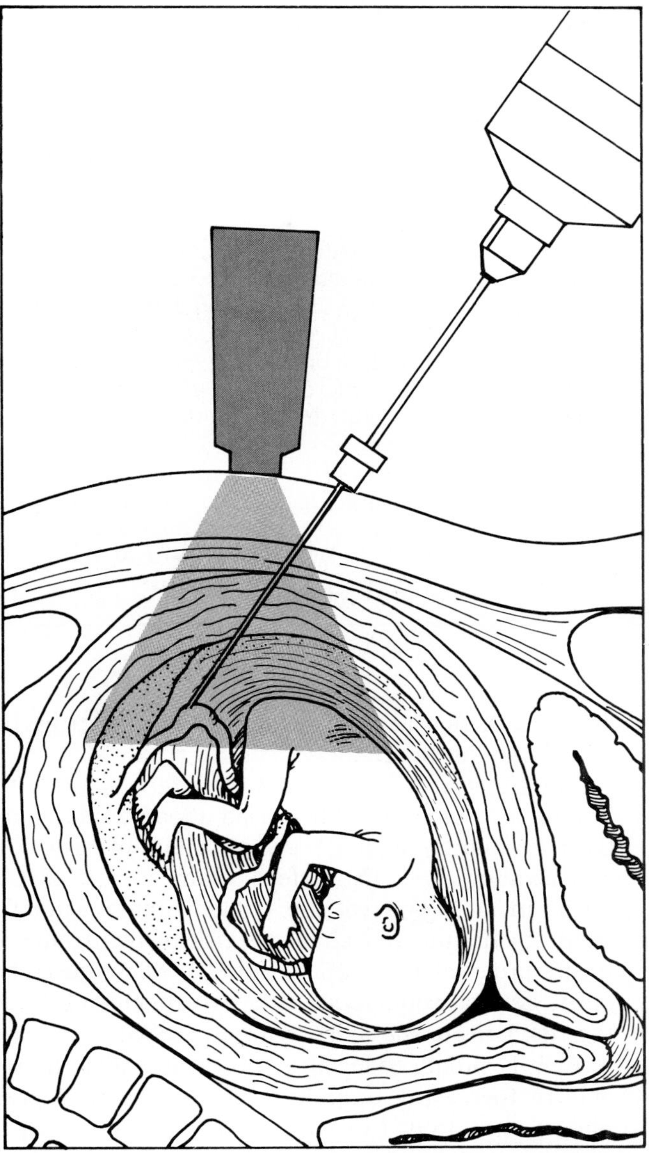

Fig. 27-10 Technique for percutaneous umbilical blood sampling guided by ultrasound.

Follow-up includes continuous fetal heart rate monitoring for several minutes up to 1 hour and a repeat ultrasound examination 1 hour later to ensure that there was no further bleeding or hematoma formation.

Chorionic Villi Sampling

Because of its advantage of earlier diagnosis than is possible with amniocentesis, transcervical **chorionic villi sampling (CVS)** has become very popular for genetic studies. Although there are risks to the fetus, the greatest advantage in this technique is that genetic diagnosis can be moved to as early as the tenth week and can produce results rapidly.

The procedure is done between 10 and 12 weeks of gestation. It involves the removal of a small tissue specimen from the fetal portion of the placenta (Fig. 27-11). At that time the placenta is a heterogenous organ in which active villus proliferation is seen (Golbus, Appelman, 1990). At this stage the chorion has differentiated into two distinct structures: (1) the chorion frondosum, which overlies the basal decidua and ultimately will become the placental site, and (2) the smooth leathery chorion laeve, from which the villi have degenerated (Wapner, Jackson, 1988). The specimen is removed either from the chorion frondosum (the preferred site) or the chorion laeve. Because chorionic villi originate in the zygote, that tissue reflects the genetic makeup of the fetus.

Real-time ultrasound is used to guide the procedure. The aspiration cannula and obturator must traverse the cervical canal, must be placed at the suitable site, and must avoid rupturing the amniotic sac. The transcervical technique is used in most CVS procedures. However, a transabdominal approach has been used and may be more widely practiced in the future because of its advantages: lower risk of uterine infection and wider window of time for safe performance.

Complications after the procedure, which rarely occur, include vaginal spotting or bleeding immediately afterward: spontaneous abortion (SAB), 0.3%; rupture of membranes, 0.1%; chorioamnionitis, 0.5%. Because of the possibility of fetomaternal hemorrhage, women with Rh negativity should receive immune globulin (RhoGAM) to avoid isoimmunization (National Institutes of Health [NIH] CVS Study Group, 1989).

If CVS is done between 56 and 66 days' gestation, an increased risk of limb anomalies has been noted

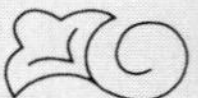 **Research Highlight** 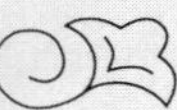

Antepartum Fetal Blood Sampling with Cordocentesis

RESEARCH ABSTRACT

Cordocentesis (PUBS)—sampling of fetal blood from an umbilical vessel under ultrasound guidance—is becoming more important in prenatal diagnosis. The results of 1011 cordocentesis procedures during a 2½-year period were analyzed. Just over one third (35%) of the procedures were done for blood group incompatibilities and intravascular transfusion. The procedure was performed for other indications in the remaining 624 cases. Amniocentesis and chorionic villus sampling (CVS) were compared with cordocentesis in detection of karyotype anomalies. The indications for cordocentesis included karyotype analysis, determination of fetal acid-base status, and diagnosis of fetal infections. In the 596 of the cases that were followed up, 190 genetic disorders were diagnosed. There were differences in detection rate of anomalies between type of procedure: with cordocentesis, 75 (39%) cases were detected; with CVS, 20 (11%) were detected; and with amniocentesis, 95 (50%). These differences were related to indications for the procedures. CVS usually was performed in cases of advanced maternal age, amniocentesis for advanced maternal age in the second trimester of pregnancy, and cordocentesis for fetal anomalies, suspected chromosomal anomalies, and advanced maternal age. Because amniocentesis was done later in pregnancy in a very high–risk group, more anomalies were detected in this group. Cordocentesis is a valuable procedure with a low complication rate. It is likely to become used more often in prenatal diagnosis.

IMPLICATIONS FOR PRACTICE

As cordocentesis becomes used more commonly in prenatal diagnosis, clients will have more questions about the procedure and its safety. Nurses need to be knowledgeable about prenatal diagnosis procedures and skillful in assisting the client and physician during the procedures. It often is left to the nurse to explain to clients exactly how procedures will be performed and what they will feel like. Nurses can do much to assist clients in reducing anxiety associated with the unknown.

RELATED RESEARCH QUESTIONS

1. What is a client's response to being informed that a prenatal diagnostic procedure is indicated?
2. Do cordocentesis, amniocentesis, and CVS differ in amount of discomfort and stress produced in the client?
3. Does an education program reduce the anxiety associated with a prenatal diagnosis procedure?
4. Does level of anxiety associated with a prenatal diagnosis procedure differ according to age and education of the mother, indication for the procedure (fetal anomalies vs. hemolytic disease), and trimester the procedure was performed?

REFERENCE

Bald R et al: Antepartum fetal blood sampling with cordocentesis: comparison with chorionic villus sampling and amniocentesis in diagnosing karyotype anomalies, *J Reprod Med* 36:655, 1991.

(Froster-Iskenius, Baird, 1989; Firth et al, 1991; Burton et al, 1992). Based on these findings, CVS may need to be restricted to 10 weeks' gestation or later.

Indications for the procedure are similar to those for amniocentesis. About 90% are performed because of advanced maternal age (Hogge et al, 1986). Other indications include biochemical and molecular assays.

Maternal Assays

ALPHA-FETOPROTEIN. The most exciting development in recent years has been the emergence of maternal serum alpha-fetoprotein (MSAFP) as a screening tool for *neural tube defects* in pregnancy. Through this technique, approximately 80% to 85% of all open neural tube defects (NTDs) can be detected early in pregnancy.

The cause of NTDs is not well understood, but it is important to note that 95% of all affected infants are born to women with no previous family history of similar anomalies. The defect occurs in 1 to 2/1000 births in most parts of the United States. After the birth of one affected child the risk of recurrence in future pregnancies is 2% to 3% (10 to 15 times) that of the general population. After two affected children, the risk rises to 6% to 8% (Burton, 1988).

AFP is produced by the fetal liver and is detectable in increasing quantities in the serum of pregnant women from 14 to 34 weeks. One must keep in mind that although amniotic fluid AFP is diagnostic, MSAFP is a screening tool only and identifies candidates for the more definitive procedures of amnio-

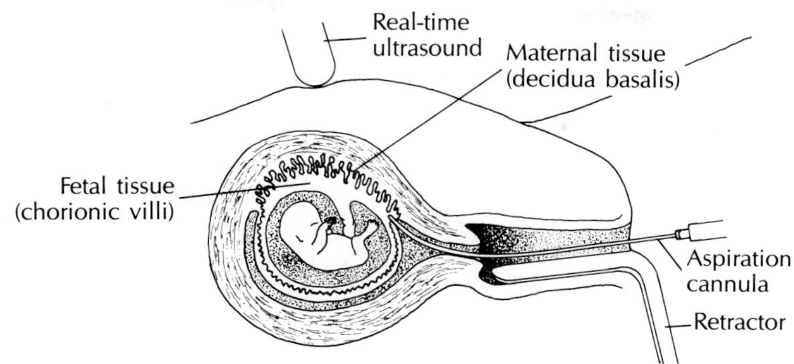

Fig. 27-11 Chorionic villi sampling. Taking sample by transcervical method. See also Fig. 7-13.

centesis and ultrasound examination. MSAFP screening can be done with reasonable reliability any time between 15 and 21 weeks' gestation (17 weeks is ideal).

Once the woman's level is determined, it is compared with normal values established by each laboratory for each week of gestation. Most use a value 2.0 to 2.5 times the normal median as abnormal (reported as multiples of the mean, or MOM). If findings are abnormal, the test should be repeated in 1 week; if two sequential MSAFP levels are elevated, the woman should be counseled regarding the significance of the findings, the nature of NTDs, and options for further testing.

The next step is ultrasound examination. In addition to NTD, the most common reason for elevated AFPs is advanced gestational age, multifetal pregnancy, unrecognized fetal demise, and severe oligohydramnios. If the fetus appears normal and of correct gestational age, an amniocentesis should be done for AFP levels (Burton, 1988). (See previous discussion of amniotic fluid AFP.)

Of interest is a convincing body of evidence that Down syndrome and probably other autosomal trisomies are associated with lower than normal levels of MSAFP and amniotic fluid AFP (Burton, 1988).

ESTRIOLS. The steroid precursor produced by the fetal adrenals is synthesized into estriols in the placenta and is excreted by the woman's healthy kidneys. Estriol levels also may be assayed in maternal serum, the preferred method if used at all. High estriol levels with a rising slope throughout pregnancy are associated with a good prognosis for the future.

Clinically, serial estriol values were most commonly determined with the presence of diabetes mellitus, hypertension, suspected IUGR, and postmaturity. These serial values were compared with a standard curve. Abnormal patterns included (1) a progressive downward slope, (2) a rapid fall (35% to 40%) of the baseline established after the last three averaged values, and (3) persistent low values.

Because of the many factors that can interfere with the results (especially urinary samples collected over a 24-hour period) and common false-positive values found with serum specimens, there has been a widespread decline in use of this technique for fetal assessment (Depp, 1990). It is mentioned here only for historical purposes because its usefulness has been superseded by more sensitive and specific tests for fetal well-being.

HUMAN PLACENTAL LACTOGEN. Human placental lactogen (hPL), also called human chorionic somatomammotropin (hCS), is produced by the syncytiotrophoblast. However, assay for this hormone is of little value in assessing placental integrity and fetal well-being. Other more accurate and reliable tests have replaced the routine assessment for hPL levels (Haesslein, 1987).

COOMBS' TEST. **Coombs' test** for Rh incompatibility is discussed at length in Chapter 38. If the maternal Coombs titer for Rh antibodies is greater than 1:8, amniocentesis for bilirubin in amniotic fluid is indicated to determine the severity of fetal anemia from hemolysis.

URINE ASSESSMENT FOR GLYCOSURIA, ACETONURIA, AND PROTEINURIA. See the index for the pages in which these findings are discussed. See Appendix D for laboratory values. Table 27-9 presents a partial list of conditions that can be diagnosed prenatally.

■ ELECTRONIC MONITORING

Indications

First- and second-trimester antenatal assessment is directed primarily at the diagnosis of fetal anomalies. The goal of third-trimester testing is to determine whether the intrauterine environment continues to be supportive to the fetus (Halle, 1992). The testing often is used to determine the timing of childbirth for clients at risk for *uteroplacental insufficiency* (the gradual decline in the delivery of needed substances by the placenta to the fetus). It has been suggested that a gradual loss of placental function occurs in which nutritive function is lost first, leading to IUGR. Subsequently, respiratory function is compromised, resulting in fetal hypoxia (Freeman, Lagrew, 1990).

Indications for both the nonstress test (NST) (or fetal activity determination [FAD]) and the contraction stress test (CST) include the following:

Maternal diabetes mellitus
Chronic hypertension
Hypertensive disorders in pregnancy
IUGR
Sickle cell disease
Maternal cyanotic heart disease
Postmaturity
History of previous stillbirth
Isoimmunization
Meconium-stained amniotic fluid at third-trimester amniocentesis
Hyperthyroidism
Collagen disease
Older pregnant woman
Chronic renal disease

There are no contraindications for the NST. Absolute contraindications for the CST are rupture of membranes, previous classic cesarean birth, preterm labor, placenta previa, or abruptio placentae. The following are considered relative contraindications for the CST: multi-fetal pregnancy, previous preterm labor, hydramnios, more than 36 weeks' gestation, and incompetent cervix (Freeman, Lagrew, 1990). As a rule, reactive patterns with the NST or negative results with the CST are associated with favorable outcomes.

Sensitivity of Parameters

LATE DECELERATION. The most sensitive indicator of fetal hypoxia is late deceleration, which is triggered by fetal chemoreceptors sensing an oxygen pressure (PO_2) of less than 20 mm Hg. This response occurs before changes in pH, baseline rate, variability, or reactivity (Adamson, Myers, 1977).

ACCELERATIONS. When the hypoxia lasts long enough for anaerobic glycolysis to cause a buildup in lactic acid, the pH falls below 7.22 and fetal heart accelerations disappear (Murrata et al, 1982). It has been hypothesized that the fetus, in a progressively deteriorating situation of hypoxemia, shows not only gradual decline in acceleration incidence but a dissociation between fetal movements and their ability to elicit accelerations in response (Ingardia et al, 1980).

VARIABILITY. FHR variability decreases as the degree of hypoxia and acidosis increases. It has been shown that when moderate FHR variability was present 30 minutes before the birth, only 2% of newborns had Apgar scores below 7 at 5 minutes (Krebs et al, 1979). With a 98% accuracy in predicting fetal well-being, the presence of normal variability is the most reassuring aspect of FHR monitoring.

Nonstress Test (Fetal Activity Determination)

The **nonstress test (NST)** is the most widely applied technique for antepartum evaluation of the fetus. The basis for the NST, or **fetal activity determination (FAD)**, is that the normal fetus will produce characteristic heart rate patterns. Acceleration of FHR in response to fetal movement is the desired outcome. In the healthy fetus with an intact CNS, 90% of gross fetal body movements are associated with FHR accelerations. This response can be blunted by hypoxia or acidosis, drugs (analgesics, barbiturates, and beta-blockers), fetal sleep, and some congenital anomalies (Sonek et al, 1990).

ADVANTAGES. These include the ease with which the NST can be performed in an out-of-hospital set-

TABLE 27-9 Partial List of Conditions Diagnosed Prenatally

Disorder	Prenatal Diagnosis
CHROMOSOMAL ANOMALIES	Chromosome analysis of cultured amniotic fluid cells
CONGENITAL DEFECTS	
Cardiac defects	Ultrasound
CNS anomalies	
Anencephaly	AFP in amniotic fluid and maternal serum, ultrasound, fetoscopy, radiography
Hydrocephaly	Ultrasound, AFP, radiography
Microcephaly	Ultrasound, radiography
Spina bifida cystica	AFP, fetoscopy, ultrasound
Gastrointestinal defects	
Diaphragmatic hernia	Amniography, ultrasound
Esophageal atresia	Amniography, fetography
Gastroschisis; omphalocele	AFP, ultrasound
Meconium ileus (cystic fibrosis)	Ultrasound, radiography
Skeletal deformities (general)	Ultrasound, radiography
Osteogenesis imperfecta	Elevated amniotic fluid pyrophosphate
FETAL INFECTIONS	
Cytomegalovirus	Cytomegalovirus from amniotic fluid
Rubella	Rubella virus from amniotic fluid
Syphilis	Radiography (fetal abnormalities)
HEMATOLOGIC DISORDERS	
Erythroblastosis fetalis	Amniotic fluid bilirubin, ultrasound, amniography, fetal blood sample
Sickle cell anemia	Fetal blood sample, DNA analysis of amniotic fluid cells
Thalassemia	DNA analysis of amniotic fluid cells, fetal blood sample
INBORN ERRORS OF METABOLISM	Amniotic fluid analysis
Argininosuccinicaciduria	C argininosuccinic acid in cultured cells, increased argininosuccinic acid levels
Combined immunodeficiency disease	Deficient adenosine deaminase activity in cultured cells
Congenital adrenal hyperplasia	Elevated 17-α-hydroxyprogesterone, Δ_4 androstenedione, and pregnanediol levels in fluid
Congenital erythropoietic porphyria	Massive amounts of porphyrin in fluid
Cystinosis	Elevated cystine in fluid
Fabry's disease	Deficient α-galactosidase activity in cultured cells
Farber disease	Deficient ceramidase activity in cultured cells
Galactosemia	Deficient galactose-1-phosphate uridyl transferase activity in cultured cells
Glutaric acidemia	Glutaric acid in fluid, deficient glutaryl-CoA dehydrogenase in cultured cells
Hyperlipoproteinemid, type II	Absence of low density lipoprotein–cell surface receptors on cultured cells
Hypophosphatasia (congenitally lethal)	Ultrasound, deficient bone and liver alkaline phosphatase isoenzyme activity in cultured cells, deficiency of total alkaline phosphatase activity in cultured cells
Krabbe's disease	Deficient cerebroside β-galactosidase activity in cultured cells
Hunter's syndrome (mucopolysaccharidosis, type II)	Deficient iduronate sulfate activity in fluid, accumulation of S-mucopolysaccharides in cultured cells
Hurler syndrome (mucopolysaccharidosis, type I)	Decreased α-L-iduronidase activity in fluid, accumulation of S-sulfate mucopolysaccharides in cultured cells

Continued.

TABLE 27-9 Partial List of Conditions Diagnosed Prenatally—cont'd

Disorder	Prenatal Diagnosis
Lesch-Nyhan syndrome	Deficient hypoxanthine-guanine phosphoribosyl transferase activity in cultured cells
Maple syrup urine disease	Deficient branched chain keto-acid decarboxylase in cultured cells
Menkes' syndrome (kinky-hair disease)	Increased incorporation of copper into cultured cells
Niemann-Pick disease	Deficient sphingomyelinase activity in cultured cells
Pompe's disease	Deficient α-1, -4-glucosidase in cultured cells
Porphyria (acute, intermittent)	Decreased activity of uroporphyrinogen I synthetase in cultured cells
Sanfilippo's syndrome	Deficient heparin sulfamidase activity in cultured cells, increased heparin sulfate in amniotic fluid
Tay-Sachs disease	Deficient β-N-acetyl-hexasaminidase A and B activity in cultured cells
Wolman disease	Deficient acid lipase activity in cultured cells
MISCELLANEOUS CONDITIONS	
Cystic fibrosis	Reduced methylumbelliferyl-guauidinobenzoate reactive proteases in amniotic fluid
Duchenne muscular dystrophy	Elevated creatine phosphokinase levels in fetal blood
Fetal sex determination	Ultrasound—fetal outline, chromosome analysis of fluid cells, elevated testosterone levels and decreased follicle-stimulating hormone levels in amniotic fluid (male fetus)
Multifetal pregnancy	Ultrasound, radiography
Tumors and cysts	Ultrasound, radiography, amniography
PLACENTAL CONDITIONS	
Abruptio placentae	Ultrasound
Blighted ovum	Ultrasound
Ectopic pregnancy	Ultrasound
Placenta previa	Ultrasound

ting, because it is noninvasive. It also is relatively inexpensive and has no known contraindications.

DISADVANTAGES. These center around the high false-positive rate for nonreactive findings as a result of fetal sleep cycles, medications, and fetal immaturity. There is slightly lower sensitivity to fetal compromise than with CST or biophysical profile.

PROCEDURE. The woman is seated in a reclining chair (or in semi-Fowler's position) to avoid supine hypotension. The FHR is recorded by Doppler transducer, and a tocotransducer is applied to detect uterine contractions or fetal movements. The nurse observes the strip chart for signs of *fetal activity* and a concurrent acceleration of FHR. If evidence of fetal movement is not apparent on the strip, the woman may be asked to depress a button on a hand-held event marker that is connected to the monitor when she feels fetal movement. The movement is then noted on the strip. Because almost all accelerations are accompanied by FM, it need not be recorded with accelerations for the test to be considered reactive (Gabbe, 1986). The test usually takes 20 to 30 minutes, but it may take longer if the fetus needs to be awakened from a sleep state.

INTERPRETATION. Generally accepted criteria for a reactive tracing are

- Two or more accelerations of 15 beats/min lasting for 15 seconds over a 20-minute period
- Normal baseline rate
- Long-term variability amplitude of 10 or more beats/min

If the test does not meet the criteria after 40 minutes, it is considered nonreactive, and a CST should be performed (Fig. 27-12 and Table 27-10).

FETAL ACOUSTIC STIMULATION. The **acoustic stimulation test** is another method of testing antepartum FHR response. The test takes approximately 10 minutes to complete, with the fetus monitored for 5 min-

TABLE 27-10 Interpretation of the Nonstress Test

Result	Interpretation	Clinical significance
Reactive	Two or more accelerations of FHR of 15 beats/min lasting 15 sec or more, associated with each fetal movement in a 20-min period	As long as twice-weekly NSTs remain reactive, most high-risk pregnancies are allowed to continue
Nonreactive	Any tracing with either no FHR accelerations or accelerations < 15 beats/min or lasting less than 15 sec throughout any fetal movement during testing period	Further indirect monitoring may be attempted with abdominal fetal electrocardiography in an effort to clarify FHR pattern and quantitate variability; external monitoring should continue, and a CST should be done
Unsatisfactory	Quality of FHR recording not adequate for interpretation	Test is repeated in 24 hr or a CST is done, depending on the clinical situation

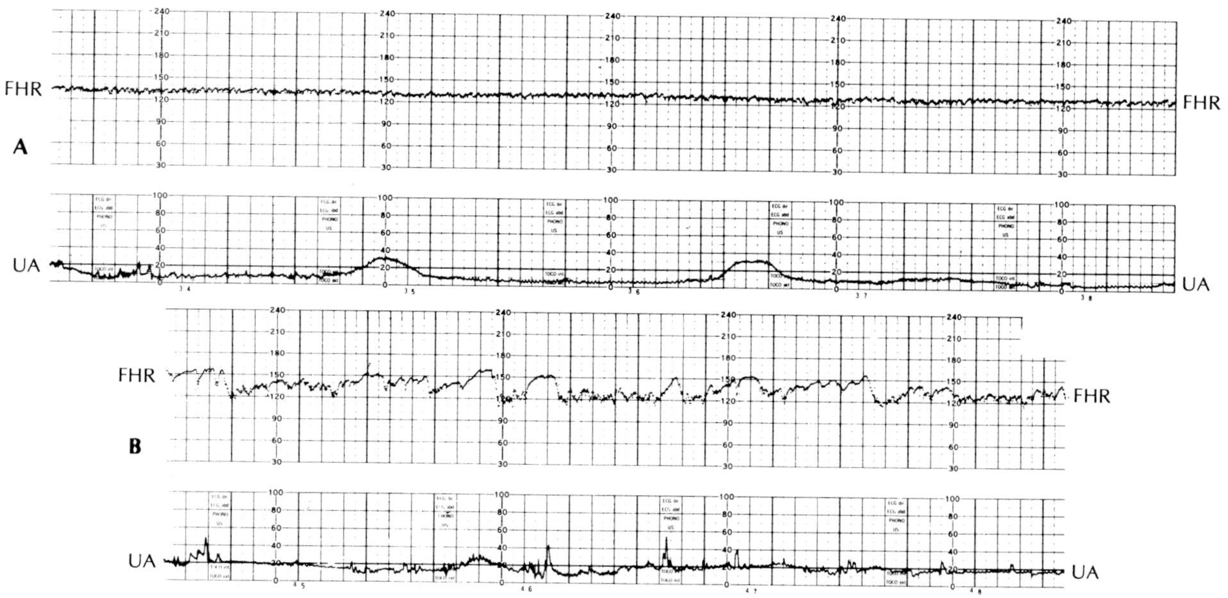

Fig. 27-12 Nonstress test. **A,** Decreased variability caused by fetal sleep cycle. **B,** Reactive nonstress test, indicative of fetal well-being, 15 minutes later.
From Perez RH: *Protocols for perinatal nursing practice,* St Louis, 1981, Mosby–Year Book.

utes before stimulation to obtain a baseline FHR. The sound source (usually a laryngeal stimulator) is then applied on the maternal abdomen over the fetal head. Monitoring continues for another 5 minutes and the chart is assessed. A reactive test is achieved if there is FHR acceleration of at least 15 beats/min for at least 120 seconds, or two accelerations of at least 15 beats/min for at least 15 seconds within 5 minutes of stimulus.

Fetal acoustic stimulation also may be applied during an NST if the baby appears to be in a sleep state. Sleutel (1990) reported that nonreactive fetuses met reactive NST criteria sooner and also exhibited greater amplitude, duration, and number of accelerations after fetal acoustic stimulation.

It is currently recommended that the NST be performed twice weekly.

Contraction Stress Test

The **contraction stress test (CST)** is one of the first electronic methods developed for assessment of fetal well-being. Devised as a graded stress test of the fetus, its purpose was to identify the fetus in jeopardy that was stable at rest but showed evidence of compromise with the introduction of stress. Uterine contractions decrease uterine blood flow and placental perfusion. If this decrease is sufficient to produce hypoxia in the fetus, a deceleration in FHR will result, beginning at the peak of the contraction and persisting after its conclusion (*late deceleration.*) In a healthy fetoplacental unit, uterine contractions usually do not produce late decelerations; when there is underlying uteroplacental insufficiency, contractions will produce late decelerations.

ADVANTAGES. The CST provides an earlier warning of fetal compromise than does the NST, and there are fewer false-positive tests.

DISADVANTAGES. In addition to the contraindications described earlier, CTS is more time-consuming and expensive than an NST. It also is an invasive procedure if exogenous oxytocin is required.

PROCEDURE. The woman is placed in semi-Fowler's position or sits in a reclining chair. She is monitored indirectly, and the nurse observes the strip for 10 minutes for baseline rate, long-term variability, and the possible occurrence of spontaneous contractions.

NIPPLE-STIMULATED CONTRACTION TEST. The nurse explains the procedure to the woman and then may apply warm, moist washcloths to both breasts for several minutes. The woman is then asked to massage one nipple for 10 minutes. An alternative approach is for her to massage the nipple for 2 minutes, rest for 2 minutes, and continue for four cycles of massage and rest. If unilateral stimulation does not achieve adequate contractions (three occurring within a 10-minute window), unilateral continuous stimulation should be tried (if the intermittent approach was used), followed by bilateral stimulation for 10 minutes. When adequate contractions are achieved or hyperstimulation occurs, stimulation should be stopped.

OXYTOCIN-STIMULATED CONTRACTION TEST. If the nipple stimulation is not successful, an oxytocin-stimulated CST should be performed. An intravenous (IV) infusion is begun with a scalp needle. The oxytocin is diluted in an IV solution, and a piggyback port infuses it into the tubing of the main IV device. The infusion is usually delivered by an infusion pump to ensure accurate dosage. The oxytocin infusion usually is begun at 0.5 mU/min. Most institutions have their own protocols, but the infusion usually is increased by 0.5 mU/min at 15 to 20-minute intervals until three uterine contractions of good quality are observed within a 10-minute period. The FHR pattern is then interpreted. The oxytocin infusion is discontinued, and the maintenance IV solution infused until such time as uterine activity has returned to the preoxytocin level. The IV device is then removed and the fetal monitor discontinued.

INTERPRETATION. If no late decelerations are observed with the contractions, the findings are considered to be negative. Repetitive late decelerations, occurring with most contractions, render the test results positive (Fig. 27-13 and Table 27-11).

NURSING ROLE IN ANTENATAL ASSESSMENT FOR RISK

In most instances, the nurse's role is that of educator and support person. This is particularly true when the woman is undergoing such examinations as ultrasound magnetic resonance imaging, CVS, PUBS, and amniocentesis. In some instances the nurse may assist the physician with the procedure.

In many antenatal settings, nurses perform NSTs and CSTs, conduct an initial assessment, and begin necessary interventions for nonreassuring patterns. These nursing actions are accomplished after additional education and training, under guidance of established protocols, and in collaboration with physicians. Client teaching, which is an integral component of this role, involves preparation for the procedure, interpretation of findings, and pyschosocial support when needed.

All women who undergo antenatal assessments are at risk for real and potential problems. The nurse must expect the woman to be anxious. With rare exceptions the tests are ordered because of suspected fetal compromise or deterioration of a maternal condition, or both. In the third trimester, pregnant women are most concerned about protecting themselves and their babies and consider themselves most vulnerable to outside influences. The label of high risk will increase this sense of vulnerability.

Most clients also exhibit a knowledge deficit in some area, whether it is related to the procedure itself, the implications of findings, or the need for further evaluation or counseling. Perinatal nurses can intervene to provide the required education. By means of a knowledge base, they can promote a positive parental self-image in these high-risk clients.

REPRODUCTIVE HEALTH HAZARDS IN THE WORKPLACE AND ENVIRONMENT

The purpose of this section is not to generate global anxiety but to alert the nurse to a line of investigation, to keep the nurse informed, and to help the nurse communicate information. Information is the foundation for decision making in personal health goals.

Potentially **harmful materials in the workplace and environment** have become an increasing concern (Ricci, 1989). Some substances adversely affect factors required for fertility. These substances have a selective effect on chromosomes, gamete formation,

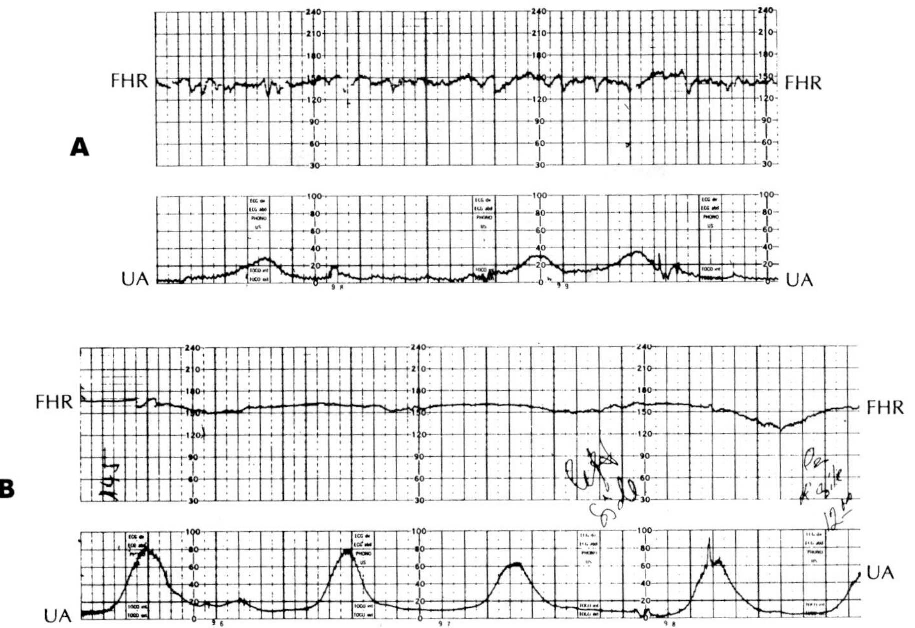

Fig. 27-13 A, Negative CST result: fetal well-being. **B**, Positive CST result: compromised fetus.
From Perez RH: *Protocols for perinatal nursing practice*, St Louis, 1981, Mosby–Year Book.

TABLE 27-11 Guide for Interpretation of the Contraction Stress Test

Result	Interpretation	Clinical Significance
Negative	No late decelerations, with a minimum of three uterine contractions lasting 40 to 60 sec within a 10-min period (Fig. 27-13, *A*)	Reassurance that the fetus is likely to survive labor, should it occur within 1 wk; more frequent testing may be indicated by the clinical situation
Positive	Persistent and consistent late decelerations occurring with more than half the contractions (Fig. 27-13, *B*)	Management lies between use of other tools of fetal assessment and termination of pregnancy; a positive test result indicates that the fetus is at increased risk for perinatal morbidity and mortality; the physician may perform an expeditious vaginal birth after a successful induction or may proceed directly to cesarean birth; the decision to intervene is determined by fetal monitoring and the presence of fetal heart rate reactivity
Suspicious	Late decelerations occurring with less than half the uterine contractions once an adequate contraction pattern has been established	NST and CST should be repeated within 24 hr; if interpretable data cannot be achieved, other methods of fetal assessment must be used*
Hyperstimulation	Late decelerations occurring with excessive uterine activity (contractions more often than every 2 min or lasting longer than 90 sec) or a persistent increase in uterine tone	
Unsatisfactory	Inadequate uterine contraction pattern or tracing too poor to interpret	

*Applies to results noted as suspicious, hyperstimulation, or unsatisfactory.

ovulation, fertilization, implantation, embryogenesis, fetal development, and parturition (see Chapter 7). Other materials affect reproduction by reducing libido (marijuana) or sexual performance (alcohol) (see Chapters 33 and 42). Substances may have a *mutagenic effect* on chromosomes at any time during the male's or female's life span. Mutagens such as plastic–vinyl chloride cause permanent genetic changes in female and male gametes. Other agents have a *teratogenic effect*. Teratogenes affect embryogenesis in the current pregnancy only. Well-known teratogens are alcohol and thalidomide (see Chapter 38 and Appendix E), rubella (see Chapters 29 and 39), and poorly controlled diabetes mellitus (see Chapter 31).

Substances that can be inhaled from the air are the most common concern. Also worrisome are materials that can be absorbed through the skin and those that can enter the body by mouth, such as lead dust that has settled on the fingers. Other potential threats arise from *physical forces:* eye stress from working at a video display terminal (VDT) all day, temperature, atmospheric pressure, oxygen content of the air, noise, vibration, acceleration, and ionizing radiation. *Social forces* that emphasize slimness and set styles of dress pose potential threats. Slimness and excessive exercise alter the woman's ovulation, high heels affect balance, and tight pants create the warm, moist environment needed for genital infections in the woman and reduced spermatogenesis in the male. Jobs that entail lifting heavy weights or working on slick floors, as well as working at high elevations or in unusual body positions, also may pose hazards to the pregnant woman or new mother (see Chapter 13) (Bond, 1986). *Emotional forces* such as severe stress affect the hypothalamic-pituitary-gonadal axis. Anovulation and irregular menstrual cycles may result.

Whether a substance or condition produces detectable effects depends in part on exposure level, dose, or length of exposure. Some individuals are more susceptible than others. Genetic factors, general health, and life-style (including smoking and diet) also can affect susceptibility to chemicals and conditions in the environment.

Nonionizing radiation in microwave ovens and ultrasound have characteristics and biologic effects different from ionizing radiation (e.g., x-rays). Nonionizing radiation in microwaves and ultrasound diagnostic equipment does *not* have sufficient energy to ionize molecules and disrupt cellular deoxyribonucleic acid (DNA) (Jankowski, 1986). There is no evidence of mutagenic or carcinogenic effects from properly constructed microwave ovens or from diagnostic ultrasound (Bond, 1986). MRI and VDTs also do *not* represent reproductive health hazards (Bond, 1986; Herbst et al, 1992; Schnorr, 1991).

Approximately 3% to 5% of all newborns have a congenital malformation, of which 1% to 2% are severe (Cunningham et al, 1989; Mattison et al, 1989). Of the 1% to 2% with severe malformations, one fourth to one third are associated with a chromosomal anomaly, and 3% are due to radiation, infection, or maternal disease. Drugs and environmental chemicals account for approximately 2% to 3% of the identifiable causes of developmental defects; however, about two thirds of all developmental malformations have no identifiable cause (Schardein, 1985; Scott et al, 1990).

Of the approximately 3000 chemicals that have been tested in experimental animals, more than 600 are developmental toxicants. Only 35, however, have been identified as causing birth defects in humans (Frankos, 1985; Schardein, 1985; Mattison et al, 1989).

The chemicals to worry about are those that come from industrial waste, landfill seepage, agricultural herbicides and pesticides, gasoline and oil, and common household solvents and cleaners (Ferguson, 1986; Shavelson, 1987; Shortridge, 1990). Methylene chloride is the most effective liquid paint and grease remover on the market. It is a common component of aerosol propellents in such products as hair spray, pesticides, paints, and lubricants. It is used in the electronic industry to clean printed circuit boards and is the solvent of choice for decaffeinating coffee. Absorbed in the body, it generates carbon monoxide, which interferes with the body's ability to pick up and deliver oxygen. Inhalation of low levels for short periods (minutes to hours) may cause dizziness, nausea, headache, and confusion. At high levels, methylene chloride may cause unconsciousness and death (Hazards, 1986). Household batteries—1½ to 2½ billion discarded by Americans each year—contain toxic metals such as lead, mercury, and cadmium.

Substances thrown out in trash cans leach out of trash dumps and landfills, polluting the ground water, and accumulate in the food chain. Drinking water may contain arsenic, benzene, cadmium, carbon tetrachloride, dioxin, lead, and vinyl chloride among others. Certain geographic areas contain greater concentrations of these pollutants than do others. Under-the-sink filtering systems filter out some of the substances (How, 1987).

Women are exposed to potentially hazardous substances in their homes and workplaces. Homemakers and domestic workers are exposed to alkalis, bleaches, detergents, and solvents that emit fumes. Fresh paint increases levels of hydrocarbons in the environment, especially if ventilation is poor. Sealers used to prevent plumbing leaks at joints often contain arsenic to retard growth of mold. This arsenic and other chemicals may be leached from plumbing systems.

People working in office buildings have displayed symptoms that have been termed the **sick-building syndrome.** Newer designs and construction to conserve energy have compromised ventilation. The result is an increase in concentrations of dust, ozone from copying machines, tobacco smoke, and hydrocarbons. Carbonless paper irritates the skin. Fumes accumulate from cleaning fluids. In some buildings the air contains levels of pollutants 50 times higher than that accepted by the Environmental Protection Agency (EPA) for outdoor air quality.

Noise is everywhere. Sound is a form of energy with the potential to damage tissues (Noise, 1986). Women report fetal startle responses to loud noises such as telephone rings and some forms of music. Some women experience excessive and extremely uncomfortable fetal movements in response to hard rock music. Newborns in intensive care nurseries show better weight gain when the noise level is controlled. Long-term damage has not been identified.

Hospital staff members are exposed to gases, x-rays, antineoplastic medications, needle accidents, and weight-related and other accidents (Munley et al 1986; Moses, 1987). Vehicle drivers breathe carbon monoxide and other combustion products of gasoline, as well as polynuclear aromatics. They also are subjected to physical stress, vibration, and accidents. Electronics assemblers are exposed to trichloroethylene, lead, tin, methylene chloride, antimony, epoxy resins, and methyl ethyl ketones. Hairdressers work with acetone, aerosol propellents (e.g., Freon), benzyl alcohol, ethyl alcohol, and hair dyes. Cigarette smoke is encountered commonly. Animal handlers, including meat cutters, inspectors, and teachers, are exposed to infections and flea and tick preparations.

Lead is a potential hazard to potters, artists, ceramists, and glass workers. Lead poisoning is still a threat (Lead, 1988). It is responsible for menstrual abnormalities, spontaneous abortion, decreased fertility in women and men, stillbirths, infants of low birth weight, and poor neurobehavioral development in children (Bellinger et al, 1987).

The impact on fetal development from male exposure to chemicals is unclear (Mattison et al, 1989). Drugs used by men frequently are excreted in the semen. Occupational exposure to drugs such as ethylene dibromide alters testicular function (Mattison, Thomford, 1987; Mattison et al, 1989). Cigarette smoking causes abnormal sperm, a decrease in sperm number, and increased chromosomal damage (Mattison et al, 1989). The number of cigarettes smoked per day determines the degree of abnormality that results.

ASSESSMENT

A complete assessment always provides a basis for research, especially when related to reproductive hazards in the home and workplace. Such careful assessment recently uncovered a peculiar finding in a population of wives of Navy aerial navigators—all reported births of females only. Study into the possible cause of this phenomenon continues.

Findings from the woman's present health status, including an extensive reproductive health history, are accumulated. Nonoccupational exposure to drugs (smoking, alcohol, "recreational" chemicals) and infection, geographic location and proximity to toxic disposal sites and industries, and partner's occupation are noted. The woman's and her partner's current and past occupational histories are vital to detection of hazards to the reproductive system. The time, length of exposure, work conditions, and symptoms related to work are identified. Partners of asbestos and agricultural workers inhale fibers and pesticides from work clothes; partners of those who work with anesthetic and other gases inhale metabolites in the worker's breath; farm workers absorb and inhale pesticides used on plants; people eat foods (fish, vegetables) from water and soil with high levels of toxic substances (Shavelson, 1987).

A toxicology screen is ordered if it is indicated. The presence and level of toxins, as well as the number and condition of blood components, may need to be assessed. If exposure of either parent to a mutagen is suspected, a karyotype may be ordered. Investigation of the cause of a defect includes a search for possible environmental agents. A retrospective approach often yields data that are difficult to validate so that an association may be suspected but not conclusive.

NURSING DIAGNOSES

Following are examples of nursing diagnoses of the woman that may emerge from assessment data:

- High risk for impaired gas exchange related to
  —Inhalation of toxic substances aided by injudicious use of chemicals, inadequate ventilation, and inappropriate disposal of chemical wastes, including equipment such as rags, brushes
- High risk for injury related to
  —Toxic substances ingested, inhaled, or absorbed through the skin

- High risk for injury related to knowledge deficit regarding
  - —Toxicity of substances in the environment
  - —Use of chemicals
  - —Avoidance of exposure
  - —Alternatives to some commonly used chemicals
  - —Safe use and disposal of chemicals
- Anxiety or grief related to
  - —Evidence of toxic exposure (e.g., impaired fertility, birth of a child with a defect)

PLANNING

Effective planning requires a worldwide effort to prevent pollution and the spread of infection. Personal and professional involvement is needed on local, state, and national levels to control hazards to reproductive health. A care plan is developed to meet the individual's needs, and the *goals* for care are stated in client-centered terms:

1. Women and men will suffer no mutagenic insults.
2. Women and men will not experience impaired fertility associated with environmental hazards to reproductive health.
3. Pregnant women will not be exposed to agents that are teratogenic to their unborn babies.
4. People will implement health practices that prevent or minimize effects of environmental hazards to reproductive health.

IMPLEMENTATION

Eight percent to 10% of birth defects occur as a result of environmental factors and may be amenable to nursing interventions (Pletsh, 1990).

Prevention should be the focus of self-care in any care plan. Several preventive measures are discussed in Chapter 13 (Bernhardt, 1990; Shortridge, 1990; Triolo, Montgomery, 1990) (e.g., exercise tips for pregnant women, client teaching for good posture and body mechanics, and standards for maternity care and employment).

Preventive measures are suggested for infection, nutrition, substance abuse, and other health-related concerns throughout this text. Cleanliness, ventilation, adherence to manufacturer's directions for use and disposal of materials, use of protective gear to shield against known and unknown hazards, and avoidance of exposure are examples of strategies to reduce risk.

In some instances safer materials can be substituted for potentially hazardous ones. Most household cleaning needs can be met with baking soda, table salt, distilled white vinegar, lemon juice, trisodium phosphate (TSP) (which does not emit fumes), a plunger, and some common sense. These substances clean drains, wash windows, degrease, prevent mold and mildew, disinfect, and scour (Dadd, 1987).

Impaired fertility and the birth of a child with a defect present special challenges to the nurse and health care team (Green, Malin, 1988). Curative and rehabilitative measures appropriate to these situations are presented in several parts of this text, especially in Chapters 29, 41, and 42.

Nurses must implement self-protective measures when working with radiation therapy (Lowdermilk, 1990). The client's room should be identified with the radioactivity logo and posted with the radiology department's precautionary protocol for the type of therapy being administered, for example, wearing gloves while handling bodily fluids. The three principles for radiation safety are time, distance, and shielding (for further discussion, see Chapter 44). A film badge or thermoluminescent dosimeter (TLD) badge must be worn to monitor the nurse's minute-by-minute exposure.

Industrial nurses must be alert to conditions in the workplace that may affect reproductive health of workers and their partners. Stress reduction through relaxation and guided imagery, as well as moderate exercise and rest, are useful (see index for these content areas).

As private citizens, nurses must become involved in their professional and political organizations to promote and support legislation to control pollution of the environment. Nurses can teach about alternative ways to clean the home and care for yards and gardens to reduce exposure to potentially harmful substances.

EVALUATION

Evaluation of short-term results is possible to some extent. The birth of a healthy baby with no apparent disorder or disease, the uncomplicated recovery of the new mother, continued fertility, and demonstration of a life-style that supports good reproductive health are some indicators that care was effective. However, the long-term effects may not be known for many years or generations.

■ SUMMARY

Assessment of risk is the focus of this chapter. Assessment by history, physical examination, and diagnostic techniques are discussed. Risk assessment identifies a population that requires special attention. Early identification of risk facilitates prospective planning and implementation of client management throughout the childbearing cycle.

Reproductive health hazards exist in the environment and workplace. The content in this chapter alerts the nurse to current information and presents a line of investigation. The information is intended to assist the nurse with decisions about personal health goals and with nursing care plans for clients and their families.

REFERENCES

Assessment For Risk Factors

Adamson D, Myers R: Late decelerations and brain tolerance of the fetal monkey to intrapartum asphyxia, *Am J Obstet Gynecol* 128:893, 1977.

American College of Obstetricians and Gynecologists: *Guidelines for perinatal care,* ed 2, Elk Grove Village, Ill, 1988, AAP and ACOG.

Aumann G, Baird M: Screening for the high-risk pregnancy. In Knuppel R, Drukker J, editors: *High risk pregnancy: a team approach,* Philadelphia, 1986, WB Saunders.

Brady J, Goldman S: Management of meconium aspiration syndrome. In Thibeault D, Gregory G, editors: *Neonatal pulmonary care,* Norwalk, Conn, 1986, Appleton-Century-Crofts.

Burton B: Elevated maternal serum alpha-fetoprotein (MSAFP): interpretation and follow up, *Clin Obstet Gynecol* 31:293, 1988.

Calhoun S: "Ask the experts": daily fetal movement counts, *NAACOG Newsletter* 17(8):6, 1990.

Depp R: Clinical evaluation of fetal status. In Scott J, et al, editors: *Danforth's obstetrics and gynecology,* ed 6, Philadelphia, 1990, JB Lippincott.

Freeman R, Lagrew, D Jr: The contraction stress test. In Eden R, Boehm F, editors: *Assessment and care of the fetus: physiological, clinical and medicolegal principles,* Norwalk, Conn, 1990, Appleton & Lange.

Gabbe S: Antepartum fetal evaluation. In Gabbe S, Nieby J, Simpson J, editors: *Obstetrics: normal and problem pregnancies,* New York, 1986, Churchill Livingstone.

Gaffney S, Salinger L, Vintzileos A: The biophysical profile for fetal surveillance, *MCN* 15:356, 1990.

Gilbert ES, Harmon JS: Antepartum and intrapartum assessment of fetal well-being. In *Manual of high-risk pregnancy and delivery: nursing perspectives,* ed 2, St Louis, 1992, Mosby–Year Book.

Golbus M, Appelman Z: Chorionic villus sampling. In Eden R, Boehm F, editors: *Assessment and care of the fetus: physiological, clinical and medicolegal principles,* Norwalk, Conn, 1990, Appleton & Lange.

Haesslein H: *Antepartum fetal assessment.* Paper presented at University of California–San Francisco, antepartum and intrapartum management conference, San Francisco, June 1987.

Halle J: Diagnostic evaluation of pregnancy. In Mattson S, Smith J, editors: *Core curriculum for maternal newborn nursing,* Philadelphia, 1992, WB Saunders.

Harvey C: Fetal scalp stimulation: enhancing the interpretation of fetal monitor tracings, *J Perinat Neonatal Nurs* 1:13, July 1987.

Hogge W, Schonberg S, Golbus M: Chorionic villus sampling: experience of the first 1000 cases, *Am J Obstet Gynecol* 154:1249, 1986.

Ingardia C et al: Prognostic components of the nonreactive nonstress test, *Obstet Gynecol* 56:305, 1980.

Kessel S, et al: Racial differences in pregnancy outcomes, *Clin Perinatol* 14:745, 1988.

Krebs H, et al: Intrapartum fetal heart rate monitoring. I. Classification and prognosis of fetal heart rate patterns, *Am J Obstet Gynecol* 133:762, 1979.

Ludomirski A, Weiner S: Percutaneous fetal umbilical blood sampling, *Clin Obstet Gynecol* 3:19, 1988.

Manning R: General principles and application of ultrasound. In Creasy R, Resnik R, editors: *Maternal-fetal medicine: principles and practices,* Philadelphia, 1989, WB Saunders.

Manning F, Harman C: The fetal biophysical profile. In Eden R, Boehm F, editors: *Assessment and care of the fetus: physiological, clinical and medicolegal principles,* Norwalk, Conn, 1990, Appleton & Lange.

Manning F, Platt L, Supos L: Antepartum fetal evaluation: development of a fetal biophysical profile, *Am J Obstet Gynecol* 136:787, 1980.

Mattison D, Angtuaco T: Magnetic resonance imaging in prenatal diagnosis, *Clin Obstet Gynecol* 31:353, 1988.

Morrison I, Olsen J: Weight-specific stillbirth and associated causes of death: an analysis of 765 stillbirths, *Am J Obstet Gynecol* 152:975, 1985.

Murrata Y, et al: Fetal heart rate accelerations and late decelerations during the course of intrauterine death in chronically catheterized rhesus monkeys, *Am J Obstet Gynecol* 144:218, 1982.

National Center for Health Statistics: Advance report of final mortality statistics, 1988, *Monthly Vital Statistics Report* 39(7) (suppl), Nov 28, 1990.

National Institutes of Health (NIH) CVS Study Group: The safety and efficacy of chorionic villus sampling for early prenatal diagnosis of cytogenetic abnormalities, *N Engl J Med* 320:609, 1989.

Nicolaides K, Thorpe-Beeston J, Noble P: Cordocentesis. In Eden R, Boehm F, editors: *Assessment and care of the fetus: physiological, clinical and medicolegal principles,* Norwalk, Conn, 1990, Appleton & Lange.

Pernoll ML, Benda GI, Babson SG: *Diagnosis and management of the fetus and neonate at risk: a guide for team care,* ed 5, St Louis, 1986, Mosby–Year Book.

Rutherford S et al: The four-quadrant assessment of amniotic fluid volume: an adjunct to antepartum fetal heart rate testing, I, *Obstet Gynecol* 70:353, 1987.

Scherwen L, Soloveno M, Weingarten C: *Nursing care of the childbearing family,* Norwalk, Conn, 1991, Appleton & Lange.

Schruefer J, Warsof S: Ultrasonographic criteria for the determination of fetal maturity, *Am J Obstet Gynecol* (in press).

Schulman H: Doppler ultrasound. In Eden R, Boehm F, editors: *Assessment and care of the fetus: physiological, clinical and medicolegal principles,* Norwalk, Conn, 1990, Appleton & Lange.

Sonek J, Reiss R, Gabbe S: Antenatal fetal assessment. In Iams JD, Zuspan FP, Quilligan EJ, editors: *Zuspan and Quilligan's manual of obstetrics and gynecology,* ed 2, St Louis, 1990, Mosby–Year Book.

Trudinger B: Doppler ultrasound assessment of blood flow. In Creasy R, Resnik R, editors: *Maternal-fetal medicine: principles and practices,* ed 2, Philadelphia, 1989, WB Saunders.

Ventura S et al: Estimates of pregnancies and pregnancy rates for the United States 1976-85, *Am J Pub Health* 78(5):506, 1988.

Wapner R, Jackson L: Chorionic villus sampling, *Clin Obstet Gynecol* 31:328, 1988.

Weinreb J, Brown C: Magnetic resonance imaging. In Eden R, Boehm F, editors: *Assessment and care of the fetus,* Norwalk, Conn, 1990, Appleton & Lange.

Environmental Hazards

Bellinger D et al: Longitudinal analyses of prenatal and postnatal lead exposure and early cognitive development, *N Engl J Med* 316:1037, 1987.

Bernhardt JH: Potential workplace hazards to reproductive health: information for primary prevention, *JOGNN* 19:53, 1990.

Bond MB: Reproductive hazards in the workplace, *Contemp OB/GYN* 28:57, March 1986.

Burton BK, Schulz CJ, Burd LI: Limb anomalies associated with chorionic villus sampling, *Obstet Gynecol* 79(5):726, Part 1, May 1992.

Cunningham FG et al: *Williams obstetrics,* ed 18, Norwalk, Conn, 1989, Appleton & Lange.

Dadd DL: Nontoxic cleaners for your home, *San Francisco Chronicle,* p C8, April 1, 1987.

Ferguson S: Birth defects and the environment—finding the connection, *CBE Environmental Rev,* p 8, Fall 1986.

Firth HV, et al: Severe limb abnormalities after chorion villus sampling at 56-66 days' gestation, *Lancet* 39:762, 1991.

Frankos VH: FCA perspective on the use of teratology data for human risk assessment, *Fundam Appl Toxicol* 5:615, 1985.

Froster-Iskenius UG, Baird PA: Limb reduction defects in over one million consecutive livebirths, *Teratology* 39:127, 1989.

Green D, Malin J: Prenatal diagnosis: when reality shatters parents' dreams, *Nursing* '88 18(2):61, 1988.

Hazards of methylene chloride, *Harvard Medical School Health Letter* 11(10):5, 1986.

Herbst AL et al: *Comprehensive gynecology, ed 2,* St Louis, 1990, Mosby–Year Book.

How to tell if your water is pure, *San Francisco Chronicle,* p C1, Feb 4, 1987.

Jankowski CF: The risks of radiation during pregnancy, *AJN* 86(3):260, 1986.

Lead poisoning still a threat, state says, *San Francisco Chronicle,* p A2, Feb 6, 1988.

Lowdermilk D: Nursing care updata: internal radiation therapy, NAACOG's *Clin Issues Perinatal Women's Health Nurs: Oncology,* 1:532, 1990.

Mattison DR, Thomford PJ: Selection of animals for reproductive toxicity studies: an evaluation of selected assumptions in reproductive toxicity testing and risk assessment. In Roloff VM et al, (editors): *Human risk assessment* —the role of animal selection and extrapolation, New York, 1987, Taylor & Francis.

Mattison DR et al: Effects of drugs and chemicals on the fetus I. Determining teratogenic risk, *Contemp OB/GYN* 33:163, March 1989.

Moses M: Reproductive health in the workplace: health workers and reproductive hazards, *Birth* 14:153, Fall 1987.

Munley AJ et al: Exposure of midwives to nitrous oxide in four hospitals, *Br Med J* 293:1063, 1986.

Noise pollution: irritant or hazard? *Harvard Medical School Health Newsletter* 11(8):1, 1986.

Pletsh P: Birth defect prevention: nursing interventions, *JOGNN* 19:482, 1990.

Schardein JL: *Chemically induced birth defects,* New York, 1985, Marcel Dekker.

Schnorr T et al: Video display terminals and the risk of spontaneous abortion, *N Engl J Med* 324:727, 1991.

Scott JR et al, (editors): *Danforth's obstetrics and gynecology,* ed 6, Philadelphia, 1990, JB Lippincott.

Shavelson L: Poisoned lives: six stories from toxic California, *Image,* p 22, July 26, 1987.

Shortridge LA: Advances in the assessment of the effect of environmental and occupational toxins on reproduction, *J Perinat Neonat Nurs* 3:1, April 1990.

Triolo PK, Montgomery LA: Occupational health hazards: implications for perinatal and neonatal nurses, *J Perinat Neonat Nurs* 3:34, April 1990.

REFERENCES—NURSING RESEARCH

Environmental Hazards

Ricci ES: Reproductive hazards in the workplace, *Nurs Res* 38:226, July/Aug 1989.

Assessment for Risk Factors

Sleutel M: Vibroacoustic stimulation and fetal heart rate in nonstress tests, *JOGNN* 19:199, 1990.

BIBLIOGRAPHY

Assessment for Risk Factors

American College of Obstetricians and Gynecologists: Antepartum fetal surveillance, *ACOG Technical Bulletin* No 107, Washington, DC, 1987, ACOG.

Arnold L et al: Infant mortality: lessons from the past, *MCN* 14:75, 1989.

Brucker M, MacMullen N: CVS: counseling your patient, *Nurse Pract* 12:34, Aug 1987.

Carey J, Seamonds J, Galligan M: Infant-death rate: rise linked to health-care cuts, *US News & World Report* p 67, Feb 24, 1986.

Cundiff J, Haubrich K, Hinzman N: Umbilical artery Doppler flow studies during pregnancy, *JOGNN* 19:475, 1990.

Dahlberg N: A perinatal center based antepartum home care program, *JOGNN* 17:30, 1988.

DiMaio M et al: Screening for fetal Down's syndrome in pregnancy by measuring maternal serum alpha-fetoprotein levels, *N Engl J Med* 317:342, 1987.

Eganhouse DJ: Fetal monitoring of twins, *JOGNN* 21(1):17, Jan/Feb 1992.

Ferguson H: Biophysical profile scoring: the fetal Apgar, *Am J Nurs* 88:662, 1988.

Fresquez ML: Advancement of the nursing role in antepartum fetal evaluation, *JPNN* 5(4):16, March 1992.

Gaffney S: Intrauterine fetal surgery: the ramifications for nurses, *MCN,* 10:250, 1985.

Gantes M et al: The use of daily fetal movement records in a clinical setting, *JOGNN* 15:390, 1986.

Gegor CL, Paine LL: Antepartum fetal assessment techniques: an update for today's perinatal nurse, *JPNN* 5(4):1, March 1992.

Goodwin L: Home fetal assessment, *JPNN* 5(4):33, March 1992.

Hammer R, Tufts M: Chorionic villi sampling for detecting fetal disorders, *MCN* 11:29, 1986.

Harmon J, Barry M: Antenatal testing, mobile outpatient monitoring service, *JOGNN* 18:21, 1989.

Jennings B: Social support: a way to a climate of caring, *Nursing Adm* 11(4):63, 1987.

Lavery JP: Ultrasound in the multifetal pregnancy, *The Female Patient* 17(5):116, May 1992.

Lehmann D, Chism J: Pregnancy outcomes in medically complicated and uncomplicated patients aged 40 years or older, *Am J Obstet Gynecol* 157:738, 1987.

Lewis C, Mocarski V: Obstetric ultrasound: application in a clinic setting, *JOGNN* 16:56, 1987.

Meizner I: Percutaneous umbilical blood sampling: a unique modality for fetal assessment, *The Female Patient* 17(5):109, May 1992.

Modica M, Timor-Tritsch I: Transvaginal sonography provides a sharper view into the pelvis, *JOGNN* 17:89, 1988.

NAACOG: *Standards for the nursing care of women and newborns,* ed 4, Washington, DC, 1991, NAACOG.

National Center for Health Statistics: Advance report of final natality statistics, 1988. *Monthly Vital Statistics Report* 39(4 suppl), Aug 15, 1990.

Owen J et al: A comparison of perinatal outcome in patients undergoing contraction stress testing performed by nipple stimulation versus spontaneously occurring contractions, *Am J Obstet Gynecol* 160:1080, 1989.

Platt L: Transvaginal ultrasound, *Contemp OB/GYN* 30 (special issue):99, Oct 1987.

Poland M, Ager J, Olson J: Barriers to receiving adequate prenatal care, *Am J Obstet Gynecol* 157:299, 1987.

Sabey PL, Clark SL: Establishing an antepartum testing unit: the nurse's role, *JPNN* 5(4):23, March 1992.

Simpson J, Elias S: Prenatal diagnosis of genetic disorders. In Creasy R, & Resnik R, editors: *Maternal-fetal medicine: principles and practices,* ed 2, Philadelphia, 1989, WB Saunders.

Sleutel M: An overview of vibroacoustic stimulation, *JOGNN* 18:447, 1989.

Stamfer MJ, Bechtel SD, Hunter DJ: Fat, alcohol selenium, and breast cancer risk, *Contemp OB/GYN* 37(Breast Health):42, June 15, 1992.

Stringer M: Chorionic villi sampling: a nursing perspective, *JOGNN* 17:19, 1988.

Environmental Hazards

Creasy RK, Resnik R: *Maternal-fetal medicine: principles and practice,* ed 2, Philadelphia, 1989, WB Saunders.

Dupre L: Safety in the workplace. I. Handling chemotherapy drugs, *Calif Nurs Rev* 10(2):12, 1988.

Fanaroff AA, Martin RJ: *Neonatal-perinatal medicine: diseases of the fetus and infant,* ed 5, St Louis, 1992, Mosby–Year Book.

Health status of Vietnam veterans. III. Reproductive outcomes and child health, *JAMA* 259(18):2715, 1988.

Heins HC: Your health pregnancy: hazards at home and on the job, *Am Baby* 53:10, March 1991.

Mattison DR et al: Effects of drugs and chemicals on the fetus. II. Antidepressants, anticonvulsants, sedatives, and more, *Contemp OB/GYN* 33:97, April 1989.

Mattison DR et al: Effects of drugs and chemicals on the fetus. III. Common OTC and prescription drugs, *Contemp OB/GYN* 33:131, May 1989.

Miller SA: Chemotherapy drug handling safety, *Calif Nurs Rev* 10(2):12, 1988.

Parkinson DK et al: Health effects of long-term solvent exposure among women in blue-collar occupations, *Am J Ind Med* 18:661, 1990.

Qian H et al: Smoking and reproductive cancer: a report from China, *Female Patient* 14:42, June 1989.

Scialli AR, Lione A: Major environmental toxicants, *Contemp OB/GYN* 34:120, Feb 1989.

Scheutzow SO: Legally speaking: protection or discrimination? A new ruling, *RN,* 54:56, July 1991.

Strohl R: External beam radiation therapy in gynecologic cancers, *NAACOG's Clin Issues Perinatal Women's Health Nurs: Oncology* 1:525, 1988.

Bibliography—Nursing Research

Affonso D, Mayberry L: Common stressors reported by a group of childbearing American women, *Health Care Women Int* 11:331, 1990.

Chez B et al: Interpretations of nonstress tests by obstetric nurses, *JOGNN* 19:227, 1990.

Patterson E, Freese M, Goldenberg R: Seeking safe passage: utilizing health care during pregnancy, *Image J Nurs Sch* 22(1):27, 1990.

chapter 27 review

Key Concepts

- A high-risk pregnancy is one in which the life or well-being of the mother or infant is jeopardized by a biophysical or psychosocial disorder coincidental with or unique to pregnancy.
- Factors that place the pregnancy and fetus/neonate at risk include anatomic, physiologic, therapeutic, environmental, and idiopathic events.
- Psychosocial perinatal warning indicators include characteristics of the parents, the child, their support systems, and family circumstances.
- Maternal and perinatal mortality for white persons is considerably lower than for other races in the United States.
- There is excellent evidence that mortality decreases when high risk is identified early and intensive care is applied.
- Diagnostic techniques include ultrasonography, MRI, PUBS, CVS, and EFM. CVS could partially replace amniocentesis for genetic diagnosis.
- Biochemical monitoring techniques involve assessment of maternal urine and blood, as well as amniotic fluid and its components.
- Electronic monitoring that results in a *reactive* NST and a *negative* CST suggest fetal well-being.
- Pollution of the environment is a serious and growing hazard to reproductive health.

Key Terms

- acoustic stimulation test (p. 800)
- alpha-fetoprotein (AFP) (p. 792)
- amniocentesis (p. 792)
- amniotic fluid assessments (p. 792)
- antepartum testing (p. 776)
- biochemical assessment (p. 792)
- biophysical profiles (BPP) (p. 789)
- biparietal diameter (BPD) (p. 785)
- chorionic villi sampling (CVS) (p. 795)
- contraction stress test (CST) (p. 801)
- Coombs' test (p. 798)
- daily fetal movement count (DFMC) (p. 791)
- Doppler ultrasound (p. 788)
- fetal activity determination (FAD) (p. 798
- fetal breathing movements (FBM) (p. 789)
- harmful materials in the workplace and environment (p. 802)
- intrauterine growth retardation (IUGR) (p. 786)
- lecithin/sphingomyelin (L/S) ratio (p. 793)
- magnetic resonance imaging (MRI) (p. 791)
- meconium-stained amniotic fluid (p. 794)
- nonstress test (NST) (p. 798)
- percutaneous umbilical blood sampling (PUBS) (p. 794)
- regionalization of health care (p. 776)
- shake test (p. 793)
- sick building syndrome (p. 805)
- ultrasound (p. 783)

Critical Thinking Exercises

1. Using Tables 27-2 and 27-3 as guides, review several clients' charts. Identify risk factors, and give rationale for each choice.
2. Role-play a nurse attending a woman undergoing CVS or amniocentesis for determination of the possibility of genetic defect. Discuss the nurse's responsibilities for client education in this situation.
3. Assist with a CST or NST. Evaluate the fetal monitor strip, and determine if it is an example of a reactive nonstress test, a nonreactive nonstress test, a positive oxytocin challenge test, or a negative oxytocin challenge test.
4. Make a list of the household chemicals used in your home. In a group seminar compile a master list. Select some examples from the list, identify their purpose, describe why they are hazardous to the reproductive health of women and men and to the developing embryo/fetus. List what alternatives can be substituted to accomplish the same purpose.

Topics for Nursing Research

- Long-term (neonatal) effects of vibroacoustic stimulation
- Adaptation of health care to meet needs of women from non-Western cultures
- Expansion of the nurse's role in antepartum testing: correlation of nurses' abilities with that of current providers
- Efficacy of daily fetal movement counts in low-risk women: establishment of minimum numbers to prevent fetal jeopardy
- Prospective and longitudinal tracing of selected hazards and their incidences and outcomes (mutagenicity, teratogenicity)
- Systematic investigation of possible reproductive hazards, including specific physical, biologic, and chemical hazards; specificity of the agent, dose, and fetal developmental stage at time of exposure

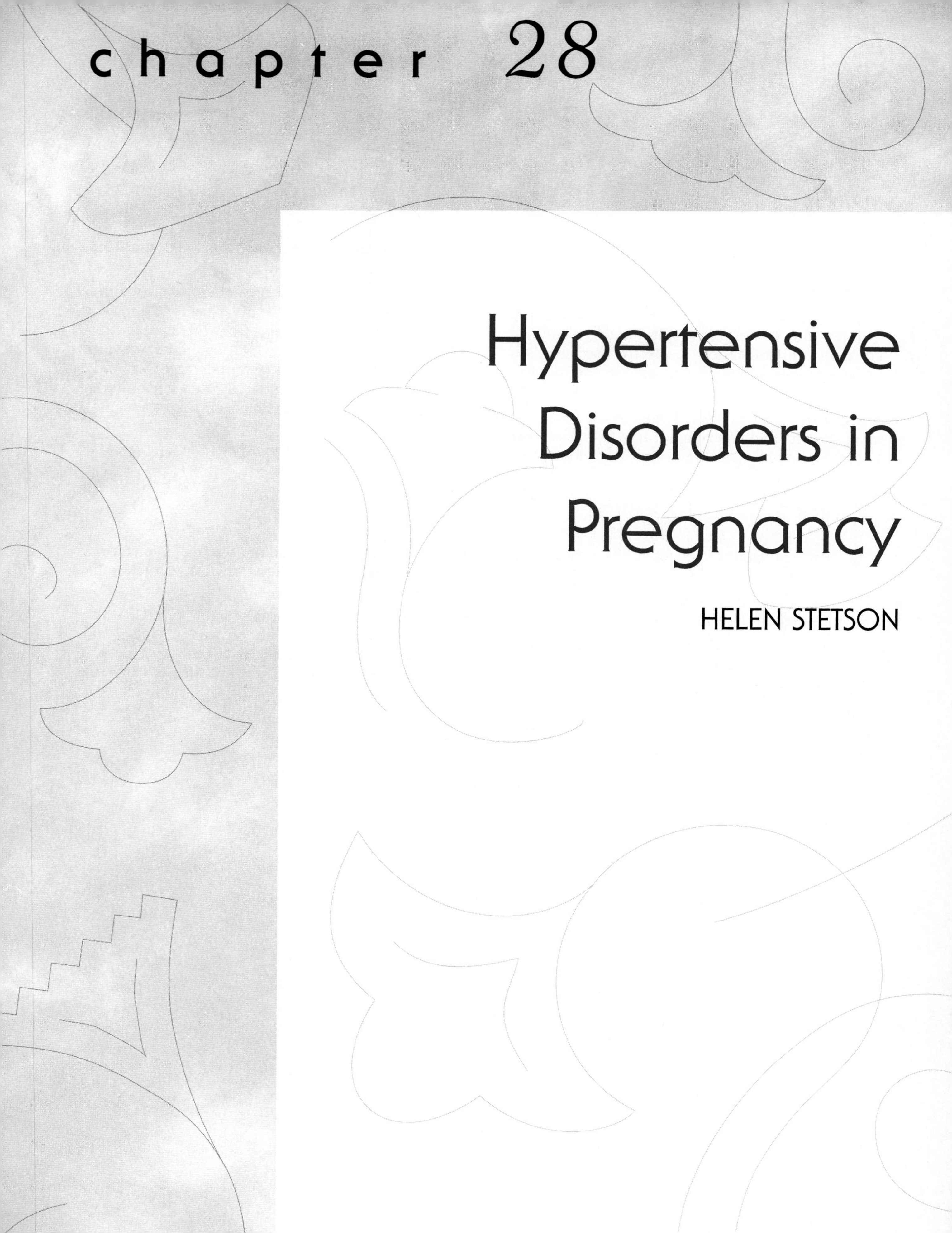

chapter 28

Hypertensive Disorders in Pregnancy

HELEN STETSON

LEARNING OBJECTIVES

- Define the key terms listed.
- Differentiate between pregnancy-induced hypertension (PIH) and concurrent hypertension.
- Review etiologic theories of PIH.
- Describe pathophysiology of PIH.
- Evaluate maternal, fetal, and newborn morbidity and mortality attributable to PIH.
- Describe the HELLP syndrome.
- List assessment techniques for PIH.
- Formulate a nursing plan of care for women with mild and severe preeclampsia.
- Summarize the management of mild and severe preeclampsia.
- Assess the use of the anticonvulsant magnesium sulfate.
- Review management of eclamptic convulsions.
- Identify topics for nursing research related to hypertensive disorders in pregnancy.

Hypertensive disorders continue to be one of the leading causes of maternal and perinatal morbidity and mortality, complicating 10% of all pregnancies. Hypertension has been noted in approximately 10% to 20% of nulliparous women. The prevalence of chronic hypertension, which varies widely in different geographic areas, is between 1% to 5% of all pregnancies (Consensus Report, 1990). Diminished placental perfusion resulting from arteriolar vasospasm that occurs with hypertension places the fetus at risk. Eclampsia (seizures) from profound cerebral effects of **pregnancy-induced hypertension (PIH)** is the major maternal hazard. Early recognition and timely intervention are vital to arrest the progression of the disorder when possible, to prevent injury to the mother, to prevent eclampsia, and to effect a safe birth.

This chapter covers classification and theories of hypertensive disorders of pregnancy and their associated predisposing factors. Pathophysiology is discussed as it affects the normal pregnant woman's organ systems. This background will provide a working basis for early identification of the onset or worsening of the hypertensive condition, as well as help guide nurses in selecting timely and appropriate nursing interventions for preventing injury to the client and baby. Preeclampsia and eclampsia are the primary focus.

■ CLASSIFICATION

Originally, hypertensive disorders of pregnancy had been called *toxemia,* but the term was inappropriately used because no known toxins are involved. The term was replaced by preeclampsia, then by pregnancy-induced hypertension, or PIH. Traditionally, preeclampsia has been classified as a hypertensive disorder, but newer findings show preeclampsia to be a multisystem disease. Hypertension is but one abnormality in a complex syndrome.

Confusion over classification continues, causing difficulties in establishing a clinical diagnosis of the specific hypertensive disorder of pregnancy. Diastolic pressure normally decreases (7 to 10 mm Hg) in early pregnancy, reaching its lowest point during midpregnancy when women usually seek care. This is problematic for women who are hypertensive before pregnancy and have greater blood pressure decreases in early pregnancy than do normotensive pregnant women. Without documentation of baseline prepregnancy or early pregnancy blood pressure values, women can be mistakenly diagnosed with preeclampsia when in fact they really have chronic hypertension.

The classic symptoms associated with preeclampsia or eclampsia, such as proteinuria, edema, and elevated blood pressure, are nonspecific and could be the result of other conditions (Consensus Report, 1990). In one study (Sibai, 1990a) a large percentage of women with eclampsia were found lacking in one or more of these symptoms. Overall, 20% of these women did not have the classic triad of symptoms. Thus it is important to consider other clinical changes as warning signs before the onset of convulsions.

The terminology classification developed by the American College of Obstetrics and Gynecology (ACOG), as well as findings from recent research, are useful for suggesting methods of evaluating and treating pregnant clients with hypertensive disorders (Consensus Report, 1990).

It is important to differentiate between hypertension that occurs before pregnancy (concurrent hypertension and pregnancy) from a pregnancy-specific condition (PIH) because each differs in its effect on the mother and fetus and its management. Women with increased blood pressure are divided into the following groups according to the ACOG committee's classification:

- Pregnancy-induced hypertension
  - Gestational hypertension
  - Preeclampsia
  - Eclampsia
- Concurrent hypertension and pregnancy
  - Chronic hypertension
  - Chronic hypertension with superimposed pregnancy-induced hypertension

Hypertension is defined as a blood pressure of 140/90 mm Hg or greater. The alternative definition is the rise in systolic blood pressure of 30 mm Hg or rise in diastolic blood pressure of 15 mm Hg greater than baseline values. This definition is considered more sensitive to individual variations such as age, race, physiologic state, dietary habits, and heredity. An elevation in blood pressure must be present on two occasions at least 6 hours apart.

Pregnancy-Induced Hypertension

Gestational hypertension is essentially a benign condition, defined as the development of hypertension after 20 weeks' gestation in previously **normotensive** women without signs of proteinuria or edema. Gestational hypertension is not accompanied by other evidence of preeclampsia or preexisting hypertension (Consensus Report, 1990; Roberts et al, 1990). The elevated blood pressure returns to baseline norms after the birth. (For a review of assessing blood pressure and a discussion of mean arterial pressure [MAP], see Chapter 8.)

Diagnosis of gestational hypertension is made retrospectively because one cannot tell whether this condition will progress to a more serious form of hypertensive disorder such as preeclampsia or eclampsia or remain benign. Thus it is important to take any rise in blood pressure during pregnancy seriously and consider it potentially dangerous.

Preeclampsia is the development of hypertension with proteinuria or edema, or both, after 20 weeks' gestation. An abnormal elevated blood pressure is the "hallmark for the diagnosis of preeclampsia" (Sibai, 1988). This is the most serious of the hypertensive complications and is life threatening to the fetus and mother if it remains unrecognized or if eclampsia develops. The potential for lethal effects on the mother and fetus warrants overdiagnosis, primarily for prevention of eclampsia (Consensus Report, 1990).

Newer research studies (Roberts et al, 1990) have found pathologic and pathophysiologic changes occurring weeks to months *before* preeclampsia actually becomes clinically evident (e.g., elevated blood pressure). By the time the disease is diagnosed, the fetus may be already compromised.

Preeclampsia ranges from a clinical spectrum of mild to severe stages and usually proceeds slowly. It may never progress beyond the mildest form, *but can progress rapidly within days or weeks to severe preeclampsia or eclampsia.*

Blood pressure must increase by at least 30 mm Hg systolic or 15 mm Hg diastolic above the woman's baseline values. If prior blood pressure measurements are unknown, readings of 140/90 mm Hg or greater after 20 weeks' gestation are considered sufficiently elevated for a preeclampsia diagnosis. **Mean arterial pressure (MAP)** in the second trimester (MAP-2), calculated as the average of all second-trimester blood pressure readings, is considered elevated at ≥90 mm Hg (e.g., 96). Third-trimester MAP (MAP-3) values ≥105 mm Hg on two occasions separated by at least 6 hours are considered abnormal (Cherry, Merkatz, 1991).

The presence of **proteinuria** distinguishes preeclampsia from gestational hypertension. Preeclampsia may be accompanied by **edema,** which is a generalized accumulation of interstitial fluid after 12 hours of bed rest or a sudden rapid weight gain of more than 2 kg (4 to 4½ lb) per week. Rapid weight gain is considered more significant. Differentiation between physiologic edema and edema associated with preeclampsia is difficult. Edema is clinically harder to assess because it can vary and can indicate other conditions. Edema no longer enters into the diagnosis of preeclampsia (Iams, Zuspan, 1990).

Eclampsia is the development of convulsion or coma with proteinuria or edema, or both. It is not caused by any coincidental neurologic disease such as epilepsy in a woman with preeclampsia.

Concurrent Hypertension and Pregnancy

Chronic hypertension is hypertension that develops before pregnancy or before 20 weeks of gestation; elevation in blood pressure is unrelated to pregnancy. Hypertension that is diagnosed for the first time during pregnancy and persists beyond day 42 postpartum also is classified as chronic hypertension (Consensus Report, 1990).

Chronic hypertension with superimposed PIH is the development of preeclampsia or eclampsia in a women with underlying hypertension. Pregnancy worsens the hypertensive condition. Prognosis is worse than with either condition alone.

Primary (essential) hypertensive disease, in which no cause can be determined, is the diagnosis in about 85% of nonpregnant, premenopausal hypertensive women. The remaining 15% of women with hypertension have secondary hypertensive vascular disease, caused by disorders such as chronic pyelonephritis or glomerulonephritis, renal artery stenosis, or coarctation of the aorta.

With chronic hypertensive disease, the physician treats the symptoms during pregnancy. The pregnancy usually is permitted to continue if the woman responds to therapy. Protracted or maternal central nervous system (CNS), cardiac, or renal complications may develop. If the woman's blood pressure reaches 200/110 mm Hg, immediate medical attention is necessary. The physician usually will order antihypertensive drugs such as hydralazine (see Table 29-3) and will assess the need for a prompt birth.

The prognosis for the pregnant woman with chronic hypertension depends on the cause, the degree of hypertension, the woman's symptoms, and her response to treatment. Whatever the cause, the fetus may be severely affected by hypertension and its sequelae (e.g., intrauterine growth retardation, abruptio placentae). Early birth may be lifesaving for the mother and fetus.

■ PHYSIOLOGY

Normal Maternal Changes

Knowledge of normal maternal physiology (see Chapter 8) is necessary to understand the pathophysiology of hypertensive disorders in pregnancy. Increases in total blood volume, cardiac output, and glomerular filtration rate (GFR) characterize maternal changes (see Chapter 8). Increased estrogen levels raise levels of renin, angiotensin II, and aldosterone. Although aldosterone exerts a sodium and water retention effect on the kidneys, progesterone blocks that effect; the normal net effect is sodium depletion. Angiotensin II stimulates a rise in blood pressure, except during normal pregnancy. During normal pregnancy, resistance to the pressor effect of angiotensin II may be related to increased levels of such vasodilator prostaglandins as PGE_2 (Friedman, 1988). Despite the increased blood volume, this decreased peripheral resistance is credited with the slight drop in maternal blood pressure during the second trimester. A return to prepregnancy blood pressure readings is expected in the third trimester (see box, below).

In dependent limbs, fluid moves from the intravascular compartment to the extravascular space. "Physiologic anemia" (normal hemodilution), results in decreased plasma colloid osmotic pressure. Mechanical pressure from the weight of the gravid uterus increases venous capillary hydrostatic pressure. The net effect is *physiologic edema* of dependent limbs during the third trimester (Gilbert, Harmon, 1992).

Changes in Normal Pregnancy

CARDIOVASCULAR

↑ Total blood volume
↓ Total peripheral resistence related to
  ↓ Hemoglobin and hematocrit (physiologic anemia)
  Vascular smooth muscle relaxation
↑ Cardiac output
↑ Clotting factors
Physiologic edema related to
  ↓ Plasma colloid osmotic pressure
  ↑ Venous capillary hydrostatic pressure (gravid uterine mechanical pressure)

RENAL

↑ GFR and renal plasma flow

ENDOCRINE

↑ Estrogen production results in
  ↑ Renin-angiotensin II—aldosterone secretion
↑ Progesterone production blocks
  Aldosterone effect (slight ↓ Na)
↑ Vasodilator prostaglandins result in
  Resistance to angiotensin II (slight ↓ BP)

BP, Blood pressure; *GFR*, glomerular filtration rate.

Physiologic edema is expected to disappear after 8 to 12 hours of bed rest.

Theories of Hypertensive Disorders

Causes of hypertension in pregnancy are multiple and have been the subject of extensive research and much speculation for decades. No known theory as yet accounts for all symptoms. Evidently PIH is somehow related to the physiologic changes of pregnancy because it disappears after the termination of pregnancy. Therefore the gravid uterus, placenta, or fetus could be the central factor in the condition.

Several major concepts that contribute to current thought about the etiology of PIH are increased vasoconstrictor tone (Gilstrap, Gant, 1990; Scott et al, 1990), abnormal prostaglandin action (Friedman, 1988), and endothelial cell activation (Creasy, Resnik, 1989; Roberts et al, 1988, 1989). Immunologic factors may play an important role (Sibai, 1991).

In part, vasospasm is the result of an increased sensitivity to circulating pressors, such as angiotensin II, and possibly an imbalance between prostacyclin and thromboxane A_2 (Consensus Report, 1990). A consistent finding in women with preeclampsia is an increased responsiveness to vasoconstrictive effects of angiotensin II. This sensitivity occurs before the onset of hypertension and as early as 23 weeks' gestation.

Generally, placental prostaglandins have been found to have potent effects on platelets and blood vessels: "imbalance [of placental prostaglandins] could significantly contribute to the increased vasoconstriction, platelet aggregation, and reduced uteroplacental blood flow characteristic of preeclampsia" (Walsh, 1990).

Recently, investigators tested the ability of aspirin (a prostaglandin inhibitor) to alter the pathophysiology of preeclampsia (Benigni et al, 1989; Schiff et al, 1989; Walsh, 1990). Investigation of the use of aspirin as a prophylactic treatment in prevention of preeclampsia and its risk-benefit ratio for the mother and baby is continuing. Other investigators are studying the use of calcium supplementation to prevent hypertension in pregnancy (see Research Highlight, p. 817).

Although speculative, the endothelial cell activation theory helps to explain the increased sensitivity to circulating pressor substances, as well as the clinical findings of vasospasm, coagulopathy, and endothelial lesions in women with preeclampsia. Endothelial cell dysfunction, believed to result from decreased placental perfusion, can account for many preeclampsia changes as follows:

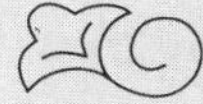 **Research Highlight** 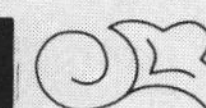

Use of Calcium to Prevent Hypertension in Pregnancy

RESEARCH ABSTRACT

Calcium supplementation has been found to lower blood pressure in nonpregnant and pregnant women. The purpose of this study was to determine whether supplementation with 2 g of calcium per day would prevent hypertensive disorders of pregnancy (gestational hypertension and preeclampsia). The subjects were 1194 women who were 20 weeks' pregnant and were obtaining prenatal care at two public hospitals (580 women) and one private hospital (614 women). Subjects were randomly assigned to either a calcium supplementation or a placebo group. None of the women, nurses, or physicians knew which tablet the woman was receiving. At each prenatal visit the blood pressure and the levels of serum total calcium, magnesium, and phosphate, as well as uric acid and urinary calcium and creatinine excretion were measured. The incidence of gestational hypertension was different for the two groups: 10.7% for the placebo group and 7.2% for the calcium group. The incidence of preeclampsia also differed: 3.9 for the placebo group and 2.6 for the calcium group. The effects were even more marked when comparisons were made among women with low baseline levels of urinary calcium; calcium supplements lowered the rate of hypertensive disorders from 13.2% in the placebo group to 7.8% in the calcium group. Women with low baseline levels of urinary calcium had the least increase in systolic and diastolic blood pressure. The incidence of complications of pregnancy was similar in the two groups. No differences in side effects were related to treatment status.

IMPLICATIONS FOR PRACTICE

A simple treatment, calcium supplementation, had a significant effect on hypertension in pregnancy. Women in the placebo group took their calcium supplement 86% of the time, and women in the calcium group took their tablets 84% of the time. Inasmuch as treatment cannot be effective unless the clients use the treatment, nurses should emphasize the importance of taking prescribed medications. Nurses can monitor use of treatments by asking clients if they are remembering to take their medications, by pill counts, and by noting side effects that may prompt clients to stop taking the medication.

RELATED RESEARCH QUESTIONS

1. What are the side effects of calcium supplementation?
2. Is there a relation between side effects of calcium supplementation and number of pills taken?
3. What factors are associated with adherence to a medication regimen?
4. Do weekly (biweekly; monthly) reminders encourage adherence to a medication regimen?

REFERENCE

Belizan JM et al: Calcium supplementation to prevent hypertensive disorders of pregnancy, *N Engl J Med* 325:1399, 1991.

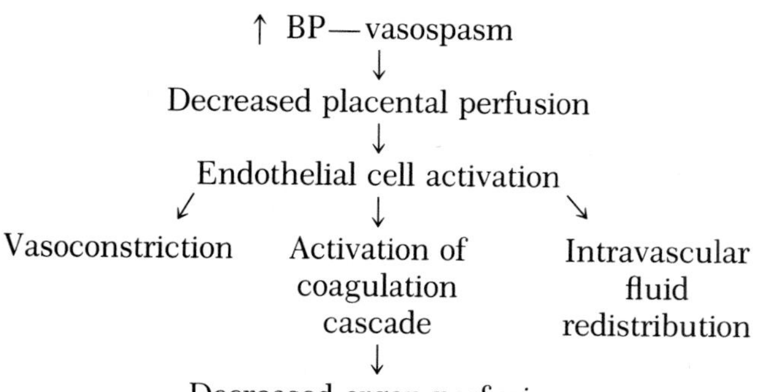

Many studies have investigated the relationship of the immune system to preeclampsia (Sibai, 1991), providing enough evidence to suggest that immunologic factors play an important role. The presence of foreign protein, the placenta, and/or the fetus may trigger an adverse immunologic response. This theory is supported by the increased incidence of PIH in first-time mothers (first exposure to fetal tissue) and in women pregnant by a new partner (different genetic material). The protective role of the immunologic response is poorly understood. It has been suggested that preeclampsia is an immune complex disease in which the maternal antibody system is overwhelmed from excessive fetal antigens in the maternal circulation. This condition seems compatible with the high incidence of preeclampsia in women exposed to a large mass of trophoblastic tissue—for example, as seen in twins (see Chapter 7) and hydatidiform moles (see Chapter 30).

Genetic predisposition may be another immunologic factor. Sibai (1991) found a greater frequency

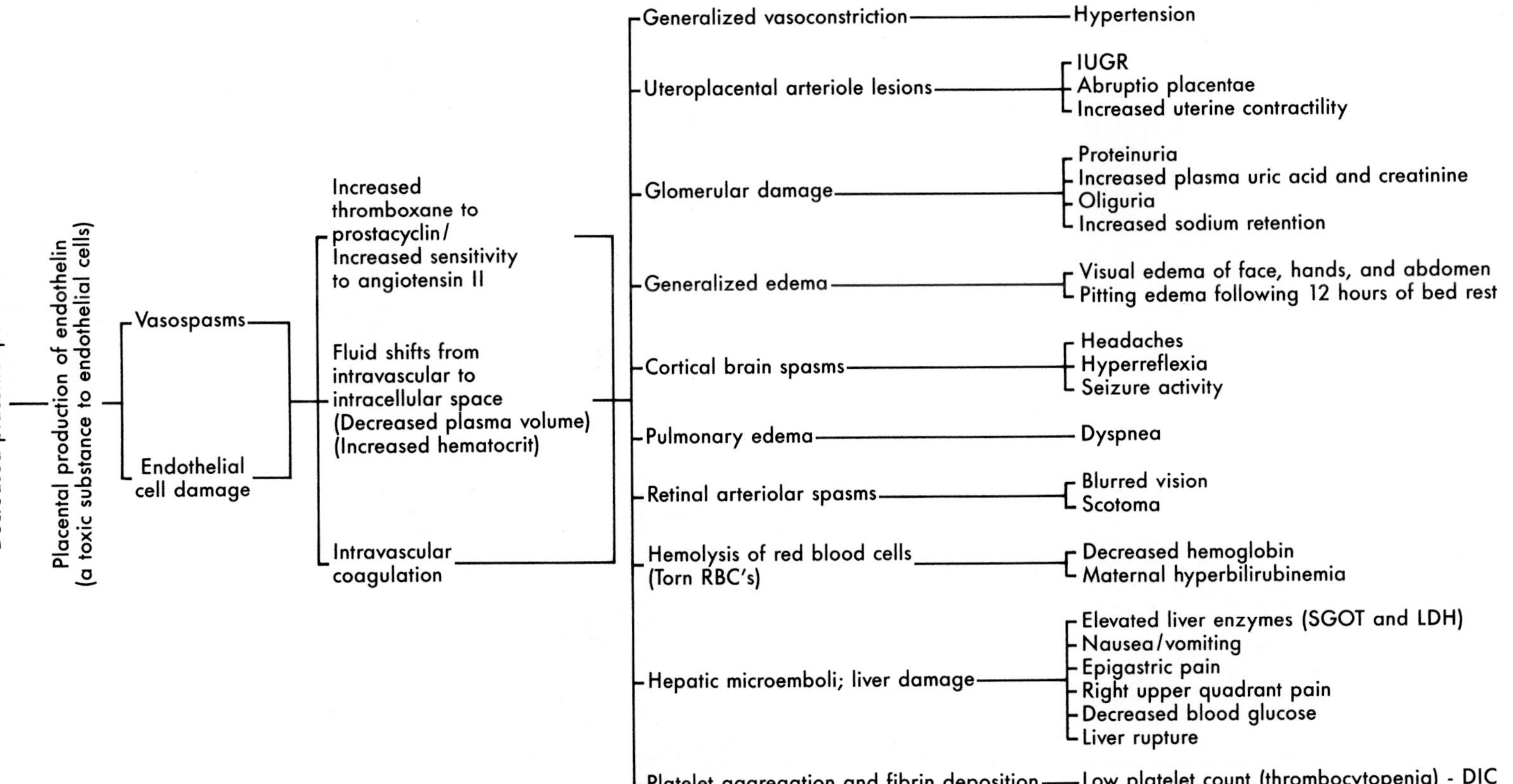

Fig. 28-1 Pathophysiology of pregnancy-induced hypertension.
Modified from Gilbert ES, Harmon JS: *High-risk pregnancy and delivery: nursing perspectives*, ed 2, St Louis, 1992, Mosby–Year Book.

of preeclampsia and eclampsia in daughters and granddaughters of women with a history of eclampsia, which suggests an autosomal-recessive gene controlling the maternal immune response. Paternal factors also are being examined (Klonoff-Cohen et al, 1989).

Diets inadequate in all nutrients, especially protein, calcium, sodium, and vitamins E and A, may be one etiologic factor in PIH. Proponents of this theory prescribe high-protein diets without caloric or sodium restriction in prevention and treatment of this disorder. In pregnancy—especially late pregnancy when the fetus has an increased protein need for body growth and functioning—the required daily allowance (RDA) for protein is increased (from 50 to 60 g/day for a singleton pregnancy). If a woman begins pregnancy with a protein deficit (as teenagers might or as women consuming a high carbohydrate diet because of low income or ignorance might) or if she has a multifetal pregnancy, her RDA for protein in pregnancy is even greater. If the woman's life-style is associated with skipping meals or with "eating on the run" (e.g., the life-style of many career-oriented women or mothers of more than three or four children), then she is at risk for a deficient protein intake. All these factors place women at greatest risk for the development of preeclampsia and eclampsia.

Pathophysiology

Studies that examine pathologic changes in organs of preeclamptic and eclamptic women have provided strong evidence that preeclampsia is very different from chronic hypertension (Creasy, Resnik, 1989; Robert et al, 1990). Pathologic changes that occur in the endothelial cells of the glomeruli (glomeruloendotheliosis) is but one example. These renal lesions are uniquely characteristic of preeclampsia, particularly in nulliparous women (85%), according to Chesley and Sibai (1988). The main pathogenic factor is not an increase in blood pressure but of *poor perfusion secondary to vasospasm.* **Arteriolar vasospasm** diminishes the diameter of blood vessels, which impedes blood flow to all organs and raises blood pressure (Consensus Report, 1990). Function in organs such as the placenta, kidneys, liver, and brain is depressed by as much as 40% to 60%. The pathophysiologic sequelae are shown in Fig. 28-1.

Impaired placental perfusion leads to early *degenerative aging of the placenta and possible intrauterine growth retardation* (IUGR) of the fetus (Fig. 28-2). It is important to recall that impaired prostaglandin synthesis (p. 816) may be a factor in PIH. Uterine activity and sensitivity to oxytocin are increased. *Therefore increased sensitivity to the effects of oxytocin must be taken into account when the drug is used for induction or augmentation of labor.*

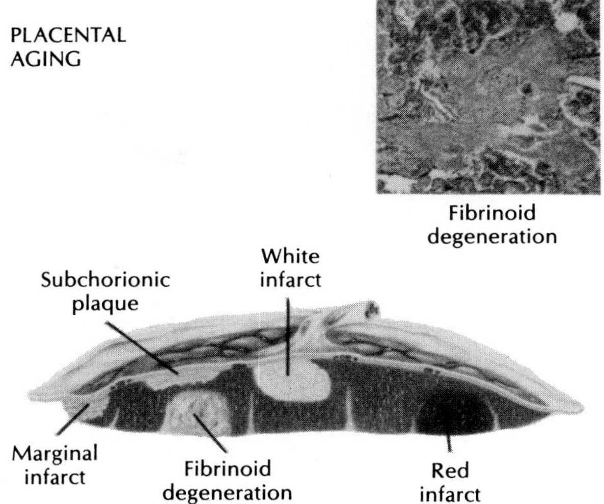

Fig. 28-2 Effects of severe pregnancy-induced hypertension on placenta, with resultant placental insufficiency.

Reduced kidney perfusion decreases the glomerular filtration rate and leads to degenerative glomerular changes. *Protein, primarily albumin, is lost in the urine.* Uric acid clearance is decreased. Sodium and water are retained. Plasma colloid osmotic pressure decreases as serum albumin levels also decrease. Intravascular volume is reduced as fluid moves out of the intravascular compartment, resulting in *hemoconcentration,* increased blood viscosity, and tissue *edema.* The hematocrit value increases as fluid leaves the intravascular space (Cunningham et al, 1989). Therefore a rising hematocrit level occurs as the condition worsens; a falling hematocrit value (to normal levels) accompanies improvement of the condition. In severe preeclampsia, blood volume may fall to or below nonpregnancy levels, severe edema develops, and *rapid weight gain* is seen (Scott et al, 1990).

Decreased liver perfusion causes impaired function. Hepatic edema and subcapsular hemorrhage, experienced by the pregnant woman as *epigastric or right upper quadrant pain,* is one sign of impending eclampsia (convulsion). Rupture of the liver is a rare but catastrophic complication (Cunningham et al, 1989). Liver enzyme levels (e.g., AST [SGOT]) rise in the wake of liver damage.

Arteriolar vasospasms and decreased blood flow to the retina lead to *visual symptoms* such as scotoma (blind spots) and blurring. The same pathologic condition leads to cerebral edema and hemorrhages, as well as increased *CNS irritability.* CNS irritability manifests as headache, hyperreflexia, positive ankle

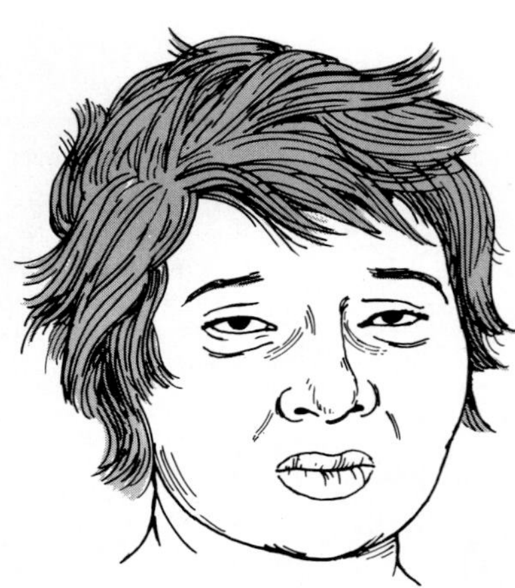

Fig. 28-3 Characteristic facies: dulled affect, periorbital edema, and puffiness of face.

clonus, and occasionally convulsions (pp. 823 and 826). Changes in **affect** (changes in emotion, mood, and altered consciousness) are typical symptoms of cerebral edema (Fig. 28-3) (Scott et al, 1990).

Debate continues whether preeclampsia contributes to or is the result of **disseminated intravascular coagulation (DIC)** or whether DIC occurs with preeclampsia.

If the hypertension is difficult to bring under control, cardiac and pulmonary complications can occur. Heart failure, a common cause of maternal death attributed to preeclampsia, is rare in young, otherwise healthy women (Scott et al, 1990). Sudden circulatory collapse and shock may occur in women with a history of repeated hypertensive pregnancies. A rapid fall in systolic blood pressure by 70 mm Hg or more is most often seen *a few hours after giving birth,* although it may occur before or during labor.

Typically, *pulmonary edema* caused by preeclampsia is associated with severe generalized edema. Intravenous (IV) fluid infusion is an iatrogenic cause of fluid overload. A weak, rapid pulse, increased respiratory rate, lowered blood pressure, and pulmonary crackles (rales) suggest *circulatory failure*. Rapid digitalization and probably diuresis with furosemide may be ordered. Pulmonary edema and congestive heart failure are virtually the only accepted indications for diuretic therapy during pregnancy (Scott, Worley, 1990). Diuretic therapy further reduces intervillous blood flow (placental perfusion), which could well cause serious fetal jeopardy. Impaired intervillous perfusion is the main cause of perinatal morbidity (illness) and mortality (death) associated with hypertension (Scott et al, 1990). *The greatest risk of pulmonary edema occurs 15 hours after birth* (Benedetti et al, 1985).

The HELLP Syndrome

The **HELLP syndrome** (*H*, hemolysis; *EL*, elevated liver enzymes; *LP*, low platelet count) represents an extension of the pathology of severe preeclampsia and eclampsia (Scott et al, 1990). The initial symptoms of the HELLP syndrome usually appear early in the third trimester. A circulating immunologic component may be the underlying cause.

For a woman to be diagnosed as having the HELLP syndrome, her platelet count must be $<100{,}000/mm^3$, her liver enzyme levels must be elevated (aspartate aminotransferase [AST] and alanine aminotransferase [ALT]), and some evidence for intravascular hemolysis must be present (schistocytes or burr cells on peripheral smear). The hemolysis that occurs accounts for the large drop in hematocrit out of proportion to blood loss that occurs in most new mothers with HELLP syndrome during the postpartum period (Weinstein, 1986). A unique form of coagulopathy (not DIC) occurs with the HELLP syndrome (for a discussion of DIC, see Chapter 30).

Recognition of the clinical and laboratory findings of the HELLP syndrome is important if early, aggressive therapy is to be initiated to prevent maternal and neonatal mortality (Weinstein, 1986; Anderson, 1987).

An unfavorable (uneffaced and undilated) cervix and the aggressive nature of this disorder support cesarean birth. Prolonged induction of labor could increase maternal morbidity. Fresh-frozen plasma may be needed if bleeding occurs and persists. The major laboratory manifestations of the disease, however, may not appear until the early postpartum period (48 to 72 hours). Delayed transfusion of packed red blood cells (RBCs) often is necessary because of the continued hemolysis. It is important to attempt to lower the blood pressure if the diastolic pressure is consistently greater than 110 mm Hg. *However, blood pressure may be normal or slightly elevated; thus it is not an adequate indicator of the severity of the disease.* ***Hypoglycemia*** may be present in the woman with the HELLP syndrome and, when the blood sugar is less than 40 mg/dL, is associated with a high maternal mortality (Egley et al, 1985).

Morbidity and Mortality

MATERNAL. The incidence of preeclampsia is approximately 7% of all pregnancies, predisposing women to potentially lethal complications such as abruptio placentae, DIC, cerebral hemorrhage, hepatic failure, and acute renal failure (Consensus Report, 1990). Maternal deaths are due predominantly to complications of abruptio placentae, hepatic rupture, and most significantly, eclampsia (Roberts et al, 1990).

In general, eclampsia is preventable and has been less common in the United States with improvement of obstetric care (Cunningham et al, 1989). A study analyzing the National Hospital discharge survey data of 400 hospitals nationwide from 1979 to 1986 showed a 36% decline in births complicated by eclampsia (Saftlas et al, 1990). However, eclampsia is still a major cause of serious maternal morbidity and maternal death worldwide (Sibai, 1990a).

Eclampsia occurs in approximately 0.05% to 0.2% of all pregnancies and in 1.5% of twin gestations (Anderson, 1987). About 8% of women with eclampsia die of the disease or its complications. The most common causes of death are intracranial hemorrhage and congestive heart failure.

PERINATAL. Preeclampsia contributes extensively to intrauterine fetal death (IUFD) (stillbirths) and perinatal mortality. The main causes of neonatal death are placental insufficiency and abruptio placentae. IUGR is common in infants of preeclamptic women as a result of poor uteroplacental perfusion (Roberts et al, 1990). One study (Sibai, 1990a) showed, over a 12-year period, perinatal mortality rates of 254 eclamptic women to be 11.8%. Neonatal deaths in this study were mainly associated with abruptio placentae and extreme prematurity.

In many parts of North America perinatal mortality as a result of eclampsia is at least 20%. This occurs mainly because of the effects of hypoxia, prematurity, or acidosis during maternal convulsion. A single maternal convulsion increases the prospect of perinatal death at least fivefold.

■ THE NURSING PROCESS

An extensive data base is essential for early identification of this potentially life-threatening disorder. The nursing process provides the framework for assessment and guides nursing care that is essential for managing this complication.

ASSESSMENT

Preeclampsia typically begins with the appearance of symptoms; however, preventive treatment needs to begin much earlier (Gavette, Roberts, 1987). A key goal is early identification of pregnant women at risk for the development of preeclampsia. Therefore each woman is assessed for high-risk factors during the first and subsequent prenatal visits.

Factors such as parity, age, and geographic location need to be taken into consideration. First-time mothers have been found to be six to eight times more susceptible than are multiparous women to the development of preeclampsia (Consensus Report, 1990). Daughters and sisters of preeclamptic women have a higher tendency to develop preeclampsia than do unrelated women. Women younger than 20 or older than 35 years of age, unmarried, and/or residing in the southern and western regions of the United States have a significantly higher incidence of preeclampsia (Saftlas et al, 1990). Race alone was not found to be a significant factor for either preeclampsia or eclampsia in this study (Saftlas et al, 1990). Teenagers, usually first-time mothers and most likely not receiving prenatal care or adequate nutrition, are at highest risk. Indirectly, lack of prenatal care delays early recognition of risk factors and preeclampsia in its earlier stages. This increases the incidence of severe disease and adverse perinatal outcome.

Obstetric conditions associated with increased placental mass such as multifetal gestation and hydatidiform moles, as well as chronic medical disorders such as hypertension, collagen vascular disease, and diabetes mellitus, lead to a greater risk for preeclampsia (Roberts et al, 1990).

Interview

The nurse reviews the woman's admission form. When the nurse and client are comfortable, the nurse begins with the interview to clarify, expand, or complete the form. Past medical history is reviewed, especially the presence of diabetes mellitus and hypertension. Family history is explored for occurrence of preeclamptic or hypertensive conditions, diabetes mellitus, or other chronic conditions. The social and experiential history provides information about the woman's marital status, nutritional status, cultural beliefs, activity level, and health habits such as smoking and alcohol consumption.

A review of systems adds to the data base for detecting blood pressure changes from baseline, abnormal weight gain and pattern of weight gain, increased signs of edema, and presence of protein in the urine. It also is important to note whether the woman is having unusual, frequent, or severe headaches, visual disturbances, and/or epigastric pain.

Physical Examination

Lack of specific, reliable diagnostic tests currently hinder early detection and treatment of preeclampsia. Mean arterial pressure (MAP) and the rollover test are additional methods for evaluating blood pressure. However, findings from various studies of the rollover test show wide disparity in sensitivity and predictive value. (The rollover test is discussed in Chapter 13.)

The ACOG committee's definition of hypertension is an increase in MAP of 20 mm Hg or, if prior blood pressure is unknown, then a MAP of 105 mm Hg (Roberts et al, 1990). Second-trimester MAP values (MAP-2) greater than 90 mm Hg may be useful in

TABLE 28-1 Differentiation of Mild and Severe Preeclampsia

	Mild Preeclampsia*	Severe Preeclampsia
MATERNAL EFFECTS		
Blood pressure	Rise in systolic blood pressure of 30 mm Hg or more; a rise in diastolic blood pressure of ≥15 mm Hg or a reading of 140/90 mm Hg × 2, 6 hr apart	Rise to ≥160/110 mm Hg on two separate occasions 6 hr apart with pregnant woman on bed rest
MAP	140/90 = 107	160/110 = 127
Weight gain	Weight gain of more than 0.5 kg (1 lb)/wk during the second and third trimesters, or a sudden weight gain of 2 kg (4-4½ lb)/wk at any time.	Same as mild preeclampsia
Proteinuria Qualitative dipstick Quantitative 24-hr analysis	Proteinuria of 300 mg/L in a 24-hr specimen or >1 g/L in a random daytime specimen of two or more occasions 6 hr apart because protein loss is variable; with dipstick, values vary from trace to 1+	Proteinuria of 5-10 g/L in 24 hr or ≥2+ protein on dipstick
Edema	Dependent edema, some puffiness of eyes, face, fingers; pulmonary rales absent	Generalized edema, noticeable puffiness of eyes, face, fingers Pulmonary edema → crackles (rales)
Reflexes	**Hyperreflexia** 3+; no ankle clonus	**Hyperreflexia** 3+ or more; ankle clonus
Urine output	Output matches intake; ≥30 mL/hr	**Oliguria:** <30 mL/hr or 120 mL/4 hr output
Headache	Transient	Severe
Visual problems	Absent	Blurred, photophobia, blind spots on funduscopy
Irritability/affect	Transient	Severe
Epigastric pain	Absent	Present
Serum creatinine	Normal	Elevated
Thrombocytopenia	Absent	Present
AST elevation	Minimal	Marked
Hematocrit	Increased	Increased
FETAL EFFECTS		
Placental perfusion	Reduced	Decreased perfusion expressed as IUGR in fetus; FHR: late decelerations
Premature placental aging	Not apparent	At birth placenta appears smaller than normal for the duration of the pregnancy. Premature aging is apparent with numerous areas of broken syncytia. Ischemic necroses (white infarcts) are numerous, and intervillous fibrin deposition (red infarcts) may be recorded

*No preeclampsia should be considered "mild" (Knuppel, Drukker, 1986; Scott et al, 1990).

identifying women at risk for preeclampsia (Gavette, Roberts, 1987; Weiner, 1987). Data from Chesley and Sibai's study (1988) suggest that MAP-2 values often are predictive of transient hypertension and thus are a sign of future chronic hypertension.

During each subsequent prenatal visit the pregnant woman is assessed for symptoms that suggest the onset of presence of preeclampsia (Table 28-1). One intent of routine assessments of blood pressure, weight, and urine of pregnant women is to promptly identify complications such as preeclampsia. Frequency of visits is determined by the initial and subsequent assessments.

Accurate and consistent *blood pressure* assessment is important for establishing a baseline and monitoring subtle changes throughout pregnancy. Many variables can influence blood pressure measurements, such as position, cuff size, arm used, and emotional state (see Chapter 8). Personnel caring for pregnant women need to be consistent in taking and recording blood pressure measurements in the standardized manner. The American Heart Association has developed a blood pressure measurement protocol (see box, below).

Phase V of the Korotkoff sounds is commonly absent in pregnant women because of the high cardiac output state. Thus it is recommended that both phases IV and V be recorded for the diastolic blood pressure. Phase IV should be used for diagnosis and clinical trials.

Observation of edema plus other assessment findings warrant additional investigation. *Edema* is assessed for distribution, degree, and pitting. If periorbital or facial edema is not obvious, the pregnant woman is asked if it was present when she awoke. As the day progresses, gravity is responsible for movement of fluid to dependent body parts. In more severe preeclampsia, facial edema is obvious. Edema may be described as dependent or pitting (Kozier, Erb, 1987).

Dependent edema is edema of the lowest or most dependent parts of the body, where hydrostatic pressure is greatest. If a person is ambulatory, this edema may first be evident in the feet and ankles. If the person is confined to bed, the edema is more likely to occur in the sacral region.

Pitting edema is edema that leaves a small depression or pit after finger pressure is applied to the swollen area. The pit is caused by movement of fluid to adjacent tissue, away from the point of pressure. Within 10 to 30 seconds the pit normally disappears. Although the amount of edema is difficult to quantitate, the method described in Fig. 28-4 may be used to record relative degrees of edema formation.

Symptoms reflecting CNS and visual system involvement usually accompany facial edema. Although it is not a routine assessment during the prenatal period, evaluation of the fundus of the eye yields valuable data. An initial baseline finding of normal *eyegrounds* assists in differentiating preexisting from new disease process (Fig. 28-5). The woman may be unable to relate other symptoms such as epigastric pain or oliguria. Respirations are assessed for rales (crackles), which may indicate pulmonary edema.

Deep tendon reflexes (DTRs) are evaluated if preeclampsia is suspected. The biceps and patellar reflexes and ankle clonus are assessed and the findings recorded (Fig. 28-6; Table 28-2). To elicit the biceps reflex a downward blow is struck over the thumb, which is situated over the biceps tendon. *Normal response is flexion of the arm at the elbow* or +2 (Table 28-2). The **patellar reflex** is elicited with the woman's legs hanging freely over the end of the examining table, or with the woman lying on her left side with the knee slightly flexed. A blow with a percussion hammer is dealt directly to the patellar tendon, inferior to the patella. *Normal response is the extension or kicking out of the leg.* To assess for hyperactive reflexes (**clonus**) at the ankle joint, the leg should be supported with the knee flexed. With one hand, the foot is sharply dorsiflexed and the position maintained for a moment. The foot is then released. *Normal (negative clonus) response* is elicited when, while the foot is held in dorsiflexion, no rhythmic oscillations (jerking) are felt. When the foot is released, no oscillations are seen as foot drops to plantar flexed position. *Abnormal (positive clonus)* response is recognized by rhythmic oscillations of one or more

Blood Pressure Measurement Protocol

1. Attempt to have woman relaxed before taking blood pressure; then measure the blood pressure with the woman in a sitting position and use the same arm for each measurement.
2. Have the arm resting on a table at heart level.
3. Use the proper cuff size.
4. Assess for approximate systolic blood pressure level using the palpation method before taking measurement.
5. Maintain a slow, steady deflation rate.
6. Take the average of two readings, at least 6 hours apart, to minimize recorded blood pressure variations across time.
7. Use accurate equipment.

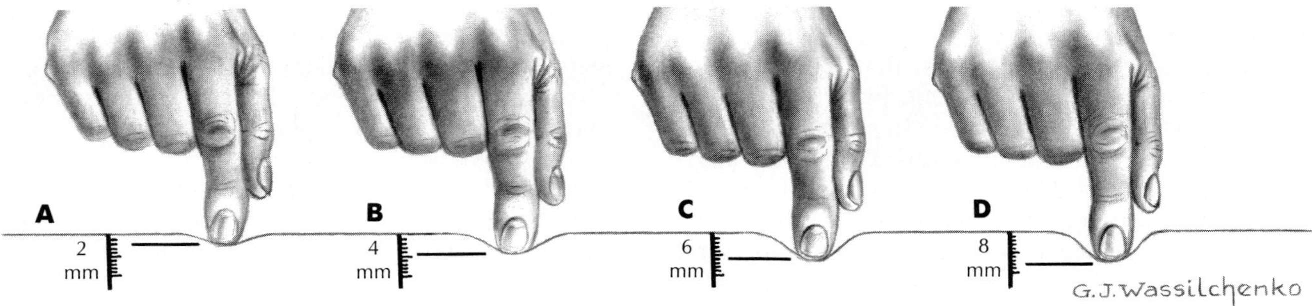

Fig. 28-4 Assessment of pitting edema: **A,** +1; **B,** +2; **C,** +3; **D,** +4.

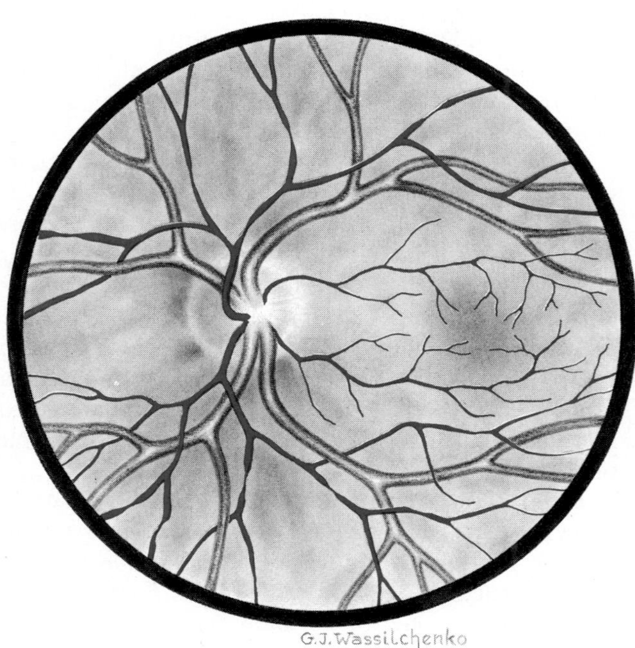

Fig. 28-5 Funduscopic evidence of severe pregnancy-induced hypertension: arteriospasm, edema, hemorrhages, arteriovenous nicking, and exudates.

TABLE 28-2 Assessing Deep Tendon Reflexes

Degree	Grading
Brisk with sustained clonus	5+
Hyperactive response (brisk with transient clonus)	4+
More than normal (brisk)	3+
Normal, active	2+
Low response (sluggish or dull)	1+
No response	0

"beats" felt when the foot is in dorsiflexion and seen as foot drops to the plantar flexed position.

The *fetal heart rate* (FHR) and rhythm are assessed inasmuch as these reflect uteroplacental sufficiency. Fetal movement and growth are determined by Leopold's maneuvers (see Chapter 17). Fundal height is measured for estimating fetal growth. Biophysical or biochemical monitoring for fetal well-being may be ordered (see Chapter 27): "As long as the fetus continues to grow in an appropriate manner, it can be inferred that the placenta and uterine blood flow [are] appropriate" (Consensus Report, 1990).

Doppler ultrasound flow studies are now being used for evaluating maternal-fetal well-being (see Chapter 27). Uteroplacental perfusion is assessed by measuring the velocity of blood flow through the uterine or umbilical arteries, or both. Doppler ultrasound of arterial blood flow is characterized as wave forms (see Fig. 27-6). Vascular resistance is estimated by comparing systolic (S) to diastolic (D) waveforms. S/D ratios do not measure perfusion.

Normally placental vascular resistance is low during pregnancy; normal S/D ratios decrease from 2.8 to 2.2 between midpregnancy and term. A systolic/diastolic ratio over 2.7 after 26 weeks may herald preeclampsia. If placental flow resistance increases, indicating poor placental perfusion, the S/D ratio increases. An S/D ratio greater than 3.0 is considered abnormal and associated with poor maternal-fetal outcomes (see Fig. 27-7, *B*). Values of 3.8 or higher have been associated with preeclampsia and IUGR (Consensus Report, 1990; Cundiff et al, 1990).

Uterine tonicity is evaluated for signs of labor and abruptio placentae. If labor is suspected, a vaginal examination for cervical changes is indicated.

During the physical examination, the pregnant woman is examined for signs of thrombocytopenia (decreased platelets). Ecchymotic areas, history of bruising with mild trauma, and bleeding from gums may reflect coagulopathy (e.g., DIC).

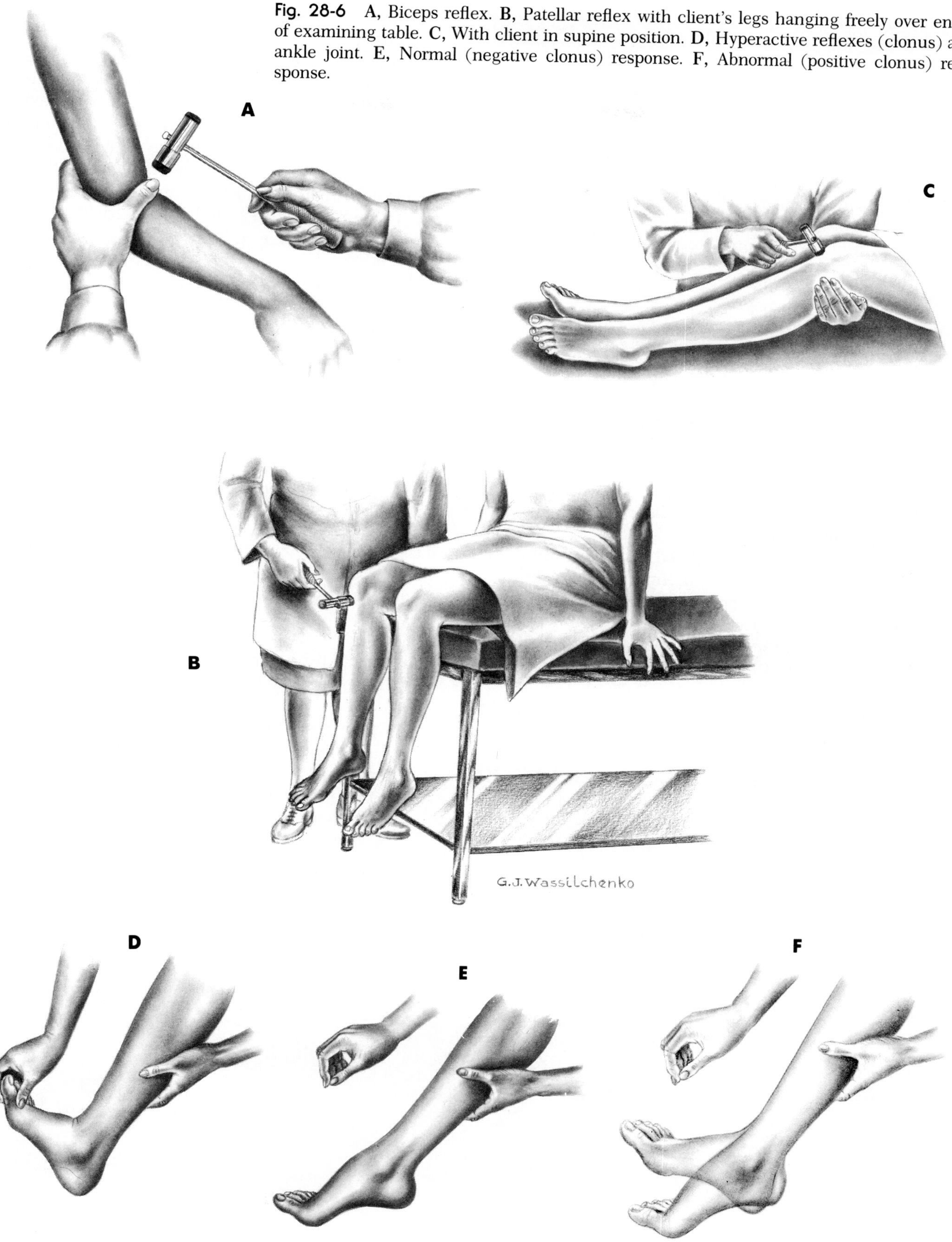

Fig. 28-6 A, Biceps reflex. B, Patellar reflex with client's legs hanging freely over end of examining table. C, With client in supine position. D, Hyperactive reflexes (clonus) at ankle joint. E, Normal (negative clonus) response. F, Abnormal (positive clonus) response.

Warning Signs

Preeclampsia

1. Rapid rise in blood pressure
2. Rapid gain in weight
3. Generalized edema
4. Quantitative increase in proteinuria
5. Epigastric pain
6. Marked hyperreflexia; especially transient or sustained ankle clonus
7. Severe headache
8. Visual disturbances
9. Oliguria with urinary output of < 120 mL in 4 hr
10. Irritability, transient mental changes
11. Nausea and vomiting, severe

Warning signs of preeclampsia are summarized in the box, above.

Eclampsia usually is preceded by various premonitory symptoms and signs, including headache, severe epigastric pain, hyperreflexia, and hemoconcentration. However, convulsions can appear suddenly and without warning in a seemingly stable woman with only minimum blood pressure elevations (Cunningham et al, 1989).

The convulsions that occur in eclampsia manifest a sequence that is frightening to observe (see box, p. 840). Increased hypertension and tonic contraction of all body muscles (e.g., arms flexed, hands clenched, legs inverted) precede the tonic-clonic convulsions (Fig. 28-7). During this stage muscles relax and contract alternately. Respirations are halted and then begin again with long, deep, stertorous inhalation. Hypotension follows, and coma ensues in 2 to 3 minutes to hours. Nystagmus and muscular twitching persist for a time. Disorientation and amnesia cloud the immediate recovery. Oliguria and anuria are notable. The seizure can recur within minutes of the first convulsion, or the woman may never experience another. Eclamptic seizures can result in tissue damage to the mother during the convulsion, especially if the side rails are not padded. During the convulsion, the mother and fetus are not receiving oxygen. Eclamptic seizures produce a marked metabolic insult to both mother and fetus.

Laboratory Tests

The nurse assists in obtaining a number of blood and urine specimens to aid in the diagnosis of preeclampsia, HELLP syndrome, or chronic hypertension. At present no known laboratory tests are available to detect the development of preeclampsia (Gavette, Roberts, 1987). However, baseline laboratory test information (e.g., hematocrit, hemoglobin, platelet count, serum creatinine, and uric acid levels) is useful in early diagnosis of preeclampsia for comparison with results obtained later in pregnancy. Changes in baseline levels help to evaluate progression and severity of disease. Close monitoring for any changes in laboratory test values is important. An initial blood specimen is obtained for the following tests to assess the disease process (e.g., DIC) and its effect on renal and hepatic functioning:

- Complete blood cell count (including a platelet count)
- Clotting studies (including bleeding time, prothrombin time, partial prothrombin time, and fibrinogen)
- Liver enzymes (AST [SGOT], ALT [SGPT])
- Chemistry panel (blood urea nitrogen, creatinine, glucose, uric acid)
- Type and screen, possible cross-match

Urine specimens may be obtained as single ran-

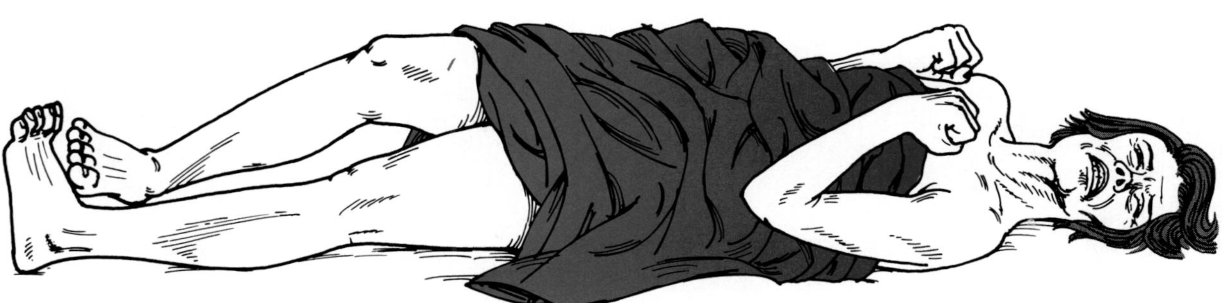

Fig. 28-7 Eclampsia (convulsions or seizures).

dom specimens or used as 24-hour collections for measuring proteinuria. Proteinuria is determined from dipstick testing of a clean-catch or catheter urine specimen. A reading greater than +1 on two or more occasions, at least 4 hours apart, should be followed by a 24-hour urine collection (Gilbert, Harmon, 1992). **Proteinuria** is defined as the excretion of 0.3 g (30 mg/dL) or greater in a 24-hour period. Proteinuria usually is a late sign in the course of preeclampsia (Consensus Report, 1990). Protein readings are designated as follows:

0	
Trace	
+1	30 mg/dL (equivalent to 300 mg/L)
+2	100 mg/dL
+3	300 mg/dL
+4	Over 1000 mg (1 g)/dL

Urine output is assessed for volume of at least 120 mL/4 hr. A 24-hour specimen is collected to measure creatinine and protein clearance.

NURSING DIAGNOSES

Nursing diagnoses are derived by carefully analyzing the assessment findings. Common nursing diagnoses for management of *mild preeclampsia* are as follows:

- Anxiety related to
  - —Preeclampsia and its effect on mother and infant
  - —Knowledge deficit regarding management (diet, bed rest)
- Ineffective individual/family coping related to
  - —Mother's restricted activity and concern over a complicated pregnancy
  - —Mother's inability to work outside the home
- Powerlessness related to
  - —Inability to prevent or control condition and outcomes

Common nursing diagnoses for management of *moderate and severe preeclampsia* are as follows:

- Altered tissue perfusion related to
  - —Preeclampsia or its complications (DIC, pulmonary edema, seizures)
- High risk for injury to fetus related to
  - —Uteroplacental insufficiency
  - —Preterm birth
  - —Abruptio placentae
- High risk for injury to mother related to
  - —CNS irritability secondary to cerebral edema, vasospasm, decreased renal perfusion
  - —Therapy
- Gas exchange impairment related to
  - —Respiratory depression
  - —Pulmonary edema
  - —Convulsion, aspiration of stomach content

PLANNING

Planning care follows medical diagnosis, choice of home or hospital management, and the woman's and family's resources. A plan is developed mutually with the client, if possible, and should be individualized and related specifically to the needs of the client and her family.

Goals/expected outcomes for care of *"mild"* preeclampsia include the following measures.

1. Woman will recognize and immediately report abnormal signs and symptoms to prevent worsening of condition.
2. Woman will adhere to the medical regimen to minimize risk to herself and her fetus.
3. Significant other(s) will become involved and supportive in woman's care and management of the disease to optimize emotional and physical outcomes.
4. Woman will be able to verbalize her fears and concerns to cope with the condition and situation.

Goals/expected outcomes for care of *moderate and severe preeclampsia* include the following measures.

1. Woman and fetus will not suffer adverse sequelae from preeclampsia or its management.
2. Woman will not experience eclampsia and the severity of its complications.
3. Fetus will not experience distress; newborn will be born in optimal condition with no adverse sequelae to maternal condition and its management.
4. Woman will give birth in optimal condition with no sequelae to her condition and its management.
5. The family will be able to cope effectively with the mother's high-risk condition, its management, and outcomes.

IMPLEMENTATION

Nursing actions will be derived from medical management, physician's directives, and nursing diagnosis.

The most effective therapy is *prevention*. Early prenatal care, identification of "at-risk" pregnant women, and recognition and reporting of physical warning signs are essential components for optimizing maternal and perinatal outcomes. The nurse's skills in assessing the client for factors and symptoms of preeclampsia cannot be overestimated.

Nurses can do much in the advocacy role. Measures should be taken to improve public education and access to antenatal care. Counseling, referral to community resources, mobilization of support systems, nutrition counseling, and information about normal adaptation to pregnancy are essential preventive components of care.

Emotional and psychologic support are essential for assisting the woman and her family in coping. The development of preeclampsia causes anxiety in the woman and her family. There is a threat to the well-being of the mother and her unborn child, and the family's expectations about pregnancy and childbirth must be altered. Such disruption in a family constitutes a crisis. The physical nature of the crisis requires the appropriate use of modern technology. The woman and her family's perception of the disease process, the reasons for it, and the care received will affect their compliance with and participation in therapy. The family will need to use coping mechanisms and support systems to help them through the experience. A plan of care for the woman suffering from preeclampsia is superimposed on the nursing care all women need during labor and the birth process.

The nursing care of women with chronic hypertensive disease is the same as that of women with preeclampsia. Preeclampsia superimposed on chronic hypertension is more difficult to manage than preeclampsia alone and carries a grave prognosis for mother and fetus. If and when cardiac involvement is diagnosed, the nursing care of the woman with cardiac disease is superimposed on the original plan. The woman and her family must be aware of the possibility of preterm birth and of the need for careful and continuous supervision during the prenatal, intranatal, and postbirth periods.

The nurse's role as educator is important in informing the woman about her condition and responsibilities in preeclampsia management, whether in the home or hospital.

Home Care for "Mild" Preeclampsia

Interventions for preeclampsia such as bed rest and diet are considered palliative (Consensus Report, 1990). The most effective therapy for preeclampsia is preventing progression of the condition and enabling the pregnancy to continue.

Home care usually supplements the general care needed in pregnancy and includes two to three weekly medical and nursing assessments at the physician's office or high-risk prenatal clinic.

Management at home can be satisfactory if preeclampsia is "mild" and fetal growth retardation is not a problem. A woman with normal Doppler velocimetry findings of the uterine artery can be monitored on an out-of-hospital basis (Farmakides et al, 1990). However, for home care to be effective, the nurse needs to assess the home environment and the client's ability to assume responsibility. In addition, the effects of illness, language, age, culture, beliefs, and support system need to be considered. The woman's support system needs to be mobilized and involved in planning and implementing her care.

Motivation, as well as readiness and ability to learn, are essential considerations for a woman who requires instruction on self-care at home. The woman with preeclampsia that is managed at home needs to be taught about the disease and its effects on the mother and baby in a manner and language she can understand. She needs to learn about the importance of bed rest and nutrition and how to monitor herself and the fetus for abnormal signs and symptoms (see teaching for self-care, below). A knowledge of the subjective and objective symptoms (see box, p. 829) that indicate deterioration of the condition is vital. If these symptoms occur, the woman must call her physician immediately.

Bed rest in the left lateral recumbent position is a standard therapy of preeclampsia and maximizes uteroplacental blood flow during pregnancy. Bed rest has been shown beneficial in decreasing blood pressure and promoting diuresis. Women with mild preeclampsia feel reasonably well; boredom from being restricted is common. Diversional activities, visits from friends, telephone conversations, and creating a pleasant environment are but a few ways in coping with boredom. Gentle exercise (e.g., range of motion, stretching, Kegel, pelvic tilts) is important in maintaining muscle tone, blood flow, regularity of bowel function, and a sense of well being.

Learning relaxation can help to reduce stress associated with the high-risk condition and to prepare the woman for labor and the birth. Progressive relaxation (see Chapter 13) studies also have shown relaxation effective in lowering blood pressures of persons with chronic hypertension as well (see box, p. 829).

The woman can be instructed in how to take her own blood pressure and keep a record of the mea-

TEACHING Learning About Preeclampsia Condition

- The cause of pregnancy-induced hypertension is not known; symptoms are believed to occur from changes in body organ functioning.
- Decreased perfusion to organs can result in symptoms of preeclampsia.
- An increase in blood pressure, edema, weight, and proteinuria indicates disease process is worsening.
- Decreased fetal movement may indicate fetal hypoxia.

TEACHING Signs and Symptoms of Preeclampsia

Notify your physician if any one or more of the following occur:

- You observe an abnormal increase in weight gain that continues even after resting up to 12 hours in bed.
- You notice an increase in edema or swelling of hands, feet, and/or face, for example. Puffy eyes, tight rings on fingers, tight shoes are some ways to tell if edema is increasing.
- You feel stomach pain or have nausea and vomiting or flulike symptoms.
- You have unusual, frequent, and/or severe headaches.
- You have visual changes such as blurred vision.

Telephone number to call:____________________

surements. Women should have formal instruction in using correct, standarized techniques (see procedure, p. 823) for obtaining accurate blood pressure measurements. A study by nurse researchers (Smith et al, 1990) evaluated the accuracy and use of four compact elecronic blood pressure monitors (purchased at a retail store) by hypertensive pregnant women. The electronic devices were found as accurate as mechanical aneroid units and easy to apply and read measurements without need for a stethoscope or another person. This is particularly advantageous for women having their blood pressure monitored on an outpatient basis.

The woman can be taught to check daily for proteinuria and weight. An initial appearance of proteinuria usually indicates progressive severity of preeclampsia. An increase in weight is associated with edema changes (see box, at right).

Because the disease has potential adverse effects on uterine blood flow, the fetus must be regularly evaluated for hypoxia. The woman should be instructed about the importance of keeping appointments for fetal monitoring tests. Explanation of the purpose of the tests and what the woman may experience during the procedures is also necessary. For home management the woman may be instructed in how to do "kick counts," a daily counting of fetal movements felt in 1 hour while resting (see Chapter 27). Fetal activity under three counts per hour is considered serious and needs to be reported. Fetal activity decreases if hypoxia develops.

Diet and fluid recommendations are much the same as for typical pregnant women. A high-protein diet and avoidance of foods high in sodium and additional salt at the table usually are recommended. Ad-

TEACHING Coping with Bed Rest

- In bed, lie on your left side (and alternate to right side as needed). This allows more blood to get to your uterus (womb) and baby.
- Increase your fluid intake to 8 glasses/day, and add roughage (e.g., bran, fruits, leafy vegetables) to your diet to decrease constipation.
- Include diversional activites such as puzzles, reading, and crafts to reduce boredom.
- Do gentle exercises such as circling your hands and feet or gently tensing and relaxing arm and leg muscles. This improves muscle tone, circulation, and sense of well being.
- Encourage family participation in your care.
- Have significant others assist you with care of the house, children, etc.
- Use relaxation to help you cope with stress. Relax your body one muscle at a time or imagine some pleasant scene, word, or image. Soothing music can also help you to relax.

TEACHING Assessing and Reporting Clinical Signs of Preeclampsia

- Report immediately any increase in your blood pressure, protein in urine, weight gain greater than 1 pound/week, or edema.
- Take your blood pressure on the same arm in a sitting position each time for consistent and accurate readings. Support arm on a table in a horizontal position at heart level.
- Use the same scale, wearing the same clothes, at the same time each day, after voiding, before breakfast, for reliable daily weights.
- Dipstick your "clean catch" urine sample for assessing proteinuria; report frequency or burning on voiding.
- Report to your physician if proteinuria is +2 or more or if you have a decrease in urine output.
- Daily assess your baby's activity. Decreased activity (three or fewer movements per hour) may indicate fetal distress.
- It is important to keep your scheduled prenatal appointments so that any changes in your or the baby's condition can be detected immediately.
- Keep a daily log/diary of your assessments for your home health care nurse, or bring it with you to your next prenatal visit.

TEACHING Nutrition

- There is no sodium restriction; however, avoid salty foods (e.g., canned foods, sodas, pretzels, potato chips, pickles, sauerkraut).
- Eat a nutritious, balanced diet. Collaborate with registered dietitian for diet best suited for individual woman (for discussion of nutrition, see Chapter 9).
- Avoid alcohol, smoking.
- Drink 8 to 10 8-ounce glasses of water per day.
- Eat foods with roughage, e.g., whole grains, raw fruits, and vegetables.

ditional protein in the diet can help to replace protein lost in the urine, as well as increase plasma colloid osmotic pressure. Pregnant women with hypertension have less plasma volume than do normotensive women; thus sodium restriction is not recommended. Women need salt for maintenance of blood volume and placental perfusion. The exception may be the woman with chronic hypertension successfully treated with low-salt diet before the pregnancy. Adequate fluid intake helps to maintain optimal fluid volume and aids in renal perfusion and filtration.

The nurse uses assessment data about the woman's diet and counsels her in areas of deficiency if needed (see box, above). Although preliminary studies show that dietary calcium supplementation decreases blood pressure, not enough data are available to recommend its use for treating hypertension (Consensus Report, 1990). The use of alcohol, smoking, and other drugs is strongly discouraged because of their harmful effects on the mother and fetus.

During the period of instruction for the woman and her family, time must be allowed for assimilation of information, questions, and concerns. A client's understanding usually is directly associated with compliance to a prescribed treatment program. Methods for enhancing learning can include visual aids, videotapes, handouts, and demonstration-return-demonstration. A case study (p. 831) and nursing plan of care (p. 832) provide guides for home management of preeclampsia.

Hospital Care for Severe Preeclampsia

If the woman's condition becomes increasingly severe, hospitalization is recommended (see Case Study, p. 834, and Care Plan, p. 835).

Severe preeclampsia is diagnosed when one or more of the following are present (Weinstein, 1986):

1. Blood pressure of at least 160 mm Hg systolic or 110 mm Hg (MAP 127 or more) diastolic on two readings 6 hours apart
2. Proteinuria of ≥5 g/24 hr
3. Oliguria ≤30 mL/hr
4. Cerebral or visual disturbances
5. Brisk (3+ or 4+) DTRS
6. Pulmonary edema or cyanosis
7. Epigastric pain

The woman also may be hospitalized for lesser degrees of hypertension but with any of the following: (1) proteinuria of 1+ or more, (2) increasing edema, (3) persistent or severe headache, (4) nausea and vomiting, (5) epigastric pain, and (6) abnormal umbilical and uterine artery Doppler velocimetry findings. In the presence of these findings, the following tests are performed: NST, biophysical profile, liver enzymes, coagulation factors, and kidney function (Farmakides et al, 1990).

Severe preeclampsia represents an obstetric emergency. Immediate and continuous care by the obstetric team is mandatory to prevent maternal and fetal morbidity or mortality. (See box, above, for hospital precautionary measures.)

The woman is admitted to either the birthing suite or to a private room on the antepartum or postpartum unit. The room must be close to staff and emergency drugs, supplies, and equipment. Noise and external stimuli must be minimized. **Seizure precautions** are taken (see box above).

Hospital Precautionary Measures

Environment
- Quiet
- Nonstimulating
- Lighting subdued

Seizure precautions
- Padded side rails
- Suction equipment tested and ready to use
- Oxygen administration equipment tested and ready to use

Call button within easy reach

Emergency medication tray immediately accessible
- Hydralazine and magnesium sulfate in or adjacent to woman's room
- Calcium gluconate immediately available in a well-labeled syringe

Emergency delivery pack accessible

CASE STUDY

Preeclampsia: Home Care

Olga is a 38-year-old gravida 3, para 0-1-1-0, at 32 weeks' gestation. She noticed feeling "puffy" and found it difficult to get into her shoes.

ASSESSMENT

During her prenatal visit, nursing assessment reveals +2 pedal edema, BP 140/90 (MAP = 107), +2 DTRs, Ø clonus, and +1 proteinuria. Olga is very concerned about her condition and that of her baby. She expresses concern about constipation and anticipates becoming very bored.

NURSING DIAGNOSIS

Assessment findings support the medical diagnosis of "mild" preeclampsia. Olga, who is responsible and highly motivated, meets the criteria for self-care at home. The nurse identifies the nursing diagnosis: High risk for injury, mother and fetus, related to worsening of preeclampsia condition.

PLANNING

A plan of care is developed with Olga's input. The nurse and Olga mutually agree on the *goal:* Olga will be able to monitor and assess herself and her fetus and immediately report any changes to her physician. The nurse sets the *expected outcomes:* Olga's self-care skill will prevent worsening of preeclampsia and ensure improvement in her condition. Through this activity she may reduce her concern about her condition and that of the baby.

IMPLEMENTATION

Nursing actions are derived from medical management of preeclampsia, physician's orders, and nursing diagnoses. Specific interventions include discussion and teaching of preeclampsia warning signs and symptoms, recording (in diary/log) of findings, measurement of blood pressure, assessment of fetal activity, testing for proteinuria, and assessment of edema and daily weight. The nurse suggests that Olga make a list of telephone numbers to call in case of emergency and post it by the telephone; provides a demonstration and observes a return demonstration; and furnishes written instructions, with illustrations in the client's language and at her level of understanding, to reinforce learning.

EVALUATION

A follow-up prenatal visit revealed that Olga brought with her a daily diary/log of her assessment findings and other significant events, could accurately verbalize signs and symptoms of preeclampsia, and demonstrate proper techniques in assessing blood pressure, fetal activity, and urine testing for protein. Fetal activity remained greater than three movements per hour, BP 130/76, bed rest was interrupted to void large amounts of urine (absence of protein), and weight decreased by 4 pounds.

CARE PLAN Preeclampsia: Home Care

GOALS	IMPLEMENTATION	RATIONALE	EVALUATION
Nursing diagnosis: High risk for injury, mother and fetus, related to not identifying a worsening of the preeclamptic condition			
Olga will be able to monitor and assess herself and her fetus and immediately report any changes to her physician.	Discuss warning signs/symptoms, and instruct Olga to notify physician immediately of any changes.	Knowledge enables Olga to become a partner in her own care; knowledge provides the basis for decision making.	Olga correctly verbalized signs/symptoms of worsening preeclampsia; written diary/log demonstrated understanding.
	Instruct Olga how to assess and record BP, fetal activity, urine for protein, edema, and daily weight; observe return demonstration.	Observing and practicing new skills increases self-confidence and provides reassurance.	Olga correctly demonstrates assessment and recording BP, fetal activity, urine testing, edema, and daily weight. Olga recorded: BP 130/76, fetal activity ≥3/hr, voiding large amounts of urine negative for protein, weight loss of 4 lb.
Nursing diagnosis: Constipation related to decreased physical activity and motility and iron supplementation			
Olga will experience bowel regularity.	Counsel concerning diet high in fiber and fluid intake (8-10 8-oz glasses) and setting a routine time for bowel movements.	A side effect of iron supplementation is constipation; roughage/fluids and regularity stimulate bowel movement.	Olga reports regular daily bowel movements without discomfort.
	Instruct/demonstrate how to do gentle exercise; observe return demonstration.	Exercise facilitates bowel regularity.	Olga reports that her friend exercises with her every morning and her husband every evening.
	Explain reasons for tendency toward constipation during pregnancy.	Hormones relax smooth muscles of bowel; decrease stomach-emptying time and bowel motility.	Olga states she understands reasons.

CARE PLAN **Preeclampsia: Home Care—cont'd**

GOALS	IMPLEMENTATION	RATIONALE	EVALUATION
Nursing diagnosis: Diversional activity deficit related to imposed bed rest			
Olga will report minimal or no boredom.	Refer to home health care nurse.	Home visit provides information regarding setting potential.	Home health nurse visit is scheduled.
	Give Olga telephone numbers of other women on bed rest and suggest she network with them.	Provides mutual support through ventilation of feelings, ideas for activity, socializing.	Olga states she looks forward to talking with others who are "in the same boat."
	Explore Olga's interests: quilt making, other handwork, crafts, reading, TV, videotapes, visits with family/friends.	Enables Olga to look at alternatives and make decisions that will best meet her needs.	Olga begins to make telephone calls as soon as she gets home.
	Discuss home management and mobilization of help from significant others and community resources.	Enables Olga to start thinking about and problem solving regarding home management.	Olga reports that her mother had offered to come whenever needed; states she has many friends.
	Teach/demonstrate/ask for return demonstration of relaxation techniques.	Provides another means of coping; empowers her in self-care.	At next visit Olga states she is not bored. Friends/husband relax with her; have set up visiting/helping schedules.

The extensiveness of health assessment on admission is governed by the severity of the woman's condition. Weight is taken on admittance and every day thereafter. An indwelling urinary catheter facilitates monitoring of renal function and effectiveness of therapy. If appropriate, vaginal examination reveals the state of the cervix. Abdominal palpation establishes uterine tonicity and fetal size, activity, and position. Electronic monitoring of the mother and fetus is initiated to determine fetal status. The nurse's skill in implementing the techniques described can be reassuring to the woman and her family.

Commonly, bed rest is ordered. The nurse's ingenuity may be called on to help the woman cope physically and psychologically with the side effects of immobility and an environment limited in stimuli and support. Thromboembolic events, which are a risk factor during normal pregnancy, pose an even greater risk with preeclampsia.

CONTROL OF BLOOD PRESSURE. The diastolic blood pressure should not be permitted to consistently exceed 100 mm Hg (Iams et al, 1990). If this occurs, IV hydralazine in 2.5 to 5 mg IV-bolus doses is given. If additional hydralazine is needed after two doses, it is administered by a constant infusion pump in which 100 mg of hydralazine (**antihypertensive agent**) (Table 28-3) is instilled into a plastic bag containing 200 mL of saline. Infusion rate is dictated by the blood pressure level and should be monitored by a pulse Doppler blood pressure cuff. If the woman is obese, a thigh blood pressure cuff is used.

The *standard of care in the United States* is the use of magnesium sulfate to control convulsions and the use of hydralazine (Apresoline, Neopresol) to control or reduce blood pressure.

Other drugs also can be used in pregnancy hypertension. These include methyldopa (Aldomet) and propranolol (Inderal). Diuretic agents are not used because they may adversely affect the fetus (see p. 836). No evidence exists that either diuretics or antihypertensive agents prevent the development of preeclampsia.

CASE STUDY

Preeclampsia: Hospital Care

Cheri Batson is a 23-year-old woman at 35 weeks' gestation with her first child. Up to this time, her pregnancy was uneventful. Since her last prenatal visit, 2 weeks ago, she gained "a lot of weight". She complains about feeling "funny" and that her rings no longer fit.

ASSESSMENT

The interview reveals that she has not been eating well because she feels nauseated and has had a dull headache for 2 days. Findings of physical examination include BP 150/98 (MAP = 115); DTRs 3+; Ø clonus; digital and facial edema; weight gain, 3 kg (6.6 lb). Urinalysis revealed proteinuria +2. Cheri was admitted to the hospital, and IV $MgSO_4$ was started.

NURSING DIAGNOSIS

Because assessment findings support the medical diagnosis of preeclampsia, the nurse identifies the nursing diagnosis: High risk for injury to mother and fetus related to CNS irritability.

PLANNING

A plan of care is developed with Cheri and her husband. The couple stated they *supported the goal* to manage her condition for the best possible outcome for her and the baby. The *expected outcome* set by the nurse is to decrease CNS irritability.

IMPLEMENTATION

Nursing actions are derived from current concepts of preeclampsia and its management. Specific interventions include establishing a baseline data base (e.g., DTRs, clonus, FHR); monitoring IV $MgSO_4$ infusion and laboratory-derived $MgSO_4$ serum levels; assessment for $MgSO_4$ toxicity; maintaining a quiet, dark environment; implementing seizure precautions.

EVALUATION

The couple state they feel relieved that the therapy was successful in controlling her condition. Cheri states she feels "much better" and has no headache. Seizures did not occur; DTRs, 2+; 0 clonus; and fetus remains stable.

CARE PLAN Preeclampsia: Hospital Care

GOALS	IMPLEMENTATION	RATIONALE	EVALUATION
Nursing diagnosis: High risk for injury to mother and fetus related to CNS irritability			
Cheri will experience decreased CNS irritability to normal levels.	Establish baseline data (e.g., DTRs, clonus).	Baseline needed to monitor effect of therapy.	Cheri's DTRs were at 2+ with no clonus.
	Monitor IV $MgSO_4$ and serum levels of $MgSO_4$.	$MgSO_4$ is an anticonvulsant that acts on the myoneural junction.	Cheri's $MgSO_4$ serum levels remained within normal range.
	Assess for $MgSO_4$ toxicity.	An overdose can decrease muscle activity, resulting in severe respiratory depression.	No $MgSO_4$ toxicity was noted.
Cheri will not convulse.	Maintain a quiet, nonstimulating, dark environment.	Strong stimuli such as bright light and loud noises can precipitate a seizure (convulsion).	Cheri experienced no seizure activity.
Nursing diagnosis: Altered tissue perfusion related to preeclampsia secondary to arteriole vasospasm			
Cheri will experience vasodilation as evidenced by diuresis and decreased edema and weight loss.	Monitor oral intake and IV $MgSO_4$ infusion. Monitor urinary output. Monitor visible edema and daily weight loss. Maintain on complete bed rest in side-lying position.	$MgSO_4$, acting on the myoneural junction, relaxes the vasospasm. This relaxation often results in increased perfusion of the kidneys, mobilization of extravascular fluid (edema), and diuresis. Bed rest maximized uteroplacental blood flow, which often reduces BP and promotes diuresis.	Cheri's periobital tissues, fingers, sacral edema is decreasing; she diureses. Cheri experiences a weight loss.
Nursing diagnosis: Fear related to threat of injury to Cheri and couple's unborn baby			
The couple will state a decrease in fear.	Keep couple informed about the management of Cheri's condition, as well as baby's status (e.g., FHR). Remain close by, listen to their fears, clarify information.	Knowledge reduces the fear of the unknown.	Couple state they do not feel as alone and different as they did before.
	Involve them in decisions about their care (e.g., comfort measures preferred, selection of oral fluid [if allowed], mouth care)	Validation that one's feelings are legitimate increases one's ability to cope and relieves stress.	Couple expresses relief that they can do something for themselves, that they have a say in matters—they don't feel so helpless.

TABLE 28-3 Pharmacologic Control of Hypertension* and Its Sequelae in Pregnancy and Labor

Medication	Target Tissue	Effects of Medication: Maternal	Effects of Medication: Fetal/Neonatal	Nursing Actions
ANTIHYPERTENSIVE*				
Hydralazine (Apresoline, Neopresol) (arteriolar vasodilators) 50-200 mg (0) per day	Peripheral arterioles: decreases muscle tone, thereby decreasing peripheral resistance Hypothalamus and medullary vasomotor center; minor decrease in sympathetic tone	Headache Flushing Palpitation Tachycardia Some decrease in uteroplacental blood flow	Minimum effects; some decrease in Po_2	Assess for effects of medications Alert mother (family) to expected effects of medications Assess BP (precipitous drop can lead to shock and perhaps to abruptio placentae) and urinary output Maintain bed rest with side rails for safety
Methyldopa (Aldomet) (used if maintenance therapy is needed): 250-500 mg orally q8h (α_2-receptor agonist)	Postganglionic nerve endings: interferes with chemical neurotransmission to reduce peripheral vascular resistance CNS: sedation	Sleepiness Postural hypotension Constipation Rare: drug-induced fever in 1% of women and positive Coombs' test in 20%	After 4 mo of maternal therapy, positive Coombs' test in infant	See Hydralazine
DIURETICS†				
Thiazides	Arteriolar smooth muscles: reduces responsiveness to catecholamines	Ineffective in preventing preeclampsia Further reduces already-present decreased plasma volume of preeclampsia Complications Fluid and electrolyte imbalance Pancreatitis Decrease in carbohydrate tolerance Hyperuricemia	Hyponatremia Thrombocytopenia	Arrange to have blood drawn to measure levels of Na, Cl, H_2O, K, and H+ to prevent hyponatremia, hypokalemia, hypochloremia, metabolic acidosis
Furosemide (Lasix): 40 mg IV	Loop of Henle	Relieves pulmonary edema Excessive use results in hypokalemia and hyponatremia	No abnormalities noted	See Thiazides

Continued.

*By midpregnancy, diastolic and systolic blood pressure normally falls by 10 to 15 mm Hg. If diastolic blood pressure is 75 mm Hg or more in second trimester and 85 mm Hg or more in third trimester, statistical increase in fetal mortality occurs.

NOTE: For obese woman, use thigh cuff or ultrasound to obtain accurate readings.

†For control of chronic hypertension, pulmonary edema, renal oliguria, acute renal failure, chronic nephrotic syndrome. If used, physician must be ready to justify action.

‡May not be appropriate for woman with severe preeclampsia or eclampsia. Use of plasma expanders and osmotic diuretics is highly controversial; they may compromise cardiac functioning.

TABLE 28-3 Pharmacologic Control of Hypertension and Its Sequalae in Pregnancy and Labor—cont'd

Medication	Target Tissue	Effects of Medication: Maternal	Effects of Medication: Fetal/Neonatal	Nursing Actions
Ethacrynic acid (Edecrin)	Similar to furosemide	Similar to furosemide	Deafness	See Thiazides
Mannitol (for impending renal failure, oliguria, DIC): 12.5-25 mg IV	Osmotic diuretic: pulls fluid into vascular bed (therefore not recommended for persons with congestive heart failure)	Increases renal plasma flow and urinary output Flushes out kidneys Reduces swelling in ischemic cells in kidney and myocardium	No known effect	See Thiazides
BLOOD VOLUME EXPANDERS				
Salt-poor, serum albumin‡	Intravascular volume	Increases blood volume		

PREVENTION OF ECLAMPSIA

MAGNESIUM SULFATE. One of the important goals of care for the woman with severe preeclampsia is preventing or controlling convulsions. **Magnesium sulfate ($MgSO_4$)**, an anticonvulsant and smooth muscle relaxant, is given to prevent convulsions. It is not a hypotensive drug. Benefits include an increase in uterine blood flow to protect the fetus and an increase in prostacyclins to prevent uterine vasoconstriction (Iams et al, 1990).

Magnesium sulfate usually is given intravenously but may be given intramuscularly. Various dosage schedules are used. For example, an initial loading dose of 4 g of magnesium sulfate in 250 mL of 5% dextrose in water may be given (infused slowly at a rate of 5 mL/30 sec). A maintenance dose follows in which magnesium sulfate is diluted in an IV solution per physician's order (e.g., 20 g $MgSO_4$ in 1000 mL of 5% dextrose in water) and administered (using an infusion pump) at a rate of 1 to 4 g/hr. The maintenance dose is administered via piggyback into the IV mainline. When magnesium sulfate is given intravenously, the effect is immediate. A therapeutic serum level (4 to 8 mg/dL) usually is maintained by a constant infusion of 2 gm/hr (Sibai, 1990b,c).

Intramuscular (IM) magnesium sulfate rarely is used because absorption rate cannot be controlled, injections are painful, and tissue necrosis can occur. The IM dose is 4 to 5 g given in each buttock (1% procaine may be ordered added to the solution to reduce injection pain) and can be followed at 4-hour intervals with IM doses of 4 to 5 g. When magnesium sulfate is given intramuscularly, levels are adequate during the first 1 to 2 hours of administration but inadequate for the next 3 to 4 hours (Sibai, 1988).

Magnesium sulfate interferes with neuromuscular impulse transmission, resulting in muscle relaxation. It reduces blood pressure by splanchnic vasodilation; therefore severe hypotension can occur. The woman's blood pressure should be monitored continuously while the drug is being administered intravenously and every 15 minutes at other times.

It is important to monitor intake and output levels carefully to avoid fluid overload from IV infusion and magnesium sulfate toxicity.

Magnesium sulfate increases sodium retention and is excreted by the kidneys. Magnesium toxicity can develop very quickly and easily in women with kidney involvement. Hourly urinary output must be measured when magnesium sulfate is administered intravenously. *The woman's urinary output must total at least 120 mL every 4 hours.* If output is less, the physician should be notified. If adequate output is not maintained, the dose should not be repeated.

A retention catheter is inserted if accurate hourly determination of urinary output is warranted. Hourly measurement is necessary when the woman is receiving a medication such as magnesium sulfate or when decreasing urinary output occurs or is suspected.

Diuresis within 24 to 48 hours is an excellent prognostic sign. It is considered evidence that perfusion of the kidney is improved as a result of relaxation of arteriolar spasm. With improved perfusion, fluid moves from interstitial spaces to the intravascular bed, and edema is reduced. Diuresis results in weight loss. In the presence of a large urinary output, the dosage of magnesium sulfate may need to be increased to 3 g/hr IV. If the volume of urine is under 100 mL/4 hr, the dosage of magnesium sulfate is reduced. The physician is notified.

Other nursing measures include having the woman lie in a left-sided position to encourage kidney perfusion and to assess the woman for affect, hydration, and other preeclamptic signs and symptoms. The nurse should notify the physician if expressions of apprehension, restlessness, and/or excitability are observed. This may indicate that the woman is unresponsive to medication.

Because *magnesium sulfate is a tocolytic agent,* its use increases the duration of labor. The nurse must be aware that if the laboring woman is receiving magnesium sulfate, the amount of oxytocin needed to stimulate labor is higher.

Early symptoms of toxicity includes nausea, a feeling of warmth, flushing, muscle weakness, and slurred speech. *Maternal toxicity has been reached when reflex activity is absent.* The drug should be discontinued immediately (Sibai, 1990b). It is imperative that patellar and brachial reflexes (Table 28-2 and Fig. 28-6) are assessed every hour if the woman is receiving a continuous IV infusion of magnesium sulfate. Reflexes are assessed before and after each IM injection of magnesium sulfate.

Adverse effects of magnesium sulfate also include respiratory paralysis. *Maternal toxicity has been reached when respirations are fewer than 12/min,* at which time the drug is withheld. The woman receiving magnesium sulfate therapy *should never be left unattended* because magnesium sulfate toxicity with respiratory arrest may occur.

The following responses to elevated serum levels of magnesium can occur:

- 4-8 mg/dL: *Therapeutic level*
- 10-12 mg/dL: Reflexes disappear
- 15-17 mg/dL: Respirations slow (below 12/min), or respiratory arrest
- 30-35 mg/dL: Cardiac arrest is possible; total paralysis

Serum levels are obtained every 4 to 6 hours and as needed.

Magnesium sulfate does not seem to affect fetal heart rate variability in a healthy term fetus and rarely is toxic in the healthy term newborn whose weight is within normal range for gestational age. However, toxic levels in the fetus can cause marked slowing of respirations and hyporeflexia after birth (Sibai, 1988). Neonatal hypermagnesemia is easily treated with calcium and exchange transfusion with citrated blood.

> **Emergency**
>
> ### Magnesium Sulfate Toxicity
>
> **SIGNS/SYMPTOMS**
>
> Respirations <12/min
> Hyporeflexia, absence of reflexes
> Urinary output <30 mL/hr
> Toxic serum levels >8 mg/dL
> Signs of fetal distress (e.g., sudden drop in FHR)
> Significant drop in maternal pulse or blood pressure
>
> **INTERVENTION**
>
> Discontinue $MgSO_4$ immediately, and change to maintenance solution.
> Call for assistance and notify physician for immediate care.
> Administer calcium gluconate or calcium chloride as ordered (e.g., 1 g for IV injection *given over 3-min period*).
> Provide frequent to continuous monitoring of DTRs, respiration rate, urine output.
> Monitor $MgSO_4$ level.

The results of a recent study (Holcomb et al, 1991) support a causal relationship between prolonged IV magnesium sulfate use and abnormal fetal bone mineralization. These radiographic bone abnormalities were absent in unexposed neonates.

Warning signs and interventions for both fetus and mother that are associated with magnesium sulfate toxicity are summarized in the emergency box above.

Antidote. The antidote for magnesium sulfate toxicity is a calcium salt such as **calcium gluconate** or *calcium chloride.* A 10-mL vial of the antidote (10% calcium gluconate, or neostigmine, pentylenetetrazol [Medrazol]) should be kept at the bedside. If needed, it is administered over 3 minutes intravenously and repeated every hour until the respiratory, urinary, and neurologic depression has been alleviated. *The maximum number of injections of a calcium salt is eight injections in a 24-hour period.*

If improvement occurs, therapy is continued until labor begins spontaneously. If the fetal age is greater than 38 weeks with a lecithin/sphingomyelin (L/S) ratio of 2:1, the presence of prostaglandin, and other indications of fetal maturity, labor may be induced (see Chapters 7 and 35). If improvement does not occur or the fetus shows signs of stress, the care for severe preeclampsia and eclampsia is initiated.

DIAZEPAM (VALIUM). One of the uses of diazepam (Valium) is its anticonvulsant effect. Its target tissues are the thalamus and hypothalamus where it has a depressant effect. It is effective in the initial management of eclamptic convulsions. Rapid IV administration may lead to apnea or cardiac arrest. There are fetal/neonatal effects as well. The presence of diazepam in the mother flattens the FHR baseline (loss of beat-to-beat variability), an important criterion in assessing fetal oxygenation. High levels in the newborn depress sucking ability, cause hypotonia, and can result in temperature instability (i.e., decreased temperature). The newborn's respiratory rate may be decreased. Nursing actions involve careful monitoring of maternal vital signs and DTRs.

BARBITURATES. Rapid-acting barbiturates such as phenobarbital sodium (0.2 to 0.3 mg IV) or amobarbital sodium (0.25 to 0.5 g IV) are the most common drugs used. Barbiturates have a CNS depressant effect; therefore they may be an adjunct in the control of seizures. Barbiturates also have a depressant effect on the fetus. Nursing actions are the same as those for diazepam.

IMMEDIATE CARE OF ECLAMPSIA. The immediate **care during a convulsion** is to ensure a patent airway. Once this has been attained, adequate oxygenation must be provided. If convulsions occur, the woman is turned onto her left side to prevent aspiration of vomitus and supine hypotension syndrome. After the convulsion ceases, food and fluid are suctioned from the glottis or trachea. $MgSO_4$ (and amobarbital sodium for recurrent convulsions) are given as ordered (Anderson, 1987). If an IV infusion is not in place, it is begun with a large-bore needle. Oxygen is administered by means of face mask or tent after convulsion ceases (masks and nasal catheters cause excessive stimulation), and suctioning is done. Oxygen rate may be up to 10 L/min (as opposed to 3 L/min advocated for continuous oxygen in chronic conditions). Time, duration, and description of convulsions are recorded, and any urinary or fecal incontinence is noted. The fetus is monitored for adverse effects. A transient bradycardia and decreased fetal heart rate variability may be present.

The woman's blood is typed and cross-matched. Blood is kept available for emergency transfusion; premature separation of the placenta, hemorrhage, and shock often occur in women with eclampsia.

Fluids are given as directed; the time, the amount, and the woman's response are noted. Determination of central venous pressure (CVP) or pulmonary arterial wedge pressure (PAWP) (Swan-Ganz catheter) may be required for accurate fluid monitoring in the presence of pulmonary edema or acute renal failure. Hospital protocols vary. Nothing by mouth (NPO) is permitted if the woman is convulsing or has symptoms of severe preeclampsia. An indwelling catheter is required for accurate measurement of urinary output. Blood sugar is evaluated by bedside fingerstick or venous draw every 1 to 8 hours as ordered. Glucose solutions are administered as ordered. To correct hypovolemia, crystalloids (0.9% saline or Ringer's lactated solution) are infused intravenously at a rate that maintains a urine output of at least 30 mL/hr, and the maternal response is recorded.

Medications (e.g., magnesium sulfate) are given as directed. The woman's response is monitored and recorded and all drugs, dosages, and times noted.

A rapid assessment of uterine activity, cervical status, and fetal status is performed. During the convulsion, membranes may have ruptured, the cervix may have dilated, and the birth may be imminent. If it is not, once the woman's seizure tendency and blood pressure are controlled, a decision should be made as to whether the birth should take place. The more serious the condition of the woman, the greater the need to proceed to the birth, which is the definitive cure for the disease. All medications and therapy are merely temporary measures (Iams et al, 1990). If fetal lungs are not mature and the birth can be delayed for 48 hours, steroids such as betamethasone (see Chapter 35) may be given. Induction of labor and vaginal or cesarean birth may be implemented, depending on the mother's and fetus' conditions.

Laboratory tests are ordered to assess for the HELLP syndrome (p. 820) and to have blood typed and cross-matched for packed cells. Other tests include determination of electrolytes, liver function battery, and complete hemogram and clotting profile, including platelets and fibrin split products (to assess for DIC).

The woman may have been incontinent of urine and stool or the membranes may have ruptured during the convulsion; she will need assistance with hygiene and a change of gown. Oral care with a soft toothbrush may be of comfort to her.

The physician or nurse explains procedures briefly and quietly. The *woman is never left alone* if the condition is severe or if she is receiving magnesium sulfate therapy. The family also is kept informed of management, rationale, and the woman's progress. Signs and symptoms are summarized in the emergency box on p. 840.

BIRTH. Preeclampsia, eclampsia, and severe hypertensive or renal disease are intensified by the continuation of pregnancy. Termination of gestation is the only practical treatment. The fetus may therefore be premature or otherwise compromised. Eclampsia

Emergency Procedure

Eclampsia (Fig. 28-7)

TONIC-CLONIC CONVULSION SIGNS

Stage of invasion: 2-3 sec; eyes fixed; twitching of facial muscles.

Stage of contraction: 15-20 sec; eyes protrude and are bloodshot; all body muscles in tonic contraction.

Stage of convulsion: Muscles relax and contract alternatively (clonic). Respirations are halted and then begin again with long, deep, stertorous inhalation. Coma ensues.

INTERVENTION

Keep airway patent, turn head to one side; place pillow under one shoulder or back, if possible.
Call for assistance.
Protect with side rails up and padded.
Observe and record convulsion activity.

AFTER CONVULSION/SEIZURE

Observe for postconvulsion coma, incontinence.
Use suction as needed.
Administer oxygen via face mask at 10 L/min.
Start IV fluids and monitor for potential fluid overload.
Give $MgSO_4$ or anticonvulsant drug as ordered.
Insert indwelling catheter.
Monitor blood pressure.
Monitor fetal and uterine status.
Expedite laboratory work as ordered to monitor kidney function, liver function, coagulation system, and drug levels.
Provide hygiene and a quiet environment.
Support and keep client and family informed.
Be prepared for birth when mother is stable.

is controlled before induction of labor is attempted inasmuch as uterine activity and sensitivity to oxytocin are increased (p. 819); then vaginal, local anesthesia or pudendal block can be administered. If labor cannot be readily induced, cesarean delivery should be performed. Abruptio placentae is associated with 20% of women with preeclampsia. Pediatric staff members should be on standby in case the newborn needs resuscitation.

EVALUATION

Evaluation is a continuous process. To be effective, it needs to be based on measurable criteria that reflect the goals of nursing care. Thus for "mild" preeclampsia, the woman will do the following:

- Recognize and immediately report abnormal signs and symptoms
- Adhere to the medical regimen
- Involve significant other(s) in her care and management of the disease
- Verbalize her fears and concerns

Outcome criteria for moderate and severe preeclampsia include the following:

- The woman and fetus will not suffer adverse sequelae from preeclampsia or its management.
- The woman will not experience eclampsia and the severity of its complications.
- The fetus will not experience distress.
- The newborn will be born in optimal condition with no adverse sequelae resulting from the maternal condition and its management.
- The woman will give birth in optimal condition with no sequelae to her condition and its management.
- The family will be able to cope effectively with the mother's high-risk condition, its management, and outcomes.

If the woman's condition does not improve, the nurse assists in care for elective birth—that is, induction of labor or cesarean birth—and the woman and family are made aware of the need for care, cause of symptoms, and prognosis. Informed consent forms are completed. If the outcome for the mother or baby is unfavorable, the family is assisted to cope with loss and grief (see Chapter 40).

■ POSTPARTUM NURSING CARE

The nursing care of the woman with hypertensive disease differs from that required in a normal postpartum period in a number of respects. The following variations in the nursing process are emphasized.

Careful ***assessment*** of the woman with a hypertensive disorder continues throughout the postpartum period. Blood pressure is measured every 4 hours for 48 hours or more frequently as the woman's condition warrants. *Even if no convulsions occurred before the birth, they may occur within this period.* Magnesium sulfate infusion may continue 12 to 48 hours after the birth. The same assessments continue until the drug is discontinued. The woman also may have a boggy uterus and a large lochia flow as a result of the magnesium sulfate therapy. This needs to be closely monitored. Diuresis should occur within 72 hours after birth.

The woman is asked to report such symptoms as headaches and blurred vision. The nurse assesses affect, alertness, or dullness. Blood pressure is reassessed before an analgesic is given for headache. NOTE: No ergot products (e.g., ergotrate, methergine) are given because they increase blood pressure.

The woman's and family's responses to labor are monitored. Regular postpartum assessment is performed.

Examples of postpartum ***nursing diagnoses*** for women with hypertensive conditions might include the following:

- Situational low self-esteem related to
  - —Inability to accept high-risk nature of the birth
- High risk for anxiety of mother related to
  - —Initial occurrence of hypertension during puerperium
- High risk for altered family processes related to
  - —Stress during high-risk postpartum period
  - —Separation from newborn if in newborn intensive care unit

Examples of mutually agreed upon ***planning*** *goals* for postpartum management of the hypertensive condition for the best possible outcome are as follows:

- The woman understands her condition and its management.
- The woman states she accepts what has happened.
- No convulsion occurs.

Implementation of postpartum care for the woman with hypertensive disease includes care related to normal involution. The woman may need to continue with medication if her diastolic blood pressure exceeds 100 mm Hg at the time of discharge. In addition, the woman and her family need opportunities to discuss their emotional response to complications. The nurse also provides information concerning the prognosis. Preeclampsia and eclampsia do not necessarily recur in subsequent pregnancies, but careful prenatal care is essential (recurrence rate is about 30%).

The nurse reaffirms the physician's advice that evaluation must be thorough during the postpartum examination to rule out chronic hypertension. The woman may need family planning for spacing of the next pregnancy and interconceptional contraceptive choices.

The expected outcomes/goals of care, set by the nurse, is ***evaluated*** as effective if the following are noted: the woman's recovery from preeclampsia is complete *or* the woman begins therapy for chronic hypertension not related to pregnancy; her self-concept is not impaired; and the infant is healthy *or* has minimum impairment. The evaluation is recorded on the woman's record so that care remains consistent after discharge.

■ SUMMARY

Hypertensive states during pregnancy constitute a physiologic risk for the woman and her fetus/newborn. This complication also imposes a psychologic risk for the woman and her family. Client teaching is central to the prevention of PIH and home care of "mild" preeclampsia. Technical skill is important in the care of women with severe preeclampsia. Knowledge of the use of magnesium sulfate as an anticonvulsant is essential. The seriousness and the unique problems posed by the HELLP syndrome challenge the nurse's assessment and care skills. Appropriate management depends on accurate differentiation of the various hypertensive states in pregnancy.

REFERENCES

Anderson GD: A systematic approach to eclamptic convulsion, *Contemp OB/GYN* 29:65, March 1987.

Benedetti TJ, Kates R, Williams V: Hemodynamic observations in severe preeclampsia complicated by pulmonary edema, *Am J Obstet Gynecol* 152:330, 1985.

Benigni A et al: Effect of low-dose aspirin on fetal and maternal generation of thromboxane by platelets in women at risk for pregnancy-induced hypertension, *N Engl J Med* 321:357, 1989.

Cherry SH, Merkatz IR: *Complications of pregnancy: medical, surgical, gynecologic, psychosocial, and perinatal,* ed 4, Baltimore, 1991, Williams & Wilkins.

Chesley LC, Sibai BM: Clinical significance of elevated mean arterial pressure in the second trimester, *Am J Obstet Gynecol* 159:275, 1988.

Consensus Report: Working Group on High Blood Pressure in Pregnancy: National high blood pressure education program working group report on high blood pressure in pregnancy, *Am J Obstet Gynecol* 163:1691, 1990.

Creasy RK, Resnik R: *Maternal-fetal medicine: principles and practice,* ed 2, Philadelphia, 1989, WB Saunders Co.

Cundiff JL, Haubrich KL, Hinzman NG: Umbilical artery Doppler flow studies during pregnancy, *JOGNN* 19:475, 1990.

Cunningham FG, MacDonald PC, Gant NF: *Williams obstetrics,* ed 18, Norwalk, Conn, 1989, Appleton & Lange.

Egley CC, Gutliph J, Bowes WA: Severe hypoglycemia associated with HELLP syndrome, *Am J Obstet Gynecol* 152:576, 1985.

Farmakides G, Coury A, Decavalas G: Pregnancy surveillance with Doppler velocimetry, *The Female Patient* 15(5):49, May 1990.

Friedman SA: Preeclampsia: a review of the role of prostaglandins, *Obstet Gynecol* 71:122, 1988.

Gilbert ES, Harmon JS: *High-risk pregnancy and delivery: nursing perspectives,* ed 2, St Louis, 1992, Mosby–Year Book.

Gilstrap LC, Gant NF: Pathophysiology of preeclampsia, *Semin Perinatol* 14(2):147, 1990.

Holcomb WL, Shackelford GC, Petrie RH: Magnesium tocolysis and neonatal bone abnormalities: a controlled study, *Obstet Gynecol* 78:611, 1991.

Iams JD, Zuspan FP, Quilligan EJ: *Zuspan and Quilligan's manual of obstetrics and gynecology,* ed 2, St Louis, 1990, Mosby–Year Book.

Klonoff-Cohen HS et al: An epidemiologic study of contraception and preeclampsia, *JAMA* 262:3143, 1989.

Knuppel RA, Drukker JE: *High-risk pregnancy: a team approach,* Philadelphia, 1986, WB Saunders Co.

Kozier B, Erb G: *Fundamentals of nursing,* ed 2, Menlo Park, Calif, 1987, Addison-Wesley.

Roberts JM et al: Preeclampsia: an endothelial cell disorder, *Am J Obstet Gynecol* 161:1200, 1989.

Roberts JM et al: *New developments in preeclampsia* (NIH Grant HP 24180), San Francisco, 1990, University of California.

Saftlas AF et al: Epidemiology of preeclampsia and eclampsia in the United States, *Am J Obstet Gynecol* 163:460, 1990.

Schiff E et al: The use of aspirin to prevent pregnancy-induced hypertension and lower the ratio of thromboxane A_2 to prostacyclin in relatively high risk pregnancies, *N Engl J Med* 321:351, 1989.

Scott JR et al: *Danforth's obstetrics and gynecology,* ed 6, Philadelphia, 1990, JB Lippincott Co.

Sibai BM: Pitfalls in diagnosis and management of preeclampsia, *Am J Obstet Gynecol* 159:1, 1988.

Sibai BM: Eclampsia. VI. Maternal-perinatal outcome in 254 consecutive cases, *Am J Obstet Gynecol* 163:1049, 1990a.

Sibai BM: Magnesium sulfate is the ideal anticonvulsant in preeclampsia-eclampsia, *Am J Obstet Gynecol* 162:1141, 1990b.

Sibai BM: Preeclampsia-eclampsia: valid treatment approaches, *Contemp OB/GYN* 35:84, Aug 1990c.

Sibai BM: Immunologic aspects of preeclampsia, *Clin Obstet Gynecol* 34:27, 1991.

Sibai BM et al: A protocol for managing severe preeclampsia in the second trimester, *Am J Obstet Gynecol* 163:733, 1990.

Walsh SW: Physiology of low-dose aspirin therapy for the prevention of preeclampsia, *Semin Perinatol* 14(2):152, 1990.

Weiner CP: The clinical spectrum of preeclampsia, *Am J Kidney Dis* 9:321, 1987.

Weinstein L: The HELLP syndrome: a severe consequence of hypertension in pregnancy, *J Perinatol* 6:316, 1986.

References—Nursing Research

Gavette L, Roberts J: Use of mean arterial pressure (MAP-2) to predict pregnancy-induced hypertension in adolescents, *J Nurse Midwife* 32:357, 1987.

Smith CV et al: Reliability of compact electronic blood pressure monitors for hypertensive pregnant women, *J Reproduct Med* 35:399, April 1990.

BIBLIOGRAPHY

Blackburn ST, Loper DL: *Maternal, fetal and neonatal physiology: a clinical perspective*, Philadelphia, 1992, WB Saunders Co.

Fanaroff AA, Martin RJ: *Neonatal-perinatal medicine: diseases of the fetus and infant,* ed 5, St Louis 1992, Mosby–Year Book.

Hill MN, Grim CM: How to take a precise blood pressure, *Am J Nurs* 91(2):38, 1991.

Hubel CA et al: Lipid peroxidation in pregnancy: new perspectives on preeclampsia, *Am J Obstet Gynecol* 161:1025, 1989.

Miles JF et al: Postpartum eclampsia: a recurring perinatal dilemma, *Obstet Gynecol* 76:328, 1990.

Musci TJ et al: Mitogenic activity is increased in the sera of preeclamptic women before delivery, *Am J Obstet Gynecol* 159:1446, 1988.

O'Brien WF: Predicting preeclampsia, *Obstet Gynecol* 75:445, 1990.

Pritchard JA, Cunningham FG, Pritchard SA: The Parkland Memorial Hospital protocol for treatment of eclampsia: evaluation of 245 cases, *Am J Obstet Gynecol* 148:951, 1987.

Rodgers GM, Taylor RN, Roberts JM: Preeclampsia is associated with a serum factor cytotoxic to human endothelial cells, *Am J Obstet Gynecol* 159:908, 1988.

Schiff et al: Low-dose aspirin does not influence the clinical course of women with mild pregnancy-induced hypertension, *Obstet Gynecol* 76:742, 1990.

Taylor RN et al: Partial characterization of a novel growth factor from the blood of women with preeclampsia, *J Clin Endocrinol Metab* 70:1285, 1990.

Shannon DM: HELLP syndrome: a severe consequence of pregnancy-induced hypertension, *JOGNN* 16:395, 1987.

Martin JN et al: Pregnancy complicated by preeclampsia-eclampsia with the syndrome of hemolysis, elevated liver enzymes, and low platelet count: how rapid is postpartum recovery? *Obstet Gynecol* 76:737, 1990.

Poole JH: Getting perspective on HELLP syndrome, *MCN* 13:432, 1988.

Remich MC, Yongkin EQ: Factors associated with pregnancy-induced hypertension, *Nurs Pract* 14:20, Jan 1989.

Bibliography—Nursing Research

Kofinas AD et al: Uterine and umbilical artery flow velocity waveform analysis in pregnancies complicated by chronic hypertension or preeclampsia, *South Med J* 83:150, 1990.

chapter 28 review

Key Concepts

- Hypertensive disorders during pregnancy are a leading cause of infant and maternal morbidity and mortality worldwide.
- The cause of PIH is unknown, and there are no known reliable tests for predicting women at risk for preeclampsia.
- Preeclampsia is a multisystem disease rather than only an increase in blood pressure.
- Failure of trophoblastic invasion of spiral arterioles is proposed as the triggering mechanism that eventually leads to vasospasm and organ ischemia; the cure is delivery of the fetus and placenta.
- The pathologic changes of preeclampsia are present long before clinical manifestations are evident, involving every organ system in the body.
- Specific high-risk factors (e.g., first pregnancy, diabetes mellitus, and twin gestation) are associated with a higher incidence of preeclampsia.
- Progression of hypertensive disorders during pregnancy are unpredictable; thus mild hypertension must be taken seriously and managed for preeclampsia.
- Once preeclampsia becomes clinically evident, therapeutic intervention is mainly palliative (e.g., bed rest, diet), which may slow the progression of the disease and allow the pregnancy to continue.
- Education is an important nursing function for early identification of preeclampsia and client/family coping.
- Home care management is an option only for women who are able to comply with the medical regimen, reliably perform self-monitoring, and immediately recognize and report abnormal signs and symptoms.
- The HELLP syndrome, which usually becomes apparent during the third trimester, can occur in women with severe preeclampsia and is considered life threatening.
- Magnesium sulfate, which is the anticonvulsive agent of choice for preventing eclampsia, requires careful monitoring of reflexes, respirations, and urinary output; its antidote, calcium gluconate, should be at the bedside.
- Intent of emergency interventions for eclampsia is to prevent self-injury, ensure adequate oxygenation, reduce aspiration risk, establish control with $MgSO_4$, and correct maternal acidemia.

Key Terms

- affect (p. 820)
- antihypertensive agent (p. 833)
- arteriolar vasospasm (p. 819)
- calcium gluconate (p. 838)
- care during a convulsion (p. 839)
- chronic hypertension (p. 815)
- clonus (p. 823)
- deep tendon reflexes (DTR) (p. 823)
- dependent edema (p. 823)
- disseminated intravascular coagulation (DIC) (p. 820)
- eclampsia (p. 815)
- edema (p. 815)
- gestational hypertension (p. 814)
- HELLP syndrome (p. 820)
- hyperreflexia (p. 822)
- magnesium sulfate ($MgSO_4$) (p. 837)
- mean arterial pressure (MAP) (p. 815)

- normotensive (p. 814)
- oliguria (p. 822)
- patellar reflex (p. 823)
- pitting edema (p. 823)
- preeclampsia (p. 815)
- pregnancy-induced hypertension (PIH) (p. 814)
- proteinuria (p. 815)
- seizure precautions (p. 830)

Critical Thinking Exercises

1. Susan F. has been diagnosed with 'mild' preeclampsia. She is resisting needed diet changes and bed rest. Role-play a nurse attempting to provide client teaching for the woman who resists dietary change and bed rest. Ask the group to suggest additional strategies.
2. Susan's condition has become worse, and she is hospitalized. She has been in a dimly lit room receiving magnesium sulfate IV for several hours for severe preeclampsia.
   a. Give rationale for dim lighting and magnesium sulfate infusion.
   b. You assess her DTRs as 0 (no response). In order of priority, list four interventions, and specify rationale for each.
3. The charge nurse alerts you to the possibility that Susan could convulse anytime during labor or early postpartum.
   a. What assessment findings would indicate that a convulsion is imminent?
   b. In order of priority, list interventions during a convulsion, and specify rationale for each.

Topics for Nursing Research*

- Educational and emotional needs of the preeclamptic woman and her family in a home or a hospital setting
- Influences of family belief system on the client's perception of her condition and care
- Evaluation of nursing interventions that promote client and family coping with the crisis of illness and hospitalization during pregnancy
- Effects of intensive therapeutic hospital management on maternal-child bonding
- Impact of nursing education on client compliance, self-care management, and early recognition of preeclampsia symptoms
- Efficacy of screening tests (e.g., MAP-2) for identification of women at risk for preeclampsia
- Efficacy of the umbilical and uterine flow velocity wave form of pregnant women with chronic hypertension or preeclampsia, or both, in predicting fetal-maternal outcomes
- Differences in MAP-2 values of normal and preeclamptic nulliparous adolescents
- Trends and patterns of the resolution of postpartum preeclampsia symptoms
- Critical time periods when women are most likely to have convulsions before and after childbirth
- Unique emotional and cognitive manifestations in women with severe preeclampsia in the hospital setting
- Factors associated with women at risk for developing preeclampsia
- Difference, if any, between traditional left side–lying position, right side–lying position, and alternating right and left sides

*Very little nursing research is available on the nature and care of hypertensive disorders during pregnancy.

chapter 29

Maternal Infections

CYNTHIA GARRETT

LEARNING OBJECTIVES

- Define the key terms listed.
- Summarize care of clients with sexually transmitted diseases.
- Summarize care of clients with human immunodeficiency virus (HIV).
- Summarize care of clients with acquired immunodeficiency syndrome (AIDS).
- Summarize care of clients with TORCH infections.
- Summarize care of clients with toxic shock syndrome (TSS).
- Summarize care of clients with vaginal infections.
- Summarize care of clients with urinary tract infections.
- Summarize care of clients with puerperal infections.
- Summarize care of clients with bacteremic shock.
- Review infection control measures to minimize nosocomial infections and occupational risk for infection.
- Identify topics for nursing research related to maternal infections.

Infections in pregnancy are responsible for significant morbidity and mortality. The direct financial costs of disease can be substantial. However, indirect costs can be as startling and are much more difficult to measure. Some consequences of maternal infection last a lifetime, such as infertility and sterility. Psychosocial sequelae may include altered interpersonal relationships and lowered self-esteem. Other conditions, such as a congenitally acquired infection, often affect a child's length and quality of life.

The focus of this chapter is general information about infectious agents that can affect the health of the mother and her child. Medical management is discussed, and the nursing process is emphasized.

Both mother and fetus must be considered in the assessment of maternal infection. In some diseases, such as tuberculosis, the fetus almost always is spared, even though the mother may be dying. With other infections, such as rubella, the fetus may be critically compromised, whereas the mother may be only slightly ill.

Pregnancy generally is regarded as an immunosuppressed condition. That a fetus is not rejected during pregnancy still remains an immunologic mystery. Altered immune responses in pregnancy may decrease maternal ability to fight infection. In addition, genital tract changes also may affect susceptibility. As pregnancy advances, vaginal walls engorge and the cervix enlarges. These intravaginal changes, accompanied by decreasing vaginal pH, may contribute to increased susceptibility (Brunham et al, 1990).

Education and counseling are important aspects of care for the prevention of maternal infections. Adolescent mothers are at high risk because of earlier onset of intercourse and increased likelihood of multiple partners. The recent trend of exchanging sex for drugs is contributing to a rise in infection rates, especially among urban, poor, and minority women (Aral, Holmes, 1990). The prevention of disease and reduction of maternal and neonatal sequelae continue to be monumental challenges.

The terms **sexually transmitted disease (STD)** and sexually transmissible infections have replaced the older designation, venereal disease. Venereal disease (VD) primarily described gonorrhea and syphilis. However, STD is a broader term, which reflects the definition of an STD as any microbe that is passed from one person to another through close, intimate contact (Spence, 1989). Although many STDs can occur (see the box at left), those infections occurring most often during pregnancy are addressed here.

Sexually Transmitted Diseases

BACTERIA

Chlamydia
Gonorrhea
Syphilis
Chancroid
Lymphogranuloma venereum
Gardnerella
Shigellosis
Salmonellosis
Genital mycoplasmas
Group B streptococci

VIRUSES

Human immunodeficiency virus
Herpes simplex virus, types 1 and 2
Cytomegalovirus
Viral hepatitis, A and B
Human papillomavirus

PROTOZOA

Trichomoniasis
Giardiasis
Amebiasis

PARASITES

Pediculosis
Scabies

FUNGI

Candidiasis

■ BACTERIAL SEXUALLY TRANSMITTED DISEASES

Chlamydia

Chlamydial infections are epidemic in the United States. *Chlamydia trachomatis,* which is the most common sexually transmitted bacterial pathogen, is responsible for substantial morbidity, personal suffering, and heavy economic burden. Estimated cost exceeds $1.5 billion per year (Schachter, 1989).

C. trachomatis is an obligatory parasite bacterium. That is, the organisms can exist only within living cells. Therefore transmission occurs by direct sexual contact or exposure at birth. There are 15 known immunotypes of *C. trachomatis* that are responsible for neonatal infections (see Chapter 39), for adult ocular and genital infections, and for lymphogranuloma venereum, a sexually transmitted disease rare in North

America (Loucks, 1986; Bourcier, Seidler, 1987; Marvin, Slevin, 1987).

Between 3 and 5 million adults are infected each year; 800,000 of these are males with urethritis. Yearly the number of cases of newborn conjunctivitis and pneumonia continues to grow. This infection is implicated in cervical dysplasia (as revealed by Papanicolaou's test), in ectopic pregnancy, and in sterility in the female. In the male it causes genital inflammation and damage to the prostate and sperm.

Morbidity resulting from chlamydial infections may even be higher. However, *C. trachomatis* is not a reportable STD. Difficulty in diagnosis, limited screening resources, and inadequate follow-up also affect disease reporting.

Definitive laboratory diagnosis is possible with tissue culture. However, it is expensive, requires skill to perform, and requires 4 to 7 days for results. There are two antigen detection methods: (1) a direct immunofluorescent test (e.g., MicroTrak) that requires a fluorescent microscope and takes 30 minutes and (2) an enzyme-linked immunosorbent assay (ELISA) test (e.g., Chlamydiazyme) that gives a color signal in 4 hours. The 30-minute test is more appropriate for screening low-risk populations, whereas the ELISA test is used for high-risk populations.

Populations at risk have been identified (Loucks, 1986; Perlman, 1986; Corbett, Meyer, 1987, Marvin, Slevin, 1987; Washington et al, 1987a, b; Centers for Disease Control [CDC], 1989). The sexually active female under 20 years of age is two to three times more likely to become infected than are women between 20 and 29. Women over 30 have the lowest rate. Women and men with multiple sexual partners are at highest risk. People who *do not* use barrier methods of birth control (condom, spermicide, diaphragm) have a higher incidence. Lower socioeconomic status may be a risk factor. Sexually active males under 20 are at high risk for urethritis. In men, the infection is linked to nongonococcal urethritis. The infection rate among homosexual males is one third that of heterosexual males. However, 4% to 8% of infected homosexual men have rectal chlamydial infection (Loucks, 1986).

The CDC guidelines recommend screening the populations at risk, treating all those who are presumably infected, and educating the medical profession and public. Combination antibiotic therapy is recommended for heterosexual men and women with gonorrhea inasmuch as 20% to 50% harbor *C. trachomatis*. Homosexual men with gonorrhea have a low incidence of concurrent chlamydia infection. Of persons infected with chlamydia, 15% of males and 26% of females also have gonorrhea. Priority groups for screening are high-risk pregnant women, adolescents, and women with multiple sexual partners (CDC, 1989).

Infections often are asymptomatic although eventual sequelae include salpingitis, ectopic pregnancy, pelvic inflammatory disease (PID), infertility, and sterility. Women usually have a history of mucopurulent discharge and bleeding resulting from inflammation and erosion of cervical columnar epithelium. **Dysuria** (painful urination) and other urinary tract discomfort, as well as **dyspareunia** (painful intercourse), also may occur.

The role of chlamydial infections in *pregnancy* and the perinatal period is under active study. Although infection is associated with tubal damage and ectopic pregnancy, the role of *C. trachomatis* in spontaneous abortion needs further investigation. In addition, preterm birth and low birth weight also have been linked to this disease, but research data are inconclusive. More recently, untreated chlamydial infections have been examined as a direct correlate of postpartum endometritis (Brunham et al, 1990).

Fetal or neonatal effects are common. Stillbirth and neonatal death are 10 times more common than in noninfected women. The newborn may acquire the infection by direct contact with an infected birth canal but may have no symptoms. **Inclusion conjunctivitis** occurs in one third of exposed newborns. Conjunctivitis appears after 3 to 4 days. Chronic follicular conjunctivitis, with conjunctival scarring and corneal neovascularization, contributes to vision sequelae. About 25% of newborns contract pneumonia and may exhibit symptoms of serious tachypnea, dyspnea, or apnea that requires hospitalization (Schachter et al, 1986).

Preferred antimicrobial treatment of urethral, cervical, and rectal chlamydia infections is with doxycycline or tetracycline. If the woman is pregnant, erythromycin is used and all sexual partners should be tested and treated. Neonatal prophylaxis is achieved with erythromycin (0.5%) ophthalmic ointment; existing neonatal infections are treated with oral erythromycin syrup.

Gonorrhea

Gonorrhea is caused by *Neisseria gonorrhoeae*, a type of diplococci bacteria. Although gonorrhea is an STD, it also is spread by direct contact with infected lesions and indirectly by transfer from inanimate objects, or **fomites.** Self-inoculation with contaminated hands is common. Secretions on fomites, such as washcloths, towels, bed linens, and clothing often are implicated. Thus this bean-shaped gram-negative organism is responsible for genitourinary, anorectal, oropharyngeal, and systemic infections.

Gonorrhea often produces only mild symptoms in women, or the diplococci may persist unsuspected in the lower genital tract. The incubation period is 2 to 5 days. Symptoms of lower urogenital tract infection includes dysuria and frequency, heavy green-yellow purulent discharge at the cervical os, cervical tenderness, vulvovaginitis, bartholinitis, dyspareunia, and postcoital bleeding. Swollen and painful Bartholin's glands and tenderness in the lymph nodes in the groin usually accompany infection. In 10% to 15% of cases, the upper urogenital tract is affected in the later stage of infection. Lower abdominal pain, cervical tenderness, fever, nausea, and vomiting are accompanying symptoms. Adnexal abscess and pelvic tenderness indicate PID. PID is implicated in ectopic pregnancy or sterility. Chronic pelvic pain and low backache may be seen. Anorectal infection is diagnosed by local inflammation, burning, and pruritus. Oropharyngeal infection may be asymptomatic or result in inflammation and sore throat. Systemic infection results in gonococcemia, skin rashes, arthritis, pericarditis, and meningitis. Gonococcal perihepatitis (Fitz-Hugh–Curtis syndrome) is discussed in Chapter 42.

After the third month of *pregnancy,* gonorrheal salpingitis rarely occurs, perhaps because with progressive pregnancy, the chorion laeve fuses with the decidua parietalis, thus obliterating the endometrial cavity. However, increasing evidence suggests that antepartum gonococcal infection may be related to preterm birth, premature or prolonged rupture of membranes, and chorioamnionitis (Brunham et al, 1990). Postnatal maternal complications of untreated gonorrhea include gonococcal endometritis, acute salpingitis, dermatitis, and arthritis.

Neonatal effects include **ophthalmia neonatorum** and pneumonia. Ophthalmitis with partial or total blindness can occur. Exposed newborns also are at risk for infection elsewhere—nose, pharynx, ears, vagina, anus, and scalp electrode site. Gonorrhea in other sites may predispose the infant to bacterial sepsis. Neonatal sepsis is characterized by temperature instability, hypotonia, poor feeding, and jaundice.

Ceftriaxone in a single dose is recommended for treatment of pregnant and nonpregnant women. Spectinomycin is the preferred alternative therapy. Among high-risk women, especially those with multiple partners, numerous STDs are common. Therefore practitioners suggest testing for and treating chlamydia and syphilis if maternal history warrants. All sexual partners should be treated and condom use encouraged for oral and genital intercourse until repeat culture findings are negative.

Erythromycin (0.5%) ophthalmic ointment is effective against gonococcal ophthalmia neonatorium. For newborns with extraocular site infection or suspected septicemia, ceftriaxone is recommended.

Syphilis

Syphilis is caused by the spirochete, *Treponema pallidum* after an incubation period of several weeks. The incidence of syphilis in the United States is increasing after a period of decline and may have serious sequelae during pregnancy.

Several methods of clinical assessment of syphilis are available:

1. Dark-field microscopic examination or direct fluorescent antibody staining of material from lesions or umbilical cord
2. Assessment of symptoms
3. Roentgenographic evidence of characteristic bone involvement
4. Serologic testing for antibodies known as reagins

Any test for antibodies may not be reactive in the presence of active infection because it takes time for the body's immune system to develop antibodies to any antigen.

Nonspecific serologic tests for nontreponemal antigens used for screening purposes are of two types: complement fixation (Kolmer, Wasserman) and flocculation (Kahn, RPR [rapid plasma reagin], Venereal Disease Research Laboratories [VDRL]). VDRL test results will not be positive until 10 to 90 days after infection; that is, 50% show positivity in 3 weeks, 90% in 6 weeks, and 100% in 13 weeks. Therefore infection may exist in the presence of a negative result from the VDRL test. If the antibodies in the newborn have been acquired from the mother, titers should drop to zero by 3 months. False-positive results may occur if the newborn has an acute infection of any kind or a collagen disease. Even in the presence of a syphilitic infection a false-negative result may occur, for example, if the mother became infected late in pregnancy. A false-positive result may occur in the presence of heroin dependence.

Specific tests for treponemal antigen are more expensive and are used for differential diagnosis. These tests include *T. pallidum* immobilization (TPI), fluorescent treponemal antibody absorption (FTA-ABS), and fluorescent treponemal antibody absorption, immunoglobulin M (FTA-ABS IgM). The FTA-ABS IgM is most specific for neonatal syphilis; a positive result is especially valuable in diagnosis of the condition in the symptom-free child. Results of the FTA-ABS IgM test may be negative, however, in the presence of active disease if infection occurred late in pregnancy and the fetus or newborn had insufficient time for an IgM response. In questionable cases the test is repeated.

NOTE: Yaws, a nonvenereal contagious disease, is caused by the spirochete *Treponema pertenue*. This spirochete is closely related to the causative organism of syphilis. Yaws is spread by contact with secretions or sores from an infected person. Both syphilis and yaws give a positive result in the serologic test for syphilis (STS). Yaws is a common disease in equatorial Africa, Hawaii, South America, and the East and West Indies. It is effectively treated with antibiotics, especially penicillin.

Early syphilis infection may be asymptomatic. During the *primary stage* chancres form at the organism entry site—perineum, labia, cervix, anus, mouth, and lips. The chancre has a red base with firm, rolled edges and is painless (Fig. 29-1, *A*). Even without treatment, chancres heal with little scarring. However, the mother is still considered infectious. The local lymphadenopathy also clears without treatment in 4 to 6 weeks.

The *secondary stage* begins about 6 weeks after healing of the primary lesions or chancres. A symmetric, nontender rash may appear anywhere over the body, including palms of hands and soles of feet. If the rash develops on the scalp, loss of hair is seen. In dark-skinned persons, hyperpigmented facial lesions are present around the nose and mouth. Characteristic white-gray genital lesions (condylomata lata) (Fig. 29-1, *B*) appear on the labia, perineum, and anus. Systemic infection causes malaise, anorexia, fever, and headache, as well as generalized lymphadenopathy. This secondary stage also clears without treatment in 2 to 6 weeks.

Latent stages appear at varying times. An early latent stage may appear up to 4 years after the primary infection. At this time, lesions reappear. For 50% to 70% of affected persons, the latent stage lasts a lifetime, during which time there is no outward evidence of disease.

The *tertiary stage* brings clinical evidence of disease throughout the body, especially bone, cardiac, and neurologic disease. Obliterative endarteritis leads to cell damage and death and to the formation of gumma nodules of dead tissue. The acronym PARESIS summarizes possible sequelae seen in the following changes: *personality, affect, reflexes, eye function, sensorium, intellect, and speech.*

Pregnancy does not alter the progression of syphilis. However, early pregnancy symptoms may mimic those of secondary syphilis and delay diagnosis. Syphilis probably continues to be a major cause of late abortion throughout the world, despite widespread success of diagnosis and treatment of this disease. Primary and secondary stages of untreated syphilis lead to stillbirth. Latent and tertiary stages of untreated syphilis lead to secondary syphilis (congenital syphilis) in the newborn (for a discussion of congenital syphilis, see Chapter 39).

Congenital syphilis occurs when the spirochetes cross the placenta after the sixteenth to eighteenth week of gestation. The following sequelae are seen: snuffles (rhinitis), rhagades (cracks, fissures around the mouth), hydrocephaly, and corneal opacity. Later, saddle nose, saber shin, Hutchinson's teeth (notched, tapered canines), and diabetes develop in untreated children. The highest risk for fetal infection occurs with recent or current secondary syphilis (Wendel, 1989). There are no residual effects if the mother is treated adequately before the fifth month. Destruction of tissue that occurs before treatment cannot be reversed, but additional tissue destruction is prevented by adequate treatment.

Unfortunately, there is a steady flow of treatment failures. One possible reason may be developing organism resistance (Guinan, 1987). A second reason may be an alteration in the immune status of the infected person (Berry et al, 1987; Johns et al, 1987; Tramont, 1987). Another possible reason is poor follow-up after treatment, leading to reinfection. Notification and treatment of sexual partners are essential, with repeat serologic testing at 3 months, 6 months, and 12 months.

Occasionally, a mother who was treated for active syphilis in the past shows a reactive titer after pregnancy. It is important to assess the adequacy of past treatment or the possibility of reinfection. In addition, the timing of syphilis treatment has a significant impact on titer results. For example, if appropriate treatment is initiated before the development of a chancre or a reactive syphilis titer, the titer results remain nonreactive. If treatment occurs after seropositive results are obtained, titer results generally become nonreactive within 6 months. When treated in the secondary stages of syphilis, clients may take 12 to 18 months to demonstrate nonreactive titers. The longer syphilis goes untreated, the longer it takes for a reactive titer to become nonreactive once treatment is begun. Some reactive titers may never convert, even though treatment is completed.

Penicillin is preferred for the treatment of syphilis. In penicillin-allergic persons, alternate choices include tetracycline or doxycycline, erythromycin, and ceftriaxone. Tetracycline is contraindicated in pregnancy because of its effects on liver function in the mother and tooth discoloration and decreased bone growth in the fetus. Another option for treatment during pregnancy (or when compliance is an issue) is penicillin desensitization followed by treatment with penicillin.

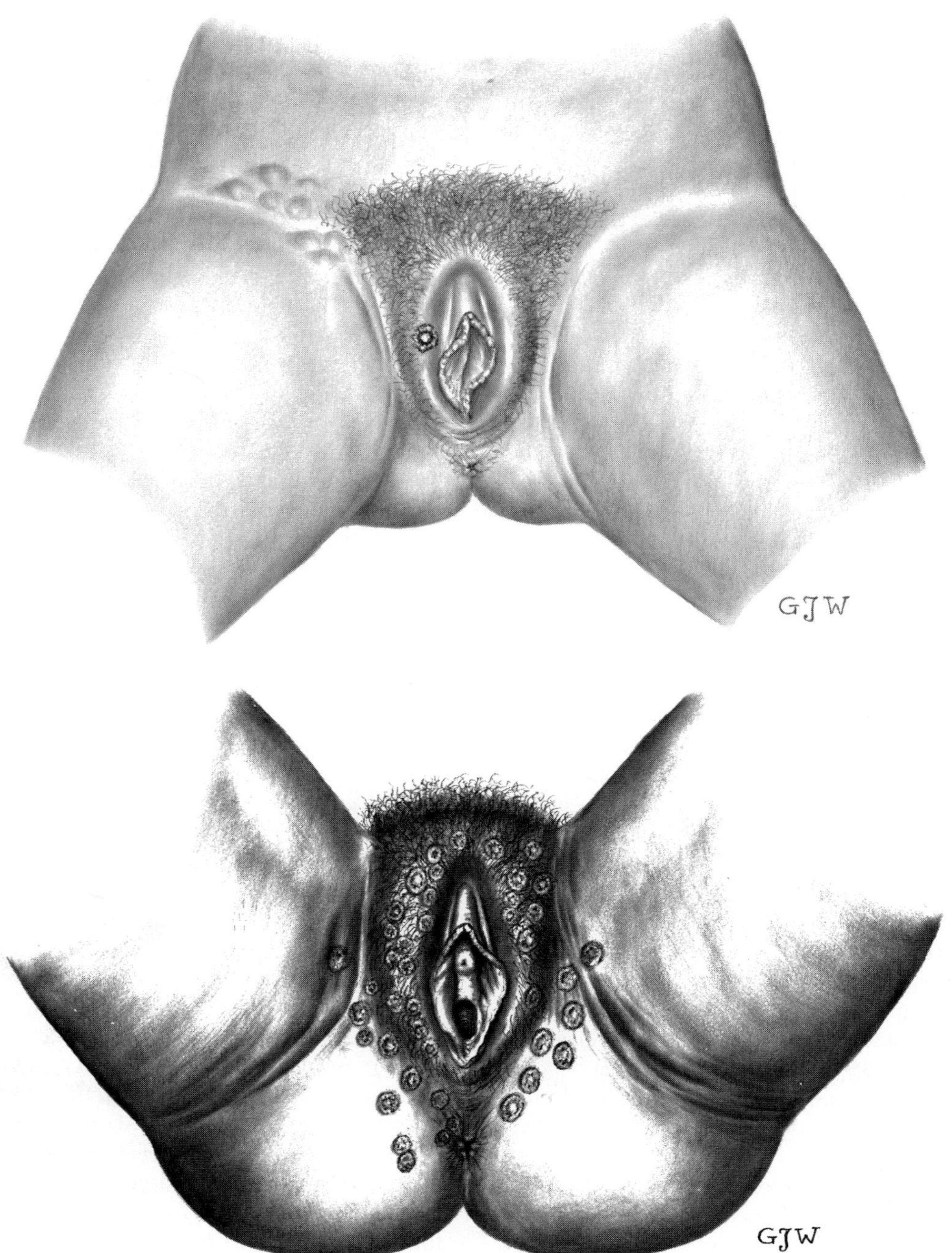

Fig. 29-1 Syphilis. **A,** Primary stage: chancre with inguinal adenopathy. **B,** Secondary stage: condylomata lata.

Pregnant women should be informed of the Jarisch-Herxheimer reaction related to penicillin therapy. General effects include fever, headache, malaise, nausea, and tachycardia. This systemic reaction to treatment may precipitate preterm labor.

Treatment of infected newborns is a priority. Congenital syphilis is rising although disagreement exists as to whether the rise is actual or merely reflects a change in disease reporting. Most states now require VDRL testing of all infants, and results determine treatment and follow-up.

Penicillin also is used to treat active congenital syphilis. In the absence of active disease, seropositive infants should show decreasing antibody titers between 3 and 6 months of age. Infants with a reactive VDRL test after 6 months should be treated.

■ VIRAL SEXUALLY TRANSMITTED DISEASES

Human Immunodeficiency Virus and Acquired Immunodeficiency Syndrome

Transmission of **human immunodeficiency virus (HIV),** a retrovirus, occurs primarily through the exchange of body fluids (e.g., blood, semen, perinatal events) (Friedland, Klein, 1987; Hecht, 1987; Landesman et al, 1987). Severe depression of the cellular immune system characterizes **acquired immunodeficiency syndrome (AIDS)** (see Chapter 6). Although the populations at high risk have been well-documented, *all* women should be assessed for the possibility of HIV exposure. HIV infection in women commonly is reported at a later stage in the disease, and they usually enter the hospital for initiation of treatment when the illness is more severe. The delay may be due in part to the occurrence of symptoms different from those of men (Shaw, 1986). Chronic vaginitis and candidiasis are common presenting problems.

Once HIV enters the body, seroconversion to HIV positivity occurs within the first 10 weeks of exposure. (Some sources note longer incubation periods, although prolonged incubation generally is the exception, not the rule.) Although seroconversion may be totally asymptomatic, it usually is accompanied by a viremic, influenza-type response to initial HIV infection. Symptoms include fever, malaise, myalgias, nausea, diarrhea, sore throat, and rash and may persist for 2 to 3 weeks.

Laboratory studies may reveal leukopenia, thrombocytopenia, anemia, and an elevated erythrocyte sedimentation rate. In addition, HIV has a strong affinity for surface-marker proteins on T lymphocytes. This affinity of HIV for T lymphocytes leads to significant T cell destruction. T helper cell titers of less than 400 cells/mm^3 are associated with a more rapid progression to AIDS (see Chapter 6).

Delay in diagnosis must be avoided when the woman is pregnant. Pregnancy is not encouraged with positive HIV status; preconceptional counseling is recommended. Exposure to the virus has a significant impact on the woman's pregnancy and newborn feeding method and on the newborn's health status (Klug, 1986). It is hypothesized that HIV from infected women is transmitted to the fetus and newborn in three ways (Friedland, Klein, 1987; Landesman et al, 1987):

1. To the fetus as early as the first trimester through maternal circulation
2. To the infant during labor and birth by inoculation or ingestion of maternal blood and other infected fluids
3. To the infant through breast milk

Frequency of in utero, intrapartum, and postpartum transmission is uncertain. Rates of maternal transmission of HIV are reported as low as 10% and as high as 70%, the most frequently reported rate being 30% (see Research Highlight, p. 854). Infants born to seropositive mothers seem to be at greater risk for an HIV infection and AIDS than do infants born to seronegative mothers who later show seroconversion.

Regardless of whether *infection* is diagnosed, the nursing process is implemented in a culturally sensitive and humane manner. "HIV infection is a biologic event, not a moral comment. It is vital to remember, to model, and to teach that [personal] reactions to particular life-styles, practices, or behaviors must not influence [the nurse's] ability to provide objective, compassionate, and effective health care to all" (Keeling, 1987).

PRENATAL PERIOD. The incidence of HIV in pregnant women is expected to increase (Minkoff, 1987). The health history, physical examination, and laboratory testing must reflect this expectation if women and their newborns are to receive appropriate care. Women who fall into the high-risk category for HIV infection include:

1. Women and/or partners from geographic areas where HIV is prevalent
2. Women and/or partners who use intravenous drugs
3. Women with persistent and recurrent STDs
4. Women who received blood transfusions between 1978 and 1985
5. Any woman who believes she may have been exposed to HIV

HIV testing should be offered to high-risk women at their initial entry into prenatal care. However, seronegativity on the first prenatal examination is not a guarantee for continued negative titers. For example, one 24-year-old woman who sought prenatal care at 8 weeks had a negative Western blot test result. However, after exposure to HIV, serum antibodies may take up to 12 weeks to develop. The Western blot test should be repeated in 1 to 2 months and late in the third trimester.

Routine prenatal tests may help to identify the woman with HIV infection (Foster, 1987; Kaplan et

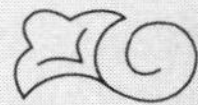 **Research Highlight** 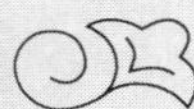

Perinatal Infection with Human Immunodeficiency Virus Type 1

RESEARCH ABSTRACT

Most infants who have AIDS and HIV type 1 (HIV-1) infections are infected by their mothers in the perinatal period. This study was conducted to determine what proportion of infants exposed to the virus are infected. The subjects were 112 of 168 seropositive mothers identified through screening of Haitian-born women giving birth at a hospital in which most of these infants are born. A group of infants born to Haitian women with seronegative results was matched with the index infants (infants of the seropositive mothers) to serve as control subjects. Infection status of 82 of the index infants was determined. Of these 82 infants, 25 (30%) were infected and 10 (40%) have died. All infants in the control group were seronegative at follow-up. Mode of birth was not associated with infection status. More than 30% of the infants were breast-fed; breast-feeding was not related to infection.

IMPLICATIONS FOR PRACTICE

Many infants born to HIV-1 seropositive mothers are or become infected. Most infants who are infected are free of symptoms at birth. Nurses must treat all infants as if they are infected and must observe universal precautions. In this study there was no relation between breast-feeding and infection status; however, it is possible that too few infants were examined to detect any differences in risk for breast-feeding. How long the mother breast-feeds also may be an important factor.

RELATED RESEARCH QUESTIONS

1. Is there a relation between breast-feeding and HIV-1 infection in infants?
2. Is there a relation between duration of breast-feeding and HIV-1 infection in infants?
3. What do nurses teach seropositive mothers about the risks of breast-feeding?
4. Is there a difference in breast-feeding success between seropositive mothers and seronegative mothers?

REFERENCE

Hutto C et al: A hospital-based prospective study of perinatal infection with human immunodeficiency virus type 1, *J Pediatr* 118:347, 1991.

al, 1987; Minkoff, 1987; Rhoads et al, 1987). Testing also can reveal gonorrhea, syphilis, prolonged and persistent episodes of herpes, *C. trachomatis,* hepatitis B, *Mycobacterium tuberculosis,* candidiasis (oropharyngeal or chronic vaginal infection), cytomegalovirus (CMV), and toxoplasmosis. About half of AIDS sufferers have elevated CMV titers. Because CMV inclusion disease poses a serious hazard to the fetus (Table 29-1), pregnant women are advised to avoid direct contact with HIV-infected persons.

History of vaccinations and immune status is documented. The titers for chickenpox and rubella are determined, and tuberculosis skin testing (purified protein derivative [PPD]) is done. Previous vaccination with Recombivax HB vaccine is noted because the vaccine once contained human blood products. (This vaccine is now free of association with human blood or blood products.)

The woman may be a candidate for receiving *Rh_o D immune globulin.* Transmission of HIV has not been traced to the Rh vaccine. The preparation process involves ethyl alcohol, which inactivates the virus. The vaccine is made from blood drawn from an identified group of regular donors. Blood used to produce the vaccine undergoes blood testing that can detect evidence of HIV (Francis, Chin, 1987; MMWR, 1987).

Some prenatal discomforts (e.g., fatigue, anorexia, and weight loss) mimic signs and symptoms of HIV infection. Differential diagnosis of *all* "pregnancy-induced" complaints and symptoms of infections is warranted. Major signs of worsening HIV infection include a weight loss of greater than 10% of prepregnancy body weight, chronic diarrhea for longer than 1 month, and fever (intermittent or constant) for longer than 1 month.

To support any pregnant woman's immune system, appropriate counseling is provided for optimum nutrition; sleep, rest, exercise; and stress reduction. If HIV infection is diagnosed, the woman is advised of the possible consequences for her infant. The woman is supported in her decision. Should she choose to continue the pregnancy, she is counseled regarding "safer sex" techniques. Use of condoms and nonoxynol 9 spermicide is encouraged to minimize further exposure to HIV if her partner is the source. Orogenital sex is discouraged. As necessary, the woman is referred for drug rehabilitation to discontinue substance abuse. Abuse of alcohol, methamphetamines (speed, crank, ice), marijuana, cocaine, nitrites (poppers, amyl), or other drugs compromise the body's immune system and increase the risk for AIDS and associated conditions.

1. HIV may require the presence of an already damaged immune system before it can cause disease.
2. Alcohol and drugs interfere with many medical and alternative therapies for AIDS.
3. Alcohol and drugs affect the judgment of the user, who may become more prone to engage in activities that place persons at high risk for AIDS or increase exposure to HIV.
4. Alcohol and drug abuse causes stress, including sleep problems, which harms immune system functioning.

Pharmaceutical treatment for HIV infection has progressed rapidly since the discovery of the virus. The primary drug approved for treatment of HIV infection is 3′ azido-3′-deoxythymidine (zidovudine, AZT, Retrovir). Although this medication shows promise for treatment of HIV infection, its use in pregnancy is limited. The potentially toxic or mutagenic effects on the fetus are unknown. Azidothymidine is being tested in some controlled studies with pregnant women who have T helper cell counts of less than 400 cells/mm^3. Other opportunistic infections that persist concurrently with HIV infection are treated with medications specific to the infection.

INTRAPARTUM PERIOD. Care of the woman in labor is not substantially altered by asymptomatic infection with HIV (Minkoff, 1987). The mode of birth is based only on obstetric considerations because the virus crosses the placenta early in pregnancy.

The primary focus is the prevention of **nosocomial** spread (infection acquired during hospitalization) of HIV and the protection of care providers. The risk of transmission of HIV is considered to be low during vaginal birth despite the exposure to the infected woman's blood, amniotic fluid, and vaginal secretions.

External electronic fetal monitoring (EFM) is preferred if EFM is needed. There is a possibility of inoculation of the virus into the neonate if fetal scalp blood sampling is done or if a fetal scalp electrode is applied. In addition, the one who performs either of these procedures is placed at risk by accidental sticks to the finger.

POSTPARTUM PERIOD. Little is known of the clinical course during the postpartum period for the woman infected with HIV. Although the immediate postpartum period has not been noted to be significant (Update, 1987), longer follow-up has revealed a high frequency of clinical illness in mothers whose children develop disease (Scott, 1985; Minkoff et al, 1987, a,b).

The newborn can be with the mother, but breastfeeding is contraindicated (see Chapter 39). Universal precautions are implemented for mother and newborn, as they are with all clients. The woman and her infant are referred to physicians who are experienced in the treatment of AIDS and associated conditions. (see nursing plan of care, p. 864).

The fetal and neonatal effects of HIV infection may not be obvious. Because the virus crosses the placenta, umbilical cord blood will show HIV antibodies whether or not the newborn is infected. Also, maternal antibodies that cross the placental barrier may be present in uninfected infants for up to 15 months. Therefore it is not until that time that HIV infection in the infant can be determined. When HIV infections become active, many of the opportunistic infections seen in adults develop in infants.

In those infants infected with HIV more than 90% have a documented neurologic or developmental abnormality. Other complications associated with HIV infection in infants include encephalopathy, microcephaly, cognitive deficits, central nervous system (CNS) lymphomas, cerebrovascular accidents, respiratory failure, and lymphadenopathy.

TORCH Infections

*T*oxoplasmosis. *o*ther infections (e.g., hepatitis), *r*ubella virus, *c*ytomegalovirus, and *h*erpes simplex viruses, known collectively as **TORCH infections,** comprise a group of organisms capable of crossing the placenta and adversely affecting the development of the fetus. Generally, all of these TORCH infections produce influenza-like symptoms in the mother. However, fetal and neonatal effects usually are much more serious. TORCH infections and their maternal, fetal, and newborn effects are outlined in Table 29-1.

TOXOPLASMOSIS. Toxoplasmosis is a protozoan infection associated with the consumption of raw meat or with poor hand washing after handling infected cat litter. Pregnant women with HIV antibodies are at risk because toxoplasmosis is one of the common accompanying opportunistic infections. The presence of toxoplasmosis can be determined with blood studies, and women in at-risk groups should have toxoplasmosis titers evaluated. Acute infection in pregnancy produces influenza-like symptoms and lymphadenopathy. Effects seen in the fetus and newborn include spontaneous abortion and neonatal parasitemia. The pharmaceutic treatment of choice for toxoplasmosis is sulfa, or clindamycin in sulfa-allergic clients.

TABLE 29-1 Maternal Infection: TORCH

Infection	Maternal Effects	Fetal or Neonatal Effects	Counseling Prevention, Identification, and Management
Toxoplasmosis (protozoa)	Acute infection: similar to influenza; lymphadenopathy	With maternal acute infection: parasitemia Less likely to occur with maternal chronic infection Abortion likely with acute infection early in pregnancy (see Chapter 42).	Avoid eating raw meat and exposure to litter used by infected cats; if cats in house, have toxoplasma titer checked If titer is rising during early pregnancy, abortion may be considered an option
Other: Hepatitis A (infectious hepatitis) (virus)	Abortion—cause of liver failure during pregnancy Fever, malaise, nausea, and abdominal discomfort	Exposure during first trimester; fetal anomalies; fetal or neonatal hepatitis; preterm birth; intrauterine fetal death	Usually spread by droplet or hand contact especially by culinary workers; γ-globulin can be given as prophylaxis for hepatitis A
Hepatitis B (serum hepatitis) (virus)	May be transmitted sexually Symptoms variable: fever, rash, arthralgia, depressed appetite, dyspepsia, abdominal pain, generalized aching, malaise, weakness, jaundice, tender and enlarged liver	Infection occurs during birth (see Chapter 42) Maternal vaccination during pregnancy should present no risk for fetus; however, data are not available. See Chapter 39 for information about vaccination of children at risk for hepatitis B	Generally passed by contaminated needles, syringes, or blood transfusions; also can be transmitted orally or by coitus, but incubation period is longer; hepatitis B immune globulin can be given prophylactically after exposure Hepatitis B vaccine recommended for populations at risk; vaccine consists of series of 3 IM doses. Populations at risk: women from Asia, Pacific islands, Haiti, sub-Africa, Alaska (women of Eskimo descent). Other women at risk include health care providers, intravenous drug users, those sexually active with multiple partners and single partner having multiple risks
Rubella (3-day German measles, virus)	Rash, fever, mild symptoms; suboccipital lymph nodes may be swollen; some photophobia Occasionally arthritis or encephalitis Spontaneous abortion	Incidence of congenital anomalies: first month, 50%; second month, 25%, third month, 10%, fourth month, 4% Exposure during first 2 months: malformations of heart, eyes, ears, or brain, abnormal dermatoglyphics Exposure after fourth month: systemic infection, hepatosplenomegaly, intrauterine growth retardation, rash At 15-20 years of age, may experience deterioration of intellect and development or may develop epilepsy	Vaccination of pregnant women contraindicated; pregnancy should be prevented for 3 months after vaccination; pregnant women nonreactive to hemagglutinin-inhibition antigen can be safely vaccinated after the birth

TABLE 29-1 Maternal Infection: TORCH—cont'd

Infection	Maternal Effects	Fetal or Neonatal Effects	Counseling Prevention, Identification, and Management
Cytomegalovirus (CMV) (a herpes virus)	Respiratory or sexually transmitted asymptomatic illness or mononucleosis-like syndrome: may have cervical discharge	Fetal or neonatal death or severe, generalized disease—hemolytic anemia and jaundice: hydrocephaly or microcephaly; pneumonitis; hepatosplenomegaly	Virus may be reactivated and cause disease in utero or during birth in subsequent pregnancies; fetal infection may occur during passage through infected birth canal; disease is commonly progressive through infancy and childhood
Herpes genitalis (herpes simplex virus, type 2 [HSV-2])	See discussion that follows cytomegalovirus		

OTHER INFECTIONS. The primary infection included in this category is hepatitis. *Hepatitis A,* or *infectious hepatitis,* is a virus spread by droplets or hands and is associated with poor hand washing after defecation. Pregnancy effects include spontaneous abortion and influenza-like symptoms—fever, malaise, nausea. If exposure to the fetus occurs in the first trimester and is untreated, possible effects include fetal anomalies, preterm birth, fetal or neonatal hepatitis, or intrauterine fetal death. Gamma globulin vaccination is given to mothers and newborns for prophylaxis.

Hepatitis B, or *serum hepatitis,* is a virus transmitted in a manner similar to that of HIV. Routes of transmission include contaminated needles, syringes or blood products, sexual intercourse, and body fluid exchange. Populations at risk for hepatitis B are noted in Table 29-1.

During pregnancy, common symptoms include fever, rash, anorexia, malaise, myalgias, and jaundice if the liver is acutely affected. Fetal and newborn effects are the same as already listed for hepatitis A. Populations at risk should be given the hepatitis B vaccine. Vaccination during pregnancy is not thought to pose risk to the fetus; neonates exposed in utero should be vaccinated after birth.

RUBELLA. Rubella, also known as German measles or 3-day measles, is a viral infection transmitted by droplets (e.g., droplets from an infected person's sneeze). Fever, rash, and mild lymphedema usually are seen in an infected mother. Consequences for the fetus are much more serious and include spontaneous abortion, congenital anomalies (referred to as congenital rubella syndrome [see discussion in Chapter 39]), and death. Vaccination of pregnant women is contraindicated because a rubella infection may develop after the vaccine is administered. As part of preconception counseling, rubella vaccine is given to women who are not rubella immune, and they are counseled to use contraception for at least 3 months after vaccination (see Chapter 6).

CYTOMEGALOVIRUS. CMV is the primary cause of congenital viral infection in the fetus and neonate and is the most common infectious cause of mental retardation. Infectious viral sources include saliva, urine, semen, breast milk, blood, and cervical/vaginal secretions. CMV also has been isolated from placental tissue. Most primary CMV infections are asymptomatic, and most women who show CMV infection in pregnancy (by positive viral titers) have a chronic or recurrent infection (Brunham et al, 1990).

Fetal and neonatal effects are severe and include hemolytic anemia, jaundice, hydrocephaly or microcephaly, and pneumonitis. Infected infants shed large amounts of the virus in saliva and respiratory secretions and in urine. Pregnant health care providers should carefully observe universal precautions to avoid exposure to droplets of infected secretions. No effective pharmaceutical treatment exists for CMV; therapies focus on treatment of symptoms.

HERPES SIMPLEX VIRUS. Herpes simplex virus type 1 (HSV-1) infections predominate during childhood. The virus is transmitted primarily by contact with *oral* secretions and causes cold sores and fever blisters. HSV-2 infections usually occur after puberty as sexual activity increases. HSV-2 is transmitted primarily by contact with *genital* secretions. Although it has been shown that HSV can survive for many hours on objects (fomites) such as doorknobs, faucets, and toilets, scientists do not believe that human infection is likely to occur through contact with such objects. Transmission occurs by close contact with a person shedding the virus. Public health experts believe that within the United States, from 10 to 40 million people carry the HSV-2. Many genital infections show a mixture of HSV-1 and HSV-2.

HSV interacts with epithelial or neuroepithelial cells and neurons. The incubation period is between 2 and 4 weeks. During the initial infection, HSV migrates to one or more sensory nerve ganglia, where it remains latent and dormant indefinitely (Fig. 29-2). An intact immune system cures the infection at the portal (place of entry). The *primary* infection involves mucocutaneous cells; recurrent infection involves stratified epithelial cells. Stressor stimuli trigger recurrent infection (Fig. 29-2). Fever, another infection, emotions, menstruation, intercourse, and ultraviolet light are some common stressors. Infections seem to be more severe in the woman during pregnancy.

HSV is diagnosed by cytologic testing and microscopic examination. A Papanicolaou smear of the lesion shows multinucleated giant cells with ground-glass nuclear appearance and cervical dysplasia. A wet-mount preparation of lesion secretions reveals polymorphonuclear leukocytes.

HSV infections may involve external genitals, the vagina, and cervix. Symptoms are more pronounced with first infections of HSV. Painful blisters form (Fig. 29-3), rupture, and then drain, leaving shallow ulcers that crust over and disappear after 2 to 6 weeks. A vaginal discharge is seen if the cervix or vaginal mucosa is involved. The woman may have fever, malaise, anorexia, painful inguinal lymphadenopathy, dysuria, and dyspareunia.

Recurrences sometimes are preceded by itching, a burning sensation in the genital area, tingling in the legs, or a slight increase in vaginal discharge. Repeated recurrence may result in keratitis, encephalitis, and possibly cervical carcinoma, although most recurrences tend to be milder and shorter in duration.

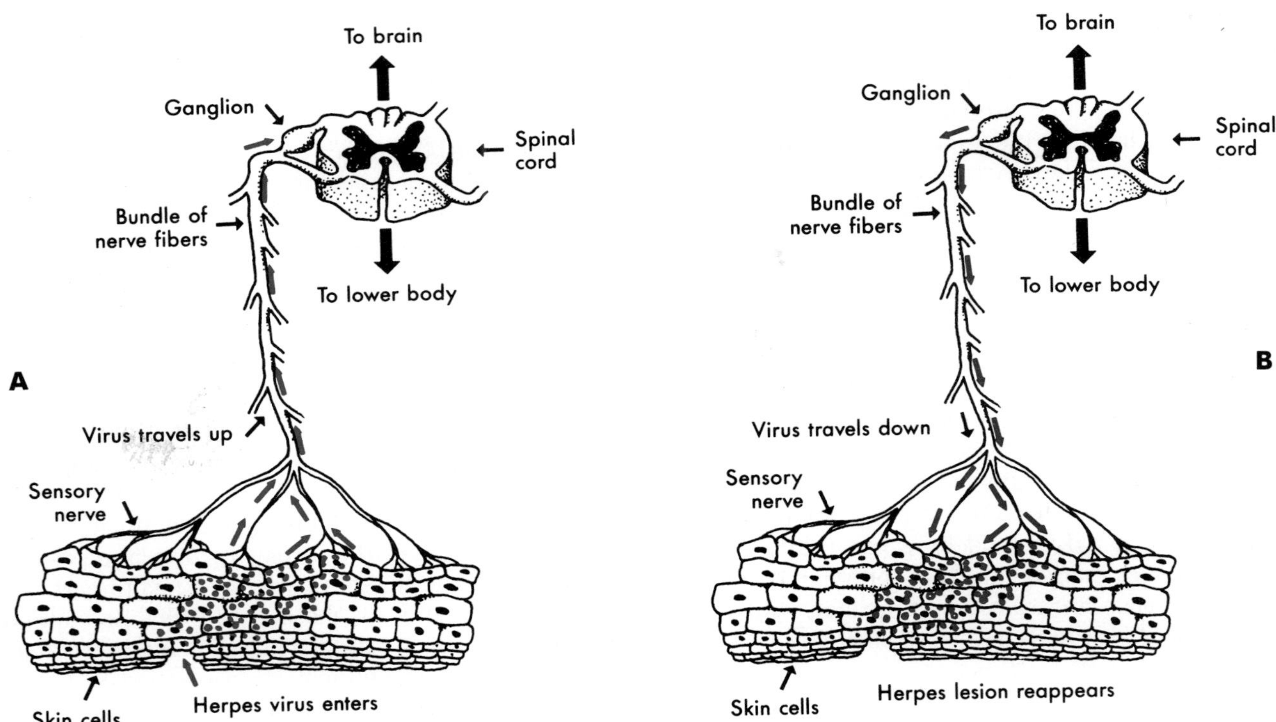

Fig. 29-2 **A,** Initial herpes infection takes place when virus (colored dots) enters cells of mucous membranes, eyes, or skin. They reproduce and travel up (colored arrows) the sensory nerves until they reach a ganglion (cluster of nerve cell bodies). There they are protected by the body's immune system, which overcomes the infection at the place of entry. **B,** Though the entry wound soon heals, when conditions allow, the virus may later travel back down the nerve pathway to reinfect skin cells again.

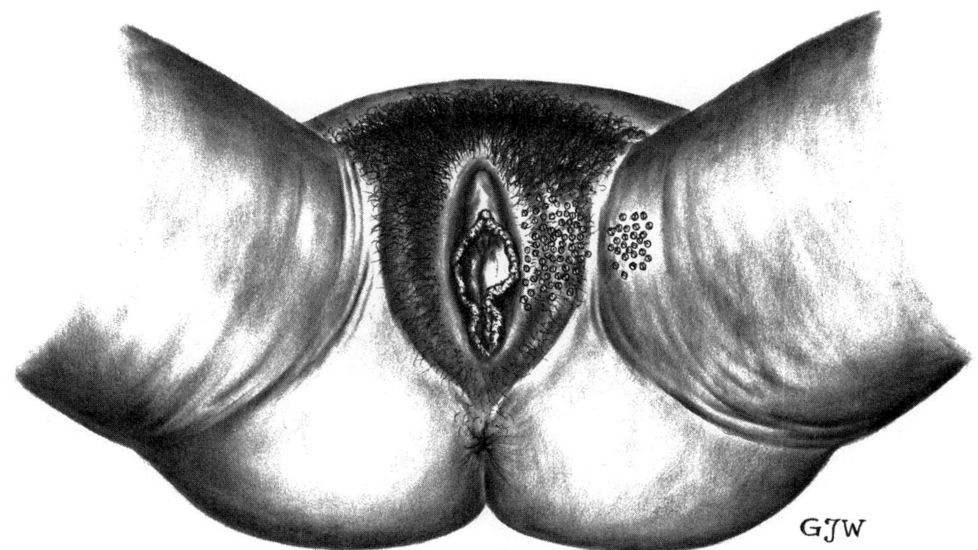

Fig. 29-3 Herpes genitalis.

The *pregnancy effects* of primary genital herpes infection include spontaneous abortion, preterm labor, and intrauterine growth retardation (IUGR). The likelihood of a poor outcome increases with advancing gestational age (Brown, Baker, 1989). The frequency and severity of recurrent infection also appear to increase with gestation (Brown et al, 1985).

The route of HSV transmission from mother to newborn is via an infected birth canal during birth. The risk of maternal-infant transmission is greater during a primary HSV-2 infection than during a recurrent episode (Corey, 1990). Cesarean birth is no longer recommended for all mothers with HSV because transplacental infection can occur. Only those mothers with clinical evidence of active lesions should give birth abdominally (Corey, 1990).

Fetal and neonatal effects are serious. Microcephaly, mental retardation, retinal dysplasia, patent ductus arteriosus, and intracranial calcification are sequelae. After intranatal infection, signs appear in 4 to 7 days. The signs include lethargy, poor feeding, jaundice, bleeding, pneumonia, convulsions, opisthotonus, bulging fontanelles, and skin and mouth lesions. Neonatal infection with disseminated disease results in 82% mortality. Survivors have CNS or ocular sequelae and face recurrence in the first 5 years of life.

Acyclovir has been used since 1977 to treat life-threatening HSV infections in adults and newborns. However, data are not clear regarding safety or efficacy in pregnancy (Brown, Baker, 1989). Treatment of symptoms consists of acetaminophen for fever and malaise and 5% lidocaine ointment, 5% acyclovir ointment, or warm soaks for lesion discomfort.

Infection control measures are an important part of treatment. Thorough hand washing should be practiced by health care providers as well as by family members. Gloves should be worn during contact with lesions or secretions. Family members with oral lesions should be discouraged from kissing the newborn. Instruction on genital hygiene and prevention of infection also should be given (see teaching box, p. 863).

Many health care centers differ on isolation policies for infants of mothers with HSV infection. In general, infants born to mothers at risk of transmitting the infection (i.e., mothers who give birth vaginally with active lesions) should be isolated by rooming-in with the mother or by enclosure in an incubator.

Health care providers with HSV infections also should take precautions. Anyone with oral HSV lesions should wear a mask if in close contact with newborns, and anyone with skin lesions (herpetic whitlow) should not give direct care until lesions are dried and crusted.

HUMAN PAPILLOMAVIRUS. **Condylomata acuminata,** sexually transmitted lesions caused by **human papillomavirus (HPV),** is the most common viral sexually transmitted infection—three times greater than genital herpes (Oriel, 1990). More than 50 HPVs infect skin and mucosal surfaces, with HPV-6, HPV-11, and HPV-16 most commonly infecting the genital tract (Ferenczy, 1987; Oriel, 1990; Shah, 1990).

Disease occurs at the entry site of the virus after

an incubation period of 2 to 3 months. *HPV is disseminated by skin-to-skin contact, not through body fluid exchange.* Exposure to the virus is by sexual contact with an infected partner; multiple partners increase the likelihood of HPV infection. Others at risk include smokers and oral contraceptive users, presumably related to the suppressive effects on the immune system. HPV is clinically significant because various types are associated with congenitally derived respiratory papillomatosis in children (see Chapter 39) and with cervical carcinoma.

Condyloma acuminatum causes dry, wartlike growths on the vulva, vagina, cervix, or rectum (Fig. 29-4). These growths may be small or large, single or multiple, or have a cauliflower appearance. Chronic vaginal discharge, pruritus, or dyspareunia can occur. Diagnosis is by colposcopy and direct visualization of the growths, by biopsy, or by presence of koilocytes (nuclear abnormalities in squamous cervical epithelium) seen in Papanicolaou smears.

In the immunocompetent person, condylomata acuminata may regress spontaneously. In many persons, however, the condition is difficult to treat. Available therapy is primarily cytotoxic or destructive. *Cytotoxic* agents are podophyllin (podophyllum resin) and 5-fluorouracil (5-FU). Podophyllin, 20% to 30% in tincture of benzoin, is used for lesions 2 cm or less in diameter, but not in the vagina or on the cervix. Petrolatum is used to protect surrounding skin because podophyllin is caustic and cytotoxic. The woman must wash the medication off after 4 hours or sooner if burning occurs. She is treated weekly for 6 weeks. Therapy may not produce a cure. The recurrence rate is 70%. *Podophyllin is not to be used during pregnancy.* The use of podophyllin during pregnancy is associated with fetal death and preterm labor. The more effective cytotoxic agent is 5-FU in 5% cream. This highly toxic agent is used for resistant condyloma. The cure rate approaches 90%. There are no systemic effects when it is administered topically inasmuch as only 5% to 6% is absorbed. Local pain and epithelial erosions are side effects of local application. Treatment with 5-FU is most effective when used in conjunction with laser therapy.

The most effective *destructive* method is a carbon dioxide laser* used with local anesthesia. It is precise and sterile and is accompanied by minimum bleeding and trauma. The treated area does not regain its normal pigmentation for several years. Post–laser therapy instruction follows.

1. Keep area clean by irrigating with warm water twice a day.
2. Dry with electric hair dryer.
3. Apply antibacterial cream twice a day.

*There is some new evidence that those women whose warts were treated with laser surgery were almost twice as likely to develop precancerous lesions as those who were not treated at all. Even more alarming was the finding that these lesions grew faster in the laser-treated women than in the control group (*San Francisco Chronicle,* Feb 1992).

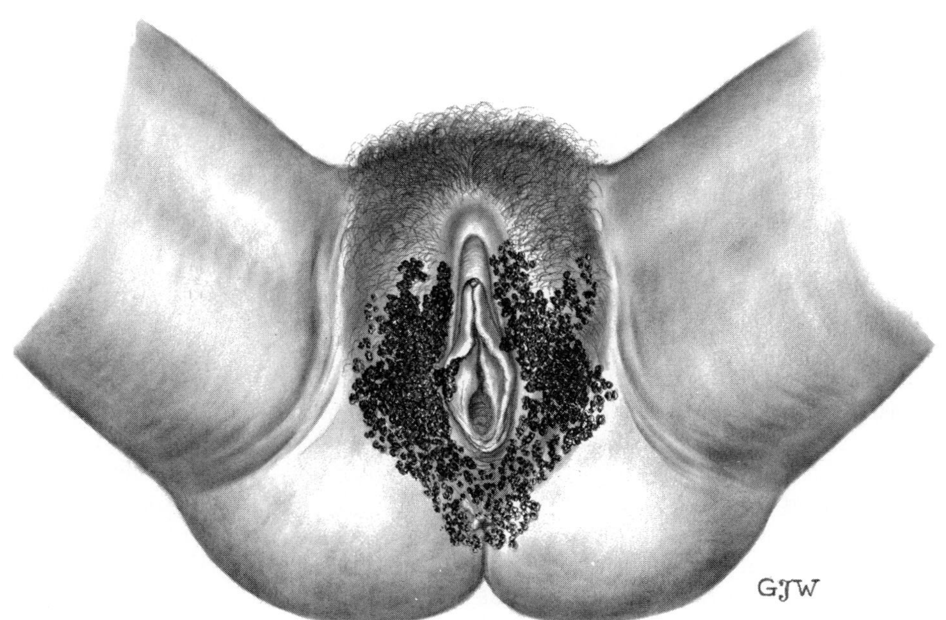

Fig. 29-4 Human papillomavirus infection. Condylomata acuminata.

4. Use gauze dressing to prevent rubbing against clothing.
5. Use lidocaine ointment 5% for discomfort.
6. Return to clinic as instructed.
7. Use latex condoms until disease is cured in the woman. Today condoms are dense enough to prevent passage of viruses (500 A° = size of HPV).

Trichloroacetic acid, 50% solution, is a destructive therapy that is somewhat safer to use than podophyllin. It can be self-applied with a cotton swab and does not need to be washed off. Cryotherapy with liquid nitrogen also is used with some success for external condyloma.

Additional therapies for the treatment of condyloma acuminatum include the antiviral substance interferon. Intralesional and intramuscular preparations have been used with varied success. However, the side effects of medication often are severe and include fever, chills, headache, myalgia, fatigue, and leukopenia.

About 30% of pregnant women harbor HPV in the genital tract (Ferenczy, 1987). *Pregnancy effects* of HPV infection include proliferation and increased friability of lesions. Many experts recommend removal of large, outward-growing lesions during pregnancy; carbon dioxide laser treatments have been used between 30 and 32 weeks' gestation. Treatment usually is followed by vaginal birth without complications (Ferenczy, 1984, 1987). Cesarean birth is indicated when the pelvic outlet is obstructed or when vaginal birth would result in excessive blood loss.

The primary *neonatal effect* of HPV infection is respiratory or laryngeal papillomatosis (see Chapter 39). The exact route of perinatal transmission is unknown, and disagreement exists as to the preferred mode of birth. Some infants born by cesarean have developed respiratory papillomatosis. However, the estimated risk of an infant developing papillomatosis after vaginal birth in a mother with active condyloma is 1/400 (Kashima et al, 1990). The mother should make an informed decision regarding vaginal or cesarean birth.

STDs present a special challenge to health care providers. Diagnosis often is difficult because multiple STDs may be present at any given time. Treatment of STDs frequently is delayed as a result of fear, concern for social stigma, and denial of or lack of knowledge about symptoms.

Bacterial STD reinfection rates are high because of failure to comply with or to complete treatment regimens. With viral STDs, once the infection enters the body, a person is always infected and the virus cycles through dormant and active phases. Follow-up after infection and treatment is crucial to avoid potentially harmful sequelae to mothers and their neonates. However, many choose to seek care only when symptoms occur.

■ NURSING PROCESS

ASSESSMENT

A comprehensive assessment focuses on some life-style issues that may be personal or sensitive. A nonjudgmental approach is essential for facilitating accurate data collection. Assessment includes the following key areas.

HISTORY. Factors that influence the development and management of STDs during pregnancy include a previous history of STD or PID, the number of current sexual partners, the amount of intercourse per week, and anticipated sexual activity through the pregnancy. Life-style choices also may affect STD in the perinatal period. Mothers who are intravenous drug users or who have partners who use intravenous drugs are at risk. Other life-style factors that increase susceptibility to STD (through suppressive effects on the immune system) include smoking, alcohol use, inadequate or poor nutrition, and high levels of fatigue or personal stress.

PHYSICAL EXAMINATION. Findings on examination vary. Some STDs may be asymptomatic. Vaginal discharge may or may not be present, and vesicles or sores may be unnoticed. Fever or pain may be mild and therefore dismissed. A thorough symptom assessment, coupled with a complete history and physical examination, is essential in identifying possible STD.

LABORATORY TESTS. Bacterial STDs are easily determined from genital tract, urine, and blood studies. Viral agents also can be cultured but less successfully. An elevated white blood cell count (WBC) may be a diagnostic help: other laboratory tests are useful depending on what other infectious agents are suspected. (The box on p. 862 describes assessment for the woman suspected of having an STD.)

NURSING DIAGNOSES

Nursing diagnoses are derived after carefully analyzing assessment findings, medical management, and physician's directives. Several examples of nursing diagnoses follow:

Assessment for the Woman at Risk for Sexually Transmitted Disease

HISTORY

Chief complaint
Description of the present illness, including symptoms, self-care treatment, use of prescribed or over-the-counter medications
Sexual history, including previous history of STD, number of current sexual partners, typical frequency of sexual activity
Life-style: use of intravenous drugs or partner who uses intravenous drugs; smoking, alcohol, poor nutrition, high level of stress
General health: date of last menstrual period, date of last Pap smear, history of contraception

PHYSICAL EXAMINATION

Inspection
Palpation

LABORATORY TESTS*

Saline wet preparation *(Trichomonas)*
Potassium hydroxide wet preparation (candidiasis, *Gardnerella*)
Urinalysis
Gonorrhea culture
Cervical culture
Herpes cervical culture
Pap smear
Complete blood cell count
VDRL test
Herpes simplex virus type 1 and 2 antibodies
Western blot—HIV
Chlamydia—culture or antigen detection test

Modified from Smith LS, Lauver D, Gray PA Jr: Sexually transmitted disease. In Fogel CI, Lauver D, editors: *Sexual health promotion*, Philadelphia, 1989, WB Saunders, p 460.
*Choice depends on specific STD.

- Pain/impaired tissue integrity related to
  —Effects of infection process
  —Scratching (excoriation) of pruritic areas
  —Hygienic practices
- Knowledge deficit related to
  —Transmission/prevention of infection/reinfection
  —Safer sex behaviors
  —Management and course of infection
- Anxiety/low self-esteem/body image disturbance related to
  —Perceived effects on sexual relationships and family processes
  —Possible effects on pregnancy/fetus
  —Long-term sequelae to infection
  High risk for altered parenting related to
  —Fear of spread to newborn

PLANNING

Planning for care of the client focuses on both physical and psychosocial needs. Avoidance of reinfection and harmful sequelae in the perinatal period is critical. Nursing care *goals* or expected outcomes are mutually derived with the woman's input. These measurable goals, stated in client-centered terms, may include the following:

1. The woman will be free of infection, or in the case of viral infection, she will experience remission or stabilization of the infection.
2. The mother will identify and be able to state the etiology, management, and expected course of the infection and its prevention.
3. The fetus/neonate will be born free of the infection or its sequelae, or, will experience minimal sequelae.

IMPLEMENTATION

Discussion of measures to avoid reinfection is essential. Topics of instruction should include proper medication administration; "safer" sex practices; genital hygiene; and principles of adequate nutrition, rest, and stress reduction (see boxes on "safer" sex, p. 863, and on genital hygiene, p. 863).

EVALUATION

Evaluation of client outcomes is a continuous process. To be effective, evaluation is based on client-centered goals identified during the planning stage of nursing care. The nurse can be reasonably assured

TEACHING "Safer" Sex

- "Safer" sex is possible only if there is no oral or genital exchange of body fluids.
- Correct use of condoms, while greatly reducing risk, is not exclusively protective.
- Use of spermicides containing nonoxynol 9 may offer additional protection.
- Select sexual partners with extreme care.
- Ask partner about past history of STDs.

TEACHING Genital Hygiene

- Wash hands before and after genital contact.
- After urination or defecation, wipe and cleanse with a single front-to-back motion and discard tissue.
- Change sanitary napkins (pads) and tampons frequently as directed and after every use of bathroom.
- Scrub and rinse tub before and after bathing.

that care was effective to the extent that goals were met; that is:

- The woman is free of infection, or her infection is stabilized and she does not become reinfected.
- The woman knows the etiology, management, and expected course of the infection and its prevention.
- The fetus/neonate is born free of the infection or its sequelae or experiences only minimal sequelae.

See case study p. 864 and nursing plan of care, p. 865

■ GENITAL TRACT INFECTIONS

Genital tract infections are among the most common medical problems in adult women. Vaginal discharge and dysuria are symptoms that cause women to seek treatment from health care providers. However, some of these infections remain asymptomatic. Anatomy predisposes women to greater risk from urogenital infection and also accounts for greater difficulty in diagnosis and treatment. Genital tract infections often are described as vaginal or urinary tract, depending on the primary sites affected.

Vaginal Infections

Any irritating vaginal discharge should be evaluated promptly and appropriate treatment initiated immediately. The three most common vaginal infections are bacterial vaginosis, candidiasis, and trichomoniasis. However, management of vaginal infections becomes more complicated if multiple organisms or agents are involved. Pediculosis pubis, threadworm, varicosities, and allergic response to perineal deodorants may obstruct the differential diagnosis and management. The discomfort imposed by these conditions challenges the woman's emotional, as well as her physical, well-being.

Infections must be distinguished from the normal vaginal discharge, leukorrhea. **Leukorrhea** is a whitish discharge. It consists of mucus and exfoliated vaginal epithelial cells as a result of hyperplasia of the vaginal mucosa such as occurs during pregnancy, at the time of ovulation, and just before menstruation. If it is copious, it can cause discomfort from maceration.

Vaginal infections may be sexually transmitted. Trichomonal vaginitis and monilial vaginitis are considered to be sexually transmitted in most but not all cases. Altered vaginal physiology during pregnancy also may precipitate **vaginitis** (inflammation of the vagina). Vaginal secretions are increased, and the vagina is less acidic during pregnancy. These conditions provide an environment that promotes microbial growth.

SIMPLE VAGINITIS. Infectious organisms such as *Escherichia coli,* staphylococci, and streptococci change the normal acidity of the vagina. A pH of 3.5 to 4.5 is needed to support Döderlein's bacillus, the vagina's main line of defense. The proximity of the urethra to the vagina predisposes the woman with vaginitis to a concurrent urethritis.

Burning, **pruritus** (itching), redness, and edema of surrounding tissues are characteristic of simple vaginitis. These symptoms are particularly discomforting during voiding and defecating.

Objectives of management of simple vaginitis are to relieve discomfort, to eradicate offending organisms and thereby foster growth of Döderlein's bacillus, and to prevent recurrence. During pregnancy, acetaminophen may be used for discomfort. Some topical creams such as hydrocortisone may relieve discomfort from tissue excoriation. Antibiotics are prescribed for treatment of specific organisms; eradication of microorganisms helps to restore vaginal acidity. Effects on the fetus from these therapies are minimal.

ATROPHIC VAGINITIS. Low estrogen levels, such as those that occur during preadolescence and lactation

CASE STUDY

Sexually Transmitted Disease

Elizabeth Cox, a 28-year-old married gravida 3, para 2-0-0-2, is at 25 weeks' gestation. She has been admitted to the antepartum unit with a primary diagnosis of pneumonia and a secondary diagnosis of chlamydial infection. Elizabeth's prenatal course is significant for a reactive HIV test at 22 weeks' gestation.

ASSESSMENT

Elizabeth states during the admission interview that she has "felt tired" for the last week and can hardly breathe. She has had vaginal discharge, tenderness, and burning for 1 week but is now concerned about her vaginal bleeding. As the nurse completes the interview, Elizabeth states: "I just don't understand why I feel so bad. I never felt this way with my other babies."

On physical assessment, the nurse observes that Elizabeth's skin is very warm and flushed but with normal skin turgor. Vital signs are temperature 101° F (39° C), pulse 110 beats/min (up from her normal rate of 80 beats/min), respirations 28/min (her usual rate is 22), and blood pressure 100/60 mm Hg (normal for her). Auscultation of Elizabeth's lungs reveals scattered basilar crackles (rales), and she reports a dry, persistent cough. Fetal heart tones are elevated to 170 beats/min.

Elizabeth is wearing a sanitary pad that shows purulent discharge containing small amounts of blood. Her labia are excoriated and tender to the touch. No uterine contractions are reported or palpated, and other physical findings are normal.

Laboratory results include a WBC of 9800/mm^3 and urine and cervical cultures that are positive for chlamydia. Chest films show findings consistent with *Pneumocystis carinii* pneumonia. (NOTE: Clients with HIV and pneumonia frequently show a "normal" WBC. Because HIV infection represents an immunosuppressed state, the WBC may drop to 2500/mm^3 in the presence of opportunistic infections.)

NURSING DIAGNOSIS

Elizabeth's history of fatigue, as well as fever, tachycardia (in mother and baby), increased respirations, and x-ray evidence of pneumonia, helps the nurse to identify the following nursing diagnosis: altered respiratory function/ineffective breathing patterns related to infection.

PLANNING

Elizabeth and the nurse develop a plan of care. Together they agree that Elizabeth's nursing care *goal* is that she will demonstrate improved respiratory function and will be less fatigued. *Expected outcomes* set by the nurse include effective respirations and resolution of infection, as evidenced by return of vital signs to normal, clear lung sounds, stable WBC count, and the client's report of how she is feeling.

IMPLEMENTATION

Nursing actions are based on the prescribed medical management, physician's orders, and the nursing diagnosis. Specific interventions include ongoing assessment of client status and vital signs, including FHR, presence and quality of cough, and lung sounds. Laboratory study results are monitored and abnormalities reported to the physician. The nurse also monitors prescribed IV therapy and administers antibiotic therapy as ordered. Adequate fluid and nutritional intake also is assessed.

EVALUATION

Goals and *expected outcomes* are used to evaluate the effectiveness of nursing interventions. Elizabeth remained on the antepartum unit for 8 days. Her fever continued to spike until the fourth hospital day. Intravenous (IV) fluid therapy continued until the fifth hospital day at which time her peripheral line was converted to a heparin lock for continued IV antibiotic therapy. By the fifth day her vital signs and the FHR were within normal limits and her WBC count had stabilized. By discharge, lung sounds were improved but not totally clear, and Elizabeth was discharged on a regimen of oral antibiotics. Her cough was present but less frequent. Elizabeth stated she felt much better than she did when she came to the hospital and was glad to be going home. On the basis of these findings, the goal set by the client and the nurse was met. (See related nursing plan of care, p. 865.)

CARE PLAN Sexually Transmitted Infections

GOAL	INTERVENTIONS	RATIONALE	EVALUATION
Nursing diagnosis: Altered respiratory function/ineffective breathing patterns related to infection*			
Elizabeth reestablishes effective breathing patterns as evidenced by return of vital signs (including FHR) to WNL for client; improved/clear lung sounds; white blood cell count WNL for client	Assess and document vital signs (including FHR). Monitor laboratory values, and report abnormalities. Assess and record presence and quality of cough or sputum; assess and record lung sounds. Administer IV therapy and antibiotics per physician's order. Accurately record intake and output.	Ongoing assessment of vital signs, respiratory conditions, and laboratory values provides data used to plan and evaluate interventions.	Elizabeth reestablishes effective breathing; her work of breathing is decreased and she states that she is less fatigued.
	Assess for adequate nutritional intake. Encourage fluid intake. Provide for sleep and rest as needed.	Adequate fluid intake, a nutritious diet, and sleep/rest are important to support recovery.	
Nursing diagnosis: Altered health maintenance related to lack of knowledge of prevention of STD			
Elizabeth's restoration of health maintenance is evidenced by her expressed understanding of STD transmission, causes, and symptoms and by her willingness to use practices to prevent STD transmission.	Assess Elizabeth's current knowledge of STD. Assess Elizabeth's readiness to learn. Provide factual information on STD transmission, causes, symptoms, and transmission. Discuss/display methods for protection during any sexual activity (see box on teaching "safer" sex, p. 863). Offer instruction in an open and nonjudgmental manner. Allow for Elizabeth's privacy. Discuss options for the notification of potentially infected sexual partners. Encourage Elizabeth to express her feelings and concerns; answer questions directly.	Assessment of Elizabeth's current knowledge provides an opportunity for the correction of misinformation and is the basis for the teaching plan. Factual, direct information, presented with consideration of educational abilities, is necessary in the prevention and treatment of STDs. An open, nonjudgmental environment facilitates learning and promotes Elizabeth's self-esteem and self-worth. Sexuality and STDs are personal and sensitive topics.	Elizabeth's restoration of health is accomplished; Elizabeth verbalizes an understanding of STD transmission, causes, and symptoms; and states intent to prevent STD transmssion.
Nursing diagnosis: Impaired tissue integrity related to irritation from vaginal discharge			
Elizabeth's tissue integrity is restored as evidenced by replacement of damaged tissue with healthy tissue.	Assess, monitor, and record characteristics of the damaged area, including color, lesions, drainage, and edema.	Information on the characteristics of the affected area establishes the basis with which to plan and evaluate interventions.	Elizabeth verbalizes understanding of hygiene and complies with prescribed treatment.

Continued.

CARE PLAN Sexually Transmitted Infections—cont'd

GOAL	INTERVENTIONS	RATIONALE	EVALUATION
	Instruct Elizabeth in genital hygiene practices (see box on teaching genital hygiene, p. 863.) Provide warm soaks or sitz baths. Instruct Elizabeth to dry the genital area with a blow dryer (with the temperature on a cool setting). Administer prescribed medications per physician's order.	Meticulous genital hygiene prevents infection of damaged tissue from other organisms. Comfort and healing are promoted.	Elizabeth's tissue integrity is restored.

FHR, Fetal heart rate; *IV*, intravenous; *WNL*, within normal limits.
*Potential complication: pneumonia as collaborative diagnosis.

and after menopause, result in a thin vaginal lining. Infection may occur from the normal vaginal flora. Antibiotics and hormone replacement therapy comprise this therapy.

CERVICITIS. Abnormal discharge may be due to an infection of the cervix and not to vaginitis. Spotting of blood between periods or after intercourse, as well as cramping during intercourse, is characteristic. Sexually transmitted gonorrhea, chlamydia, or herpetic infections are the usual infections implicated. Therapy is specific to the causative microbe.

BACTERIAL VAGINOSIS. The most common cause of vaginal symptoms among childbearing women is bacterial vaginosis, also referred to as nonspecific vaginitis. By-products of bacterial metabolism affect vaginal pH, thus altering the flora of the vagina. The predominant microorganism is *Gardnerella vaginalis*. However, vaginal fluid cultures reveal mixed organisms that also include genital mycoplasmas and anaerobes such as *Peptostreptococcus* and bacteroides. Diagnosis is based on clinical signs. The vaginal fluid pH is elevated, usually ≥4.5. The homogeneous vaginal discharge has an amine (fishy) odor when mixed with 10% potassium hydroxide. "Clue cells" are seen on microscopic examination of vaginal discharge.

The *maternal effect* of infection with this bacterium is usually a mild illness. The bacterial vaginosis is expressed by a milklike discharge. Itching, burning, and pain may be present in the vagina and around the introitus. Obstetric complications can occur, especially in untreated cases. Amniotic fluid infection, premature rupture of membranes (PROM), preterm labor and birth, and postpartum endometritis have been linked to this infection. Bacterial vaginosis also may be a risk factor for PID. *Fetal and neonatal effects* include septicemia and death.

Treatment of bacterial vaginosis is most effective with oral metronidazole. However, because of its potential teratogenic effects, metronidazole should be given only in the second and third trimester. Topical preparations of metronidazole and clindamycin also have been used to successfully treat the condition. Although sexual partners usually are treated, disagreement exists as to the actual effectiveness of treating partners.

VULVOVAGINAL CANDIDIASIS. Vulvovaginal candidiasis or candidal vaginitis occurs throughout the world, particularly in hot, subtropical climates. Most trends suggest that the disease is increasing, in part a result of the widespread use of antimicrobial agents. Similarly, the number of healthy, symptom-free women who harbor *Candida* organisms also is increasing. Several factors are noted, including pregnancy, use of high-estrogen oral contraceptives, and uncontrolled diabetes mellitus. Additional factors that precipitate candidiasis are steroid or immunosuppressive therapy; immunocompromised states (e.g., AIDS); restrictive, tight, or poorly ventilated clothing; and poor genital hygiene.

Most yeast-like organisms isolated from the vagina are *Candida albicans,* a fungus normally found in the intestines. The second most common yeast is *Torulopsis glabrata,* which accounts for approximately one fourth of candidal vaginitis (Redondo-Lopez et al, 1990). The thick vaginal discharge is irritating and pruritic. Dysuria and dyspareunia are common complaints. Speculum examination usually reveals thick, white, tenacious cheeselike patches adhering to the pale, dry, and sometimes cyanotic vaginal mucosa.

Maternal effects of vaginal candidiasis usually are not health threatening, but affected mothers may be extremely uncomfortable from the pain, itching, and vaginal discharge. Pregnancy predisposes women not only to an increased rate of infection but also to increased recurrences and increased treatment failures. Recurrent candidal vaginitis in the antepartum period necessitates screening for gestational diabetes and AIDS, if appropriate. Treatment goals include measures to relieve symptoms and topical or vaginal antifungal agents such as clotrimazole.

Fetal and neonatal effects are limited to infection acquired by direct contact from the birth canal or from the contaminated hands of caregivers. However, *Candida* organisms have been isolated from the nipples of a breast-feeding mother whose infant also was infected (Johnstone, Marcinak, 1990). Oral candidiasis, or thrush, is the most commonly seen *C. albicans* infection in newborns and usually is treated with nystatin.

TRICHOMONIASIS. *Trichomonas vaginalis* is a hearty protozoan that thrives in an alkaline milieu. The role of sexual contact in the transmission of *T. vaginalis* is well documented; trichomoniasis is prevalent in approximately 30% of sexually active women (Rein, Müller, 1990).

In symptom-free persons the infection may be identified during a routine examination or with a Papanicolaou smear. *T. vaginalis* has an affinity for mucous membranes, and 75% of infected women report a vaginal discharge that may be malodorous. This profuse, frothy discharge usually is gray or yellow-green and may stream from the vagina when a speculum is inserted.

The vaginal walls appear erythematous with small hemorrhagic sites. The vulva usually is irritated, edematous, and excoriated. Other affected sites include the urethra and Skene's glands, and common complaints include pruritus, urinary frequency, dysuria, lower abdominal pain, and dyspareunia (painful intercourse). Asymptomatic male partners may harbor *T. vaginalis* in the urogenital tract and remain a source of reinfection if untreated.

Trichomoniasis seems to have few *maternal effects* other than symptomatic discomfort. However, perinatal infection by *T. vaginalis* is the most frequent form of nonvenereal transmission of disease. *Fetal and neonatal effects* include fever and irritability. The preferred treatment, administration of metronidazole, should be administered to pregnant women only in the second and third trimesters.

GROUP B STREPTOCOCCI. Group B streptococcal bacterial infections are gaining recognition as an important factor in perinatal and neonatal morbidity and mortality. The vertical transmission rate of infection from mother to infant near the time of birth ranges between 50% and 75% (Hill, 1990). Women with preterm labor or PROM are at increased risk for maternal infection as well as neonatal infection.

Asymptomatic group B streptococcal colonization often occurs in both sexes. Group B infections may be sexually transmitted, and reinfection occurs frequently between partners. Common colonization sites include the urethra, cervix, vagina, and rectum. Sequelae of infection include vaginitis, urethritis, cervicitis, cystitis, and pyelonephritis.

Maternal effects include miscarriage, stillbirth, scarlet fever, preterm birth, fever, septicemia, and puerperal infection (see also the discussion of bacteremic shock in this chapter). *Fetal and neonatal effects* are also serious; group B streptococcal infections are the leading cause of neonatal sepsis and meningitis. Signs of sepsis generally are present within 72 hours after birth and gram-positive cocci may be isolated from the umbilicus, the ear, the rectum, blood, and tracheal and gastric aspirates. Other neonatal effects include blindness, deafness, mental retardation, learning disabilities, and death.

Treatment of group B streptococcal infections is accomplished with penicillin, ampicillin, cephalothin, or erythromycin. Prophylaxis of mothers and neonates at risk for infection also is encouraged.

■ URINARY TRACT INFECTIONS

Lower Urinary Tract Infections: Cystitis, Urethritis

Urinary tract infection (UTI) affects about 10% of pregnant women, most of these in the prenatal period. Those who have had UTIs previously are especially prone to recurrence during pregnancy. Cervicitis, vaginitis, obstruction of the flaccid ureters (particularly on the right because of pressure by the pregnant uterus against the slightly dilated flaccid ureters), vesicoureteral reflux, and the trauma of birth predispose the pregnant women to UTI, generally from *E. coli*. Women with chronic STDs, especially gonorrhea and chlamydia, also are at risk. Asymptomatic bacteriuria occurs in about 5% to 15% of all pregnant women. If untreated, pyelonephritis during gestation will develop in approximately 30% of these women. Premature labor and birth may be more common also.

Urine culture and sensitivity tests should be obtained early in pregnancy, preferably at the first visit, from a clean-catch urine specimen. Catheterization should be avoided if possible. If infection is diagnosed, treatment with an appropriate antibiotic drug for 2 to 3 weeks, together with forced fluids and urinary tract antispasmodic medication (e.g., belladonna derivatives), is recommended. Infections caused by the colon aerogenic organisms generally respond well to sulfisoxazole (Gantrisin) or nitrofurantoin. Treatment should be continued for 2 to 3 weeks until two negative cultures are obtained, and the infant should be observed for hyperbilirubinemia (see Chapter 39). Retreatment of the mother may be necessary if there is a recurrence. Acute pyelonephritis may be confused with appendicitis, cholecystitis, or preterm labor.

If infection persists or recurs, performing a urologic investigation will be necessary to identify contributory causes such as urinary tract obstruction, stones (*nephroureterolithiasis*), diverticula, tuberculosis, or poor personal hygiene. Pregnancy causes dilation of the renal hilum and calyces so that small stones often are lodged, and most of these pass painfully. Whether urinary stones form more readily during pregnancy because of urinary stasis, hypercholesterolemia, or increased calciuria and vitamin D is still debated.

Pyelonephritis

Pyelonephritis is caused by a bacterium. Some maternal infections are asymptomatic. Acute pyelonephritis is distinguished by urinary frequency, urgency, pyuria, dysuria, chills, fever, and backache. Costovertebral angle tenderness and tenderness over the affected kidney are experienced. *Fetal and neonatal effects* are serious. Acute pyelonephritis commonly is associated with preterm labor (Scott et al, 1990). The newborn is then exposed to the hazards of prematurity. Treatment with penicillin or cephalosporin and adequate hydration are warranted. Therapy with sulfonamides may cause icterus, hemolytic anemia, and kernicterus. The newborn also may be at risk for IUGR. Nitrofurantoin therapy for the mother during pregnancy may lead to megaloblastic anemia or glucose-6-phosphate dehydrogenase (G6PD) deficiency in the newborn. Acidifying the urine with high doses of ascorbic acid during pregnancy should be avoided. The fetus can become conditioned to a high vitamin C environment and develop scurvy in the neonatal period (Scott et al, 1990). The women who are most vulnerable to UTI are first-time mothers, women with difficult labors, and women with diabetes mellitus or sickle cell disease.

Glomerulonephritis

Acute glomerulonephritis is a rare complication of pregnancy. It is characterized by proteinuria, hematuria, edema, and hypertension. Treatment requires antibiotic therapy, bed rest (in side-lying or semi- to high-Fowler's position to facilitate renal perfusion), and fluid-electrolyte and dietary control. Pregnancy does not seriously affect acute early glomerulonephritis.

Women with mild, inactive glomerulonephritis generally can go through pregnancy safely. Women with progressive, chronic glomerulonephritis—that is, severe renal damage associated with proteinuria, hypertension, and an elevated blood urea nitrogen (BUN) level—do not tolerate pregnancy well. If pregnancy is not interrupted, spontaneous abortion is likely; preeclampsia and eclampsia often supervene, and fetal death may result. Cardiac or renal failure generally is the cause of maternal death.

Postpartum Urinary Tract Infections

Postnatal UTIs usually are caused by coliform bacteria. UTIs are common because of trauma to the base of the bladder and urethra and catheterization during or after labor.

Suprapubic or costovertebral angle pain, fever, urinary retention, hematuria, dysuria, or urinary frequency often signifies UTI. These symptoms indicate the need for urinalysis, urine culture, bacterial sensitivity tests, and probable wide-spectrum antibiotic therapy. Substitution of a specific antibacterial drug must await an assessment of the woman's history, response to initial therapy, and the sensitivity report.

Prompt treatment of definite UTIs is indicated. However, prophylactic therapy rarely is warranted. Most cases respond to treatment within a week. Urologic consultation is indicated if symptoms persist. Prevention of recurrence of UTI is an important part of therapy. (See Chapter 11 for information on teaching UTI prevention.)

■ NURSING PROCESS

ASSESSMENT

Prevention, diagnosis, and treatment of genital tract infections often is a complicated task. The following components provide a complete assessment.

HISTORY. Preconceptional or antenatal factors that influence the development of vaginal or UTIs include a history of chronic UTIs or kidney infection and kidney stones; chronic conditions that impair kidney function (e.g., lupus, diabetes, sickle cell disease); chronic immunosuppressive states (e.g., steroid therapy, AIDS); poor fluid and nutritional status; failure to use condoms; and poor genital hygiene. (Proper wiping and cleansing of the genital area with a single front-to-back motion is one of the most important points to communicate to clients.) Intrapartum events such as frequent catheterizations (especially with the use of epidural anesthesia); frequent vaginal examinations; prolonged second stage of labor; and birth trauma to the vagina, cervix, bladder, and urethra also may place the mother at greater risk for infection.

PHYSICAL EXAMINATION. Vaginal discharge (malodorous or not) is common on physical examination. Other physical findings include perineal edema, excoriation, erythema, and pruritus. When the urinary tract is affected, findings may include dysuria, suprapubic or costovertebral angle discomfort, backache, fever and chills, hematuria, and impaired urinary function.

LABORATORY TESTS. Definitive culture results are helpful in determining causative agents and identifying teaching needs to prevent further infections. Other laboratory data to assess include hematocrit or hemoglobin levels, WBC, proteinuria, and BUN.

NURSING DIAGNOSES

Nursing diagnoses are derived from current knowledge about UTI, medical management, and physician's directives and after carefully analyzing assessment findings. Examples of possible nursing diagnoses may include the following:

- Pain/impaired tissue integrity related to
  - —Presence of infection in lower and upper urinary tract
  - —Perineal edema and excoriation
- Altered patterns of urinary elimination related to
  - —Presence of edema and pain
  - —Impaired urinary function
- Fear/anxiety related to
  - —Possible loss of pregnancy or preterm labor/birth
  - —Knowledge deficit regarding etiology, management, course, and sequelae to infection

PLANNING

A plan of care is formulated that relates specifically to the physical and psychosocial needs of the client. *Goals* are mutually determined with the client. These measurable goals, stated in client-centered terms, may include the following:

1. The women's infection will be cured.
2. She will experience absence or improvement of pain, her edema will be relieved, and excoriated areas will heal.
3. She will experience a return to her previous urinary function and pattern of elimination with no sequelae or recurrence of infection.
4. She will state that she is less anxious because she does not lose the pregnancy or experience preterm labor/birth.
5. She can relate knowledge of etiology and prevention, management, course, and sequelae of infection.

IMPLEMENTATION

Implementation of interventions to achieve these outcomes include ongoing assessment of pain, initiation of nonpharmacologic comfort measures, and administration of analgesics as ordered. Another important aspect of care is the promotion of nutrition, hydration, rest, and genital hygiene (see teaching genital hygiene, p. 863).

Assessment of knowledge about the signs and symptoms of infection is crucial as is assessment of knowledge about treatment and sequelae of further infection. Clarification of misconceptions may be helpful, and information or counseling for the mother and her partner also is indicated (see box on teaching prevention of genital tract infections, p. 870).

EVALUATION

Evaluation of client outcomes is a continuous process. To be effective, evaluation is based on client-centered goals identified during the planning stage of nursing care. The nurse can be reasonably assured that care was effective to the extent that the goals have been met; that is:

- The woman's infection is cured.
- She experiences the absence or improvement of pain, her edema resolves, and excoriations heal.
- She experiences a return to her previous urinary function and pattern of elimination with no sequelae or recurrence of infection.
- She admits to feeling relieved that she does not lose the pregnancy or experience preterm labor/birth.
- She can relate etiology and prevention, management, course, and sequelae to infection.

TEACHING Prevention of Genital Tract Infections

- Practice genital hygiene.
- Choose underwear or hosiery with a cotton crotch.
- Avoid tight-fitting clothing (especially tight jeans).
- Select cloth car seat covers instead of vinyl.
- Limit time spent in damp exercise clothes (especially swimsuits and leotards or tights).
- Discontinue use of feminine hygiene deodorant sprays, if sensitive.
- Use condoms.
- Avoid douching.

■ POSTPARTUM INFECTIONS

Puerperal Infection

Puerperal infection (puerperal sepsis or "childbed fever") is any clinical infection of the genital canal that occurs within 28 days after abortion or childbirth. Infections may result from bacteria commonly found within the vagina *(endogenous)* or from the introduction of pathogens from outside the vagina *(exogenous)*. An episiotomy or lacerations of the vagina or cervix may open avenues for sepsis. Even more formidable, however, may be the large placental site. Here the denuded endometrium (decidua basalis) and residual blood after parturition make the uterus an ideal site for a wound infection. The virulence of infecting organisms, the woman's resistance to them, and the rapidity and specificity of therapy determine the efficacy of treatment. Puerperal sepsis occurs after about 6% of births in the United States. Fortunately body defenses generally limit the disease in most instances. Puerperal infection probably is the major cause of maternal morbidity and mortality throughout the world.

The most common infecting organisms are the numerous streptococcal and anaerobic organisms. Fulminating epidemic puerperal sepsis classically is caused by the hemolytic streptococcus. The less virulent anaerobic streptococci may be responsible for other puerperal infections. However, *Staphylococcus aureus*, gonococci, coliform bacteria, and clostridia are less common but serious pathogenic organisms that cause puerperal infection.

Commonly the infection is complicated by medical disorders such as anemia, malnutrition, or diabetes mellitus. Obstetric problems, including PROM, a long, exhausting labor, instrument birth, hemorrhage, and retention of the products of conception, increase the likelihood and severity of puerperal sepsis.

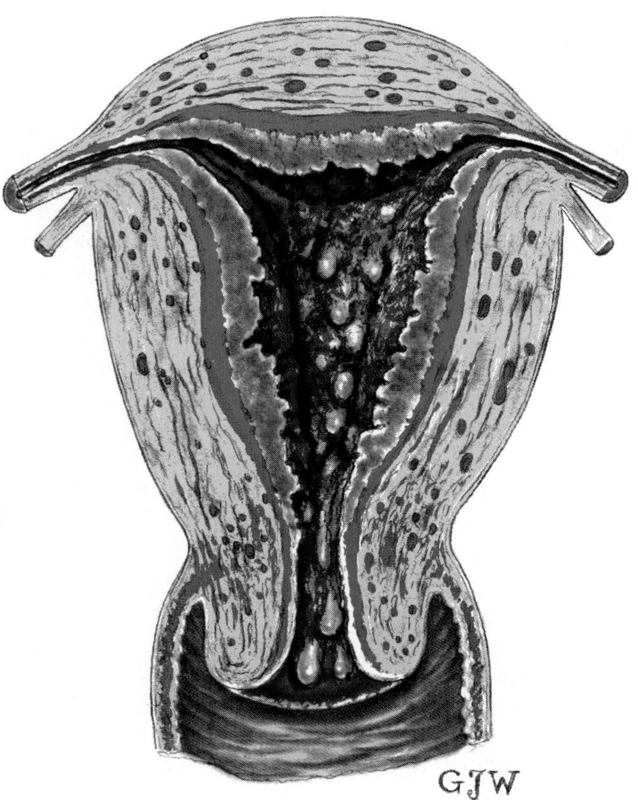

Fig. 29-5 Puerperal infection. Endometritis.

Chorioamnionitis may be the cause or the result of PROM. Chorioamnionitis may be followed by placentitis and fetal congenital pneumonia, omphalitis, or septicemia. These conditions often are caused by enteric streptococci, an aerogenic type of colon bacteria. Placentitis and chorioamnionitis may be followed by endometritis.

An *endometritis*, usually at the placental site, permits infection to begin (Fig. 29-5). Localized infection may be followed by salpingitis, peritonitis, and pelvic abscess formation. (Tubal occlusion after salpingitis is a common cause of infertility.) Septicemia may develop. Secondary abscesses may arise in distant sites such as the lungs or liver. Pulmonary embolism or septic shock, often with *disseminated intravascular coagulation* (DIC), from any serious genital infection may prove fatal. Postbirth femoral thrombophlebitis ("milk leg") may result in a swollen, painful leg and, if untreated, septic thrombophlebitis (Fig. 29-6).

CLINICAL FINDINGS. The symptoms of puerperal infection may be mild or fulminating. Any fever—that is, a temperature of 100.4° F (38° C) or more on 2 successive days, not counting the first 24 hours after birth—must be considered caused by puerperal infection in the absence of convincing proof of another

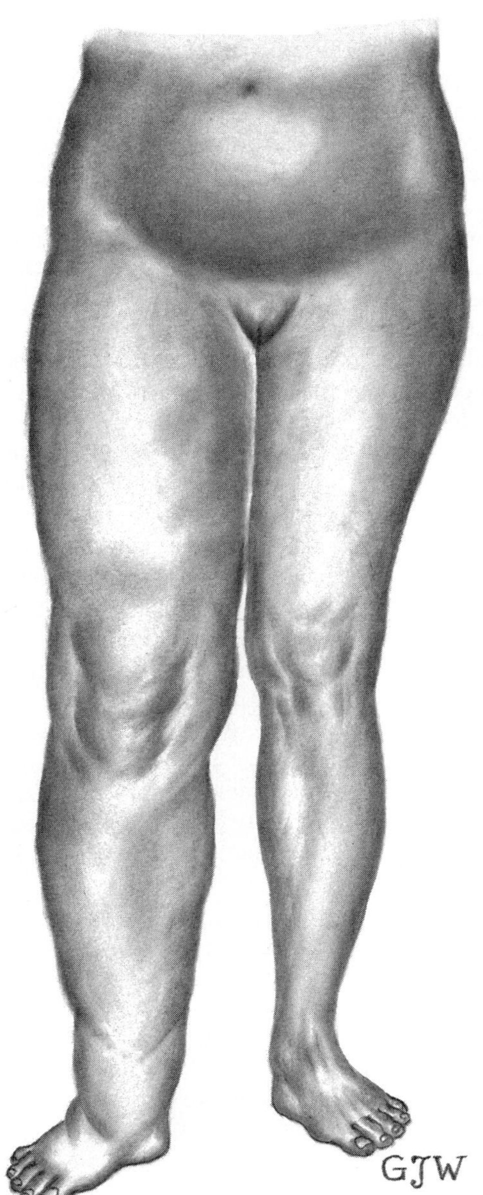

Fig. 29-6 Femoral thrombophlebitis ("milk leg").

cause. For example, a postpartum mother may show a fever and an elevated WBC count of 19,800/mm^3 as early as the second postnatal day. She also may describe symptoms of fatigue and lethargy, lack of appetite, and chills. Perineal discomfort or lower abdominal distress, nausea, and vomiting may soon develop. Foul or profuse lochia, hectic (high, spiking) fever, tachycardia, ileus, pelvic pain, and tenderness characterize critical puerperal sepsis. Without improvement, bacteremic shock or death may ensue.

LABORATORY FINDINGS. Considerable leukocytosis, a shift to the left of the differential WBC count and a markedly increased red blood cell (RBC) sedimentation rate are typical of puerperal infections. Anemia, often an accompaniment, is evidenced by reduced RBC, hemoglobin, and hematocrit values. Urine cultures usually are negative for infection. Intracervical or intrauterine bacterial cultures (aerobic and anerobic) should reveal the offending pathogens within 36 to 48 hours.

The physician also must distinguish nongenital from genital sepsis. Mastitis, respiratory and urinary tract infections, and enteritis are considered in that order of probability.

MANAGEMENT. The most effective and cheapest treatment of puerperal infection is prevention. Preventive measures include good prenatal nutrition to control anemia and intranatal hemorrhage. Good maternal hygiene is essential. Strict adherence by all medical personnel to the best aseptic techniques during the entire hospital and birth period is mandatory. Coitus after rupture of membranes is contraindicated. Dystocia or prolonged labor should be avoided, especially after leaking of amniotic fluid. Traumatic vaginal birth must be avoided, blood loss replaced, and fluid-electrolyte balance maintained.

Infection measures for cure and comfort are instituted. Fluid and electrolyte balance is vital. Broad-spectrum antibiotics are administered intravenously until the infecting organism is identified. Then organism-specific antibiotic therapy is begun. Mother-infant contact is established on the basis of the mother's levels of fatigue and discomfort. The infant's father and other family members also may provide newborn contact. Breast-feeding may continue, depending on the prescribed antibiotic regimen.

Surgical measures may be required. These include surgical procedures such as dilatation and curettage (D & C) to remove the retained products of conception, hysterectomy (if the uterus is ruptured), colpotomy to drain a pelvic abscess, or ligation or clipping of the vena cava and ovarian veins to prevent septic embolism.

The virulence of the organisms, the resistance of the woman, and her likely response to treatment are the intangibles of prognosis. Prevention, supportive therapy, and prompt massive antibiotic administration have reduced the maternal mortality in the United States to less than 0.4%. Regrettably, in developing countries the death rate may be more than 10 to 20 times this figure.

Bacteremic Shock

Critical infections, particularly those in which the causative bacteria release endotoxin, may precipitate

bacteremic (septic) shock. Pregnant women, especially those with diabetes mellitus, or women who are receiving immunosuppressive drugs are at increased risk, as are those women with endometritis during the puerperium.

High, spiking fever and chills are pathophysiologic evidence of serious sepsis. As the endotoxin suppresses antibody production, the inflammatory response falters. Increasing endotoxin damages capillary endothelia and alters permeability. Fluid leaks out, and the volume of venous blood returning to the heart is diminished. Impaired perfusion results in generalized tissue hypoxia, as well as renal and neurologic abnormalities.

An anxious mother may grow apathetic. Body temperature often falls to slightly subnormal levels. The skin becomes cool and moist. Coloring becomes pale, and the pulse becomes rapid and thready. Marked hypotension and peripheral cyanosis develop. Oliguria occurs.

Thromboplastin is released from damaged, hypoxic tissues, which initiates the coagulation cascade. Thrombocytopenia and coagulopathy (with resulting DIC) are life-threatening sequelae. (For further discussion of DIC, refer to Chapter 30.)

LABORATORY FINDINGS. Laboratory studies reveal marked evidence of infection. Blood cultures show bacteremia, usually consisting of enteric gram-negative bacilli. One such organism associated with severe bacteremic shock is *S. aureus*. *S. aureus* also causes toxic shock syndrome (TSS), an acute disease related to high-absorbancy tampon and barrier contraceptive use (Berkley et al, 1987; Wolf et al, 1987) (see p. 875, this chapter).

Additional studies may reflect hemoconcentration, acidosis, and coagulopathy. Central venous pressure (CVP) usually is low. An electrocardiogram (ECG) may show changes indicative of myocardial insufficiency. Evidence of cardiac, pulmonary, renal, and neurologic hypoxia is notable.

MANAGEMENT. Antishock treatment focuses on antimicrobial therapy, as well as oxygen support to relieve tissue hypoxia, and circulatory support to prevent vascular collapse. Heart function, respiratory effort, and kidney function are closely monitored. Prompt treatment of bacteremic shock has a good prognosis, and maternal morbidity and mortality are decreased by controlling respiratory distress, hypotension, and DIC.

Mastitis

Mastitis, or breast infection, affects about 1% of women soon after childbirth, most of whom are first-time mothers who are breast-feeding. Mastitis almost always is unilateral and develops well after the flow of milk has been established (Fig. 29-7). The infecting organism generally is the hemolytic *S. aureus*. An infected nipple fissure usually is the initial lesion, but the ductal system is involved next. Inflammatory edema and engorgement of the breasts soon obstruct the flow of milk in a lobe; regional, then generalized, mastitis follows. If prompt resolution of the septic process does not occur, a breast abscess is virtually inevitable.

Chills, fever, malaise, and local breast tenderness are noted first. Eventual localization of sepsis and axillary adenopathy are delayed developments.

Intensive antibiotic therapy (such as cephalosporins and vancomycin, which are particularly useful in staphylococcal infections), support of breasts, local heat (or cold), and analgesics are required. Lactation is maintained (if desired) by emptying the breasts every 4 hours by manual expression or breast pump. If an abscess develops, wide incision and drainage must be effected. Most women respond to treatment, and an abscess can be prevented.

Almost all instances of acute mastitis can be avoided by proper breast-feeding technique (see Chapter 22) to prevent cracked nipples. Missed feedings, waiting too long between feedings, and abrupt weaning may lead to clogged nipples and mastitis.

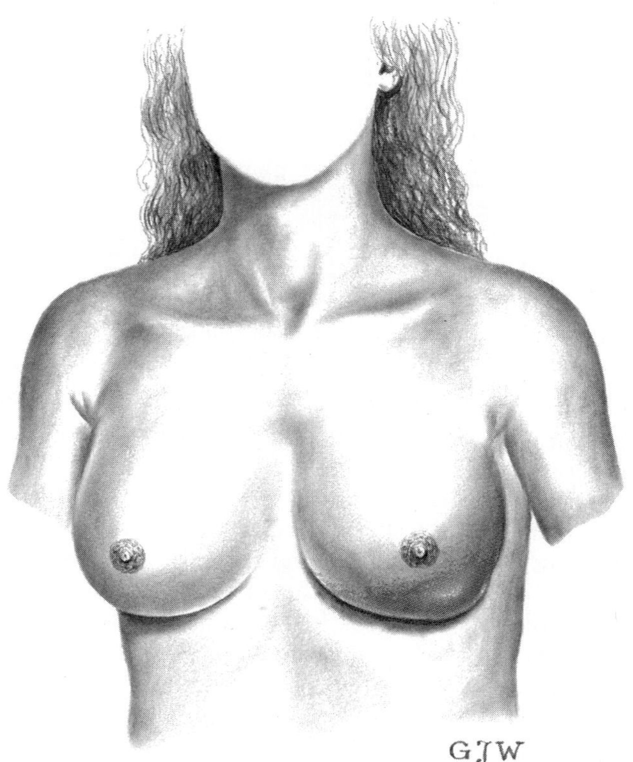

Fig. 29-7 Mastitis.

Cleanliness practiced by all who have contact with the newborn and new mother also reduces the incidence of mastitis.

Nursing Process

ASSESSMENT

The development of postpartum infections is affected by several factors. A thorough assessment may identify those at greatest risk.

HISTORY. Untreated or undertreated infections in the prenatal period may predispose mothers to postpartum infections. PROM and the length of time from rupture to birth also may be factors. Labor and birth events to assess include length of labor, type of labor and birth experience, condition of the placenta, and estimated blood loss.

PHYSICAL EXAMINATION. Signs of infection may not manifest for 24 to 48 hours. The nurse assesses for fever higher than 100.4° F (38° C), chills, and tachycardia. Abdominal or perineal discomfort, nausea, and vomiting also may develop. Foul-smelling lochia is a sign of uterine infection; other potential sites of infection include the breasts, an episiotomy or cesarean incision, and the bladder.

LABORATORY TESTS. Laboratory results that may be helpful in assessing for infection include an elevated WBC count, anemia, and positive culture results in specimens of urine, blood, the vagina, or the placenta.

NURSING DIAGNOSES

Nursing diagnoses are derived from current knowledge, medical management, and physician's directives and after carefully analyzing assessment finding. Examples of possible nursing diagnoses may include the following:

- Knowledge deficit related to
  - —Etiology, management, course, and sequelae to infection
  - —Prevention of infection
- Acute pain related to
  - —Breast engorgement
  - —Puerperal infection
- Altered family processes related to
  - —Unexpected complication to expected postpartum recovery
  - —Possible separation from newborn
  - —Interruption in process of realigning relationships after the addition of the new family member

PLANNING

A plan of care is formulated that relates specifically to the needs of the client and her family. To the extent possible, the nurse involves them all in the planning and incorporates their priorities and preferences for any actions planned. *Goals* are set in client-centered terms and prioritized in collaboration with the client and her family. Examples may include the following:

1. The mother will be able to state the etiology, management, and course of infection; she can identify measures to prevent reinfection.
2. She will describe a reduction or elimination of pain.
3. She and her family verbalize acceptance of the unexpected events; they verbalize positive coping measures (e.g., arrangement for home health care).

IMPLEMENTATION

Implementation includes continuous assessment for signs and symptoms of infection, monitoring laboratory results, administering antimicrobial agents as ordered, and providing information to the mother and family as needed. General care, such as adequate hydration, rest, and proper nutrition, also should be implemented.

EVALUATION

Evaluation of client outcomes is a continuous process. To be effective, evaluation is based on client-centered expected outcomes during the planning stage of nursing care. The nurse can be reasonably assured that care was effective to the extent that goals for care have been met; that is:

- The mother can state the etiology, management, and course of infection; she can identify measures to prevent reinfection.
- The mother describes a reduction or elimination of pain.
- The mother and her family verbalize acceptance of the unexpected events and have taken appropriate steps to meeting their new needs.

■ GENERAL INFECTIONS

Many infections place the woman at risk during the childbearing cycle. Following are some maternal infections the nurse may encounter.

COXSACKIEVIRUS B. This virus may cause mild illness in the *mother*. It is responsible for death, cardiovascular anomalies, myocarditis, and meningoencephalitis in the *fetus*.

CHICKENPOX (VARICELLA, A HERPESVIRUS INFECTION). Chickenpox is highly contagious and is transmitted by direct contact with airborne virus. A *maternal* infection may appear as herpes zoster (shingles), especially in mothers with HIV. The symptoms may be mild, with or without the characteristic vesicles. However, the severe, disseminated, epidemic type of varicella during pregnancy may be fatal for the mother (and fetus) because of necrotizing angitis (inflammation of blood and lymph vessels) and complications from varicella pneumonia.

Fetal and neonatal effects also are seen. Abortion or fetal death may occur. If maternal varicella infection occurs in the first trimester, there is a 5% to 10% chance that the fetus will develop a pattern of defects of skin, bone, and muscle known as **congenital varicella syndrome.** CNS effects include chorioretinitis and hydrocephalus. If maternal infection occurs within 20 days before birth, an infant should be considered possibly infectious and isolated from other infants (Payani, Arvin, 1986; Fox, Strangarity, 1989).

Varicella-zoster immunoglobulin (VZIG) may be given prophylactically to exposed pregnant women. Severe varicella infections, especially if complicated by pneumonia, should be treated with intravenous acyclovir or vidarabine.

INFLUENZA. Influenza is caused by a virus. *Maternal effects* can be serious if complicated by pneumonia. Abortion and preterm labor may result. *Fetal and neonatal effects* include death, preterm birth, and occasionally, anencephaly or meningomyelocele. If the woman is not pregnant, she may be given polyvalent influenza virus (attenuated live virus) vaccine.

LISTERIOSIS. Listeriosis is caused by gram-positive bacterium, *Listeria monocytogenes*. This organism is harbored in the vagina or cervix by 4% of pregnant women. Listeriosis may exhibit influenza-like symptoms. It occurs most commonly in summer or fall. Other symptoms include vaginitis, UTI, and enteritis. *Fetal and neonatal effects* are serious. This infection may result in abortion. Amnionitis or placentitis is evidenced by dirty brown amniotic fluid. With neonatal infection, generalized skin rash and meningitis is seen. Pneumonia carries a 50% mortality rate. Meningitis, which appears most often in term males, may appear later in the neonatal period. Treatment with penicillin or erythromycin usually is successful. Unfortunately the diagnosis of listeriosis often is obscure or delayed; thus the prognosis for the fetus or newborn generally is poor.

LYME DISEASE. Lyme disease is a tick-borne infection caused by the spirochete *Borrelia burgdorferi*. Infection is endemic in the Northeast, mid-Atlantic, parts of the Midwest, and West and peaks in the late spring and summer. Most infected persons develop a circular, expanding lesion (erythema chronicum migrans) at the site of the tick bite—usually groin, buttocks, axillae, trunk, upper part of the arms, and legs. Viremic symptoms, such as fatigue, headache, sore throat, fever, pain, and joint swelling also may develop, although some persons remain free of symptoms. Sequelae of untreated Lyme disease include chronic arthritis and neurologic and cardiac problems.

The spirochete of Lyme disease, which closely resembles that of syphilis, crosses the placenta. *Maternal effects* include miscarriage, preterm labor and birth, and stillbirth. *Fetal and neonatal effects* are not well documented inasmuch as Lyme disease is still relatively new and frequently misdiagnosed. Birth defects are common, especially cardiac and neurologic defects. Treatment of choice for Lyme disease during pregnancy is amoxicillin or ceftriaxone.

MALARIA. Malaria is caused by the protozoan *Plasmodium falciparum*. *Maternal effects* include chills and fever, abortion, and preterm labor. Labor may be prolonged, hazardous, fatiguing, and end in cesarean birth. There is often a recurrence during the puerperium. *Fetal and neonatal effects* occur. There is extensive involvement of the placenta. The newborn is small for gestational age (SGA) or stillborn if the maternal infection does not cause abortion. Infection occurs in 10% of newborns of infectious women. Quinine (chloroquine phosphate [Aralen]) given to the mother may be fetotoxic. In severe cases of malaria, however, use of appropriate medications may be an acceptable calculated risk.

MUMPS. Parotitis (mumps) occurs rarely in pregnant women. In the *mother*, this virus may cause abortion or preterm labor. *Fetal* death may result. Congenital malformation such as endocardial fibroelastosis may be associated with this viral infection in survivors. Prophylaxis for epidemic parotitis is possible with administration of hyperimmune mumps gamma globulin.

PARVOVIRUS. Parvovirus B-19 is associated with a mild illness of childhood known as fifth disease or erythema infectiosum. Transmission occurs by droplets, and the primary symptoms are fever and a characteristic "slapped face" rash. Outbreaks usually occur in schools in the spring; adults who work with children are at increased risk. *Maternal effects,* in addition to fever and rash, include headache, malaise, and aching, swollen joints.

Fetal and neonatal effects are more serious. Parvovirus has been recently implicated as one cause of unexplained miscarriage and stillbirth. Human parvovirus infection disrupts erythropoiesis in the fetus, leading to severe anemia, cardiac failure, nonimmune hydrops fetalis, and death. There is no treatment for parvovirus infection in mothers or infants; however, fetal blood transfusions have limited success in avoiding anemic sequelae in utero (Peters, Nicolaides, 1990).

POLIOMYELITIS. *Maternal effects* of poliomyelitis (polio) include an increased susceptibility to the polio virus during pregnancy. If the woman suffers paralysis, labor progresses normally. There is a higher incidence of mortality however. *Fetal and neonatal effects* occur. Occurrence during the first trimester may result in abortion, possible anomalies, and IUGR. Neonatal infection acquired during the passage through the birth canal may be diagnosed after the appearance of flaccid paralysis.

Prophylaxis for polio has almost eradicated this disorder in some countries. However, it is still prevalent and potentially devastating in parts of Asia and Africa. Prophylaxis for pregnant women is possible with Salk vaccine (killed virus) but *not* with Sabin vaccine (attenuated live virus). The Salk vaccine confers an immunity of about 2 years; Sabin vaccination is followed by permanent immunization (after pregnancy).

RUBEOLA. Rubeola, also known as 2-week measles, is caused by a virus. Rubeola during pregnancy is uncommon because most women have had the disease and are immune to it. Should the woman acquire rubeola during pregnancy, there are *fetal and neonatal effects*. Abortion or preterm labor may occur. The newborn may be born with a rash but generally survives, usually without developmental anomalies. Prophylactic gamma globulin may prevent the disease; measles vaccination of susceptible women before (but not during) pregnancy is recommended.

TOXIC SHOCK SYNDROME. Toxic shock syndrome *(TSS)* is a potentially life-threatening systemic disorder that has three principal clinical manifestations: fever of sudden onset, hypotension, and rash (see box above right). The erythematous macular desquamating rash is most prominent on palms and soles.

Warning Signs—Toxic Shock Syndrome (TSS)

1. Fever of sudden onset—over 102° F (38.9° C)
2. Hypotension—systolic pressure <90 mm Hg; orthostatic dizziness; disorientation
3. Rash—diffuse, macular erythrodema

The acute phase of TSS lasts about 4 to 5 days; the convalescent phase, about 1 to 2 weeks.

The CDC (1989) has established diagnostic criteria for TSS that include the aforementioned signs plus the following manifestations.

1. Involvement of three or more other organ systems:

System/Area	Manifestations
Gastrointestinal	Nausea: vomiting; diarrhea
Renal	Decreased urinary output; pyuria
Hepatic	Jaundice; abnormal values (increased transaminase)
CNS	Altered sensorium (decreased level of consciousness [LOC]); headache
Respiratory	Adult respiratory distress syndrome (ARDS)
Mucous membranes	Inflammation of vaginal, oropharyngeal, and conjunctival membranes
Muscular	Myalgia: weakness
Hematologic	Thrombocytopenia; DIC
Cardiac	Ischemic changes on ECG; decreased left ventricular contractility

2. Serologic laboratory test results for Rocky Mountain spotted fever, leptospirosis, and measles are negative. Cultures positive for *S. aureus* can be obtained from blood, urine, or stool. If primary site of infection is tampon related, positive cultures are obtained from the vagina and cervix.

A toxin (pyrogenic exotoxin C [PEC] or enterotoxin F) secreted by strains of *S. aureus* is the causative factor in TSS. About 9% of women harbor the organism normally in their vaginas; about 1% to 5% of sexually active males have urethral cultures that are positive for *S. aureus* without having the disease. Poor perineal hygiene and lack of hand washing before touching the perineal area may increase risk. Commonly associated conditions that may predispose the person to TSS by providing a portal of entry into systemic circulation include the following:

1. Menstruation
2. Chronic vaginal infection (e.g., herpes)
3. Puerperal endometritis
4. Incisional or soft tissue abscess
5. Skin infection following a bee sting
6. IV injection of heroin
7. Use of high-absorbency tampons or barrier contraceptives (e.g., sponge, diaphragm) (Berkley et al, 1987; Wolf et al, 1987)
8. Neonatal infection concurrent with maternal infection.

The population at greatest risk is women between the ages of 15 and 24 who use tampons during menstruation.

PATHOPHYSIOLOGY. The toxins may suppress synthesis of IgM antibodies. Toxin-induced injury to capillary endothelium alters capillary permeability. Fluid leaks out, and the volume of venous blood returning to the heart is diminished. Impaired tissue perfusion results in tissue hypoxia and renal and CNS abnormalities. Other problems arise from the toxin's direct damage to target organs. Tissue damage releases thromboplastin, which initiates the coagulation cascade. Thrombocytopenia and coagulopathy (e.g., DIC) are potential hazardous sequelae. In some people, impaired tissue perfusion, with its sequelae, has resulted in loss of gangrenous toes and fingers.

PROGNOSIS. Mortality is associated with TSS. In order of incidence the three causes of mortality are (1) ARDS (see Chapter 32), (2) uncontrollable hypotension, and (3) DIC.

Although most affected women have an uneventful recovery with no recurrence, some suffer adverse sequelae. Infection that does recur does so most often with the next menstrual cycle. Recurrence is most likely if the woman had not been treated with β-lactamase–resistant antibiotics. Some women have persistent abnormalities in intellectual function. Persistent problems include impaired memory, concentration, and calculation ability, abnormal ECG, and impaired cerebellar function (hyperreflexia). For a few women sequelae are more serious. Impaired renal function, neuromuscular function (vocal cord paralysis), and peripheral perfusion, especially of the hands and feet, may persist after the infection is cured.

MANAGEMENT. Early identification of TSS is essential so that appropriate therapy can be initiated. Nurses must be on the alert for this syndrome because of the increased likelihood of its occurrence in obstetric and gynecologic settings.

Nursing care involves both prevention and treatment of TSS. Preventive care focuses on client education about the relationship of TSS to the use of tampons, diaphragms, cervical caps, and contraceptive vaginal sponges (see client teaching box below). Treatment in the acute care setting may include IV fluid replacement for dehydration related to vomiting or diarrhea, administration of antibiotics, administration of transfusions for low platelet counts, and medications to treat skin rashes and hypotension (Eschenbach, 1990).

TUBERCULOSIS. Tuberculosis (TB) is caused by a gram-negative, acid-fast bacillus. Pulmonary TB does not jeopardize pregnancy, although urinary and CNS tuberculosis may. Pregnancy does not affect pulmonary tuberculosis adversely. Genital infection is rare. It may be sexually transmitted or result from primary lesions in the lungs (Fig. 29-8). Spontaneous abortion occurs in 20% of infected women. Many pregnancies are ectopic, or the woman has impaired in-

TEACHING Prevention of Toxic Shock Syndrome

General information

- Avoid the use of tampons, cervical caps, diaphragms, and contraceptive vaginal sponges during the postpartum period (6 weeks).
- Do not use any of the above if you have a history of TSS.
- Call your health care provider if you experience sudden onset of a high fever, vomiting, diarrhea, or skin rash.

Tampon use

- Insert only clean tampons with clean hands.
- Change tampons every 3 to 6 hours.
- Avoid use of superabsorbent tampons.
- Avoid overnight use of tampons by substituting other products such as sanitary napkins or minipads.

Contraceptive vaginal sponge use

- Insert only clean sponges with clean hands.
- Wet sponge with clean water only.
- Do not use the sponge during your menstrual period.

Diaphragm or cervical cap

- Insert clean diaphragm or cervical cap with clean hands.
- Do not use during your menstrual period.
- Remove within 8 hours after intercourse.

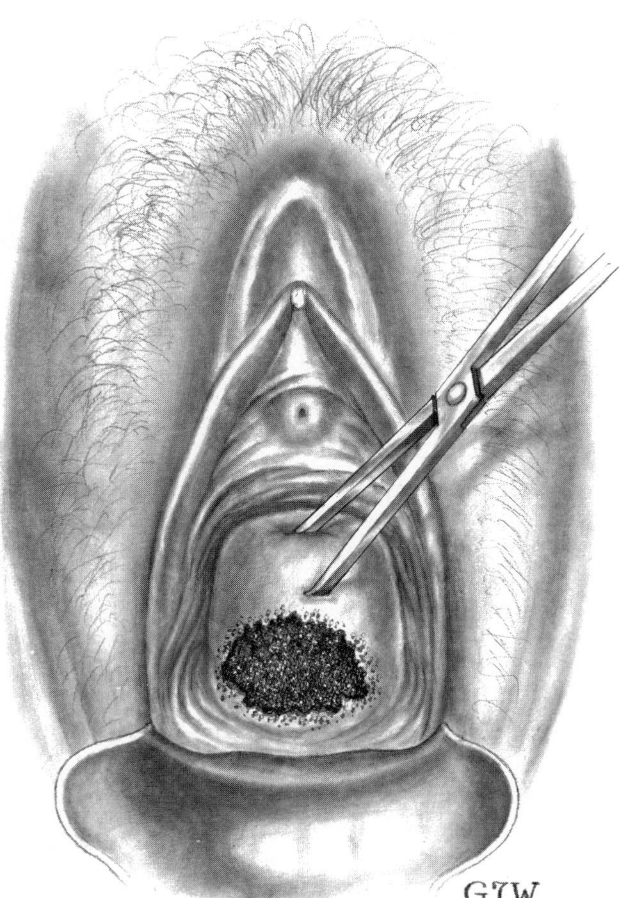

Fig. 29-8 Tuberculosis of the vaginal vault.

fertility with genital tuberculosis. Further, TB is gaining increased attention as one of the opportunistic infections seen commonly in persons with AIDs.

The outcome of *fetal* and *neonatal involvement* depends on the stage of tuberculosis infection of the mother. Congenital tuberculosis is rare. Maternal therapy with streptomycin may result in congenital nerve deafness in the neonate.

Contraception is advocated for women with active tuberculosis; pregnancy is contraindicated until the woman has been free of the disease for 1½ to 2 years. All pregnant women should be evaluated for TB (tine test or PPD) early in pregnancy and again later if suspicion of the disease exists. If results of the tine test or PPD are positive, a chest film may be indicated to rule out active disease. Some individuals who have been treated for TB will have a reactive TB test. Once the infant has been born, she or he should have no intimate contact with mother or others who may have the disease until contagion is no longer a problem. Therapeutic abortion rarely is indicated; cesarean birth is warranted only for obstetric indications.

INFECTION CONTROL

Infection control measures are essential to protect care providers and to prevent *nosocomial* infection of clients, regardless of the infectious agent. The risk of occupational transmission varies with the disease. Even if that risk is low, as it is with HIV, that any risk exists is significant to warrant *reasonable* precautions.

Precautions against airborne disease transmission are available in all health care agencies. *Universal precautions* from the CDC follow.

Universal Precautions

Medical history and examination cannot reliably identify all persons infected with HIV or other blood-borne pathogens. Thus blood and body-fluid precautions should be consistently used for everyone. This approach, previously recommended by CDC and referred to as "universal blood and body-fluid precautions" or "**universal precautions**" should be used in the care of all persons, especially those in emergency care settings in which the risk of blood exposure is increased and the infection status of the person is usually unknown.

1. All health care workers should routinely use appropriate barrier precautions to prevent skin and mucous-membrane exposure when contact with blood or other body fluids of any person is anticipated. *Gloves* should be worn for touching blood and body fluids, mucous membranes, or nonintact skin of all persons; for handling items or surfaces soiled with blood or body fluids; and for performing venipuncture and other vascular access procedures. *Gloves should be changed after contact with each client. Masks and protective eyewear or face shields* should be worn during procedures that are likely to generate droplets of blood or other body fluids to prevent exposure of mucous membranes of the mouth, nose, and eyes. *Gowns or aprons* should be worn during procedures that are likely to generate splashes of blood or other body fluids.
2. Hands and other skin surfaces should be washed immediately and thoroughly if contaminated with blood or other body fluids. Hands should be washed immediately after gloves are removed.
3. All health care workers should take precautions to prevent injuries caused by needles, scalpels, and other sharp instruments or devices during procedures; when cleaning used instruments; during disposal of used needles; and when handling sharp instruments after procedures. *To prevent needlestick injuries,* needles should not be re-

capped, purposely bent or broken by hand, removed from disposable syringes, or otherwise manipulated by hand. After they are used, disposable syringes and needles, scalpel blades, and other sharp items should be immediately placed in puncture-resistant containers for disposal; the puncture-resistant containers should be located as close as practical to the use area. Large-bore reusable needles should be placed in a puncture-resistant container for transport to the reprocessing area.

4. Although saliva has not been implicated in HIV transmission, to minimize the need for emergency mouth-to-mouth resuscitation, mouthpieces, resuscitation bags, or other ventilation devices should be available for use in areas in which the need for resuscitation is predictable.
5. Health care workers who have exudative lesions or weeping dermatitis should refrain from all direct client care and from handling client care equipment until the condition resolves.
6. Pregnant health care workers are not known to be at greater risk of contracting HIV infection than health care workers who are not pregnant; however, if a health care worker develops HIV infection during pregnancy, the infant is at risk of infection resulting from perinatal transmission. Because of this risk, pregnant health care workers should be especially familiar with and strictly adhere to precautions to minimize the risk of HIV transmission.

Precautions for Invasive Procedures

An invasive procedure is defined as surgical entry into tissues, cavities, or organs or repair of major traumatic injuries (1) in an operating or birthing room, emergency department, or out-of-hospital setting, including both physicians' and dentists' offices and (2) a vaginal or cesarean birth or other invasive obstetric procedure during which bleeding may occur. The aforementioned universal blood and body-fluid precautions, combined with the following precautions, should serve as minimum precautions for all such invasive procedures.

1. All health care workers who participate in invasive procedures must routinely use appropriate barrier precautions to prevent skin and mucous-membrane contact with blood and other body fluids of all clients. Gloves and surgical masks must be worn for all invasive procedures. Protective eyewear or face shields should be worn for procedures that commonly result in the generation of droplets, splashing of blood or other body fluids, or the generation of bone chips. Gowns or aprons made of materials that provide an effective barrier should be worn during invasive procedures that are likely to result in the splashing of blood or other body fluids. *All health care workers who perform or assist in vaginal or cesarean births should wear gloves and gowns when handling the placenta or the infant until blood and amniotic fluid have been removed from the infant's skin and should wear gloves during postnatal care of the umbilical cord.*
2. If a glove is torn or a needlestick or other injury occurs, the glove should be removed and a new glove used as promptly as client safety permits; the needle or instrument involved in the incident also should be removed from the sterile field.

Another consideration in the prevention of occupational disease transmission is that of cross-contamination. Health care providers may develop a false sense of security about the protection that gloves provide. For example, little is gained if gloves are worn to assess a newborn and those same gloved hands answer the telephone, turn on a light, or document findings on the infant's chart.

Cross-contamination of surfaces is common; awareness is essential. However, for cleaning contaminated surfaces, the following is appropriate:

- Cleanse washable surfaces with a solution of sodium hypochlorite (household bleach) and water—1 cup of household bleach to 9 cups of water. Health care institutions often purchase commercial products to disinfect.
- Remove all blood or other fluids before disinfection to avoid neutralizing the bleach solution.

SUMMARY

Infections are potentially hazardous to the woman any time, to the mother and fetus during pregnancy, and to the health care provider. The knowledgeable nurse can help the woman prevent or treat infections successfully. Overall therapeutic measures include educating the general public regarding immunization for nonimmune persons. Many states are introducing or passing laws requiring screening for rubella and chickenpox titers. Tests for exposure to syphilis are routine; populations at risk require assessment for chlamydial infection and for HIV and AIDS antibodies. Easily accessible and person-oriented (nonjudgmental) clinics should be available to all, so that people are encouraged to use them for diagnosis and treatment.

Health care providers must assume that all clients are infectious. The same procedures that protect against exposure to HIV also protect against transmission of other infectious organisms, including hepatitis B.

REFERENCES

Aral SO, Holmes KK: Epidemiology of sexual behavior and sexually transmitted diseases. In Holmes KK *Sexually transmitted diseases,* ed 2, New York, 1990, McGraw-Hill.

Berkley SF et al: The relationship of tampon characteristics to menstrual toxic shock syndrome, *JAMA* 258:908, 1987.

Berry CD et al: Neurologic relapse after benzathine penicillin therapy for secondary syphilis in a patient with HIV infection, *N Engl J Med* 316:1587, 1987.

Bourcier KM, Seidler AJ: Chlamydia and condylomata acuminata: an update for the nurse practitioner, *JOGNN* 16:17, 1987.

Brown ZA, Baker DA: Acyclovir therapy during pregnancy, *Obstet Gynecol* 73:526, 1989.

Brown ZA et al: Genital herpes in pregnancy: risk factors associated with recurrences and asymptomatic viral shedding, *Am J Obstet Gynecol* 153:24, 1985.

Brunham RC, Holmes KK, Embree JE: Sexually transmitted diseases in pregnancy. In Holmes KK et al, editors: *Sexually transmitted diseases,* ed 2, New York, 1990, McGraw-Hill.

Centers for Disease Control: 1989 *sexually transmitted diseases treatment guidelines,* Atlanta, 1989, Public Health Service.

Corbett M, Meyer JH: *The adolescent and pregnancy,* Boston, 1987, Blackwell.

Corey L: Genital herpes. In Holmes KK et al, editors: *Sexually transmitted diseases,* ed 2, New York, 1990, McGraw-Hill.

Eschenbach DA: Pelvic infections and sexually transmitted diseases. In Scott JR et al, editors: *Danforth's obstetrics and gynecology,* ed 6, Philadelphia, 1990, JB Lippincott.

Ferenczy A: Treating genital condyloma during pregnancy with the carbon dioxide laser, *Am J Obstet Gynecol* 148:9, 1984.

Ferenczy A, moderator: Symposium: treating condylomata, *Contemp OB/GYN* 30:158, March 1987.

Foster SD: Education, the best defense against AIDS: MCN focus on patient teaching, *MCN* 12:311, 1987.

Fox GN, Strangarity JW: Varicella-zoster virus infections in pregnancy, *Am Fam Physician* 39(2):89, Feb 1989.

Francis DP, Chin J: The prevention of acquired immunodeficiency syndrome in the United States, *JAMA* 257:1357, 1987.

Friedland GH, Klein RS: Transmission of the human immunodeficiency virus, *N Engl J Med* 317:1125, 1987.

Guinan ME: Treatment of primary and secondary syphilis: defining failure of three- and six- month follow-up, *JAMA* 257:359, 1987.

Hecht F: Counseling the HIV-positive woman regarding pregnancy, *JAMA* 257:3361, 1987.

Hill HR: Group B streptococcal infections. In Holmes KK et al, editors: *Sexually transmitted diseases,* ed 2, New York, 1990, McGraw-Hill.

Johns DR, Tierney M, Felsenstein D: Alteration in the natural history of neurosyphilis by concurrent infection with the human immunodeficiency virus, *N Engl J Med* 316:1569, 1987.

Johnstone HA, Marcinak JF: Candidiasis in the breastfeeding mother and infant, *JOGNN* 19:171, 1990.

Kaplan LD et al: Treatment of patients with acquired immunodeficiency syndrome and associated manifestations, *JAMA* 257:1367, 1987.

Kashima HK, Shah K, Goodstein M: Recurrent respiratory papillomatosis. In Holmes KK et al, editors: *Sexually transmitted diseases,* ed 2, New York, 1990, McGraw-Hill.

Keeling RP: AIDS education: a mandate for schools of nursing, *Dean's Notes* 9(2):1, 1987.

Klug RM: AIDS beyond the hospital: children with AIDS, *Am J Nurs* 86:1126, 1986.

Landesman S et al: Serosurvey of human immunodeficiency virus infection in parturients, *JAMA* 258:2701, 1987.

Loucks A: Chlamydia: an unheralded epidemic, *Am J Nurs* 86:920, 1986.

Marvin C, Slevin A: Chlamydia—cause, prevention, and cure, *MCN* 12:318, 1987.

Minkoff HL: Pregnant women with HIV, *JAMA* 258:2714, 1987.

Minkoff HL et al: Pregnancies resulting in infants with acquired immunodeficiency syndrome: description of the antepartum, intrapartum, and postpartum course, *Obstet Gynecol* 69:285, 1987a.

Minkoff HL et al: Follow-up of mothers and children with AIDS, *Obstet Gynecol* 87:288, 1987b.

MMWR: Penicillinase-producing *Neisseria gonorrhoeae*—United States, 1986, *JAMA* 257:1579, 1987.

Oriel D: Genital human papillomavirus infection. In Holmes KK et al, editors: *Sexually transmitted diseases,* ed 2, New York, 1990, McGraw-Hill.

Paryani SG, Arvin AM: Intrauterine infection with varicella-zoster virus after maternal varicella, *N Engl J Med* 314:1542, 1986.

Perlman D: Antibiotic found to protect unborn from a common VD, *San Francisco Chronicle,* Feb 1, 1986.

Peters MT, Nicolaides KH: Cordocentesis for the diagnosis and treatment of human fetal parvovirus infection, *Obstet Gynecol* 75:501, 1990.

Redondo-Lopez V et al: *Torulopsis glabrata* vaginitis: clinical aspects and susceptibility to antifungal agents, *Obstet Gynecol* 76:651, 1990.

Rein MF, Müller M: *Trichomonas vaginalis* and trichomoniasis. In Holmes KK et al, editors: *Sexually transmitted diseases,* ed 2, New York, 1990, McGraw-Hill.

Rhoads JL et al: Chronic vaginal candidiasis in women with human immunodeficiency virus infection, *JAMA* 257:3105, 1987.

San Francisco Chronicle: Health and fitness: a disease that can worsen with treatment, Feb 1992.

Schachter J: Why we need a program for the control of *Chlamydia trachomatis, N Engl J Med* 320:802, 1989.

Schachter J et al: Erythromycin in the routine treatment of chlamydial infections in pregnancy, *N Engl J Med* 314:276, 1986.

Scott GB et al: Mothers of infants with the acquired immunodeficiency syndrome: evidence for both symptomatic and asymptomatic carriers, *JAMA* 253:363, 1985.

Scott JR et al, editors: *Danforth's obstetrics and gynecology,* ed 6, Philadelphia, 1990, JB Lippincott.

Shah KV: Biology of human genital tract papillomaviruses. In Holmes KK et al, editors: *Sexually transmitted diseases,* ed 2, New York, 1990, McGraw-Hill.

Shaw NS: Serving your patients in the age of AIDS, *Contemp OB/GYN* 28:141, April 1986.

Spence MR: Epidemiology of sexually transmitted diseases, *Obstet Gynecol Clin North Am* 16:453, 1989.

Tramont EC: Syphilis in the AIDS era, *N Engl J Med* 316:1600, 1987.

Update: human immunodeficiency virus infection in health care workers exposed to blood of infected patients, *MMWR* 36:285, 1987.

Washington AE, Browner WS, Korenbrot CC: Cost-effectiveness of combined treatment for endocervical gonorrhea considering co-infection with *Chlamydia trachomatis, JAMA* 257:2056, 1987a.

Washington MD, Johnson RE, Sanders LL: *Chlamydia trachomatis* infections in the United States, *JAMA* 257:2070, 1987b.

Wendel GD: Early and congenital syphilis, *Obstet Gynecol Clin North Am* 16:479, 1989.

Wolf PH et al. Toxic shock syndrome, *JAMA* 258:908, 1987.

BIBLIOGRAPHY

Amsley MS: Infection protocols: parasitic disease in pregnancy, *Contemp OB/GYN* 37:31, Feb 1992.

Amsley MS: Immunization in pregnancy, *Contemp OB/GYN,* 34:15, April 1989.

Baker DA: Dangers of varicella-zoster virus infection, *Contemp OB/GYN* 35:51, April 1990.

Benoit JA: Sexually transmitted diseases in pregnancy, *Nurs Clin North Am* 23:937, 1988.

Bernstein IM, Capeless EL: Elevated maternal serum alpha-fetoprotein and hydrops fetalis in association with fetal parvovirus B-19 infection, *Obstet Gynecol* 74(3, pt 2):456, 1989.

Boodley CA, Jaquis JL: Measles, mumps, rubella, and chickenpox in the adult population, *Nurse Pract* 14(2):12, 1989.

Burnhill MS: Treating persistent and recurrent vulvovaginitis, *Contemp OB/GYN* 31:71, March 1988.

Carpenito LJ: *Nursing diagnosis: application to clinical practice,* ed 3, Philadelphia, 1989, JB Lippincott.

Centers for Disease Control: *Summary of notifiable diseases, United States, 1989,* Atlanta, 1989, Public Health Service.

Christmas JT et al: Concomitant infection with *Neisseria gonorrhoeae* and *Chlamydia trachomatis* in pregnancy, *Obstet Gynecol* 74 (3, pt 1):295, 1989.

Cohen M, Cohen H: Current recommendations for viral hepatitis, *Contemp OB/GYN* 35:56, Nov 1990.

Crombleholme W: Neonatal chlamydial infections, *Contemp OB/GYN* 36:57, Aug 1991.

DeBrow ME: Safer sex, *NSNA/Imprint Issues,* p 33, Feb/Mar, 1988.

Dinsmoor MJ: Group B streptococcus still poses a challenge, *Contemp OB/GYN* 35:93, 1990.

Eschenbach DA, Mead PB: Vaginitis: varying management appropriately, *Contemp OB/GYN* 37:25, Jan 1992.

Faden R, Geller G, Powers M: AIDS. *women, and the next generation,* New York, 1991, Oxford University Press.

Fletcher JL Jr, Gordon RC: Perinatal transmission of bacterial sexually transmitted diseases. I. Syphilis and gonorrhea, *J Fam Pract* 30:448, 1990.

Fletcher JL Jr, Gordon RC: Perinatal transmission of bacterial sexually transmitted diseases. II. Group B streptococcus and *Chlamydia trachomatis, J Fam Pract* 30:448, 1990.

Friedman-Kien AE et al: Natural interferon alfa for treatment of condylomata acuminata, *JAMA* 259:533, 1988.

Gershon A: Chickenpox: how dangerous is it? *Contemp OB/GYN* 31:41, March 1988.

Gonik B: Bacteremia and septic shock, *Contemp OB/GYN* 35:34, April 1990.

Grossman JH III: Why congenital rubella continues to occur, *Contemp OB/GYN* 35:50, Aug 1990.

Gurevich I: Counseling the patient with herpes, *RN* 53:22, Feb 1990.

Hager WD: Puerperal mastitis, *Contemp OB/GYN* 34:27, March 1989.

Harger JH: Genital herpes infections, *Contemp OB/GYN* 35:83, May 1990.

Harris JRW, Forster SM, editors: *Recent advances in sexually transmitted diseases and AIDS,* Edinburgh 1991, Churchill Livingstone.

Heins HC: Two diseases that can harm your fetus, *Am Baby,* p 18, May 1991.

Hoff R et al: Seroprevalence of human immunodeficiency virus among childbearing women: estimation by testing samples of blood from newborn, *N Engl J Med* 318:526, 1988.

Holmes KK et al: *Sexually transmitted diseases,* ed 2, New York, 1990, McGraw-Hill.

Horstmann DM: Surveillance for rubella, *Contemp OB/GYN* 34:43, April 1989.

Jiménez SLM: Measles, mumps and pregnancy, *Am Baby,* p 52, Nov 1990.

Larson E, Ropka ME: An update on nursing research and HIV infection, *Image* 23(2):4, 1991.

Lee BC: Be ready for Lyme disease in your own backyard, *RN* 52:26, April 1989.

Lee NC, Rubin GL, Grimes DA: Measures of sexual behavior and the risk of pelvic inflammatory disease, *Obstet Gynecol* 77:425, 1991.

Madinger NE, McGregor JA: Infection protocols: varicella during pregnancy, *Contemp OB/GYN* 37:83, Jan 1992.

Mangal RK, et al: Hepatitis B screening during pregnancy, *The Female Patient* 17(5):48, 1992.

Maslow AS, Bobitt JR: Herpes in pregnancy: exploring clinical options, *Contemp OB/GYN* 32:44, April 1988.

Masters WH, Johnson VE, Kolodny RC: *Masters and Johnson on sex and human loving,* Boston, 1988, Little, Brown & Co.

McGregor JA, French JI, Spencer NE: Prevention of sexually transmitted disease in women, *Obstet Gynecol Clin North Am* 16:679, 1989.

Mead PB: Parvovirus B19 infection and pregnancy, *Contemp OB/GYN* 34:56, March 1989.

Mead PB: Postpartum endometritis, *Contemp OB/GYN* 35:29, Dec 1990.

Monif GRG: Intrapartum bacteriuria and postpartum endometritis, *Obstet Gynecol* 78:245, 1991.

Mroczkowski TF: *Topics in dermatology: sexually transmitted diseases,* New York, 1990, Igaku-Shoin.

Nettina SL: Syphilis: a new look at an old killer, *Am J Nurs* 90(4):68 April 1990.

Paparone P: The summer scourge of Lyme disease, *Am J Nurs* 90(6):44, June 1990.

Parish LC, Gschnait F, editors: *Sexually transmitted diseases: a guide for clinicians,* New York, 1989, Springer-Verlag.

Pastorek JG: Antimicrobial therapy for PID, *Contemp OB/GYN* 33:31, Sept 1989.

Prober CG et al: Use of routine viral cultures at delivery to identify neonates exposed to herpes simplex virus, *N Engl J Med* 318:887, 1988.

Samra JS, Obhrai MS, Constantine G: Parvovirus infection in pregnancy, *Obstet Gynecol* 73:832, 1989.

Sever JL: TORCH infections: the list keeps growing, *Contemp OB/GYN* 33:65, March 1989.

Sever JL: Toxoplasmosis, *Contemp OB/GYN* 35:13, March 1990.

Silver RM, et al: Life-threatening puerperal infection due to Group A streptococci *Obstet Gynecol* 79(5):894, May 1992 (Part 2 of 2 parts).

Swanson JM, Chenitz WC: The prevention and management of genital herpes: a community health approach, *Community Health Nurs* 6:209, 1989.

Tillman J: Syphillis: an old disease, a contemporary perinatal problem, *JOGNN* 21(3):209, May/June 1992.

Touchstone DM, Davis DD: Consider chlamydia, *RN* 55:32, Feb 1992.

Wendel GD, Gilstrap LC III: Syphilis rise calls for accurate diagnosis, *Contemp OB/GYN* 35:37, June 1990.

White S, Larsen B: Measles in pregnancy, *Contemp OB/GYN* 35:57, Sept 1990.

Witkin SS: Chronic recurrent vaginal candidiasis, *Contemp OB/GYN* 35:56, July 1990.

chapter 29 review

Key Concepts

- Pregnancy confers no immunity against infection, and both mother and fetus must be considered when the pregnant woman contracts an infection.
- HIV is transmitted through blood, semen, and perinatal events.
- HSV interacts with epithelial or neuroepithelial cells and neurons; after an infection, the HSV migrates to one or more ganglia where it remains latent and dormant until reactivated by one or more stressors.
- *C. trachomatis* is the most common sexually transmitted bacterial pathogen in the United States and is responsible for substantial morbidity, personal suffering, and heavy economic burden.
- Young sexually active females and males who have multiple sex partners and do not practice safer sex are at greatest risk for STDs and HIV.
- STDs often occur in groups; what appear to be resistant infections actually may be multiple infections or reinfections.
- Abuse of alcohol and drugs compromises the body's immune system and increases the risk for AIDS and associated conditions.
- During the intrapartum period, a primary focus of care is the prevention of nosocomial spread of infection and the protection of care providers.
- Because medical history and examination cannot reliably identify all persons with HIV or other blood-borne pathogens, blood and body-fluid precautions should be consistently used for everyone.
- STDs and genital and perigenital infections are biologic events, for which all individuals have a right to expect objective, compassionate, and effective health care.

Key Terms

- acquired immunodeficiency syndrome (AIDS) (p. 853)
- bacteremic (septic) shock (p. 872)
- condylomata acuminata (p. 859)
- congenital varicella syndrome (p. 874)
- dyspareunia (p. 849)
- dysuria (p. 849)
- fomites (p. 849)
- human immunodeficiency virus (HIV) (p. 853)
- human papillomavirus (HPV) (p. 859)
- inclusion conjunctivitis (p. 849)
- leukorrhea (p. 863)
- mastitis (p. 872)
- nosocomial (p. 855)
- ophthalmia neonatorum (p. 850)
- pruritus (p. 863)
- puerperal infection (p. 870)
- sexually transmitted disease (STD) (p. 848)
- TORCH infections (p. 855)
- toxic shock syndrome (TSS) (p. 875)
- universal precautions (p. 877)
- urinary tract infection (UTI) (p. 867)
- vaginitis (p. 863)

Critical Thinking Exercises

You are assigned to a single woman in labor who has a history of herpes simplex virus II (HSV II). Vaginal examination reveals an active lesion that appears to be a recurrence of HSV II on the cervix. The woman is told of the finding, and a cesarean birth is planned. You notice the father of the baby appears upset and angry. As you leave the room, you overhear him ask the woman why she did not tell him that she had herpes.

1. What is your assessment of the situation? What further information do you need to verify your assumptions?
2. What are some of the effects the situation may have on the relationship between the couple?
3. Examine your personal reaction to working with this woman in light of this new information about the presence of an infection. How might these feelings affect your plan of care?
4. Formulate a plan of care, and provide a rationale for your interventions.

You are assigned to a 19-year-old mother who has tested positive for HIV. She is being discharged home with her baby.

1. Examine your personal reactions to this young mother and her baby.
2. Generate possible reactions the young woman might have to her HIV status. Compare these reactions with your own.
3. Analyze the significance of your reaction in terms of providing care to this young woman.
4. Formulate a discharge teaching plan for the woman and her family that includes care and infection control.

Topics for Nursing Research

Much of the research on perinatal infections focuses on the clinical presentation and epidemiology of diseases. Yet there are many areas that nursing should address to improve the care of mothers, infants, and their families. Suggested topics for study include the following:

- What factors influence preventive health practices (e.g., safer sex)?
- What methods are most effective in teaching women about the significance of disease prevention, especially during pregnancy?
- What factors affect compliance with treatment and partner follow-up?
- How do chronic STDs affect relationships, self-esteem, and quality of life?
- How is the course of HIV infection different in women and children?
- What are the long-term care needs of women and children with HIV?
- Can formal instruction in STD affect a decrease in low-birth-weight infants?
- What roles do fashion and exercise play in the increasing incidence and prevalence of vaginitis?

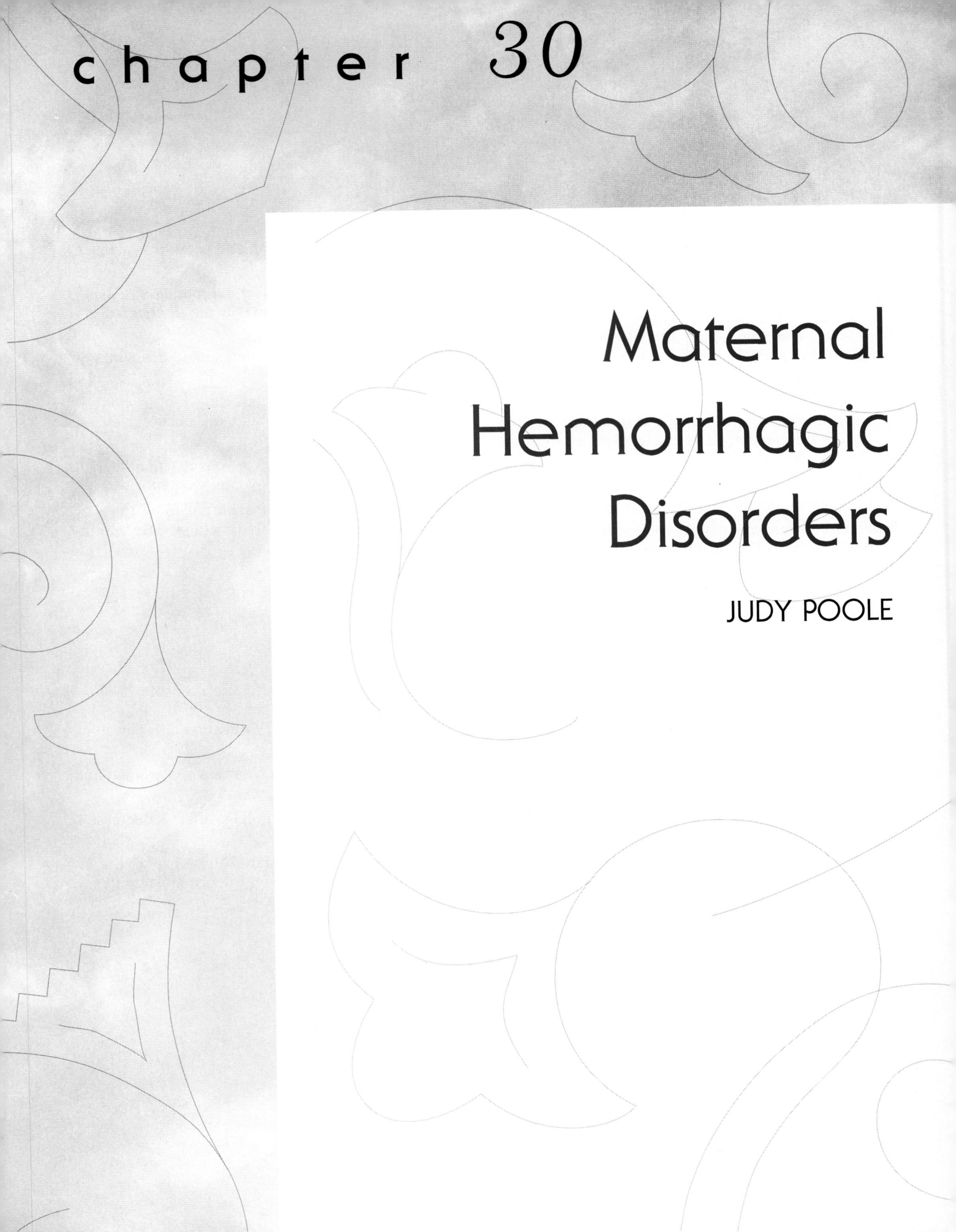

chapter 30

Maternal Hemorrhagic Disorders

JUDY POOLE

LEARNING OBJECTIVES

- Define the key terms listed.
- Review causes, signs and symptoms, possible complications, and management and care for hemorrhagic disorders during pregnancy.
- Formulate nursing diagnoses for hemorrhagic disorders during pregnancy; identify data bases and develop a nursing care plan.
- Compare abruptio placentae and placenta previa.
- Discuss clotting disorders in pregnancy with emphasis on disseminated intravascular coagulation (DIC).
- Review postbirth hemorrhage causes, signs and symptoms, possible complications, and management and care.
- Describe hemorrhagic shock and its management; discuss hazards of therapy for each disorder.
- Summarize the role of the nurse in the health care team approach to the treatment of bleeding disorders.
- Identify topics for nursing research related to maternal hemorrhagic disorders.

Hemorrhagic disorders in pregnancy are medical emergencies. Maternal mortality has decreased significantly in recent years; however, hemorrhage remains a major cause of maternal death (Suresh, Kinch, 1991). Hemorrhage was cited as the cause of death in 13% of obstetric-related deaths in the United States between 1980 and 1985 (Rochat et al, 1988). Prompt, expert teamwork on the part of the health care provider is required to save the life of the mother and infant.

The nurse must be alert to the symptoms of hemorrhage and shock and be prepared to act quickly to minimize blood loss and hasten return to normal state. Supportive care for the pregnant woman and her family includes attention to physical needs, emotional well-being, and possibly grief counseling. This chapter focuses on hemorrhagic problems in early and late pregnancy, as well as postpartum hemorrhage.

Early in pregnancy, abortion or ectopic pregnancy is the most common cause of excessive bleeding. Later, premature separation of the normally implanted placenta or placenta previa may be the cause of hemorrhage. Postbirth hemorrhage is a possibility during any childbirth experience. Specific problems that result in hemorrhage are uterine atony, lacerations of the birth canal, hematomas, episiotomy dehiscence, retained placenta, inversion of the uterus, and subinvolution of the uterus. Postbirth anterior pituitary necrosis (Sheehan's syndrome) as a result of hypovolemic shock also is discussed.

EARLY PREGNANCY BLEEDING

Bleeding during early pregnancy is alarming to the client and of concern to the health care provider. The common bleeding disorders of early pregnancy include abortion, incompetent cervix, ectopic pregnancy, and hydatidiform mole.

Spontaneous Abortion

Abortion is the termination of pregnancy before viability of the fetus. Viability is reached at about 20 to 24 weeks' gestation—a fetal weight over 500 g or a crown-rump length of 18 cm—when the fetus is able to survive in an extrauterine environment. With today's technology for newborn care, such an infant has at least a chance for survival. There are three types of abortions. *Spontaneous* abortions result from natural causes; with *therapeutic* abortions the pregnancy is interrupted deliberately for medical reasons; and *elective* abortions are performed for social reasons. This discussion includes only spontaneous abortions; for therapeutic and social abortions see Chapter 42.

An *early spontaneous abortion*, or miscarriage, is one that occurs before 16 weeks' gestation; a *late abortion* is one occurring between 16 weeks and the age of viability. The rate and cause of spontaneous abortion are difficult to determine but may be as high as 20% (Dorfman, 1991). About three fourths of these abortions occur before the sixteenth week of pregnancy, and most take place before the eighth week. More than half of all spontaneous abortions are caused by abnormal embryonic development, chromosomal defects, and inheritable disorders. Most of the other spontaneous abortions result from maternal causes such as advancing maternal age and parity, chronic infections, chronic debilitating diseases, nutrition, and recreational drug use; the reasons for the remainder are speculative (Cunningham et al, 1989). Many early pregnancies are lost for unknown reasons before the diagnosis of pregnancy is even established. The diagnosis of the type of abortion a woman is experiencing is based on the signs and symptoms present (Table 30-1 and Fig. 30-1).

CAUSES. *Recurrent, early (habitual)* spontaneous abortion is the loss of three or more previable pregnancies. The causes of recurrent early abortion may include endocrine imbalance (e.g., diabetes mellitus), infections (e.g., bacteriuria and *chlamydia trachomatis*), systemic disorders (e.g., lupus erythematosus), psychologic factors (but proof is lacking), genetic factors (about 60% of early abortions display an abnormal chromosomal makeup), and cocaine use, which has been linked to spontaneous abortion and preterm labor (Cocaine use, 1987; Cunningham, et al, 1989; Rosenak et al, 1990). An increase in maternal blood pressure and a reduction in uterine blood flow may be etiologic factors (Cole, 1987; Woods et al, 1987; Rosenak et al, 1990). (See Chapter 42 for infertility management.)

Anomalies of the reproductive tract cause second- or third-trimester pregnancy loss. Little can be done to avoid genetic causes of pregnancy loss, but prepregnancy correction of maternal disorders, immunization against infectious diseases, adequate early prenatal care, and treatment of pregnancy complications will do much to prevent abortion.

TYPES. The five types of spontaneous abortion are threatened, inevitable, incomplete, complete, and missed (Fig. 30-1). Symptoms of a *threatened abortion* (Fig. 30-1, *A*) may include spotting of blood, but the cervical os is closed. Management includes bed rest and avoiding stress and orgasm. Follow-up treatment is individualized to the woman.

TABLE 30-1 Assessing Abortion

Type of Abortion	Amount of Bleeding	Uterine Cramping	Passage of Tissue	Tissue in Vagina	Internal Cervical Os	Size of Uterus
Threatened	Slight	Mild	No	No	Closed	Agrees with length of pregnancy
Inevitable	Moderate	Moderate	No	No	Open	Agrees with length of pregnancy
Incomplete	Heavy	Severe	Yes	Possible	Open with tissue in cervix	Smaller than expected for length of pregnancy
Complete	Slight	Mild	Yes	Possible	Closed	Smaller than expected for length of pregnancy
Missed	Slight	No	No	No	Closed	Smaller than expected for length of pregnancy
Septic	Varies; usually malodorous; fever present	Varies; fever present	Varies: fever present	Varies: fever present	Usually open; fever present	Any of the above with tenderness

From Gordon RT: Emergencies in obstetrics and gynecology. In Warner CG, editor; *Emergency care: assessment and intervention*, ed 3, St Louis, 1983. Mosby–Year Book.

Inevitable (Fig. 30-1, *B*) and *incomplete* (Fig. 30-1, *C*) abortions involve a moderate to heavy amount of bleeding with an open cervical os. Tissue also may be present with the bleeding. Prompt termination of the pregnancy, usually by curettage, is the suggested treatment.

In a *complete abortion* (Fig. 30-1, *D*) all fetal tissue is passed, the cervix is closed, and there may be slight bleeding. Usually no further treatment is required.

A *missed abortion* (Fig. 30-1, *E*) refers to a pregnancy in which the products of conception have died but spontaneous abortion does not occur. It may be diagnosed when the uterus is smaller than expected for the duration of the pregnancy. There may be no bleeding or cramping, and the cervical os is closed. Treatment may include waiting up to 1 month for spontaneous abortion to occur, with frequent monitoring of the woman's clotting factors. If spontaneous abortion does not occur, the physician will terminate the pregnancy to prevent DIC or sepsis, or both, in the woman. If a missed abortion is retained for months or years and the products of conception calcify, a uterine lithopedion, or "womb stone," may be found (Fig. 30-1, *E*).

Presenting symptoms of a *septic* or infected abortion include fever and abdominal tenderness. Vaginal bleeding, which may be slight to heavy, is usually malodorous. Termination of the pregnancy, antibiotic therapy, and treatment of septic shock are initiated. Hemorrhage and sepsis (e.g., salpingitis, peritonitis) occur, especially in the induced abortion under septic conditions and in instances of neglected care. Death may follow instrumentation and perforation of the soft, slightly enlarged uterus, or septicemia or septic emboli may follow spontaneous incomplete abortion. Even mild infection may be followed by tubal occlusion and infertility.

SIGNS AND SYMPTOMS. Signs and symptoms of spontaneous abortion depend on the duration of pregnancy. Once pregnancy has been diagnosed, the presence of uterine bleeding, uterine contractions, and uterine pain are ominous signs and must be considered a threatened abortion until proved otherwise. The woman may report a heavy menstrual flow if abortion occurs before the sixth week of pregnancy. Abortion that occurs between the sixth and twelfth weeks of pregnancy will cause moderate discomfort and blood loss. After the twelfth week, abortion is

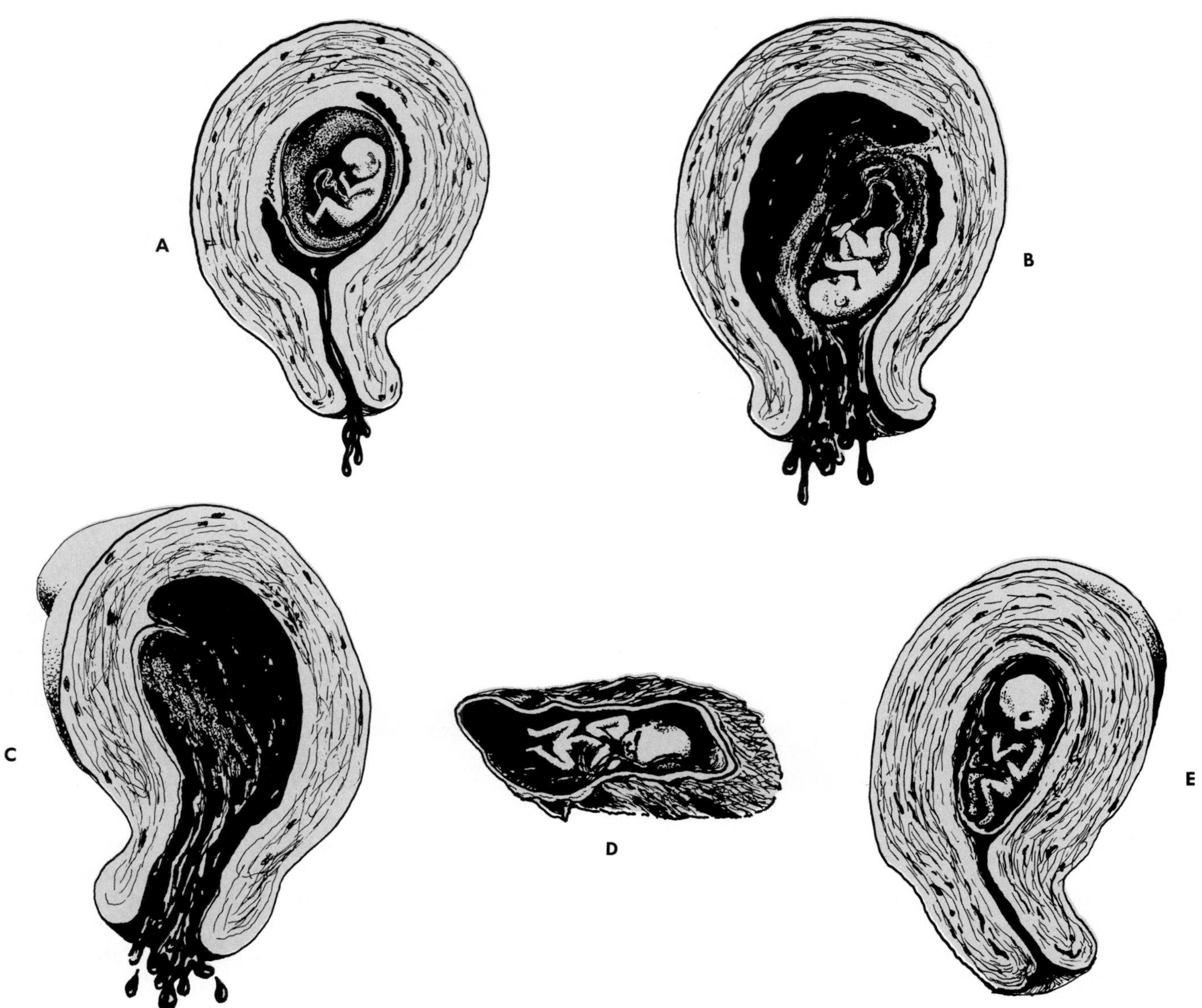

Fig. 30-1 Spontaneous abortion. **A,** Threatened. **B,** Inevitable. **C,** Incomplete. **D,** Complete. **E,** Missed.

typified by severe pain, similar to that of labor, because the fetus must be expelled.

Medical management (Table 30-2) depends on the classification of spontaneous abortion. Therefore an early accurate diagnosis of spontaneous abortion is vital.

NURSING PROCESS

ASSESSMENT

On admission to the hospital, the nurse obtains a history of the client's chief complaint, pain, bleeding, and last menstrual period (LMP) to determine the approximate length of gestation. The initial data base includes vital signs, previous pregnancies, previous pregnancy losses, type and location of pain, quantity and nature of bleeding, allergies, and emotional status (see box on p. 889). It is not uncommon for the client to be anxious and fearful of what may happen to her and to her pregnancy.

Various laboratory findings are characteristic of abortion. Results of a urine pregnancy test that are negative or weakly positive characterize abortion. With considerable or persistent blood loss, anemia is likely (hemoglobin level < 10.5 g/dL). If sepsis is present, temperature is higher than 100.4° F (38° C),

TABLE 30-2 Types of Spontaneous Abortion and Usual Management

Type of Abortion	Management
Threatened	Bed rest, sedation, and avoidance of stress and orgasm are recommended. Further treatment will depend on client's course.
Inevitable and incomplete	Prompt termination of pregnancy is accomplished usually by dilatation and curettage (D & C).*
Complete	No further intervention may be needed if uterine contractions are adequate to prevent hemorrhage and if there is no infection.
Missed	If spontaneous evacuation of the uterus does not occur within 1 month, however, pregnancy is terminated by method appropriate to duration of pregnancy (see Chapter 42). Blood clotting factors are monitored until uterus is empty. DIC and incoagulability of blood with uncontrolled hemorrhage may develop in cases of fetal death after twelfth week if products of conception are retained for longer than 5 weeks (see pp. 917 and 918 for discussion of DIC).
Septic	Immediate termination of pregnancy by method appropriate to duration of pregnancy (see Chapter 42). Cervical culture and sensitivity (C & S) studies are done, and broad-spectrum antibiotic therapy (e.g., ampicillin) is started. Treatment for septic shock is initiated if necessary.

*For a discussion of dilatation and curettage, see Chapter 42.

Assessment of Bleeding in Pregnancy

INITIAL DATA BASE

Chief complaint
Vital signs
Gravidity, parity
LMP/EDD
Pregnancy history (previous and current)
Allergies
Nausea and vomiting
Pain (onset, quality, precipitating event)
Bleeding or coagulation problems
LOC
Emotional status

EARLY PREGNANCY

Confirmation of pregnancy
Bleeding (bright or dark, intermittent or continuous)
Pain (type, intensity, persistence)
Vaginal discharge

LATE PREGNANCY

EDD
Bleeding (quantity, associated pain)
Vaginal discharge
Amniotic membrane status
Uterine activity
Abdominal pain
Fetal status/viability

EDD, Estimated date of delivery; *LMP,* last menstrual period; *LOC,* level of consciousness.

and white blood cell count (WBC) is greater than 12,000/μL. Sedimentation rate is not helpful for differential diagnostic purposes because an increased sedimentation rate is the rule with pregnancy, anemia, or infection. Endocrine studies show that human chorionic gonadotropin (hCG), estrogen, and progesterone titers are minimal or absent in established abortions.

NURSING DIAGNOSIS

Potential nursing diagnoses pertinent to early pregnancy bleeding include both physical and psychosocial aspects of care. Nursing diagnoses for the client experiencing a spontaneous abortion may include the following:

- Anxiety/fear related to
  —Unknown outcome and unfamiliarity with hospital procedures
- Fluid volume deficit related to
  —Excessive bleeding secondary to spontaneous abortion
- Acute pain related to
  —Uterine contractions
- Anticipatory grieving related to
  —Unexpected pregnancy outcome
- Situational low self-esteem related to
  —Inability to successfully carry a pregnancy to term gestation

PLANNING

The plan of care is mutually negotiated on the basis of the biophysical and psychosocial assessment of the client. The plan must relate specifically to the client's clinical and nursing diagnoses, and it must be stated in terms of measurable client behaviors. Mutually determined *goals* may include the following:

- The woman will discuss the impact of the loss on her and her family.
- The woman will identify and use available support systems.
- The woman will not develop signs and symptoms of complications.

IMPLEMENTATION

Immediate nursing care focuses on stabilization of the client. Psychosocial aspects of care focus on what this pregnancy loss means to the client and her family. Care is client- and family-centered. Careful explanations are provided as to the nature of the abortion, expected procedures, and possible future implications. The woman should be told that spontaneous abortions are common and not always related to her behavior. If the woman has a history of cigarette, alcohol, or substance abuse, she should be told of the increased risk of early pregnancy loss related to these behaviors (Deutchman, 1989; Glass, Golbus, 1989).

The nurse will reinforce explanations given by the physician and carry out appropriate orders. An intravenous (IV) line will be started, laboratory work obtained, and possibly an ultrasound scan will be performed. Laboratory tests include a complete blood count (CBC), blood typing for group and Rh factor and crossmatching, and urinalysis. Chest x-ray films and electrocardiogram evaluation are obtained if necessary. Blood, fluid, and electrolyte imbalances are corrected as soon as possible. If a dilatation and curretage (D & C) is scheduled, the nurse reinforces explanations, answers any questions or concerns, and prepares the client for surgery. D & C is a surgical procedure in which the cervix is dilated and a curette is inserted to scrape the uterine walls and remove uterine contents. Before the D & C is performed, a full history should be obtained and a general and pelvic examination should be done. General preoperative and postoperative care is appropriate for the woman requiring surgical intervention for spontaneous abortion.

Analgesics and/or anesthesia appropriate to the procedure are used. IV administration of oxytocin, 10 U in 500 mL of infusate, may be needed to induce or augment abortion. After evacuation of the uterus, 10 to 20 U of oxytocin in 1000 mL of infusate may be given to prevent hemorrhage.

Ergot products such as ergonovine, which contract the uterus and cervix, are contraindicated to avoid retention of fragments of tissue until the uterus is emptied. Retained fragments of fetal or placental tissue cause predisposition to uterine relaxation and puerperal infection. Three or four doses of ergonovine, 0.2 mg orally or intramuscularly every 4 hours, should be given if the woman is normotensive. Antibiotics are given as necessary. Transfusion may be required for shock or anemia. The woman with Rh negativity who has not developed isoimmunization is given an intramuscular injection of $Rh_o(D)$ immune globulin within 72 hours of the abortion (for further discussion, see Chapter 38).

Discharge teaching should emphasize the need for rest, and if significant blood loss occurred, iron supplementation may be ordered. Follow-up care should assess the woman's physical and emotional recovery. Referrals to local support groups should be provided (see box on p. 891).

EVALUATION

Evaluation is based on the predetermined client-centered goals. The nurse can be reasonably assured that care was effective to the degree that the goals for care have been met. That is, the woman will discuss the impact of the loss on her and her family, identify and use available support systems, and not develop signs and symptoms of complications.

Incompetent Cervix

An **incompetent cervix** is characterized by painless dilatation of the cervical os, without labor or contractions of the uterus, in the second trimester or

Discharge Teaching for the Woman after Spontaneous Abortion

- Refer to appropriate support groups, clergy, or professional counseling.
- Advise client to report any heavy, profuse, or bright red bleeding to physician.
- Reassure client that a scant, dark discharge may persist for 1 to 2 weeks.
- To reduce the risk of infection, remind woman not introduce anything into the vagina until bleeding has stopped
- Acknowledge that she has experienced a loss and that time is required for recovery. She may experience mood swings and depression.

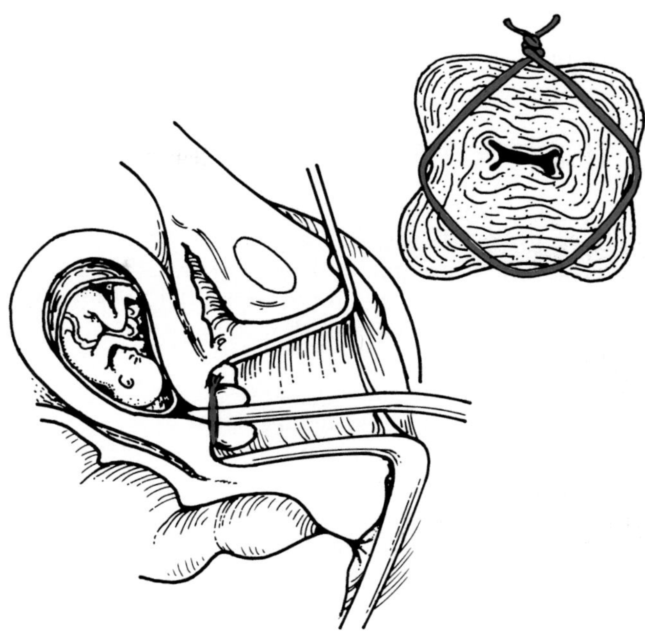

Fig. 30-2 A. Cerclage correction of incompetent cervical os. B. Cross-section view of closed internal os.

early in the third trimester of pregnancy. Miscarriage or preterm birth may result.

As many as 40% of all perinatal deaths occur in pregnancies that terminate between 20 and 28 weeks of gestation. Cervical incompetence is a major contributor to these losses. It is estimated to occur in 1/1000 births, 1/100 abortions, and 1/5 habitual abortions (Beischer, MacKay, 1986).

CAUSES. Etiologic factors include a prior history of traumatic birth, forceful D & C, or the client's mother's ingestion of diethylstilbestrol (DES) during pregnancy. Other instances may result from a congenitally short cervix or uterine anomalies.

The diagnosis of cervical incompetence is difficult and is based on clinical history. A presumptive diagnosis usually can be made if a woman manifests appreciable cervical dilatation and prolapse of the membranes through the cervix without labor. In the client with a history of repeated second-trimester spontaneous terminations, cervical incompetence should be suspected.

MEDICAL MANAGEMENT. Conservative management consists of bed rest, hydration, and tocolysis (inhibition of uterine contractions), or a cervical cerclage may be performed. Correction of the weakened cervix is possible by wedge trachelorrhaphy (removal of a wedge from the anterior segment of the cervix with closure) in the nonpregnant woman. During gestation, a McDonald **cerclage,** band of homologous fascia, or nonabsorbable ribbon (Mersilene) may be placed around the cervix beneath the mucosa to constrict the internal os of the cervix (Fig. 30-2). Successful continuation of the pregnancy to viability or beyond occurs in approximately 40% of women, provided the membranes remain intact and the cervix is not more than 3 cm dilated or more than 50% effaced at the time of correction. The suture is left in place until close to term, when it is removed and labor is allowed to begin spontaneously. This procedure must be repeated with each pregnancy.

A second method involves placement of a purse-string ligature to maintain a closed cervix during pregnancy. In the *Shirodkar* cerclage procedure, the suture remains in place permanently for the woman who anticipates future pregnancies. Births will be by cesarean.

NURSING PROCESS

ASSESSMENT

The nurse assesses the client's feelings about her pregnancy and her understanding of an incompetent cervix. It is also important to evaluate the client's support systems. Because the diagnosis of an incompetent cervix usually is not made until the woman has lost one or two previous pregnancies, she may feel guilty or at blame for this impending loss. Therefore it is important to assess for prior reactions to stresses and appropriateness of coping responses.

The client will need the support of her health care providers, as well as that of her family.

Nursing Diagnosis

Care of the client with an incompetent cervix focuses on the client's self-concept, her ability to cope with possible pregnancy loss, and her ability to understand treatment regimens. Potential nursing diagnoses include the following:

- Anxiety/fear related to
  —The threat of a lost pregnancy
- Situational low self-esteem related to
  —The inability to successfully carry a pregnancy to term
- Ineffective individual coping related to
  —The potential/actual loss of the pregnancy
- Altered family processes related to
  —A change in birth plan secondary to the potential/actual loss of the pregnancy
- Knowledge deficit related to
  —Cervical incompetence and treatment regimens
- Anticipatory grieving related to
  —The potential loss of a fetus through an incompetent cervix

Planning

As much as possible, the plan of care is mutually negotiated on the basis of the biophysical and psychosocial assessment of the client. The plan relates specifically to the client's clinical and nursing diagnoses. *Goals,* which are stated in measurable client behaviors and are client-centered, may include the following.

- The woman will verbalize her fears and concerns.
- The woman will use effective coping mechanisms in adjusting to her situation.
- The woman will be free of complications, or if complications arise she will receive prompt appropriate therapy with no sequelae.
- The woman will verbalize understanding of her condition and treatment.
- The woman will demonstrate self-care behaviors to maintain pregnancy.

Implementation

If conservative management is the treatment of choice, the client must understand the importance of bed rest at home and the need for close observation and supervision. Instruction includes the rationale for bed rest, restricting activity, and warning signs to report. The client must be instructed on the importance of taking oral tocolytic medication as prescribed, the expected response, and possible side effects. Tocolytics will be given prophylactically to prevent uterine contractions and further dilatation of the cervix. If "home monitoring" is implemented, she is taught how to apply a uterine contraction monitor and transmit the monitor tracing by telephone to the monitoring center. Nurses at the monitoring center assess the tracing for contractions, answer questions, provide emotional support and education, and report information to the client's physician (Roberts et al, 1990; Robichaux et al, 1990; Watson et al, 1990).

As the client approaches her due date, a decision is made about the route of birth. If future pregnancies are desired and Shirodkar's cerclage had been performed, cesarean birth can occur, leaving the Shirodkar band intact. If future childbearing is not desired or a McDonald cerclage is in place, the suture is released and labor is permitted. If management is unsuccessful and the fetus is born before viability, appropriate grief support should be provided (see Chapter 40 on loss and grief). If the fetus is born prematurely, appropriate anticipatory guidance and support are necessary (see Chapter 37 on preterm birth).

After placement of the cervical cerclage the client will be monitored throughout her hospital stay for the absence of contractions or signs of infection. Referrals will be made as appropriate for assistance once she is discharged home. It is important that the client understand the rationale for the treatment and the needed follow-up care.

Discharge teaching will focus on signs and symptoms of preterm labor, rupture of membranes, and infection. If home uterine monitoring is used, the client should receive her initial instructions from the home health agency before discharge.

Evaluation

The nurse can be reasonably assured that care was effective to the degree to which goals for care are met.

- The woman verbalizes her fears and concerns.
- She uses effective coping mechanisms to adjust to her condition.
- She is free of complications or if complications arise, receives prompt and appropriate therapy.
- She verbalizes understanding of her condition and treatment.
- She demonstrates self-care behaviors to maintain pregnancy.

Ectopic Pregnancy

Ectopic pregnancy is one in which the fetus is implanted outside the uterine cavity (Fig. 30-3). About 90% of ectopic pregnancies occur in the fallopian (uterine) tube, with most on the right side, for undetermined reasons. Approximately 1/100 pregnancies in the United States is ectopic, and at least three fourths of these become symptomatic and are diagnosed during the first trimester. Ectopic pregnancy is a significant cause of maternal morbidity and mortality, with maternal mortality increased 10 times that of vaginal birth and 50 times that of induced abortion (Cunningham et al, 1990).

Most extrauterine pregnancies result from abnormalities that impede or prevent the passage of the fertilized ovum through the fallopian tube (e.g., peritubal adhesions after pelvic inflammatory disease). On occasion, an ovum is fertilized within the ovary or soon after ovulation.

Ectopic pregnancy is classified according to the site of implantation (e.g., tubal, ovarian). The uterus is the only organ capable of containing and sustaining a term pregnancy. However, the rare abdominal pregnancy, with birth by laparotomy, may result in a living infant.

SIGNS AND SYMPTOMS. There are no signs or symptoms diagnostic of early ectopic pregnancy. A missed period, adnexal fullness, and tenderness may suggest an unruptured tubal pregnancy. In contrast, the following triad is associated with early ruptured extrauterine pregnancy in almost 50% of cases: amenorrhea or an abnormal menstrual period followed by slight uterine bleeding, adnexal or cul-de-sac mass, and unilateral pelvic pain over the mass. Decidua but no placental villi may be found on curettage. Additional findings of *acute rupture* may include shock out of proportion to visible blood loss, referred shoulder pain, or evidence of acute blood loss in chronic ruptured tubal pregnancy.

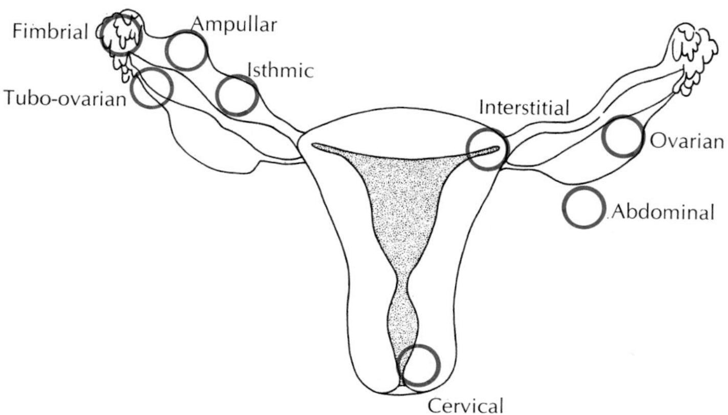

Fig. 30-3 Sites of implantation of ectopic pregnancies. Order of frequency of occurrence is ampulla, isthmus, interstitium, fimbria, tuboovarian ligament, ovary, abdominal cavity, and cervix (external os).

In *chronic ruptured* tubal pregnancy, which represents slightly more than half the total ectopic pregnancies, internal bleeding usually has been slow and the symptoms atypical or inconclusive. In addition to slight, dark vaginal bleeding, a sense of pelvic pressure or fullness; lower abdominal tenderness; flatulence; and a tense, sensitive, semicystic, perhaps crepitant, cul-de-sac mass may be felt. Slight fever, leukocytosis, and a falling hematocrit or hemoglobin level may be noted. An ecchymotic blueness of the umbilicus (**Cullen's sign**), which indicates hematoperitoneum, may develop in a neglected ruptured intraabdominal ectopic pregnancy.

MEDICAL MANAGEMENT. Hysterosalpingography (see Chapter 42) is contraindicated in suspected tubal pregnancy because it may initiate tubal rupture or hemorrhage. In possible advanced abdominal pregnancy, a sonogram showing a fetus high out of the pelvis, often in an abnormal presentation, may be diagnostic.

The differential diagnosis of ectopic pregnancy involves a consideration of numerous disorders that share many, perhaps all, the same signs and symptoms. The physician must consider uterine abortion, ruptured corpus luteum cyst, appendicitis, salpingitis, ovarian cysts, torsion of the ovary, and urinary tract infection (Table 30-3).

Prevention of ectopic pregnancy per se is impossible. The major management problem in ectopic pregnancy is hemorrhage; bleeding must be quickly and effectively controlled. Blood transfusions must be available. Laparotomy may be performed immediately after the diagnosis of ectopic pregnancy is made. Blood and clots are evacuated, and bleeding vessels are controlled. Excision of the cornua and fallopian tube is recommended if the tube is grossly involved; the ovary is conserved if possible. Hysterectomy usually is necessary for ruptured cornual or interstitial pregnancy. Ovarian pregnancy always requires loss of the ovary.

Advanced ectopic abdominal pregnancy requires laparotomy as soon as the woman is fit for surgery (Fig 30-4). If the placenta of a second- or third-trimester abdominal pregnancy is attached to a vital organ, such as the liver, no attempt at separation and removal should be made. The cord should be cut flush with the placenta and the afterbirth left in situ. Degeneration and absorption of the placenta usually occur without complication.

The diagnosis and management of ectopic pregnancy is rapidly changing as technology improves.

TABLE 30-3 Differential Diagnosis of Ectopic Pregnancy

	Ectopic Pregnancy	Appendicitis	Salpingitis	Ruptured Corpus Luteum Cyst	Uterine Abortion
Pain	Unilateral cramps and tenderness before rupture	Epigastric, periumbilical, then right lower quadrant pain; tenderness localizing at McBurney's point; rebound tenderness	Usually in both lower quadrants with or without rebound	Unilateral, becoming general with progressive bleeding	Midline cramps
Nausea and vomiting	Occasionally before, frequently after rupture	Usual; precedes shift of pain to right lower quadrant	Infrequent	Rare	Almost never
Menstruation	Some aberration; missed period, spotting	Unrelated to menses	Hypermenorrhea or metrorrhagia or both	Period delayed, then bleeding, often with pain	Amenorrhea, then spotting, then brisk bleeding
Temperature and pulse	37.2°-37.8° C (99°-100° F); pulse variable; normal before, rapid after rupture	37.2°-37.8° C (99°-100° F): pulse rapid: 99-100	37.2°-40° C (99°-104° F): pulse elevated in proportion to fever	Not over 37.2 ° C (99° F): pulse normal unless blood loss marked, then rapid	To 37.2° C (99° F) if spontaneous: to 40° C (104°F) if induced (infected)
Pelvic examination	Unilateral tenderness, especially on movement of cervix; crepitant mass on one side or in cul-de-sac	No masses; rectal tenderness high on right side	Bilateral tenderness on movement of cervix: masses only when pyosalpinx or hydrosalpinx present	Tenderness over affected ovary: no masses	Cervix slightly patulous: uterus slightly enlarged, irregularly softened: tender with infection
Laboratory findings	WBC to 15,000/μl; RBC strikingly low if blood loss large; sedimentation rate slightly elevated	WBC: 10,000-18,000/μl (rarely normal); RBC normal: sedimentation rate slightly elevated	WBC: 15,000-30,000/μl; RBC normal: sedimentation rate markedly elevated	WBC normal to 10,000/μl: RBC normal: sedimentation rate normal	WBC: 15,000/μl if spontaneous: to 30,000/μl if induced (infection); RBC normal: sedimentation rate slightly to moderately elevated

From Benson RC, editor: *Current obstetric and gynecologic diagnosis and treatment* ed 5, copyright 1984 by Lange Medical Publications Los Altos, Calif.

The use of methotrexate therapy is being explored for use in the woman with persistent ectopic pregnancy (Stoval et al, 1990). Current evidence demonstrates that laparoscopic management of ectopic pregnancies is equally safe, equally effective, and less traumatic then laparotomy and may replace laparotomy as treatment for most ectopic pregnancies (Nager, Murphy, 1991).

Prognosis varies. The success of a subsequent pregnancy depends on the woman's specific reproductive history. Ectopic pregnancy recurs in approximately 10% of women, but more than 50% of women who have had an ectopic pregnancy achieve at least one normal pregnancy thereafter.

NURSING PROCESS

ASSESSMENT

A careful history with identification of a late LMP or an actual missed period followed by slight vaginal

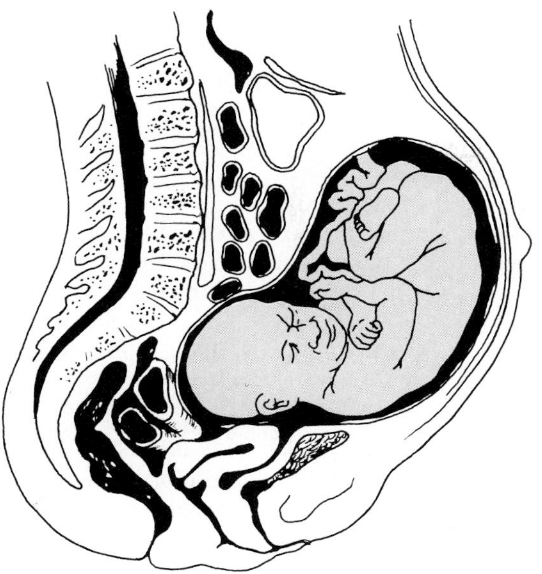

Fig. 30-4 Ectopic pregnancy, abdominal.

bleeding may be indicative. The nurse should have a high index of suspicion of the possibility of an ectopic pregnancy in the following circumstances: a woman with a history of a missed menstrual period, spotting, or pelvic pain or who has a history of pelvic infection, intrauterine device use, or tubal surgery. If the woman has internal bleeding, assessment will reveal the presence of vertigo, shoulder pain, hypotension, and tachycardia. Any woman suspected of having an ectopic pregnancy should be immediately referred to a physician for a confirmative diagnosis and medical intervention.

Physical examination reveals unilateral pain over the tube and ovary, and an adnexal mass often is palpated. Laboratory testing reveals a low hCG level. Ultrasound scanning has provided improved accuracy in preoperative diagnosis of ectopic pregnancy and has reduced the number of unnecessary laparoscopies. An appropriately timed ultrasound examination for the at-risk woman allows earlier diagnosis and a resultant reduction in the mortality and morbidity resulting from the condition (de Crespigny, 1987).

NURSING DIAGNOSIS

Potential nursing diagnoses pertinent to ectopic pregnancy include the following:

- Denial related to
  —The possibility of a tubal pregnancy
- Decreased cardiac output related to
  —Bleeding associated with a ruptured ectopic pregnancy
- Anticipatory grieving related to
  —The loss of the pregnancy

PLANNING

The plan of care is mutually determined whenever possible, on the basis of the biophysical and psychosocial assessement of the client. It must relate specifically to the client's clinical and nursing diagnoses and be stated in terms of measurable client behaviors. Some client-centered *goals* may include the following.

- The woman will discuss the impact of the loss to her and her family.
- The woman will identify and use available support systems.
- The woman will not develop signs and symptoms of complications.

IMPLEMENTATION

Once an ectopic pregnancy is suspected, the physician is notified of assessment findings. Vital signs (pulse, respirations, and blood pressure) will be taken every 15 minutes or as appropriate on the basis of the client's condition. Laboratory tests will include determination of blood type and Rh factor, CBC, and a serum pregnancy test. General preoperative and postoperative care is appropriate for the woman requiring surgical intervention for an ectopic pregnancy.

EVALUATION

The nurse can be reasonably assured that care was effective to the degree that the goals for care have been met. That is, the woman will discuss the impact of the loss to her and her family, will identify and use available support systems, and will not develop signs and symptoms of complications.

Hydatidiform Mole (Molar Pregnancy)

Hydatidiform mole (molar pregnancy) is one of three types of gestational trophoblastic neoplasms. The other two types, chorioadenoma destruens (invasive mole) and choriocarcinoma, are discussed in Chapter 44. **Gestational trophoblastic disease (GTD)**, is a condition in which trophoblastic cells covering the chorionic villi proliferate and undergo cystic changes (Cunningham et al, 1989). GTD may be benign or malignant. There are two distinct types of hydatidiform moles: complete or classic mole and partial mole, which may or may not be part of the accepted continuum of gestational trophoblastic disease (Szulman, 1984; DePetrillo et al, 1987).

Hydatidiform mole occurs in 1/1200 pregnancies in the United States, but a much higher incidence is seen in the Orient and tropical areas (Berman, Di-Saia, 1989). Most often hydatidiform moles occur in women who have undergone ovulation stimulation with clomiphene (Clomid), in women of lower socio-economic groups, and in women at both ends of the reproductive spectrum (early teens or the perimenopause). The risk of developing a second mole is four to five times higher than the risk of the first.

TYPES. The *complete mole,* or classic mole, results from fertilization of an egg whose nucleus has been lost or inactivated (Fig. 30-5, *A*). The nucleus of a sperm (23X) duplicates, resulting in the diploid number, 46XX. The mole resembles a bunch of white grapes (Fig. 30-5, *B*). The hydropic (fluid-filled) vesicles grow rapidly, causing the uterus to be larger than expected for the duration of the pregnancy. Usually, the mole contains no fetus, placenta, amniotic membranes, or fluid. Maternal blood has no placenta to receive it; therefore hemorrhage into the uterine cavity and vaginal bleeding occur. In about 90% of the 46XX diploid hydatidiform moles, a progression toward choriocarcinoma occurs. The karyotype of the *partial mole* is normal diploid, trisomic, or triploid (Fig. 30-6). Maternal genes do exist. The triploid mole usually is the result of two paternal sets and one maternal set of chromosomes (diandry), but it could result from one paternal set and two maternal sets (digyny). Triploid karyotype is either 69XXX or 69XXY. Embryonic membranes are present. The potential for malignant transformation is much less than that associated with the complete hydatidiform mole (Scott et al, 1990).

Approximately 80% of partial hydatidiform moles regress spontaneously; 15% continue as nonmetastatic gestational trophoblastic disease. Neoplasms as sequelae of a molar pregnancy develop in 50% of women with metastatic trophoblastic disease (Scott et al, 1990).

SIGNS AND SYMPTOMS. In the early stages the signs and symptoms of hydatidiform mole cannot be distinguished from those of normal pregnancy. Later, vaginal bleeding occurs in almost every case. The vaginal discharge may be dark brown (resembling prune juice) or bright red, either scant or profuse. It may continue for only a few days or intermittently for weeks. Early in pregnancy the uterus of about half the affected women is significantly larger than expected from the menstrual dates. The percentage of women with an excessively enlarged uterus increases as the length of time from the LMP increases. Approximately 25% of women will have a uterus smaller than would be expected from the menstrual dates.

Anemia from blood loss, excessive nausea and

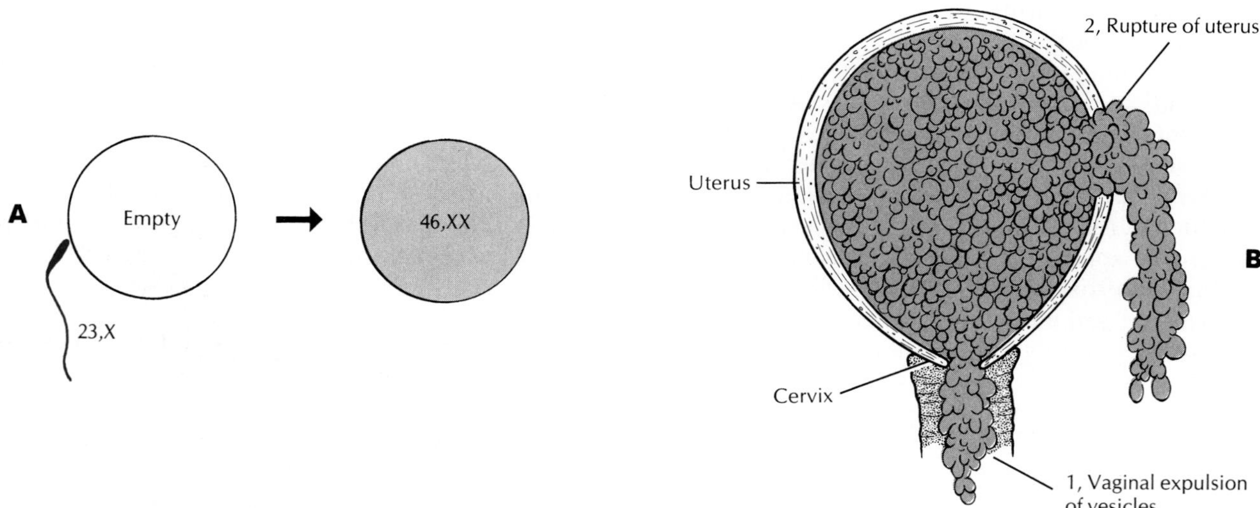

Fig. 30-5 A, Chromosomal origin of a complete mole. A single sperm (color) fertilizes an "empty" ovum. Reduplication of the sperm's 23X set gives a completely homozygous diploid 46XX. A similar process follows fertilization of an empty ovum by two sperm with two independently drawn sets of 23X or 23Y: therefore, both karyotypes of 46XX and 46XY can result. **B,** Uterine rupture with hydatidiform mole. *1,* Evacuation of mole through cervix. 2, Rupture of uterus and spillage of mole into peritoneal cavity (rare).

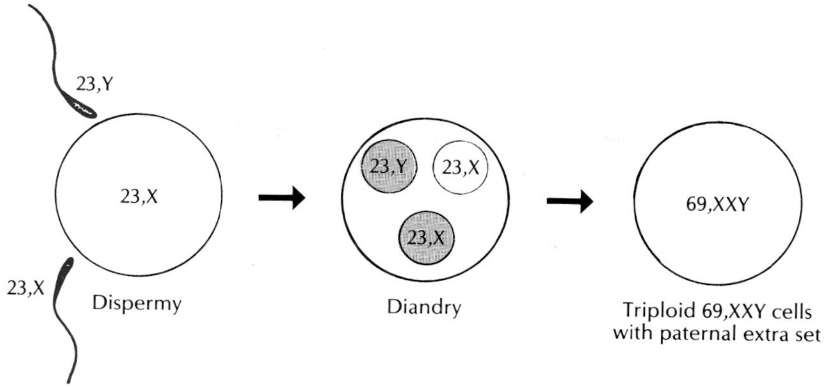

Fig. 30-6 Chromosomal origin of the triploid, partial mole. A normal ovum with a 23X haploid set is fertilized by two sperms (blue) to give a total of 69 chromosomes. A sex configuration of XXY, XXX, or XYY, is possible.

vomiting (hyperemesis gravidarum), and abdominal cramps caused by uterine distention are relatively common findings. Anemia results from intrauterine bleeding that results when molar tissue separates from the uterine wall. There is then no placenta to receive the maternal blood flow to the decidua basalis. Bleeding also may occur from trophoblastic material that has been discharged into the vagina.

Preeclampsia occurs in about 15% of cases, usually between 9 and 12 gestational weeks. In addition, symptoms of true PIH may occur before the twentieth week of pregnancy (see Chapter 28). Hyperthyroidism and pulmonary embolization of trophoblastic elements occur less commonly but are serious complications of hydatidiform mole.

MEDICAL MANAGEMENT. Many moles abort spontaneously. When hydropic vesicles are passed vaginally and the woman saves the specimen, the diagnosis can be established with certainty. The sonographic pattern of a molar pregnancy is characterized by a diffuse "snow storm" pattern (Kulb, 1990) (see Fig. 27-3). Any uncertainty in diagnosis usually is clarified by clinical history, hCG titer (although even a high titer is not considered diagnostic), and, if necessary, a repeat sonogram in 2 weeks.

Suction curettage offers a safe, rapid, and effective method of evacuation of hydatidiform mole in almost all women (Scott et al, 1990). Women who do not desire preservation of reproductive function may benefit from primary hysterectomy as the method of choice for evacuation of hydatidiform mole and concurrent sterilization. Induction of labor with oxytocic agents or prostaglandins is not recommended because of the increased risk of hemorrhage.

Follow-up management includes frequent physical and pelvic examinations, along with measurement of serum hCG levels for at least 1 year. A rising titer and an enlarging uterus may indicate choriocarcinoma. This malignant condition is treated with anticancer drugs (see Chapter 44). Therefore, to avoid confusion with signs of pregnancy, pregnancy should be avoided for 1 year. Pregnancy can then be attempted, with a low probability of recurrence of a molar pregnancy. Cure of the malignant condition is defined as a complete absence of all clinical and hormonal evidence of disease for 5 years.

NURSING PROCESS

ASSESSMENT

On the client's admission to the hospital the nurse makes an initial assessment, takes a history, and assists with the physical examination (see box on p. 889).

NURSING DIAGNOSIS

Nursing diagnoses for the woman with a molar pregnancy focus on possible consequences of the disease, rationale for treatment, contraceptive counseling, and support of the grieving process. Nursing diagnoses may include the following:

- Grieving related to
  —Loss of pregnancy
- Anticipatory grieving related to
  —Actual/perceived threat to self

- Knowledge deficit related to
  —Disease process, etiology, treatment, and outcome
- Fluid volume deficit related to
  —Excessive bleeding secondary to evacuation of uterine contents
- Anxiety/fear related to
  — Uncertainty of disease
- Situational low self-esteem related to
  — Inability to conceive a normal pregnancy

PLANNING

Whenever possible the plan of care is mutually determined with the client. The plan is based on the biophysical and psychosocial assessments of the client. It is related specifically to the client's clinical and nursing diagnoses and stated in terms of measurable client behaviors. Client-centered *goals* may include any of the following.

- The woman will verbalize understanding of the importance of following treatment and use of effective contraception.
- The woman will demonstrate minimal or no anxiety.
- The woman will use effective coping mechanisms in adjusting to pregnancy loss.
- The woman will experience minimal or no complications such as hemorrhage.

IMPLEMENTATION

The woman and her family must understand the possible consequences of the disease and the necessity for a long and tedious course of treatment. The nurse will help the client understand and cope with pregnancy loss, recognize that the pregnancy was abnormal, and accept the need to postpone a subsequent pregnancy. contraceptive counseling is provided to emphasize the importance of consistent and reliable use of the method chosen.

EVALUATION

The nurse can be reasonably assured that care was effective to the degree to which goals for care have been met.

- The woman verbalizes understanding of the importance of following treatment and uses effective contraception.
- She demonstrates minimal or no anxiety.
- She uses effective coping mechanisms in adjusting to pregnancy loss.
- She experiences minimal or no complications such as hemorrhage.

LATE PREGNANCY BLEEDING

Bleeding late in pregnancy presents an emergency situation for the nurse. Such bleeding can result in increased maternal and perinatal morbidity and mortality. Late pregnancy bleeding disorders include placenta previa, premature separation of placenta (abruptio placentae), and cord insertion and placental variations.

Placenta Previa

In **placenta previa** the placenta is implanted in the lower uterine segment. The degree to which the internal cervical os is covered by the placenta determines how placenta previa is classified (Fig. 30-7). Placenta previa often is described as *complete, total* or *central* if the internal os is entirely covered by the placenta when the cervix is fully dilated. *Partial placenta previa* implies incomplete coverage. *Marginal placenta previa* indicates that only an edge of the placenta approaches the internal os. The term *low-lying (low) implantation* is used when the placenta is situated in the lower uterine segment but away from the os (Fig. 30-8).

Gestational age and cervical dilatation and effacement affect the extent of coverage of the internal os. A better classification of placenta previa is estimation of percentage of coverage of the internal os at full di-

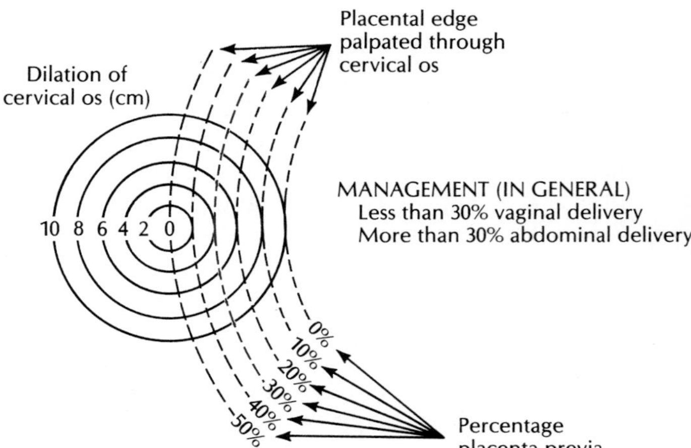

Fig. 30-7 Classification of placenta previa.
Modified from Tatum HJ, Mule JG: *Am J Obstet Gynecol* 93:768, 1965.

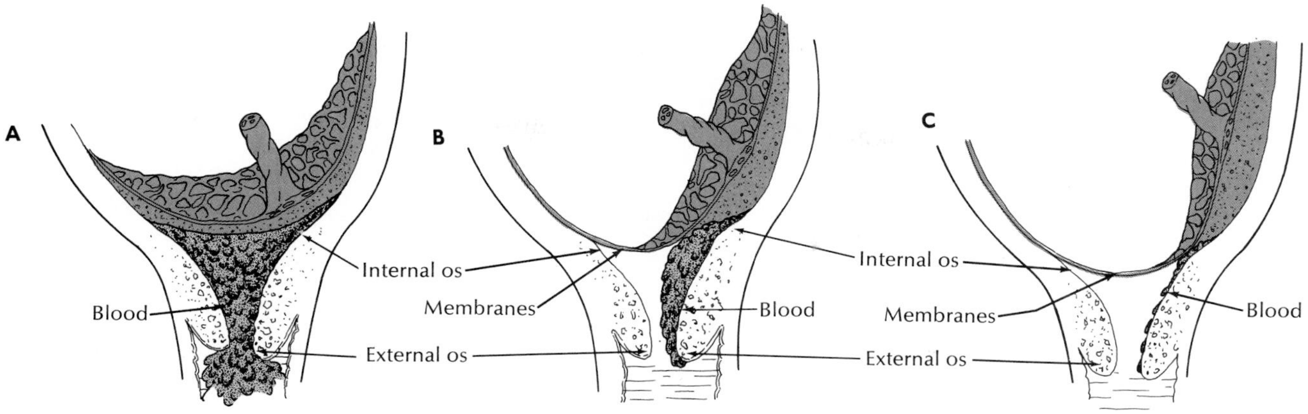

Fig. 30-8 Types of placenta previa after onset of labor. **A**, Complete, or total. **B**. Incomplete, or partial. **C**, Marginal, or low lying.

latation, which is the diameter required for birth of a mature fetus through the cervix.

In the second trimester approximately 45% of all placentas are implanted in the lower uterine segment. As the lower uterine segment elongates, the placenta seems to move upward as the uterine muscle enlarges, becoming a pelvic organ. By term, the incidence of placenta previa is 0.5% to 1%. Of the complete previas identified in the second trimester, only 1 in 12 will be a previa at term (Kulb, 1990). The recurrence rate of placenta previa is 4% to 8% (Lavery, 1990).

CAUSES. The cause of placenta previa is uncertain. Reduced vascularity of the upper segment subsequent to scarring from uterine surgery (abortion, cesarean birth), molar pregnancy, or tumor necessitating lower implantation of the placenta are plausible theories. Multifetal gestation that requires a larger surface area for placental implantation also may be a factor. Vessels of the endometrium involved in previous sites of implantation undergo changes that may reduce the blood supply to those regions, thus predisposing to low implantation in subsequent pregnancies.

The site of implantation and size of the placenta are related. Specifically, because the circulation of the lower uterine segment is less favorable than that of the fundus, placenta previa may need to cover a larger area for adequate functional efficiency, and a succenturiate or accessory lobe may be present. In placenta previa the surface area may be at least 30% greater than that of the average placenta implanted in the fundus.

MATERNAL AND FETAL OUTCOME. Maternal morbidity may occur from the placenta previa itself, the management, or the birth. Antenatal hemorrhage may be fatal or nearly fatal. Maternal morbidity is about 20% and mortality less than 1% with placenta previa. Hemorrhage occurring during the second trimester carries a poorer prognosis for pregnancy outcome than that associated with bleeding in the third trimester (Lavery, 1990). Most women will have at least one significant hemorrhage, and up to 25% will go into shock (Kulb, 1990).

Complications associated with the management of placenta previa include sepsis, surgery-related trauma to structures adjacent to the uterus, anesthesia complications, blood transfusion reactions, or overinfusion of fluids. Because of the reduced efficiency of the lower uterine segment to contract, postpartum hemorrhage may result.

Fetal risks include preterm birth, hypoxia in utero, and congenital anomalies yielding a fetal mortality rate of approximately 20%. There is no relationship between perinatal outcome and the number of bleeding episodes. However, there may be a relationship to the amount of blood lost. Infants who are small for gestational age (SGA) and intrauterine growth retardation (IUGR) have been associated with placenta previa, but the exact cause is controversial (Wolf et al, 1991). Neonatal compromise related to developmental anomalies and lingering effects of hypoxia places the newborn, up to 1 month of age, at a higher risk of death when compared with newborns of the same weight and gestational age (Kulb, 1990).

CLINICAL MANIFESTATIONS AND DIFFERENTIAL DIAGNOSIS. *Painless uterine bleeding,* especially during the third trimester, characterizes placenta previa (Table 30-4). In pregnancies complicated by a placenta previa, the first significant bleeding episode usually occurs between 29 and 30 weeks' gestation.

TABLE 30-4 Summary of Findings: Abruptio Placentae and Placenta Previa

	Abruptio Placentae			
	Marginal Separation	Moderate Separation	Severe Separation* (More Than 66%)	Placenta Previa
Bleeding: external, vaginal	Minimal	Absent to moderate	Absent to moderate	Minimal to severe and life threatening
Color of blood	Dark red	Dark red	Dark red	Bright red
Shock	Absent	Common	Very common: often sudden	Occasional
Coagulopathy	Rare	Occasional	Common	Rare
Uterine tonicity	Normal	Increased—may be localized to one region or diffuse over uterus: uterus fails to relax between contractions	Tetanic, persistent uterine contraction: boardlike uterus	Normal
Tenderness (pain)	Usually absent; if present, is localized	Increased—usually diffuse over uterus	Agonizing, unremitting uterine pain	Absent
Ultrasonographic findings:				
Location of placenta	Normal—upper uterine segment	Normal—upper uterine segment	Normal—upper uterine segment	Abnormal—lower uterine segment
Station of presenting part	Variable to engaged	Variable to engaged	Variable to engaged	High—not engaged
Fetal position	Usual distribution†	Usual distribution	Usual distribution	Commonly transverse, breech, or oblique
Concurrent hypertensive state	Usual distribution	Commonly present	Commonly present	Usual distribution

*Onset is usually abrupt: fetus usually dies.
†Usual distribution refers to the usual variations or incidence seen when there is no concurrent problem.

Approximately 10% of the clients may go to term before bleeding occurs (Lavery, 1990). At that time tearing and bleeding occur at the lower implantation site, when the lower uterine segment stretches and thins. Rarely is the first episode life threatening or a cause of hypovolemic shock. Approximately 7% of placenta previas are without symptoms and are an incidental finding on ultrasonic scans. About 3% of all cases of placenta previa are accompanied by placenta accreta, increta, or percreta (see p. 912).

The *bright-red bleeding* may be intermittent, may occur in gushes, or, more rarely, may be continuous. It may start while the woman is resting or in the midst of any activity. Fortunately, severe hemorrhage almost never occurs unless vaginal or rectal examination initiates violent bleeding before or during early labor.

The detachment of placenta previa is painless. However, if the first bleeding coincides with the onset of labor, the woman may experience discomfort because of uterine contractions.

Abdominal examination usually reveals a soft relaxed, nontender uterus of normal tone. If the fetus is in a longitudinal lie, the fundal height usually is greater than expected for gestational age because the low placenta hinders descent of the presenting fetal part. Leopold's maneuvers may reveal a fetus in an oblique or breech position or transverse lie because of the abnormal site of placental implantation.

During the third trimester, if the fetal vertex (head) is found more than 2 cm above the sacral promontory, one should suspect a low-lying to marginal placenta previa (Lavery, 1990). As a rule, fetal distress or fetal death occurs only if a significant portion of the placenta previa becomes detached from the decidua basalis or if the mother suffers hypovolemic shock.

DIAGNOSIS. At present the standard for the diagnosis of placenta previa is a transabdominal ultrasound examination. Because of technical difficulties encountered in certain circumstances, a false-negative rate of up to 7% occurs with the transabdominal approach. The error results from factors such as an engaged cephalic presentation, a posteriorly implanted placenta, maternal obesity, and compression of the lower uterine segment by an overdistended bladder. During the last few years vaginal ultrasound examination has been successfully used in these situations (Lavery, 1990). If ultrasound scanning reveals a normally implanted placenta, a speculum examination is performed to rule out local causes of bleeding (e.g., cervicitis, polyps, or carcinoma of the cervix), and a coagulation profile is obtained to rule out other causes of bleeding.

If possible, sterile vaginal speculum examination by the physician for diagnosing placenta previa should be postponed until viability has been reached (preferably after the thirty-fourth week) and after the ultrasound report is available. The vaginal examination, known as the *double-setup procedure* is a serious undertaking; it is attempted only if the physician is prepared for birth. In a double setup a sterile vaginal examination is performed in an operating room with personnel and equipment ready to effect an immediate vaginal or cesarean birth. Because manipulation of the lower uterine segment or cervix may result in profound hemorrhage, preparation for immediate birth is essential.

MEDICAL MANAGEMENT. Conservative management (e.g., bed rest to extend the period of gestation) usually is possible when the fetus is not mature. That is, initial spontaneous bleeding with a placenta previa is rarely life threatening to the mother or fetus. When fetal lung maturity (lecithin-sphingomyelin ratio [L/S] of at least 2:1) is achieved and survival is likely, the birth is accomplished.

After the diagnosis of placenta previa has been made, the woman should remain in the hospital under close supervision. At least 2 U of blood, typed and crossmatched, must be available for emergency use. A hematocrit level of at least 30% is maintained (Scott et al, 1990). The duration of pregnancy should be confirmed and, except in an emergency, birth postponed until after the thirty-sixth week. If the placenta previa is greater than 30% or if bleeding is excessive, cesarean birth is indicated, preferably with the woman under general anesthesia. If hypovolemic shock occurs, it may be very difficult to adequately replace blood loss. With placenta previa, bleeding will continue until the placenta is removed (Suresh, Kinch, 1991). Under certain conditions, vaginal birth may be possible (e.g., if the placenta previa is marginal or partial). However, the woman is given nothing by mouth (NPO) because operative birth is a possibility.

Blood loss may not cease with the birth of the infant. The large vascular channels in the lower uterine segment may continue to bleed because of the diminished muscle content of the lower uterine segment. The natural mechanism to control bleeding—the interlacing muscle bundles (the "living ligature") contracting around open vessels—so characteristic of the upper part of the uterus is absent in the lower part of the uterus. *Therefore postpartum hemorrhage may occur even if the fundus is contracted firmly.*

The location of the placental site close to the cervical os renders it more accessible to ascending infection from the vagina. Hemorrhage and anemia increase the predisposition to antenatal infection (placentitis) and postpartum (puerperal) infection.

If uterine bleeding cannot be controlled with oxytocic drugs, ligation of the hypogastric (internal iliac) arteries (see Fig. 6-12) or even hysterectomy may be necessary.

Hypovolemia must be treated without overtransfusion or overinfusion. Precise control of blood and fluid replacement necessitates continuous hemodynamic monitoring (see p. 914).

NURSING PROCESS

ASSESSMENT

With the client's admission to the hospital, the nurse begins with an assessment of the bleeding. Necessary history data include gravidity, parity, EDD, general status, bleeding (quantity, precipitating event, associated pain), vital signs, and fetal status (see box on p. 889). Abdominal assessment reveals a soft relaxed, nontender uterus of normal tone. Laboratory studies will include a CBC, determination of blood type and Rh factor, coagulation profile, and possible type and crossmatch for 2 U packed red blood cells.

NURSING DIAGNOSIS

Nursing diagnoses for placenta previa focus on alterations in hemodynamic status, knowledge deficits, fears and anxiety of the woman and her significant others, and fetal status. Potential nursing diagnoses include the following:

- Decreased cardiac output related to
  —Excessive blood loss secondary to placenta previa
- Fluid volume deficit related to
  —Excessive blood loss secondary to placenta previa
- Potential for fluid volume excess related to
  —Fluid resuscitation

- Altered peripheral tissue perfusion related to
  —Hypovolemia and shunting of blood to central circulation
- High risk for injury (fetal) related to
  —Decreased placental perfusion secondary to placenta previa
- Anxiety/fear related to
  —Maternal condition and pregnancy outcome
- Knowledge deficit related to
  —Hospitalization and treatment regimens
- Altered family process related to
  —Mother's condition and hospitalization
- Anticipatory grieving related to
  —Actual/perceived threat to self, pregnancy, or infant
- High risk for infection related to
  —Anemia, hemorrhage, placenta previa, and transfusions
- High risk for injury (mother) related to
  —Invasive monitoring procedures and treatment

PLANNING

The plan of care is mutually negotiated whenever possible. It is based on biophysical and psychosocial assessments of the client. The plan must relate specifically to the client's clinical and nursing diagnoses and should be stated in terms of measurable client behaviors. *Goals* may include the following

- The woman will identify and use available support systems.
- The woman will demonstrate compliance with prescribed activity limitations.
- The woman will not develop complications.
- The woman will carry her pregnancy to term or near term.
- The woman will give birth to a healthy infant.

IMPLEMENTATION

If conservative management is used, nursing care focuses on accurate assessments and appropriate referrals. The client will be instructed on the importance of bed rest and the need to report any further spotting or bleeding. Maternal vital signs will be assessed as indicated by the woman's condition. Serial laboratory values will be evaluated for the presence of falling hemoglobin and hematocrit levels and changes in coagulation studies. Fetal well-being will be evaluated by the use of nonstress testing, biophysical profiles, and ultrasonography. Any indication of fetal compromise will be reported immediately to the physician.

If active management is undertaken, the nurse will continuously assess maternal and fetal status while preparing the client for surgery. Laboratory studies will include CBC, DIC profile, and possible type and crossmatching for packed red blood cells. Maternal vital signs will be assessed frequently for decreasing blood pressure, rising pulse rate, changes in level of consciousness (LOC), and/or oliguria. Fetal assessment will be maintained by continuous electronic fetal monitoring (EFM) to assess for signs of hypoxia.

Emotional support for the client and her family is extremely important. If actively bleeding, the client is concerned not only for her well-being but for the well-being of her fetus. All procedures should be explained, and a support person should be present.

EVALUATION

The nurse can be reasonably assured that care was effective to the degree that goals for care have been met.

- The woman identifies and uses available support systems.
- She demonstrates compliance with prescribed activity limitations.
- She does not develop complications.
- She carries her pregnancy to term or near term.
- She gives birth to a healthy infant.

Example of a case study and a nursing plan of care are provided on pp. 903 and 904.

Premature Separation of Placenta

Premature separation of the placenta, also termed **abruptio placentae,** is the detachment of part or all of the placenta from its implantation site (Fig. 30-9). Separation occurs in the area of the decidua basalis after the twentieth week of pregnancy and before the birth of the baby.

Premature separation of the placenta is a serious event and accounts for about 15% of all perinatal deaths. Approximately one third of infants of women with premature separation of the placenta die. More than 50% of these deaths are the result of preterm birth; many others die of intrauterine hypoxia.

Abruptio placentae occurs in about 1% of all pregnancies. This problem is much more common in women with hypertension from any cause and is three times greater in women with a gravidity of more than five. Abdominal trauma is a factor in less than 5% of cases, and short cord is identified in less than 1%. Women who use *cocaine* during their preg-

CASE STUDY

Placenta Previa

Joyce is a 25-year-old healthy primigravida brought to the labor and birth room by her husband at 33 weeks' gestation with a sudden onset of painless vaginal bleeding. The admission diagnosis is probable placenta previa. After an ultrasound examination the diagnosis was changed to bleeding secondary to central previa.

ASSESSMENT

The admission interview revealed that Joyce awoke this evening and found she was bleeding. She states that the bleeding was painless and bright red and that when she got out of bed, the blood "ran down her legs." Joyce keeps asking, "What did I do to cause this?" and "Is my baby going to be OK?" Joyce states she has no history of bleeding disorders and no significant medical or obstetric history. During the physical examination the nurse notes the following vital signs: temperature 97.6° F, pulse 110 beats/min, respirations 28/min, BP 100/68 mm Hg, fetal heart rate 156/min. The uterus is soft and nontender, with no contractions palpated. Fundal height is 34 cm. On admission the peripad Joyce had worn to the hospital was noted to be two thirds saturated with dark red blood. There was no active bleeding at present. The following laboratory tests were ordered: CBC, DIC profile, bleeding time, blood type and Rh. An IV infusion was started with a 16-gauge angiocatheter to infuse at 125 mL/hr. A review of laboratory findings revealed hemoglobin 9.3 g/dL, hematocrit 27%, platelets 145,000 mm^3 with normal coagulation studies.

NURSING DIAGNOSIS

On the basis of the history of bleeding and the hemoglobin value on Joyce's admission, the nurse identifies the following nursing diagnosis as having priority: decreased cardiac output related to excessive bleeding secondary to placenta previa.

PLANNING

A plan of care, including the *goal* that takes priority, is developed with Joyce's input: Joyce's blood volume will be restored as evidenced by stable vital signs, normal hemoglobin and hematocrit values, hemodynamic stability, and absence of infection or complications.

IMPLEMENTATION

Nursing actions are derived from medical management, physician's orders, and nursing diagnosis. Specific interventions will include assessments of vital signs, signs and symptoms of onset of labor, pad count, and signs and symptoms of infection. The laboratory values will be monitored and abnormalities reported to the physician. Fetal status will be evaluated by the use of kick counts, nonstress test results, and biophysical profile. An accurate intake and output record will be maintained, with urine specific gravities noted as ordered. Continuous assessments will document the location, duration, and intensity of pain. Bleeding will be assessed for amount, color and consistency, with any increase in flow reported to the physician.

Joyce will be kept on strict bed rest. No vaginal examinations will be performed; no rectal examinations or enemas will be given. IV fluids are carefully infused; the infusion site is maintained free of infiltration and infection. Because hospitalization for an extended period is probable, the registered dietitian, the nurse, and Joyce will plan meals that are blood building (see Chapter 9).

EVALUATION

Inasmuch as Joyce's hemoglobin and hematocrit levels improved and her bleeding was minimal to absent, the goal for this first-priority nursing diagnosis was met.

nancy significantly increase the incidence of abruptio placentae (Rosenak et al, 1990; Scott et al, 1990). Women with a history of reproductive loss (abortion, preterm labor, prenatal hemorrhage, stillbirth, or neonatal death) experience premature separation of the placenta more than twice as often as does the average woman. Between 15% to 20% of women who have had a previous premature separation of the placenta will have a recurrence. If the woman has had two prior premature separations, the chance in the next pregnancy is at least 25%.

CAUSES. The primary cause of placental abruption is unknown, but several conditions have been suggested as etiologic factors: maternal hypertension, trauma, sudden uterine decompression (e.g., PROM), short umbilical cord, uterine anomaly or tumor, pressure by the enlarged uterus on the inferior vena cava, dietary deficiency and maternal use of cocaine. Maternal hypertension is the most common and has been identified in approximately half the cases of severe abruption (Lowe, Cunningham, 1990).

CARE PLAN Placenta Previa

GOALS	INTERVENTIONS	RATIONALE	EVALUATION
Nursing diagnosis: Decreased cardiac output related to excessive bleeding secondary to placenta previa			
Joyce's intravascular blood volume and cardiac output are restored as evidenced by normal pulse, blood pressure, hemodynamic values and laboratory values.	Assess and record vital signs, blood pressure, LOC, CVP/PAWP, peripheral perfusion, intake and output, and amount of bleeding. Assist physician, or initiate IV fluid therapy and/or blood replacement therapy as ordered; administer medications per physician's orders.	Accurate assessment of hemodynamic status provides a basis for planning and evaluating interventions. Restoration of vascular volume requires IV therapy and pharmaceutic interventions. Lost blood volume must be restored to prevent further complications such as infections, fetal compromise, and compromise to maternal vital organ systems.	Joyce's bleeding stops, and hemodynamic profile is restored. Her laboratory values return to normal.
Nursing diagnosis: Potential for infection related to anemia and bleeding secondary to placenta previa			
Joyce will remain physiologically safe as evidenced by absence of infection and restoration of normal laboratory values.	Assess and document vital signs, blood pressure, uterine tenderness, malodorous vaginal discharge. Monitor laboratory results for shifting of differential or rising WBC. Assess fetus for signs of intrauterine infection such as fetal tachycardia or decreasing biophysical profile scores.	Accurate assessment of subtle changes in Joyce's status can detect early signs of infection. In placenta previa, placental tissue is exposed, increasing the risk of infection.	Joyce remains afebrile, free of any signs of infection, and gives birth to a viable, mature fetus.
Nursing Diagnosis: Potential for injury (fetal) related to decreased uterine/placental perfusion secondary to bleeding			
The fetus will remain physiologically safe as evidenced by reactive nonstress test, normal biophysical profile scores, absence of late decelerations during labor, and uncompromised birth.	Monitor fetus at least daily for signs of tachycardia, decreased movement, loss of reactivity on nonstress test, and presence of late decelerations with fetal monitoring. Obtain biophysical profiles as ordered to assess for signs of intrauterine infection. Obtain ultrasonographic examination as ordered to evaluate fetal growth and amniotic fluid volume.	This fetus is at increased risk for intrauterine compromise; careful and consistent assessments will identify changes in fetal status early so that interventions can be implemented.	The fetus reached maturity (39 weeks' gestation) without compromise. At birth the infant had normal Apgar scores (9/9), cord pH (7.32), and required no resuscitation. He weighed 3345 g and went home with his family on the third postbirth day.

Abruptio placentae (premature separation)

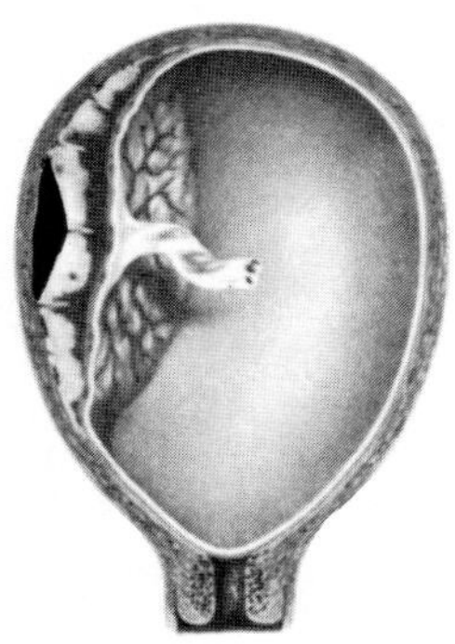

Partial separation
(concealed hemorrhage)

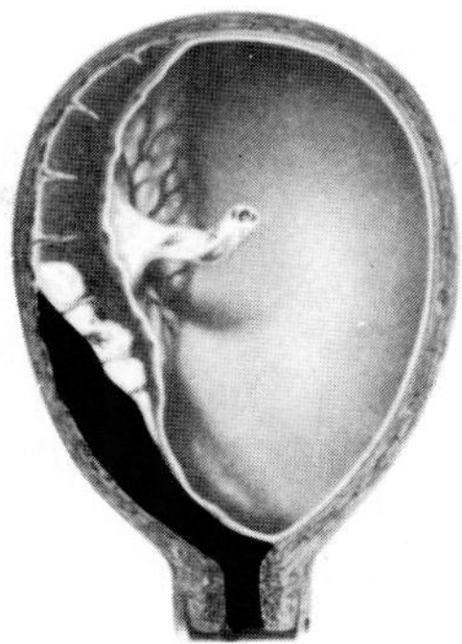

Partial separation
(apparent hemorrhage)

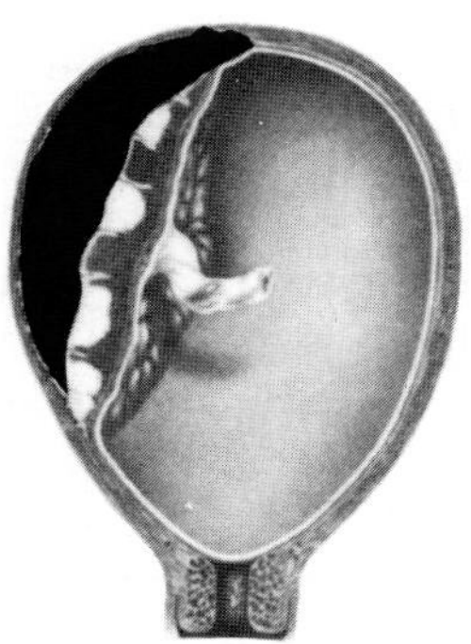

Complete separation
(concealed hemorrhage)

Fig. 30-9 Abruptio placentae. Premature separation of normally implanted placenta.
Courtesy Ross Laboratories, Columbus, Ohio.

CLASSIFICATION SYSTEMS. There are two classification systems for identifying placental abruption based on type and severity. The first classification system grades an abruption as follows (Green, 1989):

Grade 0: The client has no symptoms, but a small retroplacental clot is noted after birth. Less than 10% of the total placental surface area is detached.

Grade I: The client has vaginal bleeding, perhaps with uterine tenderness and mild tetany, but neither mother nor baby is in distress. Approximately 10% to 20% of the total placental surface area detaches.

Grade II: The client experiences uterine tenderness and tetany, with or without external evidence of bleeding. The mother is not in shock, but there is fetal distress. Approximately 20% to 50% of the total surface area detaches.

Grade III: Uterine tetany is severe, the mother is in shock, although the bleeding may or may not be revealed, and the fetus is dead. Often the mother is experiencing coagulopathy (see p. 917). Greater than 50% of the placental surface area detaches (Gilbert, Harmon, 1992). The incidence rates of grades 0/I, II, and III abruptions are 48%, 27%, and 24%, respectively.

The second system classifies abruption on the basis of signs and symptoms. In a *revealed, or overt, abruption* vaginal bleeding is evident and the client's symptoms are consistent with the amount of blood lost. Uterine tenderness and tetany, if present, are minor. In a *concealed, or covert, abruption* no bleeding is evident. Of primary importance is uterine tenderness and hypertonicity. Often fetal heart tones (FHTs) are not present. A concealed abruption is characterized by central separation of the placenta that entraps blood between the uterine wall and the placenta (a retroplacental bleed). A *mixed abruption* is a combination of the aforementioned, with bleeding, uterine tenderness, and tetany present (Kulb, 1990).

CLINICAL MANIFESTATIONS AND DIFFERENTIAL DIAGNOSIS. The separation may be partial or complete, or only the margin of the placenta may be involved. Bleeding from the placental site may dissect (separate) the membranes from the decidua basalis and flow out through the vagina; it may remain concealed (retroplacental hemorrhage); or it may do both (Fig. 30-9). Clinical symptoms vary with the degree of separation (Table 30-4).

Symptoms include uterine bleeding with a small to moderate amount of dark-red vaginal bleeding in 80% to 85% of cases. Bleeding may result in maternal hypovolemia (shock, oliguria, anuria) and coagulopathy. Mild to severe uterine hypertonicity is present. Pain is mild to severe, localized over one region of the uterus, or diffuse over the uterus with a boardlike abdomen. Extensive myometrial bleeding damages the uterine muscle. If blood accumulates between the separated placenta and the uterine wall, it may produce a Couvelaire uterus. The uterus appears purplish and copper-colored and is ecchymotic, and contractility is lost. Shock may occur and is out of proportion to blood loss. Laboratory findings include a positive Apt test result (see Chapter 27) of amniotic fluid; a fall in hemoglobin and hematocrit levels (which may appear later); and a fall in coagulation factors. Clotting defects (e.g., DIC) will develop in 10% to 30% of clients (most within 8 hours of hospital admission), as well as increased clot retraction.

DIAGNOSIS. The diagnosis of placental abruption is based on the client's history, physical examination, and laboratory studies. Abruptio placentae should be highly suspected in the client with sudden onset and intense, usually localized, uterine pain, with or without vaginal bleeding. Sonographic examination is used to rule out placenta previa; however, it is not diagnostic for an abruption. Studies have shown that a clinical diagnosis of abruption can be made by means of sonographic examination in only 25% of affected women. Negative findings on ultrasound scan do not exclude life-threatening placental abruption (Cunningham et al, 1989; Lowe, Cunningham, 1990).

Significant complications accompany moderate to severe abruptio placentae. Abruption with concealed hemorrhage carries a much greater maternal hazard because the extent of hemorrhage is not recognized, and consequently blood replacement may be too little or too late (Lowe, Cunningham, 1990). Hypovolemic shock can result in renal failure and pituitary necrosis (Sheehan's syndrome, see p. 917). Clotting defects (e.g., DIC) develop (McLaren et al, 1991). Bleeding into the myometrium causes **Couvelaire uterus,** with resulting myometrial tissue damage, increased tonicity, and inability of the uterus to relax between contractions. After the birth the uterus may feel firm, but may not be able to contract efficiently and close off bleeding sinuses; postpartum hemorrhage should be anticipated. Electronic fetal monitoring (EFM) reflects the increasing fetal distress that may finally end in fetal death. Fetal hypoxia or anoxia with possible fetal death may occur.

MEDICAL MANAGEMENT. Treatment depends on maternal and fetal status. In the presence of fetal distress, severe hemorrhage, coagulopathy, poor labor progress, or increasing uterine resting tone a cesarean birth is performed. If the mother is hemodynamically stable, a vaginal birth may be attempted when the fetus is alive and in no acute distress or if the fetus is dead.

Fluid resuscitation must be aggressive in the presence of hemorrhage. Whole blood and Ringer's lactate are infused in quantities necessary to maintain a urine output of 30 to 60 mL/hr and a hematocrit level of approximately 30% (Lowe, Cunningham, 1990).

PROGNOSIS. Maternal mortality approaches 1% in abruptio placentae; this condition remains a leading cause of maternal death. The mother's prognosis depends on the extent of the placental detachment, overall blood loss, degree of DIC, and time between the placental "accident" and birth. Fortunately, 80% to 90% of all premature separations of the placenta involve only two or three cotyledons, grades 0 and I, and therefore the prognosis generally is not grave.

Fetal prognosis is poor. At least one third of babies of mothers with a grade II or III placental separation die before, during, or soon after birth. Of those who survive, there is an increase in the absolute numbers of neurologically damaged infants.

NURSING PROCESS

ASSESSMENT

Nursing assessments include all components described for clients with spontaneous abortions and placenta previa. Additional assessments are necessary to identify an increasing fundal height, which indicates concealed bleeding.

NURSING DIAGNOSIS

Nursing diagnoses related to the care of the client with abruptio placentae focus on alterations in hemodynamic status, knowledge deficits, fears and anxiety of the woman, and fetal status. Many of the potential nursing diagnoses are the same as for placenta previa. Additional potential nursing diagnoses include the following:

- Pain related to
  —Bleeding between the uterine wall and the placenta secondary to premature separation of the placenta
- Grieving related to
  —Actual or threatened loss of infant
- Powerlessness related to
  —Maternal condition and hospitalization

PLANNING

The plan of care for the woman includes client-centered, mutually determined (whenever possible) goals that are stated in measurable client behaviors. *Goals* may include the following.

- The woman will identify and use available support systems.
- She will express relief of pain.
- She will not develop complications.
- She will give birth to a healthy infant who has not undergone fetal compromise.

IMPLEMENTATION

Careful assessments are mandatory. Information is given to the client and her family about abruptio placentae, including cause, treatment, and expected outcome. Vital signs are assessed frequently to observe for signs of declining hemodynamic status. Fetal status is continuously monitored if the fetus has survived the initial insult. Preparations are made for the birth, but it should be kept in mind that an emergency cesarean birth is always a possibility.

EVALUATION

The nurse can be reasonably assured that care was effective to the extent that the goals for care have been met. That is, the woman identifies and uses available support systems, expresses relief of pain, does not develop complications, and gives birth to a healthy infant who has not experienced fetal compromise. (For a discussion of grief and loss, see Chapter 40.)

Cord Insertion and Placental Variations

A **velamentous insertion of the cord** is a rare placental anomaly in which the cord vessels begin to branch at the membranes and then course onto the placenta (Fig. 30-10, *A*). Rupture of the membranes or traction on the cord may tear one or more of the fetal vessels. As a result the fetus may quickly bleed to death. *Battledore* (marginal) (Fig. 30-10, *B*) insertion of the cord increases the risk of fetal hemorrhage, especially after marginal separation of the placenta.

Rarely, the placenta may be divided into two or more separate lobes, resulting in *succenturiate* placenta (Fig. 30-10, *C*). Each lobe has a distinct circulation; the vessels collect at the periphery, and the main trunks unite eventually to form the vessels of the cord. Blood vessels joining the lobes may be supported only by the fetal membranes and are therefore in danger of tearing during labor or during the birth of the baby or expulsion of the placenta. During recovery of the placenta, one or more of the separate lobes may remain attached to the decidua basalis, preventing uterine contraction, increasing the risk of postpartum hemorrhage.

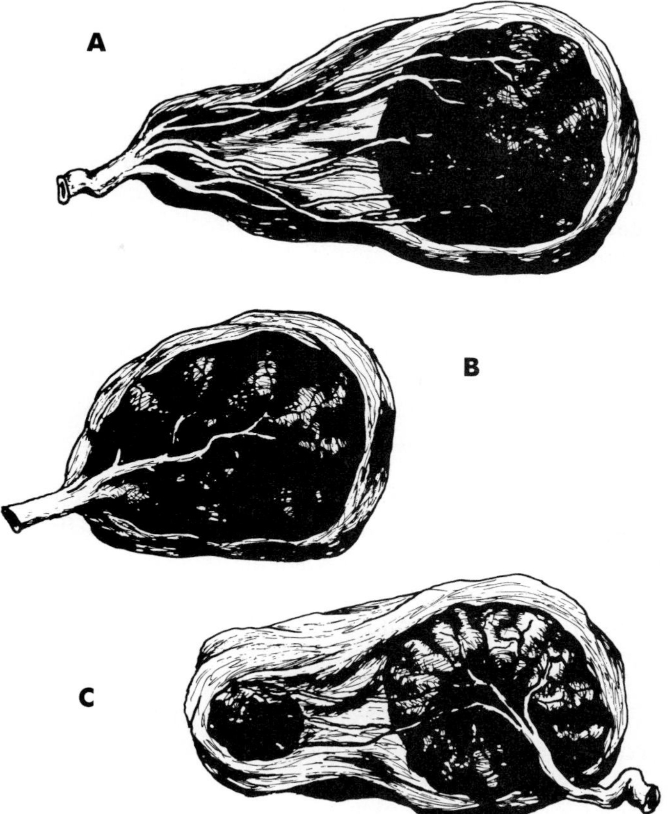

Fig. 30-10 Cord insertion and placental variations. **A**, Velamentous insertion of cord. **B**, Battledore placenta. **C**, Placenta succenturiate.

■ POSTBIRTH HEMORRHAGE

Hemorrhage is a leading cause of maternal death worldwide. Postbirth hemorrhage, traditionally the loss of 500 mL of blood or more after birth, is the most common and most serious type of excessive obstetric blood loss. Postbirth hemorrhage is a leading cause of maternal morbidity and mortality, accounting for approximately 10% of nonabortive maternal deaths. Approximately 8% of all births are complicated by postbirth hemorrhage (Murahata, 1991).

A small woman is less able to withstand the loss of blood than is a larger woman. It has been noted that the average maternal blood loss can be as much as 10% of the woman's blood volume without immediate critical consequence. Therefore a more meaningful definition of postbirth hemorrhage is the loss of 1% or more of body weight, a figure easily referable to blood volume because 1 mL of blood weighs 1 g.

Postbirth hemorrhage may be sudden and even exsanguinating. Moderate but persistent bleeding may continue for days or weeks. Postbirth hemorrhage may be early, within the first 24 hours after birth, or late, from 24 hours after birth until the twenty-eighth postpartum day.

Control of bleeding from the placental site is accomplished by prolonged contraction and retraction of interlacing strands of myometrium, the living ligature. A firm or contracted uterus does not normally bleed after childbirth unless placenta previa had existed. Therefore careful assessment of uterine tone and the maintenance of uterine contractions through manual massage or oxytocic stimulation, as needed, are important parts of postnatal care.

The most common causes of postbirth hemorrhage, in approximate order of frequency, are medical mismanagement of the third stage of labor, uterine atony, and lacerations of the birth canal. Hematologic disorders (e.g., DIC) or complications of pregnancy (e.g., inversion of the uterus, placenta accreta) may be factors in postbirth hemorrhage. Other factors may include tumors of the cervix or uterus (e.g., fibroids), medical complications of pregnancy (e.g., hyperthyroidism), or infections of the genital tract (e.g., endometritis).

Early postbirth hemorrhage almost invariably is caused by uterine atony, lacerations of the birth canal, or DIC. *Late postbirth hemorrhage* most commonly is the result of subinvolution of the placental site, retained placental tissue, or infection.

It is helpful to consider the problem of excessive bleeding with reference to the stages of labor. From birth of the fetus until separation of the placenta the character and quantity of blood passed may suggest excessive bleeding. For example, *dark blood* probably is of venous origin, perhaps from varices or superficial lacerations of the birth canal. *Bright blood* is arterial and indicates, for example, deep lacerations of the cervix. *Spurts of blood* with clots may indicate partial placental separation. *Failure of blood to clot* or remain clotted indicates coagulopathy.

The period from the separation of the placenta to its recovery is the time when excessive bleeding may occur. Commonly, this occurrence is the result of incomplete placental separation, often caused by poor management of the third stage of labor (e.g., undue manipulation of the fundus or of excessive traction on the cord). After the placenta has been recovered, persistent or excessive blood loss usually is the result of atony of the uterus (e.g., its failure to contract well or maintain its contraction) or prolapse of the uterus into the pelvis. Late hemorrhage may be the result of partial involution of the uterus and unrecognized lacerations of the birth canal.

Complications of postbirth hemorrhage are either immediate or delayed. Hemorrhagic (hypovolemic) shock (see p. 913) and death may occur from sudden, exsanguinating hemorrhage. Delayed complications provoked by postbirth hemorrhage include anemia, puerperal infection, and thromboembolism. This section focuses on immediate and delayed postbirth hemorrhage in relation to cause, management, and complications.

Immediate Postbirth Hemorrhage

UTERINE ATONY. **Uterine atony** is marked hypotonia of the uterus. Uterine atony occurs in at least 5% of births particularly in grand multiparity, with hydramnios, with a large fetus, or after the birth of twins or triplets. In such conditions the uterus is "overstretched" and contracts poorly. Other causes of atony include traumatic birth, use of halogenated anesthesia and/or magnesium sulfate, rapid or prolonged labor, chorioamnionitis, and use of oxytocin for labor induction or augmentation. Uterine atony is the principal cause of postbirth hemorrhage.

Placental separation and expulsion are facilitated by contraction of the uterus, which also prevents hemorrhage from the placental site. The corpus is, in essence, a basket weave of strong, interdigitating, smooth muscle bundles through which pass many large maternal blood vessels. If the uterus is flaccid after detachment of all or part of the placenta, brisk venous bleeding will occur and normal coagulation of the open vasculature will be impaired. In contrast, a firm, contracted uterus will not bleed because the myometrium will compress the vasculature, and resolution of the placental site can occur.

Numerous preventable problems may be responsible for uterine atony. Undesirable side effects may follow the administration of ill-chosen drugs, of very potent analgesic agents (e.g., morphine) late in the first stage of labor, and of certain anesthetics (e.g., ethyl ether) that are especially efficient smooth muscle–relaxing drugs. Mismanagement of the third stage of labor, allowing only partial separation of the placenta or retention of placental fragments, may be associated with uterine atony. Moreover, the poorly contracting uterus may have slipped deep into the true pelvis to cause chronic passive congestion of the organ, an added cause of abnormal bleeding.

MEDICAL MANAGEMENT. The first step in the treatment of uterine bleeding is to elevate and hold the uterus out of the pelvis and to massage the corpus to initiate and maintain a firmly contracted organ. The health care provider orders oxytocin, 20 to 40 *U* to 1 L crystalloid, to infuse at 10 to 15 mL/min (Zahn, Yeomans, 1990); this infusion should be continued for at least 3 or 4 hours. If the uterus fails to respond to oxytocin, methylergonovine, 0.2 mg administered intramuscularly, produces tetanic uterine contraction and is effective in treating hemorrhage from uterine atony. However, its use is contraindicated in the presence of hypertension. If methylergonovine fails or is contraindicated, prostaglandin F_{2a} becomes the oxytocic of choice. Most hemorrhage can be controlled after one or two injections of

0.25 mg intramuscularly; most failures occurred in women with chorioamnionitis (Zann, Yeomans, 1990; Baskett, Writer, 1991). Blood transfusion for the treatment of shock and blood replacement may be urgently needed.

The health care provider should hasten to palpate the interior of the uterus so that retained products of conception can be removed and possible rupture of the uterus diagnosed. If the blood being lost fails to clot, a coagulopathy (e.g., DIC) may have developed, and prompt appropriate treatment may be lifesaving.

If the procedures outlined are ineffective, surgical management may be the only alternative. Surgical management options include vessel ligation (utero-ovarian, uterine, hypogastric), angiographic embolization, and hysterectomy.

LACERATIONS OF THE BIRTH CANAL. Lacerations of the birth canal are second only to uterine atony as a major cause of postbirth hemorrhage. Therefore prevention, recognition, and prompt, effective treatment of birth canal lacerations are vitally important.

Continued bleeding despite efficient postbirth uterine contractions demands inspection or reinspection of the birth passage. Continuous bleeding from so-called minor sources may be just as dangerous as a sudden loss of a large amount of blood, although often it is ignored until shock develops. Birth canal lacerations may include injuries to the labia, perineum, vagina, and cervix.

CAUSES. Factors that influence the causes and incidence of obstetric lacerations of the lower genital tract encompass several conditions (see also discussion of lacerations in Chapter 18): operative birth; aseptic or uncontrolled spontaneous birth; congenital abnormalities of the maternal soft parts; contracted pelvis; size, abnormal presentation, and position of the fetus; relative size of the presenting part and the birth canal; prior scarring from infection, injury, or surgery; vulvar perineal and vaginal varices; and abnormalities of uterine action (for example, precipitate birth) (see Chapter 35).

Other associated problems may be abnormal tissue elasticity or friability, the presence of tumors, the general condition of the mother (e.g., exhaustion and dehydration), and the presence of complicating diseases. All these factors may exist alone or in combination.

LABIAL LACERATIONS. Extreme vascularity in the labia and periclitoral areas often results in profuse bleeding if laceration occurs. Immediate repair, by means of fine (4-0 chromic) suture on an atraumatic needle is required.

PERINEAL LACERATIONS. Lacerations of the perineum are the most common of all injuries in the lower portion of the genital tract. These are classified as first, second, third, and fourth degree (see Chapter 18). An episiotomy may extend to become either a third- or fourth-degree laceration.

VAGINAL LACERATIONS AND HEMATOMAS. Prolonged pressure of the fetal head on the vaginal mucosa ultimately will interfere with the circulation and may produce ischemic or pressure necrosis. The state of the tissues, therefore, together with the type of birth, may result in deep vaginal lacerations (for further discussion, see Chapter 18) and may result in predisposition to vaginal hematomas.

Vaginal **hematomas** occur more commonly in association with forceps rotation of a fetus in an occiputposterior position. They often are found on the same side as the occiput, perhaps because of long-continued pressure of the fetal head in one posterior quadrant of the vagina. Many vaginal hematomas occur beneath the mucosa opposite the ischial spines in the plane of the midpelvis. Therefore the physician will palpate the vaginal walls to detect a hematoma. During the postbirth period, if the woman complains of persistent perineal pain or a feeling of fullness in the vagina, a careful inspection of the vulva is made. Once the hematoma is diagnosed, treatment is initiated. The woman is returned to the birth room, where (after a suitable anesthetic has been administered) the hematoma is incised and evacuated, and deep sutures are placed for control of the bleeding.

INVERSION OF THE UTERUS. **Inversion of the uterus** (turning inside out) after birth is a potentially life-threatening complication. The incidence of uterine inversion is approximately 1/2500 births (Zahn, Yeomans, 1990). The inversion may be partial or complete. Fundal pressure and traction applied to the fundus, especially when the uterus is flaccid, may result in inversion. More specifically, the causes include straining (Valsalva's maneuver); traction on the cord before the placenta has separated; Credé's method, that is, kneading the uterine fundus in an attempt to separate an adherent placenta; and placental extraction under deep relaxing anesthesia. Although proper management of the third stage of labor prevents most cases of uterine inversions, some are unavoidable. Regardless of the precipitating factor, once they occur, prompt recognition and correction are necessary to reduce maternal morbidity and mortality.

The primary presenting sign in up to 94% of the women with uterine inversion is hemorrhage, with blood loss estimated to range from 800 to 1800 mL.

Up to 40% of these women also may suffer from shock (Zahn, Yeomans, 1990).

Prevention—always the easiest, cheapest, and most effective therapy—is especially appropriate in the avoidance of puerperal uterine inversion. *One must not pull on the umbilical cord unless the placenta has definitely separated.* Uterine inversion occasionally may recur in a subsequent birth.

Complete inversion of the uterus is obvious; a large, red, rounded mass (perhaps with the placenta attached) protrudes 20 to 30 cm outside the introitus. Incomplete inversion cannot be seen but must be felt; a smooth mass will be palpated through the dilated cervix, reducing the size of the uterine cavity by at least half.

MEDICAL MANAGEMENT. This condition requires the following interventions.

- Combat shock, which invariably is out of proportion to the blood loss. Give oxytocin intravenously to contract the uterus. Ergot products are strictly contraindicated because the cervix, as well as the uterus, will contract, and replacement of the uterine inversion may be difficult unless the cervix is severed.
- Replace the fundus of the uterus, after the woman has received tocolysis or is under deep anesthesia, by inserting and "working" first the lower uterine segment and then, finally, the fundus upward while applying traction to the cervix. Leave the placenta attached if it has not yet separated, and then manually free the placenta. Give the oxytocic as ordered. As the uterus and cervix contract, withdraw the placenta with the hand. Pack the uterus if inversion seems to recur.
- Prepare for abdominal or vaginal surgery, which may be necessary to reposition the uterus if successful manual replacement fails. Successful, prompt vaginal replacement is likely in about 75% of women.
- Give the woman blood replacement therapy as indicated. Broad-spectrum antibiotic therapy and a nasogastric tube also are initiated to minimize paralytic ileus.

NURSING PROCESS

ASSESSMENT

Postbirth hemorrhage can progress rapidly to shock; therefore the nurse must assess the client carefully and thoroughly. The client's history should be reviewed for factors that cause predisposition to postbirth hemorrhage (see box above right). The bleeding should be assessed as to color, amount, and, if possible, source. Vital signs may not be reliable indicators of shock in the immediate postpartum period because of physiologic adaptations of this period. Assessment should include evaluation for bladder distention because a distended bladder will prevent uterine contraction.

Risk Factors for Postbirth Hemorrhage

- Cesarean birth
- Birth of a large infant
- Birth assisted by forceps or vacuum extractor
- Overdistended uterus from hydramnios, multifetal gestations, large fetus
- Intrauterine manipulation/manual removal of the placenta
- Lacerations of the birth canal
- Magnesium sulfate administration during labor or postpartum
- Mutiparity
- Previous postbirth hemorrhage
- Placental abruption, retained placental fragments
- Pitocin induced/augmented labor
- Uterine atony
- Uterine inversion
- Uterine subinvolution

NURSING DIAGNOSES

Nursing diagnoses for the client experiencing postbirth hemorrhage may include the following:

- Altered tissue perfusion related to
  —Hypovolemia
- Anxiety related to
  —Perceived health status
- Body image disturbance related to
  —Birth canal injury
- High risk for infection related to
  —Hemorrhage

PLANNING

The plan of care is mutually negotiated whenever possible. It is based on biophysical and psychosocial assessment of the client. The plan must relate specifically to the client's clinical and nursing diagnoses and should be stated in terms of measurable client behaviors. *Goals* may include the following.

- The woman will identify and use available support systems.
- She will express relief of pain.
- She will not develop complications.
- She will give birth to a healthy infant who has not undergone fetal compromise.

IMPLEMENTATION

Immediate care of the client experiencing a postbirth hemorrhage includes assessment of vital signs and uterine consistency, along with administration of oxytocin. Explanations are given to the woman (and her family) regarding the rationale for procedures and the need to act quickly.

The care of the woman who has undergone lacerations of the perineum is similar to that advocated for episiotomies, that is, analgesia as needed for pain and heat or cold applications as necessary. *To avoid injury to the suture line, a woman with third- or fourth-degree lacerations is not given routine postbirth rectal suppositories or enemas.* Attention to diet and intake of fluids is emphasized, as well as oral stool softeners to assist the woman in reestablishing bowel habits.

The care of the woman experiencing an inversion of the uterus focuses on immediate stabilization of hemodynamic status. If the uterus can be replaced manually, care must be taken after the birth to avoid aggressive fundal massage.

EVALUATION

The nurse can be reasonably assured that care was effective to the extent that the goals of care have been met. If they are not met, the nurse initiates the nursing process again, beginning with assessment. The goals of care have been met if the woman identifies and uses available support systems, expresses relief of pain, does not develop complications, and gives birth to a healthy infant who has not undergone fetal compromise.

Delayed Postbirth Hemorrhage

NONADHERENT RETAINED PLACENTA. The obstetrician/midwife must recognize the normal completion of the third stage of labor, or complications may result. If the health care provider is hasty, for example, the placenta may not have an adequate opportunity to separate. If one waits too long, needless loss of blood may occur.

After birth of the baby but before recovery of the placenta, some women may have only slight bleeding, but others may have considerable blood loss. With proper management and the absence of significant bleeding, the normally implanted placenta separates with the first or second strong uterine contraction after birth of the infant. Placental separation occurs within 15 minutes in about 90% of women. Within 30 minutes after birth, an additional 5% of women will have a separated placenta. If one waits 45 minutes after birth, only another 1% or 2% will achieve placental separation. Thus if the placenta has not been recovered within 30 minutes of birth, most physicians will attempt to remove it manually.

Some obstetricians practice elective manual separation and extraction of the placenta to expedite the delivery sequence or to avoid abnormal bleeding, for example, after a twin birth. No supplementary anesthesia will be needed for women who have had regional anesthesia for birth. For other women, administration of light nitrous oxide and oxygen inhalation anesthesia or IV thiopental (Pentothal) will suffice for intrauterine exploration, placental separation, and recovery of the placenta.

If birth occurs early (fifth or sixth month), either spontaneously or by induced abortion, placental retention is the rule because of poor separation of the afterbirth. This may be caused by an immature zone of separation, weak uterine contractions, or a relatively large placenta.

Retained placenta may be the result of one of the following: partial separation of a normal placenta; entrapment of the partially or completely separated placenta by an hourglass constriction ring of the uterus; mismanagement of the third stage of labor; or abnormal adherence of the entire placenta or a portion of the placenta to the uterine wall. In all instances postbirth hemorrhage or infection may be a critical complicating factor.

ADHERENT RETAINED PLACENTA. Abnormal adherence of the placenta occurs for reasons unknown, but it is thought to result from zygote implantation in a zone of defective endometrium. There is no zone of separation between the placenta and the decidua. Abnormal adherence of the placenta is diagnosed in only about 1/12,000 births. The mother with an abnormally attached placenta is jeopardized mainly by postbirth hemorrhage leading to hypovolemic shock. Firm placental attachment is associated with increased maternal morbidity and mortality. There are no sure signs of abnormally adherent placenta during pregnancy.

Predisposing factors for abnormally firm placental attachment are scarring of the uterus such as occurs after cesarean birth, myomectomy, or vigorous curettage; endometritis associated with tuberculosis; abnormal site of implantation, such as the cervix or lower uterine segment; or malformation of the placenta.

Unusual placental adherence may be partial or complete. The following degrees of attachment are recognized:

- **Placenta accreta** (vera): slight penetration of myometrium by placental trophoblast (unusual)
- **Placenta increta:** deep penetration by placenta (rare)
- **Placenta percreta** (destruans): perforation of uterus by placenta (exceptional)

More cases of partial than complete placenta accreta occur. The true incidence is not known; however, it has been reported to be approximately 1/2000 to 3570 births (Zahn, Yeomans, 1990). At least 15% of cases of abnormally adherent placenta (all types) are associated with placenta previa. Currently being emphasized as placing the woman at increased risk is the combination of placenta previa and prior cesarean birth (Zahn, Yeomans, 1990).

In all types of abnormal adherence, placentation occurs in an area of deficient, sparse, or absent decidua. Thus the placenta develops on a surface partially or completely devoid of decidua (basalis). The uterine muscle is exposed, and invasion of the trophoblast and chorionic villi of the myometrium soon occurs. A dense fibrous area develops, together with hyalinization of neighboring uterine muscle. There is no zone of separation: no cleavage plane can be developed between the placenta and the uterine wall. Attempts to remove the placenta in the usual manner are therefore unsuccessful, and laceration or perforation of the uterine wall may result.

Bleeding with complete or total placenta accreta does not occur unless separation of the placenta is attempted. Partial placenta accreta invariably is associated with excessive intranatal or postbirth bleeding. The reason is that vessels adjacent to the adherent placenta remain open, and free bleeding prevents clotting.

When manual removal of a placenta accreta is attempted, damage to placental tissue and decidua, both rich in thromboplastin, occurs. When this substance is released in quantity into circulation, DIC may develop.

At vaginal birth the diagnosis of an abnormally adherent placenta generally is made when manual separation of a retained placenta is attempted. If the placenta will not separate readily (even a portion), immediate abdominal hysterectomy may be indicated. Persistent attempts at placental removal rarely will be successful, and fatal hemorrhage may result.

Placenta accreta or increta usually is diagnosed at cesarean birth when an abnormally adherent placenta is discovered. In such cases, especially when surgery was indicated because of placenta previa, total hysterectomy may be the best treatment. If the woman wants to have another child and is in satisfactory condition, and if hemorrhage can be controlled, the risk of not removing the uterus may be justifiable. Small retained portions of the placenta may separate or be absorbed, but infection often is a late complication. A second operation may be necessary because of later hemorrhage. After a subsequent viable pregnancy, elective repeat cesarean birth will be mandatory because another placenta accreta or increta is likely. Birth should be followed immediately by total abdominal hysterectomy.

SUBINVOLUTION OF THE UTERUS. Late postbirth bleeding may occur as a result of subinvolution of the uterus. **Subinvolution** is defined as the delayed return of the enlarged puerperal corpus to normal size and function (Cunningham et al, 1989). The causes of subinvolution include reduced circulation because of malposition, myomas, retained products of conception, infection, and gestational trophoblastic disease.

Subinvolution may complicate the puerperium because of such symptoms as pelvic discomfort or backache. There may be signs of abnormality such as leukorrhea or bleeding from an enlarged, boggy, perhaps tender uterus.

In the absence of frank bleeding, treatment is with ergonovine, 0.2 mg/4 hr for 2 or 3 days and antibiotic therapy. With hemorrhage, D & C to remove retained placental secundines and to débride the placental site for adequate healing generally is required, together with oxytocics and antibiotics.

NURSING PROCESS

ASSESSMENT

Postbirth assessments focus on uterine contractility and normal uterine involution, with special attention to risk factors. Risk factors for early onset of postbirth hemorrhage should be recognized before birth. Assessments include vital signs; uterine contractility and position; amount, color, and odor of lochia; and intake and output. Laboratory studies include evaluation of hemoglobin and hematocrit levels.

Pulse and blood pressure readings are poor indicators of postpartum hemorrhage. There is a significant lag between the onset of hemorrhage and changes in pulse and blood pressure readings (Cunningham et al, 1989). Therefore the nurse must assess thoroughly for the presence of bleeding.

Late postbirth hemorrhage may develop within several days of birth or later in the postpartum period. The client may be at home when the symptoms occur. Discharge teaching should emphasize the signs of normal involution, as well as potential complications.

NURSING DIAGNOSIS

Nursing diagnoses relevant to the care of the client experiencing a postbirth hemorrhage relate to tissue perfusion, possible complications, anxiety, and knowledge deficits. Potential nursing diagnoses include the following:

- Fluid volume deficit (immediate) related to
  —Excessive blood loss secondary to uterine atony, lacerations, or uterine inversion
- Fluid volume deficit (delayed) related to
  —Excessive blood loss secondary to retained placenta, infection, or subinvolution
- High risk for fluid volume excess related to
  —Blood and fluid volume replacement therapy
- High risk for infection related to
  —Excessive blood loss or exposed placental attachment site
- High risk for injury (maternal) related to
  —Attempted manual removal of retained placenta
  —Administration of blood products
  —Operative procedures
- Fear/anxiety related to
  —Threat to self
  —Knowledge deficit of procedures and operative management
- Alteration in parenting related to
  —Separation from infant secondary to treatment regimen
- Altered peripheral tissue perfusion related to
  —Excessive blood loss and shunting of blood to central circulation

PLANNING

The plan of care is mutually determined whenever possible. It is based on the biophysical and psychosocial assessments of the client. The plan must relate specifically to the client's clinical and nursing diagnoses and should be stated in terms of measurable client behaviors. *Goals* may include the following:

- The woman will maintain normal vital signs and laboratory values.
- She will not experience excessive bleeding and related complications.
- She will identify and use available support systems.
- She will verbalize understanding of condition, its management, and discharge instructions.

IMPLEMENTATION

Postpartum hemorrhage and shock are emergencies that are best resolved by adequate preparation. Assessment should identify risk factors, and preparations should be made in advance if possible to minimize potential blood loss. IV access should be established with a large-bore angiocatheter and fluid replacement initiated per physician's orders. Oxytocics will be employed to help maintain uterine contraction. If retained placental fragments are suspected or if surgery is required, the nurse will reinforce the physician's explanations and answer any questions or concerns of the client.

EVALUATION

The nurse can be reasonably assured that care was effective to the degree that the goals of care have been met. If they are not met, the nurse reinitiates the nursing process, starting with assessment. The goals may include that the woman maintains normal vital signs and laboratory values, does not experience excessive bleeding and related complications, identifies and uses available support systems, and verbalizes understanding of condition, its management, and discharge instructions.

■ HEMORRHAGIC SHOCK

Hemorrhage is a major threat to the mother during the childbearing cycle. **Hemorrhagic shock** may result. Shock is an emergency situation in which the perfusion of body organs may become severely compromised and death may ensue. Vigorous treatment is necessary to prevent adverse sequelae (e.g., cellular death, fluid overload, shock lung, and oxygen toxicity). A brief explanation of the physiologic mechanisms is provided to assist the nurse in implementing appropriate actions.

Physiologic Mechanisms

Physiologic compensatory mechanisms are activated in response to hemorrhage (or other trauma such as cardiac arrest). The adrenal glands release catecholamines, causing arterioles and venules in the skin, lungs, gastrointestinal tract, liver, and kidneys to constrict. The available blood flow is diverted to the brain and heart and away from other organs, including the uterus. If shock is prolonged, the continued reduction in cellular oxygenation results in an accumulation of lactic acid and acidosis (from anaerobic glucose metabolism). Acidosis (lowered serum pH) causes arteriole vasodilation; venule vasoconstriction persists. A circular pattern is established; that is, decreased perfusion, increased tissue anoxia and acidosis, edema formation, and pooling of blood further decrease the perfusion. Cellular death occurs.

Management

NURSING INTERVENTION

IMMEDIATE ACTIONS. Hemorrhagic shock often occurs rapidly. As soon as a woman exhibits the signs and symptoms of shock, the nurse stays with her and summons assistance and equipment. Nurses should have standing orders to start IV fluids and know the type of infusion to use and laboratory tests to order. While waiting for the physician, the nurse ensures a patent airway, which may include airway insertion, to facilitate oxygen administration and suction. The nurse can elevate the right hip (if left lateral position is not possible) to avoid supine hypotensive syndrome. *Trendelenburg's position (with head down and feet elevated) is not advised because this position may interfere with cardiac function.* This position should be used on physician request only.

When the physician arrives, the nurse will assist in instituting and monitoring measures to increase tissue perfusion. To maintain circulating volume it may be necessary to administer large volumes of fluid. Large amounts of crystalloids (lactated Ringer's or normal saline) will expand plasma volume; however, they will decrease the colloid oncotic pressure (COP). As COP decreases, the risk for pulmonary edema increases. To compensate for this, colloid solutions (albumin) should be used to balance the effect of volume and COP (Dorman, 1989).

MONITORING SYMPTOMS OF SHOCK. The nurse continues to monitor, assess, and record respirations, pulse, blood pressure, skin condition, urinary output, LOC, and hemodynamic parameters (central venous pressure [CVP] or left atrial wedge pressure) to evaluate effectiveness of management (Table 30-5).

Effective respiratory status is essential in that the body rids itself of excess acids by increasing the respiratory rate. Ventilatory assistance with oxygen or mechanical ventilation, or both, may be needed.

The pulse rate increases and becomes irregular as

TABLE 30-5 Symptoms of Shock

	Mild	Moderate	Severe	Irreversible
Respirations	Rapid, deep	Rapid, becoming shallow	Rapid, shallow, may be irregular	Irregular, or barely perceptible
Pulse	Rapid, tone normal	Rapid, tone may be normal but is becoming weaker	Very rapid, easily collapsible, may be irregular	Irregular apical pulse
Blood pressure	Normal or hypertensive	60-90 mm Hg systolic	Below 60 mm Hg systolic	None palpable
Skin	Cool and pale	Cool, pale, moist, knees cyanotic	Cold, clammy, cyanosis of lips and fingernails	Cold, clammy, cyanotic
Urinary output	No change	Decreasing to 10-22 mL/hr (adult)	Oliguric (less than 10 mL) to anuric	Anuric
Level of consciousness	Alert, oriented, diffuse anxiety	Oriented, mental cloudiness or increasing restlessness	Lethargic, reacts to noxious stimuli, comatose	Does not respond to noxious stimuli
CVP	May be normal (1-7 cm H_2O)	3 cm H_2O	0-3 cm H_2O	

Modified from Royce, JA: *Nurs Clin North Am* 8:377, 1973, Wagner MM, Clinical Nursing Specialist, University of Iowa Hospitals and Clinics.

shock progresses in severity. During pregnancy one early sign of bleeding may be an increase in heart rate accompanied by an *increase* in blood pressure.

In early stages of shock there will be an increase in systolic blood pressure, whereas in later stages of shock the systolic blood pressure decreases. In pregnancy blood pressure is not a sensitive indicator of impending shock. Because of the increased blood volume during pregnancy, a blood loss up to 30% can occur before signs of shock occur (Dorman, 1989). As blood is lost, there will be shunting from the peripheral circulation (including the uterus and placenta) to the central circulation. Fetal distress usually occurs before changes are seen in maternal vital signs.

Perfusion of the skin is sacrificed in the body's attempt to maintain blood flow to the heart and brain. Therefore the condition of the skin is a valuable index to the severity of shock. The nurse assesses the degree of ischemia or cyanosis of the nail beds, eyelids, and skin inside the mouth (buccal mucosa, gums, tongue). The nurse notes the degree of coolness and clamminess.

The nurse measures hourly urine output. Poor urinary output (less than 50 mL/hr) may indicate worsening of shock or inadequate fluid therapy; an increased output indicates improvement in the woman's condition.

The adequacy of cerebral perfusion may be estimated by an evaluation of the woman's LOC. In early stages of decreased blood flow the woman may complain of "seeing stars" or feeling dizzy or nauseated. She may become restless and orthopneic. As cerebral hypoxia increases, she may become confused and react slowly or not at all to stimuli. An improved sensorium is an indicator of improvement.

CVP measurement indicates the function (e.g., blood pressure) of the right side of the heart (Fig. 30-11). Normal values range between 1 and 7 cm H_2O (Clark et al, 1989). A low or falling value indicates inadequate blood volume or hypovolemia. A high or rising value indicates impaired contractility of the heart. A more precise method for evaluating hemodynamic status and heart function is the use of a **Swan-Ganz catheter.** The Swan-Ganz is a multiple-lumen pulmonary artery (PA) catheter used to measure both

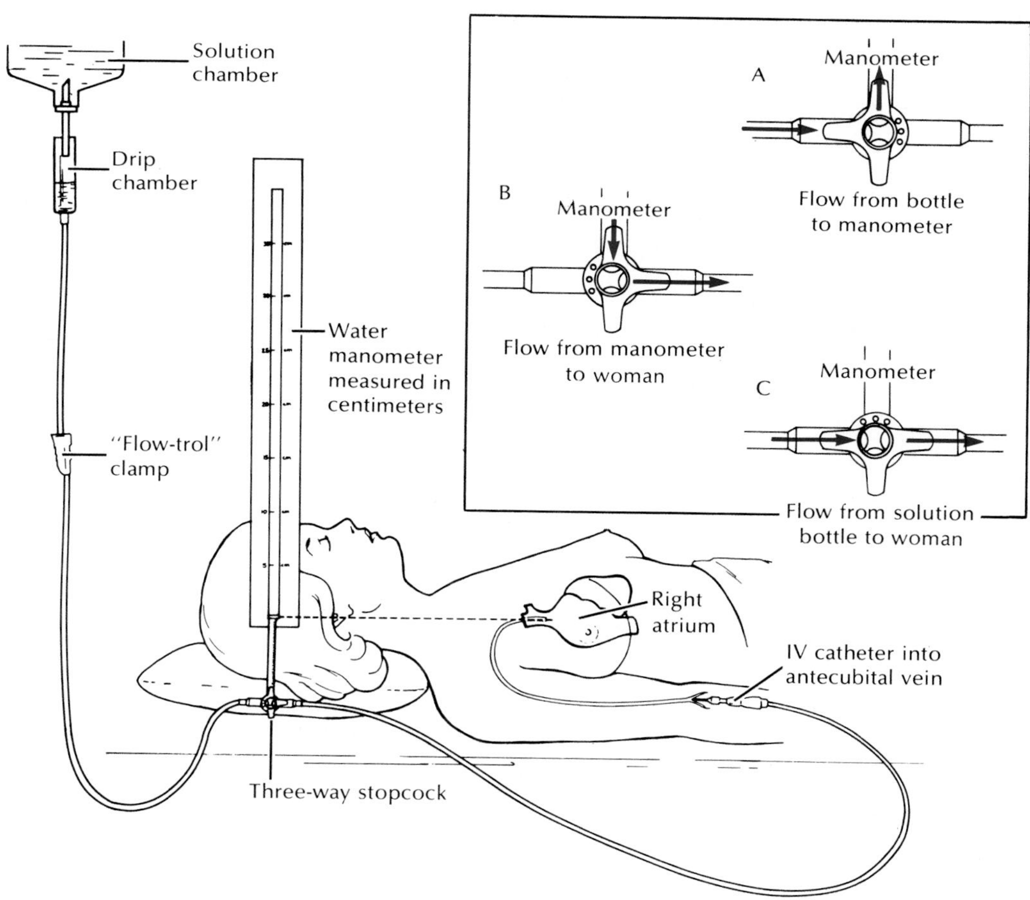

Fig. 30-11 Measurement of CVP with manometer.

right- and left-sided heart functions. By inflating the balloon at the catheter tip, one can measure the pulmonary arterial wedge pressure (PAWP), an indicator of left-sided heart function. Normal values range between 6 to 10 mm Hg during pregnancy (Clark et al, 1989). Because pulmonary edema can occur at lower wedge pressures during pregnancy, the use of a PA catheter will yield more useful information than will only CVP readings.

Anxiety is contagious. The nurse's calm, confident manner, coupled with brief, simple explanations, is an important adjunct to the interventions just discussed.

BLOOD REPLACEMENT. Blood replacement therapy is not uncommon in the management of hemorrhage (Table 30-6 and 30-7). Common clinical symptoms of inadequate intravascular volume (hypovolemia) that necessitates blood replacement include evidence of hemorrhage (loss of a large amount of blood externally or internally in a short period of time); evidence of hypovolemic shock (increasing pulse, cool clammy skin, rapid breathing, restlessness, reduced urine output); or decrease in hemoglobin and hematocrit levels below those acceptable for the trimester of pregnancy or the nonpregnant state.

Hazards of Therapy

The 24 hours after the shock period are critical. Observe for fluid overload, shock lung, and oxygen toxicity (Table 30-8). *Fluid overload* results in pulmonary and peripheral edema. *Shock lung* and *oxygen toxicity* may develop after mechanical ventilatory

TABLE 30-6 Coagulation Tests

Test	Comments
Activated partial thromboplastin time (PTT: measures intrinsic system): 25-36 sec	Screening test of choice: very sensitive, relatively easy to perform, inexpensive. All coagulation factors except proconvertin are measured.
One-stage prothrombin time (PT: Quick's test: measures extrinsic system): 9.5-11.3 sec	Test for proconvertin (VII), proaccelerin (V). Stuart-Prower factor (X), prothrombin (II), and fibrinogen deficiencies. Unfortunately, it does not measure factors necessary for earlier stages of coagulation.
Thrombin time (plasma): 10-15 sec	Test measures conversion of fibrinogen to fibrin and depends on concentration of fibrinogen or inhibitors such as fibrin split-products, antithrombins, and heparin.
Platelet count: 150,000-300,000/mm^3	**Most reliable index for DIC.**
Specific factor assays (e.g., plasma fibrinogen):195-365 mg/dL	Each of coagulation factors can be assessed by indirect clotting method using natural or synthetic factor-deficient substrates and compared with activity of normal plasma (100%). However, fibrinogen is only factor that can be measured directly by chemical method.
Bleeding time Template: 2-8 min Ivy: 1-7 min Duke: 1-3 min	Finger or earlobe puncture 5 mm deep and 2 mm wide (Bard-Parker blade No. 11) is made after antiseptic preparation of skin. Note time of puncture: touch bleeding point gently with sterile filter paper to absorb blood every 30 sec until bleeding stops.

TABLE 30-7 Replacement Clotting Factors

Infusate and Factors	Need	Risk	Expected Outcome
Fresh-frozen plasma: clotting factors	Depleted clotting factors	Hepatitis B, HIV	Increase fibrinogen to 10 mg dL per unit infused
Cryoprecipitate: I, V, VII, XIII	Fibrinogen concentration <50 mg/dL: a level of 50,000/mm^3 should be sought	Hepatitis, HIV	Increase fibrinogen 2-5 mg dL to 10 mg/dL per unit infused
Platelet concentrate; platelets	<20,000/mm^3	Rhesus isoimmunization in Rh-negative women	Increase platelet count 7500 μL per unit infused

assistance is initiated, especially if the ventilator is not maintained between 50 and 70 mm Hg. Alveolar capillary damage causes symptoms; high concentrations of oxygen are toxic to adults as well as the newborn. Irritation of mucous membranes of the upper respiratory tract, substernal pain, and cough may occur. Later neurologic symptoms include tinnitus, euphoria, confusion, and respiratory arrest.

Transfusion reactions may follow administration of blood or blood components. Even in an emergency, each unit should be checked. Complications include hemolytic reactions, febrile reactions, allergic reactions, circulatory overloading, and air embolism. Rapid transfusion with ice-cold blood can chill the heart and cause arrhythmias or arrest. It must be remembered that banked blood is calcium deficient, increasing the risk for arrhythmias.

Infection is another complication of hemorrhage. Causes may include surgical procedures, multiple pelvic examinations, anemia, and loss of the WBC component of the blood.

Postbirth Anterior Pituitary Necrosis

Postbirth anterior pituitary necrosis (**Sheehan's syndrome**) follows ischemia as a result of hypovolemic shock and DIC in about 15% of survivors of severe postbirth hemorrhage. Infarction of much or all of the anterior hypophysis causes partial or total loss of thyroid, adrenocortical, and gonadal functions. The degree of hormonal deficiency depends on the extent of gland destruction.

Women with Sheehan's syndrome fail to lactate and have a decrease in breast size. Loss of axillary and pubic hair, genital atrophy, and amenorrhea are common. Such women become apathetic and easily fatigued and can manifest altered affect (Cunningham et al, 1989).

TABLE 30-8 Hazards of Shock Therapy

Hazard	Nursing Action
Fluid overload: moist respirations, stridor, or dyspnea	Alert physician, decrease the drip rate
Shock lung: tachypnea, dyspnea, anxiety, a rise in blood pressure, cyanosis, and harsh loud breaths	Alert physician, maintain ventilator between 50 and 70 mm Hg
Oxygen toxicity: muscular twitching about the face, followed by convulsions resembling grand mal seizures.	Alert physician; take convulsion precautions

The prognosis of Sheehan's syndrome depends on the degree of residual anterior pituitary function and the supplementary therapy required. Minimum treatment requires thyroid hormone replacement, cortisone, and estrogen replacement. Infertility, reduced resistance to infection, tendency toward shock, and premature aging are problems of women with pituitary cachexia.

CLOTTING DISORDERS IN PREGNANCY

Normal Clotting

Normally a delicate balance (homeostasis) is maintained between two opposing systems, the hemostatic system and the fibrinolytic system. The *hemostatic system* is involved in the lifesaving process. This system stops the flow of blood from injured vessels, in part through the formation of insoluble fibrin that acts as a hemostatic platelet plug. The phases of the coagulation process involve an interaction of the coagulation factors; that is, each factor sequentially activates the factor next in line in the so-called cascade effect sequence. The *fibrinolytic system* refers to the process by which the fibrin is split into fibrinolytic degradation products and circulation is restored.

Clotting Problems

A history of abnormal bleeding, inheritance of unusual bleeding tendencies, and a report of significant aberrations of laboratory findings indicate a bleeding or clotting problem. For the obstetric client, bleeding disorders are suspected if the woman experiences PIH, HELLP syndrome, retained dead fetus syndrome, amniotic fluid embolism, sepsis, or hemorrhage. Determination of hemostasis is based on testing the usual mechanisms for the control of bleeding, that is, the function of platelets and the necessary clotting factors (Table 30-6).

Disseminated Intravascular Coagulation

Disseminated intravascular coagulation (**DIC**, defibrination syndrome, defibrination coagulopathy) is a pathologic form of clotting that is diffuse and consumes large amounts of clotting factors, causing widespread external or internal bleeding or both. Simply, DIC is an overzealous consumption of clotting factors (Dorman, 1989).

SIGNS AND SYMPTOMS. Physical examination reveals unusual bleeding. Spontaneous bleeding from the woman's gums or nose may be noted. Petechiae may appear around the blood pressure cuff on her arm. Excessive bleeding may occur from the site of a slight trauma (e.g. venipuncture sites, intramuscular or subcutaneous injection sites, nicks from shaving of perineum or abdomen, and injury from insertion of urinary catheter). Maternal symptoms may include tachycardia and diaphoresis. Laboratory tests reveal decreased platelets, fibrinogen, proaccelerin, antihemophilic factor, and prothrombin (the factors consumed during coagulation). Other factors should be normal. Fibrinolysis is first increased but later is severely depressed. Degradation of fibrin leads to the accumulation of fibrin-split products in the blood. Fibrin-split products have anticoagulant properties and thus prolong the prothrombin time (PT). Bleeding time is normal; coagulation time shows no clot; clot retraction time shows no clot; and partial thromboplastin time (PTT) is increased. DIC must be distinguished from other clotting disorders before therapy is initiated.

MEDICAL MANAGEMENT. The primary management of all cases of DIC involves correction of the underlying cause, for example, recovery of the dead fetus; treatment of existing infection or preeclampsia/eclampsia; or removal of abrupted placenta. Packed red blood cells may be transfused to correct anemia. Deficiencies secondary to DIC primarily involve platelets, factors V and VIII, fibrinogen, and prothrombin. Administration of fresh-frozen plasma in combination with platelet concentrates is effective in all these conditions when replacement therapy is warranted (Dorman, 1989).

Renal failure is one consequence of DIC; therefore urinary output is monitored. Urinary output must be maintained at more than 30 mL/hr. Supportive measures also include keeping the woman's right hip elevated to prevent hypotensive syndrome. Oxygen is administered by a tight-fitting rebreathing mask at 10 to 12 L/min. The emotional needs of the family are recognized and supported.

PROGNOSIS. Maternal and fetal prognosis depends on the degree and extent of the underlying disorder, as well as the response of the woman to prompt and proper treatment. Maternal risk is further increased if the fetus dies in utero.

NURSING CARE. The nurse caring for the woman at risk for DIC must be aware of the risk factors. Careful and thorough *assessment* is required, with particular attention to the signs of bleeding (e.g., petechiae, oozing from injection sites, and hematuria).

Potential *nursing diagnoses* for the woman diagnosed with or suspected of having DIC focus on alterations in hemodynamic status, knowledge deficits, fear and anxiety of the woman, and high risk for injury to the mother and fetus.

Planning care for the woman with DIC will be determined primarily by the nurse or physician on the basis of the woman's biophysical assessment findings. *Goals* may include that the woman's hemodynamic status will be corrected, that she will receive emotional support, and that she and her fetus/newborn will have no further complications.

The nurse *evaluates* care by determining the extent to which goals for care have been met. That is, the woman's hemodynamic status is corrected, she receives emotional support, and she and her fetus/newborn have no further complications.

Autoimmune Thrombocytopenic Purpura

Autoimmune thrombocytopenic purpura is an autoimmune disorder in which antiplatelet antibodies decrease the life span of the platelets. Thrombocytopenia, capillary fragility, and increased bleeding time are diagnostic. Autoimmune thrombocytopenic purpura may result in severe hemorrhage after cesarean birth or from cervical or vaginal lacerations. The incidence of postbirth uterine bleeding or vaginal hematomas also is increased.

Therapy focuses on control. Platelet transfusions are given to maintain the platelet count at 100,000/mm.^{3} Corticosteroids are given if the diagnosis is made before or during pregnancy. Splenectomy, if needed, is deferred until after the puerperium. Neonatal thrombocytopenia, a result of the maternal disease process, occurs in about 50% of the cases and is associated with high mortality.

Von Willebrand's Disease

Von Willebrand's disease, a type of hemophilia, probably is the most common of all hereditary bleeding disorders (Cunningham et al, 1989). It results from a factor VIII deficiency and platelet dysfunction. It is transmitted as an incomplete autosomal-dominant trait to both sexes. Although von Willebrand's disease is rare, it is one of the most common congenital clotting defects in American women of childbearing age. The symptoms include a familial bleeding tendency, previous bleeding episodes, prolonged bleeding time (the most important test), factor VIII deficiency (mild to moderate), and bleeding from mucous membranes. Because factor VIII increases during pregnancy, this increase may be sufficient to offset danger from hemorrhage during childbirth. However, the woman's condition should be observed for at least 1 week after childbirth. Treatment of von Willebrand's disease consists of replacement of factor VIII, if it is less than 30%, through administration of cryoprecipitate or fresh frozen plasma.

■ SUMMARY

Bleeding disorders of pregnancy are medical emergencies that demand expert teamwork on the part of the health care team. The nurse must be able to assist the physician in minimizing blood loss, in analyzing assessment findings to arrive at a correct diagnosis, and in implementing appropriate actions to maintain the pregnancy if possible, as well as provide the emergency care needed for both mother and baby. In addition, the reactions of the woman and her family need to be considered.

REFERENCES

Baskett TF, Writer WDR: Postpartum hemorrhage. In Datta S, editor: *Anesthetic and obstetric management for high risk pregnancy,* St Louis, 1991, Mosby–Year Book.

Beischer NA, McKay EV: *Obstetrics and the newborn,* ed 2, Philadelphia, 1986, Saunders.

Berman ML, DiSaia PJ: Pelvic malignancies, gestational trophoblastic neoplasia, and nonpelvic malignancies. In Creasy RK, Resnik R, editors: *Maternal-fetal medicine: principles and practice,* ed 2, Philadelphia, 1989, Saunders.

Clark SL et al: Central hemodynamic assessment of normal term pregnancy, *Am J Obstet Gynecol* 161:1439, 1989.

Cocaine use linked to infant defects, *San Francisco Chronicle,* Jan 19, 1987.

Cole HM: Cardiovascular effects of cocaine, *JAMA* 257:979, 1987.

Cunningham FG, MacDonald PC, Gant NF: *Williams obstetrics,* ed 18, Norwalk, Conn, 1989, Appleton & Lange.

de Crespigny LC: The value of ultrasound in ectopic pregnancy, *Clin Obstet Gynecol* 30:136, 1987.

DePetrillo AD et al: Symposium: gestational trophoblastic disease: an update, *Contemp OB/GYN* 29:199, Jan 1987.

Deutchman M: The problematic first-trimester pregnancy, *Am Fam Physician* 39:185, 1989.

Dorfman SF: Pregnancy for older parents. In Cherry SH, Merkatz IR, editors: *Complications of pregnancy: medical, surgical, gynecologic, psychosocial, and perinatal,* ed 4, Philadelphia, 1991, Williams & Wilkins.

Dorman KF: Hemorrhagic emergencies in obstetrics, J Perinat Neonat Nurs 3:23, Feb 1989.

Gilbert ES, Harmon JS: *High-risk pregnancy and delivery: nursing perspectives,* ed 2, St Louis, 1992, Mosby–Year Book.

Glass RH, Golbus MS: Habitual abortion. In Creasy RK, Resnik R, editors: *Maternal-fetal medicine: principles and practice,* ed 2, Philadelphia, 1989, WB Saunders.

Green JR: Placenta previa and abruptio placentae. In Creasy RK, Resnik R, editors: *Maternal-fetal medicine: principles and practice,* ed 2, Philadelphia, 1989, WB Saunders.

Kulb NW: Abnormalities of the placenta and membranes. In K Buckley, NW Kulb, editors: *High risk maternity nursing manual,* Baltimore, 1990, Williams & Wilkins.

Lavery JP: Placenta previa, *Clin Obstet Gynecol* 33:414, 1990.

Lowe TW, Cunningham G: Placental abruption, *Clin Obstet Gynecol* 33:406, 1990.

McLaren RA, Feinstein SJ, Lodeiro JG: Abruptio placentae with disseminated intravascular coagulation, *Female Patient* 16:22, July 1991.

Murahata SA: Third stage of labor and postpartum hemorrhage. In Frederickson HM, L Wilkins-Haug, editors: *Ob/gyn secrets,* St Louis, 1991, Mosby–Year Book.

Nager CW, Murphy AA: Ectopic pregnancy, *Clin Obstet Gynecol* 33:403, 1991.

Roberts WE et al: The incidence of preterm labor and specific risk factors, *Obstet Gynecol* 76(suppl 7):85, 1990.

Robichaux AG, Stedman CM, Hamner C: Uterine activity in patients with cervical cerclage, *Obstet Gynecol* 76(suppl 7):63, 1990.

Rochat RW et al: Maternal mortality in the United States: report from the maternal mortality collaborative, *Obstet Gynecol* 72:91, 1988.

Rosenak D et al: Cocaine: Maternal use during pregnancy and its effect on the mother, the fetus, and the infant, *Obstet Gynecol Surv* 45:348, 1990.

Scott JR et al: *Danforth's obstetrics and gynecology,* ed 6, Philadelphia, 1990, JB Lippincott.

Stoval TG, Ling FW, Buster JE: Reproductive performance after methotrexate treatment of ectopic pregnancy, *Am J Obstet Gynecol* 162:1620, 1990.

Suresh MS, Kinch RA: Antepartum hemorrhage. In Datta S, editor: *Anesthetic and obstetric management for high risk pregnancy,* St Louis, 1991, Mosby–Year Book.

Szulman AE: Syndromes of hydatidiform moles, *J Reprod Med* 29:788, 1984.

Watson DL et al: Management of preterm labor patients at home: does daily uterine activity monitoring and nursing support make a difference? *Obstet Gynecol* 76(suppl 7):32, 1990.

Wolf EJ et al: Placenta previa is not an independent risk factor for a small for gestational age infant, *Obstet Gynecol* 77:707, 1991.

Woods JR, Plessinger MA, Clark KE: Effect of cocaine on uterine blood flow and fetal oxygenation, *JAMA* 257:957, 1987.

Zahn CM, Yeomans ER: Postpartum hemorrhage: placenta accreta, uterine inversion, and puerperal hematomas, *Clin Obstet Gynecol* 33:422, 1990.

BIBLIOGRAPHY

American College of Obstetricians and Gynecologists: ACOG *Diagnosis and management of postpartum hemorrhage* (ACOG Technical Bulletin No 143), Washington, DC, 1990, ACOG.

Catlin A, Wetzel W:Ectopic pregnancy: clinical evaluation, diagnostic measures and prevention, *Nurs Pract* 16:38, Jan 1991.

Costa T, Job-Spira N, Fernandez H: Increased risk of ectopic pregnancy with maternal cigarette smoking, *Am J Public Health* 81:199, 1991.

Flint C: Postpartum hemorrhage at home, *Nurs Times* 84(3):47, 1988.

Luegenbiehl DL et al: Standardized assessment of blood loss, *MCN 15:* 241, 1990.

O'Sullivan M, Ricci J: Uterine rupture: management alternative, *Contemp OB/GYN* (special edition), p 83, 1988.

Perlis DW, editor: Bleeding in women, *NAACOG's Clin Issues Perinatal Women's Health Nurs* 2:283, 1991.

Robichaux AG, Stedman CM, Hamer C: Uterine activity in patients with cervical cerclage, *Obstet Gynecol* 76(supp 1):63, 1990.

Stoval TG et al: Methotrexate treatment of unruptured ectopic pregnancy: a report of 100 cases, *Obstet Gynecol* 77:754, 1991.

Trustum A: When to expect ectopic pregnancy, *RN* 54:22, Aug 1991.

Tucker R: Abruptio placenta complicated by disseminated intravascular coagulopathy. In Angelin DJ, Knapp CMW, editors: *Case studies in perinatal nursing,* Gaithersburg, Md, 1992, Aspen.

Vasilev SA, Liming PR:Ectopic pregnancy, *AORN J* 54(5):1030, Nov 1991.

chapter 30 review

Key Concepts

- Blood loss during pregnancy should always be regarded as a warning sign until ruled out by the woman's physician.
- Many spontaneous abortions occur for unknown reasons, but fetoplacental maldevelopment and maternal factors can account for others.
- The type of spontaneous abortion directs the management.
- Ectopic pregnancy is a significant cause of maternal morbidity and mortality even in developed countries.
- There are two distinctive types of hydatidiform mole: complete and partial.
- Premature separation of the placenta and placenta previa are differentiated by type of bleeding, uterine tonicity, and presence or absence of pain.
- Clotting disorders are associated with many obstetric complications.
- External fundal pressure and traction on the umbilical cord before placental separation can result in inversion of the uterus.
- Postbirth hemorrhage is the most common and most serious type of excessive obstetric blood loss.
- Hemorrhagic (hypovolemic) shock is an emergency situation in which the perfusion of body organs may become severely compromised and death may ensue.
- The potential hazards of therapeutic interventions may further compromise the woman experiencing hemorrhagic disorders.

Key Terms

- abortion (p. 886)
- abruptio placentae (p. 902)
- cerclage (p. 891)
- Couvelaire uterus (p. 906)
- Cullen's sign (p. 893)
- disseminated intravascular coagulation (DIC) (p. 917)
- ectopic pregnancy (p. 893)
- gestational trophoblastic disease (GTD) (p. 895)
- hematoma (p. 909)
- hemorrhagic shock (p. 913)
- hydatidiform mole (molar pregnancy) (p. 895)
- incompetent cervix (p. 890)
- inversion of the uterus (p. 909)
- placenta accreta (p. 912)
- placenta increta (p. 912)
- placenta percreta (p. 912)
- placenta previa (p. 898)
- retained placenta (p. 911)
- Sheehan's syndrome (p. 917)
- subinvolution (p. 912)
- uterine atony (p. 908)
- velamentous insertion of the cord (p. 907)

Critical Thinking Exercises

You are providing care for a 42-year-old nullipara admitted at 34 weeks, gestation with possible abruptio placentae. She has a history of cocaine use.

1. What are the possible reactions of the woman to the situation?
2. Examine your reactions to this assignment. What assumptions have you made? What do you need to verify?
3. Analyze assessment findings to determine appropriate nursing diagnoses.
4. Generate a plan of care for this woman.
5. Evaluate the appropriateness of the proposed interventions for this woman.

You are assigned to a 22-year-old unmarried woman threatened with the loss of her first pregnancy at 14 weeks' gestation.

1. What reactions might the woman have about her condition?
2. What assumptions can you make about this client situation?
3. Identify ways to verify or negate your assumptions.
4. How might these assumptions affect your plan of care?

Interview a woman who has experienced postpartum hemorrhage or other hemorrhagic disorder.

1. Examine her reaction to the experience.
2. Identify implications of her reactions on planning effective nursing care.
3. Propose evaluative criteria to assess effectiveness of nursing care.

Topics for Nursing Research

- Will the prophylactic use of low-dose aspirin increase the incidence and severity of bleeding during pregnancy?
- Will the increasing incidence of adolescent pregnancies and sexual activity increase the incidence of ectopic pregnancy or poor perinatal outcomes?

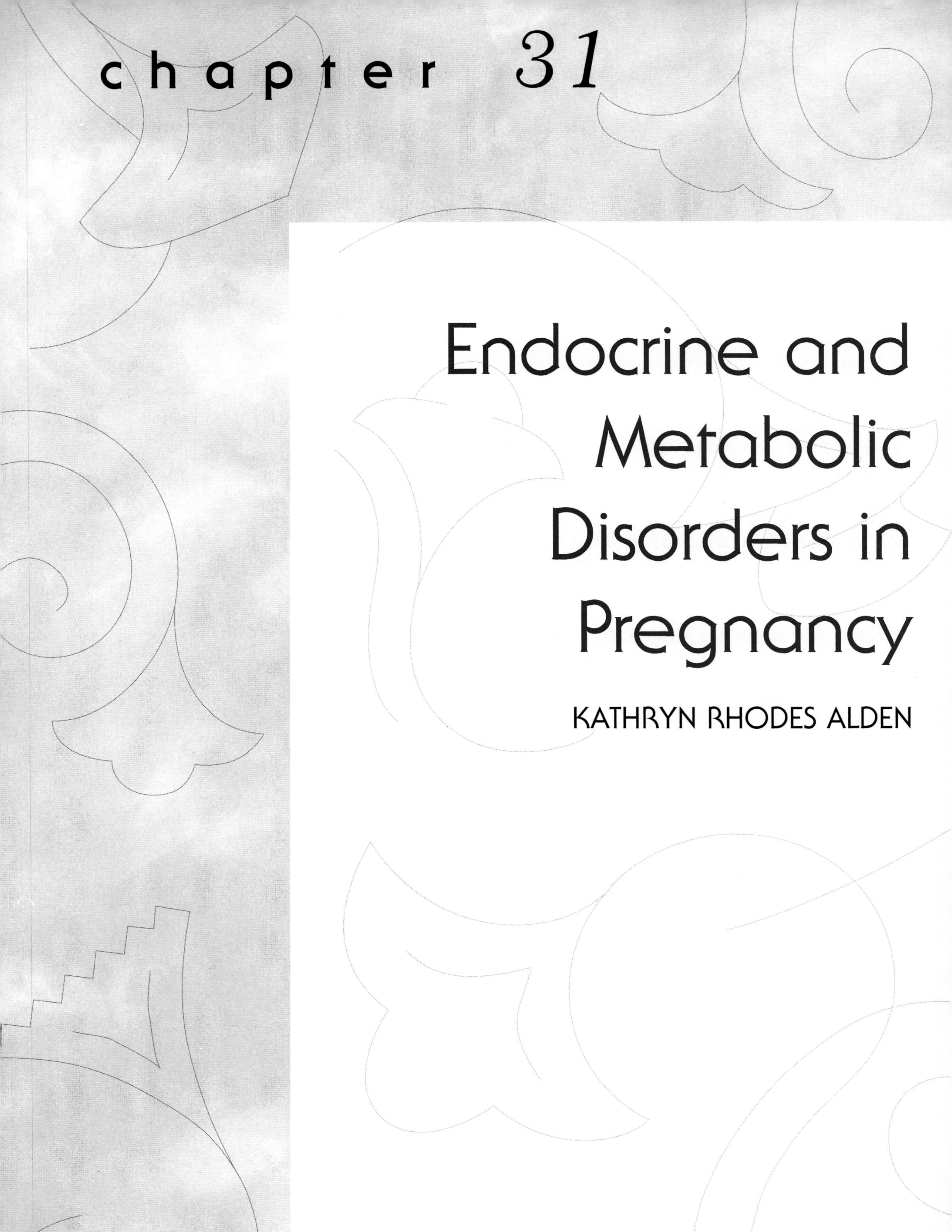

chapter 31

Endocrine and Metabolic Disorders in Pregnancy

KATHRYN RHODES ALDEN

LEARNING OBJECTIVES

- Define the key terms listed.
- Differentiate the types of diabetes mellitus and their respective risk factors in pregnancy.
- Summarize the effects of pregnancy on insulin requirements.
- Discuss maternal and fetal risks/complications associated with diabetic pregnancy.
- Discuss each step of the nursing process as it relates to diabetic pregnancy.
- Describe the significance of hyperemesis gravidarum on maternal and fetal well-being.
- Discuss each step of the nursing process as it relates to hyperemesis gravidarum.
- Explain the effects of disorders of the thyroid on pregnancy.
- Identify topics for nursing research related to endocrine and metabolic disorders.
- Describe the effects of maternal phenylketonuria on pregnancy outcome.

Endocrine and metabolic disorders complicate many pregnancies and require careful management to promote maternal and fetal well-being and positive pregnancy outcome. Diabetes mellitus is the most common endocrine disorder associated with pregnancy. Hyperemesis gravidarum and disorders of the thyroid, although encountered less often, also require careful planning for care. Phenylketonuria, an inborn error of metabolism, is a relatively new disorder in women of reproductive age, with significant implications for pregnancy outcome.

The maternity nurse is challenged to provide sound, effective care that meets the unique maternal and fetal needs prompted by these endocrine and metabolic conditions. The primary objective of nursing care must be to guide and support the woman and her family in achieving optimal outcome for both the pregnant woman and the fetus. The nurse serves as teacher, counselor, and support person to assist the woman and her family in achieving the best possible outcome and to deal with the problems and disappointments that may arise.

DIABETES AND PREGNANCY

Before the discovery of insulin in the early 1920s, diabetes and pregnancy were clearly incompatible. Many diabetic women of childbearing age were infertile or sterile, and most of those who became pregnant were unable to carry the pregnancy to term. Maternal mortality was as high as 50%, and perinatal mortality approached 65%.

Over the last 65 years, remarkable improvements have occurred in understanding and managing diabetic pregnancy. These advances in care have prompted substantial changes in maternal and perinatal outcomes. The current maternal mortality rate is approximately 0.5%; however, this rate is still five times that of nondiabetic pregnancies (Meyer, Palmer, 1990). The perinatal mortality rate has declined to less than 5%, compared with 1% to 2% in nondiabetic pregnancies (Centers for Disease Control [CDC], 1990). In well-managed cases the maternal and perinatal mortality rates are similar to those of the nondiabetic population.

Despite the advances in care, pregnancy complicated by diabetes is still considered high risk. It is managed most successfully by means of a multidisciplinary approach involving the obstetrician, internist or diabetologist, neonatologist, nurse, dietitian, and social worker. Favorable outcome of diabetic pregnancy requires commitment and active participation by the woman (and her family). She must comply with a schedule of frequent prenatal visits, strict adherence to dietary regimen, regular self-monitoring of blood glucose level, frequent laboratory evaluation, intensive fetal surveillance, and possible hospitalization (Barss, 1989).

Care of the pregnant diabetic requires that the nurse fully understand the normal physiologic responses to pregnancy, as well as the altered metabolism of diabetes. Furthermore the nurse must understand the relationship between pregnancy and diabetes to accurately assess the woman's condition, to plan for her care, and to intervene appropriately. An awareness of the psychosocial implications of diabetic pregnancy must guide the nurse in planning, implementing, and evaluating care of the woman and her family.

Pathogenesis of Diabetes Mellitus

Diabetes mellitus is a systemic disorder of carbohydrate, protein, and fat metabolism. It is characterized by **hyperglycemia** (elevated blood glucose) resulting from inadequate production of **insulin** or ineffective use of insulin at the cellular level. Insulin, produced by the beta cells in the islets of Langerhans in the pancreas, regulates blood glucose levels by enabling glucose to enter adipose and muscle cells where it is used for energy. Insulin also stimulates protein synthesis and storage of free fatty acids. When insulin is insufficient or ineffective in promoting glucose uptake by the muscle and adipose cells, glucose accumulates in the blood stream and hyperglycemia results. Hyperglycemia causes hyperosmolarity of the blood, which attracts intracellular fluid into the vascular system, resulting in cellular dehydration and expanded blood volume. Consequently, the kidneys function to excrete large volumes of urine (*polyuria*) in an attempt to regulate excess vascular volume and to excrete the unusable glucose (*glycosuria*). Polyuria, along with cellular dehydration, causes excessive thirst (*polydipsia*).

The body compensates for its inability to convert carbohydrate (glucose) into energy by burning proteins (muscle) and fats. Unfortunately, the end products of this metabolism are ketones and fatty acids, which in excess quantity produce *ketoacidosis* and *acetonuria*. Weight loss occurs as a result of the breakdown of fat and muscle tissue. This tissue breakdown causes a state of starvation that compels the individual to eat excessively (*polyphagia*).

Over time, diabetes causes significant changes in both the microvascular and macrovascular circulation. These structural changes affect a variety of organ systems, particularly the heart, eyes, and kidneys. Complications resulting from diabetes include premature atherosclerosis, retinopathy, and nephropathy.

Diabetes (types I and II) is typically regarded as a genetically determined syndrome. It usually is inherited as a recessive trait but occurs as a dominant trait in some families. Inheritance of the genetic trait (genotype) for diabetes mellitus does not necessarily mean that the individual will demonstrate diabetic glucose intolerance (phenotype). Many people with the genotype do not show any evidence of diabetes until they experience one or more of a variety of stressors, or precipitating factors. Examples of such stressors are an increase in age, normal developmental periods of rapid hormonal change (menarche, pregnancy, menopause), obesity, infection, surgery, emotional crisis, and tumor or infection of the pancreas.

Classification of Diabetes Mellitus

Although diabetes is clearly a disorder of insulin availability, it is not a single disease. The various types of diabetes mellitus and glucose intolerance can be classified by a system that was developed by the National Diabetes Data Group of the National Institutes of Health (American Diabetes Association [ADA], 1990).

TYPE I INSULIN-DEPENDENT DIABETES MELLITUS (IDDM). Formerly known as juvenile diabetes, this type is characterized by an absolute insulin-deficiency state. Its onset typically occurs in persons 30 years or younger. Persons with IDDM often experience marked alterations in blood glucose levels and are prone to ketosis.

TYPE II NON-INSULIN–DEPENDENT DIABETES MELLITUS (NIDDM). Previously known as maturity-onset diabetes, NIDDM occurs in all ages but is more common in the older overweight individual. It is associated with a lack of insulin availability or effectiveness rather than an absolute insulin deficiency. NIDDM is said to be ketosis resistant and often is controlled by diet alone.

OTHER TYPES. Formerly known as secondary diabetes, this classification refers to abnormalities in glucose tolerance after such conditions as pancreatic disease, endocrine disorders (Cushing's syndrome), drug ingestion, and cirrhosis.

IMPAIRED GLUCOSE TOLERANCE (IGT). This category refers to abnormal glucose levels intermediate between normal values and overt diabetes. Formerly known as latent, chemical, asymptomatic, or borderline diabetes, IGT may progress to actual diabetes.

GESTATIONAL DIABETES MELLITUS (GDM). Glucose intolerance of variable severity with its onset or first recognition during pregnancy is considered GDM. This definition is appropriate whether insulin is used for treatment or the diabetes persists after the pregnancy. It does not exclude the possibility that the glucose intolerance preceded the pregnancy.

Classification of Diabetes during Pregnancy

In 1949 Priscilla White proposed a system for classifying pregnancies complicated by diabetes to enable physicians to identify those diabetic women who are at greater risk during pregnancy. White's classification is based on the premise that the age of onset of diabetes, its duration, and the severity of vascular disease significantly influence perinatal outcome (White, 1978) (Table 31-1).

Although White's classification system has been used for many years, it is now recognized that with appropriate management, no major differences in outcome exist among the individual classes, except for typically poorer outcomes in classes F, H, and R. Research has repeatedly shown that the major factor influencing pregnancy outcome appears to be the degree of maternal glycemic control (Jovanovic-Peterson, Peterson, 1988).

Diabetes during pregnancy also can be classified according to whether the diabetes preceded the pregnancy or had its onset during gestation. **Pregestational diabetes** is the term for types I or II diabetes that existed before pregnancy, whereas **gestational diabetes** (GDM) refers to glucose intolerance first recognized during the pregnancy.

Metabolic Changes during Pregnancy

Normal pregnancy is characterized by complex alterations in maternal glucose metabolism, insulin production, and metabolic homeostasis. A constant supply of glucose is necessary for growth and development of the embryo/fetus. Maternal glucose is transported to the fetus by the process of facilitated diffusion. *Maternal insulin does not cross the placenta.* By the tenth week of gestation the embryo/fetus secretes its own insulin at levels adequate to use the glucose obtained from the mother.

During the first trimester of pregnancy, the pregnant woman's metabolic status is significantly influenced by the rising levels of estrogen and progesterone. These hormones stimulate the beta cells in the

TABLE 31-1 Classification of Diabetes during Pregnancy (Priscilla White)

Class	Characteristics	Implications
Glucose intolerance of pregnancy	Erroneously known as gestational diabetes. Abnormal glucose tolerance during pregnancy; postprandial hyperglycemia during pregnancy.	Diagnosis before 30 weeks' gestation important to prevent macrosomia. Treat with diet adequate in calories to prevent maternal weight loss. Goal is postprandial blood glucose <130 mg/dl at 1 hour, or <105 mg/dl at 2 hours. If insulin is necessary, manage as in classes B, C, and D.
A	Chemical diabetes diagnosed before pregnancy; managed by diet alone: any age at onset.	Management as for glucose intolerance of pregnancy.
B	Insulin treatment used before pregnancy; onset at age 20 or older; duration < 10 years.	Some endogenous insulin secretion may persist. Fetal and neonatal risks same as in classes C and D, as is management.
C	Onset at age 10-20, or duration 10-20 years.	Insulin-deficient diabetes of juvenile onset.
D	Onset before age 10, or duration > 20 years, or chronic hypertension (not preeclampsia), or background retinopathy (tiny hemorrhages).	Fetal macrosomia or intrauterine growth retardation possible. Retinal microaneurysms; dot hemorrhages, and exudates may progress during pregnancy, then regress after delivery.
F	Diabetic nephropathy with proteinuria.	Anemia and hypertension common; proteinuria increases in third trimester, declines after delivery. Fetal intrauterine growth retardation common; perinatal survival about 85% under optimum conditions; bed rest necessary.
H	Coronary artery disease.	Serious maternal risk.
R	Proliferative retinopathy.	Neovascularization, with risk of vitreous hemorrhage or retinal detachment; laser photocoagulation useful; abortion usually not necessary. With active process of neovascularization, prevent bearing-down efforts.

From Benson RC, editor: *Current obstetric and gynecologic diagnosis and treatment,* ed 5, Los Altos, Calif, 1984, Lange Medical Publications.

pancreas to increase insulin production, which promotes increased peripheral utilization of glucose and decreased blood glucose with fasting levels of 55 to 65 mg/dL (Fig. 31-1, *A* and *B*). There is a concomitant increase in tissue glycogen stores and a decrease in hepatic glucose. Throughout pregnancy, as a result of continued beta cell hypertrophy, there is an enhanced insulin response to glucose.

During the second and third trimesters, pregnancy exerts a "diabetogenic" effect on the maternal metabolic status. Because of the major hormonal changes, there is decreased tolerance to glucose, increased insulin resistance, decreased hepatic glycogen stores, and increased hepatic production of glucose. Rising levels of human placental lactogen, estrogen, progesterone, cortisol, prolactin, and insulinase increase insulin resistance through their actions as insulin antagonists. Insulin resistance is a glucose-sparing mechanism that ensures an abundant supply of glucose for the fetus. Maternal insulin requirements may double or quadruple by term gestation (Fig. 31-1, *C* to *D*).

At birth, explusion of the placenta prompts an abrupt drop in levels of circulating placental hormones, cortisol, and insulinase. Maternal tissues quickly regain their prepregnancy sensitivity to insulin. For the non–breast-feeding mother, prepregnancy insulin-carbohydrate balance usually returns in about 7 to 10 days (Fig. 31-1, *E*). Lactation utilizes maternal glucose, so that the breast-feeding mother's

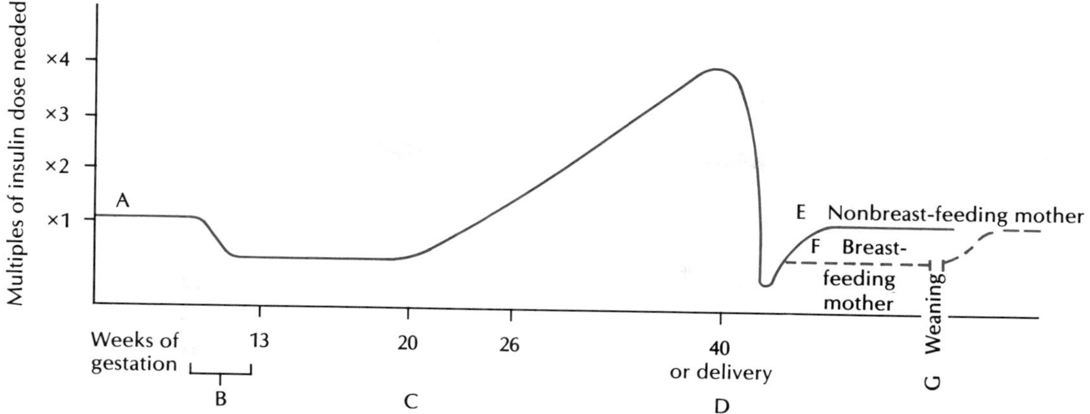

Fig. 31-1 Changing insulin needs during pregnancy caused by properties of placental hormones and enzyme (insulinase) and cortisol. **A**, gestational period characterized by nausea, vomiting, and often, decreased food intake by mother while glucose use of embryo-fetus increases. **B**, Increase in peripheral resistance to insulin (mother becomes less sensitive to insulin). **C**, Day of delivery: maternal insulin requirements drop dramatically to about prepregnancy levels; she is now very sensitive to insulin. **D**, For nonnursing mother prepregnancy insulin-carbohydrate balance usually returns in about 7 to 10 days. **E**, For nursing mother, her insulin requirements will remain low for up to 6 to 9 months. **F**, At weaning, woman's prepregnancy carbohydrate metabolism is reestablished.

insulin requirements will remain low for up to 6 to 9 months (Fig. 31-1, *F*). On completion of weaning, prepregnancy insulin requirement is reestablished (Fig. 31-1, *G*).

PREGESTATIONAL DIABETES

When a recognized diabetic becomes pregnant, she is known as a pregestational diabetic; that is, the diabetes existed before conception and will continue after the pregnancy. Pregestational diabetics may have either type I (insulin dependent) or type II (non–insulin-dependent) diabetes, which may or may not be complicated by vascular disease, retinopathy, nephropathy, or other diabetic sequelae. Type II diabetics who become pregnant typically require insulin during gestation; thus most pregestational diabetics are insulin-dependent.

The reported incidence of IDDM during pregnancy varies from 0.1% to 0.5% (Landon, Gabbe, 1988). The CDC (1990) examined data from 225 hospital-based reports in the United States, Canada, and Europe and estimated that 5/1000 pregnancies are complicated by IDDM.

The diabetogenic state of pregnancy imposed on the compromised metabolic system of the pregestational diabetic has significant implications. The normal hormonal adaptations of pregnancy affect glycemic control in the pregestational diabetic. Pregnancy also may accelerate the progress of vascular complications of diabetes.

During the first trimester, while maternal blood glucose levels normally are reduced and insulin response to glucose is enhanced, glycemic control is improved. Insulin dosage for well-controlled diabetes may need to be adjusted to avoid **hypoglycemia** (low blood glucose). An increased incidence of hypoglycemic episodes in type I diabetes occurs during early pregnancy (Meyer, Palmer, 1990). Nausea, vomiting, and cravings typical of early pregnancy result in dietary fluctuations, which influence maternal glucose levels and necessitate adjustments in insulin dosage.

As insulin requirements steadily increase after the first trimester, insulin dosage must be adjusted accordingly to prevent episodes of hyperglycemia. Insulin resistance begins as early as 14 to 16 weeks and continues to rise until leveling off during the last few weeks of pregnancy.

The long-term implications of pregnancy on the microvascular and macrovascular complications of diabetes are unclear. Progression and regression of retinopathy are common during pregnancy. Pregnancy appears to have little impact on the long-term course of diabetic nephropathy. Women with early renal nephropathy usually have successful pregnancy outcomes, although they are at increased risk for pregnancy-induced hypertension (see discussion of hypertension, Chapter 28). Little information exists about the effect of pregnancy on diabetic cardiomyopathy. In IDDM, the normal hemodynamic adjustments to pregnancy are impaired, resulting in a smaller physiologic increase in cardiac output compared with nondiabetic pregnant women. There also is increased risk of thromboembolic complications among pregnant diabetics. Thyroid dysfunction, usually hypothyroidism, is a common occurrence during diabetic pregnancy (Meyer, Palmer, 1990).

Preconceptional Counseling

Preconceptional counseling is recommended for all diabetic women of reproductive age. Under ideal circumstances the pregestational diabetic is counseled before conception to plan the optimal time for pregnancy, to establish glycemic control before conception, and to evaluate any evidence of vascular complications of diabetes. The partner of the diabetic woman should be included in the counseling process to assess the couple's level of understanding related to the effects of pregnancy on the diabetic condition and the potential complications of pregnancy as a result of diabetes. The couple also should be informed of the anticipated alterations in management of diabetes during pregnancy.

Preconceptional counseling is particularly important because it has been established that strict metabolic control before conception and in the early weeks of gestation is instrumental in decreasing the risk of congenital anomalies in the fetus (Greene et al, 1989; Rosenn et al, 1990; Steele et al, 1990; Kitzmiller et al, 1991). Research has shown that women with pregestational diabetes who participate in a preconception program have a decreased incidence of spontaneous abortion (Rosenn et al, 1991).

Oral hypoglycemic agents may exert teratogenic effects on the fetus and should be discontinued in the preconceptional period in type II diabetics who had been taking them for glucose control. These women are started on insulin before a planned pregnancy and as soon as an unplanned pregnancy is diagnosed.

Diabetic women with preexisting vascular complications are informed that pregnancy is likely to compound the problems of diabetic nephropathy, retinopathy, and other diabetic sequelae (Sheldon, 1988; Taysi, 1988; Barss, 1989).

Maternal Risks and Complications

Although maternal morbidity and mortality rates have improved significantly since the 1920s, the pregnant diabetic remains at risk for the development of complications during pregnancy. Research has demonstrated repeatedly that the best predictor of pregnancy outcome for the diabetic and her neonate is the degree of maternal glycemic control during pregnancy.

Poor glycemic control around the time of conception and in the early weeks of pregnancy is associated with an increased incidence of *spontaneous abortion* in diabetic women. Those diabetic women with good glycemic control before conception and in the first trimester appear to be no more likely than nondiabetic women to experience spontaneous abortion (Mills et al, 1988; Miodovnik et al, 1988; Greene et al, 1989; Rosenn et al, 1991).

Approximately 25% to 30% of diabetic women develop *pregnancy-induced hypertension* or *preeclampsia* during their pregnancy (see Chapter 28). The highest incidence occurs in women with preexisting vascular changes related to diabetes (Cunningham et al, 1989; Meyer, Palmer, 1990). Mimouni and Tsang (1988) reported an increased risk of preeclampsia associated with poor glycemic control during the second trimester.

Hydramnios (polyhydramnios) occurs about 10 times more often in diabetic pregnancies than in nondiabetic pregnancies. Hydramnios—amniotic fluid in excess of 2000 mL—increases the possibility of compression of maternal abdominal blood vessels (vena cava and aorta), causing supine hypotension. Maternal dyspnea may result from upward pressure on the diaphragm by the distended uterus. Premature rupture of membranes (PROM) and the onset of preterm labor is associated with hydramnios. Overdistention of the uterus because of hydramnios may increase the incidence of postpartum hemorrhage. Hydramnios also is associated with increased incidence of fetal distress, low Apgar scores, fetal anomalies, and admission to the neonatal intensive care nursery (Varma et al, 1988).

The rate of spontaneous *preterm labor* in pregnant diabetics is three times that reported in the general population (preterm labor is discussed in Chapter 35). Mimouni and Tsang (1988) have demonstrated that this is often related to poor glycemic control during the second trimester.

Infections are much more common and serious in diabetic women who are pregnant (infection is discussed in Chapter 29). Disorders of carbohydrate metabolism alter the body's normal resistance to infection. The inflammatory response, leukocyte function, and vaginal pH are all affected. Vaginal infections, particularly monilial vaginitis, are more common in pregnant diabetics. Urinary tract infections (UTIs) also are more prevalent among pregnant diabetics, possibly related to glycosuria. Infection in the diabetic is serious because it causes increased insulin resistance and may result in ketoacidosis. Stamler and associates (1990) found that the rate of postpartum infection among insulin-dependent diabetics was five times greater than among nondiabetics.

Ketoacidosis occurs most often during the second and third trimesters when the "diabetogenic" effect of pregnancy is the greatest. When the maternal metabolism is stressed by illness or infection, the diabetic woman is at increased risk for diabetic ketoacidosis (DKA). DKA also may occur because of failure to take insulin appropriately. The antecedent to DKA is hyperglycemia, caused by insulin deficiency. The result is osmotic diuresis and subsequent loss of fluid and electrolytes, hyperosmolality, volume depletion, and acidemia. Stress hormones are released, which act to impair insulin action and contribute to insulin deficiency. Consequently, decreased tissue uptake of glucose occurs, with increased production of ketones and resultant ketonemia and ketonuria. Prompt treatment is necessary to avoid maternal coma or death. Ketoacidosis occurring at any time during pregnancy can lead to intrauterine fetal death. DKA before the woman gives birth has been associated with an increased incidence of perinatal asphyxia and sudden unexplained fetal death. Perinatal mortality may be as high as 50% to 80% with maternal ketoacidosis (Gabbe, 1990; Meyer, Palmer, 1990) (Table 31-2).

Although strict glycemic control is the goal of management of diabetic pregnancy, the risk of *hypoglycemia* is increased. Early in pregnancy, when hepatic production of glucose is diminished and peripheral utilization of glucose is enhanced, hypoglycemia frequently results. Hypoglycemia during this period of organogenesis may have teratogenic effects on the fetus. Later in pregnancy, as insulin doses are

TABLE 31-2 Differentiation of Hypoglycemia (Insulin Shock) and Hyperglycemia (Diabetic Ketoacidosis)

	Hypoglycemia (Insulin Shock)	Hyperglycemia (Diabetic Ketoacidosis)
Causes	Excess insulin Insufficient food (delayed or missed meals) Excessive exercise or work Indigestion, diarrhea, vomiting	Insufficient insulin Excess or wrong kind of food Infection, injuries, illness Emotional stress Insufficient exercise
Onset	Rapid (regular insulin) Gradual (modified insulin or oral hypoglycemic agents)	Slow (hours to days)
Symptoms	Hunger Sweating Nervousness Weakness Fatigue Blurred or double vision Dizziness Headache Pallor, clammy skin Shallow respirations Normal pulse Laboratory values: Urine: negative for sugar and acetone Blood glucose: $\leq$ 60 mg/dL	Thirst Nausea or vomiting Abdominal pain Constipation Drowsiness Dim vision Increased urination Headache Flushed, dry skin Rapid breathing Weak, rapid pulse Acetone (fruity) breath odor Laboratory values: Urine: positive for sugar and acetone Blood glucose: $\geq$ 250 mg/dL
Intervention	Notify physician Give low-fat milk If orange juice is given for a fast supply of sugar, follow it later with milk If client is unconscious, 50% dextrose IV push, 5%-10% D/W IV drip, or glucagon Obtain blood and urine specimens for laboratory testing	Notify physician Administer insulin in accordance with blood glucose levels Give IV fluids such as normal saline or one-half normal saline; potassium when urinary output is adequate; bicarbonate for pH $<$ 7.0 Monitor laboratory testing of blood and urine

D/W, Dextrose in water; *IV*, intravenous.

adjusted to maintain normoglycemia, hypoglycemia also may result. Maternal symptoms of hypoglycemia, which are associated with increased epinephrine secretion, include sweating, shaking, anxiety, palpitations, and weakness. If untreated, hypoglycemia may induce central nervous system (CNS) impairment, exhibited as confusion, irritability, sleepiness, convulsions, and coma (Meyer, Palmer, 1990; Rotondo, 1990) (Table 31-2).

Fetal/Neonatal Risks and Complications

From the moment of conception the infant of a diabetic mother faces increased risk of complications that may occur during the antenatal, intrapartal, or neonatal periods (see Research Highlight below). These complications may be mild and transient but often are life threatening and may result in the infant's death. Infant morbidity and mortality associated with diabetic pregnancy are significantly reduced with strict control of maternal glucose levels before and during pregnancy.

Despite the improvements in care of diabetic pregnancy, the incidence of *congenital anomalies* among infants of insulin-dependent diabetics is from two to eight times that of the general population. Up to 50% of all perinatal deaths among infants of diabetic mothers are the result of congenital malformations (Miodovnik et al, 1988; Becerra et al, 1990; CDC, 1990). The incidence of congenital malformations is related to the severity and duration of the diabetic disease process. It also has been demonstrated that poor glycemic control before conception and in the early weeks of pregnancy—during the period of organogenesis—increases the risk of congenital anomalies (Greene et al, 1989; Rosenn et al, 1990; Steele et al, 1990; Kitzmiller et al, 1991). Research also has shown, however, that not all malformations can be prevented by strict glycemic control (Mills et al, 1988).

Anomalies commonly seen in infants of diabetic pregnancy primarily affect (1) the CNS, (2) the cardiovascular system, (3) the urinary system, and (4) the gastrointestinal system. Common abnormalities of the CNS include anencephaly, hydrocephaly, mi-

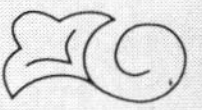
Research Highlight
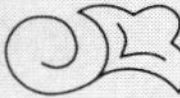

Blood Glucose Control and Birth Weight of Infants

RESEARCH ABSTRACT

The records of 133 pregnant women with type 1 diabetes cared for in one setting were reviewed. Data were not available for four women. Of the pregnancies studied, 16 ended in abortion and 2 that went beyond 28 weeks ended in stillbirths, leaving 116 subjects. The mean duration of the diabetes was 12.4 years. Data examined included blood glucose levels, glycosylated hemoglobin (Hb A_{1c}) levels, birth weight of infants, and newborn blood glucose levels. The researchers found that control of blood glucose improved over trimesters. The mean birth weight of infants was 3.27 kg; 43 (38%) babies had weights above the 90th percentile. There was no relation between birth weight and blood glucose or Hb A_{1c} levels. The Hb A_{1c} was higher in the first trimester in pregnancies that produced infants whose birth weight was above the 90th percentile. There was no correlation between maternal Hb A_{1c} or blood glucose concentration and neonatal hypoglycemia. Seven infants had congenital anomalies; two died of major abnormalities. One died of respiratory distress syndrome. There were maternal complications in 22 cases; one mother had a stroke and died 9 weeks after the birth. Labor was induced in 62% of the pregnancies, and 47 gave birth by cesarean.

IMPLICATIONS FOR PRACTICE

Diabetes in pregnancy creates risk for mothers and their neonates. The general thinking is that good glucose control before pregnancy will decrease problems during pregnancy. Women with diabetes who plan to become pregnant should seek consultation before pregnancy occurs. Nurses working with women with diabetes can provide information, support, and referral to ensure the best possible outcome for these high-risk pregnancies.

RELATED RESEARCH QUESTIONS

1. What behavioral factors are related to women's level of glucose control in pregnancy?
2. Is level of glucose control related to health locus of control?
3. Does adaptation to pregnancy differ between women with diabetes and women who do not have diabetes?
4. Does "ensuring safe passage" differ between women who have diabetes and those who do not?

REFERENCE

Peck RW et al: Birthweight of babies born to mothers with type 1 diabetes: is it related to blood glucose control in the first trimester? *Diabetic Med* 8:258, 1991.

crocephaly, and caudal regression syndrome. Congenital heart disease occurs at a rate five times that of the general population. Common heart anomalies are septal defects, transposition of the great vessels, and coarctation of the aorta. Renal agenesis, hydronephrosis, hypospadias, and undescended testes are frequently occuring urinary anomalies. Gastrointestinal abnormalities that commonly occur are duodenal atresia, imperforate anus, and malrotation of the bowel. Single umbilical artery, ear deformities, and facial clefts also occur in infants of diabetic pregnancy (Matheson, Efantis, 1989; Becerra et al, 1990; Meyer, Palmer, 1990).

Macrosomia, infant weight greater than the 90th percentile, occurs in 25% to 42% of pregnancies complicated by diabetes as compared with 8% to 14% of nondiabetic pregnancies (Jovanovic-Peterson et al, 1991). The fetal pancreas begins to secrete insulin at 10 to 14 weeks' gestation. The fetus responds to maternal hyperglycemia by secreting large amounts of insulin (hyperinsulinism). Insulin acts as a growth hormone, causing the fetus to lay down excess stores of glycogen, protein, and adipose tissue, leading to increased fetal size, or macrosomia. These infants are considered *large for gestational age* (LGA). Macrosomia is associated with dystocia (see Chapter 35), often resulting in operative vaginal birth (episiotomy and forceps), and is responsible for the increased rate of cesarean birth among diabetic mothers. The macrosomic infant may suffer from fractured clavicle, liver or spleen laceration, brachial plexus injury, facial palsy, phrenic nerve injury, or subdural hemorrhage (for further discussion, see Chapter 39). Severe *asphyxia* may occur as a result of a difficult, prolonged birth. Mimouni and associates (1988) found a positive correlation between the incidence of perinatal asphyxia and maternal hyperglycemia immediately before birth. They also recognized that those women who develop a "new" vasculopathy during pregnancy are at increased risk for perinatal asphyxia because of altered placental functioning.

Compromised uteroplacental circulation as a result of maternal vascular changes decreases the amount of oxygen available to the fetus. Consequently the fetus is subjected to a hypoxic environment that may contribute to **intrauterine growth retardation (IUGR),** resulting in a small for gestational age infant. Preterm birth, common to diabetic pregnancy, also may be related to fetal hypoxia (Matheson, Efantis, 1989; Meyer, Palmer, 1990).

Infants of diabetic mothers are at increased risk for respiratory distress related to *hyaline membrane disease*. In past years the incidence of respiratory distress was greater as many infants were born before term in an attempt to limit the chances of early fetal death. With advanced fetal surveillance techniques and improved maternal glycemic control, the incidence of preterm birth, with resultant hyaline membrane disease, has declined.

For infants of diabetic pregnancy the transition to extrauterine life often is beset with metabolic abnormalities. Within the first 30 to 60 minutes after birth, neonatal *hypoglycemia* often occurs. This is due to the effects of fetal hyperinsulinism and rapid utilization of glucose after birth. *Hypocalcemia, hypomagnesemia, hyperbilirubinemia,* and *polycythemia* occur more frequently in infants of diabetic mothers and place the neonate at increased risk (Mimouni et al, 1986). (See Chapter 39 for further discussion of these neonatal disorders.)

■ NURSING CARE OF THE PREGNANT DIABETIC WOMAN

ASSESSMENT

Interview

Whenever a pregnant diabetic woman initiates prenatal care, thorough evaluation of her health status is completed. In addition to routine prenatal assessment (see Chapter 11), the nurse obtains a detailed history regarding the onset and course of the diabetic condition, as well as the management of diabetes and the degree of glycemic control before pregnancy. Effective management of diabetic pregnancy depends on the woman's adherence to a plan of care. For the woman to care for her diabetes on a daily basis, she must have an adequate understanding of her condition and the prescribed regimen. Thus, with the initial prenatal visit, the nurse conducts a thorough assessment of the woman's knowledge regarding diabetes and pregnancy, potential maternal and fetal complications, and the plan of care. With subsequent visits, follow-up assessments are completed. Data from these assessments are used to identify the woman's specific learning needs. Brief screening tools have been developed to assist the nurse in assessing knowledge of diabetes during pregnancy (Spirito et al, 1990). The support person's knowledge of diabetes also is assessed, and teaching needs are identified.

The woman's emotional status is assessed to determine how she is coping with pregnancy superimposed on preexisting diabetes. Although normal pregnancy typically evokes some degree of stress and anxiety, pregnancy designated as "high risk" serves to compound anxiety and stress levels. Fear of maternal and fetal complications is a major concern. Strict adherence to the plan of care necessitates alterations in patterns of daily living and may be an additional source of stress.

The woman's support system is assessed to identify those persons significant to the pregnant woman and their role in her life. It is important to assess the reaction of the family/significant other to the pregnancy and the strict management plan, as well as their involvement in the treatment regimen. Socioeconomic factors also are reviewed. Any area of emotional stress is identified because such stress can precipitate complications (Zigrossi, Riga-Ziegler, 1986; Leff et al, 1991).

Physical Examination

At the initial visit a thorough physical examination is performed to assess the woman's current health status. In addition to the routine prenatal examination (see Chapter 11), specific efforts are made to assess effects of diabetes on the pregnancy and woman. A baseline electrocardiogram (ECG) is obtained to assess cardiovascular status. Evaluation for retinopathy is performed, with follow-up as needed by an ophthalmologist. Blood pressure is monitored carefully throughout pregnancy because of the increased risk for pregnancy-induced hypertension. The woman's weight gain also is monitored at each visit. Fundal height is measured, noting any abnormal increase in size for dates, which may indicate hydramnios or fetal macrosomia. Leopold's maneuvers are performed to check for fetal size and possible hydramnios.

Laboratory Tests

Routine prenatal laboratory examinations are performed (see Chapter 11). Baseline renal function is assessed with a 24-hour urine collection for total protein excretion and creatinine clearance. Routine urinalysis is performed on the initial prenatal visit and throughout the pregnancy to assess for the presence of UTI, which is common to diabetic pregnancy. At each visit, urine also is tested for the presence of glucose and ketones. Because of the risk of coexisting thyroid disease, thyroid function tests are performed (see discussion of thyroid disorders, p. 950).

For the woman with pregestational diabetes, type I or II, laboratory tests are performed to assess glycemic control. Glycemic control is evaluated on the basis of **glycosylated hemoglobin (Hb A_{1c})** levels. With prolonged hyperglycemia, some of the hemoglobin remains saturated with glucose for the life of the red cell. Therefore a test for Hb A_{1c} provides a measurement of glycemic control over time, for example, the previous 4 to 6 weeks. Regular measurements of Hb A_{1c} provide data for altering the treatment plan and lead to improvement of glycemic control (Larsen et al, 1990). Values for the measurement of Hb A_{1c}, the most commonly used index of glysosylated hemoglobin, are as follows (Corbett, 1987):

2.2%-4.8%	Nondiabetic adult
2.5%-5.9%	Good diabetic control
6.0%-8.0%	Fair diabetic control
> 8.0%	Poor diabetic control

Measurements of Hb A_{1c} are made throughout the pregnancy, at least every trimester. The physician also may elect to measure levels of fasting blood sugar and postprandial blood sugar. In addition, glucose tolerance tests, either oral or intravenous, may be performed (p. 936).

Fetal Surveillance

Diagnostic techniques for fetal surveillance often are performed during pregnancy complicated by diabetes to assess fetal growth and well-being (see Chapter 27). Efforts are made to determine the estimated date of delivery (EDD) (or confinement [EDC]). A baseline ultrasound scan is done to assess gestational age of the fetus. Follow-up ultrasound examinations are performed during the pregnancy, as often as every 4 to 6 weeks, to monitor fetal growth and development and to assess for congenital abnormalities.

Because of the greater risk for neural tube defects in diabetic pregnancies (e.g., spina bifida, anencephaly, microcephaly), measurement of maternal serum alpha-fetoprotein (AFP) is performed between 16 and 18 weeks' gestation. Elevated levels of AFP also may indicate renal agenesis, another diabetes-related anomaly.

Fetal surveillance involving fetal kick counts and nonstress testing typically begins between 28 and 30 weeks' gestation. A weekly nonstress test (NST) is performed until weeks 34 to 36, when the frequency increases to twice weekly. For the woman with vascular disease, testing may begin earlier and continue more frequently. Fetal biophysical profile monitoring often is used to evaluate fetal well-being. Fetal cardiac anomalies may be assessed by routine echocardiography. (See Chapter 27 for further discussion of fetal surveillance techniques.)

Biochemical analysis of amniotic fluid is performed to ascertain fetal lung maturity, typically in the third trimester. Amniocentesis earlier in gestation may be used to diagnose congenital anomalies (Landon, Gabbe, 1988; Barss, 1989; Matheson, Efantis, 1989; Rotondo, 1990) (see Chapter 27).

Data from all these tests identify some fetuses in jeopardy in pregnancies complicated by diabetes. The specific value of any one test is more difficult to discern. Evidence supports maternal **normoglycemia/euglycemia**— blood glucose levels within normal limits— as the key to improved perinatal survival.

Determination of Birth Date

In the past, preterm birth often was elected to avoid the risk of intrauterine death. Today most diabetic pregnancies are allowed to progress to term as long as strict glycemic control is maintained and all parameters of antepartum fetal surveillance remain within normal limits. In women with vasculopathy or poor glycemic control, who have not adhered to the program of care or who have had a previous stillbirth, elective birth to prevent late fetal death may be planned at 38 weeks provided that fetal lung maturation has been confirmed by the analysis of amniotic fluid. (For the pregnancy complicated by diabetes, fetal lung maturation is better predicted by the amniotic fluid **phosphatidylglycerol [PG]** than by the lecithin/sphingomyelin [L/S] ratio [Scott et al, 1990]). If the fetal lungs are still immature at 38 weeks, birth should be postponed as long as the results of fetal assessment remain reassuring. Amniocentesis may be repeated to monitor lung maturity. Birth despite fetal lung maturity may be essential when testing suggests fetal compromise or if the pregnant woman develops preeclampsia or pregnancy-induced hypertension, rapidly worsening retinopathy, or renal failure.

NURSING DIAGNOSES

Each woman's experience of pregnancy complicated by diabetes is unique to her and to her family. Nursing diagnoses must be carefully formulated to reflect the actual or potential altered health-related responses that can be influenced, improved, or alleviated by nursing intervention. Examples of possible nursing diagnoses for the pregestational diabetic woman follow.

Nursing diagnoses for the *antepartum period* may include the following:

- Knowledge deficit related to
  - —Diabetic pregnancy, management, and potential effects on pregnant woman and fetus
  - —Insulin effects and its administration
  - —Hypoglycemia and hyperglycemia
  - —Diabetic diet
- High risk for ineffective individual coping related to
  - —Woman's responsibility in managing her diabetes during pregnancy
- Anxiety, fear, dysfunctional grieving, powerlessness, body image disturbance, situational low self-esteem, spiritual distress, altered role performance, altered family processes related to
  - —Stigma of being labeled "diabetic"
  - —Effects of diabetes and its potentail sequelae on the pregnant woman and the fetus
- High risk for noncompliance related to
  - —Lack of understanding of diabetes and pregnancy
  - —Lack of financial resources to purchase blood glucose or urine testing supplies
  - —Insufficient funds or lack of transportation to grocery store to follow diet regimen
- High risk for injury to fetus related to
  - —Uteroplacental insufficiency
- High risk for injury to mother related to
  - —Improper insulin administration
  - —Hypoglycemia and hyperglycemia
- Altered nutrition: less or more than body requirements related to
  - —Diabetes and pregnancy

Nursing diagnoses for the *intrapartum period* may include the following:

- High risk for injury related to
  - —Hypoglycemia or hyperglycemia
  - —Preeclampsia/eclampsia
- Altered tissue perfusion related to
  - —Supine hypotension

Nursing diagnoses for the *postpartum period* may include the following:

- High risk for injury related to
  - —Fluctuating blood glucose levels after giving birth
  - —Complications of involution (hemorrhage, infection)
  - —Postpartum development of preeclampsia/eclampsia
- Ineffective individual coping, altered family processes, altered parenting, related to
  - —Newborn with sequelae to a diabetic pregnancy

PLANNING

Planning care for the diabetic pregnant woman and her family is based on identified nursing diagnoses and the plan for medical management of diabetic pregnancy. The plan is individualized, relating specifically to needs identified by the health care team and to those mutually identified by the woman, family, and the caregivers.

The *goals* (expected outcomes) of management of diabetic pregnancy include the following.

- The woman and her family demonstrate/verbalize understanding of diabetic pregnancy, the plan of care, and the importance of glycemic control.
- The woman complies with the plan of care.
- The woman achieves and maintains glycemic control.
- The woman demonstrates effective coping.
- The woman experiences no complications (i.e., maternal morbidity or mortality).
- The infant experiences no complications (i.e., perinatal morbidity or mortality).
- The family experiences mutuality and support among its members.

IMPLEMENTATION

As a vital member of the health care team ministering to the needs of the pregnant diabetic woman, the nurse assumes a variety of roles. Although normal pregnancy is a maturational crisis for most women, those pregnancies complicated by diabetes may represent a situational crisis as well because of the high-risk nature of the condition. These women require individualized, in-depth nursing care throughout the pregnancy and in the postpartum period.

Assisting the woman with stress reduction is central to the care needed by women whose pregnancies are complicated by diabetes mellitus. Increased stress contributes to elevated blood glucose levels. Stress reduction and relaxation, discussed in Chapter 13, are taught as needed. Space, privacy, and time are provided for the woman and her family to voice their feelings and questions, as well as to problem solve among themselves. In seeking to improve the woman's motivation and understanding of diabetic management, the nurse acknowledges both positive and negative feelings about the pregnancy. Providing care that is sensitive to individual needs and based on a collaborative relationship with the woman and family fosters their physical and emotional well-being (Leff et al, 1991).

Fetal surveillance techniques may identify a congenital malformation incompatible with survival. Parents need supportive care as they consider the option of early pregnancy termination (Van Putte, 1988). The early detection of serious fetal malformations allows for exploration of various options in planning the birth and immediate care of the newborn. The parents also may benefit from the time to prepare for the birth of a child with a congenital abnormality. Diagnostic tests for fetal malformations should be conducted under conditions that are both voluntary and informed (see informed consent, Chapter 4). The risks, accuracy, and limitations of the tests should be discussed. The benefits of diagnosis and the options available when a positive diagnosis is obtained should be discussed in advance.

Engaging the woman as an active participant in the plan of care maintains or enhances her self-esteem and develops her self-confidence that she will be able to care for herself and her baby. Open communication with members of the health care team is encouraged to facilitate client participation in self-care.

The nurse is most often the primary educator for the diabetic woman and her family. Through ongoing assessment, learning needs are identified. Teaching is instituted early in pregnancy and is continued thoughout the period of gestation. Adequate understanding of diabetes and pregnancy, the treatment plan, and potential complications encourage client compliance. It is only through compliance that normoglycemia can be maintained and maternal and fetal well-being are promoted.

Antepartal Nursing Care

Management of diabetic pregnancy is a complex process that requires the woman to be knowledgeable about the treatment regimen and the changes that may occur so that she may respond appropriately. Although the woman is likely to have some knowledge and experience with the various aspects of diabetic care—diet, insulin, exercise, blood glucose monitoring—she will need assistance from the nurse to understand the impact of pregnancy on diabetes to manage her care effectively.

DIET. The woman with pregestational diabetes likely has received nutritional counseling regarding management of the diabetes. Because pregnancy precipitates special nutritional concerns and needs, the woman must be educated and counseled to incorporate these changes into dietary planning. Nutritional counseling usually is provided by a registered dietitian. Pregnancy is an ideal time for the diabetic to "fine-tune" her self-management skills because self-motivation is typically high. It is essential that the woman understand the importance of maintaining normoglycemia during pregnancy.

Dietary management during diabetic pregnancy must be based on blood glucose (not urinary glucose) levels. The diet is individualized to allow for increased fetal and metabolic requirements, with consideration of such factors as prepregnancy weight and dietary habits, overall health, ethnic background and life-style, stage of pregnancy, knowledge of nutrition, and insulin therapy. The dietary goal is to provide weight gain consistent with a normal pregnancy, to prevent ketoacidosis, and to minimize widely fluctuating blood glucose levels.

Energy needs are calculated on the basis of 30 to 40 calories per kilogram of ideal body weight, with the average diet including 2200 calories (first trimester) to 2500 calories (second and third trimesters). Total calories may be distributed among three meals and one evening snack, or more commonly, three meals and at least two snacks. Meals should be eaten on time and never skipped. Snacks must be carefully planned in accordance with insulin therapy to avoid fluctuations in blood glucose levels. A large bedtime snack of at least 25 g carbohydrate with some protein is recommended. To prevent the blood glucose level from dropping too low during the night, some women find that they need an additional snack of milk and crackers or fruit.

The ratio of carbohydrate, protein, and fat is important to meet metabolic needs of the woman and the fetus. Approximately 50% of the total calories should be carbohydrate, with a minimum of 250 g/day. Simple carbohydrates are avoided; complex carbohydrates that are high in fiber content are recommended because the starch and protein in such foods help to regulate the blood glucose level as a result of more sustained glucose release. Protein intake should constitute around 20% of the total calories. Less than 30% of the daily caloric intake should come from fat, or no more than 80 g/day. Highly saturated fats are to be avoided.

In addition to sufficient calories, vitamins and minerals are necessary during pregnancy. These usually are provided as daily supplements to the diet (Landon, Gabbe, 1988; Worthington-Roberts, Williams, 1989) (see box above).

TEACHING Dietary Management of Diabetic Pregnancy

- Follow the prescribed diet plan.
- Eat a well-balanced diet, including daily food requirements for a normal pregnancy.
- Divide daily food intake among three meals and two to four snacks, depending on individual needs.
- Eat a substantial bedtime snack to prevent a severe drop in blood glucose level during the night.
- Limit the intake of fats if weight gain occurs too rapidly.
- Take daily vitamins and iron as prescribed by the physician.
- Avoid foods high in refined sugar.
- Eat consistently each day; never skip meals or snacks.
- Reduce the intake of saturated fat and cholesterol.
- Eat foods high in dietary fiber.
- Avoid alcohol and caffeine.
- Exercise regularly.

MONITORING OF BLOOD GLUCOSE LEVELS. Blood glucose testing at home is now the commonly accepted method for monitoring blood glucose levels and is the most important tool available to the woman to assess her degree of glycemic control. In addition, this monitoring provides motivation to continue the prescribed treatment plan, and the data obtained facilitate interaction with the health care team in maintaining glycemic control and minimizing fetal risk. The advent of home glucose monitoring has been credited with increasing the woman's feeling of self-control and with decreasing or eliminating hospitalizations and consequent separation from family. It presents the most accurate method to document the degree of glycemic control in an out-of-hospital setting. It enables the woman to adjust her insulin dosage on a 24-hour basis. Self-monitoring of blood glucose allows for early detection of hypoglycemia. If used before conception and early in pregnancy, home glucose monitoring may safeguard the fetus during organogenesis.

Pregestational diabetics often are familiar with self-monitoring of blood glucose levels inasmuch as this technique is typically included in the management plan for type I and some type II diabetics. However, a thorough assessment of the woman's knowledge and skill related to blood glucose testing is essential to ensure accurate monitoring of glucose levels during pregnancy. The nurse observes the pregnant woman performing the task of blood glucose monitoring to determine accuracy and comfort with the system. The family also is included in the assessment and in subsequent instruction related to blood glucose monitoring. The woman's attitudes toward self-monitoring are examined. Pregnancy demands more frequent and judicious monitoring than many women have employed previously. Willingness to comply with the monitoring schedule is essential to the management plan and affects the outcome of diabetic pregnancy.

For home blood glucose monitoring to be used effectively, the woman and her family should be knowledgeable regarding proper use of the monitoring system, when to measure blood glucose levels, and the target blood glucose ranges (see box, p. 936).

TEACHING Self-Testing of Blood Glucose Level

- Gather supplies, check expiration date, and read instructions on testing materials.
- Wash hands in warm water (warmth increases circulation).
- Select site on side of any finger. (Cleaning the site with alcohol is not necessary.)
- Pierce site with lancet.
- Drop hand down to your side; using other hand, gently squeeze finger from hand to fingertip.
- Allow blood to drop onto reagent area of strip; be sure to cover entire reagent area.
- Follow instructions for timing and wiping of excess blood.
- At proper time, read visually or on reflectance meter.
- Record your results.
- Repeat daily according to the schedule recommended by your physician and as needed for signs of hypoglycemia or hyperglycemia.
- Blood glucose levels should be as follows:

Time	Levels (mg/dL)
Before breakfast	60-90
Before lunch, dinner, bedtime	60-105
Two hours after meals	60-120
2 AM to 6 AM	60-120

Home glucose monitoring involves the use of a glucose reflectance meter, which is battery powered and determines the blood glucose level by the amount of light reflected from a reacted test strip. Using an automatic pricking device, the woman obtains a blood sample from the side of a finger (all the fingers are used in rotation). The drop of blood is placed on a glucose reagent strip. After a predetermined number of seconds, the blood is wiped or blotted from the strip. The strip is inserted into the machine and the color graph is read electronically and the results are displayed. Blood glucose levels are recorded with each measurement. (Fig. 31-2). Newer models of glucose reflectance meters incorporate memory to store a large number of readings; however, the woman is still encouraged to maintain written records of glucose levels. It is important that the monitoring equipment be checked for accuracy at intervals by comparing the woman's results on her machine with a laboratory test done at the same time. The machine also should be calibrated regularly to ensure accuracy.

Blood glucose levels are routinely measured four times a day: before breakfast, lunch, dinner, and at bedtime. Postprandial measurements, 2 hours after meals, also may be obtained. Some physicians recommend that a complete profile be obtained at least 2 days per week. This consists of eight tests per day: before meals, 2 hours after meals, at bedtime, and at 3:00 AM. Women also are encouraged to check glucose levels at any sign of hypoglycemia or hyperglycemia. Insulin dosage, diet, and other aspects of the daily management plan are adjusted in response to blood glucose levels; thus accuracy in testing and reporting is essential. When there is any readjustment in insulin dosage or diet, more frequent measurement of blood glucose is warranted; the complete profile of eight tests per day often is employed. During the second and third trimester, when insulin needs are increasing, more frequent testing is likely to be needed.

Target levels of blood glucose during pregnancy are somewhat lower than nonpregnancy values. Education of the woman and her family includes the importance of achieving and maintaining lower target values than they were used to in the nonpregnant state. The following target ranges for blood glucose levels during pregnancy are compared with nonpregnant levels (Campbell, 1988; Landon, Gabbe, 1988; Matheson, Efantis, 1989).

Time	Target Glucose Levels during Pregnancy (mg/dL)	Target Glucose Levels for Young, Healthy, Nonpregnant Type I Diabetic (mg/dL)
Before breakfast	60-90	
Before lunch, dinner, bedtime	60-105	70-130
Two hours after meals	60-120	80-150
2 AM to 6 AM	60-120	70-120

INSULIN THERAPY. Adequate insulinization is the primary factor in the maintenance of normoglycemia during pregnancy, thus ensuring proper glucose metabolism of the mother and the fetus. Insulin requirements during pregnancy change dramatically as the pregnancy progresses, necessitating frequent adjustments in insulin dosage. In the first trimester there is little or no change in prepregnancy insulin requirements; however, insulin dosage may need to be decreased because of hypoglycemia. During the second and third trimester, as a result of insulin resistance, dosage must be increased to maintain target glucose levels.

For the type I pregestational diabetic, who typically has been accustomed to one injection of intermediate-acting insulin per day, multiple daily injec-

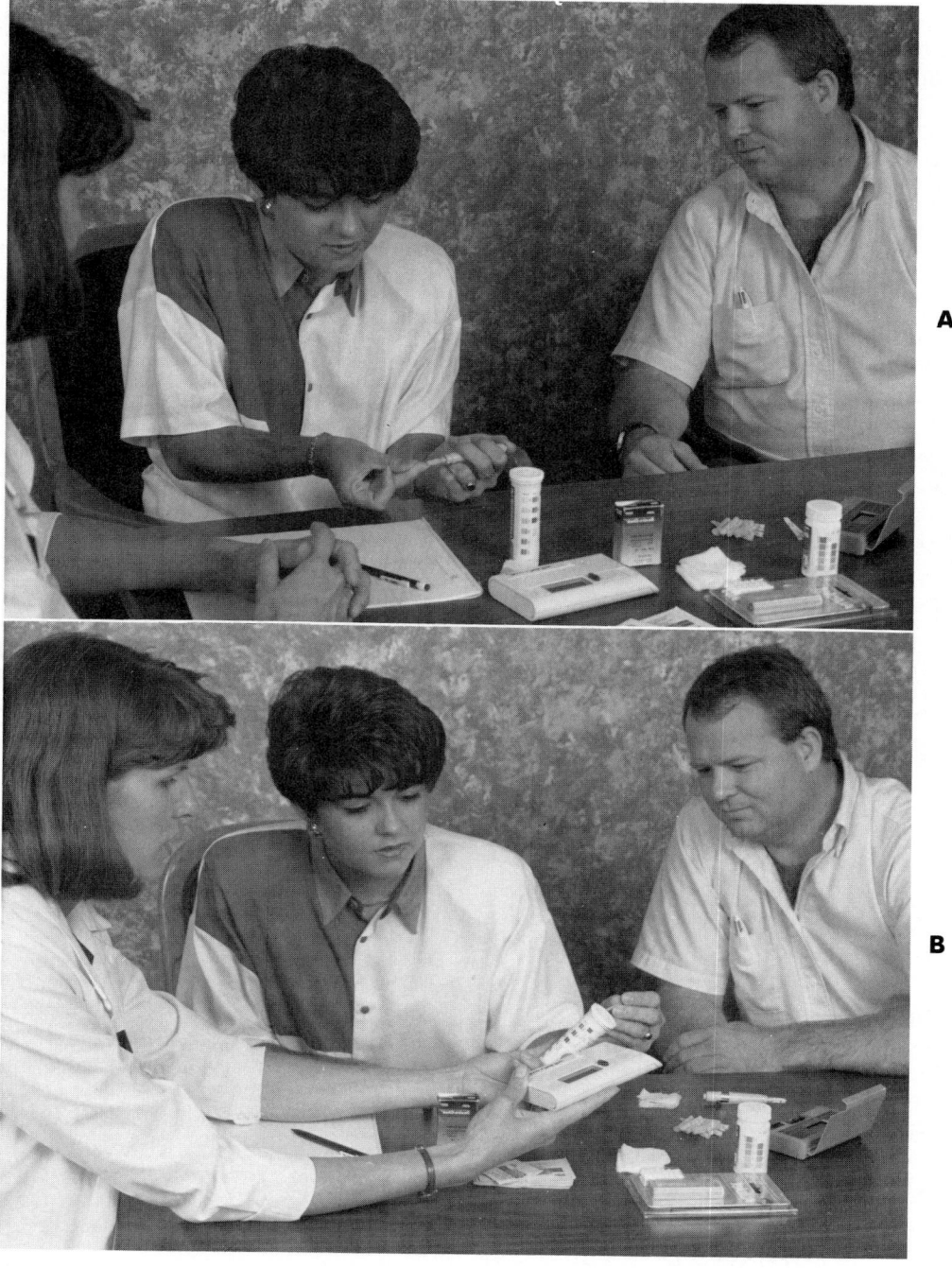

Fig. 31-2 A, Pregnant woman demonstrates how to collect a drop of blood for glucose monitoring. B, Nurse assists the woman and her husband in interpreting the glucose values displayed by the monitor.
Courtesy Jonas McKoy, University of North Carolina at Chapel Hill School of Nursing.

tions of mixed insulin are a new experience. The type II diabetic, previously treated with oral hypoglycemics, is faced with the task of learning to administer self-injections of insulin. The nurse is instrumental in education and support of pregestational diabetics with regard to insulin administration and adjustment of insulin dosage to maintain normoglycemia (see box below).

Most insulin-dependent diabetics require multiple daily injections during pregnancy. Human insulin is recommended; a combination of intermediate-acting and regular (short-acting) insulin before breakfast and at dinner time is a common regimen. Typically, the morning dose combines isophane (NPH Insulin) and regular insulin in a 2:1 ratio. Equal doses of NPH Insulin and regular insulin are administered in the evening. When fasting or postprandial glucose levels are elevated, insulin doses usually are increased by 20% and glucose levels are monitored closely for several days before further adjustments are made (Gabbe, 1990). Adjusting insulin dosage on the basis of blood glucose levels is a skill that may be unfamiliar to some pregestational diabetics. The nurse assesses the woman's understanding of this process and provides education as needed to ensure compliance.

Although subcutaneous insulin injections are most commonly used, continuous insulin infusion systems also may be employed during pregnancy. The insulin "pump" infuses insulin at a set basal rate, with a bolus dose to cover meals. The infusion tubing from this portable, battery-operated system can be left in place for several weeks without local complications (Fig. 31-3). Insulin pumps usually are reserved for women whose diabetes cannot be controlled by multiple insulin injections and who are highly motivated inasmuch as meticulous blood glucose monitoring is required. Studies have shown no significant difference in metabolic control among those women using insulin pumps and those taking multiple daily insulin injections (Burkart et al, 1988; Tomky, 1989).

EXERCISE. An essential part of the management plan for pregestational diabetes is regular exercise because exercise enhances the utilization of glucose and decreases insulin need while promoting circulation and improved muscle tone. Exercise plans are individualized and monitored closely by the health care providers. For those women with vasculopathy, only mild exercise is recommended because exercise causes a redistribution of cardiac output, which increases the potential for ischemic injury to already compromised organs. Also, women with vasculopathy typically depend completely on exogenous insulin and are at greater risk for wide fluctuations in blood glucose levels and ketoacidosis, which can be worsened by exercise (Winn, Reece, 1989).

Exercise need not be vigorous to be beneficial; 30 minutes of walking each day is satisfactory for most

TEACHING Self-Administration of Insulin

Procedure for Mixing Isophane (NPH Insulin [Intermediate-Acting] and Regular [Short-Acting] Insulin):

- Wash hands thoroughly and gather supplies. Be sure the insulin syringe corresponds to the concentration of insulin you are using.
- Check insulin bottle to be certain it is the appropriate type, and check the expiration date.
- Gently rotate (do not shake) the insulin vial to mix the insulin.
- Wipe off rubber stopper of each vial with alcohol.
- Draw back into syringe the amount of air equal to total dose.
- Inject air equal to NPH (intermediate-acting) dose into NPH vial. Remove syringe from vial.
- Inject air equal to regular insulin dose into regular insulin vial.
- Invert regular insulin bottle, and withdraw regular insulin dose.
- Without adding more air to NPH vial, carefully withdraw NPH dose.

Procedure for Self-Injection of Insulin

- Select proper injection site (remember to rotate sites).
- Cleanse injection site with alcohol.
- Pinch the skin up to form a subcutaneous pocket, and holding the syringe like a pencil, puncture the skin at a 45- to 90-degree angle. If there is a great deal of fatty tissue at the site, spread the skin taut and inject the syringe at a 90-degree angle.
- Slowly inject the insulin.
- As you withdraw the needle, cover the injection site with sterile gauze and apply gentle pressure to prevent bleeding.
- Record insulin dosage and time of injection.

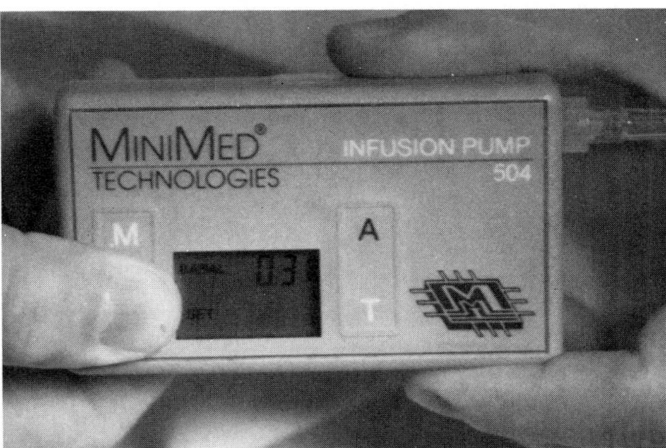

Fig. 31-3 Pregnant woman with diabetes sets the basal rate on her insulin pump.
Courtesy Jonas McKoy, University of North Carolina at Chapel Hill School of Nursing.

TEACHING **Exercise**

- Exercise plans are individualized and should be monitored by the health care provider.
- Select exercises that are enjoyable to foster regularity.
- Exercise does not have to be vigorous to be effective.
- Avoid exercising in a warm environment.
- The best time to exercise is after meals, when blood glucose is beginning to rise.
- Monitor blood glucose levels before, during, and after exercise to determine variations in glucose levels.
- Do not administer insulin into an extremity that is to be immediately involved in exercise.

pregnant women. The best time for exercise is after meals when the blood sugar is rising. If the woman exercises at a time when the insulin is peaking or engages in prolonged exercise without carbohydrate intake, hypoglycemia may result. Hyperglycemia may occur during exercise at a time when insulin action is waning. To monitor the effect of insulin on blood glucose levels, the woman can measure blood glucose before, during, and after exercise. The nurse discusses the importance of exercise with the woman and provides necessary teaching (see box above).

GENERAL CARE. Because the diabetic woman is at risk for developing infections, eye problems, and neurologic changes, general skin care and foot care are discussed. A daily bath that includes good perineal care and foot care is important. For dry skin, lotions, creams, or oils can be applied. Tight clothing should be avoided. Shoes should fit properly and are best worn with socks or stockings. Feet should be inspected regularly; toenails are cut straight across, and professional help should be sought for any foot problems. Extremes of temperature are to be avoided.

Prenatal care for the pregnant diabetic typically involves more frequent visits than for the nondiabetic pregnant woman. It is essential that the woman understand the importance of early prenatal care and the need to keep all scheduled appointments. If there is any question about glycemic control, visits are scheduled a minimum of every 2 weeks for the first 32 weeks and then weekly until the birth. At each prenatal visit the woman is given an appointment time for the next visit. Important telephone numbers are written down and given to the woman; she is encouraged to call at any time she has a question or concern.

A urine sample is checked at each visit throughout pregnancy for blood, glucose, ketones, protein, bilirubin, and pH determinations. Microscopic examination may reveal asymptomatic UTIs, which occur frequently and can cause fetal death. Women experiencing poor glycemic control are carefully assessed for infection, which may significantly alter insulin requirements.

Fetal well-being is monitored closely. The stress of frequent monitoring can be minimized somewhat through careful explanations and support and by providing a private time and space to discuss concerns.

Despite advances in home glucose monitoring, some women may require hospitalization for regulation of insulin dosage and stabilization of glucose levels. Type II diabetics who have previously taken oral hypoglycemics are changed to insulin injections to maintain normoglycemia. Hospitalization offers a controlled situation to initiate and regulate insulin therapy, while providing opportunity for intensive education in self-administration of insulin and regulation of blood glucose levels.

COMPLICATIONS. The pregnant woman is alerted to potential complications during pregnancy and is given written instructions concerning the need for prompt reporting of such problems as nausea, vomiting, and infections. It is essential that she and her family be knowledgeable about hypoglycemia and hyperglycemia, their causes, and symptoms, as well as prevention and treatment measures (Table 31-2).

To prevent complications the woman should not engage in any long-term travel without contacting the physician. Whenever she is away from home, the woman should carry along insulin, syringes, and fast-acting sugar. She should wear an identification bracelet at all times. It also is helpful to carry along an exchange list for dietary needs.

Labor and Birth (Intrapartal Care)

During the intrapartum period the pregestational diabetic must be monitored closely to prevent complications related to dehydration, hypoglycemia, and hyperglycemia. Most women use large amounts of energy (calories) to accomplish the work and manage the stress of labor and birth; however, this calorie expenditure varies with the individual. Blood glucose levels and hydration must be carefully controlled during labor. To accomplish this, an intravenous (IV) line is inserted for infusion of a maintenance fluid, usually lactated Ringer's (LR) or 5% dextrose/lactated Ringer's (D_5LR) solution. Often, D_5LR is the maintenance fluid with a piggyback of LR into the IV line to provide for additional fluid volume (e.g., when epidural anesthesia is used, a preload of IV fluid may be used to decrease chances of hypotension). Determinations of blood glucose levels are made every 1 to 2 hours while dextrose and insulin are titrated by calibrated pump to maintain blood glucose levels between 60 and 100 mg/dL. It is essential that these target glucose levels be maintained because hyperglycemia during labor can precipitate metabolic problems in the neonate, particularly hypoglycemia (Matheson, Efantis, 1989). Maternal hyperglycemia during labor also can lead to perinatal asphyxia (Mimouni et al, 1988).

For the pregestational diabetic, it is important to reduce considerably or to delete the dose of long-acting insulin given on the day of birth. Regular (short-acting) insulin is used because insulin requirements drop markedly after birth (Cunningham et al, 1989).

NOTE: For the laboring diabetic, a prescribed amount of insulin usually is mixed with 100 to 250 mL of 10% dextrose in water or normal saline for IV administration. Insulin, a protein, is attracted chemically to the plastic in the IV tubing. It leaves the solution and adheres to the lining of the tubing. Adherence to the tubing can be prevented by flushing the line first with 100 mL of normal saline and 10 U insulin, which will completely coat the lining. Then the prescribed solution of insulin is begun and will remain stable. (A protein [albumin] may be added to the solution instead; however, it is more expensive.)

During labor, continuous fetal heart monitoring is necessary. The mother should assume a side-lying position during bed rest in labor to prevent supine hypotension because of a large fetus or hydramnios. Labor is allowed to progress provided normal rates of cervical dilatation and fetal descent are maintained. Failure to progress may indicate a macrosomic infant and cephalopelvic disproportion, which necessitates cesarean birth. The woman is observed and treated during labor for diabetic complications such as hyperglycemia, ketosis, ketoacidosis, and glycosuria. A pediatrician should be present at birth to initiate proper neonatal care.

Postpartal Care

In the immediate postpartal period, insulin requirements decrease substantially because the major source of insulin resistance, the placenta, has been removed. Type I diabetics may require only one half to two thirds of the prenatal insulin dose on the first postpartum day, provided they are eating a full diet. *It takes several days after birth to reestablish carbohydrate homeostasis* (Fig. 31-1). Blood glucose levels are monitored in the postpartum period, and insulin dosage is adjusted accordingly. The insulin-dependent woman must realize the importance of eating on time even if the baby needs feeding or other pressing demands exist. Type II diabetics often require no insulin in the postpartum period and are able to maintain normoglycemia through diet alone or with oral hypoglycemics.

Possible postpartum complications include preeclampsia and eclampsia, hemorrhage, and infection. Preeclampsia occurs in approximately one fourth of all diabetic mothers. Hemorrhage is a possibility if the mother's uterus was overdistended (hydramnios, macrosomic fetus) or overstimulated (oxytocin induction). Postpartum infections such as monilial vaginitis are more likely to occur in a woman with diabetes.

Diabetic mothers are encouraged to breast-feed. In addition to the advantages of maternal satisfaction and pleasure, breast-feeding has an antidiabetogenic effect. Insulin requirements of the lactating diabetic mother are decreased because of the carbohydrate utilized in human milk production. Insulin dosage, which is decreased during lactation, must be recalculated at the time of weaning (Fig. 31-1, *F* to *G*).

The new mother needs information related to family planning and contraception. Although family planning is important for all women, it is essential for the diabetic woman to safeguard her own health and to promote optimal outcome in any future pregnancies. The woman and her partner should be informed that the risks associated with pregnancy increase with the duration and severity of the diabetic condition and that pregnancy may contribute to vascular changes associated with diabetes. Preconceptional counseling is recommended because planned pregnancy and good glycemic control are instrumental in preventing congenital anomalies and spontaneous abortion in future pregnancies.

The risks and benefits of contraceptive methods are discussed. Use of oral contraceptives by diabetic women has been controversial because of the risk of thromboembolic and vascular complications, as well as the effect on carbohydrate metabolism. Progestin-only pills and triphasic oral contraceptives are considered safer for diabetics than are combined oral contraceptives (Landon, Gabbe, 1988).

Barrier methods such as the diaphragm or condom and spermicide pose the least risk to the diabetic woman. The problem with these methods, however, is inconsistency of use, which often leads to unplanned pregnancy. Intrauterine devices are associated with an increased risk of infection, especially during the first 20 days after insertion (Farley, 1992). In the presence of significant vasculopathy, surgical sterilization may be recommended.

EVALUATION

Successful management of diabetic pregnancy involves a complex treatment plan and requires the woman's participation and commitment, as well as the direction and support of the health care team. Effectiveness of the plan of care is best measured by assessing the degree to which goals have been achieved:

- The woman and her family demonstrate/verbalize understanding of diabetic pregnancy, the plan of care, and the importance of glycemic control.
- She complies with the plan of care.
- She achieves and maintains glycemic control.
- She demonstrates effective coping.
- Neither she nor the infant experience complications.
- The family experiences mutuality and support among its members.

(See case study, p. 942, and nursing plan of care, p. 943.)

GESTATIONAL DIABETES MELLITUS

Gestational diabetes mellitus (GDM) is defined as "carbohydrate intolerance of variable severity with onset or first recognition during the present pregnancy" (ADA, 1990). Women with no prior personal history of glucose intolerance who demonstrate hyperglycemia during pregnancy are considered gestational diabetics. This definition also is inclusive of a small number of women with previously unrecognized type I or type II diabetes that is diagnosed during pregnancy. The definition of GDM is applicable to any glucose intolerance diagnosed during pregnancy whether or not insulin is used in treatment and whether or not the condition persists after the pregnancy. GDM generally is characterized by mild glucose intolerance that manifests as postprandial hyperglycemia. It most often is encountered in late pregnancy. In approximately 97% of cases, GDM disappears at the end of the pregnancy (Jovanovic-Peterson, Peterson, 1988); however, there is a high probability that it will recur in subsequent pregnancies (Philipson, Super, 1989). GDM has long-term implications in that overt diabetes will develop within 20 years after the pregnancy in approximately 60% of women with GDM if they are overweight and remain overweight. Reduction of weight to a normal range, along with good nutrition and exercise, can decrease the risk by 25% (Jovanovic-Peterson, Peterson, 1988).

GDM occurs in 2% to 6% of all pregnant women, resulting in 60,000 to 100,000 cases each year (Kaufman, 1989; Siddiq, 1989; Radak, 1991). Estimates of ethnic prevalence are variable, although Hispanics and African Americans appear to be at increased risk. Other factors known to place women at increased risk for GDM are (1) maternal age over 30, (2) obesity, or prepregnancy weight more than 20% over ideal weight, (3) family history of type II (non–insulin-dependent) diabetes, and (4) obstetric history of birth of infant larger than 9 pounds, hydramnios, or unexplained stillbirth, miscarriage, or infant with congenital anomalies (Davidson, 1989; Jovanovic-Peterson, Peterson, 1990; Radak, 1991).

The diagnosis of GDM usually is made during the second half of pregnancy. As fetal nutrient demands rise during the late second and third trimester, maternal nutrient ingestion induces greater and more sustained levels of blood glucose. At the same time, maternal insulin resistance also is increasing because of the insulin antagonistic effects of the placental hormones and insulinase, and cortisol. Consequently, maternal insulin demands rise as much as threefold. Most pregnant women are capable of increasing insulin production to compensate for the insulin resistance and to maintain normoglycemia. When the pancreas is unable to produce sufficient insulin, or if the insulin is not utilized effectively, GDM can result (Dickinson, Palmer, 1990).

Some women with GDM exhibit the classic symptoms of diabetes: excessive thirst, hunger, urination, and/or weakness. However, because approximately 70% of GDM occurs in an asymptomatic form, universal screening of all pregnant women is essential to diagnosis and treatment. The ADA recommends that all women who have not been identified as having

CASE STUDY

Pregestational Diabetes

Linda James is a 27-year-old insulin-dependent diabetic at 4 weeks' gestation. This is her first prenatal visit.

ASSESSMENT

Linda is in her second pregnancy. Her first pregnancy terminated in spontaneous abortion at 6 weeks. Because she is afraid this pregnancy will end in a "miscarriage," she is anxious to begin prenatal care and expresses the desire to learn everything she can about diabetes and pregnancy so that she can take care of herself and the unborn baby.

Diagnosed with IDDM at age 17, Linda has been on a daily injection regimen of intermediate-acting insulin. Through the years she has maintained good glycemic control most of the time, although she was hospitalized on two occasions for hyperglycemia while she was in college. She reports that lately her blood glucose levels have bordered on hypoglycemia. Linda monitors her blood glucose levels with a reflectance meter and is able to demonstrate correct technique in doing so. Her dietary regimen before pregnancy was a 2000 cal ADA diet. Because of nausea, she has found it difficult to maintain this intake since she became pregnant.

NURSING DIAGNOSIS

Because Linda has stated that she is anxious to learn all she can about diabetes and pregnancy, the nurse identifies the *nursing diagnosis:* knowledge deficit related to diabetes, its management, and potential effects on the pregnancy woman and fetus.

PLANNING

A plan of care is developed with Linda's input. The mutually agreed upon *goal* for Linda is that she will understand about diabetes during pregnancy, its management, and potential effects on herself and the fetus. The nurse sets the following *expected outcomes:* Linda will verbalize a basic understanding of diabetic pregnancy, the management plan, and potential complications. She will comply with the plan of care and she and the fetus will experience minimal or no complications.

IMPLEMENTATION

Nursing actions are derived from medical management, physician's orders, and nursing diagnosis. Specific interventions consist of assessment of Linda's knowledge regarding diabetic pregnancy and her understanding of the treatment plan. The nurse will then develop a teaching plan that includes review of pathophysiology of diabetes, explanation of the effect of diabetes on pregnancy and the effect of pregnancy on diabetes, and a description of the potential maternal and fetal complications. The nurse will discuss management of diabetic pregnancy, stressing the importance of strict adherence to the plan and the need for regular prenatal care. Linda's questions will be answered, and misconceptions will be clarified. The nurse may assist Linda in formulating questions for the physician. On completion of teaching, the nurse will assess Linda's level of understanding by asking her to repeat (paraphrase) the information. Reinforcement of teaching will continue with future prenatal visits.

EVALUATION

The expected outcomes were used to evaluate the effectiveness of the interventions. In assessing Linda's understanding of diabetic pregnancy, the nurse found that Linda was indeed very knowledgeable about IDDM but was not familiar with the effect of diabetes on pregnancy and vice versa. Therefore the nurse focused the teaching plan on addressing those issues. The teaching began with the first prenatal visit and continued on subsequent visits. Linda verbalized an adequate understanding of diabetic pregnancy and was compliant with the plan of care throughout the duration of her pregnancy.

CARE PLAN Pregestational Diabetes

GOALS	INTERVENTIONS	RATIONALE	EVALUATION
Nursing diagnosis: Knowledge deficit related to diabetes, its management, and potential effects on the pregnant woman and fetus			
Linda will verbalize understanding of diabetes, its management, and potential complications during pregnancy. Linda will comply with the plan of care. Linda and her fetus will not experience complications, or if complications occur, they will be minimized.	Assess Linda's knowledge of diabetic pregnancy and her understanding of the treatment plan. Review the pathophysiology of diabetes. Explain the effect of diabetes on pregnancy and the effect of pregnancy on the diabetes. Describe the potential sequelae of diabetes for mother and fetus. Discuss management of diabetic pregnancy. Stress the importance of strict adherence to the plan of care and the need for regular prenatal care. Encourage Linda to ask questions. Clarify misconceptions. Assist Linda in formulating questions for the physician. Ask Linda to repeat (paraphrase) information to validate her understanding.	Adequate understanding of diabetic pregnancy, its management, and potential sequelae will promote compliance with the plan of care. Understanding also helps to decrease fear and anxiety.	Linda verbalizes understanding of diabetic pregnancy, its management, and potential sequelae for herself and the fetus. Linda complies with the plan of care.
Nursing diagnosis: Fear/anxiety related to threat to maternal and fetal well-being			
Linda will identify sources of fear and anxiety. Linda will express concerns and feelings regarding diabetes and its potential sequelae for herself and the fetus. Linda will verbalize that she feels less fearful and anxious.	Promote an open, trusting relationship with Linda. Provide private area for conversation. Assess Linda's feelings regarding diabetic pregnancy. Convey acceptance of her fears and anxieties. Encourage Linda to differentiate between real and imagined threat to personal and fetal well-being. Review potential dangers to Linda and her fetus as a result of diabetes. Encourage Linda to share her concerns with the physician.	Verbalizing fears and concerns will help Linda to deal with them. It is important that fear and anxiety be reduced because they interfere with the woman's ability to cope and are a source of stress that can contribute to diabetic complications such as hyperglycemia.	Linda identifies that she is afraid this pregnancy will end in a miscarriage or that the baby may be malformed or mentally retarded. The nurse acknowledges her fears and provides her with factual information related to the chances of these problems actually occurring. Linda states she is less fearful after discussing these concerns with the nurse. Linda compiles a list of questions for the physician related to fetal risk.

Continued.

CARE PLAN **Pregestational Diabetes—cont'd**

GOALS	INTERVENTIONS	RATIONALE	EVALUATION
Nursing diagnosis: High risk for injury related to improper insulin dosage/administration			
Linda will verbalize understanding of insulin needs and insulin therapy during pregnancy, including purpose, side effects, schedule for taking, and importance of taking as prescribed. Linda will demonstrate proper technique for withdrawal and mixing of insulin. Linda will describe proper method of insulin storage. Linda will demonstrate correct technique for administering insulin. Linda and the fetus will suffer no injury from improper insulin administration.	Assess Linda's understanding of insulin needs during pregnancy and insulin dosage/administration. Explain effect of insulin on the body and purpose of insulin therapy, as well as possible side effects. Describe changing insulin needs during pregnancy. Review peak action of insulin and signs of hypoglycemia. Stress importance of following prescribed regimen. Discuss importance of administration of correct dosage with appropriate syringe. Discuss storage of insulin. Explain technique for mixing insulin in the same syringe. Demonstrate correct withdrawal and administration of insulin. Discuss site rotation, and identify sites that can be used. Explain how to adjust insulin dosage based on self-monitoring of blood glucose. Monitor Linda's self-administration of insulin until techniques are correctly demonstrated and understood.	Adequate understanding of insulin, its purpose, and effects on the body are essential to proper management of diabetes. Administration of correct dosage of insulin by proper technique will minimize complications such as hypoglycemia.	Linda verbalizes a basic understanding of insulin therapy but is not familiar with changing insulin needs during pregnancy. Although she has administered insulin to herself since her diabetes was diagnosed, she is not experienced with mixing insulins in the same syringe. She uses proper technique for withdrawal and administration of insulin but admits that she is not consistent about site rotation. After teaching is completed, Linda verbalizes understanding of the information and states she feels comfortable with insulin therapy during pregnancy.

impaired glucose tolerance before week 24 be screened for GDM between weeks 24 and 28 of pregnancy (ADA, 1990). A **glucose tolerance test (GTT)** is accomplished by administering a 50-g oral glucose load, regardless of previous meal or time of day, followed by a plasma glucose determination 1 hour later. A glucose level of 140 mg/dL or greater is considered a positive result and should be followed by a 3-hour oral GTT. The 3-hour GTT is administered after an overnight fast and at least 3 days of unrestricted diet (at least 150 g carbohydrate) and physical activity. A 100-g glucose load is given, followed by measurements of plasma glucose at 1, 2, and 3 hours. The test result is deemed positive if two or more of the following values are met or exceeded (ADA, 1985, 1990):

Fasting	105 mg/dL
1 hr	190 mg/dL
2 hr	165 mg/dL
3 hr	145 mg/dL

If only one of the values is elevated, the 3-hour (100 g) glucose tolerance test is repeated at 32 weeks. If significant risk factors are present, a repeat GTT is recommended at 32 to 34 weeks for those women

CARE PLAN Pregestational Diabetes—cont'd

GOALS	INTERVENTIONS	RATIONALE	EVALUATION
Nursing diagnosis: High risk for injury related to hyperglycemia and hypoglycemia			
Linda will verbalize understanding of hyperglycemia and hypoglycemia, including causes, symptoms, treatment, and prevention. Linda will identify the potential consequences for herself and the fetus related to hyperglycemia and hypoglycemia. Linda and her husband will promptly recognize signs and symptoms of hyperglycemia and hypoglycemia and will take appropriate measures. Episodes of hyperglycemia and hypoglycemia will be prevented or minimized.	Assess Linda's knowledge of hyperglycemia and hypoglycemia. Assess her husband's knowledge also, and include him in the teaching session. Explain causes, symptoms, treatment, and prevention of hyperglycemia and hypoglycemia (Table 31-2). Stress importance of calling the physician when signs and symptoms occur. Stress importance of carrying insulin and syringes, as well as a fast-acting sugar, when away from home. Give Medic-Alert information, and encourage Linda to wear bracelet or necklace. Discuss relationship of exercise and diet and the effect of stress.	Hyperglycemia and hypoglycemia compromise maternal and fetal well-being and must be prevented.	Linda and her husband have a basic understanding of hyperglycemia and hypoglycemia but request that the nurse review related information to ensure their understanding. At the conclusion of the teaching session, Linda and her husband state they understand the information. Linda already carries insulin and candy with her when away from home. She plans to obtain a Medic-Alert bracelet.

whose test result for the 50-g glucose test was positive but who exhibited a normal GTT (Hollander, 1988; Landon, Gabbe, 1988) (Fig. 31-4).

Maternal and Fetal Risks

As with pregestational diabetes, the key to positive pregnancy outcome for both mother and fetus is strict metabolic control instituted as early as possible during gestation. Women with GDM are at increased risk for preeclampsia and cesarean birth (Heckbert et al, 1988; Jacobson, Cousins, 1989).

The woman who maintains strict glycemic control during pregnancy, with normal fasting and postprandial glucose levels, encounters approximately the same risk of perinatal mortality as the nondiabetic woman. Women with fasting (≥105 mg/dL) and postprandial (≥120 mg/dL) hyperglycemia face the greatest risk for intrauterine fetal death and neonatal mortality. Perinatal morbidity and mortality also are higher among gestational diabetics with a history of previous stillbirth, those who develop preeclampsia, and those who were diagnosed with GDM late in pregnancy. All infants of gestational diabetics are at significant risk for fetal macrosomia, neonatal hypoglycemia, hypocalcemia, polycythemia, and hyperbilirubinemia (ADA, 1990). (For further discussion, see Chapter 39.)

The overall incidence of congenital anomalies among infants of gestational diabetics approaches that of the nondiabetic population. This is related to the fact that GDM usually develops after week 20 of pregnancy, after the critical period of organogenesis (first trimester) has passed. However, recent data in-

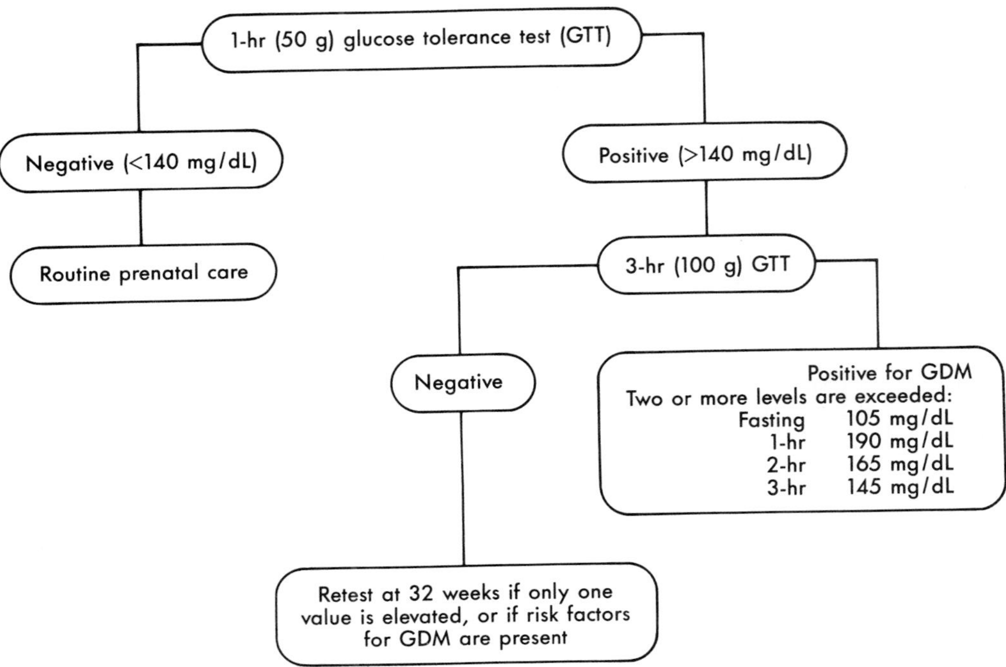

Fig. 31-4 Screening for gestational diabetes.
Modified from American Diabetes Association, 1985, 1990; Hollander, 1988; Landon, Gabbe, 1988; Gabbe, 1990.

dicate that infants of gestational diabetics who require insulin during pregnancy are approximately 20 times more likely to have major cardiovascular system defects than are infants of nondiabetic mothers (Becerra et al, 1990).

Nursing Care

In caring for the woman diagnosed as having GDM, the nursing role essentially mirrors that of pregestational diabetes. There is one distinct difference in that those nurses involved in prenatal care delivery in any setting can be instrumental in the identification of those women at risk for the development of GDM.

ASSESSMENT

In the early prenatal period a thorough history is necessary to identify any risk factors that may predispose the woman to GDM: (1) maternal age over 30, (2) obesity, or prepregnancy weight more than 20% over ideal body weight, (3) family history of diabetes, and (4) previous obstetric history that includes GDM in previous pregnancy, infant weighing more than 9 pounds or with congenital anomalies, hydramnios, or unexplained stillbirth or miscarriage. Nondiabetic women with any of the risk factors for GDM are alerted to the possibility of diabetes during pregnancy and are taught to report any symptoms that may represent onset of the condition (increased thirst, hunger, or urination; weakness). The woman is instructed regarding screening measures for GDM.

With the initial prenatal interview and during subsequent visits, assessment of physical or emotional stress, or both, is important because stress is a factor known to precipitate diabetes in the individual prone to the disease. The diagnosis of GDM often represents a crisis situation to the pregnant woman and her family. Suddenly the pregnancy is labeled "high risk," which evokes fear and anxiety related to the well-being of the mother and the fetus. Although the pregestational diabetic usually is familiar with necessary self-care skills, the gestational diabetic must learn about diabetic management and must master the skills on short notice. Because the diagnosis of GDM is often crisis oriented, there may be barriers to learning and decision making. The nurse is instrumental is assisting the woman and her family in overcoming these barriers through therapeutic communication and support, while providing the education necessary for diabetic control and self-care. Women with GDM who require insulin injections require additional support as they learn self-administration techniques (Zigrossi, Riga-Ziegler, 1986; Keohane, Lacey, 1991).

Assessment of the pregnant woman's support system is an essential part of care planning. The family's reaction to the diagnosis and the necessary treatment regimen influences the woman's emotional response to the diagnosis and her compliance with the plan of care. Sources of physical and psychosocial stress are identified, with the recommendation that stress be avoided to prevent complications such as hyperglycemia.

NURSING DIAGNOSES

Nursing diagnoses are identified on the basis of assessment data and individual response to GDM. Those diagnoses appropriate for pregestational diabetics generally apply to gestational diabetes as well (see p. 933).

PLANNING

Goals (expected outcomes) are formulated on the basis of identified nursing diagnoses and the medical plan of care. The pregnant woman and her support person(s) are involved with the nurse in the mutual establishment of goals.

In general, the goals of care for GDM are the same as for pregestational diabetes. The major difference is that the time frame for planning may be shortened with GDM because the diagnosis usually is made later in pregnancy. Planning and implementation must necessarily occur as soon as possible after diagnosis.

IMPLEMENTATION

ANTEPARTUM. When the diagnosis of GDM is made, treatment begins immediately. This allows little or no time for the woman and her family to adjust to the diagnosis before they are expected to participate in compliance with the treatment plan. This event contrasts with the pregestational diabetic who may have had years to learn about the disease and adapt to dietary modifications, self-glucose monitoring, and insulin administration. With each step of the treatment plan, it is important that the nurse and other health care providers educate the woman and her family, providing detailed and comprehensive explanations to ensure understanding, participation, and compliance with the necessary interventions. Potential complications resulting from noncompliance are discussed, while the need for maintenance of normoglycemia throughout the remainder of the pregnancy is reinforced. It may be reassuring for the woman and her family to know that the diabetic condition typically disappears when the pregnancy is over.

Dietary modification is the mainstay of treatment for GDM. There are two main goals in diet therapy: maintenance of normoglycemia and appropriate weight gain during the pregnancy. Nutritional counseling provided by a trained nutritionist is instituted as soon as possible after the diagnosis is made. The dietary program is individualized according to the woman's needs and physician's orders. A typical gestational diabetic diet includes from 2000 to 2200 calories per day consumed in three meals and three or four snacks, reduction of fat intake, exclusion of simple sugars, and increased intake of soluble dietary fiber and complex carbohydrates (Worthington-Roberts, Williams, 1989). It is desired that the woman attain an ideal weight gain of 24 to 30 pounds during pregnancy (average of 0.9 lb/wk the last two trimesters). For the pregnant obese woman whose prepregnancy weight is greater than 120% of her ideal body weight, caloric intake may be tailored to prevent excess weight gain during pregnancy while still meeting maternal and fetal requirements (Hollander, 1988) (Table 31-3).

The woman is encouraged to establish a regular program of daily *exercise*. For example, 30 minutes of walking each day may be recommended (see box on exercise p. 939).

Approximately 10% to 15% of gestational diabetics require *insulin* to maintain normoglycemia. Once the dietary regimen is implemented, weekly determinations of fasting and postprandial glucose levels are made. Indications for the initiation of insulin therapy include a fasting plasma or capillary glucose level in excess of 105 mg/dL, a postprandial plasma level greater than 120 mg/dL, or a capillary level of 140mg/dL 2 hours after a meal (ADA, 1985). A combination of regular and NPH insulin is administered in two or three injections per day, and dosage is adjusted based on self-determinations of blood glucose levels. Two thirds of the total insulin dose is administered in the morning and the remaining one third is given in the evening (Hollander, 1988; Landon, Gabbe, 1988; Chez et al, 1989) (see box on insulin administration, p. 938).

The woman and her family are taught the necessary skills to manage insulin administration. In some instances, hospitalization may be required to regulate blood glucose levels and to educate the woman on glycemic control through insulin therapy in conjunction with dietary modification.

TABLE 31-3 Sample Diet Plan: Gestational Diabetes Mellitus—2000 Calories

Distribution of Intake	Exchange	Food Allowance
Breakfast	1 milk	1 cup skim milk
	2 starches	1 slice whole wheat toast
		¾ cup dry cereal
	1 fruit	1¼ cup strawberries
	1 fat	1 tsp margarine
Morning snack	1 fruit	1 apple
Lunch	1 milk	1 cup skim milk
	2 starch	2 slices whole wheat bread
	2 meat	2 oz sliced turkey breast
	1 fruit	1 cup cubed cantaloupe
	1 vegetable	Carrot sticks
	1 fat	1 tsp mayonnaise
Afternoon snack	1 starch	3 graham crackers (2½ inches square)
Evening meal	1 milk	1 cup skim milk
	2 starch	½ cup mashed potatoes
		1 small roll
	4 meat	4 oz lean sirloin steak
	1 vegetable	½ cup cooked asparagus
		Small dinner salad
	3 fats	1 tbsp salad dressing
		2 tsp margarine
Evening snack	1 milk	1 cup skim milk
	1 starch	⅓ cup bran cereal
	1 fruit	¾ cup blueberries

Modified from American Diabetes Association/American Dietetic Association: *Exchange lists for meal planning,* Chicago, 1986, The Associations.
tbsp, tablespoon; *tsp,* teaspoon.

Periodic assessment of glycosylated hemoglobin is performed to measure the degree of glycemic control. Fasting and postprandial glucose levels usually are monitored at each weekly visit. Self-monitoring of blood glucose levels, which is a requirement for effective insulin therapy, usually is done four times daily—on rising and after meals. Those gestational diabetics managed by dietary modification alone also are taught to measure blood glucose levels. Visually read reagent strips or a glucose reflectance meter may be used for self-monitoring of blood glucose. Gestational diabetics also are taught to measure urine ketone levels on awakening, during illness, whenever a meal is delayed, and if blood glucose is above target values. If ketonuria occurs, the caloric intake of carbohydrates is cautiously increased (Jovanovic-Peterson, Peterson, 1988).

Gestational diabetics, particularly those on a regimen of insulin therapy, are at risk for developing hypoglycemia and hyperglycemia. The woman and her family are taught signs and symptoms, as well as causes, prevention and treatment measures (Table 31-2).

Women with gestational diabetes who maintain normal glucose levels are allowed to progress to term gestation but should give birth by 42 weeks. If labor cannot be safely induced at 40 weeks, biophysical assessment or nonstress tests are performed once or twice weekly. Fetal surveillance may begin at 30 weeks for those women with poor glycemic control, pregnancy-induced hypertension, history of prior stillbirth, and those who required insulin in a prior gestation. The program of fetal surveillance is similar to that employed with pregestational diabetics (Dickinson, Palmer, 1990).

INTRAPARTUM. During the labor and birth process, blood glucose levels are monitored at least every 2 hours to maintain levels at 100 mg/dL or less. Glucose levels within this range will decrease the severity of neonatal hypoglycemia. IV fluids containing glucose are not given as a bolus to the gestational diabetic, although they may be necessary as maintenance fluids.

POSTPARTUM. Approximately 97% of gestational diabetics revert to normoglycemia in the postpartum period. Four to 6 weeks after the birth a 75-g oral glucose tolerance test is performed to assess carbohydrate intolerance. Those women with abnormal results are referred to a diabetologist for follow-up (Jovanovic-Peterson, Peterson, 1988).

In planning for future pregnancies, it is important that the woman be aware that GDM is likely to recur. In addition, the woman who has experienced GDM is at risk for the development of overt diabetes. Obese women who remain overweight have a 60% chance of developing diabetes within 20 years. This risk can be reduced significantly if weight is reduced and maintained within a normal range (Jovanovic-Peterson, Peterson, 1988; Dickinson, Palmer, 1990).

■ HYPEREMESIS GRAVIDARUM

Nausea and vomiting are common complaints during pregnancy and usually are confined to the first trimester. Although these manifestations are distressing, they are typically benign, with no significant metabolic alterations or risks to the mother or fetus.

When vomiting during pregnancy becomes excessive enough to cause electrolyte, metabolic, and nutritional imbalances, the condition is termed **hyperemesis gravidarum.** Hyperemesis gravidarum occurs in approximately 3 to 4/1000 pregnancies. Although most cases are mild and resolve with time, 1/1000 pregnant women will require hospitalization as a result of severe intractable vomiting. The incidence of hyperemesis gravidarum is greater among younger women, first-time mothers, and those with increased body weight (Depue et al, 1987; Kallan, 1987).

The cause of hyperemesis gravidarum remains obscure. It is thought that high levels of estrogen may be responsible (Depue et al, 1987). Hyperemesis gravidarum often is associated with hyperthyroidism, which may be caused by elevated levels of human chorionic gonadotropin (Chin, Lao, 1988; Mori et al, 1988; Thomson et al, 1989; Chin et al, 1990). Multifetal pregnancy and trophoblastic disease (hydatidiform mole) also may be etiologic factors in hyperemesis gravidarum. Reduced gastric motility and decreased secretion of free hydrochloric acid may contribute to the condition.

Psychologic factors may be instrumental in the development of hyperemesis gravidarum. Ambivalence toward the pregnancy and conflicting feelings regarding prospective motherhood, such as body changes and life-style alterations, may cause episodes of vomiting. Women with psychologic problems whose normal reaction patterns to stress involve gastrointestinal disturbances often are affected. However, in some women, psychologic causes cannot be identified.

Nursing Care

ASSESSMENT

In extreme cases, persistent vomiting results in rapid weight loss and dehydration, which leads to fluid and electrolyte imbalances. Dehydration results in hypovolemia, which manifests as hypotension, tachycardia, increased hematocrit and blood urea nitrogen levels (BUN), and diminished urine output. Vomiting involves loss of gastric acid fluids, as well as alkaline contents from deeper within the gastrointestinal tract. This leads to the development of metabolic acidosis. Extreme maternal nutritional deprivation, or starvation, causes hypoproteinemia and hypovitaminosis. Jaundice and hemorrhage, which result from deficiencies in vitamins C and B-complex, and hypothrombinemia lead to bleeding from mucosal surfaces. The embryo or fetus may die, and the mother may die of irreversible metabolic alterations. Occasionally, severe intractable vomiting may necessitate termination of the pregnancy by therapeutic abortion to preserve the life and health of the mother.

Infants born to mothers with hyperemesis gravidarum have an increased risk of CNS malformations (Depue et al, 1987). An increased incidence of IUGR and fetal anomalies occurs in infants born to mothers who experienced weight loss and electrolyte disturbances because of excessive vomiting. Fetal death may occur as a result of severe hyperemesis gravidarum (Chin, Lao, 1988; Stellato, 1988; Gross et al, 1989).

NURSING DIAGNOSES

In collaboration with the woman, nursing diagnoses are identified on the basis of assessment data. Potential nursing diagnoses for the woman with hyperemesis gravidarum include the following:

- Fluid volume deficit related to
  - — Abnormal fluid loss secondary to vomiting
  - — Inadequate fluid intake
- Altered nutrition: less than body requirements related to
  - — Nausea and persistent vomiting
- Acute pain related to
  - — Nausea and vomiting
- Activity intolerance/fatigue related to
  - — Weakness secondary to inadequate nutrition
- Knowledge deficit related to
  - — Condition, its cause, management
  - — Potential effects on mother and fetus
- High risk for ineffective individual or family coping related to
  - — Emotional stress of condition and hospitalization
- Fear related to
  - — Effects of hyperemesis on fetal well-being
- High risk for altered family processes related to
  - — Illness of mother and separation during hospitalization
- Powerlessness related to
  - — Complication threatening pregnancy
- Altered role performance related to
  - — Unmet expectations for pregnancy
- Self-esteem disturbance related to
  - — Unmet expectations for pregnancy
- High risk for maternal/fetal injury related to
  - — Severe complications of hyperemesis

PLANNING

The plan of care for the woman with hyperemesis gravidarum is given direction from identified nursing diagnoses and the medical treatment regimen. Individualization of the plan of care is based on needs identified by the woman, her family, and the health care providers. In collaboration with the woman and her family, mutually acceptable goals are set. *Goals* for the woman with hyperemesis gravidarum might include the following.

- The woman's fluid and electrolyte balance is restored.
- The woman will resume oral intake of a nutritionally sound diet.
- The woman states that nausea has subsided.
- The woman experiences no further episodes of vomiting.
- The woman's activity tolerance is restored; she is able to resume usual activities of daily living.
- The woman and her family verbalize understanding of the condition, its management, and potential effects on her and her fetus.
- The woman and her family demonstrate effective coping and mutual support.

IMPLEMENTATION

Hospitalization often is indicated for the treatment of hyperemesis gravidarum. Conservative management includes IV hydration, vitamin supplements, sedation, antiemetics, and in some cases, psychotherapy. For more severe cases, enteral or parenteral nutrition may be necessary to correct maternal nutritional deprivation (Levine, Esser, 1988; Stellato et al, 1988; Barclay, 1990).

Nursing care of the hyperemetic woman involves implementing the medical plan of care: initiating and monitoring IV therapy, administering pharmacologic agents and nutritional supplements, and monitoring the woman's response to interventions. The nurse observes the woman for any signs of complications, such as metabolic acidosis, jaundice, or hemorrhage and alerts the physician should these occur.

Accurate measurement of intake and output, including the amount of emesis, is an important aspect of nursing care. Oral hygiene while the woman is receiving nothing by mouth, as well as after episodes of vomiting, helps to allay associated discomforts. When the woman begins to respond to therapy, limited amounts of oral fluids and bland foods such as crackers or toast are begun. The diet is advanced slowly as tolerated by the woman until she is able to consume a nutritionally sound diet. Promoting adequate rest is important for the woman with hyperemesis; the nurse can assist in coordinating treatment measures and periods of visitation to provide opportunity for rest periods.

The nurse must remain calm, compassionate, and sympathetic, recognizing that the manifestations of hyperemesis can be physically and emotionally debilitating. Concern for fetal well-being is a primary concern of the woman with hyperemesis. The nurse can provide an environment conducive to discussion of those concerns and assist the woman in identifying and mobilizing sources of support. The family is included in the plan of care whenever possible. Encouraging their participation may help to alleviate some of the emotional stress associated with hospitalization. Psychologic counseling may be needed, as well as referral to a social worker. Education of the woman and her family about hyperemesis, its causes, potential complications, and management plan is necessary at the onset of the condition because understanding will enhance compliance and influence the maternal and fetal outcome.

EVALUATION

In most instances, hyperemesis gravidarum will respond to therapy and the prognosis is good. The woman is discharged to home when fluid and electrolyte balance is restored oral intake of a nutritionally sound diet is resumed, nausea and vomiting cease, and weight gain begins. At a subsequent prenatal visit, she states she is able to resume usual activities of daily living; she understands the condition, its managment, and potential effects on her fetus; and she and her family demonstrate effective coping and mutual support. (See case study, p. 951, and nursing plan of care, p. 952.)

■ THYROID DISORDERS

The thyroid gland functions in the synthesis of triiodothyronine (T_3) and thyroxine (T_4) from circulating iodine. The balance between production and need is regulated by the hypothalamus and pituitary through the release of thyrotropin releasing factor (TRF) and thyroid-stimulating hormone (TSH).

The hormones produced by the thyroid gland are responsible for increasing the production of intracellular proteins (mostly enzymes) and energy. Consequently, the metabolic rate increases with an accelerated consumption of carbohydrates, fats, and oxygen, along with increased heat production.

CASE STUDY

Hyperemesis Gravidarium

Carolyn Scott is a 20-year-old single, first-time mother at 6 week's gestation who has been admitted to the antepartum unit with a diagnosis of hyperemesis gravidarum.

ASSESSMENT

The admission interview revealed that Carolyn has been vomiting for 2 days and has been unable to retain any food or fluids. She states that she feels "miserable." Carolyn is very concerned about the well-being of her "baby" and keeps asking "Is my baby going to die?" During the physical examination of Carolyn, the nurse notes that her eyes appear sunken, her skin turgor is poor, and oral mucous membranes are dry. Carolyn has lost 5 pounds since her last prenatal visit 2 weeks ago. Assessment of vital signs reveals a pulse rate of 98 beats/min, up from her normal rate of 76 beats/min. Her blood pressure has dropped from her usual measurement of 118/70 to 100/60 mm Hg. A review of laboratory findings reveals elevated values for hematocrit, BUN, and urine specific gravity.

NURSING DIAGNOSIS

Because Carolyn has been vomiting for 2 days and has retained no food or fluids, the nurse identifies the *nursing diagnosis:* fluid volume deficit related to abnormal fluid loss secondary to vomiting and inadequate fluid intake.

PLANNING

A plan of care is developed with Carolyn's input. The mutually agreed upon *goal* for Carolyn is that she will experience relief from vomiting and will be able to retain fluid intake. *Expected outcomes* include restoration of fluid and electrolyte balance as evidenced by normal skin turgor, moist mucous membranes, stable weight, vital signs within normal limits, and BUN, hematocrit, and urine specific gravity within normal values.

IMPLEMENTATION

Nursing actions are derived from medical management, physician's orders, and nursing diagnosis. Specific interventions include assessment of skin turgor and mucous membranes, vital signs, urine specific gravity, and daily weight. The laboratory values are monitored and abnormalities reported to the physician. An accurate intake and output record will be maintained, including emesis. The nurse monitors prescribed IV therapy and gives antiemetics as ordered. When Carolyn tolerates oral fluids, the nurse will encourage her to drink fluids that she likes.

EVALUATION

The expected outcomes were used to evaluate the effectiveness of these interventions. Carolyn was hospitalized for 1 week. IV fluids were necessary for 3 days, but she was able to tolerate a regular diet by the day of discharge. Antiemetics were effective in relieving Carolyn's discomfort from nausea and vomiting. Carolyn's blood pressure and pulse returned to her previous levels, and her skin turgor and mucous membranes returned to normal. By the end of the week, her laboratory values were within normal limits, and her urine specific gravity remained between 1.005 and 1.010. Carolyn lost 2 more pounds, but by discharge she had gained half a pound. On the basis of these findings, the goal set for Carolyn was met (see the related plan of care).

Thyroid function in pregnancy is not clearly understood (see Research Highlight, p. 953). Normal physiologic changes of pregnancy cause a mild hyperthyroid state primarily because of the effects of human chorionic gonadotropin and placental estrogen. The manifestations are seen as increased basal metabolic rate, increased cardiac output, emotional lability, heat intolerance, and absence of menses.

Hyperthyroidism

Hyperthyroidism affects approximately 1 to 2/1000 pregnancies and most often is due to Graves' disease. Clinical manifestations of hyperthyroidism are associated with increased basal metabolic rate and increased sympathetic nervous system activity. Typical symptoms include nervousness, hyperactivity, weakness, fatigue, weight loss (or poor weight gain), diarrhea, tachycardia, shortness of breath, excessive perspiration, heat intolerance, and muscle tremors. Exophthalmos and enlargement of the thyroid gland (goiter) also are common. Laboratory findings indicative of hyperthyroidism include elevated free T_4 index and increased basal metabolic rate.

Hyperthyroidism in women may be responsible for anovulation and amenorrhea, but the disease is not a

CARE PLAN Hyperemesis Gravidarum

GOALS	INTERVENTIONS	RATIONALE	EVALUATION
Nursing diagnosis: Fluid volume deficit related to abnormal fluid loss secondary to vomiting and inadequate fluid intake			
Carolyn's fluid and electrolyte balance is restored as evidenced by normal skin turgor, moist mucous membranes, stable weight, vital signs WNL for her; serum electrolytes, hemoglobin, hematocrit, and urine specific gravity are WNL. Carolyn experiences no further vomiting. Carolyn resumes adequate oral intake.	Assess and document skin turgor, condition of mucous membranes, vital signs, and urine specific gravity. Weigh daily. Monitor laboratory values and report abnormalities. Assess and record color, amount, and frequency of emesis. Maintain accurate intake and output record. Assist physician or initiate IV fluid therapy per physician's order; monitor infusion carefully. Administer antiemetics as ordered. Maintain NPO status as ordered. When oral intake is allowed, offer Carolyn's preferred liquids. Encourage oral fluids, slowly increasing amount as tolerated.	Accurate assessment of fluid and electrolyte status provides basis for planning and evaluating interventions. Restoration of fluid and electrolyte balance requires parenteral therapy until Carolyn can tolerate oral intake. Fluid and electrolyte imbalance must be corrected to prevent severe complications such as metabolic acidosis and maternal or fetal death.	Carolyn received IV fluids for 3 days until all laboratory values had returned to normal. Her skin turgor, mucous membranes, and vital signs returned to previous levels. Carolyn lost 2 more pounds, but by discharge she had gained half a pound.
Nursing diagnosis: Altered nutrition: less than body requirements related to nausea and persistent vomiting			
Carolyn will resume oral intake of nutritionally sound diet. Her nausea and vomiting will be alleviated. Carolyn describes components of nutritionally sound diet and verbalizes willingness to follow that diet. Carolyn will tolerate prescribed diet. Carolyn will gain weight appropriately during pregnancy.	Begin oral intake as ordered by physician and tolerated by Carolyn. Provide small amounts of attractively served foods to fit her preferences. Increase amounts slowly as tolerated. Monitor and document oral intake. Have dietitian consult with Carolyn in developing a meal plan that meets nutritional requirements during pregnancy and that includes a schedule of meals, as well as Carolyn's food preferences and eating environment. Discuss with Carolyn the importance of adequate nutrition during pregnancy. Verify Carolyn's understanding of nutritional information. Assess her willingness to follow the prescribed diet plan, and encourage her compliance. Monitor Carolyn's weight gain.	Adequate maternal nutrition is necessary for the health of the mother and for growth and development of the fetus.	On the third day of hospitalization, Carolyn was tolerating oral fluids and slowly progressed to a regular diet by the day of discharge. She met with the dietitian on two occasions and stated she understood the dietary regimen as well as the importance of compliance. Carolyn had begun to gain weight before discharge.

WNL, Within normal limits.

CARE PLAN Hyperemesis Gravidarum—cont'd

GOALS	INTERVENTIONS	RATIONALE	EVALUATION
Nursing diagnosis: Fear related to effects of hyperemesis on fetal well-being			
Carolyn verbalizes feelings and concerns about fetal well-being.	Convey acceptance of Carolyn's perception of fear. Encourage her to express feelings and concerns. Help Carolyn identify personal strengths and previous coping mechanisms. Provide Carolyn with information related to potential risks to fetus. Encourage Carolyn to discuss these concerns with the physician. Help her identify sources of support and mobilize support person/group of her choice. Arrange for psychology or social work consult as needed.	Acceptance of Carolyn's fears will encourage open communication regarding the source of fear. Knowledge of potential risks to fetus may help to allay her fear. Effective coping strategies are needed to enable Carolyn to deal with her illness and its effects.	Carolyn discussed her concerns with the nurse and stated that she felt relieved after discussion of the fetal risks related to hyperemesis gravidarum. Carolyn's mother was identified as her main source of support, and she was included in the discussion.

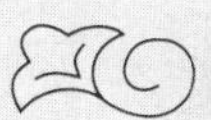 Research Highlight 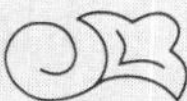

Regulation of Maternal Thyroid during Pregnancy

RESEARCH ABSTRACT

The purpose of the study was to examine maternal thyroid function and changes in function over time in a group of pregnant women. Subjects were 606 pregnant women who came to a prenatal clinic and who had no known thyroid abnormality. Mean gestational age at initial interview was 17 weeks. The women were examined again at 30 to 33 weeks' gestation and 1 to 4 days after childbirth. Biochemical measures of thyroid function included serum determinations of thyroid hormones (T_4, T_3, T_4-binding globulin [TBG], and TSH), human chononic gonadotropin (hCG), and urinary iodine concentration. Thyroid volume was estimated by ultrasonography. There was a marked increased in serum TBG and a corresponding reduction in the T_4/TBG ratio from early to late pregnancy. High hCG levels were associated with lower serum TSH and an increase in thyroid size. Serum thyroglobulin levels were increased all through pregnancy. Increased thyroid volume was common, and goiter was found in 9% of the women at the time of childbirth.

IMPLICATIONS FOR PRACTICE

Thyroid function in pregnancy is not clearly understood. In the population from which this sample was drawn, iodine intake is low. During prenatal contacts, nurses can counsel women about the necessity of adequate iodine intake during pregnancy and provide suggestions on how to achieve adequate intake.

RELATED RESEARCH QUESTIONS

1. Will an educational program increase the amount of iodine in the diet of pregnant women?
2. What are the behavioral consequences of inadequate iodine intake in pregnant women?
3. Is there a relation between cultural variations in diet and adequate intake of iodine?
4. Will a diet that includes adequate iodine reduce the number of women experiencing an increase in thyroid volume during pregnancy?

REFERENCE

Glinoer D et al: Regulation of maternal thyroid during pregnancy, *J Clin Endocrinol Metab* 71:276, 1990.

recognized cause of spontaneous abortion or fetal malformation. With inadequate control of hyperthyroidism during pregnancy, there is an increased risk of preterm birth and stillbirth. Infants of hyperthyroid mothers are often of low birth weight, and thyrotoxicosis may occur in the neonatal period. Although most cases of neonatal hyperthyroidism are transient, some may progress and ultimately impair CNS development (Chin, Kim, 1988; Davis et al, 1989).

The primary treatment of hyperthyroidism during pregnancy is drug therapy with the thiouracils. The medication of choice is propylthiouracil (PTU) in the smallest effective dosage. PTU usually is well tolerated by the mother, with infrequent side effects of nausea, vomiting, and jaundice. Leukopenia may occur as a result of thiouracil therapy; thus leukocyte counts are monitored at regular intervals. During therapy, thyroid activity is monitored every 2 weeks to prevent hypothyroidism and to adjust the medication to a minimal dosage. Thiouracils readily cross the placenta and may induce fetal hypothyroidism and goiter. Radioactive iodine must not be used in diagnosis or treatment of hyperthyroidism because it may compromise the fetal thyroid (Chin, Kim, 1988; Cunningham et al, 1989).

Surgical treatment of hyperthyroidism, subtotal thyroidectomy, may be performed during the second or third trimester. Candidates are those women with severe disease, those for whom drug therapy proves toxic, and those who are unable to adhere to the prescribed medical regimen. Postoperative hypothyroidism is common, occurring in at least 20% of hyperthyroid women. This must be treated promptly to spare the fetus. At birth, a free T_4 index determination should be made on cord blood to aid in assessing the status of the neonate.

Any maternal therapy for thyroid dysfunction may induce fetal thyroid insult. Thyroid function of the neonate should be monitored carefully to detect and treat promptly any abnormalities.

Hypothyroidism

Hypothyroidism during pregnancy is a rare phenomenon because women with this condition often are infertile. Hypothyroidism usually is due to Hashimoto's disease, thyroid gland ablation by radiation, previous surgery, or antithyroid medications. Reduced thyroid function caused by hypothalamic or pituitary failure is rare, with only a few reported cases.

Characteristic symptoms of hypothyroidism include lethargy, weakness, anorexia, weight gain, cold intolerance, mental impairment, constipation, and headache. Dry skin, thin brittle nails, alopecia, poor skin turgor, and delayed deep tendon reflexes also are common. Laboratory findings during pregnancy may reveal normal or reduced protein-bound iodine (PBI), reduced T_4 (column or D), reduced T_3 (resin), and a reduced T4 index (normal range is 0.75 to 2.5 units if T_4 by column is used; 1.3 to 5 units if T_4 [D] is used with resin T_3 uptake).

Pregnant women with hypothyroidism are at increased risk for spontaneous abortion in the first trimester. There is an increased incidence of preeclampsia and abruptio placentae among hypothyroid women, with a corresponding increase in low birth weight and stillbirth. For the most part, however, infants of hypothyroid mothers are healthy, without evidence of thyroid dysfunction (Davis et al, 1988; Cunningham et al, 1989).

Thyroid hormone supplements are used to treat hypothyroidism. Levothyroxine (Synthroid) is most often prescribed during pregnancy, beginning with the dosage of 0.05 to 0.1 mg/day and increasing to a maximum of 0.2 mg/day over several weeks. Serum TSH levels are monitored and may take up to 2 months to reach normal levels. Thyroid supplements do not cross the placenta in any appreciable amount; thus treatment of the mother is considered safe for the fetus (Chin, Kim, 1988).

Nursing Implications

The pregnant woman whose pregnancy is complicated by thyroid dysfunction often needs assistance from the nurse in coping with the discomforts and frustrations associated with symptoms of the disorder. For example, the woman with hyperthyroidism who experiences nervousness and hyperactivity concomitantly with weakness and fatigue may benefit from suggestions by the nurse to channel excess energies into quiet diversional activities such as reading or crafts. Discomfort associated with hypersensitivity to heat (hyperthyroidism) or cold intolerance (hypothyroidism) can be minimized by appropriate clothing and regulation of environmental temperatures, when possible, as well as avoidance of temperature extremes.

Nutritional counseling, in consultation with a registered dietitian, may be helpful in providing guidance for the woman in selecting a well-balanced diet. The pregnant hyperthyroid woman who experiences increased appetite and poor weight gain, as well as the hypothyroid woman who is experiencing anorexia and lethargy, need counseling to ensure adequate intake of nutritionally sound foods to meet both maternal and fetal needs.

Education of these women is essential to promote compliance with the plan of treatment. The woman is instructed regarding the disorder and its potential impact on herself and her fetus, the medication regimen and possible side effects, the need for ongoing medical supervision, and the importance of compliance (Smith, 1990).

Psychologic and emotional implications of pregnancy complicated by thyroid dysfunction are similar to those of any high-risk pregnancy. The woman is encouraged to verbalize feelings, concerns, and frustrations and is assisted in identifying support systems. The family is incorporated into the plan of care to foster mutuality and support among the members.

■ MATERNAL PHENYLKETONURIA

Phenylketonuria (PKU) is an inborn error of metabolism caused by an autosomal recessive trait that creates a deficiency in the enzyme phenylalanine hydroxylase. Absence of this enzyme results in a toxic accumulation of phenylalanine in the blood, which interferes with brain development and function. PKU is estimated to occur in about 1/10,000 to 1/15,000 infants (US Congress, Office of Technology Assessment, 1988).

Newborn screening for PKU (Appendix F), prompt diagnosis, and dietary therapy begun in the early neonatal period and continued through adolescence have made it possible for individuals to live productive lives, achieving their genetic potential for intellectual development. Because the dietary treatment of PKU does not have to be continued indefinitely, many women of reproductive age do not recall having had PKU. Others with a lesser form of PKU were never identified or treated. This has significant implications for childbearing women because it has been shown that phenylalanine has disastrous effects on the developing fetus (Worthington-Roberts, Williams, 1989).

Women with PKU have an increased risk of bearing infants with microcephaly, mental retardation, cardiac defects, and IUGR (Levy, 1987; Luke, Keith, 1990). Fetal damage can be largely prevented by a phenylalanine-restricted diet, if begun before conception and continued throughout the pregnancy. A maternal diet low in phenylalanine has questionable preventive value if begun after conception (Davidson, 1989; Luder, Greene, 1989; Pulion et al, 1990).

The key to prevention of fetal anomalies caused by PKU is the identification of women in their reproductive years who have the condition. Screening programs in the premarital period and even earlier, during school physical examinations, are possible means to identify those individuals with PKU and to *institute treatment before conception occurs*. For those women who are pregnant, a simple urine test (Phenostix) for PKU can be performed in early pregnancy (Luke, Keith, 1990).

For those women with PKU, preconceptional counseling should include discussion of potential fetal risks and the need for strict adherence to a phenylalanine-restricted diet before and during pregnancy. It should be made clear, however, that even careful and controlled management of phenylalanine levels does not ensure the birth of a normal infant. Pregnancy alternatives, such as adoption, can also be discussed (Worthington-Roberts, Williams, 1989; Hickey, Covington, 1990).

■ SUMMARY

Maternal endocrine and metabolic disorders have immediate and long-term consequences for the mother and her fetus or newborn. The woman who becomes an active participant in her care has the most potential for preventing or minimizing the adverse effects of the disorder and improving the prognosis for herself and her offspring. The tremendous strides in the management of diabetes are of value only if the woman is willing to utilize the care available. Prepregnancy care that continues throughout the childbearing experience leads to the best results for women whose pregnancies are complicated by diabetes mellitus, hyperemesis gravidarum, disorders of the thyroid, or PKU.

REFERENCES

American Diabetes Association: Summary and recommendations of the second international workshop—conference on gestational diabetes mellitus, *Diabetes* 34(suppl 2):123, 1985.

American Diabetes Association: Position statement: office guide to diagnosis and classification of diabetes mellitus and other categories of glucose intolerance, *Diabetes Care* 13 (suppl 1):3, 1990.

Barclay BA: Experience with enteral nutrition in the treatment of hyperemesis gravidarum, *Nutr Clin Pract* 5(4):153, 1990.

Barss VA: Diabetes and pregnancy, *Med Clin North Am* 73:685, 1989.

Becerra JE et al: Diabetes mellitus during pregnancy and the risks for specific birth defects: a population-based case-control study, *Pediatrics* 65:1, 1990.

Burkart W, Henker JP, Schneider HP: Complications and fetal outcome in diabetic pregnancy: intensified conventional versus insulin pump therapy, *Gynecol Obstet Invest* 26(2):104, 1988.

Campbell RG: The adult diabetic patient. In Bardin C, editor: *Current therapy in endocrinology and metabolism,* ed 3, Philadelphia, 1988, BC Decker.

Centers for Disease Control: Perinatal mortality and congenital malformations in infants born to women with insulin dependent diabetes mellitus—U.S., Canada, and Europe, 1940-1988, *JAMA* 264:437, 1990.

Chez RA et al: Meeting the challenge of gestational diabetes, *Contemp Ob Gyn* 34(3):120, 1989.

Chin NW, Kim MH: Thyroid disorders in pregnancy. In Charles D, Glover DD, editors: *Current therapy in obstetrics,* Philadelphia, 1988, BC Decker.

Chin RK, Lao TT: Thyroxine concentration and outcome of hyperemetic pregnancies, *Br J Obstet Gynecol* 95:507, 1988.

Chin RK et al: A longitudinal study of changes in erythrocyte concentration in hyperemesis gravidarum, *Gynecol Obstet Invest* 29(1):22, 1990.

Corbett JV: *Laboratory tests and diagnostic procedures with nursing diagnoses,* ed 2, Norwalk, Conn, 1987, Appleton & Lange.

Cunningham FG, Macdonald PC, Gant NF: *Williams obstetrics,* ed 18, Norwalk, Conn, 1989, Appleton & Lange.

Davidson DC: Maternal phenylketonuria, *Postgrad Med J* 65(suppl 2):510, 1989.

Davis LE, Leveno KL, Cunningham FG: Hypothyroidism complicating pregnancy, *Obstet Gynecol* 72:108, 1988.

Davis LE et al: Thyrotoxicosis complicating pregnancy, *Am J Obstet Gynecol* 160:63, 1989.

Depue RH et al: Hyperemesis gravidarum in relation to estradiol levels, pregnancy outcome, and other maternal factors: a seroepidemiologic study, *Am J Obstet Gynecol* 156:1137, 1987.

Dickinson JD, Palmer SM: Gestational diabetes: pathophysiology and diagnosis, *Semin Perinatol* 14(1):2, 1990.

Gabbe SG: Diabetes mellitus: ways of individualizing care, *Contemp Ob Gyn* 35(7):68, 1990.

Greene MF et al: First trimester HgbA and risk for major malformations and spontaneous abortion in diabetic pregnancy, *Teratology* 39:225, 1989.

Gross S, Librach C, Cecutti A: Maternal weight loss associated with hyperemesis gravidarum: a predictor of fetal outcome, *Am J Obstet Gynecol* 160:906, 1989.

Heckbert SR, Stephens CR, Daling JR: Diabetes in pregnancy: maternal and infant outcome, *Paediatr Perinat Epidemiol* 2:314, 1988.

Hickey CA, Covington C: Maternal phenylketonuria: case management as a preventive approach to chronic condition affecting pregnancy, *NAACOG's Clin Issues Perinatol Women's Health Nurs* 1(2):214, 1990.

Hollander P: Gestational diabetes, *Pract Diabetol* 7(2):14, 1988.

Jacobson JD, Cousins L: A population-based study of maternal and perinatal outcomes in patients with gestational diabetes, *Am J Obstet Gynecol* 161:981, 1989.

Jovanovic-Peterson L, Peterson C: Diabetes and pregnancy. In Bardin CW, editor: *Current therapy in endocrinology and metabolism,* ed 3, Philadelphia, 1988, BC Decker.

Jovanovic-Peterson L, Peterson C: Dietary manipulation as a primary treatment strategy for pregnancy complicated by diabetes, *J Am Coll Nutr* 9:320, 1990.

Jovanovic-Peterson L et al: Maternal postgrandial glucose levels and infant birth weight: the Diabetes in Early Pregnancy Study: The National Institute of Child Health and Human Development—Diabetes in Early Pregnancy Study, *Am J Obstet Gynecol* 64:103, Jan 1991.

Kallan B: Hyperemesis during pregnancy and delivery outcome: a registry study, *Eur J Obstet Gynecol Reprod Biol* 26:291, 1987.

Kaufman HW: Screening for gestational diabetes mellitus, *Am Fam Physician* 40(6):109, 1989.

Keohane NS, Lacey LA: Preparing the woman with gestational diabetes for self-care: use of a structured teaching plan by nursing staff, *JOGNN* 20(3):189, 1991.

Kitzmiller JL et al: Preconception care of diabetes: glycemic control prevents congenital anomalies, *JAMA* 265:731, 1991.

Landon MB, Gabbe SG: Diabetes in pregnancy. In Charles D, Glover DD, editors: *Current therapy in obstetrics,* Philadelphia, 1988, BC Decker.

Larsen ML, Horder M, Mogensen EF: Effect of long-term monitoring of glycosylated hemoglobin levels in insulin-dependent diabetes mellitus, *N Engl J Med* 323:1021, 1990.

Leff EW, Gagne MP, Jefferis SC: Type I diabetes and pregnancy . . . are we hearing women's concerns? *MCN* 16(2):83, 1991.

Levine MG, Esser D: Total parenteral nutrition for the treatment of hyperemesis gravidarum; maternal nutritional effects and fetal outcome, *Obstet Gynecol* 72:102, 1988.

Levy HL: Maternal phenylketonuria, *Enzyme* 38:312, 1987.

Luder AS, Greene CL: Maternal phenylketonuria and hyperphenylalaninemia: implications for medical practice in the United States, *Am J Obstet Gynecol* 161:102, 1989.

Luke B, Keith LG: The challenge of maternal phenylketonuria screening and treatment, *J Reprod Med* 35:667, 1990.

Matheson D, Efantis J: Diabetes and pregnancy: need and use of intensive therapy, *Diabetes Educ* 15:242, 1989.

Meyer BA, Palmer SM: Pregestational diabetes, *Semin Perinatol* 14(1):12, 1990.

Mills JL et al: Lack of relation of increased malformation rates in infants of diabetic mothers to glycemic control during organogenesis, *N Engl J Med* 318:671, 1988.

Mills JL et al: Incidence of spontaneous abortion among normal women and insulin-dependent diabetic women whose pregnancies were identified within 21 days of conception, *N Engl J Med* 319:1617, 1988.

Mimouni F et al: Perinatal asphyxia in infants of insulin-dependent diabetic mothers, *J Pediatr* 113:345, 1988.

Mimouni F, Tsang RC: Pregnancy outcomes in insulin dependent diabetics: temporal relationships with metabolic control during specific pregnancy periods, *Am J Perinatol* 5:368, 1988.

Mimouni F et al: Polycythemia, hypomagnesemia and hypocalcemia in infants of diabetic mothers, *Am J Dis Child* 140:798, 1986.

Miodovnik M et al: Periconceptional metabolic states and risk for spontaneous abortion in insulin dependent diabetic pregnancies, *J Perinatol* 5:368, 1988.

Mori M et al: Morning sickness and thyroid function in normal pregnancy, *Obstet Gynecol* 72 (3 Pt 1):355, 1988.

Philipson EH, Super DM: Gestational diabetes mellitus: does it recur in subsequent pregnancy? *Am J Obstet Gynecol* 160:1324, 1989.

Pulion DH, Macfarlane SD, Lyon IC: Maternal phenylketonuria, *NZ Med J* 103:397, 1990.

Radak JT: Why worry about gestational diabetes? *Diabetes Forecast* 44(4):27, 1991.

Rosenn B et al: Minor congenital malformations in infants of insulin dependent diabetic women: association with poor glycemic control, *Obstet Gynecol* 76(5 Pt 1):745, 1990.

Rosenn B et al: Preconception management of insulin-dependent diabetes: improvement of pregnancy outcome, *Obstet Gynecol* 77:847, 1991.

Rotondo LM: Diabetes mellitus: impact on pregnancy, *NAACOG's Clin Issues Perinat Women's Health Nurs* 1(2):133, 1990.

Scott JR et al: *Danforth's obstetrics and gynecology,* ed 6, Philadelphia, 1990, JB Lippincott Co.

Sheldon GW: Diabetes and pregnancy, *Obstet Gynecol Clin North Am* 15:379, 1988.

Siddiq YK: Management of diabetes during pregnancy, *J Med Assoc Ga* 78:745, 1989.

Smith JE: Pregnancy complicated by thyroid disease, *J Nurse Midwife* 35(3):143, 1990.

Spirito A et al: Screening measure to assess knowledge of diabetes in pregnancy, *Diabetes Care* 13:712, 1990.

Stamler EF et al: High infectious morbidity in pregnant women with insulin dependent diabetes: an understated complication, *Am J Obstet Gynecol* 163(4 Pt 1):1217, 1990.

Steele JM et al: Can pre-pregnancy care of diabetic women reduce the risk of abnormal babies? *Br Med J* 301:1070, 1990.

Stellato TA, Danziger ZL, Burkons D: Fetal salvage with maternal total parenteral nutrition: the pregnancy mother as her own control, *J Parenter Enteral Nutr* 12(40):412, 1988.

Taysi K: Preconceptional counseling, *Obstet Gynecol Clin North Am* 15:167, 1988.

Thomson JA et al: Hyperemesis gravidarum and thyrotoxicosis: a diagnostic and therapeutic problem, *Scott Med J* 34:472, 1989.

Tomky D: Tapping the full power of insulin pumps, *RN* 52(6):46, June 1989.

United States Congress, Office of Technology Assessment: *Healthy children: investing in the future,* OTA-H-345, Washington, DC, 1988, US Government Printing Office.

VanPutte AW: Perinatal bereavement crisis: coping with negative outcomes from prenatal diagnosis, *J Perinat Neonat Nurs* 2(2):12, 1988.

Varma TR et al: The relationship of increased amniotic fluid volume to perinatal outcome, *International J Gynaecol Obstet* 27:327, 1988.

White P: Classification of obstetrics diabetes, *Am J Obstet Gynecol* 130:228, 1978.

Winn HN, Reece EA: Integrating management of diabetic pregnancies, *Contemp Ob Gyn* 33(1):91, 1989.

Worthington-Roberts BS, Williams SR: *Nutrition in pregnancy and lactation,* ed 4, St Louis, 1989, Mosby–Year Book.

Zigrossi ST, Riga-Ziegler M: The stress of medical management on pregnant diabetics, *MCN* 11(5):320, 1986.

BIBLIOGRAPHY

American Diabetes Association: *Gestational diabetes: what to expect,* Alexandria, Va, 1989, The Association.

American Diabetes Association and The American Dietetic Association: *A guide for professionals: diabetes nutrition and meal planning,* Alexandria, Va, 1988, The Associations.

Balen AH, Kurtz AB: Successful outcome of pregnancy with severe hypothyroidism, *Br J Obstet Gynaecol* 197:536, 1990.

Bourgeois FJ, Duffer J: Outpatient management of women with type I diabetes, *Am J Obstet Gynecol* 163:1065, 1990.

Buckley K, Kulb NW: *High risk maternity nursing manual,* Baltimore, 1990, Williams & Wilkins.

Bunkers-Lawson T et al: A team approach: screening and management for gestational diabetes, *Diabetes Educ* 14:440, 1988.

Chin RK: Antenatal complications and perinatal outcome in patients with nausea and vomiting-complicated pregnancy, *Eur J Obstet Gynecol Reprod Biol* 33:215, 1989.

DiIoria C: The management of nausea and vomiting in pregnancy, *Nurs Pract* 13(5):23, 1988.

Drexel H et al: Prevention of perinatal morbidity by tight metabolic control in gestational diabetes mellitus, *Diabetes Care* 11:761, 1988.

Engel NS: Insulin therapy in pregnancy, *MCN* 14(1):19, 1989.

Everett WD: Screening for gestational diabetes: an analysis of health benefits and costs, *Am J Prev Med* 5(1):38, 1989.

Farley TM et al: The IUD and PID, *Lancet* 339:785, 1992.

Ferris AM et al: Lactation outcome in insulin-dependent diabetic women, *J Am Diet Assoc* 88:317, 1988.

Forsbach G et al: Prevalence of gestational diabetes and macrosomic newborns in a Mexican population, *Diabetes Care* 11:235, 1988.

Guthrie R: Maternal PKU: a continuing problem, *Am J Public Health* 78:771, 1988.

Harvey MG: Diabetic ketoacidosis during pregnancy, *JPNN* 6(1):1, 1992.

Hollander P: Gestational diabetes: the diabetes of pregnancy, *Practical Diabetology* 7(2):14, 1988.

Houston MS, Hay ID: Practical management of hyperthyroidism, *Am Fam Physician* 41:909, 1990.

Howard ED: Gestational diabetes mellitus screening tests: a review of current recommendations, *JPNN* 6(1):37, 1992.

Huffman DH, Gerber AJ: Diabetes and pregnancy: seeing patients safely through term, *Consultant* 28(6):43, 1988.

Jovanovic L: Insulin on the go, *Practical Diabetology* 7(2):10, 1988.

Klein BE et al: Does the severity of diabetic retinopathy predict pregnancy outcome? *J Diabetic Complications* 2(4):179, 1988.

Kuller JM: Effects on the fetus and newborn of medications commonly used during pregnancy, *J Perinat Neonat Nurs* 3(4):73, 1990.

Langer OL et al: Glycemic control in gestational diabetes mellitus—how tight is tight enough: small for gestational age versus large for gestational age, *Am J Obstet Gynecol* 161:646, 1989.

Lean ME, Pearson DW, Sutherland HW: Insulin management during labour and delivery in mothers with diabetes, *Diabetic Med* 7(2):162, 1990.

Leveno KG et al: Continuous subcutaneous insulin infusion during pregnancy, *Diabetes Res Clin Pract* 4:257, 1988.

Lynch BC et al: Maternal phenylketonuria: successful outcome in four pregnancies treated prior to conception, *Eur J Pediatr* 148(1):72, 1988.

Mandel SJ et al: Increased need for thyroxine during pregnancy in women with primary hypothyroidism, *N Engl J Med* 323:91, 1990.

Maresh M et al: Factors predisposing to and outcome of gestational diabetes, *Obstet Gynecol* 74(3 Pt 1):342, 1989.

Ney DM: Nutritional management of diabetes during pregnancy, *Practical Diabetology* 7(2):1, 1988.

Queenan JT: Polyhydramnios and oligohydramnios, *Contemp OB/GYN* 36(12):60, 1991.

Palmer DG, Inturrisi M: Insulin infusion therapy in the intrapartum period, *JPNN* 6(1):25, 1992.

Roberts AB, Pattison NS: Pregnancy in women with diabetes mellitus, twenty years experience: 1968-1987, *NZ Med J* 103(889):211, 1990.

Rosas T, Constantino N: Exercise as a treatment modality to maintain normoglycemia in gestational diabetes, *JPNN* 6(1):14, 1992.

Ruggiero L et al: Impact of social support and stress on compliance in women with gestational diabetes, *Diabetes Care* 13:441, 1990.

Speroff L: The IUD and PID, *Ob/Gyn Clinical Alert* 9(2):9, June 1992.

Spirito AL et al: Psychological impact of the diagnosis of gestational diabetes, *Obstet Gynecol* 73:562, 1989.

Tamaki H et al: Thyroxine requirement during pregnancy for replacement of hypothyroidism, *Obstet Gynecol* 76:230, 1990.

Waisbren SE, Doherty LB, Bailey IV: The New England Maternal PKU Project: identification of at-risk women, *Am J Public Health* 78:789, 1988.

York RA et al: Diabetes mellitus in pregnancy: clinical review, *J Perinatol* 10:285, 1990.

Bibliography—Nursing Research

Kemp VH, Hatmaker DD: Stress and social support in high-risk pregnancy, *Res Nurs Health* 12:331, 1989

Obrien ME, Gilson G: Detection and management of gestational diabetes in an out-of-hospital birth center, *J Nurse Midwife* 32(2):79, 1987.

Schroeder-Zwelling E, Hock R: Maternal anxiety and sensitive mothering behavior in diabetic and nondiabetic women, *Res Nurs Health* 9:245, 1986.

Scupholme A, Kamons AS: Validating change in risk criteria for a birth center: gestational diabetes, *J Nurse Midwife* 33(3):129, 1988.

chapter 31 review

Key Concepts

- Lack of maternal glycemic control before conception and in the first trimester of pregnancy may be responsible for fetal congenital malformations.
- Maternal insulin does not cross the placenta; the fetus begins to secrete its own insulin by the tenth week of gestation.
- After the tenth week of gestation, fetal hyperinsulinism results from maternal hyperglycemia (fetal hyperinsulinism is responsible for fetal disorders, discussed in Chapter 39).
- Maternal insulin requirements increase as the pregnancy progresses and may quadruple by term as a result of insulin resistance created by placental hormones, insulinase and cortisol.
- Poor glycemic control before and during pregnancy is responsible for maternal complications such as spontaneous abortion, infection, pregnancy-induced hypertension, and dystocia (difficult labor) caused by hydramnios and macrosomia.
- Home monitoring for glucose, multiple doses or constant infusion of insulin, and dietary counseling are being used to create a normal intrauterine environment for fetal growth and development in the pregnancy complicated by diabetes mellitus.
- In most cases, GDM is asymptomatic, thus reinforcing the need for routine screening of all pregnant women.
- The woman with hyperemesis gravidarum is discharged home when fluid and electrolyte balance is restored and weight gain begins.
- Thyroid dysfunction during pregnancy requires close monitoring of thyroid hormone levels to regulate therapy and prevent fetal insult.
- Maternal PKU results in CNS damage to the fetus that can be prevented or minimized by dietary restriction of phenylalanine before pregnancy.

Key Terms

- diabetes mellitus (p. 924)
- gestational diabetes mellitus (GDM) (p. 925)
- glucose tolerance test (GTT) (p. 944)
- glycosylated hemoglobin (Hb A_{1c}) (p. 932)
- hydramnios (p. 928)
- hyperemesis gravidarum (p. 949)
- hyperglycemia (p. 924)
- hyperthyroidism (p. 951)
- hypoglycemia (p. 927)
- hypothyroidism (p. 954)
- insulin (p. 924)
- intrauterine growth retardation (IUGR) (p. 931)
- ketoacidosis (p. 929)
- macrosomia (p. 931)
- maternal phenylketonuria (PKU) (p. 955)
- normoglycemia/euglycemia (p. 933)
- phenylketonuria (PKU) (p. 955)
- phosphatidylglycerol (PG) (p. 933)
- pregestational diabetes mellitus (p. 925)

Critical Thinking Exercises

1. Interview several diabetic mothers in the clinic and postpartum period. Determine their feelings about the number and inconvenience of prenatal visits, home care or hospitalizations before birth, tests undergone, and medication costs. In group discussion, present this information and discuss and compare the mothers' perceptions of their experiences.
   a. How did this exercise affect your perception of their experiences?
   b. Identify at least three interventions (e.g., physical care, teaching) that you would modify in a nursing plan of care because of your new perceptions. Justify your decisions and actions.
2. Develop a nursing plan of care for a woman with hyperemesis gravidarum, including psychologic considerations. Role-play how you would explain to a spouse/partner if therapy included restriction of visitors; critique, and amend your approach as needed. If this activity is implemented, discuss response of spouse/partner. What value, if any, was this exercise to you?

Topics for Nursing Research

- Development and evaluation of screening measures to assess client knowledge of diabetes during pregnancy
- Emotional response of the pregnant woman to the diagnosis and treatment of GDM
- Emotional response of the family to the diagnosis and treatment of GDM
- Evaluation of the effectiveness of nursing intervention on compliance with plan of care for diabetic pregnancy
- Identification of risk factors for noncompliance with the plan of care for diabetic pregnancy
- Nursing intervention in preconceptional counseling and education of diabetic women and adolescents
- Effectiveness of nursing intervention in treatment of hyperemesis gravidarum
- Screening for risk factors for hyperemesis gravidarum
- Emotional response (individual and family) to hyperemesis gravidarum.

chapter 32

Medical-Surgical Problems and Trauma

CAROL FOWLER DURHAM
CAROLYN F. McCAIN

LEARNING OBJECTIVES

- Define key terms listed.
- Explain the effects of selected disorders on pregnancy.
- Review the management of cardiovascular disorders in pregnant women.
- Discuss anemia during pregnancy.
- Explain the care of pregnant women with pulmonary disorders.
- Review the effect of gastrointestinal disorders on function during pregnancy.
- Review the effects of neurologic disorders on pregnancy.
- Review the care of women whose pregnancies are complicated by autoimmune disorders.
- Explain basic principles of care for a pregnant woman having abdominal surgery.
- Review assessment of the injured pregnant woman and planning for her care.
- Identify topics for nursing research related to medical-surgical problems and trauma.

The effects on pregnancy of selected preexisting medical disorders and the nursing care that can lead to their effective management are presented in this chapter. These conditions, which include disorders of the cardiovascular system, respiratory system, gastrointestinal system, integumentary system, and central nervous system, are sometimes first diagnosed during pregnancy.

Some surgical procedures and injuries and the related nursing roles also are discussed. Surgical interruption of pregnancy and surgical termination of fertility are discussed in Chapter 42.

■ CARDIOVASCULAR DISORDERS

Every pregnancy taxes the cardiovascular system of the mother (see Chapter 8). The strain is present during pregnancy and continues for a few weeks after birth. The normal heart can compensate for the increased workload so that pregnancy and birth generally are well tolerated.

If the cardiovascular changes are not well tolerated, cardiac failure can develop during the last few weeks of pregnancy, during labor, or during the postnatal period (Cunningham et al, 1989). In addition, if myocardial disease develops, if valvular disease exists, or if a congenital heart defect is large, **cardiac decompensation** (inability of the heart to maintain a sufficient cardiac output) is anticipated.

Some degree of cardiac impairment affects 0.5% to 3% of pregnant women (McKeon, Perrin, 1989). Heart disease is the leading cause of nonobstetric maternal mortality. It ranks fourth overall as a cause of maternal death. A maternal mortality rate of 37% is expected in women who have myocardial infarctions during pregnancy (Graber, 1989). A perinatal mortality of up to 50% is anticipated with persistent cardiac decompensation.

The degree of dysfunction (disability) of the woman with cardiac disease often is more important in the treatment and prognosis of cardiac disease complicating pregnancy than is the diagnosis of the valvular lesion per se. The New York Heart Association's functional classification of organic heart disease, a widely accepted standard, is as follows:

Class I: asymptomatic at normal levels of activity
Class II: symptomatic with increased activity
Class III: symptomatic with ordinary activity
Class IV: symptomatic at rest

No classification of heart disease can be considered rigid or absolute, but this one offers a basic practical guide for treatment, assuming that frequent prenatal visits, good client cooperation, and proper obstetric care occur. Medical therapy is conducted as a team approach with a cardiologist. The functional class of the disease is determined at 3 months and again at 7 or 8 months of gestation.

Spontaneous abortion is increased, and preterm labor and birth are more prevalent in the pregnant woman with cardiac problems. In addition, **intrauterine fetal growth retardation** (**IUGR**) (impeded or delayed development of the fetus) is common, probably because of low oxygen pressure (Po_2) in the mother.

A cardiac diagnosis depends on the history, physical examination, x-ray findings, and, if indicated, ultrasonogram results. The differential diagnosis of heart disease also involves ruling out respiratory problems, as well as other potential causes of chest pain.

Nursing Process during the Prenatal Period

The presence of cardiac disease makes the decision to become pregnant more difficult. Planned pregnancy requires that the woman understand the peripartum risks. In an unplanned pregnancy the nurse needs to explore the woman's desire to continue the pregnancy given all of the risks. The nurse should review with the woman any options for pregnancy termination if her cardiac status is tenuous.

ASSESSMENT

The pregnant woman with cardiac disease requires detailed assessment to determine the potential for optimal maternal health and a viable fetus throughout the peripartum period. If she chooses to continue the pregnancy, the woman's condition is assessed at weekly intervals.

INTERVIEW. The nurse solicits information from the woman regarding her personal medical history and that of her family. Special notation is made of diseases of cardiovascular significance, including congenital heart disease, rheumatic fever, valvular disease, endocarditis, congestive heart failure, angina, or myocardial infarction. It also is good practice to ascertain whether there is a history of streptococcal infections.

The nurse assesses for factors that would increase stress on the heart, such as anemia (see p. 974), infection, and edema. In reviewing the symptoms, the nurse should assess how the client is adapting to the physiologic changes of pregnancy.

In assessing the pregnant woman with a cardiovascular disorder, the nurse needs to pay special attention to the review of the cardiovascular and pulmonary systems. The nurse should determine whether the client has experienced chest pain at rest or on exertion, edema of the face, hands, or feet, hypertension, heart murmurs, palpitations, paroxysmal nocturnal dyspnea, diaphoresis, pallor, or syncope. Pulmonary symptoms such as cough, hemoptysis, shortness of breath, and orthopnea can be signs of cardiac disease.

The nurse documents all medication taken by the client—including supplemental iron—and is alert to their potential side effects and interactions.

The nurse must assess the client for undue emotional stress that might further compromise her cardiac status. Examples are depression, anxiety/fear of morbidity or mortality for herself and her fetus, financial concerns related to extended hospitalization, anger because of impaired social interaction, and feelings of inadequacy regarding her inability to meet family and household demands.

The client's cultural background may affect the amount of support that she is able to receive from significant others. Family size (number of children and extended family members in the home), as well as role expectations within the family, may be dictated by cultural norms. For the woman with cardiac impairment, this may prove to be a cause of major stress if she is unable to bear the expected number of children or if it is unacceptable to receive help with domestic chores.

PHYSICAL EXAMINATION. The routine assessment continues during the prenatal period, including monitoring weight gain and pattern of weight gain, edema, vital signs, and discomforts of pregnancy.

The client is observed for signs of cardiac decompensation, that is, progressive generalized edema, crackles (rales) at the base of the lungs, or pulse irregularity (see box above). Symptoms of cardiac decompensation may appear abruptly or gradually. Medical intervention must be instituted immediately to correct cardiac status. Unfortunately dyspnea, palpitations, syncope, and edema occur commonly in pregnant women and can mask the symptoms of a developing or worsening cardiovascular disorder. A woman's sudden inability to perform activities that she previously was comfortable doing may indicate cardiovascular decompensation.

LABORATORY/DIAGNOSTIC TESTS. Routine urinalysis and blood work (complete blood cell count and blood chemistry) are done during the initial visit. The woman with cardiac impairment requires a baseline electrocardiogram (ECG) at the beginning of her pregnancy, which permits vital diagnostic comparisons of subsequent ECGs. Echocardiograms and pulse oximetry studies may be performed as indicated. Chest films may be necessary during late pregnancy provided the abdomen is carefully shielded. In addition, fetal ultrasound, fetal movement studies, or fetal nonstress tests may be employed to determine fetal well-being.

Warning Signs—Cardiac Decompensation

PREGNANT WOMAN: SUBJECTIVE SYMPTOMS

- Increasing fatigue or difficulty breathing, or both, with her usual activities
- Feeling of smothering
- Frequent cough
- Palpitations; feeling that her heart is "racing"
- Swelling of face, feet, legs, fingers (e.g., rings do not fit anymore)

NURSE: OBJECTIVE SIGNS

- Irregular weak, rapid pulse (≥100 beats/min)
- Progressive, generalized edema
- Crackles (rales) at base of lungs, after two inspirations and exhalations
- Orthopnea; increasing dyspnea
- Rapid respirations (≥25 breaths/min)
- Moist, frequent cough
- Cyanosis of lips and nail beds

NURSING DIAGNOSES

The following examples are some prenatal nursing diagnoses that may be formulated. As always, individualization of diagnoses is vital.

- Fear related to
  —Increased peripartum risk
- High risk for ineffective individual/family coping related to
  —Woman's cardiac condition
- High risk for altered tissue perfusion related to
  —Hypotensive syndrome
- High risk for activity intolerance related to
  —Cardiac condition
- Knowledge deficit related to
  —Cardiac condition
  —Requirements to alter self-care activities
- High risk for self-care deficit related to
  —Activity intolerance
- Impaired home maintenance management related to
  —Mother's confinement to bed and/or limited activity level

PLANNING

The nursing diagnoses derived from analyses of clinical findings act as guides to the development of a plan of care. This plan addresses the specific needs of the client. Client stressors need to be limited across all four classifications of heart disease. Physiologic cardiac stress is greatest between gestation weeks 28 and 32.

CLASS I. The pregnant woman with class I heart disease should limit stress to protect against cardiac decompensation. Additional rest (at night and after meals), frequent evaluations, and the early and effective treatment of respiratory and other infections should be emphasized. Therapeutic abortion is never medically warranted.

CLASS II. A program similar to that for class I should be followed for the pregnant woman with class II heart disease. However, the woman should be admitted to the hospital near term (earlier if signs of cardiac overload or arrhythmia develop) for evaluation and treatment.

CLASS III. Bed rest for much of each day is necessary for pregnant women with class III cardiac disease. About 30% of these women experience cardiac decompensation during pregnancy. With this possibility the woman may require hospitalization for the remainder of the pregnancy. Early therapeutic abortion may be suggested, particularly in a woman who has experienced a previous cardiac failure.

CLASS IV. Because decompensation occurs even at rest in persons with class IV cardiac disease, a major initial effort must be made to improve the cardiac status of pregnant women in this category. Early therapeutic abortion, although not without risk, may be feasible with regional anesthesia in some cases. Prophylactic antibiotic therapy may be ordered with the procedure.

GOALS. The mother with cardiovascular problems faces curtailment of her activities. The restrictions can have physical and emotional implications. The community health nurse, social worker, and pediatrician are some of the resource people whose services may need to be incorporated into the plan of care. *Goals* such as the following might be appropriate.

- Woman and family verbalize understanding of the disorder, management, and probable outcome.
- Woman and family describe their role in management, including when and how to take medication, adjust diet, and prepare for and participate in treatment.
- Woman and family cope with emotional reactions to pregnancy and infant at risk.
- Woman is able to withstand the physiologic stressors of pregnancy.
- Woman is able to reach term pregnancy or the point of fetal viability.

IMPLEMENTATION

Therapy is focused on minimizing stress on the heart. Factors that increase the risk of cardiac decompensation are treated. The workload of the cardiovascular system is reduced by appropriate treatment of any coexisting emotional stress, hypertension, anemia, hyperthyroidism, or obesity.

Signs and symptoms of cardiac decompensation are reviewed during the prenatal period. The woman requires 8 to 10 hours of sleep every day and should take 30-minute naps after eating. Her activities are restricted, with housework, shopping, and exercise limited to the amount allowed for her functional classification of heart disease.

Infections are treated promptly because respiratory, urinary, or gastrointestinal tract infections can complicate the condition by accelerating heart rate and by direct spread of organisms (e.g., streptococci) to the heart structure. The woman should notify her physician at the first sign of infection or exposure to an infection. Hospitalization may be required until the infection is cured. Clients who have had valvuloplasty should receive penicillin or other antibiotic prophylaxis against bacterial endocarditis during gestation.

Nutrition counseling is necessary, optimally with the woman's family present. The pregnant woman needs a diet high in iron and protein and adequate in calories to gain weight. The iron supplements tend to cause constipation. It is important for the cardiac woman to avoid straining during defecation, thus causing a **Valsalva's maneuver** (forced expiration against a closed airway, which when released causes blood to rush to the heart and overload the cardiac system) (see also discussion on p. 368 and p. 970). Sodium intake is restricted and accompanied by careful monitoring for hyponatremia. The sodium ion, with its ability to attract and hold fluid, affects the quality and the amount of the circulating volume. The woman's intake of potassium is monitored to prevent hypokalemia. Hypokalemia is associated with heart and other muscular weakness and dysfunction.

Cardiac medications are prescribed as needed for

the pregnant woman, with attention to fetal well-being. Propranolol is considered relatively safe for use in pregnancy, but it is associated with fetal bradycardia, diminished uterine blood flow, and increased uterine irritability. Lidocaine is considered safe for use during pregnancy as long as toxic levels are avoided (McKeon, Perrin, 1989). Calcium channel blockers (e.g., diltiazem, verapamil) have been shown to be teratogenic and embryotoxic in rats and mice, but studies in pregnant women have not been adequate (Graber, 1989).

If anticoagulant therapy is required during pregnancy, *heparin* should be used because this large-molecule drug does not cross the placenta as readily as warfarin. Even though heparin is the anticoagulant of choice, its use is not without risk. Heparin use can result in maternal hemorrhage, preterm birth, and stillbirth. Oral anticoagulants, such as warfarin (Coumadin) compounds, cross to the fetus and may cause anomalies or hemorrhage in the infant. The nurse should closely monitor the woman's blood work, including clotting factors.

The woman may need to learn to self-administer heparin. She also requires specific nutritional teaching to avoid foods high in vitamin K, such as raw, deep-green and leafy vegetables, which counteract the effects of the heparin. In addition, she will require a substitute source of folic acid in her diet.

Tests for fetal maturity and well-being, as well as placental sufficiency, may be necessary. Other therapy is directly related to the functional classification of heart disease. It may be important that the nurse reinforce the need for close medical supervision. In addition, information about the management of labor and birth and the postpartum period allows the woman time to make plans for necessary extra care.

CARDIOPULMONARY RESUSCITATION OF THE PREGNANT WOMAN. Trauma, pulmonary embolism, anesthesia complications, drug overdose, hypovolemia, or septic shock may result in cardiopulmonary arrest. Preexisting disorders, such as heart or pulmonary disease, hypertension, or autoimmune collagen vascular disease, increase this risk (Troiano, 1989). Some modifications of the procedure for cardiopulmonary resuscitation (CPR) and the Heimlich maneuver are needed (Fig. 32-1). To prevent supine hypotension, the woman is positioned on a flat firm surface, with the uterus displaced laterally (manually or with a wedge or rolled towel under her right hip).

Complications may be associated with CPR of a pregnant woman. These complications may include laceration of the liver, rupture of the uterus, hemothorax, or hemoperitoneum (Troiano, 1989). Fetal complications also may occur. These include cardiac arrhythmia or asystole related to maternal defibrillation and medications; central nervous system (CNS) depression related to antiarrhythmic drugs and inadequate uteroplacental perfusion; and onset of preterm labor.

After successful resuscitation, the woman and her fetus must receive careful monitoring. She remains at increased risk for recurrent pulmonary arrest and arrhythmias (ventricular tachycardia, supraventricular tachycardia, bradycardia). Therefore her cardiovascular, pulmonary, and neurologic status should be assessed continuously. Uterine activity and resting tone must be monitored. Fetal status and gestational

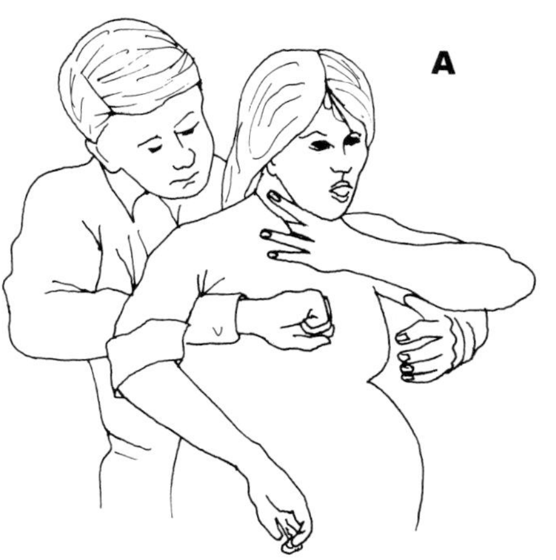

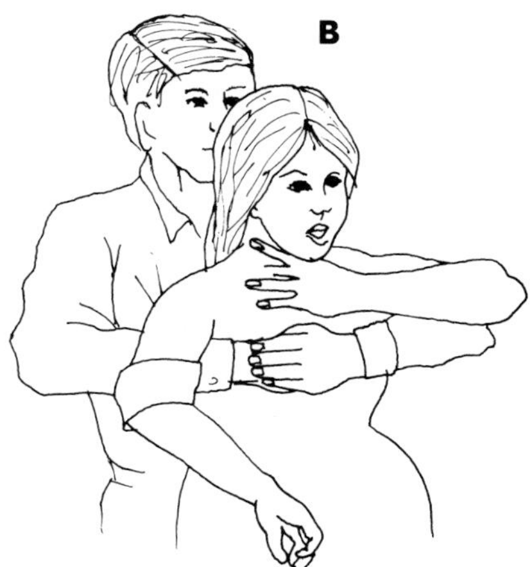

Fig. 32-1 Clearing an airway obstruction and performing chest compressions. **A,** Place top of clenched fist against middle of sternum; place other hand on top of clenched fist. Perform chest thrusts until the obstruction is expelled or woman loses consciousness. **B,** If woman is unconscious, give chest compressions as for woman without a pulse.

age should be determined. All assessment data influence both the medical and nursing plans of care.

HEART SURGERY DURING PREGNANCY. Operations for the correction of congenital or acquired heart disease should be performed before pregnancy if possible. Closed cardiac surgery, such as release of a stenotic mitral orifice, can be accomplished with little risk to mother or fetus. However, open heart surgery requires extracorporeal circulation, and under these circumstances, hypoxia may develop. As a consequence the risk of fetal damage or loss rises to 10% to 20%, thought to result from the nonpulsatile circulation created by the extracorporeal pump (Graber, 1989).

Some women who are free of symptoms after earlier cardiac surgery undergo significant deterioration during pregnancy. The normal hemodynamic demands of pregnancy compromise their cardiac status. For these clients, therapeutic abortion, if acceptable to the client and her family, is advised before the hemodynamic demands fully manifest. There is an increased incidence of spontaneous abortion, stillborns, low-birth-weight infants, and malformed fetuses to women with valvular heart disease.

EVALUATION

The nurse uses the following criteria as *overall indications* for the success of therapy.

- The woman and family verbalize understanding of the disorder, management, and probable outcome.
- The woman and family describe their role in management, including when and how to take medication, adjust diet, and prepare for treatment.
- The woman and family participate in treatment.
- The woman and family cope with emotional reactions to pregnancy and an infant at risk.
- The woman is able to tolerate the stresses imposed by pregnancy; these include increase in pulse rate by 10 beats/min, expansion of blood volume by 25%, and psychologic stress common to pregnancy and related to the heart condition.
- The woman is able to reach term pregnancy or the point of viability of the fetus.

See the case study (p. 967) and plan of care (p. 968) for a pregnant woman with heart disease.

Nursing Process during the Intrapartum Period

The intrapartum period for all pregnant women is the one that evokes the most apprehension. The woman with impaired cardiac function has additional reasons to be anxious. One of the aspects of the nurse's role is to decrease anxiety of the client and her family.

ASSESSMENT

Nursing care during the intrapartum period focuses on the promotion and maintenance of cardiac function. Assessment for signs of cardiac decompensation and fetal distress, precipitated by the stressors of labor and birth, is crucial.

INTERVIEW. If a prenatal history is unavailable and the client's condition allows, the nurse should obtain the same data as outlined in the prenatal interview (see p. 962).

In addition to the data obtained during the prenatal interview, the woman should be questioned at the onset of labor about cardiovascular manifestations since her last appointment.

Support by a significant other can decrease anxiety and physical tension and consequently the workload on the heart. The nurse needs to assess the presence of an effective labor coach and provide nursing care accordingly.

A woman's response to the stress of labor often is influenced by cultural factors. The nurse needs to be accepting of the individual's learned response to pain and help her to remain in control.

PHYSICAL EXAMINATION. During the intrapartum period, assessment includes the routine assessments for all laboring women, as well as assessments for cardiac decompensation. The latter include taking vital signs at least every 10 to 30 minutes. The color and temperature of the skin are noted. The woman is carefully watched for symptoms of emotional stress.

The physician is alerted if the pulse rate is 100 beats/min minute or greater, or if respirations are 25 breaths/min or greater. Respiratory status is checked constantly for developing dyspnea, coughing, or crackles (rales) at the base of the lungs. Pallor, cooling, and sweating may indicate cardiac shock.

LABORATORY/DIAGNOSTIC TESTS. Routine urinalysis and blood work should be completed for the intrapartum woman. Arterial blood gases (ABG) may be needed to ensure adequate oxygenation. A Swan-Ganz catheter may be inserted to accurately monitor hemodynamic status during labor and birth (see Chapter 30). ECG monitoring and continuous monitoring of blood pressure will be instituted. Continuous fetal monitoring during labor also is implemented in high-risk cases.

CASE STUDY

Childbearing Client with Heart Disease

Sarah Hargrove is a 24-year-old married woman in her first pregnancy. She has a history of rheumatic heart disease. Sarah works full time and also cares for her elderly mother-in-law who lives with Sarah and her husband. Sarah comes to the clinic for her regular prenatal visit at 28 weeks of gestation.

ASSESSMENT

Sarah complains of shortness of breath during her regular activities and of increased fatigue. She says she has trouble keeping up with her work and with household demands. Physical assessment reveals that Sarah's pulse rate is 100 beats/min, respirations are 26/min, rales are present in the base of her lungs, and there is edema of the lower extremities. A review of laboratory results reveals that hematocrit and white blood cell levels are within normal limits; urine specific gravity is increased.

NURSING DIAGNOSIS

On the basis of the physical assessment data and Sarah's complaints, the nurse identifies the *nursing diagnosis:* activity intolerance related to the effects of pregnancy (increased circulatory volume) in the presence of her cardiac condition.

PLANNING

A plan of care is developed with Sarah. The agreed-upon *goal* for Sarah is that she will monitor activity tolerance/intolerance and will take appropriate actions to avoid further development of cardiac decompensation. *Expected outcomes* are that Sarah will reduce her physical activities, sleep at least 8 hours a night, and take rest periods during the day; she will experience less shortness of breath and fatigue by the next clinic visit.

IMPLEMENTATION

Nursing actions are based on the nursing diagnosis, the medical diagnosis, and standards for care. Specific interventions include assisting Sarah with restructuring her daily routines to reduce physical activity and to include adequate sleep and rest periods, as well as teaching Sarah to assess for signs of worsening cardiac condition.

EVALUATION

The expected outcomes were used to evaluate the effectiveness of these interventions. Sarah reported getting 8 hours of sleep at night in addition to resting after meals; she reduced her hours at work and did only essential housework. She reported less fatigue and fewer episodes of shortness of breath. Although continued assessment for respiratory and/or circulatory involvement will be important for Sarah during the rest of her pregnancy, this goal was met.

NURSING DIAGNOSES

The following examples of intrapartum nursing diagnoses can be individualized according to the client's needs:

- Anxiety related to
  —Fear for infant's safety
- Fear of dying related to
  —Perceived physiologic inability to cope with the stress of labor
- High risk for impaired gas exchange related to
  —Cardiac condition
- High risk for fluid volume excess related to
  —Extravascular fluid shifts

PLANNING

On the basis of the individualized nursing diagnoses, the nurse will plan strategies to decrease the cardiac woman's physiologic and emotional stress during labor and birth to achieve *goals* such as those that follow.

- The woman verbalizes her fear over infant safety and her own mortality.
- The woman adapts to physiologic stressors of labor and birth.
- The woman is able to reach term pregnancy or the point of viability of the fetus.

IMPLEMENTATION

Anxiety is alleviated by maintaining a calm atmosphere in the labor and birth rooms. The nurse provides anticipatory guidance by keeping the woman and her family informed of labor progress and events that will probably occur. The woman's preferred method of prenatal childbirth/parent education preparation should be supported to the degree it is feasible for her cardiac condition. Nursing techniques

CARE PLAN Childbearing Client with Heart Disease

GOALS	IMPLEMENTATION	RATIONALE	EVALUATION
Nursing diagnosis: Activity intolerance related to the effects of pregnancy in the presence of cardiac condition			
Sarah will monitor activity tolerance/intolerance and will take appropriate actions to avoid further development of cardiac decompensation. Sarah will reduce physical activities, sleep at least 8 hours a night, and take rest periods during the day; she will experience less shortness of breath and fatigue by the next clinic visit.	Assist Sarah to restructure her daily activities to include adequate rest/sleep periods. Teach Sarah to assess for signs of worsening cardiac condition.	Activity is limited to the extent of the cardiac disease. Adequate rest and sleep minimize cardiac stress and conserve energy. Development of signs indicate a worsening of the client's condition.	Sarah reported getting 8 hours of sleep at night and rested after meals. Sarah reduced her work hours and did only essential housework. At her next clinic visit, Sarah reported less fatigue and shortness of breath. Sarah will continue to need close assessment for respiratory and/or circulatory impairment for the remainder of her pregnancy.
Nursing diagnosis: Ineffective individual coping related to inability to meet role expectations secondary to pregnancy and its effects on her cardiac condition			
Sarah and her family verbalize understanding of Sarah's physical limitations and identify effective coping techniques.	Encourage Sarah's husband to accompany her to clinic. Provide information about effects of pregnancy on women with cardiac disease and the need to limit activities. Encourage verbalization of feelings. Offer information about community resources.	Including family in clinic visits promotes their understanding of the client's disease and impresses on them the necessity of limiting physical activities. Information can help families determine if and how needs can be met by resources outside the family.	Sarah's husband accompanies her to clinic. He verbalizes understanding of the need for Sarah to cut back on her work hours and to have help at home. A home health aide is employed to assist Sarah's mother-in-law three times a week. Sarah states she feels supported and better able to cope with her limitations.

CARE PLAN Childbearing Client with Heart Disease—cont'd

GOALS	IMPLEMENTATION	RATIONALE	EVALUATION
Nursing diagnosis: High risk for alteration in tissue perfusion related to cardiac condition secondary to increased circulatory needs during pregnancy			
Sarah's BP, pulse, ABG and WBC values are WNL. The fetus is reactive with FHR WNL.	Monitor BP, pulse. Assess for signs of decompensation and hypoxia. Review signs of cardiac failure with Sarah. Monitor laboratory values, especially WBC, Hb/HCT, ABG. Assess FHR, perform NST as indicated. Provide information on using a modified upright position for sleeping.	Tachycardia and increased BP may indicate early heart failure/hypoxia. These are late signs of hypoxia and may indicate severe cardiac compromise. Uteroplacental insufficiency causes hypoxia, resulting in decreased fetal activity. Normal ABG values reflect adequate ventilation and oxygenation; anemia can reduce oxygen-carrying power of the blood; infections can increase the metabolic rate and oxygen needs. Eases respiratory rate by decreasing pressure of uterus on diaphragm and increases lung expansion.	Sarah's condition does not worsen. Her BP and pulse remain WNL as do her laboratory values. Sarah reports her fetus is active, and NST results are reactive. Sarah will continue weekly clinic visits for close supervision of her cardiac status and fetal status until the birth.
Nursing diagnosis: High risk for alteration (decompensation) in cardiac output related to increased circulatory volume secondary to pregnancy			
Sarah will maintain adequate perfusion and will not experience fluid overload as exhibited by stable BP, clear lung fields, and regular pulse rate between 60-100 beats/min. Sarah will exhibit no edema and will have adequate urine output.	Provide information about adequate rest, especially in the left lateral position. Assess for edema; teach Sarah to elevate her legs when sitting. Assess intake and output. Administer medications if ordered.	Tachycardia and increased BP may be related to early cardiac decompensation. Rest minimizes cardiac stress; lateral position increases uterine blood flow and also prevents supine hypotension. Elevating the legs promotes venous return. Cardiac disease may cause kidney problems (anuria, oliguria); intake and output should be about the same.	Sarah does not develop cardiac decompensation. Her BP and pulse remain WNL; her intake and output are about the same, and no oliguria is present. Sarah states that "the baby moves a lot!" and nursing assessments of FHR range from 140-150 beats/min. Sarah gets 8 hours of sleep at night and rests after meals with her feet elevated. Sarah's condition will need continued assessment for the duration of pregnancy.
The fetus will be reactive, and FHR will be in normal range.	Evaluate fetal status (FHR, daily fetal movement counts, NST results).	Fetal hypoxia can occur, causing bradycardia, tachycardia, and decreased fetal activity.	

ABG, Arterial blood gases; *BP,* blood pressure; *FHR,* fetal heart rate; *Hb,* hemoglobin; *HCT,* hematocrit; *NST,* nonstress test; *WBC,* white blood cell count, *WNL,* within normal limits.

that promote comfort, such as back massage, are used.

Cardiac function is supported by keeping the woman's head and shoulders elevated and body parts resting on pillows. Bearing down (Valsalva's maneuver) must be avoided because it reduces diastolic ventricular filling and obstructs left ventricular outflow (Scott et al, 1990). The left side–lying position usually facilitates hemodynamics during labor and birth.

Discomfort is relieved with medication and supportive care. For birth the nurse will assist in the administration of pharmacologic relief of discomfort. Epidural regional anesthesia provides better pain relief than do narcotics and causes fewer alterations in hemodynamics (Cunningham et al, 1989). *Hypotension must be avoided.*

The woman may require other types of medication (e.g., anticoagulants, prophylactic antibiotics). If evidence of cardiac decompensation appears, the physician may order deslanoside (Cedilanid-D) for rapid digitalization,* furosemide (Lasix) for rapid diuresis, and oxygen by intermittent positive pressure to decrease the development of pulmonary edema.

Beta-adrenergic agents (i.e., ritodrine and terbutaline) should not be used for tocolysis. These are associated with myocardial ischemia. Syntocinon, a synthetic oxytocin, can be used for induction of labor (see Chapter 35). This drug does not appear to cause significant coronary artery constriction in doses prescribed for labor induction or control of postpartum uterine atony.

Birth is accomplished with the woman in the left side–lying position to facilitate uterine perfusion, or if the supine position is used, a pad is positioned under the right hip to minimize the danger of supine hypotension. The knees are flexed, and the feet are flat on the bed. To prevent compression of popliteal veins and an increase in blood volume in the chest and trunk as a result of the effects of gravity, stirrups are not used. Episiotomy and the use of outlet forceps also decrease the work of the heart.

The classification of heart disease affects the management of care.

CLASS I. If there are no obstetric problems, vaginal birth is recommended. This is accomplished by use of pudendal block anesthesia with forceps to shorten the second stage of labor.

CLASS II. Penicillin prophylaxis may be ordered for nonallergic pregnant women to protect against bacterial endocarditis in labor and during the early puerperium. Mask oxygen and regional block anesthesia are important. Ergot products should not be used because they increase blood pressure. Dilute intravenous oxytocin immediately after birth may be employed to prevent postbirth hemorrhage. Tubal sterilization may be performed, but surgery is delayed several days at least to ensure homeostasis. If sterilization is not achieved, effective contraception must be provided.

CLASS III. The woman will likely be hospitalized before the onset of labor. Labor and birth are managed similarly to the plan for women with class II cardiac disease. Breast-feeding is contraindicated because lactation requires considerable energy. Sterilization should be postponed until a later date, but explicit contraceptive advice must be given.

CLASS IV. Vaginal birth by women with class IV disease is the safest approach if abortion is not performed. Maternal mortality approaches 50%; the perinatal mortality is even higher. Treatment of the pregnant woman is similar to that of women with class II disease.

EVALUATION

The nurse uses the following criteria as overall indications for the success of the intrapartum therapy.

- The woman verbalizes her fear regarding her personal and her infant's safety and mortality.
- The woman adapts to physiologic stressors of labor and birth, and such crises as congestive heart failure—the primary cause of maternal mortality in women with cardiac disease—are prevented.
- The woman gives birth to a healthy newborn.

Nursing Process during the Postpartum Period

ASSESSMENT

Monitoring for cardiac decompensation continues through the first week after birth because of hormonal shifts that affect hemodynamics. These shifts have been known to occur as late as the seventh postpartum day.

INTERVIEW. In addition to the data obtained during the prenatal and intrapartum interviews, significant

*Care must be taken with digitalization because digitalis can be highly toxic to pregnant women.

events that occurred during the course of labor and birth are added.

Routine postpartum assessments are included in the review of systems. As for any postpartum woman, routine assessment is done. These assessments include vital signs, amount and character of bleeding, uterine contractility, urinary output, pain, activity/rest pattern, diet, and daily weights.

It is important to assess the woman's support systems because activity will be curtailed until the cardiac system is recovered. The mother may not be directly involved in the infant's care for a period of time because of such factors as prematurity of the infant and the health of the mother.

The mother's/family's response to the birth and the infant needs to be observed. The woman's/couple's expectations for postpartal sexual activity and birth control need to be discussed in relation to her cardiovascular condition.

PHYSICAL EXAMINATION. As for the healthy woman, routine postpartum assessment is performed. The immediate postbirth period is hazardous for a woman whose heart function is compromised. Cardiac output increases rapidly as extravascular fluid is remobilized into the vascular compartment. At the moment of birth, intraabdominal pressure is reduced drastically; pressure on veins is removed, the splanchnic vessels engorge, and blood flow to the heart is increased. When blood flow increases to the heart, a **reflex bradycardia** may result. Fluid begins to move from the extravascular spaces into the blood stream.

Special attention is given to the woman who is at risk for cardiac decompensation. The increased intravascular fluid can cause fluid volume excess in these women. Some physicians favor the application of the abdominal binder or alternating tourniquets on the extremities to minimize the effects of this rapid change in intraabdominal pressure. Hemorrhage or infection, or both, may worsen the cardiac condition.

LABORATORY/DIAGNOSTIC TESTS. Laboratory (e.g., hemoglobin, hematocrit, and urinalysis) results are monitored, and abnormalities are reported to the physician. In addition, the woman with a cardiac condition may continue to require a Swan-Ganz catheter and ABG monitoring. The client requires frequent assessment of vital signs and strict monitoring of intake and output.

NURSING DIAGNOSES

The following nursing diagnoses that are applicable to the postpartum woman are chosen and, as always, individualized:

- Self-care deficit related to
  - —Fatigue
  - —Need for bed rest
- Situational low self-esteem related to
  - —Restriction placed on involvement in care of infant
- Ineffective breast-feeding related to
  - —Fatigue from cardiac condition
- High risk for altered parenting related to
  - —Inadequate bonding

PLANNING

Care in the postpartum period is tailored to the woman's functional capacity. Special attention to bowel and bladder elimination is required. The mother-child interactions receive special planning. The interactions should not stress the mother. Before discharge the nurse assesses the home support for the woman and infant. Preparation for discharge is carefully planned with the woman and family. Provision of help for the mother in the home by relatives, friends, and others must be addressed. If necessary, the nurse refers the family to community resources (e.g., for homemaking services). Rest and sleep periods, activity, and diet must be planned. The couple will want information about reestablishing sexual relations, contraception, and sterilization of the man or the woman (especially if the woman's condition is classified as II, III, or IV). *Goals* include those that follow.

- The woman will remain free of congestive heart failure during the postpartum period.
- The woman and her family understand the necessity of help with home management.
- The woman receives assistance with activities of daily living, breast-feeding (if allowed), and infant care.
- The woman will exhibit bonding behavior with her infant.

IMPLEMENTATION

Postpartum positioning of the woman with cardiac disease is the same as that for labor; that is, the head of the bed is elevated and the woman is encouraged to lie on her side. Bed rest may be ordered, with or without bathroom privileges. The nurse may need to help the woman meet her grooming and hygiene needs and even help her with turning in bed, eating, and other activities. Respiratory and cardiovascular sequelae to immobility, as well as boredom, must be addressed. Progressive ambulation may be permitted as tolerated. The nurse assesses the woman's affect, pulse rate, breath sounds, coughing, edema, and skin color, temperature, and dryness (e.g., pink, warm, and dry or pale, cool, and clammy) before and after walking.

Bowel movements without stress or strain are promoted with stool softeners, diet, and fluids, plus mild analgesia and local anesthetic spray. Overdistention of the bladder is prevented. A distended bladder can result in an atonic uterus and hemorrhage. Anemia may result. Anemia adds additional stress to cardiac function. However, rapid emptying of the bladder is avoided. Rapid decompression of the bladder results in a precipitous drop in intraabdominal pressure, leading to splanchnic engorgement and generalized hypotension. The woman must be protected from infection. A private room is one method to restrict traffic into her room.

The mother may direct a designated family member in the care of the infant. The mother can breastfeed if her condition warrants. That is, women in classes I and II may breast-feed; those whose functional capacity is classified as class III or IV are advised against breast-feeding.

The fed baby can be brought regularly to the mother, held at her eye level and by her lips, and brought to her fingers so she can establish an emotional bond with her baby with a low expenditure of her energy. At the same time, involving the mother passively in her infant's care helps the mother feel vitally important—as she is—to the infant's well-being (e.g., "You can offer something no one else can: provide your baby with your sounds, touch, and rhythms that are so comforting"). Perhaps the mother can be encouraged to make a tape recording of her talking, singing, or whispering, which can be played for the baby in the nursery to help the infant feel her presence and be in contact with her voice.

EVALUATION

The nurse uses the following criteria as overall indications for the success of postpartum therapy.

- The woman adapts to the physiologic stressors of pregnancy; for example, she is free of congestive heart failure during the postpartum period.
- The home situation is controlled, with assistance provided as necessary.
- The mother and family accept the limitations imposed on the woman by the presence of heart disease.
- The parent-child relationship is fostered by the family.

ASSOCIATED CARDIOVASCULAR DISORDERS

Nursing care of the woman with cardiovascular disorders combines routine peripartum care with care specific for the cardiac diagnosis. (See section on cardiovascular obstetric nursing, p. 962.) Cardiac conditions vary in their impact on pregnancy because of acuteness or chronicity. The following discussion focuses on peripartum heart failure, rheumatic heart disease, infective endocarditis, mitral valve prolapse, Marfan's syndrome, and cerebrovascular accidents.

Peripartum Heart Failure

Peripartum heart failure (failure of the heart to maintain an adequate circulation of blood) can result from an underlying chronic hypertension, previously unrecognized mitral valve stenosis, obesity, viral myocarditis, or idiopathic peripartum cardiomyopathy (Cunningham et al, 1989). In addition, anemia and infection can predispose the woman to congestive heart failure.

Peripartum heart failure from an explainable cause such as an underlying heart disease usually responds well to therapy. The typical response is rapid reversal of heart failure with furosemide (Lasix) diuresis and correction of associated obstetric complications (Cunningham et al, 1989). Within days the heart size of these women returns to normal; their long-term prognosis depends on the underlying heart disease (e.g., hypertrophic cardiomyopathy).

Cardiomyopathy, a disease of the heart muscle, can be either primary (not attributed to another disease) or secondary (heart muscle disease attributed to a known or suspected cause). Hypertrophic cardiomyopathy is an example of primary disease, and idiopathic peripartum cardiomyopathy is an example of secondary disease.

Hypertrophic cardiomyopathy (HCM) is a primary disease, classified on the basis of its structural abnormality and function. In this disorder the muscle tissue of the heart walls and the septum are hypertrophied, leaving relatively small chambers. HCM usually is asymptomatic until late adolescence or early adulthood or, more rarely, in middle age. Symptoms include angina, exertional dyspnea, dizziness, syncope, ventricular arrhythmias, S_4 gallop, and mild cardiomegaly. HCM is associated with sudden death, unrelated to functional status. HCM may be precipitated by physical or emotional stress, and the myocardial ischemia resulting from stress may promote ventricular fibrillation. Propranolol is given if symptoms develop (Cunningham et al, 1989).

Idiopathic peripartum cardiomyopathy comprises a syndrome of heart failure (1) occurring during the peripartum period, (2) with no previous history of heart disease, and (3) with no specific etiologic factors. Autoimmune factors may be implicated (Lee, Cotton, 1989). Idiopathic cardiomyopathy in nonpregnant persons results in death in more than 75% from unrelenting cardiomegaly (enlarged heart) and heart failure (Homans, 1985).

The incidence of peripartum cardiomyopathies has been reported as 1/3000 to 4000 pregnancies. It occurs more often in the multiparous woman. Maternal mortality has been estimated in the range of 30% to 60%, whereas infant mortality is approximately 10%. Clinical findings are those of congestive heart failure (left ventricular failure). Signs include breathlessness, tachyarrhythmias, and edema, with radiologic findings of cardiomegaly (Fig. 32-2). The prognosis is good if cardiomegaly does not persist after 6 months. The prognosis for women whose hearts remain enlarged after 6 months of bed rest is not as favorable. Future pregnancies usually result in some cardiac failure (50% to 88%). In subsequent pregnancy, mortality has been estimated as high as 60%. Sterilization should be considered. Oral contraceptives are contraindicated because of the risk of thromboembolism.

Medical management of cardiomyopathy during pregnancy is similar to that for a pregnant woman with myocardial ischemia. Bed rest is advocated up to 7 months, with some women requiring 20 to 22 months. The bed rest is prescribed from the onset of the disease until 3 months after the heart returns to normal size. The rationale for instituting bed rest is to decrease the heart rate, stroke volume, and arterial pressure—the overall work of the heart. Prevention and treatment of arrhythmias are major goals. Antiarrhythmic drugs or beta-adrenergic or calcium channel blockers are used. Digitalis and nitrates are contraindicated in the obstructive form of HCM.

Low sodium intake (1.5 to 2 g/day) is ordered for women with severe congestive failure. During labor, the avoidance of intravenous fluid overload is important. Because all women experience some rise in blood pressure at the onset of lactation, suppression of lactation is recommended to minimize stress.

The nursing care of clients with peripartum cardiomyopathies is essentially the same as for those with other types of cardiac problems. The use of Trendelenburg's position for relief of syncope has been demonstrated. The necessity for prolonged bed rest can pose social and economic hardships for the family; therefore referral to community resources for assistance may be necessary. Because sudden death is a

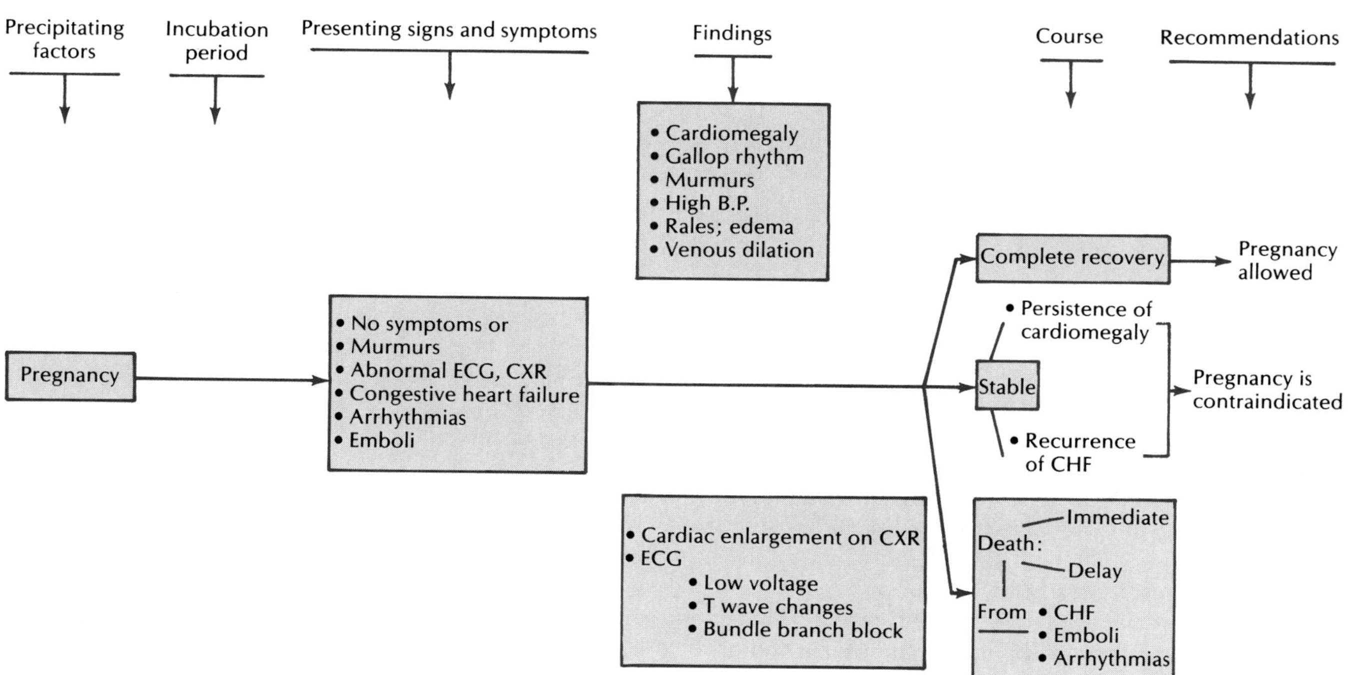

Fig. 32-2 Summary of course of peripartum cardiomyopathy.
From Veille JC: Peripartum cardiomyopathies: a review, *Am J Obstet Gynecol* 148:805, 1984.

feature of this condition, the family needs to be trained in cardiopulmonary resuscitation. Clients need to have ready access to emergency care.

Rheumatic Heart Disease

Rheumatic fever usually develops suddenly, several symptom-free weeks after an inadequately treated group A beta-hemolytic streptococcal infection. Episodes of rheumatic fever create an autoimmune reaction in the heart tissue, leading to permanent damage of heart valves (usually the mitral valve) and the chorda tendineae cordis. This damage is referred to as **rheumatic heart disease.** Rheumatic heart disease may be evident during acute rheumatic fever or discovered years later. Recurrences of rheumatic fever are common, each with the potential to increase the severity of heart damage. Heart murmurs, resulting from stenosis, valvular insufficiency, or thickening of the walls of the heart, characterize rheumatic heart disease. Abnormal pulse rate and rhythm, as well as congestive heart failure, are common.

Mitral valve stenosis accounts for 90% of rheumatic heart disease seen in pregnancy (Scott et al, 1990) and is the most important lesion hemodynamically (Brady, Duff, 1989). Even though a history of rheumatic fever may be absent, it remains the most likely cause of mitral stenosis. A tight stenosis, plus the increase in blood volume and cardiac output of normal pregnancy (see Chapter 8), may cause ventricular failure and pulmonary edema; hemoptysis may occur. Atrial fibrillation is common because of the enlarged left atrium. Cardiac failure occurs for the first time during pregnancy in 25% of women with mitral valve stenosis. Digoxin prophylaxis may be warranted. Atrial fibrillation also predisposes the woman to thromboembolism, especially in cerebral vessels (Brady, Duff, 1989), necessitating the use of heparin therapy. The care of the woman with mitral stenosis typically is managed by reducing her activity and increasing bed rest. Prophylaxis for intrapartum endocarditis and pulmonary infections usually is provided. Epidural anesthesia for labor and avoidance of intravenous fluid overload are appropriate (Cunningham et al, 1989). Mitral valvotomy during pregnancy often brings dramatic relief of congestive heart failure that has been unresponsive to medical treatment.

Infective Endocarditis

Infective endocarditis is an uncommon condition during pregnancy (Cox, Levano, 1989). However, at some hospitals the incidence in recent years has been 1:16,000 births (Cox et al, 1988). It is seen commonly in women taking illicit drugs intravenously. Bacterial endocarditis, leading to incompetence of heart valves and cerebral emboli, can result in death. Treatment is the same as for the nonpregnant woman.

Mitral Valve Prolapse

Mitral valve prolapse (MVP) is a common, usually benign, condition occurring in nearly 10% of women of reproductive age (Cunningham et al, 1989). The mitral valve leaflets prolapse into the left atrium during ventricular systole, allowing some backflow of blood. Midsystolic click and late systolic murmur are hallmarks of this syndrome. Most cases are asymptomatic. A few women have atypical chest pain (sharp and located in the left side of the chest) that occurs at rest, unrelated to exercise, and does not respond to nitrates. Clients usually are treated with beta-blockers such as propranolol (Inderal). Pregnancy usually is well tolerated unless bacterial endocarditis occurs.

Marfan's syndrome is an autosomal dominant disorder characterized by general weakness of connective tissue. About 90% of individuals with this symptom have mitral valve prolapse, and 25% have aortic insufficiency. There is an increased risk of *aortic dissection* and rupture during pregnancy, and maternal mortality is reported at 25% to 50% (Scott et al, 1990). Management during pregnancy is by restricted activity and propranolol therapy.

Cerebrovascular Accidents

Ischemia of the brain tissues, or *cerebrovascular accidents* (CVAs), occurs from occlusion of blood vessels that normally perfuse the area. It results from a cerebral hemorrhage or an embolus. Uncontrolled hypertension during pregnancy can cause cerebral hemorrhages (Cunningham et al, 1989). CVAs have been reported to occur in 1/6000 pregnancies (Simolke et al, 1991). The extent of damage depends on the location and the extent of ischemia.

■ ANEMIA

Anemia, the most common medical disorder of pregnancy, affects at least 20% of pregnant women. These women have a higher incidence of puerperal complications, such as *infection,* than do pregnant women with normal hematologic values.

Anemia results in reduction of the oxygen-carrying capacity of the blood. Because the oxygen-carrying capacity of the blood is decreased, the heart tries to compensate by increasing the cardiac output. This effort increases the workload of the heart and stresses ventricular function. Therefore anemia that occurs with any other complication (e.g. preeclampsia) may result in congestive heart failure.

An indirect index of the oxygen-carrying capacity is the packed red blood cell volume, or hematocrit level. The normal hematocrit range in nonpregnant women is 38% to 45%. However, normal values for pregnant women with adequate iron stores may be as low as 34%. This has been explained by hydremia (dilution of blood), or the physiologic anemia of pregnancy.

At or near sea level, during the first trimester, the pregnant woman is anemic when her hemoglobin level is less than 11 g/dL or her hematocrit level falls below 37%. She is anemic in the second trimester when the hemoglobin level is less than 10.5 g/dL or the hematocrit level falls below 35%; and she is anemic in the third trimester when the hemoglobin level is less than 10 g/dL or the hematocrit level is less than 33%. In areas of high altitude, much higher values indicate anemia, for example, at 1500 m (5000 ft) above sea level, a hemoglobin level less than 14 g/dL indicates anemia.

When a woman has anemia during pregnancy, the loss of blood at birth, even if minimal, is not well tolerated. She is at an increased risk for requiring blood transfusions. About 90% of cases of anemia in pregnancy are of the iron-deficiency type. The remaining 10% of cases embrace a considerable variety of acquired and hereditary anemias, including folic acid deficiency, sickle cell anemia, and thalassemia.

Nursing care of the anemic pregnant woman requires that the nurse be able to distinguish between the normal physiologic anemia of pregnancy and the disease states. (See section on physiologic anemia of pregnancy, p. 199.) During the prenatal visits the nurse should take a diet history and provide dietary teaching as appropriate. The effects of pregnancy for a woman with anemia may cause increased fatigue, stress, and financial difficulties as she copes with her activities of daily living. The nurse should assess the client's needs and provide her with appropriate resources.

Iron Deficiency Anemia

Without iron therapy even pregnant women who enjoy excellent nutrition will conclude pregnancy with an iron deficit. Diet alone cannot replace gestational iron losses. Inadequate nutrition without therapy will certainly mean iron deficiency anemia during late pregnancy and the puerperium.

Successful iron therapy during pregnancy can be carried out in most cases with oral iron supplements (e.g., ferrous sulfate, 0.3 g, three times a day). It is important to teach the woman the significance of the iron therapy (see teaching box, p. 235). In addition, it is necessary to instruct the woman in dietary ways to decrease the gastrointestinal side effects of iron. Some pregnant women cannot tolerate the prescribed oral iron. In such cases the woman should receive parenteral iron such as an iron-dextran complex (Imferon).

Folic Acid Deficiency Anemia

Folic acid deficiency anemia occurs in at least 2% of pregnant women in North America, an incidence much higher than that suspected even 5 years ago. Anemia compromises the women's defenses, making her more vulnerable to urinary tract infections and hemorrhage.

Poor diet, cooking with large volumes of water, or home canning of food (especially vegetables) may lead to folate deficiency. Also, malabsorption may play a part in the development of anemia caused by a lack of folic acid.

During pregnancy the recommended daily intake is 150 μg folic acid. In folate deficiency, a dosage of about 5 mg/day orally for several weeks should ensure a remission. A generous maintenance dose each day should prevent a relapse. Because iron deficiency anemia may also accompany folate deficiency, augmented iron intake should be provided.

Sickle Cell Hemoglobinopathy

Sickle cell hemoglobinopathy is a disease caused by the presence of abnormal hemoglobin in the blood. Sickle cell trait (SA hemoglobin pattern) is sickling of the red blood cells (RBCs) but with a normal RBC life span and usually causes only mild clinical symptoms. Sickle cell anemia (sickle cell disease) is a recessive, hereditary, familial hemolytic anemia that affects those of African-American or Mediterranean ancestry. These individuals usually have abnormal hemoglobin types (SS or SC). Persons with sickle cell anemia have recurrent attacks (crises) of fever and pain in the abdomen or extremities beginning in childhood. These attacks are attributed to vascular occlusion (from abnormal cells), tissue hypoxia, edema, and RBC destruction. Crises are associated with normochromic anemia, jaundice, reticulocytosis, positive sickle cell test, and the demonstration of abnormal hemoglobin (usually SS or SC).

Almost 10% of African Americans in North America have the sickle cell trait, but less than 1% have sickle cell anemia. The anemia often is complicated by iron and folic acid deficiency.

Pregnancy usually results in a worsening of most aspects of the disease (Scott et al, 1990). The anemia that occurs in normal pregnancies may aggravate sickle cell anemia and bring on more crises. Pregnant women with sickle cell anemia are prone to pyelonephritis, leg ulcers, bone infarction, cardiopathy, congestive heart failure, and preeclampsia. Urinary tract infection (UTI) and hematuria are common. An aplastic crisis may follow serious infection. Medical therapy, including transfusions to maintain the hematocrit level at least at 30%, is essential. Cesarean birth is warranted only for obstetric indications. Oral contraceptives are contraindicated.

Table 32-1 identifies some potential problems faced by the woman with sickle cell disease and some preventive and maintenance interventions.

TABLE 32-1 Sickle Cell Disease: Potential Problems, Prevention, and Maintenance

Potential Problem	Prevention and Maintenance
1. Inadequate oxygen to meet needs of labor and prevent sickling	1. a. Monitor Hb level and HCT to maintain Hb at ≥ 7 g and HCT at ≥ 20% b. Have typed and cross-matched blood available c. Assist with transfusions d. Administer oxygen continuously during labor e. Coach for relaxation and to lessen anxiety (see Chapter 13)
2. Infection resulting from anemia: urinary tract infection, pyelonephritis, pneumonia	2. a. Continue actions as under No. 1 b. Maintain adequate hydration c. Administer antibiotics, as ordered d. Maintain strict asepsis e. Encourage frequent voiding to keep bladder empty
3. Sequestration crisis caused by need for and destruction of RBCs	3. Administer folic acid supplement (15-30 mg) to decrease erythropoietic demands and reduce probability of capillary stasis
4. Crisis caused by hypoxia, hypotension, acidosis, dehydration, exertion, sudden cooling, low-grade fever	4. a. Continue actions as under No. 1 b. Avoid supine hypotension c. Maintain adequate hydration d. Maintain comfortable room temperature: use warm blankets or cool cloths as needed e. Assist with analgesia and anesthesia
5. Pseudotoxemia (hypertension, and proteinuria; *no* large weight gain); often accompanies bone pain crisis	5. a. If true PIH occurs, care is the same as for PIH (see Chapter 28) b. Monitor blood pressure and urine c. Administer heparin, as ordered
6. Thrombophlebitis (from increased blood viscosity)	6. a. Monitor for positive Homans' sign b. Initiate bed rest if Homans' sign is positive or if reddened, warm areas, or a lump are found c. Maintain adequate hydration d. Administer heparin, as ordered e. Apply warm compresses f. Apply antiembolism stockings
7. Congestive heart failure	7. a. Assess pulse, respiratory rate q15min b. Auscultate for rales frequently c. Place in semirecumbent position d. Administer oxygen and medications (e.g., digitalis, antibiotics, diuretics, analgesics) e. Prevent bearing down; reassure woman about low forceps birth under anesthesia (local or regional)
8. Pulmonary infarction (hemoptysis, cough, temperature to 102° F [38.9° C], friction rub)	8. Assess for this possible complication to facilitate early diagnosis
9. Postpartum hemorrhage (resulting from heparin therapy)	9. Administer ordered oxytocic medication

Hb, Hemoglobin; *HCT*, hematocrit; *PIH*, pregnancy-induced hypertension; RBCs, red blood cells.

Thalassemia

Thalassemia (Mediterranean or Cooley's anemia) is a relatively common anemia in which an insufficient amount of hemoglobin is produced to fill the RBCs. Thalassemia is a hereditary disorder that involves the abnormal synthesis of the α- or β-chains of hemoglobin. β-Thalassemia is the more common variety in the United States and often is diagnosed in persons of Italian, Greek, or southern Chinese descent. The unbalanced synthesis of hemoglobin leads to premature RBC death, resulting in severe anemia. Thalassemia major is the homozygous form of the disorder; thalassemia minor is the heterozygous form.

Thalassemia major may complicate pregnancy. Preeclampsia is more common in women with thalassemia major. Thalassemia major may be associated with low-birth-weight infants and increased fetal wastage. Placental weight often is increased, perhaps secondary to maternal anemia. The frequency of fetal distress from hypoxia is greater than in control women. Therefore pregnant women with thalassemia major should be monitored more closely than normal pregnant women.

Regular transfusion may be necessary. Folic acid should be given to avoid folate deficiency. Partial exchange transfusion may be warranted in severe thalassemia. Splenectomy may be necessary if enlargement and pain occur. Women with thalassemia major may die of chronic infection or progressive hepatic or cardiac failure—the result of excessive iron deposition—because much of the hemoglobin that is present is precipitated in the form of hard crystals.

Persons with *thalassemia minor* have a mild, persistent anemia, but the RBC level may be normal or even elevated. However, no systemic problems are caused by the anemia that is a part of the minor form of the disease. Thalassemia minor must be distinguished principally from iron deficiency anemia.

Pregnancy will neither worsen thalassemia minor nor will it be compromised by the disease. The anemia will not respond to iron therapy. Prolonged parenteral iron can lead to harmful, excessive iron storage. Infants born to parents with thalassemia will inherit the disorder. Persons with thalassemia minor should have a normal life span despite a moderately reduced hemoglobin level.

■ PULMONARY DISORDERS

As pregnancy advances and the uterus impinges on the thoracic cavity, any pregnant woman may experience increased respiratory difficulty. This difficulty will be compounded by pulmonary disease.

A pregnant woman with a pulmonary disorder requires assessment, planning, and interventions specific to the disease process, in addition to the routine peripartum care. The nurse also must be alert to pulmonary complications precipitated by the pregnancy.

Bronchial Asthma

Bronchial asthma is an acute respiratory illness caused by allergens, marked change in ambient temperature, or emotional tension. In many cases the actual cause may be unknown. A family history of allergy is likely in about 50% of all persons with asthma. In response to stimuli, there is widespread but reversible narrowing of the hyperreactive airways, making it difficult to breathe. The clinical manifestations are expiratory wheezing, productive cough, thick sputum, and/or dyspnea.

Fewer than 1% of pregnant women have this disorder. The effect of pregnancy on asthma is unpredictable. Physiologic alterations induced by pregnancy do not make the pregnant women more prone to asthmatic attacks. Asthma increases the incidence of abortion and preterm labor, but the fetus per se is unaffected. In severe cases, asthma may be life threatening for the pregnant women. The prognosis for both mother and fetus will be good in most cases.

Therapy for bronchial asthma has two objectives: (1) relief of the acute attack and (2) prevention or limitation of later attacks. In all persons with asthma, known allergens should be eliminated and a comfortable home temperature maintained. Respiratory infections should be treated and mist or steam inhalation employed to aid expectoration of mucus. Bronchial asthma therapy is initiated. Acute episodes may require steroids, aminophylline, oxygen, and correction of fluid-electrolyte imbalance. Precautions specific for obstetrics include the following:

- Do not use morphine in labor because it may cause bronchospasm; meperidine (Demerol) usually will relieve bronchospasm.
- Avoid or limit the use of ephedrine and corticotropin (pressor drugs) in preeclampsia and eclampsia.
- Choose vaginal birth with use of local or regional anesthesia, whenever possible.

Adult Respiratory Distress Syndrome

Adult respiratory distress syndrome (ARDS), or shock lung, occurs when the lungs are unable to maintain levels of oxygen and carbon dioxide within normal limits. Marked tachycardia, dyspnea, and cyanosis that do not respond to nasal oxygen or intermittent positive pressure breathing are the most noted signs. ARDS is not a condition specific to pregnancy; it also can result from chest trauma, drug ingestion, or pneumonia. When ARDS is associated with pregnancy, pulmonary embolism, disseminated intravascular coagulation (DIC) (see Chapter 30), and aspiration pneumonia are the precipitators.

The postpartum incidence of ARDS is not affected by the means of birth but by the amount of trauma experienced during pregnancy and birth. It also may occur after spontaneous or medically induced abortion.

Laboratory reports are important in identifying the origin of acute pulmonary problems. The important observations for the nurse to note are vital signs, signs of thrombophlebitis, and hemorrhage. During the postpartum period, apprehension, distended neck veins, cyanosis, diaphoresis, or pallor provide clues. Mental confusion or disorientation also may be noted.

Temperature elevation may indicate the development of thrombophlebitis. The pulse rate increases to compensate for respiratory insufficiency of any origin. The severity of the pulmonary problem increases as the pulse rate rises. An initial rise in blood pressure occurs as cardiac output increases in an attempt to supply the tissue with oxygen. When lung damage is severe, the blood pressure drops.

Respiratory changes are the most important indicators of ARDS. The rate, depth, respiratory pattern, symmetry of chest movement, and use of accessory muscles should be noted; therefore observation of respiratory characteristics after activity is important. If there is any indication of abnormality, respirations are counted for a full minute; an error of plus or minus 4 may be highly significant. On auscultation, crackles (rales), rhonchi, wheezes, or a pleural friction rub should be reported, especially when they have occurred since an earlier normal assessment. The pregnant woman should be positioned for breathing comfort. Oxygen and emergency equipment should be available. The woman should be reassured and coached in relaxation techniques so that her anxiety is lessened.

The lower extremities need to be checked for swelling, pain, inflammation, venous distention, and Homans' sign. If thrombophlebitis is suspected, the woman should be maintained on bed rest. Sudden movement or straining can dislodge a clot and lead to pulmonary embolism.

Alterations in vein distensibility have been noted, possibly because of softening of collagen induced by hormonal influences. The combination of vein distensibility and obstruction of venous blood return from the lower extremities (caused by fetal pressure on veins, especially in the last trimester) predisposes a woman to pooling of blood. In addition, hypercoagulation and pooling may lead to thrombophlebitis. Thrombophlebitis can result in ARDS (emboli from thromboembolism cause obstruction in the pulmonary circulation).

It has been noted that during pregnancy there is an increase in some of the coagulation factors. This increase in coagulation results in shortening of the partial thromboplastin time (PTT). This state predisposes the woman to an increase in rapidity of blood clotting and an increased tendency to form blood clots (hypercoagulability). Petechiae, ecchymosis, hematuria, and epistaxis are important indications of DIC. Replacement of clotting factors and heparin therapy may be required for DIC. Sources of trauma should be identified and eliminated so that outside causes of hemorrhage are avoided.

Aspiration pneumonia can be caused by changes in the gastrointestinal system during pregnancy. Progesterone has been known to relax smooth muscles. When the resting tone is lowered, the cardiac sphincter becomes weak and reflux of the stomach contents can easily occur. Increased intraabdominal pressure (because of fetal growth) further predisposes the mother to gastric reflux.

Food eaten as long as 24 to 48 hours before labor can be vomited and then aspirated. Aspiration of solid foods and liquids may cause bronchial obstruction leading to bronchoconstriction, which in turn can result in ARDS. Large particles can be removed by coughing, suctioning, or bronchoscopy, but liquids are harder to remove. The hydrochloric acid in the aspirated stomach contents may cause an asthmatic-like syndrome with necrotizing bronchitis. For this reason an antacid is given preoperatively as a prophylactic measure.

This syndrome carries a high rate of mortality. The prognosis is good if the woman is otherwise healthy and if ventilatory support can be maintained until the underlying disease can be treated (Cunningham et al, 1989).

Cystic Fibrosis

Improvements in diagnosis and treatment of cystic fibrosis have allowed an increasing number of females to survive to adulthood. Most are infertile; however, pregnancy is not uncommon. The pregnancy is often complicated by chronic hypoxia and frequent pulmonary infections. Women with cystic fibrosis show a decrease in their residual volume during pregnancy, as do normal pregnant women. However, persons with cystic fibrosis are unable to maintain vital capacity. Presumably, the pulmonary vasculature cannot accommodate the increased cardiac output of pregnancy. The results are decreased oxygen to the myocardium, decreasing cardiac output, and an increase in hypoxemia. Increased maternal and perinatal mortality is related to severe pulmonary infection.

During labor, monitoring for fluid and electrolyte balance is required. The amount of sodium lost through sweat can be significant, and hypovolemia can occur. Conversely, if the woman has any degree of cor pulmonale, she must be guarded against fluid overload. Oxygen is freely given during labor. Epidural or local anesthesia is the method of choice for birth.

The woman should know that her child will be heterozygous for cystic fibrosis, even if it is not homozygous. This in turn is likely to increase the genetic pool in the community (Creasy, Resnick, 1989).

The baby of a woman with cystic fibrosis should be breast-fed only after the sodium content of her milk has been estimated. It may be as high as 280 mmol/L (Creasy, Resnik, 1989).

■ GASTROINTESTINAL DISORDERS

Compromise of gastrointestinal function during pregnancy is apparent to all concerned. Obvious physiologic alterations, such as the greatly enlarged uterus, and less apparent changes, such as hormonal differences and hypochlorhydria (deficiency of hydrochloric acid in the stomach's gastric juice), require understanding for proper diagnosis and treatment. Gallbladder disease and inflammatory bowel disease are two gastrointestinal disorders that may occur during pregnancy.

Cholelithiasis and Cholecystitis

Women are four times more likely to have **cholelithiasis** (presence of gallstones in the gallbladder) than are men (Creasy, Resnik, 1989). Maternal adaptation significantly alters gallbladder function (Scott et al, 1990). Pregnancy seems to make the woman more vulnerable to gallstone formation. Decreased muscle tone allows gallbladder distension, thickening of the bile, and prolonged emptying time. Increased progesterone levels result in a slight hypercholesterolemia. However, **cholecystitis** (inflammation of the gallbladder) does not commonly occur during pregnancy.

Generally, gallbladder surgery should be postponed until the puerperium. Impaction of a stone in the cystic or common bile duct during pregnancy may require immediate cholelithotomy or cholecystectomy. Meperidine (Demerol), morphine, or atropine alleviates ductal spasm and pain.

Inflammatory Bowel Disease

Inflammatory bowel disease can be acute or chronic. Infection or antibiotic therapy can induce acute inflammation of the bowel. Chronic inflammatory bowel disease can be classified as *regional enteritis* (Crohn's disease) or *ulcerative colitis*.

Chronic inflammatory bowel diseases are prone to periods of exacerbation and remission. The cause is unknown. The clinical manifestations for this chronic disorder are liquid diarrhea, urgency of defecation, and crampy lower abdominal pain. Blood, mucus, and/or pus may be seen in the stool.

In regional enteritis, fertility is decreased. The chronic intraabdominal inflammatory process is the most likely cause of altered fertility (Creasy, Resnik, 1989). Fertility does not seem to be altered in women with ulcerative colitis.

Treatment and therapy are the same for the pregnant woman as for the nonpregnant woman. Medications include sulfasalazine and prednisone. Folic acid and vitamin supplementation is especially important because of the problems with malabsorption and malnutrition associated with chronic inflammatory bowel disease.

The effect of inflammatory bowel disease on pregnancy is minimal unless there is marked debilitation, whereupon spontaneous abortion, fetal death, or preterm birth may occur. In general, when pregnancy coincides with active ulcerative colitis, most women will experience a severe exacerbation of the disease. When pregnancy occurs during a period of inactivity of the disorder, a flareup is unlikely.

■ INTEGUMENTARY DISORDERS

Dermatologic disorders induced by pregnancy (see Chapter 8) include melasma (chloasma), herpes gestationis, noninflammatory pruritus of pregnancy, vascular spiders, palmar erythema, and pregnancy granuloma (including epulides). Skin problems generally aggravated by pregnancy are acne vulgaris (acne) (in the first trimester), erythema multiforme, herpetiform dermatitis (fever blisters and genital herpes), granuloma inguinale (Donovan bodies), condylomata acuminata (genital warts), neurofibromatosis (von Recklinghausen's disease), and pemphigus. Dermatologic disorders usually improved by pregnancy include acne vulgaris (in the third trimester), seborrhea dermatitis (dandruff), and psoriasis. An unpredictable course during pregnancy may be expected in atopic dermatitis, lupus erythematosus, and herpes simplex.

Therapeutic abortion or early birth may be justified for some dermatologic conditions. These conditions include disseminated lupus erythematosus, neurofibromatosis, and herpes gestationis. Herpes gestationis (*not* a viral-induced disorder) is a rare but serious dermatologic disease. This is a blistering disease of pregnancy. It usually occurs as an extremely pruritic widespread eruption. The lesions vary from erythematous and edematous papules to large, tense bullae (Fig. 32-3). Prednisone usually brings prompt relief and inhibits development of new lesions. Where the skin heals, the healed sites are not scarred but usually are hyperpigmented; the process may recur in subsequent pregnancies (Cunningham et al, 1989).

Isotretinoin (Accutane), commonly prescribed for cystic acne, is highly teratogenic. There is a risk for craniofacial, cardiac, and CNS malformations in exposed fetuses.

Explanation, reassurance, and commonsense measures should suffice for normal skin changes (see Chapter 8). In contrast, disease processes during and soon after pregnancy may be extremely difficult to diagnose and treat.

NEUROLOGIC DISORDERS

The pregnant woman with a neurologic disorder needs to deal with potential teratologic effects of prescribed medications, changes of mobility during pregnancy, and ability to care for the baby. The nurse should be aware of all drugs the client is taking and the associated potential for producing congenital anomalies. As the pregnancy progresses, the woman's center of gravity shifts and causes balance and gait changes. The nurse needs to advise the woman of these expected changes and to suggest safety measures as appropriate. Familial and community resources should be assessed to provide child care for the neurologically impaired woman.

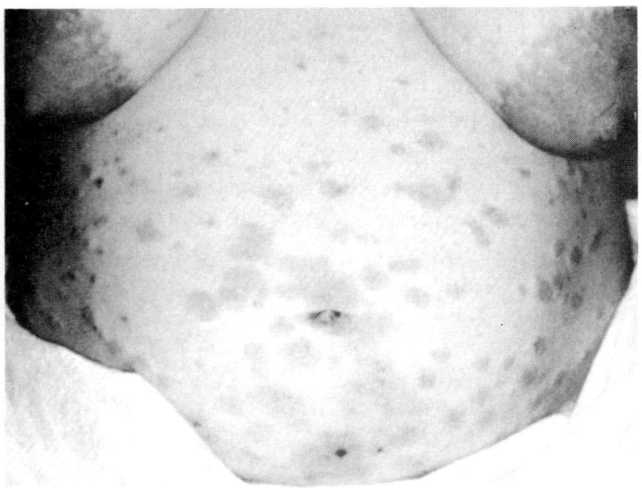

Fig. 32-3 Herpes gestationis (disorder is *not* virus-induced).
Cunningham FG, MacDonald PC, Gant NF: *Williams obstetrics*, ed 18, Norwalk, Conn, 1989, Appleton & Lange.

Epilepsy

Epilepsy may result from developmental abnormalities or injury. Epilepsy seriously complicates about 1/1000 gestations. Convulsive seizures may be more frequent or severe during complications of pregnancy, such as edema, alkylosis, fluid-electrolyte imbalance, cerebral hypoxia, hypoglycemia, and hypocalcemia. On the other hand, the effects of pregnancy on epilepsy are unpredictable.

The differential diagnosis of epilepsy vs. eclampsia may pose a problem. Epilepsy and eclampsia can coexist. However, a history of seizures and a normal plasma uric acid level, as well as the absence of hypertension, generalized edema, or proteinuria, point to epilepsy. Electroencephalography rarely is diagnostic.

Pregnancy usually alters pharmokinetics. In addition, nausea and vomiting may interfere with ingestion and absorption of medication. Diazepam (Valium) crosses the placenta and accumulates in fetal circulation. Cleft lip or cleft palate or other malformations may be associated with its use (Mattison et al, 1989). Although diazepam or chlordiazepoxide (Librium) are safe analeptic drugs, they may cause respiratory depression in the newborn. Phenytoin (Dilantin) and its analogues may be fetotoxic (see Chapter 39).

Grand mal seizures can be controlled by intravenous sodium amobarbital or magnesium sulfate. Epilepsy is not an indication for therapeutic abortion or cesarean birth.

Multiple Sclerosis

Multiple sclerosis, a patchy demyelinization of the spinal cord and CNS, may be a viral disorder. Multiple sclerosis is more common during the childbearing years. It may occasionally complicate pregnancy, but exacerbations and remissions are unrelated to the pregnant state. For this reason, medically indicated therapeutic abortion is illogical. The burden of pregnancy and subsequent child care may warrant early interruption of pregnancy and sterilization in extreme cases. Nursing care of the pregnant woman with multiple sclerosis is similiar to the care of the normal pregnant woman. Women with multiple sclerosis occasionally may have an almost painless labor.

The character of uterine contractions is unaffected by the disease, however. The incidence of multiple sclerosis in the offspring is about 3% to 5% (Birk, Rudick, 1989).

Bell's Palsy

An association between idiopathic facial paralysis and pregnancy was first cited by Bell in 1830. Bell's palsy occurs in about 1 in 2000 pregnancies. Incidence peaks during the third trimester and the puerperium (Cherry, Merkatz, 1991; McGregor et al 1987). A causative relationship does not seem to exist between the appearance of Bell's palsy and any of the complications of pregnancy.

No effects of maternal Bell's palsy have been observed in infants. Maternal outcome is generally good. Electromyography and nerve conduction velocity studies are useful in predicting the outcome. Evidence of a complete block in conduction carries a worse prognosis. Loss of taste also carries a less favorable prognosis. Steroids sometimes are prescribed for the condition, but they do not hasten recovery. In most affected women, 90% or more of facial function can be expected to return (Cunningham et al, 1989; Scott et al, 1990). Supportive care includes prevention of injury to the exposed cornea, facial muscle massage, careful chewing and manual removal of food from inside the affected cheek, and reassurance that return of total neurologic function is likely.

Spinal Cord Injuries

As women with spinal cord injury (SCI) enter the childbearing process, it is essential that nurses be prepared to help these women have a positive experience throughout the perinatal period. The ability to achieve pregnancy is not affected by SCI; as for all women a correlation exists between a positive self-image and role definition.

There is no physiologic reason that prevents SCI women from achieving a normal pregnancy. Fertility is not impaired by their injury, and no greater incidence of spontaneous abortion or fetal abnormalities occurs among this population (Young et al, 1983). However, the SCI woman must deal with her own expectations regarding parenting, the expectation of her significant others, and the perceived expectation of both the medical profession and society. SCI women receive a variety of responses to their impending or confirmed pregnancy from their family, as well as from the medical profession.

Physiologically the SCI woman encounters many of the same problems that pregnant women generally experience. All women have urinary frequency during their pregnancy. This is more of a problem for SCI women because of their alteration in voiding methods (Blackburn, Loper, 1992). Some SCI women use an indwelling catheter, some catheterize themselves at specific intervals, and others use the Credé method for bladder emptying. Generally the increased urine production of pregnancy forces the women to increase the number of times they void daily, which increases the number of times they must transfer and undress themselves. Pressure on the bladder by the enlarging uterus increases the incidence of incontinence. Most SCI women find that a padding system is needed, especially during the third trimester. The most common materials used for padding are disposable diapers, either infant or adult size, and sanitary napkins. Many SCI women are unable to return to their prepregnant level of bladder functioning and must continue to wear padding after the birth of the baby.

The alteration of bladder functioning increases the SCI woman's susceptibility to bladder and kidney infections. SCI women generally experience an increase in the number and frequency of UTIs beginning in the second trimester and continuing through birth. Treatment of the UTI demands knowledge of the tetratologic effects of the antibiotics.

Constipation is another problem for the pregnant woman. The SCI woman has developed a bowel program as part of her routine of daily living. This usually includes either stool softeners or bulk-producing medication. During pregnancy the bowel program must be altered to accommodate the hormonal effect, slowing of the gastrointestinal tract, and pressure from the enlarging uterus on the intestinal tract. Adaptations used during pregnancy to combat constipation include increasing the frequency and the amount of stool softeners or bulk producers, increasing the frequency of bowel movements, adding more roughage to the diet, and maintaining a high fluid intake.

The need to use the bathroom more frequently is just one of the mobility problems that the SCI woman encounters. SCI women use the prone position to sleep to relieve pressure on the ischial spines and gluteal muscles and to straighten joints. As a pregnancy progresses, it becomes impossible for the SCI woman to lie prone. This necessitates more frequent repositioning during the night and often involves the significant other more dramatically in the caregiving. Transfers to and from the wheelchair, bathroom, bed, and car become more difficult as the pregnancy progresses. This difficulty in transfering threatens to hinder the woman's independence.

It has been assumed that because SCI women have impaired sensation, they will not be able to tell when they are in labor. Although they may not experience labor in the same manner as do other women, they are so in tune with their bodies that they know when something is happening. Some sense their abdomen tightening, others have increased spasms, others have a rhythmic need to void or defecate, and still others who had sparing (incomplete cord damage with occasional areas of remaining sensation) experience menstrual-like cramps or actual labor. Women who are injured at the level of T5 or above may correlate increasing symptoms of autonomic dysreflexia with labor (Blackburn, Loper, 1992).

Autonomic dysreflexia results from hyperstimulation of the splanchic nerves and loss of central control over the sympathetic spinal reflexes. It may manifest by sweating, flushing, a pounding headache, pilomotor erection, and severe hypertension. The symptoms are more prevalent at the end of the first stage of labor and all of the second stage as perineal pressure and distention occur. The headache and increased blood pressure must not be confused with pregnancy-induced hypertension. The most common treatment for dysreflexia is epidural anesthesia and/or birth of the baby. Verduyn (1986) cautions against the use of oxytocin for the induction of labor in women prone to dysreflexia unless the physician and/or the labor and birth nurse are versed in the recognition and treatment of autonomic dysreflexia. He discusses four cases in which the use of oxytocin for the induction of labor, in the absence of qualified personnel, had disastrous results.

The SCI woman experiences no trouble with a vaginal birth even though she has no ability to push. Uterine contractions, plus a relaxed perineum, facilitate a vaginal birth. The indications for a cesarean birth are the same for an SCI woman as for any other woman.

After the birth the SCI woman must be assisted with perineal hygiene. The nurse should check the perineum carefully because the woman has decreased or absent perineal sensation. Heat lamps must be used with extreme caution inasmuch as the possibility of unnoticed burning exists. Long sanitary napkins, without the use of sanitary belts, are ideal to absorb lochia and to prevent pressure areas.

The SCI woman also needs additional help in providing care to her newborn. Paraplegic and quadriplegic women have let-down reflexes and can breastfeed successfully (Blackburn, Loper, 1992). Her concerns regarding her ability to care for the newborn often are verbalized during pregnancy. The nurse can be instrumental in helping her problem solve and plan for the care of the infant. SCI mothers express appreciation for those nurses who take extra time to help problem solve infant care needs.

SCI women have been highly imaginative in developing adaptive equipment for the safety and care of their children. Some of the adaptations include redesigning the crib so that the side can be raised and the baby moved directly onto the mother's lap. Mothers also have designed special equipment to pick a baby up from a playpen or the floor. In addition to worrying about the physical care of their children, the mothers worry about how the child will adapt to her disability. The children of SCI parents tend to be accepting of their parents' disability and frequently educate their classmates regarding the functional ability of their parents.

AUTOIMMUNE DISORDERS

Autoimmune disorders comprise a large group of diseases that disrupt the function of the immune system of the body. In these types of disorders, the body develops antibodies that attack its normally present antigens. Autoimmune disorders have a predilection for women in their reproductive years; therefore associations with pregnancy are not uncommon (Scott et al, 1990). Pregnancy may affect the disease process. Some disorders adversely affect the course of pregnancy or are detrimental to the fetus. Autoimmune disorders include rheumatoid arthritis, systemic lupus erythematosus, hyperthyroidism, myasthenia gravis, and immunologic thrombocytopenic purpura. Autoantibodies from rheumatoid arthritis do not cross the placenta; those of the other disorders do. The woman with immunologic thrombocytopenic purpura may give birth to a child who demonstrates thrombocytopenia. Petechiae and bleeding into the gastrointestinal and genitourinary tracts and into the brain may be evident. If the mother has myasthenia gravis, the newborn may exhibit a weak cry, sucking mechanism, and facial muscles and may have respiratory problems. Thyrotoxicosis is probable in the newborn of the mother with hyperthyroidism.

Rheumatoid Arthritis

Most women with rheumatoid arthritis (RA) find that the severity of symptoms decreases during pregnancy. For this reason many affected women attempt to become pregnant as often as possible; however, many are subfertile because of the RA. During pregnancy, women with RA experience an increase in α_2-glycoprotein. In addition, total plasma and free cortisol (especially estrogens and progesterone) show an increase. This combination apparently leads to depressed cellular immunity (Persellin, 1981). Women in whom the rheumatoid factor (autoantibodies found in the synovial fluid) decreases during pregnancy report improvement in their symptoms. Researchers are now investigating the possibility of a positive effect on RA associated with the use of oral contraceptives.

The woman with RA needs to be informed of the positive and negative aspects that accompany pregnancy. She must be cautioned that although symptoms may subside during pregnancy, she should anticipate a return of her symptoms after giving birth. Exacerbations often recur about a month after birth.

Management of RA during pregnancy includes an appropriate balance of rest and exercise, heat and physical therapy, and salicylates. Aspirin probably remains the safest and most useful antiinflammatory drug in these women. Mild hemostatic changes in the newborn, an increase in the average length of gestation, and possibly premature closure of the ductus arteriosus are attributed to maternal ingestion of large doses of aspirin.

Systemic Lupus Erythematosus

One of the most common serious disorders of childbearing age, **systemic lupus erythematosus (SLE),** is a chronic multisystem inflammatory disease. The condition is not rare; more than 250,000 persons are known to have SLE, with an estimated 50,000 new cases per year. Although the antibody may be formed in response to a virus, a familial tendency seems to be involved.

The vague early symptoms, such as fatigue, may be overlooked. Eventually all organs become involved. The condition is characterized by a series of exacerbations and remissions.

If the diagnosis has been established and the woman desires a child, she is advised to wait for 2 years. At that time, if the disease has been controlled well on low doses of corticosteroids, pregnancy may be reasonably considered (Scott et al, 1990; Blackburn, Loper, 1992). Postpartum exacerbation may represent a rebound phenomenon as suppression of cell-mediated activity, normal during pregnancy, is terminated. Oral contraceptives are contraindicated; diaphragms and condoms are the preferred methods of fertility management if pregnancy is desired in the future. Sterilization is suggested if no more children are wanted. The outlook for persons with SLE has improved markedly in the past few years. Persons diagnosed with SLE have a 5-year survival rate of more than 90%, and more than 80% survive for 10 years or more.

The effect of pregnancy on SLE seems inconsistent. The rate of spontaneous abortion is high. Maternal complications correlate with the degree of cardiac or renal involvement (Scott et al, 1990; Blackburn, Loper, 1992). Renal failure, hypertension, and death are associated with diffuse proliferative lupus glomerulonephritis. When the kidneys are involved, women are subject to superimposed preeclampsia, stillbirths, preterm birth, and small-for-gestational age infants. However, if the disease is stable during pregnancy, the risk that the disease will worsen with gestation is only slight.

The relationship of immunosuppressive drugs (such as corticosteroids) and infection must be acknowledged. Infection is now a leading cause of death among persons with SLE.

Although the antibodies cross the placenta, their amount varies so that the effect on the fetus also varies. The most severely affected newborns suffer from discoid lupus, anemia, neutropenia, thrombocytopenia, and congenital complete heart block.

Myasthenia Gravis

Myasthenia gravis, an autoimmune motor (muscle) end plate disorder that involves acetylcholine use, affects the motor function at the myoneural junction. Muscle weakness, particularly of the eyes, face, tongue, neck, limbs, and respiratory muscles, results. The peak prevalence of myasthenia gravis is about 25 years of age. Pregnancy may complicate the disorder, although some women experience a remission during gestation. Pregnancies in women with this disease can be carried to safe birth if certain precautions are taken. Moreover, congenital myasthenia gravis is rare. Therefore the disorder is not an indication for therapeutic abortion.

The nurse and physician should be alert to symptoms, which include easy fatigue, intermittent double vision, upper eyelid drooping, and facial muscle weakness. In more serious cases, upper arm weakness and breathing difficulty occur. Infections may precipitate onset or relapse and must be treated aggressively during pregnancy.

Women with myasthenia gravis usually tolerate labor well, because they already have some degree of muscle relaxation. Meperidine is the obstetric analgesic of choice. Local anesthesia is preferred. Oxytocin may be given, but scopolamine and muscle relaxants (e.g., magnesium sulfate) are contraindicated. After birth, women must be carefully supervised, because relapses often occur during the puerperium.

Occasionally an infant born to a mother with severe myasthenia gravis also shows myasthenic signs sufficient to require neostigmine treatment for 1 to 2 months. Complete recovery of the infant is the rule. However, infants born with the disorder do not have as good a prognosis as do infants born without the disorder.

■ ABDOMINAL SURGERY DURING PREGNANCY

The need for immediate abdominal surgery occurs as frequently among pregnant women as among nonpregnant women of comparable age. However, diagnosis is more difficult in the pregnant woman. An enlarged uterus and displaced internal organs may prevent adequate palpation and may alter the position of the surgical procedure.

Differential diagnosis includes consideration of obstetric complications (e.g., ectopic pregnancy and premature separation of the placenta) and the onset of labor. Mild leukocytosis and increased serum values of alkaline phosphatase and amylase are characteristic of pregnancy, as well as surgical intraperitoneal processes. Rising or abnormally high laboratory values warrant suspicion. X-ray evaluation, a valuable adjunct to diagnosis, is contraindicated, particularly in the first trimester, except in extreme cases. The surgeon is confronted with both a surgical and an obstetric problem.

Laparotomy or laparoscopy may be required. Hazards of these procedures include abortion and premature labor. However, surgical or anesthetic intervention does not affect the incidence of congenital malformations.

Appendicitis

Acute suppurative appendicitis complicates about 1/1000 pregnancies. This disorder poses the following special problems during gestation.

1. Appendicitis is more difficult to diagnose during pregnancy. The appendix is carried high and to the right, away from McBurney's point, by the enlarged uterus (Fig. 32-4).
2. Appendiceal rupture and peritonitis occur two to three times more often in pregnant women than in nonpregnant women.
3. Maternal and perinatal morbidity and mortality are greatly increased when appendicitis occurs during pregnancy.

Most cases of acute appendicitis occur during the first 6 months of gestation, with decreasing frequency through the third trimester, labor, and puerperium. The differential diagnosis of appendicitis during pregnancy is complicated by gastrointestinal or genitourinary problems that may be confused with appendicitis. A high level of suspicion is important in the diagnosis of appendicitis.

Appendectomy before rupture is extremely important. Antibiotic therapy before rupture is of questionable value; after rupture it may be lifesaving. Therapeutic abortion is never indicated in appendicitis. Ce-

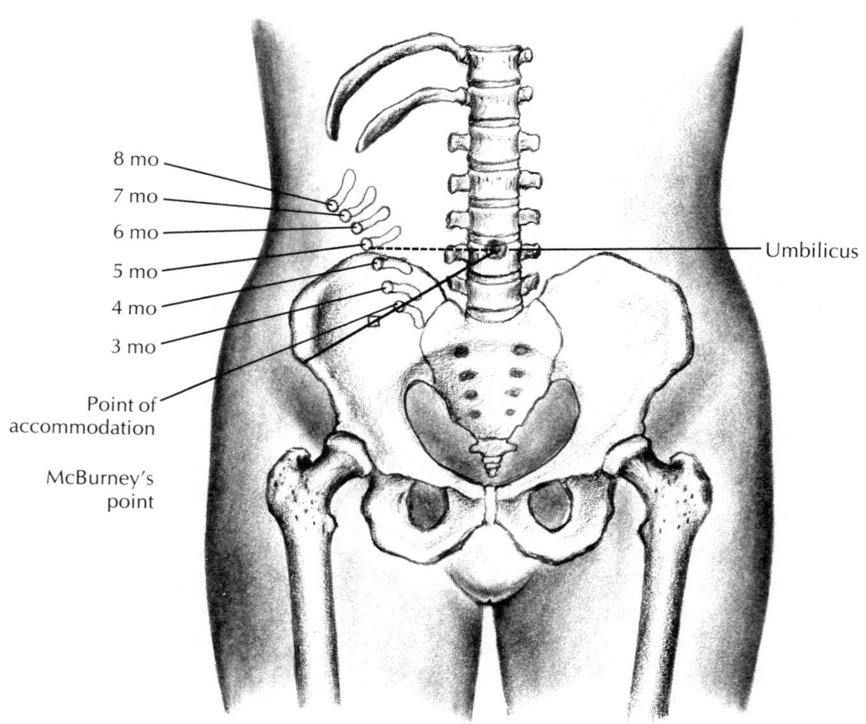

Fig. 32-4 Change in position of appendix during pregnancy.

sarean birth at or near term may be justified in association with appendectomy.

Maternal mortality increases to about 10% in the third trimester and is about 15% when appendicitis develops during labor. Perinatal mortality is approximately 10% with unruptured appendicitis but is at least 35% with peritonitis.

Intestinal Obstruction

Although intestinal obstruction (adynamic ileus) is not common during pregnancy, any woman with a laparotomy scar is more likely to have intestinal obstruction during gestation. Adhesions as a result of previous surgery or pelvic inflammatory disease, an enlarging uterus, and displacement of the intestines are etiologic factors.

Persistent cramplike, abdominal pain, vomiting, auscultatory rushes within the abdomen, and "laddering" of the intestinal shadows on x-ray films aid in the diagnosis of intestinal obstruction. Immediate surgical intervention is required for release of the obstruction. Pregnancy rarely is affected by the surgery, assuming the absence of complications such as peritonitis. Cesarean birth is not indicated in intestinal obstruction.

Abdominal Hernias

The incidence of abdominal hernias and related incarceration of the bowel is reduced during pregnancy despite permanent enlargement of umbilical or incisional hernial rings. Displacement of a nonadherent bowel by the enlarging uterus and its shielding of so-called weak areas of the abdominal wall are responsible. In fact, temporary spontaneous reduction of some abdominal wall hernias occurs during gestation. In contrast, however, the uncommon irreducible or adherent hernias may become incarcerated as pregnancy progresses.

Straining or bearing down during the second stage of labor may be contraindicated for women with hernias. Therefore low forceps-assisted birth may be planned. Abdominal hernia is not an indication for cesarean birth; herniorrhaphy should be performed between pregnancies.

Gynecologic Problems

Ovarian cysts and twisting of ovarian cysts or adnexal tissues may occur. Pregnancy predisposes a woman to ovarian problems, especially during the first trimester. Conditions include retained or enlarged cystic corpus luteum of pregnancy, ovarian cyst, and bacterial invasion of reproductive or other intraperitoneal organs.

Laparotomy or laparoscopy may be required to discriminate between ovarian problems and early ectopic pregnancy, appendicitis, or other infectious processes.

Nursing Process

ASSESSMENT

Fetal vital signs and activity and uterine contractility (labor may have begun) are monitored, and constant vigilance for symptoms of impending obstetric complications is maintained. The woman and her family may have heightened concerns regarding effects of the procedure and medication on fetal well-being and the course of pregnancy. The extent of presurgery assessment is determined by the immediacy of surgical intervention and the specific condition that requires surgery (Phipps et al, 1991).

Some causes of vital sign changes early in the postoperative phase are listed in Table 32-2.

TABLE 32-2 Some Causes of Vital Sign Changes in Early Postoperative Phase

Increase	Decrease
Temperature	
Stress reaction (low-grade fever)	Cold operating room and recovery room
Pulse rate	
Jarring during transfer Shock, hemorrhage Hypoventilation Acute gastric dilation Pain Anxiety Cardiac arrhythmias	Digitalis overdose Cardiac arrhythmias
Respiratory rate	
Hypoventilation: poor positioning, right chest or upper abdominal dressing, obesity, gastric dilation	Drugs: anesthetics, narcotics, sedatives
Blood pressure	
Anxiety (↑ systolic) Pain	Jarring during transfer Severe pain Cardiac arrhythmias Shock: fluid loss, hemorrhage, acute gastric dilation

From Phipps WJ et al: *Medical-surgical nursing: concepts and clinical practice*, ed 4, St Louis, 1991, Mosby–Year Book.

NURSING DIAGNOSES

Nursing diagnoses vary with the surgical condition and the immediacy of surgical intervention. Nursing diagnoses may include the following:

- Knowledge deficit related to
  —Surgical condition
  —Surgical procedure
  —Recovery
  —High risk for sequelae for woman and fetus
- High risk for injury related to
  —Effects of postoperative immobility
- Anxiety related to
  —Surgery on woman and effects on fetus
- Spiritual distress related to
  —High risk status

PLANNING

The preoperative and postoperative plans for care incorporate consideration for the family's and woman's concern for the fetus, as well as for the woman. *Goals* for care vary with each client. However, the following general goals apply in all situations.

- The woman's and her family's spiritual care needs are met.
- The woman and family understand the condition, rationale for surgical intervention, expected outcome, and postoperative course and management.
- Maternal-fetal-placental unit well-being is maintained.
- Mother and fetus/neonate suffer no adverse sequelae.
- Mother complies with scheduled postoperative follow-up care.

IMPLEMENTATION

Preoperative care for a pregnant woman differs from that for a nonpregnant woman in one significant aspect: the presence of at least one other person, the fetus. Procedures such as preparation of the operative site and the time of insertion of IV lines and urinary retention catheters vary with the physician and the facility. However, in every instance there is a total restriction of solid foods and liquids or a clear specification of the type, amount, and time at which clear liquids may be taken before surgery. Food by mouth is restricted for several hours before a scheduled procedure. Even if she has had nothing by mouth—but more important, if surgery is unexpected—the woman is in danger of vomiting and aspirating, and special precautions are taken before anesthetic is administered (see Chapter 35).

General preoperative observations and ongoing care are the same as for any surgery, with the addition of fetal surveillance. In addition, a notation of fetal heart rate and status is important.

Most recovery rooms have special forms that provide a checklist for assessing the client's postoperative status and progress. General observations and ongoing care pertinent to postoperative recovery are initiated. This includes maintaining fluid and electrolyte balance by diligent attention to intake and output. The nurse promotes physical and emotional rest through the appropriate use of nurse-ordered comfort measures and physician-ordered medications and procedures. If intrauterine pregnancy continues, monitoring of fetal heart rate and activity, as well as uterine activity, is continued (see Chapter 16).

Client safety remains an important component of care. The family is called on to assist in maintaining client safety through orientation of the woman (and her family and friends) to the need to use side rails, to call for assistance in getting out of bed, to protect the IV infusion and incision sites, and to cleanse the perineum.

DISCHARGE PLANNING. Planning for discharge begins when the pregnant woman first enters the health care delivery system. The extent to which the goals of care can be met before surgery is reviewed, and adjustments are made accordingly. For example, if the surgery was an emergency such as for appendicitis, there is little time for preoperative preparation. After the woman has recovered from the effects of surgery, the nurse needs to take time to encourage her to voice her fears, concerns, and questions. She may have questions regarding the effect of the surgery and anesthesia on the fetus. If she is unable to express these concerns to the physician, the nurse acts as client-advocate and informs the physician.

The participation of the woman and her family in discharge planning is necessary to individualize the care to fit with the available family support systems, the home situation, and the facilities. If the woman is to perform some type of treatment or exercises at home, the family member or friend who will be caring for her is included when she is taught these activities, and her mastery is evaluated. The woman may be demonstrating symptoms of grief and loss, and her participation in discharge planning may be minimal. She may need assistance coping with these feelings (see Chapter 40).

The woman may need referral service to various community agencies for evaluation of the home situ-

Topics for Discharge Teaching

- Care of incision site
- Diet and elimination related to gastrointestinal function
- Signs and symptoms of developing complications: wound infection, thrombophlebitis, pneumonia
- Equipment needed and technique for assessing temperature
- Recommended schedule for resumption of activities of daily living
- Treatments and medications ordered
- List of resource persons and their telephone numbers
- Schedule of follow-up visits

ation, child care, home health care, and financial or other assistance. All arrangements for her return home and for convalescent care should be completed as early as possible before her expected date of discharge. (See box for discharge teaching topics, above.)

EVALUATION

The nurse can be reasonably assured that care has been effective if the goals of care have been achieved.

- The woman's and her family's spiritual care needs are met.
- The woman and her family understand the condition, rationale for surgical intervention, expected outcome, and postoperative course and management.
- Maternal-fetal-placental unit well-being is maintained.
- Mother and fetus/newborn suffer no adverse sequelae.
- Mother complies with scheduled postoperative follow-up care.

TRAUMA DURING PREGNANCY

Minor injury during pregnancy is a common occurrence; most trauma (more than 50%) occurs during the third trimester. A change in the woman's center of gravity, as well as other changes in pregnancy, are responsible for syncope, loss of balance, and general clumsiness. Discomfort such as a contracting uterus or vigorous fetal movement may be distracting while the woman is driving or working. The leading cause of death in women of reproductive age is trauma—not neoplasms or obstetric complications (Daddario, 1989). Trauma care, or care of the physical injury, needs to focus on the mother and the fetus.

Nursing Process

ASSESSMENT

The woman's condition is the initial concern. The injury sustained determines the type and extent of assessment conducted. Attention is focused first on the basic ABCs: airway, breathing, and circulation. The woman's abdomen is assessed for ruptured uterus and for uterine activity. The fetus is then assessed for heart rate and activity. An individualized health assessment is performed. When available, the woman's prenatal record is reviewed.

Findings from the injury must not be confused with the normal physiologic changes during pregnancy. The usual signs of organ rupture—for example, guarding, rebound tenderness, and rigidity—may be only responses to stretching of the abdominal wall. An examination of the woman in a supine position results in hypotension and a systolic value as low as 80 mm Hg; changing her position to left lateral or simply moving the fetus raises the systolic value to more than 100 mm Hg. A "silent" abdomen, a sign of bowel trauma, may be a normal finding because of the decreased motility that occurs during pregnancy. Delayed emptying time of the stomach during pregnancy poses a threat of vomiting and possible aspiration if the woman has eaten within the last several hours.

During pregnancy the woman may sustain a significant blood loss (approximately a 30% reduction of circulating blood volume) without the usual signs and symptoms of hypovolemia. Pelvic blood vessels (retroperitoneal and parametrial arteries) enlarge greatly during pregnancy; thus they are damaged and perhaps rupture more easily as a result. The large uterus can compartmentalize and hide hemorrhage originating in the liver and spleen. A rapid pulse may reflect only the usual increase of 10 to 15 beats/min, or it may be a sign of hypovolemia.

Laboratory and diagnostic tests are determined by the type of injury. Appropriate blood studies include tests for serum amylase and blood gases; baseline bleeding profile; and complete blood cell count, typing, and cross-matching. In normal pregnancies a white blood cell count of 18,000/mm^3 in the last trimester and 25,000/mm^3 during labor is usual; these same values also indicate intraabdominal hemorrhage. DIC can complicate severe trauma, placental abruption, and sepsis.

An indwelling urinary bladder catheter for drainage facilitates management of fluid therapy and aids diagnosis (Fig. 32-5). For example, difficulty in passing the catheter suggests urethral disruption, and hematuria suggests a ruptured bladder. The catheter also provides access for retrograde cystogram x-ray examination.

Intraperitoneal hemorrhage must be detected. Radiology, real-time ultrasound, and computed tomography scan are useful diagnostic modalities. The physician places a peritoneal lavage catheter for detecting intraperitoneal hemorrhage. The procedure is performed through a small incision into the peritoneum, with the woman under local anesthesia. The test result is positive for bleeding if the aspirate exceeds 10 mL nonclotting blood or if, after instillation

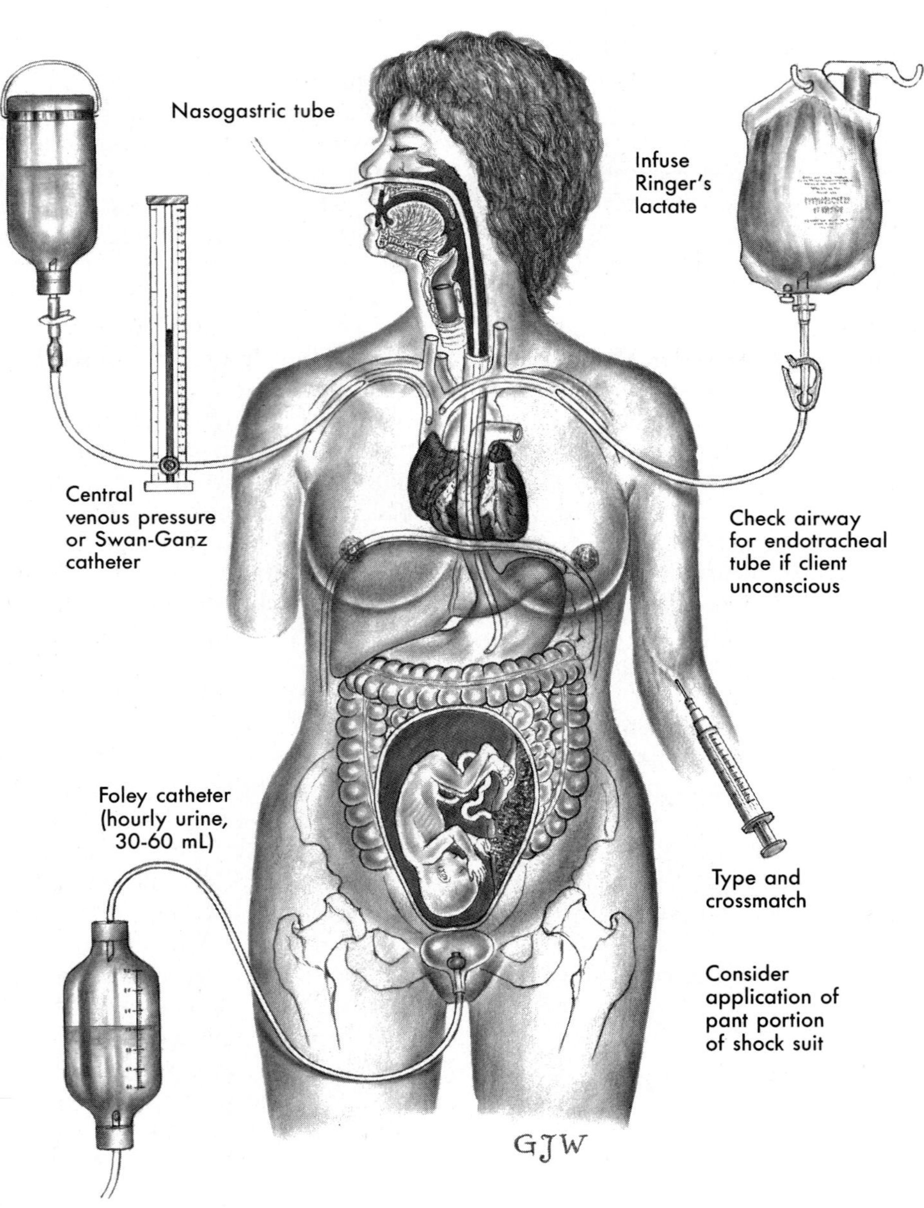

Fig. 32-5 Summary of technique used for resuscitation. Trauma care should begin in field where injury occurred, always with attention to basic ABCs: airway, breathing, and circulation.

of 1 L lactated Ringer's solution, bloody fluid is recovered. Radiographic studies may be necessary to guide management.

NURSING DIAGNOSES

The nursing diagnoses are formulated from assessment findings. Examples of possible nursing diagnoses include the following:

- Anxiety, fear related to
  —Uncertainty of outcome for the woman and fetus
- Knowledge deficit related to
  —Inadequate pretreatment preparation time
- High risk for injury related to
  —Recent food intake before need for anesthesia
- High risk for decreased cardiac output related to
  —Reduced circulatory volume
- High risk for decreased tissue perfusion related to
  —Decreased oxygenation secondary to hemorrhage

PLANNING

Mutual planning may not be possible in all situations. The pregnant woman and family are included in planning at the earliest possible time.

Goals, which are derived from the injury, its management, and its course, are based on the woman's and family's individual needs. The following goals provide examples.

- The woman's injuries resulting from accidents are diagnosed and treated accurately and rapidly.
- The woman and fetus sustain no permanent adverse sequelae.
- The woman and family grieve appropriately.
- The woman's injuries are prevented through prenatal education on safety in view of normal maternal adaptations.

IMPLEMENTATION

Intervention begins with prevention. The woman is counseled to discontinue activities requiring balance and coordination, to use car seat restraints appropriately, to recognize early adverse symptoms, and to seek therapy immediately. If the woman is hospitalized only for observation, she is involved in assessment for signs and symptoms of complications.

Immediate trauma care consists of attention to the ABCs (Fig. 32-5). While hypoxia and hypovolemia are being corrected, the woman should be transferred to a trauma center with obstetric and neonatal back-up, if possible. During transfer, attendants must remember the aortocaval (supine hypotension) syndrome. The woman should be positioned on her side, or the uterus should be displaced laterally by a uterine displacer or by a pillow placed under the woman's right hip. Hypotension must be avoided to prevent compromise of cardiac output followed by decrease of blood flow to the uterus.

A nasogastric tube is inserted, if indicated, because delayed gastric emptying time and increased intestinal transit time increase the risk of vomiting and aspiration. Mouth care and reassurance are used to counter any irritation caused by the tube. Fluid and electrolyte replacement is instituted and monitored. Oxygen needs are met.

Penetrating abdominal wounds, internal hemorrhage, and ruptured uterus are all indications for immediate surgical intervention. Wounds high in the abdomen have most likely penetrated a vital structure because organs such as the bowel, liver, and spleen have been displaced upward by the enlarging uterus (Fig. 32-5).

POSTTRAUMATIC UTERINE AND FETAL SURVEILLANCE. When the mother's condition has been stabilized, attention is turned toward monitoring the fetus and monitoring for preterm labor and placental abruption. Usually, if these complications occur, they happen within 24 to 48 hours after the accident.

In case of minor trauma the woman is hospitalized and evaluated for the following: vaginal bleeding, uterine irritability, abdominal tenderness, abdominal pain or cramps, evidence of hypovolemia, a change in or absence of fetal heart rate, fetal activity, leakage of amniotic fluid, and the presence of fetal cells in maternal circulation.

After injury, if placental abruption (abruptio placentae) is to occur, it usually manifests within 48 hours. Uterine rupture can occur at the site of a previous scar or over the site of implantation, which is weakened by increased vascularity at the site. Expulsion of the uterine contents into the abdominal cavity may occur and usually is followed by massive hemorrhage.

EVALUATION

The nurse can be assured that care has been effective if the goals of care have been achieved.

- The woman's injuries are diagnosed and treated accurately and rapidly.
- The woman and fetus sustain no permanent adverse sequelae.
- The woman and family grieve appropriately.

- The women's injuries are prevented through prenatal education on safety in view of normal maternal adaptations.

■ SUMMARY

Pathophysiology, medical treatment, and nursing care of several disorders have been presented in this chapter. These disorders have immediate and long-term consequences for the mother and her fetus or newborn. As always, sensitivity to the woman and her family during the childbearing experience that is complicated by a physical disorder is as important as expert technologic assistance. Nursing care of the pregnant woman with a medical or surgical complication presents a challenge that offers the potential for fulfillment on both a professional and personal level.

REFERENCES

Cardiovascular Disorders

Brady K, Duff P: Rheumatic heart disease in pregnancy, *Clin Obstet Gynecol* 31:21, 1989.

Cox SM, Leveno KJ: Pregnancy complicated by bacterial endocarditis, *Clin Obstet Gynecol* 31:48, 1989.

Cox SM et al: Bacterial endocarditis: a serious pregnancy complication, *J Reprod Med* 33:671, 1988.

Cunningham FG, MacDonald PC, Gant NF: *Williams obstetrics,* ed 18, Norwalk, Conn, 1989, Appleton & Lange.

Graber EA: When an OB patient has coronary disease, *Contemp OB/GYN* 33:56, June 1989.

Homans DC: Peripartum cardiomyopathy, *N Engl J Med* 312:1432, 1985.

Lee W, Cotton DB: Peripartum cardiomyopathy: current concepts and clinical management, *Clin Obstet Gynecol* 31:54, 1989.

McKeon VA, Perrin KO: The pregnant woman with myocardial infarction: nursing diagnosis, *Dimens Crit Care Nurs* 8(2):92, 1989.

Scott JR et al: *Danforth's obstetrics and gynecology,* ed 6, Philadelphia, 1990, JB Lippincott Co.

Simolke GA, Cox SM, Cunningham FG: Cerebrovascular accidents complicating pregnancy and the puerperium, *Obstet Gynecol* 78:37, 1991.

Troiano NH: Cardiopulmonary resuscitation of the pregnant woman, *J Perinat Neonat Nurs* 3(2):1, 1989.

Medical Disorders

Birk KA, Rudick RA: Caring for the OB patient who has multiple sclerosis, *Contemp OB/GYN* 34:58, Jan 1989.

Blackburn ST, Loper DL: *Maternal, fetal and neonatal physiology: a clinical perspective,* Philadephia, 1992, WB Saunders Co.

Cherry SH, Merkatz IR: *Complications of pregnancy: medical, surgical, gynecologic, psychosocial, and perinatal,* ed 4, Baltimore, 1991, Williams & Wilkins.

Creasy RK, Resnik R: *Maternal-fetal medicine: principles and practice,* ed 2, Philadelphia, 1989, WB Saunders Co.

Cunningham FG, MacDonald PC, Gant NF: *Williams obstetrics,* ed 18, Norwalk, Conn, 1989, Appleton & Lange.

Mattison DR et al: Pharmacology: effects of drugs and chemicals on the fetus, *Contemp OB/GYN* 33:97, April 1989.

McGregor JA, Guberman A, Goodlin R: Idiopathic facial nerve paralysis (Bell's palsy) in late pregnancy and the early puerperium, *Obstet Gynecol* 69:435, 1987.

Persellin RH: Inhibitors of inflammatory and immune responses in pregnancy serum, *Clin Rheum Dis* 7:769, 1981.

Scott JR et al: *Danforth's obstetrics and gynecology,* ed 6, Philadelphia, 1990, JB Lippincott Co.

Verduyn WH: Spinal cord injured women, pregnancy and delivery, *Paraplegia* 24:231, 1986.

Young BK, Kutz M, Klein SA: Pregnancy after spinal cord injury: altered maternal and fetal responses to labor, *Obstet Gynecol* 62:59, 1983.

Surgery during Pregnancy

Phipps WJ, Long BC, Woods NF: *Medical-surgical nursing: concepts and clinical practice,* ed 4, St Louis, 1991, Mosby–Year Book.

Injuries during Pregnancy

Daddario JB: Trauma in pregnancy, *J Perinat Neonat Nurs* 3(2):14, 1989.

BIBLIOGRAPHY

Baker ER et al: Risks associated with pregnancy in spinal cord–injured women, *Obstet Gynecol* 80(3) (Part 1):425, Sept 1992.

Mitchell PJ, Bebbington M: Myasthenia gravis in pregnancy, *Obstet Gynecol* 80(2):178, August 1992.

Cardiovascular Disorders

Brown CE, Wendel GD: Cardiac arrhythmias during pregnancy, *Clin Obstet Gynecol* 31:89, 1989.

Guidelines for cardiopulmonary resuscitation and emergency cardiac care, JAMA 268(16):2171, 1992.

McColgin SW, Martin JN, Morrison JC: Pregnant women with prosthetic heart valves, *Clin Obstet Gynecol* 31:76, 1989.

Nolan TF, Hankins GD: Myocardial infarction in pregnancy, *Clin Obstet Gynecol* 31:68, 1989.

Porter KB, Knuppel RA: Uses of pulse oximetry during pregnancy, *Contemp OB/GYN* 31:47, June 1988.

Roth CK, Riley B, Cohen SM: Intrapartum care of a woman with aortic aneurysms, *JOGNN* 21(4):310, July/Aug 1992.

Schmidt J, Boilanger M, Abbot S: Peripartum cardiomyopathy, *JOGNN* 18:465, 1989.

Yeomans ER, Hankins GD: Cardiovascular physiology and invasive cardiac monitoring, *Clin Obstet Gynecol* 31:2, 1989.

Medical Disorders

Aldrete JA, Santos EG: Recognizing aspiration pneumonitis, *Contemp OB/GYN* 35(3):61, March 1990.

Bag S et al: Pregnancy and epilepsy, *J Neurol* 236:311, 1989.

Birk K et al: The clinical course of multiple sclerosis during pregnancy and the puerperium, *Arch Neurol* 47:738, 1990.

Buehler BA et al: Prenatal prediction of the fetal hydantoin syndrome, *N Engl J Med* 322:1567, 1990.

Dombroski RA: Autoimmune disease in pregnancy, *Med Clin North Am* 73:605, 1989.

Donaldson JO: The pregnant epileptic: fetal risks from anticonvulsant therapy, *JAMA* 264:1044, 1990.

Goldstein J, Kappy KA: Pharmacology: nonrheumatoid arthritis during pregnancy, *Contemp OB/GYN* 34:89, Jan 1989.

Hayashi RH: Responding to respiratory emergencies, *Contemp OB/GYN* 37:75, Feb 1992.

Lavery JP: Treating asthma in pregnancy, *Contemp OB/GYN* 36:121, June 1991.

Lowe TW, Cunningham FG: Adult respiratory distress syndrome, *Contemp OB/GYN* 35:49, Sept 1990.

MacMullen NJ, Brucker MC: Pregnancy made possible for women with cystic fibrosis, *MCN* 14:196, 1989.

Magil B, Machol L: Caring for pregnant patients with sickle cell disease, *Contemp OB/GYN* 33:214, March 1989.

Petri M: Outcomes encouraging in mothers with lupus, *Contemp OB/GYN* 31:103, March 1988.

Resnik R: Managing SLE during pregnancy, *Contemp OB/GYN* 35:67, June 1990.

Thorton NG, Dewis M: Multiple sclerosis and female sexuality, *Can Nurse* 85:16, April 1989.

Thorton YS: Caring for the myasthenic OB patient, *Contemp OB/GYN* 31, Feb 1988.

Thorton YS: The sometimes perilous rashes of pregnancy, *Emerg Med* 20:171, March 15, 1988.

Surgery during Pregnancy

Tarkington MA, Gilbert RN, Bresette JF: Reducing iatrogenic ureteral injury, *Contemp OB/GYN* 37:93, Feb 1992.

Injuries during Pregnancy

Dunn PA et al: Assessing a pregnant woman after trauma, *Nursing 90* 20:53, Dec 1990.

Field DR et al: Maternal brain death during pregnancy: medical and ethical issues, *JAMA* 260:816, 1988.

Howard JC, Nyari DM: Traumatic fetal death, *Dimens Crit Care Nurs* 8:217, 1989.

Pearlman MD, Tintinalli JE, Lorenz RP: Blunt trauma during pregnancy, *N Engl J Med* 323:1609, 1990.

chapter 32 review

Key Concepts

- The stress of the normal maternal adaptations to pregnancy on a heart whose function is already taxed may cause cardiac decompensation.
- Anemia, the most common medical disorder of pregnancy, affects at least 20% of pregnant women.
- The chance of developing adult respiratory distress syndrome increases with the amount of trauma experienced during pregnancy or birth.
- Autoimmune disorders (e.g., systemic lupus erythematosus, myasthenia gravis) show a predilection for women in their reproductive years; therefore associations with pregnancy are not uncommon.
- Trauma during pregnancy has the potential to affect both the mother and the fetus; assessment after trauma is more difficult because of the normal physiologic changes of pregnancy.
- In the pregnant woman, an enlarged uterus, displaced internal organs, and altered laboratory values may confound differential diagnosis when the need for immediate abdominal surgery occurs.
- Preoperative care for a pregnant woman differs from that for a nonpregnant woman in one significant aspect: the presence of at least one other person, the fetus.

Key Terms

- adult respiratory distress syndrome (ARDS) (p. 977)
- autoimmune disorders (p. 982)
- cardiac decompensation (p. 962, 963)
- cholecystitis (p. 979)
- cholelithiasis (p. 979)
- hypertrophic cardiomyopathy (HCM) (p. 972)
- idiopathic peripartum cardiomyopathy (p. 973)
- infective endocarditis (p. 974)
- intrauterine fetal growth retardation (IUGR) (p. 962)
- Marfan's syndrome (p. 974)
- mitral valve prolapse (MVP) (p. 974)
- mitral valve stenosis (p. 974)
- peripartum heart failure (p. 972)
- reflex bradycardia (p. 971)
- rheumatic heart disease (p. 974)
- sickle cell hemoglobinopathy (p. 975)
- systemic lupus erythematosus (SLE) (p. 983)
- Valsalva's maneuver (p. 964)

Critical Thinking Exercises

You are assigned to a woman who has a history of Class III heart disease (New York Heart Association classification). She has come to the clinic, where she is diagnosed to be at 8 weeks' gestation. She has a two-year-old at home and her husband, who is not present today, thinks she is healthy and does not need any help with household or child care activities during pregnancy.

1. Examine the options for this woman given this situation. What are the pros and cons of each?
2. Select one option.
   a. Justify your choice.
   b. Identify nursing diagnoses.
   c. Formulate a plan of care.

Mrs. S was admitted to the ICU after sustaining multiple injuries in an automobile accident. She is at 30 weeks' gestation and is being maintained on life support measures to keep the fetus alive until it can be delivered as close to term as possible.

Mr. S has been at his wife's side since she was admitted.

1. What are the critical issues to be addressed by the nursing staff in this situation?
2. How can the wishes of the husband/family be incorporated into the care of Mrs. S?
3. What are the pros and cons of maintaining Mrs. S on life support for the sake of the fetus?
4. Examine what your reactions would be if you were asked to care for Mrs. S.

Topics for Nursing Research

- What are the effects of cardiovascular disease on mother-infant bonding and family structure?
- What are the stressors and coping strategies of women who become pregnant after cancer treatment?

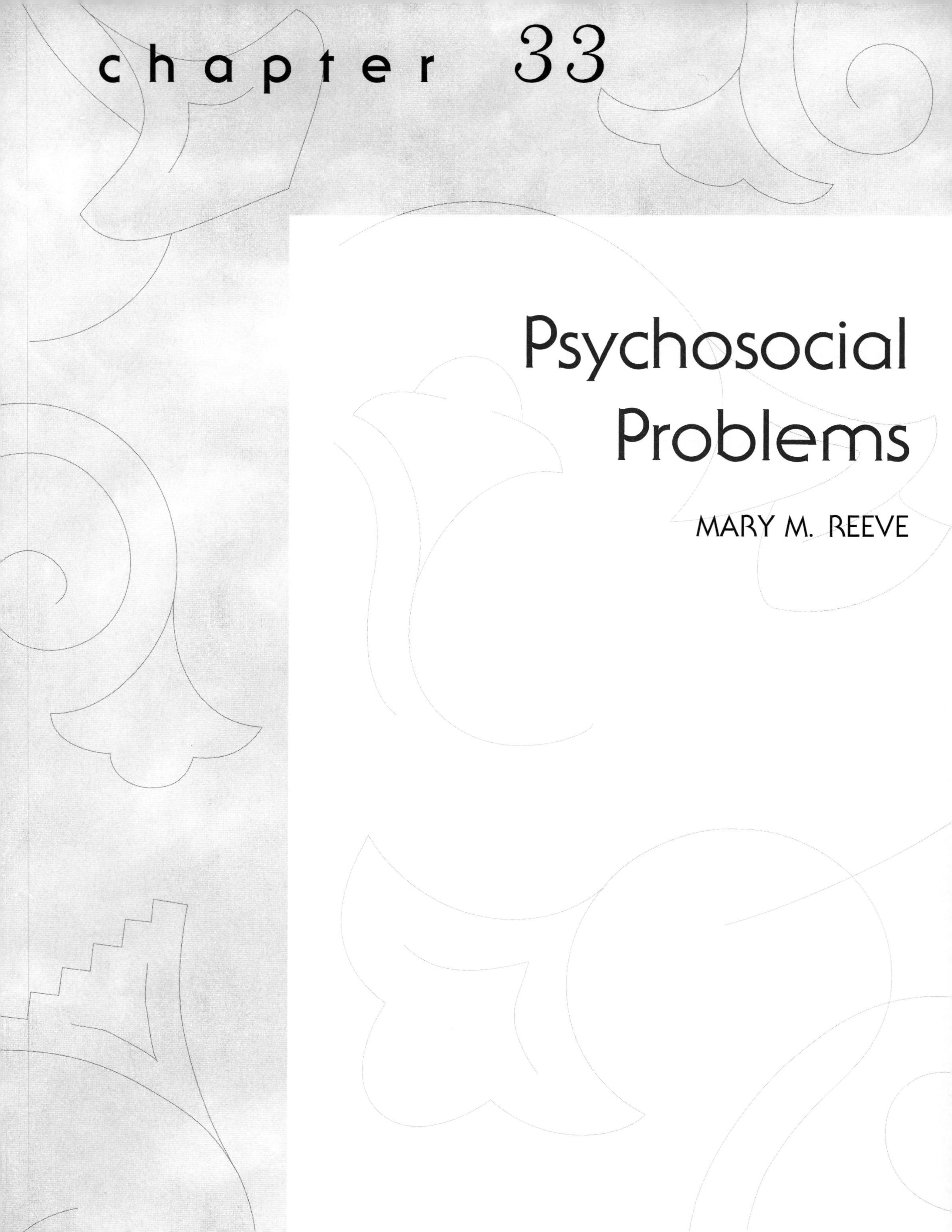

chapter 33

Psychosocial Problems

MARY M. REEVE

LEARNING OBJECTIVES

- Define the key terms listed.
- Review the care of women experiencing emotional complications during the childbearing cycle.
- Discuss the care of pregnant women who use, abuse, or are dependent on drugs such as alcohol, opioids, and cocaine.
- Assess the effects of poverty on the childbearing cycle.
- Identify topics for nursing research related to psychosocial problems.

Psychosocial conditions have implications for the health of the mother and newborn. These conditions can interfere with family integration and restrict attachment to the newborn. Some may threaten the safety and well-being of the mother and newborn. This chapter explores emotional disorders, psychoactive substance use (drug dependency), and poverty. The nursing process with affected women and their families is emphasized.

EMOTIONAL COMPLICATIONS

Mental health problems can complicate pregnancy, childbirth, and the puerperium. Developmental and personality disorders generally have an onset in childhood or adolescence. They usually persist into adulthood (Stuart, Sundeen, 1991). Mental retardation, autism, and disruptive behavior disorders are examples. Mental health disorders generally predate pregnancy. Sleep and arousal disorders, schizophrenic disorders, delusional (paranoid) disorders, and anxiety disorders are a few behavioral categories.

Pregnancy per se is not a cause of psychiatric illness. The psychologic and physical stresses relating to pregnancy or to the new obligations of motherhood may, however, bring on an emotional crisis (Affonso, 1984). The principal emotional disturbances complicating gestation are mood (affective) disorders and schizophrenia. Organic mental syndromes and disorders (non–substance-induced) also may be seen. The mood disturbances include depression or depression with manic episodes (bipolar disorders). Paranoia or other disorganizational problems may characterize schizophrenic disorders. Toxic delirium associated with substance abuse, excessive analgesia, or serious metabolic disorders is not common. Rarely, psychosis secondary to alcoholism or syphilis may complicate both prenatal and postnatal progress. Psychoactive substance-induced organic mental disorders are seen more often today. They are discussed later in this chapter.

No one single factor has been isolated as responsible for precipitating postpartum mental illness. Emotional illnesses arising during the puerperium are diagnosed by their initial features: affective, schizophrenic, or organic. Those illnesses that do not meet the criteria for any of these disorders are designated "postpartum psychoses" (American Psychiatric Association, 1987).

Mood (Affective) Disorders

Although the cause of **affective disorders** is unknown, the family history may reveal that one or more adults have had this problem. Moreover, women who have psychiatric complications during the course of pregnancy often have had similar crises previously. More than 50% of pregnancy-related mental illnesses are affective reactions. Of these, about 10% are prenatal manic or depressive states; the remainder occur in the postnatal period. Younger women seem more prone to manic reactions, but depression is the more common problem for most women.

Rejection of the infant, often caused by abnormal jealousy, is a prominent feature of affective disorders. The mother may be obsessed by the notion that the offspring may take her place in her partner's affections. In other instances, guilt regarding aversion to pregnancy, attempted abortion, or other personal conflicts may be the basic problem.

Manic reactions often occur during the first or second week of the puerperium, perhaps after a brief depression. Agitation, excitement, and volubility (ready and continuous flow of words; talkativeness), often with rhyming or punning, develop. The woman becomes disinterested in personal care and food. Because dehydration or exhaustion may occur, prompt and effective supportive treatment is essential.

Psychiatric therapy may include a tranquilizer with a significant sedative effect, for example, promethazine (Phenergan). Lithium may be given later for more prolonged control. Psychotherapy is essential. The usual duration of the manic state is 1 to 3 weeks. The prognosis for mother and infant is good after initial separation and gradual reunion.

Depressive reactions are far more common than manic reactions. The stress of pregnancy is both biologic and psychologic. During the postpartum period, women often experience many emotional reactions (Laizner, Jeans, 1990). Four aspects after birth demand significant coping abilities: physical adjustment, initial insecurities, support systems, and loss of previous identity. Some mothers are unable to adjust and become depressed or experience other emotional upheaval (Nicolson, 1990). The emotional disorders of the postpartum period can be grouped into three categories: postpartum blues, nonpsychotic postpartum depression, and postpartum psychosis.

POSTPARTUM BLUES. **Postpartum blues** are usually transient and may affect 75% to 80% of women giving birth (Hansen, 1990; Jones 1990). The blues may elicit crying spells, feelings of loneliness or rejection, anxiety, confusion, restlessness, exhaustion, forgetfulness, and inability to sleep (Hansen, 1990; Jones, 1990). These reactions may occur any time after birth but often manifest on the third or fourth day and peak between the fifth and fourteenth postpartum day. Diagnosing and categorizing the blues have been difficult because of the lack of standard assessment instruments. However, Kennerley and Gath (1989a) describe a reliable and valid new instrument that measures the seven symptoms of postpartum blues: mood swings, feeling "low," anxiety, feeling overemotional, tearfulness, fatigue, and confused or muddled thinking.

Predisposing factors of postpartum blues may include biologic changes, stress, normal responses, or social or environmental causes. Biologic theorists have studied the hormonal fluctuations and attribute some affective reactions to changes in progesterone, estradiol, cortisol, and prolactin levels (Harris et al, 1989; Majewska et al, 1989; and Ehlert et al, 1990). Stress theory supporters propose that any stressful event (e.g., surgery) can trigger reactions such as the blues (Iles et al, 1989). Others view the blues as a normal physiologically based response that increases mothering instincts and protectiveness toward the infant (Majewski et al, 1989). Social and environmental issues such as strained marital and family relations, a history of premenstrual syndrome (PMS), anxiety, fear of labor and depression during the pregnancy, and poor social adjustment may be predisposing factors (Kennerley, Gath, 1989b).

POSTPARTUM DEPRESSION. The frequency of **postpartum depression** varies from 5% to more than 25% (Daw, 1988; Steiner, 1990). The criteria for classifying postpartum depression vary but often are limited to affective syndromes that occur within 6 months of childbirth. The depressive episode may be minor, or it may be major without psychotic features (Jones, 1990; Troutman, Cutrona, 1990). Loss of sexual interest and fatigue occur commonly in all postpartum women. However, those experiencing depression also demonstrate poor concentration, feelings of guilt, loss of energy, and lack of interest in usual activities (Hopkins et al, 1989). The symptoms of postpartum depression last longer than the blues. In addition, the woman may experience weight changes (loss or gain), social withdrawal, inability to cope, and concern about mothering skills to care for the infant. If major depression continues, hospitalization may be required. Support from groups—as well as individual therapy and administration of psychotropic drugs such as trifluoperazine (Stelazine), fluoxetine (Prozac), and bupropion (Wellbutrin)—may be needed (Busch, Perrin, 1989; Harding, 1989; Taylor, 1989; Martell, 1990).

Predisposing factors may be hormone-related, stress-related, or infant-related. As with postpartum blues, some researchers have identified a link between hormonal levels and postpartum depression (Harris et al, 1989; Smith et al, 1990). Prolactin and progesterone levels are found to be significantly related to depression. Environmental and family stress issues may be linked to postpartum depression (see Research Highlight, p. 998). Women who experience depression often have fewer support systems, more stressful life events, and poor personal resources with which to combat these events. Predictive factors for postpartum depression that may assist the nurse in assessing potential problems include low income, absence of a confidant for support, meager or absent social support, and stressful life events (e.g., single parenthood, divorce, or recent death of a parent or child) (Auerbach, Jacobi, 1990; Stein et al, 1989). There may be a correlation between the infant's behavior and the mother's depression. Maternal depression is associated with a range of adverse outcomes for the newborn, such as newborn irritability (Zuckerman et al, 1990) and low birth weight (McAnarney, Stevens-Simon, 1990). Infants who had a difficult temperament and were unpredictable and less adaptable often had mothers who were depressed. However, the mothers rarely attributed their depression to the infant but blamed themselves for their lack of skill in providing for the baby (Whiffen, Gotlib, 1989).

POSTPARTUM PSYCHOSIS. The most severe depression is that of **postpartum psychosis.** Symptoms often begin as postpartum blues or postpartum depression. Delusions, hallucinations, confusion, delirium, and panic may occur (Metz et al, 1988). The woman may manifest symptoms resembling schizophrenia or acute brain syndrome (Steiner, 1990). Hospitalization for several months usually is required. Suicide or danger to the infant, or both, are the greatest hazards of postpartum psychosis (Goldstein, 1989; Hamilton, 1989).

Schizophrenia

Schizophrenic reactions, now suspected of being a disorder of cerebral metabolism, affect adolescents and younger adults rather than older persons. Abnormal personality features are common. Unusually shy, retiring, hypersensitive, or overly suspicious women are prone to **schizophrenia.** A sudden onset of delusions or hallucinations may alter a seemingly well-accepted normal pregnancy. The symptoms indicate the woman's inability to adjust to and cope with her new obligations as a mother.

The partner and infant are totally rejected. Hostility toward the significant other and the medical staff is obvious. The woman abandons reality and totally retreats into her own world. The mother completely neglects her infant. Suicide is unlikely. A phenothi-

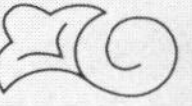 **Research Highlight** 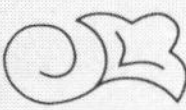

Factors in Postpartum Depression: Onset and Recovery

RESEARCH ABSTRACT

The purpose of this study was to examine the role of psychosocial variables that affect onset of and recovery from postpartum depression. The participants were 730 pregnant women recruited from clinics and private practices of obstetricians. They were assessed during pregnancy, with follow-up for 1 month after childbirth. Data were collected by means of standard tools for depression, depressive symptoms, marital distress, dysfunctional attitudes, quality of parental relationships, stress, and coping. Of the total sample, 75 were depressed and 655 were not depressed at the initial assessment. An additional 32 were diagnosed as depressed at the postpartum assessment.

Women who became depressed after childbirth had higher scores in depressive symptoms, higher levels of stress, and lower levels of marital satisfaction. They used escape-avoidance to cope and perceived less caring from their own mothers and fathers than did women who were not depressed. They also perceived their infants as more bothersome and difficult to care for. Of the women who were depressed during pregnancy, 54 had recovered by the postpartum assessment. Depressed women who recovered reported less stress and more marital satisfaction. Although results were statistically significant, the variables studied accounted for only 12% of the variance in the diagnosis of postpartum depression. Other factors, yet unidentified, have significant effects on depression after childbirth.

IMPLICATIONS FOR PRACTICE

Preexisting depression, stress, and marital satisfaction are factors associated with postpartum depression. Nurses working with pregnant women should assess these factors and provide suggestions for reducing stress and coping with symptoms of depression. Suggestions for obtaining support from the partner or family can be discussed. Appropriate referrals may be necessary.

RELATED RESEARCH QUESTIONS

1. Will an educational program help women to identify stressors in their lives and learn ways to cope with the stress?
2. Will an educational program help women to obtain support from their partners or family?
3. Is there an association between complications of pregnancy and postpartum depression?
4. Is there a relation between depression in pregnancy and maternal-infant interaction?

REFERENCE

Gotlib IH et al: Prospective investigation of postpartum depression: factors involved in onset and recovery, *J Abnorm Psychol* 100:122, 1991.

azine type of tranquilizer, for example, chlorpromazine (Thorazine), will be useful. Transfer of the woman to a psychiatric hospital usually is necessary. A good prognosis is likely with the first psychotic episode, especially if it occurs unexpectedly during the puerperium.

ASSESSMENT

Recognition of the symptoms of depression is essential for the perinatal nurse. The nursing care plan must reflect the expected behavioral responses of the particular disorder. The individualized plan is based on the woman's characteristics and her specific circumstances. The woman's partner, the father of the baby, or other family member also may be experiencing emotional upheaval.

NURSING DIAGNOSES

Nursing diagnoses relevant to any emotional illness that complicates pregnancy may include the following:

- High risk for injury to fetus related to
  - —Psychotropic medication
  - —Maternal suicide
- High risk for injury to newborn related to
  - —Unmet needs (e.g., hygiene, nutrition) and safety precautions
  - —Mother's poor impulse control
- Ineffective family coping related to
  - —Increased care needs of mother-fetus/newborn
- Impaired home maintenance management related to
  - —Increased care needs of mother-fetus/newborn

- High risk for altered parenting related to
  - —Lack of supervised opportunities for attachment to infant
- High risk for altered growth and development of infant related to
  - —Lack of intellectual stimulation
- —Unmet needs (hygiene, nutrition) and safety precautions

PLANNING

Planning focuses on the mother's dependency needs, attachment to the infant, family integration, parenting skills and care of the infant, and home maintenance management. Supervision of the mother and family in the home is a prime concern (Martell, 1990). Client-centered *goals* include the following:

- The mother's and infant's physical well-being will be maintained.
- The mother and family will cope effectively.
- Each family member will continue healthy growth and development.

IMPLEMENTATION

Community resources such as the community health nurse, homemaker service, or foster care are utilized as necessary. Discharge planning, carefully developed with the family in collaboration with a hospital-community health care team, is vital.

PRENATAL HOSPITALIZATION. In-hospital psychiatric treatment often is required to treat psychotic pregnant women. Maternal physiologic adaptations and fetal movement often result in intensification of delusional ideas in the schizophrenic woman. Women with bipolar mood (affective) disorders may respond well during pregnancy and childbirth. After the birth, however, these women are prone to worsening of psychotic symptoms and depression (Spielvogel, Wile, 1986). Hospitalized women present treatment challenges in three areas: psychotropic medication, legal sanctions, and management in an acute hospital setting. A brief overview of these difficulties is given here. Psychiatric texts must be consulted for specific details.

PSYCHOTROPIC MEDICATIONS. All psychotropic medications pass through the placenta to the fetus and through breast milk to the infant. The risks of medication are weighed against the risks of maternal agitation and potentially self-destructive behavior. Infants exposed to psychotropics between 8 and 10 weeks' gestation show a higher rate of congenital anomalies (5.4%) than does the population with no such exposure (3.2%) (Edlund, Craig, 1984). A higher perinatal death rate and an increased incidence of an extrapyramidal syndrome consisting of "tremors, hypertonia, weakness, and poor sucking and other reflexes" complicate the neonatal period (Hauser, 1985). Medication dosage is balanced between the mother's needs and fetal response determined by nonstress tests (NST). Some medications may be behavioral teratogens with short- and long-term effects (Cook et al, 1990).

Bipolar affective disorders often are treated with *lithium*. A high incidence of fetal cardiovascular abnormalities is linked to lithium taken during the first trimester. Maternal shifts in fluid balance may require doubling the lithium dose to achieve a therapeutic level (Spielvogel, Wile, 1986). Fetal lithium toxicity may cause polyhydramnios. Fetal toxicity can result if the lithium dose is not decreased by at least 50% 1 week before birth—if the date can be correctly anticipated. Regardless of dose and the mother's plasma level, the neonate may show signs of toxicity: cyanosis, lethargy, low Apgar scores, and absent Moro's reflex (Krause et al, 1990).

LEGAL SANCTIONS. Women with mental health problems who can provide self-care may be unable to care for themselves *and* the fetus. Hospital care may be mandated during pregnancy. Delusions about the pregnancy and its medical monitoring may necessitate legal intervention. Other legal issues arise closer to the birth. These issues surround the care of the mother and her infant and fertility management (Spielvogel, Wile, 1986).

IN-HOSPITAL MANAGEMENT. Schizophrenic pregnant women often experience an intensification of their disorder. These women usually remain ambivalent toward the fetus and resist examination and procedures. Because they seem unaware of signs of labor, staff members must be keenly alert to behavioral and physical indicators of labor. Even though disorganization often diminishes, specific delusions may persist. The new mother may not be able to be close to her baby or to recognize or meet the baby's needs.

Pregnant women with bipolar affective disorders usually respond well to pregnancy, the fetus, and the birth. The new mother's responses may not be consistent or appropriate to the baby, however. After the birth, psychotic symptoms or depression worsens. Mothers need to be supervised carefully when visiting with their babies to ensure their safety.

POSTPARTUM MENTAL ILLNESS. In caring for a woman experiencing postpartum depression, the nurse must be aware of the effect on the family. If the mother is feeling inadequate, is unable to cope with herself or the infant, is withdrawn, or is severely fatigued, the family is affected. Stressors are magnified, which can result in isolation of the mother and family, a change in relationship with the partner, or a negative impact on parenting. The nurse must be alert for these signs of dysfunction and be prepared to help promote attachment between mother and baby, referral of the mother and family for support services and counseling, and assisting the family is prioritizing and performing necessary family functioning (Martell, 1990).

Most treatment programs for postpartum depression tend to be reactive rather than predictive. Nicolson (1990) reports that a more effective approach would be to assess postnatal depression not as an individual illness or vulnerability but more as a normal grief reaction and part of every postnatal profile. Interpretation by the mother of her experience may be the key to more appropriate treatment. Nurses could help mothers recognize that the experience is not always happy, positive, and a gain rather than a loss. Many mothers grieve over the loss of their former selves (figures, life-styles, sexual attractiveness) and go through an upheaval and extreme stress. The nurse can help the mother to acknowledge her new self and new role and accept the knowledge that depression and a grief reaction may be normal and not permanent.

The nurse's role varies with the type of postpartum depression. With the baby blues or mild depression, the nurse can refer the woman to peer support groups or workshops that may help her with specific problems such as assertiveness. In more severe depression a nurse practitioner or psychiatric specialist could provide specialized counseling, or a referral for psychiatric counseling may be needed. In the most extreme cases, in-hospital management may be required.

The onset of postpartum psychosis usually is abrupt and occurs within days of childbirth. The symptoms center around the mother's relationship with the baby. The mother's response may be of an overprotective or of a rejecting nature (Hurt, Ray, 1985). The mother may be convinced that someone is trying to take her baby from her and will clutch it protectively. Or she may believe that the baby is dead or defective or that God is caring for it and so the baby does not need care.

The presenting symptoms form the basis for management. A major depressive condition is one that continues for more than 2 weeks and includes at least four of the following symptoms: change in appetite, change in sleep, psychomotor agitation, loss of interest in usual activities, decrease in sexual drive, increased fatigue, feelings of guilt or worthlessness, slowed thinking or impaired concentration, and possible suicidal ideation (American Psychiatric Association, 1987). Schizophrenia-like symptoms are treated with psychotropic medications. Lithium may be prescribed with or without psychotropic medications for bipolar affective disorders. A phenothiazine type of tranquilizer, for example, chlorpromazine (Thorazine), will be useful. Depression may be treated with psychotherapy and electroconvulsive therapy if suicidal or infanticidal thoughts are identified. Women may need assistance for alterations in patterns of sleep-rest, self-care (basic hygiene), nutrition and fluid balance, elimination, self-esteem, and family coping and processes. Discharge planning focuses on preparation for meeting the demands of an infant while the mother is still integrating her experience with psychosis, supporting the partner, and exploring the effects of the illness on their family (Hurt, Ray, 1985).

The mother's depression or psychosis prevents her from engaging in the mutual interaction with the baby that is needed for acquaintance and subsequent attachment (bonding). If the mother wants to breastfeed, nurses can assist with the same techniques used for any new mother. It is important to maintain and support the maternal role (Auerbach, Jacobi, 1990). Within the hospital setting the reintroduction of the mother and baby can occur at the mother's own pace. During these interactions the mother's readiness to care for the baby after discharge is evaluated. The interactions are carefully supervised and guided. A schedule is set for increasing hours over 3 to 4 days, culminating in the infant's admission to the unit for an overnight stay. The overnight stay allows the mother to experience the infant's being there and giving up sleep for the baby, a situation difficult for new mothers under ideal conditions. During this time the nurses observe the woman for **attachment,** or **bonding behaviors.** Attachment behaviors are defined as eye-to-eye contact (*en face* position), physical contact of holding, touching, cuddling, talking to the baby and calling the baby by name, as well as initiating care for the baby when appropriate. A staff member is assigned to keep the baby within sight at all times. Indirect teaching, praise, and encouragement are designed to bolster the mother's self-esteem and self-confidence. Staff work with the father is provided concurrently. Administrative and clinical support in the psychiatric unit has facilitated comprehensive care to women who develop a psychosis in the puerperium and to their families.

A good prognosis is likely with the first psychotic

episode, especially if it occurs unexpectedly during the puerperium. The child probably will never suffer from schizophrenia, despite speculation regarding hereditary tendencies.

EVALUATION

Evaluation is based on the client's progress toward meeting the goals established (p. 999). The nurse can be assured that care has been effective if the physical well-being of the mother and infant is maintained, the mother and family are able to cope effectively, and each family member continues in a healthy growth and development pattern.

■ PSYCHOACTIVE SUBSTANCE USE

The use of **psychoactive** (mind-altering) **substances** is pandemic. In this discussion, substance abuse is defined as the use of any mind-altering agent to such an extent that it interferes with the individual's biologic, psychologic, or sociocultural integrity (Stuart, Sundeen, 1991). Interference with biologic integrity might be exemplified (during pregnancy) in poor nutrition leading to poor weight gain, anemia, and a predisposition to infection and pregnancy-induced hypertension. Poor hygiene and multidrug use may compound and confuse the signs and symptoms (Frank et al, 1988; Silverman, 1989; Little et al, 1990; Lynch, McKeon, 1990). Some drugs (morphine, heroin, diazepam, and others) induce platelet disorders that predispose the woman to hemorrhage (Scott et al, 1990). Psychologic consequences may include acute psychosis in a pregnant teenager who has been taking phencyclidine (PCP) or the inability of a new mother to attach to her infant (see discussion of emotional disturbances). Expectant and new mothers using psychoactive substances receive negative feedback from society, as well as from health care providers who condemn them for endangering the unborn and the newborn infant and who may withhold support. **Drug dependence (addiction)** is the physical or psychologic dependence, or both, on a substance. Pregnant women who are drug dependent often do not seek prenatal care until labor begins (Burkett et al, 1990; Cordero, Custard, 1990). Pregnant women often have little understanding of the effects of these substances on themselves, their pregnancies, or on their babies. They will take the drug just before seeking admission; therefore withdrawal symptoms can be delayed for 6 to 12 hours. **Withdrawal** refers to the psychologic and physical symptoms that occur after removal of the substance in the substance-dependent person.

The care of the substance-dependent pregnant woman is based on historic data, symptoms, physical findings, and laboratory results. As a result of the woman's defensiveness and frequent denial, history taking has to be done in a sensitive and competent manner.

The woman dependent on a drug tends to exhibit a passive response to life and its responsibilities. She may show a high degree of depression. Substance use has meant a way for her to relieve psychologic distress, to encourage social interaction, and to blunt the feelings of loneliness and emptiness that are part of depression. Pregnancy usually is not planned. It occurs as an "accidental" phenomenon. It may serve as a positive event, confirming her worth as a woman.

After birth, however, the woman is faced with the parental tasks of caring for and nurturing a completely dependent infant and of forming a warm, close, intimate relationship with the child. Care of the woman addicted to a drug offers a tremendous nursing challenge. The difficulty of this challenge soon becomes apparent. The demands of motherhood are being made of a person who is herself dependent and arrested at the stage of taking and receiving rather than giving. Most substance-dependent persons are unable to establish positive intimate relationships and lack a meaningful support system.

With the advent of very early discharge, often within 24 hours after birth, assessment becomes extremely difficult and an increasing challenge to health care professionals. The mother's ability to care for her infant after discharge from the hospital should be assessed by frequent observations, including some in the home setting.

This discussion focuses on the use and abuse of alcohol, heroin, cocaine, and methamphetamine. Many other substances are abused. The care needed by the individual varies with the particular circumstances of that individual and the substance abused. However, the nursing process is similar for all.

Alcohol

Identification of the woman with an alcohol problem may be difficult. Denial of the problem or its consequences is almost universal and a key element of the disease. Underreporting of alcohol use in pregnancy is a major concern of health care workers (Little et al, 1988). A concerned, nonjudgmental, matter-of-fact approach is used in the hope that the woman admits a problem if it exists. Inability to form positive relationships often results from manipulative behavior. A low tolerance for frustration or anxiety and ex-

TABLE 33-1 Psychoactive Substance Effects

Drug	Psychologic Signs	Physiologic Signs
ALCOHOL		
Intoxication	Mood lability or change Impaired attention or memory Irritability Talkativeness	Slurred speech Flushed face Incoordination, unsteady gait Nystagmus
Withdrawal	Anxiety Depressed mood or irritability Maladaptive behavior	Nausea and vomiting Malaise or weakness Hyperactivity Coarse tremor of hands, tongue, eyelids Orthostatic hypotension
COCAINE ("CRACK")		
Intoxication	Psychomotor agitation Elation Grandiosity; talkativeness Hypervigilance Maladaptive behaviors	Tachycardia Pupillary dilation Hypertension Perspiration; chills Nausea; vomiting
Withdrawal	Depressed mood Disturbed sleep Increased dreaming	Fatigue Headache Convulsions (seizure)
HEROIN		
Intoxication	Euphoria, dysphoria Psychomotor retardation Apathy Maladaptive behavior Impaired attention or memory	Pupillary constriction Drowsiness Slurred speech
Withdrawal	Insomnia	Lacrimation, rhinorrhea Pupillary dilation Sweating Diarrhea Yawning Mild hypertension Tachycardia Fever
METHAMPHETAMINE ("ICE")		
Intoxication	Hyperactivity Insomnia Restlessness Irritability Aggressiveness	Tachycardia, palpitations Tachypnea Nausea, vomiting Constipation Impotence
Withdrawal	Depression Increased sleeping Lethargy	Headache Nausea, vomiting Muscle pain Weakness
PHENCYCLIDINE (PCP)	Euphoria Psychomotor agitation Increased anxiety Emotional lability Grandiosity Sensation of slowed time Synesthesias Maladaptive behaviors	Vertical or horizontal nystagmus Hypertension Increased heart rate Numbness Decreased response to pain Ataxia; dysarthria

pressions of guilt related to alcoholic behavior patterns may be evident. Physical signs and symptoms also may be present (Table 33-1). During withdrawal, central nervous system (CNS) agitation is expressed as fatigue, insomnia, agitation, restlessness, and belligerence. Bruises, rashes, and other injuries may be observed. Poor physical hygiene and malnutrition are potential problems, especially in the chronic alcohol abuser. Assessment for maternal and fetal well-being follows the protocols discussed for other clients. Women who smoke, are unmarried, less educated, and younger (i.e., under 25 years of age) are at the highest risk for alcohol abuse in pregnancy and should be the prime targets of educational efforts of health workers.

Cocaine

The cocaine abuser often has a constellation of cocaine-related problems: family problems, employment difficulties, various health issues, psychologic stress, guilt, and anger (Landry, Smith, 1987). Coexisting psychiatric disorders cloud differential diagnosis. For example, schizophrenics display excessive dopamine levels in some areas of the brain. Decreased amounts of *norepinephrine* and *serotonin* have been implicated in persons with biologically based depression. Dysfunction of serotonin metabolism is seen in manifestations of violence, rage, and maladaptive behavior. Cocaine raises norepinephrine and serotonin levels rapidly and then depletes them abruptly. The biochemical systems of norepinephrine, serotonin, and dopamine play a vital role in mood regulation and mental health; all three systems are affected by cocaine.

The effects of cocaine are similar to those of amphetamines (p. 1004), with short-term CNS stimulation. There is a blockage of re-uptake of catecholamines, resulting in a high level of catecholamines. This leads to the hyperaroused stated found in cocaine abusers (Janke, 1990).

The increase in the use of cocaine and the even more addictive "crack" among childbearing women has been phenomenal in the past few years (Tracy, 1988). Crack is cocaine mixed with baking soda and heated until it reaches its purest form. It is sold in the form of "rocks," which are smoked in pipes. Whereas its use may cross all cultural groups, its inexpensiveness and availability are naking it the drug of choice among poorer populations (Lynch, McKeon, 1990). Because crack is highly addictive, it poses new problems to health care providers who may first see the pregnant addict in the labor and birthing area.

Diagnostic protocol to distinguish between drug use and drug addiction requires considerable knowledge and is beyond the scope of this text. An appropriate plan of care is designed depending on the diagnosis (i.e., substance use problems or addiction disease) (Landry, Smith, 1987). The focus of this section is the identification of the pregnant cocaine user and the effects of cocaine on the pregnancy. The care of the cocaine-affected newborn is addressed in Chapter 39.

The nurse or physician takes a history of the drug abuse (95% also are addicted to heroin or methadone), type of drug and mode of administration, and participation (if any) in drug programs; assesses the woman's feelings and plans for this pregnancy (infant); and determines the expected date of the birth. The social worker or psychiatric social worker is brought in to evaluate the woman's social, economic, home, and ethnic problems; welfare requirements; and educational or vocational status and needs.

MEDICAL COMPLICATIONS. Pregnancy is compromised by cocaine-related medical complications that are encountered by the infrequent, as well as frequent, high-dose user. A variety of less serious medical problems is seen, including lack of energy, insomnia, nasal sinus problems, nose bleeds, sore throat, and decreased libido. More serious problems develop as general health deteriorates. The nasal septum perforates. Cardiovascular stress increases and tachycardia, systemic hypertension, ventricular arrhythmias, sudden coronary artery spasm, and myocardial infarction develop. Cocaine-associated complications also include liver damage, intestinal ischemia, seizures, hemorrhagic bronchitis, headache, and death. Needle-borne diseases such as hepatitis B and acquired immunodeficiency syndrome (AIDS) are common. "Tracks," septic phlebitis, cellulitis, and superficial abscesses are seen in intravenous drug users. Many users are poorly nourished and commonly have sexually transmitted diseases (STDs). Pulmonary disease with acute pulmonary edema is a commonly encountered complication. A **toxicology** (urine) **screen** (for the presence of abused substances) or other laboratory tests for liver damage and anemia may be ordered when drug use is suspected. An assessment of the woman's support system adds valuable data for developing a plan of care. The presence of any of the medical complications, results of laboratory tests, or signs and symptoms of intoxication or withdrawal (Table 33-1) assist in the identification of substance use problems and addictive disease.

Cocaine users typically mediate the side effects of cocaine by a CNS depressant such as alcohol (Landry, Smith, 1987; Matera et al, 1990). Thus the woman and her fetus are exposed to the risks of cocaine and alcohol. In some areas of the United States it is estimated that 10% of pregnant women use cocaine (Lynch, McKeon, 1990).

Cocaine produces tachycardia and a rise in blood pressure by increasing the levels of catecholamines (Woods et al, 1987). During pregnancy, uterine blood vessels are maximally dilated, but they vasoconstrict readily in the presence of catecholamines. Separation of the placenta (abruption) or acute onset of preterm labor, with long, hard contractions and precipitous birth after intravenous cocaine administration, probably is secondary to acute spasm of uterine blood vessels (Woods et al, 1987; Janke, 1990; Adams et al, 1990; Chisum, 1990). Use of the drug during pregnancy can lead to small-for-gestational-age neonates and fetal death (Woods 1987; Chasnoff, 1989). Neonate addiction is discussed in Chapter 39.

Heroin

Assessment of heroin use is similar to that for alcohol and cocaine use. Interview and open discussion may disclose the problem and its extent (e.g., length of addiction, amount needed in cost per day). Physical examination reveals intravenous tracks, cellulitis, and surface abscesses at the administration sites. Further assessment of the peripheral vascular system may reveal burning paresthesia or decreased or absent peripheral pulses (or both) in the extremity used for self-injection. Signs of STDs and urinary tract infections often are present.

Laboratory tests are ordered for toxicology, STDs, hepatitis B, and antibodies to human immunodeficiency virus (HIV). Determinations of blood urea nitrogen, serum creatinine, total protein levels, albumin-to-globulin ratio, total iron-binding capacity, hemoglobin, and hematocrit values are obtained. Chest x-ray study may be ordered for pulmonary disease. Hilar lymphadenopathy in 95% of addicted persons, pulmonary edema, bacterial pneumonia, and foreign body emboli (from the substances used to "cut" street drugs) may be revealed.

Initial and serial ultrasound studies are used to determine gestational age because amenorrhea, common among drug users, precludes dating by history of last menstrual period. However, nonstress and stress testing are not significantly helpful in assessing fetal well-being. The addicted fetus is nonreactive. Estriol measurements are inaccurate. The heroin-addicted woman is more likely to experience premature rupture of membranes and preterm labor (Ney et al, 1990).

Methamphetamine

The active metabolite of methamphetamine is amphetamine, a CNS stimulant. Powdered methamphetamine is known as "speed" and "meth." Methamphetamine-exposed pregnant women have higher rates of preterm births and neonates with intrauterine growth retardation and smaller head circumferences than those of a drug-free comparison group (Oro, Dixon, 1987). Neonatal behavioral patterns are altered. They are characterized by abnormal sleep patterns, poor feeding, tremors, and hypertonia. These behaviors are seen if the fetus was exposed to cocaine, methamphetamine, or their combination (Oro, Dixon, 1987; Cook et al, 1990). The addition of cocaine significantly increases the rate of placental hemorrhage and stillbirth. Other neonatal behaviors include state disorganization and decreased sleep. Feeding may be prolonged and accompanied by disorganized rooting and sucking. Tube feeding may be required. Withdrawal symptoms may be treated with phenobarbital or opium tincture (Paregoric).

ICE. The crystalline form of methamphetamine is known as "ice." This smokable form is odorless. It gives users a very long steady high, is more addictive than heroin, and is more potent than "crack" cocaine ("Ice," 1989). Ice enables a person to go without rest or food for 24 hours, only to "crash" for the next 24 hours. Common signs include tachycardia, tachypnea, paranoid illusions, and violent behavior. Symptoms of amphetamine abuse appear after 2 years of use: paranoia and delusional, irrational, and illogical behavior. Convulsions, coma, and death follow overdose (New drug, 1989).

The drug is very popular with young women who want to lose weight rapidly and with teenagers who want to stay up all night. Drug dependency has serious consequences for the pregnant woman. The drug causes convulsions in the mother and the newborn. Other effects on the fetus/newborn are thought to be similar to those experienced by the fetus/newborn exposed to powdered methamphetamine.

Marijuana

Marijuana can be smoked in cigarettes, pipes, or water pipes or mixed into food and eaten. It provides an intoxicating and sensory-distorting "high." Marijuana smoke has the characteristics of tobacco smoke and has similar dangers (Cook et al, 1990). Marijuana readily crosses the placenta. Both cigarettes and marijuana increase carbon monoxide levels in the mother's blood, which can reduce oxygen in fetal blood. Research findings regarding marijuana effects on pregnancy are inconsistent. That is, maternal use did not consistently increase the incidence of spontaneous abortion or stillbirths. Neonatal effects also vary and may include altered sleep and arousal patterns and tremulousness. Reasons for the inconsistent results may reflect variations in composition of the drug, other maternal factors (e.g., life-style, health), problems of unreporting of marijuana use, or methodologic issues (Cook et al, 1990). Women who abuse marijuana are more likely to bear children with features compatible with fetal alcohol syndrome. This finding supports the possibility that marijuana may have a synergistic effect on alcohol and other substances (Cook et al, 1990). Marijuana rapidly passes into breast milk. Because the effects on the newborn of marijuana-contaminated breast milk are unknown, breast-feeding by these mothers is not recommended. Postnatal effects of prenatal exposure to marijuana have not as yet been identified.

Phencyclidine

PCP is a synthetic drug known by various names (peace pill, angel dust, hog). Its effects are unpredictable and include hostility, aggressiveness, and other bizarre behavior (Cook et al, 1990). Because some effects mimic schizophrenia, a user may be admitted to a psychiatric unit. After use, it persists in the brain and body fat for an extended period. It crosses the placenta and tends to be found in higher concentration in fetal tissue than in maternal tissue. Inasmuch as PCP tends to be used in various combinations of alcohol, cocaine, and marijuana, specific effects on pregnancy, the fetus, and the neonate have not been identified (Fico, Vanderwende, 1988; Cook et al, 1990).

ASSESSMENT

Each client is assessed for signs and symptoms of psychoactive substance use through interview, physical examination, and laboratory tests (see discussions of substances and Table 33-1). Psychologic and physiologic symptoms are described and reported.

NURSING DIAGNOSES

The following are examples of nursing diagnoses formulated from the assessment data:

- High risk for fluid volume deficit and altered nutrition: less than body requirements, related to
  - —Effects of excessive use of psychoactive drugs
- High risk for injury to self, fetus, or newborn related to
  - —Sensory effects of drug
- High risk for infection related to
  - —Life-style
  - —Dehydration and malnutrition
  - —Method of administration of drug or effects of drug
- Self-care deficit, bathing/hygiene related to
  - —Effects of substance
- Denial, related to
  - —Lack of understanding of disease process
  - —Effects of psychoactive drug on developing fetus and pregnancy
- Ineffective individual coping related to
  - —Lack of support system
  - —Low self-esteem
  - —Lack of healthy mechanisms for recognition and release of anger
- High risk for violence related to
  - —Maintenance of drug habit
  - —Effects of substance used

PLANNING

Planning for care must be accomplished with recognition of the woman's life-style and habits. The ideal long-term goal would be total abstinence. However, the woman may be unable to face that level of commitment at this time. The thought of giving up the substance forever is anxiety provoking. It is rare for a substance-dependent person to stop use of that substance suddenly. Short-term goals are necessary. The woman must participate in the decision-making process in formulating the goals. It is particularly important that the goals be phrased so that it is clear that the woman has responsibility for her behavior. The *goals* are written into a contract signed by the woman and the nurse (or physician). One copy is kept by the woman.

SHORT-TERM GOALS

- Woman's physiologic status is stabilized.
- Woman keeps appointments for prenatal and postpartum care for herself and her infant.
- Fetal effects are minimized; baby remains safe and receives care.

LONG-TERM GOAL

- Woman voluntarily becomes involved in long-term medical, social (e.g., Alcoholics Anonymous, withdrawal [methadone] program), psychiatric, and vocational rehabilitation.

IMPLEMENTATION

A multidisciplinary approach is needed to plan for the care of the expectant mother. In increasing numbers, pregnant psychoactive drug users are seen on maternity units. Hospitals are reporting an increase of three to four times as many drug-related births since 1985 (Janke, 1990). The needs of these mothers present special challenges to nurses. A standardized nursing care plan may be best developed by the total team of nurses on the maternity unit. A starting point in the development of a care plan may need to be a values clarification experience. It is not uncommon for nurses to harbor negative feelings about the behavior of psychoactive drug users. Collaboration with psychiatric nurses may be necessary to strengthen the maternity nurse's therapeutic potential with these clients. Comprehensive care involves many organizations, child protective services, human resource agencies, and the community health department (Mondanaro, 1987).

The need for *biologic support* may be related to overdose, withdrawal, allergy, or toxicity. Physical deterioration results from the harmful effects of drugs, including conditions such as malnutrition, dehydration, and various infections. The acute physical condition takes priority over the woman's other health needs.

Interactive interventions are initiated as soon as appropriate. The intervention is directed toward reducing the stressors that apply to each individual and is identified in the nursing diagnoses. Examples of interactive interventions include group support, client education, or individual counseling. Psychiatric nurses are skilled in intervening in denial, dependency, manipulation, and anger. Other required skills include establishing behavioral contracts and increasing self-esteem. The primary focus of care is the woman. Usually she is already acutely aware of the dangers to the fetus resulting from her behavior. Emphasis on the fetus's well-being instead of on her own may add to her guilt, frustration, and low self-esteem.

Social support systems are mobilized. Family counseling, self-help groups, transitional living programs, and community treatment programs are involved. Some social service agencies remove the child from the home. Others focus on assisting troubled parents in learning to solve their problems with the child in the home. Employee assistance programs are now available in many industries, including hospitals (Clemmer, 1987).

Labor room nurses need to work out a standardized plan for care. Typically the woman displays poor control over her behavior and a low threshold for pain, which is especially noticeable when she is in labor. Increased dependency needs are apparent. **Intoxication** or withdrawal signs and symptoms of the mother and fetus (Table 33-1) may challenge staff members. Staffing should be sufficient to ensure strict surveillance of visitors to prevent unsupervised drug administration. (See case study, p. 1007, and nursing plan of care, p. 1008.)

Advice regarding breast-feeding is individualized. All abused substances appear in breast milk, some in greater amounts than others. Some substances (e.g., methadone) may cause newborn depression and failure to thrive (Chasnoff, 1987; Chaney, 1988). The baby's eating and safety needs must of course be considered. Breast-feeding necessitates a closeness between the mother and child, and the baby may be more irritable and difficult to console. These women, who are already in a fragile state with depleted energy reserves and coping capability, commonly experience severe emotional decompensation. This can be aggravated by breast-feeding and care of the infant, which are exhausting under ideal circumstances. For some women the need to breast-feed and care for the infant provides the impetus to break the drug dependency habit. Community health agencies may be mobilized for home supervision or guidance in antepartum and infant care or for putting the infant up for adoption. Day/night-center care programs or halfway houses may be indicated.

The substitution of methadone for heroin is still a controversial issue. If women withdraw from heroin during pregnancy, blood flow to the placenta is impaired. To prevent this, methadone is used to assist in withdrawal from heroin. Some experts advocate complete withdrawal without methadone use, despite the risk of interrupted blood flow to the placenta. Others contend that use of methadone to withdraw from heroin is good for the mother; however, methadone withdrawal for the infant may be worse after birth (Edeline et al, 1988; Silverman, 1989).

Discharge planning should begin with the first contact with the woman. If the woman is to be discharged to the care of her parents, several nursing actions may be employed. The client is involved in decision making whenever possible. The mother is involved with the care of her infant when she is willing. Mother-child attachment is promoted. Angry, argumentative encounters between the mother and nurse are avoided; the nurse needs to respond with patience, sympathy, consistency, and at times, with firmness. The mother's positive maternal responses and feelings are supported even if she is relinquishing her infant for adoption.

EVALUATION

Evaluation is difficult because the long-range effects cannot be projected. Short-term positive achievements are indicators of success (e.g., if the mother keeps her appointments or improves her nu-

CASE STUDY

Cocaine Abuse during Pregnancy

Joy Taylor is a 19-year-old, single, primigravida who is at 32 weeks' gestation. She is admitted to the perinatal unit in preterm labor (PTL) and admits to "occasional" snorting of cocaine.

ASSESSMENT

Admitting history included the following data: Joy has tried to stop use of cocaine during her pregnancy but still "binges" at least every weekend and sometimes during the week. Joy states, "I know I shouldn't use it, but everyone was, and I was so upset that Joe was gone!" The baby's father has just left her without providing any emotional or financial support. She will soon have to quit her job as a receptionist and rely on welfare and food stamps. Her vital signs are all elevated above her normal baseline: pulse 108 beats/min, respirations 20/min, temperature 99° F, blood pressure 140/98 mm Hg. She has gained only 15 pounds during her pregnancy. Her pupils are dilated, and she seems agitated. The monitor displays a fetal heart rate (FHR) of 158 beats/min, and the fetus is active. Joy is experiencing mild contractions every 5 to 6 minutes. Her blood and urine test results are negative for infection and preeclampsia.

NURSING DIAGNOSIS

The assessment findings support several nursing diagnoses. The diagnosis that takes priority at this time is high risk for injury to the fetus related to preterm labor.

PLANNING

Joy needs considerable assistance from the nurse to plan care necessary for her immediate problem and for the remainder of her pregnancy. Joy and the nurse mutually agree that the *goal* that takes priority is to stop the preterm labor. The *expected outcomes* set by the nurse include tocolysis of labor (see Chapter 35) and helping Joy to increase her ability to cope so that she will be able to carry her pregnancy to full term without further use of cocaine.

IMPLEMENTATION

Nursing actions are derived from the medical management and physician orders, as well as nursing orders based on nursing diagnoses. The first goal is to stop the PTL. Specific interventions during tocolysis include continuous assessment of the status of the mother and fetus (e.g., contractions, FHR, fetal activity, signs and symptoms of toxicity to the tocolytic drug being used). The nurse will manage the intravenous administration of tocolytic drugs to suppress labor (see Chapter 35), encourage bed rest, and prepare Joy for discharge. Discharge planning must include how to take the tocolytic medication and how to recognize and report any toxicity and recurrence of preterm labor contractions. A trusting relationship must be developed so that the nurse can help Joy work on life-style issues that are interfering with the progress of her pregnancy. A referral to a community health nurse (CHN) is needed for follow-up of her status, including use of oral tocolytics and emotional support.

EVALUATION

Joy's preterm labor is suppressed and does not recur. Joy is able to express some positive aspects about herself and is making plans to change her current life-style to help in carrying her pregnancy to full term. (See nursing plan of care.)

trition and personal hygiene or learns to diaper the baby). It is not reasonable to expect to see evidence of significant strides, such as complete abstinence from drugs and assumption of mature adult behaviors within a short period.

■ POVERTY

The very poor—the social class of persons who consistently live at or below the poverty level—are in a perpetual state of despair. Their limited skills give them no bargaining power in the job market. Education needed to improve their status is beyond them. The poor desire a better life for their children but are trapped in a circular pattern that perpetuates their condition. Their powerlessness to control their fate or condition is a source of fatalism and resignation that is characteristic of the group in general. This fatalistic attitude is a significant impediment to occupational and educational aspirations and to seeking health care. A newer phenomenon in today's eco-

CARE PLAN Cocaine Abuse During Pregnancy

GOAL	IMPLEMENTATION	RATIONALE	EVALUATION
Nursing diagnosis: High risk for injury to fetus related to preterm labor (PTL)			
Joy's preterm labor will be suppressed.	Monitor IV tocolytic therapy. Monitor maternal and fetal status for response to therapy.	Close monitoring is essential to determine effectiveness and to identify early signs of toxicity.	Joy's PTL is suppressed without occurrence of toxicity.
	Encourage decision making about bed rest, diversion, hygiene.	Shows respect for Joy's ability to make decisions so that she will feel less powerless.	Joy is able to comply with bed rest.
	Prepare Joy for discharge: provide education in oral administration and in recognition of recurrence of PTL; what and how to report; resource persons to call as needed.	Knowledge provides a basis for decision making; process assists in developing new coping skills; nurse's trust helps Joy develop self-esteem that may carry over into other facets of her life.	Joy takes oral medication as instructed; PTL does not recur.
Nursing diagnosis: Ineffective individual coping related to lack of support system			
Joy will express positive attitude toward self.	Encourage recognition of personal strengths.	Decreases reliance on inappropriate peer dominance.	Joy is able to use positive "I" statements.
Joy will carry pregnancy to term without use of cocaine.	Help develop problem-solving strategies.	Encourages involvement in planning care and activities.	Joy helps develop appropriate plan of care for full-term birth.
	Explore resources for decreasing use of substances.	Joy will need help and support to "kick the habit" and remain drug free for rest of pregnancy and as new mother.	Joy attends rehabilitation program; discusses problem issues with clinic nurse and/or CHN, and remains drug free for remainder of pregnancy.
Nursing diagnosis: Nutrition, less than body requirements related to drug use/lack of knowledge			
Mother (and fetus) will maintain adequate nutritional status.	Counsel Joy on nutrition for pregnant client and fetus.	Joy has poor understanding of nutritional requirements for pregnancy.	Joy's nutritional status and intake are appropriate for third trimester.
	Mutually develop meal plan to include schedule, environment, likes/dislikes.	Substance abusers often forget to eat or acknowledge personal preferences.	Joy follows meal plan and includes personal preferences in meal selection.

nomic situation is that of the "new" poor who are educated but have lost their jobs as a result of economic and social conditions. These persons comprise an entirely different group of clients with whom the nurse may work.

The term **poverty** implies both visible and invisible impoverishment. **Visible poverty** refers to lack of money or material resources, which includes insufficient clothing, poor sanitation, and deteriorating housing. **Invisible poverty** refers to social and cultural deprivation such as limited employment opportunities, inferior educational opportunities, lack of (or inferior) medical services and health care facilities, and an absence of public services (Spector, 1979).

Factors Related to Poverty

One factor that notably affects women is *employment and wage discrimination*. Poverty and undue stress are responses to the discrimination and exploitation that women experience in the workplace. Most seriously affected are the swelling numbers of single-parent families headed by women (Griffith-Kenney, 1986).

Throughout the United States are groups of people, geographically segregated, who constitute what is known as "pockets of poverty." They are seen in the dense urban areas, such as the ghettos, and many rural areas, especially those that are geographically isolated from needed facilities and services. The nonurbanized regions identified as poverty areas in the United States are Appalachia, the deep South, the lower Southwest, and northern New England (Spector, 1979).

Certain *ethnic or racial groups* are overrepresented in the impoverished population. The most obvious of these are African Americans, Mexican Americans, Mexican immigrants, and Native Americans.

Migrant Families

Migrant farm workers and their families are among the most disadvantaged groups. The low position of these families on the economic scale and their rootless, mobile existence subject them to inadequate sanitation, substandard housing, social isolation, and lack of educational opportunities and medical services. This is especially harmful to the mothers and children. Health care generally is inadequate. Families are apt to live in a number of localities in the course of a year, without continuity of whatever health care is available. Pesticides and herbicides have been identified as mutagenic and teratogenic. Because both parents work in the fields, both are exposed to potential mutagens; the women may be exposed to teratogens during pregnancy. Accident rates are high, and meals may be erratic.

Some migrants have a home base to which they return at the end of a growing season; others travel continuously, migrating north in summer and south in winter. With most there is little if any integration into the dominant culture; therefore migrant groups suffer social isolation. Groups who travel together, especially those with the same ethnic background, develop a cohesiveness and form their own set of values and customs. Sometimes a migrant family will leave the migration stream and become a part of a permanent community. However, this involves adaptation to a new environment and life-style that can be stress provoking to these families.

Preventive Health Care

The vulnerability of economically and socially deprived persons in our society to health problems is apparent across the spectrum of health care from prevention to rehabilitation. Preventive health care is more than the prevention of disease states. It involves those factors in a person's life that protect the individual and allow for growth and development of potential. Adequate clothing and shelter, proper nutrition, education, a safe environment—all taken for granted by the economically advantaged—are noticeably lacking in the health experience of many low-income groups.

The concept of preventive health often is missing. The development of a concept of preventive health begins in childhood as the child is directed and encouraged to "eat your dinner and grow up to be a strong boy," "brush your teeth," "go to the doctor for a checkup," and "get enough sleep." These repeated admonitions eventually result in a concept of health care that includes prevention as well as cure. For women who have experienced this indoctrination, acceptance of the necessity for prenatal care comes more readily. For those women who have gone to a physician only when they were very ill, the relative health of the pregnant state precludes full use of care available. For some low-income women a choice between prenatal care (preparation for birth) and providing their families with necessities results in their foregoing prenatal care.

In some communities clinics have been established specifically for high-risk mothers and their infants. Adolescent mothers and preterm infants make up a large part of the client population at these clinics. Although prevention of the problem is probably the best approach, follow-up care is of great importance. Helping mothers develop parenting skills will do much to promote the optimum growth and development of these disadvantaged children.

In England, Olds and Kitzman (1990) demonstrated a marked improvement in health-related behaviors during pregnancy with home visitation programs and education. Nursing and nurse-researchers are in the forefront of efforts to provide care for childbearing families. The Children's Defense Fund recently reported that the increasing maternal and infant mortality rates can be blamed in part on poor health care related to poverty and lack of medical insurance and publicly financed health services (*San Francisco Chronicle*, 1990).

The national concern over infant mortality and access to health care has led to an increase in some areas of medicaid assistance for prenatal care. However, increased medicaid coverage alone cannot increase use of early prenatal care or improve birth outcomes. Reasons include the difficulties in enrolling in the medicaid program, lack of additional social support, and reluctance of many health care providers to accept medicaid clients. A newly restructured system may be necessary to address the multiple issues involved rather than only an increase in financial aid (Guyer, 1990; Piper et al, 1990).

The following are additional explanations for delayed care: (1) lack of acceptance of pregnancy (denial of or unwanted pregnancy, psychologic problems of depression, or anxiety); (2) fear of hospitals or health care workers, problems with making and keeping appointments, and feeling that there was no need for prenatal care; (3) financial issues such as lack of knowledge of availability of care; and (4) family responsibilities, including conflict with the father, baby-sitting problems, other family crises, or geographic moves (Young et al, 1989). Parity, availability of clinics, and public transportation may be more important than financial barriers (St. Clair et al, 1990).

Reproductive Experience

Low-income women tend to begin reproducing at an earlier age and end at a later age than do other women. In addition, they have many pregnancies, and these are adversely affected by the close spacing of gestations. In 1970, Birch and Gussons described this phenomenon as "too young, too old, and too often." This has not changed in recent years. Maternal age and parity are implicated in perinatal mortality. There is increased risk to the fetus, infant, and mother when the mother is at either extreme of age or parity. The quality of prenatal care has a significant impact on birth weight and optimal birth outcomes (Poland et al, 1990). Preterm birth, low birth weight, and their complications remain the chief causes of perinatal mortality. Low-income mothers are more likely to give birth to preterm infants than are mothers in the population at large. Social support, often unavailable to the poor, is essential to enable persons to cope with life's stresses. There is a correlation between life stresses during pregnancy and the pregnancy outcome (Norbeck, Anderson, 1989).

PREGNANCY OUTCOMES. The differences in pregnancy outcomes related to socioeconomic class have been well documented for more than half a century. Studies have consistently demonstrated a relationship between economic class and maternal and infant morbidity and mortality. These discrepancies have been of major concern to nursing groups as they have attempted to improve the health and well-being of all individuals in society.

COMPLICATIONS. Low-income mothers are more predisposed to illness and obstetric complications during pregnancy. Obstetric complications such as placenta previa, abruptio placentae, and placental insufficiency often result in preterm births, intrauterine growth retardation, and low-birth-weight or small-for-gestational-age newborns and subsequent infant difficulties (Wen et al, 1990). Many obstetric complications have life-threatening consequences for the mother as well as for the infant. Examples of complications include hemorrhage, cardiac disease, or uncontrolled infection.

The problems faced by low-income mothers have direct implication for nursing service. Much of our current knowledge could be used to minimize or prevent the occurrence of the problems. One of the prerequisites to providing assistance to the low-income mother is to find better and more effective ways to deliver safe and meaningful care to her.

Infants born to homeless women are at very high risk as a result of poor prenatal care and nutritional status of the mother, low birth weight, inadequate infant nutrition, and respiratory and ear infections (Damrosch et al, 1988). Nurses must realize that they cannot provide all the solutions needed for the problems of homelessness and poverty. However, a connection exists between health and other conditions that affect those involved. Nurses can assist families by helping them to improve their self-esteem and develop and use skills that will help them to move out of the poverty cycle. Peer and professional support can be great assets for these families, as can information on stress management. Nurses can help most by using their influence to develop and shape political policies that deal with the issues of the poor and homeless (Berne et al, 1990). Primary, secondary, and tertiary measures must be included in the care of these clients. Involvement of the family, interdisciplinary team support, and community resources are all required to provide long-term care for both the mother and newborn.

■ SUMMARY

Modern perinatal care requires knowledge of mental health and psychiatric nursing concepts, as well as a multitude of concerns involved in the care of emotionally disturbed women and substance abusers. In addition to understanding the issues of primary, secondary, and tertiary perinatal care for these clients, the nurse must address the problems of those clients experiencing poverty, homelessness, and migrant family status.

REFERENCES

Emotional Complications

Affonso D: Postpartum depression. In Fields P, editor: *Recent advances in perinatal nursing*, New York, 1984, Churchill Livingstone, Inc.

American Psychiatric Association: *Diagnostic and statistical manual of mental disorders*, ed 3, Washington, DC, 1987, The Association.

Auerbach KG, Jacobi AM: Postpartum depression in the breastfeeding mother, NAACOG's *Clin Issues Perinatal Women's Health Nurs* 1(3):375, 1990.

Busch P, Perrin K: Postpartum depression: assessing risk, restoring balance, *RN* 52:46, 1989.

Cook PS et al: *Alcohol, tobacco, and other drugs may harm the unborn*, DHHS Pub No (ADM)90-1711, Rockville, Md, 1990, US Public Health Service.

Daw JL: Postpartum depression, *South Med J* 81:207, 1988.

Edlund MJ, Craig TJ: Antipsychotic drug use and birth defects: an epidemiologic reassessment, *Compr Psychiatry* 25:32, 1984.

Ehlert U et al: Postpartum blues; salivary cortisol and psychological factors, *J Psychosom Res* 34:319, 1990.

Goldstein RL: The psychiatrist's guide to right and wrong. III. Postpartum depression and the "appreciation" of wrongfulness, *Bull Am Acad Psychiatry Law* 17:121, 1989.

Hamilton JA: Postpartum psychiatric syndromes, *Psychiatr Clin North Am* 12:89, 1989.

Hansen C: Baby blues: identification and intervention, *NAACOG's Clin Issues Perinatal Women's Health Nurs* 1(3):369, 1990.

Harding JJ: Postpartum psychiatric disorders: a review, *Compr Psychiatry* 30:109, 1989.

Harris B et al: The hormal environment of postnatal depression, *Br J Psychiatry* 154:660, 1989.

Hauser LA: Pregnancy and psychiatric drugs, *Hosp Community Psychiatry* 36:817, 1985.

Hopkins J, Campbell S, Marcus M: Postpartum depression and postpartum adaptation: overlapping constructs? *J Affective Disord* 17:251, 1989.

Hurt LD, Ray CP: Postpartum disorders: mother-infant bonding on a psychiatric unit, *J Psychosoc Nurs* 23(2):15, 1985.

Iles S, Gath D, Kennerley H: Maternity blues: a comparison between post-operative women and post-natal women, *Br J Psychiatry* 155:363, 1989.

Jones LC: Postpartum emotional disorders, *ICEA Rev* 14(4):21, Nov 1990.

Kennerley H, Gath D: Detection and measurement by questionnaire, *Br J Psychiatry* 155:356, 1989a.

Kennerley H, Gath D: Maternity blues: association with obstetric, psychological and psychiatric factors, *Br J Psychiatry* 155:367, 1989b.

Krause S, Ebbesen F, Lange AP: Polyhydramnios with maternal lithium treatment, *Obstet Gynecol* 75(3):504, 1990.

Laizner AM, Jeans ME: Identification of predictor variables of postpartum emotional reactions, *Health Care Women Int* 11:191, 1990.

Majewski MD, Ford-Rice F, Falkey G: Pregnancy-induced alterations of GABAA receptor sensitivity in maternal brain: an antecedent of postpartum blues? *Brain Res* 482:397, 1989.

Martell LK: Postpartum depression as a family problem, *MCN* 15:90, March/April 1990.

McAnarney ER, Stevens-Simon C: Maternal psychological stress/depression and low birth weight. Is there a relationship? *Am J Dis Child* 144(7):789, 1990.

Metz S, Sichel F, Goff C: Postpartum panic disorder, *J Clin Psychiatry* 49:278, 1988.

Nicolson P: Understanding postnatal depression: a mother-centered approach, *J Adv Nurs* 15(6):689, 1990.

Smith R et al: Mood changes, obstetric experiences, and alterations in plasma cortisol beta-endorphin and corticotrophin releasing hormone during pregnancy and the puerperium, *J Psychosom Res* 34:53, 1990.

Spielvogel A, Wile J: Treatment of the psychotic pregnant patient, *Psychosomatics* 27(7):487, 1986.

Stein A et al: Social adversity and perinatal complications: their relation to postnatal depression, *Br Med J* 2928:1073, 1989.

Steiner M: Postpartum psychiatric disorders, *Can J Psychiatry* 35:89, 1990.

Stuart GW, Sundeen SJ: *Principles and practice of psychiatric nursing*, ed 4, St Louis, 1991, Mosby–Year Book.

Taylor E: Postnatal depression: what can a health visitor do? *J Adv Nurs* 14:877, 1989.

Troutman B, Cutrona C: Nonpsychotic postpartum depression among adolescent mothers, *J Abnorm Psychol* 99:69, 1990.

Whiffen V, Gotlib I: Infants of postpartum depressed mothers: temperamental and cognitive status, *J Abnorm Psychol* 98:274, 1989.

Zuckerman B et al: Maternal depressive symptoms during pregnancy and newborn irritability, *J Dev Behav Pediatr* 11(4):190, April 1990.

Psychoactive Substance Use

Adams C, Eyler FD, Behnke M: Nursing interventions with mothers who are substance abusers, *J Perinat Neonat Nurs* 3:43, April 1990.

Burkett G, Yasin S, Palow D: Perinatal implication of cocaine exposure, *J Reprod Med* 35(1):35, Jan 1990.

Chaney NE et al: Cocaine convulsions in a breast-feeding baby, *J Pediatr* 112:134, 1988.

Chasnoff IJ: Cocaine intoxication in a breast-fed infant, *Pediatrics* 80:836, 1987.

Chasnoff IJ: Cocaine, pregnancy, and the neonate, *Women Health* 15(3):23, March 1989.

Chisum GM: Nursing interventions with the antepartum substance abuser, *J Perinat Neonat Nurs* 3:26, April 1990.

Clemmer J: When an addicted nurse comes back to work, *RN* 50(10):62, Oct 1987.

Cook PS et al: *Alcohol, tobacco, and other drugs may harm the unborn*, DHHS Pub No (ADM)90-1711, Rockville, Md, 1990, US Public Health Service.

Cordero L, Custard M: Effects of maternal cocaine abuse on perinatal and infant outcome, *Ohio Med* 86:410, 1990.

Edelin KC et al: Methadone maintenance in pregnancy: consequences to care and outcome, *Obstet Gynecol* 71:399, 1988.

Fico TA, Vanderwende C: Phencyclidine during pregnancy: fetal brain levels and neurobehavioral effects, *Neurotoxicol Teratol* 10:349, 1988.

Frank DA et al: Cocaine use during pregnancy: prevalence and correlates, *Pediatrics* 82:888, 1988.

"Ice" drug now used at work, officials say, *San Francisco Chronicle*, Oct 25, 1989.

Janke JR: Prenatal cocaine use: effects on perinatal outcome, *J Nurse Midwife* 35:74, March/April 1990.

Landry M, Smith DE: Crack: anatomy of an addiction, II, *Calif Nurs Rev* 9(3):28, 1987.

Little BB et al: Patterns of multiple substance abuse during pregnancy: implications for mother and fetus, *South Med J* 83:507, 1990.

Lynch M, McKeon VA: Cocaine use during pregnancy: research findings and clinical implications, *J Obstet Gynecol Neonat Nurs* 19:285, 1990.

Matera C et al: Prevalence of use of cocaine and other substances in an obstetric population, *Am J Obstet Gynecol* 163:797, 1990.

Mondanaro J: Strategies for AIDS prevention: motivating health behavior in drug dependent women, *J Psychoactive Drugs* 19(2):143, 1987.

New drug "Ice" called worse peril than crack, *San Francisco Chronicle,* Aug 31, 1989.

Ney JA: The prevalence of substance abuse in patients with suspected preterm labor, *Am J Obstet Gynecol* 162:1562, 1990.

Oro AS, Dixon SD: Perinatal cocaine and methamphetamine exposure: maternal and neonatal correlates, *J Pediatr* 111:571, 1987.

Scott JR et al: *Obstetrics and gynecology,* ed 6, Philadelphia, 1990, JB Lippincott Co.

Silverman S: Combinations of drugs taken by pregnant women add to problems in determining fetal damage, *JAMA* 261:1694, 1989.

Stuart GW, Sundeen SJ: *Principles and practice of psychiatric nursing,* ed 4, St Louis, 1991, Mosby–Year Book.

Tracy CE: Women suffer most from drugs, *The Philadelphia Inquirer,* p 7E, Nov 27, 1988.

Woods JR, Plessinger MA, Clark KE: Effect of cocaine on uterine blood flow and fetal oxygenation, *JAMA* 257:957, 1987.

Poverty

Berne AS et al: A nursing model for addressing the health needs of homeless families, *Image* 22:8, Jan 1990.

Birch HG, Gussons JD: *Disadvantaged children: health, nutrition, and failure,* New York, 1970, Harcourt Brace & World.

Damrosch SP et al: On behalf of homeless families, *MCN* 13:259, July/Aug 1988.

Griffith-Kenney J: *Contemporary women's health: a nursing advocacy approach,* Menlo Park, Calif, 1986, Addison-Wesley.

Guyer B: Medicaid and prenatal care: necessary but not sufficient, *JAMA* 264:2264, 1990.

Norbeck JS, Anderson NJ: Psychosocial predictors of pregnancy outcomes in low-income black, hispanic and white women, *Nurs Res,* 38:204, July/Aug 1989.

Olds D, Kitzman H: Can home visitation improve the health of women and children at environmental risk? *Pediatrics* 86:108, 1990.

Piper JM, Ray WA, Griffin MR: Effects of Medicaid eligibility expansion on prenatal care and pregnancy in Tennessee, *JAMA* 264:2219, 1990.

Poland ML et al: Quality of prenatal care: selected social, behavioral, and biomedical factors, and birth weight, *Obstet Gynecol* 75:607, 1990.

San Francisco Chronicle, Dec 21, 1990.

Spector RE: *Cultural diversity in health and illness,* New York, 1979, Appleton-Century-Crofts.

St Clair PA et al: Situational and financial barriers to prenatal care in a sample of low-income, inner-city women, *Public Health Rep* 105:264, 1990.

Wen SW et al: Intrauterine growth retardation and preterm delivery: prenatal risk factors in an indigent population, *Am J Obstet Gynecol* 162:213, 1990.

Young C et al: Maternal reasons for delayed prenatal care, *Nurs Res* 38:242, July/Aug, 1989.

BIBLIOGRAPHY

Emotional Complications

Auerbach KG, Jacobi AM: Postpartum depression in the breastfeeding mother, *NAACOG's Clin Issues Perinatal Women's Health Nurs* 1:375, 1990.

Beck CT: The lived experience of postpartum depression: a phenomenological study, *Nurs Research* 41(3), May/June 1992.

Berchtold N, Burrough M: Reaching out: depression after delivery support group network, *NAACOG's Clin Issues Perinatal Women's Health Nurs* 1:385, 1990.

Boyer DB: Prediction of postpartum depression, *NAACOG's Clin Issues Perinatal Women's Health Nurs* 1:359, 1990.

Casiano ME: Outpatient medical management of postpartum psychiatric disorders, *NAACOG's Clin Issues Perinatal Women's Health Nurs* 1:395, 1990.

Comitz S, Comitz G, Semprevivo DM: Postpartum psychosis: a family's perspective, *NAACOG's Clin Issues Perinatal Women's Health Nurs* 1:410, 1990.

Curry MA: Stress, social support, and self-esteem during pregnancy, *NAACOG's Issues Perinatal Women's Health Nurs* 1:303, 1990.

Driscoll JW: Maternal parenthood and the grief process, *J Perinat Neonat Nurs* 4:1, Feb 1990.

Fisher LY: Nursing management of the pregnant psychotic patient during labor and delivery, *JOGNN* 17:25, Jan/Feb 1988.

Flager S, Nicoll L: A framework for the psychological aspects of pregnancy, *NAACOG's Clin Issues Perinatal Women's Health Nurs* 1:267, 1990.

Gross D: Implications of maternal depression for the development of young children, *Image* 21:103, 1989.

Hansen CH: Baby blues: identification and intervention, *NAACOG's Clin Issues Perinatal Women's Health Nurs* 1:369, 1990.

Heaman M: Psychosocial aspects of antepartum hospitalization, *NAACOG's Clin Issues Perinatal Women's Health Nurs* 1:333, 1990.

Jordan PL: First-time expectant fatherhood: nursing care considerations, *NAACOG's Clin Issues Perinatal Women's Health Nurs* 1:311, 1990.

Killien MG: Working during pregnancy: psychological stressor or asset? *NAACOG's Clin Issues Perinatal Women's Health Nurs* 1:325, 1990.

Kumar R: An overview of postpartum psychiatric disorders, *NAACOG's Clin Issues Perinatal Women's Health Nurs* 1:351, 1990.

Lagerlof JM: Maternal fetal "conflict": balancing our values, *Calif Nurs Rev,* p 34, Jan/Feb 1988.

Lederman RP: Anxiety and stress in pregnancy: significance and nursing assessment, *NAACOG's Clin Issues Perinatal Women's Health Nurs* 1:279, 1990.

Lohr JB, Bracha HS: Can schizophrenia be related to prenatal exposure to alcohol: some speculations, *Schizophr Bull* 15:595, 1990.

Malasanos L et al: Assessment of mental status. In Malasanos L, Barkkauskas V, Stottenberg-Allen K: *Health assessment,* ed 4, St Louis, 1990, Mosby–Year Book.

Mercer RL: Postpartum depression, *NURSEweek,* Sept 2, 1991.

Muller ME: Binding-in: still a relevant concept? *NAACOG's Clin Issues Perinatal Women's Health Nurs* 1:297, 1990.

Olshansky EF: Psychosocial implications of pregnancy after infertility, *NAACOG's Clin Issues Perinatal Women's Health Nurs* 1:342, 1990.

Semprevivo DM, McGrath J: A select psychiatric mother and baby unit in Britain: implications for care in the United States, *NAACOG's Clin Issues Perinatal Women's Health Nurs* 1:402, 1990.

Taylor E: Postnatal depression: what can a health visitor do? *J Adv Nurs* 14:877, 1989.

Psychoactive Substance Use

Abel EL, Sokol R: Fetal alcohol syndrome is now the leading cause of mental retardation, *Lancet* 2:1222, 1986.

Barbour BG: Alcohol and pregnancy, *J Nurse Midwife* 35:78, March/April 1990.

Bauchner H et al: Risk of sudden infant death syndrome among infants with in utero exposure to cocaine, *J Pediatr* 113:831, 1988.

Chasnoff IJ et al: Maternal cocaine use and genitourinary tract malformations, *Teratology* 37:201, 1988.

Chasnoff IJ et al: Temporal patterns of cocaine use in pregnancy, *JAMA* 261:1741, 1989.

Cox SM et al: Bacterial endocarditis, a serious pregnancy complication, *J Reprod Med* 33:671, 1988.

Ernhart CB et al: Underreporting of alcohol use in pregnancy, *Alcoholism* 12:506, 1989.

Levy M, Koren G: Obstetric and neonatal effects of drugs of abuse, *Emerg Med Clin North Am* 8:633, 1990.

MacGregor SN et al: Cocaine abuse during pregnancy: correlation between prenatal care and perinatal outcome, *Obstet Gynecol* 74:882, 1989.

Mastrogiannis DS: Perinatal outcome after recent cocaine usage, *Obstet Gynecol* 76:8, 1990.

NAACOG: Pregnancy and alcohol: a hazardous mix, *NAACOG Newsletter* 15:1, March 1988.

NAACOG: Caring for cocaine mothers and babies, *NAACOG Newsletter* 16:1, Oct 1989.

Neerhof MG et al: Cocaine abuse during pregnancy: peripartum prevalence and perinatal outcome, *Am J Obstet Gynecol* 16:633, 1989.

Pitts K, Weinstein L: Cocaine and pregnancy—a lethal combination, *J Perinatol* 10:180, 1990.

Rhodes AM: Maternal liability for fetal injury, *Mat Child Health* 15:41, Dec 1990.

Ronkin S et al: Protecting mother and fetus from narcotic abuse, *Contemp OB/GYN* 31:178, March 1988.

Silverman S: Scope, specifics of maternal drug use, and effects on fetus are beginning to emerge from studies, *JAMA* 261:1688, 1989.

Smith J: The dangers of prenatal cocaine use, *MCN* 13:174, May/June 1988.

Zuckerman B et al: Effects of maternal marijuana and cocaine use on fetal growth, *N Engl J Med* 320:762, 1989.

Poverty

Barnes LP: The illiterate client: strategies in patient teaching, *MCN* 17(3):127, May/June 1992.

Berchtold N, Burrough M: Reaching out: depression after delivery support group network, *NAACOG's Clin Issues Perinatal Women's Health Nurs* 1:385, 1990.

Casiano ME: Outpatient medical management of postpartum psychiatric disorders, *NAACOG's Clin Issues Perinatal Women's Health Nurs* 1:395, 1990.

Duncan GJ, Hoffman SF: Teenage welfare receipt and subsequent dependence among black adolescent mothers, *Fam Plann Perspect* 22:16, Jan 1990.

Ginzberg E: Access to health care for hispanics, *JAMA* 265:238, 1991.

Grossman LK, Harter C, Kay A: The effect of postpartum lactation counseling on the duration of breast-feeding in low-income women, *Am J Dis Child* 144:471, 1990.

Keltner BR, Tymchuk AJ: Reaching out to mothers with mental retardation, *MCN* 17(3):136, May/June 1992.

Kumer R: An overview of postpartum psychiatric disorders, *NAACOG's Clin Issues Perinatal Women's Health Nurs* 1:351, 1990.

Lia-Hoagberg B et al: Barriers and motivators to prenatal care among low-income women, *Soc Sci Med* 30:487, 1990.

Moleti CA: Caring for socially high-risk pregnant women, *MCN* 13:24, Jan/Feb 1988.

Raskin VD, Richman JA, Gaines C: Patterns of depressive symptoms in expectant and new parents, *Am J Psychiatry* 147:658, 1990.

Schneck ME et al: Low-income pregnant adolescents and their infants: dietary findings and health outcomes, *J Am Diet Assoc* 90:555, 1990.

Suitor CW, Gardner JD, Feldstein ML: Characteristics of diet among a culturally diverse group of low-income pregnant women, *J Am Diet Assoc* 90:543, 1990.

Wasserman GA et al: Psychosocial attributes and life experiences of disadvantaged minority mothers: age and ethnic variations, *Child Dev* 61:566, 1990.

chapter 33 review

Key Concepts

- Psychosocial problems that may complicate childbearing can interfere with family integration and restrict bonding with infant.
- Involvement of the family, an interdisciplinary team approach, and community resources are required to provide long-term care for both the mother and the neonate.
- Values clarification for the health care workers may be necessary to assist them in providing nonjudgmental care for substance abusers.
- Low-income mothers are more predisposed to intercurrent illness and obstetric complications during the childbearing cycle.
- The nurse must be aware of community health resources for low-income clients.

Key Terms

- affective disorders (p. 996)
- attachment (bonding) behaviors (p. 1000)
- depressive reactions (p. 996)
- drug dependence (addiction) (p. 1001)
- intoxication (p. 1002, 1006)
- invisible poverty (p. 1008)
- manic reactions (p. 996)
- postpartum blues (p. 996)
- postpartum depression (p. 997)
- postpartum psychosis (p. 997)
- poverty (p. 1008)
- psychoactive substances (p. 1001)
- schizophrenia (p. 997)
- toxicology screen (p. 1003)
- visible poverty (p. 1008)
- withdrawal (drug) (p. 1001)

Critical Thinking Exercises

1. Visit a high-risk, part-pay, or county-supported clinic. Assess the risk factors for the clients.
   a. What is the reproductive history for the low-income client?
   b. What nursing actions may alleviate potential complications for the low-income client? Justify your answers.
   c. What criteria must the client meet to be eligible for service?
2. Through research of charts from medical records and interviews, determine what percentage of the women giving birth at your hospital have had no prenatal care.
   a. Compare risk factors identified in these women to those found in women who sought care early in the prenatal period and had excellent prenatal supervision.
   b. Make and check inferences based on data.

Topics for Nursing Research

- Relationship between the birth of low-birth-weight infants and postpartum depression or paternal depression
- Relationship between stress factors of pregnancy and birth and maternal depression or paternal depression
- Instrument development for screening and data gathering about the use of alcohol and other substances during pregnancy
- Educational methodology to enable the pregnant woman to refrain from substance abuse during pregnancy
- Benefits and risks to mother and infant from the use of methadone
- Effective interventions to increase compliance with health care by women who abuse substances

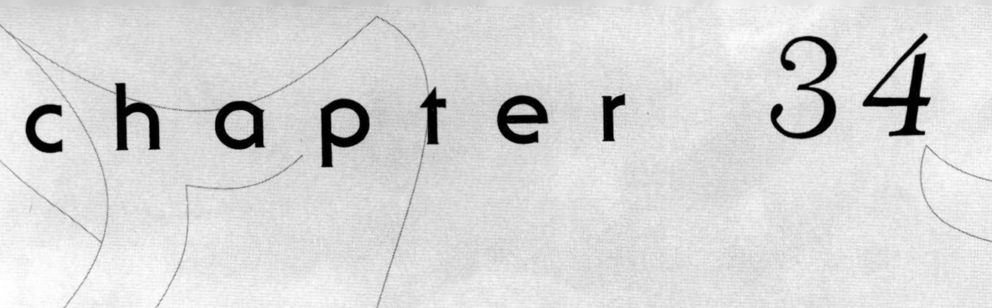

chapter 34

Adolescent Sexuality, Pregnancy, and Parenthood

PHYLLIS A. JOHNSON

LEARNING OBJECTIVES

- Define the key terms listed.
- Discuss dynamics of adolescent sexual development.
- Examine the incidence and cost of adolescent pregnancy and parenthood.
- Discuss societal and cultural factors related to adolescent sexual activity.
- Compare the developmental tasks of adolescence, pregnancy, and parenthood.
- Identify teaching strategies for discussing sexuality and contraception.
- Compare the nutritional needs of the nonpregnant, pregnant, and lactating adolescent.
- Compare a nursing plan of care for the adolescent who elects to terminate the pregnancy and one who opts to carry to term.
- Compare a nursing plan of care for the adolescent who gives birth and chooses to keep the baby and the one who opts to release the baby for adoption.
- Discuss nursing process with the adolescent father.
- Discuss nursing process with the adolescent's parent (the grandparent-to-be).
- Identify topics for nursing research related to adolescent sexuality, pregnancy, and parenthood.

The term *adolescent* comes from the Latin *ad alescere,* which means "to grow up." Within this developmental phase, physical, social, and psychologic issues are interwoven that create unique characteristics, behaviors, and needs. Each year more than 1 million American teenagers become pregnant. The United States has one of the highest rates of teen pregnancy in the developed world. The public cost of teenage childbearing calculates to approximately $4.65 billion that is spent annually through Aid to Families with Dependent Children (AFDC) for families headed by women who become parents as adolescents (McAnarney, Greydanus, 1989). A variety of factors explain the epidemic proportion of adolescent sexual activity in our society. The belief, held by some, that government financial support encourages parenthood is a myth.

Health strategies planned and implemented on the basis of an understanding of adolescent development will have a higher probability of success. Health professionals who work with adolescents need to understand the cognitive-developmental levels, the cultural environment, the value systems, and the biologic functioning of adolescence if comprehensive health care strategies are to be successfully planned and implemented. The nurse's own value system and professional response to teenage sexual behavior, contraception, pregnancy, abortion, birth, and parenting will influence health outcomes for this population and the generations to follow.

Behaviors associated with the major causes of adolescent morbidity and mortality share a common theme: **risk taking**—that is, intentional behaviors with uncertain outcomes (Irwin, 1989). Teens say they take risks because they are enjoyable, because the risks do not seem that great, and because everybody else is taking them.

The high incidence of adolescent pregnancy means that most perinatal nurses will at some time care for pregnant adolescents or their infants. This chapter is designed to provide some of the information necessary to improve the health of this population.

■ ADOLESCENCE AND DEVELOPMENT

Adolescence is that period of an individual's transformation from a child to an adult (for further discussion, see Chapter 6). It is the period of development during which the individual asks and answers the question, "Who am I?"

A major task of the adolescent is to develop decision-making abilities (Fig. 34-1). The level of cognitive development influences **sexual decision making** with regard to sexual activity vs. abstinence, pregnancy vs. contraception, pregnancy maintained vs. abortion, and parenthood vs. adoption. Sexual decision making is more a function of cognitive-developmental level than of age. The nurse must understand

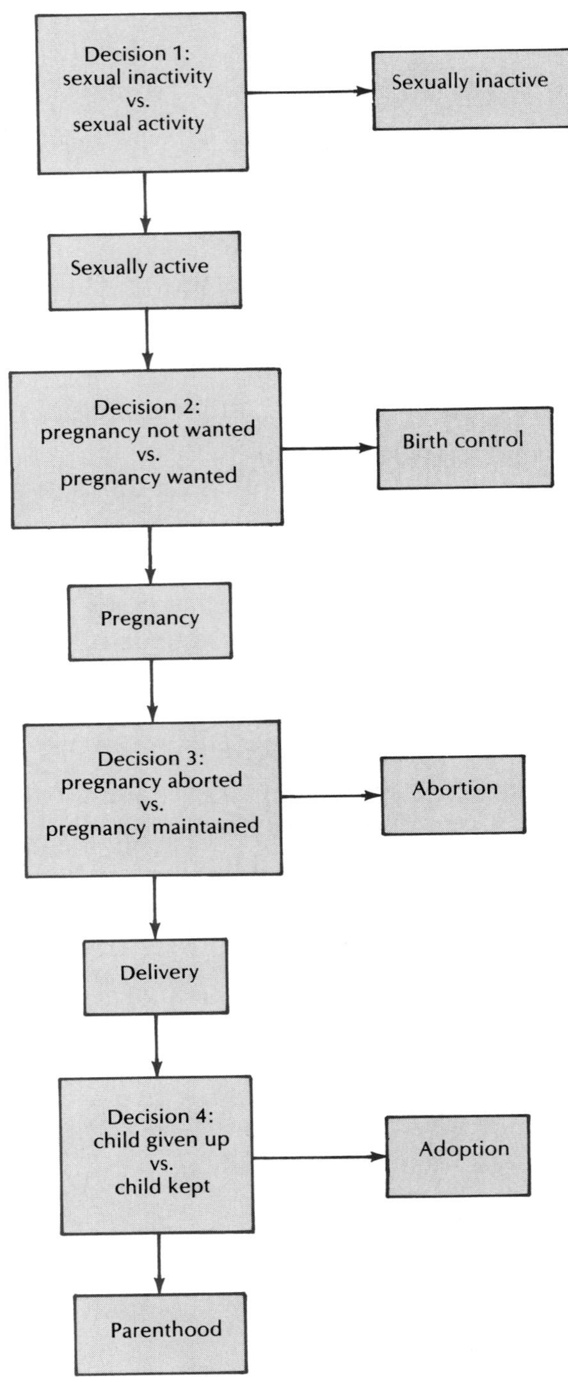

Fig. 34-1 Decision tree for adolescent sexual decision making.
From Kreipe RE. In McAnarney E, editor: *Premature adolescent pregnancy and parenthood,* New York, 1983, Grune & Stratton, Inc. Reprinted by permission.

these processes to assist adolescents in developing more effective reasoning about sexuality and in adopting more responsible behavior.

A major characteristic of adolescence is establishing an identity. The combination of dramatic bodily changes, sexual maturation, movement from concrete to abstract thought, and emancipation from parents and growing involvement with peers can create a sense of confusion about who one is. The peer group functions as the mechanism by which the female adolescent can alleviate her anxieties about separating from her parents and becoming an adult. Identity formation provides the ego strength and sex-role identity to engage in sexual intimacy with another individual without losing one's own identity (Erikson, 1968).

Developmental Tasks of Adolescence

Developmental tasks of adolescence must be accomplished before the child can become a mature adult. The tasks vary from culture to culture and with individual adolescents and their goals. These tasks include (1) acceptance of body image, (2) acceptance of sexual identity, (3) developing a personal value system, (4) preparation for making a living, (5) independence from parents, (6) developing decision-making ability, and (7) development of an adult identity. Thus adolescence is characterized by the onset of the physical changes of puberty and the psychosocial development of the ego, which helps the individual achieve a sense of self.

Adolescent female development is characterized by physical development, behaviors and concerns approximating chronologic age (see box at right). However, each adolescent is different and develops at her own rate. In addition to biologic changes, the adolescent's development is influenced by the family, the larger society, the peer group, religion, and socioeconomic condition. The period of adolescence may be divided into three stages: early, middle, and late. The higher the developmental level, the greater the readiness to accept responsibility for self and others. Early adolescents (10 to 14 years) have only a vague sense of self and are more interested in girl-friend relationships than those with the opposite sex. *Early adolescents are unable to relate their own behavior to consequences of that behavior*. Even though they engage in sexual activity, they do not think a pregnancy will result. Middle adolescents (15 to 16 years) struggle with feelings of dependency vs. independence as peers replace parents; they are more likely to demonstrate wide variations in their emotions. Magical thinking increases risk-taking behavior. Early and middle adolescents learn and retain information but are incapable of applying the information to their lives. They frequently operate by trial and error without considering the consequences.

Late adolescents (17 to 19 years) have a firmer sense of self. Their love relationships are more secure. They can clearly relate abstract information to their own lives. Effective interaction with the adolescent requires an understanding of the level of psychosocial development and tasks of this age-group.

One of the major challenges of adolescence is the establishment of sexual identity (for further discussion, see Chapter 6). Sexual identity refers to an individual's inner sense and self-perception of femaleness and maleness, which develop over time. The onset of puberty produces drastic changes in physical growth, normal functioning, and sexual tension. Sexual tension subsides with behavior such as masturba-

Adolescent Development

Early Adolescence (10 to 14 years)

1. Thinking is concrete.
2. Major interests are in same-sex peers, but a beginning interest in the opposite sex is emerging.
3. There are conflicts with parents.
4. The adolescent behaves as a child one minute and as an adult the next.

Middle Adolescence (15 to 17 years)

1. Peer group acceptance is a major issue and determines self-esteem.
2. The adolescent engages in daydreams, fantasies, and magical thinking.
3. The adolescent struggles for independence from parents.
4. The adolescent exhibits idealistic and narcissistic behaviors.
5. The adolescent exhibits emotional lability, frequent outbursts, and mood swings.
6. Heterosexual relationships are important.

Late Adolescence (17 to 21 years)

1. The adolescent begins to go steady.
2. The adolescent develops abstract thinking.
3. The adolescent begins to develop plans for the future.
4. The adolescent seeks emotional and financial independence from parents.
5. Love is part of intimate, heterosexual relationships.
6. Decision-making ability has developed.
7. A firm sense of self as an adult is developed.

tion, sexual intercourse, or the unconscious equivalent (e.g., nocturnal emission). These experiences are new to the young adolescent. Group pressure from peers may be a strong force in either encouraging or discouraging sexual experimentation. Such pressure may override parental wishes.

Whether the adolescent uses self-denial or engages in sexual pleasure (sexual behavior) also depends on the adolescent's values, perceived external controls, and self-identity. The type of family interaction was not found to be associated with delaying adolescent sexual activity (Casper, 1990).

Cognitive and Moral Development

Cognitively, the very young pregnant adolescent is a concrete thinker with limited or nonexistent reasoning ability. She is unable to conceptualize what could "possibly" happen. She fails to relate how the sex act tonight can result in the birth of a child in 9 months. Only through abstract thinking (formal operations) will she be able to solve problems by evaluating "if-then" alternatives. The development of morality depends on cognitive development. Most young adolescents follow rules for the purpose of gaining approval from others (conventional level of morality). As late adolescents mature cognitively and gain life experiences with right and wrong, they develop their own personal moral code (postconventional morality) (Kohlberg, 1980).

The transition from child to adult is accomplished by completing the three processes of (1) the biologic development of puberty (2) the cognitive-developmental level, and (3) the psychosocial development that is adolescence. The ages given are averages or approximations that can be used as guides, *but each adolescent must be assessed individually* to ascertain her or his maturational status.

Adolescence is a developmental process that must be completed; it cannot be skipped. Life events may force a young person into adult roles before completing the adolescent period, but an adolescent cannot change the prescribed order and "grow up" because he or she is soon to be a parent.

Physiologic Development

The neuroendocrine interaction of hormones stimulates the onset of puberty. As the brain matures, stimulation of the hypothalamus leads to secretion of gonadotropin-releasing hormones. These hormones induce the anterior pituitary to release gonadotropins (follicle-stimulating hormone and luteinizing hormone), which stimulate the gonads to mature and release ova in the female and to produce and release sperm in the male. This prepares the adolescent for reproduction. The release of growth hormone-releasing hormone from the hypothalamus triggers the onset of rapid physical growth (Greydanus, Shearin, 1990). This accelerated growth, which occurs approximately 2 years earlier in females than in males, continues over a 3-year period. Physical size should not be used as the basis for planning care. The nurse should assess all parameters of adolescent development, that is, the influence of the peer group and the family situation before health interventions are undertaken. The levels of understanding, teaching methods, teaching priorities, and support systems required for the individual adolescent are determined by interaction of these factors.

■ ADOLESCENT SEXUALITY

Effective approaches to solving the problem of adolescent pregnancy begin with a definition of the problem. Redefining adolescent pregnancy as a social problem "of" society rather than "in" society may lead to more comprehensive solutions. There is a pervasive moralism in American society that adolescent sexual activity is unacceptable. Sex outside marriage, irrespective of age, is unacceptable to many individuals. In the United States, opinions differ as to whether the major issue in adolescent pregnancy is a lack of access to contraception or one of inappropriate premarital sexual activity. Some parents, as well as other adults, are concerned that providing sex education and contraceptives would be giving permission for or encouraging sexual activity.

Sexuality is an integral component of personal identity that evolves and matures throughout a person's life span. Sexuality is not synonymous with sex. Sexuality is the interaction of biology, personal psychology, and environmental factors. Biologic functioning refers to the individual's ability to give and receive pleasure and to reproduce. **Psychologic sexual self-concept and identity** refers to the individual's internal meaning of sexuality, such as body image, identification of being male or female, and learning masculine or feminine roles. The third component, the sociocultural values or rules, helps to shape how individuals relate to the world and how they choose relationships of shared sexuality with other persons.

Sexual Behavior

Many adolescents in the United States are sexually active and at risk of pregnancy. Nationally, 57% of teens reported they have sex (Centers for Disease Control, 1991). In addition, 22% of high school students in the United States reported they had had at least four sex partners. About 63% of all cases of sexually transmitted diseases occur among persons younger than 24 years of age (Tyre et al, 1990).

The media (television, music, movies, radio, videos, print) influence adolescents' ideas about sexuality. Sexual themes and activity have increased 103% in soap operas since 1980 (Fine et al, 1990). The conflicting messages the adolescent receives from these various sources create pressure on those who do not wish to be sexually active. One reason young adolescents are sexually active is the earlier onset of menarche, which occurs today between the ages of 10 and 12 years, along with increased sexual desires (McAnarney, Hendee 1989a). A study of 14-year-old African-American pregnant girls revealed that sexual decision making was related to four key factors: attempt to establish a relationship based on trust, a belief in their lack of vulnerability to become pregnant, family structure, and their beliefs about the alternatives available once pregnancy had occurred (Pete, Desantis, 1990).

Risk-taking behaviors must be considered within the dynamics of adolescent development and today's society. Although there are many healthy, happy adolescents who enjoy an active sex life and are responsible and aware of the implications of their sexual expression, *the United States has one of the highest rates of adolescent pregnancy and childbearing in the industrialized world.* In 1981 the adolescent pregnancy rate in the United States was 96/1000; in The Netherlands it was 14/1000 (McAnarney, Hendee, 1989a). The greatest increase in live births per 1000 women is in adolescents 14 years and younger (US Department of Health and Human Services, 1988). Almost half of today's 14-year-olds will become pregnant before the age of 20. Most young girls have their first sexual encounter in the home. The most frequent season for the initiation of sexual intercourse is during the summer months.

Adolescent males express their sexuality in diverse ways. The average age at first intercourse for males is 15.7 years. Male adolescents in particular brag about their sexual conquests. An adolescent may not want to carry the stigma of being the only virgin in the group. As inexperienced adolescents listen to tales of sexual adventures, they have no way of knowing that many stories are invented to impress the listener; thus many become sexually active, not from sexual desire but from the need to belong to the group (Adler et al, 1990).

Sexually experienced adolescents are unlikely to abstain from continued sexual activity. In very young adolescents, sexual abuse or incest must be suspected (McAnarney, Hendee, 1989a). For most adolescents sexual activity is experimental. Knowledge of the dynamics of development is particularly important for those who counsel teenagers, because these are the very processes by which adolescents develop more effective reasoning about sexuality and thus initiate change in behavior.

Contraception

Adolescents who are sexually active often do not use contraceptives consistently and correctly. Adolescents are sexually active an average of 15 months before initiating regular contraceptive use. Most of these young women discontinue its use within the first year after its initiation (White, Kellinger, 1989). They "forget" to take pills or hide them. They "do not want pills to pollute their bodies." Young boys often carry condoms in their wallets merely as a symbol. Adolescents say they do not use contraceptives because (1) they do not feel they will get pregnant and (2) they did not anticipate having intercourse. Many girls are afraid they will be considered "bad girls" if they use contraceptives.

Because of the inability of adolescent males to think abstractly or to take another's perspective, they may have difficulty understanding the importance of the use of contraceptives. Adolescent females frequently romanticize their boyfriends' decision not to use contraceptives by perceiving unprotected intercourse as affirming love or commitment. In advising teenagers about contraception, the nurse should consider the adolescent's level of maturity and motivation to avoid pregnancy, moral and religious beliefs, frequency of intercourse, regularity of menses, and risk of contracting sexually transmitted diseases.

More adolescents use oral contraceptives than condoms, the second most popular method. Young teens and women in their early twenties have the lowest risk of severe complications from oral contraceptive use. There is no evidence that even young adolescents of 13 or 14 years have any special problems with oral contraceptives. Earlier concerns that oral contraceptives cause premature epiphyseal closure have been disproved. Nevertheless, it is preferable that the young adolescent has had up to 12 months of regular menstrual cycles before initiating the use of oral contraceptives. Adolescents should be educated about all methods, including abstinence. The method chosen should reflect the teen's lifestyle. The simultaneous use of oral contraceptives and condoms will help to protect adolescents from sexually transmitted diseases.

Abortion

Approximately 39% of all adolescent pregnancies are terminated by induced abortion, and approximately one third of all abortions in the United States are performed on adolescents (McAnarney, Hendee,

1989a). The educational level of the adolescent's parent is a factor in whether she will have an abortion. This is true for African Americans, Caucasians, and Hispanics. The higher the level of education of the adolescent's parent, the less likely the pregnancy will be carried to term (Cooksey, 1990). Teenagers who have more than one abortion during adolescence may have needs that require referral for psychologic counseling. Because of their developmental status, teenagers usually need more intensive counseling than do adult women in coping with an abortion. If the issue is not adequately resolved, adolescents may have problems later in life with sexuality and parenting issues. Nurses may need to refer the adolescent for counseling under either of these conditions. The physical and psychologic consequences of abortion among adolescents are unclear because of a lack of scientific studies and follow-up investigations.

Sex Education

Past **sex education** strategies have focused on reproductive anatomy and physiology and on teaching behaviors typical of middle-class American family life. More recently, sex education has focused on addressing problems of human sexuality faced by teenagers. For example, programs have focused on helping teens to "say no." Opponents of school-based sex education programs believe that explicit discussions about sexuality increase teenagers' sexual activity and undermine the role of the parents. Proponents, however, cite the absence of such discussions by parents and the failure to supply adolescents with needed information as barriers to preventing adolescent pregnancy. The roles of the family, church, and the school are complex and controversial with regard to sex education.

Parents may not involve themselves in sex education for several reasons: (1) they may not have adequate information; (2) they may be uncomfortable with the topic of sex; and (3) adolescents may be uncomfortable when parents discuss sex. Some parents find it difficult to acknowledge that their "child" is a sexual person with sexual feelings and behaviors. Parental refusal to discuss sexual behavior with a female adolescent may cause her to keep sexual activity a secret and may interfere with the adolescent's efforts to seek help. With older adolescent girls, the partner's home was the most frequent location for sexual encounters. National surveys of parents reveal greater support for inclusion of comprehensive sex education in school curricula and at earlier ages for today's youth (Gasiorowski, 1988; Donovan, 1989; Rosoff, 1989; Centers for Disease Control, 1991).

Sex education programs should begin before puberty (some suggest as early as kindergarten) and provide adolescents with experience in personal decision-making and practice in applying the information to their lives. Programs should address how to handle peer pressure, should focus on both females and males, and should involve parents to enhance parent-adolescent communication and to strengthen family ties. Community institutions (e.g., churches, local lay groups, and professional groups) also should be involved to lend support to the programs. Such support may be in the form of financial help or volunteers. These programs must be based on a set of values that are explicitly communicated (Lockhart, Wodarski, 1990). As yet, systematic research on the effects of sex education are inconclusive.

Sexually Transmitted Diseases and Human Immunodeficiency Virus

The incidence of sexually transmitted diseases (STDs) has risen among teenagers more rapidly than in the general population (Brown, 1989). Young adolescents are at lowest risk of sexual exposure to human immunodeficiency virus (HIV) unless they are sexually abused by an adult who is HIV positive or who has acquired immunodeficiency syndrome (AIDS). Teenaged prostitutes and delinquents are at greater risk. Teenagers who may have acquired HIV through transfusion for treatment of hemophilia or other blood-related conditions should be counseled about the potential for infecting a sexual partner (McAnarney, 1988). The highest incidence of gonorrhea and syphilis has occurred in the 15-to 19-year age group. Mortality of children 15 years and younger from HIV infection is greater than 70%. It is predicted that the HIV incidence will increase significantly in the adolescent population.

■ ADOLESCENT PREGNANCY

Pregnancy in adolescence interrupts work on identity formation and developmental tasks. Trying to accomplish the developmental tasks of pregnancy and the developmental tasks of normal adolescence simultaneously may be overwhelming. The psychologic burden may lead to depression and to postponement in attaining an adult identity.

Primary, secondary, and tertiary prevention are needed in the prevention of adolescent pregnancy. *Primary* intervention includes, but is not limited to, teaching young children about sexuality. In addition, our society must address inequities in opportunities that place females and minority groups at higher risk for becoming victims of social problems. Comprehensive health care services for adolescents must be available. *Secondary* prevention must include accessible contraceptive services for sexually active teens. Finally, *tertiary* prevention must include easily accessible prenatal care, family planning, and follow-up care for infants and children of adolescents (McAnarney, Hendee, 1989b).

Many risk factors are associated with teenage pregnancy. They include low socioeconomic status, minority status, being raised in a single-parent household, being raised in a neighborhood characterized by a high incidence of these factors, and having low educational attainment and occupational aspirations. Adolescents who become pregnant before completion of high school are on average 2 years behind grade level at the time of pregnancy. Thus school failure may be a contributing factor to adolescent pregnancy. The adolescents at highest risk for pregnancy are those younger than 16 years of age (McAnarny, Hendee, 1989b).

Developmental Tasks of Pregnancy

The adolescent faces certain **developmental tasks of pregnancy,** which include the following:

1. *Accepting the biologic reality of pregnancy.* Most adolescents do not expect to become pregnant. They may deny it until the signs are so obvious they can no longer be ignored by family members. It is common for teenagers to diet and wear constricting clothes to hide their condition and to succeed in hiding the pregnancy until it is quite advanced, sometimes until the birth. The level of denial in some teenagers and their families can be quite high.

Young and associates (1989) found in their study that concealment of the pregnancy was the primary reason younger adolescents failed to seek prenatal care before the third trimester, whereas poor motivation frequently was the reason given by the older adolescents (18 to 19 years).

2. *Accepting the reality of the unborn child.* The adolescent may accept only the fantasy of having a cute, happy, healthy baby to dress up and play with like a doll. The idea of the infant's growth and development into an older child is not a reality to the adolescent.

3. *Accepting the reality of parenthood.* Being a parent implies being loving, concerned, and capable of providing the nurturing care an infant needs. Although there usually is a *desire* to be a good mother, young adolescents (mother and father) have limited life experiences, their own need to grow and develop, and little ability to cope with abstractions and to solve problems. The amount and type of support available to adolescents can significantly influence the accomplishment of these tasks.

Cultural Influences

The pregnancy rate for poor and low-income minority adolescents is high. Poverty and societal racism have a harmful effect on family and community life. Minority youth become sexually active at earlier ages and have less access to birth control information than do Caucasian adolescents. The lack of social and family support, nurturance, and supervision of the adolescent (as may occur in single-family households)—coupled with fewer opportunities to accomplish social and educational goals—places these individuals at high risk for pregnancy. Adolescents have cultural differences in their knowledge of sexuality (Scott et al, 1988) and in their beliefs about pregnancy and prevention (Horn, 1983) based on their cultures. For example, Native Americans believed that intrauterine devices (IUDs) were undesirable because they might mark the baby if pregnancy occurred. African-American teens considered birth control pills as well as IUDs unacceptable, whereas the beliefs and preferences of Caucasian teens varied along religious lines. Mexican-American and Central/South American females were more likely to use effective birth control than were Puerto Rican, Cuban, and other Hispanic subjects (Durant et al, 1990).

Nurses must be aware of differences in cultural beliefs if open communication is to occur. When these beliefs are assessed and incorporated into a plan of care, more effective programs for pregnancy prevention may result and more appropriate care provided.

Family Reactions to Adolescent Pregnancy

One of the most difficult tasks of the pregnant adolescent is telling her parents that she is pregnant. The adolescent may not talk about her pregnancy until it is obvious. Her mother usually is the first to find out and may attempt to prevent the adolescent's father from discovering his daughter's pregnancy.

Initial reactions of grandparents-to-be to the news usually are shock, anger, shame, guilt, and sorrow. The nurse must assess any disharmony that is occurring in the family and assist family members in adapting to the pregnancy (or other options). The stereotype of the poor family accepting the pregnant daughter and her newborn unequivocally is not verified. Mothers of poor African-American pregnant adolescents often are angry and disappointed because they wanted their daughters to have a better chance in life than they have had.

Adolescent Fathers

Teenage fathers are more likely to be children of teenage parents than are their peers who are not fathers. Consequently they may not view pregnancy as a disruption to their young lives. In some low-income communities the capacity of adolescents to impregnate is viewed with a sense of pride and as a sign of manhood (Esman, 1990).

Adolescent fathers are more likely to be poorer and less educated than adolescent males who do not become fathers at an early age. Contrary to popular belief that pregnant adolescent couples have transient relationships, many of these relationships tend to be ongoing. According to Elsters and associates (1989) fewer than 9% knew their partner less than 6 months before conception; more than 50% had known their partner for 2 years or longer. Most adolescent fathers try to provide some support for their partners (e.g., money, gifts, transportation) (Sander, Rosen, 1989) (see Research Highlight at right). They also want to be involved in the decision-making process concerning the mother's options regarding the pregnancy (Robinson, 1988). However, families of the adolescent couple frequently exclude the adolescent father from the decision-making process because of anger about the pregnancy or because they believe that he is not capable of making a decision. Frequently, however, adolescent fathers feel that their partners do not really need them for support and thus they do not believe they are neglecting them.

Over time, contact diminishes significantly for unmarried couples and if married, marital satisfaction tends to be low. This is true for adolescent couples from various ethnic groups. The nurse should assess the adolescent couple's relationship in planning care for the pregnant adolescent (and the father).

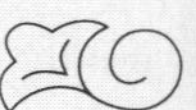 **Research Highlight** 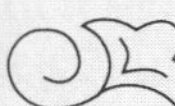

Parental Responsibility of Unwed Adolescent Fathers

RESEARCH ABSTRACT

This study investigated factors related to the willingness of adolescent fathers to take parental responsibility for their children. The subjects were 43 African-American unmarried adolescent fathers who were recruited from a community health center. Data were collected with a demographic (including factors such as age education) questionnaire, the Offer Self-Image Questionnaire, and questionnaires that were developed by the researcher to measure parental responsibility, role expectations, and perceived role expectations of the adolescent's parents and his partner. The researcher found that the adolescent's role expectations and self-image influenced his parental responsibility. Neither his partner's nor his parents' role expectations influenced his willingness to assume parental responsibility.

IMPLICATIONS FOR PRACTICE

This study aids in understanding issues related to adolescent fatherhood. Many adolescent fathers are involved in parenting. Their efforts can be encouraged. Nurses can assist in fostering a positive self-image, which may lead to more willingness of the father to take responsibility for his children. By providing assistance to adolescent fathers, nurses also are supporting the mothers and their children.

RELATED RESEARCH QUESTIONS

1. Are there racial and ethnic differences in parental responsibility in adolescent fathers?
2. Will an educational program to increase self-image result in adolescent fathers assuming more parental responsibility?
3. What are factors that influence adolescent fathers to assume parental responsibility?
4. Is there a relation between the quality of relationship between the adolescent father and the mother of his child and assumption of parental responsibility by the father?

REFERENCE

Christman K: Parental responsibility of African-American unwed adolescent fathers, *Adolescence* 25:645, 1990.

Legal Issues Related to Pregnant Adolescents

EMANCIPATED MINORS. Minors who are married, who are in the military service, or who are living away from home and are self-supporting may be considered legally emancipated from their parents. These minors are considered mature enough to consent to their own medical care, and their parents have no legal liability to pay the bill for health care services.

CONFIDENTIALITY. The constitution protects an adolescent's right to privacy. Health care information about adolescent clients is to be kept confidential. However, parents who give consent for and pay for their children's health care are entitled to be informed about that care. They also are entitled to request and receive the adolescent's medical records. The nurse who cares for adolescents should be familiar with federal law and state statutes.

CONTRACEPTION AND ABORTION. In most states it is legal to provide contraceptive services to minors. The role of the nurse is to determine that the minor understands the risks associated with the contraceptive, as well as the chance of pregnancy associated with the recommended contraceptive.

Laws regarding a minor's consent to abortion are complex and vary across states. Some state statutes may require *parental consent;* others require *parental notification* before an unemancipated minor may obtain an abortion. Sterilization law also varies among the states. Some states prohibit the elective sterilization of any person younger than 18 years of age. Usually the request and consent must be in writing. Federal law prohibits federal reimbursement for any sterilization of a person younger than 21 years of age (42 Code of Federal Regulations, 1989). It is each nurse's responsibility to be aware of these laws, and to refer adolescent clients to legal counsel, if necessary, to ensure that their client's rights are protected.

RETAINING CHILD CUSTODY. Infants born to unmarried adolescent mothers are classified as illegitimate. Illegitimate children have the same social and legal rights from both parents as those of children of marriages. The mother can authorize or refuse medical treatment for the infant.

ADOPTION. State law determines the procedures for adoption. Adoption options available to the mother include the following: agency vs. private adoption and arrangements such as closed adoption (no sharing of any identifying information between parties and no possibility of meeting in the future) to a very open adoption (in which the birth mother may visit her child and the adoptive family regularly), as well as any combination of these options. The nurse should assess the mother's understanding of her adoption options.

■ ADOLESCENT PARENTHOOD

The transition to parenthood may be difficult for adolescent parents. Coping with the **developmental tasks of parenthood** often is complicated by the unmet developmental needs and tasks of adolescence. These new parents may experience difficulty accepting a changing self-image and adjusting to new roles related to the responsibilities of infant care. They may feel "different" from their peers, excluded from "fun" activities, and forced prematurely to assume an adult social role. The conflict between their own desires and the demands of the infant and the low tolerance of frustration typical of adolescence further contribute to the normal psychosocial stress of childbirth.

Some differences between adolescent and adult mothers have been observed. For example, adolescents, although providing warm and attentive physical care, appear to use less verbal interaction than do older parents and tend to be less responsive to their infants than are older mothers. Although some observations suggest that some adolescents may use more aggressive behaviors, child abuse has not been documented. The fact that teens and adult mothers view their infants differently (e.g., teens view them as more fussy) and may respond to them inappropriately is caused by their limited knowledge of child development. For example, adolescents often expect too much of their children too soon.

Developmental Tasks of Parenthood

The developmental tasks of parenthood include (1) reconciling the imagined with the actual child, (2) becoming adept in caregiving activities, (3) being aware of the infant's needs, and (4) establishing oneself and one's infant as a family.

Although it is biologically possible for the young female teen to become a parent, her egocentricity and concrete thinking interfere with her ability to parent effectively. The very young adolescent is inexperienced and unprepared to recognize early signs of illness, potential danger, or household hazards. Children may be inadvertently neglected. Infants of adolescents are nine times more likely to die as a result of accidents and violence than are infants of older mothers (McAnarney, Greydanus, 1989). The higher rates of infant mortality are attributed to the inexperience, lack of knowledge, and immaturity of the adolescent mother, resulting in her inability to recognize a problem and obtain necessary resources. Nevertheless, in most instances, with adequate support and developmentally appropriate teaching, effective parenting can be learned by adolescents.

Maintaining a relationship with the baby's father is beneficial for the mother and the child. Involvement of the father is related to appropriate maternal behaviors (Ruff, 1990) and the mother's increased sense of confidence and security, as well as a healthy sense of trust, self-esteem, and social skills in the child (Sander, Rosen, 1989).

The Extended Family

Childbearing in poor families often occurs without the supporting presence of the newborn's father. For very young adolescents, another member of the family may assume a significant role in the care of the infant. Frequently the baby's grandmother supports, coaches, or supervises the adolescent in her maternal role. Often the grandmother assumes the primary caretaker role if she considers the adolescent too immature or lacking in judgment to assume the role. However, Stevens (1984) found that very young, low-income African-American mothers who assumed parenting responsibilities became skilled in child care if they had grandmothers who were knowledgeable about child rearing.

RISKS AND CONSEQUENCES OF PREGNANCY

The effects of young maternal age on obstetric and neonatal outcome often are difficult to separate from the influence of low socioeconomic status, race, educational disadvantage, substance abuse, crowding, STD, marital status, and lack of social support. The young adolescent is at higher risk for each of these confounding variables, and the increased risk during pregnancy may be related to the variable, not the age. Nevertheless, because young maternal age is associated with a higher risk of adverse maternal and neonatal outcomes, the relationship between age and pregnancy outcomes is addressed.

Physiologic Maternal Risk

In the past it was believed that young adolescents were more likely than adults to experience pregnancy-induced hypertension and cephalopelvic disproportion. A higher incidence of abruptio placentae in early adolescents also has been reported. However, adolescents who receive early and adequate prenatal care should be at no greater risk of experiencing an adverse obstetric outcome than are adult women of a similar sociodemographic background. Pregnancy-induced hypertension is thought to be related to the fact that very young mothers (under 16 years old) are more likely to be African American and first-time mothers. Earlier reports of an increased risk of cephalopelvic disproportion among pregnant adolescents, compared with adults, have not been confirmed in more recent studies (McAnarney, Hendee, 1989a).

Iron deficiency anemia is a problem in all pregnant women. The adolescent who begins her pregnancy already anemic, however, is at increased risk and must be followed up closely and carefully counseled regarding nutrition during pregnancy. Other problems seen in adolescents are *cigarette smoking* and *substance abuse*. Fetal damage from maternal smoking or drug use may already have occurred by the time pregnancy is confirmed.

Physiologic Neonatal Risk

As maternal age increases, the risk of having a low-birth-weight infant decreases. Compared with infants born to older women, those born to mothers younger than 15 years of age are more than twice as likely to weigh less than 2500 g at birth and are nearly three times more likely to die within the first 28 days of life (Lee, Corpuz, 1988). Multiparous adolescents are more likely to bear low-birth-weight infants and have infants who are at greater risk of dying within the first 28 days of life than are primiparous adolescent and adult women. The higher mortality rate is primarily a result of the higher incidence of low-birth-weight infants. Prenatal care appears to reduce this morbidity and mortality. Young adolescent parents experience higher postneonatal mortality rates, higher rates of sudden infant death syndrome (SIDS), and a greater number of childhood illnesses and injuries. These occurrences are probably related to the lack of supervision by the adolescent.

Socioeconomic Risks

Many adolescents who become pregnant drop out of school. Teen pregnancy remains the major cause for female adolescents to terminate their education prematurely. Leaving school early is associated with unemployment and poverty. Thus adolescent parents often fail to complete their basic education, have fewer opportunities for employment and career advancement, and have limited earning potential. More young mothers than older mothers live in families with annual incomes near the poverty level. Payments from AFDC rarely provide adequate support for the optimal development of young children. Adolescent mothers tend to have more children than desired, and their children tend to be more closely spaced. All these factors result in limited resources that can impair optimal parenting.

The incidence of abandonment, abuse, separation, and divorce is two to four times higher among adolescents married in their teens than among those married in their twenties. In addition to the stress of the transition to marriage, this family instability is related to other variables, including low level of education, low level of employment, and lack of support systems.

The Very Young Pregnant Adolescent

The pregnant adolescent younger than 14 years of age (the very young pregnant adolescent) is most at risk for problems in pregnancy and childbirth. The incidence of low-birth-weight infants, infant mortality, and abortion are two to three time higher in this age-group than for women older than 25 years of age (McAnarney, 1988; National Center for Health Statistics, 1988; U.S. Department of Health and Human Services, 1988; U.S. Department of Health and Human Services, 1989; National Center for Health Statistics, 1990).

The very young adolescent is at particular risk because she enters prenatal care later than do older adolescents and women. Late presentation for care may result in inadequate time before the birth to attend to correctable problems. The very young pregnant adolescent is at higher risk for each of the confounding variables (already mentioned) associated with poor pregnancy outcomes and for those conditions associated with first pregnancy (e.g., pregnancy-induced hypertension). Similarly, for example, operative birth in young adolescents is related to low birth weight rather than cephalopelvic disproportion. The increased risk during pregnancy is related to the variables, cited not to age per se. When prenatal care is given early and consistently, and confounding variables (e.g., socioeconomic factors) are accounted for, very young pregnant adolescents are at no greater risk (nor are their infants) than older pregnant women. The role of the nurse in reducing risks and consequences of adolescent pregnancy is thus twofold: first, to encourage early and continued prenatal care and, second, to refer the adolescent, if necessary, for appropriate social support services, which can help reverse a negative socioeconomic environment.

■ NURSING PROCESS WITH SEXUALLY ACTIVE ADOLESCENTS

When adolescent choices include engaging in sexual activity, the adolescent is at risk for a variety of health problems. The nurse can work effectively with the sexually active adolescent to achieve optimal health outcomes. The nursing process can be used to accomplish this goal.

ASSESSMENT

A thorough health history *interview* (including menstrual, sexual, and dietary factors), with review of systems, complete physical examination (including breast and pelvic examination), and laboratory tests, should be conducted. In addition, assessment of the psychosocial (e.g., sexual identity, body image, self-concept), cognitive-developmental stage, and support systems is essential. Careful assessment is needed to identify learning and care needs. The health history interview should be conducted in a quiet, private room with the adolescent fully clothed. An unhurried, nonjudgmental attitude will facilitate client relaxation. The interview begins with nonthreatening questions.

After rapport is established with the client, more sensitive questions may be asked. The nurse should be aware of culturally unacceptable verbal and nonverbal responses. The nurse should use direct language such as "sexual intercourse," not "making love." A **sexual history** is essential. It should include knowledge and use of safer-sex practices, use of contraceptives, sources of sex education, knowledge of and history of STDs, number of sexual partners, satisfaction with sexual partner, types and frequency of sexual contacts, techniques of sexual intercourse, and satisfaction with sex. An adolescent with more than one sex partner is more at risk for STDs.

A thorough *physical examination* is essential. The nurse should be alert for possibilities of sexual abuse in the young adolescent. Because the young adolescent has very little experience with what normal bodily functions are, STDs may go unnoticed and unreported to health care providers for treatment. Heavy menstrual bleeding or other abnormal bleeding in adolescents may be related to abortion, trauma, endocrine diseases, infection, or other causes, such as taking oral contraceptives incorrectly or even correctly (Hilliard, Rebar, 1990).

A pelvic examination is essential for any teenager who is sexually active and for those considering oral contraceptives. During puberty the vaginal epithelium is thin. Therefore it is more vulnerable to irritation and infection. Contact vaginitis can result from perfumed soap, powders, sprays, and tight jeans or other garments. Adolescent girls are modest and usually will be very tense during the pelvic examination. The pelvic examination is considered distasteful and anxiety provoking. It is even more threatening if sexual abuse has occurred. Before a first pelvic examination, instruction in relaxation techniques is helpful. Lidocaine ointment may be used as a lubricant. The anxious adolescent client may feel more comfortable using a mirror so she can participate in the examination. An appropriate goal is to help the adolescent feel in control and avoid embarrassment. The adolescent should be asked to decide whether her mother remains in the room or leaves during the examination. If the adolescent finds the examination too painful and is truly unable to cooperate, an examination under anesthesia may be necessary (Hilliard, Rebar, 1990).

Although true breast disease is uncommon in adolescent girls, anxiety about symptoms such as swelling is common. Breast examination findings in teenagers frequently are hormone-related and commonly occur during the surge of puberty. Swelling of the breasts also may occur during pregnancy and with substance abuse. The teenager should be reassured that breast swelling will abate spontaneously when the hormone surge regresses (Beach, 1990).

Common *laboratory studies* include complete blood cell count, rubella antibody test, HIV antibody test, urinalysis, urine culture and sensitivity, Papanicolaou (Pap) test, wet smear, cervical culture, hemoglobin and hematocrit levels, blood typing, cultures for gonorrhea and chlamydia, and serology testing for syphilis.

NURSING DIAGNOSES

After a review of assessment findings from the interview, physical examination, and laboratory/diagnostic tests, appropriate nursing diagnoses are formulated. Examples of nursing diagnoses that may apply include the following:

- Body image disturbance related to
  — Lack of knowledge regarding puberty changes
- Knowledge deficit related to
  — Sexually transmitted diseases
- High risk for pregnancy complications related to
  — Unsafe sexual practices

PLANNING

A nursing plan for care is based on the adolescent's health care needs. The goals for care, mutually determined by the adolescent and the nurse, are stated in client-centered terms. Examples of possible *goals* include the following.

- The adolescent will experience a therapeutic relationship with health care providers.
- The adolescent will be able to relax (or experience without trauma) during pelvic examination.
- The adolescent will understand the menstrual cycle.
- The adolescent will dispel myths and misunderstanding regarding contraception and sexual behaviors.
- The adolescent will identify safer sex behaviors.

IMPLEMENTATION

Health education must be conducted at the primary, secondary, and tertiary levels of prevention. Health education at the *primary prevention* level includes providing information about good hygiene and STDs. *Secondary prevention* includes education about appropriate health protective barriers during sex. *Tertiary prevention* includes proper treatment of current STDs and prevention of sequelae and further exposure. Health education strategies need to be creative and developmentally, culturally, educationally, and linguistically appropriate. Education should be appropriate for low-risk groups, high-risk groups, and parents or partners of low- or high-risk groups. Adolescents, because of their risk-taking behavior, are expected to be the next group hardest hit by the HIV epidemic. On the basis of the nursing diagnoses, the nurse may need to refer the adolescent to a nurse practitioner, physician, counselor, social worker, or legal services.

Oral contraceptives do not reduce the risk of contracting STDs. However, they can reduce by 50% the risk that certain STDs, such as gonorrhea and chlamydial infection, will escalate into pelvic inflammatory disease.

The condom, when used with a spermicide, is the next-best contraceptive choice for teens, second only to oral contraceptives. In addition to preventing pregnancy, the latex condom and spermicide help protect against STDs.

Adolescents frequently misuse and misunderstand the "rhythm" method, more accurately called the *fertility-awareness method*. They often miscalculate the approximate midpoint between menstrual periods, abstain during what they consider to be the fertile days, and believe this makes them "safe." The adolescent needs to be taught the complex process of determining her individual fertility status so that she abstains from sexual intercourse for the full amount of time considered "unsafe." This method is even less effective for adolescents who have irregular menstrual cycles (Tyre et al, 1990).

EVALUATION

The nurse can be reasonably assured that care has been effective if the goals of care have been met. That is, the adolescent experiences a therapeutic relationship with health care providers; is able to relax during pelvic examinations; understands the menstrual cycle; dispels myths and misunderstandings regarding contraception and sexual behaviors; and identifies safer sex behaviors.

■ NURSING PROCESS DURING PREGNANCY

Many interacting biologic and social factors affect the quality of human reproduction, and these in turn are influenced by the preconceptional, maternal, and neonatal care that is made available. The adolescent and her offspring are particularly vulnerable to the risks inherent in pregnancy and parenthood. This is a result of circumstances characteristic of her age-group, such as cognitive-developmental level, psychologic immaturity, economic dependency, delayed medical care, and lack of political power and influence. The multifaceted and complex needs of the adolescent are most effectively addressed by means of a multidisciplinary team of nurses, physicians, registered dietitians, and social workers.

ASSESSMENT

Interview

A thorough health history, with a review of systems and sexual history, is warranted (see p. 1027). Before pregnancy the very young adolescent usually has received care only from a pediatric health care provider. The nurse needs to elicit the health status of the adolescent male parent (American Academy of Pediatrics, 1989). If possible, it should be determined if the adolescent is the victim of sexual abuse or incest, the most common cause of pregnancy in those younger than 15 years of age.

Immunization status should be assessed. Immunizations such as those against diphtheria, tetanus (after 10 years), poliomyelitis, measles, mumps, and rubella need to be renewed. Tuberculosis is increasing in low-income populations as poor economic conditions increase crowding and homelessness. Vision and dental screening also must be considered. Vaginal bleeding early in pregnancy may be mistaken for menstrual bleeding and delay the diagnosis of pregnancy. Thus, dating the pregnancy according to the last menstrual period only may lead to inaccurate dating and result in a delay of prenatal care.

NUTRITION ASSESSMENT. Nutrition assessment is essential. Prepregnancy weight for height is a determinant of gestational weight gain. Some other maternal characteristics associated with an increased risk of low gestational weight gain ($<$ 7 kg, or 16 lb) and preterm births occur in combination. These include low family income, African-American race, young age, unmarried status, and low educational level (Institute of Medicine, 1990). Diet evaluation by use of 24-hour recall provides a base for assessing the nutrients consumed by the young adolescent and can be easily obtained in any setting. The very young adolescent also should be asked about athletic participation, dance classes, and other vigorous activity that could alter her calorie requirements. The adolescent is at greater nutritional risk because of the high fat content of food served at school cafeterias and the consumption of large amounts of fast foods. Beverage intake also should be assessed. Adolescents may inadvertently consume excessive amounts of caffeine in soft drinks and other beverages. In addition to food and beverages, life-style behaviors such as frequent dieting, abuse of alcohol, smoking, and substance abuse affect nutritional status and should be assessed.

Current studies show significant substance abuse among pregnant adolescents, with indications of underestimation of use (Kokotailo, Adger, 1991). Young adolescents are most likely to drink on weekends with the intent of "getting drunk." Thus the pattern of substance abuse should be assessed. Weekend binge drinking patterns are of concern in relation to fetal alcohol syndrome.

Nutritional needs for the young adolescent (12 to 14 years old) will be higher than those of the woman whose growth has been completed. Although the recommended daily allowance (RDA) is based on chronologic age, it provides the best available figures to use if the pregnant female is growing. A high proportion of pregnant teens, particularly low-income teens (Schneck et al, 1990), are nutritionally at risk and require nutrition intervention early and throughout their pregnancies. Hematocrit values of adolescents show them to be at risk for nutritional anemia. Adolescents' diets tend to be inadequate, particularly in iron and folic acid (Jackson, Mathur, 1991).

Health care providers should use specific, reliable procedures for obtaining and recording weight and height and should implement them consistently in classifying women according to weight for height, setting weight gain goals, and monitoring weight gain over the course of pregnancy (Institute of Medicine, 1990).

PSYCHOSOCIAL STATUS. Psychosocial screening includes assessment for response to pregnancy, depression, or suicide. In addition, the nurse should assess the adolescent's cognitive-developmental level, literacy, problem-solving ability, time orientation, body image, dependency, and peer and partner relationships.

KNOWLEDGE BASE AND PERCEIVED NEEDS. The adolescent is assessed for her knowledge of reproduction, sexual functioning, and her own sexuality. Basic knowledge of these factors is important to help the pregnant adolescent understand more readily the additional changes during pregnancy. Assessment of perceived learning needs reveals valuable information that may be used as the basis for planning and intervention.

SUPPORT SYSTEMS. Emotional support, particularly from the family of origin, is extremely important to the pregnant adolescent. Persons in the support system, particularly the parents, boyfriend, or husband, can significantly influence pregnancy outcome. The nurse must assess how the pregnant adolescent perceives her role and the roles and level of support from others in her support system.

Many pregnant teenagers come from socially and economically deprived families. Appropriate use of health care resources and compliance with preventive health care measures may not be part of their health value system. The nurse can assist those adolescents at risk to begin to change their own behavior so that use of the health care delivery system and its resources enhance health and well-being.

Physical Examination

Physical assessment is the same as that for the sexually active adolescent (see p. 1027). In the presence of severe pleuritic pain with upper right-quadrant tenderness under the rib cage, the young sexually active female is assessed for Fitz-Hugh–Curtis syndrome. This syndrome accompanies perihepatitis that is secondary to gonococcal or nongonococcal pelvic inflammatory disease (PID).

Careful determination of baseline blood pressure is necessary because teenagers have lower systolic and diastolic pressures than do older women. A teenager could be in serious jeopardy for eclampsia with a blood pressure reading of 140/90mm Hg.

Laboratory Tests

Screenings should include the following: hemoglobin and hematocrit levels, white blood cell count and differential, electrophoresis, blood type, Rh factor, and irregular antibody rubella titer; VDRL and fluorescent treponemal antibody absorption test (FTA-ABS); urinalysis, urine culture, and renal function tests (blood urea nitrogen), creatinine, electrolytes, creatinine clearance, and total protein excretion; Pap smear, vaginal or rectal smear for *Neisseria gonorrhoeae* beta-streptococcal and chlamydial infections; tuberculin skin testing; and cardiac evaluation: electrocardiogram, chest x-ray film, and echocardiogram. Adolescent pregnancies should be dated by both ultrasound scanning and Dubowitz assessment (Stevens-Simon et al, 1991).

NURSING DIAGNOSES

The information gathered during the assessment, along with laboratory data, is analyzed and provides the basis for formulating nursing diagnoses. Nursing diagnoses relevant to the pregnant adolescent might include the following:

- High risk for fetal injury related to
  —Inadequate placental perfusion secondary to preeclampsia
- Knowledge deficit related to
  —Nutritional needs of the mother and fetus during pregnancy
  —Infant growth and development
- Altered health maintenance related to
  —Socioeconomic deficits

PLANNING

The plan of care reflects the adolescent mother's need for increased surveillance, compliance with health care measures, and feelings of personal and social integrity. The care begins as early as possible in the prenatal period and extends through the formative period of the new family.

Whenever possible *goals* for care are mutually determined. These goals may include the following:

- The adolescent will receive early and continued prenatal care.
- She will receive comprehensive medical, psychosocial, parenting, and social services, preferably in one setting.
- She will receive creative, developmentally appropriate health care delivery to maximize the use of services.
- She will experience a physically safe and emotionally satisfying pregnancy and promote optimum health for her child.
- She will acquire knowledge and skills that enhance decision-making abilities.
- She will have increased awareness and make effective use of support systems.

Goals also are set mutually with grandparents and the father of the adolescent's baby if appropriate.

IMPLEMENTATION

It is important that health care professionals who work with pregnant adolescents have come to terms with their own sexuality so they can maintain a nonjudgmental approach. They should be genuinely interested in the adolescent—enthusiastic, warm, caring individuals able to view adolescents as young persons worthy of respect and dignity. Nurses need to be able to listen and to respond with honest answers. If possible, the nurse should be available to the adolescent by telephone. An environment of trust will enable the adolescent to discuss her true feelings and enable the health care professional to determine the adolescent's real problems and set realistic goals. Knowledge of adolescent development will allow the nurse to accept normal adolescent behavior, rather than view it as "acting out."

Nurses need to be adept in using a variety of teaching strategies. Group discussions meet the adolescent's strong need for peer contact and acceptance. However, because of the immaturity of the participants, the nurse will likely need to act as leader. Anonymous questions and pretests can be used to identify knowledge deficits or belief in myths. Demonstrations by the nurse, with return demonstrations by the teen, facilitate the assessment of the teenager's abilities. It is important to use simple, concrete, direct language. Teenage slang should be used by nurses only if it is part of their usual vocabulary. Correct terminology for body parts and direct answers to questions communicate respect. Because early adolescents have short attention spans, stimulation of more than one of the senses through use of multimethod approaches and active participation by the adolescent are helpful. For example, the use of visual models, films, charts, and role playing helps to reinforce learning and fits with the concrete way early adolescents think (Fig. 34-2). Written instructional materials such as brochures and visual teaching aids should be attractive, bright in color, and contain more pictures than words. The comic book format may appeal to the very young adolescent. The adolescent is more likely to read materials that resemble regular school assignments.

Because the young adolescent is narcissistic, focusing on the needs of the fetus tends to be less successful than focusing on the needs of the adolescent. Nurses need to help the adolescent improve her decision-making ability, explore the risks and consequences of her actions, and assume responsibility for her behavior. Some of the techniques used to encourage growth in these areas include having the adolescent select a menu, choose appropriate types of clothing for the infant for a certain temperature, and discuss solutions to real problems. The nurse also can assist the adolescent in separating herself from her baby so that she can see the child's unique needs. Information relative to child development and to infant caregiving is basic to this goal.

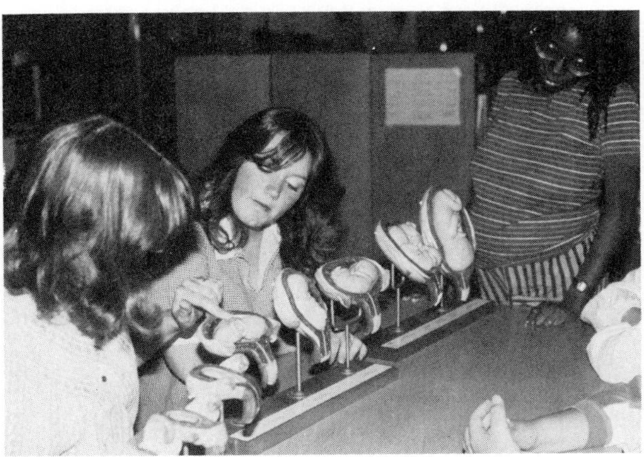

Fig. 34-2 Teenage expectant mothers learn about maternal adaptations to pregnancy.
Courtesy Marjorie Pyle, RNC, Lifecircle, Costa Mesa, Calif.

Prenatal Care

The adolescent is considered to be at risk during her pregnancy, and an increased number of prenatal visits should be scheduled. Significant effort should be made to encourage prompt clinic attendance; missed appointments should be followed up by telephone calls or personal contacts.

Adolescents are likely to obtain more adequate care if the prenatal site is attractive and inviting and if special efforts are made to register and retain them in care (Cartoof et al, 1991). The content of prenatal classes is chosen with the adolescent's needs and developmental level in mind. Maternal adaptation during pregnancy should be discussed, using concrete examples of "what to do" and "what not to do." Prenatal education requires creativity, flexibility, humor, and at times, ego strength. The nurse should avoid treating the adolescent as a child. Nevertheless, typical content and methods of presentation for adult women may be ineffective for adolescents. For example, if the teen has no partner, she may be "turned off" by films that depict a loving couple.

SUPPORT AND INFORMATION GROUPS. The prenatal care services already discussed are offered predominantly in clinics or in hospitals. In addition to these services, a variety of self-help groups are available for pregnant teens and their families. The programs vary in structure and content depending on the organization or agency sponsoring the program. Examples of group types include those that focus on the pregnant adolescent and her self-care, teen parenting (which teens and their infants may attend together) (Fig. 34-3), and others such as support groups for parents (of the pregnant teen) who learn how to cope and adapt to the experience (Fig. 34-4). Generally, group meetings are held on a weekly or monthly basis. Some hospitals or communities that do not currently offer such programs for adolescents may begin by designing their own or by purchasing prepackaged ones. Many of the prepackaged materials also include directions for staff training and technical assistance. For adolescents who receive little parental, partner, or peer support, as well as those

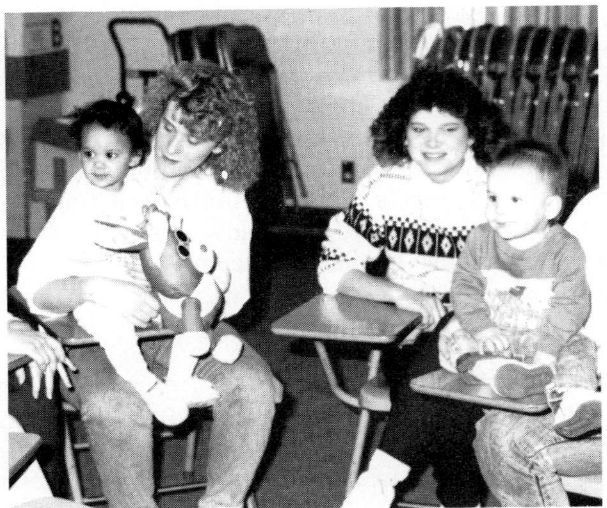

Fig. 34-3 A meeting of pregnant and parenting adolescents belonging to the support and information group. Courtesy Young Parents Young People (St. Louis, Mo.).

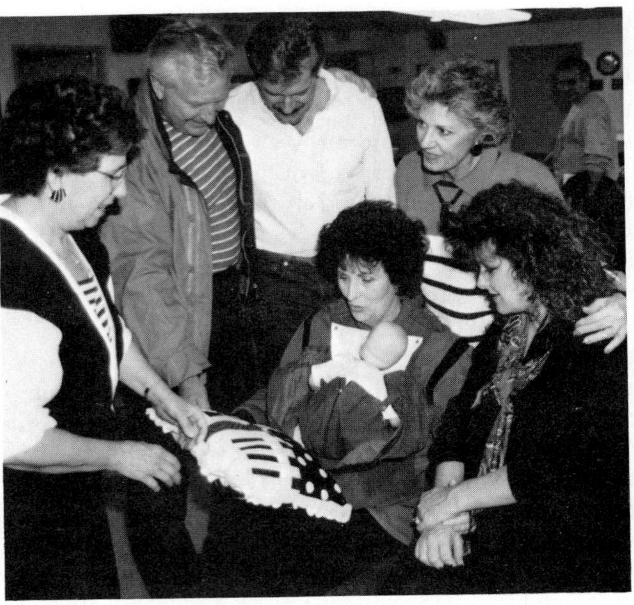

Fig. 34-4 Grandparent classes help grandparents-to-be to update their knowledge and skill, such as teaching about infant stimulation (pillow is designed for infant stimulation). Grandparents discuss how best to help the adolescent with the developmental tasks of adolescence, pregnancy, and parenthood.
Courtesy Marjorie Pyle, RNC, Lifecircle, Costa Mesa, Calif.

who may have all these supports, such programs have proved highly effective in helping teens and their families cope with the experiences associated with pregnancy and parenting.

NUTRITION COUNSELING. The purpose of nutrition counseling is to increase the adolescent's knowledge of nutrients and ability to plan, select, and prepare optimally nutritive foods for herself and her family. The nutritional needs of the teen can best be met by consumption of foods with a high concentration and balance of nutrients (Table 34-1). The nutritional needs of the mature (15 years and older) pregnant adolescent approach those required by pregnant adults. Additional amounts of vitamins, minerals, and calories are needed to meet growth needs of the pregnant adolescent and her infant and to correct deficiencies resulting from inadequate intake of nutrients before, during, and after pregnancy. Iron supplements are needed to provide for the growing muscle mass and blood volume increase in the pregnant teen (Story, 1990). Most adolescent females consume at least one snack per day, with a range of one to seven snacks daily. Snacks contribute more than "empty calories." Nutrients found in many of the snacks eaten by adolescent females were found to contribute approximately half the RDA of riboflavin, vitamin C, and thiamin.

As an integral part of health care programs for pregnant teenagers, the nutrition consultant must be skillful in establishing rapport and developing a relationship that promotes effective client counseling in the nutritional aspects of reproduction. Counseling should include setting a weight gain goal together with the pregnant adolescent, preferably at the initial prenatal examination, and explaining why weight gain is important. Additional strategies include building on cultural practices; categorizing nutrition practices as beneficial, neutral, or harmful; and reinforcing those practices that are positive and promoting change only in those that are harmful. Having pizza for breakfast occasionally is acceptable. Counseling should extend to the postpartum period to ensure a significant and lasting effect on the future of the parents and child.

Because energy expenditure for pregnant adolescents is so variable, the best assurance of adequate intake is a satisfactory weight gain. The recommended range of total weight gain and pattern of gain should be based mainly on prepregnancy weight for height. For women with a normal prepregnancy body mass index, a recommended gain at the rate of approximately 0.4 kg (<1 lb) per week in the second and third trimesters of pregnancy is advised (Institute of Medicine, 1990). Young adolescents and African-American

TABLE 34-1 Sample Menus for Pregnant Adolescents

	Day 1	Day 2
Breakfast	1 cup unsweetened ready-to-eat cereal with 1 cup 2% milk ¾ cup orange juice	2 pancakes, 1 medium waffle, or 1 slice French toast 2 Tbsp syrup 1 cup 2% milk
Snack	1 blueberry muffin 1 cup 2% milk	2 graham crackers 1 6-oz can apple juice
Lunch	1 cheeseburger (fast food) 1 banana Carrot sticks 1 cup 2% milk	3 slices pizza 1 apple Small salad 1 Tbsp dressing 1 cup 2% milk
Snack	1 apple 3 Tbsp peanut butter Caffeine-free soda*	½ cup cottage cheese dip Raw vegetables Caffeine-free soda*
Dinner	1 cup spaghetti with meat sauce Salad 2 Tbsp dressing 1 roll ½ cup chocolate pudding 1 glass water†	3 oz baked chicken 1 cup rice 1 cup green beans 1 roll 1 ice cream sandwich 1 glass water†
Snack	1 slice angel-food cake ½ cup fresh or frozen fruit, no sugar added	3 cups popcorn 1 glass ginger ale
	Kilocalories = 2515‡	Kilocalories = 2568‡

*Sample diets should include foods that clients normally consume and therefore provide teaching opportunities about better choices (example: cola vs. caffeine-free drink).
†Encourage adequate water consumption daily—6 to 8 glasses.
‡Kilocalorie calculations are based on the maximum allowance for growth; however, the best indication that a pregnant adolescent is eating sufficient kilocalories is to monitor weight gain throughout pregnancy. If inadequate or excess weight gain occurs, consultation with a registered dietitian is recommended.

women are encouraged to target their weight gain for the higher end of the appropriate range. Weight gain recommendations begin at 40 pounds for an underweight young adolescent, 35 pounds for an adolescent of normal weight, and 25 pounds for an overweight adolescent. Ferrous iron (30 mg daily) is recommended for all pregnant women. If the young adolescent has an inadequate diet, she may need multivitamins and folate. If the adolescent consumes less than 600 mg calcium (698 mg in two cups of milk) daily, calcium supplementation (600 mg daily) is indicated (Institute of Medicine, 1990).

Adolescents frequently are beginning pregnancy with depleted body reserves or are still growing. Additional intake is probably not required during the first trimester. Young adolescents may require higher intakes throughout their pregnancy. In general, pregnant adolescents should consume not less than 2000 calories per day; in many cases, higher intakes are needed. Table 34-2 includes recommended caloric intake for pregnant and lactating adolescents.

The young mother who improves her own and her family's dietary patterns is building the foundation for a healthier beginning for generations to follow. Referral to the women, infants, and children program (WIC) or other food supplementation programs may ensure that nutritious food is available in the home during pregnancy and the infant's first year.

NEWBORN FEEDING. Many adolescents initially respond negatively to the idea of breast-feeding. Fear of permanent alteration in the breasts, a view of breast-feeding as "dirty," other misconceptions, or a lack of role models contribute to the failure to choose breast-feeding as an option. Peer reactions or negative responses from the spouse or boyfriend are other factors. Thus formula-feeding is often the feeding method chosen. The nurse may help the adolescent weigh the realities of breast-feeding, such as 24-hour commitment, against the realities of continuing her education. For successful breast-feeding the adolescent's family and school must work together. When

TABLE 34-2 Recommended Daily Dietary Allowance in Calories (Kilocalories)* for Females

Age (yr)	Weight kg	Weight lb	Height cm	Height in	Calories per kg	Calories per day
11-14	46	101	157	62	47	2200
15-18	55	120	163	64	40	2200
19-24	58	128	164	65	38	2200
25-50	63	138	163	64	36	2200
51+	65	143	160	63	30	1900
Pregnant						
First trimester						+0†
Second trimester						+300‡
Third trimester						+300‡
Lactating						
First 6 mo						+500§
Second 6 mo						+500§

From Subcommittee on the Tenth Edition of the RDAs, Food and Nutrition Board, Commission on Life Sciences, National Research Council—10th rev ed: *Recommended dietary allowances,* Washington, DC, 1989, National Academy Press.
*Based on light to moderate activity.
†If weight is at or above standard for height and age.
‡Based on pregnancy gain of 12.5 kg and infant birth weight of 3.3 kg.
§Plus 650 calories if weight is below standard for age and height.

identified counseling needs are beyond the nurse's scope, the adolescent is referred to a counselor who deals effectively with teenagers.

Labor and Birth

The very young adolescent may be frightened of needles, pelvic examinations, noises from other women in labor or from equipment, and birth rooms. Single, private rooms should be provided when possible. The adolescent in labor should have the support of a knowledgeable coach, whether husband, friend, parent, or nurse. Many teenagers come to labor lacking preparation; they are fearful and often alone. If they are admitted early in the first stage, teaching about relaxation with contractions, ambulation, side-lying positions, and comfort measures can be accomplished. The adolescent is more concerned with how the baby will get out than with fetal well-being. Even though she may show an intense response to the contractions, the adolescent is trusting and will follow suggestions. Labor often progresses quickly. Anticipatory guidance and explanation of all procedures before they are administered should always be a component of the nurse's care. Many adolescents keep their infants and are responsive to staff members' sharing in their delight about the infant. For these young parents, efforts to promote parent-child attachment are particularly important (see Research Highlight, p. 1035).

Postpartum Care

Physically, the adolescent mother requires the same care as any woman who has given birth. Explicit directions for self-care and infant care are required. Most adolescents view the care of the infant as their primary area of concern. The need for continued assessment of the new mother's parenting abilities during the postbirth period is essential. In addition, continued support should be provided by involving grandparents (Fig. 34-5) or other family members, through home visits, and group sessions for discussion of infant care and parenting problems. Outreach programs concerned with self-care, parent-child interactions, child injuries, and instances of failure to thrive, as well as those that provide prompt and effective community intervention, prevent more serious problems.

Postpartum contraception is a high priority in very young adolescents. The risk of repeat pregnancy in adolescence is very high, and all the accompanying risks of adolescent pregnancy increase with each subsequent pregnancy. Almost universally, postpartum adolescents will say they will never have sex again and therefore "need no birth control." Nevertheless adolescents need to leave the hospital with barrier methods (foam and condoms) and the knowl-

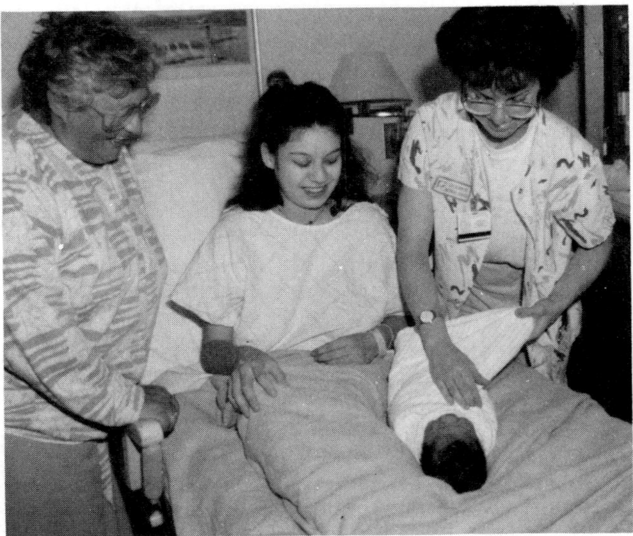

Fig. 34-5 Role modeling by the nurse and grandparent supports the adolescent's transition into parenthood. Courtesy Marjorie Pyle, RNC, Lifecircle, Costa Mesa, Calif.

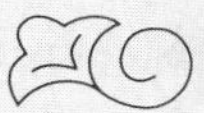 **Research Highlight** 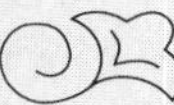

Social Support, Self-Esteem, and Maternal-Fetal Attachment in Adolescents

RESEARCH ABSTRACT

The purpose of this study was to examine relationships among self-esteem, social support, and maternal-fetal attachment in adolescents. The sample consisted of 90 primiparous adolescents from a variety of ethnic backgrounds. The adolescents were living in residential maternity homes. The instruments used for data collection were the Coopersmith Self-Esteem Inventory, Norbeck's Social Support Questionnaire, Cranley's Maternal-Fetal Attachment Scale, and a background questionnaire. No significant relationships were found among self-esteem, social support, and maternal-fetal attachment. In a multiple regression analysis, four variables were significant predictors of maternal-fetal attachment. The variables were whether the pregnancy was planned, intent to keep the baby, functional support, and total network.

IMPLICATIONS FOR PRACTICE

Assessment of whether the pregnancy was planned, whether the adolescent intends to keep the baby, and what types of support are available can be assessed by the nurse while taking a history. Extra nursing support may be necessary for those adolescents with unplanned pregnancies and little support. The nurse can provide anticipatory guidance in how to increase the supportive network and direct adolescents to resources to meet financial, child care, and housing needs.

RELATED RESEARCH QUESTIONS

1. Do supportive networks differ among racial and ethnic groups?
2. Does maternal-fetal attachment differ between adolescents who plan to keep and those who plan to relinquish their infants?
3. Do self-esteem and maternal-fetal attachment vary by age?
4. Does an educational program increase the number of members in the supportive network and the quality of the support provided?

REFERENCE

Koniak-Griffin D: The relationship between social support, self-esteem, and maternal-fetal attachment in adolescents, *Res Nurs Health* 11:269, 1988.

edge of how and when to use them. Very young adolescents may be shy or embarrassed about touching their genitals to use the barrier method. In addition, they will not likely anticipate intercourse. For these reasons some health care providers send adolescents home on a regimen of oral contraceptives. This practice is controversial because of the increased risk of thromboembolic disease in the immediate postpartum period (first 4 weeks). Thus the decision must be based on the individual adolescent and her life situation. Adolescent males need to be considered and included in any interventions in sexuality education, family planning, and parent education.

The adolescent will need support if she is contemplating the option of adoption for her child. Health professionals need to avoid using phrases that give negative connotations to the adoption process. Phrases such as "put up for adoption" and "give up for adoption" imply a callous, uncaring, insensitive biologic parent. Neither should the terms "real or natural parents" be used exclusively for genetic parents. The adoptive parents are the "real parents" because they care for the child. Neutral language such as "arranging for an adoption," "biologic parent" or "birth mother," and "adoptive parent" are preferred. The mother is given the option of either remaining on the postpartum floor or transferring to another unit. She is assured that she will have as much access to the baby as she desires.

Grief results from change or actual or perceived loss. The adolescent may experience grief brought on by the contemplation of adoption, giving birth to a preterm infant who may be in the intensive care unit, or the death of the infant. The nurse can help the birth mother move through the grieving process. The adolescent who gives birth to a preterm infant or one who is small for gestational age may find it extremely difficult to reconcile this tiny, scrawny infant with her fantasized "Gerber" baby. She may experience fear over the thought of caring for the child introduced to her in the intensive care unit. The confidence and trust in her abilities gained during the prenatal period may be replaced with feelings of being overwhelmed and incompetent. The consequent alienation of mother and infant may never be overcome. Intensive teaching and continuous support programs are essential if both the young mother and her vulnerable infant are not to be estranged.

Many young mothers pattern their practice on what they themselves experienced. It is vital, therefore, to determine the kind of support that those close to these young mothers are able or prepared to give and the kinds of community aid that can supplement this support. The adolescent may have conflict with dependency vs. independency issues as she performs her mothering role within the framework of her family of origin. The adolescent's family of origin also may need assistance in adapting to their new roles.

Nursing Process with the Adolescent Father

Nursing care includes the father of the child. As with the mother the nurse must be aware of the male adolescent's cognitive-developmental levels, values, and culture. The more successful outreach programs address cultural diversity in teenage fathers (Hendricks, 1988).

The adolescent father, as well as the adolescent mother, is faced with immediate developmental crises: completing the developmental tasks of adolescence and making a transition to parenthood and, sometimes, to marriage. These transitions can be stressful. The nurse can initiate interaction with the adolescent father by asking his pregnant partner to bring the father to the clinic with her so that he may participate in the birth. With the pregnant teen's agreement, the father also may be contacted directly. Data needed for inclusion of the young father in all aspects of the care are based on assessment of four areas: (1) the couple's relationship, (2) levels of stress, concern, and coping, (3) educational and vocational goals, and (4) the level of health education knowledge. Adolescent fathers (as all fathers) need support to discuss their emotional responses to the pregnancy. The nurse's nonjudgmental attitude is essential for open communication. The father's feelings of guilt, powerlessness, or bravado should be recognized because of their negative consequences for both parents and child. Counseling needs to be reality oriented. Topics such as finances, child care, parenting skills, and the father's role in the birth experience need to be discussed. Teenage fathers also need knowledge of reproductive physiology and birth control options.

The adolescent mother's partner, as well as her family, affects how she will deal with her pregnancy, labor and birth, and subsequent parenthood. The adolescent partner may continue to be involved in an ongoing relationship with the young mother. In many instances he plays an important role in the decisions she faces in pregnancy. He may influence her decision to continue the pregnancy, to have an abortion, to keep the child, or to place the child for adoption.

The nurse supports the young father by helping him develop realistic perceptions of his role as "father to a child." The nurse encourages his use of coping mechanisms that are not detrimental to his, his partner's, and his child's well-being. The nurse enlists support systems, parents, and professional agencies on his behalf. Encouraging mutual responsibility for birth control is a constant necessity.

EVALUATION

Perinatal nurses need to evaluate the care they provide to the adolescent client to assess the effectiveness of their nursing actions. Nurses can be reasonably assured that care was effective to the extent that the goals of care have been met:

- The adolescent will receive early and continued prenatal care.
- She will receive comprehensive medical, psychosocial, parenting, and social services.
- She will receive creative, developmentally appropriate health care.
- She will experience a physically safe and emotionally satisfying pregnancy and promote optimum health in this child and any future children.
- She will acquire knowledge and skills that enhance decision-making abilities.
- She will have increased awareness and make effective use of support systems (e.g., grandparents, baby's father, friends).

NURSING PROCESS FOR PARENTHOOD

Carrying the pregnancy to term and keeping the baby is one option in adolescent sexual decision making. Parenting ability is based on a parent's sensitivity to the infant's needs. Many factors can affect sensitivity, including stress, level of cognitive development, knowledge, infant responses, and support systems. The adolescent mother's age and grade in school influence her behavior toward her infant. Even though there are many books and much advice on the topic of parenting, no household precisely fits the description of those portrayed in books. Nor are the suggestions and recommendations always appropriate. Thus, parenting is a complex process that depends to a large degree on the decision-making ability of the parent within her own unique situation.

ASSESSMENT

Assessment of parenting abilities should include the following: the ability to empathize with the child, the adolescent's self-concept, definition of and identification with the maternal role, ability to problem solve and consider the child within the context of the future, and the adolescent's support system. Ability to perform caregiving tasks such as feeding, stimulation, diapering, and nurturance of well and sick infants also should be assessed.

The adolescent's ability to function in a mothering role is affected by the level of stress she is experiencing. Adolescents are exposed to many stresses as they undertake the tasks and responsibilities of parenthood, a role that is best assumed by adults who are financially and educationally secure. Because stress can affect the quality of functioning, making the adolescent insensitive to the needs of others, the nurse should assess the type of stressors, the adolescent's reactions to the actual or perceived stress, her problem-solving ability, and the adolescent's support system.

NURSING DIAGNOSES

Many different nursing diagnoses may evolve from the assessment data. Examples of nursing diagnoses that may apply include the following:

- Anxiety or ineffective individual coping related to
  - —Inadequate knowledge of the labor and birth process
  - —Lack of support from significant others/family
- Situational low self-esteem related to
  - —Perception of behavior or performance during labor and birth
  - —Judgmental attitude of those who surround the adolescent during labor and birth
- Pain related to
  - —Lack of knowledge of self-care techniques
- Impaired communication related to
  - —Age difference between her and her health care providers
- Family coping, potential for growth related to
  - —Individualized nursing plan of care
  - —Involvement of grandparents and significant others

PLANNING

Mutual goals are developed on the basis of the adolescent's health care needs. *Goals* are stated in client-centered terms and may include the following:

- The adolescent mother responds appropriately to her newborn's cues.
- The adolescent mother states she is pleased with her family's support.
- The adolescent mother makes positive statements about her infant and herself as a mother.
- The adolescent mother learns child care and self-care techniques.

IMPLEMENTATION

Because adolescents may resent the attention paid to the new baby, the nurse needs to demonstrate to the adolescent that she is still important. This will help establish the trust and cooperation necessary for future interaction and teaching. Before discussing topics about the care of the infant, the nurse should inquire about the adolescent and her friends, school, and social life and allow her to discuss her feelings and responses to the labor and birth process. Nurses can act as role models for adolescent parents in caring for themselves and their infants. Areas of particular importance for the mother are healthy life-styles, cleanliness, and good eating habits. The nurse's physical assessment skills can be taught to the parent so that she becomes more knowledgeable about her child's needs. Very young adolescents lack the expertise and maturity to provide 24-hour a day care to a child. The high-risk, low-birth-weight, or preterm infant requires even more care from his or her mother than does a normal infant.

The adolescent's egocentricity makes it difficult for her to separate her own thoughts, feelings, and needs from those of the baby. She may attribute very sophisticated thought processes to the infant. It is not uncommon for the adolescent to make statements such as "He doesn't like breast milk,". "He is just crying to get attention," or "She is just doing that to make me stay home." The adolescent may try to feed her infant foods that she (the adolescent) likes —for example, pizza, soda, or potato chips,—thereby placing the child in danger of choking. The nurse must attempt to demonstrate in a concrete manner the infant's limited physical and cognitive abilities. Listing specific foods that should and should not be fed to the infant would be helpful.

Because adolescent mothers tend to be less sensitive and less communicative with their infants, interventions that emphasize verbal and nonverbal communication skills between mother and child are important. Because of the adolescent's own cognitive level, such intervention strategies must be concrete and specific. The neonatal behavioral assessment scale developed by Brazelton (1973) is widely used to help parents become aware of the infant's methods to communicate need and satisfaction and to see the newborn as an interactive partner. Physical self-care and infant care are essential topics that must be covered in very direct language. For some, good hygiene is a topic that needs to be covered in depth. Demonstrations of baby care techniques, with return demonstrations, are essential.

Because other family members may share or take on the primary caretaker role of the infant (with or without the permission of the adolescent mother), it is important to assess the adolescent's feelings about the situation and to facilitate discussion about such arrangements with the family to increase open communication and a positive experience for all involved.

EVALUATION

Nurses can be reasonably assured that care has been effective to the extent that the goals of care have been met.

- The adolescent mother responds appropriately to her newborn's cues.
- She states that she is pleased with her family's support.
- She makes positive statements about herself as a mother and about her infant.
- She learns child-care and self-care techniques.

A case study below, and nursing plan of care, p. 1039, provide examples of nursing care of the pregnant adolescent.

SUMMARY

The significant increase in adolescent pregnancy is both a problem *in* and *for* society. There are no universally agreed on solutions. The nurse plays a significant role in influencing the outcomes of health for these clients. Successful outcomes are based on care that is developmentally appropriate, compassionate, and creative and that takes into account physiologic, socioeconomic, cultural, and social factors.

CASE STUDY

Teenage Pregnancy

Jane Brady is a 16-year-old, single primigravida who is at 28 weeks' gestation. Despite encouragement to bring a support person to the clinic with her, she always comes alone. Jane's parents are divorced, and she lives with her mother and older sister.

ASSESSMENT

The admission interview revealed that Jane has missed several prenatal care clinic appointments. Jane states that she has no transportation to the clinic because her mother and sister both work full-time. Her mother and sister have expressed interest in assisting with child care, but Jane says, "Sometimes I want to keep the baby and sometimes I don't." On questioning, the nurse discovers that Jane has several close friends but feels embarrassed and different around her peers at school with her "big belly." During Jane's physical examination the nurse notes that her blood pressure has remained within her usual range of 100/70 to 106/72 mm Hg. Her pulse is 76 beats/min, and her laboratory tests are within normal limits.

NURSING DIAGNOSIS

On the basis of the assessment data, the nurse can formulate a number of nursing diagnoses. One nursing diagnosis takes priority: high risk for injury (maternal and fetal) related to inadequate prenatal supervision.

PLANNING

A plan of care is developed with Jane and her family's input. The mutually agreed on *goals* for Jane include that (1) she will have a safe and healthy pregnancy and birth, (2) she will develop an improved self-concept and actively participate in developing her plan of care, and (3) she will make an informed decision about keeping her infant or arranging for an adoption.

Expected outcomes set by the nurse include the following: (1) Jane attends all scheduled prenatal care appointments and has a safe and healthy pregnancy and birth; (2) Jane discusses her concerns and feelings and actively participates in school activities with her peers and with the nursing plan of care; and (3) Jane makes an informed decision regarding parenthood or adoption.

IMPLEMENTATION

Nursing actions are derived from nursing diagnoses and physician's management. Specific interventions include assessments of problems surrounding missed prenatal appointments and monitoring of vital signs and laboratory values. The nurse encourages Jane's participation in problem solving and achievement of her educational and support needs. The nurse assists Jane and her family to formulate an informed decision about parenthood or adoption.

EVALUATION

The expected outcomes were used to evaluate the effectiveness of these interventions. Jane verbalized understanding of the need for prenatal care and attended all remaining scheduled prenatal visits accompanied by a support person. Jane discussed her concerns and feelings about herself and the pregnancy and participated in problem-solving exercises focused on identified issues. Jane continued her education and decided to arrange for an adoption of the baby. She and her family stated they felt good about the decision.

CARE PLAN Teenage Pregnancy

GOALS	IMPLEMENTATION	RATIONALE	EVALUATION
Nursing diagnosis: High risk for injury (maternal and fetal) related to several missed prenatal appointments			
Jane attends all scheduled prenatal care appointments and has a safe and healthy pregnancy and birth.	Identify transportation problems to the clinic and suggest solutions. Schedule appointments around school activities. Examine feelings or concerns about the prenatal visits. Create safe stable environment. Provide consistent caregiver. Explain the need to closely monitor the pregnancy.	Accurate identification and elimination of barriers to prenatal care increase the probability of optimal pregnancy outcome.	Jane attends her scheduled prenatal visits. Jane identifies her feelings. Jane verbalizes understanding of the need for prenatal care.
Nursing diagnosis: Situational low self-esteem related to altered body image and altered role performance due to pregnancy and middle-stage adolescence			
Jane will discuss her feelings and concerns and actively participate in school activities with peers and with the nursing plan of care.	Take unhurried time discussing Jane's concerns and feelings. Encourage Jane to discuss her thoughts with her close friends. Identify Jane's goals in life and suggest ways to meet those goals (Who am I?). Encourage participation in known problem solving. Compliment Jane on her general appearance, verbalization of fears, and participation in care. Identify with Jane her support system, including outside resources (AFDC, WIC, home health care, child care, psychologists, guidance counselors, tutors). Refer to guidance counselor if Jane needs tutoring to achieve educational needs. Encourage Jane to choose one person who will attend prenatal care, assist in childbirth, and participate in child care activities with her.	The adolescent's developmental need for a sense of identity is enhanced by the nurse's caring attitude and the involvement of the support system.	Jane discusses concerns and feelings. Jane participates in problem-solving. Jane continues her education during pregnancy. Jane brings a support person to prenatal visits. Jane appears clean and well-groomed. Jane utilizes community resources as needed.

Continued.

CARE PLAN Teenage Pregnancy—cont'd

GOALS	IMPLEMENTATION	RATIONALE	EVALUATION
Nursing diagnosis: High risk for ineffective individual coping related to knowledge deficit for making a decision regarding parenthood and adoption issues			
Jane will make an informed decision. Jane will increase her problem-solving skills as evidenced by her identifying several options for action and choosing from among them.	Evaluate Jane's feelings regarding parenthood and adoption and avoid sending verbal or nonverbal messages that will influence her. Discuss the pros and cons of parenthood and adoption with Jane. Encourage questions, and answer honestly. Clarify misconceptions. Suggest solutions to problems such as financial support or educational needs that may be of concern to Jane in evaluating parenthood. Refer Jane to a licensed adoption agency for specific questions surrounding the adoption process. Encourage Jane to discuss the decision with her family, but stress that she alone can make the decision. Evaluate Jane's feelings regarding seeing her child after birth or knowing its sex if adoption is chosen. Until adoption papers are signed, Jane should know that she can change her decision.	Exploring feelings and providing accurate, honest information will enhance the adolescent's ability for optimal decision-making.	Jane makes an informed decision regarding parenthood or adoption. Jane's problem-solving skills increase.

REFERENCES

Adler N et al: Adolescent contraceptive behavior: an assessment of decision processes, *J Pediatr* 116:463, 1990.

American Academy of Pediatrics, Committee on Adolescence: Care of adolescent parents and their children, *Pediatrics* 83:138, 1989.

Beach R: Breast exam: protect, reassure, educate, *Contemp OB/GYN* 35:41, Feb 1990.

Brazelton TB: *Neonatal behavioral assessment scale,* London, 1973, Spastics International Medical Publication.

Brown H: Recognizing common STDs in adolescents, *Contemp* OB/GYN 33:47, March 1989.

Cartoof V, Klerman L, Zazueta V: The effect of source of prenatal care on care-seeking behavior and pregnancy outcomes among adolescents, *J Adolesc Health* 12:124, 1991.

Casper L: Does family interaction prevent adolescent pregnancy? *Fam Plann Perspect* 22:109, March 1990.

Centers for Disease Control: *Survey: teen health and sex habits,* Atlanta, Sept 1991, The Centers.

Cooksey E: Factors in the resolution of adolescent premarital pregnancies, *Demography* 27:207, Feb 1990.

Donovan P: *Risk and responsibility: teaching sex education in America's schools today,* New York, 1989, Alan Guttmacher Institute.

Durant R et al: Contraceptive behavior among sexually active Hispanic adolescents, *J Adolesc Health Care* 11:490, 1990.

Elsters A, Lamb M, Kimmerly N: Perceptions of parenthood among adolescent fathers, *Pediatrics* 83:758, 1989.

Erikson E: *Identity, youth, and crisis,* New York, 1968, WW Norton.

Esman A: *Adolescence and culture,* New York, 1990, Columbia University Press.

Fine G, Mortimer J, Roberts D: Leisure, work and the mass media. In Feldman S, Elliott G, editors: *At the threshold: the developing adolescent,* Cambridge, Mass, 1990, Harvard University Press.

42 Code of Federal Regulations, 441.250-441.259, 1989.

Gasiorowski J: *Adolescent sexuality and sex education: a handbook for parents and educators,* Dubuque, Ia, 1988, Wm C Brown Co.

Greydanus D, Shearin R: *Adolescent sexuality and gynecology,* Philadelphia, 1990, Lea & Febiger.

Hendricks L: Outreach with teenage fathers: a preliminary report on three ethnic groups, *Adolescence* 23(91):711, 1988.
Hilliard P, Rebar R: Abnormal uterine bleeding needs a special approach, *Contemp OB/GYN* 35:51, May 1990.
Institute of Medicine: *Nutrition during pregnancy,* part I, Weight gain; part II. Nutrient supplements, Washington, DC, 1990, National Academy Press.
Irwin C: Risk-taking behaviors during the second decade of life. *Proceedings from the 1989 Adolescent Health Coordinators Conference,* Washington, DC, 1989, National Center for Education in Maternal and Child Health.
Jackson E, Mathur K: Adolescent pregnancy: effects of nutrients on hematocrit and birth weight, *J SC Med Assoc* 87:8, Jan 1991.
Kohlberg L: Stage and sequence: the cognitive developmental approach to socialization. In Nadien MB, editor: *The child's psychosocial development: from birth to adolescence,* Wayne, NJ, 1980, Avery Publishing Group.
Kokotailo P, Adger J: Substance use by pregnant adolescents, *Clin Perinatol* 18:125, 1991.
Lee K, Corpuz M: Teenage pregnancy: trend and impact on rates of low birth weight and fetal, maternal, and neonatal mortality in the United States, *Clin Perinatol* 15:929, 1988.
Lockhart L, Wodarski J: Teenage pregnancy: implications for social work practice, *Fam Ther* 17:29, Jan 1980.
McAnarney E: Early adolescent motherhood: crisis in the making. In Levine M, McAnarney R, editors: *Early adolescent transitions,* Lexington, Mass, 1988, Lexington Books.
McAnarney E, Greydanus D: Adolescent pregnancy and abortion. In Hofman A, Greydanus D, editors: *Adolescent medicine,* Norwalk, Conn, 1989, Appleton & Lange.
McAnarney E, Hendee W: Adolescent pregnancy and its consequences, *JAMA* 262:74, 1989a.
McAnarney E, Hendee W: The prevention of adolescent pregnancy, *JAMA* 262:78, 1989b.
National Center for Health Statistics: *Natality statistics,* Washington, DC, 1988, US Department of Health and Human Services.
National Center for Health Statistics: *Advance report of the monthly vital statistics,* Washington, DC, 1990, US Department of Health and Human Services, Public Health Service.
Robinson B: Teenage pregnancy from the father's perspective, *Am J Orthopsychiatry* 58:46, 1988.
Rosoff J: Sex education in the schools: policies and practice, *Fam Plann Perspect* 21:52, March/April 1989.
Sander J, Rosen J: Teenage fathers: working the neglected partner in adolescent childbearing, *Fam Plann Perspect* 21:6, Jan/Feb 1989.
Schneck M et al: Low-income pregnant adolescents and their infants: dietary findings and health outcomes, *J Am Diet Assoc* 90:555, 1990.
Scott C et al: Hispanic and black American adolescents' beliefs relating to sexuality and contraception, *Adolescence* 23:667, 1988.
Stevens J: Black grandmothers' and black adolescent mothers' knowledge about parenting, *Dev Psychol* 20:1017, 1984.
Stevens-Simon C, Roghman K, McAnarney E: Early vaginal bleeding, late prenatal care, and misdating in adolescent pregnancies, *Pediatrics* 87:838, 1991.
Story M, editor: *Nutrition management of the pregnant adolescent—a practical reference guide* (March of Dimes) Washington, DC, 1990, US Department of Health and Human Services, US Department of Agriculture.
Tyre L, Rothbart B, Anderson K: Helping adolescents make the right contraceptive choice, *Contemp OB/GYN* 35:37, March, 1990.
U.S. Department of Health and Human Services: *Health, United States, 1987,* Pub No PHS 88-1232, Hyattsville, Md, 1988, National Center for Health Statistics.
U.S. Department of Health and Human Services: *1989,* Public Health Service 29, 1990.
Young C et al: Adolescent third-trimester enrollment in prenatal care, *J Adolesc Health Care* 10:393, 1989.

References—Nursing Research

Horn B: Cultural beliefs and teenage pregnancy, *Nurs Pract* 8:35, 1983.
Pete J, Desantis L: Sexual decision making in young black adolescent females, *Adolescence* 25(97):145, 1990.
Ruff C: Adolescent mothering: assessing their parenting capabilities and their health education needs, *J Natl Black Nurses Assoc* 4:55, Jan 1990.
White J, Kellinger K: Teenagers' perceptions of unplanned adolescent pregnancies and oral contraceptive use, *J Am Acad Nurse Pract* 1:55, Feb 1989.

BIBLIOGRAPHY

American Academy of Pediatrics, Committee on Adolescence: Adolescent pregnancy, *Pediatrics* 83:132, 1989.
Atwater E: *Adolescence,* Englewood Cliffs NJ, 1988, Prentice Hall.
Bernards N, Hall L, editors: *Teenage sexuality: opposing viewpoints,* St Paul, Minn, 1988, Greenhaven Press.
Brooks-Gunn J, Furstenberg F: Adolescent sexual behavior, *Am Psychologist* 44:249, 1989.
Christmon K: Parental responsibility of African-American unwed adolescent fathers, *Adolescence* 25(49):645, 1990.
Church C: Neonatal implications of adolescent pregnancy, *NAACOG's Clin Issues Perinatal Women's Health Nurs* 2:245, 1991.
Glanville C: Implementing negotiating strategies into teen parenting programs, *J Natl Black Nurses Assoc* 4:45, Jan 1990.
Herr K: Adoption vs. parenting decisions among pregnant adolescents, *Adolescence* 24(96):795, 1989.
Hofman A, Greydanus D: *Adolescent medicine,* ed, 2 Norwalk, Conn, 1989, Appleton & Lange.
Katchadourian H: Sexuality. In Feldman S, Elliott G, editors: *At the threshold: the developing adolescent,* Cambridge, Mass, 1990, Harvard University Press.
Machol L: Helping teens avoid unplanned pregnancy, *Contemp OB/GYN* 34:96, April 1989.
Reedy N: The very young pregnant adolescent, *NAACOG's Clin Issues Perinatal Women's Health Nurs* 2:209, 1991.
Rhodes A: Options and issues for pregnant adolescents, *MCN* 13:427, 1988.
Scholl T et al: Maternal weight gain, diet and infant birth weight: correlations during adolescent pregnancy, *J Clin Epidemiol* 44:423, 1991.
Troutman B, Cutrona C: Nonpsychotic postpartum depression among adolescent mothers, *J Abnorm Psychol* 99:69, Jan 1990.
Turner R, Grindstaff C, Phillips N: Social support and outcome in teenage pregnancy, *J Health Soc Behav* 31:43, Jan 1990.

Bibliography—Nursing Research

Cooper C, Dunst C, Vance S: The effect of social support on adolescent mothers' styles of parent-child interaction as measured on three separate occasions, *Adolescence* 25(97):49, 1990.
Degenhart-Leskosky S: Health education needs of adolescent and nonadolescent mothers, *JOGNN* 18:238, 1989.
Hutchinson S: Adolescent mothers' perceptions of newborn infants and the mother's use of coping behaviors: a descriptive study, *J Natl Black Nurses Assoc* 4:14, Jan 1990.
Jones M, Mondy L: Prenatal education outcomes for pregnant adolescents and their infants using trained volunteers, *J Adolesc Health Care* 11:434, 1990.

chapter 34 review

Key Concepts

- Adolescents see their world in far different terms than do adults: their major tasks are the development of cognitive ability and identity formation.
- Cognitive development influences sexual decision making.
- Increasingly, poverty, life-style, and risk-taking behaviors are implicated in adolescent morbidity, with associated sequelae of pregnancy and other major health problems.
- Physiologic consequences and personal and public costs of adolescent pregnancy and parenthood are staggering.
- The adolescent's perception of pregnancy and parenthood is individual and depends on many variables.
- The developmental tasks of adolescents are interrupted by pregnancy.
- Poor nutrition and poverty have been implicated in physiologic consequences to the adolescent mother and her fetus and newborn.
- Adolescents' reactions to perceived stress depend on the quality of their support systems, their self-esteem, and their skill in problem identification and problem solving.
- The adolescent's knowledge of child development usually is limited.
- Standard approaches to prenatal and postpartum teaching are not appropriate or appealing for most adolescents.

Key Terms

- adolescence (p. 1018)
- developmental tasks of adolescence (p. 1019)
- developmental tasks of parenthood (p. 1025)
- developmental tasks of pregnancy (p. 1023)
- psychologic sexual self-concept and identity (p. 1020)
- risk taking (p. 1018)
- sex education (p. 1022)
- sexual decision making (p. 1018)
- sexual history (p. 1027)
- sexuality (p. 1020)

Critical Thinking Exercises

You are assigned to care for Lisa, a 14-year-old girl who is pregnant and attending the prenatal clinic for the first time.

1. Identify your feelings about adolescent pregnancy. What assumptions did you make about Lisa? How can you verify or negate these assumptions?
2. Examine pregnancy from the adolescent's viewpoint, using theory from this chapter. Determine where your perceptions differ.
3. Design a teaching plan to meet adolescent cognitive levels and learning needs on the topic of prenatal care.
4. Observe attitudes of the staff in the prenatal clinic toward adolescents. Analyze the impact of these attitudes on services provided to adolescents.

Topics for Nursing Research

- What are the long-term effects of various sex education programs on teenagers' knowledge, attitudes, and levels of sexual activity?
- What are the motivations for abstinence in female and male virgins?
- What is the effect of the nurse's age and gender on adolescent male and female participation in pregnancy-related programs?
- What are the "resiliency" factors of very low-income adolescents who do not become sexually active?
- What is the impact of new reproductive technology on the use and incidence of adolescent pregnancy?

chapter 35

Labor and Birth at Risk

DEITRA LEONARD LOWDERMILK

LEARNING OBJECTIVES

- Define key terms listed.
- Identify assessments for women experiencing different types of dystocia.
- Formulate nursing diagnoses based on assessment of dystocia.
- Describe interventions for different types of abnormal labor and birth problems related to dystocia: trial of labor, induction of labor, forceps-assisted birth, vacuum extraction, cesarean birth, and vaginal birth after cesarean.
- Discuss criteria for evaluating nursing care of clients experiencing dystocia.
- Compare nursing assessment and management of clients with preterm labor at home and in the hospital setting.
- Describe assessment and management of clients experiencing postterm pregnancy.
- Identify topics for nursing research related to labor and birth at risk.

When there are complications during labor and birth, perinatal morbidity and mortality increase. Some complications are anticipated, especially if the mother is identified at high risk during the antepartum period; others are unexpected or unforeseen. It is crucial for nurses to understand the normal birth process to prevent and detect deviations from normal and to implement nursing measures when complications arise. Optimum care of the laboring woman, fetus, and family experiencing complications is possible only when the nurse and other members of the obstetric team use their knowledge and skills in a concerted effort for the provision of care.

This chapter focuses on the different types of labor and birth problems related to dystocia, preterm labor and birth, and postterm pregnancy. The discussion of interventions for dystocia includes trial of labor, induction of labor, forceps-assisted birth, vacuum extraction, cesarean birth, and vaginal birth after cesarean. The discussion of care of the woman experiencing preterm labor includes home and hospital assessment and management. The discussion of the woman experiencing postterm pregnancy includes assessment strategies and management during labor and birth.

■ DYSTOCIA

Dystocia is defined as long, difficult, or abnormal labor and is caused by various conditions associated with the five essential factors of labor (see Chapter 14). Dystocia can be caused by any of the following:

1. *Dysfunctional labor,* resulting in ineffective uterine contractions or maternal bearing-down efforts (the powers)
2. *Alterations in the pelvic structure* (the passage)
3. *Fetal causes,* including abnormalities of presentation or position, anomalies, excessive size, and number of fetuses (the passenger)
4. *Maternal position* during labor and birth
5. *Psychologic responses* of the mother to labor related to past experiences, preparation, culture and heritage, and support system

These five factors are interdependent. Interactions among the factors and how they influence labor progress must be considered in assessing the woman for an abnormal labor pattern. Dystocia is suspected when there is a lack of progress in the rate of cervical dilatation, a lack of progress in fetal descent and expulsion, or an alteration in the characteristics of uterine contractions.

Dysfunctional Labor

Dysfunctional labor is described as abnormal uterine contractions that prevent normal progress of cervical dilatation, effacement (primary powers), and/or descent (secondary powers).

PRIMARY UTERINE DYSFUNCTION. Dysfunction of uterine contractions can be further described as primary or secondary. The woman who is experiencing *primary dysfunctional labor,* or **hypertonic uterine dysfunction,** often is an anxious first-time mother who is having painful contractions that are out of proportion to their intensity and that do not cause cervical dilatation or effacement. These contractions usually occur in the latent stage (cervical dilatation <4 cm) and usually are uncoordinated and frequent (Fig. 35-1). The force of the contraction may be in the midsection of the uterus rather than in the fundus, and the uterus may not completely relax between contractions (Koontz, 1988).

Women experiencing hypertonic uterine dysfunction may be exhausted and express concern about loss of control because of the intense pain and lack of progress. Management of primary uterine dysfunction is by **therapeutic rest,** which is achieved through the administration of effective analgesics such as morphine or meperidine to reduce the pain

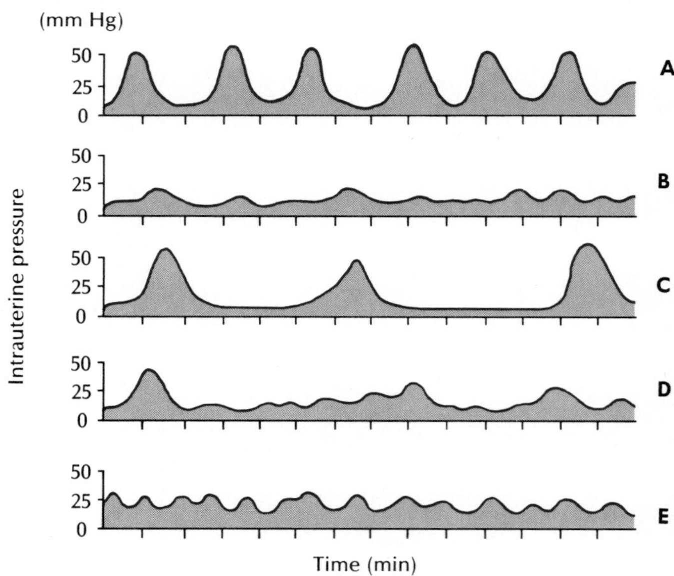

Fig. 35-1 Uterine contractility patterns in labor. **A,** Typical normal labor. **B,** Subnormal intensity, with frequency greater than needed for optimum performance. **C,** Normal contractions but too infrequent for efficient labor. **D,** Incoordinate activity. **E,** Hypercontractility.

and encourage sleep. Often these women will awaken with normal uterine activity.

Precipitous labor is defined as labor that lasts less than 3 hours from onset of contractions. Hypertonic uterine contractions may result in precipitous labor, characterized by tetanic-like contractions. Because labor is rapid, maternal and fetal complications can occur. Maternal complications include uterine rupture, lacerations of the birth canal, amniotic fluid embolism, and postpartum hemorrhage. Fetal complications include hypoxia caused by decreased periods of uterine relaxation between contractions and intracranial hemorrhage related to rapid birth (Cunningham et al, 1989). Erb-Duchenne palsy also has occurred with precipitous labor (Acker et al, 1988).

The second and more common type of uterine dysfunction is *secondary uterine inertia,* or **hypotonic uterine dysfunction.** The woman, who may be in her first or a subsequent pregnancy, initially makes normal progress into the active stage of labor; then the contractions become weak and inefficient or stop altogether (Fig. 35-1). The uterus is easily indentable even at the peak of contractions. Fetopelvic disproportion and malpositions are common causes.

Women experiencing hypotonic uterine dysfunction may become exhausted and are at risk for infection. Medical management usually includes ruling out fetopelvic disproportion, followed by augmentation of dysfunctional labor with oxytocin (Bowes, 1989) (p. 1057).

SECONDARY POWERS. Secondary powers, or bearing-down efforts, are compromised by large amounts of analgesic. Anesthesia may block the bearing-down reflex and alter the effectiveness of voluntary efforts. Exhaustion from lack of sleep or long labor and fatigue from inadequate hydration and food affect the woman's voluntary efforts. Maternal position can work against the forces of gravity, as well as decrease the contraction's strength and efficiency. Gravity adds 10 to 35 mm Hg to the pressure exerted by the presenting part (Fenwick, Simkin, 1987). Table 35-1 summarizes dysfunctional labor.

Alterations in Pelvic Structure

PELVIC DYSTOCIA. **Pelvic dystocia** can occur with contractures of the pelvic diameters that reduce the capacity of the bony pelvis, including the inlet, midpelvis, outlet, or any combination of these planes. Pelvic contractures may be caused by congenital abnormalities, maternal malnutrition, neoplasms, and lower spinal disorders. Immature pelvic size predisposes some adolescent mothers to pelvic dystocia. Pelvic deformities may be the result of automobile or other accidents.

Inlet contracture occurs in 1% to 2% of term births and is diagnosed when the diagonal conjugate is less than 11.5 cm. The incidence of face and shoulder presentation increases. These presentations prevent engagement and fetal descent, thereby increasing the risk of prolapse of the umbilical cord. Inlet contracture is associated with maternal rickets and a flat pelvis. Weak uterine contractions may be noted during the first stage of labor.

Midplane contracture, the most common cause of pelvic dystocia, is diagnosed when the sum of the interischial spinous and posterior sagittal diameters of the midpelvis is 13.5 cm or less. Fetal descent is arrested (transverse arrest of the fetal head) because the head cannot rotate internally. Cesarean birth is the usual management, but vacuum extraction has been used safely if the cervix is fully dilated. Midforceps-assisted birth usually is avoided because of increased perinatal mobidity associated with this intervention.

Outlet contracture exists when the interischial diameter is 8 cm or less. It rarely occurs without midplane contracture. Outlet contracture is associated with a long, narrow pubic arch and an android pelvis (see Fig. 14-14). Fetal descent is arrested. Maternal complications include extensive perineal lacerations during vaginal birth because the fetal head is pushed posteriorly.

SOFT TISSUE DYSTOCIA. **Soft tissue dystocia** results from obstruction of the birth passage by an anatomic abnormality other than that of the bony pelvis. The obstruction may result from placenta previa (low-lying placenta) that partially or completely obstructs the internal os of the cervix (see Chapter 30). Other causes, such as leiomyomas (uterine fibroids) in the lower uterine segment, ovarian tumors, and a full bladder or rectum, may prevent the fetus from entering the pelvis. Occasionally, *cervical edema* occurs in labor when the cervix is caught between the presenting part and the symphysis, preventing complete dilatation.

Bandl's ring, a pathologic retraction ring (see Fig. 14-15), is associated with prolonged rupture of membranes and protracted labor (Cunningham et al, 1989).

Fetal Causes

Dystocia of fetal origin may be caused by anomalies, excessive size and malpresentation, malposition, or multifetal pregnancy. Complications associated with dystocia of fetal origin include neonatal as-

TABLE 35-1 Dysfunctional Labor: Primary and Secondary Powers

Hypotonic Uterine Dysfunction	Hypertonic Uterine Dysfunction	Inadequate Voluntary Expulsive Forces
DESCRIPTION		
Cause may be contracture and fetal malposition, overdistention of uterus (twins), or unknown (primary powers) (Fig. 35-1)	Usually occurs before 4 cm dilatation; cause not yet known, may be related to fear and tension (primary powers) (Fig. 35-1)	Involves abdominal and levator ani muscles Occurs in second stage of labor; cause may be related to conduction anesthesia, heavy analgesia, exhaustion
CHANGE IN PATTERN OF PROGRESS		
Contractions decrease in frequency and intensity Uterus easily indentable even at peak of contraction Uterus relaxed between contractions (normal)	Pain out of proportion to intensity of contraction Pain out of proportion to effectiveness of contraction in effacing and dilating the cervix Contractions increase in frequency Contractions uncoordinated Uterus is contracted between contraction (basal hypertonus), cannot be indented	No voluntary urge to push or bear down or inadequate/ineffective pushing
POTENTIAL MATERNAL EFFECTS		
Infection Exhaustion Psychologic trauma	Loss of control related to intensity of pain and lack of progress Exhaustion	Spontaneous vaginal birth prevented
POTENTIAL FETAL EFFECTS		
Fetal infection Fetal and neonatal death	Fetal asphyxia with meconium aspiration	Fetal asphyxia
MEDICAL MANAGEMENT		
Rule out fetopelvic disproportion Oxytocic stimulation of labor (p. 1056)	Analgesic (e.g., morphine, meperidine) if membranes not ruptured or fetopelvic disproportion not present Relief of pain permits mother to rest; when she awakens, normal uterine activity may begin	Coach mother in bearing down with contractions Position mother in favorable position for pushing Low forceps or vacuum extraction if assistance for vaginal birth is needed Cesarean birth only if fetal distress occurs

phyxia, fetal injuries or fractures, and maternal vaginal lacerations. Although spontaneous vaginal birth is possible, fetal dystocia often leads to low forceps, vacuum extraction, or cesarean births.

ANOMALIES. Gross ascites, abnormal tumors, myelomeningocele, and hydrocephalus are fetal anomalies that can cause dystocia. These anomalies can affect the relationship of fetal anatomy to the maternal pelvic capacity, resulting in failure of the fetus to descend through the birth canal.

CEPHALOPELVIC DISPROPORTION. **Cephalopelvic disproportion** (CPD) related to excessive fetal size (4000 g [8 lb 13½ oz] or more) occurs in about 5% of term births. Excessive fetal size, or macrosomia, is associated with maternal diabetes mellitus, obesity, multiparity, or the large size of one or both parents. Shoulder dystocia, a condition in which the head is born but the anterior shoulder cannot pass under the pubic arch, can occur with macrosomia. When this occurs in a vaginal birth, the mother must be placed in a position to free the shoulders. The McRoberts maneuver, a maneuver in which the mother's legs are flexed with her knees on her abdomen, may be implemented (Mashburn, 1988). This maneuver causes the sacrum to straighten, and the symphysis pubis rotates toward the mother's head; the angle of pelvic inclination is decreased, freeing the shoulder (Fig. 35-2).

MALPOSITION. The most common fetal malposition is persistent occipitoposterior position (right occipitoposterior [ROP] or left occipitoposterior [LOP]; see Fig. 14-5), occurring in about 25% of all labors. Labor is prolonged, especially the second stage; the mother complains of severe back pain from the pressure of the fetal head against her sacrum. Counterpressure to the sacral area and frequent position changes may decrease the pain. The hands and knees or lateral position has been used to facilitate rotation of the fetus from a posterior to an anterior position (Lehrman, 1985; Fenwick, Simkin, 1987). Because the fetus usually will rotate spontaneously, birth may be accomplished by use of low forceps or manual rotation.

FETAL MALPRESENTATION. **Breech presentation** is the most common example of malpresentation, occurring in 3% to 4% of all births and up to 25% of preterm births. There are four main types of breech presentation: frank breech (thighs flexed, knees extended), complete breech (thighs and knees flexed), incomplete breech, in which the foot extends below buttocks, and incomplete breech, in which the knee extends below buttocks (Fig. 35-3). Breech presentations are associated with multifetal gestation, pre-

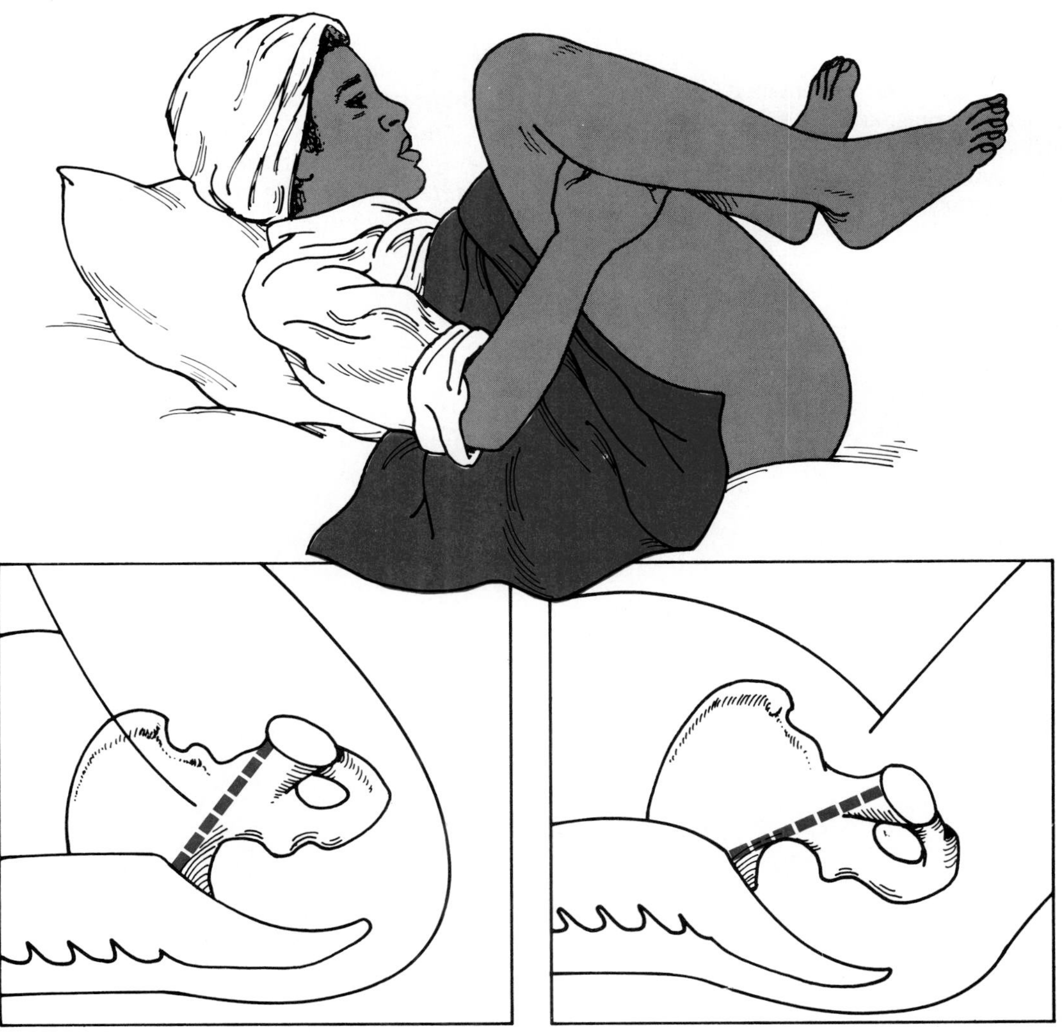

Fig. 35-2 McRoberts maneuver.
Modified from Gabbe S, Niebyl J, Simpson J: *Obstetrics, normal and problem pregnancies,* New York 1986, Churchill Livingstone.

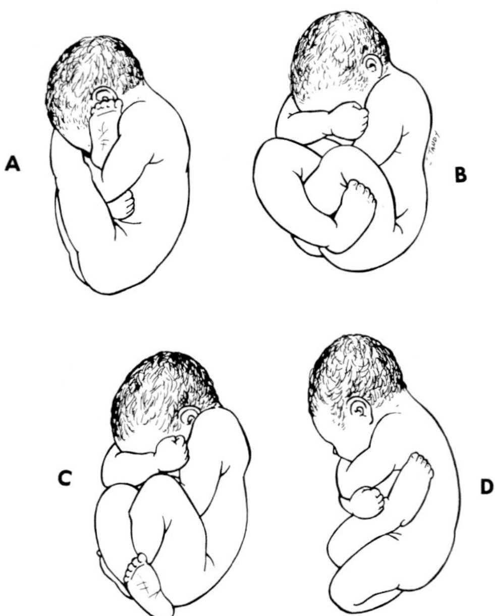

Fig. 35-3 Types of breech presentation. **A,** Frank breech: thighs are flexed on hips; knees are extended. **B,** Complete breech: thighs and knees are flexed. **C,** Incomplete breech: foot extends below buttocks. **D,** Incomplete breech: knee extends below buttocks.

term birth, fetal and maternal anomalies, hydramnios, and oligohydramnios. Diagnosis is made by abdominal palpation and vaginal examination and usually is confirmed by ultrasound scan.

During labor, fetal descent may be slow because the breech is not as good a dilating wedge as the fetal head, but labor usually is not prolonged. There is a risk of prolapsed cord if membranes rupture in early labor. Presence of meconium in amniotic fluid is not necessarily a sign of fetal distress because it results from pressure on the fetal abdominal wall as it traverses the birth canal. Fetal heart tones are best heard at or above the umbilicus. Vaginal birth is accomplished by mechanisms related to emergence of the buttocks and lower extremities (Fig. 35-4). Piper forceps sometimes are used to deliver the head (Fig. 35-10).

Breech presentation births are associated with birth trauma, asphyxiation, preterm birth, and congenital anomalies, resulting in higher neonatal and perinatal morbity and mortality rates and neurologic abnormalities later in life than occur in vertex presentation births (Englinton, 1988). Alternatives to vaginal birth of the fetus in breech presentation are *external cephalic version* (turning the fetus to a vertex presentation by exerting pressure on the fetus externally through the maternal abdomen) and *cesar-*

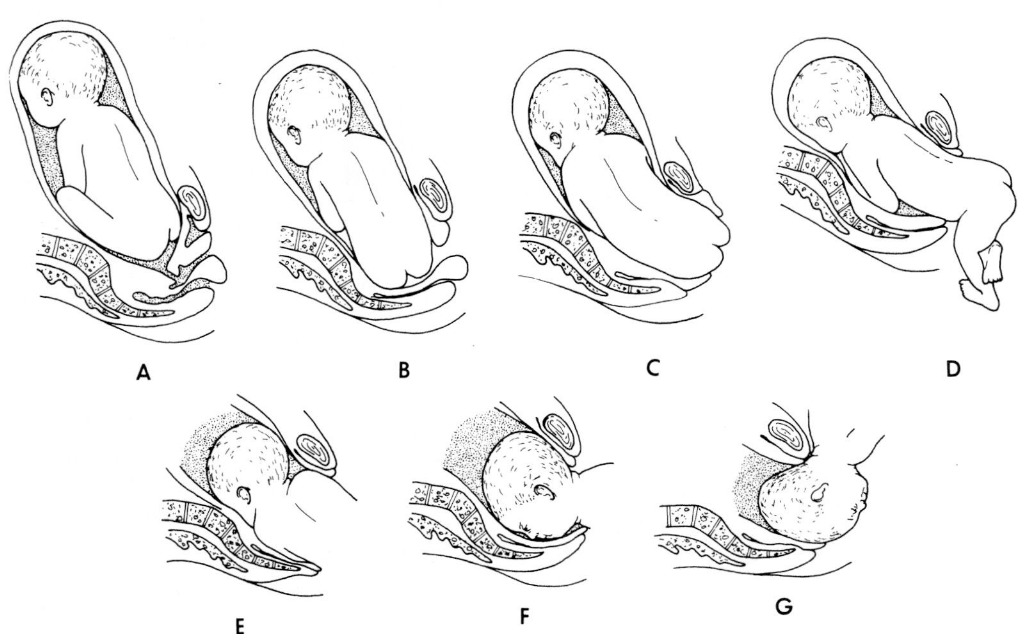

Fig. 35-4 Mechanism of labor in breech position. **A,** Breech before onset of labor. **B,** Engagement and internal rotation. **C,** Lateral flexion. **D,** External rotation or restitution. **E,** Internal rotation of shoulders and head. **F,** Face rotates to sacrum when occiput is anterior. **G,** Head is born by gradual flexion during elevation of fetal body.

ean birth (birth of the fetus through an abdominal incision).

Although opinions vary, cesarean birth (p. 1060) is commonly performed for women with fetuses estimated to be larger than 3800 g (8 lb 6 oz) or smaller than 2000 g (4 lb 4 oz) if labor is ineffective or complications occur (Bowes, 1989). Although cesarean birth reduces the risks to the fetus, maternal risks are increased. External cephalic version (p. 1055) also is not without risks and is not always successful. Women with a breech presentation late in pregnancy need to be informed about the options of birth, as well as the risks associated with each.

Face and brow presentations (Fig. 35-5) are uncommon and are associated with fetal anomalies, pelvic contractures, and fetopelvic disproportion. Vaginal birth is possible if the fetus flexes to a vertex presentation, although forceps often are used. Cesarean birth is indicated when the presentation persists, if there is fetal distress, or if labor progress stops.

Shoulder presentations (the fetus is in a transverse lie) usually require cesarean birth, although external cephalic version may be attempted after 38 weeks' gestation (Cunningham et al, 1989).

MULTIFETAL PREGNANCY. **Multifetal pregnancy** is the gestation of twins, triplets, quadruplets, or more infants (see Chapter 7). Infants of multifetal pregnancies account for 2% to 3% of all viable births and are associated with more complications, including dysfunctional labor, than are single births. The high incidence of complications and risk of perinatal mortality are primarily related to low-birth-weight infants resulting from preterm birth and intrauterine growth retardation. In addition, fetal complications such as congenital anomalies and abnormal presentations can cause dystocia and increased incidence of cesarean birth. For example, only half of all twin pregnancies will have both fetuses presenting in the vertex position, the most favorable for vaginal birth; one third may present as one twin in vertex and one in breech. To accomplish a vaginal birth of both twins, an intrapartum external version may be attempted for the twin in a a nonvertex position when the presenting twin's position is vertex. If the presenting twin is not in a vertex position, a cesarean birth usually is performed (Fig. 35-6) (Acker, Sachs, 1989; Adams, Chervenak, 1990).

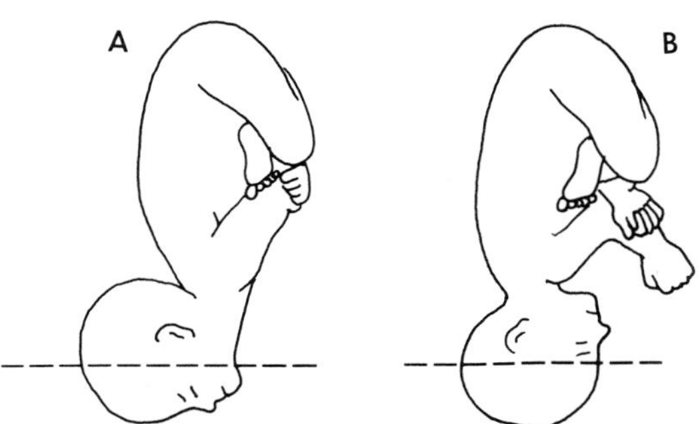

Fig. 35-5 Extension of normally flexed head. Face (**A**) and brow (**B**) presentations.

Position of the Mother

The functional relationships between the uterine contractions, the fetus, and the mother's pelvis are altered by maternal positioning. In addition, positioning can provide either a mechanical advantage or disadvantage to the mechanisms of labor by altering the effects of gravity and the relationships among body parts that are significant to labor progress (Fenwick, Simkin, 1987). Discouraging maternal movement or restricting labor to the recumbent or lithotomy position may compromise labor. The incidence of dystocia is increased, resulting in increased need for augmentation of labor, use of forceps, vacuum extraction, and cesarean birth (Andrews, Chrzanowski, 1990).

Psychologic Response

Hormones released in response to stress can cause dystocia. Sources of stress vary for each individual, but pain and the absence of a support person are two accepted factors. Confinement to bed and restriction

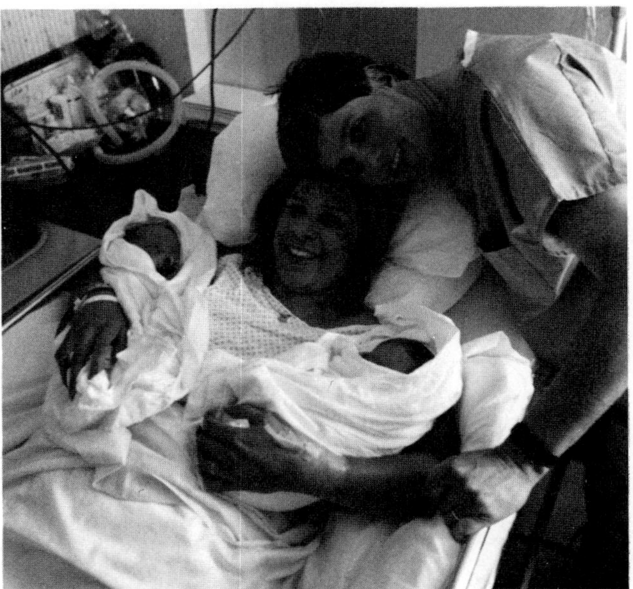

Fig. 35-6 Cesarean birth of twins.

of maternal movement add a potential psychologic stress to compound the physiologic stress of immobility in the unmedicated laboring woman. When anxiety is excessive, it can inhibit normal cervical dilatation, resulting in **prolonged labor** and increased pain perception. Anxiety also causes increased levels of stress-related hormones (β-endorphin, adrenocorticotropic hormone [ACTH], cortisol, and epinephrine). The labor-inhibiting effects of excessive levels of these hormones are well documented (Simkin, 1986) and may be associated with dystocic labor patterns (Liu, 1989).

Abnormal Labor Patterns

Abnormal labor patterns occur in 8% of pregnancies, with the highest incidence among nulliparous women (Friedman, 1989). These patterns may result

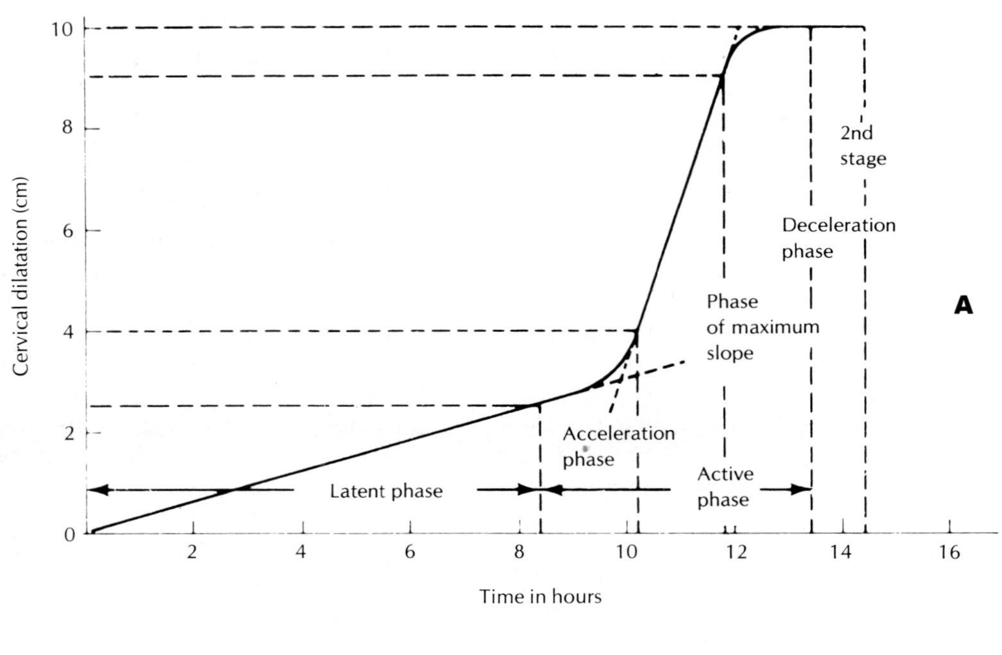

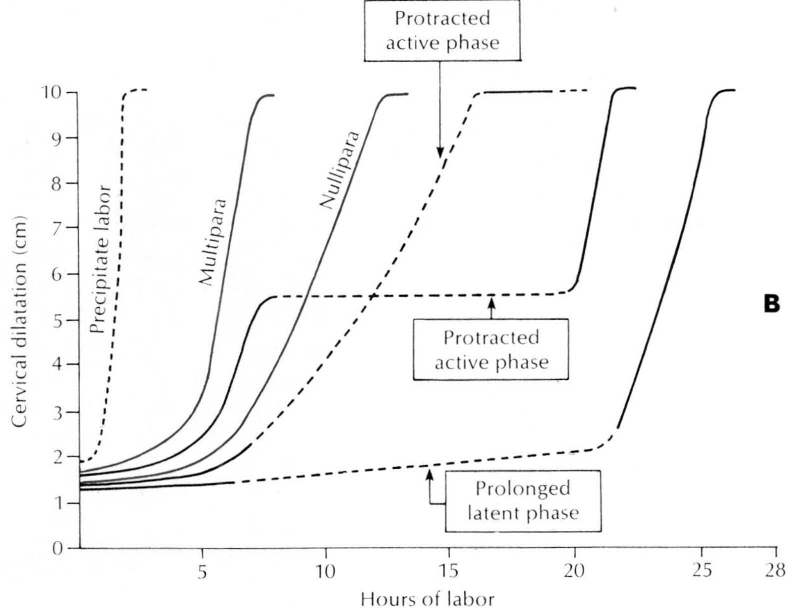

Fig. 35-7 A, Partogram of a normal labor. B, Major types of deviation from normal progress of labor may be detected by noting dilatation of cervix at various intervals after labor begins. If a woman exhibits an abnormal labor pattern as depicted by broken lines, physician should be notified immediately.

from the various causes previously described: ineffective uterine contractions, pelvic contractures, cephalopelvic disproportion, abnormal fetal presentations or position, early use of analgesics, conduction anesthesia, and anxiety and stress. Progress in either the first or second stage of labor can be protracted (delayed) or arrested. Abnormal progress can be recognized when cervical dilatation is plotted on a labor graph and compared with a normal labor curve. Fig. 35-7, *A*, is a graphic representation of normal labor progress of a first-time mother.

The *latent phase* includes that portion of the first stage between the onset of labor contractions and the acceleration in rate of cervical dilatation. The upswing in the curve denotes the onset of the *active phase* of the first stage of labor, which is divided into an acceleration phase, a phase of maximum slope, and a deceleration phase. Compare these normal phases with Fig. 35-7, *B*, which shows major types of deviation from normal progress of labor. These can be detected by noting the dilatation of the cervix at various intervals after labor begins. If a woman exhibits an abnormal labor pattern as depicted by the broken lines, the health care provider is notified.

Six abnormal labor patterns have been identified and classified by Friedman (1989) according to cervical dilatation and fetal descent. A prolonged latent phase is one that exceeds 20 hours or longer in nulliparous women and 14 hours or longer in the multiparous woman. The active phase of labor can be complicated by protraction disorders (no progress). In a protracted active phase, the cervix dilates less than 1.2 cm/hr in the nulliparous woman and less than 1.5 cm/hr in the multiparous woman. Arrest of the active phase is determined when neither the nulliparous nor multiparous woman demonstrates progress for more than 2 hours.

Descent of the presenting part also can be protracted or arrested in the active phase of labor. A protracted descent pattern is one in which the rate of descent is less than 1 cm/hr in the nulliparous woman and less than 2 cm/hr in the multiparous woman. Arrest of descent is the lack of progress for more than 1 hour in both nulliparous and multiparous women. Failure of descent is a lack of descent of the presenting part during the deceleration phase and the second stage.

Fetal mortality increases sharply after 15 hours of the active first stage of labor. Maternal morbidity and mortality may occur as a result of uterine rupture, infection, serious dehydration, and postpartum hemorrhage. A long difficult labor also can have an adverse psychologic effect on the mother, father, and family. Management of prolonged labor depends on the cause and can include therapeutic rest, augmentation with oxytocin, forceps birth, vacuum extraction, and cesarean birth (Bowes, 1989). A summary of normal and prolonged labor patterns, with medical management strategies, is given in Table 35-2.

Nursing Process

ASSESSMENT

Risk assessment is a continuous process. Review of the initial *interview* conducted at the woman's admission to the labor unit and ongoing observations of her psychologic response to labor reveal factors that can cause dysfunctional labor: for example, anxiety or fear, presence of a complication of pregnancy, or previous labor complications. The initial *physical assessment* data and ongoing assessments provide information about the frequency, duration, and intensity of uterine contractions, cervical status, fetal heart rate (FHR), presentation and station of the fetus, and status of membranes. *Laboratory data* such as scalp pH can identify fetal distress; ultrasound findings can identify potential dysfunctional labor problems related to the fetus or maternal pelvis. All these assessments contribute to accurate identification of potential and actual nursing diagnoses related to dystocia and maternal-fetal compromise.

NURSING DIAGNOSES

Nursing diagnoses vary with the type of dystocia, as well as with the individual needs of the woman and her family. Potential or actual nursing diagnoses that might be identified for clients experiencing dystocia include the following:

- Anxiety related to
  - —Slowed labor progress
- Pain related to
  - —Dystocia
  - —Obstetric procedures
- High risk for fetal injury related to
  - —Fetal compromise
- High risk for maternal injury related to
  - —Interventions implemented for dystocia
- Powerlessness related to
  - —Loss of control
- High risk for infection related to
  - —Rupture of membranes, operative procedures
- Fatigue related to
  - —Prolonged labor
- Fear related to
  - —Real or potential threat to self or fetus

TABLE 35-2 Labor Patterns in Normal and Abnormal Labor

NORMAL LABOR

1. Dilatation: continues
   a. Latent phase: <4 cm and low slope
   b. Active phase: >5 cm or high slope
   c. Deceleration phase: ≥9 cm
2. Descent: active at ≥9 cm dilatation
3. Normal labor progresses rapidly; multiparous women faster than nulliparous women

Pattern	Abnormal Prolonged Labor		Preferred Treatment	Possible Treatment
	Nulliparas	Multiparas		
1. Prolonged latent phase	>20 hr	>14 hr	Therapeutic rest	Oxytocin/cesarean birth
2. Protracted active-phase dilatation	<1.2 cm/hr	<1.5 cm/hr	Close observation	Oxytocin
3. Secondary arrest: no change	≥2 hr	≥2 hr	Oxytocin if CPD is not present	Rest
Protracted descent	<1 cm/hr	<2 cm/hr	Cesarean birth if CPD is present	Cesarean birth, forceps birth, vacuum extraction
Arrest of descent	≥1 hr	≥½ hr	Cesarean birth if CPD is present	Cesarean birth, forceps birth, vacuum extraction
Failure of descent: no change during deceleration phase and second stage			Cesarean birth	Not applicable

Based on Bowes, 1989; Cunningham et al, 1989; Friedman, 1989; Sokol, Brindley, 1990
CPD, Cephalopelvic disproportion.

- Impaired tissue integrity related to
  —Operative procedures
- High risk for altered parenting related to
  —Unplanned cesarean birth
- Altered sensory perception overload related to
  —Numerous interventions for dystocia
- Ineffective individual coping related to
  —Disappointment
  —Pain
  —Fear
  —Exhaustion
  —Lack of support system
- Knowledge deficit related to
  —Procedures, positioning, relaxation techniques, etc.
- Situational low self-esteem related to
  —Inability to labor and give birth as expected
- Fluid volume excess related to
  —Intravenous infusion with oxytocin
- Fluid volume deficit related to
  —NPO status

PLANNING

Nursing diagnoses provide direction for care. During this important step, goals are set in client-centered terms, and the goals are prioritized. Nursing actions are selected with the client, as appropriate, to meet the goals.

Goals (expected outcomes) for the woman who is experiencing dystocia include those that follow.

- She will understand the causes and treatment of dysfunctional labor.
- She will utilize positive patterns of coping to maintain a positive self-concept.
- She will demonstrate diminished or minimal anxiety.
- She will express relief of pain.
- She will experience labor and birth with minimal or no complications such as infection, injury, or hemorrhage.
- She will give birth to a healthy infant who has not experienced fetal distress.

IMPLEMENTATION

Nurses assume many caregiving roles when labor is complicated. Knowledge of medical management for each condition is essential to implementing the nursing process. This knowledge enables the nurse to work collaboratively with the physician and to meet the client's knowledge and emotional needs. Interventions include external cephalic version, trial of labor, induction/augmentation with oxytocin, amniotomy, and operative procedures such as forceps-assisted birth, vacuum extraction, and cesarean birth.

EXTERNAL CEPHALIC VERSION. **External cephalic version** (ECV) is the attempt to turn the fetus from a breech or shoulder presentation to a vertex presentation for birth. ECV may be attempted in a labor and birth setting after 37 weeks' gestation. Before it is attempted, ultrasound scanning is used to determine the fetal position, to rule out placenta previa, and to assess the amount of amniotic fluid, the fetal age, and the presence of any anomalies. A nonstress test is performed to ensure fetal well-being. Informed consent is obtained. The ECV is accomplished by gentle, constant pressure accompanied by continuous fetal heart surveillance (Fig. 35-8). A tocolytic agent, such as ritodrine or terbutaline (p. 1074), may be given intravenously to relax the uterus and facilitate the maneuver. Ultrasound may be used to identify potential problems such as cord entanglement and placental separation (Englinton, 1988).

During an attempted ECV, the nurse continuously monitors the FHR, especially for bradycardia, checks maternal vital signs frequently, and assesses the client's level of comfort because the procedure may cause discomfort. After the procedure is completed, the nurse continues to monitor maternal vital signs, uterine activity, and FHR and assesses for vaginal bleeding until the client's condition is stable.

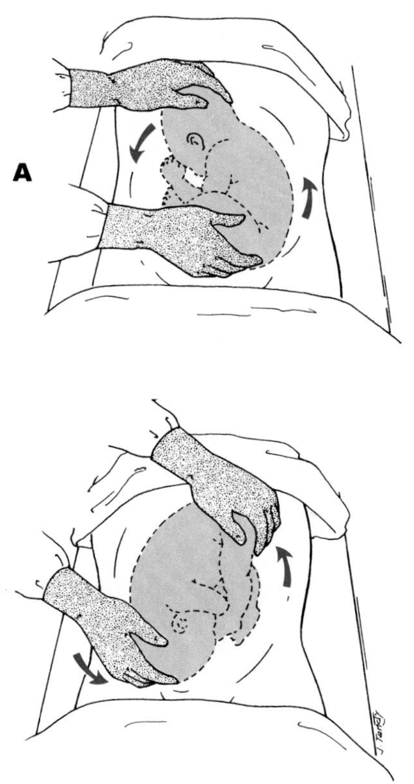

Fig. 35-8 External version of fetus from breech to vertex presentation. This must be achieved without force. **A,** Breech is pushed up out of pelvic inlet while head is pulled toward inlet. **B,** Head is pushed toward inlet while breech is pulled upward.

TRIAL OF LABOR. A **trial of labor** (TOL) is a reasonable period (4 to 6 hours) of active labor. It allows assessment of the possibility of a safe vaginal birth for the mother and infant. TOL may be initiated when the mother's pelvis is of questionable size or shape, when she wishes to have a vaginal birth after a previous cesarean birth, and when the fetus shows an abnormal presentation. Fetal sonography and/or maternal pelvimetry is used before a TOL to rule out fetopelvic disproportion. The cervix must be soft and dilatable. During TOL, the woman is evaluated for active labor, including adequate contractions, engagement and descent of the presenting part, and effacement and dilatation of the cervix. Induction of labor seldom is implemented.

The nurse assesses uterine activity, cervical changes, maternal vital signs, and fetal status during this TOL. If maternal or fetal complications are identified, the nurse is responsible for initiating appropriate actions, including notifying the obstetrician, and evaluating and documenting the maternal or fetal response to the interventions.

INDUCTION OF LABOR. **Induction of labor** is the initiation of uterine contractions before their spontaneous onset for the purpose of bringing about the birth. Induction may be indicated for a variety of medical and obstetric reasons, including pregnancy-induced hypertension, diabetes mellitus and other maternal medical problems, postterm gestation, suspected fetal jeopardy (e.g., intrauterine growth retardation), logistic factors such as rate of rapid birth, distance from the hospital, and fetal death. Under such conditions the risk of birth to the mother or fetus is less than the risk of continuing the pregnancy (Dunn, 1990).

Both chemical and mechanical methods are used to induce labor. Intravenous oxytocin and amniotomy are the most common methods used in the United States. Less commonly used methods of induction include nipple stimulation, ingestion of castor oil, soapsuds enema, stripping of membranes, and acupuncture (Tal et al, 1988; ACOG, 1991). Prostaglandin (PG) E (PGE_2) gel and other agents such as relaxin also are used but have not yet been approved by the U.S. Food and Drug Administration (FDA) for this purpose (NAACOG, 1988; Jacobs, 1989).

Success rates for induction of labor are higher when the cervix is favorable, or inducible. A rating system such as the **Bishop score** (Table 35-3) can be used to evaluate inducibility. For example, a score of 9 or more on this scale indicates the cervix is soft, anterior, 50% effaced, and dilated 2 cm or more; the presenting part is engaged. Labor should be successful. An unfavorable score is less than 5.

CERVICAL RIPENING METHODS. Different **prostaglandins** (hormones) have been applied to the cervix before induction to induce or "ripen" (soften and thin) the cervix (for further discussion of PGs, see Chapter 6). PGE_2 gel is under review by the FDA as a cervical ripening agent in the United States (ACOG, 1991). The drug is made by mixing PGE_2 vaginal suppositories with a gel substance. The gel may be administered through a catheter into the cervical canal or applied to a diaphragm that is placed next to the cervix. Additional doses may be reapplied every 4 to 6 hours, with two to three doses usually being sufficient. Oxytocin induction usually is not started until 4 to 6 hours later to avoid hyperstimulation (Rayburn, 1989). Side effects of PGE_2, which include vomiting, fever, diarrhea, and hyperstimulation of the uterus, are uncommon with gel applications (Henderson, Lichter, 1989; Jacobs, 1989; Sinquefield, 1989; Sokol, Brindley, 1990).

Nursing assessments after the gel has been administered are similar to those performed for women whose labor is induced with oxytocin (p. 1057).

TABLE 35-3 Bishop Score

	Score			
	0	1	2	3
Dilatation (cm)	0	1-2	3-4	5-6
Effacement (%)	0-30	40-50	60-70	80
Station (cm)	−3	−2	−1	+1
Cervical consistency	Firm	Medium	Soft	
Fetal position	Posterior	Midline	Anterior	

AMNIOTOMY. **Amniotomy** (artificial rupture of membranes [AROM]) can be used to stimulate labor when the condition of the cervix is favorable. Labor usually begins within 12 hours of the rupture; however, if amniotomy does not stimulate labor, prolonged rupture may lead to infection. For this reason, amniotomy often is used in combination with oxytocin induction. Before the procedure, an explanation of what to expect is given to the mother; she also is assured that the procedure is painless for her and the fetus. The membranes are ruptured with an amnihook or other sharp instrument; amniotic fluid is allowed to drain slowly. The fluid is assessed for color, odor, and consistency (i.e., absence of meconium or blood). The time of rupture is recorded. The FHR is assessed before and after the procedure to detect changes that may indicate presence of cord compression or prolapse. The client's temperature should be checked at least every 4 hours to rule out possible infection. If the temperature is 100° F (37.8° C), hourly temperature assessments are indicated. Comfort measures such as changing the client's underpads frequently should be implemented, since the amniotic fluid will continue to leak from the vagina after rupture of membranes.

OXYTOCIN. **Oxytocin** is a hormone normally produced by the posterior pituitary gland that stimulates uterine contractions. Oxytocin may be used either to induce the labor process or to augment a labor that is progressing slowly because of inadequate uterine contractions. It also can be used to assess fetal response to the stress of labor contractions (oxytocin challenge test [OCT]); see Chapter 27.

The *indications* for oxytocin induction of labor may include, but are not limited to, the following:

- Slowing of progress of labor
- Management of abortion—to stimulate the uterus to pass the conceptus
- Prolonged rupture of membranes
- Prolonged pregnancy (42 to 43 weeks)
- Preterm birth in diabetic mother or mother with severe isoimmunization
- Severe preeclampsia, abruptio placentae, or fetal death necessitating termination of the pregnancy artificially
- Multiparous women with a history of precipitate labor who live a long distance from the hospital

The management of stimulation of labor is the same regardless of indication. Because of the potential dangers associated with the use of injectable oxytocin in the prenatal and intranatal periods, the FDA has issued restrictions on its use.

Contraindications to oxytocic stimulation of labor include, but are not limited to, the following:

Fetopelvic disproportion
Fetal distress
Placenta previa
Prior classic uterine incision or uterine surgery
Active genital herpes infection

Oxytocin can present hazards to both mother and fetus. Maternal hazards include tumultuous labor and tetanic contractions, which may cause premature separation of the placenta, rupture of the uterus, laceration of the cervix, or postbirth hemorrhage. These complications can cause infection, disseminated intravascular coagulation, and amniotic fluid embolism. Women also may become anxious or fearful if the induction is not successful because of concerns they may have about the method of birth.

Fetal hazards include fetal asphyxia and neonatal hypoxia from too frequent and prolonged uterine contractions, physical injury, and prematurity, if the estimated date of birth is inaccurate.

Initiation of induction or augmentation of labor with oxytocin is the responsibility of the health care provider, although the medication often is administered by a nurse. A written protocol for the preparation and administration of oxytocin should be established by the obstetric department in each institution. Until recently, the aim of induction with oxytocin was to achieve a contraction pattern that simulated the active phase of labor as quickly as possible. Recent research on uterine tolerance to oxytocin has shown that lower doses given at longer intervals are as effective as previous protocols and are less likely to cause uterine hyperstimulation and dysfunctional labor (Curtis, Safransky, 1988; Mercer et al, 1991).

After the woman has been evaluated for induction, the following recommended procedures are performed in a labor and birth setting (NAACOG, 1988):

- A primary intravenous infusion of a physiologic electrolytic fluid is started. Intravenous medications other than oxytocin can be administered through this line. The nurse explains the procedure, the rationale, and what to expect (uterine contractions will be stronger and will occur more often and more regularly).
- A secondary intravenous infusion containing dilute oxytocin (usually 10 U/1000 mL) is added to the main line. This line should be connected close to the primary venipuncture site. No medication except oxytocin should be given through this line. Oxytocin should be administered through a pump delivery system to ensure accurate dose and safe administration.
- Oxytocin is administered according to prescribed orders or protocol. Initial dosages of 0.5 to 1 mU/min, with increases of 1 to 2 mU/min, are administered at 30- to 60-minute intervals until the desired contraction pattern is achieved. That is, contractions are of 40 to 60 seconds' duration and 2½ to 4 minutes apart; intensity is 50 to 75 mm Hg if intrauterine pressure is being monitored internally.
- Once the cervix is dilated 5 to 6 cm and labor is established, the oxytocin dose can be reduced by similar decrements.
- Usually no more than 20 mU oxytocin per minute are needed to achieve progressive cervical dilatation. In many cases, less than 4 mU/min are needed (Sokol, Brindley, 1990).
- The FHR; uterine resting tone; and frequency, duration, and intensity of contractions are monitored continuously (electronic fetal-maternal monitoring is suggested); and maternal blood pressure and pulse are monitored at 30- to 60-minute intervals and/or when doses are changed.
- The nurse assesses intake and output to prevent water intoxication. The intravenous intake usually is limited to 1000 mL in 8 hours (125 mL/hr); urine output should be 120 mL or more in 4 hours.
- The nurse also assesses for side effects of nausea, vomiting, headache, or hypotension.
- *Oxytocin is discontinued immediately and the physician notified of uterine hyperstimulation or nonreassuring FHR.* With the latter, other nursing interventions, such as administration of oxygen by face mask and positioning the woman on her left side, are implemented immediately (see emergency box, p. 1058).
- Documentation of maternal and fetal assessments is necessary in the medical record and on the fetal monitor tracing. In addition, the woman and her support persons are kept informed of her progress.

AUGMENTATION. Augmentation of labor is the stimulation of uterine contractions after labor has started spontaneously yet progress is unsatisfactory. Augmentation usually is implemented for hypotonic dysfunctional labor. The procedures and nursing assessments used are the same as those used for oxytocin induction of labor.

Some physicians advocate active management of labor, that is, intervention with augmentation of labor as soon as labor is not progressing at least 1 cm/hr. Advocates of active management indicate that intervening early with aggressive use of oxytocin (increases of 6 mU/min) shortens labor (usually 12 hours or less) and reduces the incidence of cesarean birth (Akoury et al, 1988; Turner et al, 1988). This practice is currently under study in the United States to determine its effectiveness and impact on perinatal morbidity and mortality. Nurses who participate in

EMERGENCY

Uterine Hyperstimulation with Oxytocin

SIGNS

Uterine contractions >90 sec, occurring in intervals <q2min
Uterine pressure above 75 mmHg
Fetal distress
- Bradycardia
- Tachycardia
- Heart irregularity
- Late decelerations
- Decreased variability

INTERVENTIONS

Maintain woman on left side.
Turn off oxytocin; keep maintenance IV line open; increase rate.
Start oxygen via face mask.
Notify physician/midwife.
Continue monitoring of FHR and uterine activity.
Document responses to actions.

these studies will be administering higher doses of oxytocin than is currently practiced. Therefore, closer attention to uterine activity and fetal status is imperative.

The procedure on p. 1059 summarizes the nursing responsibilities for induction of labor by amniotomy and oxytocin administration.

FORCEPS-ASSISTED BIRTH. A **forceps-assisted birth** is one in which two instruments with curved blades are used to assist in the birth of the fetal head. The cephalic-like curve of the forceps commonly used is similar to the shape of the fetal head. A pelvic curve of the blades conforms to the pelvic axis. The blades are joined by a pin, screw, or groove arrangement. These locks prevent the forceps from compressing the fetal skull. Maternal indications for forceps-assisted birth include the need to shorten the second stage in dystocia (difficult labor) or to correct the mother's deficient expulsive efforts (e.g., she is tired or she has been given spinal or epidural anesthesia), as well as to reverse a dangerous condition (e.g., cardiac decompensation).

Fetal indications include birth of a fetus in distress, in certain abnormal presentations, or in arrest of rotation, as well as to deliver an aftercoming head in a breech presentation (Dennan, 1989).

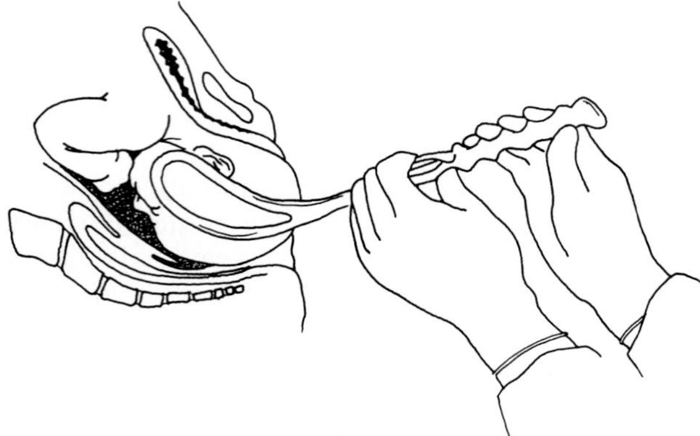

Fig. 35-9 Outlet forceps extraction of the head.

Certain conditions are required for a successful forceps-assisted birth. The woman's cervix must be fully dilated to avoid lacerations and hemorrhage. The presenting part must be engaged, and a vertex presentation is desired. Membranes should be ruptured so that the position of the fetal head can be determined and that a firm grasp of the forceps on the head during birth can be ensured. Cephalopelvic disproportion (CPD) should not be present. To avoid lacerations and injury the woman's bladder should not be distended (Sokol, Brindley, 1990).

There are different definitions of forceps applications. According to ACOG (1988a), *outlet* forceps are appropriate when the fetal scalp is visible on the perineum without manually separating the labia (Fig. 35-9). There must be no more than a 45-degree rotation from an occiput anterior or occiput posterior position. Outlet forceps are used to shorten the second stage of labor. *Low* forceps is the term used when forceps are applied to the fetal head that is at least at +2 station. Rotation may be more than 45 degrees. *Midforceps* are defined as forceps applied when the fetal head is engaged (no higher than station 0) but above a +2. There are no circumstances when forceps should be applied to an unengaged presenting part.

NURSING CONSIDERATIONS. The nurse obtains forceps designated by the physician (Fig. 35-10). The FHR is checked, reported, and recorded *before* forceps are *applied*. The mother is informed that the forceps blades fit like two tablespoons around an egg. The blades come over the baby's ears. The FHR is rechecked, reported, and recorded *before traction* is applied after application of forceps. Compression of the cord between the fetal head and the forceps would cause a drop in FHR. The physician would then remove and reapply the forceps.

After birth, the mother is assessed for vaginal and

Procedure for Induction of Labor

Apply fetal and maternal electronic monitor before beginning induction.
Explain technique, rationale, and reactions to expect:
- Route and rate: what "piggyback" is for
- Reasons for use:
  Induce labor
  Improve labor
- Reactions to expect concerning the nature of contractions. Intensity of contraction increases more rapidly, holds the peak longer, and ends more quickly. The contractions will begin to come regularly and more often.
- Monitoring to anticipate:
  Maternal: BP, P, uterine contractions, uterine tone
  Fetal: heart rate, activity
- Success to expect: a favorable outcome will depend on inducibility of the cervix (Bishop score of 9 or more)

Position woman in side-lying position.
Prepare solutions and administer according to prescribed orders with pump delivery system:
- Infusion pump and solution is set up
- Piggyback solution is connected to IV line
  —Solution with oxytocin is flagged with a medication label
  —Begin induction at 0.5-1.0 mU/min
  —Increase dose 1-2 mU/min at intervals of 30-60 min

Maintain dose when:
- Intensity of contraction results in intrauterine pressures of 50 to 75 mm Hg (by internal monitor)
- Duration of contraction is 40 to 60 sec
- Frequency of contractions is 2½ to 4-min intervals

Assess intake and output; limit IV intake to 1000 mL/8 hr; output should be 120 mL or more q4h.
Monitor for nausea, vomiting, headache, hypotension.
Discontinue use of oxytocin per hospital protocol; keep maintenance line open.
Discontinue infusion of oxytocin, keep maintenance line open, and notify physician if *warning signs* occur:
- *Contractions*—excessive intrauterine pressure >75 mm Hg, duration >90 sec, and frequency > q2min
- *Fetal distress*—fetal bradycardia, tachycardia, or heart irregularity

Keep woman and family informed.

For amniotomy

Position woman on bedpan or fracture pan.
Person performing procedure puts on gloves and inserts first two fingers of one hand into cervix until membranes are identified.
Amnihook or Allis clamp is inserted alongside fingers, and membranes are torn and hooked by the instrument.
Assess FHR.
Assess color, odor, and consistency of fluid.

Charting

- *Medication:* kind, amount, time of beginning, increasing dose, maintaining dose, and discontinuing medication in client record and on monitoring strip
- *Reactions of mother and fetus:*
  —Pattern of labor
  —Progress in labor
  —FHR
- *Signs of maternal or fetal stress*

BP, Blood pressure; *IV*, intravenous; *P*, pulse.

cervical lacerations (bleeding occurs even with a contracted uterus) and urine retention, which may result from bladder injuries. The infant should be assessed for bruising or abrasions at the site of the blade applications, facial palsy resulting from pressure of the blades on the facial nerve, and subdural hematoma. Newborn and postpartum caregivers should be informed that a forceps-assisted birth was performed.

VACUUM EXTRACTION. **Vacuum extraction** is a birth method involving the attachment of a vacuum cup to the fetal head, using negative pressure. It is a popular alternative to forceps birth in Europe and is gaining popularity in the United States. Indications for use are similar to those for outlet forceps, but it is especially appropriate in cases of failure to rotate and arrest of second stage of labor (Galvan, Broekhuizen, 1987). Prerequisites for use include a vertex presentation, ruptured membranes, and absence of fetopelvic disproportion.

The woman is prepared for a vaginal birth in the lithotomy position to allow for sufficient traction. The cup is applied to the fetal head, and a caput develops inside the cup as the pressure is initiated (Fig. 36-11). Traction is then applied to facilitate descent of the fetal head. As the head crowns, an *episiotomy*

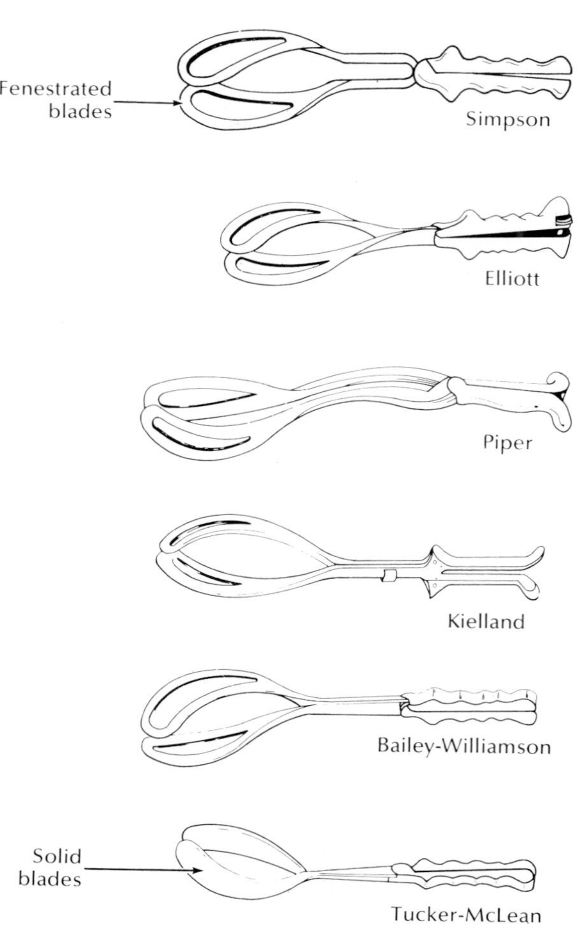

Fig. 35-10 Types of forceps. Piper forceps are used to assist delivery of the head in breech birth.

is performed if necessary and the vacuum cup is released and removed after birth of the head. If vacuum extraction is not successful, a forceps or cesarean birth will be performed.

Risks to the newborn include cephalhematoma, scalp lacerations, and subdural hematoma. Maternal complications are uncommon but can include perineal, vaginal, and cervical lacerations.

NURSING CONSIDERATIONS. The nurse's role for the woman who has given birth by use of vacuum extraction is one of support person and educator. The nurse can prepare the woman for birth and encourage her to remain active in the birth process by pushing during contractions. Also, the FHR should be assessed frequently during the procedure. After birth, the newborn should be observed for signs of infection at the application site and cerebral irritation (e.g., poor sucking, listlessness). The parents may need to be reassured that the caput succedaneum will begin to disappear in a few hours. Neonatal caregivers should be alerted that the birth was by vacuum extraction.

CESAREAN BIRTH. **Cesarean birth** is the birth of a fetus through a transabdominal incision of the uterus. Although the myth persists that Julius Caesar was delivered in this manner, the derivation of the term is more likely from the Latin word *caedo* meaning "to cut." Whether cesarean birth is planned (elective) or unplanned (emergency), the loss of the experience of giving birth to a child in the traditional manner may have a negative effect on a woman's self-concept. An effort is made to maintain the focus on the *birth* of a child rather than on the operative procedure. The mother experiences abdominal rather than vaginal birth.

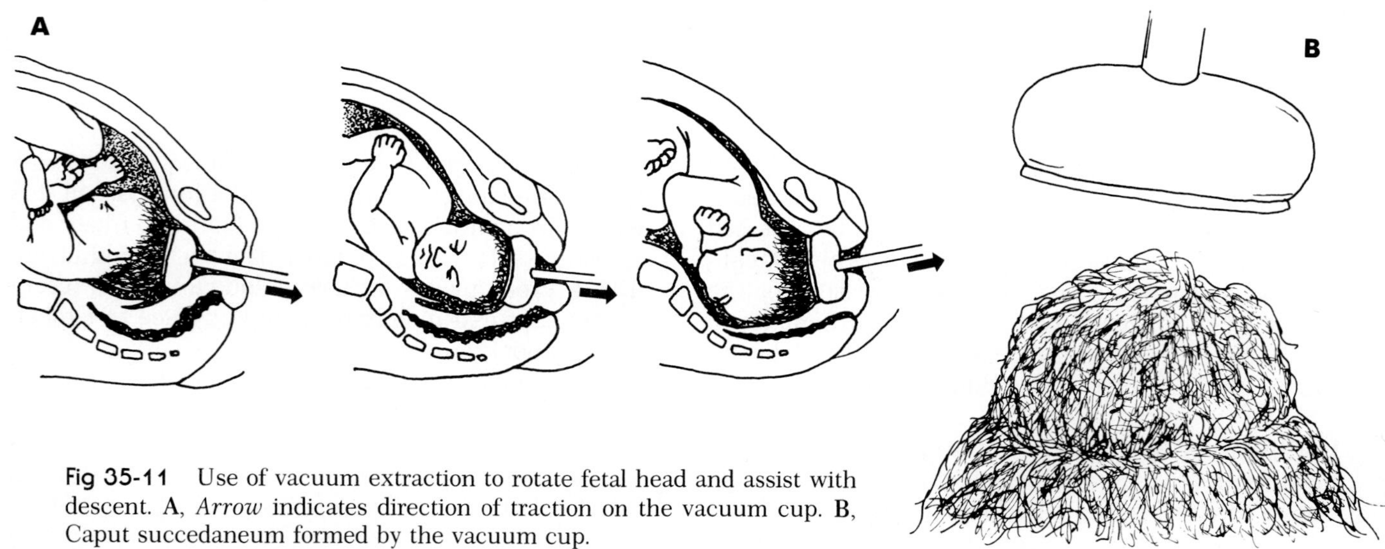

Fig 35-11 Use of vacuum extraction to rotate fetal head and assist with descent. **A**, *Arrow* indicates direction of traction on the vacuum cup. **B**, Caput succedaneum formed by the vacuum cup.

The basic purpose or use of cesarean birth is to preserve the life or health of the mother and her fetus. The use of cesarean birth is based on evidence of maternal or fetal stress. Maternal and fetal morbidity and mortality have decreased since the advent of modern surgical methods and care. However, cesarean birth still poses threats to the health of both mother and infant. The technique of cesarean surgery has changed. Today incisions into the lower uterine segment rather than into the muscular body of the uterus permit a more effective healing.

The incidence of cesarean births has increased dramatically in the last 25 years. From the mid-1960s to the late 1980s, the cesarean birth rate has increased from less than 5% to more than 24% (Graves, 1990), or about one fourth, of all births. Reasons cited for this increase include increased use of electronic fetal monitoring, an increase in the number of first-time pregnancies, as well as pregnancy at an older age, and the high incidence of repeat cesarean births (Martel et al, 1987; Silver, Wolfe, 1989; Dunn, 1990). There are institutional differences in primary cesarean birth rates (see Research Highlight below).

INDICATIONS. There are few absolute indications for cesarean birth. Today most are performed primarily for the benefit of the fetus. Four diagnostic categories are responsible for 75% to 90% of the cesarean births: dystocia, repeat cesarean, breech presentation, and fetal distress (Marieskind, 1989). Other indications for the procedure include active herpes viral infection, prolapsed umbilical cord, medical complications such as pregnancy-induced hypertension, placental abnormalities such as placenta previa and premature separation (abruption), malpresentations such as shoulder presentation, and fetal anomalies such as hydrocephaly.

SURGICAL TECHNIQUES. The two main types of cesarean operation are *classic* and *lower segment* cesarean births. Classic cesarean birth rarely is performed today. It may be used when rapid birth is necessary and in some cases of shoulder presentation and placenta previa. The incision is vertical into the upper body of the uterus (Fig. 35-12, *A*). The procedure is associated with a higher incidence of blood loss, infection, and uterine rupture in subsequent pregnancies than is lower segment cesarean birth.

Lower segment cesarean birth can be performed through a vertical (Sellheim) or transverse (Kerr) incision (Fig. 35-12, *B* and *C*). The transverse incision

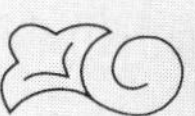 **Research Highlight** 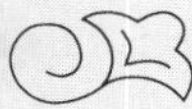

Institutional Differences in Primary Cesarean Birth Rates

RESEARCH ABSTRACT

The purpose of this study was to determine if there were differences in primary cesarean birth rates in a maternity center staffed by certified nurse-midwives who had physician back-up, as compared with a university teaching hospital staffed by resident and attending physicians. The sample included 796 women who received care in a maternity center and 804 women who received care in the university teaching hospital, all in 1977 and 1978. Demographic data (such as age and education) were similar for both groups. Data, taken from medical records, included information from the first prenatal visit to discharge after the birth. The researchers found a significantly lower primary cesarean birth rate at the maternity center. Contracted pelvis, fetal malpresentation, and placental bleeding were associated with cesarean birth at both institutions. At the university hospital, cesarean birth also was associated wth preeclampsia, fetal distress, primiparity, and maternal age. Fetal outcome did not differ between the two institutions except that more infants born at the university hospital had low Apgar scores.

IMPLICATIONS FOR PRACTICE

Different styles of managing labor and birth had significant differences on primary cesarean rates. Consumers should be aware that cesarean birth rates may differ depending on the setting. Health care providers need to examine their own management styles to see if appropriate, safe changes can be made.

RELATED RESEARCH QUESTIONS

1. What are factors associated with lower cesarean birth rates in a birthing center?
2. Does use of electronic fetal monitoring increase the cesarean birth rate?
3. Does a woman's motivation to avoid a cesarean birth affect the likelihood of her having one?
4. Is the cesarean birth rate associated with the years of experience of the physician?

REFERENCE

Garuffi G, Strobino DM, Paine LL: Investigation of institutional differences in primary cesarean birth rates, *J Nurse Midwife* 35:274, Sept/Oct 1990.

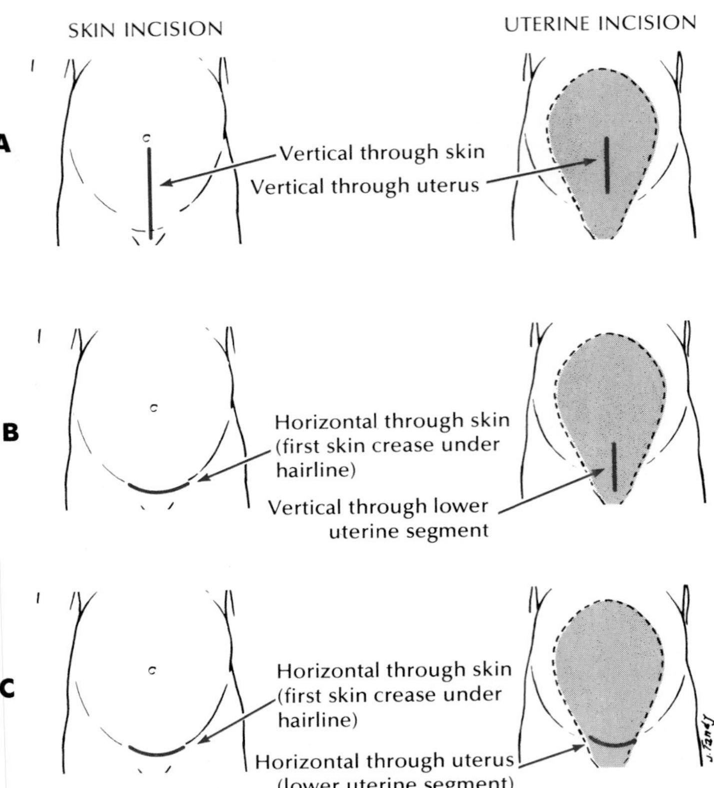

Fig. 35-12 Cesarean birth: skin and uterine incisions. **A,** Classic: vertical incisions of skin and uterus. **B,** Low cervical: horizontal incision of skin; vertical incision of uterus. **C,** Low cervical: horizontal incisions of skin and uterus.

is more popular because it is easier to perform, is associated with less blood loss and fewer postoperative infections, and is less likely to rupture in subsequent pregnancies (Cunningham et al, 1989; Dunn, 1990). Vaginal birth after cesarean is contraindicated with classic incisions.

COMPLICATIONS/RISKS. Cesarean births are not without complications, both for the mother and fetus. Maternal complications occur in 25% to 50% of births and include aspiration, pulmonary embolism, wound infection, wound dehiscence, thrombophlebitis, hemorrhage, urinary tract infection, injuries to bladder or bowel, and complications related to anesthesia. There also is a risk that the fetus will be born prematurely if gestational age is not accurately assessed and that fetal injuries can occur during the surgery (Dunn, 1990). In addition, the woman is at economic risk because the cost of cesarean birth is higher than that of vaginal birth and a longer recovery period may require additional expenditures.

Many women who experience a cesarean birth speak of the feelings that interfere with their maintaining an adequate self-concept. These feelings include fear, disappointment, frustration at losing control, anger (the "why me" syndrome), and loss of self-esteem related to a change in body image. Success in mothering activities and in the recovery process can do much to restore these women's self-esteem. Some women see the scar as mutilating, and worries concerning sexual attractiveness may surface. Some men are fearful of resuming intercourse because of the fear of hurting their mates. Parents will wonder if a cesarean birth was absolutely necessary. Such feelings may surface even years later.

ANESTHESIA. Spinal, epidural, and general anesthetics are used for cesarean births. Since the 1970s, epidural blocks have increased in popularity because women have wanted to be awake for and aware of the birth experience. However, the choice of anesthetic depends on several factors. The mother's medical history or present condition, such as a spinal injury or hemorrhage, may contraindicate the use of regional anesthesia. Time is another factor, especially if there is an emergency and the life of the mother or infant is at stake. Then general anesthetic will most likely be used. The woman herself is a factor. She may not know all the options or have fears about "a needle in her back" or being awake and feeling pain. The woman needs to be fully informed about the risks and benefits of the different types of anesthesia (see Chapter 15) so that she can participate in the decision whenever there is a choice.

ELECTIVE CESAREAN BIRTH. Women face elective (scheduled) cesarean birth when labor is contraindicated (e.g., placenta previa) or when birth is necessary but labor is not inducible (e.g., hypertensive states that cause a poor intrauterine environment that threatens the fetus). These women share with other first-time surgical clients the same apprehensions concerning surgery. These anxieties are coupled with the uncertainty of being able to cope with child care after a major operation.

Women electing to have repeat cesarean birth have time for psychologic preparation. The psychologic response of these women may differ. Some may have disturbing memories of the conditions preceding the initial surgical birth and their experiences in the postoperative recovery period. They may face the added burden of care of an infant while recovering from a surgical operation with great concern. Other women elect the repeat cesarean birth because they can exert more *control* over events than if a trial of labor fails and an unplanned cesarean birth is necessary.

EMERGENCY CESAREAN BIRTH. Women having emergency cesarean births share with their families abrupt changes in their expectations for birth, postbirth care, and the care of the new baby at home. This may be an extremely traumatic experience. The woman usually approaches surgery tired and discouraged after a fruitless labor. She is worried about her own and the infant's condition. She may be dehydrated, with low glycogen reserves. All preoperative procedures must be done quickly and competently. The time for explanation of procedures and of operation is short. Because maternal and family anxiety levels are high, much of what is said is forgotten or perhaps misconstrued. After surgery, time must be spent reviewing the events preceding the operation and the operation itself to ensure that the woman understands what has happened. Fatigue is often noticeable in these women. They need much supportive care.

PRENATAL PREPARATION. Concerned professional and lay groups in the community have established councils for cesarean birth to meet the needs of these women and their families. Such groups advocate the inclusion of preparation for cesarean birth in all parenthood preparation classes. No woman can be guaranteed a vaginal birth, even if she is in good health and there is no indication of danger to the fetus before the onset of labor. Every woman needs to be aware of and prepared for this eventuality. The unknown and unexpected are ego weakening.

Childbirth educators stress the importance of emphasizing the similarities as well as differences between cesarean and vaginal birth. Also, in support of the philosophy of family-centered birth, many hospitals have policies that permit fathers to share in these births as they have in vaginal ones. Women undergoing cesarean birth agree that the continued presence and support of their partners have helped them respond positively to the entire experience (Fawcett, Henklein, 1987).

CARE DURING CESAREAN BIRTH. The goal for the woman and her family is family-centered care for a cesarean birth. The *preparation* of the woman for cesarean birth is the same for either elective or emergency surgery. The obstetrician discusses the need for the cesarean birth and the prognosis for mother and infant with the woman and her family. The anesthesiologist assesses the woman's cardiopulmonary system and presents the options for anesthesia. Informed consent is obtained for the procedure.

Maternal vital signs and blood pressure and FHR continue to be assessed per hospital routine until the operation begins. Physical preoperative preparation usually includes an abdominal-mons shave or clipping of pubic hair (Gallup, 1988), inserting a retention catheter to keep the bladder empty, and administration of prescribed preoperative medications. An antacid often is prescribed to prevent aspiration of gastric secretions into the client's lungs. Intravenous fluids will be started to maintain hydration and to provide an open line for administration of blood or medications if needed. Prophylactic antibiotics may be ordered to reduce the incidence of endometritis (Duff, 1988). Blood and urine samples are collected and sent to the laboratory for analysis. Laboratory tests, usually ordered to establish baseline data, include a complete blood cell count and chemistry, type and cross-matching, and urinalysis.

Dentures and nail polish are removed, but removal of jewelry may be optional depending on hospital policies. If the client wears glasses and is going to be awake, the nurse should make sure her glasses accompany the client to the operating room so she can see her infant. If the client wears contact lenses, the nurse can find out whether they can be worn for the birth.

During preoperative preparation the support person is encouraged to remain with the woman as much as possible to provide continuing emotional support (Shearer et al, 1988). During the preoperative preparation the nurse provides essential information about the procedures. Although the nursing actions may be carried out quickly when the cesarean birth is unplanned, verbal communication, particularly explanations, is important. Silence can be frightening to the woman and her support person. The nurse's use of touch can communicate feelings of care and concern for the client.

The nurse can assess the woman's and her partner's perceptions about the cesarean birth. As the woman expresses her feelings, the nurse may identify potential for disturbance in self-concept during the postpartum period.

If there is time before the birth, the nurse can teach the woman about postoperative expectations, pain relief, turning, coughing, and deep breathing.

Once the woman has been taken to surgery her care becomes the responsibility of the obstetric team, surgeon, anesthesiologist, pediatrician, and surgical nursing staff (Fig. 35-13). If possible, the father, gowned appropriately, accompanies the mother to the surgical unit and remains close to her so that he can continue to provide support and comfort.

The nurse who is circulating may assist with positioning the woman on the birth (surgical) table. It is important to position her so that the uterus is displaced laterally to avoid compressing the inferior vena cava, which causes decreased placental perfusion (Bowes, 1989).

A

B

C

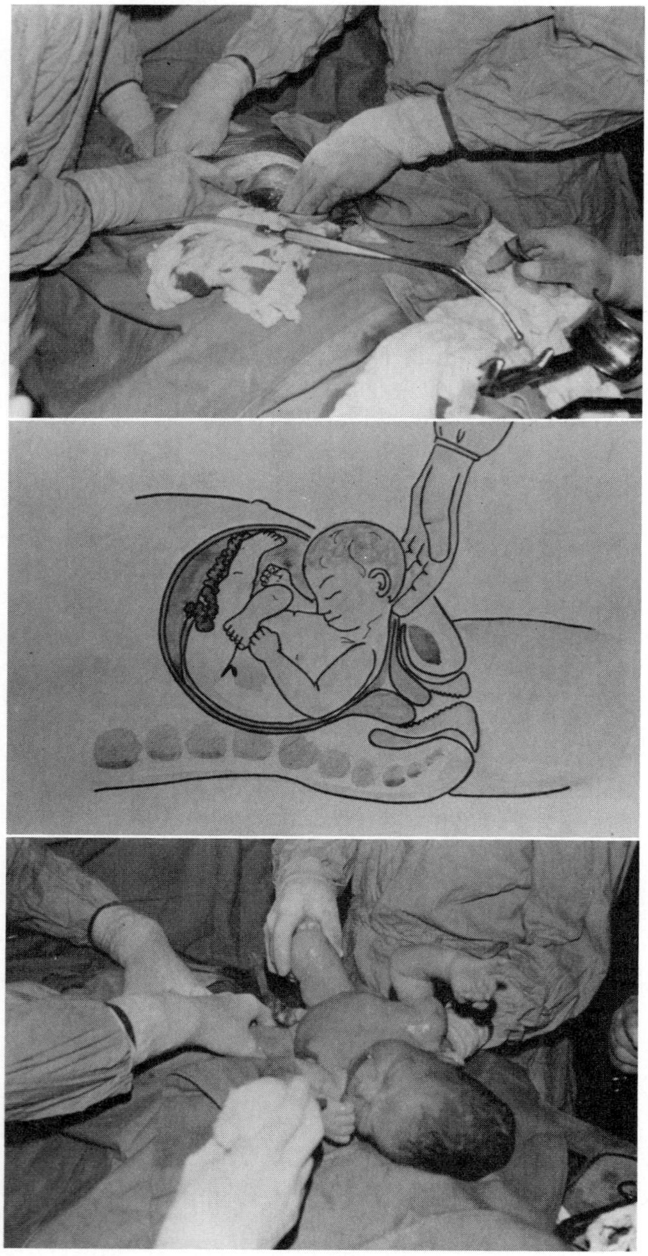

Fig. 35-13 Cesarean birth. **A,** "Bikini" incision has been made, the muscle layer is separated, the abdomen entered, the uterus has been exposed and incised; suctioning of amniotic fluid continues as head is brought up through the incision. Note small amount of bleeding. **B,** Graphic representation of head being brought up through the uterine incision. **C,** A quick assessment while neonate's mouth and nares are suctioned with bulb syringe; note extreme molding of head resulting from cephalopelvic disproportion.
Courtesy Marjorie Pyle, RNC, Lifecircle, Costa Mesa, Calif.; B illustrated by Pam Mizell RN.

If the father is not allowed or chooses not to be present, the nurse can stay in communication with him and give progress reports when possible. If the mother is awake during the birth, the nurse can tell her what is happening and provide support. The mother may be anxious about the sensations she is experiencing, such as cold solutions used to prepare the abdomen and pressure or pulling during the actual birth of the infant. She also may be apprehensive because of the bright lights, unfamiliar equipment present, and masked and gowned personnel in the room.

Care of the infant is delegated to a pediatrician and a nurse who is skilled in neonatal resuscitation, because these infants are considered to be at risk until there is evidence of physiologic stability after the birth.

A crib with resuscitative equipment is readied before surgery. Those responsible for care are expert in resuscitative techniques, as well as in observational skills for detecting normal infant responses. After birth, if the infant's condition permits, the baby can be given to the father to hold. If the mother is awake, she can see and touch the baby (Fig. 35-14). The bonding attachment processes can continue uninterrupted. The infant whose condition is compromised is transported immediately to the nursery for observation and appropriate interventions. In some institutions the father may accompany the infant; if not, personnel keep the family informed of the infant's progress, and parent-infant contacts are initiated as soon as possible.

If the family-oriented approach is not feasible, the family is directed to the surgical waiting room. The physician reviews with the family members the condition of the mother and child after the birth is completed. Family members may accompany the infant as she or he is transferred to the nursery. This gives the family an opportunity to see and admire the new baby.

POSTPARTUM CARE. The care of the woman after cesarean birth combines surgical and obstetric nursing. Once surgery is completed, the mother is transferred to a recovery room or back to her labor room. Nursing assessments in this immediate postbirth period include degree of recovery from anesthesia effects, postoperative and postbirth status, and degree of pain. A patent airway is maintained, and the woman is positioned to prevent possible aspiration. Vital signs are taken every 15 minutes for 1 to 2 hours, or until stable. The condition of the incisional dressing, the fundus, and the amount of lochia are assessed, as well as intake and output. The woman will be helped to turn and do deep breathing and leg exercises. Medications for pain may be administered.

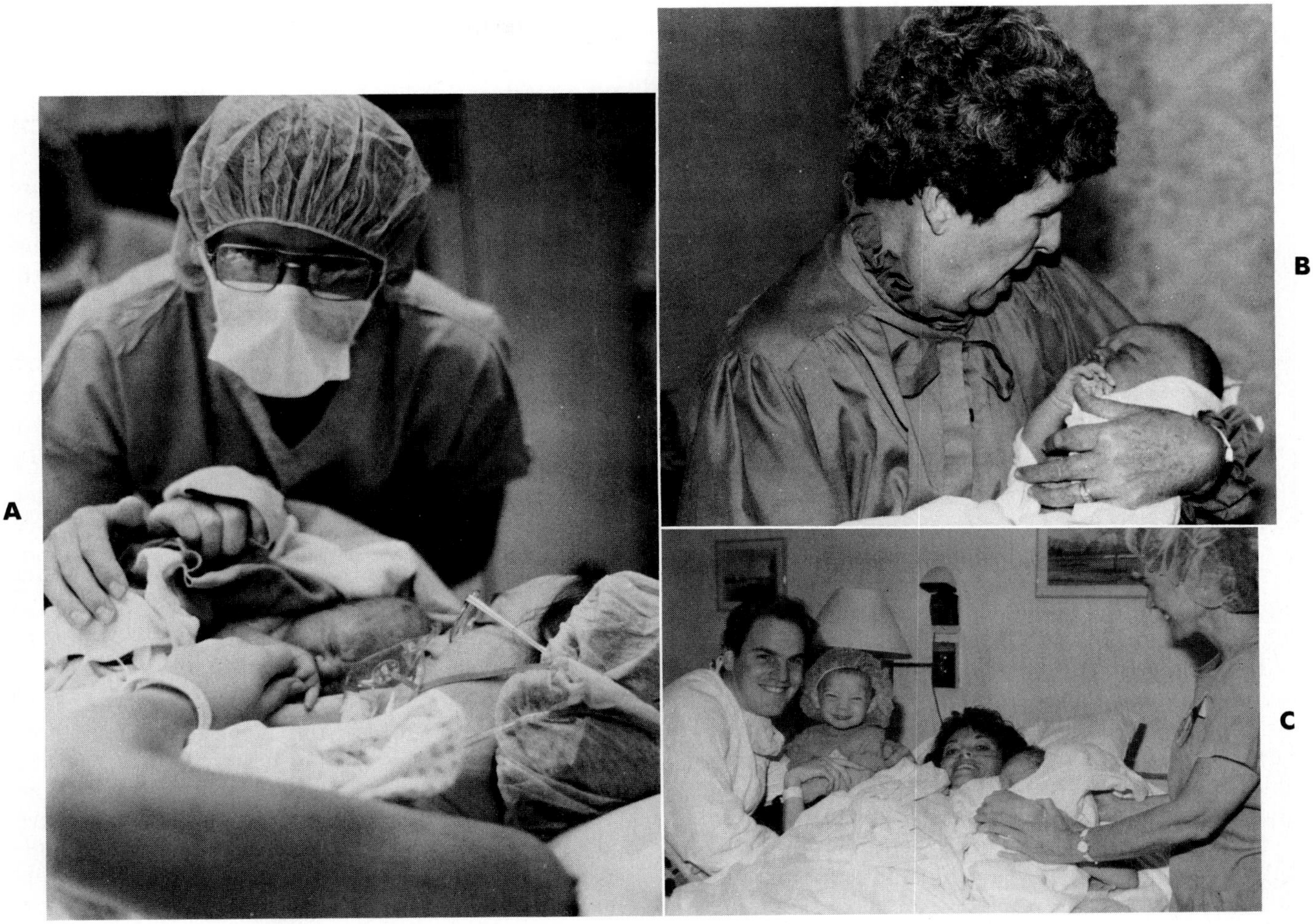

A

B

C

Fig. 35-14 **A,** Parents and their newborn. Physician is manually removing placenta and suctioning remaining amniotic fluid and blood from uterine cavity and closing uterine incision, peritoneum, muscle layer, fatty tissue, and finally the skin, while new family is sharing some private time. **B,** Grandmother begins bonding and attachment as mother's postsurgery recovery begins. **C,** Older siblings are reassured by a visit with mother after surgery; this provides the older sibling an introduction to the new member of the family while being held in the security of his father's arms.
A and B courtesy Barbara Kalmen, Edwards Air Force Base, Calif.; C courtesy Marjorie Pyle, RNC, Lifecircle, Costa Mesa, Calif.

If the baby is present, the mother and father are given some time alone to facilitate bonding and attachment with the infant. Breast-feeding can be initiated if the mother feels like trying. The woman usually is transferred to the postpartum unit after 1 to 2 hours, or when her condition is stable.

The attitude of the nurse and other health team members can influence the woman's perception of herself after a cesarean birth. The caregivers should stress that the woman is a new mother first and a surgical client second. This attitude will help the woman perceive herself as having the same problems and needs as other new mothers.

Physiologic concerns the first few days may be dominated by pain at the incision site and from intestinal gas and the need for pain relief. Pain medications usually are ordered every 3 to 4 hours, but patient-controlled analgesia (PCA) or epidural narcotics may be ordered instead. Other comfort measures such as position changes, splinting the incision with pillows, heat to the abdomen, and relaxation techniques may be implemented. Ambulation and avoid-

TEACHING Postpartum Pain Relief after Cesarean Birth

Incisional

Splint incision with a pillow when moving or coughing.
Use relaxation techniques such as music, breathing, and dim lights.
Apply a heating pad to the abdomen.

Gas

Walk as often as you can.
Do not eat or drink gas-forming foods, carbonated beverages, or whole milk.
Do not use straws for drinking fluids.
Lie on your left side to expel gas.

ing gas-forming foods and carbonated beverages may relieve gas pains. (See teaching box above.)

Daily care includes perineal care, breast care, and routine hygienic care, including showering after the dressing has been removed. During each shift the nurses assesses vital signs, incision, fundus, and lochia. Breath sounds, bowel sounds, Homans' sign, and urinary and bowel elimination also are assessed.

During the postpartum period the nurse can provide care that meets psychologic and teaching needs of mothers who have had cesarean births. The nurse can explain postpartum procedures to help the woman cooperate in her recovery from surgery. The nurse also can help the woman plan care and visits from family and friends that will provide adequate rest periods. Information and assistance with infant care can facilitate adjustment to the mothering role. The father can be included in infant teaching sessions, as well as explanations about the woman's recovery. The couple should be encouraged to express their feelings about the birth experience. Some parents are angry, frustrated, or disappointed about not having a vaginal birth. Some women express feelings of low self-esteem or negative self-image. It may be helpful to have the nurse who was present during the birth visit and help fill in "gaps" about the experience.

Discharge teaching includes information about diet, exercise and activity restrictions, breast care, sexual activity and contraception, medications, signs of complications (see teaching box, above right), and infant care. The nurse assesses the need for continued support or counseling to facilitate the mother's emotional recovery from the birth. Referral to support groups or to community agencies may be indicated.

TEACHING Signs of Postoperative Complications after Discharge

Report the following signs to your doctor:
- Fever greater than 100.4° F (38° C)
- Painful urination
- Lochia heavier than a normal period
- Wound separation
- Redness or oozing at the incision site
- Severe abdominal pain

VAGINAL BIRTH AFTER CESAREAN. The incidence of primary cesarean birth is 17.4% (National Center for Health Statistics, 1989). Indications for primary cesarean birth, such as dystocia, breech presentation, or fetal distress, often are nonrecurring. Therefore a woman who has had a cesarean birth may subsequently become pregnant and not have any contraindications to labor and vaginal birth.

The continued practice of "once a cesarean, always a cesarean" no longer is recommended by most obstetricians. A trial of labor and **vaginal birth after cesarean (VBAC)** are now recommended as routine procedures by ACOG (1988b) for women who have had one previous cesarean birth by low transverse incision. Studies have shown that such vaginal birth is relatively safe (Lavin et al, 1982), with only a 0.5% risk of uterine rupture through a lower uterine segment scar (Knuppel, Drukker, 1986). Labor and vaginal birth are not recommended if contraindications, such as a previous fundal classic cesarean scar or evidence of cephalopelvic disproportion, are present.

According to Scott et al (1990), 60% to 75% of women can give birth vaginally after a trial of labor (p. 1055), which is recommended for women who meet the requirements for VBAC. During the antepartal period, the woman should be given information about VBAC and encouraged to choose it as an alternative to repeat cesarean if no contraindications occur. VBAC support groups and prenatal classes can help prepare the woman psychologically for labor and vaginal birth.

This labor should occur in a hospital facility that has the equipment and personnel available within 30 minutes from the time a decision is made for cesarean birth to the beginning of the procedure. Ideally, the woman is admitted to the labor and birth unit at the onset of spontaneous labor. In the latent phase of labor, the nurse encourages normal activities such as ambulation. In the active phase of labor, FHR and uterine activity usually are monitored electronically and intravenous access such as a heparin lock may be established. Collaboration among the woman in labor, the nurse, and the physician often results in a successful VBAC (Fig. 35-15).

There is no evidence that administering oxytocin to induce or augment labor or the use of epidural anesthesia is contraindicated, although some physicians may not elect these procedures (Flamm et al, 1987, 1988).

Attention should be given to the woman's psychologic, as well as physical, needs during the trial of labor. Anxiety can inhibit release of oxytocin, delaying labor progress and leading to failure and repeat cesarean birth. The nurse can encourage the woman to use breathing and relaxation techniques and to change position to promote labor progress. The husband or support person can be encouraged to provide comfort measures and emotional support. If a trial of labor fails, the woman will need support, as well as encouragement to express her feelings about once again not achieving her desired outcome.

EVALUATION

To evaluate the effectiveness of nursing care for a woman experiencing dystocia, the nurse reviews the goals and expected outcomes that were met and assesses the woman's and the family's level of satisfaction with the care received. Expected outcomes include the following.

- The woman will demonstrate an understanding of the causes and treatment of dysfunctional labor.
- She will express decreased anxiety and fear about her condition and the status of the fetus.
- She will not exhibit signs of complications such as infection, hemorrhage, and fetal distress.
- She will verbalize decreased pain.
- She will state satisfaction with her participation in decision making about care options.
- She will verbalize positive feelings about herself.
- She will give birth to a healthy infant.

See the case study, p. 1068, and plan of care, p. 1069, for a woman experiencing dystocia.

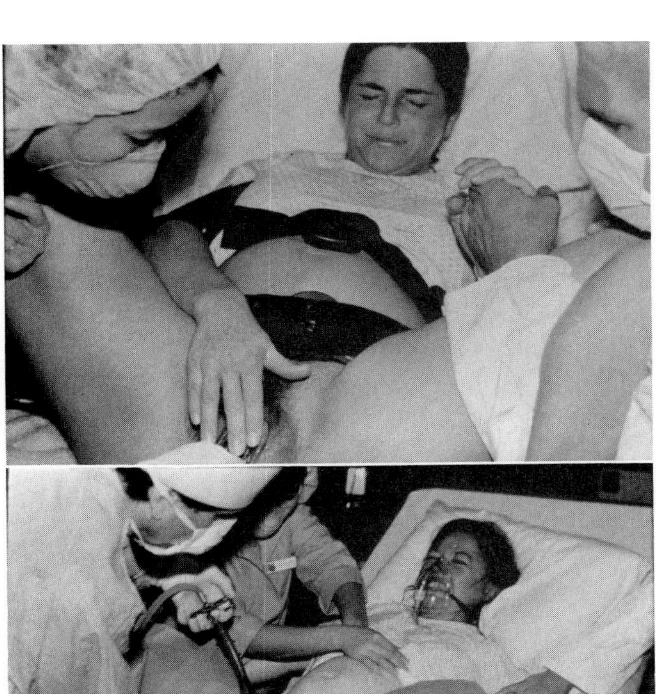

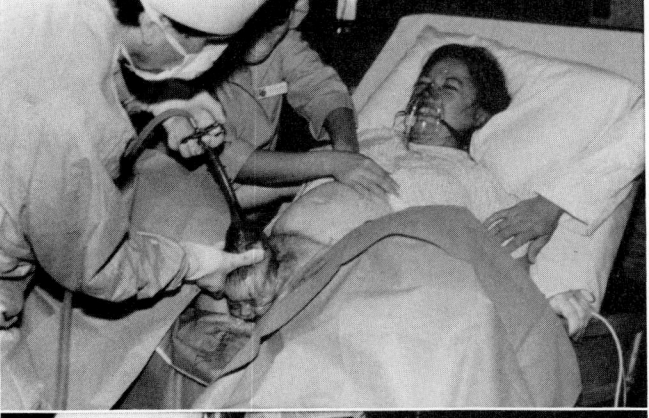

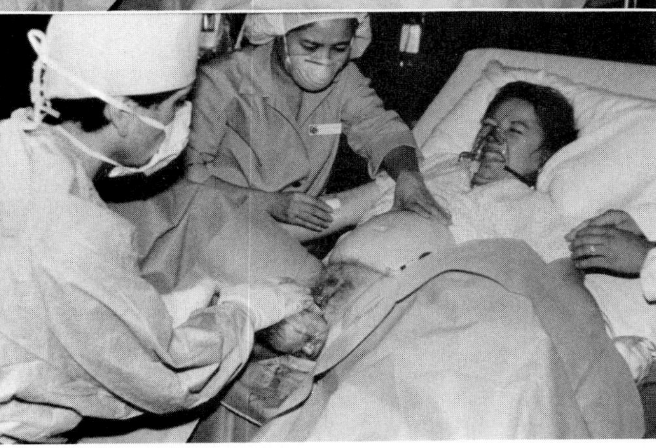

Fig. 35-15 **A**, Electronic monitors remain in place as mother bears down during second stage of labor; her hand on the emerging head provides encouragement. **B**, Physician assisting birth with vacuum extractor. Note scar from previous cesarean birth. **C**, Mother continues to receive oxygen until complete birth of baby.
Courtesy Marjorie Pyle, RNC, Lifecircle, Costa Mesa, Calif.

CASE STUDY

Client with Dysfunctional Labor

Maggie Vadis is a married, 21-year-old nullipara at 38 weeks' gestation who has been admitted to the labor unit in active labor. She is accompanied by her husband Tom.

ASSESSMENT

The interview with Maggie reveals that she attended childbirth preparation classes and is planning to use the breathing and relaxation techniques to cope with labor. She states that her "water broke" 4 hours ago and that there was a gush of clear fluid. Maggie's physical examination reveals that her cervix is dilated 5 cm, 90% effaced; the fetus is at station 0; mild uterine contractions are occurring every 4 to 6 minutes and lasting 40 seconds; and FHR is 148 beats/min, with good beat-to-beat variability and accelerations with fetal movements. A review of laboratory findings reveals a hematocrit of 35%; urine is negative for protein, glucose, and ketones.

After 3 hours, assessment of Maggie reveals no change in labor pattern or in cervical dilatation. Maggie is showing signs of fatigue. Augmentation of labor with intravenous oxytocin was prescribed and implemented. After 2 hours of augmentation, Maggie is crying and asking for something for the pain and is no longer using her breathing and relaxation techniques.

NURSING DIAGNOSIS

Because no labor progress has occurred in more than 3 hours, the nurse identifies the *nursing diagnosis:* high risk of maternal injury related to dysfunctional labor.

PLANNING

A plan of care is developed with Maggie and Tom's input. The agreed-on *goal* for Maggie is that her labor pattern will be sufficient to produce cervical dilatation and that birth will be accomplished without maternal complications. *Expected outcomes* set by the nurse include labor progress, as evidenced by progressive cervical dilatation; no signs of infection as evidenced by vital signs within normal limits; and vaginal discharge clear and without foul odor.

IMPLEMENTATION

Nursing actions are based on the nursing diagnosis, the medical orders, and standards for care. Specific interventions will include assessing the uterine contractile pattern manually or electronically, encouraging position changes or ambulation, encouraging Maggie to void every 1 to 2 hours, monitoring for progressive cervical dilatation and effacement, monitoring vital signs, especially temperature, checking odor and color of vaginal discharge, and administering oxytocin as ordered. The nurse also will monitor intake and output and assess for dehydration.

EVALUATION

The expected outcomes were used to evaluate the effectiveness of these interventions. Maggie's vital signs remained within normal limits, and her vaginal discharge was clear and without a foul odor. After receiving oxytocin, Maggie's contractions were 3 minutes apart, lasting 40 seconds and of moderate intensity. Her cervix changed from 5 to 6 cm in 1 hour; however, Maggie had to have a cesarean birth because of fetal distress before she was fully dilated. Both she and her male infant were in satisfactory condition after the birth. On the basis of these findings, the goal set for Maggie was met.

CARE PLAN Client with Dysfunctional Labor

GOALS	IMPLEMENTATION	RATIONALE	EVALUATION
Nursing diagnosis: High risk of maternal injury related to dysfunctional labor			
Labor pattern is sufficient to produce dilatation, and birth is accomplished without maternal complications.	Assess frequency of uterine contractions. Encourage ambulation or position changes. Encourage Maggie to void every 1 to 2 hours. Monitor for progressive cervical dilatation and effacement. Administer oxytocin as ordered. Monitor intake and output. Assess for dehydration.	Early recognition of dysfunctional labor pattern may prevent complications; actions may stimulate uterine activity and normal labor pattern.	Maggie's vital signs remain within normal limits; signs of infection do not develop. Maggie's labor does not progress satisfactorily; her labor is augmented with oxytocin. Although complications do not develop, Maggie gives birth by cesarean because of fetal distress.
Nursing diagnosis: Ineffective coping related to prolonged labor, pain, and fatigue			
Effective coping techniques are identified and used.	Encourage relaxation and position changes. Give factual information about what is happening. Offer comfort measures such as massage and warm blankets. Acknowledge reality of pain.	Relaxation and decreased level of anxiety facilitate positive coping with situation. Providing information and support may enhance coping.	Maggie again tries to use relaxation techniques and states that back massage is somewhat helpful. She continues to complain of pain. Other interventions are needed.
Nursing diagnosis: Anxiety related to lack of progress and feelings of failure and the need for induced labor			
Anxiety is diminished or managed. Maggie verbalizes feelings of vulnerability and participates in the decision-making process.	Give encouragement; keep informed of progress. Provide information about procedures. Encourage verbalization of feelings. Present options in care when possible. Listen to Maggie's comments that may indicate loss of self-esteem.	Reassurance and information can decrease anxiety, enhance understanding; may increase client's feelings of being in control of situation.	Maggie states she understands reason for labor augmentation and feels less anxious.
Nursing diagnosis: Pain related to intensity of uterine contractions			
Maggie's pain will be managed or relieved effectively.	Encourage use of relaxation techniques. Review breathing techniques. Encourage position changes. Provide comfort measures. Provide quiet environment. Administer pain medications as ordered.	Breathing and relaxation techniques, comfort measures, quiet environment, and pain medications may decrease pain or enhance client's coping response to pain.	Maggie states pain is decreased after implementation of comfort measures and analgesia.

Continued.

CARE PLAN Client with Dysfunctional Labor—cont'd

GOALS	IMPLEMENTATION	RATIONALE	EVALUATION
Nursing diagnosis: High risk for fetal injury related to hypoxia			
Fetal distress will not occur or will be managed, and infant will be born safely.	Assess reaction of FHR to contractions, noting decelerations or bradycardia If fetal distress occurs, turn off oxytocin, position Maggie on left side, start oxygen, and notify physician.	Assessment will determine fetal well-being; hypoxia is prevented or managed.	Fetal distress does occur; male infant is born by cesarean birth in satisfactory condition; resuscitation is not needed. Tom and Maggie hold infant in the recovery unit.

PRETERM LABOR AND BIRTH

Preterm birth is that which occurs after week 20 but before the end of the week 37 of gestation. The overall incidence of preterm birth in the United States ranges from 250,000 to 400,000 per year, or approximately 9% (Creasy, Merkatz, 1990). Preterm birth is responsible for almost two thirds of infant deaths; one half of these deaths are associated with infants who weigh 1500 g or less.

The infant born before term does not possess the growth and development necessary for uncomplicated adjustment to extrauterine life. Her or his prospects for survival or good health may be severely compromised. For those who survive, the emotional and financial costs to families and health care systems are phenomenal. The neonatal intensive care cost for one low-birth-weight infant is estimated to be $14,000 to $30,000 but can be as high as $100,000 (Office of Technology Assessment, 1988; Tokos, 1990). The cost for long-term care and special education for preterm infants born with severe physical and neurologic handicaps is estimated to be greater than $100,000.

Etiologic Factors

In approximately two thirds of preterm births, no definite cause can be identified. However, one third of preterm labors occur after premature rupture of membranes (PROM). Other complications of pregnancy that also are associated with preterm labor include multifetal gestation, hydramnios, incompetent cervix, premature separation of the placenta, and certain infections such as polynephritis and chorioamnionitis (Andersen, Merkatz, 1990).

Risk factors for preterm birth are similar to those for preterm birth but may not have a direct etiologic role in preterm labor. Risk factors for low birth-weight infants have been identified and categorized by the Institute of Medicine (1985). These risk factors are useful to health care workers in identifying women who may be at risk for preterm labor (see box, p. 1071).

African-American women are twice as likely as Caucasian women or other noncaucasian women (Hispanic, Native American, Japanese) in the United States to give birth to a low-birth-weight infant. A high risk for preterm labor is common in women who are younger than 20 or older than 34 years of age, unmarried, and of low socioeconomic status and educational level.

Women who have certain medical risks before pregnancy are at greater risk for preterm labor, especially previous preterm birth or previous abortion. Uterine anomalies and specific medical conditions such as hypertension and diabetes mellitus are associated with higher preterm birth rates. Risks associated with the current pregnancy include pregnancy-induced hypertension, placental problems, anemia, and fetal anomalies.

Poor nutrition, smoking more than 10 cigarettes a day, alcohol or substance abuse, or both, and lack of prenatal care are among maternal habits and activities that increase the risk of a preterm birth. The impact of work and stress also may affect the rate of preterm birth, although more study is needed.

Uterine irritability and events that trigger uterine contractions—such as sexual activity, progesterone deficiency, inadequate plasma volume, and certain infections such as chlamydia—may be involved in the onset of preterm labor. However, the impact of these factors is not clearly understood (Main, 1988; Bennett, Botti, 1989; Brustman et al, 1989).

Nursing Process

Obstetric management of preterm birth involves early detection of preterm labor, suppressing uterine activity, and improving intrapartum care of the fetus destined to be born early.

All pregnant women are screened according to risk factors associated with preterm labor at their initial prenatal visit. Many risk-scoring systems have been developed to assist in identifying women who might be at high risk for preterm labor. Women are assessed at 22 to 26 weeks of gestation. Those who are considered at high risk are followed up more closely, for example, on a weekly basis. They receive education in the symptoms of preterm labor (see guidelines in Chapter 13) and instruction in palpation, timing, and reporting of uterine contractions.

Home uterine monitoring with an ambulatory tokodynamometer device (Fig. 35-16) may be implemented to detect excessive uterine contractions before they can be perceived by the woman herself. The woman records uterine activity twice a day; the data are transmitted by telephone to the hospital or to a monitoring service for analysis. Appropriate therapy is instituted if labor is suspected (Hill et al, 1990). Although some studies show that the use of home uterine activity monitoring is associated with lower incidence of preterm birth, others speculate that the decrease is related to more frequent contact with health care providers (Iams et al, 1988; Creasy, Merkatz, 1990; Hill et al, 1990). Continued study is needed.

Risk Factors for Preterm Labor

DEMOGRAPHIC RISKS

Race (African American)
Age (<17, >34 yr)
Low socioeconomic status
Unmarried
Low education level

MEDICAL RISKS

Previous preterm labor or birth
Second-trimester abortion (more than two spontaneous or therapeutic)
Uterine anomalies
Medical diseases (e.g., diabetes, hypertension)
Current pregnancy risks
- Multifetal pregnancy
- Hydramnios
- Poor weight gain
- Placental problems (e.g., placenta previa, abruptio placentae)
- Anemia
- Infections (e.g., pyelonephritis, recurrent UTIs)
- Incompetent cervix
- Spontaneous premature rupture of membranes
- Hyperemesis
- Fetal anomalies

BEHAVIORAL AND ENVIRONMENTAL RISKS

Poor nutrition
Smoking (more than 10 cigarettes a day)
Alcohol and other substance abuse
DES exposure and other toxic exposures
Little or no prenatal care

POTENTIAL RISK FACTORS

Stress
Uterine irritability
Events triggering uterine contractions
Cervical changes before onset of labor
Inadequate plasma volume expansion
Progesterone deficiency
Infections (e.g., mycoplasma, *Chlamydia trachomatis*)

DES, Diethylstilbestrol; *UTIs*, urinary tract infections.

NURSING DIAGNOSES

The common nursing diagnoses for the woman with preterm labor include the following:
- Knowledge deficit related to
  —Recognition of preterm labor and/or management of preterm labor
- High risk for maternal or fetal injury related to
  —Preterm labor and birth
- Anxiety related to
  —Possible preterm birth
- Impaired physical mobility related to
  —Prescribed bed rest
- Anticipatory grieving related to
  —Potential loss of fetus
- Situational low self-esteem related to
  —Inability to carry pregnancy to term

PLANNING

The nurse develops a plan of care based on whether the woman's care is managed at home or in the hospital. Common *goals* (expected outcomes) include those that follow.

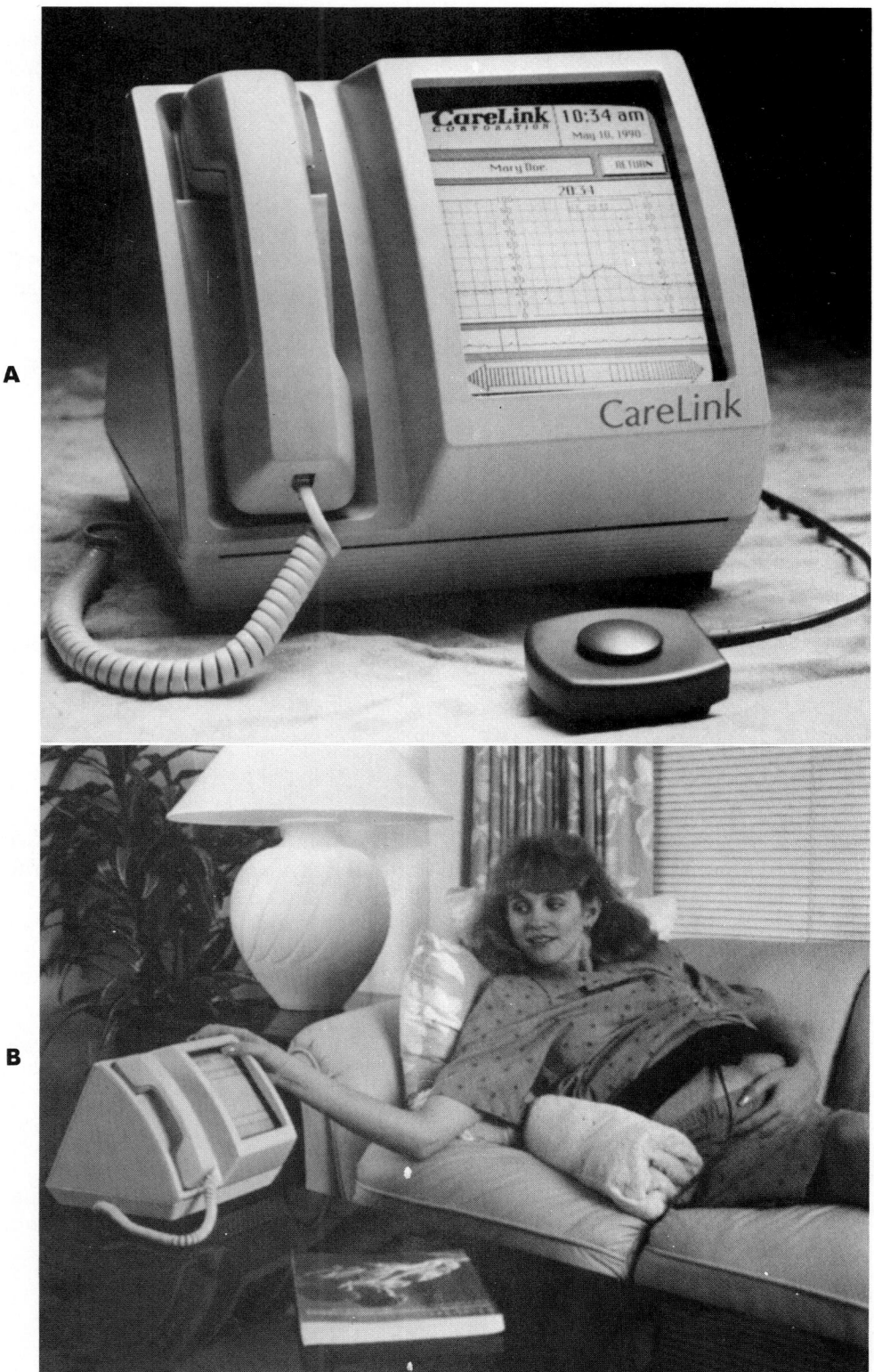

Fig. 35-16 Home uterine activity monitoring. A, Recording unit and transmitter. B, Tokodynamometer in place at center of abdomen below umbilicus.
Courtesy Carelink Home Perinatal Services.

- The woman will demonstrate compliance with prescribed activity limitations or medication schedules, or both.
- She will not experience complications from prescribed drug management.
- She will carry pregnancy to term or near term.
- She will give birth to a healthy mature infant.

IMPLEMENTATION

Pregnant women should be taught to notify the physician or midwife if they have symptoms of preterm labor, particularly uterine contractions occurring more frequently than every 10 minutes (see Research Highlight below). If the woman is active, it may be helpful if she lies on her left side and drinks fluids to increase blood flow to the uterus, to correct myometrial hypoxia, and to decrease uterine activity. If the woman continues to have uterine contractions after 1 hour of implementing these interventions, she usually is instructed to come to the office or hospital for further evaluation. The woman is placed on her left side, and an external fetal and uterine monitor is applied to assess uterine activity and FHR. An intravenous fluid may be started to provide additional hydration. A sterile speculum examination usually is performed to obtain cervical and/or vaginal cultures

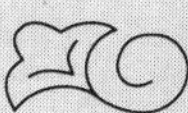 **Research Highlight** 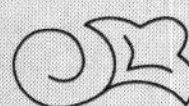

Home Uterine Monitoring to Prevent Preterm Birth

RESEARCH ABSTRACT

The purpose of this study was to assess the effectiveness of an educational program to prevent preterm birth and to determine if adding home uterine monitoring would improve results. Before 28 weeks of gestation, 251 women, identified with risk factors for preterm labor, were randomly assigned to one of two groups: home monitoring group or education-palpation group. Women in both groups transmitted 1-hour monitor tracings to a central location. Only in the home monitoring group, however, were the tracings analyzed and used in client management. All participants were contacted by a nurse for a minimum of 5 days each week.

A group of 143 women with the same preterm risk factors who had given birth in the previous 30 months was selected from the same agency to serve as the standard against which to measure outcomes. Four subjects dropped out of the study. There were 189 twin and 201 singleton gestations among the women. There were no differences in outcomes between the singleton and twin pregnancies. In the singleton gestations the preterm risk factors were similar among groups. The incidence of preterm birth was less in the education-palpation group than in the standard-care group. There was no difference between the education-palpation and the home uterine monitoring groups. More women in the experimental groups than in the standard care group were seen while suppression of preterm labor was possible; therefore neonatal outcome was significantly improved. In the twin gestations there were no demographic differences among groups. The incidence of preterm labor was the same in the three groups, but the incidence of preterm birth was decreased in both experimental groups. Infants in the home-monitoring group had the best neonatal outcome.

IMPLICATIONS FOR PRACTICE

Most women in whom preterm labor develops seek care after rupture of membranes or when the cervix is dilated; thus tocolysis is unsuccessful. Home uterine monitoring is an important adjunct to the treatment of women at risk for preterm labor and aids in its detection while tocolysis is still possible. In this study, participants also had frequent contact with a nurse. With the singleton pregnancies, it was difficult to determine whether the nurse, the home uterine monitoring, or a combination of the two was the effective component. In the twin pregnancies the participants already were receiving frequent nursing contact. Addition of home uterine monitoring improved outcomes. Women at risk for preterm labor must receive education in symptoms of preterm labor and directions about when to seek care.

RELATED RESEARCH QUESTIONS

1. Does home uterine monitoring or frequent nursing contact improve outcome in singleton pregnancies at risk for preterm labor?
2. Does weekly electronic monitoring improve detection of preterm labor?
3. Do women with singleton gestations perceive contractions more accurately than do women with twin gestations?
4. Does teaching pregnant women without known risk factors for preterm labor to palpate contractions weekly reduce the incidence of preterm labor?

REFERENCE

Dyson DC et al: Prevention of preterm birth in high risk patients: the role of education and provider contact versus home uterine monitoring, *Am J Obstet Gynecol* 164:756, 1991.

to detect the presence of an infection such as beta streptococcus. A clean-catch or catheterized urine specimen is obtained and examined for the presence of a urinary tract infection. A cervical examination is performed to assess for dilatation or effacement, or both.

The diagnosis of preterm labor includes both uterine and cervical changes in effacement or dilatation, or both (Andersen, Merkatz, 1990). If uterine activity subsides and dilatation and effacement do not change from the initial examination, the woman may be discharged to home. She may be given instructions regarding limitations of activities (see teaching box at right) and medications for prevention of preterm labor. If labor continues, care will continue in the hospital setting until the woman's condition is stable and she can go home, either on a regimen of restricted activity or medications, or both, to prevent recurrence of preterm labor or until birth.

SUPPRESSION OF UTERINE ACTIVITY. If uterine contractions persist, or if cervical changes occur, tocolytic treatment may be used to stop labor. **Tocolytic agents** are drugs that inhibit uterine contractions. *Toko-* and *toco-* are Greek roots referring to obstetrics; *-lytic* is also Greek and means "to break down" or stop. The agents used include β-adrenergic drugs such as ritodrine or terbutaline and magnesium sulfate (Andersen, Merkatz, 1990).

RITODRINE. *Ritodrine (Yutopar)* was the first, and remains the only, β-sympathomimetic drug approved by the FDA for use in the United States to inhibit preterm labor (Cunningham et al, 1989). Ritodrine acts on type II β-adrenergic receptors, which cause uterine muscle relaxation, vasodilation, bronchodilation, and muscle glycogenolysis. Decrease in serum potassium levels may cause arrhythmias. The initial dose usually is given intravenously, followed by intramuscular or oral therapy, or both, after the client's condition is stabilized. The dose is determined by the physician and the woman's response to the medication.

Contraindications for use include maternal diseases such as cardiovascular disease, severe preeclampsia, severe antepartum hemorrhage, chorioamnionitis, and hyperthyroidism. Fetal death and gestational age of less than 20 weeks confirmed by ultrasound scan are two fetal-related contraindications.

A delay of preterm birth has potential *beneficial effects* for the fetus. In addition, the tocolytic agents available usually are able to delay birth long enough for the use of glucocorticoids to effect fetal pulmonary maturation.

Cardiopulmonary complications are possible. Therefore careful assessment and monitoring are essential. Because of the possible cardiopulmonary effects, an electrocardiogram may be ordered before the treatment. A cardiac monitor for the mother may be indicated to maintain continuous assessment for *tachycardia* and *arrhythmia* (see emergency box below).

TERBUTALINE. *Terbutaline (Brethine)* is another β-adrenergic agent often used for preterm labor. Administration and contraindications are similar to those described for ritodrine, although terbutaline is more frequently given subcutaneously or orally.

Prolonged and continuous high-dose treatment with ritodrine and terbutaline causes desensitization of β-adrenergic receptors; preterm labor usually re-

TEACHING Home Management of Preterm Labor

Remain on bed rest on your left or right side as instructed.
Assess for fetal activity daily.
Monitor for uterine contraction activity daily.
Practice relaxation techniques.
Eat well-balanced meals.
Drink 8 to 10 (8 oz) cups of fluids a day.
Report rupture of membranes, bleeding, signs of labor (menstrual-like cramps, pelvic pressure, low backache, uterine contractions) to your physician or midwife.
Avoid or limit activities that could stimulate labor, as instructed (e.g., sexual intercourse, breast stimulation).
Take medications as prescribed. Report side effects to physician/midwife.
Keep appointments with physician/midwife.

Data from Brustman et al, 1989; Johnson, 1989; Robertson, 1989.

EMERGENCY

Pulmonary Edema Caused by Ritodrine Therapy

SIGNS

Dyspnea
Crackles (rales)

INTERVENTIONS

Discontinue drug immediately.
Start oxygen.
Give diuretics as ordered.
Restrict fluids.

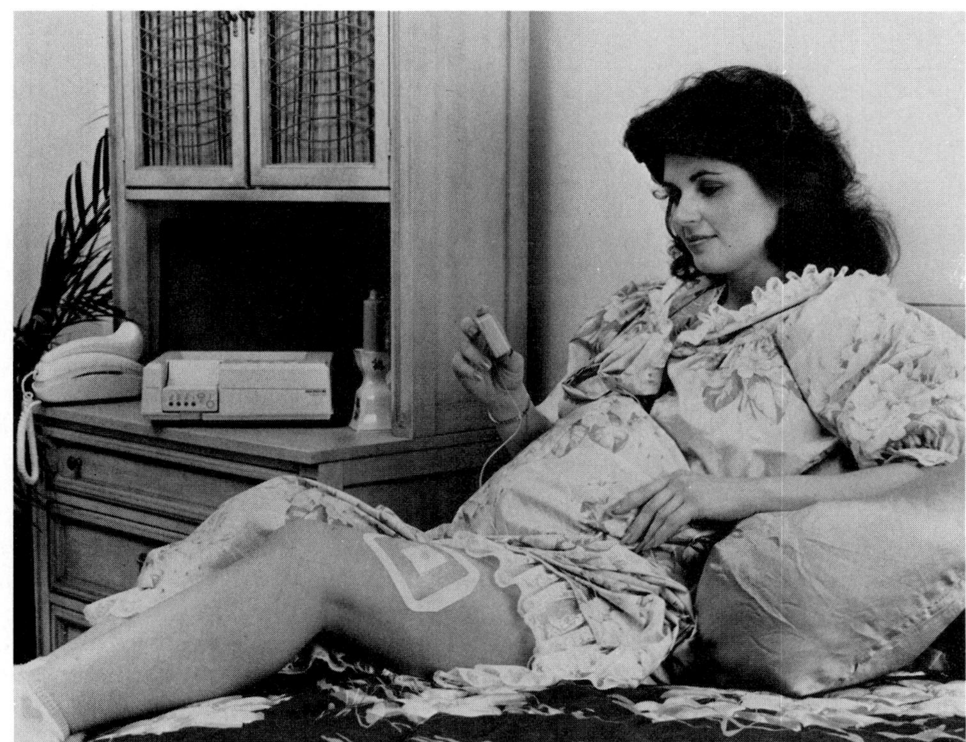

Fig. 35-17 Subcutaneous terbutaline pump attached to client.
Courtesy Healthdyne Perinatal Services, Marietta, Ga.

curs as a result of tocolytic breakthrough. The use of subcutaneous terbutaline by pump infusion for long-term tocolysis has been reported to be effective in preventing this recurrence (Iams et al, 1988). The pump therapy decreases desensitization by delivering a continuous low-dose infusion, with intermittent bolus doses at times when uterine activity is known to occur in the individual client. The average daily dose by pump is 3 to 4 mg terbutaline administered subcutaneously; a daily oral dose is 30 to 60 mg (Gill et al, 1989; Sala, Moise, 1990).

Women who use the terbutaline pump (Fig. 35-17) require instruction in the operation of the pump and self-injection techniques. In addition, they need to know the signs of preterm labor, how to palpate uterine contractions, recognize warning signs and symptoms of terbutaline toxicity (see box, p. 1076), and follow activity precautions. Nursing assessments for women who are at home or in the hospital may include determinations of vital signs, weight gain, lung function, FHR and fetal movement, fundal height, urine checks for glucose, protein, and ketones, cervical examination to detect changes, uterine activity monitoring, gastrointestinal function, deep tendon reflexes and edema, and psychosocial adaptation (Gill et al, 1989). Uterine monitoring and nursing support for preterm labor clients at home are available (see Research Highlight, p. 1077).

Nursing Considerations. Nursing interventions for clients receiving ritodrine or terbutaline depends on whether the drug is administered intravenously, subcutaneously, or orally. Before intravenous therapy, the woman usually receives hydration with 500 mL isotonic crystalloid over 30 minutes. The drug is then administered via pump infusion. The dose is increased in increments as ordered, using the minimum amount of the drug that will stop uterine contractions. After 12 to 24 hours of successful therapy, oral therapy usually is instituted (ACOG, 1989a).

During intravenous therapy, the nurse monitors uterine activity and FHR continuously. FHR should not exceed 180 beats/min. Maternal vital signs, including blood pressure, are assessed per protocol; pulse should not exceed 140 beats/min. Breath sounds are assessed and lungs auscultated every 8 to 12 hours. The nurse assesses the client for other signs of drug side effects, such as fluid overload, pulmonary edema, and cardiac arrhythmias. If any are noted, the medication is stopped and the physician/midwife is notified. An *antidote,* a beta-blocking agent such as *propranolol (Inderal),* may be prescribed. The maximum intravenous fluid rate is 125

Warning Signs—Side Effects of Terbutaline

MATERNAL
Central Nervous System

Severe dizziness, drowsiness, headache, nervousness, restlessness

Blood Pressure

Severe hypertension

Heart Rate

Continuous palpitations, chest pain, tachycardia ≥140 beats/min

Musculoskeletal

Severe muscle cramps and weakness

Gastrointestinal

Continuous nausea and vomiting

Respiratory

Pulmonary edema

Metabolic

Hyperglycemia, hypokalemia

FETAL
Tachycardia

≥180 beats/min

mL/hr. Blood samples may be drawn for laboratory analysis of glucose and potassium levels to detect hypokalemia or hyperglycemia. The client is maintained on bed rest in a side-lying position to optimize placental perfusion and to decrease pressure on the cervix. Intake and output and daily weights are monitored to detect overhydration. The woman should be told about the potential side effects to prevent undue stress if they occur (Caritis et al, 1988).

If the woman is on an oral or a subcutaneous therapy regimen, maternal vital signs and FHR, fetal activity, and uterine activity are assessed per hospital routine or as ordered. Medications need to be given on time every 4 to 6 hours to prevent recurrence of uterine activity.

MAGNESIUM SULFATE. *Magnesium sulfate* is known to decrease uterine activity. It is being used as a tocolytic agent because it is safer for the woman than ritodrine. It usually is given intravenously, but intramuscular and oral routes may be used (Andersen, Merkatz, 1990). However, if administered orally, magnesium oxide or gluconate is used; the main side effect is diarrhea (Caritis et al, 1988; Creasy, 1989).

For intravenous therapy, the woman usually receives hydration with 500 mL isotonic crystalloid over a 30-minute period preceding therapy. Magnesium sulfate is mixed with normal saline, and a 4-g dose is infused over a 20-minute period. The drug is then infused via a pump at 1 to 2 g/hr and increased per protocol (usually 0.5 g/hr every 15 to 30 minutes) until contractions stop. After 12 hours of successful therapy, oral tocolytic therapy is started. Intravenous therapy with magnesium sulfate usually has been used for tocolysis for brief periods (less than 3 days), but long-term tocolysis (more than 10 days) has been reported. Research findings suggest that magnesium sulfate can be given safely as long as clinically indicated for preterm labor (Dudley et al, 1989).

NURSING CONSIDERATIONS. Nursing assessments during intravenous administration of magnesium sulfate therapy include monitoring blood pressure, pulse, and respiratory rates; checking deep tendon reflexes; measuring intake and output; assessing level of consciousness; and checking laboratory results for therapeutic levels of magnesium (4-8g/dL) and calcium levels for hypocalcemia. Calcium gluconate should be available to reverse serious side effects. (For further discussion of magnesium sulfate, see Chapter 28.) Uterine activity and FHR also are monitored.

OTHER DRUGS. Other drugs that are being investigated for treatment of preterm labor include prostaglandin antagonists (indomethacin, nonsteroidal inflammatory agents [naproxen], and salicylates) and calcium channel blockers (nifedipine). Although these drugs are effective in relaxing the uterus, concern about potential effects on the fetus and bleeding have limited their use (Brown, 1989; Creasy, 1989).

PROMOTION OF FETAL LUNG MATURITY. Respiratory distress syndrome (RDS) is common in small preterm infants who have fetal lung immaturity (for further discussion, see Chapter 37). The incidence and severity of RDS has been found to be reduced if glucocorticoids (e.g., betamethasone) are administered to the mother at least 24 to 48 hours before the birth.* The fetus must be at less than 34 weeks of gestation. The administration must be made at least 24 hours before birth and no longer than 7 days before birth. Neither the use of tocolytics nor steroidal therapy is universally recommended for preterm labor after premature rupture of membranes (Andersen, Merkatz, 1990).

---

*ALERT: The woman who has received tocolytics, as well as glucocorticoids to stimulate fetal lung maturity, is at risk for cardiac decompensation. Therefore the nurse must be vigilant in monitoring the woman for signs of cardiac decompensation (see signs, p. 963).

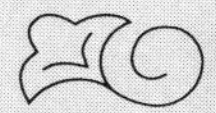 **Research Highlight** 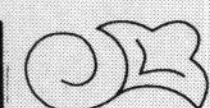

Uterine Monitoring and Nursing Support for Preterm Labor Clients at Home

RESEARCH ABSTRACT

The management of preterm labor clients at home with daily uterine monitoring and daily nursing support was compared with standard care in achieving term birth. Sixty-seven clients who had been treated successfully in a hospital were randomly assigned to one of two groups: daily home monitoring and nursing support or standard care. Both groups of clients received instruction on palpation of contractions and signs and symptoms of preterm labor.

Clients in the monitoring/nursing group used an ambulatory tokodynamometer for 1 hour each morning and evening. A nurse telephoned them each day to assess signs and symptoms of preterm labor. If increased uterine activity was detected, the clients were instructed to void, increase their oral fluid intake, and monitor uterine activity for 1 hour while resting. Increases in uterine activity were treated with tocolysis at home.

Clients in the standard care group contacted their physician if they noted preterm labor symptoms or noted four or more contractions that did not diminish with oral hydration and rest for 1 hour. They received tocolysis as necessary.

Preterm labor recurred in 15 (45%) of the monitoring/nursing group and in 19 (56%) of the standard care group. This difference was not statistically significant. No one in the monitoring/nursing groups—but six (32%) in the standard care group—gave birth at the first recurrence of preterm labor. This resulted in a significant difference in the rate of preterm birth: seven (46%) in the monitoring/nursing group and 16 (84%) in the standard care group. Home uterine monitoring and nursing support were effective in reducing the incidence of preterm birth.

IMPLICATIONS FOR PRACTICE

Home uterine monitoring is becoming increasingly common for clients experiencing preterm labor. Nurses will care for these clients in in-hospital settings until uterine contractility is reduced. They will be responsible for preparing clients for home monitoring. This preparation includes signs and symptoms of preterm labor and use of home monitoring equipment. Nurses also will be responsible for home care of these clients. It is important for nurses to be knowledgeable about the technical aspects of such monitoring and also about the psychosocial implications of a diagnosis of preterm labor and the changes in patterns of daily living necessitated by the diagnosis.

RELATED RESEARCH QUESTIONS

1. What is a client's response to home uterine monitoring?
2. What is a family's response to home uterine monitoring?
3. Does ability to follow a home uterine monitoring regimen vary with age, education, socioeconomic status, or parity?
4. What factors distinguish Braxton Hicks contractions from preterm labor contractions?

REFERENCE

Watson DL et al: Management of preterm labor patients at home: does daily uterine activity monitoring and nursing support make a difference? *Obstet Gynecol* 76(suppl 1):32S, 1990.

CARE DURING PRETERM LABOR AND BIRTH. If labor cannot be stopped, the physician or midwife makes every attempt to help the mother give birth to the preterm infant safely and without trauma. During labor, drugs such as narcotics or barbiturates that can depress the fetus are avoided. Epidural analgesia is commonly used during labor, but pudendal block or local anesthetic may be administered for the birth instead. An episiotomy often is performed to shorten the second stage of labor and to reduce excessive pressure on the fragile fetal head. The route of birth is controversial, but cesarean birth may be performed for malpresentation and maternal or fetal distress (Andersen, Merkatz, 1990).

Parental concern for the well-being of the infant is apparent during labor. Parents need to be aware of the interest and support of staff members. However, false assurance of fetal health must be avoided. For some parents the reality of the situation is not appreciated until they see their daughter or son in the intensive care unit. For others who experience fetal or neonatal death, the loss intensifies once the stress of labor and childbirth is over (see Chapter 40).

During the postpartum period physical care of the mother is similar to that required after any vaginal birth. However, the family will be very anxious concerning the health and prognosis of their infant (Sammons and Lewis, 1985). Nursing care of the preterm infant involves not only medical and nursing personnel but also the participation of the parents (see Chapter 37). The nurse must be aware of the impact that preterm birth may have on family dynamics (Richardson, 1987). Parents must accept that the infant has special needs, and they must learn to meet these needs before discharge so that they will have more realistic expectations when they are at home (Weingarten et al, 1990).

EVALUATION

Evaluation of the effectiveness of nursing care for women with preterm labor is based on the goals. Expected outcomes are that the woman verbalizes understanding of her treatment, complies with her prescribed treatment, develops no complications related to drug therapy, and gives birth at or near term to a healthy, mature infant.

POSTTERM LABOR AND BIRTH

Postterm birth is the birth of an infant beyond the end of week 42 of gestation, or 294 days from the first day of the last menstrual period. The incidence of postterm gestation is estimated to be between 3.5% and 15%; only about 4% of pregnancies terminate after 43 weeks (Resnik, 1989; Spellacy, 1990).

Maternal risks are related to the birth of an excessively large infant. The woman is at increased risk for dysfunctional labor, induction of labor, forceps-assisted birth, lacerations related to vaginal birth, and cesarean birth (Boyd et al, 1988; Spellacy, 1990).

Fetal risks appear to be twofold. The first is related to the possibility of birth trauma and asphyxia through fetopelvic disproportion. The second risk is believed to result from the compromising effects on the fetus of an "aging" placenta. Spellacy (1990) notes that placental function decreases after 40 weeks of gestation and amniotic fluid volume declines to approximately 250 to 300 mL. Oligohydramnios is associated with fetal distress related to cord compression. If placental insufficiency is present, there is a high incidence of fetal distress during labor. Neonatal problems may include asphyxia, meconium aspiration syndrome, and respiratory distress. Postterm babies also have increased mortality, increased feeding and sleeping problems, more illness, and low developmental and mental scores (Asher et al, 1988; Beckmann, 1990; Spellacy, 1990).

The management of postterm pregnancy is still controversial. Induction of labor at 42 weeks is suggested by some authorities. Others allow pregnancy to proceed to 43 weeks as long as tests of fetal well-being are performed and results are normal. Antepartum assessments for postterm pregnancy may include daily fetal movement counts (at least 10 in a 12-hour period) and abdominal girth measurements (to detect oligohydramnios). Nonstress and stress tests may be performed at least weekly. The biophysical profile (p. 789) may be the best indication of fetal well-being because it combines nonstress testing with real-time ultrasound scanning to assess fetal movements, fetal breathing movements, and amniotic fluid volume (AFV). Determining the amount of AFV is critical because decreased AFV has been associated with fetal distress in postterm pregnancies (Spellacy, 1990).

Cervical checks are performed weekly after 40 weeks' gestation to assess if the condition of the cervix is favorable for induction (>5 on the Bishop score) (Table 35-3). Amniocentesis or amnioscopy may be performed to detect meconium in the amniotic fluid (Resnik, 1989; Spellacy, 1990) (also see Chapter 27).

TEACHING Postterm Gestation

Perform daily fetal movement counts.
Assess for signs of labor.
Call your physician or midwife if your membranes rupture.
Keep appointments for fetal assessment tests or cervical checks.
Come to the hospital soon after labor begins.

Nursing Considerations

During the postterm period the woman is encouraged to assess fetal activity daily, assess for signs of labor, and to keep appointments with her physician or midwife (see teaching box above). The woman should be instructed to go to the hospital soon after labor begins.

Labor of a woman with a postterm fetus should be monitored for signs of fetal distress. The woman is encouraged to come to the hospital in early labor so the fetus can be monitored electronically for more accurate assessment of the FHR pattern. Fetal scalp pH sampling may be obtained for fetal distress or if meconium is present in the amniotic fluid. Accurate assessment of the woman's labor pattern also is important because dysfunctional labor is common in this complication (Spellacy, 1990).

Emotional support is essential for the postterm woman and her family. A vaginal birth is anticipated, but the couple should be prepared for a forceps-assisted birth (or vacuum extraction) or for cesarean birth if complications arise.

■ SUMMARY

Complications during birth have both physical and emotional sequelae. The mother faces life-threatening hazards. Prolonged and difficult labor can be physically debilitating. The consequent fatigue may interfere with initial interactions with her newborn. Memories of a difficult birth can resurface years later as a stress factor in subsequent births. The family will be faced with long-term grief reaction if the infant suffers disability. If death of either mother or infant occurs, the family, as it was, no longer exists. During this time of crisis, parents need the best possible medical and nursing care that our technically and psychologically knowledgeable society can offer.

REFERENCES

Acker DB et al: Risk factors for Erb-Duchenne palsy, *Obstet Gynecol* 71:389, 1988.

Acker DB, Sachs BP: Twin gestation in labor. In Cohen WR et al, editors: *Management of labor,* ed 2, Rockville, Md, 1989, Aspen.

Adams DM, Chervenak FA: Intrapartum management of twin gestation, *Clin Obstet Gynecol* 33:42, 1990.

Akoury HA et al: Active management of labor and operative delivery in nulliparous women, *Am J Obstet Gynecol* 158:255, 1988.

American College of Obstetricians and Gynecologists (ACOG committee opinion, Committee on Obstetrics): *Maternal and fetal medicine,* No 59: *Obstetric forceps,* Washington, DC, 1988a, ACOG.

American College of Obstetricians and Gynecologists (ACOG committee opinion): No 64: *Guidelines for vaginal delivery after a previous cesarean birth,* Washington, DC, Oct 1988b, ACOG.

American College of Obstetricians and Gynecologists: Technical bulletin No 133: *Preterm labor,* Washington, DC, 1989a, ACOG.

American College of Obstetricians and Gynecologists: Technical bulletin No 137: *Dystocia,* Washington, DC, 1989b, ACOG.

American College of Obstetricians and Gynecologists: Technical bulletin No 157: *Induction and augmentation of labor,* Washington, DC, 1991, ACOG.

Andersen HF, Merkatz IR: Preterm labor. In Scott JR et al: *Danforth's obstetrics and gynecology,* ed 6, Philadelphia, 1990, JB Lippincott.

Asher RH et al: Assessment of fetal risk in postdate pregnancies, *Am J Obstet Gynecol* 158:259, 1988.

Bennett NL, Botti JJ: New strategies for preterm labor, *Nurs Pract* 14(4):27, April 1989.

Bowes WA: Clinical aspects of normal and abnormal labor. In Cohen WR et al, editors: *Management of labor,* ed 2, Rockville, Md, 1989, Aspen.

Boyd ME et al: Obstetric consequences of postmaturity, *Am J Obstet Gynecol* 158:334, 1988.

Brown JJ: Calcium channel blockers for tocolysis. In Parer JJ, editor: *Antepartum and intrapartum management,* Philadelphia, 1989, Lea & Febiger.

Brustman LE et al: Changes in the pattern of uterine contractility in relationship to coitus during pregnancies at low and high risk for preterm labor, *Obstet Gynecol* 73:166, 1989.

Caritis SN et al: Pharmacologic treatment for preterm labor, *Clin Obstet Gynecol* 31:635, 1988.

Creasy RK: Preterm labor and delivery. In Creasy RK, Resnik R: *Maternal-fetal medicine: principles and practice,* ed 2, Philadelphia, 1989, WB Saunders.

Creasy RK, Merkatz IR: Prevention of preterm birth: clinical opinion, *Obstet Gynecol* 76(suppl 1):2s, 1990.

Cunningham FG, McDonald PC, Gant NF: *Williams obstetrics,* ed 18, Norwalk, Conn, 1989, Appleton & Lange.

Curtis P, Safransky N: Rethinking oxytocin protocols in the augmentation of labor, *Birth* 15(4):199, April 1988.

Dennan PC: *Dennan's forceps deliveries,* ed 3, Philadelphia, 1989, FA Davis.

Dudley D, Gagnon D, Varner M: Long-term tocolysis with intravenous magnesium sulfate, *Obstet Gynecol* 73:373, 1989.

Duff P: Antibiotic prophylaxis. In Phelan JP, Clark SL, editors: *Cesarean delivery,* New York, 1988, Elsevier.

Dunn LJ: Cesarean section and other obstetric operations. In Scott JR et al, editors: *Danforth's obstetrics and gynecology,* ed 6, Philadelphia, 1990, JB Lippincott.

Englinton GS: External version in modern obstetrics. In Phelan JP, Clark SL, editors: *Cesarean delivery,* New York, 1988, Elsevier.

Fawcett J, Henklein J: Antenatal education for cesarean birth: extending a field test, *JOGNN* 16:61, Jan/Feb 1987.

Fenwick L, Simkin P: Maternal positioning to prevent or alleviate dystocia in labor, *Clin Obstet Gynecol* 30:83, Jan 1987.

Flamm BL et al: Oxytocin during labor after previous cesarean section: results of a multicenter study, *Obstet Gynecol* 70:709, 1987.

Flamm BL et al: Vaginal birth after cesarean section: results of a multidimensional study, *Am J Obstet Gynecol* 158:1079, 1988.

Friedman EA: Normal and dysfunctional labor. In Cohen WR et al, editors: *Management of labor,* ed 2, Rockville, Md, 1989, Aspen.

Gallup DG: Opening and closing the abdomen. In Phelan JP, Clark SL, editors: *Cesarean delivery,* New York, 1988, Elsevier.

Galvan BJ, Broekhuizen FF: Obstetric vacuum extraction, *JOGNN* 16:242, July/Aug 1987.

Gill P, Smith M, McGregor C: Terbutaline by pump to prevent recurrent preterm labor, *MCN* 14:163, May/June 1989.

Graves EJ: 1988 summary: National hospital discharge summary. In *Advance data from vital and health statistics,* No 185, Hyattsville, Md, 1990, National Center for Health Statistics.

Henderson CE, Lichter ED: Induction of labor. In Cohen WR et al, editors: *Management of labor,* ed 2, Rockville, Md, 1989, Aspen.

Hill WC et al: Home uterine activity monitoring is associated with a reduction in preterm birth, *Obstet Gynecol* 76(suppl 1):13s, 1990.

Iams JD, Johnson FF, Creasy RK: Prevention of preterm birth, *Clin Obstet Gynecol* 31:599, 1988.

Institute of Medicine (Committee to Study the Prevention of Low Birthweight): *Preventing low birthweight,* Washington, DC, 1985, National Academy Press.

Jacobs MM: Prostaglandins for cervical ripening. In Parer JJ: *Antepartum and intrapartum management,* Philadelphia, 1989, Lea & Febiger.

Johnson FF: Assessment and education to prevent preterm labor, *MCN* 14:157, May/June 1989.

Knuppel RA, Drukker JE: *High-risk pregnancy: a team approach,* Philadelphia, 1986, WB Saunders Co.

Koontz WL: Abnormal labor. In Phelan JP, Clark SL, editors: *Cesarean delivery,* New York, 1988, Elsevier.

Lavin JP et al: Vaginal delivery in patients with a prior cesarean section, *Obstet Gynecol* 59:135, 1982.

Lehrman E: Birth in the left lateral position, *J Nurse Midwife* 30:193, July/Aug 1985.

Main DM: Epidemiology for preterm birth, *Clin Obstet Gynecol* 31:521, 1988.

Marieskind H: Cesarean section in the United States: has it changed since 1979? *Birth* 16:196, 1989.

Martel M et al: Maternal age and primary cesarean rates: a multivariate analysis, *Am J Obstet Gynecol* 156:305, 1987.

Mashburn J: Identification and management of shoulder dystocia, *J Nurse Midwife* 33:225, Sept/Oct 1988.

Mercer B, Pilgrim P, Sibai B: Labor induction with continuous low-dose oxytocin infusion: a randomized trial, *Obstet Gynecol* 77:659, 1991.

NAACOG: The nurse's role in the induction/augmentation of labor, *OGN Nursing Practice Resource,* Jan 1988 (PO Box 71437, Washington, DC 20024-1437).

National Center for Health Statistics: *Vital and health statistics: detailed diagnosis and procedures, National Hospital Discharge Survey, 1987* (Series 13, No 100) Washington, DC, March 1989, US Department of Health and Human Services.

Office of Technology Assessment: *Healthy children: investing in the future,* Washington, DC, Feb 1988, Congress of the United States.

O'Grady JP: A role exists for vaginal instrument delivery, *Contemp OB/GYN* 35(special issue):49, 1990.

Porreco RP: Once a cesarean, always a cesarean? In Phelan JP, Clark SL, editors: *Cesarean delivery,* New York, 1988, Elsevier.

Rayburn W: Prostaglandin E_2 gel for cervical ripening and induction of labor: an initial analysis, *Am J Obstet Gynecol* 160:529, 1989.

Resnik R: Postterm pregnancy. In Creasy RK, Resnik R, editors: *Maternal-fetal medicine: principles and practice,* ed 2, Philadelphia, 1989, WB Saunders.

Richardson P: Women's important relationships during pregnancy and the preterm labor event, *West J Nurs Res* 9:203, 1987.

Robertson PA: Optimizing the quality of life in preterm labor. In Parer JJ: *Antepartum and intrapartum management,* Philadelphia, 1989, Lea & Febiger.

Sala DJ, Moise KJ: The treatment of preterm labor using a portable subcutaneous terbutaline pump, *JOGNN* 19:108, March/April 1990.

Scott JR et al: *Danforth's obstetrics and gynecology,* ed 6, Philadelphia, 1990, JB Lippincott.

Sammons WA, Lewis JM: *Premature babies: a different beginning,* St. Louis, 1985, Mosby–Year Book.

Shearer E, Shiono P, Rhoads G: Recent trends in family centered maternity care for cesarean birth families, *Birth* 15:3, Jan 1988.

Silver L, Wolfe SM: Unnecessary cesarean section: how to cure a national epidemic, Washington, DC, 1989, Public Citizens Health Research Group.

Simkin P: Stress, pain and catecholamines in labor. I. A review, *Birth* 13(8):234, 1986.

Sinquefield G: Clinical practice exchange: use of prostaglandin in nurse-midwifery practice, *J Nurse Midwife* 34:137, May/June 1989.

Sokol RJ, Brindley BA: Practical diagnosis and management of abnormal labor. In Scott JR et al, editors: *Danforth's obstetrics and gynecology,* ed 6, Philadelphia, 1990, JB Lippincott.

Spellacy WN: Postdate pregnancy. In Scott JR et al, editors: *Danforth's obstetrics and gynecology,* ed 6, Philadelphia, 1990, JB Lippincott.

Tal Z et al: Breast electrostimulation for the induction of labor, *Obstet Gynecol* 72:671, 1988.

TOKOS: *Strategies to prevent preterm birth,* 1990, TOKOS Medical Corp, San Diego, Ca.

Turner MJ, Brassil M, Gordon H: Active management of labor associated with a decrease in the cesarean rate of nulliparas, *Obstet Gynecol* 71:150, 1988.

References—Nursing Research

Andrews CM, Chrzanowski: Maternal position, labor, and comfort, *Appl Nurs Res* 3:7, Jan 1990.

Beckmann CA: Postterm pregnancy: effects on temperature and glucose regulation, *Nurs Res* 39:21, Jan/Feb 1990.

Liu YC: The effects of the upright position during childbirth, *Image* 21(1):14, Jan 1989.

Weingarten CT et al: Married mothers' perceptions of their premature or term infants and the quality of their relationships with their husbands, *JOGNN* 19:64, Jan/Feb 1990.

BIBLIOGRAPHY

American College of Obstetrics and Gynecologists: Technical Bulletin No 130: *Diagnosis and management of postterm pregnancy,* Washington, DC, 1989, ACOG.

Adamsons K, Wallach RC: Treating preterm labor with diazoxide, *Contemp OB/GYN* 31:161, Jan 1988.

Culp RE, Osofsky HJ: Effects of cesarean delivery on parental depression, marital adjustment, and mother-infant interaction, *Birth* 16(2):53, 1989.

Few B: Indomethacin for treatment of premature labor, *MCN* 13(2):93, March/April 1988.

Hansell RS, McMurray KB, Huey GR: Vaginal birth after two or more cesarean sections: a five year experience, *Birth* 17(3):146, 1990.

Hartikainen-Sorri A, Sorri M: Occupational and sociomedical factors in preterm birth, *Obstet Gynecol* 74:13, 1989.

Herbst AL et al: *Comprehensive gynecology,* ed 2, St Louis, 1992, Mosby–Year Book.

Kosasa TS et al: Evaluation of the cost-effectiveness of home monitoring of uterine contractions, *Obstet Gynecol* 76(suppl 1):71s, 1990.

Nageotte M et al: Prophylactic amnioinfusion in pregnancies complicated by oligohydramnios: a prospective study, *Obstet Gynecol* 77:677, 1991.

Neilson JP, Mutambira M: Coitus, twin pregnancy, and preterm labor, *Am J Obstet Gynecol* 160:416, 1989.

Phelan JP, Clark SL, editors: *Cesarean delivery,* New York, 1988, Elsevier.

Scott JR: Mandating trial of labor after cesarean delivery: an alternative viewpoint, *Obstet Gynecol* 77:811, 1991.

Symposium: Alternatives to cesarean section, *Contemp OB/GYN* 31:191, Jan 1988.

Tucker SM et al: *Patient care standards: nursing process, diagnosis, and outcome,* ed 4, St Louis, 1988, Mosby–Year Book.

Watson DL et al: Management of preterm labor patients at home: does daily uterine activity monitoring and nursing support make a difference? *Obstet Gynecol* 76(suppl 1):32s, 1990.

Bibliography—Nursing Research

Cahill CA: Beta-endorphin levels during pregnancy and labor: a role in pain modulation, *Nurs Res* 38:200, July/Aug 1989.

Driscoll M et al: Prevention of preterm labor project in a public hospital: breaking down barriers to prenatal care, *J Perinat Neonat Nurs* 4(3):44, 1990.

Fortier JC: The relationship of vaginal and cesarean birth to father-infant attachment, *JOGNN* 17:128, March/April 1988.

Freda MC, Damus K, Merkatz I: What do pregnant women know about preventing preterm birth? *JOGNN* 20:140, March/April 1991.

Gennaro S: Postpartal anxiety and depression in mothers of term and preterm infants, *Nurs Res* 37:82, March/April 1988.

Kearney M, Cronenwett L: Perceived perinatal complications and childbirth satisfaction, *Appl Nurs Res* 2:140, May/June 1989.

Kearney M, Cronenwett L, Reinhardt R: Cesarean delivery and breast feeding outcomes, *Birth* 17:97, Feb 1990.

Monahan PA, DeJoseph JF: The woman with preterm labor at home: a descriptive analysis, *J Perinat Neonat Nurs* 4:12, April 1991.

Thomas L et al: The effects of rocking, diet modifications, and antiflatulent medication on postcesarean section gas pain, *J Perinat Neonat Nurs* 4(3):12, 1990.

Zahr L: Correlates of mother-infant interaction in premature infants from low socioecomic backgrounds, *Pediatr Nurs* 17:259, 1991.

chapter 35 review

Key Concepts

- Dystocia results from differences in the normal relationships among any of the five essential factors of labor.
- The differences between dystocia and eutocia relate to changes in the pattern of progress in labor.
- The functional relationships between the uterine contractions, the fetus, and the mother's pelvis are altered by maternal positioning.
- Uterine contractility is increased by oxytocin and prostaglandin and is decreased by tocolytic agents.
- All expectant parents benefit from learning about operative obstetrics (e.g., use of forceps, cesarean birth) and preterm labor during the prenatal period.
- The basic purpose of cesarean birth is to preserve the life or health of the mother and her fetus.
- Unless contraindicated, vaginal birth is possible after previous cesarean birth.
- The pregnant woman and her family can be taught to treat preterm labor at home with bed rest, tocolytics, and avoidance of activities that stimulate the uterus.
- In-hospital treatment for preterm labor involves the use of tocolytics and pharmacologic stimulation of lung maturity.
- Postterm birth poses a risk to both the mother and the fetus.

Key Terms

- amniotomy (p. 1056)
- augmentation of labor (p. 1057)
- Bishop score (p. 1056)
- breech presentation (p. 1049)
- cephalopelvic disproportion (CPD) (p. 1048)
- cesarean birth (p. 1060)
- dysfunctional labor (p. 1046)
- dystocia (p. 1046)
- external cephalic version (ECV) (p. 1055)
- forceps-assisted birth (p. 1058)
- hypertonic uterine dysfunction (p. 1046)
- hypotonic uterine dysfunction (p. 1047)
- induction of labor (p. 1055)
- multifetal pregnancy (p. 1051)
- oxytocin (p. 1056)
- pelvic dystocia (p. 1047)
- postterm birth (p. 1078)
- precipitous labor (p. 1047)
- preterm birth (p. 1070)
- prolonged labor (p. 1052)
- prostaglandins (p. 1056)
- soft tissue dystocia (p. 1047)
- therapeutic rest (p. 1046)
- tocolytic agents (p. 1074)
- trial of labor (TOL) (p. 1055)
- vacuum extraction (p. 1059)
- vaginal birth after cesarean (VBAC) (p. 1066)

Critical Thinking Exercises

1. You are assigned to a woman experiencing preterm labor at 32 weeks' gestation. Her previous labor was also preterm and the infant died at three days of age. This is the woman's third admission for preterm labor this pregnancy.
   a. What impact might her history have on the nursing care she receives this time?
   b. What approach to this woman will best meet her needs for this admission?
   c. Discuss pros and cons of home management for prevention of preterm birth for this woman.
   d. Develop a plan of care for prevention of preterm birth based on the above discussion.
2. You are preparing a woman for an unplanned cesarean birth for failure to progress.
   a. Examine possible reactions of the woman to this situation. How would these affect the effectiveness of nursing care?
   b. Examine your feelings as you think about how to prepare the woman for surgery. How would these feelings affect your care?
   c. How would your preparation differ from preparing a woman for a planned cesarean? Explain differences in postpartum needs between the woman who had a planned cesarean and the woman who experienced an unplanned one.
3. You are assigned to a woman who is experiencing prolonged labor.
   a. What assessments are important in this situation?
   b. Analyze the assessment data to determine nursing diagnoses.
   c. Generate a plan of care for the woman with prolonged labor. Justify your choices of interventions.
   d. Provide evaluative criteria to demonstrate a caring approach to the problem was implemented.

Topics for Nursing Research

The focus of nursing research must be the identification of effective nursing interventions for clients at risk for intrapartum complications and ways to promote preventive health care practices. The following topics provide study suggestions.

- What are effective maternal positions to prevent dysfunctional labor?
- What is the impact of stress, work, rest, diet, or personal habits on preterm labor?
- Are frequent nursing assessments as effective as use of home uterine-activity monitoring devices for decreasing the number of preterm births?
- What is the impact of nursing education for promoting compliance with long-term bed rest and tocolysis in clients at risk for preterm labor?
- What are the differences in educational and emotional needs of the client and her family in the home and hospital setting?
- Does early discharge after cesarean birth affect the woman's functional status?
- What is the efficacy of monitoring techniques in preventing preterm labor?
- What are factors associated with choosing healthy life-styles?
- What are some intervention models to decrease risk of preterm labor (e.g., improved nutrition, decreased or abstinence from alcohol intake)?
- What is the efficacy of nontraditional methods of labor induction (e.g., castor oil, acupuncture)?

unit 7

Newborn Complications

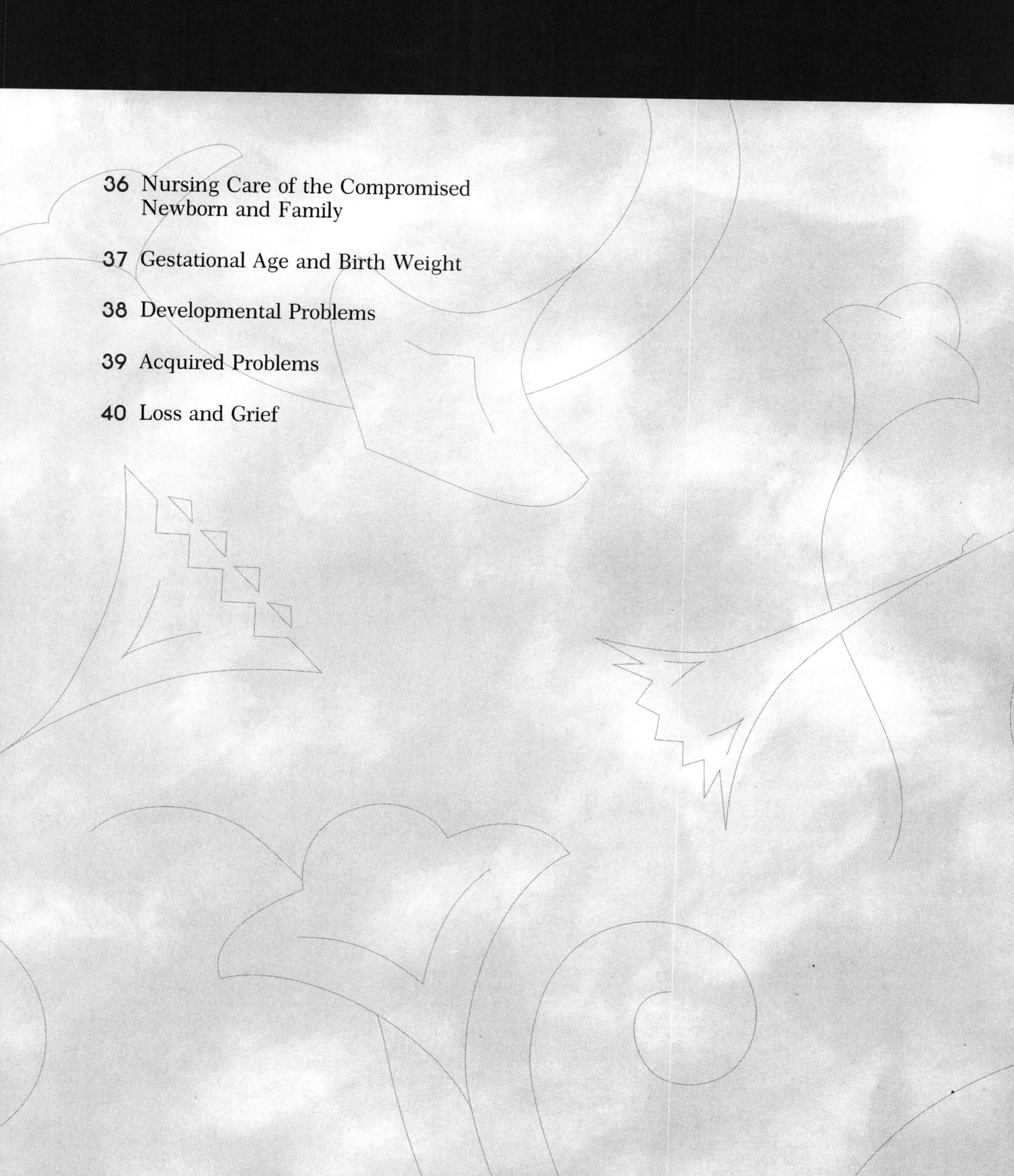

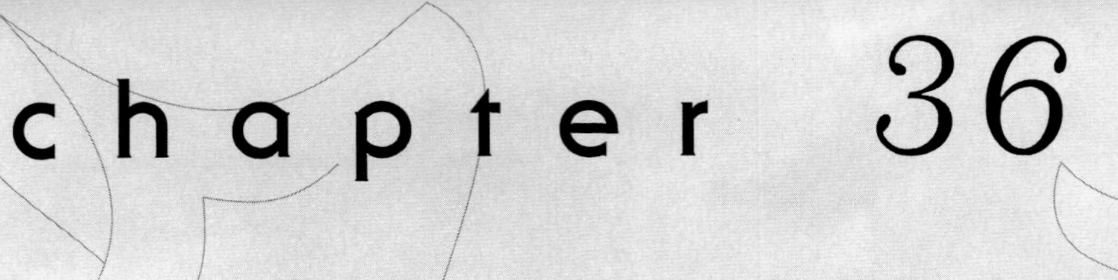

Nursing Care of the Compromised Newborn and Family

SUE A. JOINES

LEARNING OBJECTIVES

- Define the key terms listed.
- Outline the assessment of an infant at risk.
- Develop a nursing plan of care for an infant with respiratory distress.
- Explain the importance of temperature support and regulation.
- Discuss nursing care related to nutrition, feeding, and elimination.
- Describe procedures for meeting the nutrient and fluid needs of infants at risk.
- Explore the emotional aspects of care of the high-risk infant and the family.
- Compare and contrast the "kangaroo method" and the technologic approaches to thermoregulation.
- Develop a discharge plan for the infant at risk.
- Identify topics for nursing research related to nursing care of the compromised newborn.

The **high-risk neonate** is an infant whose intact survival is in jeopardy. Health care must support this neonate's basic functioning while compensating for its inadequacies. Assessment and supportive care are complicated by the infant's inability to speak and by the infant's nonspecific, generalized responses to dysfunctional problems. Assessment rests heavily on history provided by the mother and obstetric team, as well as current levels of knowledge regarding gestational age and disorders of the neonate. Planning and implementation of the nursing process with the high-risk infant focus on maintaining physiologic systems. The manner in which nursing care is provided can influence the health care team to keep the family's childbearing experience in focus, while providing support for the compromised high-risk neonate.

Care of the high-risk infant has become highly specialized and is beyond the scope of this text.* Subsequent chapters in this text include nursing care of infants with specific risk factors. The discussion in this chapter focuses on factors that place the newborn at high or moderate risk (see Table 27-2 and box, p. 783), as well as general concepts relevant to the care of the high-risk infant. Topics include the newborn with respiratory distress, temperature support and regulation, nutrition and elimination, emotional aspects of care, and transport to a regional center.

A case study and nursing plan of care for a compromised neonate are presented on pp. 1089 and 1090.

■ NURSING CARE OF THE NEWBORN WITH RESPIRATORY DISTRESS

Any newborn with respiratory difficulty is in jeopardy.† The infant's response to prompt, appropriate treatment is directly related to the cause of the respiratory problem, the degree of maturity, and other medical problems.

Breathing is a new experience for the infant. In priority of care, it ranks second only to the control of massive hemorrhage. Because of its high priority and its challenging nursing aspects, considerable space in the birth room is devoted to initiating and maintaining respirations.

The alert nurse often is the pivotal factor in functional or dysfunctional survival of the infant in respiratory distress. The degree of alertness and informed observation places the nurse in a preventive, curative, and rehabilitative role.

ASSESSMENT

Respiratory distress can be present at birth or develop in the first few hours of life (Urrutia, 1991). Nonstressed newborn infants establish normal respiratory rates and rhythms and they are pink and vigorous with good muscle tone, but some still develop respiratory distress. Respiratory difficulty may occur suddenly, as with aspiration or tension pneumothorax. In these cases the infant exhibits cyanosis and retractions.

More commonly, respiratory difficulty follows a progressive sequential pattern: the *respiratory rate* initially may increase without a change in rhythm. Flaring of the nares and expiratory grunt also are early signs of respiratory distress. The *apical pulse* increases in rate. *Retractions,* depending on the cause, may begin as subcostal, suprasternal, and clavicular retractions (Fig. 36-1). The *color* changes from pink to circumoral pallor, to circumoral cyanosis, and then to generalized cyanosis; acrocyanosis deepens. *Respiratory effort* and deepening distress are indicated by the following events (Fig. 36-2):

1. Chin tug (chin is pulled down [mouth opens wider] as auxiliary muscles of respiration are activated)

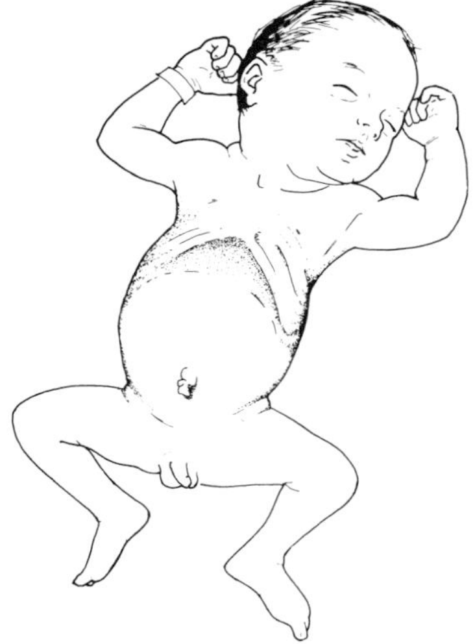

Fig. 36-1 Retraction: substernal, subcostal, and intercostal retractions are evident.
Courtesy Ross Laboratories, Columbus, Ohio.

*See References and Bibliography. Most facilities have developed modular study guides and manuals for procedures and for laboratory values and their management.

†See discussion in Chapter 21 on techniques for providing the neonate with suctioning, oxygen therapy, and resuscitation.

CASE STUDY

Compromised Neonate

Christie was born at 33 weeks' gestation. She is her parents' first baby. This pregnancy was planned and uncomplicated until contractions began at 33 weeks' gestation. When the contractions began, the mother's health care provider instructed her to empty her bladder, drink two 8-oz glasses of liquid, and lie down. When the contractions continued, she was instructed to have her husband drive her to the emergency unit, where the health care provider met her. On arriving at the emergency unit, the mother experienced gross rupture of membranes. It was immediately apparent that meconium was present. The electronic monitor tracing established current fetal well-being. Because of the presence of meconium (an indicator of possible fetal distress), labor was permitted to continue, and Christie was born 4 hours after rupture of membranes.

ASSESSMENT

The prenatal record revealed none of the usual risk factors for preterm labor or premature rupture of membranes. At the mother's request, an unmedicated, vaginal birth was attempted and achieved. Christie's Apgar score was 4 at 1 minute. Christie responded to the resuscitation efforts of the intensive care nursery (ICN) team, and her 5-minute Apgar score was 8.

Christie received initial intubation. Although meconium aspiration had occurred, it was determined to be thin meconium and not seen below the level of the vocal cords. After this initial stabilization, Christie was taken to the ICN, where her birth weight was recorded as 2013 g (4 lb 7 oz) (AGA for 33 weeks).

Christie's parents were holding each other and crying as she was being resuscitated and taken to the ICN. Christie's father asked and was permitted to accompany her to the ICN. Christie's mother was tearful, but her health care provider was in the process of repairing her episiotomy and she was therefore unable to accompany her daughter to the ICN.

NURSING DIAGNOSES

On the basis of the assessment findings, several nursing diagnoses are possible. Of three primary diagnoses related to airway clearance, thermoregulation, and fluid volume, airway clearance takes priority:

- High risk for ineffective gas exchange related to
  —Immaturity
  —Inadequate airway clearance

PLANNING

As possible, the nurse involves the client in planning care. However, in this case, it is not possible, and the nurse identified the following goal: Christie will maintain effective gas exchange with a clear airway (as evidenced by auscultation of breath sounds).

IMPLEMENTATION

On arrival to the ICN, Christie was placed in a prewarmed incubator with a servocontrol mechanism. She initially required CPAP and then oxygen by hood with intermittent suctioning. First Christie was weaned from CPAP to oxygen by hood and then off of the oxygen altogether, according to the hospital's procedure.

EVALUATION

Throughout her stay in the ICN, Christie's gas exchange was adequate, and her airway was kept clear with suctioning as needed (breath sounds clear after each suctioning).

2. Abdominal seesaw breathing patterns (see Figs. 20-2, *B*, and 36-2)
3. Increased number of apneic episodes

If the newborn is hypoxic, the *temperature* may begin to drop. (Any sudden changes in environmental temperature can precipitate apneic episodes [Merenstein, Gardner, 1989].) An accurate and timely *blood pressure* reading can assist in early diagnosis of cardiorespiratory disease and in monitoring fluid therapy. Blood pressure readings are obtained by the Doppler method or electronic monitor. A blood pressure cuff of appropriate size must be used. A too-wide cuff results in a false low reading; an overly narrow cuff will give a falsely elevated reading. For the newborn a cuff of about 2.5 to 3 cm (1 in) wide and 7.5 cm (3 in) long usually is adequate (Fig. 36-3, p. 1092).

The stethoscope should have a pediatric-sized diaphragm for maximum skin contact and localization of sounds. The stethoscope is applied with firm pressure but not so much pressure that transmission of sound and vibrations is compromised.

CARE PLAN Compromised Neonate

GOAL	IMPLEMENTATION	RATIONALE	EVALUATION
Nursing diagnosis: High risk for ineffective gas exchange related to immaturity and inadequate airway clearance			
Christie will maintain effective gas exchange and a clear airway (as evidenced by auscultation of breath sounds).	Provide CPAP; wean to hood oxygen, with intermittent suction as necessary.	Provide oxygen in least invasive manner possible. Support infant's oxygen needs without the adverse sequelae of oxygen therapy.	Christie's oxygen needs are met; She experienced no adverse sequelae of oxygen therapy. Her breath sounds are clear to auscultation, before and after suction.
Nursing diagnosis: High risk for ineffective thermoregulation related to immaturity			
Christie will maintain a normal skin temperature of 97°-98° F (36.1°-36.7° C).	Place in prewarmed incubator with servocontrol mechanism. Affix thermistor probe. Assess incubator function. Assess environmental contributors to cold stress (incubator near fans, windows, doorways, drafts). Complete tactile and visual assessment for symptoms of decreased body temperature.	Prevent cold stress from contact with cold/nonfunctional equipment and environment. Monitor infant to be able to respond promptly to altered body temperature (acrocyanosis, cold extremities). The preterm infant is particularly sensitive to fluctuations in environmental temperatures and is least able to cope with these physiologically (i.e., is unable to generate heat to elevate body temperature by crying, flexion, increase in activity, or by shivering—for further discussion, see p. 1097).	Christie's skin temperature is maintained between 97° and 98° F (36.1° and 36.7° C).
Nursing diagnosis: High risk for fluid volume deficit or overload related to immaturity			
Christie will receive adequate nutrition (nutrients, fluids, and electrolytes) without experiencing: respiratory distress, hypoglycemia, abdominal distention, or trauma to the tissues of the gastrointestinal tract, constipation, or diarrhea.	Provide nourishment: TPN	TPN provides adequate nourishment for growth and healing while the infant is unable to tolerate enteral feedings.	Christie's nourishment is adequate, and she does not experience the adverse sequelae of fluid deficit or overload.
	Gavage	Gavage provides enteral feedings when the infant is too weak to suckle all or part of the feeding.	
	Nipple/breast	Breast-feeding provides age-appropriate nourishment for the infant and aids in the prevention of NEC (see Chapter 37). For further discussion of the benefits of breast-feeding, see Chapter 22.	Mother states she feels good that she is contributing to the care of the infant.

CARE PLAN Compromised Neonate—cont'd

GOAL	IMPLEMENTATION	RATIONALE	EVALUATION
	Encourage nonnutritive sucking.	Decreases oxygen requirements, promotes quiet rest, and helps prepare infant for nipple feeding.	Christie is quiet and still during gavage procedure and has a coordinated suck and swallow reflex when nipple/breast feeding is instituted.

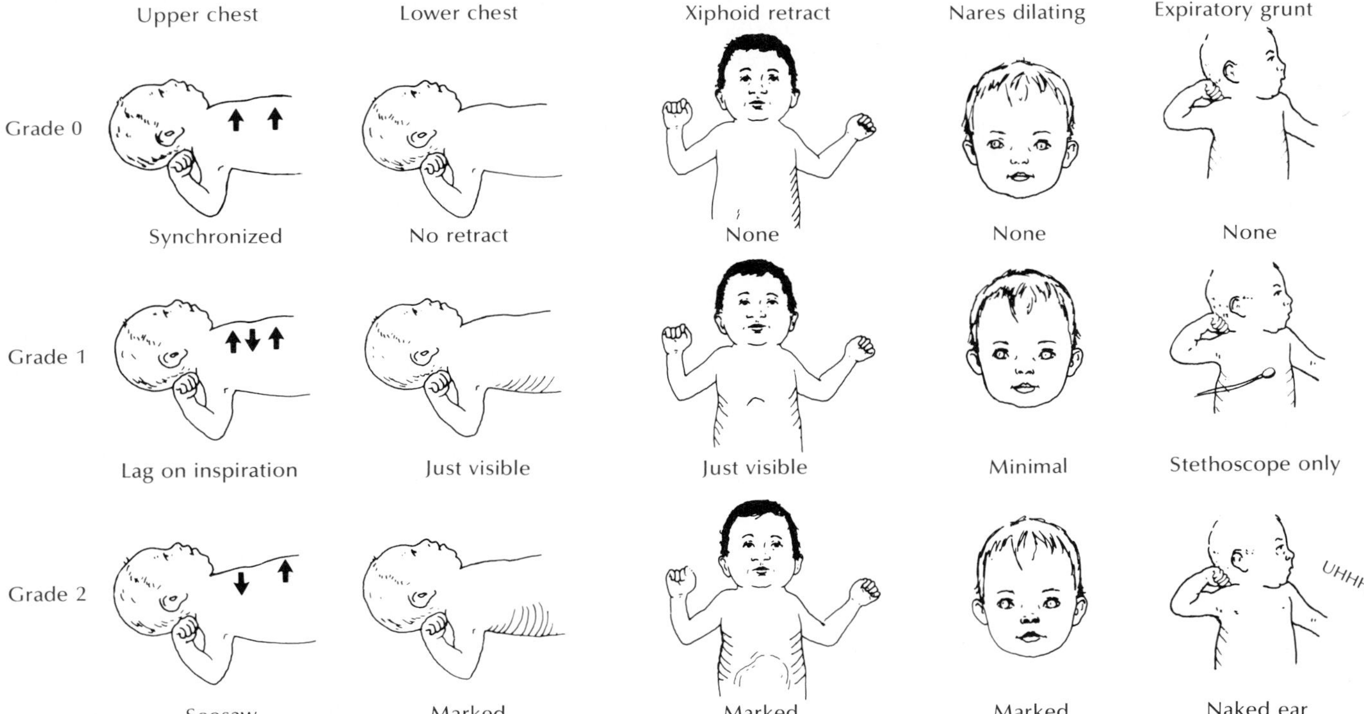

Fig. 36-2 Observation of retractions. Silverman-Anderson index of respiratory distress is determined by grading each of five arbitrary criteria: *grade 0* indicates no difficulty; *grade 1,* moderate difficulty; and *grade* 2, maximum respiratory difficulty. Retraction score is sum of these values; total score of 0 indicates no dyspnea, whereas total score of 10 denotes maximum respiratory distress.
Modified from Silverman W, Anderson D: *Pediatrics* 17:1, 1956.

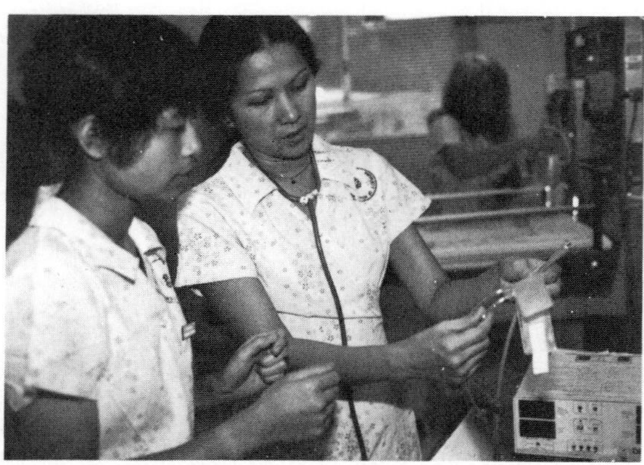

Fig. 36-3 Preparing to assess a newborn's blood pressure electronically.

The Doppler instrument and electronic monitoring device (on a biometric console) are more accurate methods for determining blood pressure. However, this type of equipment is not available in all hospitals or community health settings.

The monitor displays the systolic and diastolic value, the mean systolic/diastolic pressure (the reading is midway between the diastolic and systolic pressures), and the newborn's heart rate. The existing standard normal range for the mean pressure for infants weighing 2500 g (5½ lb) or more is 30 to 60 mm Hg.

NURSING DIAGNOSES

Some possible nursing diagnoses follow:

- Impaired gas exchange related to
  - —Immaturity
- Ineffective airway clearance related to
  - —Newborn anatomy, immobility, and increased secretions
  - —Meconium aspiration
  - —Immaturity or congenital disorder
  - —Respiratory depression secondary to narcosis or acidosis
- Ineffective breathing pattern related to
  - —Immaturity
  - —Cold stress
- High risk for altered nutrition related to
  - —Inadequate intake, retention, or utilization of nutrients
- High risk for altered parenting related to
  - —Infant's physical condition at birth

PLANNING

During the planning step, *goals* are established to meet the unique needs of the high-risk newborn. The goals are prioritized, and nursing actions are selected to meet these goals. Whenever possible, goals are established with the client and are phrased in client-centered terms. For example, the expected outcome is that the infant will achieve the following:

- Maintain adequate gas exchange
- Maintain a clear airway
- Maintain an effective respiratory pattern
- Not suffer from unidentified congenital anomalies
- Maintain adequate nutritional intake to support metabolic needs of repair, maintenance, and growth

The parent(s) will achieve the following:

- Perceive the infant as potentially normal (if this is medically substantiated)
- Begin bonding and attachment to the infant
- Correctly demonstrate use of the bulb syringe, positioning of infant for feeding by breast or bottle, and techniques for managing the choking or gagging infant.

IMPLEMENTATION

Supportive Measures

The newborn's respiratory efforts must be supported by careful positioning. When the infant is supine, the arms are at the sides, flexed, and slightly abducted. Diapers, if used, must be wrapped and secured loosely. The prone position,* as an alternative to supine and lateral positions, has been shown to decrease respiratory effort, increase arterial oxygen pressure (PaO_2), and diminish the work of respiration.

Suctioning assists the infant in maintaining a patent airway. It is vital that nurses maintain proficiency and currency in suctioning techniques (see Research Highlight, p. 1093). An unobstructed airway assists the newborn's breathing by improving ventilation. (See discussion of suctioning procedures in Chapter 21.)

A *thermoneutral environment* is essential for metabolic homeostasis. Cold stress is detrimental to the well-being of any infant but is of particular concern for the infant with respiratory distress. (For a discus-

*The American Academy of Pediatrics is expected to comment about the prone position within a few months.

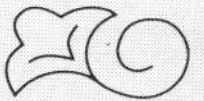 **Research Highlight** 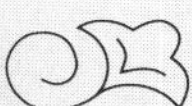

Neonatal Endotracheal Suctioning Practices

RESEARCH ABSTRACT

The purpose of this research was to determine the current procedures used by neonatal nurses for endotracheal suctioning of newborn infants. A questionnaire designed by the researchers was mailed to 354 centers that care for infants who need mechanical ventilator assistance. The researchers requested that the questionnaire be completed by a staff nurse who had at least 2 year's experience in providing direct client care in a neonatal intensive care unit. A total of 203 usable questionnaires (57.3%) were returned.

The data were analyzed in relation to 13 research questions. Taking vital signs, performing postural drainage, instilling irrigant, and providing hyperoxygenation were the routine actions taken during the suctioning process for an intubated infant. Of the nurses who administer hyperoxygenation, 65.5% routinely do so before suctioning and 66.7% routinely do so afterward. Most respondents (87.7%) said the percentage of oxygen used varied on the basis of the infant's need. Criteria for hyperoxygenation were the infant's past response to suctioning, current appearance, or a decrease in transcutaneous oxygen pressure ($tcPo_2$) during the suctioning process. Some (41.9%) nurses routinely perform hyperventilation before suctioning, and more (61%) nurses do so after suctioning. The amount of hyperventilation varies with the needs of the infant and the current ventilator settings. Few (9.4%) nurses use hyperinflation before suctioning. The amount of secretions determines the frequency of suctioning. Postural drainage, percussion, and vibration are always performed before suctioning by 32.5% and sometimes by 52.2% of nurses. Almost all (91.6%) of the nurses use 0.9% sodium chloride to irrigate the endotracheal tube. Most nurses (80.3%) apply negative pressure for fewer than 5 seconds. Only 12.3% of the nurses use a suction catheter of the recommended size where the suctioning process is performed with the endotracheal tube in place. The researchers concluded that there was a great deal of variation in suctioning practices. Some practices are supported in the research literature (hyperoxygenation), and others are not (rate of hyperventilation). Further research is recommended.

IMPLICATIONS FOR PRACTICE

There is limited research that supports the safety of various endotracheal suctioning practices. Some available research findings are being used to guide clinical practice. When such findings document the safety and efficacy of procedures, they should be used in practice. For example, the literature supports hyperoxygenation before suctioning; however, in this sample only 65% of the nurses routinely used it. It is important for nurses to read the current literature and examine their practice in relation to the reported findings.

RELATED RESEARCH QUESTIONS

1. What is the optimum ratio of the outside diameter of a suction catheter to the inside diameter of the endotracheal tube?
2. Will an education program increase the use of in-line suction adapters?
3. What is the appropriate hyperventilation rate to use before suctioning?
4. How accurate are nurses in assessing adverse effects of infant suctioning by means of observational cues as compared with the use of $tcPo_2$ values?

REFERENCE

Tolles CL, Stone KS: National survey of neonatal endotracheal suctioning practices, *Neonatal Network* 9(2):7, Feb 1990.

sion of thermogenesis and the prevention of cold stress, see Chapter 21.)

Nutrition and Feeding

Nutrition and feeding of the infant in respiratory distress are as much a challenge for the nurse as for the infant. The extra work of breathing taxes the infant's energy reserves and demands greater caloric intake. For the infant in respiratory distress, neither breast- nor bottle-feeding are appropriate, and gavage feeding may be indicated. The newborn in severe respiratory distress may receive all feedings by gavage (see p. 1102). For the infant who does not tolerate gavage feeding, parenteral fluids, or total parenteral nutrition may be required. For the convalescent infant in no respiratory distress who can bottle-feed, a soft nipple with an adequate opening is used (e.g., when the bottle is inverted, fluid should drip at 1 drop per second). Some infants can be put to the breast, whereas others must be fed breast milk or formula by bottle and nipple. The mother of a high-risk infant who wishes to breast-feed must receive supportive guidance. (For discussion of breast-feeding, see Chapter 22.) The provision of correct information regarding expression and storage of breast milk is essential to the safe collection of milk for the high-risk infant (Wilks, Meier, 1988; Beckholt, 1990).

Whether breast- or formula-feeding is used, the nurse remains close by during feedings provided to the infant by the parent. The nurse provides assistance, support, and encouragement for the parent(s). As necessary, the nurse clears the airway before and during feedings. The nurse demonstrates a calm approach in caring for the choking or gagging infant. The nurse demonstrates the use of the bulb syringe, positioning of the infant, and burping techniques in an organized and composed manner. As appropriate, parents are supported in their independent attempts to use the bulb syringe and to feed and burp the infant.

Oxygen Therapy

Oxygen therapy may be lifesaving, but its administration must be carefully monitored, as with any medication. Indications for the use of oxygen include clinical criteria substantiated by biochemical data (arterial oxygen pressure [Pa_{O_2}] <60 mm Hg). Clinical criteria include increased respiratory effort, respiratory distress with apnea, central cyanosis, and hypotonia.

Periodic breathing is a respiratory pattern commonly seen in preterm infants. Infants in periodic respiration demonstrate cycles of respiratory pauses of 5 to 10 seconds in length, followed by 10 to 15-second periods of compensatory rapid respirations. Periodic respirations are not to be confused with apnea. **Apnea** is a 10- to 15-second *cessation* of respiration. Apnea commonly is associated with cyanosis, pallor, hypotonia, or bradycardia. Causes of apnea include prematurity, infection, impaired oxygenation, metabolic disorders, drugs, thermal instability, gastroesophageal reflux, and intracranial abnormalities (Fanaroff, Martin, 1992).

In assessment of the high-risk newborn, color is an important indicator of status in the respiratory, cardiovascular, and central nervous systems. Although acrocyanosis is a normal finding in the neonate, cyanosis of the lips, mouth (circumoral), or mucous membranes of the newborn indicates an underlying problem (cardiac, pulmonary, or central nervous system) (Merenstein, Gardner, 1989).

Indiscriminate use of oxygen may be hazardous. An important principle to remember is that "no concentration of oxygen has been proved to be safe. A concentration that is therapeutic for one infant may be toxic for another" (Merenstein, Gardner, 1989). Complications occurring as a result of oxygen therapy include retinopathy of prematurity, previously called *retrolental fibroplasia* (see Chapter 37), and bronchopulmonary dysplasia (see Chapter 37). (For a general discussion of oxygen therapy, see Chapter 21.)

The oxygen concentration administered to an infant is carefully controlled in amount, temperature, and humidity. Some incubators have an automatic cut-off mechanism when ambient oxygen reaches a preset level. These controls do not replace the intermittent (hourly) or continuous monitoring of the oxygen levels. Oxygen delivered to an infant is warmed and humidified to prevent cold stress and drying of respiratory mucosa.

To minimize the risk of either hyperoxic or hypoxic insults to a sick infant, decisions regarding the concentration of oxygen administered are based on the results of periodic assessment, including clinical observation (color, respiratory effort, and activity), oxygenation (laboratory values such as Pa_{O_2}, hemoglobin, and arterial blood gas), and telemetry (transcutaneous oxygen monitoring or pulse oximetry) (Merenstein, Gardner, 1989).

TRANSCUTANEOUS OXYGEN PRESSURE MONITOR. Historically, methods of measuring oxygenation have included invasive techniques such as umbilical artery catheterization, as well as radial and temporal puncture or catheterization. A noninvasive technique that can provide continuous measurement of oxygen tension is the **transcutaneous oxygen pressure (tcP_{O_2}) monitor.** The electrodes of this monitor are applied (according to manufacturer's directions) to hairless, greaseless sites, in air-tight contact with the skin. To avoid skin breakdown under the electrodes, site selection is limited to non–pressure-bearing areas (e.g., infant must not lie on top of electrode). Electrode sites are changed every 2 to 4 hours.

There are two limitations to the use of tcP_{O_2} monitors. One, tcP_{O_2} monitor electrodes are warmed to 42° to 45° C, which can artificially inflate the measurement of tcP_{O_2} (Whitney, 1990). Two, tcP_{O_2} monitors the amount of oxygen dissolved in plasma, which is only 3% to 5% of the total amount of oxygen traveling through the blood stream. The pulse oximeter assesses the other 95% to 98% of the oxygen present, that which is bound to hemoglobin (Spyr, Preach, 1990).

PULSE OXIMETER. An oxygen saturation monitor (**pulse oximeter**), measures oxygen carried by hemoglobin. As with the tcP_{O_2} monitor, this method allows for continuous assessment of oxygenation. A sensor, applied to the infant's finger, toe, or wrist, detects the amount of light (from the light source) that passes through a vascular bed (Merenstein, Gardner, 1989). The monitor reads the amount of light absorbed by the oxygen-carrying hemoglobin and converts this into the saturation value. A normal oxygen saturation level is between 95% to 100%. Steps are taken to improve oxygenation as soon as levels begin to drop, even at 95%. As saturation levels fall below 90% (approximately equal to a PaO_2 of 60 mm Hg), hemoglobin carries less oxygen to be released; thus tissues become hypoxic (Spyr, Preach, 1990; Sonnesso, 1991).

WEANING FROM OXYGEN. Respiratory assistance is slowly withdrawn as the infant's status improves. The infant is ready to be weaned from respiratory assistance when (1) arterial blood gases are maintained within normal limits, (2) respiratory effort is present, and (3) muscle tone improves and activity increases and is tolerated (as evidenced by oxygen saturation).

Weaning occurs in a stepwise and gradual manner, and only as the infant tolerates the decreased ventilatory or oxygen settings, or both. As the infant on receiving intermittent mandatory ventilation (IMV) gradually increases spontaneous respirations, the mechanical ventilation required is decreased. From mechanical ventilation the infant may be transferred to continuous positive airway pressure (CPAP), and then extubated and placed under a hood. Throughout the weaning process, oxygen levels are monitored by means of $tcPO_2$ or a pulse oximeter (oxygen saturation monitor) (see p. 1094).

The goal of weaning is withdrawal of all oxygen; however, some infants do not achieve this before discharge from the hospital. Throughout the weaning process the health care providers assess for symptoms that indicate the infant is not tolerating the weaning process: increased pulse, respiratory distress, and cyanosis. When these symptoms occur, oxygen is increased and weaning proceeds more slowly. If weaning is not possible, the underlying cause may be bronchopulmonary dysplasia, patent ductus arteriosus, or central nervous system (CNS) damage (Merenstein, Gardner, 1989).

Methods of Oxygen Administration

Depending on the requirements of the infant, varying methods are used to deliver oxygen.

HOOD. If the infant's oxygen requirement exceeds 30%, oxygen can be administered by a hood. The hood is a clear plastic cover, sized to fit over the head and neck of the infant, avoiding the overdilution of oxygen. Within the hood the infant receives the correct amount of oxygen. At the same time the infant is protected from fluctuations in the ambient concentration of oxygen such as occur when the portholes of the incubator are opened (Fig. 36-4). Hood size is determined by the size of the infant: the plastic should not come in contact with the skin of the neck, nor should the hood be large enough for the infant to slip out from under it (Merenstein, Gardner, 1989).

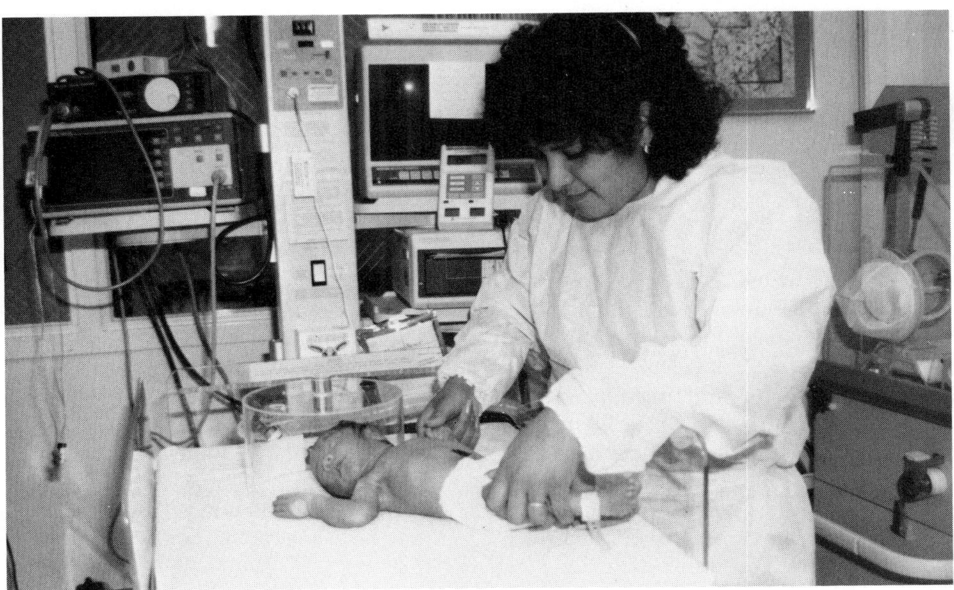

Fig. 36-4 Mother interacting with her baby by touch. Note use of oxygen hood and overhead warmer in place of incubator.
Courtesy Marjorie Pyle, RNC, Lifecircle, Costa Mesa, Calif.

CONTINUOUS POSITIVE AIRWAY PRESSURE. **Continuous positive airway pressure (CPAP)** (also called *continuous distending pressure*) is used for infants who are unable to maintain adequate PaO_2 despite the use of oxygen via hood. CPAP is the continuous infusion of oxygen under a preset pressure. This pressure increases alveolar volume by preventing the alveoli from collapsing on expiration. CPAP can be administered via nasal cannula or endotracheal tube and increases functional residual capacity, improves oxygenation, and decreases pulmonary shunting. Implemented early enough, CPAP may prevent the need for mechanical ventilation (Merenstein, Gardner, 1989).

MECHNICAL VENTILATION. **Mechanical ventilation** is required if hood and CPAP delivery are ineffective in providing adequate oxygenation. Mechanical ventilation is indicated for infants with (1) blood gas values that indicate severe hypoxemia or severe hypercapnia and/or (2) the following clinical conditions: apnea with bradycardia, ineffective respiratory effort, shock and asphyxia, or idiopathic respiratory distress syndrome (IRDS) in infants smaller than 1000 g (Merenstein, Gardner, 1989).

Ventilator settings are individualized to the infant's needs. The ventilator can be set to provide a predetermined amount of oxygen to the infant during spontaneous respirations and also will provide mechanical ventilation in the absence of spontaneous respirations (i.e., by IMV). By means of IMV in combination with continuous distending pressure, the infant receives positive end-expiratory pressure (PEEP). With the use of the ventilator to deliver continuous distending pressure without IMV, the infant receives CPAP (Merenstein, Gardner, 1989).

Other ventilatory settings include the following:

- *Peak inspiratory pressure* —level of pressure to

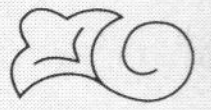 **Research Highlight** 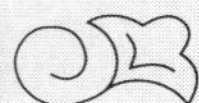

Evaluation of Manometer Use in Manual Ventilation of Infants

RESEARCH ABSTRACT

There is variation in the proficiency level of nurses who work in neonatal intensive care units (NICUs) in the performance of manual ventilation of infants. The purpose of this study was to determine whether nurses could accurately deliver the prescribed level of peak inspiratory pressure (PIP) during manual ventilation of infants with and without a manometer and whether the number of years of work experience made a difference in their proficiency. Subjects were a convenience sample (one easily available) of 60 registered nurses who worked in a large NICU. The nurses had from 1 to 26 years experience.

Data were collected during specified suctioning times. Each nurse was observed once while performing manual ventilation. Peak airway pressures were measured during manual ventilation with an apparatus that provides real-time hard-copy recordings of pressures. An observer recorded each time the nurse looked at the manometer while performing manual ventilation. The researchers found that all the nurses checked the manometer at some time during ventilation. The nurses provided prescribed PIP 78.01% of the time when using the manometer as compared with 41.40% when not using the manometer. This difference was statistically significant. More experienced nurses used the manometer less than did the less experienced nurses. The relation between years of experience and accuracy in delivering PIP was not statistically significant.

IMPLICATIONS FOR PRACTICE

Because the accuracy of delivering PIP to these very fragile infants varied so much when the manometer was not used, it is important that standards of care be established to decrease risk to infants during manual ventilation. In-service programs to help staff members maintain their proficiency should be provided. A system of peer review and evaluation could be instituted to ensure that a safe level of practice is maintained.

RELATED RESEARCH QUESTIONS

1. Does the ability to control PIP when manually ventilating an infant differ with the size of the infant?
2. Will a yearly in-service program and evaluation improve the proportion of time a nurse delivers the prescribed PIP?
3. What factors are associated with the ability to control PIP when manually ventilating an infant?
4. Is there a relation between hand size, grip strength, and accuracy in delivering PIP when manually ventilating an infant?

REFERENCE

Howard-Glenn L, Koniak-Griffin D: Evaluation of manometer use in manual ventilation of infants in neonatal intensive care units, *Heart Lung* 19:620, 1990.

be present on inspiration; precision in mechanical ventilation is essential (see Research Highlight, p. 1096).

- *Rate* —how often the ventilator is to deliver the specified volume of oxygen to the infant, equivalent to the number of breaths per minute
- *Inspiration/expiration ratio* —quantitatively, the amount of time spent in inspiration compared with expiration
- *Mean airway pressure* —the amount of pressure exerted on the airway throughout the respiratory cycle (Merenstein, Gardner, 1989)

Another means of oxygen administration that may reduce the incidence of pulmonary tissue damage (**barotrauma**) which can occur with traditional ventilatory methods is called *high-frequency oscillation,* or jet ventilation (Gordin, 1989). Barotrauma from conventional methods of ventilation is a major contributing factor in chronic pulmonary disease. Jet ventilation provides comparatively smaller volumes of oxygen at a significantly higher rate than do traditional mechanical ventilators and therefore decreases the intrathoracic pressure (Merenstein, Gardner, 1989). High-frequency ventilation is becoming a more common treatment modality, especially for IRDS, and is the subject of various clinical trials (Gerhardt et al, 1989).

EXTRACORPOREAL MEMBRANE OXYGENATION. **Extracorporeal membrane oxygenation** (ECMO) makes use of cardiopulmonary bypass for the purpose of oxygenation of the infant's blood outside the body through a membrane oxygenator (Polin, Fox 1992). This membrane oxygenator serves as a lung to decrease the workload of the infant's own lungs while healing injury created by hyperoxia and barotrauma during ventilation. Blood flows out of the body from the right internal jugular through a catheter to the membrane oxygenator. From the oxygenator, blood returns to the infant through the right common carotid artery or the femoral vein. Although relatively new, ECMO has been successful in the treatment of various acute and chronic lung diseases, including meconium aspiration syndrome and persistent pulmonary hypertension (Merenstein, Gardner, 1989).

EVALUATION

The nurse can be reasonably assured that care of the infant was effective if the goals for care have been met:

- The infant's respiratory function provides adequate gas exchange and a clear airway.
- The infant does not suffer from unidentified congenital anomalies.
- The infant's nutritional intake is adequate to provide for the metabolic needs of repair, maintenance, and growth.

The nurse can be reasonably assured that nursing interventions were effective in support of the parents of a high-risk infant, if the following goals are met.

- The parents perceive the infant as potentially normal (if this is medically substantiated).
- The parents begin bonding and attachment to the infant.
- The parents demonstrate skill in using the bulb syringe, positioning of infant for feeding, breast- or formula-feeding, and techniques for managing the choking or gagging infant.

TEMPERATURE SUPPORT AND REGULATION

Cold Stress

The concept of an optimum thermal environment for neonates evolved during the 1960s. This idealized setting, called the *neutral thermal environment,* is one in which an infant can maintain a normal body temperature while producing only the minimum amount of heat generated from basal life-sustaining metabolic processes. The importance of maintaining neutral thermal conditions is greatest in the youngest, most immature infants, whose ability to generate additional heat in a heat-losing environment may be minimal. The ability to increase metabolic rate in these infants may be hampered further by impaired gas exchange in the lungs or by restriction of caloric intake, or both (Fanaroff, Martin, 1992).

NOTE: Infants are alerted to cold stress when thermal receptors in the skin are stimulated. The face is particularly sensitive, and even when the infant's body is warm, cooling of the face will cause a responsive rise in metabolic rate. Conversely, warming of the facial skin when the body is cold suppresses cold stress–induced hypermetabolism (Fanaroff, Martin, 1992).

On sensing heat loss, the infant attempts to minimize the loss and increase heat production. Heat loss from the skin is minimized by vasoconstriction and flexion of the extremities to decrease the area of exposed skin surface. Heat is produced by increasing physical work (e.g., crying, becoming hyperactive) and increasing metabolism. In a heat-losing environment, even the healthy term infant's stores of substrate such as glycogen and fat can be depleted, and acidosis and, eventually, exhaustion occur (Fig. 36-5). (See also Chapter 20.)

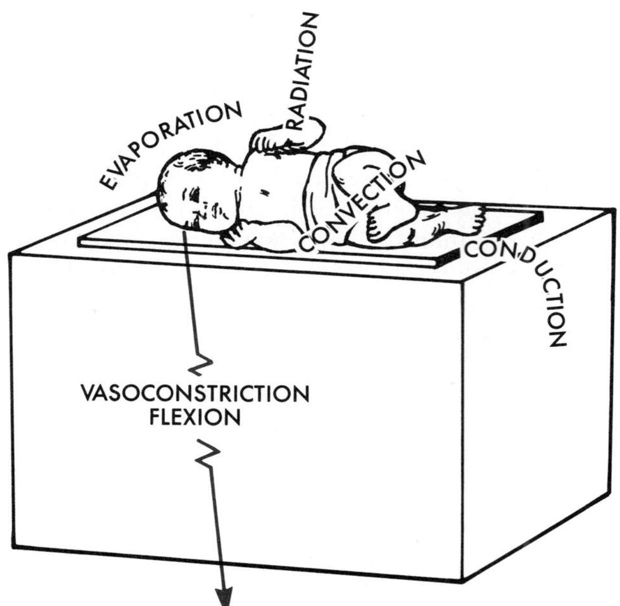

Fig. 36-5 Infant's response to cold stress.
From Fanaroff AA, Martin RJ: *Neonatal-perinatal medicine: diseases of the fetus and infant*, ed 5, St Louis, 1992, Mosby–Year Book.

ASSESSMENT

In the non–cold-stressed neonate, measuring *axillary temperature* is the safest, most practical means of monitoring deep body temperature. However, in the cold-stressed neonate, metabolism of brown fat in the axillary area may result in misleadingly high readings. (For extensive discussion of thermogenesis, see Chapter 20.)

A temperature-monitoring thermistor probe or transducer taped to the skin is designed to provide accurate temperature readings for the newborn under an overhead radiant heat source or in an incubator with a servocontrol mechanism. When only a single skin temperature is to be sensed, the thermistor probe is attached to the skin over the liver or between the umbilicus and the pubis. Least-favored attachment sites are over bony prominences (one of the least vasoreactive body regions) or extremities (one of the most vasoreactive regions). False temperature measures will occur if the probe is covered by diapers or blankets or artificially cooled by a stream of cold oxygen (Fanaroff, Martin, 1992).

Skin temperature usually decreases first in the cold-stressed infant. Therefore the infant's body and extremities are touched to assess for coolness or warmth. The infant is also assessed for physiologic signs of **cold stress.** The stronger, more mature infant responds by increased physical activity and crying. In other infants, respiratory rate often increases. Color changes may be noted in any infant. These include deepening acrocyanosis, appearance of generalized cyanosis, and mottling of the skin (cutis marmorata) (Plate 18). In a male with descended testes, the cremasteric reflex is activated; that is, on exposure to cold, the testes are pulled up into the inguinal canal.

The sigmoid colon bends at a right angle to itself at a depth of 3 cm. Inserting a rectal thermometer to a depth of less than 5 cm (2 in) will not accurately reflect core temperature (Fanaroff, Martin, 1992; Merenstein, Gardner, 1989). Insertion of the thermometer to 5 cm to obtain an accurate reading risks perforation of the rectum. Rectal perforation carries a mortality of approximately 70% in reported cases (Merenstein, Gardner, 1989). Therefore routine use of a glass rectal thermometer or an electronic probe is contraindicated for the neonate, even after rectal patency has been demonstrated.

NURSING DIAGNOSES

Nursing diagnoses related to thermoregulation include the following:

- Ineffective thermoregulation related to
  - —Immaturity
  - —Poorly controlled environment (temperature of room, equipment, warmer, or Isolette; location of warmer, Isolette, or bassinet)
- High risk for apnea, hypoglycemia, and/or acidosis related to
  - —Cold stress

PLANNING

During the important planning step, *goals* are prioritized and stated in client-centered terms. Whenever possible, the parents are included in this process. Nursing actions are selected so that the infant will be able to meet these goals:

- Maintain skin temperature between 97° to 98° F (36.1° and 36.7° C) (for discussion of thermoneutral environment, see Chapter 21)
- Keep free from the sequelae of cold stress (sclerema, oxygen deprivation to tissues, metabolic acidosis, hypoglycemia, abnormal blood gas values, and CNS dysfunction)
- Keep free from apneic episodes
- Minimize initial weight loss, and then gain weight appropriately

IMPLEMENTATION

Nursing care is implemented to prevent or minimize cold stress. The first action a nurse takes to support thermoregulation is quickly drying the infant with a prewarmed, absorbent blanket, taking particular care to dry and cover the head (21% of the infant's total surface area). Then the damp blanket is removed from contact with the infant. To help maintain the newborn's temperature, the infant is placed skin-to-skin with the mother (see p. 1108 for further discussion). The nurse helps protect the infant from cold air blowing directly over the face inasmuch as receptors in facial skin are extremely sensitive to cold.

When assessments or interventions are necessary, the unwrapped infant is placed in a prewarmed incubator with a servocontrol mechanism, in a radiant warmer, or on a warm surface. The infant's head is kept covered with a hooded blanket or a cap. The use of stockinette caps is discouraged because they do not prevent heat loss (Greer, 1988). A layer of plastic wrap can help protect against drafts while the infant is under a radiant heat source (Fig. 36-6). All surfaces and materials that touch the infant must be warm, including the nurse's hands. Oxygen and air are warmed before they are administered to the neonate.

Warmers and incubators are maintained in operative condition. The nurse understands how to operate the equipment (warmers and incubators) used within the particular facility. This equipment is assessed for function and then prewarmed before it is used for an infant. If an incubator is used, portholes are kept closed. Warmers and incubators are kept away from windows, fans, and air-conditioning units (sources of drafts, heat, and cold).

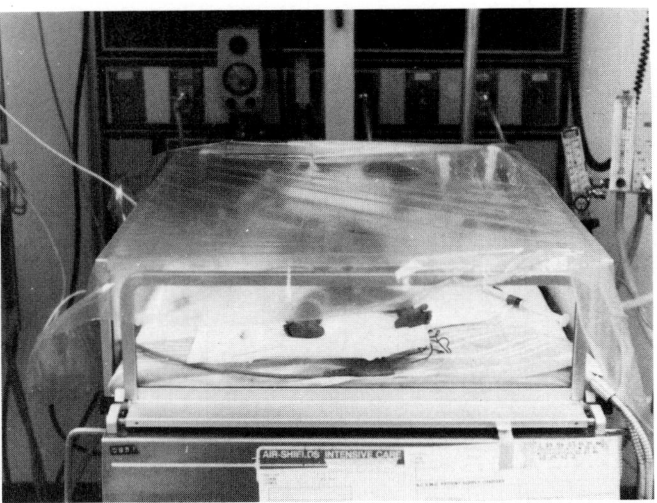

Fig. 36-6 Infant under plastic wrap to ensure a draft-free environment.
Photograph by Anne Kunke, San Jose, Calif.; from Whaley LF, Wong DL: *Nursing care of infants and children*, ed 4, St Louis, 1991, Mosby–Year Book.

The nurse sets the thermostat of the radiant warmer or incubator with servocontrol mechanism and applies the probe to the anterior portion of the abdomen. The probe is reapplied if it becomes wet or detached. Periodically the infant's axillary temperature is assessed and compared with the reading on the display panel. Both the axillary and display panel temperature readings are documented. Abdominal skin temperatures are maintained between 97° to 98° F (36.1° and 36.7° C), and axillary temperature is maintained at 97.7° F (36.5° C). Any rise in temperature above 99° F (37.3° C) or drop below 96.7° F (35.9° C) is reported. The nurse modifies the environment (clothes, blankets, thermostat settings) to return the infant to the desired body temperature.

Warming the Hypothermic Infant

Rapid changes in body temperature may cause apnea and acidosis in the neonate. Therefore the warming process occurs over 2 to 4 hours.* The nurse places the infant in an incubator with a servocontrol mechanism and sets the thermostat at 2° F (1.2° C) above skin temperature, even if the skin temperature is lower than normal. The thermistor probe is taped to the skin of the right upper quadrant of the anterior abdomen. When the skin temperature reaches the predetermined temperature, the incubator temperature is reset. The process is repeated until a skin temperature of 97.7° F (36.5° C) is achieved.

Weaning the Infant from the Incubator

The incubator weaning process is accomplished slowly over a period of hours or days. The nurse assists the infant through the following measures: (1) the infant is dressed in a diaper and shirt; (2) the incubator temperature is lowered, and the temperature readings of both the infant and incubator are recorded; and (3) the infant's response is assessed. This procedure is repeated until the incubator temperature equals the room temperature and the infant's skin temperature is 97.7° F (36.5° C). Then the infant is wrapped in a blanket, the incubator port-

*Rapid warming is elected by some authors (e.g., Kaplan, Eidelman, 1984).

holes are opened, and the infant's response is reassessed. The infant can be placed in an open bassinet if the axillary temperature is adequate.

EVALUATION

The nurse can be reasonably assured that care of the infant was effective if the goals have been met.

- The infant's skin temperature is maintained between 97° to 98° F (36.1° and 36.7° C).
- The infant is free from sequelae of cold stress.
- The infant does not experience apneic episodes.
- The infant's initial weight loss is minimal, and then the infant begins to gain weight.

NUTRITION AND ELIMINATION

Within the category of infants labeled high-risk, low-birth-weight newborns compose the largest subgroup. Of the low-birth-weight infants, one third are small for gestational age (SGA), and two thirds are preterm and appropriate for gestational age (AGA). SGA newborns also may be preterm.

Fulfilling the nutritional needs of high-risk infants is an important aspect of care. The infant's immediate and long-term status depends on nutrition. Effectively meeting the infant's individualized nutritional requirements will provide for growth and healing. For example, the SGA infant's glycogen stores are inadequate. Symptomatic or asymptomatic hypoglycemia may result if this infant is without nourishment for an extended time. Left untreated, hypoglycemia may cause serious damage to carbohydrate-dependent brain cells (see Chapter 37).

Providing enteral (via gastrointestinal route) nourishment to the high-risk infant is not always possible. Early enteral feeding for the infant with a low Apgar score is avoided. This is associated with the development of necrotizing enterocolitis (NEC) in the asphyxiated neonate (see Chapter 37). For this reason, many high-risk infants are initially maintained on parenteral nutrition.

Caloric, nutrient, and fluid requirements of the infant at risk may be greater than those of the term, normal newborn for many reasons. Preterm or dysmature (malnourished) newborns often have limited stores of nutrients and fluids. Further depletion of stores can occur as a result of one or a combination of the following factors:

- Birth asphyxia
- Increased respirations or respiratory effort
- Insensible fluid loss by evaporation (with radiant heat or phototherapy)
- Hypothermic environment
- Vomiting, diarrhea, and dysfunctional absorption from the gastrointestinal tract
- Growth demands (i.e., preterm newborn's growth rate approximates that of fetal growth during the last trimester, at least two times that of a term infant after birth)

Additional losses occur as a result of the inability of the renal system to concentrate urine and maintain an adequate rate of urea excretion, as well as by an inadequate response to antidiuretic hormone.

ASSESSMENT

General Observations

Weight is measured and recorded daily. Weight loss or rate of weight gain is calculated. Oral feedings are provided when possible. Documentation of feedings includes the following:

1. Type of feeding (breast or bottle)
2. Qualitative evaluation of suckling—strength and duration
3. Amount of breast milk or formula taken (if bottle-fed, record number of calories per 30 mL)
4. Presence of cyanosis (circumoral or general)
5. Presence of abdominal distention (Fig. 36-7) (record the time, degree, and effect on respirations)
6. Occurrence of vomiting or regurgitation (record

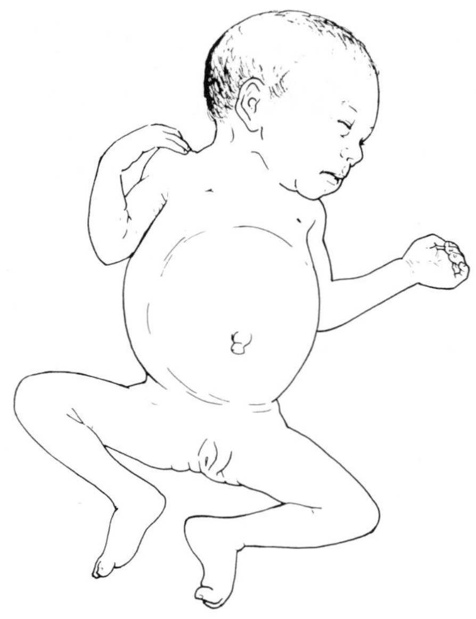

Fig. 36-7 Sudden abdominal distention.
Courtesy Ross Laboratories, Columbus, Ohio.

the color, amount, time in relation to feeding, character [forcefulness or associated with a burp], and presence of mucus in vomitus)
7. Time required for feeding

If feeding is done by gavage, the amount of residual feeding is assessed (undigested or partially digested breast milk or formula) by aspirating the stomach contents before initiating the feeding. After the gavage procedure, the following factors are recorded: (1) amount and quality of residual (presence of undigested feeding or mucus), (2) the size of the feeding tube, (3) the route of tube insertion (orogastric or nasogastric), (4) the amount of breast milk or formula given, and (5) the presence of cyanosis, distention, or vomiting.

Regardless of birth weight, the neurologic or physical status of the infant may prevent enteral feedings. Parenteral fluids and nutrients, including **total parenteral nutrition (TPN),** are provided for the infant who is unable to suck because of either developmental reasons (lack of coordinated suck and swallow reflex) or respiratory problems (on mechanical ventilation), as well as to help prevent NEC in the asphyxiated neonate.

TPN is ordered by the physician per hospital protocols. TPN orders must specify the desired electrolytes and nutrients per milliliter, as well as the milliliters of fluid per kilogram of body weight per hour (rate of infusion). The nurse assesses the type of fluids being given, rate per minute, and the infusion site. The care used in starting the infusion, the subsequent nursing care, and the contents of the infusate are factors in determining how long each infusion site will be used (Fanaroff, Martin, 1992).

Nourishment Types and Schedules

The formula type and feeding schedule of the infant at risk are based on the assessment of the following:

- Infant's birth weight
- Pattern of weight gain or loss
- Estimated gestational age (presence or absence of pharyngeal coordination or suck and swallow reflex is assessed for all infants ≤36 weeks—normally present at 32 to 34 weeks' gestation [Fanaroff, Martin, 1992])
- Physical condition (presence or absence of bowel sounds, abdominal distention, or bloody stools [Zeimer, George, 1990]; strength of suckle; presence and degree of respiratory distress and/or apneic episodes, if any; residual from previous feeding, if being fed by gavage)
- Fatigability
- Malformations
- Renal function
- Laboratory values (nitrogen balance, electrolyte balance, glucose, serum bilirubin)

Depending on the results of this assessment, the mode of feeding (breast, bottle, gavage, parenteral), the volume, and the type of formula (number of calories per milliliter and nutrient mix) are adjusted. Whether fed by breast, bottle, gavage, or total parenteral nutrition, the infant is evaluated for tolerance of the solute and fluid load.

Elimination patterns are assessed. Frequency of urination, as well as amount, color, and specific gravity are monitored. The amount, frequency, and character of stools are assessed. The infant's bowel movements are assessed, and the following are documented: constipation, diarrhea, loss of fats (steatorrhea), guaiac test results, and pH.

Weight and Fluid Loss and Gain

As much as 80% to 85% of the preterm infant's (28 to 34 weeks) body weight consists of water as compared with 70% in the term infant. Most of this water occupies the extracellular fluid compartment. Greater fluid demands to meet increased cellular metabolic processes (e.g., from stress, repair, or growth) predispose the newborn to weight and fluid losses. Even with the early fluid and nutrition intake, the preterm infant's weight and fluid losses seem exaggerated. Inadequate fluid intake (by delayed administration or insufficient volume) contributes to the preterm infant's weight and fluid losses.

Insensible water loss (IWL) represents evaporative losses that occur largely through the skin. Approximately 30% of this IWL is from the respiratory tract, and most of this is prevented by humidified oxygen-enriched gases that are used for respiratory support in sick infants. Total IWL ranges anywhere from 1.75 to 3.6 mL/kg/hr. The quantity is influenced by gestational age, postpartum age, weight, use of radiant warmer or incubator, and other factors.

The limits of acceptable weight loss are as follows. During the neonate's first 3 days of extrauterine life, the preterm infant can lose up to 12% of birth weight. For the term, AGA infant, a weight loss of up to 10% is acceptable. Weight loss of up to 15% is acceptable for infants weighing 4500 g (9 lb 14 oz) or more. For dysmature SGA infants a loss of up to 5% is acceptable.

After the first 3 days, a preterm newborn's loss or gain during each 24-hour period should not exceed 2% of the previous day's weight.

The following examples illustrate how to calculate weight loss and gain:

EXAMPLE 1

Day 4 1750 g
Day 5 1730 g
20 g loss

$$\frac{20}{1750} = \frac{x\%}{100\%}$$

$$1750x = 2000$$

$$1750\overline{)2000.00}\ \text{quotient } 1.1$$

$$x = 1.1\%\ \text{weight loss}$$

EXAMPLE 2

Day 4 1750 g
Day 5 1790 g
40 g gain

$$\frac{40}{1750} = \frac{x\%}{100\%}$$

$$1750x = 4000$$

$$1750\overline{)4000.00}\ \text{quotient } 2.3$$

$$x = 2.3\%\ \text{weight gain}$$

If a weight loss is calculated, the nurse investigates and assesses for the following: increased stooling and/or voiding, increased evaporative losses, inadequate volume or incorrect fluid administration, and problems of malabsorption. The nurse reports and records these findings and continues to assess the infant by (1) blood glucose determinations, (2) increased frequency of infant and incubator temperature assessments, (3) monitoring fluid administration (volume and type), (4) urine output, and (5) specific gravity determination.

If a weight gain is calculated, the nurse investigates and assesses for overfeeding or fluid retention. The nurse reports and records these findings and continues to assess the infant by (1) blood glucose determinations, (2) fluid administration monitoring (volume and type), (3) urine output, and (4) specific gravity determination.

NURSING DIAGNOSES

Examples of nursing diagnoses related to nutrition and elimination include the following:

- Altered nutrition, less than body requirements, related to
  —Dysmaturity
- Fluid volume deficit or overload related to
  —Immaturity or neonatal disorder
- Ineffective breathing pattern related to
  —Sudden abdominal distention

PLANNING

During the important planning step, goals are set in client-centered terms. Parents are encouraged to be involved to the extent to which they feel ready. Goals are prioritized, and nursing actions selected to meet these goals.

The infant will achieve the following goals:

1. Maintain adequate nutrition (nutrients, fluids, and electrolytes) without experiencing
   a. respiratory distress
   b. hypoglycemia
   c. abdominal distention
   d. trauma to the tissues of the gastrointestinal tract, constipation, or diarrhea
2. Have need for nonnutritive sucking fulfilled
3. Receive adequate feedings to provide for
   a. metabolic requirements
   b. sufficient energy to perform physical activity
   c. losses through gastrointestinal and urinary tracts
   d. growth and maintenance of a consistent pattern of weight gain

The parents will achieve the following goals:

1. Begin to participate in the feeding process as appropriate for the infant's and parents' capabilities
2. By discharge, independently demonstrate the feeding method appropriate for the particular infant (breast, bottle, gavage, or gastrostomy)

IMPLEMENTATION

Oral Feeding

For the infant with adequate strength and gastrointestinal function, the nurse attempts to provide the prescribed nourishment by the oral route. Oral feedings are initiated with sterile water. Breast milk or formula may be fed by nipple, intermittent gavage, or by continuous flow with a pump and feeding tube (inserted into the stomach or jejunum). If the infant is able to breast-feed, the nurse assists the mother, providing support and help, as necessary. Throughout the feeding (breast, bottle, or gavage), the newborn is observed to assess how the procedure is tolerated.

The use of breast milk or formula and the type of artificial nipple selected are specific to the needs of the infant. The physician orders the quantity of breast milk or type of formula in terms of the nutritional needs of the infant. The different types of commercial formula vary in calories, protein, and mineral content (see Chapter 22). The type of nipple selected ("preemie," regular, orthodontic) depends on the infant's ability to master the specific type of nipple and a consideration of the energy resources the infant can expend on the process.

Gavage Feeding

Gavage feeding is a method of providing nourishment to the infant who is (1) compromised by respiratory distress, (2) too immature to have a coordinated suck and swallow reflex, or (3) easily fatigued by suckling (Fig. 36-8). With gavage feeding, breast milk or formula is given to the infant by way of a nasogastric tube. This spares the infant the work of suckling. Gavage feeding can be done with an intermittently placed tube, or continuously with an indwelling catheter. The formula may be supplied intermittently by syringe, with gravity-controlled flow, or continuously via infusion pump.

The nasogastric or orogastric route can be used to place the gavage feeding tube. The orogastric route is preferred because most infants are preferential nose breathers. However, some infants do not tolerate this tube placement. In these cases, use of a small nasogastric feeding tube can help provide nutrition for an infant who would otherwise gag or vomit or for one who is learning to suckle during the gavage feeding (Merenstein, Gardner, 1989).

To determine the necessary length of the gavage tube, the tip is placed at the corner of the infant's mouth or the tip of the nose, extended to the lobe of the ear, then down to either the tip of the xiphoid process or halfway between the xiphoid process and the umbilicus (Fig. 36-8, *A*). This length is marked with a piece of tape or by noting the corresponding black mark on the feeding tube. The tube is then lubricated with sterile water and inserted gently (to avoid tissue trauma) through the mouth (or nare) (Fig. 36-8, *B*). The tube is guided down the esophagus until the predetermined mark is reached.

The correct placement of the tube is assessed before instillation of any fluid. Two techniques are used. In the first, a small amount of air (0.5 to 1 mL in preterm or very small infants) is injected into the tube with a syringe while the nurse simultaneously listens with a stethoscope over the stomach area. Sounds of gurgling or growling will be heard if the tube is properly situated in the stomach. However, it is possible to hear the air entering the stomach even when the tube is positioned above the gastroesophageal (cardiac) sphincter (Metheny et al, 1990; Whaley, Wong, 1991). The nurse pulls back on the plunger to aspirate stomach contents, which indicates proper placement. However, aspiration of respiratory secretions may be mistaken for stomach contents. In addition, absence of fluid is not necessarily evidence of improper placement. The stomach may be empty, or the tube may not be in contact with stomach contents. Incorrect placement can leave the tube in the trachea (infant usually will gag, cough, or become cyanotic) or in the esophagus rather than the stomach. Correct tube placement in the stomach is also verified by syringe aspiration of stomach contents (previous feeding or mucus) (Weibley et al,

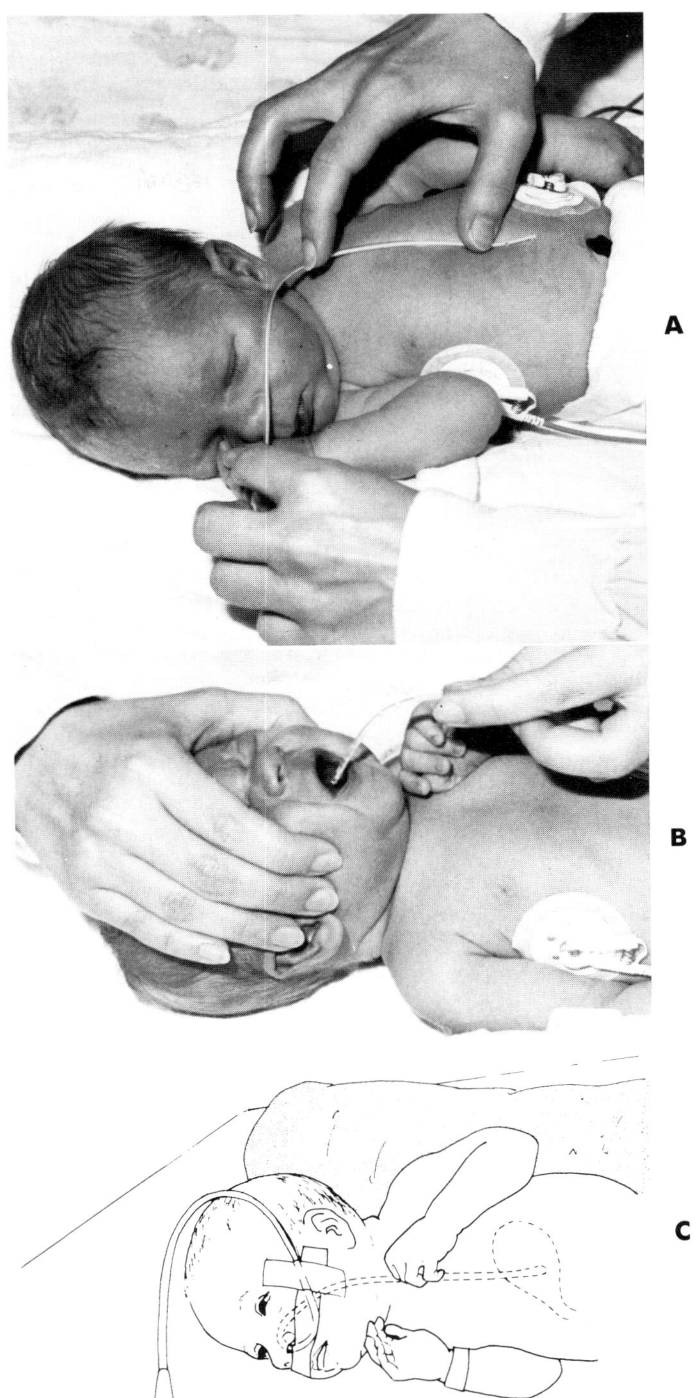

Fig. 36-8 Gavage feeding. **A,** Measurement for gavage feeding from tip of nose to earlobe and to midpoint between end of xiphoid process and umbilicus. Adhesive tape may be used to mark the correct length on the tube. **B,** Insertion of gavage tube using orogastric route. **C,** Indwelling gavage tube, nasogastric route. After feeding by orogastric or nasogastric tube, infant is propped on right side for 1 hour to facilitate emptying of stomach into small intestine. Note rolled towel for support. (See also Fig. 21-2.)

1987; Metheny et al, 1990). This aspiration is completed gently while the tube is rotated to avoid trauma to the gastric mucosa (Merenstein, Gardner, 1989). Once correct placement is determined, the tube is taped in place. The tube is stabilized by holding or taping it to the cheek, not to the forehead, because of possible damage to the nostril* (Fig. 36-8, C) (Whaley, Wong, 1991).

To begin the feeding, the nurse removes the plunger of a 30-mL syringe and connects this to the gavage tube. While crimping the feeding tube, the nurse pours the specified amount of breast milk or formula into the barrel of the syringe. The nurse then releases the crimp in the tube and allows the feeding to flow by gravity (the higher the syringe, the faster the rate of flow). The infant usually will tolerate the feeding better if the rate approximates that of an oral feeding (about 1 mL/min).

*Adhesive tape is best removed by applying a water-soaked cotton ball to the tape, then lifting the tape *carefully* while applying pressure on the skin directly beneath the tape.

Overfeeding of the high-risk neonate is avoided. Overfeeding can lead to distention, with apnea, or to vomiting, with subsequent aspiration. Assessment for overfeeding is performed by measuring the residual gastric aspirate before the feeding is initiated. If residual contents are present, the residual is refed to the infant and that volume is subtracted from the feeding.

When the prescribed volume has been delivered, the nurse crimps or pinches the tube and removes the syringe. The gavage tube is capped (or the nurse continues to pinch it) and removed in one steady motion. Capping the tube (or pinching it off) prevents breast milk or formula from leaking from the tube and being aspirated during removal of the tube.

After the feeding the infant is burped and positioned to avoid aspiration should vomiting occur. Documentation of the procedure includes (1) amount and quality of residual (from previous feeding), (2) size of feeding tube, (3) type and quantity of fluid provided (sterile water, breast milk, or formula), and (4) infant's response to the procedure.

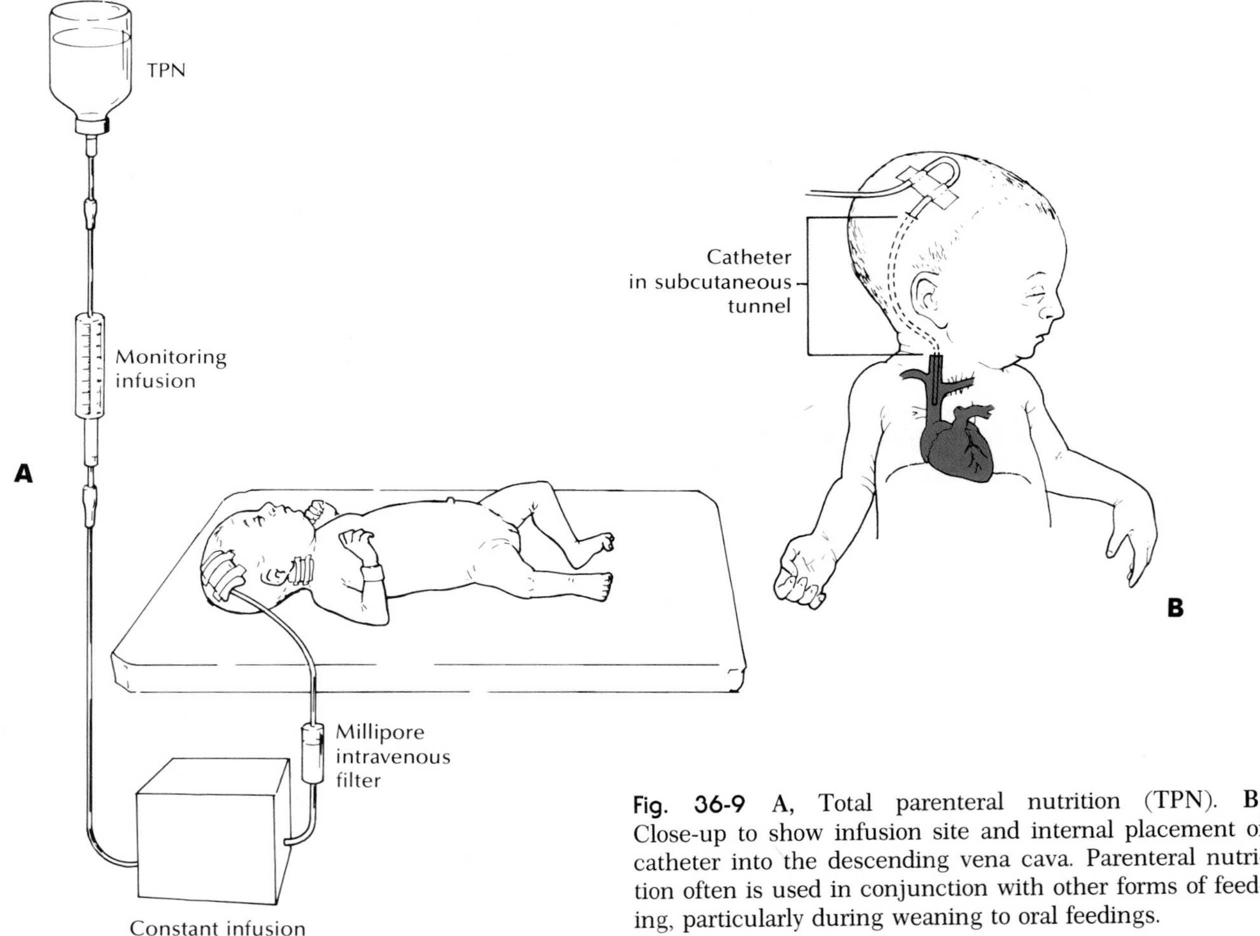

Fig. 36-9 **A,** Total parenteral nutrition (TPN). **B,** Close-up to show infusion site and internal placement of catheter into the descending vena cava. Parenteral nutrition often is used in conjunction with other forms of feeding, particularly during weaning to oral feedings.

Parenteral Fluids and Nutrition

Supplemental parenteral fluids are indicated for the infant who is unable to obtain sufficient fluids or calories by oral or gavage feeding (Fig. 36-9). On the other hand, TPN is indicated for the infant who (1) requires mechanical ventilation, (2) requires surgical repair for gastrointestinal anomalies or obstruction, (3) suffers from chronic diarrhea, (4) has malabsorption syndrome, or (5) is unable to receive any nutrition by the oral or gavage routes.

For the infant receiving parenteral fluids or TPN, the nurse assesses and documents the following: (1) type and infusion rate of solution, (2) functional status of infusion equipment, including tubing and infusion pump (double-checks rate with visual count of drop rate), (3) condition of infusion site, and (4) the infant's responses.

While caring for the infant receiving parenteral fluids or TPN, the nurse secures and protects the insertion site (Fig. 36-10), following the principles of asepsis and inspects the infusion site for signs of infiltration (Fig. 36-11). The nurse repositions the infant frequently (every 2 to 4 hours) to maintain body alignment and protect the infusion site.

Nonnutritive Sucking

If the infant is nourished via the gavage or the parenteral route, **nonnutritive sucking** is encouraged. Allowing the infant to suckle on a pacifier during gavage or between oral feedings results in improved oxygenation, decreased energy expenditure with less restlessness, and faster attachment to the nipple when oral feedings are initiated (Gill et al, 1988).

Advancing Infant Feedings

On the basis of the assessment data collected by the nurse, as the infant's weight gain and physical condition improve, the physician will order the advanced feeding. From the infant's perspective, feedings are advanced from passive (parenteral and gavage) to active (nipple and breast-feeding).

The infant is gradually weaned off parenteral nutrition. On the basis of the infant's tolerance, nourishment given by gavage is increased while parenteral fluids and nutrients are decreased. From gavage feedings the infant progresses to bottle-feeding, breast milk, or formula. As the infant is increasingly able to suckle breast milk or formula, the amount of fluid fed by gavage is decreased. Often during this transition the infant is provided nourishment by both nipple and gavage feeding to ensure receipt of the prescribed volume and nutrient intake. For the formula-fed infant, oral feedings can be further advanced by increasing the number of calories per 30 mL (maximum of 24 calories per 30 mL).

For infants weighing less than 1800 g (4 lb), feedings are advanced very slowly and with caution. If feedings are advanced too rapidly, the infant may experience vomiting (with risk of aspiration), diarrhea, abdominal distention (especially with residual vol-

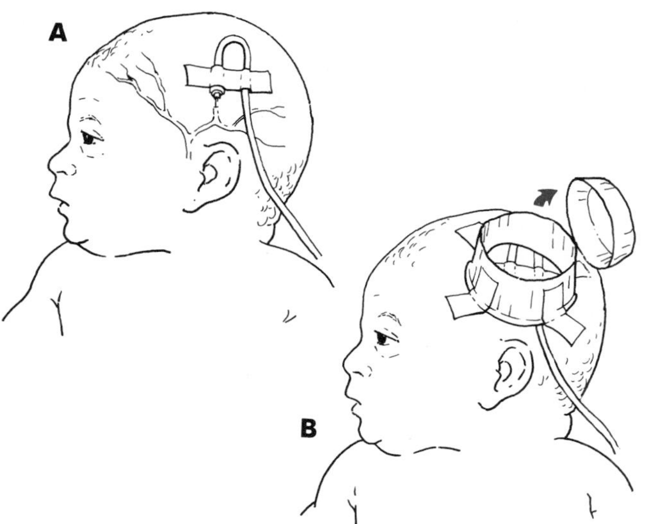

Fig. 36-10 A, Venipuncture of scalp vein. B, Paper cup protecting venipuncture site.

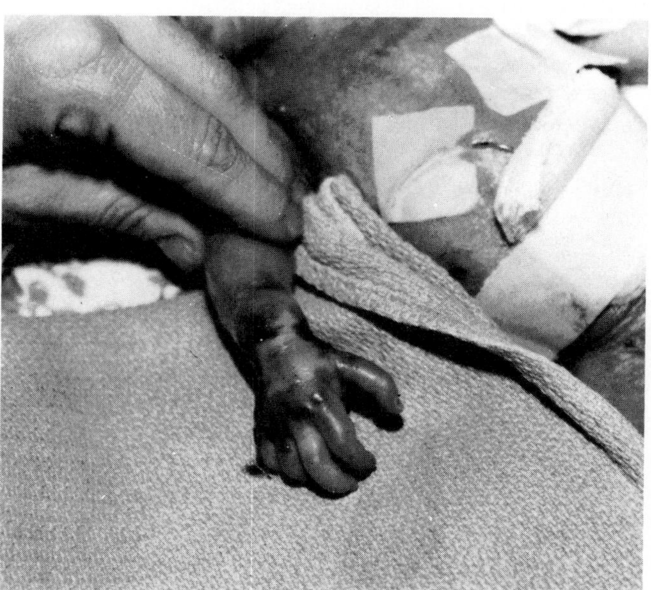

Fig. 36-11 Intravenous infiltration in small infant can cause severe ischemia.
Courtesy Mount Zion Hospital and Medical Center, San Francisco, Calif.

ume >2 mL), and apneic episodes. In the high-risk infant, rapid advancement of feedings may cause fluid retention with cardiac embarrassment or pronounced diuresis with resultant hyponatremia.

To the degree they are ready and able, the nurse involves the parents in meeting the nutritional needs of the infant. As the time of discharge nears, the parents are instructed in the appropriate method of feeding, as well as the assessments pertaining to that method (e.g., tolerance of feedings, gavage tube placement).

Feeding the Newborn with Cleft Lip and Palate

The baby born with a cleft lip and palate may be normal in every other way. Surgical repair on the lip usually is performed soon after birth if possible to assist parents in the attachment process with their newborn. The palate usually is repaired some months later (see discussion, Chapter 38). The nurse may be called to feed the newborn during the early neonatal period or to teach the parent to do so.

Feeding the infant offers a special challenge to nurses, and the process is often time-consuming and laborious. Aspiration is one of the major concerns. Feeding with breast milk is far less dangerous if aspirated than if formula is used. Clefts of lip or palate reduce the infant's ability to suck, which interferes with compression of the areola or nipple and usually renders both breast-feeding and formula-feeding difficult. Liquid taken into the mouth has a tendency to escape via the cleft through the nose. Feeding usually is best accomplished with the infant's head in an upright position, either held in the nurse's hand or cradled in the arm (Whaley, Wong, 1991).

The type of feeding equipment and rate of feeding must be individualized for each infant. Normal nipples often are unsuitable for these infants, who are unable to generate the suction required; therefore special nipples or other feeding devices are needed. These nipples either cover the defect or carry the fluid beyond the defect (Fig. 36-12).

Because of their difficulty generating suction and occluding the oral cavity, these infants have a tendency to swallow more air than do infants with normal oral cavities. Consequently, the infant must be fed slowly and burped more frequently and may require more frequent feedings.

During the feeding the nurse or parent should interact with the infant, talking and making eye contact. Interaction is needed to stimulate psychosocial development in the infant and to facilitate bonding and attachment. The nurse who provides a role model for this behavior may facilitate the parent's acceptance of the newborn with this developmental defect.

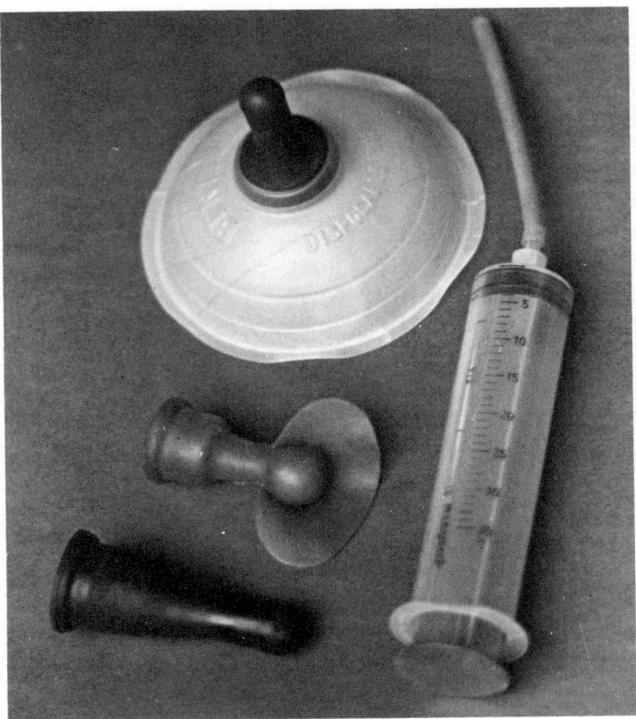

Fig. 36-12 Some devices used to feed infant with cleft palate. *Clockwise,* Lamb's nipple, flanged nipple, special nurser, and syringe with rubber tubing (Breck feeder). From Whaley LF, Wong, DL: *Essentials of pediatric nursing,* ed 4, St Louis, 1993, Mosby–Year Book.

Feedings that extend beyond 20 to 30 minutes can deplete the infant's energy (Curtin, 1990). When the infant has trouble with nipple feeding, either a rubber-tipped medicine dropper, Asepto syringe, or Breck feeder often provides an efficient, safe feeding device. Gavage feedings may be needed occasionally to supplement oral feedings.

EVALUATION

The nurse can be reasonably assured that the care of the infant was effective if the goals for care have been met.

- The infant receives adequate nutrition (nutrients, fluids, and electrolytes) without experiencing respiratory distress, hypoglycemia, abdominal distention, trauma to the tissues of the gastrointestinal tract, constipation, or diarrhea.
- The infant's need for nonnutritive sucking is fulfilled.

- The infant receives adequate feedings to provide metabolic requirements and sufficient energy for physical activity, to counter losses through gastrointestinal and urinary tracts, and to supply constituents for growth to maintain a steady pattern of weight gain.
- The parents begin to participate in the feeding process as appropriate for the infant's and parents' capabilities.
- By discharge the parents are able to demonstrate independently the feeding method appropriate for the particular infant (breast, bottle, gavage, or gastrostomy).

EMOTIONAL ASPECTS OF CARE

Preterm, sick, and convalescent infants have at least the same emotional and developmental needs as the term infant. Events in the sick infant's life are distinctly different from those of the normal term infant. The experiences of the sick infant include "sensory deprivation of normal stimuli that the preterm infant would have experienced in the womb and that term babies would have experienced at home with their families" (Merenstein, Gardner, 1989). Compared with the normal term infant, the high-risk infant experiences physical distress related to procedures performed by the primary caregivers (e.g., venipunctures for intravenous therapy, nasogastric tube insertion for feedings, having electrodes taped to and removed from the skin, and heel-stick punctures for blood samples).

The infant's vision is altered by the oxygen hood, and the infant is bombarded by high levels of auditory input from the machinery providing oxygen and suction. In addition, the infant is unable to establish diurnal and nocturnal rhythms because of constant exposure to the bright overhead lights in the intensive care nursery. Given this life experience, particular attention must be paid to meeting the emotional and developmental needs of these infants.

Inadequate attention to emotional and developmental needs may cause the infant to develop signs of anxiety and tension, the result of being exposed to life-support measures while being separated from the constant presence of one mothering, comforting person. Cues of anxiety and tension in the neonate can include the following:

- Failure to thrive (slow or absent recovery, growth, or weight gain)
- Looking away from or to the side of the caregiver's face
- Absent, weak, or infrequent crying (as if to say, "What's the use?")

Sound

Infants in incubators are exposed to continuous noise levels of 50 to 86 decibels (dB), with frequent peaks that can reach and exceed levels of 90 to 100 dB. Each new piece of life-support equipment used can add 15 to 20 dB to the background noise. The American Academy of Pediatrics (AAP) Committee on Environmental Hazards has recommended that efforts be directed toward reducing noise levels to less than 70 dB in nurseries (Miller et al, 1974). Drugs commonly used for infants such as ethacrynic acid (Edecrin), furosemide (Lasix), and the aminoglycides streptomycin, kanamycin, neomycin, gentamicin, and tobramycin are known from animal studies to potentiate noise-induced hearing loss (Bergman et al, 1985).

Sounds, especially impact sounds, can cause some infants to become hypoxic as part of a startle response (Long et al, 1980). These sounds can be produced during care activities such as opening and closing incubator doors or can result when equipment alarms are activated. Noise can be reduced by asking personnel to provide care more quietly, to talk quietly, to play music quietly, and so on. One must assess the degree to which all of the beeping sounds from heart rate monitors are really helpful. Because low-pressure respirator alarms are especially loud, they can be silenced during airway suctioning and other care (Fanaroff, Martin, 1992).

Light

Lighting in nurseries, the colors used to paint walls, the decorations, and the windows are examples of environmental factors designed to suit the observational and psychologic needs of adults who provide infants with care and their parents and families. Daylight-simulating illumination helps caregivers observe color and other changes that occur in sick infants. However, it is not clear whether this type of illumination is otherwise beneficial or harmful to the infants. Recent data about high-intensity lighting suggest that a link exists between background nursery light levels and the occurrence of retinopathy of prematurity in preterm human infants (Glass et al, 1985). More research is needed to sort out these effects and to arrive at meaningful recommendations for nursery illumination.

Communication Patterns

Infants communicate their needs and ability to tolerate sensory stimulation (from their caregivers or the environment). For nurses and parents of these high-risk infants, knowledge of these cues is essential. Although the full-term infant may thrive on stimulation, the caregiver of the high-risk neonate understands that this same stimulation can cause the physical symptoms of stress and anxiety.

The infant who needs or wants attention demonstrates what Brazelton terms "care-eliciting behaviors" (Brazelton in Merenstein, Gardner, 1989). These behaviors that indicate **readiness for interaction** include crying, following the caregiver visually, and smiling. On the other hand, the infant who is overstimulated demonstrates withdrawal.

The infant experiencing overstimulation takes steps to decrease the intensity of the stimulation. **Cues of overstimulation** include a number of behaviors: the infant looks away from the face of the caregiver or may hiccough, gag, or regurgitate the feeding. The infant may exhibit the startle reflex or develop an irregular respiratory rate and an increased heart rate (Harris, Milford, 1986).

To limit unnecessary environmental stimulation to the neonate, caregivers can implement the following interventions.

- Swaddle and prop the infant in positions of comfort.
- Organize care of the infant to provide for extended periods of undisturbed rest/sleep.
- Place a "do not disturb" sign on the incubator as a reminder to provide the infant time to rest.
- Arrange a folded blanket over the incubator to provide a shield from the bright overhead lights and to muffle sound if items are set on the incubator (such as formula bottles, chart, other equipment).

Infant Stimulation

A sense of trust develops as the infant learns the feel, sound, and smell of the same parenting persons, who provide comfort (e.g., removes painful stimuli, including hunger and wet or soiled clothing). The infant soon learns that cries bring attention from the mothering person.

For the healthy, term infant, this parenting occurs at home by the same person(s). For the high-risk infant, hospital care cannot duplicate the home environment, but caregivers can provide the infant a modified parenting experience. In the technologic environment of the NCIU, the nursing focus should be on the infant first and the equipment second. The possibilities of developing an environment sensitive to the emotional and developmental needs of the high-risk neonate are limited only by the bounds of human creativity.

Infant stimulation must be individualized on the basis of the nurse's interpretation of the infant's cues and responses. When the neonate is ready for stimulation, the nurse has many options.

- Timing of treatments can be planned to provide tactile stimulation by stroking the infant's skin.
- As possible, the parents are encouraged to touch and hold the infant, even if it is only through the portholes.
- Mobiles and decals that can be changed frequently may be placed inside the incubator.
- The nurse responds to the infant's efforts to cry by offering reassurance, providing for nonnutritive sucking (offering a pacifier), stroking the infant's back, and talking to the infant.
- When the infant can tolerate being out of the incubator, even for short periods, the caregiver (nurse or parents), or both can cuddle, rock, sing to, and talk to the infant. These activities are beneficial especially during feedings (breast, bottle, gavage, or gastrostomy).
- As possible, the parent(s) hold the infant for burping after feedings.
- In the nursery, conversation and noise are kept as low as possible. Wind-up musical toys can be placed in the incubator.
- If the infant is fed by gavage or gastrostomy, nonnutritive sucking is encouraged (see p. 1105). This will help the infant associate this pleasant, self-gratifying, and self-initiated activity with the comforting feeling of a filling stomach.
- The newborn can be held *en face* with the caregiver (parent or nurse). Eye contact is maintained while the caregiver talks or sings to the infant.
- If the infant is receiving phototherapy, the protective eye patches are removed periodically when the lights have been turned off (e.g., during feeding) so the infant can see the caregiver's face for the short, comforting sessions.

In summary, infants respond to their environments. For the high-risk neonate, a stressful environment taxes the energy stores necessary for recovery and growth. The NICU environment can be modified to provide developmentally supportive care. To promote respiratory and feeding status, decrease morbidity, improve behavioral organization, and shorten hospitalization, nurses need to provide high-risk infants with care that (1) times interventions with the sleep/wake cycles of the infant, (2) limits light and noise levels, and (3) uses the infant's behavior during medical, nursing, or social interventions as cues for stress (Becker et al, 1991).

Skin-to-Skin or Kangaroo Care

In Western technologic societies, to help preterm infants maintain thermoregulation, external heat sources are used (e.g., incubators and radiant warmers). It is known that cold stress depletes stores of energy necessary for repair, maintenance, and growth. With this technologic approach to thermoregulation, these high-risk infants are separated from their mothers.

An alternative to technology and maternal-infant separation is skin-to-skin care, also called **kangaroo care.** That is, the infant, dressed only in a diaper, is placed directly onto the mother's bare chest and is then covered with the mother's clothing or a warmed blanket, or both (Fig. 36-13). In this upright, prone position, the mother's body temperature functions as an external heat source to support the infant's temperature regulation (Anderson, 1989).

Kangaroo care was originally developed in Bogota, Colombia, where radiant warmers and incubators were in severely short supply. The program using skin-to-skin care originated from severe economic problems but is based on a deep respect for natural processes. In this program, preterm infants in satisfactory condition, no matter how small, remain with the mother 24 hours a day.

Programs similar to the one developed in Colombia have now been developed in England, The Netherlands, and Sweden. Not surprisingly, infants treated with kangaroo care have dramatically positive outcomes. These infants maintain their temperatures and oxygenation levels, have fewer episodes of crying, apnea, and periodic respirations. These infants are alert and quiet longer (when positive parent-infant interactions with eye contact occurs) and have slightly higher heart rates (a good sign because bradycardia can be a concern). Hospital stay for these infants is shorter than for the infants treated with the traditional radiant warmer or incubator (Anderson, 1989).

Other positive results include a thermal synchrony (as infant's temperature decreases, mother's temperature increases). Mothers involved in skin-to-skin care (1) are more inclined to breast-feed than are other mothers, (2) develop a greater milk supply, and (3) breast-feed longer than mothers not involved in kangaroo care (Anderson, 1989). Infants receiving kangaroo care do not develop the "pathologic flat" head. In addition, the upright position decreases the risk of regurgitation and aspiration.

This "new" method of providing for the thermoregulation needs of the high-risk infant is becoming more accepted in Western health care. For parents and infants the positive research findings are numerous. These positive effects, combined with the decreased length of hospital stay, demonstrate that the use of this humanistic treatment method can be expanded within Western medical-nursing care.

ENVIRONMENTAL HAZARDS

Sound, light, and other stimulation may constitute environmental hazards for the sick newborn. Infants respond to stimulation not only socially but also with

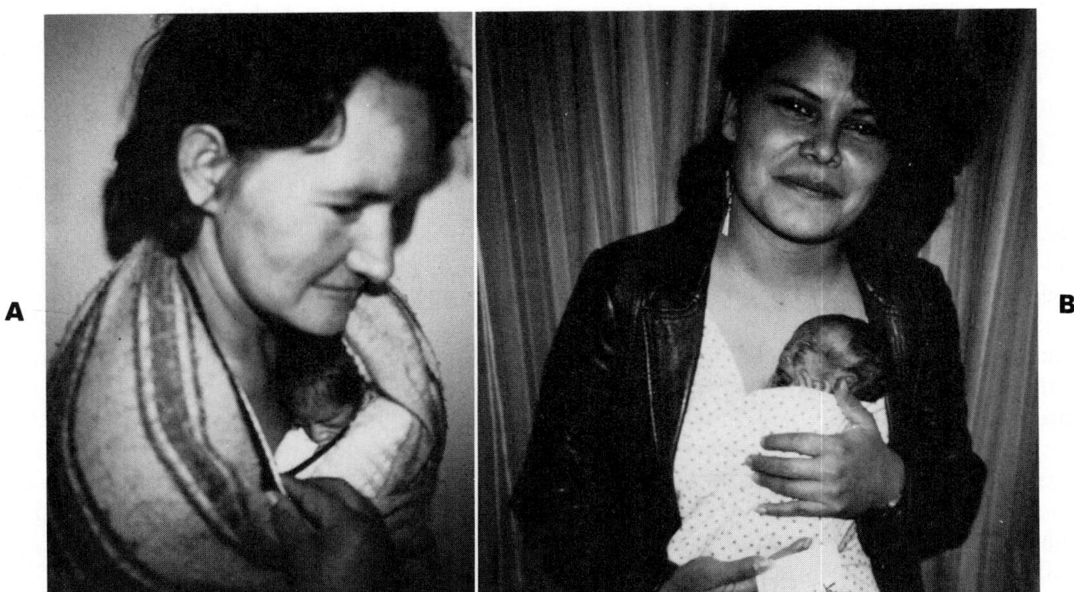

Fig. 36-13 The kangaroo method. **A,** Infant snuggled inside wrap. **B,** Infant inside mother's blouse in skin-to-skin contact (originally used in Bogota, Colombia, South America).
Courtesy Vivian Wahlberg, RN, CM, Dr Med Sc, Karolinska, Stockholm.

a variety of autonomic responses, some of which may be detrimental to the sick neonate. It is rare to analyze quantitatively the composition of nursery or incubator air. The report by Waffarn and Hodgman (1979), in which 18 of 42 infant incubators were found to contain detectable concentrations of mercury vapor, suggests that such studies may be appropriate.

Metal pipes and plastic tubing are used to deliver gases to an incubator, into a head hood, or directly into an infant's lungs. Because of soldered and glued joints, protectively coated surfaces, and other sources of contamination, the air can contain oils, lead, cadmium, bismuth, mercury, and various other residues of organic and metallic salts (Hamel et al, 1976). The gases can also contain microorganisms. Many of these contaminants can be eliminated by using appropriate filters. However, the success of any filtering system must be confirmed by laboratory testing.

As more studies are generated to evaluate the health impact of radiation, ultraviolet light, microwaves, and other environmental agents, the specific susceptibility of infants to these potential hazards should be considered in research designs. The lack of existing awareness that radiation may be a hazard is suggested each time an infant's pelvis is included in a roentgenographic field when only a chest film is ordered. It also is seen whenever a portable roentgenogram is taken in a nursery and the adults, concerned about their own exposure, step out of the range of the x-ray unit or shield themselves with protective lead aprons while not preventing possible exposure of the naked infant in the next incubator. More data are needed about potential environmental hazards in the nursery (Fanaroff, Martin, 1992).

■ DISCHARGE PLANNING

Discharge planning for the high-risk infant begins on admission to the NICU. The goals for nursing and medical care include meeting the criteria for discharge. These criteria include "adequate weight gain, adequate caloric intake, thermal stability in an open crib, and cardiorespiratory stability with controlled or resolved apnea" (Damato, 1991).

Throughout hospitalization the discharge planning nurse gathers information from all of the health care team members: the family, primary nurses, physicians, social services. This information will determine the infant's and family's preparedness for discharge.

As the care-learning needs of the infant's parents are assessed, steps are taken to eliminate knowledge deficits. As necessary, information is provided about infant care, especially in relation to the particular infant's needs (e.g., gavage or gastrostomy feeding, use of oxygen or suction). Parent education includes opportunities for parents to provide return demonstration of their increasingly independent skills in caring for their infant. Instruction in infant cardiopulmonary resuscitation (CPR) is provided before discharge.

Referrals for appropriate resources are made before discharge. Social service involvement is especially important for young or psychosocially high-risk parents (those with substance abuse, mental illness). Social services can provide parents information regarding financial assistance (Aid to Families with Dependent Children, Medicaid, Crippled Children's Program, Social Security Disability).

Parents are referred to appropriate programs for infants with special problems (Down syndrome, spina bifida, or cerebral palsy). Parents are referred to community resources for assistance with special medical needs (gavage feedings, tracheostomy or colostomy care, oxygen). Referrals are made for home care nurse/home health assistance as appropriate (some medical insurance covers these services). These health care providers can provide actual nursing activities, as well as some relief from the emotional burden of caring for an infant with medical problems. Some hospitals offer programs for infant stimulation and development to which parents and infants are referred as necessary.

The discharge planning nurse can develop a current directory of special programs and social, community, and funding resources for parents of high-risk infants. Although the parent may not perceive the need for the resources at the time of discharge, the telephone numbers can be saved for use later.

■ TRANSPORT TO A REGIONAL CENTER

When hospitals are not equipped to care for the mother and fetus or newborn at high risk, transfer to a specialized perinatal or tertiary care center is arranged. If the birth of a compromised neonate is anticipated, maternal transport is arranged. Ideally, this transport occurs with the fetus in utero. This has two distinct advantages: (1) mother-infant attachment is facilitated (separation is avoided) and (2) neonatal morbidity and mortality are decreased. For a variety of reasons it is not always possible to transport the mother before the birth (e.g., imminent birth and lack of prior diagnosis). Therefore it is necessary for physicians and nurses to have the necessary skills and equipment for accurate diagnosis and emergency intervention to stabilize the client's physical condition and to maintain it until transport can be carried out. (For discussion of surgical emergencies of the newborn, see Chapter 38; for specific maternal conditions, see Index.)

Parents of infants who have been transported to regional centers need special support. The birth of a compromised infant, especially one that needs transport to a regional center, causes extreme parental stress. The parents often are grieving the loss of the anticipated birth of the ideal infant. They are fearful of the possible eventual outcomes for the infant. Parents will require a great deal of support as they deal with the technologic world in which they find themselves and their infant. With the infant attached to "high-tech" equipment with wires and tubes, it is sometimes difficult for the parents to actually see the infant.

Before transport to the regional care center, high-risk infants are stabilized. Attention is given to the following basic areas (Sandman, 1989):

- Thermoregulation
- Oxygen/ventilation needs
- Acid-base balance
- Fluid needs
- Glucose needs
- Vital signs

During transport to a regional perinatal center, the following general categories of supplies, equipment, and medications should be available.*

MATERNAL AND FETAL/NEONATAL NEEDS

- Oxygen and equipment for maintaining a clear airway and supporting adequate gas exchange
- Intravenous equipment and solutions for meeting hydration needs, for administering medications, for transfusion of blood or blood products, and for obtaining blood samples
- Equipment for monitoring vital signs and blood pressure
- Blood-drawing supplies
- Supplemental source of electricity

ADDITIONAL MATERNAL SUPPLIES

- Stretcher with approved restraints or safety belts; linen
- Eclampsia tray: supplies, medications, and equipment
- Delivery pack
- Electronic fetal monitor

*Carefully outlined and specific guidelines are provided in NAACOG-OGN Nursing Practice Resource: *Maternal-neonatal transport*, No 8, June 1983. (The Nurses Association of the American College of Obstetricians and Gynecologists, 409 Twelfth Street, SW, Washington, DC, 20024-2191, 202/638-0026.)

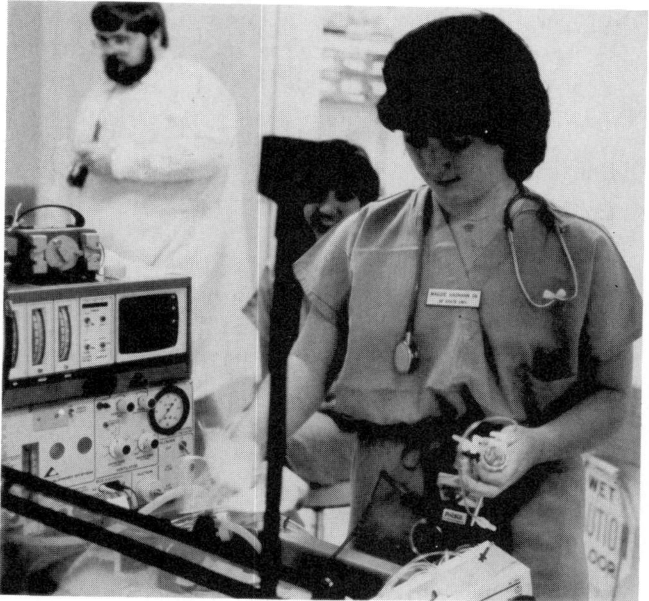

Fig. 36-14 Preparing a total life support system for transport of compromised newborns to regional center for postpartum care.

ADDITIONAL SUPPLIES FOR NEONATE NEWBORN

- Transport unit with total life support and monitoring capacity (Fig. 36-14)
- Thoracotomy tray and thoracentesis set

A FAMILY'S GRIEF

Anticipatory Grief

Anticipatory grief has been defined as the anticipation of a future loss (Fulton, Gottesman, 1980; Siegel, Weinstein, 1983). (For extensive discussion of loss and grief, see Chapter 40.) Some researchers have found that advanced warning and the opportunity to experience some anticipatory grief before the death can help facilitate the bereavement process after the death. Anticipatory grief is stimulated by the reality of life situations families face. Parents whose child is in an ICU or has a debilitating disease will experience anticipatory grief. There is an alteration in relationships, a change in life-style, and a very real threat to their hopes and dreams for the future with their loved one. There will be grief responses for what has already been lost, as well as over those losses that occur on a daily basis: progressive debilitation, increasing dependency, uncertainties of what the future might bring, loss of control, and so on.

An important task for families facing the illness, dying, and, ultimately, death of their loved one is to balance the physical and emotional demands of caring for their child as they cope with the accompanying stress and yet avoid detachment before death actually occurs (Futterman et al, 1972). The family with a seriously or terminally ill member has several tasks. The family needs to cope with the member's condition, but they also need to take care of themselves. Cohen and Cohen (1981) identified family coping tasks:

- Denial vs. acceptance of the illness
- Establishing relationships with caregivers
- Meeting the needs of the dying person
- Regulating affect
- Negotiating additional familial relationships
- Coping with the postdeath phase

During the illness or hospitalization, or both, the family begins to experience how the present illness foreshadows the absence of their loved one in the future (Rando, 1986). Going home and finding an empty nursery portrays to the family glimpses of what their life will be like without their child.

In anticipatory grief there should be continued involvement of family members with their loved one. Parents still need to direct their attention, energy, and caregiving activities toward the ill or dying child. Parents, as well as other family members and friends, fluctuate between hope for a miracle and a concrete awareness of the reality of their impending loss. In some sense they may not believe that their child will die, but they find themselves thinking about what kind of monument they would like, how they will act at the funeral, or what clothes they will wear (Weiss, 1988).

Family members should not become detached from their loved one before the death. Premature detachment is an issue of complicated anticipatory grieving. Families may feel that "getting over" the pain of loss will be made much easier if they take a step backward, away from their loved one.

Professionals can help families by involving them in their loved one's care, providing privacy for resolving issues of unfinished business, answering questions, and preparing them for the inevitability of the dying experience.

Sudden vs. Anticipated Loss

The sudden and unexpected death of an infant is very difficult for parents. There is not time to anticipate the loss. Because most children's deaths are sudden and unexpected, such as in the case of pregnancy loss or perinatal loss, parents may experience a delayed grief response. Immediately they are asked to make decisions regarding organ donation, autopsy, and funeral arrangement—things they might never have thought of before in relation to their family. The physical and emotional trauma felt by families in this instance may have a debilitating effect that may prolong their grief (Parkes, Weiss, 1983; Rando, 1984; Miles, Perry, 1985; Sanders, 1989).

Rando (1986b) identified the following characteristics of the death that will influence the parents' grief response:

- The situation surrounding the death
- The timeliness of the death
- The parent's perception of the preventability of the death
- Whether the death was sudden, unexpected, or anticipated
- The length of illness before death
- The amount of the parent's anticipatory grief and involvement with the child

Research findings vary regarding the grief responses of families when the death is anticipated rather than sudden and unexpected. Some have determined a definite qualitative difference between the type of losses (Sanders, 1982-1983; Rando, 1983). Families who experienced chronic, long-term illness and sudden deaths had more difficult adjustments to their loss than those families whose loss was anticipated over a shorter time. Unanticipated bereavement can lead to "an inability to believe that anything can work out well," which can result in a kind of low-level clinical depression in persons who before their loss reacted quite differently to life's events (Weiss, 1988).

The need for follow-up after a loss is important to determine the family's well-being and need for referral or support, or both.

Parental Grief

Although the mourning process is similar for all bereaved persons, parents have unique issues to deal with in the death of a child. The reality of the loss violates one of the basic laws of nature: parents should precede their children in death. Parents face other issues as well, such as how to continue to function in the role of parent. Coping with one's grief while parenting surviving children can be an extremely difficult task for bereaved parents. However, many parents have stated that it has been their surviving children who have pulled them through (Scrimshaw, March, 1984). For parents who are parents without a child, the physical and emotional feelings of grief, wanting/needing to be a parent, and lack of support from society can make them feel isolated and alone (Knapp, Peppers, 1980; Limbo, Wheeler, 1986).

Rando (1986a) describes several reactions of bereaved parents:

- *The avoidance phase.* Parents may be confused and dazed, unable to comprehend what has happened. There is a desire to avoid the terrible acknowledgement that their child is dead.
- *The confrontation phase.* This is a time of intense emotions, during which the perception of the loss is the most acute. It is a time defined as "angry sadness." Extreme emotions are felt: fear and anxiety, anger, guilt, separation and longing, depression, and obsession. During this phase, parents search for meaning, experience grief attacks, identification with the deceased child, and neglect of other relationships. They also have physiologic manifestations. Parents may experience aching arms, waking in the night to a child crying, may feel their dead child needs them, and may have disturbing dreams that reveal their feelings of vulnerability, loss, and uncertainty (Knapp, Peppers, 1980; Miles, 1985).
- *The reestablishment phase:* The physical, emotional, and social responses to grief gradually decline as the parent begins to reenter and become involved in everyday life.

SUMMARY

In caring for the high-risk neonate, the nurse's role includes assessment, planning, implementation, and evaluation of the following: establishing and maintaining a thermoneutral environment, maintaining adequate oxygenation while preventing complications of oxygen administration, and ensuring adequacy of nutritional intake (via oral, gavage, or parenteral routes) and elimination to maintain weight within normal limits (without significant weight loss or gain). For hospitals without the capability to care for the high-risk maternity client or neonate, transport to a tertiary care center is arranged for these clients with special needs. Until transport can be effected, medical and nursing care is directed to stabilize and maintain the client's condition as just outlined.

With adequate attention to the emotional and developmental needs of high-risk infants, nurses can help establish positive attachment behaviors and avoid emotional and developmental problems for the family. From birth to discharge, the care of the compromised neonate is complex and provides a nursing challenge.

REFERENCES

General

Anderson GC: Skin to skin: kangaroo care in western Europe, *Am J Nurs* 89:(5):661, May 1989.

Beckholt AP: Breastmilk for infants who cannot breastfeed, *JOGNN* 19:216, May/June 1990.

Bergman I et al: Cause of hearing loss in the high-risk premature infant, *J Pediatr* 106:95, 1985.

Curtin G: The infant with cleft lip or palate: more than a surgical problem, *J Perinat Neonatal Nurs* 3:80, March 1990.

Damato EG: Discharge planning from the neonatal intensive care unit, *J Perinat Neonat Nurs* 5:43, Jan 1991.

Fanaroff AA, Martin RJ, editors: *Neonatal-perinatal medicine: diseases of the fetus and infant,* ed 5, St Louis, 1992, Mosby–Year Book.

Gerhardt T et al: Pulmonary function in preterm infants whose lungs were ventilated conventionally or by high-frequency oscillation, *J Pediat* 115:121, 1989.

Glass P et al: Effect of bright light in the hospital nursery on the incidence of retinopathy of prematurity, *N Engl J Med* 313:401, 1985.

Gordin P: High-frequency jet ventilation for severe respiratory failure, *Pediatr Nurs* 15:625, 1989.

Hamel AJ, Deane RS, Paquette RD: Compressed air and oxygen supply lines as a source of contamination of respiratory therapy equipment, *Items and Topics* 22:8, 1976.

Harris M, Milford C: (1986). Is intensive care too intensive? *Nurs Insights* 1:5, March 1986.

Kaplan M, Eidelman AT: Improved prognosis in severely hypothermic newborn infants treated by rapid rewarming, *J Pediatr* 105:468, 1984.

Long JG, Lucey JF, Philip AGS: Noise and hypoxemia in the intensive care nursery, *Pediatrics* 65:143, 1980.

Merenstein GB, Gardner SL: *Handbook of neonatal intensive care,* ed 2, St Louis, 1989, Mosby–Year Book.

Miller RW et al: Noise pollution: neonatal aspects (Committee on Environmental Hazards, American Academy of Pediatrics), *Pediatrics* 54:476, 1974.

Polin RA, Fox WW: *Fetal and neonatal physiology,* Philadelphia, 1992, WB Saunders Co.

Sandman K: Emergency stabilization of the critically ill neonate, *Crit Care Nurse* 8:14, June 1989.

Sonesso G: Are you ready to use pulse oximetry? *Nursing 91,* p 60, Aug 1991.

Spyr J, Preach MA: Pulse oximetry: understanding the concept, knowing the limits, *RN,* p 38, May 1990.

Urrutia NL: Sorting the complexities of respiratory distress syndrome, *MCN* 16:308, Nov/Dec 1991.

Waffarn F, Hodgman JE: Mercury vapor contamination of infant incubators: a potential hazard, *Pediatrics* 64:640, 1979.

Whaley LF, Wong DL: *Nursing care of infants and children,* ed 4, St Louis 1991, Mosby–Year Book.

Wilks S, Meier P: Helping mothers express milk suitable for preterm and high-risk infant feeding, *MCN* 13:121, March/April 1988.

Zeimer MM, George C: (1990). Breastfeeding the low-birthweight infant, *Neonatal Network* 9:33, April 1990.

References—Nursing Research

Becker PT et al: Outcomes of developmentally supportive care for very low birth weight infants, *Nurs Res* 40:150, 1991.

Gill NE et al: Effect of nonnutritive sucking on behavioral state in preterm infants before feeding, *Nurs Res* 37:347, 1988.

Greer PS: Head coverings for newborns under radiant warmers, *Nurs Res* 17:265, 1988.

Metheny N et al: Effectiveness of the auscultatory method in predicting feeding tube location, *Nurs Res* 39:262, 1990.

Weibley TT et al: Gavage tube insertion in the premature infant, *MCN* 12:24, 1987.

Whitney JD: The measurement of oxygen tension in tissue, *Nurs Res* 39:203, 1990.

References—A Family's Grief

Cohen MS, Cohen EK: Behavioral family systems interventions in terminal care. In Sebel HJ, editor: *Behavior therapy in terminal care: a humanistic approach,* Cambridge, Mass, 1981, Ballinger.

Fulton R, Gottesman DJ: Anticipatory grief: a psychosocial concept reconsidered, *Br J Psychiatry* 137:45, 1980.

Futterman EH, Hoffman I, Sabshin M: *Parental anticipatory mourning,* New York, 1972, Columbia University Press.

Knapp R, Peppers L: *Motherhood and mourning,* New York, 1980, Praeger.

Limbo RK, Wheeler SR: *When a baby dies: a handbook for healing and helping,* LaCrosse, Wis, 1986, Lutheran Hospital.

Miles MS: Emotional symptoms and physical health in bereaved parents, *Nurs Res* 34:76, 1985.

Miles MS, Perry K: Parental responses to sudden accidental death of a child, *Crit Care Q* 8:73, Jan 1985.

Parkes CM, Weiss RS: *Recovery from bereavement,* New York, 1983, Basic Books.

Rando TA: Investigation of grief and adaptation in parents whose children have died from cancer, *J Pediatr Oncol* 8:3, 1983.

Rando TA: *Grief, dying and death,* Champaign, Ill, 1984, Research Press.

Rando TA: A comprehensive analysis of anticipatory grief: perspectives, processes, promises, and problems. In Rando TA, editor: *Loss and anticipatory grief,* Lexington, Mass, 1986a, Lexington Books.

Rando TA, editor: *Parental loss of a child,* Champaign, Ill, 1986b, Research Press.

Sanders CM: Effects of sudden vs. chronic illness death on bereavement outcome, *Omega* 13:227, 1982-1983.

Sanders CM: *Grief, the mourning after: dealing with adult bereavement,* New York, 1989, Wiley Interscience.

Scrimshaw SCM, March DMS: I had a baby sister but she only lasted a day, *JAMA* 25:732, 1984.

Siegel K, Weinstein L: Anticipatory grief reconsidered, *J Psychosoc Oncol* 1:61, 1983.

Weiss S: Is It possible to prepare for trauma? *J Palliative Care* 4:70, Jan 1988.

BIBLIOGRAPHY

Brooten D: RN follow-up plan helps high-risk infants, *Am Nurse,* Feb 1988.

Crane LD et al: Effects of transcutaneous carbon dioxide tension in neonates with respiratory distress, *J Perinatol* 10:35, Jan 1990.

Gordin P: Assessing and managing agitation in a critically ill infant, *MCN* 15:26, 1990.

Keating SB, Kelman GB: *Home health care nursing: concepts and practice,* Philadelphia, 1988, JB Lippincott Co.

Ludington-Hoe SM, Hadeed AJ, Anderson GC: Physiologic responses to skin-to-skin contact in hospitalized premature infants, *J Perinatol* 11:19, Jan 1991.

Moss JR, Craft MJ: Accurate assessment of infant emesis volume, *Pediatr Nurs* 16:455, 1990.

Roberts PM, Jones MB: Extracorporeal membrane oxygenation and indications for cardiopulmonary bypass in the neonate, *JOGNN* 19:391, Sept/Oct 1990.

Snow LS, Fry ME: Formula feeding in the first year of life, *Pediatr Nurs* 16:442, 1990.

Thomas KA: How the NICU environment sounds to a preterm infant, *MCN* 14:249, July/Aug 1989.

Turner BS: Maintaining the artificial airway: current concepts, *Pediatr Nurs* 16:487, 1990.

Young LY, Creighton DE, Suave RS: The needs of families of infants discharged home with continuous oxygen therapy, *JOGNN* 17:187, May/June 1988.

Zink L, Willett L, Leuschen MP: (1991). Predicting outcome of care in the neonatal intensive care unit, *J Perinatol* 11:152, Feb 1991.

Bibliography—Nursing Research

Abrams L et al: Effect of peripheral IV on neonatal axillary temperature measurement, *Pediatr Nurs* 15:630, 1989.

Beckmann C: Postterm pregnancy: effects on temperature and glucose regulation, *Nurs Res* 39:21, 1990.

Brooten D et al: Anxiety, depression, and hostility in mothers of preterm infants, *Nurs Res* 37:213, 1988.

Brown L et al: Very low birth-weight infants: parental visiting and telephoning during initial infant hospitalization, *Nurs Res* 38:233, 1989.

Deiriggi P: Effects of waterbed flotation on indicators of energy expenditure in preterm infants, *Nurs Res* 39:140, 1990.

Harrison LL, Leeper JD, Yoon M: Effects of early parent touch on preterm infants' heart rates and arterial oxygen saturation levels, *J Adv Nurs* 15:877, 1990.

Medoff-Cooper B, Delivoria-Papadopoulos M, Brotten D: Serial neurobehavioral assessments in preterm infants, *Nurs Res* 40:94, 1991.

Medoff-Cooper B, Weininger S, Zukowsky K: Neonatal sucking as a clinical assessment tool: preliminary findings, *Nurs Res* 38:162, 1989.

Meier P: Bottle- and breast-feeding: effects on transcutaneous oxygen pressure and temperature in preterm infants, *Nurs Res* 37:316, 1988.

Thomas K: The emergence of body temperature biorhythm in preterm infants, *Nurs Res* 40:98, 1991.

Wright S, Norton C, Kesten K: Retention of infant CPR instruction by parents, *Pediatr Nurs* 15:37, Jan 1989.

chapter 36 review

Key Concepts

- Identification of risk situations affecting mother and infant is vital to plan adequate care.
- High-risk infants have special problems caused by immaturity, alterations in functioning of systems, and metabolic balances.
- Parents need help to accept, care for, and take home infants who require care for risk conditions.
- The alert nurse often is the pivotal link between functional and dysfunctional survival for the infant in respiratory distress.
- A thermoneutral environment is essential for metabolic homeostasis.
- For the infant receiving supplemental oxygen, periodic laboratory measurements and close clinical observation are essential for making appropriate adjustments in care to minimize the risk of both hyperoxic and hypoxic insults.
- The extent to which nutritional needs are met is directly related to the infant's immediate and long-range well-being.
- The aim of transporting high-risk infants to regional centers is to provide access to the required level of care.
- Parents need assistance with real or anticipated loss and grief.

Key Terms

- anticipatory grief (p. 1111)
- apnea (p. 1094)
- barotrauma (p. 1097)
- cold stress (p. 1098)
- continuous positive airway pressure (CPAP) (p. 1096)
- cues of overstimulation (p. 1108)
- extracorporeal membrane oxygenation (ECMO) (p. 1097)
- gavage feeding (p. 1102)
- high-risk neonate (p. 1088)
- infant stimulation (p. 1108)
- kangaroo care (p. 1109)
- mechanical ventilation (p. 1096)
- nonnutritive sucking (p. 1105)
- oxygen therapy (p. 1094)
- pulse oximeter (p. 1094)
- readiness for interaction (p. 1108)
- respiratory distress (p. 1088)
- total parenteral nutrition (TPN) (p. 1101)
- transcutaneous oxygen pressure ($tcPO_2$) monitoring (p. 1094)

Critical Thinking Exercises

1. "Buddy up" with an ICN nurse for 1 clinical day. The clinical observation day should follow an orientation to the ICN so that the student can focus on the experience to be described.
   a. Why is this suggestion made?
   b. What implications underlying this suggestion can you apply to parents viewing their infant in the ICN for the first time?
2. Choose any of the following:
   a. Observe a complete physical assessment. Compare with the routine physical assessments in the well-baby nursery.
   b. Describe the infant's willingness to interact with caregivers and to engage in eye-to-eye contact. Note your reactions to the neonate. Discuss implications for nursing care of the neonate and family, based on your findings.
   c. Calculate the percentage of weight gain and loss for three high-risk neonates. Identify probable causes and describe nursing actions.
   d. Observe nursing care related to maintenance of respirations, temperature, and nutrition and elimination.
3. Choose an infant at high risk. Identify ethical issues involved. Discuss the identified issues (using content regarding ethical issue decision making in Chapter 5) from the following perspectives:
   a. As the professional nurse working with the baby and family.
   b. As the parent.
   c. As the taxpayer.
   d. As a legislator who must decide how best to allocate funds among a variety of community needs.

Topics for Nursing Research

- Replicate study temperature maintenance in the neonate (under radiant warmer and in open bassinet) under the following conditions: (1) no head covering, (2) stockinette head covering, (3) lined cap (cotton, polyester fill, polyester and cotton terry), and (4) other.
- Compare the efficacy and safety of temperature taking by the following routes: (1) axillary, (2) rectal, and (3) tympanic membrane.

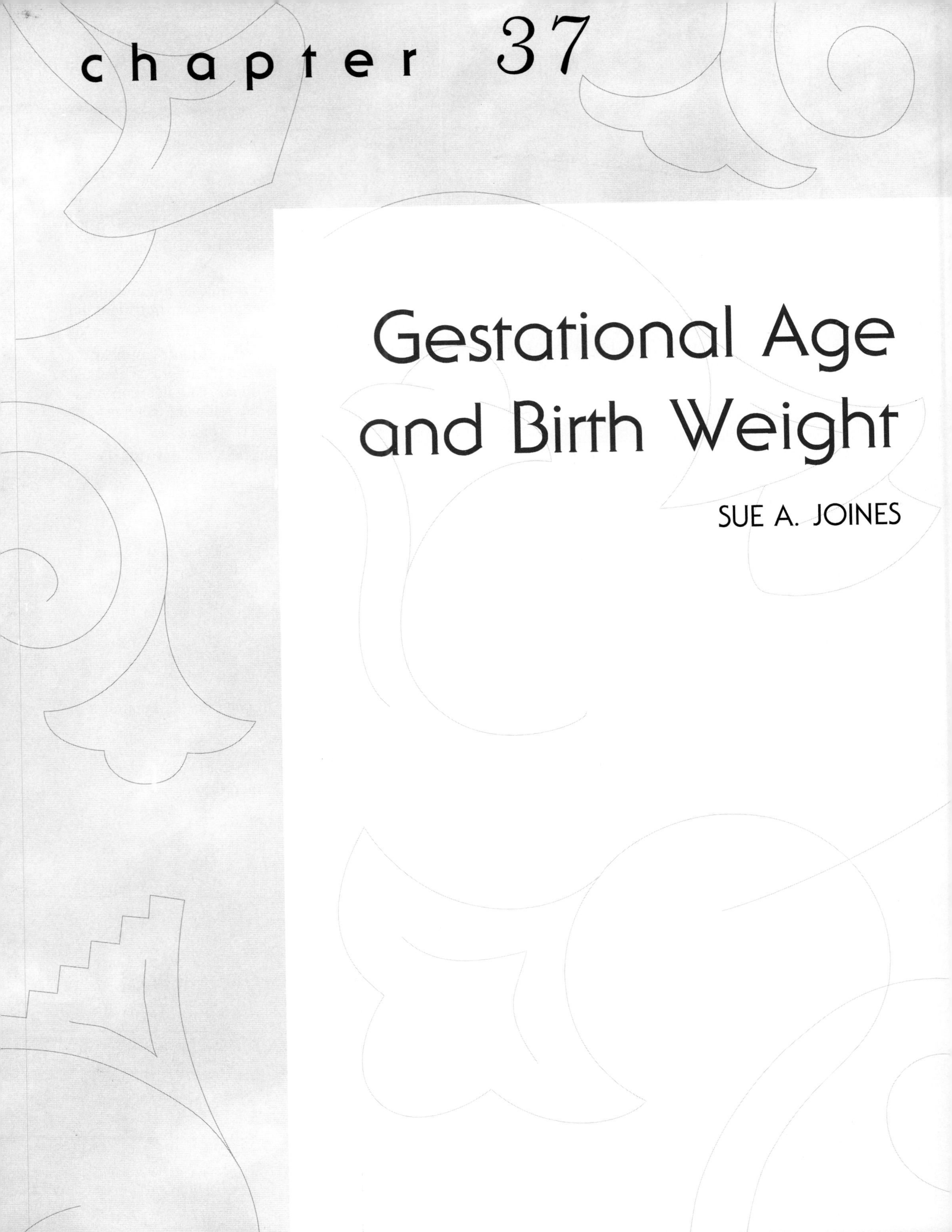

chapter 37

Gestational Age and Birth Weight

SUE A. JOINES

LEARNING OBJECTIVES

- Define the key terms listed.
- Describe preterm, term, postterm, and postmature neonates.
- Assess newborn infants according to gestational age and birth weight.
- Rate newborn infants according to the physical maturity scale and the neuromuscular maturity scale.
- Explain respiratory distress syndrome (RDS) and treatment measures.
- Review prematurity and oxygen therapy.
- Discuss retinopathy of prematurity (ROP), bronchopulmonary dysplasia (BPD), and predisposition of preterm newborns to these problems.
- List the signs and symptoms of perinatal asphyxia.
- Describe meconium aspiration syndrome.
- Examine nursing care of parents of infants at risk because of gestational age and birth weight.
- Identify topics for nursing research related to gestational age and birth weight.

Assessment for gestational age and birth weight is an important consideration because these factors are closely associated with perinatal morbidity and mortality. Modern technology has contributed significantly to improved health and overall survival of infants at risk because of gestational age or birth weight. However, the survival of infants born significantly before term has resulted in the development of conditions that may negatively affect the quality of their lives. These conditions include necrotizing enterocolitis, bronchopulmonary dysplasia, and retinopathy of prematurity. Classification of newborns according to *gestational age* is as follows:

Preterm or premature. Born before completion of 37 weeks' gestation, regardless of birth weight

Term. Born between the beginning of the week 38 and the end of week 42 of gestation

Postterm (postdate). Born after completion of week 42 of gestation

Postmature. Born after completion of week 42 of gestation, having undergone the effects of progressive placental insufficiency

The cause of preterm and postterm birth is largely unknown. It is known, however, that the incidence of preterm birth is highest among low socioeconomic groups. This is likely a result of the lack of comprehensive prenatal health care. Other factors found to be associated with preterm birth include preeclampsia, multifetal pregnancy, and placental accidents.

The *birth weight* of the newborn has a normal range for each gestational week (Figs. 37-1 and 37-2). Variations in weight may occur in the preterm, term, postterm, or postmature newborn. Classification of newborns by weight is as follows:

Large for gestational age (LGA). Weight is above the 90th percentile (or two or more standard deviations above the norm) at any week.

Appropriate for gestational age (AGA). Weight falls between the 10th and 90th percentile for infant's age.

Small-for-gestational age (SGA). Weight is below the 10th percentile (or two or more standard deviations below the norm).

Low birth weight (LBW). Weight of 2500 g or less at birth. These newborns are considered to have had either less than the expected rate of intrauterine growth or a shortened gestation period. Preterm birth and LBW commonly occur together (e.g., <32 weeks and <1200 g birth weight). **Intrauterine growth retardation (IUGR)** is the term used to describe the fetus whose rate of growth does not meet expected norms.

Common causes of LGA newborns include glucose intolerance of pregnancy, true maternal diabetes mellitus, maternal overnutrition, and heredity. SGA newborns may be affected by maternal smoking, hypertensive states, undernutrition, anemia, or nephritis. In addition, the birth of an SGA newborn may be associated with multifetal gestation, a discordant twin pregnancy, or congenital anomalies. High altitude, rubella, or intrauterine infection may predispose a woman to the birth of an SGA newborn. Fetal malnutrition, IUGR, and chronic fetal distress are other processes that may result in the birth of SGA infants.

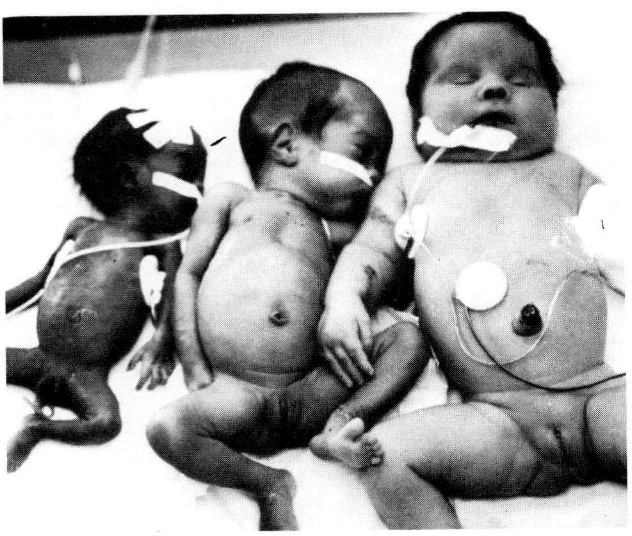

Fig. 37-1 Three babies of same gestational age, with weights of 600, 1400, and 2750 g, respectively, from left to right. Their weights are plotted in Fig. 37-2 at points *A*, *B*, and *C*.
From Korones SB: *High-risk newborn infants: the basis for intensive nursing care,* ed 4, St Louis, 1986, Mosby–Year Book.

Infant Mortality and Morbidity

Preterm birth is responsible for almost two thirds of infant deaths. The infant born before term does not possess the growth and development necessary for uncomplicated adjustment to extrauterine life, and prospects for survival or good health may be severely compromised. Infants weighing more than 2500 g (5½ lb) and born after 37 weeks of pregnancy have the best prospects of survival. There is a dramatic reduction in mortality in infants, regardless of weight, who are born after the week 36 of gestation. The prognosis for LBW infants weighing more than 1800 g (4 lb) is more favorable than for those weighing 1500 to 1800 g (3 to 4 lb). The mortality is less

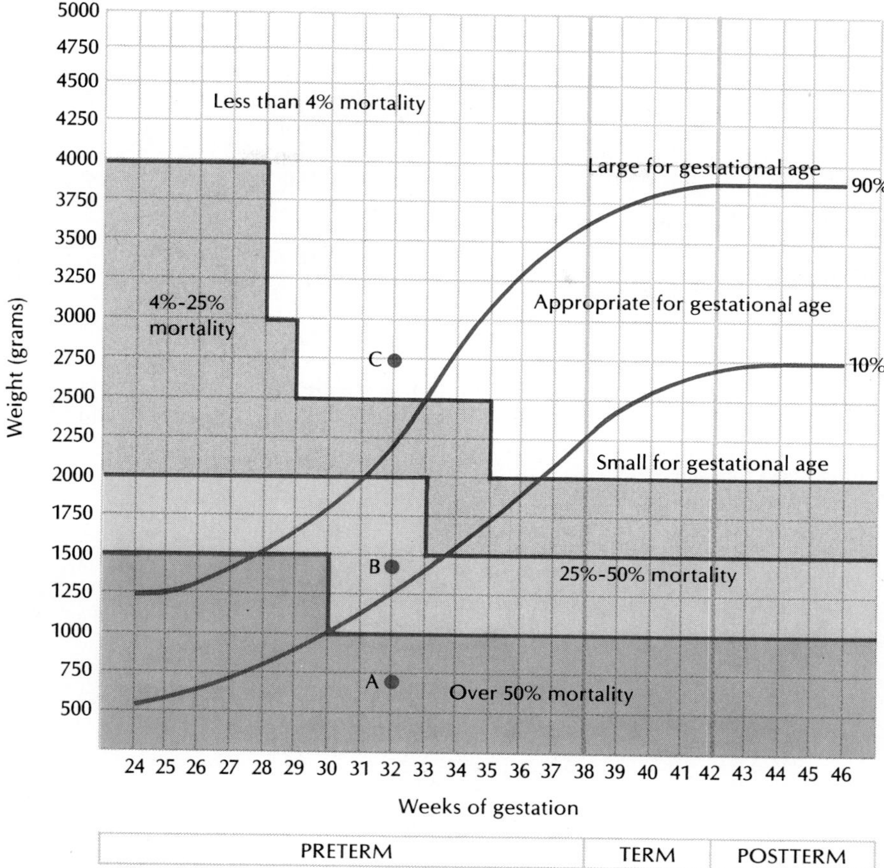

Fig. 37-2 Intrauterine growth status for gestational age and according to appropriateness of growth. Weights of infants shown in Fig. 37-1 are plotted at points *A*, *B*, and *C*. Courtesy Mead Johnson & Co, Evansville, Ind; modified from Battaglia FC, Lubchenco LO: *J Pediatr* 71:59, 1967.

than 5% if the pregnancy has progressed to 35 weeks and the fetus weighs more than 2000 g (4½ lb).

Children and adults who were LBW infants are more likely to have major problems such as cerebral palsy, mental retardation, sensory and cognitive disabilities, and a diminished ability to successfully adapt socially, psychologically, and physically to an increasingly complex environment (Fanaroff, Martin, 1992). In addition to the human tragedy, the fiscal impact of this problem on our society is estimated to be in the billions of dollars each year.

PRETERM INFANT

The preterm infant is at risk because of immaturity of organ systems and lack of reserves. The morbidity and mortality rate for preterm infants is higher by three to four times than that of older infants of comparable weight. The potential problems and care needs of the preterm infant of 2000 g differ from those of the term, postterm, or postmature infant of equal weight (Philip, 1987).

Preterm infants are at a distinct disadvantage when they face the transition from intrauterine to extrauterine life. *The degree of disadvantage depends primarily on their level of maturity*. Physiologic disorders and anomalous malformations affect their response to treatment as well. In general, the closer they are to the normal term infant in gestational age and birth weight, the easier will be their adjustment to the external environment.

ASSESSMENT

Gestational Age

Physical assessment procedures to determine gestational age are based on the method devised by

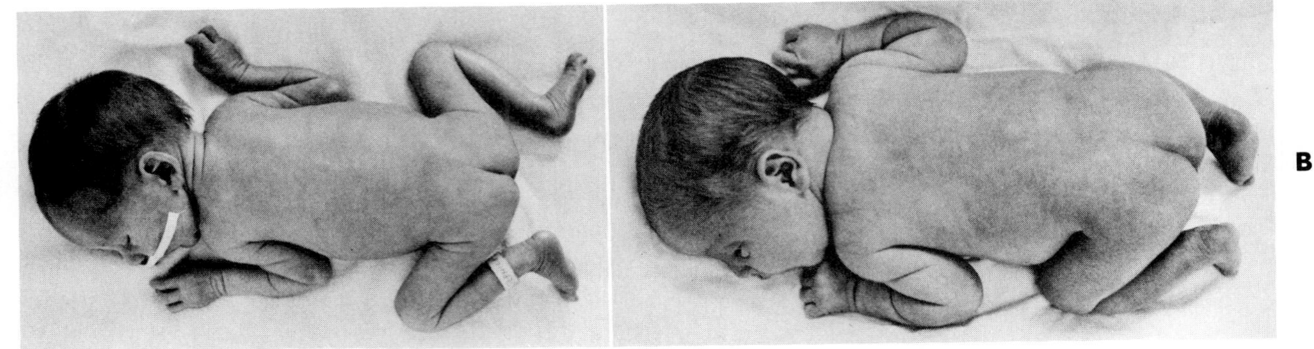

Fig. 37-3 A, In prone position, preterm infant lies with pelvis flat and legs splayed like a frog's. B, Normal full-term infant lies with his limbs flexed, pelvis raised, and knees usually drawn under abdomen.
Courtesy Mead Johnson & Co, Evansville, Ind.

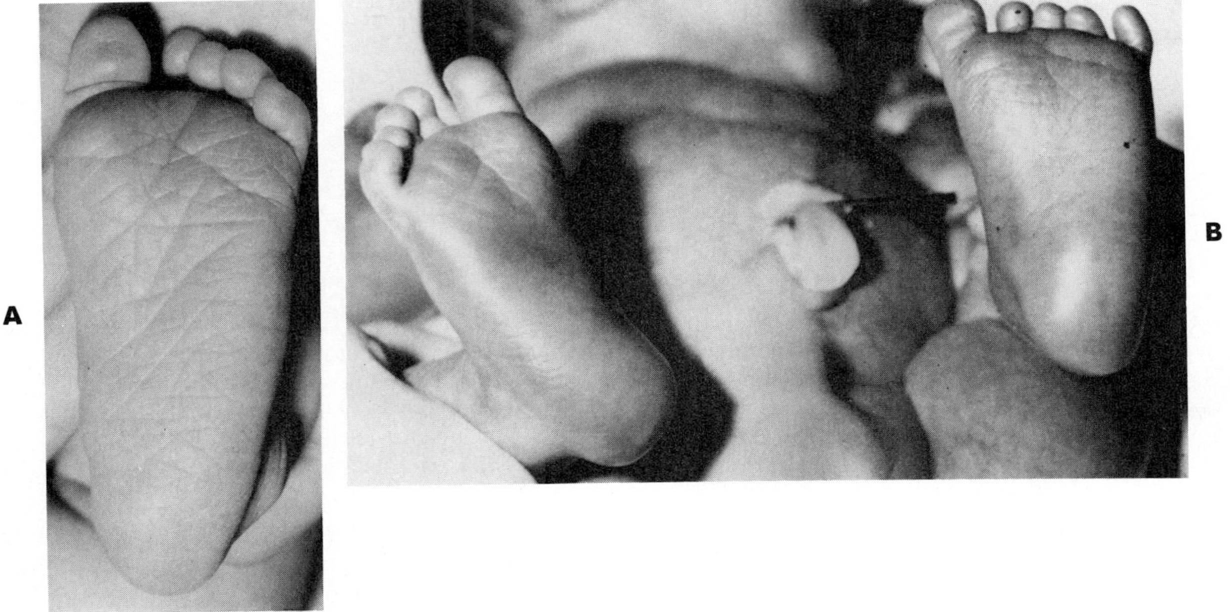

Fig. 37-4 A, Normal sole creases of full-term newborn. B, Sole of foot of preterm infant. As infant loses interstitial fluid after birth, creases become apparent even in preterm infants. Therefore assessment should be performed in first 2 hours after birth.

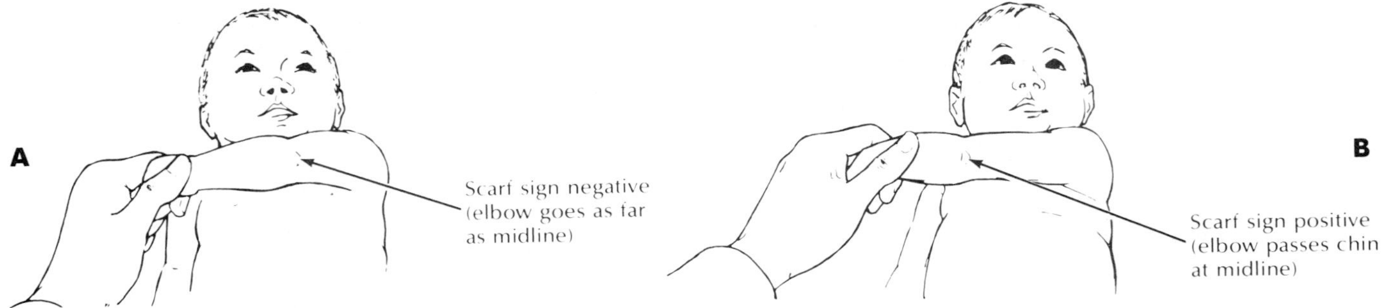

Fig. 37-5 Assessment of gestational age in term newborn (A) and preterm newborn (B).

Dubowitz and associates (1970). Ideally the tests are performed between 2 and 8 hours of age. For the first hour the infant is recovering from the stress of birth, and this is reflected in muscle movements; for example, the arm recoil is slower in a fatigued infant. After 48 hours some responses change significantly. The plantar creases on the soles of the feet appear to increase in number and become visible as the skin loses fluid and dries. See Figs. 37-3 to 37-7 and Tables 37-1 (**physical maturity,** p. 1124) and 37-2

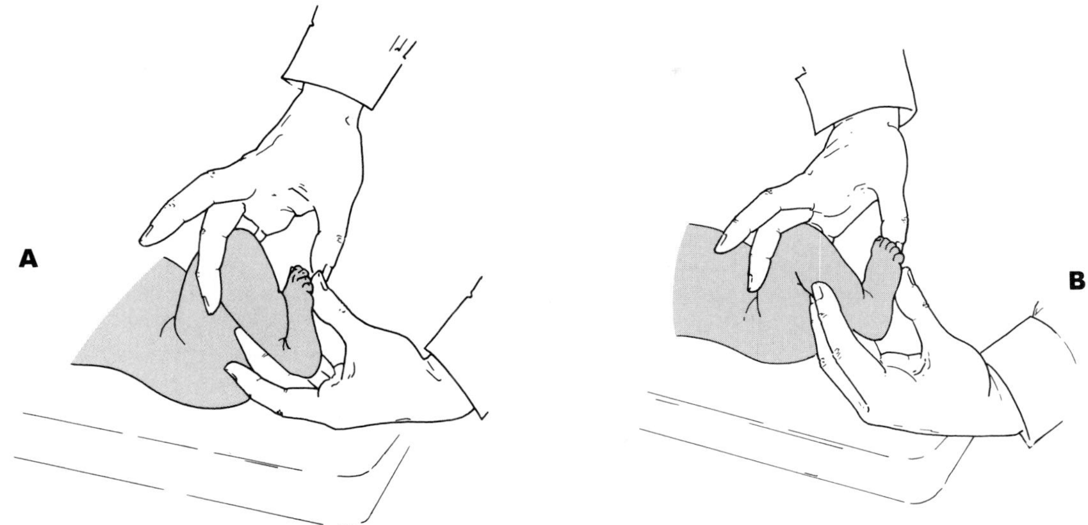

Fig. 37-6 Ankle dorsiflexion. **A,** Angle of 0 degrees in term newborn. **B,** Angle of 20 degrees in the preterm newborn.

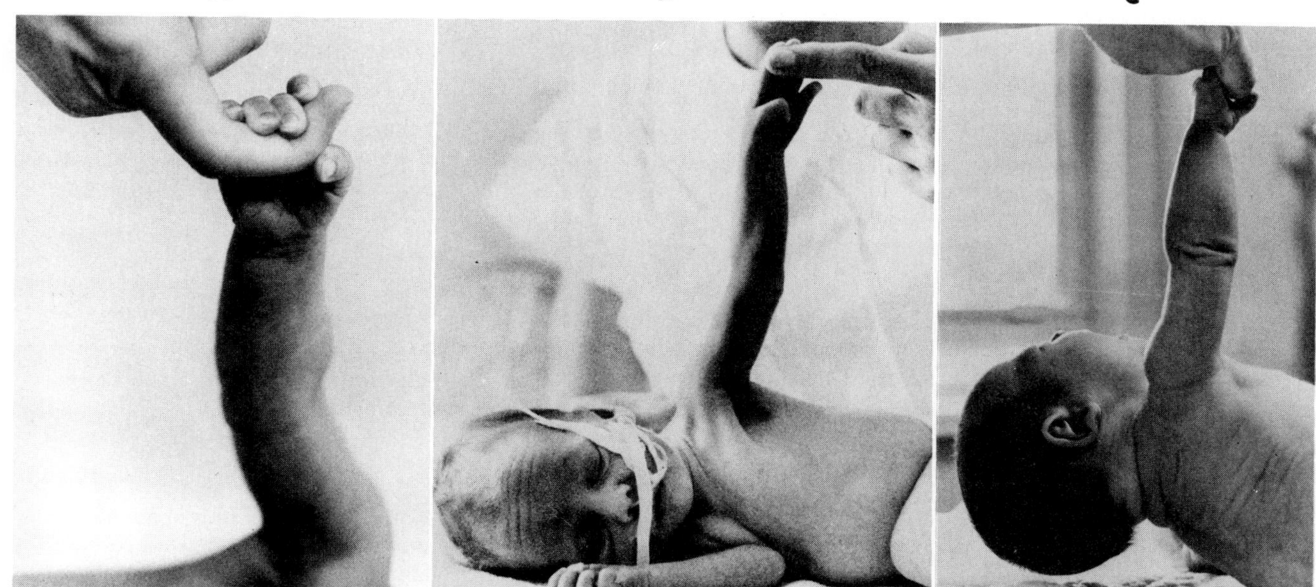

Fig. 37-7 **A,** Primitive grasp reflex present in all normal neonates usually weakens and disappears after 3 months. When palm is stimulated by finger, infant will grasp it. Full-term infant reinforces grip as finger is drawn upward. Dorsum of hand should not be touched because this excites opposite reflex, and hand opens. **B,** Grasp reflex present in preterm infant is distinct from that noted in term infant. Grip can be obtained and arm drawn upward, but when traction is applied, grip opens and there is much less muscle tension. **C,** Once grasp is obtained in term infant, grip is reinforced when the arm is drawn upward. There is progressive tensing of muscles until baby hangs momentarily.
B and C courtesy Mead Johnson & Co, Evansville, Ind.

TABLE 37-1 Elaboration of Physical Maturity Scales

Criterion	Findings and Assigned Scores: 0	1	2	3	4	Infant Score*
Skin						———
Edema	Edema evident over hands and feet; pitting seen over tibia	Pitting edema over tibia	No edema obvious	—	—	
Texture and opacity	Gelatinous, transparent; veins seen especially over abdomen	Visible veins; thin, smooth	Few larger veins seen, especially over abdomen; medium-thick smooth skin	Veins rarely seen; some thickening, superficial cracking	No vessels; parchmentlike, thick, cracking; if leathery, very cracked, and wrinkled, give score of 5	
Color	Dark red (infant is quiet for evaluation)	Pink	Pale pink	Pale; pink mainly over palms, soles, lips, and ears		
Lanugo	None	Abundant over body; long; thick	Thinning, especially over lumbosacral area	Bald areas; thinning over other areas	Mostly bald of lanugo; at least half of back bald	———
Plantar creases	No creases seen	Faint red marks on upper half of sole	Red marks obvious over more than upper half; deeper lines over less than one third	Indentations noticeable over more than one third; lines seen over two thirds	Creases cover entire sole (Fig. 37-4)	———
Breast	Nipple barely perceptible; no palpable breast tissue	Flat, smooth areola present around well-defined nipple; some breast tissue	Stippled areola but edge flat; 1-2 mm breast bud	Stippled areola with edges raised; 3-4 mm breast bud	Full areola; 5-10 mm breast bud; may have breast milk	———
Ear Form Cartilage	Pinna flat, soft, easily folded	Slight incurving of pinna; soft, easily folded; slow recoil	Well-incurved pinna; soft; ready recoil	Upper pinna well curved; formed and firm to edge; instant recoil	Thick cartilage; ear stiff	———
Genitals						———
Male	No testes in scrotum and no rugae over scrotum	—	Testes descending; few rugations	Testes within scrotum, good rugae	Scrotum pendulous with rugae covering scrotum	
Female	Prominent clitoris and labia minora; labia majora do not cover labia minora	—	Labia majora and labia minora equally prominent	Labia majora appear large; labia minora, small	Labia majora completely cover clitoris and labia minora	
					TOTAL	———

*Highest score possible = 25.

(**neuromuscular maturity** below) for the clinical estimation of gestational age. Fig. 37-8 is an example of the recording of **newborn maturity rating and classification**.

Potential Problems of Preterm Newborn

An accurate assessment of gestational age is a good indicator of the problems a preterm newborn is likely to experience (Philip, 1987). In assessing the preterm infant, the health care provider follows a systematic approach. The response of the preterm infant to extrauterine life is different from that of the term infant. Knowing the physiologic basis of these differences helps the nurse assess these infants, understand the response of the preterm infant, and determine which potential problems are most likely to occur.

ESTIMATION OF GESTATIONAL AGE BY MATURITY RATING

Symbols: X - 1st Exam O - 2nd Exam

NEUROMUSCULAR MATURITY

	0	1	2	3	4	5
Posture						
Square Window (Wrist)	90°	60°	45°	30°	0°	
Arm Recoil	180°		100°-180°	90°-100°	< 90°	
Popliteal Angle	180°	160°	130°	110°	90°	< 90°
Scarf Sign						
Heel to Ear						

PHYSICAL MATURITY

	0	1	2	3	4	5
SKIN	gelatinous red, trans-parent	smooth pink, visible veins	superficial peeling &/or rash, few veins	cracking pale area, rare veins	parchment, deep cracking, no vessels	leathery, cracked, wrinkled
LANUGO	none	abundant	thinning	bald areas	mostly bald	
PLANTAR CREASES	no crease	faint red marks	anterior transverse crease only	creases ant. 2/3	creases cover entire sole	
BREAST	barely percept.	flat areola, no bud	stippled areola, 1–2 mm bud	raised areola, 3–4 mm bud	full areola, 5–10 mm bud	
EAR	pinna flat, stays folded	sl. curved pinna, soft with slow recoil	well-curv. pinna, soft but ready recoil	formed & firm with instant recoil	thick cartilage, ear stiff	
GENITALS Male	scrotum empty, no rugae		testes descend-ing, few rugae	testes down, good rugae	testes pendulous, deep rugae	
GENITALS Female	prominent clitoris & labia minora		majora & minora equally prominent	majora large, minora small	clitoris & minora completely covered	

Gestation by Dates ______________ wks

Birth Date __________ Hour __________ am pm

APGAR __________ 1 min __________ 5 min

MATURITY RATING

Score	Wks
5	26
10	28
15	30
20	32
25	34
30	36
35	38
40	40
45	42
50	44

SCORING SECTION

	1st Exam=X	2nd Exam=O
Estimating Gest Age by Maturity Rating	______ Weeks	______ Weeks
Time of Exam	Date ______ Hour ______ am pm	Date ______ Hour ______ am pm
Age at Exam	______ Hours	______ Hours
Signature of Examiner	______ M.D.	______ M.D.

Fig. 37-8 Newborn maturity rating and classification.
From Mead Johnson & Co, Evansville, Ind. Scoring section adapted from Ballard JL et al: *Pediatr Res* 11:374, 1977.
Figures modified from Sweet AY: Classification of the low-birth-weight infant. In Klaus MH, Fanaroff AA: *Care of the high-risk infant*, Philadelphia, 1977, WB Saunders.

TABLE 37-2 Elaboration of Neuromuscular Maturity Scales*

Criterion	Method of Assessment	0
Posture (Fig. 37-3)	Position: supine Activity: quiet Assessment: extension and flexion of arms, hips, legs	Complete extension
Square window (wrist)†	Position: supine Method: with thumb supporting back of arm below wrist, apply gentle pressure with index and third fingers on dorsum of hand; do not rotate infant's wrist Assessment: angle formed between hypothenar eminence and forearm	Very premature (<30 wk) 90°
Arm recoil	Position; supine Method; flex forearms on upper arms for 5 sec; pull on hands to full extension and release Assessment: degree of flexion	No recoil; arms remain extended 180°
Popliteal angle	Position: supine; pelvis on flat, firm surface Method: flex leg on thigh; then flex thigh on abdomen; holding knee with thumb and index finger, extend leg with index finger of other hand behind ankle Assessment: degree of angle behind knee	Complete extension; very premature 180°
Scarf sign (Fig. 37-5)	Position: supine Method: support head in midline with one hand; pull hand to opposite shoulder Assessment: position of elbow in relation to midline	Elbow to opposite arm like scarf around neck
Heel to ear	Position: supine, pelvis is kept flat on surface Method: pull foot up toward ear on same side; do not hold knee Assessment: distance of foot from ear and degree of extension of knee	Toes touch ear; leg completely extended (180°)

X, First examination; *O*, second examination.

*Compare combined scores for physical and neuromuscular maturity to the "maturity rating" scores and read estimated weeks of gestational age. Estimate of gesta-
appropriate graphs. All three measurements should fall within same approximate range, for example, all within SGA, LGA, or AGA. If one measurement is excessively

†Counterpart: ankle dorsiflexion (Fig. 37-6).

Finding and Assigned Scores					Infant Score	
1	2	3	4	5	X	0
Extension of arms; slight flexion of hips, legs	Extension of arms	Slight flexion of arms; full flexion of legs	Complete flexion	—	______	______
Premature (30-35 wk) 60°	Premature (30-35 wk) 45°	Maturing (35-38 wk) 30°	Term: hand lies flat on ventral surface of forearm 0°	—	______	______
—	Some recoil; sluggish response 100°-180°	Maturing (35-38 wk) 90°-100°	Brisk recoil to complete flexion <90°	—	______	______
Premature (30-35 wk) 160°	Premature (30-35 wk) 130°	Maturing (35-38 wk) 110°	Maturing (35-38 wk) 90°	Extension is resisted <90°	______	______
Elbow beyond midline of thorax	Elbow just beyond midline	Elbow at midline	Elbow does not reach midline	—	______	______
Toes almost reach face (130°)	Knees flexed (110°)	Knees flexed (90°)	Knees flexed; popliteal angle is less than 90°	—	______	______

NEUROMUSCULAR MATURITY TOTALS ______ ______
PHYSICAL MATURITY TOTALS ______ ______
(see Table 37-1)
COMBINED SCORE ______ ______
(see Fig. 37-8 for maturity rating)

tional age obtained is accurate only to plus or minus 2 weeks. After gestational age is estimated, infant's length, weight, and head circumference are entered on large (falling into LGA range) and other two fall into SGA range, growth deviation should be assessed.

RESPIRATORY FUNCTION. Just as with the term infant, initial assessment will begin with respiratory function, observing the infant's ability to make the pulmonary transition from intrauterine to extrauterine life. The preterm infant is likely to have difficulty making this transition because of numerous deficits in the respiratory system:

- Decreased number of functional alveoli
- Deficient surfactant levels
- Smaller lumen in the respiratory system
- Greater collapsibility or obstruction of respiratory passages
- Insufficient calcification of the bony thorax
- Weak or absent gag reflex
- Immature and friable capillaries in the lungs

In combination, these deficits severely hinder the infant's respiratory efforts and result in respiratory distress or apnea. The health care provider needs to be prepared to provide oxygen and ventilation, as necessary (Merenstein, Gardner, 1989).

CARDIOVASCULAR FUNCTION. After respiratory assessment the health care provider assesses the cardiovascular system and its ability to provide perfusion to essential tissues and organs. The health care provider must be prepared to intervene if symptoms of hypovolemia or shock, or both, are present. These symptoms include decreased blood pressure, slow capillary refill, and continued respiratory distress despite provision of oxygen and ventilation.

MAINTAINING BODY TEMPERATURE. As a result of numerous factors, the preterm infant is susceptible to temperature instability. *Heat loss is great because of the large surface area in relation to body weight.* Other factors include the following:

- Minimal insulating subcutaneous fat
- Limited stores of ***brown fat*** (an internal source for generation of heat present in normal term infants)
- Decreased or absent reflex control of skin capillaries (shiver response)
- Inadequate muscle mass activity (therefore the preterm infant will be unable to produce its own heat)
- Friable (easily damaged) capillaries
- Immature temperature-regulation center in the brain

To contend with the preterm infant's temperature instability, the health care provider performs ongoing assessment of temperature and provides a regulated, external source of heat.

CENTRAL NERVOUS SYSTEM FUNCTION. The preterm infant's central nervous system (CNS) is susceptible to injury from various sources:

- Birth trauma with damage to immature structures
- Bleeding from fragile capillaries
- Impaired coagulation process, including prolonged prothrombin time
- Recurrent anoxic episodes
- Predisposition to hypoglycemia

The nurse assesses CNS function by checking the infant's ability to coordinate its suck and swallow and by monitoring for impairment in the CNS control of respiratory and cardiovascular systems (apnea and bradycardia) (Merenstein, Gardner, 1989).

MAINTAINING ADEQUATE NUTRITION. Maintenance of adequate nutrition in the preterm infant is complicated by problems of intake and of metabolism. With regard to intake the preterm infant has the following disadvantages: weak or absent suck, swallow, and gag reflexes, a small stomach capacity, and weak abdominal muscles. The preterm infant's metabolic functions are weakened by a limited store of nutrients, a decreased ability to digest proteins or absorb nutrients, and immature enzyme systems.

The nurse provides ongoing assessment of the infant's ability to take in and digest nutrients. The health care provider needs to be prepared to provide nourishment to the preterm infant by means other than the oral route (e.g., gavage or intravenous).

MAINTAINING RENAL FUNCTION. The preterm infant's immature renal system is unable (1) to adequately excrete metabolites and drugs, (2) to concentrate the urine, or (3) to maintain balances in acid-base, fluids, or electrolytes. The nurse assesses intake and output, as well as specific gravity; monitors laboratory values for acid-base and electrolyte balance; and observes for symptoms of drug toxicity.

MAINTAINING HEMATOLOGIC STATUS. Compared with the term infant, the preterm infant is predisposed to hematologic problems as a result of the following factors:

- Increased capillary friability
- Increased tendency to bleed (low plasma prothrombin levels)
- Slowed development of red blood cells
- Increased hemolysis
- Loss of blood from frequent laboratory tests

The nurse assesses for any evidence of bleeding, observing for symptoms of disseminated intravascular coagulation (DIC) (bleeding from puncture sites, gastrointestinal tract, CNS, or skin) (Merenstein, Gardner, 1989).

RESISTING INFECTION. The preterm infant is at increased risk for infection because of a shortage of stored maternal immunoglobulins, an impaired ability to make antibodies, and a compromised integumentary system (thin skin and fragile capillaries).

Growth and Development Potential

Although it is impossible to predict with complete accuracy the growth and development potential of each preterm newborn, some findings support an anticipated favorable outcome (Bennett et al, 1983). The growth and development landmarks are corrected for gestational age.

The age of a preterm newborn is corrected by adding the gestational age and the postnatal age. For example, if an infant was born at 32 weeks' gestation 4 weeks ago, the infant would be considered 36 weeks of age. The child's **corrected age** 6 months after the birth date is 4 months. Responses are evaluated against the norm expected for a 4-month-old infant.

Favorable findings that support the prediction of a growth and development pattern within the norm include certain measurable factors. At *discharge from the hospital,* which usually occurs between 37 and 40 weeks after the woman's last menstrual period (LMP), the infant exhibits the following characteristics. (1) The baby is able to raise the head when prone and is able to hold the head parallel with the body when tested for head lag response. (When the infant is pulled up by the hands, the infant's head lags, but then the head and chest will be in line as the upright position is reached. This alignment will be held momentarily before the head falls forward [pull-to-sit or traction reflex]). In addition, the infant (2) cries with vigor when hungry, (3) shows appropriate weight gain and pattern of weight gain according to growth grid, and (4) has neurologic responses appropriate for corrected age. Also, the retinas appear normal.

At *39 to 40 weeks* the infant is able to focus on the examiner's or parent's face and is able to follow with her or his eyes.

At the *corrected ages of 6 and 12 months* the infant is assessed again for age-appropriate responses. The infant who displays any of the following behaviors may have problems: was and continues to be a poor eater; is irritable; displays sensory, perceptual, intellectual, or motor deviations in development; or displays or develops hypertonia or hypotonia.

These behaviors must be interpreted with caution, and the infant requires reevaluation by an interdisciplinary team at frequent intervals. Parents will need continued support and attention should these signs appear. Minor behavioral deviations also are diagnosed so that the parents can be assisted in their understanding and acceptance of the child. Deviations such as clumsiness, varying degrees of incoordination, slowness in reading and writing, and similar problems may be distressing to the child, parents, and other family members.

Parental Adaptation to Preterm Infant

Parents who experience the preterm birth of their infant have a different experience from parents giving birth to a full-term infant (Sammons, Lewis, 1985). Because of this difference, parental attachment and adaptation to the parental role also will be different. Table 37-3 summarizes the key differences in the two experiences.

PARENTAL TASKS. Parents face a number of psychologic tasks before effective relationships and parenting patterns can evolve. These tasks include the following:

- *Anticipatory grief over the potential loss of an infant.* The parent grieves (see Chapter 40) in preparation for the infant's possible death, although the parent clings to the hope that the child will survive. This begins during labor and lasts until the infant dies or shows evidence of surviving.
- *Acceptance by the mother of her failure to give birth to a healthy, full-term infant.* Grief and depression typify this phase, which persists until the infant is out of danger and is expected to survive.
- *Resumption of the process of relating to the infant.* As the baby begins to improve—gains weight, feeds by nipple, and is weaned from the incubator—the parent can begin the process of developing attachment to the infant that was interrupted by the infant's precarious condition at birth (Als, Brazelton, 1981).
- *Learning how this baby differs in special needs and growth patterns.* Another parental task is to learn, understand, and accept this infant's caregiving needs and growth and development expectations (Sammons, Lewis, 1985).
- *Adjusting the home environment to the needs of the new infant.* Grandparents and siblings also react to the birth of the preterm infant. Parents must reconcile the grief of grandparents and the bewilderment and anger of brothers and sisters at the disproportionate amount of parental time absorbed by the newborn.

PARENTAL RESPONSES. Two different approaches noted by Newman (1980) are *coping through commitment* and *coping through distance.* With the first approach parents take each day as it comes, recognizing and accepting the lessened responses of their infant and noting the gradual progress in their child's condition. With the second approach the parents pull away from emotional attachment to the infant; they

TABLE 37-3 Differences in Experiences of Term and Preterm Delivery

Term Delivery	Preterm Delivery
The parents have gone through the full developmental process of a 40-week pregnancy.	The parents have not completed the psychological and emotional growth of a 40-week-gestation pregnancy.
The infant is healthy and has the physiologic, motor, and state control and social capacities common to full-term infants.	The infant is small, immature, often physically unattractive, and sick.
The parents have an enormous surge of emotion postpartum, which is derived from a combination of feelings of achievement and pride in their own success and fulfilled expectations about the intactness and healthiness of their infant.	The parents are often overwhelmed by feelings of failure, loss, fear, and sadness.
Full-term infants in the first 1 to 2 hours after birth have a period of alert time during which they open their eyes, look around, breast-feed, and generally behave like or exceed most parent's fantasies of a little baby.	The infant has none of the cute, appealing behaviors of a full-term infant. The infant is not alert, does not suck, and may be too sick to be held at all.

From Sammons W, Lewis J: *Premature babies: a different beginning,* St Louis, 1985, Mosby–Year Book.

postpone becoming attached until the infant is in better health.

Parents have been observed to progress through stages as they spend more time with their infants. In the first stage they maintain an *en face* position, stroking and touching their infant (Figs. 37-9 and 37-10). In the second stage they assume some child care activities—feeding, bathing, changing the infant. In the third stage the infant becomes a person and is seen as a whole child (Schraeder, 1980). Sosa and Grua (1982) reported a personal communication with Brazelton in which he correlated parental behaviors with the previously noted three stages. In the first stage parents ask about *chemical data,* such as "What is his bilirubin today?" In the second stage they note their baby yawning, sneezing, hiccoughing, *reflexes* that mark their infant as human. At this time the infant is still not "claimed." In later stages they note their infant's *responses* to them and begin to feel that "this child is mine" and part of their family. Parents take on the role of advocate for their child.

INFANT RESPONSIVENESS. The preterm infant's states of consciousness are more labile than the term infant's. The quiet alert state is less evident and unpredictable. Field (1979) noted that if a mother concentrated her interactions on imitation of the infant's behavior, the infant was increasingly attentive and interested. Too-active an involvement in child care tended to result in the infant's becoming disinterested and glancing away (gaze aversion). One young mother noted that "gentle stroking of her infant's head caused him to look at her." (She also reported that even at age 7 years, gentle head stroking calmed her child.)

PARENTING DISORDERS. The incidence of physical and emotional abuse is three times greater toward the infant who, because of preterm birth or illness, was separated from the mother for a period of time after birth (Fomufod, 1976). Physical abuse includes varying degrees of poor nutrition and poor hygiene. Emotional abuse ranges from subtle to outright dislike of the child. There may be preferential treatment for brothers and sisters, nagging, extremely high expectations of the child, and other types of overt or covert negative parental responses.

Factors surrounding the birth may predispose parents to subconsciously or overtly reject the child. These factors might include parental pain and anxiety, a heavy financial burden for the infant's care, unresolved anticipatory grief, threat to self-esteem, or unwanted pregnancy. The goal of the helping professionals is to reduce the incidence of child abuse and neglect.

GROWTH IN THE PARENTAL ROLE. Parents go through a number of phases of adjustment as they become the "real" parents of the preterm infant (Sammons, Lewis, 1985). These phases of adjustment, which include grieving and bereavement, bonding and attachment, and adapting to the role of parent, parallel the parental tasks noted on p. 1129. Parents of preterm infants often are deprived of the fulfillment of their expectations of the labor and birth

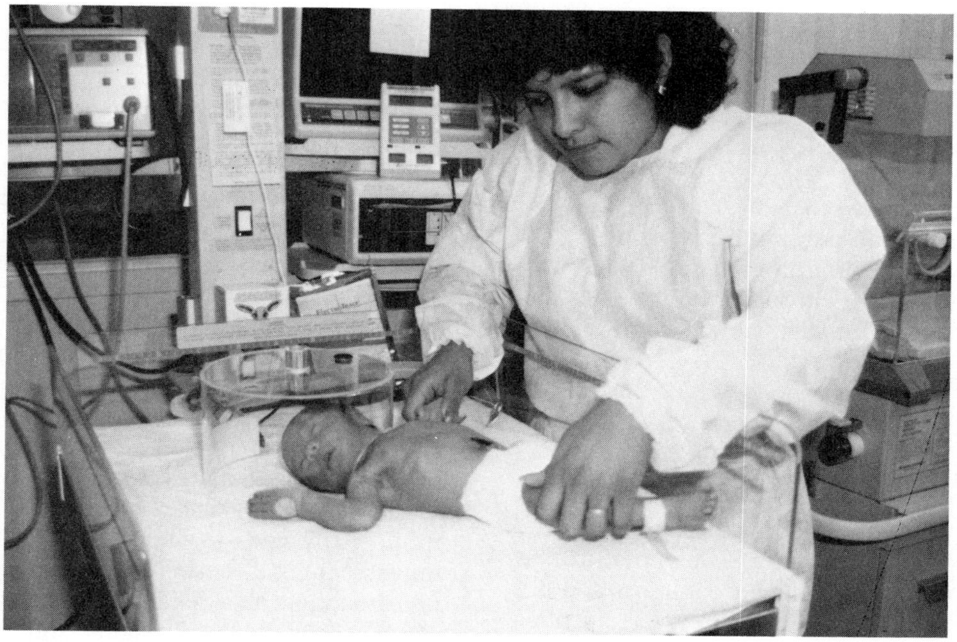

Fig. 37-9 Mother interacting with her baby by touch. Oxygen hood and overhead warmer are being used in place of incubator.
Courtesy Marjorie Pyle, RNC, Lifecircle, Costa Mesa, Calif.

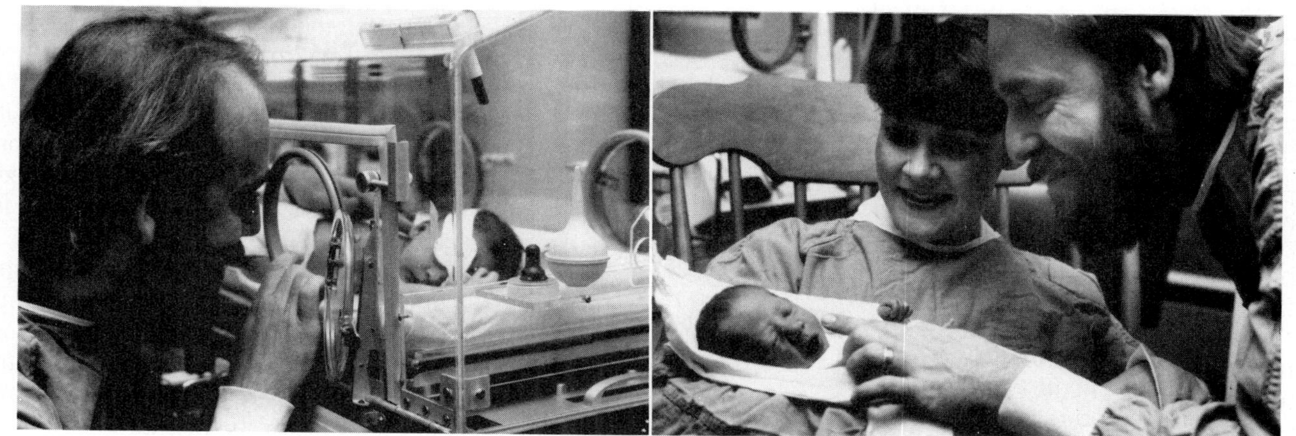

Fig. 37-10 Father interacts with his baby. **A**, Stroking baby's back. **B**, Touching baby with fingertip.

processes and grieve the loss of their fantasy infant (for further discussion, see Chapter 40). The bonding and attachment process is delayed and complicated by separation, anxiety, and lack of intimacy. While parents are adapting to their new role, the preterm infant moves away from total dependence on staff members and equipment. The infant becomes progressively more accessible to parents; that is, she or he is out of the incubator and equipment is removed. As the infant achieves these medical milestones, the parents actively participate in caregiving, experience joy at the baby's increased awake time and increased responsiveness, and start to use the baby's name—not just "it," "he," or "she."

NURSING DIAGNOSES

To formulate nursing diagnoses, the nurse must analyze data obtained from continuous monitoring of the infant and from observation of and discussions with the parents. The diagnoses may be physical, cognitive, or psychologic, for example:

- Ineffective breathing pattern related to
  - —Inadequate chest expansion, secondary to infant's position
- Parental anxiety related to
  - —Knowledge deficit regarding infant's cues
  - —Knowledge deficit regarding feeding the infant
- Situational low self-esteem related to
  - —Parent's feelings of inadequacy in caring for the infant

PLANNING

The nursing plan of care for the preterm infant is dictated by the physiologic needs of immature systems, often involving emergency treatments and procedures. During this time, nursing care is a critical element in the infant's chances for survival. In addition to meeting the infant's physical needs, nursing care is planned in conjunction with parents to promote parent-infant attachment and interaction. *Goals* are presented in client-centered terms.

The infant will achieve the following:

- Maintain physiologic functioning
- Maintain adequate nutrition
- Experience no or minimal hematologic problems
- Not develop infection
- Not develop retinal problems
- Not suffer trauma to immature musculoskeletal system
- Experience parent-infant attachment

The parents will achieve the following:

- Perceive the child as potentially normal (if this is medically substantiated)
- Provide care comfortably
- Experience pride and satisfaction in the care of the infant
- Organize their time and energies to meet the love, attention, and care needs of the other members of the family as well as their own

IMPLEMENTATION

The best environment for fetal growth and development is in the uterus of a healthy, well-nourished woman for 38 to 42 weeks. The extrauterine environment of the preterm newborn must approximate a healthy intrauterine environment for the normal sequence of growth and development to continue. The provision of such an environment is the basis for care of the preterm infant. Medical and nursing personnel and respiratory therapists work as a team to provide the intensive care needed. The nurse acts as a constant presence in the infant's support system.

Admission of a preterm newborn to the intensive care nursery usually is an emergency situation. A rapid initial evaluation is made to ascertain the need for lifesaving treatment. Resuscitative measures are started in the birthing room. The newborn's need for warmth and oxygen is ensured during transfer from the birthing room to the nursery.

Nursing actions are based on knowledge of the *physiologic problems* (p. 1125) imposed on the preterm infant and on the infant's need to conserve energy for repair, maintenance, and growth. Nursing care is conscientiously centered on the continuous assessment and analysis of physiologic status. Nurses fulfill many roles in providing the intensive and extended care that these infants require. Nurses continuously gather data regarding the infant's physiologic status. They make decisions and initiate therapies based on their interpretation of these data. In addition, nurses are the support persons and teachers during the first phase of the parents' adjustment to the birth of the preterm infant.

The nurse-to-infant ratio depends on the assessment and intervention needs of each compromised infant. The ratio can vary from one infant per nurse (for the severely compromised infant) to as many as eight infants per nurse (for infants ready for transfer to the general care nursery). Hospitals not equipped to care for high-risk infants arrange for their immediate transfer to specialized centers (see p. 1110 for transport preparation).

The nurse uses many technologic support systems to monitor body responses and maintain body function in the infant (Hansen, 1982). Gentle touch, concern for the traumatic effects of harsh lighting, and control of machinery noise are interwoven with the technical skill of the nurse in the intensive care nursery.

Physical Care

The preterm infant's *environmental support* consists of the following:

- Incubator or overhead heat panel and plastic bubble cover over infant to control for body temperature
- Air or oxygen administration, depending on infant's cardiopulmonary and circulatory status
- Electronic monitors as needed for observation of respiratory and cardiac functions
- Flotation mattress and restraints and props (bolsters, rolled linens) for positioning infant to facil-

itate physiologic functioning and to maintain skin integrity and correct body alignment
- Protection from noise (see discussion of infant stimulation in next section).

Metabolic support consists of measures such as the following:
- Parenteral fluids to assist in supporting nutrition, normal arterial blood gas (ABG) levels and acid-base homeostasis
- Parenteral fluids to facilitate antibiotic therapy if sepsis is a concern
- Blood specimen analyses to monitor ABG levels, pH, blood glucose, and sepsis.

Infant Stimulation

Although a preterm infant responds differently to **infant stimulation** than does the term infant, they continue to benefit from touch as long as it is adjusted to the developmental and tolerance level of the particular infant. Both procedural and social stimulation can be used to provide the least amount of distress to the infant. For example, cycled lighting has beneficial effects on preterm infants (see Research Highlight below). These infants need tactile stimulation provided with slow, sure motions. In changing the infant's position, the nurse supports the head and holds the infant's limbs close to the body. This type of supportive manipulation provides stimulation while reducing motor disorganization. At age 34 to 36 weeks since LMP the infant will respond in an alert state to visual and auditory stimuli. At age 36 to 40 weeks since LMP infants are much more capable of tolerating stimulation from caregivers and parents.

Caregivers and parents can use varied approaches to soothe the distressed infant. These include talking to the infant, controlling the infant's arms across the chest with the palm of the caregiver's hand, swaddling the infant to reduce the self-distressing effects of startle reflexes, holding and rocking the infant in

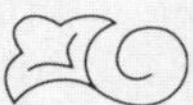 **Research Highlight** 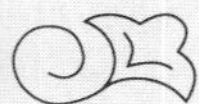

Effects of Cycled Light on Preterm Infants

RESEARCH ABSTRACT

There is concern about effects of the neonatal intensive care environment on the development of preterm infants. This study used data collected for another study and compared the effects of cycled lighting (turning lights off for a portion of a 24-hour day) with continuous lighting. There were nine infants born at or before 34 weeks' gestation in each group. All infants were in incubators with attached cardiorespiratory monitors. The infant's nurse made the decision when to turn the lights off and on. Data were collected over a 24-hour period using time-lapse videorecordings. The camera was placed over the incubator. Cardiorespiratory data were collected from a Hewlett-Packard monitor.

In the cycled lighting group the infants were in dimmed lighting for an average of 10.7 hours. These infants had lower heart rates and lower motor activity when the lights were dimmed than when the lights were on. There were no day-night differences in heart rate or activity in the infants in continuous lighting. During the day there were no differences between the two groups in activity level or respiratory rate, but heart rate was lower for the group in cycled lighting. During the night, when the lights were dimmed for the cycled group, activity and heart rate were lower for the cycled group; there were no differences in respiratory rate. Infants in the cycled group had longer periods of quiet inactivity that resembled quiet sleep.

IMPLICATIONS FOR PRACTICE

Decreasing light levels may facilitate rest and help to conserve energy in preterm infants. When the lights were dimmed, activity and noise from staff members also decreased. Nurses can provide an environment that helps preterm infants to develop neurobehavioral organization. This allows the infants to conserve energy and to respond appropriately to their parents.

RELATED RESEARCH QUESTIONS

1. Does cycled light promote adaptation to the home environment?
2. Do male and female infants differ in their responses to cycled light?
3. Does cycled light promote growth as measured by weight gain?
4. What are the effects of cycling light in response to the sleep-wake cycle of infants?

REFERENCE

Blackburn S, Patteson D: Effects of cycled light on activity state and cardiorespiratory function in preterm infants, *J Perinat Neonat Nurs* 4:47, April 1991.

an upright position, and offering a pacifier (Merenstein, Gardner, 1989).

Infant Feeding

The preterm infant may be fed by breast, bottle, or gavage. For the infant that requires gavage feeding, **nonnutritive suckling** of a pacifier during the gavage procedure (see Chapter 36) may facilitate earlier transition to nipple feeding. In addition, these infants may have a better weight gain, experience fewer complications, and be discharged sooner (Gill et al, 1988). Caution is used in selecting pacifiers for newborns in the hospital or the home. Makeshift pacifiers have been implicated in hazardous aspirations (Milluncheck, McArtor, 1986). Ten deaths related to aspiration of baby bottle nipples were reported to the Consumer Product Safety Commission between 1975 and 1983. Nurseries and parents should buy only *one-piece pacifiers*.

The following criteria are used for initiating nipple feedings (Merenstein, Gardner, 1989):

- Coordinated sucking, swallowing, and breathing
- Adequate gag reflex (usually established by 34 to 36 weeks)
- Respiratory function that allows unlabored suckling (<60 respirations per minute with oxygen <30% to 40%)
- Steady weight gain

Parent Education: Cardiopulmonary Resuscitation

Sudden infant death syndrome (SIDS) is 8 to 10 times more likely to develop in preterm infants than in term infants. Further, infants discharged from a neonatal intensive care unit are about twice as likely to die unexpectedly during the first year of life as are infants in the general population (Rehm, 1983). Instruction in cardiopulmonary resuscitation (CPR) is "mandatory for parents of infants who are more likely to experience a life-threatening episode of apnea, bradycardia, or choking. Infants identified as being at risk include those who are premature, have had a documented episode of apnea or bradycardia, have had episodes of choking, [and] have breathing difficulty . . ." (Wright et al, 1989). Before taking the infant home, parents must be able to administer CPR (see Chapter 21). The telephone number to be dialed in case of emergency should be posted near the phone.

Support of Parents

The nurse as support person and teacher shapes the environment and makes the caregiving more responsive to the needs of parents and child. Nurses are instrumental in helping parents learn who their infant is and to recognize behavioral cues in her or his development.

As soon as possible the parents should see and touch the infant so they can begin to acknowledge the reality of the event and reaffirm the infant's true appearance and condition. They will need encouragement to begin working through the psychologic tasks imposed by the preterm birth.

A nurse or physician should be present when the parents visit the infant for the following reasons:

- To help them "see" the infant rather than focus on the equipment. The significance and function of the apparatus that surround the infant should be explained to them.
- To explain the characteristics normal for an infant of their baby's gestational age. In this way parents do not compare their child with a full-term healthy infant.
- To encourage the parents to express their feelings about the pregnancy, labor, and birth and the experience of having a preterm infant.
- To assess the parents' perceptions of the infant to determine the appropriate time for them to become actively involved in care.

Parents who have negative feelings about the pregnancy or the infant at risk need support. Their feelings can be acknowledged as valid, including the burden they are experiencing financially and emotionally and their understandable feelings toward the infant. (See preceding discussion on parenting disorders.)

Soon after the birth, the parents are given the opportunity to meet the infant in the *en face* position, to touch the infant, and to see her or his favorable characteristics. As soon as possible, depending primarily on her physical condition, the mother is encouraged to visit the nursery at will and help with the infant's care. When she cannot be physically present, staff members devise appropriate methods to keep the family in almost constant touch with the newborn.

Some hospitals have instituted a parents' club for parents of infants in intensive care nurseries. These clubs encourage parents experiencing the same anxiety and grief to share their feelings. An "older" member often takes over a new member and provides additional support. Incorporating these actions into the infant's care plan acknowledges and supports nature's design by engaging and maintaining a bond between the mother and infant. This ensures the infant the continued care needed for physical and emotional survival at the optimum level.

Early discharge of some preterm infants is possible. The nurse's assessment, counseling, and teaching skills are invaluable for the success of home follow-up of infants after early hospital discharge.

EVALUATION

Multidimensional evaluation of the care given preterm infants and their families is required (Montgomery, Williams-Judge, 1986). In some families the infant dies despite all medical and nursing knowledge and skill. In other families the sequelae of preterm birth result in infants who will face lifetime disability. For these families evaluation criteria relate to the concepts of loss, grief, and self-concept (see Chapter 40). For many other infants and families the immediate threat to well-being is overcome by intensive neonatal care.

The nurse can be reasonably assured that care was effective if the following *goals* are met regarding the *physical aspects of care*.

- Respirations are initiated and maintained.
- Body temperature is maintained.
- The infant is adequately nourished.
- CNS trauma is prevented or minimized.
- Infection is prevented
- Renal function is supported.
- Hematologic problems are prevented or minimized.
- Musculoskeletal problems are prevented or minimized.
- Retinal damage is prevented or minimized.

The nurse can be reasonably assured that care was effective if the following *goals* are met regarding *psychosocial aspects of care*.

- The mother retains a positive self-concept as a woman, mother, and sexual being.
- The mother, father/partner, and family perceive the child as potentially normal (if this is medically substantiated); provide the child with realistic care comfortably; and experience pride and satisfaction in the care of the child.
- The parents are able to organize their time and energy to meet the needs for love, attention, and care of all family members, including themselves.

A case study and care plan follow.

CASE STUDY

Preterm Newborn

Michael was born at 32 weeks' gestation. His sister, born at full term, is now 3 years old. His mother's pregnancy was uneventful until labor contractions and spontaneous rupture of membranes occurred at 32 weeks' gestation; no tocolysis was attempted because of the rapid progress of labor.

ASSESSMENT

The mother's prenatal record was not significant for factors often associated with preterm labor. Amniotic fluid was clear with white flakes of vernix, and the lecithin/sphingomyelin ratio was 2.5:1. Michael experienced a nonmedicated, spontaneous, vaginal birth. His Apgar scores were 7 at 1 minute and 8 at 5 minutes. He weighed 2098 g (4 lb 10 oz) (AGA for 32 weeks). He was taken to the neonatal intensive care unit (NICU) for recovery and observation. Both parents were tearful to see their small son and watch him being taken by the pediatrician and intensive care nurse to the NICU. His mother asked when they could see him again and if she could breast-feed him as she had done with his sister.

NURSING DIAGNOSIS

On the basis of the assessment findings, several nursing diagnoses are possible. The nursing diagnosis that takes priority at this time is identified: high risk for ineffective breathing pattern related to inadequate chest expansion secondary to infant's positioning.

PLANNING

Goals are developed with client input whenever possible, which is not the case in this situation. The nurse identifies the following goals: Michael will maintain adequate respiratory function as evidenced by ABGs within normal limits (i.e., carbon dioxide pressure [Pco_2] 33 to 48 mm Hg; oxygen pressure [Po_2] 50 to 70 mm Hg); skin color pink, absence of respiratory distress (e.g., grunting, nasal flaring, retractions), and breath sounds clear to auscultation.

IMPLEMENTATION

Michael is maintained in a variety of side-lying positions, with good body alignment maintained by use of bolsters or rolled linens. His head is extended slightly on the neck to achieve a "sniffing" posture. A flotation mattress is used.

EVALUATION

Michael did not require supplemental oxygen or suctioning; his ABGs remained within normal limits on room air, and his color remained pink. Michael did not experience respiratory distress, and his breath sounds were clear.

CARE PLAN Preterm Newborn

GOALS	IMPLEMENTATION	RATIONALE	EVALUATION
Nursing diagnosis: High risk for ineffective breathing pattern related to inadequate chest expansion secondary to infant's position			
Michael will maintain adequate respiratory function as evidenced by ABGs within normal limits (Pco_2 33-48 mm Hg; Po_2 50-70 mm Hg); skin color pink; absence of respiratory distress (e.g., grunting, nasal flaring, retractions); breath sounds clear to auscultation.	Michael is maintained in a variety of side-lying positions with good body alignment maintained by use of bolsters or rolled linens.	Promotes postural drainage and avoids fluid accumulation in dependent tissues; prevents problems of immobility (e.g., pneumonia).	Michael did not require supplemental oxygen or suctioning. His ABGs were within normal limits, and his color remained pink.
	His head is extended slightly to achieve a "sniffing" posture.	In sniffing posture, trachea is opened to its maximum; hyperextension reduces the tracheal diameter.	Michael did not experience respiratory distress, and his breath sounds remained clear.
	A flotation mattress is used.	Promotes longer periods of quiet sleep, fewer active awake states, and fewer periods of agitation (Deiriggi, 1990).	
Nursing diagnosis: High risk for inadequate thermoregulation related to immature temperature regulation center in the brain, large body surface in relation to body weight, and minimal subcutaneous and brown fat stores			
Michael's temperature will be maintained as evidenced by axillary temperature between 95.9°-99.1°F (36.5°-37.3°C)	Michael is placed unwrapped in prewarmed incubator, under radiant warmer or plastic bubble wrap. All things coming in contact with Michael's skin are kept warm (including nurse's hands and oxygen).	An external source of heat and avoidance of contact with cold air or objects prevent cold stress, with subsequent energy and caloric expenditure.	Michael's axillary temperature was maintained within normal limits.
	The thermistor probe is placed in contact with the skin of the abdomen (avoiding bony prominences and liver), and the portholes to the incubator are closed (if it is used).	Readings from the probe enable caregiver to regulate the environmental temperature. Placing probe over bony prominences or liver may result in artificially elevated temperatures.	Michael was placed in an open bassinet at 12 hours of age.

Respiratory Distress Syndrome

Respiratory distress syndrome (RDS), idiopathic respiratory distress syndrome, and hyaline membrane disease all refer to the lung disorder seen almost exclusively in preterm infants, although it occasionally affects a term infant. This condition appears to occur as a result of underdevelopment of the lungs (Whaley, Wong, 1991).

Infants who are born before 30 weeks' gestation or who weigh less than 1200 g are at highest risk for RDS. In addition, male infants are twice as likely to have RDS as their female counterparts (Merenstein, Gardner, 1989).

The cause of RDS remains unknown. The primary components contributing to the development of RDS are atelectasis and persistent (or regression to) fetal circulation. It has yet to be determined which condition occurs first, but each appears to contribute to the other (Merenstein, Gardner, 1989).

Surfactant, a surface-active phospholipid, acts to prevent alveoli from collapsing at the end of expira-

CARE PLAN **Preterm Newborn—cont'd**

GOALS	IMPLEMENTATION	RATIONALE	EVALUATION
Nursing diagnosis: High risk for parental anxiety related to preterm birth, separation, and breast-feeding			
Parents will be able to see, touch, and feed Michael in the NICU.	Michael's parents are encouraged to stay with him in NICU and actively participate in all aspects of care possible; they hold and examine him *en face;* his mother breast-feeds him. The nurses explain the equipment being used; discuss his behavioral cues and physical characteristics; encourage parents to express their feelings about the pregnancy, labor, and birth; discuss their feeding decisions; facilitate milk expression and storage by providing equipment and/or referral for lactation consultation.	Actions support the parents in the first phase of their adjustment to the preterm neonate, that is, learning who their newborn is and how to recognize and respond to his cues. Seeing and holding him reaffirms the reality of the birth, appearance and condition of their infant. Parents with negative perceptions about the pregnancy or newborn are at risk and need additional support from health care providers. Breast-feeding is supported and encouraged because it provides antibodies, nutrients, and warmth and facilitates bonding and attachment (Meier, 1988; Wilks, Meier, 1988; Zeimer, George, 1990).	Both parents visit Michael for extended periods, holding him and calling him by name. Michael's mother breast-feeds him during the day and uses the milk expression equipment at night, storing the milk appropriately. Initially, Michael lost 71 g (2.5 oz) (under 10%), then steadily began to gain weight. Michael is discharged home at 2211 g (4 lb 14 oz), with parents performing all aspects of his care.

tion. The lack of surfactant may be the basis for development of RDS in the preterm infant. RDS is less commonly seen in infants exposed to intrauterine stressors where surfactant is more rapidly produced (e.g., maternal diabetes [classes C, F, and R], heroin-addicted mothers, and hypertensive conditions during pregnancy) (Merenstein, Gardner, 1989).

A deficiency in surfactant forces the infant to work to reexpand the lungs with each inspiration. The result is fatigue, depletion of energy reserves, hypoxia and hypercapnia, progressive atelectasis, and diminishing lung compliance (or increasing "stiffness"). Factors that impair the production of surfactant are hypoxia, acidosis, and reduced pulmonary blood circulation. Thus a vicious cycle is established. The normal newborn expends more calories and consumes more oxygen to breathe than does the adult. For the infant in respiratory distress this expenditure may be as much as six times that of the normal term newborn. The development of RDS is diagrammed in Fig. 37-11.

RDS may be present at birth or develop over a period of hours. Symptoms will appear as deviations in respiratory rate and effort. Initially, grunting and nasal flaring are evident. Subsequently, tachypnea (≥60 respirations/per minute) and retractions provide further evidence of the effort the infant must expend to maintain lung expansion. Hypotension and shock may be evident. Apneic periods replace expiratory grunting.

Cultures of blood, urine, and cerebrospinal fluid are obtained to rule out sepsis. Blood specimens are collected to assess for hypoglycemia, hypocalcemia, ABG values, and pH (Whaley, Wong, 1991). Chest films assist in ruling out congenital anomalies, pneumonia, and pneumothorax (Merenstein, Gardner, 1989).

The infant with RDS requires expert nursing care. The infant needs a thermoneutral environment to maintain body temperature between 95.9° to 99.1° F (36.5° to 37.3° C). Ambient oxygen concentration may need to be increased; ventilator assistance may be necessary to assist gas exchange. Calories, nutrients, and fluids may be administered via parenteral routes. Mechanical ventilation for respiratory acidosis and sodium bicarbonate for metabolic acidosis may be used. Blood is replaced milliliter for milliliter if an excessive amount is lost, usually as a result of samples taken for laboratory analysis. Serum bilirubin levels are controlled by phototherapy or exchange transfusion, or both. Low serum albumin levels, hypoxia, and acidosis interfere with the albumin's binding to bilirubin and therefore subject these infants to kernicterus at low serum bilirubin levels (10 mg/dL or less; see Chapter 38).

The following respiratory therapies are used for RDS. *Oxygen* (60% or less) is administered by means of a hood (Fig. 37-9). *Continuous positive airway pressure* (CPAP) may be administered by means of an intratracheal tube, face mask, nasal prongs, or hood. *Continuous negative pressure* may be needed. It is provided by a respirator that works in the same manner as CPAP but exerts negative pressure on the newborn's body while the head is exposed. The newborn may breathe room air or an air-oxygen mix by means of a mask or prongs. *Intermittent positive end-expiratory pressure* (PEEP), in which assisted ventilation is used to increase end-expiratory pressure, prevents alveolar collapse (Whaley, Wong, 1991).

An additional therapy is the use of *extracorporeal membrane oxygenation (ECMO)*. ECMO sometimes is used in conjunction with a modified heart-lung machine (Bartlett et al, 1985). (For further discussion of ECMO, see Chapter 36.)

An even more recently developed treatment for RDS is the administration of an artificial surfactant or surfactant from an exogenous source. The surfactant is given at birth before the first breath or after diagnosis of RDS (Miller, Armstrong, 1990). The effect persists up to 72 hours. This treatment has been shown to reduce the respiratory complications of RDS (Glickman-Ioli, Richardson, 1990; Whaley, Wong, 1991). Adverse effects of artificial surfactant have been minimal to absent in the acute care of infants.

Oxygen-Associated Complications

Bronchopulmonary dysplasia (BPD) and retinopathy of prematurity (ROP) are diseases of preterm birth secondary to oxygen therapy (Bancalari, Gerhardt, 1986). Both conditions are relatively "new" disorders, recognized since the advent of methods of administering high concentrations of oxygen beginning in the 1940s. Although oxygen therapy may be lifesaving and occasionally must be given in high concentrations for extended periods, it also is potentially hazardous and must be administered cautiously. In addition to BPD and ROP, other conditions have become apparent. The mechanical creation of positive pressure in the lungs has increased the incidence of "air leaks." Use of oxygen apparatuses also has resulted in nasal, tracheal, or pharyngeal perforation or inflammation (Whaley, Wong, 1991).

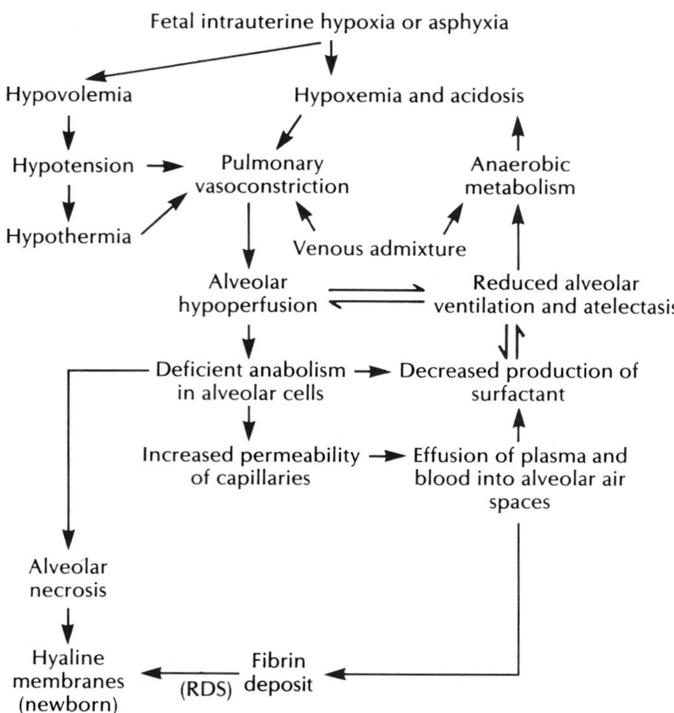

Fig. 37-11 Development of respiratory distress syndrome. Courtesy A. Hacket, Stanford University Medical Center, Stanford, Calif.

BRONCHOPULMONARY DYSPLASIA. Bronchopulmonary dysplasia (BPD) is a common concomitant of lung disorders in infants, primarily preterm infants, in which focal areas of emphysema develop in the lungs. The cause is unknown, but the condition may develop as a sequela to alveolar damage caused by lung disease, use of high oxygen concentrations, and the prolonged use of CPAP or PEEP (Bancalari, Gerhardt, 1986).

Symptoms of respiratory distress, tachypnea, and increased effort appear. It is difficult to wean the infant from the positive pressure ventilator. This finding may be the first indication of the disease process.

The first sign that the infant is recovering from BPD is a decreasing dependence on oxygen therapy. Recovery may take several months. The mortality rate is between 30% and 50%; death may occur after the infant has been discharged from the hospital.

RETINOPATHY OF PREMATURITY. The retinal changes in **retinopathy of prematurity (ROP)** were first described in 1942. Originally ROP was considered a disorder caused by prolonged exposure to high levels of oxygen. ROP is now thought to be a complex, multicausal disease of preterm birth (Whaley, Wong, 1991). Judicious use of oxygen therapy and monitoring of arterial oxygen pressure (PaO_2) levels have reduced the incidence of ROP, but the disease has not been eliminated.

Prevention of ROP is a fundamental concept for the nursing care of infants receiving oxygen. Close monitoring of oxygen regulation and infant status will facilitate therapeutic and safe oxygen administration. The most crucial period for toxic levels to occur is during the recovery phase from RDS and other respiratory distress. The exact level at which PaO_2 becomes toxic and causes ROP is unknown.

Oxygen tensions that are too high for the level of retinal maturity initially result in vasoconstriction. After oxygen therapy is discontinued, neovascularization occurs in the retina and vitreous, with capillary hemorrhages, fibrotic resolution, and possible retinal detachment. Cicatricial (scar) tissue formation and consequent visual impairment may be mild or severe. The entire disease process in severe cases may take as long as 5 months to evolve. Examination by an ophthalmologist before discharge and a schedule for repeat examinations thereafter are recommended for the parents' guidance.

NECROTIZING ENTEROCOLITIS. Necrotizing **enterocolitis** (NEC) is an acute inflammatory disease of the gastrointestinal mucosa, commonly complicated by perforation. This often fatal disease appears in about 5% of newborns in intensive care nurseries. Although the cause of NEC is unknown, the following factors contribute to its development: immaturity, hypoxemia (postbirth), high-solute feedings, excessive amounts of feedings, **perinatal asphyxia** (commonly a historical antecedent), and bacterial or viral gastrointestinal infection (Merenstein, Gardner, 1989).

Recent research suggests that reversal of perinatal asphyxia (p. 1142) within 30 minutes may prevent gastrointestinal tract insult and thus prevent the initiation of NEC pathophysiology. After 30 minutes, distribution of cardiac output tends to be directed more toward the heart and brain and away from the abdominal organs. Therefore prompt birth of the intrauterine-asphyxiated fetus or ventilation of the asphyxiated newborn may be beneficial to the gastrointestinal tract, as well as to other organs.

The onset usually is between 4 and 10 days. In the full-term infant the onset almost always is within the first 10 days. In the preterm infant the onset may be delayed up to 30 days. Signs of developing NEC are nonspecific, which is characteristic of many neonatal disease processes. Abdominal distention, often to the point of "shining," is probably the most common and regularly encountered sign. The infant's color is poor. Apneic periods increase. Commonly there are gastric residuals of 2 mL or more before feedings. The stool may show occult blood (positive guaiac test result). Diagnosis is confirmed by x-ray examination.

Treatment is supportive. Oral or tube feedings are discontinued to rest the gastrointestinal tract. Parenteral therapy (often by total parenteral nutrition [TPN]) is begun. NEC is an infectious disease; therefore control of infection is imperative. Antibiotic therapy may be instituted, and surgery is performed when necessary. Therapy may be prolonged, and recovery may be delayed by adhesions, complications of bowel resection, and intolerance of oral feedings.

■ POSTTERM AND POSTMATURE INFANTS

Postterm, or *postdate,* infants are those whose gestation is prolonged beyond 42 weeks, regardless of birth weight. These infants may be LGA or SGA, but most often their weight is AGA. Commonly these infants have little vernix caseosa other than in the skin creases, and that may be stained yellow or green. The cause of **prolonged pregnancy** is unknown. Certain groups are more likely to have gestations longer than 42 weeks, including first-time mothers, multiparous women (four or more children), and women with a history of a postdate pregnancy.

Postmaturity implies progressive placental insufficiency, resulting in a dysmature newborn. It is important to note that *not all postterm infants are postmature.*

In the SGA postterm infant, fetal malnutrition and hypoxia occur as a result of deteriorating metabolic exchange in the aging placenta. The depletion of subcutaneous fat produces the wasted appearance of the dysmature infant.

Perinatal mortality is significantly higher in the postterm fetus and neonate. During labor and birth, increased oxygen demands of the postmature fetus cannot be met. Insufficient gas exchange by the postmature placenta causes an increased incidence of intrauterine hypoxia and subsequent meconium aspiration. Of all the deaths of postterm newborns, one half occur during labor and birth, about one third occur before the onset of labor, and one sixth occur during the puerperium.

ASSESSMENT

When a pregnant woman is 2 weeks past her estimated date of delivery (EDD), one of the following possibilities exists.

- The pregnancy is not prolonged; therefore there is no threat to the fetus.
- The pregnancy is prolonged, but the placenta continues to function efficiently, and there is no threat to the fetus.
- The pregnancy is prolonged, and there is acute placental failure with threat to the fetus.
- The pregnancy is prolonged, there has been chronic placental insufficiency, and the threat to the fetus continues.

For safe birth of the fetus, it becomes important to determine whether prolonged pregnancy actually has developed and whether there is any evidence of fetal jeopardy. Data for determining fetal gestational age are obtained from several sources and correlated (see Chapters 20 and 27).

HISTORY AND INTERVIEW. Verification of the last menstrual period (LMP) is important to the diagnosis of prolonged pregnancy. A correlation of the LMP with the estimated duration of pregnancy at two of the earliest obstetric examinations may lead to substantiation or recalculation of the EDD (see p. 302).

If the dates are accurate but the uterus is larger than expected for the duration of pregnancy, hydramnios or multifetal pregnancy may be the cause. If the dates seem correct but the size of the fetus is disparate, fetal compromise such as IUGR may be the problem, particularly when it occurs in association with preeclampsia.

The woman's medical status is reappraised. Diabetic women and women who have glucose intolerance of pregnancy have large babies, and this may confuse the estimate of gestational age. Amniocentesis to ascertain the true gestational age is advised.

PHYSICAL EXAMINATION. Reviewing the prenatal record precedes the physical examination. Results may support the diagnosis of prolonged pregnancy. The following findings suggest that the infant will be postmature:

- Maternal weight loss in the last weeks of pregnancy (3 lb [1.3 kg] or more a week)
- Reduced rate of uterine and fetal growth
- Palpation of a hard fetal head; lack of cephalic molding; high arrest of the fetal head
- Meconium staining of the amniotic fluid
- Oligohydramnios or decreased amniotic fluid (less than 300 mL)

DIAGNOSTIC TESTS. Two serial *ultrasound examinations* and measurement of the *fetal biparietal diameter* (for further discussion, see Chapter 27) should be accomplished 2 weeks apart after the twentieth week. This may confirm or reestablish the EDD. However, the EDD cannot be calculated when the *initial* biparietal diameter measures 9.5 cm or more (term size).

The fetal monitoring will include fetal activity determination, weekly estimate of fetal weight, nonstress test (NST) or oxytocin challenge test (OCT), and biophysical profile (see Chapter 27).

ASSESSMENT OF THE NEWBORN. Most postterm and postmature infants are oversized but otherwise normal, with advanced development and bone age.

A postmature infant will have some but not necessarily all of the following physical characteristics:

- Generally has normal skull, but reduced dimensions of rest of body make skull look inordinately large
- Dry, cracked skin (desquamating), parchmentlike at birth
- Nails of hard consistency extending beyond fingertips
- Profuse scalp hair
- Subcutaneous fat layers depleted, leaving skin loose and giving an "old person" appearance
- Long and thin body contour
- Absent vernix
- Often meconium staining (golden-yellow to green) of skin, nails, and cord
- May have an alert, wide-eyed appearance symptomatic of chronic intrauterine hypoxia

NURSING DIAGNOSES

The postmature infant's size and condition will determine whether the nursing diagnoses suitable for the "normal" newborn or those formulated for the preterm infant are appropriate. Examples include the following:

- Ineffective airway clearance related to
  —Meconium aspiration syndrome
- High risk for hypothermia related to
  —Depleted stores of subcutaneous fat
- High risk for injury (permanent disability) related to
  —Birth trauma
- High risk for injury secondary to hypoglycemia related to
  —Depleted glycogen stores

PLANNING

Physiologic problems of postmaturity are reflected in the plan of care. *Immediate goals* are that the newborn will initiate and maintain respirations, will not experience CNS trauma or infection, and if there is birth trauma, it will be identified and treated promptly without sequelae. The *long-term goal* is that the infant will not experience adverse effects of postmaturity.

IMPLEMENTATION

Immediate care is similar to that given to preterm infants (Affonso, Harris, 1980). Procedures to support physiologic function (e.g., respiration, body temperature, nutrition) are discussed in Chapters 21 and 36.

Medical Management

After confirmation of prolonged pregnancy the health care practitioner determines the protocol for birth. A *trial of labor* by induction may be ordered (see Chapter 35).

The postmature fetus (AGA or SGA) may not tolerate the stress of labor well because of increasing placental insufficiency. Indices of fetal jeopardy are late fetal heart rate deceleration patterns, with a slow return to the baseline rate, meconium-stained amniotic fluid, oligohydramnios, and a fetal scalp blood pH of 7.2 or less. Cephalopelvic or fetopelvic disproportion complicates some postterm labors. The oversized fetus may be exposed to excessive trauma during vaginal birth, such as fractures and intracranial hemorrhage, and to asphyxia during labor (see Chapter 39 for birth trauma).

If induction is unsuccessful, if labor is unsatisfactory, or if fetal distress develops, cesarean birth is performed.

Nursing Care

During the antepartum period the nurse contributes to the assessment for identification of a prolonged pregnancy and often conducts nonstress tests to monitor fetal well-being. Identification and management of maternal reactions are important components of the nursing care plan. Emotional response of the woman can reflect feelings of fatigue, frustration, and anger as the pregnancy "never seems to end." She may experience negative feelings about her ability to cope and her "normality as a woman." Fears for the safety of her baby and the baby's future development can arise.

Intrapartum nursing care of the fetus is the same as for all other labors (see Unit III). It may be similar to that needed for fetopelvic disproportion and dystocic labor (see Chapter 35). Parental fears are recognized, and support is offered. After birth the neonate is assessed in the same manner as all newborns (see Chapter 20).

EVALUATION

The nurse can be assured that care was effective when the short-term goals for care have been met. That is, the newborn initiated and maintained respirations, did not experience CNS trauma or infection, and if there was a birth trauma, it was identified and treated promptly without sequelae. Evaluation of the degree to which the long-term goal is achieved is delayed beyond the period of infancy.

■ SMALL-FOR-GESTATIONAL-AGE, INTRAUTERINE GROWTH RETARDED, AND DYSMATURE INFANTS

Infants whose birth weight falls below the 10th percentile expected at term, for reasons other than heredity, are considered at high risk (mortality greater than 10%) (Korones, 1986).

Various conditions can affect and impede growth in the developing fetus. The cause, severity, and the gestational age at which the insult occurs determine how fetal growth is affected and what problems will be present in the newborn. Conditions occurring in the first trimester, which affects all aspects of fetal growth (infections, teratogens, and chromosomal abnormalities), result in *symmetric* IUGR. Conditions causing symmetric growth retardation will result in a short, SGA infant, usually with a smaller head circumference and reduced brain capacity.

Growth retardation in later stages of pregnancy, as a result of maternal or placental factors, results in *asymmetric* growth retardation (with respect to gestational age, weight will be ≤10th percentile whereas length and head circumference will be ≥10th percentile). Asymmetric growth retardation occurs as a result of the fetus receiving inadequate supplies of oxygen and nutrients (placental insufficiency). Conditions that cause placental insufficiency include "maternal hypertension (preeclampsia and essential hypertension), smoking, malnutrition (undernutrition) and varied forms of maternal vascular and renal diseases" (Creasy, Resnik, 1989). Infants with asymmetric IUGR have the potential for normal growth and development. Abnormal fetal size may indicate an adaptive response, with diminished fetal weight-sparing brain growth (Warshaw [1985] in Creasy, Resnik, 1989).

ASSESSMENT

Several physical findings are characteristic of the *growth-retarded neonate:*

- Generally has normal skull, but reduced dimensions of rest of body make skull look inordinately large
- Reduced subcutaneous fat
- Loose and dry skin
- Diminished muscle mass, especially over buttocks and cheeks
- Sunken abdomen (scaphoid) as opposed to being normally well rounded
- Thin, yellowish, dry, and dull umbilical cord (normal cord is gray, glistening, round, and moist)
- Sparse scalp hair
- Wide skull sutures (inadequate bone growth)

SGA infants are likely to experience perinatal asphyxia, meconium aspiration syndrome, hypoglycemia, and heat loss.

Perinatal Asphyxia

Commonly, SGA infants have been exposed to chronic hypoxia for varying periods before labor and birth. Labor is a stressor to the normal fetus; it is an even greater stressor for the growth-retarded fetus. The chronically hypoxic infant is severely compromised by even a normal labor and has difficulty compensating after birth. The alert, wide-eyed appearance of the newborn is attributed to prolonged prenatal hypoxia. Appropriate management and resuscitation are essential for the depressed infant.

The birth of SGA babies with perinatal asphyxia may be associated with a maternal history of heavy cigarette smoking; preeclampsia; low socioeconomic status; multifetal gestation; gestational infections such as rubella, cytomegalovirus, and toxoplasmosis; advanced diabetes mellitus; and cardiac problems. When a woman with this background arrives in labor, the nursing staff must be alert to and prepared for possible perinatal asphyxia. Sequelae to perinatal asphyxia include meconium aspiration syndrome and hypoglycemia.

Meconium Aspiration Syndrome

Intrauterine passage of meconium is a common indication of fetal stress. This stress, fetal asphyxia, or another cause promotes peristalsis, and meconium is expelled into the amniotic fluid. Continued intrauterine stress or the stress of birth causes the fetus to make respiratory efforts that draw the meconium-stained amniotic fluid into the respiratory passages. This process results in **meconium aspiration syndrome**. This sticky, tarlike stool clings to the walls of alveoli and impairs respiratory function. Meconium aspiration causes physical obstruction of the airways and hinders gas exchange. Meconium fosters the growth of virulent pathogens within the respiratory tract because it is a good medium for bacterial growth (Merenstein, Gardner, 1989). Symptoms of respiratory distress syndrome are common after meconium aspiration.

Hypoglycemia

Stressed infants are at risk for the development of **hypoglycemia** (Merenstein, Gardner, 1989). Stress may include perinatal asphyxia and IUGR. Definitions of hypoglycemia vary for the term and the preterm infant. Within the first 3 days of life, hypoglycemia is defined as a blood glucose level of less than 40 mg/dL in the term infant or less than 25 mg/dL in the preterm infant.

Symptoms of hypoglycemia include cyanosis, apnea, tachypnea, and irregular respirations and diaphoresis. CNS symptoms can include jitteriness, weak cry, lethargy, floppy posture, convulsions, or coma. Diagnosis is confirmed by blood glucose determinations by laboratory or by on-unit visual methods with reagent strips such as Chemstrip-BG or Dextrostix.

Heat Loss

As a result of a number of factors, SGA infants require particular attention to maintain thermoneutrality. These infants have less muscle mass, less brown fat (an internal fuel source for generation of heat found in large amounts in normal term infants), less heat-preserving subcutaneous fat, and little ability to control skin capillaries. Nursing considerations focus on maintenance of thermoneutrality to support recovery from perinatal asphyxia; cold stress jeopardizes recovery from asphyxia.

NURSING DIAGNOSES

Analysis of assessment findings will determine suitable nursing diagnoses such as the following examples:

- Impaired gas exchange related to
  - —Meconium aspiration
- High risk for injury related to
  - —Hypoglycemia
- Ineffective thermoregulation related to
  - —Reduced subcutaneous fat

—Increased surface area in relation to body weight (mass)
—Diminished muscle mass
- High risk for altered parenting related to
—Physical appearance and condition at birth

PLANNING

The nursing plan of care for the SGA infant is similar to that for the preterm infant. *Goals* are established with clients and, whenever possible, are stated in client-centered terms.

The infant will have the following outcomes:

- Maintain physiologic functioning
- Maintain adequate gas exchange
- Maintain blood glucose levels within normal range and experience no episodes of hypoglycemia
- Maintain effective thermoregulation
- Begin bonding and attachment to parents

The parents will have the following outcomes:

- Perceive the infant as potentially normal (if this is medically substantiated)
- Provide care comfortably
- Experience pride and satisfaction in the care of the infant
- Organize their time and energies to meet the love, attention, and care needs of the other members of the family as well as their own
- Begin bonding and attachment to the infant

IMPLEMENTATION

Care of the SGA infant is based on the clinical problems present. The nursing care related to those problems is the same as for the preterm infant (see Implementation, p. 1132).

Gas exchange is supported by maintaining a clear airway (for discussion of suctioning, see p. 589) and preventing cold stress (for discussion of oxygen administration and ventilation, see p. 1094). Hypoglycemia is treated with oral feedings (e.g., breast, formula, dextrose solution) per hospital protocol. Parenteral infusions may be necessary. An external heat source is used until the infant's temperature is stabilized (p. 1099). Nursing support of parents is similar to that given to parents of preterm infants (p. 1134).

EVALUATION

The nurse can be reasonably assured that care was effective when the goals have been met. That is, the infant maintained physiologic functioning, adequate gas exhange, blood glucose levels within normal range, and normal temperature; and began bonding and attachment to the parent(s). The parents perceive the infant as potentially normal (if this is medically supported), provide care comfortably, experience pride and satisfaction in the care of the infant, organize their time and energies to meet the love, attention, and care needs of the other members of the family as well as their own, and have begun bonding and attachment to the infant.

LARGE-FOR-GESTATIONAL AGE INFANTS

The LGA, or oversized, infant traditionally has been one who weighs 4000 g (8 lb 13 oz) or more at birth. About 10% of newborns are of this weight, and about 2% weigh 4500 g (9 lb 15 oz) or more. Most of these newborns have other proportionately larger measurements. Many are born well after the estimated date of delivery (EDD). Better maternal health and nutrition probably are responsible for this greater growth during recent generations.

Maternal pelvic diameters have not kept pace with these changes; thus fetopelvic disproportion often occurs, particularly in obese women, women who gain 16 kg (35 lb) or more during gestation, and diabetic women, who are prone to have large babies. Birth trauma, especially associated with breech or shoulder presentation, is a serious hazard for the oversized neonate. Asphyxia or CNS injury, or both, also may occur.

A biparietal diameter greater than 10 cm verified by fetometry (ultrasound or x-ray examination), a uterine fundal measurement (McDonald's rule) greater than 42 cm in the absence of hydramnios, and only average or smaller interior pelvic diameters are frequent findings. All pregnancies of longer than 42 weeks' gestation are carefully evaluated. All large fetuses are monitored during a trial of labor, and preparation is made for a cesarean birth if fetal distress or poor progress of labor occurs.

Prognosis for the mother may entail lacerations to the birth canal if operative vaginal birth is permitted. Cesarean birth usually is indicated, particularly with borderline cephalopelvic disproportion or in breech presentation, even in multiparous women who have given birth to oversized fetuses. LGA newborns may be preterm, term, or postterm; children of diabetic (or prediabetic) mothers; and postmature.

Each of these categories has special concerns. Regardless of coexisting potential problems, *the oversized infant is at risk by virtue of size alone.*

Any one or a combination of injuries discussed in nursing actions for LGA infants may occur in normal- or small-sized infants. In addition to the large size of the infant, factors that predispose to birth trauma include the following (birth trauma is discussed in Chapter 39):

- Preterm labor and birth
- Length of labor
- Size and shape of maternal pelvis
- Fetal presentation, attitude, and lie

ASSESSMENT

The nurse assesses the LGA infant for gestational age, hypoglycemia and trauma from the vaginal or cesarean birth (see Chapter 39, acquired problems).

NURSING DIAGNOSES

The nursing diagnoses are based on the type of condition the newborn has experienced. Diagnoses are individualized, and may include any of the following:

- High risk for injury related to
  - —Hypoglycemia
  - —Cephalopelvic disproportion and vaginal birth
  - —Operative birth (e.g., forceps- or vacuum-assisted birth; cesarean birth)
- High risk for altered parenting related to
  - —Difficult labor and birth
  - —Physical appearance and condition at birth
  - —Permanent sequelae from birth trauma (e.g., Erb's palsy)

PLANNING

Planning for care and goal setting depends on the LGA infant's condition. *Goals* include:

- The neonate will not experience hypoglycemia.
- The neonate will not experience birth trauma, and, if present, it will be identified and managed in a timely manner.
- The parents will begin the bonding and attachment process.

IMPLEMENTATION

Blood glucose levels are monitored, and hypoglycemia is corrected. Specific birth injuries, if present, are treated appropriately.

EVALUATION

The nurse can be reasonably assured the goals for care of the LGA infant were achieved if hypoglycemia is treated and blood glucose levels are within normal limits, if birth trauma is managed with minimal or absent sequelae, and if parents begin the bonding and attachment process.

■ SUMMARY

Infants whose gestational age and birth weight fall outside those parameters defined as normal are considered to be at risk. The survival and well-being of the infant depend on the collaborative efforts of the medical and paramedical team. The nurse's skills in observing and recording often form the foundation for early diagnosis and appropriate treatment of medical and surgical conditions. Furthermore the nurse's role in facilitating the development of a positive parent-child relationship cannot be overemphasized.

REFERENCES

Affonso D, Harris T: Postterm pregnancy: implications for mother and infant, challenge for the nurse, *JOGNN* 9:139, 1980.

Als H, Brazelton TB: A new model of assessing the behavioral organization in preterm and full term infants, *J Am Acad Child Psychiatry* 20:239, 1981.

Bancalari E, Gerhardt T: Bronchopulmonary dysplasia, *Pediatr Clin North Am* 33:1, 1986.

Bartlett, RH et al: Extracorporeal circulation in neonatal respiratory failure: a prospective randomized study, *Pediatrics* 76:479, 1985.

Bennett FC, Robinson NM, Sells CJ: Growth and development of infants weighing less than 800 grams at birth, *Pediatrics* 71:319, 1983.

Creasy RK, Resnik R: *Maternal-fetal medicine: principles and practice,* ed 2, Philadelphia, 1989, WB Saunders Co.

Dubowitz LMS et al: Gestational age of the newborn, *J Pediatr* 77:1, 1970.

Fanaroff AA, Martin RJ: *Neonatal-perinatal medicine: diseases of the fetus and infant,* ed 5, St Louis, 1992, Mosby–Year Book.

Field TM: Interaction patterns of preterm and term infants. In Field TM, editor: *Infants born at risk,* Jamaica, NY, 1979, Spectrum Publications.

Fomufod AK: Low birthweight and early neonatal separation as factors in child abuse, *J Natl Med Assoc* 68:106, 1976.

Glickman-Ioli J, Richardson MJ: Giving surfactant to premature infants, *AJN* 90(3):59, 1990.

Hansen FH: Nursing care in the neonatal intensive care unit, *JOGNN* 11:17, 1982.

Korones SB: *High-risk newborn infants: the basis for intensive nursing care,* ed 4, St Louis, 1986, Mosby–Year Book.

Merenstein GB, Gardner SL: *Handbook of neonatal intensive care,* ed 2, St Louis, 1989, Mosby–Year Book.

Miller EP, Armstrong CL: Surfactant replacement therapy—innovative care for the premature infant, *JOGNN* 19:14, 1990.

Milluncheck E, McArtor R: Fatal aspiration of a make-shift pacifier, *Pediatrics* 77:369, 1986.

Montgomery LA, Williams-Judge S: An anticipatory support program for high-risk parents, *Neonatal Network* 5:33, Aug 1986.

Newman L: Parents' perceptions of their low birth weight infants, *Pediatrician* 9:182, 1980.

Philip A: *Neonatology: a practical guide,* ed 3, Philadelphia, 1987, WB Saunders Co.

Rehm R: Teaching cardiopulmonary resuscitation to parents, *MCN* 8:411, Nov/Dec 1983.

Sammons W, Lewis J: *Premature babies: a different beginning,* St Louis, 1985, Mosby–Year Book.

Schraeder BD: Attachment and parenting despite lengthy intensive care, *MCN* 5:37, 1980.

Sosa R, Grua P: Perinatal responses to normal and premature birth experiences, *J Calif Perinat Assoc* 2:36, 1982.

Whaley LF, Wong, DL: *Nursing care of infants and children,* ed 4, St Louis, 1991, Mosby–Year Book.

Wilks S, Meier P: Helping mothers express milk suitable for preterm and high-risk infant feeding, *MCN* 13:121, March/April 1988.

Zeimer MM, George C: Breastfeeding the low-birthweight infant, *Neonatal Network* 9:33, Dec 1990.

References—Nursing Research

Deiriggi PM: Effects of waterbed flotation on indicators of energy expenditure in preterm infants, *Nurs Res* 39:140, May/June 1990.

Meier P: Bottle- and breast-feeding: effects on transcutaneous oxygen pressure and temperature in preterm infants, *Nurs Res* 37:36, Jan/Feb 1988.

Gill NE et al: Effect of nonnutritive sucking on behavioral state in preterm infants before feeding, *Nurs Res* 37:347, Nov/Dec 1988.

Wright S, Norton C, Kesten K: Retention of infant CPR instruction by parents, *Pediatr Nurs* 15:37, Jan 1989.

BIBLIOGRAPHY

Anderson GC: Current knowledge about skin-to-skin (kangaroo) care for preterm infants, *J Perinat* 11:216, 1991.

Beckholt AP: Breast milk for infants who cannot breastfeed, *JOGNN* 19:216, 1990.

Bullock LF, McFarlane J: The birth-weight/battering connection, *AJN,* p 1153, Sept 1989.

Consolvo CA: Producing videos for home use by parents of high-risk infants, *MCN* 15:178, May/June 1990.

Crane LD et al: Effects of position changes on transcutaneous carbon dioxide tension in neonates with respiratory distress, *J Perinat* 10:35, 1990.

Damato EG: Discharge planning from the neonatal intensive care unit, *J Perinat Neonat Nurs* 5:43, Jan 1991.

Ladden M: The impact of preterm birth on the family and society: psychologic sequelae of preterm birth, *Pediatr Nurs* 16:515, 1990.

Lieberman E, Ryan KJ, Schoenbaum SC: The association of interpregnancy interval with small for gestational age births, *Obstet Gynecol* 74:1, 1989.

Ludington-Hoe SM, Hadeed AJ, Anderson GC: Physiologic responses to skin-to-skin contact in hospitalized premature infants, *J Perinat* 11:19, 1991.

Merritt TA et al: Impact of surfactant treatment on cost of neonatal intensive care: a cost benefit analysis, *J Perinat* 10:416, 1990.

Roberts PM: NEC: etiology, treatment, prevention, and nursing care, *Crit Care Nurse* 10(4):38, 1990.

Weaver KA, Anderson GC: Relationship between integrated sucking pressures and first bottle-feeding scores in premature infants, *JOGNN* 17:113, 1988.

Bibliography—Nursing Research

Becker PT et al: Outcomes of developmentally supportive nursing care for very low birth weight infants, *Nurs Res* 40:150, 1991.

Beckman CA: Postterm pregnancy: effects on temperature and glucose regulation, *Nurs Res* 39:21, 1990.

Brown LP et al: A sociodemographic profile of families of low birthweight infants, *West J Nurs Res* 11:520, 1989.

Brown LP et al: Very low birth-weight infants: parental visiting and telephoning during initial infant hospitalization, *Nurs Res* 38:233, 1989.

Gennaro S et al: Concerns of mothers of low birthweight infants, *Pediatr Nurs* 16:459, 1990.

Harrison LL, Leeper JD, Yoon M: Effects of early parent touch on preterm infants' heart rates and arterial oxygen saturation levels, *J Adv Nurs* 15:877, 1990.

Harrison MJ: A comparison of parental interactions with term and preterm infants, *Res Nurs Health* 13:173, 1990.

McCain GC: Parenting growing preterm infants, *Pediatr Nurs* 16:467, 1990.

Miles MS: Parents of critically ill premature infants: sources of stress, *Crit Care Nurs Q* 12(3):69, 1989.

Mitchell SH, Najak ZD: Low-birthweight infants and rehospitalization: what's the incidence? *Neonatal Network* 8:27, Sept 1989.

Newman CB, McSweeney M: A descriptive study of sibling visitation in the NICU, *Neonatal Network* 9(4):27, 1990.

chapter 37 review

Key Concepts

- Preterm infants are at risk for problems related to the immaturity of organ systems.
- Nurses who work with preterm infants have an important role: to observe for respiratory distress and other early symptoms of physiologic functioning problems.
- Parental adaptation to preterm infants is different from that of parents who have given birth to full-term infants.
- Nurses have a vital role in facilitating the development of a positive parent-child relationship.
- Nurses' skills in interpreting data, making decisions, and initiating therapy in newborn intensive care units are crucial to the infant's survival.
- Parents need special instruction (e.g., CPR, oxygen therapy, suctioning) before they take a high-risk infant home.
- SGA infants are considered at high risk as a result of fetal growth retardation.
- The high incidence of fetal distress among postmature infants is related to progressive placental insufficiency.

Key Terms

- appropriate for gestational age (AGA) (p. 1120)
- bronchopulmonary dysplasia (BPD) (p. 1138)
- corrected age (p. 1129)
- hypoglycemia (p. 1142)
- infant stimulation (p. 1133)
- intrauterine growth retardation (IUGR) (p. 1120)
- large for gestational age (LGA) (p. 1120, 1143)
- low birth weight (LBW) (p. 1120)
- meconium aspiration syndrome (p. 1142)
- necrotizing enterocolitis (NEC) (p. 1139)
- neuromuscular maturity (p. 1123, 1125)
- newborn maturity rating and classification (p. 1125)
- nonnutritive suckling (p. 1134)
- perinatal asphyxia (p. 1139, 1142)
- physical maturity (p. 1123, 1124)
- prolonged pregnancy (p. 1139)
- postmature (p. 1120, 1139)
- postterm (postdates) (p. 1120, 1139)
- premature (p. 1120, 1121)
- preterm (p. 1120, 1121)
- respiratory distress syndrome (RDS) (p. 1136)
- retinopathy of prematurity (ROP) (p. 1138)
- small for gestational age (SGA) (p. 1120, 1141)
- term (p. 1120)

Critical Thinking Exercises

1. For several infants, perform and record assessment for gestational age. Determine the gestational age of one or more infants. Verify your conclusions.
2. Assist with the care of a compromised infant in the special care nursery.
   a. Identify the infant's physical characteristics. Compare with that for the "normal" term infant.
   b. Observe the interactions between the parents and the infant. Make and check inferences based on data. Are your inferences plausible?
   c. Develop a nursing plan of care for the infant's most urgent problem and compare with the plan for a "normal" term infant.
   d. Develop a nursing plan of care for supportive care for the parents. Compare with a similar plan for the parents of a "normal" term infant.

Topics for Nursing Research

- How do the educational needs of mothers of preterm, term, postterm, and postmature newborn infants differ?
- What is the interrater reliability for nurses' estimation of gestational age?
- Is there a relationship between the manner in which parents address the preterm infant (it; he/she; name) and their readiness to take on an active caregiving role?
- LGA infants: effect of temperature and glucose regulation.
- Reliability of the criteria of behavioral characteristics that determine the date of discharge (p. 1129)—that is, are the behavioral characteristics used to determine discharge date (p. 1129) of the preterm infant reliable indicators of preparedness for discharge?

chapter 38

Developmental Problems

PHILOMENA WHELAN

LEARNING OBJECTIVES

- Define the key terms listed.
- Discuss assessment of the newborn for hyperbilirubinemia.
- Develop a nursing plan of care for the prevention, identification, and management of hyperbilirubinemia in any newborn.
- Compare Rh and ABO incompatibility.
- Explain nursing management to prevent the pathologic consequences of hyperbilirubinemia.
- Review prenatal diagnosis of neonatal disorders.
- Present assessment strategies during the postnatal period to aid in diagnosis of congenital disorders.
- Describe preoperative and postoperative nursing care of the newborn.
- Develop a nursing plan of care for parents of a newborn with a defect or disorder.
- Describe each congenital disorder presented in this chapter, and identify the priority of nursing care for each.
- Identify topics for nursing research related to developmental problems.

■ HYPERBILIRUBINEMIA

The yellow discoloration of the skin and other organs caused by accumulation of bilirubin is termed **jaundice** or *icterus*. Jaundice in the newborn, a common sign of potential trouble, is caused primarily by unconjugated bilirubin, a breakdown product of hemoglobin (Hb), after its release from hemolyzed red blood cells (RBCs). The challenge of neonatal jaundice is to distinguish physiologic jaundice from a serious clinical pathologic condition.

A variety of etiologic factors cause hyperbilirubinemia. The main focus of this section is **isoimmune hemolytic disease** of the newborn secondary to Rh or ABO incompatibility.

Rh Incompatibility

Soon after the Rh factor was reported, it was found that erythroblastosis fetalis, hydrops fetalis, and icterus gravis—variations of hemolytic disease of the newborn—are the results of the hemolysis of fetal Rh-positive RBCs by specific antibodies from an Rh-negative mother. Between 10% and 15% of Caucasian couples and about 5% of African-American couples have Rh incompatibility. It is rare that an Oriental couple will be similarly affected. Not all Rh-positive men are homozygous for the Rh factor, nor will all children of Rh-positive men with Rh-negative partners be Rh positive. About 50% of the progeny of Rh-positive men who are heterozygous will be Rh positive; the remainder will be Rh negative (see Fig. 7-4). Rh-negative offspring are in no danger because they are compatible with their mothers.

During pregnancies with an Rh-positive fetus, there usually is no effect on the fetus as a result of isoimmunization. Placental separation allows the transfer of fetal blood to maternal circulation, which stimulates maternal antibody production. Effects of sensitization are seen in subsequent pregnancies with an Rh-positive fetus when the maternal antibodies to Rh-positive RBCs enter the fetal circulation.

Severe Rh incompatibility results in marked fetal hemolytic anemia. The placenta clears the released blood pigments fairly well, however, so that only in extreme cases (such as icterus gravis) is the fetus icteric (yellow, or jaundiced). The *marked anemia* leads to cardiac decompensation, cardiomegaly, hepatomegaly, and splenomegaly. Edema, ascites, and hydrothorax develop. Severe anemia may lead to hypoxia. Intrauterine or early neonatal death may occur.

Once birth has occurred, the erythroblastotic newborn becomes icteric (in severe cases, within 30 minutes after birth) because it cannot excrete the considerable residue of RBC hemolysis. Yellowish pigmentation of cerebrobasal nuclei, hippocampal cortex, and subthalamic nuclei often develop (kernicterus).

ABO Incompatibility

ABO incompatibility is more common than Rh incompatibility, but the effects generally are less severe in the affected infant. ABO incompatibility occurs when the fetal blood type is A, B, or AB and the maternal type is O. Naturally occurring anti-A and anti-B antibodies are transferred across the placenta to the fetus. First-born infants may be affected. The newborn may show a weakly positive direct **Coombs' test** result. Cord bilirubin usually is less than 4 mg/100 mL, and any resulting hyperbilirubinemia usually can be treated with phototherapy as discussed on p. 599 and Fig. 21-11. Exchange transfusions are required only in occasional cases. Ongoing hemolysis may cause anemia, jaundice, and kernicterus and justifies serial hematocrit studies until the infant is stable.

Kernicterus

Kernicterus refers to bilirubin encephalopathy that results from the deposit of bilirubin, especially within the brainstem and basal ganglia. The yellow staining (jaundice of the brain tissue) and necrosis of neurons result from toxic levels of unconjugated bilirubin. Unconjugated bilirubin is readily capable of crossing the blood-brain barrier if not bound to protein because of its high lipid solubility. Kernicterus may occur in certain newborns with no apparent clinical jaundice but is generally directly related to the total serum bilirubin level. In a full-term infant, a serum bilirubin level of 20 mg/dL is considered the upper limit before brain damage begins.

Only one sequela in survivors is specific: **choreoathetoid cerebral palsy.** Other sequelae, such as mental retardation and serious sensory disabilities, may reflect hypoxic, vascular, or infectious injury that often is associated with kernicterus. About 70% of newborns who develop kernicterus die in the neonatal period.

The perinatal events that reinforce the development of hyperbilirubinemia also increase the likelihood that kernicterus will develop, even in the presence of mild to moderate unconjugated hyperbilirubinemia. These perinatal events include hypoxia, asphyxia, acidosis, hypothermia, hypoglycemia, bacterial infection, certain medications, and hypoalbuminemia. These conditions interfere with conjugation or compete for albumin-binding sites.

Clinical manifestations of kernicterus commonly first appear between 2 and 6 days after birth. *Kernicterus is never present at birth.* Symptoms change as the disease process progresses. Four phases are recognized:

1. *Phase one.* The newborn is hypotonic and lethargic and exhibits a poor sucking reflex and depressed or absent Moro's reflex (some infants die during this phase).
2. *Phase two.* The newborn develops spasticity and hyperreflexia, often manifests opisthotonos, has a high-pitched cry, and may be hyperthermic. Convulsions may occur.
3. *Phase three.* At about 7 days of age, the newborn's spasticity lessens and may disappear.
4. *Phase four.* After the first month of life, sequelae develop (e.g., spasticity, athetosis, partial or complete deafness, or mental retardation).

ASSESSMENT

Prenatal Events

Risk factors from the prenatal record are identified. The severity of physiologic jaundice differs greatly between *Oriental* and other ethnic populations. The mean serum levels of unconjugated bilirubin in Chinese, Japanese, Korean, Eskimo, and Native American full-term newborns are between 10 and 14 mg/dL, or approximately double those for Caucasian populations. The incidence of bilirubin toxicity also is increased (Fanaroff, Martin, 1992). African-American newborns demonstrate a lower incidence of hyperbilirubinemia than do Caucasian newborns.

Maternal infections often precede neonatal hyperbilirubinemia. Bacterial (e.g., syphilis), viral (e.g., rubella), and protozoal (e.g., toxoplasmosis) infections have a direct association. Maternal ingestion of sulfonamides or salicylates close to birth affect the newborn's ability to remove bilirubin. Medical conditions such as *maternal diabetes mellitus* predispose the newborn to hyperbilirubinemia (Pernoll et al, 1986).

Maternal blood type and Rh place the woman at risk for *isoimmunization. Women who are Rh negative* are at risk for developing antibodies to the Rh factor, a process called isoimmunization or sensitization. To develop antibodies, the mother will need to have been inoculated with Rh-positive RBCs. Therefore the woman's history is investigated for events that can lead to inoculation. These events include (1) transfusion with Rh-positive blood, which causes immediate sensitization of the woman, (2) spontaneous or elective abortions after 8 or more gestational weeks, (3) previous pregnancy(s) with an Rh-positive fetus, (4) amniocentesis for any reason, and (5) premature separation of the placenta (the last often is difficult to identify).

Hematopoiesis (formation and development of blood cells) begins in the embryo during the sixth week after conception (i.e., during the eighth week after the last menstrual period [LMP]). Therefore a woman who has experienced one or more abortions 2 months or more since her LMP or has given birth has received inoculations of fetal blood generally at the time of placental separation.

During amniocentesis, the needle may cause localized damage to the single layer of cells that separates maternal and fetal circulation in the placenta, thus allowing some fetal RBCs into maternal circulation.

If any of these events have occurred, the woman's record is checked for documentation of prophylaxis for isoimmunization (e.g., Rho immune globulin). The postnatal course of a previous infant also is assessed for evidence of maternal isoimmunization. Rh-negative women who receive prenatal care have blood drawn to screen for the presence of antibodies to antigens such as the Rh factor (see p. 1150) (i.e., the Hemantigen screen and Coombs' test). The *Hemantigen test* also screens for other less common RBC antigens such as Kell, Duffy, and Kidd. Fortunately, serious fetal damage from these factors is unlikely.

Periodically during the pregnancy of Rh-negative women, the results of *indirect Coombs' tests* are reviewed. In this test the maternal blood serum is mixed with Rh-positive RBCs. The test result is positive (maternal antibodies are present) if Rh-positive RBCs agglutinate (clump). The dilution of the specimen of blood at which clumping occurs (if it does occur) determines the titer (level of maternal antibodies). The titer determines the degree of maternal sensitization (isoimmunization). If the titer reaches 1:16, an amniocentesis for delta optical density (ΔOD) analysis is performed to confirm Rh incompatibility (Perry, et al, 1986). ΔOD is a spectrophotometric (color) analysis test (see Chapter 27). This test determines the amount of bilirubin in the amniotic fluid. Fetal hemolysis is signified by rising bilirubin levels, which may suggest the need for an intrauterine transfusion or termination of the pregnancy. *Maternal blood type O,* as well as maternal diabetes mellitus, also may place the newborn at risk (see p. 1150).

Perinatal Events

The perinatal record is reviewed for conditions that are associated with increased RBC destruction in the newborn and that may increase susceptibility (particularly of the immature infant) to the neurotoxic effect of bilirubin by (1) enhancing its passage across the blood-brain barrier and (2) reducing cellular integrity (Fanaroff, Martin, 1992). These factors include (1) perinatal asphyxia with a pH under 7.20, (2) an unstable physiologic condition of the newborn indicated by an Apgar score of 3 or less at 5 minutes, (3) hypothermia (temperature less than 95° F [35° C]), (4) deterioration of the infant's condition as indicated by clinical signs, (5) hypoglycemia (also leads to acidosis), and (6) maternal infection leading to neonatal sepsis.

All these conditions adversely affect metabolism. Compromised metabolism in the neonate delays or interferes with bilirubin conjugation into a water-soluble form for excretion in urine and stool. Although the precise effects of these insults are undetermined, the increased risk to the newborn may be sufficient to justify treatment at lower levels of bilirubin.

Postnatal Events

The infant who has severe **erythroblastosis fetalis** initially may exhibit yellow-stained vernix or umbilical cord. The infant may have *hydrops fetalis*. Signs of this manifestation of severe hemolytic anemia include edema, pleural and pericardial effusions, and ascites, all of which indicate cardiac failure (many of these infants are stillborn). Placental enlargement is seen with severe disease. The placenta may weigh as much as one half to three fourths of the neonate's weight. Hepatosplenomegaly commonly is identified.

Preterm birth, low birth weight (LBW), and immaturity affect the newborn's ability to process bilirubin. *Immaturity* of, or defects in, the *glucuronyl transferase enzyme system* delays or interferes with the conjugation of bilirubin. Hepatic cell damage caused by infection or drugs also interferes with that enzyme system.

Sequestered blood accounts for elevated bilirubin levels. Blood is sequestered (trapped or confined) in cephalhematomas, ecchymoses, and hemangiomas. As the blood is hemolyzed, levels of serum bilirubin rise.

Neonatal Jaundice

Approximately 50% of all full-term newborns are visibly jaundiced during the first 3 days of life. Serum bilirubin levels less than 5 mg/dL usually are not reflected in visible skin jaundice. Every newborn is assessed for jaundice and hyperbilirubinemia. Findings are assessed from physical and behavioral examination and laboratory tests. Jaundice appears first on the head and then progresses downward to the lower extremities, that is, cephalocaudal progression. The *blanch test* assists in differentiating cutaneous jaundice from skin color. The test is performed by applying pressure with the thumb over a bony area (e.g., forehead) for several seconds to empty all the capillaries in that spot. If jaundice is present, the blanched area will look yellow before the capillaries refill. The conjunctival sacs and buccal mucosa are assessed, especially in darker-skinned infants. It is preferable to assess for jaundice in daylight because of the possible distortion of color from artificial lighting, reflection from nursery walls, and the like.

The nurse notes the infant's behavior. Changes in feeding and sleeping patterns, pallor, and dark color of stools and urine accompany hyperbilirubinemia. Neurologic signs of kernicterus are presented on p. 1151.

Laboratory results add to the data base. Blood type, Rh factor, levels of hemoglobin and hematocrit, and Coombs' test results identify maternal-fetal RBC incompatibility and erythroblastosis fetalis.

Physiologic **hyperbilirubinemia** (jaundice, p. 537) occurs in the healthy full-term newborn who was not exposed to perinatal complications (such as hypoxia). It manifests by a progressive increase in serum levels of unconjugated bilirubin from 2 mg/dL in cord blood to a mean peak of 5 to 6 mg/dL between 60 to 72 hours of age in Caucasian and African-American infants. Oriental infants may show a rise of 10 to 14 mg/dL between 72 and 120 hours of age. A rapid decline in unconjugated bilirubin level to 2 mg/dL is seen by the fifth day of life in Caucasian and African-American newborns and by the seventh to tenth day of life in Oriental newborns.

Physiologic jaundice is more severe in preterm infants, with a mean peak of serum bilirubin of 10 to 12 mg/dL by the fifth day of life. This delay in reaching the maximum concentration as compared with the full-term infant is related primarily to the delay in hepatic activity in the preterm infant. In certain high-risk LBW infants, mean peak levels of unconjugated bilirubin of 10 to 12 mg/dL may be associated with bilirubin encephalopathy (kernicterus). Thus all visible jaundice in preterm infants should be monitored and investigated (Fanaroff, Martin, 1992).

Pathologic hyperbilirubinemia cannot be defined solely in terms of serum concentrations of unconjugated bilirubin. Pathologic hyperbilirubinemia refers to that level of serum bilirubin which, if left untreated, can result in lesions in the brain tissue (kernicterus), renal tubular cells, intestinal mucosa, and pancreatic cells.

Criteria that support the diagnosis of hyperbilirubinemia and warrant further investigation include the following signs (Merenstein, Gardner, 1989; Fanaroff, Martin, 1992):

1. Serum bilirubin concentrations greater than 4 mg/dL in cord blood
2. Clinical jaundice evident within 24 hours of birth
3. Total serum bilirubin levels increasing more than 5 mg/dL in 24 hours and/or increasing at a rate of 0.5 mg/dL/hr or greater over a 4- to 8-hour period
4. Full-term newborn: serum bilirubin level greater than 13 to 15 mg/dL at any time and/or clinical jaundice lasting more than 10 days
5. Preterm newborn: serum bilirubin level greater than 10 mg/dL at any time, although all visible jaundice, even with serum bilirubin levels as low as 5 mg/dL, should be carefully monitored, especially if it lasts more than 14 to 21 days

Blood from the umbilical cord is sent to the laboratory to establish the blood type and Rh status. Occasionally an Rh-positive infant is wrongly typed as Rh-negative because of so-called blocking antibodies covering the affected newborn's RBCs.

A *direct Coombs' test* is performed with *neonatal cord blood*. The neonate's RBCs are "washed" and mixed with Coombs' serum. The test result is positive (maternal antibodies are present) if the infant's RBCs agglutinate. The dilution of the specimen of blood at which agglutination occurs (if it does occur) determines the titer of maternal antibodies in fetal serum. The titer determines the degree of maternal sensitization. If the titer is 1:64, an exchange transfusion is indicated.

Increased erythropoiesis with many nucleated RBCs is seen in hemolytic anemia of a progressive type. Hypoglycemia may be present and is treated to avoid additional central nervous system (CNS) insult.

Transcutaneous bilirubinometry is a screening test for neonatal jaundice that is based on the relationship between the yellow color of the skin and total serum bilirubin level. This rapid, noninvasive transcutaneous procedure uses a spectrophotometric hand-held fiberoptic instrument that illuminates the skin and measures the intensity of its yellow color. The intensity of color is then displayed as a number that correlates with serum bilirubin concentration; it is *not* an absolute estimate of total bilirubin. This test is a screen for those jaundiced newborn infants with rising bilirubin levels whose condition may need further diagnostic investigation.

The small probe of the bilirubinometer is applied firmly against the newborn's skin over a bony surface of the forehead or the sternum. The photoprobe is held against the skin with enough pressure to blanch the skin. Then a pulse of light is transmitted through the skin to the subcutaneous tissues, and the reflected color is recorded within a few seconds.

Skin pigmentation *does affect* the readings. Correlations between transcutaneous bilirubin index and serum bilirubin levels have been established for Japanese infants, American Caucasian infants, and African-American infants at term. The different values for the preterm or LBW newborn of each racial group are not yet available. The instrument is not suitable for monitoring the newborn during or immediately after phototherapy or exchange transfusion.

NURSING DIAGNOSES

Following are examples of nursing diagnoses for newborns at risk from hyperbilirubinemia:

- High risk for injury to neurons and cells in the kidney, pancreas, and intestine related to
  —Hyperbilirubinemia
- Impaired gas exchange related to
  —Hemolytic anemia
- High risk for fluid volume deficit related to
  —Phototherapy
- High risk for parental anxiety related to
  —Hyperbilirubinemia, its management, and potential sequelae
- Impaired skin integrity related to
  —Increased stooling while under phototherapy
- Ineffective thermoregulation (increased, decreased) related to
  —Phototherapy

PLANNING

Hospital protocols for care of hyperbilirubinemia are developed as a collaborative effort of the health care team. The health care team utilizes hospital protocols or standards in individualizing care for the infant and parents. *Goals* for care are stated in client-centered terms, as in the following examples.

- The infant's prenatal and perinatal risk factors are identified, and intervention is implemented where appropriate.
- The infant does not develop hyperbilirubinemia and its sequela, kernicterus.
- The infant has minimal or no sequelae from hyperbilirubinemia and its treatment.
- Parents understand newborn's condition, therapies, and possible sequelae.

IMPLEMENTATION

Preventive Measures

Prevention of hyperbilirubinemia is the primary focus of care. Although the nurse is not responsible for typing and cross-matching blood and blood products, the nurse plays a major role in the correct administration of those products. Most hospitals require that before blood products are administered, two nurses check the product to be administered against the physician's order and the woman's blood type and Rh status.

Prenatal control of diabetes mellitus, prevention of infection, avoidance of sulfonamides and aspirin (when possible), and prevention of preterm birth reduce perinatal risks. Prevention of or prompt appropriate therapy for perinatal asphyxia, acidosis, cold stress, sepsis, and hypoglycemia will decrease the newborn's risk of severe hemolytic disease and of susceptibility to neurotoxicity of bilirubin. Early feeding is initiated to stimulate the gastrocolic reflex to remove bilirubin through stooling (see Chapter 22).

Prophylaxis for Rh isoimmunization is now available. **Rh_O (D) immune globulin (RhIg)** administration can prevent the more severe forms of isoimmune hemolytic disease that result from Rh_OD^u group incompatibility. Prophylaxis for Rh isoimmunization involves the use of Rh_O (D) immune globulin (RhoGAM) as a preventive measure against Rh isoimmunization. It is not a treatment for Rh-negative women who are already sensitized because it has no effect against antibodies already present in the maternal blood stream. An injection of Rh_O (D) immune globulin provides passive immunity. It prepares RBCs that contain the Rh antigen for lysis by phagocytes before the woman's immune system is activated to produce antibodies.

*Rh immune globulin is administered intramuscularly in the following amounts to Rh-negative women whose Coombs' test results are negative** (Queenan, 1991):

- 50 μg after chorionic villus sampling
- 300 μg after
  - —Spontaneous or elective (induced) abortion after 8 weeks' gestation
  - —Ectopic pregnancy
  - —Amniocentesis
  - —At 28 weeks' gestation
  - —Within 72 hours of preterm or term birth of Rh-positive infant
- More than 300 μg after
  - —Large transplacental hemorrhage
  - —Mismatched blood transfusion

Jaundice may not be apparent before the baby is discharged. Therefore parents need to learn how to identify jaundice and to know when to notify the physician, midwife, or nurse practitioner (Locklin, 1987).

Curative Measures

Hyperbilirubinemia occurs in approximately 50% of normal newborns. *Phototherapy* by bili lights or phototherapy blanket (Shibley, 1991) is conducted in the normal newborn nursery, usually for physiologic hyperbilirubinemia (see discussion on p. 599 and Fig. 22-11). (See case study, p. 1155, and nursing plan of care, p. 1156, for hyperbilirubinemia.)

Some fetuses are candidates for **intrauterine transfusion.** The transfusion is accomplished by infusing Rh_O (D)-negative and usually group O RBCs into the peritoneal cavity or the umbilical vein of the fetus. Only blood that is negative for cytomegalovirus (CMV), hepatitis, and human immunodeficiency virus (HIV) is used (Perry et al, 1986). The RBC transfusion counteracts the anemia and prevents cardiac decompensation. A second transfusion is administered 10 days later, followed by transfusions every 3 weeks until birth.

Exchange transfusion may be required in the immediate neonatal period for the following reasons:

- To reduce serum bilirubin levels
- To improve oxygen-carrying capacity of the blood by
  - —Removing RBCs that are destined for hemolysis by circulating antibodies
  - —Correcting the anemia
  - —Removing antibodies (or other causative agents) responsible for hemolysis
- To correct acidosis

An exchange transfusion is accomplished by alternately removing a small amount of the infant's blood and replacing it with a like amount of donor blood. Depending on the infant's size, maturity, and condition, amounts of 5 to 20 mL at a time are slowly exchanged. The total amount of blood exchanged approximates 170 mL/kg of body weight (80 mL/lb) or 75% to 85% of the infant's total blood volume. During the procedure, staff members observe infection control precautions for invasive procedures (see Chapter 29).

When the transfusion is completed, the nurse continues to closely observe and record the infant's behavior for 24 to 48 hours. The infant's heart rate, respirations, blood pressure, temperature, and pedal

*NOTE: *RhIg is* never *given to an infant or father.*

CASE STUDY

Hyperbilirubinemia

Bret Jackson is a preterm infant born after 34 weeks of gestation to a 26-year old mother who came to the hospital in active labor (9 cm dilatation). Spontaneous vaginal birth resulted, and Bret's Apgar scores were 6 and 8.

ASSESSMENT

Brenda Jackson's prenatal record reveals no infection, diabetes, or history of hemoglobinopathies. Her blood type is A+. Perinatal events were within normal limits: no asphyxia, no hypothermia, and no hypoglycemia. Jaundice became evident at 36 hours of age. Laboratory bilirubin level was 9.7 mg/dL.

NURSING DIAGNOSIS

On the basis of observation of jaundice, 34 weeks' gestation, and bilirubin level of 9.7 mg/dL, the nursing diagnosis, was identified: high risk for injury related to hyperbilirubinemia.

PLANNING

The nurse sets the *goal* for the infant. Stated in client-centered terms, Bret's hyperbilirubinemia is treated promptly and he will demonstrate no signs of kernicterus.

IMPLEMENTATION

The nurse will maintain phototherapy as ordered (see discussion on p. 599 and p. 601). Eye patches are in place and as much skin surface as possible is exposed to the light. The infant is removed from under the lights to be fed and cuddled for no longer than 1 hour. The infant's position is changed frequently, good skin care is provided, urination and stooling are noted, and fluid loss caused by the phototherapy is replaced. The nurse continues to observe for signs of kernicterus. The nurse ensures that the strength of the bili lights is tested (according to hospital and manufacturer policy) while the infant is receiving phototherapy.

EVALUATION

Bret's bilirubin levels decline with treatment, and he demonstrates no signs of kernicterus at the time of discharge and during subsequent visits to the pediatrician.

pulses are monitored. The infant is observed for lethargy, jitteriness, convulsions, presence of dark urine, and edema. In addition, the nurse monitors the infant to prevent hemorrhage from the infusion site and to detect and treat promptly any complications of blood transfusion, such as heart failure, hypocalcemia, acute hypercalcemia, hyperkalemia, hypernatremia, hypoglycemia, acidosis, sepsis, shock, thrombus formation, and transfusion mismatch reaction (Wise, Nolan, 1990).

Rehabilitative Measures

Planning for rehabilitative measures is necessary if kernicterus occurs. The family will need the services of many community resources to care for the affected child. An interdisciplinary approach that includes social services must be taken.

EVALUATION

On a short-term basis the nurse can consider nursing care to be effective to the degree that goals for care are met.

- The infant's prenatal and perinatal risk factors are identified and intervention is implemented when appropriate.
- The infant does not develop hyperbilirubinemia and its sequela, kernicterus.
- The infant suffers minimal or no sequelae from hyperbilirubinemia and its treatment.
- The parents understand the newborn's condition, therapies, and possible sequelae.

Should the goals not be met, the nurse reassesses the situation and develops a new plan of care.

CONGENITAL ANOMALIES

The desired and expected outcome of every wanted pregnancy is a normal, functioning infant with good intellectual potential. Fulfillment of this hope depends on numerous factors, both hereditary and environmental. Probably all human characteristics have a genetic component, including those that produce undesirable symptoms or unwelcome physical abnormalities that impair the fitness of the individual. Some diseases occur through the action of a single gene or the combined action of many genes in-

CARE PLAN Hyperbilirubinemia

GOALS	IMPLEMENTATION	RATIONALE	EVALUATION
Nursing diagnosis: High risk for injury related to hyperbilirubinemia			
Bret's hyperbilirubinemia is treated promptly; bilirubin levels will begin to decrease immediately. Bret will show no signs of kernicterus.	Maintain phototherapy as ordered: keep eyes patched and ensure that patches do not slip; expose as much skin surface as possible to the lights (p. 600). Remove the lights for periods of no longer than 1 hour to be fed and cuddled; change position often; provide good skin care; note urine and stool pattern; replace fluid loss. Observe for signs of kernicterus.	Eye shields could cause upper airway obstruction and apnea, as well as direct injury to eye from shield or lights. Continuous therapy is more effective in reducing bilirubin levels. Periodic removal of infant from therapy does not diminish therapy effectiveness and allows for sensory stimulation and time for bonding with parents.	Bret's bilirubin levels decline with treatment, and he demonstrates no signs of kernicterus at discharge or at subsequent visits to pediatrician. Bret suffers no injuries from the treatment, e.g., excoriated buttocks from stools, abrasion from eye shields.
Nursing diagnosis: Ineffective thermoregulation (increased/decreased) related to phototherapy/immaturity			
Bret's body temperature will remain stable.	Provide environment that will maintain axillary temperature at 97.7°-98.6° F (36.5°-37° C). Use radiant warmer or Isolette if indicated. Check temperature every 3 hours and as needed.	Exposure of large skin surface may compromise thermoregulation (see p. 601).	Bret's temperature remains between 97.7°-98.6° F (36.5°-37° C).
Nursing diagnosis: Anxiety related to knowledge deficit regarding hyperbilirubinemia, its treatment, and possible complications			
Parents learn about Bret's condition, therapies, and possible sequelae.	Explain the different causes of hyperbilirubinemia and their potential sequelae. Explain the treatment modalities.	Knowledge increases one's sense of control and enhances coping, provides a basis for decision making, and increases parents' self-confidence.	Parents verbalize understanding of instruction.
Parents participate in maintaining the treatment regimen.	Encourage parents to take an active role in the treatment plan (e.g., keeping eye patches in place and full skin exposed to light while under phototherapy). Encourage questions, feelings, or concerns.		Parents participate in maintaining the treatment regimen.

herited from the parents; others are the result of the action of the environment on the genetic composition of the individual. A disease or disorder that can be transmitted from generation to generation is termed *genetic* or *hereditary* (see Chapter 7). A **congenital** disorder is one that is present at birth and can be caused by genetic or environmental factors, or both.

Each year 250,000 infants are born with significant structural and functional disorders. Major congenital defects are now the leading cause of death in infants younger than 1 year of age in the United States. With the fall in other causes of neonatal mortality, these defects now account for about 20% of those deaths.

The seriousness of this community health problem is reflected in the more than 6 million hospital days and $200 billion a year allocated to the care and treatment of these neonates. Prevention and detection procedures are being improved continuously. Methods of promoting the availability of these services to populations at risk challenge the community health care systems. An interdisciplinary team approach is vital in providing holistic care: surgery, rehabilitation, and education of the child and social, as well as psychologic and financial, assistance to the parents. Parental disappointment and disillusion and any negative feelings the nurse may have toward (or stigmatization of) the infant's disorder add to the complexity of nursing care.

ASSESSMENT

Prenatal Diagnosis

Refined testing procedures have become available to monitor the development of the fetus. Prenatal diagnostic techniques such as amniocentesis, ultrasound, alpha-fetoprotein measurements, chorionic villi sampling, percutaneous umbilical cord blood sampling, and gene probes contribute to the data base (see Chapter 27). Although they comprise a valuable adjunct to prenatal care, these tests do not achieve 100% accuracy in detecting congenital defects (see Table 27-9) (Lemna et al, 1990; Wolfe et al, 1990; Zacharias, 1990; Brambati et al, 1991; Greene, Benacerraf, 1991; Wenstrom et al, 1991).

Some women choose to continue the pregnancy after positive identification of a congenital problem. The prenatal record is reviewed for documentation of parental wishes for the level of aggressive management acceptable for the infant's care.

Despite the status and availability of current technology, not all congenital disorders are or can be anticipated. The historic and medical information in the prenatal record is reviewed for factors that are associated with congenital disorders. These factors include various medical, surgical, and social conditions and their treatments (see Chapter 39), maternal infection (see Chapter 29), maternal endocrine and metabolic disorders (see Chapter 31), and infection and drug dependence in the newborn (see Chapter 39).

Perinatal Diagnosis

Many congenital anomalies require intervention soon after birth. Careful observations in the birth room or nursery will identify most of these conditions.

VOLUME OF AMNIOTIC FLUID. An excessive amount of amniotic fluid, **hydramnios,** is commonly associated with congenital anomalies in the newborn. The infant should be examined closely at the earliest possible time. In the presence of hydramnios, any of the following may be suspected:

1. Cephalocaudal malformations, such as hydrocephalus, microcephaly, anencephaly, and spina bifida
2. Orogastrointestinal malformations, such as cleft palate, esophageal atresia with or without a tracheal fistula, pyloric stenosis, volvulus, and imperforate anus
3. Miscellaneous conditions, such as Down syndrome, congenital heart disease, deformed extremities, and infants of diabetic or prediabetic mothers
4. Preterm birth

Oligohydramnios (an insufficient amount of amniotic fluid) is associated primarily with those anomalies of the urinary tract that prevent normal micturition in utero. As a rule, renal agenesis or renal dysplasia is involved.

1. Urethral stenosis also has been reported to be associated with oligohydramnios.
2. Anomalies of the earlobes, rather than agenesis of the ear, sometimes are associated with renal abnormalities and are not direct results of oligohydramnios.
3. Potter's syndrome (renal agenesis) is the classic example of an association between oligohydramnios and renal anomalies. It includes atypical facies that involves abnormal earlobes.

Postnatal Diagnosis

An Apgar score and minimal assessment are completed for all neonates after birth (p. 493). Any deviations from normal are reported to the physician immediately.

RESPIRATORY SYSTEM. Screening for congenital anomalies of the respiratory tract is necessary even for the infant who is apparently normal at birth. Respiratory distress at birth or shortly thereafter may be the result of lung immaturity or anomalous development. Congenital laryngeal web and bilateral choanal atresia (Fig. 38-1) are readily apparent at birth. Both require emergency surgery. Respiratory distress caused by diaphragmatic hernia and tracheoesophageal fistula appear immediately or may be delayed, depending on the severity of the defect.

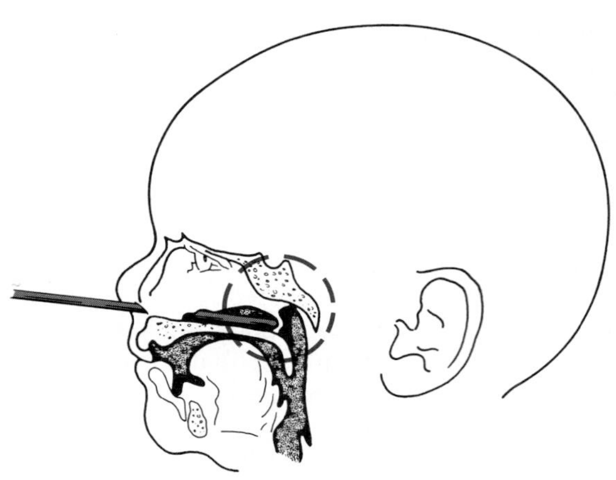

Fig. 38-1 Choanal atresia. Posterior nares are obstructed by membrane or bone either bilaterally or unilaterally. Infant becomes cyanotic at rest. With crying, newborn's color improves. Nasal discharge is present. Snorting respirations often are observed with increased respiratory effort. Newborn may be unable to breathe and eat at same time. Diagnosis is made by noting inability to pass small feeding tube through one or both nares.
Courtesy Ross Laboratories, Columbus, Ohio.

NEUROLOGIC SYSTEM. Neurologic signs may reflect hidden congenital anomalies, as well as numerous other conditions. Many neonatal responses are nonspecific. Each sign, such as high-pitched cry, hypotonia, jitteriness, low-set ears, and microcephaly or hydrocephaly, must be evaluated carefully before appropriate therapy can be instituted.

Some **neural tube defects** are obvious at first glance. The three main defects are anencephaly, spina bifida (which includes occult and visible meningocele and myelomeningocele), and encephalocele (p. 1167). These are defects in midline closures. If a neural tube defect is identified, the infant may have one or more of the other malformations in this group: cleft lip and palate, tracheoesophageal fistula, and diaphragmatic hernia.

CARDIOVASCULAR SYSTEM. Congenital cardiovascular disorders are divided into two major types: cyanotic and noncyanotic. Severe congenital cardiovascular disorders often are evident immediately after birth, for example, severe cyanotic heart disease (Fig. 38-2). These infants usually are transferred directly to special nurseries or pediatric units. Some problems, such as a small patent ductus arteriosus or a minimal coarctation of the descending aorta, become apparent only as the infant is exposed to stresses such as growth demands of later infancy and early childhood or to infection. In about 75% of cases, cardiovascular anomalies are unexpected.

Cardiovascular defects occur in 4 to 10/1000 births (Hoffman, 1990). Congenital heart disease is implicated in approximately 50% of deaths from malformations during the first year of life. The etiologic factors are still unclear, although a familial tendency is evident in many cases. Coexisting congenital defects are common in newborns with cardiovascular anomalies. Maternal diseases such as rubella, alcoholism, and insulin-dependent diabetes during pregnancy, as well as maternal age over 40 years, have been implicated. Symptoms characteristically are first evident after the umbilical cord is severed. The infant's *cry* is weak and muffled or loud and breathless. The newborn may be *cyanotic*. Cyanosis usually is generalized, increases in the supine position, and often is unrelieved by oxygen. Cyanosis usually deepens with crying. The gray dusky color may be mild, moderate, or severe. Other infants may be *acyanotic* and pale, with or without mottling on exertion (such as crying).

The newborn's *activity level* varies from restless to lethargic. The infant may be unresponsive except to pain. The arms may be flaccid while the infant is being fed. *Posturing* is significant. Hypotonia and flaccidity may be evident, even during sleep. There may be hyperextension of the neck or opisthotonos. The newborn may be dyspneic when supine. Persistent *bradycardia* (below 120 beats/min or less than 30 beats/min from the normal baseline for 10 minutes or more [Tucker, 1988]) or persistent *tachycardia* (160 beats/min or more) may be noted. The cardiac rhythm may be abnormal, and cardiac murmurs are heard in some infants. Signs of congestive heart failure, diminished cardiac output, and decreased tissue perfusion may be evident.

Respirations are counted when the newborn is asleep. Findings may include tachypnea (60 respirations per minute or more), retractions with nasal flaring or tachypnea, and dyspnea with diaphoresis or grunting. Diaphoresis is an uncommon response in the normal newborn. Respirations may be gasping, followed in 2 or 3 minutes by respiratory arrest without prompt treatment. Grunting may occur with or without exertion.

These findings must be reported immediately. Newborns showing these types of signs require prompt definite diagnosis and immediate appropriate therapy in a tertiary care neonatal intensive care unit or pediatric unit.

GASTROINTESTINAL SYSTEM. Screening for gastrointestinal tract malformations is performed on a routine basis for all infants. Abdominal wall defects are apparent at birth. Omphalocele is discussed on p. 1165. Intestinal obstruction, which occurs in about 1 in 3000 newborns, may occur in the presence of diaphragmatic hernia (p. 1164). A scaphoid (sunken) abdomen usually indicates a diaphragmatic hernia. A distended abdomen is particularly noteworthy in H-type tracheoesophageal fistula. These conditions require immediate surgery and are discussed later in this chapter.

Other malformations are apparent when further assessment is made. Malformations such as esophageal atresia and imperforate anus are discussed on pp. 1165 and 1166.

UROGENITAL SYSTEM. Careful notation of perinatal events and observations such as oligohydramnios and absence of voiding aid in the identification and confirmation of existing congenital anomalies. In cases of ambiguous genitals (p. 1171), there is an urgent association between the parent-child relationship and the identification of the infant's sex. The identity of the newborn must be established as quickly as possible to facilitate initiation of a positive parent-child relationship. Assessment to determine a gender assignment consists of several studies (Whaley, Wong,

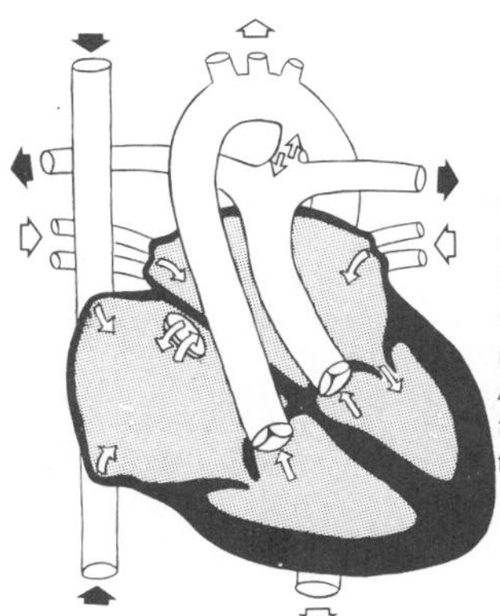

Complete transposition of great vessels

The anomaly is an embryologic defect caused by a straight division of the bulbar trunk without normal spiraling. As a result, the aorta originates from the right ventricle, and the pulmonary artery from the left ventricle. An abnormal communication between the two circulations must be present to sustain life.

Fig. 38-2 Congenital heart abnormalities. Courtesy Ross Laboratories, Columbus, Ohio.

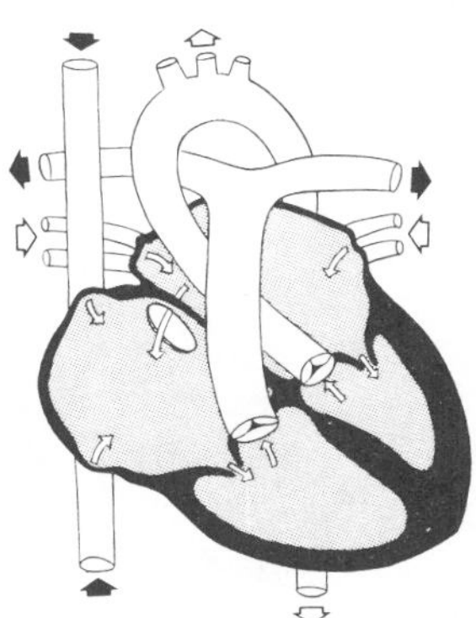

Atrial septal defects

An atrial septal defect is an abnormal opening between the right and left atria. Basically, three types of abnormalities result from incorrect development of the atrial septum. An incompetent foramen ovale is the most common defect. The high ostium secundum defect results from abnormal development of the septum secundum. Improper development of the septum primum produces a basal opening known as an ostium primum defect, frequently involving the atrioventricular valves. In general, left to right shunting of blood occurs in all atrial septal defects.

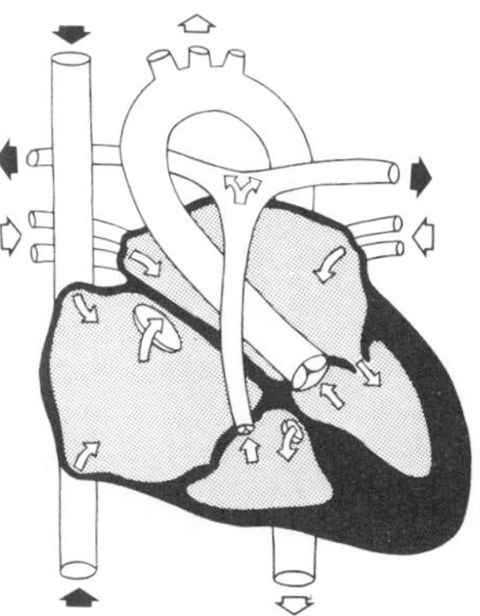

Tricuspid atresia

Tricuspid valvular atresia is characterized by a small right ventricle, large left ventricle, and usually a diminished pulmonary circulation. Blood from the right atrium passes through an atrial septal defect into the left atrium, mixes with oxygenated blood returning from the lungs, flows into the left ventricle, and is propelled into the systemic circulation. The lungs may receive blood through one of three routes: (1) a small ventricular septal defect, (2) patent ductus arteriosus, (3) bronchial vessels.

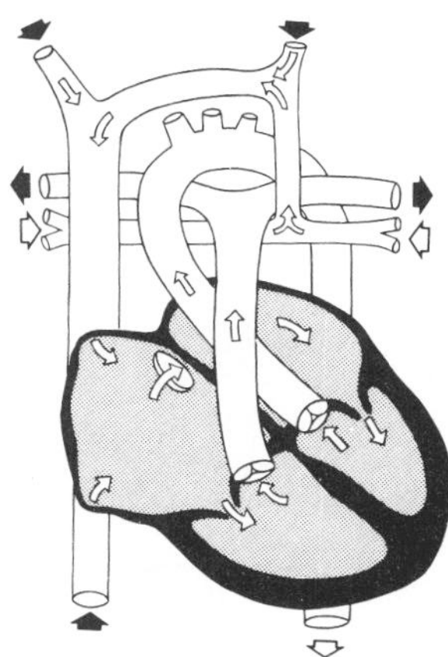

Anomalous venous return

Oxygenated blood returning from the lungs is carried abnormally to the right heart by one or more pulmonary veins emptying directly, or indirectly, through venous channels into the right atrium. Partial anomalous return of the pulmonary veins to the right atrium functions the same as an atrial septal defect. In complete anomalous return of the pulmonary veins, an interatrial communication is necessary for survival.

Continued.

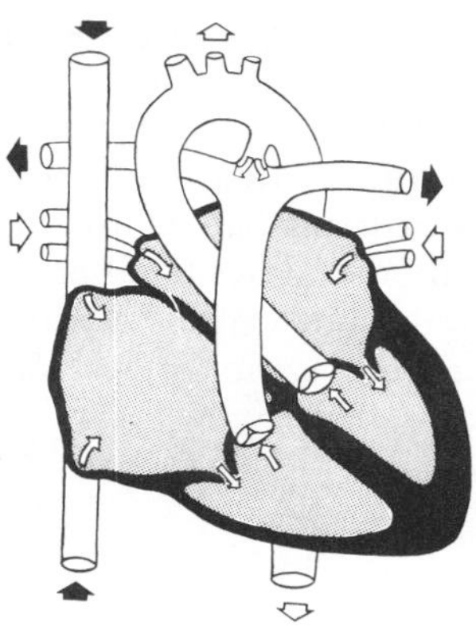

Patent ductus arteriosus

The patent ductus arteriosus is a vascular connection that, during fetal life, short circuits the pulmonary vascular bed and directs blood from the pulmonary artery to the aorta. Functional closure of the ductus normally occurs soon after birth. If the ductus remains patent after birth, the direction of blood flow in the ductus is reversed by the higher pressure in the aorta.

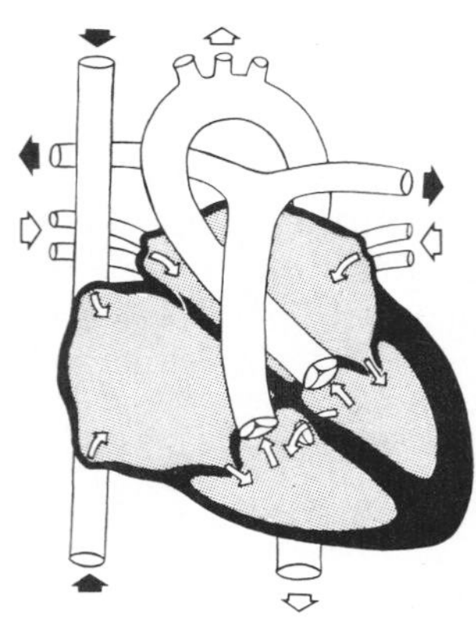

Ventricular septal defects

A ventricular septal defect is an abnormal opening between the right and left ventricle. Ventricular septal defects vary in size and may occur in either the membranous or muscular portion of the ventricular septum. Due to higher pressure in the left ventricle, a shunting of blood from the left to right ventricle occurs during systole. If pulmonary vascular resistance produces pulmonary hypertension, the shunt of blood is then reversed from the right to the left ventricle, with cyanosis resulting.

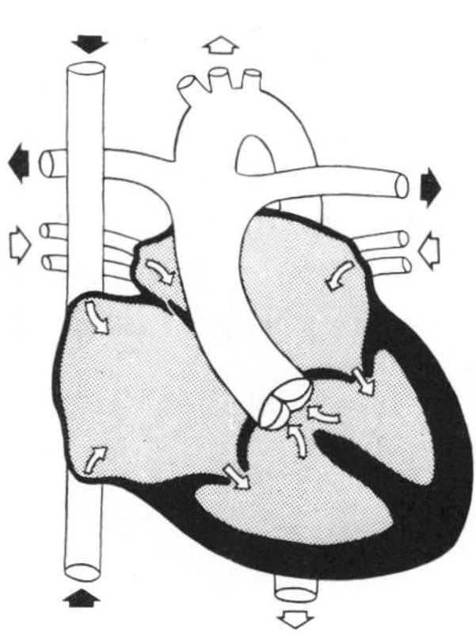

Truncus arteriosus

Truncus arteriosus is a retention of the embryologic bulbar trunk. It results from the failure of normal septation and division of this trunk into an aorta and pulmonary artery. This single arterial trunk overrides the ventricles and receives blood from them through a ventricular septal defect. The entire pulmonary and systemic circulation is supplied from this common arterial trunk.

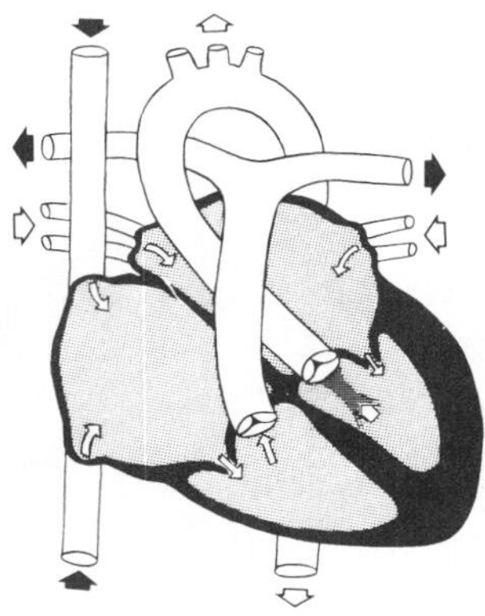

Subaortic stenosis

In many instances, the stenosis is valvular with thickening and fusion of the cusps. Subaortic stenosis is caused by a fibrous ring below the aortic valve in the outflow tract of the left ventricle. At times, both valvular and subaortic stenosis exist in combination. The obstruction presents an increased work load for the normal output of the left ventricular blood and results in left ventricular enlargement.

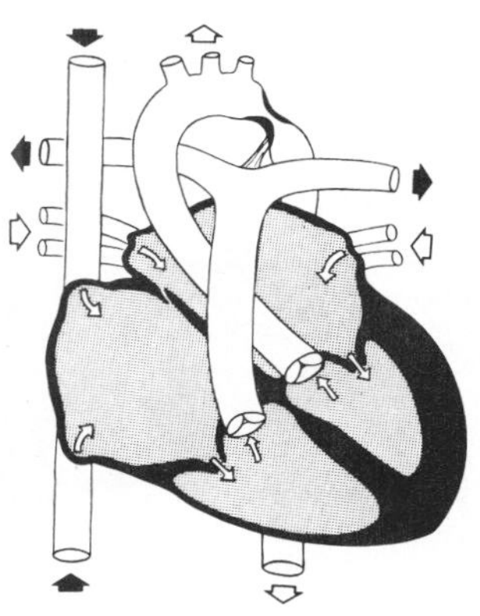

Coarctation of the aorta

Coarctation of the aorta is characterized by a narrowed aortic lumen. It exists as a preductal or postductal obstruction, depending on the position of the obstruction in relation to the ductus arteriosus. Coarctations exist with great variation in anatomic features. The lesion produces an obstruction to the flow of blood through the aorta causing an increased left ventricular pressure and work load.

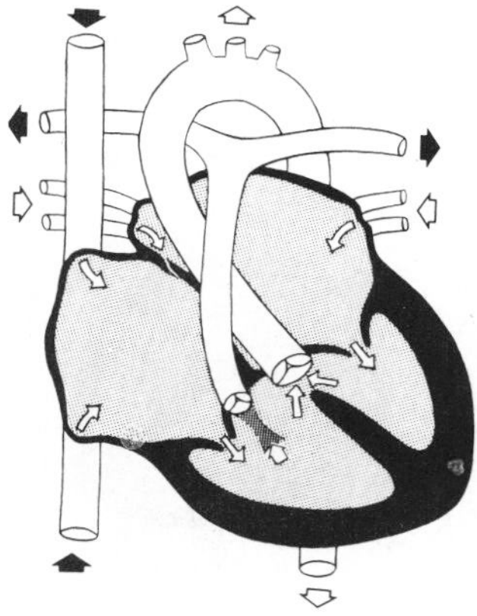

Tetralogy of Fallot

Tetralogy of Fallot is characterized by the combination of four defects: (1) pulmonary stenosis, (2) ventricular septal defect, (3) overriding aorta, (4) hypertrophy of right ventricle. It is the most common defect causing cyanosis in patients surviving beyond two years of age. The severity of symptoms depends on the degree of pulmonary stenosis, the size of the ventricular septal defect, and the degree to which the aorta overrides the septal defect.

Fig. 38-2, cont'd Congenital heart abnormalities.
Courtesy Ross Laboratories, Columbus, Ohio.

TABLE 38-1 Common Autosomal Aberrations

Syndrome	Chromosomal Abnormality and Nomenclature	Average Incidence* (Live Births)	Major Clinical Manifestations
Cri-du-chat	Deletion of short arm of a B (no. 5) chromosome—46,XY,5p-	1:50,000	Distinctive weak, high-pitched mew-like cry resembling the cry of a cat; small head; hypertelorism; failure to thrive; severe mental retardation—profound with age
Trisomy 13 (Patau's)	Trisomy of a group D (no. 13) chromosome—47,XY,13+	1:4000 to 1:15,000	Multiple anomalies, including cleft lip and palate (frequently bilateral); ear malformations; microphthalmia; polydactyly; eye defects; mental retardation; early death
Trisomy 18 (Edwards')	Trisomy of a group E (no. 18) chromosome—47,XY,18+	1:3500-8000	Deformed and low-set ears; micrognathia; rocker-bottom feet; overlapping (index over third) fingers; prominent occiput; hypertelorism; failure to thrive and early death; mental retardation
Trisomy 21 (Down)	Trisomy of a group G (no. 21) chromosome—47,XY,21+ (trisomy); 46XY,D—G-, (Dq-Gq) + (translocation); 46,XY/47,XY,21 + (mosaic)	1:70†	Brachycephaly with flat occiput; inner epicanthal folds; small ears, nose, and mouth with protruding tongue; muscular hypotonia; broad, short hands with stubby fingers and simian palmar crease, broad stubby feet with wide space between big and second toes; mental retardation; variable life expectancy

Modified from Whaley LF, Wong DL: *Nursing care of infants and children,* ed 4, St Louis, 1991, Mosby–Year Book.
*Data from Nora JJ, Fraser FC: *Medical genetics: principles and practice,* ed 3, Philadelphia, 1989, Lea & Febiger.
†Risk related to maternal age: age 30 years = 1:1500; age 35 years = 1:300; age 40 years = 1:100; age 45 years = 1:25. Previously 50% were born to mothers over 35 years of age; now only 20% are born to women in that age-group, in large part because of the availability of prenatal diagnosis.

1991): history (e.g., ingestion of steroids, relatives with ambiguous genitalia); physical examination; chromosomal analysis (results available in 2 to 3 days); endoscopy, ultrasonography, and radiographic contrast studies; biochemical tests (e.g., 17-ketosteroids); and laparotomy or gonad biopsy.

Exstrophy of the bladder or the cloaca is rare (p. 1170).

Some infants have multiple congenital anomalies. A syndrome refers to a recognized pattern of malformations. The most familiar is Down syndrome (Table 38-1; Figs. 38-3 and 7-3). Diagnosis is confirmed early in the neonatal period.

Five congenital anomalies require emergency surgery. These conditions and other malformations are presented under Implementation in this chapter. Although the surgery is the physician's responsibility, considerable nursing care is involved.

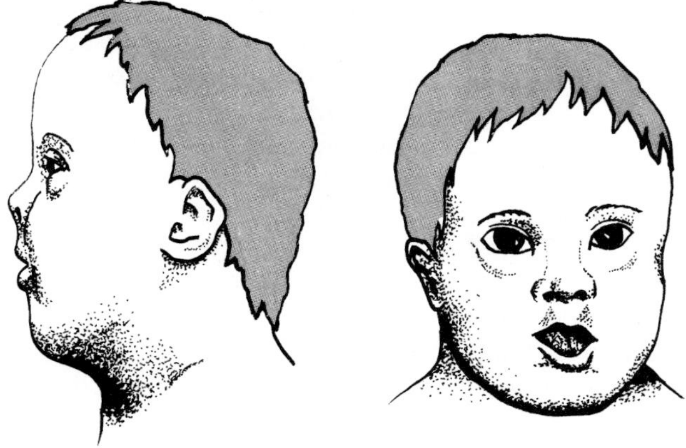

Fig. 38-3 Clinical features of Down syndrome.

Genetic Diagnosis

Most diagnostic procedures for detection of genetic disorders are implemented after birth at any time from the postnatal period through adulthood. The number and variety of these tests are too extensive to include here; therefore only those employed most frequently in the newborn period will be discussed.

BIOCHEMICAL TESTS. The most widespread use of postbirth testing for genetic disease is the routine screening of newborns for inborn errors of metabolism such as phenylketonuria (PKU) (see Chapter 7 and Appendix D), which is mandatory in most states in the United States. **Inborn errors of metabolism** is a term applied to a large group of disorders caused by a metabolic defect that results from the absence of or change in a protein, usually an enzyme, because of gene action (p. 159). These defects can involve any substrate produced from protein, carbohydrate, or fat metabolism. Inborn errors of metabolism are recessive disorders and, as such, require that the individual receive a defective gene from each parent. The parents usually are unaffected because their normal, dominant gene directs the synthesis of sufficient protein to meet their metabolic needs under normal circumstances. With new biochemical techniques it is now possible to detect the presence of the abnormal gene in an increasing number of these disorders.

PKU results from a deficiency of the enzyme phenylalanine dehydrogenase. The test for PKU is not valid until the newborn has ingested an ample amount of the amino acid phenylalanine, a constituent of both human and cow milk (see Chapter 22). The child with this disorder will have blond hair, blue eyes, and fair skin. A diet low in phenylalanine is ordered to prevent the severe mental retardation and bizarre behavior seen in untreated cases.

Galactosemia, caused by a deficiency of the enzyme galactose-1-phosphate uridyltransferase, results in the inability to convert galactose to glucose. Galactosemia can be detected by measuring blood levels of galactose in the urine of affected newborns who have ingested milk containing galactose. Failure to thrive, mental retardation, cataracts, jaundice, hepatomegaly, and cirrhosis of the liver are manifestations in untreated cases. Therapy consists of the elimination of galactose from the diet.

In recent years many states in the United States have required routine screening for *hypothyroidism.* Thyroxine (T_4) is measured from a drop of blood obtained from a heel stick at 2 to 5 days of age. At this time the normally expected increase in T_4 is lacking in newborns with hypothyroidism. Cretinism develops in untreated affected individuals. The same blood sample can be used to test for all three of these metabolic disorders—PKU, galactosemia, and hypothyroidism (see Fig. 21-17).

CYTOLOGIC STUDIES. In most instances disorders resulting from chromosomal abnormalities can be diagnosed by clinical manifestations alone. Occasionally an infant is born whose clinical appearance is only suggestive of a problem. In these cases cytologic studies more often are carried out to confirm or to rule out a tentative diagnosis. Sometimes all that is required are sex chromatin or fluorescent staining techniques. These stains can be prepared from any cells in the body. The most easily obtained and therefore the most commonly used are mucosal cells scraped from the inside of the cheek, which are placed on a glass slide, prepared, and stained (buccal smear).

Preparation of a karyotype (see Fig. 7-1) requires cells in the process of cell division. The most commonly used cells are those obtained from bone marrow, skin, or peripheral blood. The cells are grown in culture media. Division is arrested at the stage when cells are best visualized, then stained, photographed, and arranged in a karyotype for assessment. A karyotype also is requested in cases in which the sex of the infant is in doubt because the assignment of a gender constitutes a social emergency (p. 1170).

Two examples of chromosome abnormalities are Turner's and Klinefelter's syndromes (p. 158). The child with *Turner's syndrome* is a female with the genetic designation of 45,X. She will have short stature, webbed neck, low posterior hairline, shield-shaped chest with widely spaced nipples, and lymph edema of hands and feet. This female is sterile. The child with *Klinefelter's syndrome* is a male whose genetic designation may be 47,XXY or 48,XXYY. This male is tall with long legs, has hypogenitalism, and is sterile. He may have deficient male secondary sexual characteristics and may demonstrate aberrant behavior.

DERMATOGLYPHICS. The pattern formed by dermal ridges early in development is largely genetically determined by many genes on many chromosomes. Therefore addition or deletion of genetic material will produce alterations in the loops, swirls, and arches of the finger and toe prints, in the palm lines, and in the flexion creases on palms of the hands and soles of the feet. Characteristic dermatoglyphic patterns have been noted in almost all the chromosomal abnormalities such as Down syndrome (see simian line, Figs. 38-4 and 7-3,*B*). Certain fingerprint patterns may be found in persons who have cardiac valvular problems later in life.

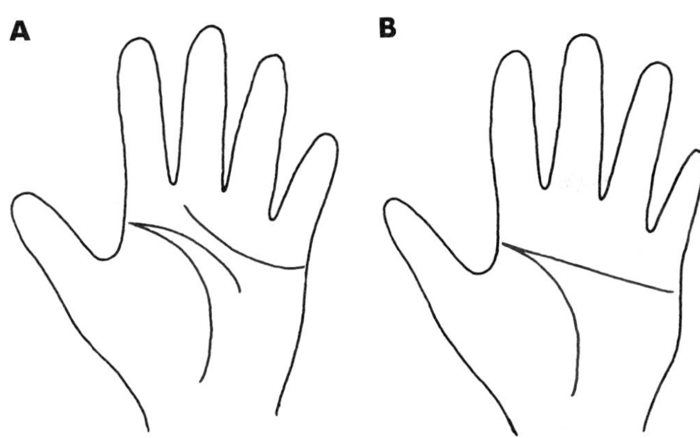

Fig. 38-4 Examples of flexion creases on palm. **A**, Normal. **B**, Simian crease.

Many other diagnostic studies may be performed in the neonatal period to detect or rule out genetic defects, for example, x-ray studies for a variety of structural defects of bone and for gastrointestinal, renal, and neurologic disorders. Meconium ileus in the newborn often is the first manifestation of cystic fibrosis.

PARENTAL RESPONSES. Parental responses are carefully assessed. Signs and symptoms of initial grief responses are expected (see Chapter 40). The family's understanding of the information presented to them is assessed on an ongoing basis. The family's comprehension of the proposed management and risks, as well as alternative courses of action, is evaluated. The family's feelings about proposed management and their role in care after therapy are explored. The family's emotional, social, and financial resources must be considered.

NURSING DIAGNOSES

Following are examples of nursing diagnoses to direct the care of newborns with congenital abnormalities.

NEWBORN

- High risk for injury or death related to
  —Presence of a congenital disorder
- High risk for infection related to
  —Anomaly or its treatment
- High risk for impaired gas exchange, nutrition, or mobility related to
  —Congenital anomaly
- High risk for altered growth and development related to
  —Inborn error of metabolism

PARENTS/FAMILY

- Dysfunctional grieving or spiritual distress related to
  —Birth of a child with a defect
- High risk for ineffective individual/family coping related to
  —Birth of a child with a defect
- Knowledge deficit related to
  —Cause, management, alternative courses of action, community resources, prognosis, care needed by child after discharge
- Anxiety related to
  —Uncertainty of prognosis or ability to care for child
- High risk for altered parenting related to
  —Birth of a child with a disorder or defect

PLANNING

Planning for the care of a newborn with a congenital defect begins before the birth of the infant. Hospital protocols and standards of care are established so that definitive and prompt therapy is facilitated. Parents are involved in the plan for care to the extent possible. For some disorders, a collaborative health team approach that includes specialists (e.g., orthodontists, physical therapists, geneticists) and community services representatives is needed.

Goals are stated in client-centered terms for the newborn and parents.

- The newborn's disorder is recognized, and appropriate therapy is initiated promptly.
- The newborn suffers no adverse sequelae from the disorder or its management.
- The parents understand the newborn's condition and its management and possible sequelae, as well as the anticipated prognosis.
- The parents choose a course of action commensurate with their family's values and goals.

IMPLEMENTATION

General Preoperative and Postoperative Care

The newborn withstands the stress of surgery surprisingly well, provided it is performed as soon after birth as feasible and the facilities available for care are adequately equipped and staffed. The medical-nursing team must be specially trained to anticipate and meet the newborn's physiologic needs. The surgical team consists of the radiologist, surgeon, anesthesiologist, and nurse. Diagnostic studies are kept to a minimum, and consideration of the newborn's immaturity is kept in mind. Preoperative activities include stabilization of the infant and administration of antibiotics. Other activities relate to specific anomalies such as orogastric tube placement and abdominal decompression, management of open lesions, and monitoring specific measurements and fluid and electrolyte balance.

The infant is transported to the operating room in an incubator with a self-contained power pack for the continuous provision of warmth. The infant is accompanied by an intensive care nursery nurse. Preanesthesia preparation includes hydration, administration of preoperative medications (usually minute amounts of atropine), insertion of an endotracheal tube, and gastric emptying.

During the operation, blood loss is constantly monitored. Blood is replaced milliliter for milliliter because the newborn's remarkable ability to maintain blood circulation through vasoconstriction means that vital signs remain unaltered until sudden and complete collapse occurs as the compensatory system is overtaxed. Temperature is maintained by positioning the infant on a thermal mattress and draping suitably.

Once the operation is completed, the infant is returned to the intensive care nursery. The first hour after the procedure is a crucial one; constant surveillance of recovery from the anesthesia is imperative. Body temperature is maintained between 97° and 98° F (36.1° and 36.7° C); optimum temperature is 97.6° F (36.5° C). An open airway is maintained by means of positioning of the head, suctioning, and use of high humidity. Postoperative mechanical ventilation is required for most newborns.

Oxygen dosage is prescribed on the basis of arterial blood gas values (such as oxygen pressure) as measured by arterial blood samples or pulse oximeter. Fluid-electrolyte balance is monitored. Intravenous replacement is given as ordered. Postural drainage and percussion are ordered as necessary. The infant is turned from side to side to equalize pressure areas. An indwelling gastric catheter attached to intermittent suction removes gastric secretions and prevents their possible aspiration. The nurse should assess the neonate's pain and take appropriate actions.

Common Surgical Emergencies

The following five congenital anomalies account for more than 90% of surgical emergencies of the newborn: diaphragmatic hernia, tracheoesophageal anomalies, omphalocele, intestinal obstruction, and imperforate anus.

DIAPHRAGMATIC HERNIA. Diaphragmatic hernia is the most urgent of the neonatal emergencies. Incomplete embryonic development of the diaphragm allows herniation of abdominal viscera into the thoracic cavity (Fig. 38-5). The defect and herniation may be minimal and easily repairable, or the defect may be so extensive that the viscera present in the thoracic cavity during embryonic life prevented the normal development of pulmonary tissue. Most cases involve a posterolateral defect, usually on the left. The extent of the defect and the severity and timing of the symptoms determine the seriousness of the problem.

Signs that are suspicious of extensive diaphragmatic herniation can be assessed by the nurse. Signs include the following: constant respiratory distress from birth that becomes increasingly severe as bowels fill with air, heart sounds heard in right side of the chest, large or asymmetric chest contour, dullness to percussion on affected side, bowel sounds heard in thoracic cavity, and diminished breath sounds.

Preoperative activities include positioning the infant with head and chest higher than the abdomen, abdominal decompression, and the prevention of crying in the infant.

Prompt surgical repair is imperative after correction of acidosis, insertion of a nasogastric tube and aspiration, and oxygen therapy. The prognosis de-

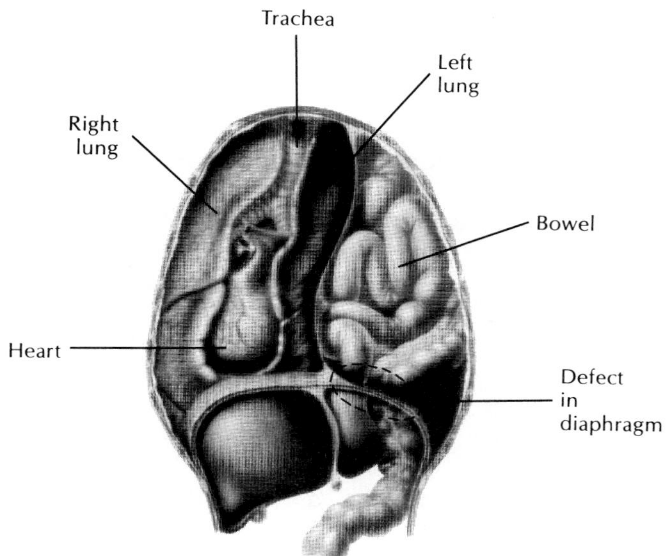

Fig. 38-5 Diaphragmatic hernia.
Courtesy Ross Laboratories, Columbus, Ohio.

pends largely on the degree of pulmonary development and the success of diaphragmatic closure. Prognosis in severe cases is guarded. Extracorporeal membrane oxygenation (ECMO) may be indicated after surgery in infants who do not respond to conventional medical therapy for circulatory and respiratory complications (Polin, Fox, 1992).

TRACHEOESOPHAGEAL ANOMALIES. **Esophageal atresia** is an urgent congenital anomaly. Various types are recognized, depending on the presence or absence of an associated *tracheoesophageal fistula,* the site of the fistula, and the point and degree of esophageal obstruction (Fig. 38-6). Moderate hydramnios is common with esophageal atresia and tracheoesophageal fistula. About half of these newborns have associated anomalies, including congenital heart defects and genitointestinal malformations.

The following signs are suspicious for atresia, with or without tracheoesophageal fistula: excessive oral secretions with drooling, progressive respiratory distress as unswallowed secretions spill over into trachea, and feeding intolerance. In feeding intolerance, choking, coughing, and cyanosis follow even a small amount of fluid taken by mouth. Soon after the first feeding is initiated, there is regurgitation of unaltered formula (unmixed with stomach secretions or bile).

Nursing actions are supportive. In the presence of excessive oral secretions and respiratory distress, *the infant should not be fed orally* before a physician is consulted. In the presence of abdominal distention, the newborn is placed in semi-Fowler's position, and the head is raised 30 degrees or more (infant seat may be used). This position facilitates respiratory efforts and discourages reflux (spillage) of stomach secretions into the respiratory tree, with resultant chemical bronchitis and pneumonitis. On physician's order or per standing orders, a suction tube is inserted into the blind pouch, and the tube is connected to low, intermittent suction.

Surgical correction of the anomaly is mandatory. After the surgery, oropharyngeal suctioning is permitted only to a length of 8 cm or to the length of the endotracheal tube if one is present. This prevents damage to the anastomosis from the catheter. Pacifiers are not permitted because sucking increases secretions. The prognosis depends on the degree of maturity of the newborn and the presence of a fistula or pneumonia.

OMPHALOCELE. **Omphalocele** is a herniation noted at birth in which part of the intestine protrudes through a defect in the abdominal wall at the umbilicus (Fig. 38-7). Failure of migration of the midgut in embryonic development probably is responsible for omphalocele. The protruding bowel is covered only by a thin, transparent membrane composed of amnion.

Prompt closure of defects of less than 5 cm in diameter usually is successful. Larger defects may re-

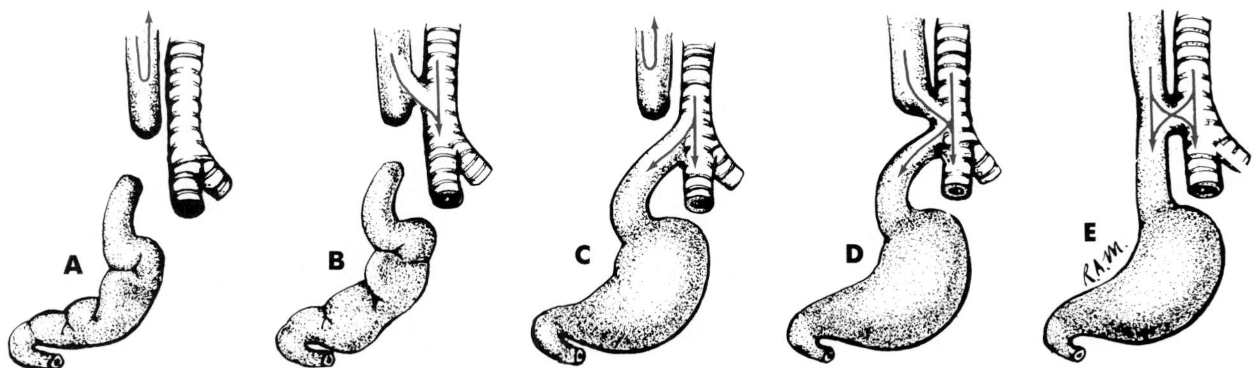

Fig. 38-6 Congenital atresia of esophagus and tracheoesophageal fistula. **A,** About 8%. Upper and lower segments of esophagus end in blind sac. **B,** Less than 1%. Upper segment of esophagus ends in atresia and connects to trachea by fistulous tract. Infant may drown with first feeding. **C,** About 87%. Upper segment of esophagus ends in blind pouch; lower segment connects with trachea by small fistulous tract. **D,** Less than 1%. Both segments of esophagus connect by fistulous tracts to trachea. Infant may drown with first feeding. **E,** About 4%. Esophagus is continuous but connects by fistulous tract to trachea; known as *H-type*.
From Whaley LF, Wong DL: *Nursing care of infants and children,* ed 4, St Louis, 1991, Mosby–Year Book.

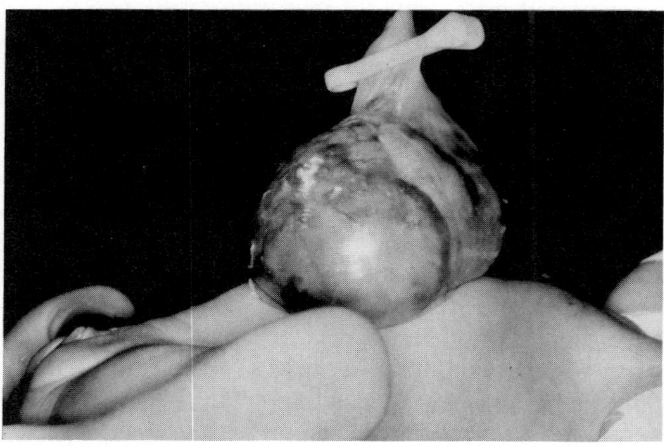

Fig. 38-7 Omphalocele containing liver.
Courtesy John R Campbell, MD, University of Oregon Health Sciences Center, Portland, Ore.

quire closure in stages. The general prognosis is related to associated anomalies.

There usually is only a short time span between the infant's birth and surgical intervention. Planning support for the parents is an essential aspect of nursing care. In addition to the usual preoperative orders, preparation of the infant for surgery includes insertion of an orogastric tube, aspiration of stomach contents, insertion of an intravenous line in an upper extremity, immediate administration of antibiotics, and protection of the defect from infection, rupture, and drying. The omphalocele is covered with sterile towels or sponges that are kept moist with sterile saline solution warmed to body temperature. The sponges are enclosed in plastic wrap to prevent heat and moisture loss.

INTESTINAL OBSTRUCTION. Congenital jejunal or ileal obstruction is suspected when distention and bile-stained or fecal vomiting occur in a newborn in the first 24 to 48 hours of life. Normal meconium stool is not passed. Although this condition is uncommon, preterm infants and those with other anomalies may be affected.

Nursing care is supportive.

- Stop oral feedings and monitor intravenous therapy and electrolyte replacement (see p. 1105).
- Prevent aspiration, and suction gastric contents on physician's order (indwelling catheter to low, intermittent suction may be ordered).
- Place infant in semi-Fowler's position to facilitate respiration.

Prompt surgery usually provides good results.

IMPERFORATE ANUS. **Imperforate anus** is a term used to describe a wide variety of congenital disorders that are more common in male than in female infants (Fig. 38-8). About 85% of affected girls will have developed a small fistula (Fig. 38-9), but this is rare in boys. The obstruction may be of the low type (anal membrane) or the high type (anal or rectal atresia).

Because lifetime continence may depend on coexisting sacral anomalies and proper corrective surgery, a pediatric surgeon is consulted at once. Surgery may be as simple as an incision of an anal membrane. With anorectal agenesis, a prompt colostomy will be necessary.

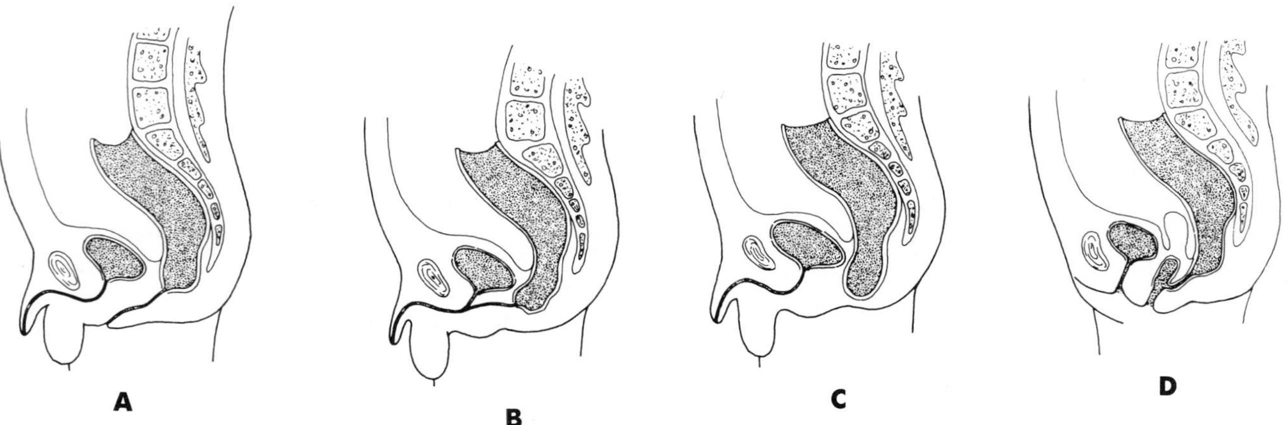

Fig. 38-8 Types of imperforate anus. Anal sphincter muscle may be present and intact. **A,** High lesion opening onto perineum through narrow fistulous tract. **B,** High lesion ending in fistulous tract to urinary tract. **C,** Low lesion in bowel passes through puborectal muscle. **D,** High lesion ending in fistulous tract to vagina.

Fig. 38-9 A, Imperforate anus; fourchette fistula. Note meconium draining through fistula. Arrow indicates meconium exiting via fistulous tract. B, Imperforate anus with rectopectal penile fistula *(arrow)*.
Courtesy John R Campbell, MD, University of Oregon Health Sciences Center, Portland, Ore.

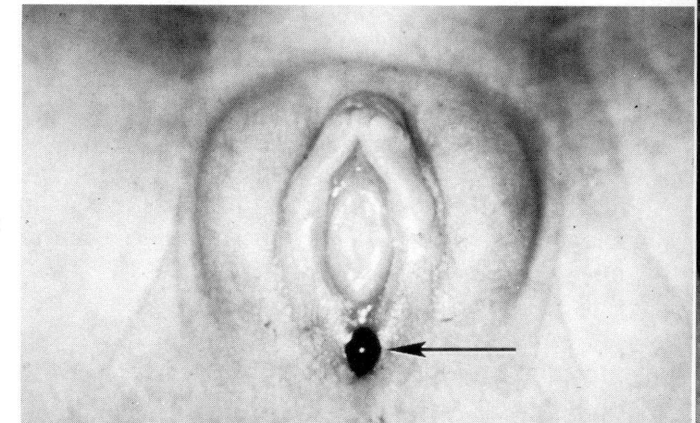

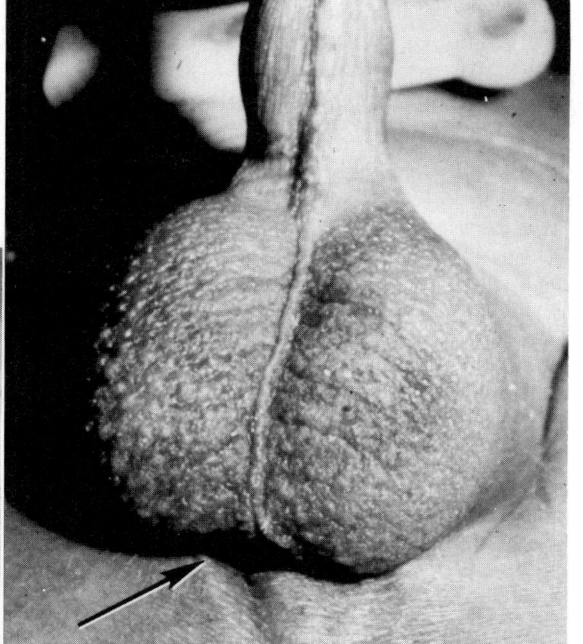

Common Malformations

MENINGOMYELOCELE. **Meningomyelocele,** a neural tube defect, is a herniation of part of the meninges (containing cerebrospinal fluid [CSF] and CNS tissue) through a defect in the vertebral column or skull. The defect often occurs in the lower portion of the back (Fig. 38-10). In the accompanying spinal malformation, **spina bifida,** the meningomyelocele extrudes through the opening of the spinal column. The opening is the result of a congenital absence of one or more vertebral arches. Occasionally a familial history (5% recurrence rate) of this anomaly is identified. Most cases are of unknown (infectious?) origin. A *meningocele* is also a herniation of the meninges. A meningocele contains CSF but does not contain CNS tissue (cord or nerve roots). Prenatal diagnosis of neural tube defects (meningomyelocele, meningocele, anencephaly) is now possible (see Chapter 27).

If the neonate is born with a large defect, the nurse aids in preventing the rupture and infection of any meningomyelocele sac before surgery. Protection of the defect includes the following actions.

1. Position infant with care.
   a. Position infant prone or side-lying with rolled towels to prevent pressure or injury to defect, thereby preventing portal of entry for infectious agents.
   b. Change position every hour to prevent pressure areas.
   c. If physician permits infant to be held, exercise caution to avoid injury to defect.
2. Provide skin care: skin around defect is cleansed and dried carefully to prevent breakdown, which would establish a portal of entry for infectious agents. Apply physician-ordered dressings, ointments, and so on.

The nurse assists in the diagnosis of a hidden defect (e.g., *spina bifida occulta*) (Fig. 38-10, *B*). The nurse assesses neurologic function and notes the following: paralysis of lower extremities, flaccidity and

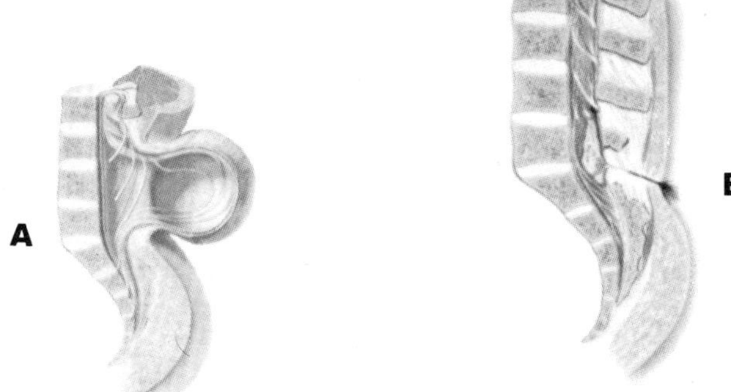

Fig. 38-10 A, Myelomeningocele. Note absence of vertebral arches. B, Dermal sinus tract with dermoid cyst, often associated with spina bifida occulta. Note also tuft of hair.

spasticity of muscles below defect, and sphincter control (character and number of voidings and stools; leakage of urine and stool).

Surgical repair often can be performed in the neonatal period. If other anomalies, such as hydrocephalus, are present, delayed correction may be elected. Permanent impairment of neuromuscular function below the level of the defect depends on the amount of CNS tissue involved. In severe cases, voluntary and involuntary functions are absent. The prognosis is guarded. Only about 60% of cases are operable. Many of these children die or achieve only partial function. Hydrocephalus ultimately develops in virtually all of these infants.

The parents will need considerable support and instruction regarding the infant's care. In some instances parents may require assistance in placing the child in a special care facility.

CONGENITAL HYDROCEPHALUS. Congenital **hydrocephalus** is macrocephaly caused by abnormal enlargement of the cerebral ventricles and skull. This disorder has many causes. Head enlargement is the result of increased intraventricular CSF pressure. This condition is accompanied by enlargement of the head, prominence of the forehead, "setting sun" sign of the eyes, atrophy of the brain, weakness, and convulsions as the condition worsens. Congenital hydrocephalus is encountered in approximately 1/2000 fetuses (about 12% of all malformations). Several types are known. Spina bifida occurs in approximately one third of infants born with hydrocephalus.

Surgery usually is performed soon after birth. If surgical shunting is not accomplished, increasing intracranial pressure—evidenced by palpably widening fontanelle and sutures, lethargy, irritability, vomiting, or high-pitched shrill cry—results in irreversible neurologic damage.

Nursing actions appropriate to the needs of a newborn with hydrocephalus include careful documentation of ongoing observations. Meticulous skin care is necessary to prevent pressure areas and infection of the skin of the head. Lamb's wool, sheepskin, or a flotation mattress is used under the infant. Frequent position changing and keeping the newborn clean and dry help maintain skin integrity and health.

The newborn's heavy head is supported carefully when being held or turned. The method, amount, and frequency of feeding are chosen to accommodate the infant's tolerance and energy level. Care is taken to prevent vomiting and subsequent aspiration. Nonnutritive sucking, touching, and cuddling needs are met.

Damaged or destroyed brain tissue cannot be restored. Spontaneous arrest of hydrocephalus may occur, but often surgical shunting may be required to eliminate excess CSF. Despite arrest of the process, serious mental retardation and neurologic sequelae are common.

ANENCEPHALY AND MICROCEPHALY. **Anencephaly** and **microcephaly** are congenital fetal deformities in which the head is considerably smaller than normal. In anencephaly there is complete or partial absence of the brain and of the overlying skull. Because the pituitary gland is absent or vestigial, the adrenal cortex is diminutive (for lack of adrenocorticotropic hormone [ACTH] stimulation). About 70% of anencephalic infants are girls. This condition commonly is accompanied by hydramnios. The cause of anencephaly is unknown, but multiple environmental factors have been postulated. A 3% recurrence rate has been noted in familial histories. Anencephaly is incompatible with life; warmth and fluid are provided until the neonate's death, which usually occurs before the end of the first 24 hours after birth.

In microcephaly the head generally is well formed but small. X-ray exposure of the woman may result in fetal microcephaly. Rubella, CMV, and perhaps other infectious processes are the causes in some cases. Microcephalic infants require specific nursing care and medical observation to appraise the extent of psychomotor retardation that almost always accompanies this abnormality. The nurse's supportive role with parents is considerable.

CLEFT LIP OR PALATE. **Cleft lip or palate** is a common congenital midline fissure, or opening, in the lip or palate; one or both deformities may occur (Fig. 38-11). The incidence is approximately 1/700 Caucasian newborns and 1/2000 African-American newborns. Polygenetic factors are causative in some cases, but fetal viral infection, maternal corticosteroid therapy, radiation, dietary influence, and hypoxia have been associated factors. The combination of cleft lip and palate affects more male than female infants.

Treatment requires special feeding techniques, for example, the use of uniquely designed nipples (p. 1106). The cleft lip is repaired before palate repair and may be performed soon after birth if the newborn is free of infection, in good condition, and weighs at least 2500 g (5 lb 9 oz). Some clinicians suggest that lip repair (Fig. 38-12, *A*) is best undertaken when the infant weighs 4500 g (10 lb) or more because more tissue is available. Advantages of earlier labial (lip) repair include facilitating a positive parent-child relationship and permitting the infant to learn to use and strengthen musculature around the mouth. Infants with palatolabial fissures often look grotesque and repulsive to the parents. After initial

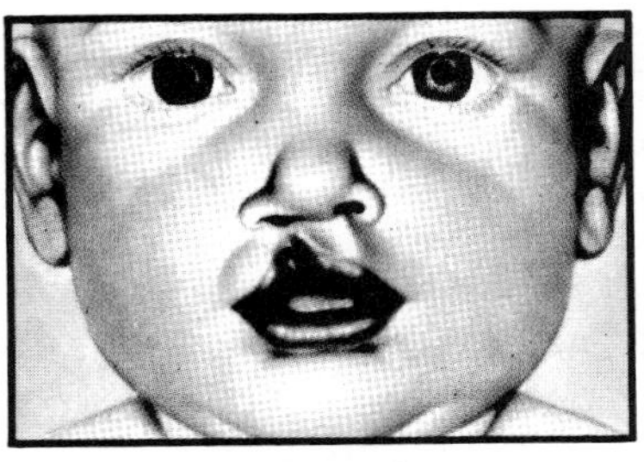

Unilateral incomplete (notch in vermilion border)

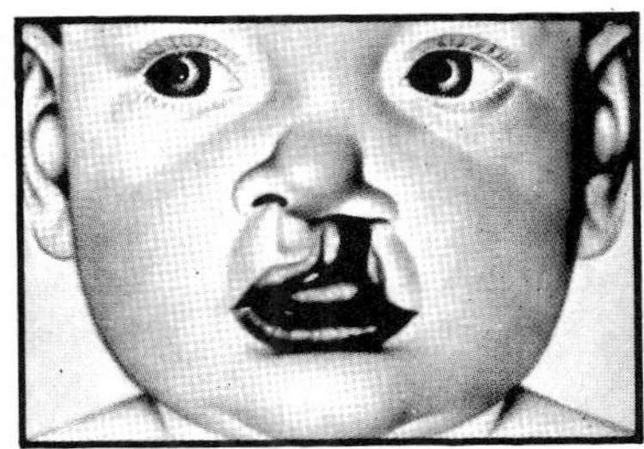

Unilateral complete

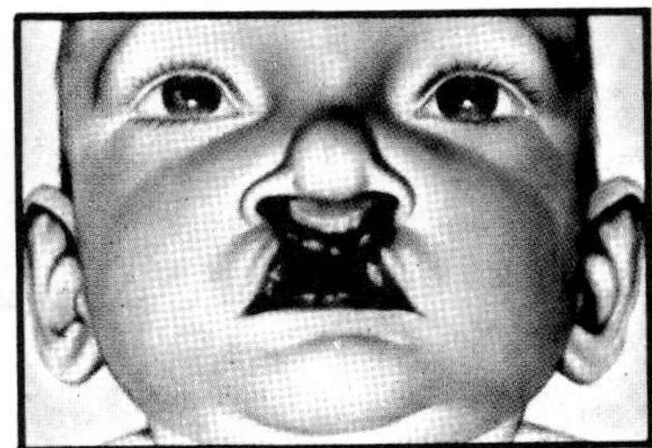

Bilateral complete

A

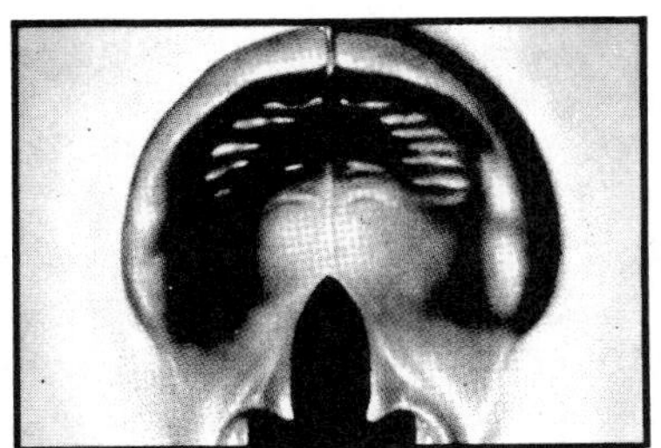

Soft palate only

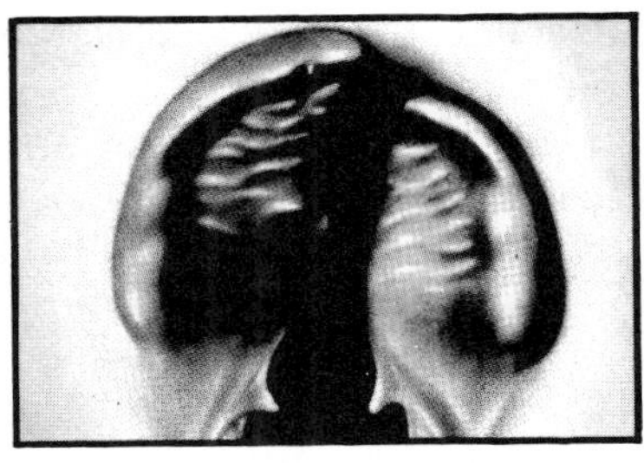

Unilateral complete

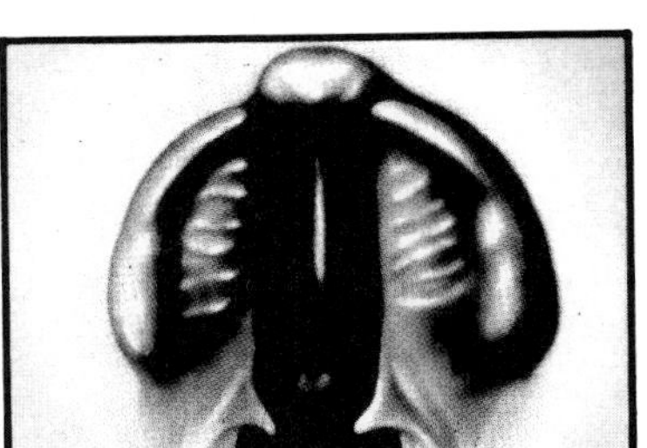

Bilateral complete

B

Fig. 38-11 A, Cleft lip. B, Cleft palate.
Courtesy Ross Laboratories, Columbus, Ohio.

A

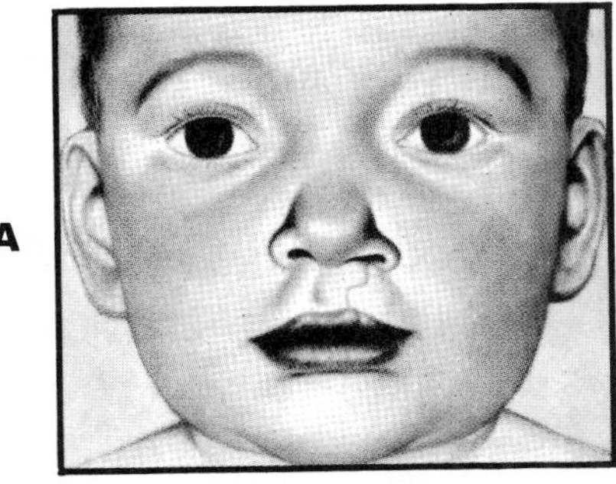

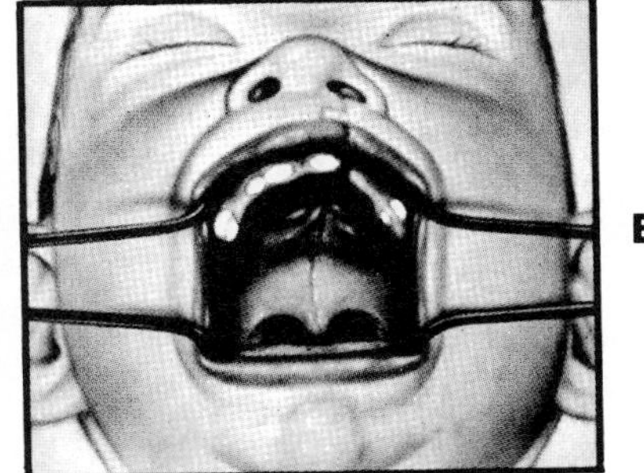

B

Fig. 38-12 Surgical repair of unilateral complete cleft lip (**A**) and of unilateral complete cleft palate (**B**).
Courtesy Ross Laboratories, Columbus, Ohio.

labial repair and with collaborative health team support, the mother commonly is able to assume responsibility for the newborn's care until palatal repair is feasible (Fig. 38-12, *B*). Repair usually occurs between 16 and 24 months of age (9 kg [20 lb] body weight or more). The plastic surgeon, pediatrician, orthodontist, hospital and community nurses, speech therapist, and social worker comprise the collaborative health team that has made possible the effective treatment available today. Until repair of the palate is performed, a prosthesis is fitted to aid the infant's feeding and speech development and to reduce respiratory tract infections.

MUSCULOSKELETAL DISORDERS. The two most common musculoskeletal deviations seen in the neonatal period are congenital dysplasia of the hip and congenital clubfoot. Both conditions are easily recognized. Early detection and definitive treatment are mandatory for successful correction. Delay makes repair more difficult and prognosis less favorable.

CONGENITAL HIP DYSPLASIA. Also known

as *congenital dislocation of the hip,* **hip dysplasia** is an often-hereditary disorder occurring more commonly in girls (Fig. 38-13) because of the structure of the pelvis. In this condition the acetabulum is abnormally shallow. The head of the femur becomes dislocated upward and backward to lie on the dorsal aspect of the ilium. The pressure of the displaced femoral head may form a false acetabulum on the ilium. A stretched joint capsule results, and ossification of the femoral head is delayed.

Before dislocation occurs, reduced movement, splinting of the affected hip, limited abduction, and asymmetry of the hip may be noted. After dislocation, all these signs will be present, together with the external rotation and shortening of the leg. A clicking sound may be noted on gentle forced abduction of the leg (Ortolani's sign, Fig. 20-12), and a bulge of the femoral head is felt or seen (Fig. 38-13, *B*). X-ray films will reveal a deformity in congenital dysplasia of the hip.

Treatment involves pressing the femoral head into the acetabulum to form an adequate socket before ossification is complete. Several abduction devices such as the following are available.

- Thick diapers abduct and externally rotate leg and flex hip (pin anterior flaps of diapers under posterior flaps). Double or triple disposable diapers also can be used.
- The Pavlik harness is worn continuously for 3 to 6 months.
- A spica cast is used to maintain abduction, extension, and internal rotation when a stable reduction cannot be maintained with other devices (Schaming et al, 1990).

TALIPES EQUINOVARUS. Talipes equinovarus, or clubfoot, is a congenital fixed deformity in which the foot is twisted out of shape or position. The heel is turned inward from the midline of the leg, the sole of the foot is flexed at the ankle joint, and the Achilles tendon is shortened.

Before the infant is 2 months old, often during the first days of life, successive plaster casts are applied first to correct the heel inversion and adduction of the forefoot and later, the equinus deformity. The prognosis depends on the extent of the deformity and the response to progressive orthopedic treatment.

PHOCOMELIA. **Phocomelia,** or "seallike limbs," is a developmental anomaly typified by absence of the arms or legs, or both, or stunting of the extremities. In the early 1960s the drug *thalidomide* was implicated as the causative agent for the limb deformities of many thousands of infants, especially in Germany. As a result the U.S. Food and Drug Administration tightened its regulations governing drug approval. Painfully apparent was evidence that drugs ingested during pregnancy may have tragic implications for fetal development. Thalidomide (and perhaps imipramine [Tofranil]) is a cause of this condition. Sporadic cases of congenital amputation or stunting are of unknown cause. The child born with these deformities requires special care.

Supportive care of the parents must begin at the birth of the child and continue for years. After the initial grief reaction, the parents need information regarding the rehabilitative and psychosocial components of their child's care. (Grief and loss are discussed in Chapter 40.)

POLYDACTYLY. Extra digits on the hands or feet occur occasionally (Fig. 38-14). In some instances **polydactyly** is hereditary. If there is little or no bone involvement, the extra digit is tied with silk suture soon after birth. The finger falls off within a few days, leaving a small scar. When there is bone involvement, surgical repair is indicated.

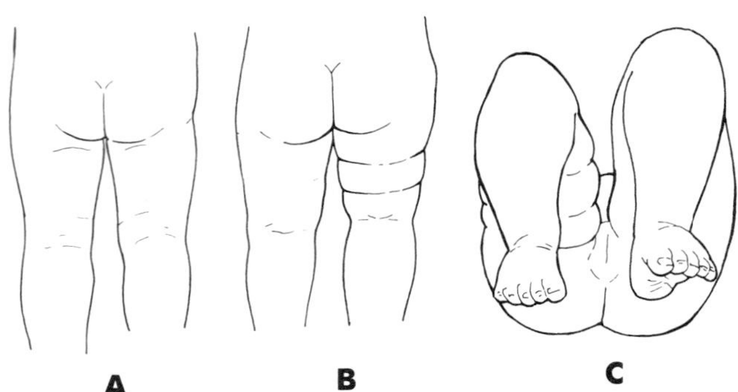

Fig. 38-13 Congenital dysplasia of hip. **A**, Normal gluteal and popliteal skin creases. **B**, Abnormal skin creases and asymmetry of skin folds. **C**, Apparent shortening of femur. Femur head is displaced.
Courtesy Ross Laboratories, Columbus, Ohio.

GENITOURINARY TRACT ANOMALIES. Abnormally low-set or misshapen ears may indicate other, often genitourinary, anomalies (such as renal agenesis) (see Fig. 20-26).

EXSTROPHY OF THE BLADDER. Exstrophy of the bladder (Fig. 38-15) is a rare congenital anomaly of unknown cause. With this anomaly a separation of the symphysis pubis and anterior abdominal wall structures results in exteriorization of the bladder trigone and surrounding mucosa. The exposed mucosa is deep red, has numerous folds, and is sensitive to touch. A direct passage of urine to the outside occurs. Associated anomalies, such as undescended testes, inguinal hernia, absence of the vagina, or bowel defects, should be sought. Surgical correction, often elimination of the bladder and construction of an ileal conduit, rarely is justified in the

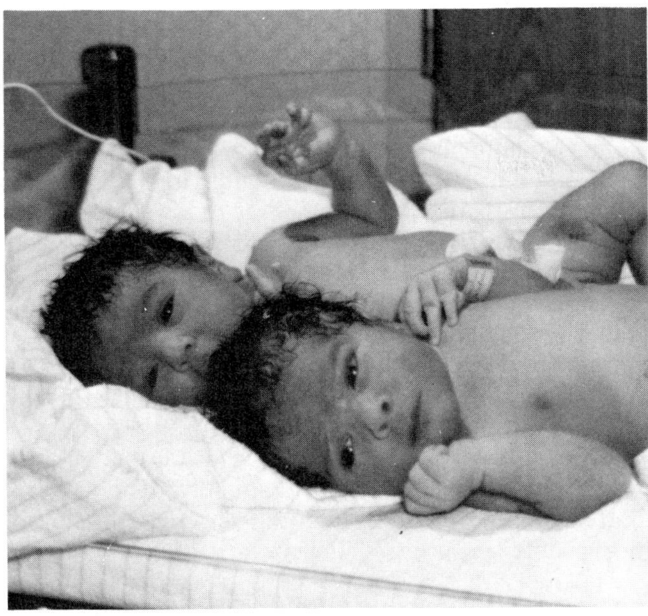

Fig. 38-14 Polydactyly: supernumerary digits of both hands of both identical twin girls. Since no bone is involved, the extra digits are tied off with silk suture soon after birth. Most common congenital anomaly of upper extremity and is occasionally seen in conjunction with other congenital malformation.
Courtesy Marjorie Pyle, RNC, Lifecircle, Costa Mesa, Calif.

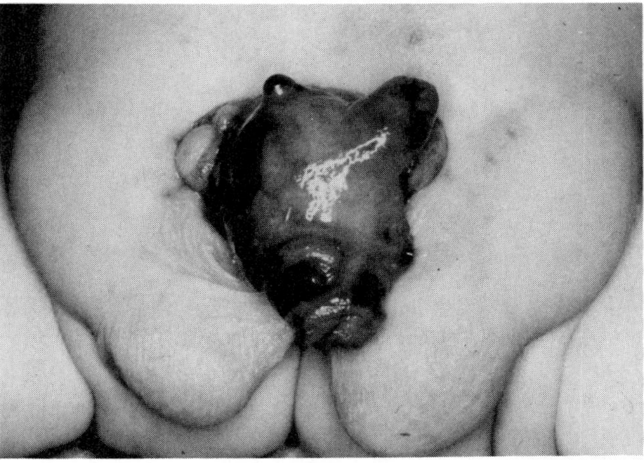

Fig. 38-15 Exstrophy of bladder.
Courtesy Edward S Tank, MD, Division of Urology, University of Oregon Health Sciences Center, Portland, Ore.

neonatal period. A prosthesis for collection of the urine and protection of the bladder may be employed.

Nursing management in the presence of exstrophy of the bladder focuses on the prevention of urinary tract infection and ulceration of adjacent skin from the constant seepage of urine. The child's touching and cuddling needs are met. Parents require considerable support and teaching to care for the defect if surgery is scheduled when the infant is several weeks or months of age.

HYPOSPADIAS AND EPISPADIAS. Hypospadias is a developmental anomaly in which the urethral meatus is placed lower than normal. In a male infant the meatus opens in the midline of the undersurface of the penis or on the perineum. In a female infant the meatus opens into the vagina. This condition tends to be hereditary.

Epispadias, also occurring in both sexes but predominating in boys, is a congenital absence of the upper urethral wall. In girls it often is associated with exstrophy of the bladder. In boys the meatal opening is located anywhere along the dorsum (upper side) of the penis.

Most instances of hypospadias are minor and require no corrective surgery. Pronounced defects require extensive urethroplasty. If needed, surgery is completed before the boy enters school so that he can urinate from a standing position like other boys. The more serious defects often coexist with other, multiple anomalies.

Nursing management of the physical care of the infant with hypospadias is the same as that for the normal infant. Should urethroplasty be required, circumcision is not performed because the foreskin is used in the surgical procedure. The parents are taught how to care for the urethral meatus and foreskin to prevent infection and to promote cleanliness.

SEXUAL AMBIGUITY. Sexual ambiguity in the newborn (Fig. 38-16) often is discovered by the nurse, who usually is the first one to perform a physical assessment.

Erroneous or abnormal sexual differentiation may be a genetic aberration (e.g., congenital adrenal hypoplasia), or it may be caused by maternal problems (such as steroid sex hormone therapy for threatened abortion). It is imperative to establish the genetic sex and the sex of child rearing as soon as possible. Early determination of genetic sex is important to permit the surgical correction of anomalies before an individual or social pattern is set. Prompt consultation with a surgeon who is experienced in the area of intersexuality should be arranged without delay. Meanwhile parents need supportive care as they await the decision.

TERATOMA. Teratoma, a solid or semisolid neoplasm, is composed of the three embryonal tissue types (ectoderm, mesoderm, endoderm). A teratoma in the newborn may occur in the skull, mediastinum,

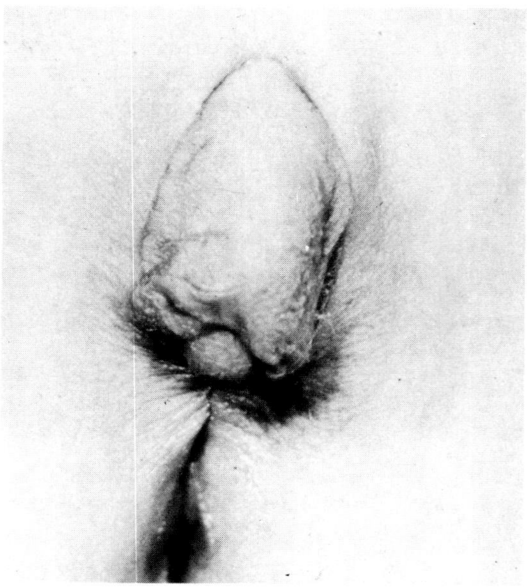

Fig. 38-16 Ambiguous external genitals (e.g., structure can be an enlarged clitoral hood and clitoris or a malformed penis).
Courtesy Edward S Tank, MD, Division of Urology, University of Oregon Health Sciences Center, Portland, Ore.

or abdomen. A solid or semisolid tumor in the sacral area also may prove to be a teratoma. It is protected by sterile dressings before surgical removal. Many teratomas diagnosed in the newborn are malignant. If the lesion cannot be removed entirely by surgery, x-ray therapy and chemotherapy are used. Long-term survival rate for infants with sacrococcygeal teratoma is 85% after surgical removal in the neonatal period. The survival rate is only 50% if surgery is delayed until the infant is more than 1 month old. Rectal and anal function can always be preserved.

Genetic Disease

At the present time there is no cure for genetic disease, although therapies can be implemented to prevent or reduce the harmful effects of a few disorders. Structural defects sometimes can be modified to produce normal or near-normal function. Research is continually being carried out in genetic engineering in the hope that methods can be devised to influence or change the genes directly, thereby preventing the disease process. (For discussion of ethics, see Chapter 4.) However, at this time the major thrust in therapy is modification of the internal or external environment to minimize the effects of the disease. Rapid advances in the field of plastic and reconstructive surgery have reduced the impact of many functional and cosmetically displeasing physical defects. In some hereditary disorders, supplying the missing product that cannot be synthesized prevents the undesirable effects, for example, thyroid extract for hereditary cretinism, corticosteroids for adrenogenital syndrome, insulin for diabetes mellitus, and administration of missing blood factors for the hemophilias.

Diet modification may be required for infants with some inborn errors of metabolism. For example, a low phenylalanine diet reduces the harmful effects of that protein in PKU. Some female children successfully treated for PKU are now of reproductive age and present unique management challenges to caregivers (p. 1162). Other examples are substitution of lactose-free products for milk fed to infants and children with galactosemia and the use of a diet low in branched-chain amino acids for infants and children with maple syrup urine disease.

PARENTAL SUPPORT. Clarifying information is an important nursing function. A newly diagnosed disorder often implies the implementation of a therapeutic regimen. For example, the disorder in question may be an inborn error of metabolism such as PKU or galactosemia that requires consistent and rigid adherence to a diet. The family may need help to secure the necessary formula and counseling from dietetic services. The importance of maintaining the diet, especially keeping an adequate supply of special preparations and avoiding unauthorized substitutions, must be impressed on the family.

Referral to appropriate agencies is another essential part of the follow-up management. Many organizations and foundations help provide services and equipment for affected children, for example, the Cystic Fibrosis Foundation and the Muscular Dystrophy Association. Early Infant Stimulation Foundation programs are available for a child with Down syndrome. There also are numerous parent groups with whom the family can share experiences and derive mutual support in coping with similar problems. Nurses need to become familiar with services available in their community that provide assistance and education to families with these special problems (see Appendix H).

Probably the most important of all nursing functions is providing *emotional support* to the family during all aspects of the care of the child born with a defect or disorder (Stringer et al, 1991). Feelings that are generated under the real or imagined threat posed by a genetic disorder are as varied as the persons being counseled. Responses may include all stress reactions, such as apathy, denial, anger, hostility, fear, embarrassment, grief, and loss of self-esteem (see Chapter 40).

Parents benefit from seeing before and after pictures of other babies born with the same defect. Coupled with other verbal and nonverbal supportive care, this visual reassurance is effective. Parents can be referred to other parents (or organizations of parents such as the Cleft Palate Club) for continuing mutual support.

Guilt and self-blame are universal reactions. Many look on the disorder as a stigma—especially if the disorder is visible to others. Knowledgeable persons involved with the family often are able to dispel fears and even absolve the family from guilt simply by explaining the random nature of cell division and segregation. Parents may derive comfort from knowing that everyone carries defective genes, which, when combined with the same genes in a partner, can produce undesirable consequences. Old wives' tales, superstitions, and long-held misconceptions are all factors that may influence a client's reaction to a disorder. Obstacles such as religious beliefs, intellectual level, and prior attitudes toward the disease affect the way in which families respond.

The attitude of other family members and relatives can have a significant impact on some persons—especially situations in which the blame can be pinpointed (such as a dominant or an X-linked disorder). Recessive disorders are less likely to cause blaming because both partners carry the defective gene. Unfortunately most families tend to view a congenital disorder as shameful. Its presence in a family may cause altered plans for marriage or childbearing even when the probability of recurrence is no more than a random risk. The way a family views the probability of recurrence varies tremendously. For example, one family will consider a 10% risk as reassuring, whereas another may consider it too great a risk to contemplate marriage or childbearing.

The nature of a newborn's condition also influences the way families respond to a disorder. Factors such as the severity or chronicity of a disease, the age of onset, the threat of early death, a lengthy period of deterioration, presence or absence of pain, mental retardation, or cosmetic disfiguration all determine the impact a condition has on a family. One family may risk having a child with a disorder that produces a minor defect or even an early death but will not risk having a child with a lifelong physical or mental disability.

Sometimes counselors and other health personnel create barriers through their own attitudes toward a specific disease. It is often difficult to be nonjudgmental and objective in all instances. Nurses may intentionally or unintentionally influence families in making decisions. This is especially true when the client's intellectual level makes it difficult or impossible for that person to comprehend the ramifications of a situation. Even persons who can repeat information accurately often fail to grasp its significance in their case. Families may pressure the nurse to make decisions for them with questions such as, "What would you do if you were me?"

Families and individuals need ongoing education, guidance, and support (Sammons, Lewis, 1985; Johnson, 1986). They should be given the facts and possible consequences and all the assistance they need in problem solving, but the final decision regarding a course of action must be their own.

EVALUATION

Care is evaluated by assessing the degree to which goals have been met. On a short-term basis, care has been effective if the following outcomes occur.

- The newborn's disorder is recognized and appropriate therapy is initiated promptly.
- The newborn suffers no adverse sequelae to the disorder or its management.
- The parents understand the newborn's condition, its management, and possible sequelae, as well as the anticipated prognosis.
- The parents choose a course of action commensurate with their family's values and goals.

If the goals have not been met, the nurse reassesses the situation and develops a new plan of care.

SUMMARY

Most infants make the transition from intrauterine to extrauterine life with little difficulty. For some, however, birth is complicated by many factors. Hyperbilirubinemia and congenital abnormalities place the newborn in jeopardy for intact survival.

The survival and well-being of these high-risk infants depend on advanced and often aggressive-nursing and medical management and a suitably controlled environment. The parents of the high-risk infant may experience feelings of lowered self-esteem and self-worth and alienation from the infant. Thus the nurse plays a vital role in the care of both the high-risk newborn and the parents.

REFERENCES

Brambati B et al: Genetic diagnosis before the eighth gestational week, *Obstet Gynecol* 77:318, 1991.

Fanaroff AA, Martin RJ, editors: *Neonatal-perinatal medicine: diseases of the fetus and infant,* ed 5, St Louis, 1992, Mosby–Year Book.

Greene MF, Benacerraf BR: Prenatal diagnosis in diabetic gravidas: utility of ultrasound and maternal serum alpha-fetoprotein screening, *Obstet Gynecol* 77:520, 1991.

Hoffman JI: Congenital heart disease: incidence and inheritance, *Pediatr Clin North Am* 37:31, 1990.

Johnson SH: *Nursing assessment and strategies for the family at risk: high-risk parenting,* ed 2, Philadelphia, 1986, JB Lippincott Co.

Lemna WK et al: Mutation analysis for heterozygote detection and the prenatal diagnoses of cystic fibrosis, *N Engl J Med* 322:291, 1990.

Locklin M: Assessing jaundice in full-term newborns, *Pediatr Nurs* 13:15, 1987.

Merenstein GB, Gardner SL: *Handbook of neonatal intensive care,* ed 2, St Louis, 1989, Mosby–Year Book.

Pernoll ML, Benda GI, Babson SG: *Diagnosis and management of the fetus and neonate at risk: a guide for team care,* ed 5, St Louis, 1986, Mosby–Year Book.

Perry SE, Parer JT, Inturrisi M: Intrauterine transfusion for severe isoimmunization, *MCN* 11:182, 1986.

Polin RA, Fox WW: *Fetal and neonatal physiology,* vol 1 and 2, Philadelphia, 1992, WB Saunders Co.

Queenan JT: High-risk pregnancy: Rh and other blood group immunizations, *Contemp OB/GYN* 36:25, July 1991.

Sammons WA, Lewis JM: *Premature babies: a different beginning,* St Louis, 1985, Mosby–Year Book.

Schaming D et al: When babies are born with orthopedic problems, *RN.*, 1990.

Shibley B: Phototherapy at home, *NURSEweek,* p 12, Jan 7, 1991.

Stringer M et al: Establishing a prenatal genetic diagnosis: the nurse's role, *MCN* 16:152, 1991.

Tucker SM: *Pocket guide to fetal monitoring,* St Louis, 1988, Mosby–Year Book.

Wenstrom K et al: Magnetic resonance imaging of fetuses with intracranial defects, *Obstet Gynecol* 77:529, 1991.

Whaley LF, Wong DL: *Nursing care of infants and children,* ed 4, St Louis, 1991, Mosby–Year Book.

Whaley LF, Wong DL: *Essentials of pediatric nursing,* ed 4, St Louis, 1993, Mosby–Year Book.

Wise BV, Lawrence-Nolan LA: A risk of blood transfusions for premature infants, *MCN* 15:96, March/April 1990.

Wolfe HM et al: Maternal obesity: a potential source of error in sonographic prenatal diagnosis, *Obstet Gynecol* 76:339, 1990.

Zacharias JF: The new genetics, *JOGNN* 19:122, March/April 1990.

Resources for Down Syndrome

The National Association for Down's Syndrome, Dept N83, Box 63, Oak Park, IL 60303, and the Down's Syndrome Congress, Dept N83, 1640 W Roosevelt Rd, Chicago, IL 60608. For additional help, contact national and local associations for the mentally retarded.

BIBLIOGRAPHY

Baker M: Jennifer's life is a success story, *RN* 53:30, Feb 1990.

Creasy R, Resnik R: *Maternal-fetal medicine: principles and practice,* Philadelphia, 1989, WB Saunders Co.

Cullen MT, Athanassiadis AP, Romero R: Prenatal diagnosis of anterior parietal encephalocele with transvaginal sonography, *Obstet Gynecol* 75:489, 1990.

Danilowicz D: Update on patent ductus arteriosus, *Hosp Med* 25:53, Aug 1989.

Dolfus C et al: Infant mortality: a practical approach to the analysis of the leading causes of death and risk factors, *Pediatrics* 86:176, 1990.

Erlen JA: Anencephalic infants as sources of organs: issues and implications for nurses, *JOGNN* 19:249, 1990.

Gaston M: Screening newborns for sickle cell disease, *Contemp OB/GYN* 33:203, 1989.

Hanson-Smith B: *Nursing care planning guides for childbearing families,* Baltimore, 1989, Williams & Wilkins.

Hobbins JC: Diagnosis and management of neural-tube defects today, *N Engl J Med* 324:690, 1991.

Holzgreve W, Miny P: Prenatal diagnosis and management of fetal tumors. I. Sacrococcygeal teratoma, *Female Patient* 14:48, Sept 1989.

Keating SB, Kelman GB: *Home health care nursing: concepts and practice,* Philadelphia, 1988, JB Lippincott Co.

Killam W, Miller R, Seeds J: Extremely high maternal serum alpha-fetoprotein levels at second-trimester screening, *Obstet Gynecol* 78:257, 1991.

Larson DR: Ethics: should anencephalic neonates be organ donors? *AORN J* 47:778, 1988.

Luthy DA et al: Cesarean section before the onset of labor and subsequent motor function in infants with meningomyelocele diagnosed antenatally, *N Engl J Med* 324:662, 1991.

Monteagudo A, Reuss L, Timor-Tritsch I: Imaging the fetal brain in the second and third trimesters using transvaginal sonography, *Obstet Gynecol* 77:27, 1991.

O'Brien GD: Limits of ultrasound screening for anomalies, *Contemp OB/GYN* 34:51, Jan 1989.

Pletsch PK: Birth defect prevention: nursing interventions, *JOGNN* 19:482, 1990.

Suchy S, Yeager M: Down syndrome screening in women under 35 with maternal serum hCG, *Obstet Gynecol* 76:20, 1990.

Bibliography—Nursing Research

Brown L et al: Transcutaneous bilirubinometer: an instrument for clinical research, *Nurs Res* 39:241, 1990.

Jones MA: Identifying signs that nurses interpret as indicating pain in newborns, *Pediatr Nurs* 15:76, 1989.

Van Cleve L: Parental coping in response to their child's spina bifida, *J Pediatr Nurs* 4(3):172, 1989.

chapter 38 review

Key Concepts

- Hyperbilirubinemia has a variety of etiologic factors, including maternal-fetal Rh and ABO incompatibility.
- Erythroblastosis fetalis leads to anemia, edema, and cytotoxic effects of unconjugated bilirubin.
- Injection of Rh_O(D) immune globulin to Rh-negative and Coombs'-negative women bestows passive immunity and minimizes the possibility of isoimmunization.
- An Rh-negative woman receives Rh-positive RBCs from the fetus through disruption of the cellular layer separating fetal and maternal circulation and through an erroneous blood transfusion.
- Neonatal exchange transfusion with type O, Rh-negative RBCs serves to treat anemia and acidosis and to remove bilirubin, maternal antibodies, and fetal RBCs that are beginning to hemolyze.
- Perinatal events such as hypoxia and cold stress increase the neonate's susceptibility to neurotoxic effects of bilirubin.
- Major congenital defects are now the leading cause of death in term neonates born to mothers who had good perinatal care.
- Hydramnios and oligohydramnios are associated with many congenital anomalies.
- Current technology permits prenatal diagnosis of many congenital anomalies and disorders.
- The curative and rehabilitative problems of a child with a congenital disorder are often complex, requiring a multidisciplinary approach to care.
- Supportive care to parents must begin at birth or at diagnosis and continue for years.

Key Terms

- ABO incompatibility (p. 1150)
- anencephaly (p. 1168)
- choreoathetoid cerebral palsy (p. 1150)
- cleft lip or palate (p. 1168)
- congenital (p. 1156)
- Coombs' test (p. 1150, 1153)
- diaphragmatic hernia (p. 1164)
- epispadias (p. 1171)
- erythroblastosis fetalis (p. 1152)
- esophageal atresia (p. 1165)
- exchange transfusion (p. 1154)
- hip dysplasia (p. 1170)
- hydramnios (p. 1157)
- hydrocephalus (p. 1168)
- hyperbilirubinemia (p. 1152)
- hypospadias (p. 1171)
- imperforate anus (p. 1166)
- inborn errors of metabolism (p. 1162)
- intrauterine transfusion (p. 1154)
- isoimmune hemolytic disease (p. 1150)
- jaundice (p. 1150)
- kernicterus (p. 1150)
- meningomyelocele (p. 1167)
- microcephaly (p. 1168)
- neural tube defects (p. 1158)
- omphalocele (p. 1165)
- phocomelia (p. 1170)
- polydactyly (p. 1170)
- Rh_O (D) immune globulin (RhIg) (p. 1154)
- teratoma (p. 1171)

Critical Thinking Exercises

You have been assigned to care for Emilie Gibson, an 18-year-old unwed mother who has just given birth to a son John with a cleft lip and palate. You are bringing the baby to the mother for the first time.

1. Identify your feelings about the infant and his physical defect.
2. Anticipate how the mother is likely to react to this encounter.
3. What would your thoughts and feelings be as you carry this infant to his mother?
4. What communication techniques (including body language) will you employ to project an attitude of acceptance of the baby to the mother?

   When she looks at John, Emilie says, "Isn't he ugly? God must be punishing me for being sinful."

5. What is your nursing diagnosis, or diagnoses, at this time?
6. What evaluative criteria for the nursing care of this mother will you establish?
7. What nursing actions would you select and implement? Justify your choices.

   Emilie had an uneventful postpartum physical recovery, and she has shown a positive attitude toward John. She was discharged on her third postpartum day, but John remained in the nursery for an additional 10 days because of poor weight gain. She visited daily and assisted in his care.

8. Devise a plan for teaching Emilie how to care for John, including teaching aids and evaluative criteria.

Topics for Nursing Research

- Which colors and lighting in nurseries would improve the nurse's ability to detect jaundice early and to determine its extent?
- Home phototherapy: compare the results of using bili lights vs. the phototherapy blanket in decreasing bilirubin levels.
- Can dermatoglyphics be used for assessment in the neonatal period to identify infants at risk for particular chronic diseases?

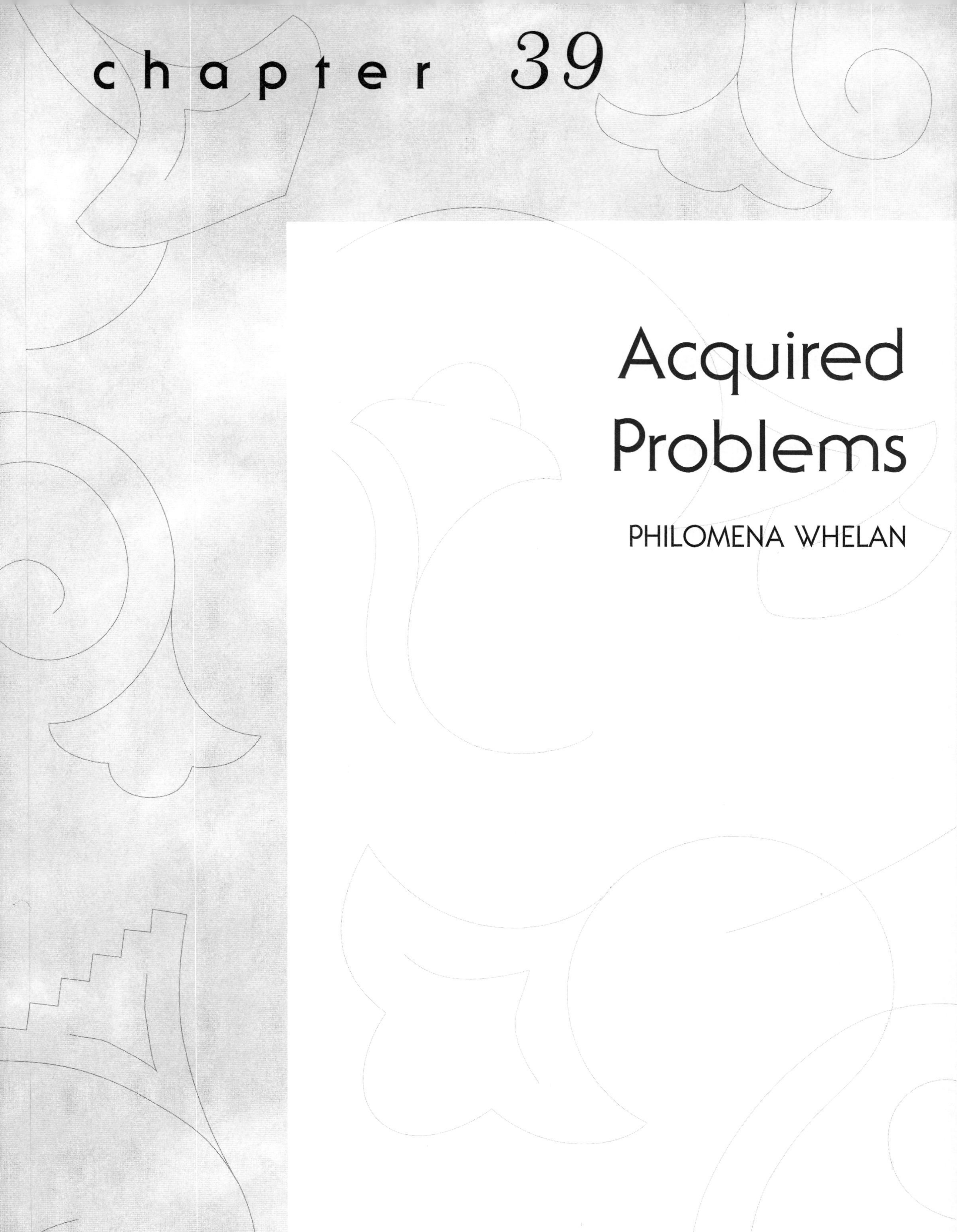

chapter 39

Acquired Problems

PHILOMENA WHELAN

LEARNING OBJECTIVES

- Define the key terms listed.
- Describe assessment of infants for birth trauma and for sequelae of a diabetic pregnancy.
- Develop nursing care plans for each of the conditions commonly seen in infants of diabetic mothers.
- Summarize the care of the newborn with soft tissue, skeletal, and nervous system injuries.
- Describe in detail the assessment of a newborn for infection.
- Formulate nursing diagnoses for the infant and family for each type of infection.
- Review implementation and evaluation of care of affected infants and their families.
- Describe the assessment of a newborn for drug dependence.
- Summarize general nursing care of the drug-dependent newborn.
- Assess the effects of alcohol, heroin, methadone, marijuana, cocaine, phencyclidine, and smoking on the fetus and newborn.
- Develop a care plan for the drug-dependent newborn and family.
- Identify topics for nursing research related to acquired problems.

This chapter deals with acquired problems of the newborn. Acquired problems refer to those conditions caused by environmental factors rather than genetic circumstances. The focus is on care of birth trauma, the infant of a diabetic mother, neonatal infections, and effects of maternal substance abuse.

■ BIRTH TRAUMA

Birth trauma (injuries) is physical injury sustained by a neonate during labor and birth. The significance of birth injuries is most accurately assessed by review of recent mortality data. These data show a steady decline in fatal birth injuries. In 1981 birth injuries ranked sixth among major causes of neonatal mortality, resulting in 23.8 deaths per 100,000 live births. In 1984 birth injuries caused 8.9 deaths per 100,000 live births, falling to eighth among leading causes. As of 1988 birth injuries continued to rank eighth but caused 4.6 deaths per 100,000 live births, a reduction of approximately 50% in 4 years. This ongoing improvement has been attributed to refinements in obstetric techniques, increased use of cesarean birth for births that would be difficult vaginally, and decreased use of vacuum extraction and version and extraction. Despite this decrease, birth injuries still represent an important source of neonatal morbidity. Therefore the clinician should consider the broad spectrum of birth injuries in the differential diagnosis of neonatal clinical disorders (Fanaroff, Martin, 1992).

In theory, most birth injuries may be avoidable, especially if careful assessment of risk factors and appropriate planning of birth occur. The use of ultrasonography allows antepartum diagnosis of macrosomia, hydrocephalus, and unusual presentations. To avoid significant birth injury controlled elective cesarean birth can be chosen for some pregnancies (Merenstein, Gardner, 1989). A small percentage of significant birth injuries may be unavoidable despite skilled and competent obstetric care—as in especially hard or prolonged labor or with an abnormal presentation (Fanaroff, Martin, 1992). Some injuries cannot be anticipated until the specific circumstances are encountered during childbirth. Emergency cesarean birth may provide a last-minute salvage, but in these circumstances the injury may be truly unavoidable. The same injury might be caused in several ways. Thus a cephalhematoma could result from an obstetric technique such as forceps birth or vacuum extraction, or the same injury may be caused by pressure of the fetal skull against the maternal pelvis.

Many injuries are minor and resolve readily in the neonatal period without treatment. Other traumas require some degree of intervention. A few are serious enough to be fatal. The nurse's contributions to the welfare of the newborn begin with early observation and accurate recording. The prompt reporting of signs that indicate deviations from normal permits early initiation of appropriate therapy.

ASSESSMENT

Several factors predispose an infant to birth injuries (Fanaroff, Martin, 1992; Merenstein, Gardner, 1989). *Maternal* factors include uterine dysfunction that leads to prolonged or precipitous labor, preterm or postterm labor, and cephalopelvic disproportion. Injury may result from dystocia caused by *fetal* macrosomia, multifetal gestation, abnormal or difficult presentation (not caused by maternal uterine or pelvic conditions), and congenital anomalies. *Intrapartum events* that can result in scalp injury include the use of intrapartum monitoring of fetal heart rate (FHR) and collection of fetal scalp blood for acid-base assessment. *Obstetric birth techniques* can cause injury. Forceps birth, vacuum extraction, version and extraction, and cesarean birth are all potential contributory factors. Often more than one factor is present, and the multiple predisposing factors may be related to a single maternal disease.

The Apgar score may alert the caregiver to birth injuries. Flaccid muscle tone, regardless of cause, increases the risk of joint dislocations and separation during the birth process. Flaccid tone in extremities may be traced to nerve plexus injuries or long-bone fractures. A weak or hoarse cry is characteristic of laryngeal nerve palsy as a result of excessive traction on the neck during birth. Marked bruising of the skin may preclude accurate assessment for color.

A complete physical assessment of the newborn is performed soon after birth (see Chapter 20). The birth of large-for-gestational-age (LGA) newborns may be preterm, term, postmature, or postterm; LGA neonates also may be born to diabetic (or prediabetic) mothers (see Figs. 37-1 and 37-2). Each of these categories has special concerns. Regardless of coexisting potential problems, the oversized infant or the infant too large for the maternal pelvis is at risk by virtue of size alone. Birth trauma, especially associated with breech or shoulder presentation, is a serious hazard for the oversized neonate. Asphyxia or central nervous system (CNS) injury, or both, also may occur before or during birth. Because evidence of birth injury may not be apparent at the initial examination, assessment continues during each contact with the neonate.

NURSING DIAGNOSES

The nursing diagnoses will depend on the particular injury incurred. Thus the following list represents examples only.

PARENTS

- Anxiety related to knowledge deficit regarding
  - —The injury
  - —Cause of injury
  - —Management and therapy
  - —Prognosis
- Anticipatory grieving related to
  - —Possible sequelae of the birth injury
- Spiritual distress related to
  - —Occurrence of birth injury

CHILD

- Potential for impaired physical mobility related to
  - —Brachial plexus injury
- Potential impaired gas exchange related to
  - —Diaphragmatic paralysis (partial or complete)
- Pain related to
  - —Injury

PLANNING

Meeting the unique needs of the birth-injured newborn requires constant vigilance. Goals are established and prioritized. Nursing actions are selected in terms of the particular disorder and individual needs of the infant and family.

The overall *goals* for care of infants with birth trauma are as follows.

1. The newborn suffers no or only minimal sequelae of trauma.
2. The infant receives prompt and appropriate treatment.
3. The parents initiate and maintain a positive parent-child relationship.
4. The parents'/family's educational needs regarding the injury and its management are met.

IMPLEMENTATION

Soft Tissue Injuries

Caput succedaneum is a localized edematous swelling of the scalp that persists for a few days after birth and then disappears. It has no pathologic significance (see Fig. 20-6, *A*).

Cephalhematoma is a collection of blood from ruptured blood vessels between the periosteum and surface of the parietal bone (see Fig. 20-6, *B*, and discussion 540). The swelling may appear unilaterally or bilaterally, usually is minimal or absent at birth, increases over the first 3 days of life, and disappears gradually in 2 to 3 weeks. Occasionally hyperbilirubinemia may result from breakdown of the accumulated blood.

Subconjunctival (scleral) and retinal hemorrhages result from rupture of capillaries caused by increased intracranial pressure during birth. They clear within 5 days after birth and usually present no problems. However, parents need reassurance about their presence.

Erythema, ecchymoses, petechiae, abrasions, lacerations, and *edema* of buttocks and extremities may be present. Localized discoloration may appear over presenting or dependent parts. Ecchymoses and edema appear as bruises anywhere on the body. They can appear on the presenting part from the application of forceps. They can result from manipulation of the infant's body during birth.

Bruises and ecchymoses over the face may be the result of face presentation (Fig. 39-1). The skin over the entire head may be ecchymotic and covered with

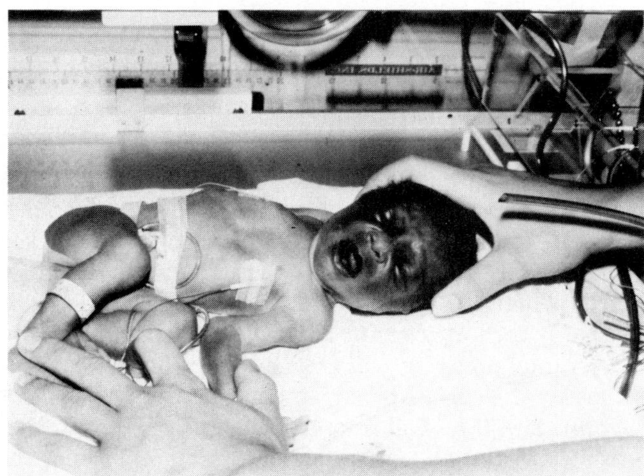

Fig. 39-1 Marked bruising of the entire face of 1490-g female born vaginally after face presentation. Less severe ecchymoses were present on the extremities. Despite use of phototherapy from the first day, icterus resulting from breakdown of the accumulated blood was noted on the third day, and exchange transfusions were required on the fifth and sixth days.
From Fanaroff AA, Martin RJ, editors: *Neonatal-perinatal medicine: diseases of the fetus and infant,* ed 5, St Louis, 1992, Mosby–Year Book.

petechiae caused by a tight nuchal cord. Petechiae, or pinpoint hemorrhagic areas, acquired during birth may extend over the upper portion of the trunk and face. These lesions are benign if they disappear within 2 days of birth and no new lesions appear. Ecchymoses and petechiae may be signs of a more serious disorder, such as *thrombocytopenic purpura*. If they do not disappear spontaneously in 2 days, the physician is notified. To differentiate hemorrhagic areas from skin rashes and discolorations, the nurse blanches the skin with two fingers. Because extravasated blood remains within the tissues, petechiae and ecchymoses do not blanch.

Trauma as a result of dystocia occurs over the presenting part; forceps injury occurs at the site of application of the instrument. Forceps injury commonly has a linear configuration across both sides of the face, outlining the placement of the forceps. The affected areas are kept clean to minimize the risk of secondary infection. These injuries usually resolve spontaneously within several days with no specific therapy. The increased use of padded forceps blades may reduce the incidence of these lesions significantly (Fanaroff, Martin, 1992).

Accidental lacerations may be inflicted with a scalpel during cesarean birth. These cuts may occur on any part of the body but most often are found on the scalp, buttocks, and thighs. Usually they are superficial, needing only to be kept clean. Butterfly adhesive strips will hold the edges of more serious lacerations together. Rarely, sutures are needed.

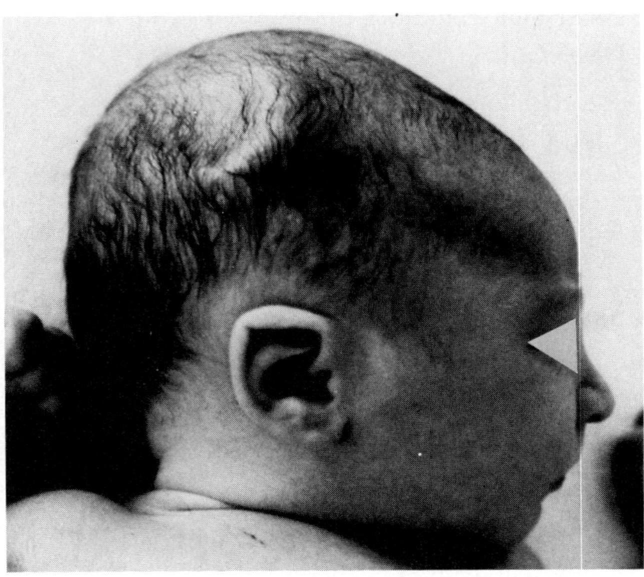

Fig. 39-2 Depressed skull fracture in a full-term male born after rapid (1 hour) labor. The infant was delivered by occiput-anterior presentation after rotation from occiput-posterior position.

From Fanaroff AA, Martin RJ, editors: *Neonatal-perinatal medicine: diseases of the fetus and infant,* ed 5, St Louis, 1992, Mosby–Year Book.

Skeletal Injuries

The newborn's immature, flexible *skull* can withstand a great degree of deformation (molding) before fracture results. Considerable force is required to fracture the newborn's skull. Location of the fracture determines whether it is insignificant or fatal. If an artery lying in a groove on the undersurface of the skull is torn as a result of the fracture, increased intracranial pressure will ensue (see p. 1184). Unless a blood vessel is involved, linear fractures (which account for 70% of all fractures for this age-group) heal without special treatment. The soft skull may become indented without laceration of either the skin or the dural membrane. These depressions, or "ping-pong ball" indentations, may occur during difficult births from pressure of the head on the bony pelvis (Fig. 39-2). They also can occur as a result of injudicious application of forceps.

The *clavicle* is the bone most often fractured during birth. Generally the break is in the middle third of the bone. Dystocia, particularly shoulder impaction, may be the predisposing problem. *Limitation of motion of the arm, crepitus of the bone, and the absence of Moro's reflex on the affected side are diagnostic.* Except for use of gentle rather than vigorous handling, there is no accepted treatment for fractured clavicle, and the prognosis is good. The figure-of-8 bandage appropriate for the older child should not be used for the newborn.

The *humerus* and *femur* are other bones that may be fractured during a difficult birth. Fractures in newborns generally heal rapidly. Immobilization is accomplished with slings, splints, swaddling, and other devices.

The parents need support in handling these infants because they often are fearful of hurting them. Parents are encouraged to practice handling, changing, and feeding the affected newborn under the guidance of nursery personnel. This will increase their confidence and knowledge and facilitate attachment. A plan for follow-up therapy is developed with the parents so that the times and arrangements for therapy are workable and acceptable to them.

Peripheral Nervous System Injuries

Erb-Duchenne paralysis (**brachial paralysis** of the upper portion of the arm) is the most common type of paralysis associated with a difficult birth (Fig. 39-3).

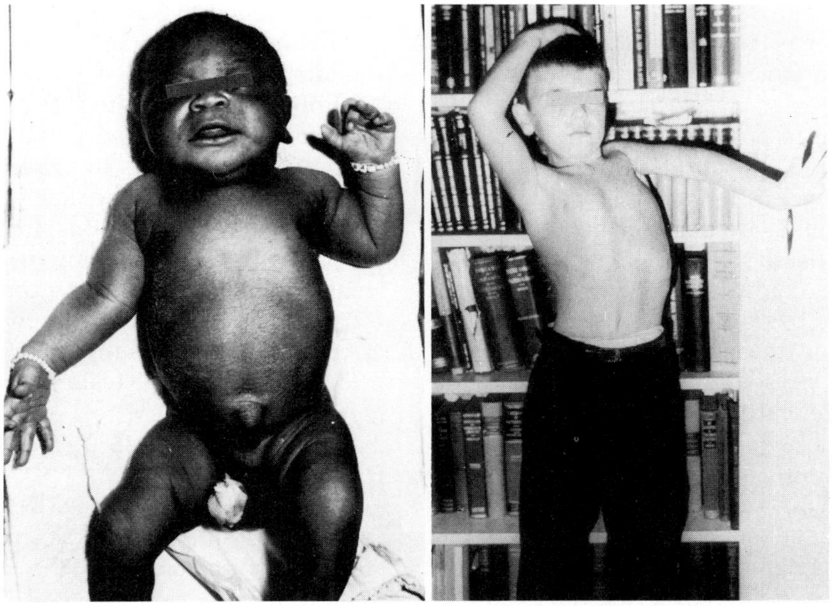

Fig. 39-3 A, Erb-Duchenne paralysis in newborn infant. Moro's reflex was absent in right upper extremity. Recovery was complete. B, Residual of Erb-Duchenne paralysis. Left arm was short; it could not be raised above level shown.
From Shirkey HC, editor: *Pediatric therapy*, ed 6, St Louis, 1980, Mosby–Year Book.

Injury to the upper plexus results from stretching or pulling the shoulder away from the head. Typical symptoms are a flaccid arm with the elbow extended and the hand rotated inward, absence of Moro's reflex on the affected side, sensory loss over the lateral aspect of the arm, and an intact grasp reflex.

Treatment consists of intermittent immobilization, proper positioning, and exercise to maintain the range of motion of joints. Gentle manipulation and range-of-motion exercises are delayed until about the tenth day to prevent additional injury to the brachial plexus.

Immobilization may be accomplished with a brace or splint or by pinning the infant's sleeve to the mattress. The infant should be positioned for 2 or 3 hours at a time as follows (Fig. 39-4).

- Abduct the arm 90 degrees.
- Externally rotate the shoulder.
- Flex the elbow 90 degrees.
- Supinate the wrist with the palm directed slightly toward the face (Fig. 39-4).

The arm should be freed periodically for good skin care. About the tenth day, gentle massage and range-of-motion exercises are begun to prevent contractures.

Damage to the lower plexus, *Klumpke's palsy*, is less common. With lower arm paralysis, the wrist and hand are flaccid, the grasp reflex is absent, deep tendon reflexes are present, and dependent edema

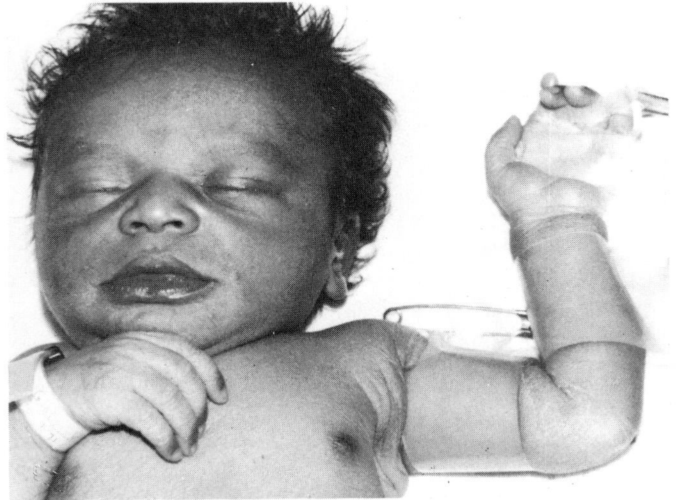

Fig. 39-4 Recommended corrective positioning for treatment of Erb-Duchenne paralysis. Note abduction and external rotation at shoulder, flexion at elbow, supination of forearm, and slight dorsiflexion at wrist.
From Behrmann RE, editor: *Neonatology: diseases of the fetus and infant*, St Louis, 1973, Mosby–Year Book.

and cyanosis may be apparent (in the affected hand). Treatment consists of placing the hand in a neutral position, padding the fist, and gently exercising the wrist and fingers.

Parents are taught to position and immobilize the arm or wrist or both. They can gently massage and manipulate the muscles to prevent contractures while the arm is healing. If edema or hemorrhage is responsible for the paralysis, the prognosis is good and recovery may be expected in a few weeks. If laceration of the nerves has occurred and healing does not result in return of function within a few months (3 to 6 months or 2 years at the most), surgery may be indicated; however, little or no function will develop.

Facial paralysis (Fig. 39-5) generally is caused by pressure on the facial nerve during birth. The face on the affected side is flattened and unresponsive to the grimace that accompanies crying or stimulation, and the eye will remain open. Moreover, the forehead will not wrinkle. Often the condition is transitory, resolving within hours or days of birth. Permanent paralysis is rare.

Treatment involves careful, patient feeding, prevention of damage to the cornea of the open eye, and supportive care of the parents. Commonly the infant looks grotesque, especially when crying. Feeding may be prolonged, with the milk flowing out of the newborn's mouth around the nipple on the affected side. The mother will need understanding and sympathetic encouragement while learning how to feed and care for the infant, as well as how to hold and cuddle the baby.

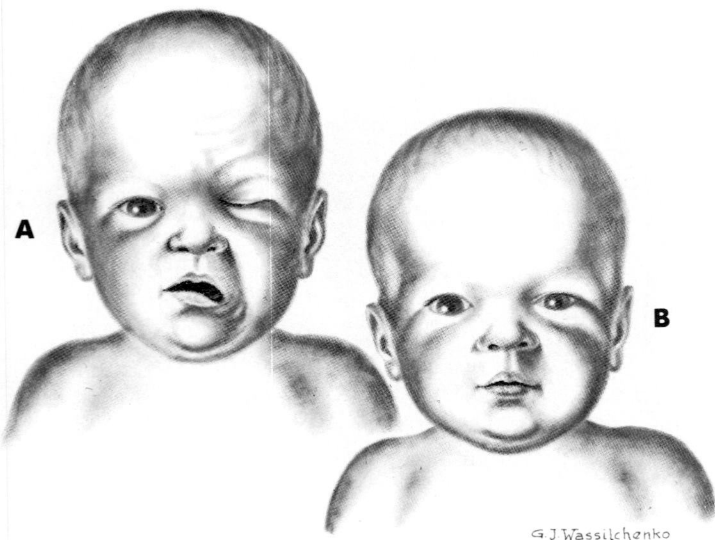

Fig. 39-5 **A,** Paralysis of right side of face 15 minutes after forceps birth. Absence of movement on affected side is especially noticeable when infant cries. **B,** Same infant 24 hours later.
From Whaley LF, Wong DL: *Nursing care of infants and children,* ed 4, St Louis, 1991, Mosby–Year Book.

Phrenic nerve injury almost always occurs as a component of brachial plexus injury. Injury to the phrenic nerve results in diaphragmatic paralysis. Cyanosis and irregular thoracic respirations, with no abdominal movement on inspiration, are characteristic of paralysis of the diaphragm. Babies with diaphragmatic paralysis usually require mechanical ventilatory support, at least for the first few days after birth. Occasionally this support is essential for several weeks until corrective surgery can be performed.

Central Nervous System Injuries

All types of **intracranial hemorrhage (ICH)** occur in newborn infants. ICH as a result of birth trauma is more likely to occur in the full-term, large infant. The frequency and degree of severity of ICH are different in the newborn than in older children or adults. In the newborn more than one type of hemorrhage can and does frequently occur (Fanaroff, Martin, 1992; Whaley, Wong, 1991).

Subdural hemorrhages (hematomas), life-threatening collections of blood in the subdural space, most often are produced by the stretching and tearing of the large veins in the tentorium of the cerebellum, the dural membrane that separates the cerebrum from the cerebellum. When this type of bleeding has occurred, common history includes a nulliparous mother, with the total labor and birth occurring in less than 2 or 3 hours, a difficult birth involving high or midforceps application, or an LGA infant. Subdural hematoma occurs only infrequently today because of recent improvements in obstetric care. However, it is especially serious because of its inaccessibility to aspiration by subdural tap (Fanaroff, Martin, 1992; Whaley, Wong, 1991).

Subarachnoid hemorrhage, the most common type of ICH, occurs in term infants as a result of trauma and in preterm infants as a result of hypoxia. Small hemorrhages are the most common. Bleeding is of venous origin, and underlying contusion also may occur (Whaley, Wong, 1991).

The clinical presentation of hemorrhage in the full-term infant can vary considerably. In most cases symptoms are absent, and hemorrhaging is diagnosed only because of abnormal findings on lumbar puncture (e.g., red blood cells in the cerebrospinal fluid). Occasionally the infant appears normal initially and then has seizures on the second or third day of life, followed by no apparent sequelae. In contrast, the initial clinical manifestations of neonatal subarachnoid hemorrhage may be the early onset of alternating depression and irritability, with refractory seizures (Fanaroff, Martin, 1992).

Intracerebellar hemorrhage, although infrequent, may occur in low-birth-weight infants in association with perinatal trauma and asphyxia. At present the exact causes are not fully understood. The clinical picture is characterized by severe progressive apnea, a falling hematocrit level, and death (Fanaroff, Martin, 1992).

In general, nursing care of an infant with intracranial hemorrhage is supportive and includes monitoring of ventilatory and intravenous therapy, observation and management of seizures, and prevention of increased intracranial pressure (ICP). Minimum handling to promote rest and reduce stress should guide nursing care (Whaley, Wong, 1991).

Spinal cord injuries almost always result from breech births, especially difficult ones in which version and extraction were used. Brow and face presentations, dystocia, preterm birth, maternal nulliparity, and precipitous birth also have been identified as predisposing factors in these types of injuries. Stretching of the spinal cord, usually by forceful longitudinal traction on the trunk while the head is still firmly engaged in the pelvis, is the most common mechanism of injury. This injury rarely is seen today because cesarean birth often is used for breech presentation (Fanaroff, Martin, 1992).

Clinical manifestations depend on the severity and location of the injury. High cervical cord injuries are more likely to cause stillbirths or rapid death of the neonate. Lower lesions cause an acute spinal cord syndrome. Common signs of spinal shock include flaccid extremities, diaphragmatic breathing, paralyzed abdominal movements, atonic anal sphincter, and distended bladder. Therapy is supportive and usually unsatisfactory. Infants who survive present a therapeutic challenge that requires combined treatment from many health care providers, including the pediatrician, neurologist, neurosurgeon, urologist, psychiatrist, orthopedist, nurse, physical therapist, and occupational therapist. Parents need to understand fully the implications of severe injury to the spinal cord and the overwhelming implications it presents for the family (Merenstein, Gardner, 1989; Fanaroff, Martin, 1992).

EVALUATION

The nurse can be assured that care has been effective if the goals for care have been met. That is, the newborn suffers no or only minimal sequelae of trauma and the injury receives prompt and appropriate therapy. In addition, the parents initiate and maintain a positive parent-child relationship, and the educational needs of parents and family regarding the injury and its management are met. On a long-term basis, care has been effective if no residual adverse sequelae of birth injury occur as the child grows and develops.

INFANTS OF DIABETIC MOTHERS

No single physiologic or biochemical event can explain the diverse clinical manifestations seen in the **infants of diabetic mothers (IDMs)** or **infants of gestational diabetic mothers (IGDMs).** A better understanding of maternal and fetal metabolism, resulting in stricter control of maternal diabetes and improved obstetric and neonatal intensive care, has led to a decrease in perinatal mortality in diabetic pregnancy from over 10% to under 4% in the last 25 years. Congenital anomalies are observed in IDMs two to six times more often than in the general population (Creasy, Resnik, 1989; Cherry, Merkatz, 1991). The mechanism of the process that leads to problems from conception through birth is as follows.

In early pregnancy, fluctuations in blood glucose levels and episodes of ketoacidosis are believed to cause congenital anomalies. Later in pregnancy, when the mother's pancreas cannot release sufficient insulin to meet increased demands, maternal hyperglycemia results. The high levels of glucose cross the placenta and stimulate the fetal pancreas to release insulin. The combination of the increased supply of maternal glucose and other nutrients and increased fetal insulin results in excessive fetal growth called *macrosomia*. **Hyperinsulinemia** accounts for most of the problems seen. In addition, poor diabetic control, maternal vascular involvement, or superimposed maternal infection adversely affects the fetus. *Normally, maternal blood has a more alkaline pH than does fetal blood* (with its excess of carbon dioxide). This phenomenon encourages exchange of oxygen and carbon dioxide across the placental membrane. When the maternal blood is more acidotic than the fetal blood, no carbon dioxide or oxygen exchange occurs at the level of the placenta. The mortality for the unborn baby resulting from an episode of maternal ketoacidosis may be as high as 50% or more (Fanaroff, Martin, 1992). There is some indication that some neonatal conditions—macrosomia, hypoglycemia, hypocalcemia, hyperbilirubinemia, and perhaps fetal lung immaturity—may be eliminated or the incidence decreased by maintaining control over maternal glucose levels within narrow limits (Creasy, Resnik, 1989).

Perinatal management focuses on maternal hydration-calorie-insulin balance, adequate fetal perfusion and oxygenation, and prevention of maternal stress. Fetal hypoxia and acidosis can initiate or aggravate respiratory distress syndrome (RDS). Careful assessment of labor identifies a dystotic labor early so that appropriate interventions may be implemented for a safe vaginal or abdominal birth. Infusions given to the mother that contain dextrose require insulin to minimize the risk of fetal postnatal hypoglycemia and hyperbilirubinemia (Polin, Fox, 1992).

Once the infant is born, the same management principles apply for the conditions already described and those that follow, whether they occur in the IDM or any other newborn. These conditions include macrosomia and birth trauma, congenital anomalies, hypoglycemia, hypocalcemia, lung immaturity (RDS), hyperbilirubinemia, hyperviscosity of blood, and cardiomyopathy.

ASSESSMENT

The mother's health and obstetric record is reviewed (see Chapter 11). Observation and physical examination of the newborn reveal the conditions associated with pregnancies complicated by diabetes mellitus. Appropriate laboratory tests are performed.

Macrosomia

At birth the typical LGA infant has a round, cherubic ("tomato" or cushingoid) face, chubby body, and plethoric, or flushed, complexion (Fig. 39-6). These are the characteristics of **macrosomia.** The infant has enlarged viscera (hepatosplenomegaly, splanchnomegaly, cardiomegaly) and increased body fat (Fig. 39-7). The placenta and umbilical cord are larger than average. The brain is the only organ that is not enlarged. IDMs may be LGA but physiologically immature.

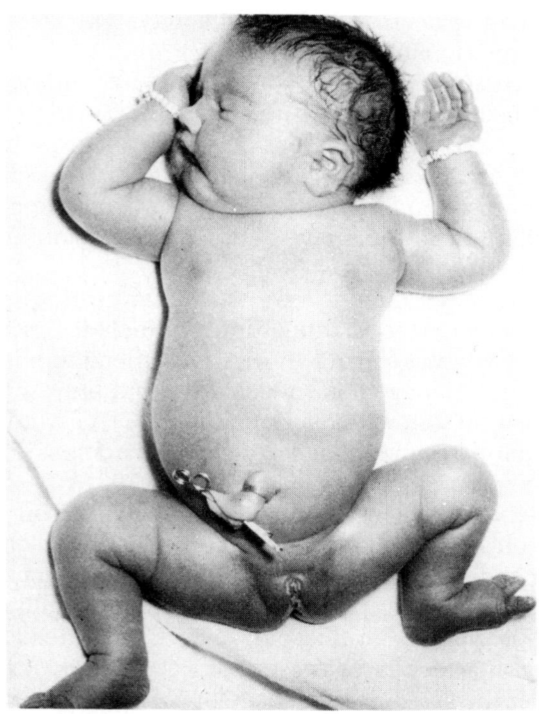

Fig. 39-6 "During their first 24 or more extrauterine hours they lie on their backs, bloated and flushed, their legs flexed and abducted, their tightly closed hands on each side of their head, the abdomen prominent and their respiration sighing. They convey a distinct impression of having had so much food and fluid pressed upon them by an insistent hostess that they desire only peace so that they may recover from their excesses."
From Shirkey HC, editor: *Pediatric therapy,* ed 6, St Louis, 1980, Mosby–Year Book, Quotation in Whaley LF, Wong DF: *Essentials of Pediatric Nursing,* ed 3, St Louis, 1989, Mosby–Year Book.

Insulin has been implicated as the primary growth hormone for intrauterine development. Maternal diabetes results in elevated maternal levels of amino acids and free fatty acids along with hyperglycemia. As the nutrients cross the placenta, the fetal pancreas responds by producing insulin to match the fuel supply. The resulting accelerated protein synthesis, together with a deposition of excessive glycogen and fat stores, is responsible for the typical macrosomic infant. This is the infant most at risk for the neonatal complications of hypoglycemia, hypocalcemia, hyperviscosity, and hyperbilirubinemia. *The excessive amounts of metabolic fuels presented to the fetus from the mother and the consequent fetal hyperinsulinism are now understood to represent the basic pathologic mechanism in the diabetic pregnancy* (Fanaroff, Martin, 1992).

Macrosomia (LGA infants) is particularly common in class A, B and C diabetic pregnancies. Clinical efforts can focus only on the control of maternal plasma glucose concentrations. With good prenatal care and control of diabetes mellitus, the incidence of macrosomia can be decreased. The excessive size of these infants can and often does lead to dystocia because of fetopelvic disproportion. These infants, who may be born vaginally or by cesarean birth after a trial of labor, may incur birth trauma.

Birth Trauma and Perinatal Asphyxia

Birth injury (resulting from macrosomia or method of birth) and perinatal asphyxia occur in 20% of IGDMs and 35% of IDMs. Examples of birth trauma include cephalhematoma; paralysis of the fa-

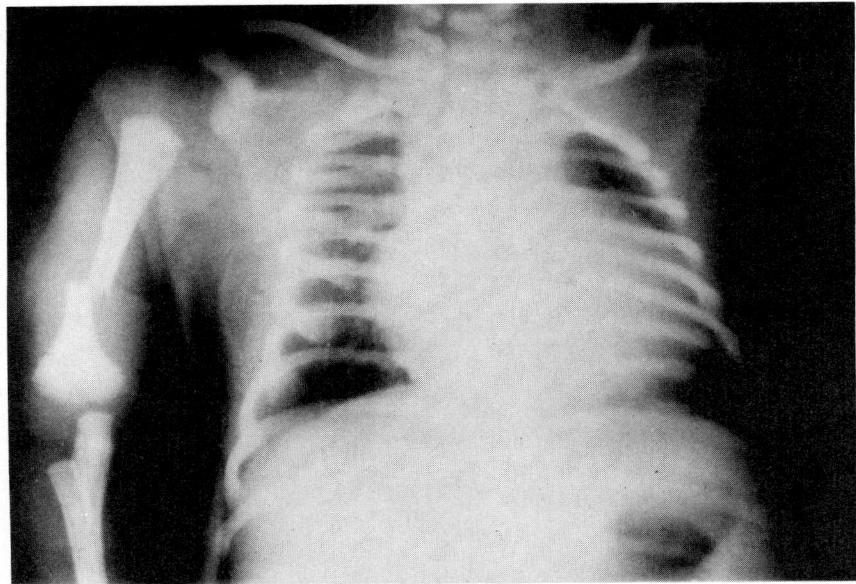

Fig. 39-7 Chest roentgenogram of a vaginally born full-term infant (4.7 kg) of a diabetic mother. The infant had cardiomegaly, hepatomegaly, congested lung fields, and fractures of the right humerus and left clavicle.
From Fanaroff AA, Martin RJ, editors: *Neonatal-perinatal medicine: diseases of the fetus and infant,* ed 5, St Louis, 1992, Mosby–Year Book.

cial nerve (seventh cranial nerve) (Fig. 39-5); fracture of the clavicle or humerus; brachial plexus paralysis, usually Erb-Duchenne (upper right arm) (Fig. 39-3) paralysis; and phrenic nerve paralysis, invariably associated with diaphragmatic paralysis.

Congenital Anomalies

Congenital anomalies occur in about 7% to 10% of IDMs. Their incidence is two to four times that for normal infants. The incidence is greatest among the small-for-gestational-age (SGA) newborns. Intrauterine growth retardation (IUGR) leading to SGA infants is seen in IDMs with severe vascular disease. The most commonly occurring anomalies involve the CNS (anencephaly, encephalocele, meningomyelocele, hydrocephalus) and caudal regression syndrome (sacral agenesis, with weakness or deformities of the lower extremities, malformation and fixation of the hip joints, and shortening or deformity of the femurs) (Fig. 39-8); tracheoesophageal fistula; and congenital heart malformations or cardiomyopathy. Hypertrichosis on the pinnae has been added to the list of characteristic clinical features (Fanaroff, Martin, 1992).

Neonatal small left colon syndrome occurs in some IDMs and IGDMs. This syndrome is suspected when failure to pass meconium, abdominal distention, and

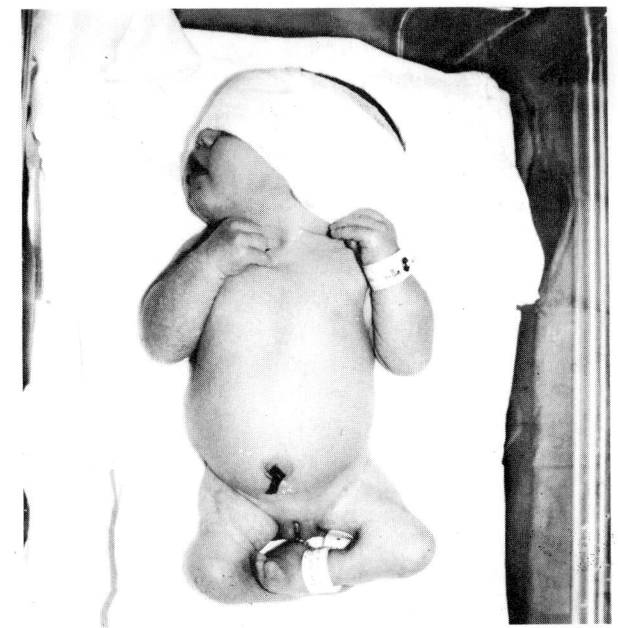

Fig. 39-8 Infant of diabetic mother with caudal regression syndrome (sacral agenesis).
From Fanaroff AA, Martin RJ, editors: *Neonatal-perinatal medicine: diseases of the fetus and infant,* ed 5, St Louis, 1992, Mosby–Year Book.

bile-stained vomitus are noted. Contrast enemas show a markedly diminished caliber of the left colon from the splenic flexure. The syndrome is transient (Fanaroff, Martin, 1992).

Cardiomyopathy

The incidence of congenital heart lesions in these infants is five times higher than in the general population. Other lesions include transposition of the aorta and pulmonary artery, ventricular septal defects, and coarctation of the aorta. Maternal diabetic control is correlated with the incidence of lesions. Poor control is defined as maternal blood glucose greater than 300 mg/dL, with glycosuria, ketonuria, or occasional ketoacidosis. Good control is defined as the maintenance of maternal blood glucose between 100 and 120 mg/dL. Careful diabetic management, especially in the second and third trimesters, decreases the severity of these lesions.

All IDMs need careful observation for **cardiomyopathy;** 30% to 50% of IDMs have cardiomegaly or congestive heart failure within 7 days of birth. Two types of cardiomyopathy can occur. Thus clinicians must be alert to correctly identify the type of lesion so that appropriate therapy is instituted. Both types are associated with respiratory symptoms and congestive heart failure.

Hypertrophic cardiomyopathy (HCM) is characterized by a hypercontractile and thickened myocardium. The ventricles are decreased in size, and the mitral valve is poorly functioning, which results in an outflow tract obstruction. In *nonhypertrophic cardiomyopathy (non-HCM)* the myocardium is poorly contractile and overstretched. The ventricles are increased in size, and there is no outflow obstruction. HCM is treated with a β-adrenergic blocker (such as propranolol to decrease contractility and heart rate). A cardiotonic is used to treat non-HCM (e.g., digoxin to increase contractility and decrease heart rate). The abnormality usually resolves in 3 to 12 months (Fanaroff, Martin, 1992).

Hypoglycemia and Hypocalcemia

In hypoglycemia and hypocalcemia, separation of the placenta suddenly interrupts the constant infusion of glucose. The high level of circulating glucose at the time the umbilical cord is severed falls rapidly in the presence of fetal hyperinsulinism. *Asymptomatic* or symptomatic hypoglycemia occurs within the first 1 to 3 hours after birth. Hypocalcemia occurs in 30% of IDMs. In addition, hypocalcemia is associated with preterm birth, birth trauma, and perinatal asphyxia. Symptoms of hypocalcemia, a prevalent finding in IDMs and IGDMs, are similar to those of hypoglycemia, but they occur between 24 and 36 hours of age. However, hypocalcemia must be considered if therapy for hypoglycemia is ineffective.

Respiratory Difficulty

IDMs or IGDMs manifest a greater incidence of RDS than is found in normal infants of comparable gestational age. Synthesis of surfactant may be delayed because of the high fetal serum level of insulin (Philip, 1987). Fetal lung maturity, as evidenced by a *lecithin/sphingomyelin (L/S) ratio of 2 to 1, is not reassuring if the mother has diabetes mellitus or gestation-induced diabetes mellitus*. For the infants of such mothers, an L/S ratio of 3:1 or more, or the presence of **phosphatidylglycerol** in the amniotic fluid, is more indicative of adequate lung maturity.

Respiratory distress without RDS also occurs. Transient tachypnea or "wet lung" syndrome is a cause of respiratory distress (Fanaroff, Martin, 1992).

Hyperbilirubinemia

Hyperbilirubinemia develops in 50% of newborns of 32 to 34 weeks' gestation, and 15% of infants born at 37 weeks' gestation manifest this condition. Many newborns are plethoric because of polycythemia. *Polycythemia* increases blood viscosity, thereby impairing circulation. In addition, this increased number of red blood cells to be hemolyzed increases the potential bilirubin load that the newborn must clear. The excessive red blood cells are produced in extramedullary foci (liver and spleen) in addition to the usual sites in bone marrow. Therefore both liver function and bilirubin clearance may be adversely affected.

NURSING DIAGNOSES

Following are examples of nursing diagnoses.

NEWBORN

- High risk for injury related to
  - —Metabolic effects of maternal condition
  - —Hypoglycemia, hypocalcemia, hyperbilirubinemia, hyperviscosity of blood
  - —Birth trauma
- High risk for ineffective gas exchange related to
  - —Lung immaturity
  - —Cardiomyopathy
- Ineffective thermoregulation related to
  - —Physiologic immaturity

PARENTS/FAMILY

- Anxiety, fear, or powerlessness related to
  —Uncertainty regarding neonate's prognosis
- Self-esteem disturbance related to
  —Experience of an "abnormal" pregnancy and compromised neonate
- Anxiety related to knowledge deficit regarding
  —Neonate's condition, management, and prognosis

PLANNING

Ideally, planning for the IDM begins during the antenatal period. Pediatric staff members are present at the birth. For each child an individualized plan of care is developed. *Goals* for the newborn may include the following:

1. The newborn will experience a birth without trauma or injury.
2. The newborn will experience a neonatal period without sequelae of trauma or pregnancy complicated by maternal diabetes mellitus.

Goals for the family may include:

1. The family will understand diabetes mellitus or the birth injury.
2. The family will willingly comply with management.
3. If the newborn exhibits a disorder or dies, the family initiates the grieving process.

IMPLEMENTATION

Implementation of care depends on the neonate's particular problems. General care of the compromised newborn is addressed in Chapter 36. If the maternal blood glucose level was well controlled throughout the pregnancy, the infant may require only monitoring. Because euglycemia is not always possible, the nurse must promptly recognize and treat any consequences of maternal diabetes that arise. The most common problems IDMs experience that require intervention include birth trauma and perinatal asphyxia (p. 1139), respiratory distress syndrome (p. 1136), difficult metabolic transition, including hypoglycemia and hypocalcemia (p. 1142), as well as congenital anomalies (p. 1156). (See case study below , and nursing plan of care, p. 1190, for IDMs.)

CASE STUDY

Infant of a Gestational Diabetic Mother

Jason, born at 38 weeks' gestation by elective cesarean, is the first child for Judy Miller. Jason weighed 8 lb 10 oz (4763 g) at his birth 30 minutes ago. Judy's gestational diabetes mellitus was only moderately well controlled.

ASSESSMENT

A review of the prenatal record revealed that amniocentesis yielded an L/S ratio of 3:1, with the presence of phosphatidylglycerol. Results from the initial physical examination included the following: Apgar scores of 8 at 1 minute and 9 at 5 minutes of age; LGA; no apparent congenital anomalies or birth trauma; and no meconium aspiration (amniotic fluid clear; skin, nails, and cord clear). Currently, Jason is under a radiant warmer with a thermistor probe attached. The parents have many questions. Jason starts to gag.

NURSING DIAGNOSIS

Assessment findings suggest that several diagnoses are possible. One takes priority: altered breathing pattern related to secretions in airway after cesarean birth.

PLANNING

Planning of interventions is based on current knowledge of the effects of maternal gestational diabetes and cesarean birth on the fetus and neonate. The goal for care is identified: infant will maintain an open airway and show no signs of respiratory distress.

IMPLEMENTATION

Resuscitation and oxygen administration equipment is available and within easy reach. Jason was under an overhead radiant heat panel with a thermistor probe. He was positioned on his side. The nurse suctioned his mouth and nose for clear fluid. He responded with a clear lusty cry; breath sounds remain clear and there are no signs of respiratory distress. The nurse continues to care for Jason as if he were a preterm neonate despite his large size and weight, until his respiratory maturity is well established.

EVALUATION

The nurse can be reasonably assured that care has been effective when Jason cried lustily and demonstrated no signs of respiratory distress; breath sounds remained clear.

CARE PLAN **Infant of a Gestational Diabetic Mother**

GOALS	IMPLEMENTATION	RATIONALE	EVALUATION
Nursing diagnosis: Altered breathing pattern related to secretions in airway after cesarean birth			
Jason will maintain open airway and show no signs of respiratory distress.	Ensure availability of resuscitation and oxygen equipment.	Saves time in event of respiratory distress.	Jason maintains an open airway, and respiratory distress is prevented.
	Regard infant as preterm regardless of birth weight/size until gestational age and respiratory maturity are established.	Lung maturity is delayed if pregnancy is complicated by diabetes.	
	Monitor closely for signs of respiratory distress, per hospital protocol.	Early identification is necessary for timely intervention.	
	Maintain body temperature; prevent cold stress.	Cold stress can result in respiratory distress.	
	Position Jason on side, with head slightly lower and neck slightly extended.	Facilitates mucus drainage and prevents aspiration of mucus from nasopharynx.	
	Suction mouth and nose as needed.		
Nursing diagnosis: High risk for injury related to hypoglycemia/hypocalcemia secondary to maternal gestational diabetes			
Jason will maintain acceptable blood glucose levels and remain free from signs of hypoglycemia/hypocalcemia.	Assess for blood glucose levels per hospital protocol; for a term infant, levels of 35 mg/dL are within normal limits for first 3 days.	Jason's hyperinsulinism can lead rapidly to hypoglycemia after birth when maternal supply through the placenta stops.	Jason's blood glucose remained well above 35 mg/dL at each testing.
	Observe for and report signs of hypoglycemia.	Hypoglycemia can result in brain damage.	Jason did not show any signs of hypoglycemia.
	If suck/swallow reflexes are intact, feed per hospital protocol.	Maintains blood glucose within normal limits; prevents aspiration.	
	Assess for hypocalcemia if therapy for hypoglycemia is ineffective (e.g., nervousness continues despite adequate blood glucose level).	Hypocalcemia jeopardizes neonatal well-being; e.g., edema, apnea, intermittent cyanosis, abdominal distention and tetany can occur.	Jason had no episodes of hypocalcemia.

EVALUATION

The nurse can be assured that care has been effective if the goals of care are achieved. That is, the newborn has a birth without trauma or injury and a neonatal period without sequelae of trauma or pregnancy complicated by maternal diabetes; the family has an understanding of diabetes or any birth injury and they willingly comply with management; and if the newborn exhibits a disorder or dies, the family initiates the grieving process.

■ NEONATAL INFECTIONS

Sepsis (presence of microorganisms or their toxins in the blood or other tissues) continues to be one of the most significant causes of neonatal morbidity and mortality. The newborn infant is uniquely susceptible to infection. Maternal immunoglobulin (Ig) M does not cross the placenta. IgA and IgM require time to reach optimum levels after birth. Phagocytosis is less efficient. Serum complement levels are inadequate. Serum complement (C1 through C6) is in-

CARE PLAN Infant of a Gestational Diabetic Mother—cont'd

GOALS	IMPLEMENTATION	RATIONALE	EVALUATION
Nursing diagnosis: Anxiety (grieving, powerlessness, situational low self-esteem, spiritual distress, ineffective individual or family coping, altered family processes) related to having a newborn with a disorder or a potential disorder			
Parents will verbalize understanding of effects of maternal diabetes on their child's well-being. Parents will verbalize feelings and concerns regarding their infant.	Explain effects of maternal diabetic condition on newborn. Explain all procedures to parents. Answer questions and correct misconceptions. Encourage open communication. Demonstrate child care activities. Observe parent-infant interactions. Schedule appointments for laboratory studies and follow-up physical examination. Refer to outside resources (child care, homemaker, clergy, home health).	Knowledge relieves fear of the unknown and supports coping and self-esteem. Encouraging and answering questions demonstrates respect and understanding for parents. Fosters parent-infant bonding/attachment.	Parents verbalize understanding of instructions. Parents express feelings and concerns about their infant. Parents learn how to care for their child. Parents express love for infant, call him by name, and participate in his care.

volved in immunologic reactions, some of which kill or lyse bacteria and enhance phagocytosis. Dysmaturity seen with IUGR and preterm and postterm birth further compromises the neonate's immune system. Special precautions for preventing infection, as well as prompt recognition when it occurs, are necessary for optimum management of newborn care. Newborn infections may be acquired in utero, during birth, during resuscitation, and nosocomially (Fanaroff, Martin, 1992).

Prenatal acquisition occurs by organisms placentally transferred directly into the fetal circulatory system and from infected amniotic fluid (e.g., herpes simplex virus [HSV], cytomegalovirus [CMV], rubella). Microorganisms ascend from the vagina and pass through the cervix. The membranes become infected and possibly rupture. Infection of the fetal skin and respiratory or gastrointestinal tract may result.

During birth, contact with an infected birth canal can result in generalized or local infection. The upper airway and gastrointestinal tract are again the principal pathways for generalized infections. The conjunctiva and oral cavity are the usual sites of local infection.

Postnatal infection may be acquired during resuscitation, usually from contamination of indwelling catheters or endotracheal tubes. Nursery-acquired infections may be transferred to the infant by hands of personnel or spread from contaminated equipment. The umbilicus is a receptive site for cutaneous infection leading to sepsis (Fanaroff, Martin, 1992).

Certain pathogens may cause abortion, stillbirth, intrauterine infection, congenital malformations, and acute disease. These pathogens also may cause chronic infection, with subtle manifestations that may be recognized only after a prolonged period. It is important to recognize the manifestations of infections in the neonatal period—not only to treat the acute infection and to prevent nosocomial infections in other infants but also to anticipate effects on the subsequent growth and development of the infant.

Septicemia refers to a generalized infection in the blood stream. Septicemia, a common type of sepsis, affects between 1/500 to 1/1600 newborns. Pneumonia, the most common form of neonatal infection, is one of the leading causes of perinatal death (Fanaroff, Martin, 1992). Bacterial meningitis affects one in 2500 live-born infants. Gastroenteritis is sporadic, depending on epidemic outbreaks. Local infections such as conjunctivitis and omphalitis occur commonly, but incidence rates are unavailable. (Incidence rates of specific infections are given in the text when available.) Infection continues to be a significant factor in fetal and neonatal morbidity and mortality.

ASSESSMENT

The *prenatal record* is reviewed for risk factors associated with and signs and symptoms suggestive of infection. Maternal vaginal or perineal infection may be transmitted directly to the infant during passage through the birth canal. Psychosocial history and history of sexually transmitted diseases (STDs) may strongly suggest possible human immunodeficiency virus (HIV), hepatitis B, or CMV infection.

The *perinatal events* also are reviewed. Premature rupture of membranes (PROM) may be caused by maternal or intrauterine infection (see Research Highlight below). Ascending infection may occur after prolonged rupture of membranes, prolonged labor, or intrauterine fetal monitoring. Resuscitation that requires intubation and deep suctioning may result in infection. The newborn's gestational age, maturity, birth weight, and gender all affect the incidence of infection. Sepsis occurs about twice as often and results in a higher mortality rate in male than in female infants. The newborn is assessed for skin abscesses, rashes, cellulitis, and other indications of infection.

During the *postnatal period* the time of onset of suspicious signs is noted. Onset within the first 48 hours of life is more commonly associated with prenatal or perinatal predisposing factors. Onset after 2 or 3 days more commonly reflects disease acquired at or subsequent to birth (Fanaroff, Martin, 1992).

The earliest clinical signs of neonatal sepsis are characterized by a lack of specificity. The nonspecific signs include lethargy, poor feeding, poor weight gain, or irritability. Or the nurse or parent may simply note that the infant is just not doing as well as before. Differential diagnosis may be difficult because signs of sepsis are similar to signs of noninfectious neonatal problems such as anemia or hypoglycemia. Additional clinical and laboratory information and appropriate cultures supplement the findings described.

Primary or secondary involvement of any organ system adds to the clinical signs. Hypothermia is as

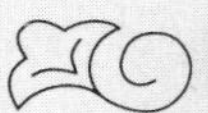 **Research Highlight** 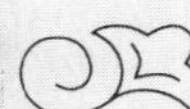

Premature Rupture of Membranes and Sepsis in Preterm Neonates

RESEARCH ABSTRACT

The purpose of this study was to determine whether PROM was associated with sepsis in preterm infants; 507 preterm singleton infants, born alive from pregnancies in which PROM had occurred, were matched with preterm infants in which PROM had not occurred. The variables for which the infants were matched were gestational age, ethnicity, gender, and date of birth. The authors used data from medical records. They matched pairs of infants: one with PROM and one not exposed to PROM. The researchers found that more infants exposed to PROM had sepsis and infection than did infants unexposed to PROM. PROM was not associated with neonatal mortality. When the PROM occurred more than 48 hours before birth, the infants were more likely to have sepsis and infection. The most important factors in decreasing risk of infection in PROM births was a birth weight of more than 1500 g and gestation of more than 33 weeks.

IMPLICATIONS FOR PRACTICE

PROM poses a significant risk of infection for preterm infants. Neonates born after PROM merit close observation for signs of infection and sepsis. Because mortality rates did not increase when membranes had been ruptured longer than 48 hours, preterm birth should be delayed until gestation is greater than 33 weeks and the infant weighs more than 1500 g. Frequent assessment of neonates born after PROM is essential.

RELATED RESEARCH QUESTIONS

1. What factors in addition to PROM are associated with sepsis?
2. What are responses of parents to PROM?
3. What are responses of parents to the decision to delay birth after PROM?
4. How accurate are nurses in their detection of signs of infection in neonates?

REFERENCE

Levine CD: Premature rupture of the membranes and sepsis in preterm infants, *Nurs Res* 40:36, Jan/Feb 1991.

common as hyperthermia (fever) in response to infection. Tachypnea or apnea, cyanosis, tachycardia or bradycardia, and hypotension may be noted. Focal neurologic signs, tremors, seizures, or a full (bulging) fontanelle are seen in septic newborns even without meningitis. Other signs may be vomiting, abdominal distention, diarrhea, jaundice, pallor, or petechia. Necrotizing enterocolitis may develop (p. 1139). Jaundice occurs within the first 24 hours in the absence of hemolytic disease. Hemorrhage may be an associated sign in sepsis, which may be preceded or accompanied by focal infections such as omphalitis or conjunctivitis or by skin abscesses.

Laboratory studies are performed. Specimens for cultures include samples of blood, umbilical cord stump, nasopharynx or oropharynx, ear canals, skin, cerebrospinal fluid (CSF), stool, and urine. Increased direct (conjugated) bilirubin levels may be found, especially if the infecting microorganism is gram negative. Complete blood cell count with differential is performed to determine the presence of anemia, increased white blood cell count, or decreased red blood cell count (an ominous sign). C-reactive protein may or may not be elevated.

Vigilant assessment (e.g., parenteral fluid infusion) continues during and after treatment. The newborn continues to be assessed for sequelae to septicemia. Before the advent of antibiotics, 90% of newborns with sepsis died. Antibiotic therapy decreased mortality to between 13% and 45% depending on the causative organism.

Sequelae to septicemia include meningitis, pyarthrosis, and septic shock. **Meningitis,** a common sequela, may be evidenced by a bulging anterior fontanelle (see discussion of signs of increased intracranial pressure, p. 1184). Systemic antibiotics may not diffuse into CSF. Intrathecal (within the subarachnoid space) infusion of a drug such as polymyxin may be initiated.

Pyarthrosis, which may affect any joint, usually localizes in the hips. Limitation in joint movement is one of the few signs of this condition.

Septic shock results from the toxins released into the blood stream. The most common sign is a drop in blood pressure—a vital sign commonly overlooked in the care of the newborn. Other signs are rapid, irregular respirations and pulse (similar to septicemia in general).

NURSING DIAGNOSES

Any number of nursing diagnoses are possible, depending on the infant's gestational age and birth weight, the organ systems involved, and the nature of the infection. Following are examples of nursing diagnoses.

NEWBORN

- High risk for infection related to
  - —Need for resuscitation or inhalation therapy
  - —Need for indwelling umbilical catheters, total parenteral nutrition (TPN), parenteral fluids
  - —Intrauterine electronic fetal monitoring
  - —Male gender
  - —Dysmaturity, IUGR, gestational age
- Ineffective thermoregulation related to
  - —Infection
- Impaired tissue integrity related to
  - —Need for multiple supportive measures (e.g., biometric monitoring, TPN, inhalation therapy)
- Pain related to
  - —Need for multiple supportive measures

PARENTS/FAMILY

- Anxiety, fear, or anticipatory grieving related to
  - —Uncertainty about child's prognosis
- High risk for altered parenting related to
  - —Separation of parent and child
  - —Feelings of inadequacy in caring for the child
  - —Inability to breast-feed
- Powerlessness or spiritual distress related to
  - —Perinatal events or newborn infant's condition
- Anxiety related to knowledge deficit regarding
  - —Newborn's condition, its course, and management

PLANNING

Planning begins with the development of standards for preventive measures in nurseries and protocols for diagnosis and treatment of infections. Individual assessment findings are utilized to plan care for each infant. Parents and family are encouraged to participate in planning. *Goals* include the following.

1. The newborn remains free of sepsis.
2. The newborn's early signs of sepsis are recognized, and appropriate therapy is instituted.
3. If therapy is necessary, the newborn suffers no harmful sequelae.
4. Parents begin bonding and attachment to newborn.
5. Parents maintain self-esteem.
6. Staff members establish caring relationship with parents to foster their trust and to encourage continuing, active, positive interactions of family with members of health care system.

IMPLEMENTATION

Preventive Measures

Virtually all controlled clinical trials have demonstrated that effective hand washing is responsible for the prevention of nosocomial infection in nursery units (Fanaroff, Martin, 1992). Nursing is directly or indirectly responsible for minimizing or eliminating environmental sources of infectious agents in the nursery. Measures to be taken include universal precautions (see Chapter 29), careful and thorough cleaning, frequent replacement of used equipment (e.g., changing intravenous tubing per hospital protocol, cleaning resuscitation and ventilation equipment), and disposal of excrement and linens in an appropriate manner. Overcrowding must be avoided in nurseries.

The skin, its secretions, and normal flora are natural defenses that protect against invading pathogens. The American Academy of Pediatrics suggests that the risks and benefits of different skin care techniques be evaluated for the effect each technique has on the skin, whether the cleansing agent is absorbed or is toxic, and if the agent changes the skin flora and may promote infectious problems. Initial cleansing is delayed until the newborn's temperature has stabilized. Sterile cotton sponges (not gauze) soaked with warm water may be used to remove blood and meconium from the neonate's face, head, and body. A mild nonmedicated soap (in single-use container or in a small bar reserved for a single newborn) can be used with careful water rinsing. The vernix caseosa is left in place. No single method of cord care has been shown to prevent colonization and subsequent disease. Alcohol, triple dye, or an antimicrobial agent is applied locally (Frigoletto, Little, 1988).

Curative Measures

Breast-feeding or feeding the newborn breast milk from the mother is encouraged. Protective mechanisms exist in breast milk. Colostrum contains agglutinins that are active against gram-negative bacteria. Human milk contains iron-binding protein that exerts a bacteriostatic effect on *Escherichia coli*. Human milk also contains macrophages and lymphocytes. The vulnerability of infants to common mucosal pathogens such as respiratory syncytial virus may be reduced by passive transfer of maternal immunity in colostrum and breast milk. (See discussion of necrotizing enterocolitis, p. 1139; also see Chapter 22 for assisting mothers with breast-feeding, maintenance of lactation until the newborn can breast-feed, and expression and storage of breast milk.)

The mother's knowledge of the importance of her breast milk for the compromised newborn and her active involvement in this aspect of care benefit her in several ways. Bonding with the infant is facilitated. Self-concept and self-esteem are enhanced. Coping skills may be strengthened. If the infant dies, the mother's healthy grieving may be facilitated. If the mother cannot breast-feed or provide breast milk, the nurse provides support during the mother's formula-feeding or other activity with the infant. The parents' activity with the infant is supported and appropriately guided and praised to achieve the benefits desired.

Emphasis is placed on following reliable surveillance to identify infection in newborns so that prompt isolation and appropriate therapy are instituted.

Eye and umbilical cord prophylaxis is discussed in Chapter 21. Monitoring intravenous infusion rate and administering antibiotics are the nurse's responsibility. It is important to administer the prescribed dose of antibiotic within 1 hour after it is prepared to avoid loss of drug stability. If the intravenous fluid the infant is receiving contains electrolytes, vitamins, or other medications, the nurse should check with the hospital pharmacy before adding antibiotics. The antibiotic (or other medication) may be deactivated or may form a precipitate. Instead, a piggyback solution of the prescribed fluid is attached with a three-way stopcock to the needle at the infusion site. The nurse should remember to include the number of milliliters of fluid used from the piggyback bottle when calculating the newborn's intake.

Care must be taken in suctioning secretions from the newborn's oropharynx or trachea. These secretions may be infected. Mouth suction–activated devices other than new Delee device (Fig. 21-4) should never be used. Although no cases of virus transmission via this route have been documented, enough concern exists to make it seem prudent to use wall or bulb suction devices.

Isolation procedures are implemented according to hospital policy as indicated. Isolation protocols are changing rapidly, and the nurse is urged to participate in continuing education and in-service programs to remain up-to-date.

Rehabilitative Measures

Rehabilitative measures vary with the individual needs of the neonate. Some newborns will need to be weaned from ventilatory support systems. Those who suffer sequelae such as mental retardation and epilepsy will require a knowledgeable family and supportive community resources. Other children will require corrective care for problems with dentition, vision, and hearing.

EVALUATION

The nurse can be reasonably assured that care was effective if the goals for care are achieved.

- The newborn remains free of sepsis.
- The newborn's early signs of sepsis are recognized and appropriately treated.
- If therapy is necessary, the newborn suffers no harmful sequelae.
- Parents begin bonding and attachment to newborn and maintain self-esteem.
- Staff members establish caring relationship with parents to foster their trust and to encourage continuing, active, positive interactions of family with members of health care system.

TORCH Infections

The occurrence of certain maternal infections during early pregnancy is well known to be associated with various congenital malformations and disorders (see Chapter 29 and 38). The most common and best understood infections are represented by the acronym **TORCH,** for *t*oxoplasmosis, *o*ther, *r*ubella virus, *c*ytomegalovirus, and *h*erpes simplex (see box below). Herpes simplex may result in a severe, often fatal systemic illness in newborns. Survivors of herpetic infection may have residual neurologic defects and chorioretinitis. The other congenital infections also may result in an encephalopathy with various anomalies, including microcephaly, chorioretinitis, intracranial calcifications, microphthalmos, and cataracts. To a certain extent the varied clinical manifestations of these infections overlap, but a specific diagnosis can be made by the constellation of clinical findings, as well as specific antibody studies (Fanaroff, Martin, 1992).

TORCH Infections Affecting Newborns

T Toxoplasmosis
O Other: syphilis, varicella, group B β-hemolytic streptococcus, chlamydial infections, hepatitis B, HIV
R Rubella
C CMV infections or cytomegalic inclusion disease (CMID)
H Herpes simplex

TOXOPLASMOSIS. Toxoplasmosis is a multisystem disease caused by the protozoan *Toxoplasma gondii.* Cats who hunt infected birds and mice harbor the parasite and excrete the infective oocysts in their feces. Human infection follows hand-to-mouth contact, such as after disposal of cat litter or after handling or ingesting raw meat from cattle or sheep that grazed in contaminated fields.

About 30% of women who contract toxoplasmosis during gestation transmit the disease to their offspring. The mother often has no symptoms. The diagnosis of toxoplasmosis in the newborn is supported by elevated levels of cord blood serum IgM.

More than 70% of affected newborns are free of symptoms. The clinical features of toxoplasmosis resemble cytomegalic inclusion disease in mother and infant. Both diseases are responsible for serious perinatal mortality and morbidity: 10% to 15% die; 85% have severe psychomotor problems or mental retardation by 2 to 4 years; and 50% have visual problems by 1 year.

Severe toxoplasmosis is associated with preterm birth, growth retardation, microcephaly or hydrocephaly, microphthalmos, chorioretinitis, CNS calcification, thrombocytopenia, jaundice, and fever. Some clinical manifestations do not develop until later in life.

Treatment of toxoplasmosis during pregnancy is problematic. Pyrimethamine is the first-choice drug against *T. gondii*. However, it may be teratogenic, especially during the first trimester (Fanaroff, Martin, 1992). Sulfonamide therapy is effective, but the drug must be discontinued before birth and even-exchange transfusion of the newborn may be necessary to avoid kernicterus. This may occur because sulfa drugs have a greater albumin-binding affinity than does bilirubin, which may rise after birth to critical levels. The newborn may be treated with pyrimethamine, as well as oral sulfadiazine, but folinic acid supplement will be required to prevent anemia. Regrettably, encysted (intramuscular) forms of *T. gondii* cannot be eradicated by any therapy and they may cause recurrence of the disease.

HEPATITIS B VIRUS INFECTION. Hepatitis B virus (HBV), the most common etiologic agent of viral hepatitis, is implicated in 24% to 40% of cases. HBV infection during pregnancy is *not* associated with an increase in malformations, stillbirths, or IUGR; however, there is about a 32% increase in risk for preterm birth (Fanaroff, Martin, 1992). The transmission rate of HBV to the newborn is as high as 90% (Hodson, Truog, 1989). Transmission occurs transplacentally, serum to serum, and by contact with contaminated urine, feces, saliva, semen, or vaginal secretions during birth. Infants are most commonly infected during birth or in the first few days of life. The rate of transmission is highest when the mother contracts the virus immediately before birth. Transmission may possibly occur through breast milk, but antigens also develop in formula-fed infants at the same or higher rate. Diagnosis is made by viral culture of amniotic fluid, as well as the presence of hepatitis B surface antigen and IgM in the cord or baby's serum.

Neonatal and fetal effects are serious. Preterm birth exposes the neonate to the problems of prematurity. Infants may be symptom-free at birth or show evidence of acute hepatitis with changes in liver function. Infants are at high risk for chronic hepatitis, cirrhosis of the liver, or liver cancer even years later (Fanaroff, Martin, 1992).

Infants whose mothers have antibodies for hepatitis B surface antigen (HBsAg) or who have developed hepatitis during pregnancy or the postpartum period should be treated with hepatitis B immune globulin (HBIG), 0.5 mL intramuscularly, as soon as possible after birth—within the first 12 hours of life. Concurrently, but at a different site, the vaccine also should be given (Fanaroff, Martin, 1992). The second dose of vaccine is given at 1 month, and the third dose is given at 6 months. The vaccine should protect the child for up to 9 years. After the newborn has been cleansed thoroughly and has received the vaccine, breast-feeding may be allowed.

The Public Health Service defines women at high risk for hepatitis B as those who are Indochinese refugees, of Asian descent, or born in Haiti or South Africa; women with a history of liver disease; women who have occupational exposure to the HBV, such as laboratory technologists, nurses, and physicians; and women who work with mentally retarded individuals. Intravenous drug abusers, prostitutes, and household contacts of hepatitis B carriers also are at high risk (Merenstein, Gardner, 1989).

Studies of universal screening for hepatitis B infection in pregnant women indicate that 0.8% of women in the United States have HBsAg antibodies in pregnancy. Fewer than 50% of these women have risk factors for hepatitis B infection. Several analyses have demonstrated the cost effectiveness of universal screening, and in 1988 the Centers for Disease Control (CDC) recommended that all pregnant women be screened for HBsAg at an early prenatal visit (Fanaroff, Martin, 1992).

SYPHILIS. Congenital and neonatal syphilis has reemerged in recent years as a significant health problem.

Fetal infestation with the spirochete *Treponema pallidum* is blocked by Langhans' layer in the chorion until this layer begins to atrophy between 16 and 18 weeks' gestation. If spirochetemia is untreated, it will result in fetal death by midtrimester abortion or stillbirth in one of four cases. All newborns in whom the infection occurs before 7 months' gestation are affected. Only 60% are affected if the infection occurs late in pregnancy. If maternal infection is treated adequately before the eighteenth week, newborns seldom demonstrate signs of the disease. Although treatment after the eighteenth week may cure fetal spirochetemia, pathologic changes may not be prevented completely.

Because the fetus becomes infected after the period of organogenesis (first trimester), maldevelopment of organs does not result. Congenital syphilis may stimulate preterm labor, but there is no evidence that it causes IUGR. Stigmas of congenital syphilis (Fig. 39-9) may include inflammatory and destructive changes in the placenta; in organs such as the liver, spleen, kidneys, adrenal glands; and in bone covering and marrow. Disorders of the CNS, teeth, and cornea may not become evident until several months after birth.

ASSESSMENT. The most severely affected newborns may be ***hydropic*** (edematous) and ***anemic,*** with enlarged liver and spleen. Hepatosplenomegaly probably is the result of extramedullary hematopoietic activity stimulated by the severe anemia.

In some cases signs of congenital syphilis do not appear until late in the neonatal period. In these newborns early signs, such as poor feeding, slight hyperthermia, and snuffles, may be nonspecific. ***Snuffles*** refers to the copious clear serosanguineous mucous discharge from the obstructed nose. A mucopurulent discharge indicates secondary infection, usually by streptococci or staphylococci.

By the end of the first week of life, in untreated cases a copper-colored maculopapular ***dermal rash*** appears. The rash is characteristically first noticeable on the palms of the hands, soles of the feet, the diaper area, and around the mouth and anus. The maculopapular lesions may become vesicular and confluent and extend over the trunk and extremities. ***Condylomas*** (elevated wartlike lesions) may be seen around the anus. Rough, cracked mucocutaneous lesions of the lips heal to form circumoral radiating scars known as ***rhagades.***

Other involvement results in exfoliation (separation, flaking) of nails and loss of hair. Iritis and choroiditis are characteristic of infection of the eyes.

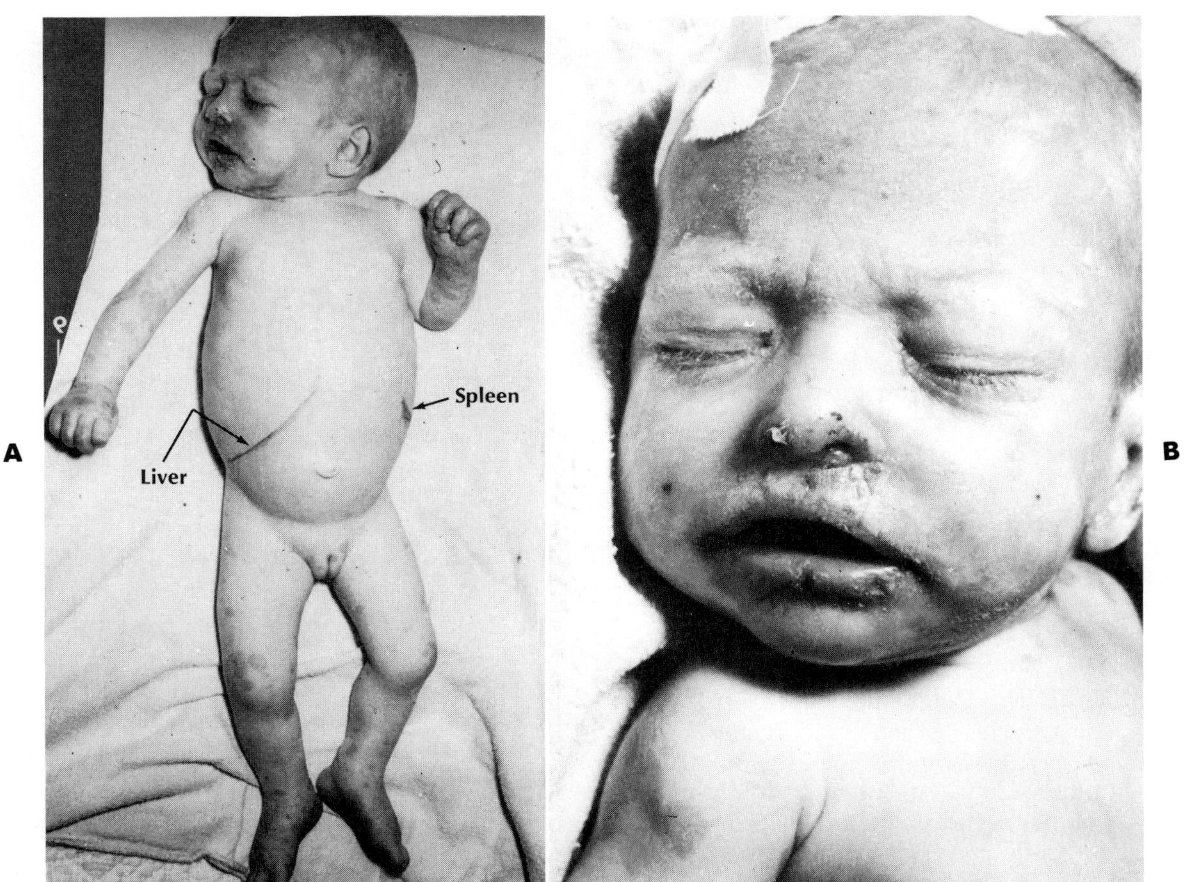

Fig. 39-9 Early congenital syphilis apparent at birth, which corresponds to secondary syphilis in the adult. (Late congenital syphilis, corresponding to tertiary syphilis, becomes apparent after 2 years of age.) **A,** Cutaneous lesions of congenital syphilis. Lines drawn on body indicate hepatosplenomegaly. No destruction of bridge of nose (common finding in congenital syphilis) is noted on this infant. **B,** Rhinitis (snuffles) resulting in rhagades and excoriation of upper lip. Red-colored rash is around mouth and on chin.
From Shirkey HC, editor: *Pediatric therapy,* ed 6, St Louis, 1980, Mosby–Year Book.

Nephrotic syndrome secondary to renal infection; hepatitis with ***jaundice,*** lymphadenopathy, inflammation of the pancreas, testes, and colon; and a pseudoparalysis of the extremities may be noted. Laboratory tests may show a pleocytosis (usually lymphocytosis) and elevated CSF protein levels.

By 3 months of age, in 90% of infants (treated or untreated), periostitis and metaphyseal osteochondritis may be demonstrated by roentgenographic studies. These bone lesions generally disappear by 10 months of age whether or not the infant receives antibiotic treatment.

After the physician determines that congenital syphilis is possible, the CSF (obtained by lumbar puncture) is examined by means of the fluorescent treponemal antibody absorption (FTA-ABS) test (see Chapter 29). If results are inconclusive, the physician probably will opt to treat the child as if the disease existed.

MEDICAL MANAGEMENT. If the mother had been adequately treated before giving birth and serologic testing of the newborn does not show syphilis, generally the newborn is not treated with antibiotics. In this case the newborn is checked for antibody titer (received from the mother via the placenta) every 2 weeks for 3 months, at which time the test result should be negative. Some physicians recommended antibiotic therapy for asymptomatic or inconclusive cases.

For antibiotic treatment to be effective, an "adequate" blood level must be maintained for an "adequate" period of time. Suggested medication protocol in the presence of symptomatic systemic disease differs from author to author and from physician to physician. After 12 hours of antibiotic therapy, the child's condition is not considered contagious. It generally is accepted that erythromycin is the substitute antibiotic of choice for newborns sensitive to penicillin.

PROGNOSIS AND SEQUELAE. In general, treatment of syphilis is more effective if it is begun early rather than late in the course of the disease. However, a recurrence rate of 5% can be expected. Even adequate treatment of congenital syphilis after birth does not always prevent late (5 to 15 years after initial infection) complications. Potential complications include neurosyphilis, deafness, Hutchinson's teeth (notched incisors), saber shins, joint involvement, saddle nose (depressed bridge), gummas (soft, gummy tumors) over the skin and other organs, and interstitial keratitis (inflammation of the cornea). The failure of therapy with the persistence of spirochetes in the eyes is not unusual. Antibiotics penetrate ocular tissue poorly. Congenital syphilis during early childhood rarely causes death.

RUBELLA INFECTION. Congenital rubella infection is a major concern. The last epidemic in the United States occurred in 1964 and 1965. Of the 30,000 affected pregnancies, 20,000 resulted in infants with **congenital rubella syndrome,** and 10,000 fetal deaths or therapeutic abortions were recorded (Fanaroff, Martin, 1992). Since vaccination was begun in 1969, congenital rubella cases have been reduced drastically. Rubella immunity should be confirmed in all women before pregnancy (for further discussion, see Chapter 11). Confirmation is determined either by verification of rubella immunization or by serologic determination of rubella-specific IgM in cord or neonatal serum because history of rubella infection is unreliable. Diagnosis is possible with viral cultures of amniotic fluid, placenta or neonatal throat, urine, or spinal fluid.

Congenital rubella is not a static disease. More than two thirds of infected infants show no apparent involvement at birth, but consequences develop years later. Central and peripheral *hearing defects,* the most common result, appear to be progressive after birth. The major teratogenic effects of rubella involve the *cardiovascular* system (pulmonary artery hypoplasia, patent ductus arteriosus, and coarctation of the aortic isthmus) and *cataract* formation. Multiple other abnormalities commonly occur. These disorders include intrauterine and postnatal growth retardation, thrombocytopenic purpura (Fig. 39-10), dermal erythropoiesis, interstitial pneumonia, bony radiolucencies, retinopathy, and hepatosplenomegaly. Severe infections may result in fetal death. Delayed effects manifest as thyroid dysfunction, diabetes mellitus, growth hormone deficiency, and progressive rubella panencephalopathy (Fanaroff, Martin, 1992).

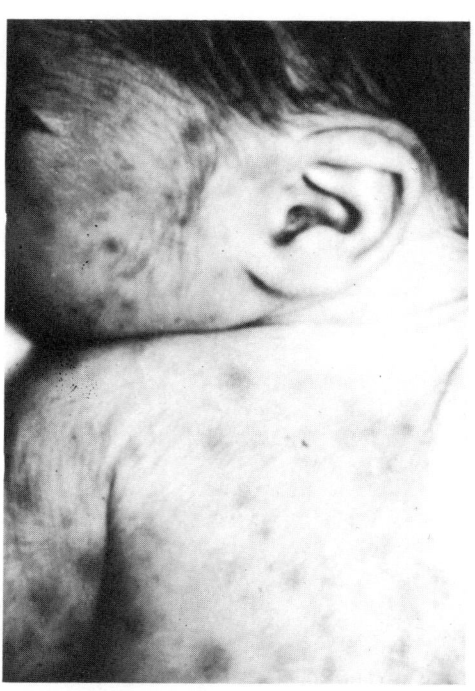

Fig. 39-10 Newborn with congenital rubella syndrome, showing multiple purpuric lesions over face, trunk, and upper arm.
From Fanaroff AA, Martin RJ, editors: *Neonatal-perinatal medicine: diseases of the fetus and infant,* ed 5, St Louis, 1992, Mosby–Year Book.

The risk of a congenitally infected infant varies with the gestational age of the fetus when maternal infection occurs. Anomalies are most severe if the mother contracts the virus during the first trimester.

The rubella virus has been cultured in babies for 1 to 1½ years after their birth. These infants are a serious source of infection to susceptible individuals, particularly potentially or actually pregnant women. Extended pediatric isolation is mandatory until the noncontagious stage of rubella has been reached. (The newborn should be isolated until pharyngeal mucus and urine are free of virus.)

For vaccination during the puerperium for women who are nonimmune for rubella, see Chapter 25. The use of Rh immune globulin may not interfere with effective rubella immunization.

CYTOMEGALOVIRUS INFECTION. Cytomegalic inclusion disease (CMID) is a disorder caused by one or more of at least six strains of CMV. CMV is deoxyribonucleic acid (DNA) virus of the herpes family. Maternal viremia during pregnancy may result in abortion, stillbirth, or congenital or neonatal CMID in a live-born infant. It is the most common cause of congenital viral infections in humans, occurring in 1% of all newborns (Fanaroff, Martin, 1992). It is always a severely crippling disease of the infant.

Maternal infection with CMV may begin as a mononucleosis-like syndrome. However, in most adults the onset of the disease is uncertain and, in fact, may be asymptomatic. It may remain subclinical for years. Respiratory transmission is the major vector, but the virus has been recovered from semen, vaginal secretions, urine, or feces, as well as from bank blood. Maternal CMID may be diagnosed serologically. Many women have antibody evidence of CMID. Women at risk for CMV infection include those who work in, or have children in, day-care centers, institutions for the mentally retarded, or certain health fields (nursery, dialysis, laboratories, oncology).

The newborn with classic, full-blown CMID displays IUGR and has microcephaly. The neonate also has a petechial rash, jaundice, and hepatosplenomegaly. Anemia, thrombocytopenia, and hyperbilirubinemia are to be expected. Intracranial, periventricular calcification often will be noted on x-ray films. Inclusion bodies ("owl's eye" figures) in cells sedimented from freshly voided urine or in liver biopsy specimens are typical. Elevated levels of cord blood IgM are suggestive of disease. The virus may be isolated from urine or saliva of the newborn. Differential diagnosis includes other causes of jaundice, syphilis (positive VDRL findings), toxoplasmosis (positive Sabin-Feldman dye test result), hemolytic disease of the newborn (positive Coombs' test reaction), or coxsackievirus infection (positive culture).

Despite the extensive, endemic nature of the disease in women and men and its potential for havoc in perinatal life, critically affected newborns are only occasionally born. Milder forms of the disease often may result when the fetus is affected late in pregnancy. CMV can be transmitted through breast milk while the mother is experiencing acute CMV syndrome. Severe mental and physical handicaps mark virtually all infants who survive CMID.

Infants without symptoms at birth are at risk for late sequelae. Hearing loss may not be apparent until after the first year of life. Chorioretinitis, microcephaly, mental retardation, and neuromuscular deficits may occur by 2 years of age. Some children are at risk for a defect in tooth enamel, resulting in severe caries.

No reasonable prevention or specific therapy exists for mother or infant (Fanaroff, Martin, 1992). Repeated pregnancies may be complicated by CMV infection. CMV can be passed from infected infants to a fetus. Pregnant health care personnel who have contact with infants suspected of having CMV must be sure to maintain strict universal precautions.

HERPES SIMPLEX VIRUS INFECTION. HSV infections among newborns are being diagnosed more frequently. HSV infection is estimated to occur in as many as 1/2000 to 5000 births (Fanaroff, Martin, 1992).

The herpes viruses belong to a group of DNA viruses that cause latent infection, last for the lifetime of the individual, and result in periodic recurrences. Pregnancy increases both the frequency of infection and the persistence of the virus. The newborn may acquire the virus by any of four **modes of transmission:**

- Transplacental infection
- Ascending infection by way of the birth canal
- Direct contamination during passage through an infected birth canal
- Direct transmission from infected personnel or family

Transplacental transmission of HSV infection to the newborn may occur during maternal viremia. However, an ascending transcervical infection first involves the intact fetal membranes, causing chorioamnionitis. This infection then is likely to be the *cause* of rupture of membranes rather than the sequel to their rupture. Ascending transcervical infection of intact membranes may account for the triple rate of spontaneous abortions in the first 20 weeks of gestation with genital HSV infections, the development of neonatal infections despite cesarean birth with intact membranes, and the high rate of preterm birth (Brown et al, 1987). Transcervical infection can be accelerated by fetal monitoring electrodes. The electrodes break the fetal skin barrier and increase the risk of infection. However, most infants show no evidence of infection in utero.

Congenital infection is rare. Congenital infection is marked by in utero destruction of normally formed organs. Affected infants are growth retarded. They have severe psychomotor retardation, with intracranial calcifications, microcephaly, hypertonicity, and seizures. They suffer eye involvement, including microphthalmos, cataracts, chorioretinitis, blindness, and retinal dysplasia. Some infants have patent ductus arteriosus, limb anomalies, and recurrent skin vesicles, with a short life expectancy.

Most infants are infected directly during passage through the birth canal. The risk of infection during vaginal birth in the presence of genital herpes has not been clearly delineated. It may be as high as 40% to 60%, with active infection at term. Primary maternal infections after 32 weeks' gestation carry a higher risk for the fetus and newborn than do recurrent infections (Fanaroff, Martin, 1992). The transmission rate of chronic vaginal herpes from the pregnant woman to her newborn is low, 8% or less (Bennett, 1987; Prober, 1987). Passive intrauterine immunity to herpes may be responsible. If the mother is symptom-free at birth, detectable infection may not be found in the infant.

Postnatal acquisition of the virus and spread within a nursery have been documented by DNA analysis. Both the mother and father, as well as maternal breast lesions, have been implicated in neonatal infections. There also is concern regarding symptomatic and asymptomatic shedding among hospital personnel. Nursery personnel with cold sores should practice strict hand washing and wear a mask, but there is no evidence to require their actual removal from the nursery unless they have a herpetic whitlow (primary herpes simplex infection of the terminal segment of a finger) (Frigoletto, Little, 1988; Fanaroff, Martin, 1992).

Clinically, neonatal HSV infections are classified as disseminated infection, encephalitis, and localized infection of the skin, eye, or mouth.

Disseminated infections may involve virtually every organ system, but the liver, adrenal glands, and lungs are predominantly involved. Affected infants exhibit initial symptoms usually in the first week of life but sometimes in the second week, with signs of bacterial sepsis or shock. Clinical manifestations include skin vesicles in about 50% of infants (Fig. 39-11). Death results from progression of CNS involvement, respiratory distress and pneumonitis, shock, disseminated intravascular coagulation (DIC), and bleeding. Overall, the mortality rate without antiviral therapy is 82%.

Encephalitis may occur as a component of disseminated disease. Blood-borne seeding of the brain results in multiple lesions of cortical hemorrhagic necrosis. It also can occur alone or in association with oral, eye, or skin lesions. In the second to fourth week of life, brain involvement usually manifests. Only 60% of the infants have skin lesions, and the CSF of fewer than 50% will reveal the virus. Lethargy, poor feeding, irritability, and local or generalized seizures may be the presenting manifestations. Almost half the infants die of neurologic deterioration as late as 6 months after onset, and virtually all survivors have severe sequelae, including microcephaly and blindness (Fanaroff, Martin, 1992).

Localized HSV infections most commonly occur with skin findings or, rarely, with isolated oral cavity lesions. CNS or disseminated disease will develop in 70% of the infants with skin vesicles. Ocular involvement, which can occur alone, may be secondary to either HSV-1 or HSV-2. Ocular disease may not be discovered for months. Microphthalmos, cataracts, optic atrophy, and corneal scarring may result from chorioretinitis, keratitis, and retinal hemorrhage (Fanaroff, Martin, 1992).

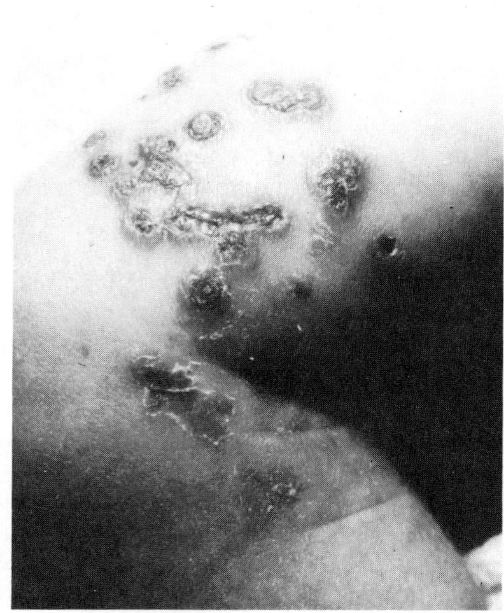

Fig. 39-11 Neonatal herpesvirus infection.
From Fanaroff AA, Martin RJ, editors: *Neonatal-perinatal medicine: diseases of the fetus and infant,* ed 5, St Louis, 1992, Mosby–Year Book.

MANAGEMENT. Care of all newborn infants begins with parental prevention of genital infections. Spermicidal foams kill the virus, and condoms offer some protection against direct contact with lesions in the sexual partner. Although maternal ingestion of oral or intravenous acyclovir shortens the viral shedding time, its effect on fetal safety is unknown. Therefore this agent is not recommended during pregnancy (Fanaroff, Martin, 1992).

Antepartum maternal cultures and antibody screening do not predict the infant's risk of exposure to HSV at birth. The best time and route of birth are still controversial factors. There is consensus that infants should be born by cesarean surgery when an active herpes infection is present at the onset of labor and the amniotic membranes have been ruptured less than 4 hours, regardless of whether the infection is primary or recurrent. Because of the possibility of transplacental and ascending transcervical infection, the mother must be informed that even cesarean birth gives no guarantee that the baby will be free from infection (Fanaroff, Martin, 1992). Fetal scalp monitors are avoided.

During the postpartum period the nurse's main function is to teach the mother about the disease—recognition of lesions and prevention of its transmission during care of the infant. Initially all infants should be isolated. Until the results of the maternal cultures are determined to be negative, both gown and gloves should be worn by persons in contact with these infants (Fanaroff, Martin, 1992).

The newborn's eyes, oral cavity, and skin are inspected carefully for the presence of any lesions. Cultures are obtained from the mouth, the eyes, and any possible lesions. Circumcision is delayed until the infant is discharged. The infant may be discharged with the mother if the infant's cultures are negative for the virus. The mother is advised about the need for weekly pediatric appointments throughout the first month. As long as there are no suspicious lesions on the mother's breasts, breast-feeding is allowed. For the infant at risk, prophylactic topical eye ointment (vidarabine) is ordered to be administered for 5 days for prevention of keratoconjunctivitis. There are no current recommendations for prophylactic systemic therapy. Each case should be considered individually. Blood, urine, and CSF specimens should be cultured when indicated clinically. If herpetic lesions first occur after 6 weeks of life, the risk of dissemination and severe illness is very low (Fanaroff, Martin, 1992).

Therapy includes general supportive measures, as well as treatment with vidarabine or acyclovir. Use of hyperimmune globulin has not been beneficial, but vidarabine inhibits both cellular and viral replication. A multicenter study has demonstrated that with vidarabine therapy the mortality rate of infants with disseminated disease decreased from 90% to 70% and in infants with CNS disease, from 50% to 15%. The earliest possible institution of therapy at 30 mg/kg/day is recommended. The dose should be given over 12 hours for 14 days. Continuing therapy may be required in case of recurrence. Ophthalmic ointment should be administered simultaneously (Fanaroff, Martin, 1992).

Acyclovir has now become the most commonly used drug for neonatal infections. It is considered to be a safe drug because only viral replication is inhibited, although long-term sequelae are not yet known. Acyclovir is easier to administer and has been demonstrated to be more effective than vidarabine for herpes encephalitis. Clinical trials indicate no significant differences in outcome between the two drugs. The current recommended dose of acyclovir is 10 mg/kg/day intravenously every 8 hours for at least 14 days (Fanaroff, Martin, 1992).

Chlamydial Infection

Chlamydia trachomatis is an intracellular bacterium that causes *neonatal conjunctivitis* and pneumonia. The conjunctivitis (congestion and edema), with minimal discharge, develops 5 days to 2 weeks after birth. If chlamydial disease is not treated, chronic follicular conjunctivitis, with conjunctival scarring and corneal neovascularization, may result. Newborns with pneumonia exhibit prolonged staccato cough, tachypnea, mild hypoxemia, and eosinophilia (Merenstein, Gardner, 1989).

If prenatal screening reveals infection with *C. trachomatis*, antepartum treatment of the mother with erythromycin or sulfisoxazole appears to improve pregnancy outcome. The newborn also is treated with oral erythromycin for 2 to 3 weeks, along with irrigation of the eye with saline or buffered ophthalmic solution daily. Topical antibiotic is not necessary. Silver nitrate is not effective against *C. trachomatis*, but erythromycin or tetracycline ointment may prevent ophthalmic infection (Fanaroff, Martin, 1992).

Human Immunodeficiency Virus—Acquired Immunodeficiency Syndrome

Maternal infection with the retrovirus HIV is discussed in Chapter 29. The focus of this discussion is the newborn at risk for infection with HIV. Although the transmission rate of HIV infections has been reported by some authors to be as high as 50% to 60% in infants born to mothers infected with HIV, most researchers cite a transmission rate between 20% and 35% (Merenstein, Gardner, 1989; Cherry, Merkatz, 1991). Pediatric acquired immunodeficiency syndrome (AIDS) accounts for 2% of reported AIDS cases in the United States, and 80% of these children acquired infection in the perinatal period. The incidence is likely to increase. The blood supply in the United States is now screened for HIV, thus decreasing the chance of transmission by this route. However, the number of women of childbearing age infected with HIV is increasing. The populations at risk for acquiring HIV have been identified (see Chapter 29).

Transmission of HIV from the mother to the infant occurs transplacentally at various gestational ages, perinatally via maternal blood and secretions, and postnatally through breast milk (Pyun et al, 1987; Fanaroff, Martin, 1992).

Routine screening and counseling of all pregnant women is sparking considerable controversy (Landesman et al, 1987; Frigoletto, Little, 1988). The CDC has issued guidelines for counseling and antibody testing (Public Health Service guidelines, 1987). Several issues are being debated regarding routine screening. Many issues touch the core of the social fabric of the United States. They include the populations who have been identified to be at risk, including victims of child abuse; the adequacy and availability of social services, education, and health care systems; the volatile issue of therapeutic abortion; the option of avoiding future pregnancies (Facing, 1987); and the reliability of current tests for HIV.

DIAGNOSIS. *Diagnosis* of HIV infection in the newborn is the subject of intense research. Pyun et al (1987) studied specific antibody responses by the neonate. Pregnant women infected with HIV produce IgG antibodies. The IgG crosses the placenta to the fetus. Therefore cord blood is positive for antibody when tested by enzyme-linked immunosorbent assay (ELISA) or Western blot techniques. Because of their physiologically depressed immune response, newborns generally produce a less vigorous and more limited antibody response to HIV infection.

Every baby born to a mother who is seropositive for HIV will have HIV antibody at birth. Uninfected infants lose this maternal antibody during the first 8 to 15 months of life. Most infected infants begin to develop their own antibody and remain seropositive (Harnish et al, 1987; Johnson et al, 1987; Cherry, Merkatz, 1991; Fanaroff, Martin, 1992). Other tests are being sought to diagnose HIV infection at birth. So far, none have been completely reliable. The presence of HIV in the newborn currently must be verified either by culture or by demonstration of the presence of antigen (Harnish et al, 1987). Pyun et al (1987) were able to demonstrate the early appearance of anti-HIV antibody of the IgM and later of the IgG3 class, suggesting perinatal infection.

The occurrence of an **opportunistic infection** in the newborn may alert the caregiver to the presence of HIV infection or assist in the confirmation of the diagnosis of HIV infection. In pediatrics the presence of lymphoid interstitial pneumonitis is now considered a criterion for diagnosis (Fanaroff, Martin, 1992). The presence of oral candidiasis (thrush) that is refractory to treatment with topical antifungal agents carries a high index of suspicion for HIV infection (Prenatal, 1987).

Before 1 year of age, infected infants usually manifest symptoms similar to those seen in adults. These signs include lymphadenopathy, hepatosplenomegaly, chronic diarrhea, interstitial pneumonitis, and persistent thrush. In addition, infants have failure to thrive, recurrent severe bacterial infections, and occasionally recurrent enlargement of the parotid glands. *Pneumocystis carinii* has occurred in 70% and Kaposi's sarcoma in 5% of affected children. Viral infection caused by CMV and Epstein-Barr virus is commonly observed in children with AIDS. Bacterial sepsis also may be an initial manifestation (Fanaroff, Martin, 1992).

Infants who exhibit signs of HIV infection at birth tend to die within a month. The disease progression has been slower and the mortality lower in infants with a later onset.

MANAGEMENT. *Management* begins by implementing universal precautions and precautions for invasive procedures (see Chapter 29) to prevent further transmission of HIV (Public Health Service guidelines, 1987; Fanaroff, Martin, 1992). Circumcision in males is avoided. Umbilical cord stumps are cleaned meticulously every day until healing is complete. Therapy includes prophylactic gamma globulin, antimicrobial medications specific for the infections encountered, and corticosteroids in the presence of lymphoid interstitial pneumonitis. Zidovudine (AZT; formerly azidothymidine) and ribavirin cross the brain barrier and may result in increase in weight and in the number of helper T lymphocytes. For general care of the compromised newborn, see Chapter 36.

Counseling regarding the care of the women themselves, the family's care of the infant, and future pregnancies challenges the caregiver. Mothers with HIV infections should not breast-feed. Self-care involves avoiding at-risk behaviors during sexual encounters, avoiding substance abuse (see Chapter 33), and avoiding future pregnancies. Regardless of proved risks and mass media education, "safer sex" practices have not been implemented by many persons for a variety of reasons, including denial (Leishman, 1987). The public health community has become aware that women who know they carry HIV antibody still become pregnant for many reasons. These include denial of risk, desire to have a family despite the risk, and many more complex sociocultural considerations (Prenatal, 1987).

Some parents are opting to place the infected infants in foster homes despite the low risk for transmission among members of the same household. Social services are required in these cases. If the parent chooses to keep the infant, home health care is arranged. For more information and updated information, parents are offered the following resource: the National AIDS Hotline, 1-800-342-AIDS.

The family must be counseled about vaccinations. Children with symptomatic or asymptomatic HIV infection should receive all routine vaccines except oral polio virus vaccine. The family should be advised that household contacts should not receive oral polio vaccine because the virus can be transmitted to the immunocompromised child. Inactivated poliomyelitis vaccine can be given (Whaley, Wong, 1991).

Candidiasis

Candida infections, also known as moniliasis, are not uncommon in the newborn. *Candida albicans,* the organism usually responsible, may cause disease in any organ system. It is a yeastlike fungus (producing yeast cells and spores) that can be acquired from a maternal vaginal infection during birth, by person-to-person transmission, or from contaminated hands, bottles, nipples, or other articles. It usually is a benign disorder in the neonate, often confined to the oral and diaper regions (Whaley, Wong, 1991).

Candidal diaper dermatitis appears on the perianal area, inguinal folds, and lower portion of the abdomen. The affected area is intensely erythematous, with a sharply demarcated, scalloped edge, frequently with numerous satellite lesions that extend beyond the larger lesion. The source of the infection is through the gastrointestinal tract. Treatment consists of applications of an anticandidal ointment, such as nystatin (Mycostatin), with each diaper change. The infant also may be given an oral antifungal preparation to eliminate any gastrointestinal source of infection (Whaley, Wong, 1991).

Oral candidiasis (**thrush** or mycotic stomatitis) is characterized by the appearance of white plaques on the oral mucosa, gums, and tongue. The white patches are easily differentiated from milk curds; the patches cannot be removed and tend to bleed when touched. In most cases the infant does not seem to be discomforted by the infection. A few newborns seem to have some difficulty swallowing.

Infants who are sick, debilitated, or receiving antibiotic therapy are more susceptible. Those with conditions such as cleft lip or palate, neoplasms, and hyperparathyroidism seem to be more vulnerable to mycotic infection.

The objectives of management are to eradicate the causative organism, to control exposure to *C. albicans,* and to improve the infant's resistance. Interventions include maintenance of scrupulous cleanliness to prevent reinfection (nursing personnel, parents, others.) Good hand-washing technique is always essential. Clean surfaces should be provided for newborns (the newborn is never placed directly on sheets on which the mother has been sitting). Proper cleanliness of the equipment and environment is ensured. If the infant is breast-feeding, the mother also is treated with topical nystatin. The compromised newborn's physiologic function (see Chapter 36) must be supported.

Medications are administered as ordered. Aqueous solution of gentian violet (1% to 2%) is applied with a swab to oral mucosa, gums, and tongue. (Guard against permanent stain on skin, clothes, equipment. Warn parents about purple staining of baby's mouth.)

Nystatin is instilled into the newborn's mouth with a medicine dropper after the infant is given sterile water to wash out any residual milk. Nystatin also may be swabbed over mucosa, gums, or tongue.

To give oral medication by medicine dropper the infant's head is positioned to the side or the infant is supported in a semi-Fowler's position. The dropper is inserted into the oral cavity so that the tip rests against the cheek, alongside the tongue. After the infant begins to suck on the dropper, the nurse squeezes the rubber end slowly until the dropper is empty.

Gonorrhea

The incidence of gonococcal infection in pregnant women has ranged from 2.5% to 7.3% in recent studies (Fanaroff, Martin, 1992). With this high incidence, it is not surprising that neonatal infection with *Neisseria gonorrhoeae* occurs frequently. After rupture of membranes, ascending infection can result in orogastric contamination of the fetus. The organism also may invade mucosal surfaces such as the conjunctiva (ophthalmia neonatorum), rectal mucosa, and pharynx. Contamination may occur as the infant passes through the birth canal, or it may occur postnatally from an infected adult. Neonatal gonococcal arthritis, septicemia, meningitis, vaginitis, and scalp abscesses also can develop.

Endocervical cultures for *N. gonorrhoeae* should be obtained routinely during pregnancy and appropriate treatment instituted when necessary to prevent fetal-neonatal infection. The newborn with a mild infection often recovers completely with appropriate treatment (see Chapter 29). Occasionally infants die of overwhelming infection in the early neonatal period.

■ SUBSTANCE ABUSE

Certain maternal behaviors result in perinatal risk. Maternal habits hazardous to the fetus and newborn are drug addiction, smoking, and alcohol abuse. Occasional withdrawal reactions have been reported in newborns of mothers who use to excess such drugs as barbiturates, alcohol, or amphetamines. Serious reactions are seen in newborns whose mothers abuse psychoactive drugs (see Chapter 33) or are treated with methadone. Almost 50% of pregnancies of women addicted to opioids result in LBW infants who are not necessarily preterm. Alcohol is a teratogen. Maternal ethanol abuse during gestation creates a readily identifiable fetal alcohol syndrome (FAS).

The adverse effects of exposure of the fetus to drugs are varied. They include transient behavioral changes such as fetal breathing movements or irreversible effects such as fetal death, IUGR, structural malformations, or mental retardation. Some maternal drug use is for the pharmacologic control of disease processes (e.g., insulin) or for symptomatic relief of benign problems (e.g., aspirin). It has been shown that 92% to 100% of all obstetric clients take at least one physician-prescribed drug, and 65% to 80% also take self-prescribed drugs. In addition to the therapeutic use of drugs, the nontherapeutic use of drugs—such as alcohol, nicotine, or narcotics—poses threats to fetal well-being. Critical determinants of the effect of the drug on the fetus include the specific drug, the dosage, the route of administration, the genotype of the mother or fetus, and the timing of the drug exposure (see Chapter 33). Figs. 39-12 and 7-6 show critical periods in human embryogenesis and the teratogenic effects of drugs.

ASSESSMENT

Assessment of the newborn requires a review of the mother's prenatal record. A medical and social history of drug abuse and detoxification is noted. Some obstetric problems are seen in pregnancies complicated by substance abuse. The obstetric events include PROM, amnionitis, preterm labor, precipitous labor, abruptio placentae, placenta previa, and spontaneous abortion. Perinatal and neonatal mortality and morbidity also occur. There is an increase in stillbirths and in the births of newborns who have IUGR or are LBW preterm.

The woman who is addicted to narcotics may have infections that compound the risk to the infant. These infections include hepatitis, septicemia, and STDs, including AIDS (Niebyl, 1988).

The nurse often is the first to observe the signs of drug dependence in the newborn. The nurse's observations help the physician differentiate between drug dependence and other conditions, such as tracheoesophageal fistula, CNS disorder, sepsis, hypoglycemia, and electrolyte imbalance.

The newborn is assessed by means of the guidelines discussed in Chapter 20. The newborn's gestational age and maturity are noted (p. 1123). In utero exposure to some drugs results in observable malformations or dysmorphism (abnormality of shape). Neonatal behavior may arouse suspicion. Lethargy, decreased visual alertness and auditory response to the Brazelton neonatal behavioral assessment scale, or withdrawal symptoms are noted. Urine screening may be used to identify substances abused by the mother. Because many women are multidrug users, the newborn infant initially may exhibit a confusing complex of signs.

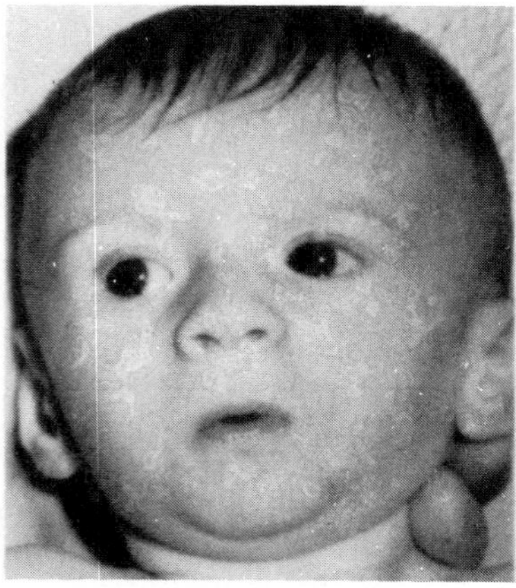

Fig. 39-12 Fetal alcohol anomaly.
Courtesy Dr. Charles Linder, Medical College of Georgia. From Goodman RM, Gorlin RJ: *Atlas of the face in genetic disorders*, ed 2, St Louis, 1977, Mosby–Year Book.

NURSING DIAGNOSES

Nursing diagnoses, which depend on the assessment findings, are tailored to the individual needs of the newborn and the family. Following are examples of nursing diagnoses.

NEWBORN

- High risk for infection related to
  - —Maternal risk behaviors
  - —PROM
- Altered growth and development related to
  - —Effects of maternal substance abuse
- Sleep pattern disturbance related to
  - —Drug withdrawal

PARENTS

- Actual or potential altered parenting related to
  - —Continuation of substance abuse or detoxification program
  - —Guilt about infant's condition
  - —Inability to cope with care needs of a special infant
- Anxiety related to knowledge deficit regarding
  - —Care needs of an affected infant
- High risk for violence, self-directed or directed toward infant related to
  - —Drug-dependent life-style

PLANNING

Planning for care of the newborn presents a challenge to the health care team. Parents are included in the planning for the newborn's care and also are encouraged to plan for their own care. A multidisciplinary approach is needed that includes home health or community resource personnel (e.g., regulatory agencies such as child protective services).

Goals are stated in client-centered terms and include the following:

- The newborn suffers no adverse sequelae to drug withdrawal.
- The infant's malformations and dysfunction are identified, and appropriate curative and rehabilitative measures are instituted.
- Parents come to terms with the newborn's condition and its management.

IMPLEMENTATION

Education and social support to prevent the abuse of drugs provide the ideal approach. However, given the scope of the drug abuse problem, total prevention is unrealistic.

Nursing care of the drug-dependent newborn involves supportive therapy for fluid and electrolyte balance, nutrition, infection control, and respiratory care. Medications are given as ordered. The newborn's narcotic withdrawal signs may require a schedule of weaning from the drug. Phenobarbital—6 mg/kg/24hr administered intramuscularly—or 2 mg given orally four times a day for 3 or 4 days may be ordered. The dose is reduced by one third every 2 days for about 2 weeks, at which time treatment is discontinued. Paregoric may be ordered: 2 to 4 drops/kg orally every 4 to 6 hours initially to as much as 20 to 30 drops/kg orally every 4 to 6 hours, depending on the symptoms.

Swaddling, holding, reducing stimuli, and feeding as necessary may be helpful in easing withdrawal.

Drug dependence in the newborn is physiologic, not psychologic. Thus a predisposition to dependence later in life is not thought to be a factor. However, the psychosocial environment in which the infant is raised may create a tendency to addiction.

The mother requires considerable support. Her need for and her abuse of drugs result in a decreased capacity to cope. The newborn's withdrawal signs and decreased consolability stress her coping abilities even further. Home health care, treatment for addiction, and education are important considerations. Sensitive exploration of the woman's options for the care of her infant and herself and for future fertility management may help her see that she has choices. This approach helps communicate respect for the new mother as a person who can make responsible decisions.

EVALUATION

Final evaluation may not be possible. Short-term *goals* include the following examples.

- The newborn suffers no adverse sequelae to drug withdrawal.
- The infant's malformations and dysfunction are identified, and appropriate curative and rehabilitative measures are instituted.
- The parents come to terms with the newborn's condition and its management.

However, both the infant and the parent have long-term needs. The extent to which goals are met may not be known for years.

Alcohol

Reference to the association between fetal malformation and maternal alcoholism can be found in Greek and Roman mythology. Laws in Carthage and Sparta forbade consumption of alcohol by couples on their wedding night to prevent the conception of children with defects. Documentation of the **fetal alcohol syndrome (FAS)** can be found in the literature since the early part of the eighteenth century. The incidence of FAS in the United States is about 2.2/1000 live births and worldwide it is 1.9/1000 births. Milder effects may be seen in as high as 23 to 29/1000 births (Abel, Sokol, 1988; Niebyl, 1988; Barbour, 1990).

According to Barbour (1990) FAS is a set of symptoms that includes prenatal and postnatal growth retardation and CNS malfunctions, including mental retardation. Infants born to social or modest drinkers may exhibit *fetal alcohol effects (FAE)*. These effects run the gamut from learning disabilities and behavioral problems to speech or language problems and hyperactivity. Often these problems are not detected until the child goes to school and learning problems become evident.

Predictable abnormal patterns of fetal and neonatal morphogenesis are attributed to severe, chronic alcoholism in women who continue to drink heavily during pregnancy. The pattern of growth deficiency begun in prenatal life persists after birth, especially in the linear growth rate, rate of weight gain, and growth of head circumferences. Table 39-1 summarizes the risks associated with maternal alcohol ingestion.

Ocular structural anomalies are common findings (Fig. 39-13). Limb anomalies and a variety of cardiocirculatory anomalies, especially ventricular septal defects, pose problems for the child. Mental retardation (IQ of 79 or below at 7 years of age) and fine motor dysfunction (poor hand-to-mouth coordination, weak grasp) add to the handicapping problems that maternal alcoholism can impose. Genital abnormalities are seen in daughters of alcohol-addicted mothers. Two thirds of newborns with FAS are girls; the cause of this altered sex birth ratio is unknown. Severe and chronic alcoholism (ethanol toxicity), not maternal malnutrition, is responsible for the severity and consistency of postnatal performance problems (Fanaroff, Martin, 1992). High alcohol levels are lethal to the developing embryo. Lower levels cause brain and other malformations. Long-term prognosis (no studies are available as yet) is discouraging even in an optimum psychosocial environment, when one considers the combination of growth failure and mental retardation.

Alcohol effects, however, depend not only on the amount of alcohol consumed but on the interaction of quantity, frequency, type of alcohol, and other drug abuse. Other drugs such as cigarettes, caffeine, and marijuana may potentiate the fetal effects of alcohol consumption during gestation (Fanaroff, Martin, 1992).

The newborn of a mother who abuses alcohol is faced with a number of clinical problems. Identification of the problems leads to the medical diagnosis of FAS. The newborn may suffer respiratory distress related to preterm birth, neurologic damage, and a "floppy" epiglottis and small trachea. Tracheoepiglottal anomalies may cause cardiopulmonary arrest. Other disorders include recurrent otitis media and hearing loss. Craniofacial features may be important in diagnosing craniofacial and oral anomalies, dental development abnormalities, and long-term bodily growth patterns (Jackson, Hussain, 1990). Feeding difficulties are related to preterm birth, poor sucking ability, and possible cleft palate. The newborn may exhibit brain dysfunction, microcephaly, and grand mal seizures.

TABLE 39-1 Risks Associated with Maternal Alcohol Ingestion

Amount of Alcohol	Risks
Two or more drinks daily includes:	IUGR
2 mixed drinks, 1 oz liquor each	Immature motor activity Increased rate of anomalies
2 glasses of wine, 5 oz each	Decreased muscle tone
2 beers, 12 oz each	Poor sucking pressure Increased rate of stillbirths Decreased placental weight
Five or more drinks on occasion	Increased risk of structural brain abnormalities
Six or more drinks daily	FAS

From McCarthy P: *Am J Primary Health Care* 8:34, 1983. Copyright the Nurse Practitioner: The American Journal of Primary Health Care.

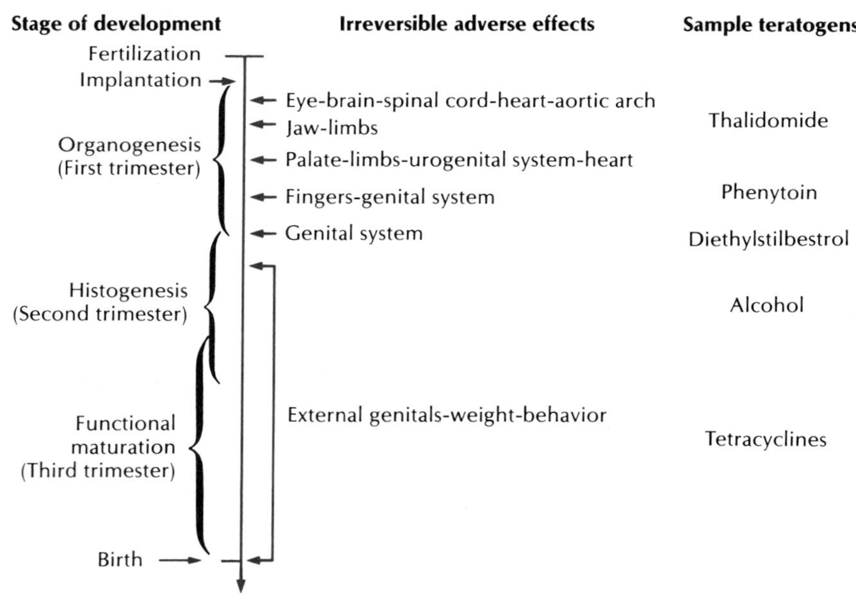

Fig. 39-13 Critical periods in human embryogenesis.
From Fanaroff AA, Martin RJ, editors: *Neonatal-perinatal medicine: diseases of the fetus and infant,* ed 5, St Louis, 1992, Mosby–Year Book.

Long-term effects into childhood may include impaired visual-motor perception and performance, lowered IQ scores, and delayed receptive and expressive language (Hill et al, 1990), as well as reduced capacity to process and store factual data (Becker et al, 1990). FAS follows the infant into childhood and adulthood with continuing negative results. It is now recognized as one of the leading causes of mental retardation in the United States. Although the distinctive facial features of the infant tend to become less evident, the mental capacities never become normal. Long-term effects of the disorder persist, manifested in low IQ scores, poor ability in mathematics, distractability, and poor judgment (Streissguth et al, 1991).

Nursing care involves many of the same strategies used for the care of preterm infants (Chapter 37). Special efforts are made to involve the parents in their child's care and to encourage opportunities for parent-child attachment. The application of the nursing process to the care of a newborn with FAS is presented in the case study below and the nursing plan of care (p. 1208).

Children placed in a warm, caring environment with understanding caregivers who can deal with the infant's hyperirritability can be helped to lead a more normal existence than their condition might warrant (Barbour, 1989). These caregivers provide extensive cuddling and human contact and can deal with the eating problems that commonly lead to a diagnosis of *failure to thrive.*

Heroin

Heroin crosses the placenta. Of infants born to heroin-addicted mothers, 50% are LBW and 50% are SGA. Heroin may have a direct growth-inhibiting effect on the fetus. There is an increased rate of stillbirths but not of congenital anomalies.

Detoxification is not advised before 14 weeks' gestation because of a potential risk of spontaneous abortion. Neither is it advised after the thirty-second week because of possible withdrawal-induced fetal distress (Niebyl, 1988).

Heroin withdrawal occurs in 50% to 75% of infants born to addicted mothers, usually within the first 24 to 48 hours of life. The signs depend on the length of maternal addiction, the amount of drug taken, and the time of injection before birth. The infant whose mother is taking methadone may not demonstrate signs of withdrawal until a week or so after birth. The symptoms of newborns whose mothers used heroin or methadone are similar in nature. Initially the infant may be depressed. The **withdrawal syndrome** may consist of a combination of any of the following signs. The newborn may be jit-

CASE STUDY

Fetal Alcohol Syndrome

Albert was born 3 hours ago. His birth weight was 5½ lb (2464 g). His mother, age 24, drank heavily during the pregnancy.

ASSESSMENT

Albert exhibits clinical problems of FAS: microcephaly, hypotonia, irritability, poor suck, and increased respiratory effort. Both his mother and father are anxious to care for their baby.

NURSING DIAGNOSIS

Many nursing diagnoses are possible; however, one takes priority at this time: ineffective breathing pattern related to FAS.

PLANNING

Parents and nurse mutually agree on the *goals:* Albert will maintain a patent airway, and he will be able to maintain adequate ventilation by his own effort. The nurse sets an additional *expected outcome:* parents will cope effectively with Albert's needs.

IMPLEMENTATION

The nurse places Albert in a position in which he exhibits least distress (prone or side lying) and places him on a cardiopulmonary monitor. His mouth and nose are suctioned as needed. The nurse ensures that resuscitative and oxygen administration equipment is readily available. Before Albert is discharged, his parents learn cardiopulmonary resuscitation (CPR) and are referred to a home health care nurse.

EVALUATION

The nurse can be reasonably assured that care was effective when the goals for care are met. That is, Albert maintains a patent airway and adequate ventilation through his own respiratory effort; his parents begin to participate in his care; his mother accepts an appointment with a social worker; and a visit from a home health care nurse is set.

CARE PLAN Fetal Alcohol Syndrome

GOALS	IMPLEMENTATION	RATIONALE	EVALUATION
Nursing diagnosis: Ineffective breathing pattern related to FAS			
Albert will maintain a patent airway. Albert will be able to maintain adequate ventilation by his own respiratory effort.	Have resuscitative equipment available. Place Albert on cardiopulmonary monitor (set close alarm limits). Place Albert in position where he exhibits least distress (prone or side). Suction mouth and nose as necessary. Implement seizure precautions.	Hypotonia and poor suck predispose Albert to distress from diminished ability to handle secretions and fluids; seizures may occur as Albert withdraws from alcohol.	Albert maintains a patent airway. Albert maintains adequate ventilation through his own respiratory effort. Albert has no seizures.
Nursing diagnosis: Altered nutrition, less than body requirements, related to irritability and poor suck			
Albert will ingest and retain nutrients sufficient for growth.	Elevate Albert's head during and after feeding. Feed in small frequent amounts. Evaluate different nipples for feeding. Burp well after feeds. Feed by oral gavage as necessary. Obtain daily weight; maintain strict intake and output. Keep suction ready to use; aspirate nares as circumstances require.	Engages gravity to help fluids move downward to gastrointestinal tract. Prevents overfilling of stomach to diminish chance of aspiration. Compensates for infant's poor suck. Diminishes chance of aspiration. Provides nourishment as needed. Evaluates feeding method. Diminishes chance of aspiration.	Albert takes and retains enough nutrients for growth.
Nursing diagnosis: Altered family processes related to need to care for and love a child with a handicap, as well as lack of knowledge of infant's special needs and expected sequelae			
Albert will be successfully cared for by his parents. Parents will learn about infant's special needs. Parents will begin process of bonding and attachment to Albert.	Encourage frequent parental visits to the special care nursery, and promote physical contact with Albert. Teach parents about Albert's anomalies and their possible sequelae. Help parents verbalize their concerns. Be realistic when discussing Albert's potential for future development. Involve the parents in Albert's care (diapering, holding, bathing). Refer to outside resources (e.g., infant developmental/stimulation programs). Introduce parents to CPR skills; observe return demonstration.	Parent-child bonding and attachment are essential for well-being of parent and child. Knowledge and practice increase parents' self-confidence and perhaps self-esteem and sense of some control over the situation. Mobilization of community resources provides reassurance.	Parents learn about Albert's anomalies and their possible effects on the child's future. Parents recognize and eventually accept Albert's handicaps. Parents verbalize their concerns. Parents learn child-care activities. Parents utilize community resources as needed.

tery and hyperactive. Commonly the newborn's cry is shrill and persistent. The infant may yawn or sneeze frequently. The tendon reflexes are increased, but the Moro's reflex is decreased. The neonate may exhibit poor feeding and sucking, tachypnea, vomiting, diarrhea, hypothermia or hyperthermia, and sweating. In addition, an abnormal sleep cycle, with absence of quiet sleep and disturbance of active sleep, has been described in these infants (Fanaroff, Martin, 1992).

If withdrawal is not treated, vomiting, diarrhea, dehydration, apnea, and convulsions may develop. Death may follow. Therapy is individualized. Dehydration and electrolyte imbalance are prevented or treated. Usually one of the following drugs is ordered: phenobarbital, paregoric (compound tincture of opium), or diazepam, singly or in combination.

The long-term effect on these newborns is now being studied. Researchers have found that "many serious" mental and physical problems are evident in the child's first few months of life, as well as "numerous indications . . . [of] serious abnormalities in the brain structure that will not be revealed until later years" (Howard, 1986).

Methadone

Methadone, a synthetic opiate, has been the therapy of choice for heroin addiction since 1965. By blocking the euphoric effects, it reduces the craving for heroin. It does cross the placenta. An increasing number of infants have been born to methadone-maintained mothers, who seem to have better prenatal care and a somewhat better life-style than those taking heroin (Fanaroff, Martin, 1992).

There is some question as to the benefits of methadone therapy during pregnancy because of its effect on the fetus (see Chapter 33). In one study (Davis, Templer, 1988) children exposed to methadone in utero demonstrated more pathologic problems and scored significantly lower on IQ testing than did those who had been exposed to heroin. These findings question the benefits of methadone treatment for pregnant heroin abusers and the related ethical issues. Multiple drug abuse, however, is a problem for many. The drugs include alcohol, barbiturates, tranquilizers, and other psychoactive drugs. Many are heavy smokers as well. Methadone withdrawal occurs in about 70% to 90% of newborns born to these women.

Methadone withdrawal resembles heroin withdrawal syndrome but tends to be more severe and prolonged. In addition, the incidence of seizures is higher. Seizures usually occur between days 7 and 10. The infants exhibit a disturbed sleep pattern similar to that seen in heroin withdrawal. The newborns have higher birth weight, usually appropriate for gestational age. No increased incidence of congenital anomalies is seen.

Late-onset withdrawal occurs at 2 to 4 weeks and may continue for weeks or months. A higher incidence of sudden infant death syndrome (SIDS) also has been reported in these infants. This factor is important for perinatal nurses who coordinate follow-up care for the infant and education for the mother or other caregiver. That is, community health nurses need to know about the potential for withdrawal symptoms to occur.

Therapy for methadone withdrawal is similar to that for heroin withdrawal. The few available follow-up studies of these infants reveal a higher incidence of hyperactivity, learning and behavior disorders, and poor social adjustment (Fanaroff, Martin, 1992).

Marijuana

Marijuana is believed to be the most abused drug in the United States, with an estimated 20 million users. It crosses the placenta. Its use during pregnancy may result in a shortened gestation and a higher incidence of precipitate labor (less than 3 hours) (Niebyl, 1988). Some investigators have found a higher incidence of meconium staining (Niebyl, 1988; Fanaroff, Martin, 1992). No increased incidence of congenital complications or effects on the infant's growth and physical parameters specific to marijuana use alone have been identified. However, the use of marijuana with alcohol results in decreased birth weight and a fivefold increase in risk for FAS. Compounding this issue is multidrug use, especially among adolescents, thus combining the harmful effects of marijuana, tobacco, alcohol, and cocaine. Long-term follow-up studies on exposed infants are needed.

Cocaine

Cocaine is another commonly abused drug among all social classes. It is the most powerfully addictive drug available (see Chapter 33). It is often used with other drugs such as marijuana and alcohol. Its use is blamed for a higher incidence of spontaneous abortion and abruptio placentae secondary to frequent episodes of vasospastic hypertension. It crosses the placenta and is found in breast milk.

Infants born to cocaine-abusing mothers show a high rate of perinatal morbidity, IUGR, microcephaly, preterm birth, cerebral hemorrhage or infarction, and congenital anomalies (Chasnoff, 1989).

Cocaine-dependent newborns often experience a significant and agonizing withdrawal syndrome that can last 2 to 3 weeks. The withdrawal signs have some of the same characteristics as heroin withdrawal. Irritability, marked nervousness, rapid changes in mood, and hypersensitivity to noise and external stimuli characterize the infant's behavior. These neonates exhibit poor feeding, irregular sleep patterns, tachypnea, tachycardia, and often diarrhea. Chasnoff et al (1989) identified significant depression in interactive behavior and a poor organization response to environmental stimuli.

The infants exposed to cocaine typically are lethargic, almost catatonic. They have visual attention problems in that they are unable to focus on their parent's face. These children often have been subjected to numerous small strokes because of abrupt changes in their mothers' blood pressure during pregnancy. Renal problems, lack of coordination, developmental retardation, and perhaps visual problems may be related. There may be an increased risk for SIDS (Chasnoff et al, 1989; Bauchner et al, 1988).

Phencyclidine (Angel Dust)

Phencyclidine (PCP) is one of the most dangerous of the available abused drugs. It may have extremely unpredictable, bizarre, and violent effects, especially when combined with crack (cocaine free base) (a combination known as "space base") (see Chapter 33). PCP increases the risk of injury to the user and therefore also to her passively dependent fetus. The user may be unaware that she is ingesting PCP because it commonly is misrepresented as another drug of abuse or mixed with other drugs.

PCP crosses the placenta and is found in breast milk. Literature about newborns is limited. The infants exposed to PCP appear to be alert, active babies. "Their mothers often think they are smarter. They hold their heads up faster. . . . But, in fact, it is abnormal behavior. Although we aren't sure why, the tone of the muscles in the head is of the kind that we see in [children with] cerebral palsy," a disorder of the CNS characterized by spastic paralysis or other forms of defective motor ability (Bean, 1986).

Miscellaneous Substances

Methamphetamine ("ice") is one of the most potent stimulants available (for discussion of maternal use, see p. 1004). It is used commonly by adolescents and young adults. The fetal and neonatal effects of maternal use of methamphetamines in pregnancy are not well known. The effects appear to be dose related. LBW, preterm birth, and perinatal mortality may be consequences of higher doses used throughout pregnancy. Newborns may be drowsy and jittery and may experience respiratory distress soon after birth. Lethargy may continue for several months, along with frequent infections and poor weight gain. Emotional disturbances and delays in gross and fine motor coordination may be seen during early childhood.

Phenobarbital is another commonly abused drug in all social classes. It crosses the placenta readily and is subsequently found in high levels in the fetal liver and brain. Because of its slow metabolic rate, when withdrawal does occur, onset is generally at 2 to 14 days after birth and duration is about 2 to 4 months. Irritability, crying, hiccoughs, and sleepiness mark the initial response. During the second stage the infant is extremely hungry, regurgitates and gags frequently, and demonstrates episodic irritability, sweating, and a disturbed sleep pattern.

Treatment consists of swaddling, frequent feedings, and protection from noxious external stimuli. If there is no improvement with the use of these methods, the newborn should be given phenobarbital and then slowly withdrawn from this drug after control of symptoms (Fanaroff, Martin, 1992).

Caffeine has not been implicated as a teratogen in humans. After controlling for smoking and other habits (including alcohol consumption), demographic characteristics, and medical history, Linn et al (1982) found no relationship between caffeine consumption and any adverse outcomes of pregnancy (Niebyl, 1988). The FDA (1980) suggests that "prudence dictates that pregnant women and those who may become pregnant avoid caffeine-containing products or use them sparingly."

Tobacco

Cigarette smoking in pregnancy has been found to be associated with birth weight deficits of up to 250 g for a full-term neonate (Fanaroff, Martin, 1992). Maternal cigarette smoking is implicated in 21% to 39% of LBW infants. The rate of preterm birth is increased. Nicotine and continine, the two pharmacologically active substances in tobacco, are found in higher concentrations in infants whose mothers smoke. These substances can be secreted in breast milk for up to 2 hours after the mother has smoked. Cigarette smoke contains more than 2000 compounds, including carbon monoxide, dioxin, cyanide, and cadmium. Long-term studies show residual effects beyond the neonatal period (Niebyl, 1988). Deficits in growth, in intellectual and emotional development, and in behavior have been documented.

The **fetal tobacco syndrome** is a diagnostic term applicable to infants who fit the following criteria (Nieberg et al, 1985):

1. The mother smoked five or more cigarettes a day throughout pregnancy.
2. The mother had no evidence of hypertension during pregnancy, specifically (a) no preeclampsia and (b) documentation of normal blood pressure at least once after the first trimester.
3. The newborn has symmetric growth retardation at term (up to or greater than 37 weeks), defined as (a) a birth weight less than 2500 g and (b) a ponderal index ([weight in g]/[length in m]) greater than 2.32.
4. There is no other obvious cause of IUGR (e.g., congenital infection or anomaly).

Pregnant women need to be aware of the harmful effects of smoking on their unborn baby's health. Mothers (and all others) need to refrain from smoking near the newborn infant. There is an increasing concern over second-hand smoke and its potential effects on infants. Several studies have reported a positive association between maternal smoking and SIDS (Niebyl, 1988). It is not clear whether this association reflects in utero exposure or passive exposure postnatally, or both.

■ SUMMARY

The newborn with acquired problems presents a challenge to the health care team. The nurse must have sound knowledge about conditions that place the newborn at risk, including problems related to birth trauma, diabetic mother, neonatal infections, and substance abuse. Constant vigilance, prompt reporting, and timely therapy are necessary to prevent serious sequelae as a result of the disorder and its therapy.

The outcome for infants born to addicted mothers depends on the interrelationships among many factors. These factors include intrauterine drug exposure, often of multiple drugs, and the emotional, familial, and environmental instability associated with drug use. Nurses must be aware of the commonly abused drugs and the effects on the neonate and the family. The nurse also must be aware of legal and ethical issues but avoid a judgmental approach to caring for these clients.

The parents and other family members need a sensitive, thoughtful nurse to help them cope with the stress that arises from birth and care of a compromised newborn. The complex care of clients with multiple problems requires an interdisciplinary approach that includes team members from the community and home health agencies, as well as from acute care settings, for both short-term and long-term support.

REFERENCES

Birth Trauma

Fanaroff AA, Martin RJ: *Neonatal-perinatal medicine: diseases of the fetus and infant,* ed 5, St Louis, 1992, Mosby–Year Book.

Merenstein GB, Gardner SL: *Handbook of neonatal intensive care,* ed 2, St Louis, 1989, Mosby–Year Book.

Whaley LF, Wong DL: *Nursing care of infants and children,* ed 4, St Louis, 1991, Mosby–Year Book.

Infants of Diabetic Mothers

Cherry SH, Merkatz IR: *Complications of pregnancy: medical, surgical, gynecologic, psychosocial, and perinatal,* ed 4, Baltimore, 1991, Williams & Wilkins.

Creasy R, Resnik R: *Maternal-fetal medicine: principles and practice,* ed 2, Philadelphia, 1989, WB Saunders Co.

Fanaroff AA, Martin RJ: *Neonatal-perinatal medicine: diseases of the fetus and infant,* ed 5, St Louis, 1992, Mosby–Year Book.

Philip A: *Neonatology: a practical guide,* ed 3, Philadelphia, 1987, WB Saunders Co.

Polin RA, Fox WW: *Fetal and neonatal physiology,* vols 1 and 2, Philadelphia, 1992, WB Saunders Co.

Neonatal Infections

Bennett EC: Sexually transmitted diseases: current approaches, *NAACOG Newsletter* 14:1, Aug 1987.

Brown AA et al: Effects on infants of a first episode of genital herpes during pregnancy, *N Engl J Med* 317(2):1249, 1987.

Cherry SH, Merkatz IR: *Complications of pregnancy: medical, surgical, gynecologic, psychosocial, and perinatal,* ed 4, Baltimore, 1991, Williams & Wilkins.

Facing the complex issues of pediatric AIDS: a public health perspective, *JAMA* 258:2736, 1987 (editorial).

Fanaroff AA, Martin RJ: *Neonatal-perinatal medicine: diseases of the fetus and infant,* ed 5, St Louis, 1992, Mosby–Year Book.

Frigoletto FD, Little GA: *Guidelines for perinatal care,* ed 2, 1988, American Academy of Pediatrics and American College of Obstetricians and Gynecologists.

Harnish DG et al: Early detection of HIV infection in a newborn, *N Engl J Med* 316:272, 1987.

Hodson WA, Truog WE: *Critical care of the newborn,* ed 2, Philadelphia, 1989, WB Saunders Co.

Johnson JP, Nair P, Alexander S: Early diagnosis of HIV infection in the neonate, *N Engl J Med* 316:273, 1987.

Landesman S et al: Serosurvey of human immunodeficiency virus infection in parturients, *JAMA* 258:2701, 1987.

Leishman K: Heterosexuals and AIDS: the second stage of the epidemic, *Atlantic Monthly,* p 39, Feb 1987.

Merenstein GB, Gardner SL: *Handbook of neonatal intensive care,* ed 2, St Louis, 1989, Mosby–Year Book.

Prenatal care and HIV screening, *JAMA* 258:2693, 1987 (letter to editor).

Prober CG: Low risk of herpes simplex virus infections in neonates exposed to the virus at the time of vaginal delivery to mothers with recurrent genital herpes simplex virus infections, *N Engl J Med* 316:240, 1987.

Public Health Service guidelines for counseling and antibody testing to prevent HIV infection and AIDS, *MMWR* 36:509, 1987.

Pyun KH et al: Perinatal infection with human immunodeficiency virus: specific antibody responses by the neonate, *N Engl J Med* 317:611, 1987.

Whaley LF, Wong DL: *Nursing care of infants and children,* ed 4, St Louis, 1991, Mosby–Year Book.

Substance Abuse

Abel EL, Sokol RJ: Incidence of fetal alcohol syndrome and economic impact of FAS-related anomalies, *Drug Alcohol Depend,* 1988.

Barbour BG: Is fetal alcohol syndrome completely irreversible? *MCN* 14:44, 1989.

Barbour BG: Alcohol and pregnancy, *J Nurse Midwife* 35:78, March/April 1990.

Bauchner H et al: Risk of sudden infant death syndrome among infants with in utero exposure to cocaine, *J Pediatr* 113:831, 1988.

Bean Y: Report of ongoing research on the infants of mothers using cocaine and PCP, *Los Angeles Times,* Jan 1986.

Becker M, Warr-Leeper GA, Leeper HA: Fetal alcohol syndrome: a description of oral motor, articulatory, short-term memory, grammatical, and semantic abilities, *J Commun Disord* 23:97, 1990.

Chasnoff IJ: Cocaine, pregnancy, and the neonate, *Women Health* 15:23, March 1989.

Chasnoff IJ et al: Prenatal cocaine exposure is associated with respiratory pattern abnormalities, *Am J Dis Child* 143:583, 1989.

Davis DD, Templer DI: Neurobehavioral functioning in children exposed to narcotics in utero, *Addict Behav* 13:275, 1988.

Food and Drug Administration: Caffeine and pregnancy, *FDA Drug Bull* 10:19, 1980.

Hill RM, Hegemier S, Tennyson LM: The fetal alcohol syndrome: a multihandicapped child, *Neurotoxicology* 10:585, 1990.

Howard J: Report of ongoing research on the infants of mothers using cocaine and PCP, *Los Angeles Times,* Jan 1986.

Jackson IT, Hussain, K: Craniofacial and oral manifestations of fetal alcohol syndrome, *Plast Reconstr Surg* 85:505, 1990.

Linn S et al: No association between coffee consumption and adverse outcomes of pregnancy, *N Engl J Med* 306:141, 1982.

Nieberg L et al: The fetal tobacco syndrome, *JAMA* 253:2998, 1985 (commentary).

Niebyl JR: *Drug use in pregnancy,* ed 2, Philadelphia, 1988, Lea & Febiger.

Streissguth AP et al: Fetal alcohol syndrome in adolescents and adults, *JAMA* 265:1961, 1991.

BIBLIOGRAPHY

Birth Trauma

Brooten D: RN follow-up plan helps high-risk infants, *Am Nurse,* Feb 1988.

Troy P et al: Sibling visiting in the NICU, *AJN* 88:68, 1988.

Infants of Diabetic Mothers

Baxi L, Collins MH, Timor-Tritsch IE: Early detection of caudal regression syndrome with transvaginal scanning, *Obstet Gynecol* 75(part 2):486, 1990.

Hoskins SK: Nursing care of the infant of a diabetic mother: an antenatal, intrapartal, and neonatal challenge, *Neonatal Network* 9:39, Dec 1990.

Mills JL et al: Lack of relation of increased malformation rates in infants of diabetic mothers to glycemic control during organogenesis, *N Engl J Med* 318:671, 1988.

Neonatal Infections

American Academy of Pediatrics, American College of Obstetricians and Gynecologists: *Guideline of perinatal care,* ed 2, Oak Grove Village, Ill, 1988, American Academy of Pediatrics.

Boland MG, Czarniecki L: Starting life with HIV, *RN* 54, Jan 1991.

Boucher FD: Infants and the HIV virus, *MCCPOP Newsletter,* Fall 1988.

Bromberg MH, Hsia LS: Rubella in the perinatal period, *J Perinat Neonat Nurs* 1:24, April 1988.

Cohen SP: Bacterial sepsis in the very low birth weight infant, *J Perinat Neonat Nurs* 1:66, April 1988.

Demarini D, Tsang RC: What causes neonatal hypocalcemia? *Contemp OB/GYN* 35:107, May 1990.

Gershon A: Chickenpox: how dangerous is it? *Contemp OB/GYN* 31:41, March 1988.

Gordin PC: Candida infection in the very low birth weight infant, *J Perinat Neonat Nurs* 1:47, April 1988.

HIV infection and childhood sexual abuse, *JAMA* 259:2235, 1988 (letter).

Ippolito C, Gives RM: AIDS and the newborn, *J Perinat Neonat Nurs* 1:78, April 1988.

Karthas NP, Chanock S: Clinical management of HIV infection in infants and children, *Fam Community Health,* Aug 1990.

Klein ME: Hepatitis B virus: perinatal management, *J Perinat Neonat Nurs* 1:12, April 1988.

Laga M et al: Prophylaxis of gonococcal and chlamydial ophthalmia neonatorum: a comparison of silver nitrate and tetracycline, *N Engl J Med* 318:653, 1988.

Marecki MA: *Chlamydia trachomatis:* a developing perinatal problem, *J Perinat Neonat Nurs* 1:1, April 1988.

McIntosh K: Congenital syphilis—breaking through the safety net, *N Engl J Med* 323:1339, 1990.

Meintz SL, Lynch RD: The human right of bonding for warehoused "AIDS babies," *Fam Community Health,* Aug 1989.

Queenan JT: A success story for today, *Contemp OB/GYN* 33:9, May 1989.

Samson LF: Perinatal viral infection and neonates, *J Perinat Neonat Nurs* 1:56, April 1988.

Stear LA, Elinger SS: Understanding acquired immunodeficiency syndrome: implications for pregnancy, *J Perinat Neonat Nurs* 1(4):33, 1988.

Symanski ME: Action stat! Neonatal sepsis, *Nursing 91* 21:33, April 1991.

Substance Abuse

Amaro H, Zuckerman B, Cabral H: Drug use among adolescent mothers: profile of risk, *Pediatrics* 84:144, 1989.

Cordero L, Custard M: Effects of maternal cocaine abuse on perinatal and infant outcome, *Ohio Med* 36:410, 1990.

Eliason MJ, Williams JK: Fetal alcohol syndrome and the neonate, *J Perinat Neonat Nurs* 3:64, April 1990.

Giacoia GP: Cocaine in the cradle: a hidden epidemic, *South Med J* 83:947, 1990.

Hadeed AJ, Siegel SR: Maternal cocaine use during pregnancy: effects on the newborn infant, *Pediatrics* 84:205, 1989.

Kennard MJ: Cocaine use during pregnancy: fetal and neonatal effects, *J Perinat Neonat Nurs* 3:53, April 1990.

Lewis KD, Bennett B, Schmeder NH: The care of infants menaced by cocaine abuse, *MCN* 14:324, 1989.

Little BB et al: Cocaine abuse during pregnancy: maternal and fetal implications, *Obstet Gynecol* 73:157, 1989.

Little BB et al: Failure to recognize fetal alcohol syndrome in newborn infants, *Am J Dis Child* 144:1142, 1990.

Petitti DB, Coleman C: Cocaine and the risk of low birth weight, *Am J Public Health* 808:25, 1990.

Sullivan KR: Maternal implications of cocaine use during pregnancy, *J Perinat Neonat Nurs* 3:12, April 1990.

Zuckerman B et al: Effects of maternal marijuana and cocaine use on fetal growth, *N Engl J Med* 320:762, 1989.

Bibliography—Nursing Research

Levine CD: Premature rupture of the membranes and sepsis in preterm neonates, *Nurs Res* 40:36, 1991.

Oro AS, Dixon, SD: Waterbed care of narcotic-exposed neonates: a useful adjunct to supportive care, *Am J Dis Child* 142:186, 1988.

chapter 39 review

Key Concepts

- A small percentage of significant birth injuries may be unavoidable and occur despite skilled and competent obstetric care.
- The same birth injury may be caused in several ways.
- The nurse's primary contribution to the welfare of the newborn begins with early observation, accurate recording, and prompt reporting of signs that indicate deviations from normal.
- Metabolic abnormalities of diabetes mellitus in pregnancy adversely affect embryonic and fetal development.
- Prepregnancy planning and good diabetic control, coupled with strict diabetic control during pregnancy, may prevent the embryonic/fetal/neonatal conditions associated with pregnancies complicated by diabetes mellitus.
- Regardless of the infant's disorder or condition, the care provider must remember that the newborn belongs to a family that also has many needs.
- Infection in the newborn may be acquired in utero, during birth, during resuscitation, and from within the nursery.
- The best known and most common maternal infections during early pregnancy that are associated with various congenital malformations are represented by the acronym TORCH.
- Transmission of HIV from the mother to the infant occurs transplacentally at various gestational ages, perinatally via maternal blood and secretions, and through breast milk.
- The nurse often is first to observe signs of drug dependence in newborns, as well as to acquire information from the maternal history.
- Providing high-quality perinatal care to a varied population with multiple conditions is complicated by the special needs of high-risk drug-dependent clients.
- Signs and symptoms of infant withdrawal vary in time of onset depending on the drug involved.
- Rehabilitative measures must be included in the plan for care for the newborn and the parent to offer the infant an opportunity for optimum growth and development after discharge.

Key Terms

- birth trauma (injuries) (p. 1180)
- brachial paralysis (p. 1182)
- caput succedaneum (p. 1181)
- cardiomyopathy (p. 1188)
- cephalhematoma (p. 1181)
- congenital rubella syndrome (p. 1198)
- facial paralysis (p. 1184)
- fetal alcohol syndrome (FAS) (p. 1205)
- fetal tobacco syndrome (p. 1210)
- hyperinsulinemia (p. 1185)
- infant of diabetic mother (IDM) (p. 1185)
- infant of gestational diabetic mother (IGDM) (p. 1185)
- intracranial hemorrhage (ICH) (p. 1184)
- macrosomia (p. 1186)
- meningitis (p. 1193)
- mode of transmission (p. 1199)
- opportunistic infection (p. 1202)
- phosphatidylglycerol (p. 1188)
- phrenic nerve injury (p. 1184)
- sepsis (p. 1190)
- septicemia (p. 1191)
- septic shock (p. 1193)
- subconjunctival (scleral) and retinal hemorrhages (p. 1181)
- thrush (p. 1203)
- TORCH infection (p. 1195)
- withdrawal syndrome (p. 1207)

Critical Thinking Exercises

1. Review and discuss the medical and nursing records of infants who experienced birth injury or whose mothers experienced a diabetic pregnancy. Identify the findings that identified the particular risk(s) to the infants. Discuss the nursing and medical management of the infants. Compare with text.
2. Role-play the interactions of a nurse with the parents of a child born with syphilis or other STD, or born to a mother who is HIV-positive or has AIDS.
3. Repeat the above exercise. The newborn is dependent on heroin, methadone, cocaine, or methamphetamine.
4. Complete an assessment of community resources within the neighborhood that offer services to infants compromised by infection and drug dependence and their families. Identify services needed but not readily available or accessible. Justify your recommendations.
5. Discuss social changes that may support the prevention of infection and drug addiction. Consider the mass media, advertising, and other factors.

Topics for Nursing Research

- Identify optimal protocol for assessing vital signs for the infant with various disorders, for example, the infant of a diabetic mother.
- Identify incentives to encourage women with substance abuse problems to obtain prenatal care early in pregnancy.

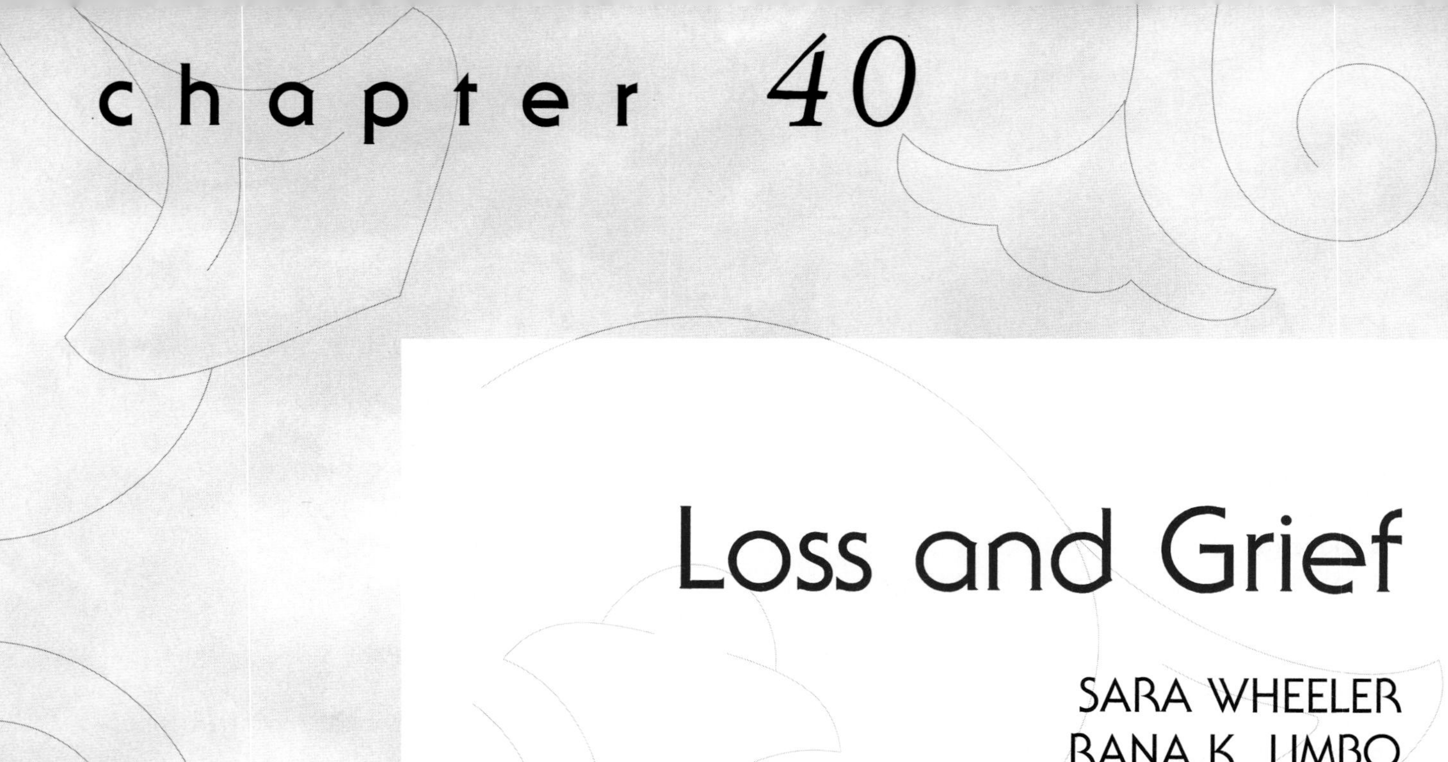

Loss and Grief

SARA WHEELER
RANA K. LIMBO
BONNIE K. GENSCH

LEARNING OBJECTIVES

- Define the key terms listed.
- Relate pregnancy and parenting tasks to unexpected outcomes during the childbearing cycle.
- Describe the bereavement process, including physiologic, psychologic, social, and cultural responses to loss.
- Formulate an example of an appropriate nursing diagnosis related to grief.
- Describe strategies in caring for families who have experienced a loss during the childbearing cycle.
- Develop criteria to evaluate nursing care for grieving families.
- Develop possible responses the nurse might use in communicating with clients who have experienced loss and grief.
- Identify topics for nursing research related to loss and grief.

During pregnancy, new roles and relationships begin to develop among the mother, father, siblings, extended family, friends, and the expected baby. The childbearing process is one of giving up and letting go of previous life-styles, body image, and relationships, as well as taking on new roles and responsibilities and learning how to love someone before one has met them. Before and during pregnancy, parents imagine what or who the baby will look like, how their lives will be changed, and what the birth experience will be like. However, the reality of the childbirth experience rarely matches the parents' dreams and hopes.

There are life crises that can be superimposed on the experience of childbearing when a family experiences infertility, preterm labor or birth, a cesarean birth, any perception of loss of control during their birthing experience, birth of a baby whose gender is not preferred, the birth of a child with a handicap, a maternal death and/or the death of the baby during pregnancy or shortly after (Limbo, Wheeler, 1986b). All of these situations have a common denominator: they are losses of what was hoped for, dreamed about, or planned.

Certainly from the perspective of health care providers, the seriousness of these crises varies. But, from the perspectives of the parents, the perceived loss may be the most terrible thing that has ever happened to them. They never thought that, instead of celebrating life, they would be mourning at a birth. They are among those who have experienced a loss and are **bereaved.** The feelings and emotions associated with bereavement are called grief responses to loss.

The statistics on losses in the childbearing years in the United States are grim. Approximately 750,000 babies die from **miscarriage,** a pregnancy that ends before 20 weeks' gestation. There are approximately 30,000 **stillbirths,** babies who die in utero and are born after 20 weeks' gestation or weigh 350 g or more, depending on the state laws regarding stillbirth. A baby born showing signs of life such as respiratory effort, heart rate, a pulsating cord or muscle irritability is considered a **newborn death,** regardless of number of weeks of gestation. Newborn deaths account for some 30,000 deaths a year. More than 1.4% of all pregnancies result in **ectopic pregnancy,** a pregnancy that takes place outside of the uterus, usually in a fallopian tube. The cesarean birth rate is around 19% nationwide, with some areas being as high as 45%. There is no accounting of the number of pregnancies terminated for genetic reasons (therapeutic abortion or medical interruption of a pregnancy). Approximately 3% of all live newborns are placed for adoption. Also, 1 of 100,000 births will result in a maternal death (ACOG, 1989; Borg, Lasker, 1981; Cunningham, MacDonald, Gant, 1989).

When an individual or family perceives that they have experienced a loss, the role of the nurse is critical. Nurses must be prepared to put aside their own values and beliefs and meet each family member at the point of their need. Their needs are based on the perception each family member has regarding his or her personal loss. In many instances the nurse is also grieving.

A sound theoretic framework of grief theory, communication skills, and caring can help the nurse reach out to grieving families and individuals and provide anticipatory guidance, support, and information. This creates an environment in which individuals and families have the opportunity to feel able to make decisions and not feel out of control, alone, or isolated.

■ THEORETIC FRAMEWORK FOR PRACTICE

Uncomplicated Bereavement

When an individual experiences the loss of a relationship, hopes and dreams for the future end. Reestablishing life without that particular relationship involves a process called **uncomplicated bereavement** or mourning. The subsequent feelings and emotions are called **grief responses.** This process may be a brief, unconscious experience—perhaps a sigh when looking at a daughter when a son was hoped for—or, for others, mourning may last days, months or years. The intensity and length of grief responses depend on the perception of the loss, age, religious beliefs, the life changes brought on by the loss, personal ability to cope with the loss, and support systems (Carter, 1990; Sanders, 1989). Bowlby and Parks (1970) described the characteristics of grief and the bereavement process in their research on separation and loss. Their work was further developed by Davidson (1984) in his research with more than 1200 mourners over a 10-year period. The four dimensions of mourning were identified.

The first dimension is **shock and numbness.** Parents feel stunned with disbelief, panic, distress, and/or anger. This experience can be interrupted by outbursts of emotion. It is difficult to make decisions during this time, and normal functioning is impeded. This phase predominates during the first 2 weeks after a loss. Parents feel as though they are in a bad dream and that they will wake up and everything will be all right.

Searching and yearning can be identified by feelings of restlessness, anger, guilt, and ambiguity. Parents yearn for what could have been and search for the answer for why the loss occurred. This phase is present at the time of the loss and peaks 2 weeks to 4 months after the loss. Parents have said that their arms ache to hold a baby, they wake to the sound of a baby crying, and they have disturbing dreams. They are preoccupied with thoughts about what happened, how they caused it to happen, and the event of the death itself.

Disorganization is identified when mourners turn from testing what is real to an awareness of the reality of the loss. Feelings that occur include depression, difficulty in concentrating on work or solving problems, and a general sense of not feeling well about oneself physically and emotionally. This phase peaks around 5 to 9 months after the loss and slowly subsides. Many parents feel that they will never get over the loss or that they are losing their minds, and they may feel or become physically ill.

Reorganization occurs when the mourner is better able to function at home and work with an increase in self-esteem and self-confidence. The mourner has the ability to cope with new challenges and has placed the loss in perspective. During this phase, parents laugh and begin to enjoy the simple pleasures of life without feeling guilty. Reorganization begins to peak some time after the first year as parents begin to move on with their lives. Families have said they will never forget the baby who died, but they have resumed a "normal" life.

Both men and women express feeling loss of control and loss of self-esteem when unexpected outcomes have been perceived as more than a disappointment. The physical, emotional, and social grief responses to loss encompass many feelings and emotions (see box at right).

Mourning is not a neat and orderly process that moves smoothly from one dimension to another. All of the dimensions of bereavement exist at the same time with one or more predominating at any given moment. There is much movement back and forth among and between the dimensions. The bereaved reveal their mourning through their language, intensity and duration of grief responses, and ability to regain their lives without that which was lost.

Anticipatory grief occurs when families have knowledge of an impending loss, such as when a baby is admitted to a neonatal intensive care unit (NICU) with problems or when a diagnosis of an anencephalic baby is made by ultrasound. The baby is still alive, but the prognosis is poor. Being able to anticipate the loss gives families an opportunity to plan, feel more in control of their situation, and be able to say good-bye in a special way. However, some individuals or family members may distance or detach themselves from the experience or their loved one as a way of preventing or avoiding the pain of loss and grief.

Signs and Symptoms of Grief

PHYSICAL EFFECTS

- Exhaustion
- Loss of appetite
- Sleeping problems
- Lack of strength
- Weight loss
- Headaches
- Blurred vision
- Breathlessness
- Palpitations
- Weight gain
- Aching arms
- Restlessness

EMOTIONAL AND/OR PSYCHOLOGIC EFFECTS

- Denial
- Guilt
- Anger
- Resentment
- Bitterness
- Depression
- Time confusion
- Irritability
- Sadness
- Sense of failure
- Concentration on problems
- Failure to accept reality
- Preoccupation with deceased

SOCIAL EFFECTS

- Withdrawal from normal activity
- Isolation (emotional and physical) from spouse, family, or friends

Tasks of Mourners

Worden (1991) identified four tasks of mourners. In order for the woman and her family to adapt to the loss of their baby or loved one, they should accomplish these tasks:

- Accepting the loss
- Working through the pain
- Adjusting to the environment
- Moving on

Accepting the reality of the loss occurs when the woman and family come to grips with the reality of the loss. Their baby has died, and their lives have changed. Accepting the loss occurs when the woman and family realize the baby has died. Seeing, holding, touching, and memorializing are all ways in which the bereaved can perceptually confirm the baby's death. It is important for the woman and family to tell their stories about the events, the experiences, and the feelings surrounding the loss in order to cognitively and emotionally understand that the baby has died. Caregivers need to use the words "dead" and "died" rather than "lost" or "gone" to assist the bereaved in accepting the reality. This task relates to the first two initial phases of grief.

Working through the pain of grief means that the mourner must feel and express the intense emotions of grief. Not all parents and families experience the same intensity of pain, but it is unlikely that they will experience the death of a baby and not experience some feelings of grief. Society generally tends to minimize grief surrounding the death of a baby because no real social relationship with or attachment to the baby existed, but the familial bonds that develop can be strong. Mothers, fathers, and siblings often develop images of and relationships with an unborn baby even in early pregnancy. Often society equates age and visibility of a relationship with how much mourning is appropriate.

Families who experience a perinatal loss may suppress or deny their feelings because it seems on the surface to be more socially acceptable. The nurse can be instrumental in preparing the woman and family for reactions from others once they leave the hospital or clinic setting. Whether or not a supportive social network is available, a perinatal bereavement support group can help the parents work through their pain by nonjudgmentally sharing feelings (see National Perinatal Bereavement Support Groups, Appendix H). To deny the pain of grief will lead sooner or later to physical and emotional illness. Unfortunately, it is more acceptable in our society to be treated for physical problems rather than emotional ones. When no physical reasons for illness can be found, complicated bereavement may be the source.

Being able to adjust to the environment after the loss means learning how to accommodate the changes the loss has wrought. The loss of a baby means not being able to fulfill the role of mother, father, sibling, or other family members. The bereaved must cope with issues such as deciding what to do about the nursery or the baby clothes, going back to work, parenting other children, getting pregnant again, and handling insensitive family members and friends.

Detachment must occur if the parents are to adapt to their loss. Over time, the bereaved can adjust their view of how the loss has affected their lives. This does not mean they have forgotten about their baby. It means that as the weeks and months go by, they have an opportunity to develop a new perspective, different feelings, and various ways of coping.

Moving on with life, or reorganization, allows the bereaved to love and live again. Once more being able to enjoy things that gave pleasure previously, being able to nurture oneself and others, developing new interests, and reestablishing relationships are all signs of "moving on." For some women and families, the birth of a subsequent child is necessary for them to move on with their lives. A bereaved parent never forgets the precious child, and the memories become bittersweet.

Bittersweet grief (Kowalski, 1984) refers to the memories that linger after the loss has occurred (see "To Jessica," above, and "Bittersweet grief," p. 1221). This grief occurs when someone is reminded about the loss. This can happen typically during birthdays, death days, anniversaries, school events, changes in the seasons, and the month when the loss occurred. The bereaved possess conscious and unconscious psychologic triggers that unexpectedly may remind them of their loved one and the events surrounding the loss.

To Jessica

The candles are lit,
    but no song will be sung.
No laughter, no glee, of my little one
    who would have been three.
If you only knew the plans that would be
    made by your dad and me.
The cake to be baked . . .
The presents wrapped . . .
    and all the funny party hats.
The pictures taken by your dad,
    of course,
As loving friends fill the house.
All of this is not meant to be,
since you were taken away from me.
    No birthday cake . . .
    No presents unwrapped . . .
    No pictures of you in your party hat.
But the candles are lit,
    Never to go out.
For they burn forever in my heart.

Caring

Swanson-Kauffman's (1986, 1988, 1990) research on women and their families who have experienced miscarriage, loss of one of a set of twins, or hospitalization of their newborn in NICUs has identified a theoretic framework for caring for the bereaved who experience perinatal loss. The framework identifies five components in a caring concept:

Bittersweet Grief

To Jessica Mayo -- on Her 11th Birthday
Sunday, November 18, 1990
"The child born on the Sabbath Day,
is bonny and blithe and good and gay."
Sundays are special days.
. . . a day of rest, a day to play.
A day to reflect on days past.
. . . a day to thank God for all that we bless.
I bless your memory.
I wish you were here.
On your eleventh birthday I still want to share.
. . . Your dreams of the future.
. . . Our memories past.
My baby's first cry.
My daughter's first laugh.
I was told you were an angel in heaven above.
Eleven years later, I'm an expert . . .
At long-distance love.
On your third birthday I wrote my first poem to you.
Eight years later, it's still true
". . . no birthday cake,
no presents unwrapped . . .
no pictures of you in your party hat.
But the candles are lit,
Never to go out
For they burn forever in my heart.
Love, Mom"
Kathie Rataj Mayo
1990

- Knowing
- Being with
- Doing for
- Enabling
- Maintaining belief

Knowing implies that the nurse has taken the time to ask questions of the bereaved to better understand what the perception and meaning of the loss is to the woman and her family.

Being with refers to how the nurse conveys acceptance to the woman and her family and how the nurse is able to understand the various feelings and perceptions each family member may have.

Doing for refers to the activities performed by the nurse that provide for the physical care, comfort, and safety of the woman and her family. This may include offering pain medication, sitz baths, maintaining the patency of the IV, postpartum checks, and back rubs.

Enabling requires the nurse to offer the woman and her family options for their care. The nurse must first understand how each family member perceives the loss and what it means to that family member. Offering information, anticipatory guidance, choices for decision making, and support during hospitalization and after discharge helps the family feel more in control of the situation. Enabling raises their self-esteem and allows them to feel more comfortable in asking for options based on their needs for memories and closure rather than what the nurse thinks their needs are.

Maintaining belief refers to the nurse encouraging the woman and her family to believe in their own ability to "pick up the pieces" and begin to heal. The nurse should avoid cliché treatment of the bereaved; rather, the nurse should spend time with the family members in order to see their inner strengths and coping abilities and to point them out to the family.

■ NURSING CARE

The critical intervention time is the period of immediate crisis after the loss. The goal of the nurse is to provide care, support, information, and anticipatory guidance as a help to decision making. The family usually does not expect the loss to occur. The sudden and unexpected nature of the loss contributes to the family's lack of experience and knowledge concerning grief responses and the mourning process, and, more importantly, it obscures the family's need later for positive memories of this tragic time in their lives. It is the nurse's responsibility to be:

1. Knowledgeable about grief
2. Aware of what families might need or appreciate for future memories
3. Able to create a nonjudgmental environment in which families can express their feelings and emotions, make decisions based on needs, and feel support for those decisions

ASSESSMENT

Families who experience a loss may have a variety of feelings and responses. Assessment of the feelings, the perception of the loss, and the events surrounding the loss is important. In supporting bereaved families, it is immaterial how the nurse or others view the event. Feelings of loss and grief are real. The bereaved should not be made to feel guilty or hurt because of feelings they may or may not have, nor should they feel that their needs for support, information, and decision making are unmet because their loss was perceived by others as unimportant.

Some people view an early pregnancy as the union of cells, others visualize a baby, and still others are wrapped up in the thrill of being pregnant. There appears to be a time when cognition and emotion join, and acceptance of the pregnancy means "pregnant with baby" (Limbo, Wheeler, 1986a,b). The point when this occurs varies for each man, woman, and child. Assessing family members' perception of the loss and their perception of the events surrounding the loss is crucial before intervention, especially in the instance of miscarriage, ectopic pregnancy, stillbirth, newborn death, and loss of the "perfect" child.

Helpful questions to ask when assessing the perception of loss might include:

- When did you find out you were pregnant?
- Who have you told about your pregnancy?
- What plans had you made for this pregnancy?
- When was your due date?

The key word to listen for is "baby." The language people choose to use in expressing the perception of the event reveals what they believe they have lost and what it is they are grieving over. In other losses, such as adoption, cesarean birth, ectopic pregnancy, infertility, **blighted ovum** (a pregnancy where the fetus does not develop), and death of the mother, questions that help describe the importance of the event, the lost relationship, and the meaning of the experience help the nurse to determine the perception of the event.

Attention should be paid to family members' verbal and nonverbal responses when they were questioned about the event. Questions to ask include:

- Did they cry?
- Were their verbalizations anger, guilt, or disbelief?
- What did their faces look like when they were telling their story?
- Did they look at you when you asked them questions?
- Was it hard to get their attention?
- How did they answer your questions?
- Did they have a hard time answering even the simplest questions?
- Did their answers make sense?

Answers to these questions are indications of their grief response. Ability or inability to respond to open-ended questions are all clues that help the nurse decide the kind and amount of intervention needed at any given time.

Pregnancy and birth bring about many changes in role expectations, relationships, and self-perception. The perceptions of loss associated with pregnancy and birth may be any or all of the following:

- Feelings of being out of control
- Decrease in self-esteem
- Concerns about fertility or ability to bear children
- Changes in relationships with others, specifically the father of the baby and the woman's mother
- Changes in body image
- Changes in role expectations
- Loss of precious baby or "perfect" child

Again, listening for the words used to describe the experience can help the nurse formulate an appropriate nursing diagnosis and plan of care before intervention.

NURSING DIAGNOSES

Nursing diagnosis may include physiologic and psychosocial problems related to grieving or problems occurring in the grieving process. Examples of nursing diagnoses include the following:

- Powerlessness related to
  - —Hospitalization
  - —Inability to care for self
  - —Inability to communicate
  - —Lack of knowledge
- Sleep-pattern disturbance related to
  - —Grieving process
  - —Anticipatory grief
- Spiritual distress related to
  - —Loss of baby, mother, or "perfect child"
  - —Loss of self-esteem
- Alteration in family processes related to
  - —Loss of family member (i.e., mother or baby, or birth of child with a disorder)
  - —Dissatisfaction over loss of control
  - —Inability to make decisions
  - —Anxiety for not achieving a pregnancy (infertility)
  - —Acting-out behaviors, depression, apathy, or anxiety
  - —Social isolation

PLANNING

During this important step in the nursing process, expected outcomes are based on the mutual goals chosen by the client and the case manager. The goals are prioritized. Nursing actions are then selected to meet the expected outcomes.

Goals may include the following:

1. Family members are able to share their experiences and their feelings of powerlessness, loss

of self-esteem, and changes in their relationships.

2. The woman and her family receive anticipatory guidance, emotional support, and information about the grieving process, their specific responses, and feelings.
3. The woman and her family show increasing independence in making decisions regarding their plan of care.
4. The family's religious and cultural beliefs, rituals, and decisions are respected (see box below).
5. The woman and her family are able to use family and community resources for support.
6. The woman and her family can express satisfaction with their health care professionals.

When these individual goals are met, the ultimate expected outcome—positively integrating the perceived loss experience within the individual and family—can, over time, be met. The family's experience during hospitalization can either become a positive memory or a haunting memory that can last a lifetime. The overall nursing goal is to create a nonjudgmental atmosphere that provides a listening ear, anticipatory guidance, support, and information to help with decision making at the time of the loss and during any follow-up contact after hospitalization.

Cultural and Religious Aspects of Death

BURIAL

Cremation is forbidden, discouraged, or allowed under unusual circumstances for Baha'is, Roman Catholics, Jews, and members of the Christian and Missionary Alliance, Church of Jesus Christ of Latter-Day Saints, and Greek Orthodox Church.

Cremation is customary for Hindus and Unitarian Universalists.

EMBALMING

The body is not to be embalmed, unless required by state law, for Jews and Baha'is.

SACRAMENTS

Baptism is performed only if the baby is living, for most Protestant and Roman Catholic Churches.

Rituals in preparing the body for burial are performed in Judaism, Hinduism, and Islam.

SPECIAL MEMENTOS

Picture taking may be in conflict with beliefs of some cultures, such as Native American, Indian, Eskimo, Amish, Hindu, or Moslem. It would be important to offer a choice for these families. Within the culture as a whole, this may not be acceptable, but within a family it may be a desired memento.

IMPLEMENTATION

Mothers, fathers, and extended families look to the medical and nursing staff for support and understanding during their time of loss (see Research Highlight, p. 1224). They take cues from their health care providers to determine what to do and what their behavior or responses to their loss should be. Many families do not know what they need at the time of loss. Their hopes, dreams, self-esteem, and role expectations have been shattered. However, all families can choose from offered options once they have had time to consider what their needs might be. It is the rare mother and family who know exactly what they need and are willing to verbalize or demand their needs. When a mother or family is able to verbalize their needs, it is extremely important for the nurse to respond positively to that need. The nurse should do everything possible to see that the need is met. Otherwise that unmet need may be the basis of "if only's" that can plague the mother, father, and other family members for a lifetime. Unmet needs can be the foundation for the development of complicated bereavement.

Regardless of the specific loss experienced, all families need the listening ear of the nurse. Therapeutic communication and counseling techniques help the mother, father, and other family members express their feelings and emotions, understand their responses to the loss, and empower them to make decisions.

Communication and Counseling Techniques

Listening is the single most important communication technique nurses have in providing support, care, and understanding. To be a good listener, the nurse should be seated comfortably in a chair positioned at a 45-degree angle about 2 to 4 feet from the person talking. The nurse's facial expression and demeanor should be one of concern and caring.

Ask the bereaved only one question at a time. Leaning forward, nodding your head, and saying "Uh-huh" or "Tell me more" is encouragement enough for the bereaved to tell their story. The use of silence many times gives the bereaved the opportunity to collect their thoughts and to respond to your

Research Highlight 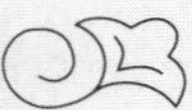

Mothers' Views of Nursing Interventions in Perinatal Grief

RESEARCH ABSTRACT

There are recommendations for nursing care for bereaved parents in the nursing literature. How helpful are these recommendations? The purpose of this study was to describe mothers' perceptions of nursing support during grieving. Thirty mothers whose infants had died between 17 and 41 weeks' gestation were interviewed by telephone between 3 and 9 weeks after delivery. The questionnaire had 15 limited-response and three open-ended questions. The items included interventions currently in use at the data collection site and others obtained from the literature. The most helpful interventions were those that acknowledged the baby including viewing, education about delivery room care, the neonatal unit, funeral arrangements, and emotional responses. Information about sibling coping and a support group was perceived as helpful by fewer mothers. A perinatal grief booklet and support for the baby's father were viewed as helpful by most. Talking with a nurse and receiving spiritual support were helpful. The most important nursing interventions were to stay with the mother and provide attention.

IMPLICATIONS FOR PRACTICE

This research corroborates current literature about what is helpful for mothers who are grieving the loss of an infant. Viewing infants even though they were macerated or had anomalies was helpful for these mothers. This should reassure nurses about the appropriateness of providing viewing opportunities for parents. Careful explanation of the appearance of the infant should occur. Taking time to stay with grieving mothers is essential.

RELATED RESEARCH QUESTIONS

1. What interventions for grieving do fathers perceive as helpful?
2. Do parents' perceptions of what is helpful in grieving for the loss of a newborn differ from what they perceive as helpful after the death of an older infant?
3. Does perception of nursing interventions for grief vary according to culture and ethnicity?
4. Does previous experience of loss affect parents' perceptions of nursing interventions for grief?

REFERENCE

Sexton PR, Stephen SB: Postpartum mothers' perceptions of nursing interventions for perinatal grief, *Neonatal Network* 9(5):47, 1991.

question. Grief responses in the initial days of crisis makes it difficult for individuals to concentrate on what is being asked, to think what the question means, and to respond to the question.

Listen patiently while people tell their story of loss or grief. When necessary, ask questions that help people talk specifically about their grief and the experiences surrounding the loss. Encourage the bereaved to talk about their loved one and what their loss means to them. Resist the temptation to give advice or to use clichés in offering support to the bereaved (see box on p. 1225).

Nurses need to become more comfortable with their own feelings of grief and loss to effectively support and care for the bereaved. It is all right to cry with bereaved families and to share the moment with them; it is not all right to be more emotional than the bereaved, thus placing them in the role of comforter.

Worden (1991) identified several counseling techniques the nurse might want to use in helping the family share and express their grief.

ACTUALIZE THE LOSS. Ask the bereaved questions that help them in expressing the experience of the loss. Make sure to use the name of their baby and, in the case of a death, see the baby before speaking with family members. Questions might include:

"Tell me about your labor and delivery with Lucas."

"When did you know you were miscarrying?"

"What was the most significant thing you remember about Jessica's funeral?"

"Who does Angela resemble in your family?"

HELP THE SURVIVORS IDENTIFY AND EXPRESS FEELINGS. The feelings and emotions of expressed grief can seem overwhelming to the health care professionals who are caring for the bereaved. The feelings of anger, guilt, and sadness are paramount in the early days and months following a loss. When the bereaved are expressing anger, it can be helpful to identify the feeling by simply saying "You sound angry" or "You look angry. Where is this anger coming

What to Say and What Not to Say

WHAT YOU CAN SAY

"I'm sad for you."
"How are you doing with all of this?"
"This must be hard for you."
"What can I do for you?"
"I'm sorry."
"I'm here, and I want to listen."

WHAT NOT TO SAY

"You're young, you can have others."
"You have an angel in heaven."
"This happened for the best."
"Better for this to happen now, before you knew the baby."
"There was something wrong with the baby anyway."
Calling the baby a "fetus" or "it."

from?" Being willing to sit down and talk with them about their anger can help them move past those feelings into their underlying feelings of powerlessness and helplessness.

The bereaved have many questions surrounding their loss, such as: "What did I do?" "What caused this to happen?" "Do you think I should have or could have done_______?" These are all examples of searching and yearning. Part of the grief process for the bereaved is to figure out what happened, what their role was in the loss, why them, and why their baby. The nurse must recognize that the answers to these questions should be answered by the bereaved; it is part of their healing. When a bereaved mother asks, "Do you think that I shouldn't have painted the baby's room? Did that cause my baby to die?", an appropriate response to her might be, "I understand that you need to find an answer for why your baby died. What are some of the other things you've been thinking about?"

Giving the bereaved advice or answering their questions does not help them through the grief process, and many times there are no definite answers why this terrible thing has happened to them. Nurses can speculate, but for the most part they do not know "why."

Being with people when they are terribly sad, crying, or sobbing can be extremely difficult. The initial impulse is to touch them or to hand them a tissue. Although this may seem supportive at the time, the expression of emotion may be stopped or stifled. The bereaved will make it clear when they are ready for a tissue by wiping their eyes or nose, raising their head to look around, or reaching for a tissue themselves.

Careful assessment before using *touch as a therapeutic technique* is important. If touch is used inappropriately, the bereaved will stiffen, pull away, look at where they were touched, or stop expressing feelings and emotions (for further discussion of cultural and ethnic use of touch, see Chapter 3).

In caring for the bereaved, the nurse should have a presence of self—the willingness to be alongside and quietly supporting the bereaved in whatever expression of feelings or emotions are appropriate for them. It is this presence that leaves families with the feeling that they were cared for.

PROVIDE TIME TO GRIEVE. At the time of loss, families become unaware of time frames (e.g., change of shift). When families are pushed or rushed into making decisions, in most cases they will make a decision based on the health care system's need to move things along, not theirs. Nurses should be sensitive to a family's need to spend time with the baby. Providing time to see and hold their baby privately, making arrangements for their baby to be returned to them for further viewing, and not processing consent forms for autopsy or removal from the hospital offers the family the opportunity to further accept the reality of the loss and say good-bye.

INTERPRET NORMAL FEELINGS. Many parents feel that they are losing control when they express the normal feelings and emotions of grief, they are going crazy with the thoughts that plague them about their loved one, or they are totally out of touch when a loss occurs. It is essential for the nurse to verbally reassure and educate bereaved parents about grief process including the physical, social, and emotional responses of individuals and families. Offering reading material on grief process, miscarriage and ectopic pregnancy, responses of family and friends, talking with children, planning a special good-bye, and the differences in how men and women grieve are all examples of the grief education needs of bereaved families.

Offering health teaching on the bereavement process alone is not enough. In the initial days following a loss, it is difficult for parents to cognitively understand what they have been told as well as to remember what has been said. During hospitalization or contact with the nurse, a combination of written material and verbally sharing information can help provide the bereaved with an understanding of their own and others' grief. After discharge, other strategies for providing information and education on grief process include: follow-up phone calls to families the nurse has cared for; offering bereaved families the chance to talk with other bereaved parents in one-on-one support over the phone; referral to a perinatal bereavement support group offering mutual self-help; and sharing a bibliography that identifies books and articles on loss, grief, and perinatal bereavement.

ALLOW FOR INDIVIDUAL DIFFERENCES. Grief is very personal and private. How people respond to loss and grief depends on elements such as age, sex, culture, religion, socioeconomic status, how others around them respond to their loss, and how they coped with prior losses. Within a family, the nurse may observe many different responses. Typically, men want to protect their partner from further pain, or parents and grandparents want to protect their children from more hurt. The underlying feelings of powerlessness and helplessness can be hidden behind expressions of anger, resistance to ideas, overcontrol of situations, or blame. These feelings can leave the partner or grandparent feeling isolated and alone when in fact it is their concern for their loved one that perpetuates the expression of such feelings. The nurse can respond to the underlying feelings by:

1. Recognizing what a difficult time this is for the mother, father, parent, grandparent, or child.
2. Acknowledging how hard it must be for them to feel so responsible for making sure everything and everyone is cared for.
3. Eventually asking them about their own hopes, dreams, and subsequent feelings of loss.

These communication techniques can help the nurse move the resistive person to a position of support where his or her needs also can be met.

Families should be asked at least three times during their hospitalization when important decisions need to be made. This gives them the opportunity to change their mind, to express their needs to each other, and to make a decision based on their needs as individuals and as family members.

Physical Comfort

Coping with loss and grief after childbirth can be an overwhelming experience for the woman and her family. Many times these families request to be moved away from the maternity unit. Their baby has died, and for them, the thought of being on the same unit with other mothers and babies is more than they want to handle. Other mothers, however, may want to remain on the maternity unit, where the staff nurses are better prepared to meet their physical and emotional needs. It should be the mother's choice where to spend the postpartum stay.

When a mother does choose to move to another floor, it is the nurse's responsibility to ensure that her needs for pain medication and for physical assessment of breasts, fundus, lochia flow, and perineum are continued. This may be done through in-service education of nursing staff on units where the bereaved mother and her family are transferred by perinatal nurses or through consultation with the perinatal clinical nurse specialist. Also, the nurse caring for the family at the time of the loss should visit the family after transfer so the family will not feel forgotten.

The physical needs of a bereaved mother are the same as any mother who has given birth. The cruel reality for many bereaved mothers is that their milk may come in although there is no baby to breastfeed, afterpains remind them of their emptiness, and gas pains feel as if there is still a baby moving inside them. Many struggle with the frustration of having to go through all the pain of childbearing only to be discharged home with empty arms. "What was this for?" they wonder. "All they did is cut me up and take my baby from me. I got nothing for all of this pain and suffering when they wheeled me out."

A bereaved mother must have her physical needs met after childbirth; providing postpartum checks, sitz baths, perineal care, pain medication, and information about inhibiting lactation, afterpains, lochia flow, and sexuality after a loss can play a major role in keeping her from thinking that she is not worthy or that she "did not do it right." Hands-on interventions such as help with getting out of bed the first few times, bathing, answering call lights as soon as possible, and performing back massages convey caring in a tangible way. Being sensitive to the needs of the father/partner, such as offering another meal tray, juice, a place to sleep, and perhaps a shower in the mother's room shows that the nurse understands their needs to be together in this crisis.

The grieving process makes it difficult for the bereaved to sleep. Their appetites may be nonexistent or voracious. Adequate rest, diet, and fluids must be offered to replenish the family's physical strength. Discharge instructions, verbal and written, should include the need for food from the five basic food groups, a decrease in food or fluids that contain caffeine, a limit of alcohol consumption and nicotine, an increase in fluid intake to at least a quart a day, regular exercise, and tips on how to rest when unable to sleep. Suggestions for helping the bereaved rest or sleep at night might include taking a warm bath or drinking milk before bedtime, limiting alcohol or nicotine after noon, listening to restful music, and trying relaxation exercises, a nightly walk before bedtime, massage, or, when necessary, sleeping medication. It is recommended that sleeping medication be used every third night to allow the bereaved to do their needed grief work without becoming sleep deprived. Sleep deprivation, poor nutrition, and inadequate fluids can be the forerunner to the development of a clinical depression, which can complicate their mourning process.

Options for Memories

Families need to be involved in the decision-making process. The decisions they make during the loss will be their memories for a lifetime. Offering a choice to parents implies they have the freedom to choose. Choices or options need to be offered in a gentle manner. Parents should not be rushed, pushed, or feel forced to make a decision their health care provider feels would be best for them. In the initial phases of grief, families need to be asked questions at least three times. Shock and numbness make it difficult for them to fully understand the ramifications of the option, let alone making the decision. Time and an environment sympathetic to the needs of grieving families offer them the opportunity to change their mind and not feel bad or as if they have inconvenienced someone.

Nurses walk a fine line between offering the bereaved what they have a right to and making them feel guilty for not wanting to choose those options. Communicating with parents that options are their right, not their obligation, is vitally important.

SEEING AND HOLDING. One of the first options discussed is whether the family wants to see their baby or, in the case of miscarriage and ectopic pregnancy, the products of conception. A statement such as "Some parents have found it helpful to see their baby (or the products of conception)" gives the parents permission to do what might seem odd or distasteful. Responses can vary greatly among family members and between someone who experiences a miscarriage and ectopic pregnancy and someone who experiences stillbirth or newborn death.

Parents appreciate explanations about how their baby looks (i.e., red, peeling skin like a bad sunburn; dark discoloration similar to bruises; molding of the head that makes the head look soft and swollen; or any defects). This helps them in knowing what to expect. The nurse should make the baby look as good as possible. Remember, parents see their baby through eyes very different from those of health care professionals. Bathing the baby, applying lotion to the baby's skin, combing hair, placing identification bracelets on the arm and leg, dressing the baby in a diaper and special outfit, sprinkling powder in the baby's blanket, and wrapping the baby in a pretty blanket conveys to the parents that their baby is cared for the same as any baby in the nursery. The olfactory senses are greatly heightened in the bereaved. The use of powder and lotion stimulates the parents' senses and provides pleasant memories of their baby.

Caring for a baby who has died can be a difficult task for the nurse. It can be made more difficult if the baby has been dead for several days or weeks in utero, before birth. It may be helpful to have a colleague help in making the baby look as good as possible and in taking pictures. In some cases decapitation or dismemberment has occurred. Consultation with a local funeral director can help the nurse prepare the baby to meet his or her parents. If the baby has been in the morgue, he or she can be placed underneath a warmer for 20 to 30 minutes and wrapped in a warm blanket before being brought to the parents. Cold cream rubbed over stiffened joints can help reposition the baby.

When bringing the baby to the parents, it is important to treat the baby as one would a live baby. Holding the baby close, touching a hand or cheek, using the baby's name, and talking with the parents about the special features of their child convey that it is all right for them to do likewise. If a baby has a congenital anomaly, the nurse can desensitize the family by having a perfect hand or foot showing as they approach the parents. Help them explore the baby's body as they desire, pointing out family resemblances or characteristics you find especially endearing.

Be sure to offer the parents time alone. Parents will need to know when the nurse will return and how to call should they need anything. It is difficult to predict how long and how often parents will need to be with their baby. These moments are the only ones they will have to parent their child while their child's physical presence is still with them. Some parents need only a few minutes; others, hours; and still others, days.

A rocking chair can be a soothing place for parents to sit while holding their baby. When parents are ready to return their baby to the nursery, morgue, or the funeral director, they will tell the nurse. It is extremely painful for some parents to say good-bye to their baby. They will tell the nurse they are ready verbally and nonverbally. Being sensitive to their need to accept the loss and cope with the reality of death is essential for their healing.

KNOWING THE BABY'S SEX/NAMING THE BABY. This is an option that can be offered whether or not the sex can be determined. Genetic studies are an option to determine the cause of death as well as the sex of the baby. Naming the baby is an important decision that parents can make. In choosing a name, the baby is made a member of their family, the loss is more real, and it makes it easier for the baby to be remembered in a special way. If the sex of the baby cannot be determined and the parents would like to name their baby, they could choose a special name for their baby, a name already chosen for the sex of the child they hoped for, or a unisex name.

AUTOPSY/ORGAN DONATION. An autopsy can be instrumental in determining the cause of death. For some families this information is helpful in understanding why their loss occurred, processing their grief, and perhaps preventing another loss. Other parents may feel their baby has been through enough. They prefer not to have further information about the cause of death. Also, some religions will prohibit the choice of autopsy for parents.

Options for the type of autopsy are available to parents, such as an autopsy excluding the head. Parents may need plenty of time to make this decision. There is no need to rush them unless there was evidence of contagious disease or maternal infection at the time of death.

Organ donation can be an aid to grieving and an opportunity for the family to see something good come from this experience. The physician is usually the first to offer this opportunity to the family. Organ donation from a baby can occur if the baby was born alive and at 36 weeks' gestation or more. The parents may be offered the opportunity to donate the baby's eyes; currently, all eye tissue from infants is used for research purposes.

BATHING AND DRESSING. When possible, families should be given the opportunity to bathe, dress, and anoint their baby. This can be a very symbolic ritual for many families. Some babies' skins are fragile and may crack or ooze when touched. Parents can still apply lotion with cotton balls, sprinkle the powder, tie ribbons, fasten the diaper, place amulets, medallions, rosaries, or special toys/mementos in their baby's hand or next to their baby. They may want to do other parenting responsibilities, such as combing hair, wrapping the baby in a blanket, placing the baby in a bassinet, or carrying their baby to the nursery. They may have special clothes at home or they may want to purchase a special outfit in which to dress their baby.

PRIVACY. If at all possible, the mother should be admitted to a private room. This offers her and her partner an opportunity to have special time together, with their baby and with other family members. Marking the door to the room with a special card alerting hospital staff that this family has experienced a loss can be a helpful reminder and can prevent embarrassment for the staff and uncomfortable feelings for the family (see Fig. 40-1).

VISITATION WITH OTHER FAMILY MEMBERS OR FRIENDS. Families need to be offered the opportunity to invite their children, grandparents, extended family members, and friends to visit with them during hospitalization and to see and hold their baby. This affords others the opportunity to become acquainted with the baby, to understand the parents' loss, to offer their support, and to say good-bye.

This experience helps parents explain to their surviving children who their brother or sister was and what death means, and it offers the children answers to their questions in a concrete manner, thus helping the children express their grief. Involving extended family and friends enables the parents to rely on the people who will support the family at the time of loss and in the future.

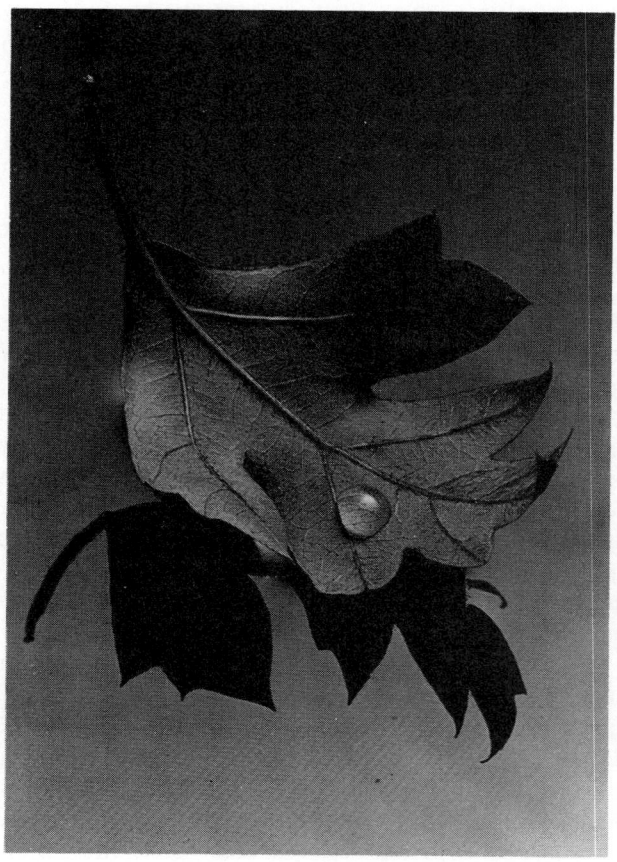

Fig. 40-1 Door card for room of mother who has experienced perinatal loss.
© Resolve Through Sharing, La Crosse, Wisc.

LOCK OF HAIR. A lock of hair may be an important keepsake for the parent's memories. Parents need to be asked first for permission before cutting a lock of hair. Hair can be removed from the nape of the baby's neck where it is not noticeable.

RITUALS OF REMEMBRANCE. Meeting the spiritual aspect of many families' needs at the time of a loss can be important to their care. Support from the clergy is an option that should be offered to all parents. Parents may wish to have their own pastor, priest, rabbi, or spiritual leader contacted, or, they may wish to see the hospital's chaplain. They also may choose neither option.

Members from the clergy may offer the parents the opportunity for baptism, when appropriate. Other rituals that may be offered are: a blessing, naming ceremony, adoption ceremony, last rites, ritual of the sick, memorial service, a prayer, or just their physical presence as a spiritual representative.

FUNERAL ARRANGEMENTS. Parents should be given information about the choices for the final disposition of their baby, regardless of gestational age. In the instance of a baby under 20 weeks' gestation, many hospitals will offer to make the final disposition arrangements. Babies under 20 weeks' gestation are considered to be products of conception. Embryos, fallopian tubes removed with an ectopic pregnancy, tissue from a pregnancy obtained during a dilatation and curettage, and babies under 20 weeks' gestation are all considered tissue or pathology. In most states, if a baby is over 20 weeks and 1 day of gestation or is born alive, it is the parents' responsibility to make the final arrangements for their baby.

All states have laws that govern what constitutes a live birth. In most states a "live birth" is considered to be any products of conception expelled from a woman that show any signs of life. Signs of life are considered to be any muscle irritability, respiratory effort or heart rate regardless of gestational age. All nurses should be knowledgeable about their state's laws regarding what constitutes a live birth, what forms need to be completed and filed in the case of fetal death, stillbirth, or neonatal death, transportation of the deceased and the role of the funeral director in working with bereaved families.

Final disposition of all identifiable babies, regardless of gestational age, includes burial or cremation. Depending on the cemetary's policies, casketed babies or the ashes from cremated babies can be buried in a special place designated for babies, at the foot of an already-deceased relative, in a plot by themselves, in a mausoleum, or scattered in a designated area. Many states have regulations about where cremated bodies can be scattered. A local funeral director or a state's vital statistics bureau should have information about the state's rules, codes, and regulations regarding live births, burial requirements, transportation of the deceased by parents, and cremation.

In making final arrangements for their baby, parents may want a special service. They may choose to have a service in the hospital chapel, visitation at a funeral home or their home, a funeral service, or a graveside service. Parents can make any of these services as special, personal, and memorable as they would like. They can choose special music, poetry, or prose written by others or themselves.

At the funeral home, parents may want to hold their infant again, take pictures, dress their baby, and position their baby in the casket. All of these things are possible with a supportive funeral director who understands the needs of the bereaved parents.

SPECIAL MEMORIES. Parents need tangible mementos of their baby. This again allows for actualizing the loss. Parents may want to bring in a baby book already purchased. Special memory books, cards, and information on grief and mourning are available through national perinatal bereavement organizations for purchase by parents, hospitals, or clinics.

The nurse should record the baby's weight, length, and head circumference. Footprints and handprints should be taken and placed with the other information on a special card, memory book, or baby book. Sometimes it is difficult to obtain good handprints or footprints. Using alcohol or acetone on the palms or soles first can help the ink adhere to make the prints clearer, especially for small babies. When making prints, have a hard surface underneath the paper to be printed. Place the baby's heel or palm down first, roll the foot or hand forward, and keep the toes and fingers extended. It may be helpful to have a partner in doing this procedure. If the print does not turn out, trace around the baby's hands and feet. This distorts the actual size. A form of plaster of paris can also be used to make an imprint of the baby's hand or foot.

Any article that comes in contact with or is used in caring for the baby should be saved, placed in a sealable bag, and given to the parents. Articles should not be washed or cleaned beforehand because the odor will be removed and the parents will not be able to note the scent of their baby. Some examples of articles parents have appreciated receiving are the tape measure used to measure the baby, lotions, combs, clothing, hats, blankets, pacifiers, crib cards, and identibands. Identibands should be placed on the baby before being given to the parents. The identibands help the parents remember the size of the baby and enable them to directly touch something their baby touched.

PHOTOGRAPHS. Pictures are the most important memento a parent can have. Photographs should be taken in any instance where there is an identifiable baby (Fig. 40-2). It does not matter how tiny, what the baby looks like, or how long the baby has been deceased. Nor does it matter what other nursing staff members think about pictures being taken.

Pictures should be taken by an instant print camera, as well as a 35-mm camera. Every effort should be made to make the baby look as good as possible. Pictures should include close-ups of the baby's face, hands, and feet. In some of the pictures the baby should be clothed in a hat or gown and wrapped in a blanket. Photos should also be taken of the baby unclothed. If there are any congenital anomalies, close-ups of the anomalies should also be taken. Flowers, blocks, stuffed animals, or toys can also be placed in the background to make the picture more special and more like a portrait. The parents or siblings may also want to have their picture taken holding the baby. Keeping a camera nearby and taking pictures when parents are spending special time with their baby can make wonderful memories later.

Some parents may have their own camera or video camera with them and would like the nurse to record them holding or parenting their baby during bathing, dressing, or diapering. Asking families in advance what special times they want to record (before knowledge of the baby's death) can help make the most special memories for the family.

Taking the Baby to the Morgue

Before being placed in the morgue, the baby's skin should be prepared by gently putting cold cream on the eyelids, hands, and face to keep the skin from dehydrating during refrigeration. The baby should be undressed, placed on a large smooth blanket, positioning the hands and arms at the baby's sides, above the shoulder (as babies are seen in the nursery), and wrapped carefully to avoid making impressions on the face. If the baby is too large for the casket, the arms may need to be positioned on the chest.

When taking the baby to the morgue, the nurses should hold babies close to their chest, with the face covered. Walking in a purposeful manner and not making eye contact with anyone along the way should keep curious individuals from asking questions. Should the nurse be approached, a response such as "Baby is not seeing any visitors today" will keep people from being further interested. Nurses may want a colleague to accompany them to the morgue, mainly for their own support at that time.

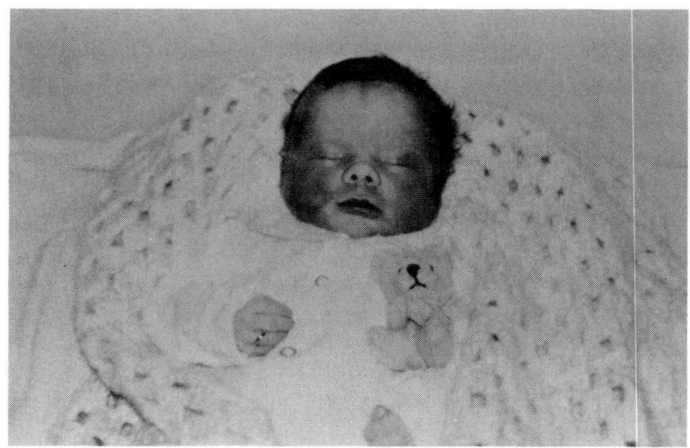

Fig. 40-2 Miranda—Full-term newborn death.
Used with permission, La Crosse Lutheran Hospital, La Crosse, Wisc.

Documentation

Many hospitals have a checklist to use in providing care, mobilizing members of the multidisciplinary health care team, communicating options the family has chosen, and keeping track of all the details in meeting the needs of bereaved parents (Limbo, Wheeler, Gensch, 1988). (See box on p. 1231.) This checklist may or may not be a permanent part of the chart. Documentation in the nursing notes of the primary concerns, grief responses, health teaching, health care advice, and referrals for the mother or any other family members is essential for continuity and consistency of care.

Follow-up after Discharge

Follow-up phone calls after a loss occurs are important. The grief of the mother and her family doesn't end with discharge, but rather really begins once they return home, attend the funeral, and start to live life without their baby. The calls are made to let the parents know they are still thought of and cared about. The calls are made at predictable, difficult times such as the first week at home, 1 month to 6 weeks later (parents should be invited to attend a support group at this time), 4 to 6 months after the loss, the expected date of delivery, and at the anniversary of the death. Families who experienced a miscarriage/ectopic pregnancy or preterm birth appreciate a phone call on their expected date of delivery (EDD). The calls are an opportunity for parents to ask questions, share their feelings, seek advice, and receive information to help them in processing their grief.

A grief conference is an opportunity for families to sit down with their health care providers and receive information about the baby's autopsy report, genetic studies, or just to ask questions they have been wanting to ask since their baby's death. Parents appreciate the opportunity to review the events of their hospitalization, to go over their chart with their physician, and to talk with those who cared for them during hospitalization. The grief conference gives health care professionals the opportunity to assess how the family is coping with their loss, to provide additional information/education on grief, and to share their own feelings and experiences with the family.

EVALUATION

The evaluation of nursing care is made more difficult because of the shock and numbness of the bereavement process and the varied grief responses of the parents and other family members during hospitalization. Families need time to make decisions, the opportunity to change their minds, information on grief responses and the bereavement process, and the caring support of the nursing staff to ensure that

Resolve Through Sharing®
CHECKLIST FOR ASSISTING PARENT(S)
EXPERIENCING
MISCARRIAGE/ECTOPIC PREGNANCY

RTS Counselor ______	Date ______
Mother's Name ______	Age ______ Due Date ______
Date of Beginning of Miscarriage ______	Date of Surgery ______
# of Miscarriages ______ # of Children ______	Religion ______
Address ______	Occupation ______
Phone Number ( ) ______	Marital status ______
Father's Name ______	Age ______ Occupation ______
Address ______	Phone Number ( ) ______
Baby's Name ______	Sex ______
Support people available ______	Children's names: ______
Problem areas ______	Physician ______
O.K. to send written material to home address ☐Yes ☐No	

Date	Time	See Miscarriage Protocol RTS Manual Sec. II p. 21-22	Comments	Initials
		Notify/Assign RTS counselor ☐Yes ☐No		
		Pastoral Care ☐Yes ☐No		
		Offered: ☐Blessing ☐Memorial Service ☐Naming Ceremony		
		Asked: "Would you like someone with you now?" ☐Yes ☐No		
		D&C/Surgical procedure discussed ☐Yes ☐No		
		Saw baby or tissue ☐Mother ☐Father		
		Touched and/or held baby ☐Mother ☐Father		
		If RH negative, RhoGAM given within 72 hrs ☐Yes ☐No		
		Patient's room flagged with door card ☐Yes ☐No		
		Photos taken: ☐35 mm ☐Polaroid ☐Given to Parents ☐On file		
		Footprints & handprints/weight & length: ☐Given to Parents ☐On file		
		Grief process discussed ☐Yes ☐No		
		Incongruent grief discussed ☐Yes ☐No		
		Grief packet given ☐Yes ☐No		
		Info Brochure given to parents re: RTS PSG ☐Yes ☐No		
		Name/business card given ☐Yes ☐No		
		Regular OB/Midwife notified ______ ☐Memo ☐Vervally		
		Childbirth Educator notified ______ ☐Yes ☐No		
		Telephone number verified ☐Yes ☐No Optimal call time ______		
		Preg & Inf Loss Card sent to RTS Secretary ☐Yes ☐No		
		Given option to transfer from Maternity Unit ☐Yes ☐No		
		Genetic Studies ordered/Kevin Josephson, Genetic Associate notified 2771 or 783-6321 ☐Yes ☐No		
		Sex determination desired (tissue in NS only) ☐Yes ☐No		
		Would like another parent to call: ☐Yes ☐No ☐Ask Later Parent contact: ______		
		Follow-up calls: eg. ☐1 wk, ☐3 wk, ☐4 mo, ☐due date/anniv date		

Forms for burial or cremation of:

a) Products of Conception - 2 copies of "Request for Return of Products of Conception to Patients" (1 copy-chart, 1 copy-lab). Obtain forms from Histology.

b) Identifiable Baby less than 20 wk or less than 350 gm - 2 copies of "Request for Return of Products of Conception to Patients" (1-chart, 1-lab). "Notice of Removal" #DOH 5043 - Responsible party for burial signs this form (either parent or a funeral director). Pink copy goes to responsible party. "Final Disposition of a Human Corpse" #DOH 5045 is required for any age identifiable baby that goes across state lines.

Note: Some cemeteries may require a "Final Disposition of Human Corpse" report for their own record keeping.

Continued.

Resovle Through Sharing®
CHECKLIST FOR ASSISTING PARENT(S)
EXPERIENCING
STILLBIRTH OR NEWBORN DEATH

Mother's Discharge Date: ______	Religion: ______
Mother's Name: ______	Age ___ Gr___ Para ___ L.C. ___ Due Date ______
Address: ______	Previous Loss: ______
Phone Number: ( ) ______	Date/Time Delivered: ______
Father's Name: ______	Date/Time Death: ______
Address: ______	Baby's Name: ______ Sex: ___
Phone Number: ( ) ______	Children's Name(s): ______ Age: ___
Optimal call time:	______ Age: ___
RTS Counselor: ______	______ Age: ___
Unit: ______ Ext ______	Support People: ______
Regular OB MD/Midwife: ______	Attending MD &/or Pediatrician ______

Date	Time	Follow Protocol in RTS manual Sec. II, P. 3-8	Comments	Initials
		Notify/Assign RTS counselor ☐Yes ☐No		
		Pastoral Care notified: ☐Yes ☐No		
		Communications notified: ☐Yes ☐No		
		Saw baby when born and/or after delivery ☐Mother ☐Father		
		Touched and/or held baby ☐Mother ☐Father ☐Siblings ☐Grandparents ☐Friends		
		Offered private time with their baby: ☐Yes ☐No		
		Baptism offered: (use seashell as vessel, give to parents) ☐Yes ☐No		
		Remembrance of Blessing offered: ☐Yes ☐No ☐given to parents		
		Given option to transfer off Maternity Unit: ☐Yes ☐No		
		Patient's room flagged with door card: ☐Yes ☐No		
		Autopsy: ☐Yes ☐No Genetic Studies: ☐Yes ☐No Genetic Associate notified: (see note) ☐Yes ☐No		
		Regular Physician/Midwife notified of death: ☐Yes ☐No Memo sent to Physician/Midwife: ☐Yes ☐No		
		Section of Fetal Monitor Strip: ☐Given to Parents ☐On file		
		ID Bands/Crib Cards/Tape Measure: ☐Given to Parents ☐On file		
		Footprints/Handprints/Weight/Length recorded on "In Memory Of" sheet: ☐Given to Parents ☐On file		
		Lock of hair offered: ☐Yes ☐No ☐Given to Parents ☐On file		
		Mementos (clothing, hat, blanket, pacifier, crib cards, basin, thermometer, silk flower) ☐Given to Parents ☐On file		
		Complimentary birth certificate: ☐Given to Parents ☐On file		
		Resolve Through Sharing Photos taken: (clothed, unclothed, w. props, family photo) 1) Polaroid - 3 or more ☐Given to Parents ☐On file 2) 35 mm (6-12 pictures) ☐Given to Parents ☐On file 3) Medical photos: ☐Yes ☐No		

Note: Genetic Associate, Kevin Josephson, ext. 2771 or home 783-6321. Medical Media is available 8-4:30 weekdays for photos (or "on call" nights and weekends if needed for medical photos).

their needs are anticipated and met. Gathering mementos and saving them until the parents are ready to have them, ensuring an opportunity for parents to spend as much time with their baby as desired, and creating precious memories are all important to families healing after a loss. However, it is just as important to respect family systems, culture, and religious practices and to support families when they choose to do things "their way."

The evaluation of nursing care should rest on building an environment in which families can express their grief as well as their needs. The goal for nursing care is to meet individual family members at the point of need and to provide information for decision making and support once family decisions have been made.

A case study and nursing plan of care is shown on pp. 1234 and 1235.

Date	Time		Comments	Initials
		Informed about postponing funeral until mother is able to attend: ☐Yes ☐No		
		Services/Funeral arrangements, options discussed: ☐Self-transport ☐Gravesite service ☐Visitation ☐Hospital chapel ☐Cremation ☐Funeral home ☐Burial at foot or head of relative's grave ☐Specific area for babies in cemetery		
		Funeral arrangements made by: ☐Mother ☐Father Discussed: ☐Seeing baby at funeral home ☐Taking pictures there ☐Providing outfit/toy for baby ☐Dressing baby at funeral home		
		Grief information packet given to: ☐Mother ☐Father		
		Discussed grief process/incongruent grief with: ☐Mother ☐Father		
		Discussed grief conference: ☐Yes ☐No		
		RTS Parents Support Group brochure given to: ☐Mother ☐Father		
		RTS business card given to: ☐Mother ☐Father		
		Pregnancy & Infant Loss Card sent to RTS secretary: ☐Yes ☐No		
		Follow-up calls: 1 week: ... 3 weeks: ... Due date: ... 6-10 months: ... Anniversary date: ...		
		Grief conference planned with parents: Date ____ Time ____ Place ____ Letter of confirmation sent: ☐Yes ☐No		
		Parent Support Group, first meeting attended: Date: ____ Follow-up meetings attended: Dates ____		
		Would like another parent to call: ☐Yes ☐No ☐ask later Parent contact: ____		

Forms: Report of Fetal Death #5402 Rev. 12-86 for ≥ 20 week or 350 gm wt. or more (Photocopy and save for parents)
Autopsy if ordered LLH 40-04P
Record of Death LLH 40-459 if SB or NB death
Genetics Protocol (folder) if ordered - follow checklist front of folder
Notice of Removal of a Human Corpse from an Institution #5043 Rev. 11/86-SB or NB death
Final Disposition form #5045 Rev. 11/86 for SB or NB transported across state lines by parents or for family burial (see note)
If funeral home involved - Final Disposition will be completed by them.
Original Certificate of Death (for NB death only) #5040 Rev. 6-84
Note: If a live birth (NB) death occurs, parent should go to courthouse with Original Certificate of Death and R.D. will assist with forms for Family Burial. A copy of death certificate can be obtained from courthouse for $5.

■ OTHER LOSSES

Perinatal Diagnoses with a Negative Outcome

Early prenatal diagnostic tests such as ultrasonography, chorionic villi sampling, and amniocentesis can determine the well-being of the embryo/fetus. Reasons for doing prenatal testing might include a history of chromosomal abnormality in the family; three or more miscarriages (recurrent spontaneous abortions); maternal age; lack of fetal growth, movement, or heartbeat; diabetes mellitus, or other chronic illnesses.

If the physician's diagnosis is 99% sure that the baby has a serious genetic defect that would lead to an impending death in utero or after birth (such as a congenital anomaly incompatible with life or a genetic disorder with severe mental retardation), the choice of medical interruption of a pregnancy or therapeutic abortion may be offered. The subject of abortion is controversial and may prevent parents from sharing this decision with other family members or friends. This of course limits their support systems after their loss.

The decision to terminate pregnancy paves the way to a variety of feelings such as guilt, despair, sadness, and anger; the nurse's role is to be a good listener. It is important to assess how these families feel about the experience and to offer options for their memories as appropriate. The healing can take place after a family's needs are met and feelings are expressed. The parent who decides to continue the pregnancy will require emotional support as well. Remember, parents may be grieving not only because of the loss of the perfect child but the loss of expectations for their child's future.

CASE STUDY

Fetal Death: 20 Weeks' Gestation

Ann, age 27, is a first-time mother at 20 weeks' gestation who was admitted to labor and delivery after complaining of severe abdominal cramping and leaking small amounts of pink vaginal discharge. Ann and her husband, John, are placed in a private labor room. As the nurse enters the room she hears Ann state, "I don't want to lose this baby—I feel so close to it now that I have felt it move—I'm scared." After several unsuccessful trials of drug therapy to cease labor, and the cessation of the FHR, Ann is being prepared for her imminent delivery. She has been crying and her husband has been holding her hand. He has said nothing about his feelings, but has expressed his concern for Ann.

ASSESSMENT

The situation is assessed as persistent preterm labor despite drug therapy at 20 weeks' gestation. There are no FHTs at this time, and parents have been informed of their baby's death. Ann is scared and upset. Her husband is at her bedside, listening and supporting Ann. He has not shared his feelings yet. They would like Ann's mother to be called and want someone from pastoral care to support "them" at this time. They have no understanding of the labor and delivery process and are unsure if they want to see or hold the baby after birth. Neither Ann nor John have experienced any prior losses.

NURSING DIAGNOSIS

Ann and John have not attended childbirth education classes, nor had they anticipated the death of their baby before hospitalization. Three nursing diagnoses are appropriate at this time:

- Anxiety related to lack of knowledge of the labor and delivery process
- Powerlessness related to loss and grief
- High risk for ineffective individual (or family) coping related to death of a baby

PLANNING

A plan of care is developed with Ann and John's input. The mutually agreed-upon *goal* is to prepare them for the experience of labor and delivery and to offer information for decision making regarding seeing and holding the baby. The *expected outcomes* set by the nurse are that Ann and John will work together for a positive birth experience, they will verbalize their perceptions of loss, their concerns about seeing and holding their baby and will make a decision based on their needs some time during hospitalization.

IMPLEMENTATION

Introduce yourself and immediatedly indicate your awareness of the situation, perhaps saying, "This looks like a very difficult and sad time for both of you." Notify Ann's mother and request pastoral care as soon as possible. Encourage and assist verbalization of feelings of both parents. Be aware of your own nonverbal messages. Provide physical care, and meet the dependency needs of both parents in a thoughtful and unhurried manner. Act as an advocate to the physician regarding parent's questions concerning cause of death and expected events during and after labor and delivery. Fill in gaps in information, and clarify misconceptions. Prepare the parents for the following: What to expect during labor and delivery (e.g., stages, relaxation, breathing exercises, sensations of pushing, and pushing); How John can support Ann (e.g., ice chips, massage, breathing with her, and encouragement); document in chart and checklist options family has chosen; options at the time of delivery (e.g., seeing and holding the baby, what the baby will look like, and private time). If the mother, father, or others (with parent's permission) wish to see and/or hold baby:

1. Prepare family for viewing.
2. Make baby look as good as possible.
3. Provide identiband and bathe, dress, and wrap infant (ask if family would like to do this).
4. Provide for privacy, (i.e., mark door, and stay nearby if needed).
5. Take pictures, footprints, and handprints; record baby's vital statistics and save articles used in caring for the baby.
6. Let family know they can have baby with them anytime day or night.

EVALUATION

The goals were used to evaluate the effectiveness of these interventions. Ann verbalized her needs to the nurse or through her husband. John stayed at her bedside and supported her by rubbing her back, holding her hand, and offering her ice chips. After discussion of what the baby would look like after birth, Ann and John decided they wanted to see the baby. After birth, Ann, John, and Ann's mother held the baby. They named their daughter "Emily Ann." Pastoral care offered a blessing. Both Ann and John verbalized their appreciation of having pictures, footprints, and the memory sheet filled out with Emily's vital statistics.

CARE PLAN Fetal Death: 20 Weeks' Gestation

GOALS	IMPLEMENTATION	RATIONALE	EVALUATION
Nursing diagnosis: Anxiety and fear related to lack of knowledge of the labor and delivery process			
Ann and John will be able to cope with the labor and delivery process.	Explain labor and delivery phases, including pushing and what to expect physically and emotionally. Explain comfort measures for support person to use in caring for the mother, such as ice chips, back massage, and encouragement. Discuss options at the time of delivery.	Prenatal fear of loss of control during labor can be avoided by preparing a mother and her significant other for the process.	Ann and John worked well together during labor and delivery. He held her hand and helped her to breathe.
Nursing diagnosis: Powerlessness related to loss and grief			
Parents will be able to express their needs and make decisions regarding the loss of their baby.	Offer family options for decision making. Provide information when needed and time to make decisions. Use therapeutic communication and counseling skills to support the family's grief responses and help with decision making	Acceptance of the loss is the first task of mourners. Shock and numbness make it difficult to make decisions Offering information and time to make decisions can help to raise self-esteem and promote feelings of some control over the situation.	They spent 2 hours with their baby in recovery and asked to have her brought to them in postpartum unit.
Nursing diagnosis: High risk for ineffective individual (family) coping related to death of baby			
Ann and family will be able to cope with the loss and experience uncomplicated bereavement.	Mobilize family's identified support systems, such as grandmother and chaplain Secure tangible mementos such as footprints, handprints, and pictures. Follow-up after discharge can include phone calls, grief conference, and referral to support group.	Involving family, friends, and clergy mobilizes support for the bereaved parent at the time of the loss and after. Mementos are a tangible memory of their baby and their loss. Follow-up is crucial for the bereaved family not to feel alone and isolated after a loss.	Ann's mother came in to support Ann and John. She saw her granddaughter. Pastoral care offered a blessing. The baby is named Emily Ann. Ann and John verbalized appreciation for their mementos.

Loss of One or More in a Multiple Birth

The death of a baby or babies in a multiple birth during pregnancy, labor, and delivery or after birth requires parents to parent and grieve at the same time. It imposes a very confusing and ambivalent induction into parenthood (Swanson-Kauffman, 1988). Parents feel they cannot do anything right. They cannot parent their surviving child with all the joy and enthusiasm of new parents; their surviving child reminds them of their loss. They cannot give over completely to grieve in the manner they would want to because the surviving child demands their attention. These parents are at high risk for parenting, as well as developing complicated bereavement. They might repress their grief to parent their surviving child, or they may be overwhelmed in their grief and may be unable to parent the surviving child.

It is important to help the parents acknowledge

the dual nature of their situation. They should be treated as bereaved families, and all the options discussed previously should be offered. Pictures should be taken of the babies together and separately. Parents should be offered the opportunity to hold all of their babies in their arms and have private time to say good-bye to the baby who has died.

Bereaved parents should be warned that well-meaning family members or friends may say, "Well at least you have ____" implying that there should be no grief because they are so lucky to have one. Parents need to be able to anticipate insensitivity to their loss and to share with those people that they do not feel that way. By simply setting a boundary on what their feelings are, they are able to acknowledge their baby who died and then have an opportunity to share more about their feelings if they so choose.

Bereaved parents of twins have special problems in coping with their life without their anticipated "extra special" family, telling their surviving child about their twin, dealing with the possibility of that child's feelings of survivor guilt, and deciding on how to celebrate birthdays, death days, or special holidays.

Adolescent Grief

Adolescent pregnancy accounts for approximately 20% of all births in the United States (ACOG, 1989). Adolescent participants have been included in the samples of research done in all areas of perinatal bereavement. This indicates that adolescents do grieve the loss of their babies during pregnancy or shortly after (Bright, 1987; Schodt, 1982).

Lederman (1984) highlighted the significance of the relationship of the pregnant woman to her mother. Many mothers and health care professionals may feel the adolescent's loss of her baby was for the best. Adolescents may not feel the same way and may be grieving the loss of a much-wanted, needed baby.

The first step for the nurse in caring for a bereaved adolescent should be to acknowledge the significance of giving birth no matter what age the mother might be. Second, the nurse should make additional efforts in developing a trusting relationship in working with an adolescent. Third, the nurse should offer all of the options, anticipatory guidance, support, and information to meet the adolescent at the point of her need. It may take longer for adolescents to process their grief because of their level of cognitive and psychoemotional maturation. Being patient, saving mementos, and giving adolescents information on how they can contact the nurse should they have any need is important in helping the adolescent accept the reality of the loss and process their grief.

Maternal Death

It is extremely rare for a woman to die in childbirth, but **maternal death** does happen. Families may be faced with not only mourning the death of a wife and mother, but also the death of the baby. Or, they may be faced with parenting a baby without a surviving mother. "Death of the mother completely disrupts the family structure and often leaves the father with the care of a baby at a time when his emotional reserves are lowest" (Johnson, 1986). The same bereavement process and tasks need to be accomplished for the surviving partner, children, grandparents, other family members, and friends for them to heal after such a devastating loss.

The nursing care of families at this time is similar to what has already been described. Options need to be offered, memories will be made, and mementos will need to be obtained and held for the family until they are ready for them. These families are at high risk for developing complicated bereavement and dysfunctional parenting of the surviving baby and other children in the family. Referral to social services to help the family mobilize support systems, as well as for counseling, can help combat potential problems before they develop and can be beneficial not only at the time of the loss, but in the future.

■ COMPLICATED BEREAVEMENT

Working with the bereaved in the weeks and months after a loss occurs requires knowledge of how to identify **complicated bereavement.** The difficulties an individual or a family experience may be in the grieving of the loss itself or an exacerbation of prior problems that were simply intensified during mourning. Referral to a competent therapist is part of one's professional responsibility to the family experiencing complicated bereavement.

Those who need referrals often experience:

- Symptoms of anxiety or depression that interfere with functioning in any of the three major areas of life: family, work, or physical health
- Persistent thoughts of suicide, which become almost constant, expression of serious suicidal intent, or the development of a plan
- Feelings of being "stuck" in searching and yearning, which is evident by persistent anger, guilt, or obsessive thinking about the loss
- Abuse of mood-altering chemicals
- Relationship difficulties (partner, children, family, friends, or coworkers)

It is the responsibility of a qualified mental health professional to distinguish between uncomplicated bereavement or an adjustment disorder with depressed mood and a major depression. However, there are certain symptoms that can signal the likelihood of major depression, something for which a person should be immediately referred:

- Loss or gain of 15% of one's body weight
- Inability to maintain or initiate basic living activities, including care of surviving children
- Persistent suicidal thoughts with or without intent or plan
- Reclusiveness

These are all red flags for depression. An individual experiencing uncomplicated bereavement who does not have a major depression feels better over time, is sad but functional, and can perform the usual activities of daily living, though not with as much enthusiasm and energy as before the loss.

Finding a mental health professional to consult with is imperative for the nurse doing bereavement follow-up. That person could be anyone who does therapy and is knowledgeable about bereavement and the referral process. Bereavement complications seem to be worked with best by a strong individual therapist with knowledge of family systems or a marriage and family therapist who also does good individual work.

Families should be told about the therapy process.

1. A change in symptoms should occur within four sessions; otherwise there is something wrong with the therapist, therapy, or the mix of client and therapist.
2. All therapists should be willing to discuss with a client their professional degrees, experience, particular strengths, and how they usually work with a similar client.
3. The client should have input into the treatment plan, know what the goals of therapy are, and know approximately how long it will take to accomplish them (i.e., is the therapist thinking about 4 to 6 weeks, or 6 to 12 months?).

Going for therapy is a big step for people. It is helpful to know that the highest number of cancellations and "no shows" in a therapist's practice are first visits. Anything the nurse can do for a family or individual to help with that major hurdle would be helpful. However, it is also important to remember that for whatever reason, people may have symptoms but may not be ready to work on their issues.

SUMMARY

The effectiveness of nursing care can be more difficult to assess when working with families who have experienced a loss. Integrating grief responses to loss and the mourning process into their life experiences takes considerable time and energy. It is important for the nurse to remember that mementos, experiences in parenting their child, and parents' participation in decision-making do not take away grief. Rather, those opportunities build a foundation from which to move forward in mourning without regret. Families usually do not thank the nurse for their care. They may be grateful at a later date. The initial grief feelings of shock and numbness coupled with early discharge leave families feeling overwhelmed and unsure of what to do next, unsure of where to go, unaware or acutely aware of the expectations others may have of them, and unable to cope with social amenities.

Nurses must rely on the hope that they have created a trusting, nonjudgmental, and safe environment in which the family is offered the opportunity and time to decide what their needs are, to what extent they want them met, who will participate in meeting those needs, and, when needed, the opportunity to change their minds about what they will need for their memories. Follow-up after discharge is crucial for both the family and the nurse to evaluate care received in the hospital, and it is an important means of offering continuous, supportive care, which can be evaluated over time.

REFERENCES

ACOG: American College of Obstetricians and Gynecologists Fact Sheet, 1989.

Borg S, Lasker J: *When pregnancy fails,* Boston, 1981, Beacon Press.

Bowlby J, Parkes CM: Separation and loss within the family. In Anthony EJ, Koupernik C, editors, *The child and his family,* New York, 1970, Wiley.

Bright P: Adolescent pregnancy and loss, *MCN* 16:1, 1987.

Cunningham FG, MacDonald PC, Gant NF: *Williams obstetrics,* ed 18, New York, 1989, Appleton-Lange.

Davidson GW: *Understanding mourning,* Minneapolis, 1984, Augsburg Publishing House.

Johnson SH: *Nursing assessment and strategies for the family at risk: high-risk parenting,* ed 2, Philadelphia, 1986, JB Lippincott.

Lederman R: *Psychosocial adaptation to pregnancy,* Englewood Cliffs, NJ, 1984, Prentice Hall.

Limbo RK, Wheeler SR: *When a baby dies: a handbook for healing and helping,* La Crosse, Wis, 1986a, Lutheran Hospital.

Limbo RK, Wheeler SR: *Coping with unexpected outcomes, NAACOG Update Series* 5(3):1, 1986b.

Limbo RK, Wheeler SR, Gensch BK: *Resolve through sharing counselor's certification manual,* La Crosse, Wis, 1988, Lutheran Hospital.

Sanders CM: *Grief, the mourning after: dealing with adult bereavement,* New York, 1989, Wiley Interscience.

Schodt C: Grief in adolescent mothers after an infant death, *Image* 14:20, 1982.

Swanson-Kauffman KM: Caring in the instance of unexpected early pregnancy loss, *Top Clin Nurs* 8(2):37, 1986.

Swanson-Kauffman KM: There should have been two: nursing care of parents experiencing perinatal death of a twin, *J Perinat Neonat Nurs* 2(2):78, 1988.

Swanson-Kauffman KM: Providing care in the NICU: sometimes an act of love, *Adv Nurs Science* 13(1):1990.

Worden WJ: *Grief counseling and grief therapy: a handbook for the mental health practitioner,* New York, 1991, Springer.

References—Nursing Research

Carter S: Themes of grief, *Nurs Res* 38:6, 1989.

Kowalski K: *Perinatal death: an ethnomethodological study of factors influencing perinatal bereavement,* unpublished doctoral dissertation, Denver, 1984, University of Colorado.

BIBLIOGRAPHY

Arnold J: Grieving, *NSNS/Imprint* Feb/March:43, 1990.

Costello A, Gardner SL, Merenstein GB: Perinatal grief and loss, *J Perinatol* 8(4):361, 1988.

Furrh CB, Copley R: One precious moment. *Nursing 89,* p 52, Sept 1989.

Green D, Malin J: When reality shatters parents' dreams. *Nursing 88,* p 64, Feb 1988.

Hainsworth M: Women in grief, *Persp Psych Care* 24(3/4):85, 1987/88.

Henshaw SK, Van Vort J: Teenage abortion, birth and pregnancy statistics: an update, *Fam Plan Pers* 21(2):85, 1989.

Hutti MH: A quick reference table of interventions to assist families to cope with pregnancy loss or neonatal death, *Birth* 15(1)33, 1988.

Ilse S, Furrh CB: Development of a comprehensive follow-up care plan after perinatal and neonatal loss, *J Perinat Neonat Nurs* 2(2):23, 1988.

Krone C, Harris CC: The importance of infant gender and family resemblance within parents' perinatal bereavement process: establishing personhood, *J Perinat Neonat Nurs,* 2(2):1, 1988.

Limbo RK, Wheeler SR: Women's response to the loss of their pregnancy through miscarriage: a longitudinal study, forum newsletter, *Assoc Death Educ Couns* 10(4):1-2, 1986.

Murray J, Callan VJ: Predicting adjustment to perinatal death, *Br J Med Psych* 61:237, 1988.

Ransohoff-Alder M, Berger CS: When newborns die: do we practice what we preach? *J Perinatol* 9(3):311, 1989.

Smith AC, Borgers SB: Parental grief response to perinatal death, *Omega* 19(3):203, 1988.

Theut SK et al: Perinatal loss and parental bereavement, *Am J Psych* 146(5):635, 1989.

Wilson AL, Soule DJ, Fenton LJ: The next baby: parents' responses to perinatal experiences subsequent to a stillbirth, *J Perinatol* 5:188, 1988.

Zeanah CH: Adaptation following perinatal loss: a critical review, *J Am Acad Child Adolesc Psychiatry* 28:467, 1989.

Bibliography-Nursing Research

Carter SL: Themes of grief, *Nurs Res* 38(6):354, 1989.

Cowan ME, Murphy SA: Identification of postdisaster bereavement risk predictors, *Nurs Res* 34(2):71, 1985.

Demi AS, Miles MS: Bereavement, *Annu Rev Nurs Res* 4:105, 1986.

Gifford BJ, Cleary BB: Supporting the bereaved, *AJN* (2):49, 1990.

Gilbert KB: Interactive grief and coping in the marital dyad, *Death Studies* 13:605, 1989.

Hutti MH: An examination of perinatal death literature: implications for nursing practice and research, *Health Care for Women International* 5:387, 1984.

Page-Lieberman J, Hughes CB: How fathers perceive perinatal death, *MCN* 15:320, 1990.

Reed K: Influence of age and parity on the emotional care given to women experiencing miscarriages, *Image* 22(2):89, 1990.

chapter 40 review

Key Concepts

- Parental and infant attachment can begin before pregnancy with many hopes and dreams for the future.
- The gestational age of the baby does not influence the severity of the grief response or bereavement process.
- When a baby dies, all members of a family are affected, but no two family members will grieve in the same way.
- When birth becomes death, the role of the nurse is critical in caring for the woman and her family regardless of the woman's age.
- An understanding of grief responses and the bereavement process is fundamental in the implementation of the nursing process.
- Careful assessment of each family member's perception of the loss is important before intervention.
- Therapeutic communication and counseling techniques can help families identify their feelings, feel comfortable in expressing their grief, and understand their bereavement process.
- Follow-up after discharge is an essential component in providing care to families who have experienced a loss.
- Nurses need to be aware of their own feelings of grief and loss in order to provide a nonjudgmental environment of care and support for bereaved families.

Key Terms

- anticipatory grief (p. 1219)
- bereaved (p. 1218)
- bittersweet grief (p. 1220)
- blighted ovum (p. 1222)
- complicated bereavement (p. 1236)
- disorganization (p. 1219)
- ectopic pregnancy (p. 1218)
- grief responses (p. 1218)
- maternal death (p. 1236)
- miscarriage (p. 1218)
- mourning (p. 1219)
- newborn death (p. 1218)
- reorganization (p. 1219)
- searching and yearning (p. 1218)
- shock and numbness (p. 1218)
- stillbirth (p. 1218)
- uncomplicated bereavement (p. 1218)

Critical Thinking Exercises

1. Interview labor-delivery nurses who in their work have experienced the birth of an imperfect child or an unexpected fetal death. What were their feelings? What were the behaviors of staff persons? Who assisted the parents?
   a. After viewing a film on death and grieving, discuss the kinds of behavior the group observed of the grieving person.
   b. Invite a speaker from a local support group to describe her or his work with parents and families.
   c. Develop a role-playing situation wherein a student acts as a nurse assisting parents of an imperfect child. Anticipate meetings with older children, families, and friends.
2. Compare and contrast the grieving process as it might affect the family experiencing the fetal death of a perfect child and the family whose child is born with a defect.

Topics for Nursing Research

- Adolescent grief after a perinatal loss
- Subsequent pregnancy after a loss
- Subsequent parenting after a loss
- Grief in placing a baby for adoption
- Effectiveness of perinatal bereavement self-help support groups
- Grief after a medical interruption of a pregnancy
- When one of a set of twins dies: The parenting and grieving experience
- Siblings' grief after perinatal loss
- Effect of a perinatal loss on the subsequent child
- Cultural responses to perinatal loss
- The phenomena of bittersweet grief
- The experience of miscarriage: does everybody grieve?
- Nurse's perceptions of perinatal loss and the subsequent effect on client care

unit 8

Women's Health

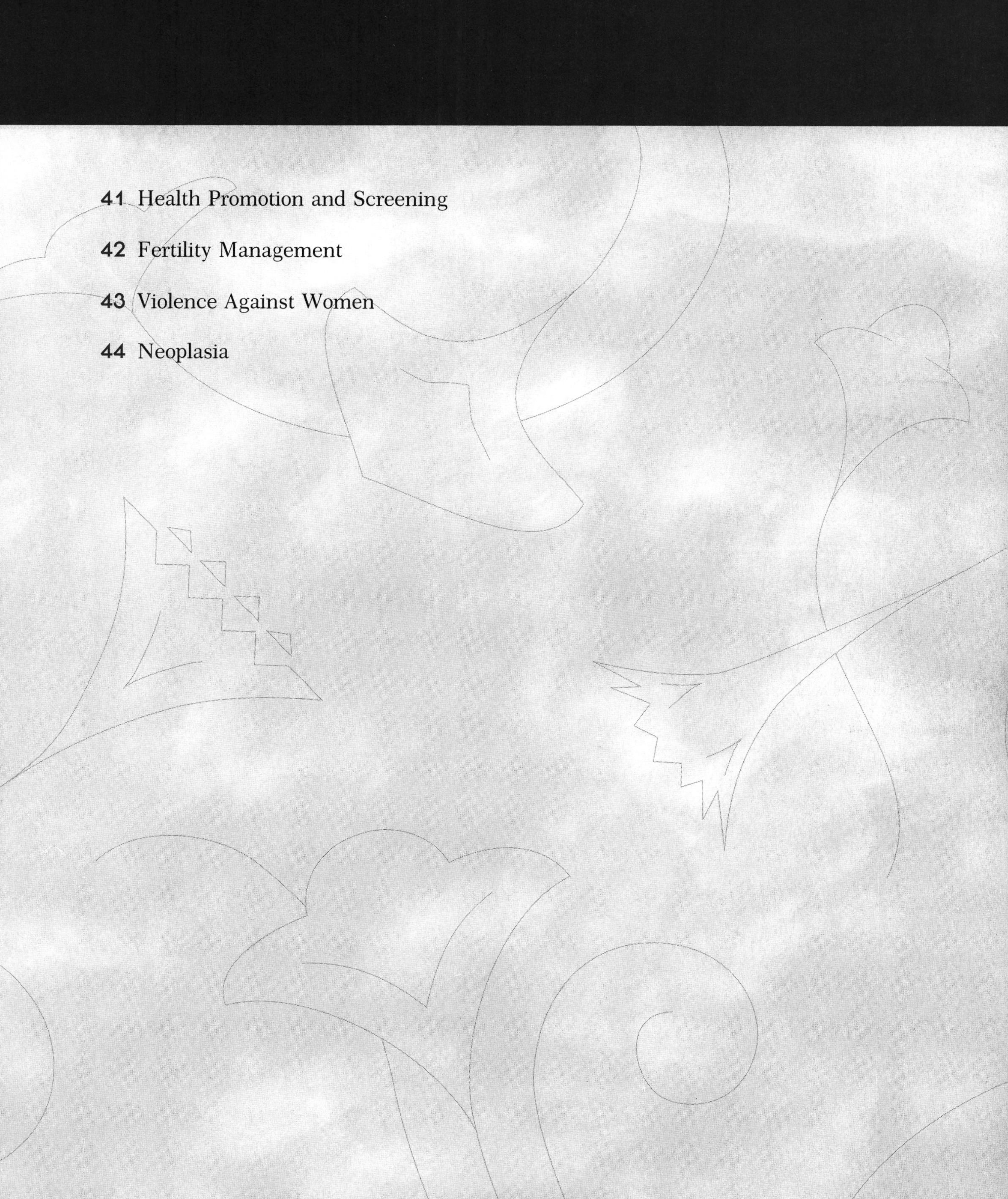

chapter 41

Health Promotion and Screening

EDNA B. QUINN

LEARNING OBJECTIVES

- Define the key terms listed.
- List factors influencing a woman's contact with the health care system.
- Outline the schedule for women's health promotion and screening.
- Identify reasons women enter the health care delivery system.
- Explain how well women's health assessment varies with culture, age, physical handicaps, and family abuse.
- Review important considerations in screening for cervical cancer.
- Review client teaching of breast self-examination.
- Describe sequelae associated with injuries of the birth canal.
- Develop a nursing care plan for the woman with primary dysmenorrhea.
- Outline client teaching about premenstrual syndrome.
- Relate the pathophysiology of endometriosis to associated symptoms.
- Develop an assessment guide for women experiencing the climacterium.
- Develop a nursing care plan for the woman experiencing the postclimacterium.
- Suggest community resources helpful to women of all ages.
- Identify topics for nursing research related to health promotion and screening.

This chapter deals with those aspects of women's health promotion and screening not covered elsewhere in this text or in basic physical assessment texts. It highlights assessment of older women, abused women, and women with disabilities. Cultural considerations in gynecologic care are included, and concerns related to screening for breast and cervical cancer are discussed. The most common problems associated with the menstrual cycle, long-term sequelae of childbirth trauma, and difficulties during the climacteric and postclimacteric periods associated with normal changes in the reproductive and genitourinary systems are also discussed.

In the reproductive years, health promotion takes place for most women in prenatal and family planning care settings. Their care is discussed elsewhere in this text. It is assumed that the reader is familiar with the health history and the gynecologic examination (details of history taking and gynecologic physical assessment are found in Chapters 6 and 11). Newborn through adolescent assessment is discussed in pediatric nursing texts.

■ WELL WOMAN HEALTH CARE

The rising expectations of women, as well as profound changes in the family, society, and sexual behavior, make women's health promotion a challenging field. For years the traditional medical system, either consciously or unconsciously, oppressed and exploited women "for their own good" (Ehrenreich, English, 1978). In the 1970s, many women sought alternatives to what they perceived as insensitive and sexist treatment, and the women's self-help movement was born. Groups of women established and ran their own clinics, providing services and educational programs. Women in the movement were determined to learn more about their own bodies, and they demanded the right to make decisions regarding their health care in active participation with care providers.

Today "a host of alternative health care systems have emerged in response to the perceived inattention of the traditional medical community to wellness issues" (Stotland, 1990, p. 7). Women are continuing to question and change the traditional system. The American Nurses Association has made women's health issues a priority for 1992, focusing on two major concerns: the lack of women in scientific studies and the lack of research on diseases that disproportionately affect women, such as breast cancer and osteoporosis. Space does not permit a detailed discussion of the women's health movement and the issues that gave rise to it, but nurses should understand this historical background for women's health care.

Health promotion and disease prevention are directed toward screening for disease or environmental hazards and maintaining and enhancing wellness. A major thrust of care is educating women about the impact that life-style has on health status and the risks involved if they abuse their health.

The fact that most women are interested in participating in decision-making and self-care gives the nurse a unique opportunity. As a change agent and client advocate intent on promoting "enabling" behaviors, the nurse can increase women's knowledge and self-esteem so that they will become active and satisfied participants in their own health care.

■ NURSING PROCESS

Nursing is an interactive process that involves establishing relationships within the broad goal of maintaining and enhancing health. Clients are able to sense genuine concern and caring. The nurse must not act authoritarian but should provide support, counsel, and information, enabling the woman to make informed, competent decisions about her health care. Support and reassurance begins with the woman's first contact with the entire health care staff.

It is often the nurse's responsibility in health promotion to coordinate the client's care according to set guidelines and protocols, such as the U.S. Preventive Services Task Force's Guide to Clinical Preventive Services (1989). A nurse often takes the history, orders diagnostic tests, interprets test results, makes referrals, and calls the attention of the physician to problems that require medical attention. Nurses functioning in the extended role perform the physical assessment, including the gynecologic examination, in well women.

Guidelines should be applied with an awareness of common problems in different populations and respect for the unique qualities of each client.

Nursing diagnoses are based on the assessment and are negotiated with the client. They generate client-centered goals for interventions, such as educational strategies, counseling, appropriate referrals, and evaluation of outcomes.

ASSESSMENT

SCHEDULE FOR SCREENING. Protocols may recommend periodic visits every 1 to 3 years, depending on the age and risk status of the client. Annual visits that include history, height and weight, blood pressure, clinical breast exam, pelvic exam, and Papanicolaou smear (Pap test) are the norm. The American Cancer Society recommends a baseline screening mammography for women between ages 35 and 40, and then one every 1 to 2 years until age 50. Mammography is advised every year for women beginning at age 50. Recent research indicates it substantially reduces deaths from breast cancer in women over 40 (Denny, Koren, Wisby, 1989). The following laboratory and diagnostic procedures are ordered at the discretion of the clinician: hemoglobin, nonfasting total blood cholesterol, fasting plasma glucose, urinalysis for bacteria, VDRL and other screening tests for sexually transmitted diseases, tuberculin skin test, hearing, electrocardiogram, fecal occult blood, and bone mineral content.

REASONS FOR ENTERING THE HEALTH CARE SYSTEM. Many women first enter the health care delivery system for a Pap test or contraception. Visits to the gynecologist, nurse-practitioner, or nurse-midwife may be their only contact with the system unless they become ill. Some women postpone examination until a specific need arises, such as pregnancy, pain, abnormal bleeding, or incapacitating vaginal discharge. Embarrassing signs and symptoms, such as urinary incontinence, dyspareunia (painful intercourse), and annoying vaginal discharge, are often only elicited by sensitive interviewing and careful examination. Other women report a minor symptom as a "ticket" for entering the health care system when other motives for seeking care, either conscious or unconscious, underlie their primary complaint. It is not uncommon for serious concerns (fear of pregnancy, sexually transmitted disease, or cancer; sexual functioning; or perimenopausal events) to surface during the interview.

Health care needs will vary with culture and religion, age, and personal differences. The changing status and roles of women, socioeconomic status, and personal circumstances contribute to differences in the health behavior of women. Women of higher socioeconomic status are more likely to recognize the need for care and seek preventive services (Fogel, Woods, 1981). Employment outside the home, physical disability, a change in residence, separation or divorce, single parenthood, and widowhood affect women's ability to seek care.

THE INTERVIEW. The data base should be collected in an unhurried manner, with questions phrased in a sensitive, nonjudgmental manner. Body language should match verbal communication. The nurse must recognize the woman's *vulnerability* and assure the woman of *strict confidentiality*. For many women, modesty and fear of the unknown make the assessment—the interview, the physical examination, and particularly the pelvic examination—an ordeal. Even in this age of "enlightenment," many women are uninformed, misguided by myths, or afraid to appear stupid by asking questions about sexual and reproductive functioning.

Areas to explore with all women include social support, economic resources, exercise and recreational activity, sleep patterns, sexuality, alcohol and drug intake, and use of the health care system.

CULTURAL CONSIDERATIONS. Recognition of signs and symptoms of disease, as well as deciding when to seek treatment, are influenced by *cultural perceptions*. Every society has culture-specific beliefs and extensive prescriptions regarding sexuality and reproduction.

In the United States, premarital sexual activity, often with multiple partners or partners of the same or opposite sex, has become increasingly acceptable, contributing to the increased incidence of unplanned pregnancy, sexually transmitted diseases, and cervical dysplasia and neoplasms. On the other hand, in many other cultures, knowledge of sexual matters is limited, and explicit graphic reproduction of the genitals is forbidden. The reputation and status of the entire family may rest on the woman's marital fidelity and premarital virginity (Laffin, 1975). Therefore, to ensure an intact hymen (or proof of virginity) tampons and douches are avoided, and medical examination of the vaginal vault is limited to a one-finger internal examination and the use of the smallest available speculum (see Fig. 11-4). A female attendant should always chaperone the pelvic examination when the examiner is male.

THE OLDER WOMAN. The older woman can present a challenge in taking a history. Multiple chronic and debilitating health problems often overlap with the process of aging, and signs and symptoms of disease may be less dramatic, producing only vague complaints. Confusion, for example, may be the only symptom of an infection or cerebrovascular accident. Older people are at greater risk of developing painful conditions or injuries, but pain may be an unreliable symptom. They seem to lose pain perception or experience pain differently. If many conditions present simultaneously, the cause of pain may be difficult to isolate (Witte, 1989).

Some women fail to report symptoms because they fear the complaint will be attributed to old age or that nothing can be done. They may have lived with a chronic condition for so long that they have come to accept the symptoms as part of daily life. Denny, Koren, Wisby (1989) reported that one third of women seen in nurse-managed clinics for the elderly in Chicago suffered from stress incontinence and had never sought help.

The tendency for multiple problems to be treated with many drugs puts the older person at risk for iatrogenic disorders. A complete medication history is essential, with special attention to the interaction of drugs, diseases, and the aging process.

Functional assessment should be included as part of the older woman's history. In the review of systems, the nurse needs to ask about self-care activities such as walking, getting out of bed, getting to the bathroom, bathing, combing the hair, dressing, and eating. Questions about driving a car or using public transportation, dialing the telephone, hanging up clothes, getting groceries, and preparing meals should also be included. It is important to assess whether the client is able to take medications correctly.

THE WOMAN WITH A DISABILITY. Clients with serious physical or emotional disorders—the deaf, the blind, the depressed, the physically disabled, the mentally retarded, and the brain injured—must all be respected and fully involved in the assessment to the limit of their ability. The nurse should communicate directly with the client with a disability, maintaining eye contact; it is best to learn about the disability from the client. When the family is available, they can often advise on communication techniques used successfully at home. If there is a language barrier, a translator should be used. A translator who signs may be available for the deaf, but most deaf people read, write, and read lips, so that an interviewer who speaks and enunciates each word slowly and in full view may be understood. The blind can usually hear, and the nurse should avoid two common pitfalls with these clients—trying to communicate with gestures, and talking louder in hopes of being understood (care providers also tend to speak louder when trying to communicate with non–English-speaking clients).

Clients with emotional problems may not be able to give a reliable history, but their points of view and attitudes should be obtained from *them* to the extent possible. The client's record and, when necessary, the family and other health professionals involved in care, must be consulted.

ABUSED WOMEN. When seeing any woman, the nurse must keep in mind the possibility that violence against the woman may have occurred (for further discussion, see Chapter 43). Abuse is a life-threatening health problem that affects millions of women and their children. Many care providers defer questions about family violence because they are unaware of the extent of the problem or they find it difficult to ask about violence. Just as they learn to ask other intimate questions, nurses can learn to inquire about this problem. Help depends on early detection and intervention. Fear, guilt, and embarrassment keep many women from giving information about family violence. Clues in the history (e.g., numerous injuries and stress-related symptoms) and evidence on physical examination of injuries, such as burns or lacerations, should alert the nurse to the problem. Assessment requires a detailed history of the woman's investment in her situation and active listening. The nurse helps the woman formulate a plan: What referral options (local agencies and shelters) can help her? If she plans to return home, how will she manage? The nurse's goal is to empower the woman; she needs to gain a feeling of control over her life, to set her own goals and make her own decisions. Misinformation and resorting to legal avenues can be dangerous. It is important for the nurse to communicate two messages: (1) that the nurse is deeply concerned and (2) that the woman does not deserve to be abused (King, 1989).

CONCLUDING QUESTIONS. At the conclusion of the interview, the nurse should ask, "Is there anything else you think would be important for me to know?" If several complaints are mentioned in the history, it is often useful to ask, "What problem concerns you most?" With vague, complicated, or contradictory histories, it may be helpful to ask, "What do you think is the matter with you?"

PHYSICAL EXAMINATION. Physical examination may not always include a pelvic exam. Regardless of whether a complete gynecologic examination is indicated, an atmosphere conducive to privacy, with respect for the client's dignity and culture, should be provided. Basic content on the physical examination is found in Chapter 11. Since the most critical parts of the examination are the breast examination and the Papanicolaou (Pap) smear included in the pelvic examination, this chapter will focus on them.

BREAST SELF-EXAMINATION (BSE). The breast examination provides an ideal opportunity to teach or review BSE. Monthly BSE is recommended, but most women practice it far less often, and some women do not perform it at all. Nursing research indicates that positive attitudes toward the BSE, social influences, and the stated intention to perform BSE correlate well with the behavior (Lierman et al, 1990) (see Research Highlight, p. 1249). The nurse should explore these influences and encourage the client to verbalize (and thereby reinforce) her intention to per-

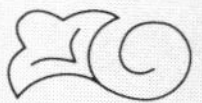 **Research Highlight** 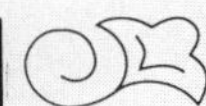

Adherence to Breast Self-Examination in Older Women

RESEARCH ABSTRACT

The purpose of this study was to examine the relations between parts of a modified theory of reasoned action and to explore differences in these model parts between older women who perform breast self-examination (BSE) frequently and those who perform BSE infrequently. The theory of reasoned action assumes that people are rational and that they can control their behavior. Behavior will not always be reasonable, but it will be logical. The theory states that the intention to perform is the best predictor of behavior. Ninety-three volunteers from 52 to 90 years of age participated in the study. Questionnaires were distributed in 12 women's church groups. The questionnaires were completed anonymously and returned in stamped, self-addressed envelopes. The response rate was 60%. The questionnaires were developed by the researchers and measured behavior, behavioral intention, affect, attitude, social norm, personal normative belief, and facilitating factors. The researchers found that during the previous 6 months, the frequency of BSE ranged from 0 (13%) to 6 or more (29.4%). The intention to perform ranged from −3 (7.5%) to +3 (14%). Intention to perform BSE and BSE performance were strongly correlated (.75). Attitude was more strongly related than social norm with intention and BSE performance. In addition, women who thought breast cancer would have a great effect on their lives performed BSE less often. There were significant differences between groups (frequent and infrequent BSE performers) on all study variables.

IMPLICATIONS FOR PRACTICE

Women who performed BSE infrequently thought it was difficult, not necessary, a waste of time, and hard to remember. They also lacked confidence in their ability to perform BSE correctly and were more fearful of reporting a lump to a physician. Frequent performers had significant social support for the examinations. The differences between the two groups indicate there is a need for professional instruction in BSE. Nurses should encourage infrequent performers to enlist their social network to support their performance of BSE.

RELATED RESEARCH QUESTIONS

1. Will an educational program directed at a woman's social network increase her frequency of BSE?
2. Is there a relation between the size of a woman's breast and the frequency and accuracy of BSE?
3. Is there a relation between sexual preference and frequency of BSE?
4. Is there a relation between frequency of BSE and perceptions of the breasts as sexual organs as compared to perceptions of the breasts as organs for nourishment?

REFERENCE

Lierman LM, Kasprzyk D, Beloliel JQ: Understanding adherence to breast self-examination in older women, *West J Nurs Res* 13(1):46, 1991.

form BSE monthly. Return demonstration is essential; this allows for correction where there is error, and reinforcement of the woman's confidence in self-care ability (Fig. 41-1).

Nemcek (1990) found that difficulty in remembering when to perform BSE, fear of finding a lump, perceived inability to recognize lumps, and embarrassment were barriers to BSE in a study of 95 African-American women. For each woman, barriers must be assessed and strategies to overcome them must be individualized. The extra time these efforts take may save a life. Breast cancer is the leading cause of cancer deaths in women, but when the tumor is localized, the survival rate approaches 100% (Nemcek, 1990). Most tumors are discovered by the woman herself.

PELVIC EXAMINATION. The gynecologic examination does not differ markedly from the rest of the physical examination except that it is a more intimate and invasive procedure and requires specialized skills and greater sensitivity on the part of the examiner. A positive attitude can do much to make it less threatening. Women need procedure-specific, concrete, objective information along with self-care instructions during stressful medical procedures (Barsevick, Lauver, 1990).

PAPANICOLAOU SMEAR. How frequently Pap smear screening should be performed is debatable. The American College of Obstetricians and Gynecologists recommends yearly Pap smears as a result of the risk of false negatives and rare rapid growing cervical cancers. The American Cancer Society recommends a Pap smear every 3 years in women who have had two consecutive negative tests a year apart, and no further routine smears in women over 60 who have had regular screening (Denny, Koren, Wisby,

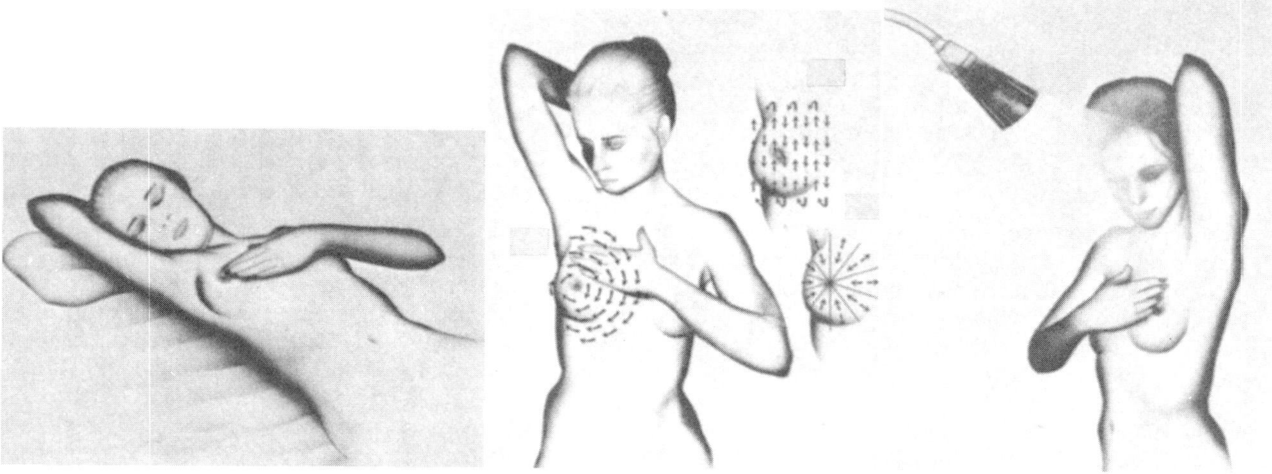

Fig. 41-1 Breast self-examination instructions (used with permission of American Cancer Society).

1989; Wheat, Mandelblatt, Kunitz, 1988). Elderly women who have not been screened, African Americans, lower socioeconomic groups, and more sexually active women are at higher risk for cervical carcinoma. A woman exposed to diethylstilbestrol (DES) in utero should have a Pap smear twice a year (Clay, 1990).

It is often the nurse who communicates the results of the Pap test. Learning about an abnormal Pap smear over the telephone can be terrifying. Fear can immobilize a client so that she does not return for treatment. Before the examination the nurse should explain the purpose of the smear and that early cellular changes that could become cancerous can be treated with a 100% cure rate.

A woman with a Pap smear indicating infection should be treated and the smear repeated in 3 months. Results showing kilocytosis (indicating human papillomavirus [HPV]) or squamous and endocervical atypia must be referred to a gynecologist. Follow-up may include endocervical curettage, colposcopy, and biopsy. **Cervical intraepithelial neoplasia (CIN)** requires colposcopy. CIN risk factors include sexual intercourse before age 21, multiple sexual partners, smoking one or more packs of cigarettes per day, and history of HPV. CIN is classified into categories I, II, and III according to severity. Dysplasia (disordered growth) is the term given to all disorders that are considered precancerous (Clay, 1990) (Table 41-1).

Health promotion and screening include being sure the client knows the American Cancer Society's seven warning signs (see box on p. 1251).

TABLE 41-1 Pap Smear Classification

Old Terminology	Current Terminology	Characteristics
Class I	Within normal limits	Minimal or no inflammation; no malignant cells
Class II	Inflammatory atypia	Inflammation; mild atypia
Class III	Cervical intraepithelial neoplasia	
Mild dysplasia	CIN Grade I	Abnormal nucleus; normal cytoplasm
Moderate dysplasia	CIN Grade II	Abnormal nucleus; minimal cytoplasm abnormalities
Severe dysplasia Carcinoma *in situ*	CIN Grade III	Abnormal chromosome and cytoplasm; abnormal cells predominate; many undifferentiated cells

From Beal MW: Cervical cytology, *NAACOG's Clinical Issues in Perinatal and Women's Health Nursing* 1(4):475, 1990.

TEACHING **Cancer's Seven Warning Signals**

1. Change in bowel or bladder habits
2. A sore that does not heal
3. Unusual bleeding or discharge
4. Thickening or lump in breast or elsewhere
5. Indigestion or difficulty in swallowing
6. Obvious change in wart or mole
7. Nagging cough or hoarseness

If you have a warning signal, see your doctor.

NURSING DIAGNOSES

Nursing diagnoses are based on assessment data and are unique to each client. For example, nursing diagnoses for a new client who is out of work and admits she does not perform BSE would include:

- High risk for anxiety related to
  - —Unfamiliar environment
  - —Uncertainty about health status
  - —Cost of health care
  - —Fear of breast cancer
- High risk for knowledge deficit related to
  - —Health promotion
  - —Self-care measures
  - —Female anatomy and physiology
  - —Warning signs of cancer

PLANNING

The plan of care is mutually negotiated, based on the biopsychosocial assessment of the client. It must relate specifically to the client's clinical and nursing diagnoses and be stated in terms of measurable client behaviors. Common *goals* might include:

- The client will experience less fear and anxiety as evidenced by verbal expression of relief, relaxed facial expression, and statement of intention to perform BSE.
- The client will demonstrate a change in health-related behavior as evidenced by statement of the importance of BSE, statement of when BSE should be performed, and demonstrating the ability to correctly perform BSE.

IMPLEMENTATION

Once a nursing diagnosis is confirmed and goals are mutually established with the client, nursing interventions are implemented. Interventions are directed toward goal achievement. In health promotion and screening, most interventions relate to education, support, and referral. Examples of nursing interventions include:

- Orient the client to the clinic routines, environment, and equipment.
- Promote trust by friendly, calm, and unhurried rapport.
- Encourage the client to express her concerns.
- Teach relaxation techniques and coping skills.
- Teach the benefits of BSE and BSE schedule.
- Perform breast examination; teach and observe return demonstration.
- Elicit the client's intention to perform BSE.

EVALUATION

Evaluation is probably the most neglected or misunderstood step in the nursing process. Nurses often evaluate interventions rather than objectives set with the client, and they assume that because they have done everything they intended to do, goals have been met. The final analysis is not how well the nurse has performed, but whether the client's goals have been met. Each goal must be specifically evaluated. In the examples above, if the client is still anxious or fearful, or if she is unable to perform BSE, then the process must be reevaluated: Were nursing diagnoses based on adequate data? Were they accurate? Were objectives mutually negotiated, appropriate, and realistic? Were interventions appropriate? Nurses must constantly evaluate their practice in terms of client outcomes.

COMMON MENSTRUAL DISORDERS

Common menstrual disorders that have a negative effect on the quality of the lives of women and their families are discussed in this chapter (refer to Chapter 6 for a review of the normal menstrual cycle and endocrine physiology and Chapter 42 for conditions associated with infertility).

Hypogonadotropic Amenorrhea

Hypogonadotropic amenorrhea reflects a problem in the central hypothalamic-pituitary axis. In rare instances, a pituitary lesion or genetic inability to produce follicle-stimulating hormone (FSH) and luteinizing hormone (LH) is at fault. A diagnostic workup (Chapter 42), including thyroid-stimulating hormone (TSH) and prolactin levels, x-rays or CT scan of the sella turcica, and a progestational challenge, is done to determine the cause.

Hypogonadotropic amenorrhea most commonly results from hypothalamic suppression as a result of two principal influences: *stress* (in the home, school, or workplace) or a *critical body fat-to-lean ratio* (underweight for height, rapid weight loss, and eating disorders such as anorexia nervosa or bulimia, or strenuous exercise such as competitive athletics or dancing, especially ballet). Menstrual regularity requires the maintenance of weight and body fat above a critical level.

The history often reveals a weight-conscious woman engaging in significant physical exercise and concerned with control over her own body. She may weigh less than 115 lb and may have lost 10 lb or more through exercising. The serious female athlete may have an adequate weight but a reduced proportion of body fat. Peripheral levels of endorphins increase with strenuous exercise and are believed to have a suppressive effect on the hypothalamus. A loss of calcium from the bone, comparable to that seen in postmenopausal women, may occur with this type of amenorrhea.

If counseling is ineffective in altering the client's life-style of exercise and weight control, **hormone replacement therapy (HRT)** may be indicated. Yearly reevaluation for return of normal menstrual function is necessary. HRT does not protect against pregnancy if normal function returns; therefore, caution is advised. Therapy usually includes conjugated estrogen for days 1 through 24 of each month (starting with the first calendar day of the month) and medroxyprogesterone acetate (Provera) for days 10 through 24. Withdrawal bleeding usually occurs on day 27.

Dysmenorrhea

Dysmenorrhea or painful menstruation is one of the most common gynecologic problems in women of all ages. It is estimated that American women lose 1.7 million working days each month because of dysmenorrhea. It affects about 35% of all older adolescents, 25% of college students, and 60% to 70% of single women 30 to 40 years old (Shaver et al, 1987).

PRIMARY DYSMENORRHEA. **Primary dysmenorrhea** occurs in the absence of organic disease, usually appearing from 6 months to 2 years after menarche. It often improves by age 25 or following pregnancy with vaginal delivery. Psychogenic factors may influence symptoms, but symptoms are definitely related to ovulation and do not occur when ovulation is suppressed. Nursing research indicates that affected women apparently view menstruation as a normal event and have positive perceptions of their general health (Shaver et al, 1987). During the luteal phase and subsequent menstrual flow, prostaglandin F_2 alpha ($PGF_2\alpha$) is secreted. Excessive release of $PGF_2\alpha$ increases the amplitude and frequency of uterine contractions and causes vasospasm of the uterine arterioles, resulting in ischemia and cyclic lower abdominal cramps. Systemic responses to $PGF_2\alpha$ include backache, weakness, sweats, gastrointestinal symptoms (anorexia, nausea, vomiting, and diarrhea), and central nervous system symptoms (dizziness, syncope, headache, and poor concentration) (Heitkemper et al, 1988). Cycle-related differences in serum cortisol, urine catecholamines, and self-reported anxiety have also been reported (Heitkemper et al, 1991). The cause of excessive prostaglandin release is unknown.

For some women, heat (heating pad or hot bath), massage, distraction, exercise, and sleep are sufficient to relieve primary dysmenorrhea. Heat relieves ischemia by decreasing contractions and increasing circulation. Orgasm may bring relief by reducing tension and increasing a sense of well-being, increasing menstrual flow, and relieving pelvic vasocongestion. Diet changes to decrease salt and increase natural diuretics, such as asparagus or parsley, may help reduce edema and related discomforts.

Several over-the-counter (OTC) preparations—analgesics, nonsteroidal antiinflammatory drugs (NSAIDs), and diuretics—are available. Cope and Midol contain both aspirin and caffeine; Midol also contains cinnamedrine, a mild uterine relaxant. Many products contain pamabrom (similar to caffeine in its diuretic effect) and pyrilamine maleate, an antihistamine with sedative and analgesic properties. Aspirin, acetaminophen (recommended dosage, 650 mg every 4 hours not to exceed 4000 mg in a 24-hour period), and ibuprofen (Motrin, Advil, Nuprin), an NSAID, in doses of 200 to 400 mg every 4 to 6 hours, work by inhibiting prostaglandin synthesis. Other **prostaglandin-synthesis inhibitors** include naproxen (Naprosyn and Anaprox) and mefenamic acid (Ponstel). They are most effective if started several days before menses. Exposing an early unsuspected pregnancy to drugs must be avoided (Sohn, Korberly, Tannenbaum, 1986; Lublanezki, Fischer, 1987).

As a last resort for intractable dysmenorrhea, surgery may be indicated. Approximately 70% of clients who undergo presacral neurectomy or sympathectomy obtain relief.

SECONDARY DYSMENORRHEA. **Secondary dysmenorrhea** is associated with organic pelvic disease, such as endometriosis, pelvic inflammatory disease, cervical stenosis, uterine or ovarian neoplasms, or uterine polyps. An IUD can also be a cause. Secondary dysmenorrhea may be misdiagnosed as primary dysmenorrhea or may be confused with complications of early pregnancy. Treatment must be directed toward the underlying cause.

Premenstrual Syndrome

Symptoms of **premenstrual syndrome (PMS)** begin in the luteal phase about 7 to 10 days before menses and end with the onset of menses. There may be a heightened sense of creativity and increased mental and physical energy. Negative symptoms are related to edema (abdominal bloating, pelvic fullness, edema of the lower extremities, breast tenderness, and weight gain) or emotional instability (depression, crying spells, irritability, panic attacks, and impaired ability to concentrate). Headache, fatigue, and backache are common complaints (Hsia, Long, 1990). A small percentage of women find PMS so incapacitating that normal activities are disrupted for several days during each cycle. A lack of understanding of PMS may result in poor self-esteem and stress relationships to the breaking point.

The cause of PMS is unknown. Theories include progesterone deficiency, prolactin and prostaglandin excesses, and dietary deficiencies. PMS has a significant psychosocial component.

There is little agreement on management. A careful, detailed history and daily log of symptoms and mood fluctuations spanning several cycles may give direction to a plan of management. Counseling, in the form of support groups or individual/couple counseling, may be helpful (see Research Highlight, below). Medications, such as prostaglandin inhibitors or diuretics for edema, and a well-balanced diet, low in caffeine and sodium or with naturally diuretic foods, may ease symptoms. Exercise and vitamin supplements are often recommended (see case study, p. 1254, and plan of care for PMS, p. 1255).

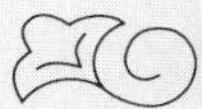 **Research Highlight** 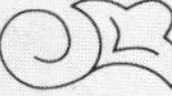

Effects of a Premenstrual Syndrome Education Program

RESEARCH ABSTRACT

The purpose of this study was to determine the effects of an education program on the symptoms of premenstrual syndrome. Participants were 47 women who reported moderate to severe premenstrual symptoms. Data were collected using the menstrual symptomatology questionnaire (MSQ), a menstrual symptom diary (MSD), and forms for demographic data and an inventory of life-style. After recording symptoms for 1 month in the MSD, participants were randomly assigned to control and experimental groups. The diaries were kept for 2 more months. The experimental group attended two 45-minute classes on the premenstrual syndrome. Content of the class included suggestions for changes in diet, exercise, stress management, and hormone therapy. The researcher found that the experimental group had lower anxiety, fewer appetite symptoms, and less severe edema symptoms. Experimental group participants had fewer days of premenstrual symptoms.

IMPLICATIONS FOR CLINICAL PRACTICE

Educational programs are effective in reducing anxiety and other symptoms. Nurses should take every opportunity to provide information and reassurance for their clients with problems. They can prepare educational materials for the client to read on her own and to refer to as necessary.

RELATED RESEARCH QUESTIONS

1. Are written education materials as effective as a class in reducing premenstrual symptomatology?
2. What is the relation between health locus of control and premenstrual symptomatology?
3. What are the effects of keeping a diary on premenstrual symptomatology?
4. What are the effects of premenstrual symptomatology on the significant other?

REFERENCE

Seideman RY: Effects of a premenstrual syndrome education program on premenstrual symptomatology, *Health Care for Women International* 11(4):491, 1990.

CASE STUDY

Premenstrual Syndrome (PMS)

Michele Brown is a 24-year-old nursing student who identified herself as having premenstrual syndrome (PMS) by filling out a questionnaire given to her by the gynecology clinic director where she was doing her clinical experience.

ASSESSMENT:

Michele indicated that she exhibits the following symptoms approximately 10 days before her menstruation begins: temporary water weight gain, breast tenderness, depression and moodiness, and craving for sweets.

NURSING DIAGNOSIS:

Because Michele experiences a temporary weight gain every month, the nurse identifies the following nursing diagnosis: fluid volume excess related to hormonal influence and fluid retention 10 days before menstruation.

PLANNING:

Michele and the nurse mutually agree on a plan of care and the following *goal:* Michele will experience a decrease in weight gain caused by water retention. The *expected outcome* is a reduction in premenstrual edema and weight gain.

IMPLEMENTATION:

Nursing actions are derived from medical management, physician's orders, and nursing diagnoses. Specific interventions include asking Michele to reduce or eliminate both salty foods and added salt at the table. The nurse will weigh Michele and assess for edema once in the first half of the cycle to obtain baseline data; Michele will check her weight at home on this day to validate the accuracy of her scales and then record her weight on a daily basis for 10 days before her next period is expected. If these measures are not effective, pharmaceutical preparations or natural diuretic foods (p. 1252) will be considered.

EVALUATION:

The expected outcomes were used to evaluate the effectiveness of the interventions. Michele had no increase in weight and no edema during the premenstrual period, indicating that the goal was met. See the following related Plan of Care.

Endometriosis

Endometriosis is characterized by the presence and growth of endometrial tissue outside of the uterus, including both glands and stroma. It may be implanted on the ovaries, cul-de-sac, uterosacral ligaments, rectovaginal septum, sigmoid colon, round ligaments, pelvic peritoneum, or urinary bladder (Fig. 41-2, p. 1256). A chocolate cyst is a cystic area of endometriosis in the ovary. The dark coloring of the contents of the cyst is caused by old blood.

Ectopic endometrial tissue responds to hormonal stimulation in the same way that the uterine endometrium does. During the proliferative and secretory phases of the cycle, the endometrium grows. During or immediately after menstruation, the tissue bleeds, resulting in an inflammatory response with subsequent fibrosis and adhesions to adjacent organs. Scar tissue and distortion or blockage of surrounding organs may result.

The exact number of women with endometriosis is unknown, but 5% to 15% of women who undergo pelvic surgery are observed to have endometriosis. The condition usually develops in the third decade of life and worsens with repeated cycles, or it may remain asymptomatic and undiagnosed, eventually disappearing during the climacterium. However, women who have symptoms require medical management and nursing intervention.

Several theories to account for the cause of endometriosis have been suggested. The most accepted theory is *transtubal migration or retrograde menstruation*. According to this theory, endometrial tissue is regurgitated or mechanically transported from the uterus during menstruation to the fallopian tubes and into the peritoneal cavity, where it implants on the ovaries and other organs. The *coelomic metaplasia doctrine* is a theory that accounts for the diversity of sites, including the lungs, lymphatics, and blood vessels, where endometrial tissue may appear. The ovary, peritoneum, and pleura derive from coelom. These organs, according to this theory, retain genetic material capable of developing endometrium. Other theories include the *lymphatic spread mechanism theory,* in which endometrial tissue is carried by lymph to extrauterine sites; the *hematogenous route*

CARE PLAN Premenstrual Syndrome (PMS)

GOALS	INTERVENTIONS	RATIONALE	EVALUATION
Nursing diagnosis: Fluid volume excess related to hormonal influence and fluid retention 10 days before menstruation as evidenced by water weight gain			
Michele relates a decrease in gain caused by water retention.	Encourage Michele to: reduce or eliminate salty foods and added salt at the table. Consider pharmaceutical preparations or natural diuretic foods.	Sodium retains fluid in the tissues. To prevent or minimize premenstrual water weight gain, Michele must decrease salt intake or enhance diuresis.	Michele will show a reduction in water weight gain and edema premenstrually.
Nursing diagnosis: Pain, breast discomfort related to influence of hormones and chemicals in diet			
Michele relates less breast discomfort.	Decrease caffeine intake. Wear a comfortable supporting bra.	Interventions prevent or minimize breast tenderness.	Michele reports a decrease in breast tenderness.
Nursing diagnosis: Situational low self-esteem related to hormonal changes before menses as evidenced by self-report of depression and moodiness			
Michele will relate less emotional distress.	Encourage Michele to: Monitor vitamin intake. Avoid alcohol and tobacco. Get plenty of exercise. Talk about feelings with someone close. Join a support group. Monitor feelings and coping strategies in a daily log. Engage in enjoyable activities: social events and jogging or other sports.	Interventions serve to decrease or prevent depression and mood swings.	Michele verbalizes an understanding of information presented and experiences less depression. Michele's log reflects improved coping ability. Michele reports feeling better about herself; she attends support group.
Nursing diagnosis: Altered nutrition: high risk for more than body requirements related to hormone-related change in carbohydrate metabolism			
Michele relates decreased intake of foods high in simple sugars (glucose).	Encourage Michele to: Reduce intake of simple sugars, candy, pastries, table sugar. Eat small, frequent meals and nutritious snacks (e.g., fruit and cheese); maintain a balanced diet.	Interventions serve to minimize wide fluctuations in blood sugar levels	Michele reduces intake of simple sugars, substituting more fresh fruit and vegetables and protein foods.

theory, in which endometrial tissue is transported by the circulatory system to extrauterine sites; and the *surgical implantation theory,* in which endometrial tissue is implanted in scar tissue during pelvic surgery (e.g., cesarean birth).

Symptoms vary among women and change over time. The major symptom is secondary dysmenorrhea. Women also complain of pain on defecation around the time of the menstrual cycle, pelvic heaviness, or pain radiating into the thighs. Less common symptoms include pain on exercise or during intercourse as a result of adhesions, and abnormal bleeding—hypermenorrhea, menorrhagia, or premenstrual staining—possibly as a result of ovarian adhesions that have disrupted normal ovarian hormone production.

Impaired fertility may result from adhesions around the uterus that pull the uterus into a fixed, retroverted position. Adhesions around the fallopian tubes may prevent the spontaneous movement that

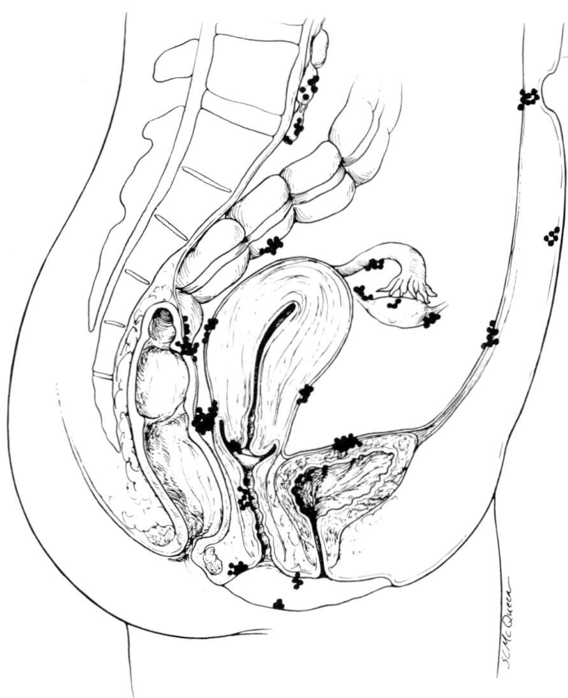

Fig. 41-2 Common sites of endometriosis.
From Droegemueller W et al: *Comprehensive gynecology*, St Louis, 1987, Mosby–Year Book.

carries the ovum to the uterus or blocks the fimbriated ends. Approximately 30% to 45% of women with endometriosis are infertile, compared with only 12% of women in the general population.

Treatment is based on the severity of symptoms and the goals of the woman or couple. Women without pain who do not want to become pregnant need no treatment. Women with mild pain who may desire a future pregnancy may require analgesics. Those who have severe pain and can postpone pregnancy may be treated with low estrogen-to-progestin–ratio oral contraceptives to shrink endometrial tissue. Another treatment method is danazol (Danocrine), a mildly androgenic synthetic steroid that suppresses FSH and LH secretion. Most women note relief from pain within 6 weeks. Danazol is continued for 9 months; when it is discontinued, menstruation returns.

Danazol can produce side effects that can cause the drug to be discontinued. These include masculinizing traits in the woman (which often disappear when treatment is discontinued), weight gain, edema, decreased breast size, oily skin, hirsutism, deepening of the voice, decreased libido, vasomotor symptoms (e.g., hot flushes), atrophic vaginitis, emotional lability, and seborrhea. Migraine headaches, dizziness, fatigue, and depression are also reported.

Danazol should never be prescribed when pregnancy is suspected, and contraception should be used with it since ovulation may not be suppressed. Danazol can produce pseudohermaphroditism in female fetuses. The drug is contraindicated in women with liver disease and should be used with caution in women with cardiac and renal disease. Because it is an expensive drug, danazol may not be available to all women. The recommended dosage is 400 to 800 mg a day for 6 to 9 months, and one 200-mg tablet costs about $2.00.

Recently a gonadotropin-releasing hormone (GnRH) agonist (Nafarelin) has shown promise of being an effective alternative to danazol. GnRH agonists suppress gonadotrope responsiveness to GnRH, thereby inhibiting the secretion of gonadotropic hormones and the production of ovarian hormones. Clinical trials indicate that Nafarelin is as effective as danazol, with fewer side effects, in the treatment of endometriosis when 200 to 400 μg are administered twice daily. Because it is destroyed by digestive enzymes, it must be used either intranasally or subcutaneously (Few, 1988).

Endometriosis may not be cured by hormonal treatments, and pain may return within 3 to 9 months for 38% of women when treatment is discontinued. Pregnancy may well be a "treatment" for endometriosis—both pregnancy and lactation are excellent prophylaxis in the presence of endometriosis because they suppress menstruation and cause ectopic endometrial tissue to shrink. Relief from pain may persist for years following pregnancy.

Surgical intervention, most commonly laparoscopy or laparotomy with bowel wedge resection, may be appropriate for some women. It is possible to lyse adhesions, resect implants, and cauterize or use a laser via the laparoscope. Endometriosis recurs within 5 years in 40% of women electing conservative surgery; persistent pain may be a result of missed disease (Petersen, Rhoe, 1988). There is a 50% improved fertility rate following surgery.

During the climacterium, endometrial tissue atrophies, and endometriosis ceases to be a problem. However, women who use HRT for problems associated with menopause should be aware that endometriosis can be reactivated during this therapy.

ASSESSMENT

In addition to taking a careful menstrual, obstetric, sexual, and contraceptive history, the nurse should explore the woman's perceptions of her condition, cultural or ethnic influences, experiences with other caregivers, life-style, and patterns of coping. The amount of pain experienced and its effect on daily activities should be evaluated. Home remedies and prescriptions to relieve discomfort are noted. A symptom diary, in which the client records emotions, behaviors, physical symptoms, diet, and exercise and rest patterns, is a useful diagnostic tool.

NURSING DIAGNOSES

Examples of nursing diagnoses for women experiencing menstrual disorders include:

- High risk for ineffective individual or family coping related to
  - —Insufficient knowledge of the cause of the disorder
  - —Emotional and physiologic effects of the disorder
- Knowledge deficit related to
  - —Self-care
  - —Available therapy for the disorder
- High risk for body image disturbance related to
  - —Menstrual disorder
- High risk for low self-esteem related to
  - —Others' perception of her discomfort
  - —Inability to conceive
- Pain related to
  - —Menstrual disorder

PLANNING

After data collection and review, mutual goals are established and a plan of care is developed. *Goals* may include:

1. The client will verbalize her understanding of reproductive anatomy, etiology of her disorder, medication regimen, and diary use.
2. The woman (couple) understands and accepts her emotional and physical responses to her menstrual cycle.
3. The woman (couple) develops personal goals that benefit her (them) emotionally and physically.
4. The woman (couple) chooses appropriate therapeutic measures.
5. The woman (couple) adapts successfully to the condition if cure is not possible.

IMPLEMENTATION

During the history and diagnostic workup, the clinician's concern and acceptance of the woman's symptoms as valid are in themselves therapeutic. Data from the daily log of emotional status, subjective feelings, and physical state are correlated with physiologic changes. If the woman has a male partner, both the woman and her partner keep separate logs that include how each perceives the other's responses day by day. Through the log, feelings are vented, problems are identified and clarified, insights occur, and possible solutions begin to develop. The clinician facilitates insights and suggests therapeutic options. The woman (couple) makes choices considered best for her (them).

Nurses need to discuss the options available to women with menstrual disorders. They must understand basic information about the anatomy and physiology, pathophysiology, psychologic impact, and treatment for the condition.

Support groups are an important resource. Nurses can use a local women's center or clinic to bring together women who want to learn more about their condition and support each other.

EVALUATION

Disorders associated with menstruation disrupt the quality of life for affected women and their families. Reviewing the monthly diary provides a basis for evaluation and further revision of the nursing care plan. The nurse can be assured that care has been effective when the woman reports improvement in the quality of her life, skill in self-care, and a positive self-concept and body image. See p. 1258 for a case study and p. 1259 for a plan of care for a client with endometriosis.

■ NORMAL CLIMACTERIUM AND POSTCLIMACTERIUM

Most women can expect to live into their ninth decade. Changes that accompany aging, especially those associated with the climacterium, can be a source of anxiety. **Climacterium** refers to the period of a woman's life when she passes from the reproductive to the nonreproductive stage with regression of ovarian function.

Premenopause is the first phase of the climacterium when fertility decreases and menses become irregular. Irregular cycles may last a few months or a few years. Troublesome symptoms, such as vasomotor instability, fatigue, headaches, and emotional disturbances, may appear during this phase.

Menopause (*meno*-month; *pause*-stop) is the point at which menstruation ceases. Using the word to mean a stage, similar to the climacterium, is incorrect. The average age for menopause is 51.4, but 10% of women stop menstruation by age 40 and 5% do not stop until 60. Surgical menopause occurs with hysterectomy and bilateral oophorectomy.

CASE STUDY

Endometriosis

Terry Smith is a 28-year-old married woman who is referred to the clinic nurse for instruction and counseling after seeing the physician. A tentative diagnosis of endometriosis has been made. Danazol, 400 mg BID, is prescribed, and a laparoscopy to confirm the diagnosis is scheduled.

ASSESSMENT

Terry complains of heavy menstrual periods, accompanied by severe pelvic and abdominal pain that may radiate down her thighs or may be accompanied by a sensation of pelvic fullness. Her pain has gradually worsened over time. Terry reports that she and her husband have a strong relationship, but there is a lot of tension: "We both are under a lot of stress." She confides that she has painful intercourse (dyspareunia) and no longer enjoys sexual relations. "We just can't be spontaneous," she adds. She and her husband would like to have a child, but she has been unable to conceive, although she has been married 3 years. She states, "I feel like such a failure. I'm trying to get pregnant, and it's not working." Terry reports that she has been feeling tired and weak. "I come home from work and just collapse." Her hemoglobin is 10.5 g. Terry asks, "What will this prescription do for me?" She appears anxious and states, "I'm scared of what the doctor is going to do. I'm afraid of what he is going to find and that there is nothing he can do."

NURSING DIAGNOSIS

Because she has reported severe dysmenorrhea, the nurse identifies the following *nursing diagnosis:* pain related to endometriosis.

PLANNING

A plan of care is mutually negotiated with the *goal* or *expected outcome* that Terry's pain will be eliminated or minimized.

IMPLEMENTATION

Specific interventions include assessing the location, type, and duration of pain and the history of Terry's discomfort; teaching about analgesics and comfort measures for pain relief; and teaching about danazol.

EVALUATION

The expected outcome was used to evaluate the effectiveness of the nurse's interventions. On the subsequent visit, Terry reported that dysmenorrhea was no longer a problem since she was not having menses, and pain with sexual relations was less. Based on these findings, the goal set for Terry was met. See the following related plan of care.

Perimenopause, roughly the same period as the climacterium, includes premenopause, menopause, and at least 1 year after menopause.

Postmenopause is the phase following menopause, when symptoms associated with decreased ovarian hormones, such as vaginal atrophy and osteoporosis, can develop.

Symptomatology: Climacterium

Approximately 20% of women never experience symptoms. Most women experience mild or moderate symptoms and rarely require medical attention, and a few women have severe symptoms.

VASOMOTOR INSTABILITY. *Vasomotor instability* is the most common disturbance of the climacterium. During the perimenopause women experience changeable vasodilation and vasoconstriction as **hot flushes** (flashes) and night sweats. A hot flush is a sudden sensation of warmth of varying duration and intensity, in the head, neck, and chest. It is preceded by an increase in peripheral skin temperature, heart rate, circulating cortisol, norepinephrine, adrenocorticotropic hormone (ACTH), and LH levels. FSH and estradiol do not increase.

Mild flushes do not interfere with daily activities; the sensation of heat is brief and bearable. *Moderate* flushes cause discomfort, with noticeably elevated temperature resembling fever, accompanied by perspiration. *Severe* flushes produce intense feelings of heat and extreme discomfort that interfere with activities of daily living. Women report they feel as if they are suffocating and seek relief by opening windows, removing outer layers of clothing, and fanning themselves. Vasoconstriction may immediately follow, producing chills. Blood pressure usually remains the same throughout the episode.

Hot flushes can occur often throughout the day, and may continue for several months or years. Several factors can precipitate an episode, including crowded or warm rooms, alcohol, hot drinks, spicy

CARE PLAN **Endometriosis**

GOALS	INTERVENTIONS	RATIONALE	EVALUATION
Nursing diagnosis: Pain related to endometriosis			
Terry's pain is relieved or minimized.	Assess location, type, and duration of pain and history of discomfort. Give analgesics PRN.	After pain is assessed and diagnosis is established, interventions to assist with pain relief are implemented.	Terry's pain is localized and minimized.
Nursing diagnosis: Knowledge deficit related to condition and treatment			
Terry's knowledge needs are met.	Teach about endometriosis and comfort measures and use and side effects of medications.	Knowledge dispels the unknown and empowers the client to become a partner in her care.	Terry understands condition and uses medication and comfort measures correctly.
Nursing diagnosis: Body image disturbance and self-esteem disturbance related to symptomatology of diagnosis			
Terry's self-esteem is maintained.	Provide time to discuss feelings. Refer to support group.	Interventions promote positive body image and self-esteem.	Terry reports she feels positive about herself.
Nursing diagnosis: Anxiety related to diagnosis			
Terry reports decreased anxiety.	Discuss feelings and concerns about diagnosis. Provide support and realistic hope. Teach about endometriosis and treatment.	Ventilation of feelings and knowledge about the cause and management can decrease anxiety.	Terry's anxiety is decreased through understanding. Terry verbalizes understanding of information presented.

foods, and proximity to a source of heat (Scharbo-DeHaan, Brucker, 1991).

Night sweats, characterized by profuse perspiration and heat radiating from the body during the night, are another form of vasomotor instability experienced by many women. Sleep may be interrupted nightly, since bed clothes and linens may be soaked. Many women complain of not being able to go back to sleep. Other perimenopausal symptoms associated with fluctuations of vasoconstriction or vascular spasms include dizziness, numbness and tingling in fingers and toes, and headaches.

EMOTIONAL DISTURBANCES. Mood swings, irritability, anxiety, and depression are often associated with perimenopause. Women complain of feeling more emotionally labile, nervous, or agitated, with less control of their emotions. Physiologic and biochemical changes, midlife stress, and cultural messages influence emotional stability.

Rapidly changing hormones may cause postpartum mood swings and precipitate postpartum depression. Women often associate mood swings and irritability of the climacterium with feelings they experienced during and immediately after pregnancy. The biochemical process that underlies variations in emotional responses in the climacterium is unknown, however. Estrogen replacement therapy (ERT) has been recommended to relieve symptoms, but the large number of emotional symptoms experienced suggest that there are other causes for emotional disturbances during the climacterium.

Midlife stress related to the many changes that women in their 40s and 50s experience may aggravate attempts to cope with menopause. Dealing with teenage children, having teenagers leave home, helping aging parents, becoming widowed or divorced, and grieving for friends and family who are ill or dying are among the many stresses that increase the woman's risk of serious emotional problems.

The ability to cope with any stress involves three factors: the person's perception or understanding of the event, her support system, and coping mechanisms. Nurses counseling women in the climacterium must therefore assess how much information about the climacterium the woman has, her perception of stressful experiences, whom she can depend on for help, and her repertoire of coping skills.

Cultural messages also influence emotional status during perimenopause. Many women have accepted childbearing and childrearing as their major role in life, and the inability to bear children is a significant loss. Others see menopause as the first step to old age and associate it with a loss of attractiveness, physical ability, and energy. Western culture values youth and physical attractiveness; the wisdom gained from life experience is not valued, and the elderly suffer a loss of status, function, and role. There are no rituals to give older women a special place and function. In cultures where postmenopausal women gain status, such as India, the Far East, and the South Pacific Islands, depression among menopausal women is not observed. Western women, however, may have little to compensate for the losses they experience. For women who perceive menopause as a time of loss, depression is likely to occur.

For other women, menopause is not a loss or a symbol of losses, but a relief. In a study by Anderson et al, (1987) women believed they gained more than they lost in menopause. Menopause was a relief from the fear of pregnancy, the hassle of menstruation, and the inconveniences of contraception. It was rare for a woman, whether employed or unemployed, to express sadness or regret that her children had left home.

In spite of a strong cultural message that youth is valued above age, women who value themselves adjust well to menopause. There is no evidence of an increase in depression or psychosis in menopausal women (McKeon, 1989).

FATIGUE AND HEADACHES. Fatigue is another common problem during menopause, affecting more than 40% of menopausal women in a British study (Howie, 1987). Its cause is unknown. A small number of women suffer from headaches during the perimenopause. Women who have experienced headaches during the premenstrual phase state that these become worse during the climacterium.

Symptomatology: Postclimacteric Period

Symptoms that occur in the postmenopausal phase are related to genital atrophy and osteoporosis.

GENITAL ATROPHY. As estrogen levels decrease, the vaginal epithelium thins. There is an increase in the vaginal pH, resulting in dryness, burning, irritation, and dyspareunia. In some women, the shrinking of the uterus, vulva, and distal portion of the urethra leads to disturbing symptoms, including urinary frequency, dysuria, uterine prolapse, stress incontinence, and constipation.

Itching around the vulva occurs as the vulva becomes thinner, less elastic, and more prone to irritation and inflammation. Women complain of an intense, constant itch that worsens after scratching.

Dyspareunia (painful intercourse) can occur because the vagina becomes smaller, vaginal walls become thinner and dryer, and lubrication during sexual stimulation takes longer. Intercourse becomes painful and may result in postcoital bleeding. Women may decide to forgo intercourse altogether.

Urinary frequency occurs sometimes after menopause because the distal portion of the urethra, which has the same embryologic origin as the reproductive organs, shortens and shrinks. Irritants have easier access to the urinary tract with its shorter urethra and may cause frequency and cystitis. Urine culture results in postmenopausal women may be negative for pathogens.

Urinary incontinence and *uterine displacement* are two other common findings during this period. These conditions are discussed on pp. 1269 and 1270. *Constipation* or pain during bowel movements may indicate that a rectocele is present (see p. 1267).

Not all women experience symptoms of genital atrophy. Endogenous estrogen has been found to provide stimulation a decade after menopause. Hormone replacement therapy (HRT) often brings relief.

OSTEOPOROSIS. **Osteoporosis** is an age-related reduction in bone mass associated with an increased susceptibility to fractures (Reed, Birge, 1988). Normally there is a dynamic balance between bone formation (osteoblastic activity) and bone resorption (osteoclastic activity). Since one of the functions of estrogen is to stimulate the osteoblasts, the postmenopausal drop in estrogen levels causes an imbalance between bone formation and resorption. Old bone deteriorates faster than new bone is formed, resulting in a slow thinning of the bones.

Estrogen is also required for the conversion of Vitamin D into calcitonin, which is essential in the absorption of calcium by the intestine. A reduced calcium absorption from the gut, in addition to the thinning of the bones, places postmenopausal women at risk for problems associated with osteoporosis.

Approximately one in four women is affected. During the first 5 to 6 years after menopause, women lose bone six times more rapidly than men. By the time women reach age 80, they have lost 47% of their trabecular bone, concentrated in the vertebrae, pelvis and other flat bones, and in the epiphyses. Women at risk are likely to be Caucasian or Asian, small boned, and thin (obese women have higher estrogen levels resulting from the conversion of androgens in adipose tissue; mechanical stress from extra weight also helps preserve bone mass). A family history of the disease is common. The influences of heredity, race, and sex may be a result of differences in peak bone mass. African-American women are not at risk, possibly because of the greater initial bone density of the African-American race (Madson, 1989).

Low calcium intake is a risk factor, particularly during adolescence and into the third and fourth decade when peak bone mass is attained (Chesnut, 1989; Johnston, Longcope, 1990). A high protein or caffeine intake increases calcium excretion, causing a systemic acidosis that stimulates bone resorption. Smoking also leads to acidosis and decreases estrogen production. Excessive alcohol interferes with calcium absorption and depresses bone formation. A greater phosphorus than calcium intake, which occurs with soft drink consumption, causes bone loss. Other risk factors include steroid therapy and disorders such as hypogonadism and hyperthyroidism (Madson, 1989).

The first sign of osteoporosis is often loss of height resulting from vertebral fracture and collapse (Fig. 41-3). Back pain, especially in the lower back, may or may not be present. Later signs include "dowager's hump," in which the vertebrae can no longer support the upper body in an upright position, and fractured hip, in which the fracture often precedes the fall. Damage to the vertebrae usually precedes bone loss in the hip by an average of 10 years (Reed, Birge, 1988).

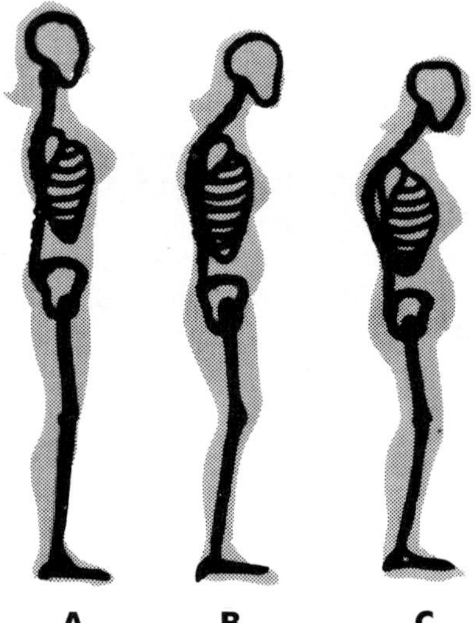

Fig. 41-3 Skeletal changes secondary to osteoporosis assessed by height and body shape at **A**, age 55; **B**, age 65; and **C**, age 75.

Radiographic techniques to identify women at risk are imprecise, expensive, and have not been approved for screening by third-party payers. Osteoporosis cannot be detected by x-ray examination until 30% to 50% of the bone mass has been lost, and routine screening is not warranted (Morley et al, 1988). Computerized axial tomography (CAT scan) can identify bone loss in amounts of 2% to 3%. A blind study relating height loss to x-ray examination in 65 women indicated that 75% of women who had lost 2 or more inches had osteoporosis on x-ray examination; only 21% of those who lost less than 2 inches had osteoporosis on x-ray examination ($p < .001$). A negative test, however, does not rule out early bone loss (Reed, Birge, 1988).

Hormone Replacement Therapy (HRT)

Estrogen replacement therapy (ERT) increases serum levels of calcitonin, which prevents bone resorption, maintains bone density, and decreases the risk of fracture (Barrett-Connor, Wingard, Criqui, 1989). This reduction in osteoporosis occurs if ERT is begun within 3 years of menopause. ERT should therefore be started as soon as possible after menopause, when bone loss is accelerated, and continued for life if acceptable to the woman. (McKeon, 1990; Youngkin, 1990). The dose needed to prevent osteoporosis is 0.625 mg of conjugated equine estrogen.

With any drug there is a benefit to risk ratio. ERT is still controversial, but many authorities recommend treatment for all women without contraindications at the time of menopause (McKeon, 1990). ERT should be prescribed only if the woman understands the risks and benefits of therapy and agrees to careful follow-up (Madson, 1989).

The type of estrogen used for postmenopausal ERT is much less potent than ethinyl estradiol used in oral contraceptives and has fewer serious side effects. It is unlikely that ERT causes hypertension, gallbladder disease, or an increased incidence of thrombophlebitis or thromboembolism in postmenopausal women who use estrogen, as compared with control subjects.

CORONARY HEART DISEASE. Postmenopausal women are at risk for coronary artery disease because of changes in lipid metabolism; there is a decline in serum levels of high-density lipoprotein (HDL) cholesterol and an increase in low-density lipoprotein (LDL) levels. In contrast to the increased risk of myocardial infarction in women over age 35 taking oral contraceptives, numerous studies indicate that postmenopausal ERT is associated with reduced cardiovascular morbidity and mortality (Barrett-Connor, Wingard, Criqui, 1989). ERT has a protective effect, even in women who smoke (Matthews et al, 1989).

NEOPLASTIC EFFECTS. The breast and endometrium are target tissues of estrogen, and estrogen is contraindicated in women with a history of breast or endometrial malignancies. Carcinoma of the breast may exist for as long as 8 years before it is palpable. Therefore a mammogram must be obtained for all women before ERT, and the importance of regular SEB and follow-up should be emphasized.

Studies to determine an association between estrogen use and breast cancer have been controversial as a result of methodologic problems. Although the risk appears to be minimal, caution is advised. In a recent prospective study of a cohort of 121,700 female nurses, a significant increase in breast cancer associated with current or recent use of postmenopausal hormones was found. Past users were at no increased risk, which suggests that ERT may increase the risk of breast cancer, but this effect is reversible within two years of discontinuing therapy (Colditz et al, 1990). Bergkvist et al (1989) found an increased risk of breast cancer with estradiol and also with combined estrogen-progestin postmenopausal therapy.

Long-term unopposed estrogen therapy (estrogen without progestin) to prevent osteoporosis increases the risk of developing endometrial cancer five times (Barrett-Connor, Wingard, Criqui, 1989). The risk of developing cancer decreases with progestogen added for 12 to 14 days at the beginning of each month. Several authorities recommend that women without a uterus not be given progestins because of the positive effects of unopposed estrogen on lipids (Charles, 1989; McKeon, 1990). Intramuscular and once-a-week oral estrogen regimens are available, but they result in higher initial blood levels than oral estrogens. Daily medication appears safer. Transdermal estradiol, in the form of a patch applied twice a week to the skin, provides a relatively constant level of estrogen (Whitehead et al, 1990). Some women develop skin irritation in the area of the patch or injection.

Conjugated estrogens available in cream and suppository form are often prescribed to relieve genitourinary problems such as urinary frequency, vaginal pruritus, and dyspareunia resulting from atrophy of reproductive tissue.

Decisions with regard to taking estrogen alone or in combination with progestin must be made after weighing the benefits and risks of each protocol. Cancer is a serious threat, but heart disease is a more common cause of mortality (see box below).

SEXUALITY. Sex does not end with menopause. However, women and their partners may change their expression of sexuality during and after menopause, depending on physical changes, changes in the partner, and cultural myths and messages (McKeon, 1989).

Physical changes occur after menopause. There is progressive atrophy of the reproductive tissues, especially the breasts and labia, which flatten out as a result of loss of subcutaneous fat. The vagina is less expansive, and the vaginal walls are thinner and with-

TEACHING Hormone Replacement Therapy

- Menopause, the permanent cessation of menses, occurs spontaneously about age 51.
- In most women, the loss of ovarian function and subsequent fall in estrogen production results in vasomotor flushes, genitourinary symptoms, mood changes, and osteoporosis.
- To prevent these problems experts recommend estrogen-progestin replacement therapy for women who have no contraindications to estrogen.
- Hormone replacement therapy (HRT) should be continued indefinitely (which may mean lifelong treatment) for women who are at high risk for osteoporosis; high-risk factors include advanced age; Caucasian or Asian race; thin, small-framed body; history of low calcium intake; early menopause; sedentary life-style; nulliparity; cigarette smoking; and diet high in protein, phosphate, alcohol, or caffeine.
- ERT decreases the risk of cardiovascular disease in older women, but increases the risk of endometrial cancer. Adding a progestin to therapy greatly decreases this risk but also reverses the protective influence of estrogen in cardiovascular disease. It is not known whether ERT increases the risk of breast cancer; ERT is contraindicated in women at high risk for breast cancer.
- The benefits of estrogen replacement therapy (ERT) outweigh the risks for most women. HRT, combined with general health promotion strategies, enhances health and well-being.

out rugae. During intercourse, vaginal lubrication is decreased. As a result, it takes longer to reach orgasm, and intercourse may be painful.

There is no way to prevent the inevitable aging process that the body undergoes. For people who see aging as loss, sexuality may become difficult to incorporate into what they perceive to be a less attractive identity. The fear of rejection is always present.

Changes in the male partner may influence whether he continues to want sex. As men age, they too, take longer to reach orgasm; erections take longer to occur and are less firm. Men may believe they are becoming impotent or ill and give up sexual activity, viewing it as too frustrating. Women may believe their partners are losing interest in them. Couples may need counseling to understand these changes. Libido is not changed by shifts in hormones, and the capacity for orgasm is not decreased.

The lack of available male partners has a devastating effect on sexual expression. Women outlive men, and older widowed and divorced women have fewer opportunities to develop relationships because they are less sought after. In counseling older women who do engage in intercourse, the nurse cannot assume that new or nonmonogamous partners are HIV-free and should inform clients of their risk for HIV infection and the need to use condoms (Whipple, Scura, 1989).

As long as women are able to bear children, some accept intercourse as part of their responsibility as wives. When menopause frees them from this duty they may choose to forgo intercourse. For other women, libido may increase without the fuss of contraception, fear of pregnancy, or interruption from menses.

ASSESSMENT

A thorough health history, physical examination, and laboratory tests are essential to distinguish pathologic states from the normal climacterium. Personal or familial history of breast or uterine cancer, hypertension, thrombophlebitis, liver or gallbladder disease, undiagnosed uterine bleeding, or other acute or chronic disease are noted, as are hysterectomy and bilateral oophorectomy.

Recent changes in menstrual history help to identify the phase of the climacterium the woman is experiencing, and risk factors for osteoporosis are identified.

The woman's perception of this stage of life, ethnic and cultural factors, and knowledge and concerns about sexuality and care available are all recorded.

NURSING DIAGNOSES

Following are examples of nursing diagnoses for women experiencing a normal climacterium:

- Knowledge deficit related to
  - —Menopause
- Family coping, potential for growth related to
  - —Receiving information about the condition, its management, and prognosis
  - —Emotional support
- High risk for altered growth and development related to
  - —Insufficient knowledge of climacterium
- High risk for pain related to
  - —Regression of ovarian function
- High risk for injury related to
  - —Osteoporosis
- High risk for sexual dysfunction related to
  - —Changes associated with the climacterium
- High risk for low self-esteem related to
  - —Physical and emotional changes during the climacterium

PLANNING

Planning requires knowledge of the climacterium and great sensitivity. Planning should take place collaboratively with the woman and her spouse/partner and family members as necessary. Informed consent regarding ERT, weight-bearing exercise, and calcium supplements is a major concern because treatment may involve considerable expense, inconvenience, and side effects (Bartlett, 1989). Mutually negotiating goals to ensure the client's compliance is extremely important. *Goals* are stated in terms of client behaviors:

- The woman will explain the physical and emotional changes associated with menopause.
- The woman's symptoms will not interfere with daily activities.
- She will not develop osteoporosis or will experience only minimal effect.
- The woman and family will cope effectively with events of the climacterium.
- The woman and family will view the climacterium as a normal developmental phase instead of a deficiency disease.
- The woman will report concerns about changes associated with menopause and treatment.
- The woman will participate in decision making about the plan of care.
- The woman will adhere to the plan of care.

IMPLEMENTATION

Most women know little about menopause, and old wives' tales and misinformation can cause anxiety. They need to know what to expect, why it happens, and what measures will help make them more comfortable. Women appreciate the opportunity to discuss their symptoms. They need to know that their symptoms have a normal physiologic basis and that other women experience similar complaints.

Treatment must be individualized for the specific woman. There is a need for menopause clinics, where research on the effects of various treatments can be developed and evaluated and where care by the various specialty groups involved in care, such as endocrinology, radiology, psychosocial resources, exercise physiology, and nutrition, can be effectively coordinated. Women's support groups are also needed.

SEXUAL COUNSELING. Nurses must give accurate information on matters such as appropriate contraception, sexuality, and the physiology of menopause and should offer support and nonjudgmental guidance. Clients need advice about contraception, since ovulation may not cease for a year after the last menstrual cycle and menopausal women can still become pregnant. Birth control pills and IUDs may not be recommended for women after age 40. The nurse's attitude toward sex and the older adult is important. Negative attitudes can reinforce the client's misgivings about maintaining an active and satisfying sex life. The nurse can reassure the couple grieving over lost youth and attractiveness that the desire for sex into old age is a natural one and that the body has the capacity for sexual satisfaction. Only minor adjustments may be required. The nurse can suggest specific remedies, such as vaginal water-soluble lubricants to relieve dyspareunia, and refer couples to a counselor or physician for problems beyond the scope of nursing practice.

Prolonged hospitalization of an elderly partner may have a significant impact on the couple's sexual relationship. They may have difficulty renewing sexual activity when the separation is over; the nurse should discuss this with them. In the event that a couple is admitted to a nursing home, the nurse should encourage placement of the couple together.

MIDLIFE SUPPORT GROUPS. Nurses need to be familiar with local resources and direct women to classes that supply appropriate information and support. They can encourage women to develop a supportive network with other women with whom they can share their concerns.

Recently women's centers and clinics have started support groups and classes for women who want to discuss menopause and other midlife events. If no group or class is available in the community, nurses need to consider starting one.

ALTERNATIVE METHODS OF MANAGEMENT. There are many women who cannot or will not take ERT. A progestogen is the next best therapy; it provides significant relief from hot flushes and may also decrease excretion of calcium, but it will not prevent vaginal or urethral atrophy (Herbst et al, 1991). Some women can obtain relief from other products.

Bellergal-S tablets, composed of phenobarbital, ergotamine tartrate, and belladonna, may eliminate or significantly reduce symptoms related to autonomic nervous system activity. Phenobarbital, a barbiturate, is a sedative that may have side effects, especially drowsiness. It can also be addictive, and this must be considered if a woman plans to take the tablet for a long time. Bellergal-S is contraindicated for women with peripheral vascular disease, coronary heart disease, hypertension, impaired hepatic or renal function, sepsis, glaucoma, or hypersensitivity to any of the drug's components. *Clonidine* is generally used for hypertensive clients but at smaller doses than those used for lowering blood pressure. It has been found effective in reducing the number of hot flushes experienced.

Vitamin E is a popular alternative among women who do not take HRT. Women who take vitamin E regularly report relief from hot flushes, leg cramps, and loss of energy. Vitamin E is found in a variety of foods, including spinach, peanuts, wheat germ, vegetable oils, and soybeans, or may be taken as a supplement. Dosage varies widely depending on the clinician; between 50 and 400 IU can be taken daily during meals without any ill effects (Nachtigall, 1977).

Certain plants used in Chinese *herbal medicine*, European folk medicine, and Native American medicine may have properties that relieve hot flushes. Genseng and dong quai are Oriental herbs that some women use to prevent hot flushes. Some of the herbs and roots that have been used traditionally were included in Lydia Pinkham's Vegetable Compound (1819-1883). Its popularity among Victorian women may be accounted for in part by the alcohol (18%) used to preserve the herbs in solution (Burton, 1949). After estrogen became available, the compound lost popularity, but it is available today with the following ingredients: jamaica dogwood, pleurisy root, black cohosh, life root, licorice, dandelion, and gentian. Licorice has been found to contain vegetable estrogens. Other plants (e.g., pussy willow, sarsaparilla, wild cherry, and yucca) also contain estrogen or can be converted to estrogen by the body. Claims for herbal remedies have not been substantiated by scientific research.

Muscle tone around the reproductive organs decreases after menopause. *Kegel exercises* strengthen these muscles, improve tone, and, if practiced regularly, help prevent prolapsed uterus and stress incontinence. This is a low-cost, effective, noninvasive intervention to control symptoms. However, symptoms return if exercises are discontinued (Ferguson et al, 1990) (see Kegel exercises, Chapter 11).

K-Y Lubricating Jelly and coconut oil are two examples of *water-soluble lubricants* that provide relief from painful intercourse. They may be applied directly to the vulva and the penis. Oil-based lubricants such as petroleum jelly (Vaseline) should not be used because they clog vaginal glands, which can then be sites for bacterial infection.

Fluid intake should be increased and *infection* prevented. Another consequence of genital atrophy is urinary frequency and dysuria, often associated with asymptomatic bacteriuria. Older women may not experience typical symptoms (cramping, pain, or burning on urination). The nurse should encourage a daily intake of at least eight glasses of water to decrease urine concentration and the growth of bacteria. This simple measure may prevent serious infection. Most urinary tract infections are limited to the urethra and the bladder, but occasionally the kidneys are involved. Signs of serious infection include fever, chills, vomiting, and costovertebral angle (CVA) tenderness (pain in the back over the kidneys) (see prevention of urinary tract infections, Chapter 11).

PREVENTION OF COMPLAINTS ASSOCIATED WITH OSTEOPOROSIS. HRT is the only well-documented prevention of osteoporosis. Two antiresorptive agents may hold promise for future treatment: *Calcitonin* is effective in preventing and treating osteoporosis, but must be given subcutaneously and is therefore impractical; *Etidronate disodium* has been shown to reduce fractures by half and significantly increase bone mass. It is poorly absorbed and must be given on an empty stomach, followed by 2 hours of fasting (Johnston, Longcope, 1990; Storm et al, 1990; Watts et al, 1990). The following may retard the disease.

CALCIUM. The role of calcium supplementation in treating osteoporosis is controversial, but it appears to retard bone loss from cortical bone and may have an impact on reducing the incidence of fractures. Its effect is less dramatic than ERT (Birge, Dalsky, 1989; Heaney, 1989; Riggs, 1989; Shangraw, 1989; Dawson-Hughes, 1990).

Although calcium cannot reverse loss of bone mass or prevent fractures, calcium supplementation may retard the development of osteoporosis after menopause. Oral calcium should be taken daily as early as premenopause. The recommended dose is 1.5 g daily, usually taken at bedtime. However, calcium supplements are best taken with meals because of the increase in acid secretions and extended time in the stomach. At least 8 ounces of water to increase solubility is recommended. Calcium is most commonly available as calcium carbonate, calcium lactate, and calcium phosphate. Over half of the calcium preparations on the market are useless because they do not dissolve; "Tums" are most soluble (Shangraw, 1989). Mineral supplements are not classified as drugs by the FDA and are therefore not regulated. Calcium is not recommended for women with kidney disease because it may lead to hypercalcemia. Vitamin D may be recommended as a supplement because it aids in calcium absorption.

NUTRITION. Foods high in calcium and low in phosphorus are recommended. Excessive protein should be avoided. Fat-free milk and yogurt are good sources of calcium and vitamin D. It is difficult to eat other foods that contain calcium (sesame seeds, spinach, greens, broccoli, and seaweed) in quantities sufficient to meet daily requirements. Women should avoid excessive alcohol, soft drinks, and coffee. Efforts should be made to increase bone mass in adolescent women.

EXERCISE AND SAFETY. Exercise alone cannot prevent or reverse osteoporosis, but recent data indicate that weight-bearing exercise, such as walking and stair-climbing 30 to 60 minutes a day, may delay bone loss and increase bone mass at any age (Riggs, 1989). The nurse should help women plan an exercise program. Examples of exercises are available from the National Osteoporosis Foundation (Fig. 41-4). Two registered nurses in an urban center in Virginia manage a walking club that has grown from a small network to more than 1800 members (Moore, 1989).

Osteoporosis-related fractures are often related to falls, and accident prevention, including proper storage of articles and correction of poor lighting and loose carpeting, should be discussed with the older woman (see box on p. 1266).

EVALUATION

The nurse can be reasonably assured that care was effective to the degree that the goals of care have been met. That is, the woman explains the physical and emotional changes associated with menopause,

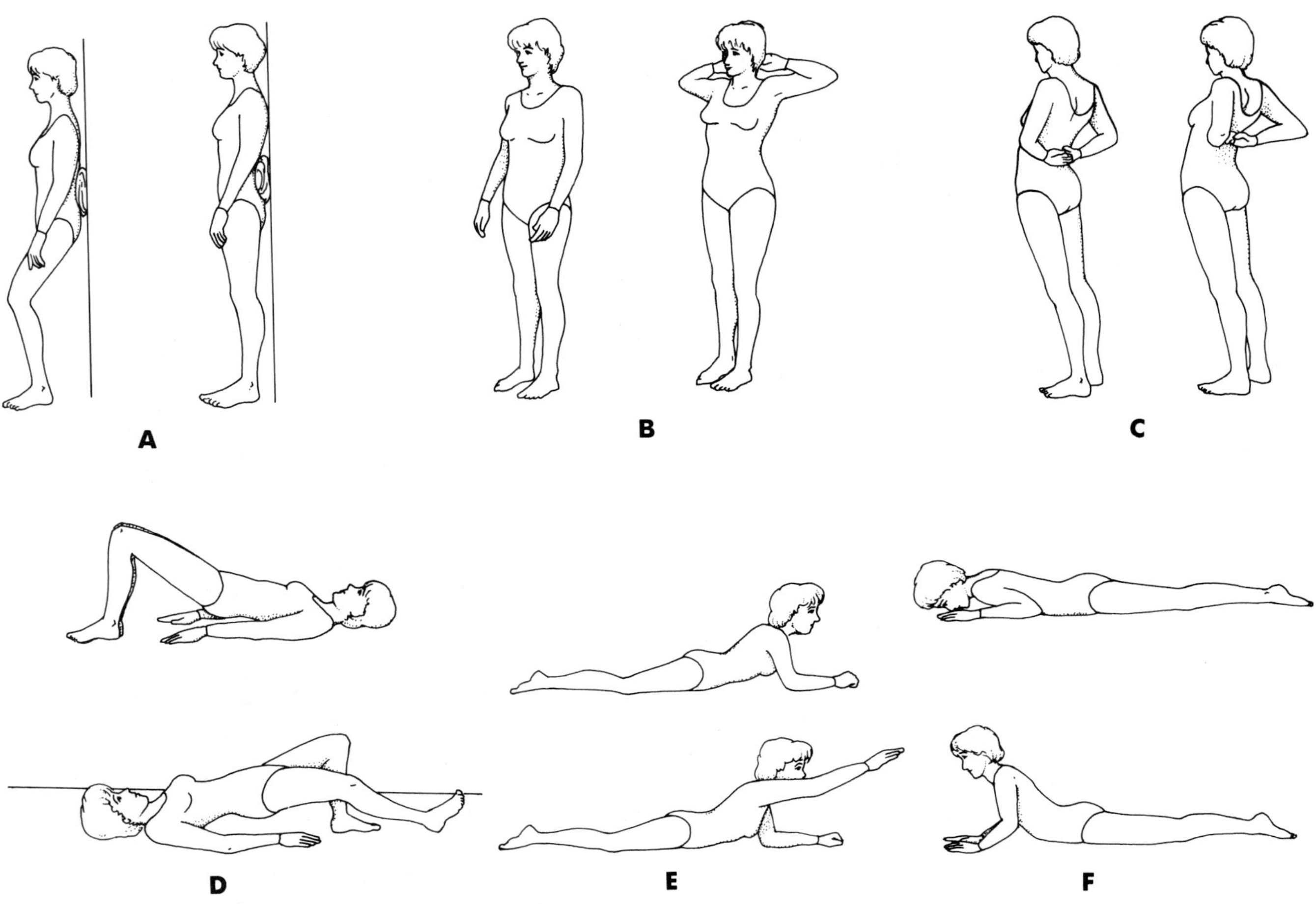

Fig. 41-4 **A**, Wall standing and pelvic tilt. **B**, Isometric posture correction. **C**, Standing back bend. **D**, The bridge. **E**, The elbow prop. **F**, Prone press-ups with deep breathing.
From "Boning Up on Osteoporosis" with special permission from the National Osteoporosis Foundation.

TEACHING Prevention of Osteoporosis

- Osteoporosis is primarily a disease that affects postmenopausal women. It is characterized by lower back pain, a loss of height, and fractures of the back and hip. More women die each year from complications of osteoporosis than from cervical and breast cancer combined.
- Postmenopausal women naturally lose bone mass when the ovaries stop producing estrogen, which is necessary for calcium metabolism. Risk factors for osteoporosis include a family history of the disease, small build, early menopause, nulliparity, long-term low intake of dairy products, high intake of soft drinks and caffeine, smoking, alcoholism, inadequate exercise, and certain diseases and medications such as phenytoin (Dilantin), furosemide (Lasix), and corticosteroids.
- Estrogen replacement therapy (ERT) can be prescribed to prevent fractures from osteoporosis. The risks and benefits of ERT must be weighed on an individual basis with the physician.
- Significant bone loss can be prevented by a well-balanced diet, including 200 to 400 IU of vitamin D and 1500 mg of calcium a day, and regular weight-bearing exercise. Good sources of calcium are dairy products, fish, oysters, tofu, dark-green leafy vegetables, and whole-wheat bread.
- Supplements of vitamin D and calcium can be prescribed, but the body cannot use them without the right balance of other vitamins and minerals.
- Eliminating environmental hazards in the home can decrease the risk of falls.
- Weight-bearing exercise 30 to 60 min/day may delay bone loss and increase bone mass.

does not let the symptoms interfere with daily activities, does not develop osteoporosis, copes effectively with events of the climacterium, views the climacterium as a normal developmental phase, reports concerns about changes associated with menopause and its treatment, participates in decision-making about her plan of care, and adheres to the plan of care.

SEQUELAE OF CHILDBIRTH TRAUMA

Alterations in Pelvic Support

The term **pelvic relaxation** refers to the weakening and lengthening of fascial supports of the pelvic organs. In most cases it is the delayed but direct result of childbearing. Although extensive damage may be noted and repaired shortly after birth, symptoms related to pelvic relaxation most often appear during the perimenopausal period, when the effects of ovarian hormones on pelvic tissues are lost and atrophic changes begin. Pelvic trauma, stress and strain, and the aging process are contributing causes. Neither exercise nor rest will correct the problem or restore normal anatomic relations and physiologic function.

Generally, symptoms of pelvic relaxation relate to the structure involved: urethra, bladder, uterus, vagina, cul-de-sac, or rectum. The most common complaints are pulling and dragging sensations, pressure, protrusions, fatigue, and low backache. Symptoms may be worse after prolonged standing or deep penile penetration during intercourse. Urinary stress incontinence may be present.

During distention of the birth canal, levator ani bundles separate, and the fascia is stretched. Although external damage may be minimal or not visible, extensive damage may have occurred in the deep supporting structures. When lacerations occur in the levator muscles, the muscle fibers contract so that the muscle separates and retracts laterally, eliminating the perineal body and normal support of the rectum.

Permanent defects in support, such as rectocele and cystocele, may occur in childbirth regardless of obstetric management and also in women who have never been pregnant. **Rectocele** is the herniation of the anterior rectal wall through the relaxed or ruptured vaginal fascia and rectovaginal septum; it appears as a large bulge that may be seen through the relaxed introitus (Fig. 41-5). Rectoceles may be small and produce few symptoms, but some are so large that they protrude outside of the vagina when the woman stands. Symptoms are absent when the woman is lying down. A rectocele causes a disturbance in bowel function, the sensation of "bearing

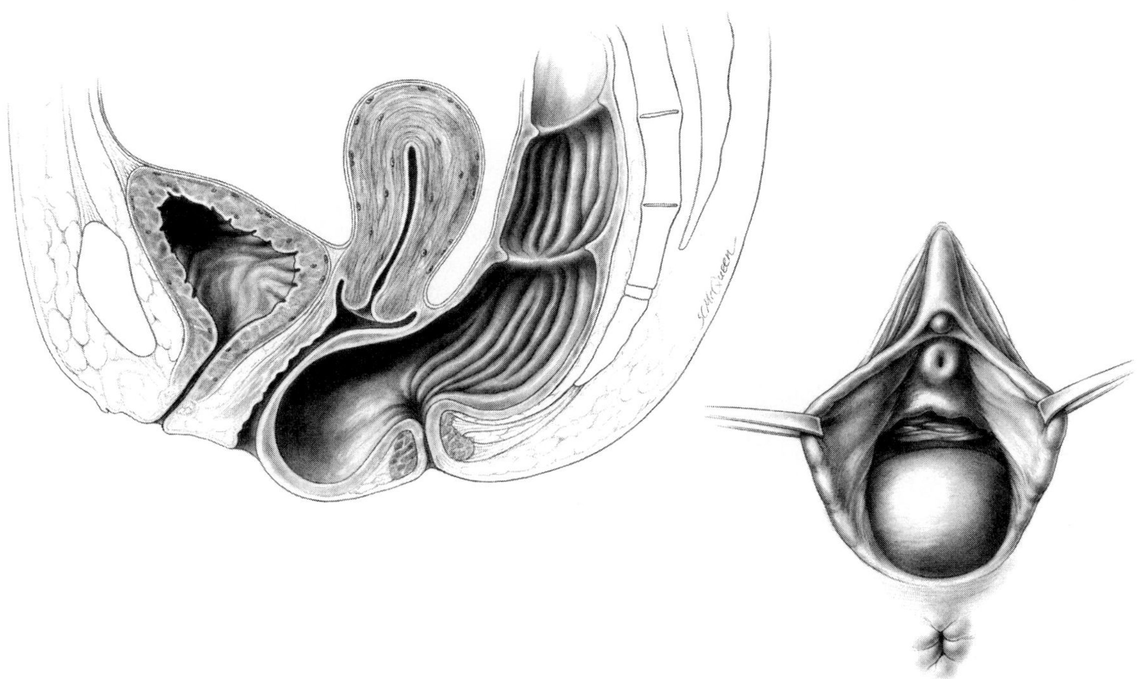

Fig. 41-5 Side and direct views of rectocele.
Redrawn from Symmonds RE: Relaxations of pelvic supports. In Benson RC, editor: *Current obstetric and gynecologic diagnosis and treatment,* ed 5, Los Altos, Calif, 1984, Lange Medical Publications.

down" or that the pelvic organs are falling out. With a very large rectocele, it may be difficult to have a bowel movement. Each time the woman strains during bowel evacuation, the feces are forced against the thinned rectovaginal wall, stretching it more. Some women facilitate evacuation by applying digital pressure vaginally to hold up the rectal pouch. Rectoceles are usually repaired surgically.

Enterocele (Fig. 41-6), or posterior vaginal hernia, is the herniation of the peritoneum of the posterior cul-de-sac between the uterosacral ligaments into the rectovaginal septum. The sacculation contains loops of small bowel but no rectum. This condition is commonly seen with uterine prolapse and after vaginal hysterectomy for relaxation. The woman may be unaware of the problem or complain of pressure or a bearing-down or dragging sensation with low backache. Enterocele is diagnosed during a rectovaginal examination as an increased thickness of the rectovaginal septum or perception of pressure on the examiner's fingertip when the woman is asked to increase intraabdominal pressure by coughing. The defect is closed surgically through the vagina by approximating the uterosacral ligaments and the levator muscles in the middle.

With fetopelvic disproportion, prolonged labor, or a precipitate birth, structures of the vesical and vaginal walls are stretched and may be injured. The bladder neck and urethra may be compressed between the presenting part and the pubic bones or forced downward ahead of the presenting part. Since soft-tissue damage usually occurs behind an intact vaginal epithelium, there is nothing visible to repair. Cystocele, urethrocele, and vaginal prolapse are possible sequelae.

Cystocele (Fig. 41-7) is the protrusion of the bladder downward into the vagina that develops when supporting structures in the vesicovaginal septum are injured. Anterior wall relaxation gradually develops over time—often after several babies. When the woman stands, the weakened anterior vaginal wall cannot support the weight of the urine in the bladder; the vesicovaginal septum is forced downward, the bladder is stretched, and its capacity is increased. With time the cystocele enlarges until it protrudes into the vagina. Complete emptying is difficult because the cystocele sags below the bladder neck. Cystocele is often accompanied by rectocele, and the bladder descends when the uterus prolapses. The woman may complain of a bearing-down sensation or a protrusion of a mass from the vagina.

Cystocele is recognized as a bulging of the anterior wall of the vagina. Unless the bladder neck and urethra are damaged, urinary continence is unaffected. Women with large cystoceles complain of having to push upward on the sagging anterior vaginal wall to be able to void. Recurrent cystitis and ascending urinary tract infection may develop. Surgical support is

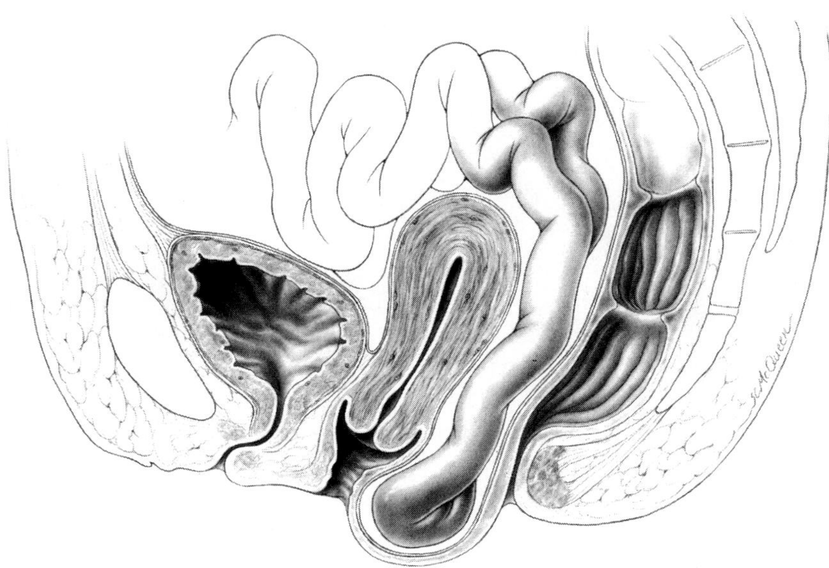

Fig. 41-6 Lateral view of enterocele and prolapsed uterus.
Redrawn from Symmonds RE: Relaxations of pelvic supports. In Benson RC, editor: *Current obstetric and gynecologic diagnosis and treatment,* ed 5, Los Altos, Calif, 1984, Lange Medical Publications.

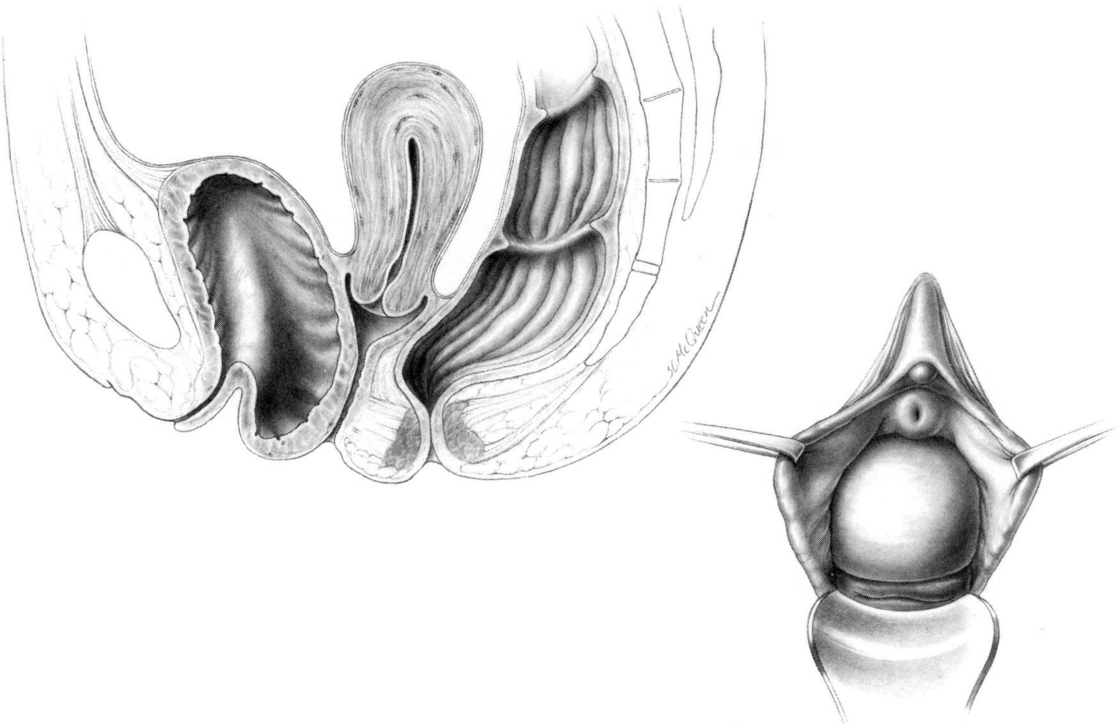

Fig. 41-7 Side and direct views of cystocele.
Redrawn from Symmonds RE: Anatomy of the female reproductive system. In Benson RC, editor: *Current obstetric and gynecologic diagnosis and treatment,* ed 5, Los Altos, Calif, 1984, Lange Medical Publications.

accomplished through the vagina. Plication (taking a fold, tuck, or running stitch to gather material together) of the bladder wall reduces the cystocele.

Urethrocele is a herniation of the paravaginal fascia under the urethra that allows the urethra to protrude into the vagina. The condition may be asymptomatic, or the woman may complain of a vaginal protrusion or stress urinary incontinence if there is relaxation of fascial supports in the area of the posterior urethrovesical angle.

Vaginal prolapse is an uncommon but greatly distressing condition that may occur after vaginal or abdominal hysterectomy. It must be repaired surgically.

Causes of *vaginal atresia* include faulty repair of a laceration, failure to perform a needed repair, and anterior and posterior colporraphy. Injury usually occurs along a lateral wall in the upper third of the vagina. Palpation reveals a sharp, annular, constricting band of tissue. Surgical correction usually involves incising some annular bands of tissue or using graduated obturators to dilate a constricting band in the lower one third of the vagina.

URINARY INCONTINENCE. Many women experience uncontrollable leakage of urine as a result of childbirth injury. Conditions that disturb urinary control include **stress urinary incontinence,** due to sudden increases in intraabdominal pressure (such as that due to sneezing or coughing); *urge incontinence,* caused by disorders of the bladder and urethra, such as urethritis and urethral stricture, trigonitis, and cystitis; *neuropathies,* such as multiple sclerosis, diabetic neuritis, and pathologic conditions of the spinal cord; and *congenital and acquired urinary tract abnormalities.*

Stress urinary incontinence may follow injury to bladder neck structures. A sphincter mechanism at the bladder neck compresses the upper urethra, pulls it upward behind the symphysis, and forms an acute angle at the junction of the posterior urethral wall and the base of the bladder (Fig. 41-8). To empty the bladder, the sphincter complex relaxes and the trigone contracts to open the internal urethral orifice and pull the contracting bladder wall upward, forcing urine out. The angle between the urethra and the base of the bladder is lost or increased if the supporting pubococcygeus muscle is injured; this change, coupled with urethrocele, causes incontinence. Urine spurts out when the women is asked to bear down or cough in the lithotomy position.

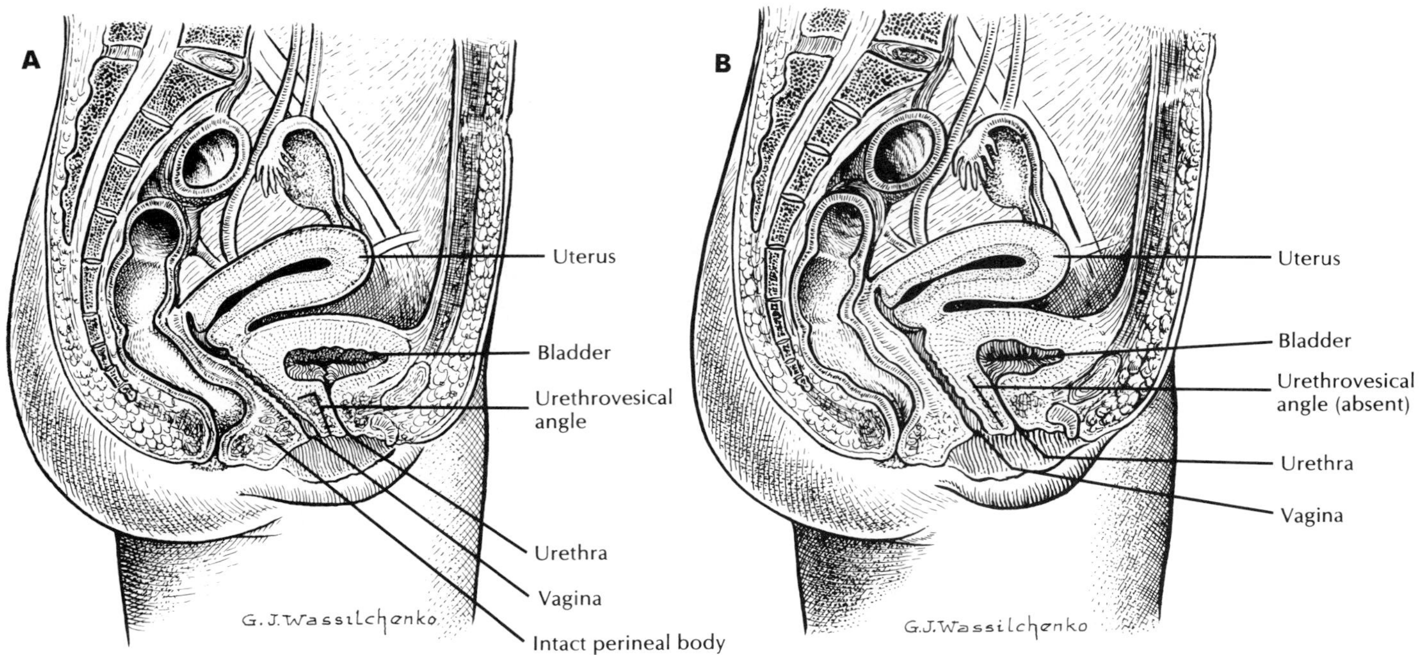

Fig. 41-8 Urethrovesical angle. **A**, Normal angle. **B**, Widening (absence) of angle.

Mild stress incontinence can be relieved by Kegel exercises (see Chapter 11) 80 to 100 times a day. HRT may improve urinary control for postmenopausal women, but surgical correction is often indicated to relieve symptoms.

INJURIES TO PELVIC JOINTS. Separation of the *symphysis pubis* occurs to some degree during birth. If forcible extraction or delivery of a large baby occurs, serious injury is likely. The woman suffers severe pain on movement in the symphysis pubis and *sacroiliac joints*. Palpation reveals tenderness over the symphysis, wide separation of the ends of the pubic bones, and unusual mobility (several centimeters) of the bone ends when she shifts her weight from one foot to the other.

UTERINE DISPLACEMENT. **Uterine prolapse** occurs when the cardinal ligaments (see Fig. 6-7) that support the uterus and vagina do not return to normal after delivery and when the relationship of the axis of the uterus to that of the vagina is altered (Fig. 41-9). Cystocele and rectocele almost always accompany uterine prolapse, causing it to sag even further backward and downward into the vagina. There are varying degrees of prolapse—with procidentia (complete prolapse), the cervix and body of the uterus protrude through the vagina and the vagina is inverted. Transvaginal surgical correction of severe prolapse to correct the cystocele and rectocele, return the uterus to its normal position, shorten the elongated cervix, and shorten the cardinal ligaments is indicated. When surgery is contraindicated (e.g., in aged and debilitated women) a **pessary** may be inserted to support the uterus (Fig. 41-10, *A*).

Retroversion, the most common simple displacement of the uterus, may be congenital or a sequel to childbirth. *Lateral displacement* may signal adnexal disease such as a large ovarian tumor, inflammation, or scar tissue.

Normally the round ligaments hold the uterus in anteversion, and the uterosacral ligaments pull the cervix backward and upward (see Figs. 6-5, 6-6, and 6-9). By 2 months postpartum these ligaments should return to normal length, but in approximately one third of women, the uterus remains retroverted. This condition is rarely symptomatic, but conception may be difficult because the cervix points toward the anterior vaginal wall and away from the posterior fornix, where seminal fluid pools after coitus. Infrequently, chronic pelvic congestion, accompanied by posterior prolapse of the tubes and ovaries into the cul-de-sac, results from retroversion of the uterus. Symptoms may include deep pelvic and low back pain, difficulty with elimination, exaggeration of premenstrual tension, and dyspareunia.

Slight prolapse

Normal

Marked prolapse (procidentia)

Fig. 41-9 Depiction of prolapse of uterus.

Redrawn from Symmonds RE: Relaxations of pelvic supports. In Benson RC, editor: *Current obstetric and gynecologic diagnosis and treatment,* ed 5, Los Altos, Calif, 1984, Lange Medical Publications.

A

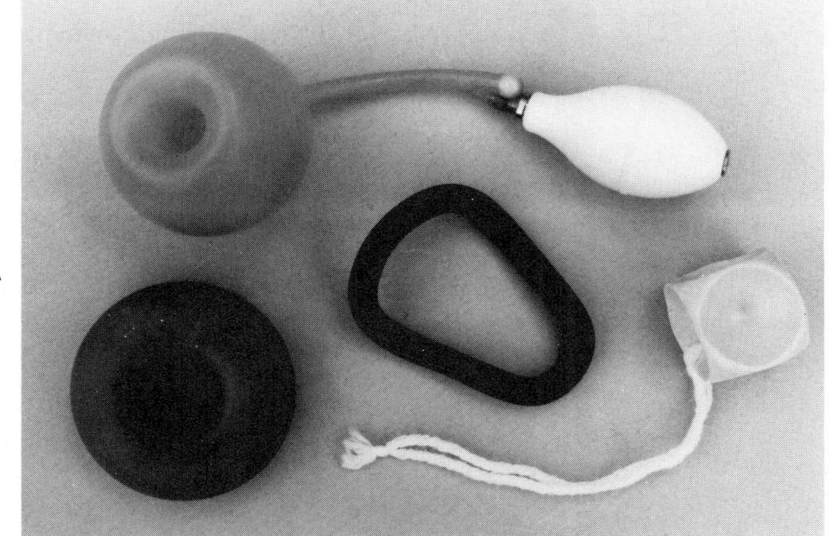

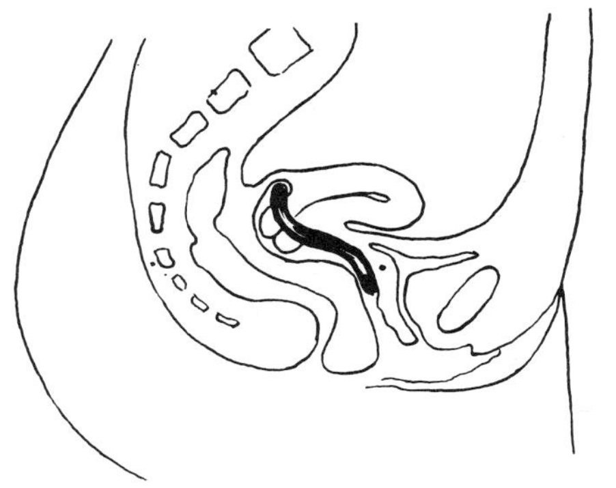

B

Fig. 41-10 **A,** Examples of pessaries (Smith-Hodge, donut, inflatable types). **B,** Pessary in place to hold cervix well backward and upward in pelvis.

A from Droegemueller W, et al: *Comprehensive gynecology,* St Louis, 1987, Mosby–Year Book. B from Beacham DW, Beacham WD: *Synopsis of gynecology,* ed 10, St Louis, 1982, Mosby–Year Book.

Insertion of a pessary (Fig. 41-10, *B*) to replace the uterus in the anterior position may confirm that symptoms were related to malposition of the uterus. Usually a pessary is used only for a short time; it can lead to pressure necrosis and vaginitis. Good hygiene is important; some women can be taught to remove the pessary at night, cleanse it, and replace it in the morning. If the pessary is always left in place, regular douching to remove increased secretions and frequent checkups are indicated. After a period of treatment, most women are free from symptoms and do not require the pessary. Surgical correction is rarely indicated.

GENITAL FISTULAS. A **fistula** is an abnormal communication between one hollow viscus and another, or from one hollow viscus to the outside. Genital fistulas may occur between the bladder and the genital tract (e.g., vesicovaginal); between the ureter and the vagina (ureterovaginal); and between the rectum or sigmoid colon and other structures (e.g., enterovesical). They may be a result of a congenital anomaly, gynecologic surgery, obstetric trauma, cancer, radiation therapy, gynecologic trauma, or infection.

Vesicovaginal fistula, the most common urinary tract fistula, forms in the anterior vaginal wall (Fig. 41-11). It is usually a result of injury near the uterovesical junction during radical hysterectomy for cancer. Urine is lost through the vagina, resulting in partial or complete incontinence. A transvaginal surgical repair is possible in most cases.

Rectovaginal fistula is most often caused by an infection in the episiotomy, a suture placed through the rectal wall during repair, or an unrecognized rectal injury during childbirth. Fistulas may also be a result of extension of cervical cancer or radiation therapy. Surgical repair is possible but is often complicated by infection, which delays healing or causes the repair to break down.

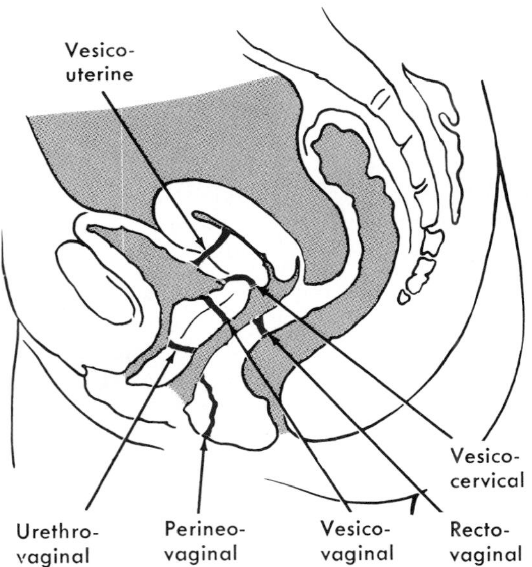

Fig. 41-11 Types of fistulas that may develop in vagina, uterus, and rectum.
From Phipps WJ et al: *Medical-surgical nursing: concepts and clinical practice,* ed 3, St Louis, 1991, Mosby–Year Book.

ASSESSMENT

Assessment for sequelae to childbirth trauma and uterine displacement focuses primarily on the genitourinary tract, the reproductive organs, bowel elimination, and psychosocial and sexual factors. A complete health history, physical examination, and laboratory tests are done to support the appropriate medical diagnosis. The nurse needs to assess the woman's knowledge of the disorder, its management, and possible prognosis.

NURSING DIAGNOSES

Following are examples of possible nursing diagnoses:

- Constipation or diarrhea related to
  —Anatomic changes
- Pain related to
  —Relaxation of pelvic support and/or elimination difficulties
- Ineffective coping related to
  —Changes in body image
- Altered family processes or interpersonal relationships related to
  —The woman's anatomic and functional changes
- High risk for injury related to
  —Lack of skill in self-care procedures
  —Lack of understanding of the rationale for the need to comply with therapy
- Social isolation, spiritual distress, body image disturbance, or low self-esteem related to
  —Changes in anatomy and function
- Anxiety related to
  —Surgical procedure

PLANNING

Goals are mutually negotiated and stated in client-centered terms. Possible *goals* are:

1. The client will be able to state possible childbirth sequelae and symptoms and participate in yearly physical examinations that facilitate early diagnosis and corrective intervention.
2. The client will use good hygiene and will practice measures to prevent problems related to pelvic support alterations.
3. The client will accept change in body functions without loss of positive body image, self-concept, and self-esteem.
4. The client will cooperate with medical and surgical interventions successful in the repair of anatomic defects and control of reproductive and genitourinary tract dysfunction.

IMPLEMENTATION

Nursing care of the woman with pelvic relaxation problems or a fistula requires great sensitivity because the woman's reactions are often intense. She may become withdrawn or, conversely, hostile because of embarrassment about odors and soiling of her clothing beyond her control. Occasionally the woman becomes so accustomed to the odors that she is no longer aware of them. The nurse must use tact in suggesting hygienic practices that reduce odor. Commercial deodorizing douches are available, or noncommercial solutions, such as chlorine solution (1 teaspoon of chlorine household bleach to 1 quart of water) may be used. The chlorine solution is also useful for external perineal irrigation. Sitz baths and thorough washing of the genitals with unscented, uncolored, mild soap and warm water help. Sparse dusting with deodorizing powders such as sodium borate can be useful. Hygienic care is time consuming and must be repeated frequently throughout the day; protective pads or pants must be worn. All of these activities are demoralizing to the woman and frustrating to her and her family.

If a rectovaginal fistula is present, high enemas, given before leaving the house, provide temporary relief from oozing of fecal material in the preoperative period.

Much of the nurse's efforts with these problems are directed toward participating in a team effort to prepare the woman for surgery. Preoperative teaching involves the primary nurse, operating room nurse, surgeon, and anesthesiologist. The nurse in the health promotion setting is usually most aware of the client's living circumstances, physical limitations, and social problems and therefore may be best suited to coordinate continuity of care.

EVALUATION

Care can be evaluated as effective if the anatomic defect is repaired and function is restored. If function cannot be fully restored through surgery, medication, or other therapy, goals are evaluated related to self-care in compliance with the medical regimen, regaining or maintaining self-esteem, and satisfactory family and interpersonal processes.

■ SUMMARY

Nurses have an important role to play in health promotion and screening. They may see women from different cultural backgrounds, women with disabilities, and women of different age groups, particularly older women. Understanding the various reasons women enter the system for gynecologic health care and the unique concerns and fears they bring will enhance holistic care and contribute to keeping clients in the system. Using the nursing process as a framework for practice, the nurse performs a careful nursing assessment, involves the woman—and family, as appropriate—in goal setting and planning, and provides teaching, counseling, and referrals. Care is evaluated to ensure that cliented-centered goals are met. Common problems seen in younger women include menstrual disorders, such as hypogonadotropic amenorrhea, dysmenorrhea, premenstrual syndrome, and endometriosis. Guidance and support is provided during the climacterium and postclimacterium to dispel myths and foster self-esteem and self-care. Problems encountered in older women include osteoporosis and late sequelae to childbirth trauma—conditions involving pelvic support problems, urinary incontinence, and genital fistulas.

REFERENCES

Anderson E et al: Characteristics of menopausal women seeking assistance, *Am J Obstet Gynecol* 156(2):428, 1987.

Barrett-Connor EL: The risks and benefits of long-term estrogen replacement therapy, *Public Health Rep* 104 suppl:62, Sept-Oct 1989.

Barrett-Connor EL, Wingard DL, Criqui MH: Postmenopausal estrogen use and heart disease risk factors in the 1980s: Rancho Bernardo, Calif., revisited, *JAMA* 261(14):2095, 1989.

Bartlett EE: Patient counseling for osteoporosis prevention, *Public Health Rep (US)* 104 suppl:84, Sept-Oct 1989.

Beal MW: Cervical cytology, *NAACOG: Clinical Issues in Perinatal and Women's Health Nursing* 1(4):470, 1990.

Bergkvist L et al: The risk of breast cancer after estrogen and estrogen-progestin replacement, *N Engl J Med* 321:293, 1989.

Birge SJ, Dalsky G: The role of exercise in preventing osteoporosis, *Public Health Rep* 104 suppl:54, Sept-Oct 1989.

Burton J: *Lydia Pinkham is her name,* New York, 1949, Farrar, Strauss & Co.

Charles AG: Estrogen replacement after menopause? *Postgrad Med* 85:99, 1989.

Chesnut CH: Is osteoporosis a pediatric disease? Peak bone mass attainment in the adolescent female, *Public Health Rep* 104 suppl:50, Sept-Oct 1989.

Clay LS: Midwifery assessment of the well woman: the Pap smear, *J Nurs Midwif* 35(6):341, 1990.

Colditz GA et al: Prospective study of estrogen replacement therapy and risk of breast cancer in postmenopausal women, *JAMA* 264(20):2648, 1990.

Dawson-Hughes B, Dallal GE, Krall EA: A controlled trial of the effect of calcium supplementation on bone density in postmenopausal women, *N Engl J Med* 323(13):878, Sept 1990.

Denny MS, Koren ME, Wisby M: Gynecological needs of elderly women, *J Gerontol Nurs* 15(1):33, 1989.

Ehrenreich B, English D: *For her own good: 150 years of the experts' advice to women,* New York, 1978, Anchor Press.

Ferguson K et al: Stress urinary incontinence: effect of pelvic muscle exercise, *Obstet Gynecol* 75:671, 1990.

Few BJ: Treating endometriosis with nafarelin, *MCN* 13(5):323, 1988.

Fogel CI, Woods NF: *Health care of women: a nursing perspective,* St Louis, 1981, Mosby–Year Book.

Heaney RP: The calcium controversy: finding a middle ground between the extremes, *Public Health Rep* 104 suppl:36, Sept-Oct 1989.

Herbst AL et al: *Comprehensive gynecology,* ed 2, St Louis, 1991, Mosby–Year Book.

Howie C: Sparing the flushes, *Nurs Times* 83(49):51, 1987.

Hsia LSY, Long MH: Premenstrual syndrome: current concepts in diagnosis and management, *J Nurs Midwif* 35(6):351, 1990.

Johnston CC, Longcope C: New treatments for osteoporosis, *Lancet* 335(8697):1065, 1990.

Kain CD, Reilly N, Schultz ED: The older adult: a comparative assessment, *Nurs Clin North Am* 25(4):833, 1990.

King MC, Ryan J: Abused women: dispelling myths and encouraging intervention, *Nurse Pract* 14(5):47, 1989.

Laffin J: *The Arab mind considered: a need for understanding,* New York, 1975, Paplinger Publishing.

Lichtman R: Perimenopausal hormone replacement therapy: review of the literature, *J Nurs Midwif* 36(1):30, 1991.

Lublanezki N, Fischer RG: OTC-menstrual pain preparations, *Pediatr Nurs* 13(6):435, 1987.

McKeon VA: Cruel myths and clinical facts about menopause, *RN* 52(6):52, 1989.

McKeon VA: Estrogen replacement therapy: current guidelines for education and counseling, *J Gerontol Nurs* 16(10):6, 1990.

Madson S: How to reduce the risk of postmenopausal osteoporosis, *J Gerontol Nurs* 15(9):20, 1989.

Matthews KA et al: Menopause and risk factors for coronary heart disease, *N Engl J Med* 32(10):641, 1989.

Moore SR: Walking for health: a nurse-managed activity, *J Gerontol Nurs* 15(7):26, 1989.

Morley JE et al: UCLA geriatric grand rounds: osteoporosis, *J Am Geriatr Soc* 36(9):845, 1988.

Nachtigall L: *The Lila Nachtigall Report,* New York, 1977, GP Putnam's Sons.

Petersen N, Rhoe J: Endometriosis: obtaining relief via "near-contact" laparoscopy, *AORN J* 48(4):700, 1988.

Riggs L: Nutrition/exercise panel summary, *Public Health Rep* 104 suppl:34, Sept-Oct 1989.

Scharbo-DeHaan M, Brucker MC: The perimenopausal period: implications for nurse-midwifery practice, *J Nurs Midwif* 36(1):9, 1991.

Shangraw R: Factors to consider in the selection of a calcium supplement, *Public Health Rep* 104 suppl:46, Sept-Oct 1989.

Sohn C, Korberly B, Tannenbaum R: Menstrual products, *Handbook of Nonprescription Drugs* 17:371, 1986.

Storm T et al: Effect of intermittent cyclical etidronate therapy on bone mass and fracture rate in women with postmenopausal osteoporosis, *N Engl J Med* 322(18):1265, 1990.

Stotland NL: Social change and women's reproductive health care, *Women's Health Issues* 1(1):4, 1990.

U. S. Preventive Services Task Force (National Health Information Center, USDHS): *Guide to clinical preventive services,* Baltimore, 1989, Williams & Wilkins.

Watts NB et al: Intermittent cyclical etidronate treatment of postmenopausal osteoporosis, *N Engl J Med* 323(2):73, 1990.

Wheat ME, Mandelblatt JS, Kunitz G: Pap smear screening in women 65 and older, *J Am Geriatr Soc* 36(9):827, 1988.

Whipple B, Scura KW: HIV and the older adult: taking the necessary precautions, *J Gerontol Nurs* 15(9):15, 1989.

Whitehead MI et al: Transdermal administration of oestrogen/progestagen hormone replacement therapy, *Lancet* 335(8685):310, 1990.

Witte M: Pain control, *J Gerontol Nurs* 15(3):33, 1989.

Youngkin EQ: Estrogen replacement therapy and the estraderm transdermal system, *Nurs Pract* 15(5):19, 1990.

References—Nursing Research

Barsevick AM, Lauver D: Women's informational needs about colposcopy, *Image J Nurs Sch* 22(1):23, 1990.

Heitkemper MM et al: Gastrointestinal symptoms and bowel patterns across the menstrual cycle in dysmenorrhea, *Nurs Res* 37(2):108, 1988.

Heitkemper M et al: GI symptoms, function, and psychophysiological arousal in dysmenorrheic women, *Nurs Res* 40(1):20, 1991.

Lierman LM et al: Predicting breast self-examination using the theory of reasoned action, *Nurs Res* 39(2):97, 1990.

Nemcek MA: Health beliefs and breast self-examination among black women, *Health Values* 14(5):41, 1990.

Reed AT, Birge SJ: Screening for osteoporosis, *J Gerontol Nurs* 14(7):18, 1988.

Shaver JF et al: Menstrual experiences: comparisons of dysmenorrheic and nondysmenorrheic women, *West J Nurs Res* 9(4):423, 1987.

BIBLIOGRAPHY

Albanese JA, Nutz PA: *Mosby's nursing drug cards,* ed 2, St Louis, 1991, Mosby–Year Book.

Ballinger CB: Psychiatric aspects of the menopause, *Br J Psychol* 156:773, 1990.

Blanchard DS: What women can do to protect against osteoporosis, *RN* 53(10):60, 1990.

Budoff PW: *No more hot flashes and other good news,* New York, 1983, GP Putnam's Sons.

Brucker MC, Scharbo-DeHaan M: Breast disease: The role of the nurse-midwife, *J Nurs Midwif* 36(1):63, 1991.

Carter CL et al: A prospective study of reproductive, familial and socioeconomic risk factors for breast cancer using NHANES I data, *Public Health Rep* 104(1):45, 1989.

Cervato PL: Piecing together the osteoporosis puzzle, *RN* 53(4):77, 1990.

Clinical Practice Committee, American Geriatrics Society Board of Directors: Screening for cervical carcinoma in elderly women, *J Am Geriatr Soc* 37(9):885, 1989.

Cohen SM, Hollingsworth AO, Rubin M: Another look at psychologic complications of hysterectomy, *Image J Nurs Sch* 21(1):51, 1989.

Cooper K: *Preventing osteoporosis,* New York, 1989, Bantam Books.

Cummings SR et al: Appendicular bone density and age predict hip fracture in women: the study of osteoporotic fractures research group, *JAMA* 263(5):665, 1990.

Daly FA, Futrell M: Retirement attitudes and health status, *J Gerontol Nurs* 15(1):29, 1989.

Delaney J et al: *The curse: a cultural history of menstruation,* New York, 1976, New American Library.

Devor M et al: Estrogen replacement therapy and venous thrombosis, *Am J Med* 92:275, 1992.

Dickson GL: The metalanguage of menopause research, *Image J Nurs Sch* 22(3):168, 1990.

Dignan M et al: The role of focus groups in health education for cervical cancer among minority women, *J Community Health* 15(6):369, 1990.

Ebersole P, Hess P: *Toward healthy aging: human needs and nursing response,* ed 3, St Louis, 1990, Mosby–Year Book.

Giger JN, Davidhizar RE: *Transcultural nursing: assessment and intervention,* St Louis, 1991, Mosby–Year Book.

Hunter M: The South-East England longitudinal study of the climacteric and postmenopause, *Maturitas* 14:117, 1992.

Jackson KD: Endometrial ablation with rollerball electrode, *AORN* 54(2):265, Aug 1991.

Jones DY, Schatzkin KA, Brinton LA: A prospective study of reproductive, familial and socioeconomic risk factors for breast cancer using NHANES I data, *Public Health Rep* 104(1):45, 1989.

Koster A: Change-of-life anticipations, attitudes, and experiences among middle-aged Danish women, *Health Care Women Internatl* 12:1, 1991.

Krause N: Perceived health problems, formal/informal support, and life satisfaction among older adults, *J Gerontol Nurs* 45(5):33, 1990.

Lichtman R, Papera S, editors: *Gynecology: well woman care,* Norwalk, Conn, 1990, Appleton & Lange.

Lang N: *Quality of health care for older people in America: a review of nursing research,* Kansas City, 1991, ANA.

McElmurry BJ, Huddleston DS: Self-care and menopause: critical review of research, *Health Care for Women International* 12:15, 1991.

McKinlay SM, et al: The normal menopause transition, *Maturitas* 14:102, 1992.

Matthews KA et al: Influences of natural menopause on psychological characteristics and symptoms of middle-aged healthy women, *J Consult Clin Psych* 58:345, 1990.

Nachtigall LE, Nachtigall LB: Protecting older women from their growing risk of cardiac disease, *Geriatrics* 45(5):24, 1990.

National Research Council Diet and Health: *Implications for reducing chronic disease risk,* Washington, DC, 1989, National Academy Press.

Ojeda L: *Menopause without medicine: feel healthy, look younger, live longer,* Claremont, Calif, 1989, Hunter House.

Phipps WJ et al: *Medical-surgical nursing: concepts and clinical practice,* ed 4, St Louis, 1991, Mosby–Year Book.

Robie PW: Cancer screening in the elderly, *J Am Geriatr Soc* 37(9):888, 1989.

Rubin MM, Lauver D: Assessment and management of cervical intraepithelial neoplasia, *Nurs Pract* 15(9):23, 1990.

Sandelowski M: *Women, health, and choice,* Englewood Cliffs, NJ, 1981, Prentice-Hall.

Scully D, Bart P: A funny thing happened on the way to the orifice: women in gynecology textbooks, *Am J Soc* 78:1045, 1973.

Seidel H et al: *Mosby's guide to physical examination,* ed 2, St Louis, 1991, Mosby–Year Book.

Sevel F: Designing effective health promotion and disease prevention programs: a course model, *Health Values* 14(1):32, 1990.

Slemenda CW et al: Predictors of bone mass in perimenopausal women. A prospective study of clinical data using photon absorptiometry, *Ann Intern Med* 112(2):96, 1990.

Speroff L: A clinical point of view: menopause is a normal event, *OB/GYN Clinical Alert* 9(3):23, July 1992.

Taplin S, Anderman C, Grothaus L: Breast cancer risk and participation in mammographic screening, *AJPH* 79(11):1494, 1989.

Tilyard M et al: Treatment of postmenopausal osteoporosis with calcitriol of calcium, *N Engl J Med* 326(6):357, 1992.

Tucker SM et al: *Patient care standards, nursing process, diagnosis and outcome,* ed 5, St Louis, 1992, Mosby–Year Book.

Utian WF: *Managing your menopause,* Englewood Cliffs, NJ, 1991, Prentice Hall.

Yu L et al: The ISQ-P tool: measuring stress associated with incontinence, *J Gerontol Nurs* 15(2):9, 1989.

Bibliography—Nursing Research

Quinn AA: A theoretical model of the perimenopausal process, *J Nurse Midwif* 36(1):25, 1991.

Schank MJ, Lough MA: Maintaining health and independence of elderly women, *J Gerontol Nurs* 15(9):1989.

Speake DL, Cowart ME, Stephens R: Healthy lifestyle practices of rural and urban elderly, *Health Values* 15(1):45, 1991.

Trice LB: Meaningful life experience to the elderly, *Image J Nurs Sch* 22(4):248, 1990.

Walker S et al: A Spanish language version of the health-promoting lifestyle profile, *Nurs Res* 39(5):268, 1990.

chapter 41 review

Key Concepts

- Gynecologic disorders diminish the quality of life for affected women and their families.
- Premenstrual syndrome (PMS), no longer considered a purely psychologic problem, is a disorder that begins approximately 7 to 10 days before menses and ends with the onset of menses.
- Endometriosis is characterized by secondary amenorrhea, dyspareunia, abnormal uterine bleeding, and infertility.
- The climacterium is a normal developmental phase during which a woman passes from the reproductive to the nonreproductive stage.
- During the climacterium, women seek care for symptoms that arise from vasomotor instability, emotional disturbances, fatigue, genital atrophy, and changes related to sexuality.
- Osteoporosis, a progressive loss of bone mass that results from decreasing levels of estrogen after menopause, can be prevented or minimized with hormone replacement therapy.
- Estrogen increases calcitonin levels to prevent bone resorption and maintain bone density. The role of calcium supplementation and exercise, without HRT, in maintaining bone density is controversial.
- Sexuality and the ability for sexual expression continue after menopause.
- Pelvic relaxation and lengthening of fascial supports are most often the delayed sequelae of childbirth trauma, but they may be seen in young or childless women.

Key Terms

- cervical intraepithelial neoplasm (CIN) (p. 1250)
- climacterium (p. 1257)
- cystocele (p. 1268)
- endometriosis (p. 1254)
- enterocele (p. 1268)
- estrogen replacement therapy (ERT) (p. 1261)
- fistula (p. 1272)
- health promotion (p. 1246)
- hormone replacement therapy (HRT) (p. 1252)
- hot flush (flash) (p. 1258)
- hypogonadotropic amenorrhea (p. 1251)
- menopause (p. 1257)
- osteoporosis (p. 1260)
- pelvic relaxation (p. 1267)
- pessary (p. 1272)
- premenstrual syndrome (PMS) (p. 1253)
- primary dysmenorrhea (p. 1252)
- prostaglandin-synthesis inhibitor (p. 1252)
- rectocele (p. 1267)
- secondary dysmenorrhea (p. 1252)
- stress urinary incontinence (p. 1269)
- urethrocele (p. 1268)
- uterine prolapse (p. 1270)

Critical Thinking Exercises

1. Interview a woman with PMS to determine her responses to the condition.
   a. What are her perceptions about how others view her condition?
   b. Examine how her responses compare to theoretic responses as well as your own perceptions.
   c. Analyze the woman's responses to identify positive and negative aspects of PMS.
   d. Formulate a plan of care using the data from the interview.
2. You are assigned to a clinic where women are assessed and treated for menopausal symptoms.
   a. What are some generalizations about women and menopause?
   b. What are your perceptions about women who have numerous complaints/symptoms that they attribute to menopause?
   c. What impact could these perceptions have on providing care to menopausal women?
   d. How can nurses effect a positive change in the care of midlife and older women?

Topics for Nursing Research

- Pap smear screening in elderly women: more clearly defining high-risk subsets of the elderly. Screening for long-term-care facility residents.
- The use of nurse practitioners and midwives in Pap smear screening and colposcopy clinics: cost effectiveness and outcomes.
- Women's perceptions of women's health problems: menstruation, endometriosis, and PMS.
- The nurse's role in preventing osteoporosis.
- The relationships among place of residence, income, education, health beliefs, and health practices.
- Health values and health practices among African American women and other cultural groups.
- Evaluation of health promotion strategies.
- Data about symptoms and perceptions about menopause derived from women in the community who are not seeking care vs. self-selected women who do seek care.
- Psychologic needs of women undergoing pelvic surgery.

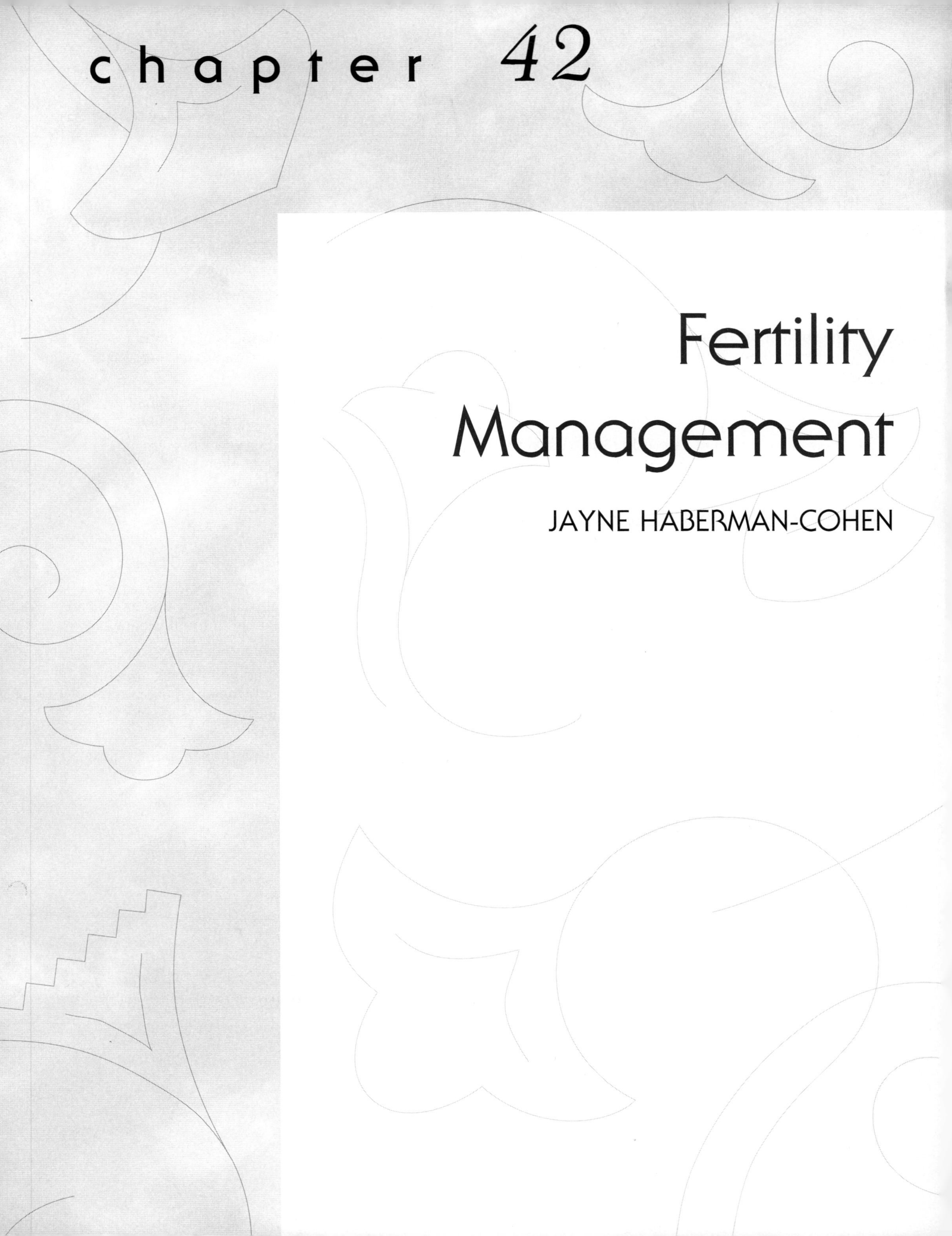

chapter 42

Fertility Management

JAYNE HABERMAN-COHEN

LEARNING OBJECTIVES

- Define the key terms listed.
- List common causes of impaired fertility.
- Discuss the psychologic impact of impaired fertility.
- List common diagnoses and treatments for impaired fertility.
- Describe the different methods of contraception.
- State the advantages and disadvantages of commonly used methods of contraception.
- Explain the common nursing interventions that facilitate contraceptive use.
- Evaluate the alternatives available to a woman experiencing an unplanned pregnancy.
- Describe the techniques used for surgical interruption of pregnancy.
- Develop a nursing care plan for surgical intervention of pregnancy.
- Recognize the various ethical and legal considerations of impaired infertility, control of fertility, and termination of fertility.
- Identify topics for nursing research related to fertility management.

This chapter addresses several fertility-related issues, associated tests, and common therapies. The reproductive spectrum is addressed, covering everything from impaired fertility to voluntary control of fertility to surgical interruption of pregnancy.

■ IMPAIRED FERTILITY

The inability to conceive and bear a child comes as a surprise to 15% to 20% of otherwise healthy adults (Evans et al, 1989). It is difficult to be denied the experiences of pregnancy and birth, parenthood, and the expression of love through the care and nurturing of another human being. Disturbance in one's sexual self concept is often experienced. Couples requesting assistance with impaired fertility have already decided that they want a child. They seek acceptance and assistance from the nurse and physician in coping with and possibly resolving this problem.

The traditional definition of **impaired fertility** is the inability to conceive after at least 1 year of unprotected intercourse. Impaired fertility is the inability to conceive and also the inability to give birth to a live infant. A contemporary definition does not consider a time limit. It is the inability to conceive or carry to live birth at a time the couple has chosen to do so.

Impaired fertility is *primary* if the woman has never been pregnant or the man has never impregnated a woman. It is *secondary* if the woman has been pregnant at least once but has not been able to conceive again or sustain a pregnancy.

Sterility implies that conception is not possible and the cause cannot be remedied. The incidence of impaired fertility seems to be increasing. An estimated one out of every six couples in the United States is involuntarily childless (Willson, Carrington, 1987). Probable causes include the trend to delay pregnancy until later in life when fertility decreases naturally, the increase in pelvic inflammatory disease, and the increase in substance abuse. Environmental agents (e.g., pesticides and lead) negatively affect both male and female reproductive systems (Mattison et al, 1990). Diagnosis and treatment of impaired fertility require considerable physical, emotional, and financial investment over an extended period. Frank (1990b) found that personal beliefs, physician advice, and emotional stress are the critical factors influencing infertility treatment decisions. Men tend to make decisions based on potential side effects and women on the potential effectiveness of treatment (Frank, 1990a).

The attitude, sensitivity, and caring nature of those who are involved in the assessment of impaired fertility lay the foundation for the client's ability to cope with the subsequent therapy and management. All members of the health team must respect the clients' rights to privacy and the confidentiality of client records.

RELIGIOUS CONSIDERATIONS. Civil laws and religious proscriptions about sex must always be kept in mind by the clinician. For example, the Orthodox Jewish husband and wife may face infertility investigation and management problems because of religious laws that govern marital relations. According to Jewish law the couple may not engage in marital relations during menstruation and through the following 7 "preparatory days." The wife then is immersed in a ritual bath (Mikvah) before relations can resume. The 5 menstrual days and 7 preparatory days collectively are called the "nida state." Any vaginal bleeding of physiologic origin marks the beginning of the nida state. Fertility problems can arise when the woman has a short cycle (i.e., a cycle of 24 days or less, when ovulation would occur on day 10 or earlier). Small doses of estrogen may delay ovulation to allow for the time needed to complete the nida state. Other procedures that induce bleeding may delay intercourse for another 12 days to allow for the nida state. Thus Orthodox Jewish clients, as well as observant Catholics, may at times question proposed diagnostic and therapeutic procedures because of religious proscriptions. These clients are encouraged to consult their rabbi or priest for a ruling.

Other religions teach that a marriage can be annulled if a woman is found to be infertile, though the reverse is not true if a man is found to be infertile. Religious influences over fertility and hence impaired fertility account for many of the sociocultural attitudes displayed toward childless couples (Menning, 1977).

PSYCHOSOCIAL CONSIDERATIONS. Within the United States, feelings connected to impaired fertility are many and complex.* The origin of some of these feelings are myths, superstitions, misinformation, or "magical" thinking about the cause of infertility. Other feelings arise from the need to undergo many tests and examinations and from being "different" from others.

Menning (1977) and Speroff et al (1983) have tried to debunk some common myths. These myths include:

1. *Infertility has a psychologic origin.* For 80% to

*See Chapter 6 for psychosocial aspects and Chapter 40, Loss and Grief.

90% of all cases of impaired fertility, there is a discernible physiologic explanation.

2. *Adopting improves a couple's chance of conceiving.* No significant increase in conception has been found among couples with impaired fertility who had adopted compared with couples who had not adopted.
3. *Being infertile is a sexual disorder.* For most couples, impaired fertility is not related to their ability to perform sexual intercourse.
4. *It is immoral to wish to bear children and to actively pursue that goal.* For those who wish to have children, their impaired fertility is an involuntary barrier to their choice of parenthood.

Veevers' report (1973) on the social meaning of parenthood and nonparenthood provides further insight into the psychosocial impact of impaired fertility. The extent to which a society perceives nonparenthood as unnatural, as an avoidance of responsibility, a rejection of gender role, a sign of immaturity, or a hindrance to positive marital adjustment is the extent to which couples with impaired fertility may perceive their society as being nonsupportive. Under such circumstances, infertile couples might have problems not only in accepting their impaired fertility but also in discussing their feelings with health care providers.

CULTURAL CONSIDERATIONS. Worldwide, cultures continue to employ symbols and rites that celebrate fertility. One fertility rite that persists today is the custom of throwing rice at the bride and groom. Other fertility symbols and rites include the passing out of congratulatory cigars, candy, or pencils by a new father and baby showers held in anticipation of a child's birth. Last, but not least, is the American image of motherhood. Mothers and motherhood are paid homage, especially in the communications media of the United States. It is no wonder that Mother's Day is the busiest day for telephone companies and one of the busiest for florists.

The person without children in Samoa is pitied. According to Brownlee (1978), in many cultures a woman's inability to conceive may be due to her sins, to evil spirits, or to the fact that she is an inadequate person. The virility of a man in some cultures remains in question until he demonstrates his ability to reproduce by having at least one child.

Determination of a culturally defined cause for sterility is usually accompanied by a culturally proposed solution for the problem. These proposed solutions may or may not be effective. For example, Vietnamese men thought sterility was caused by loss of sperm during wet dreams or through daytime discharge (Coughlin, 1965). Tonics consisting of licorice, aconite, and ginseng might be used to counteract the effect. Certain foods such as cereal were to be eaten, and substances such as alcohol were to be avoided.

In most cultures, responsibility for impaired fertility is usually attributed to the woman. If infertility is believed to be caused by a misplaced uterus, methods are used to replace it. A Samoan woman may go to a bush doctor who will massage the abdomen over the uterus with oil and attempt to put it back in place (Clark, Howland, 1978).

For Mexican-American women and others who subscribe to heat/cold balance and imbalance theories, barrenness is considered to result from having a "cold womb" (Clark, 1970). The cold womb may be heated through external and internal means. Clark (1970) describes two methods used by Mexican-American women. One method requires a barren woman to sit over a washtub of hot water, to which rosemary is added, so that the vapors warm the womb. The other method attempts to build up body heat over a period of 3 days. This is done by avoiding cold foods and water, using a belladonna plaster over the sacral area, and ingesting cathartic pills and hot chocolate. For further discussion of cultural aspects of care, see Chapter 3.

Factors Associated with Infertility

The couple is a "biologic unit" of reproduction. Many factors, both male and female, contribute to normal fertility. A normally developed reproductive tract is essential. Normal functioning of an intact hypothalamic-pituitary-gonadal axis supports gametogenesis—the formation of sperm and ova. The life span of the sperm and ovum is short. Although sperm remain viable in the female's reproductive tract for 48 hours or more, probably only a few retain fertilization potential for more than 24 hours. Ova remain viable for about 24 hours, but the optimum time for fertilization may be no more than 1 to 2 hours (Cunningham, MacDonald, Gant, 1989). It is likely that viable sperm may need to be present in the uterine tube at the time of ovulation for optimum fertilization (Cunningham, MacDonald, Gant, 1989). Thus timing of intercourse becomes critical.

The male must produce sperm that are normal, adequate in number, and motile. Accessory glands must provide supportive secretions to the sperm to form semen. The tube system to the urethra must be patent. Ejaculation must deposit semen around the cervix at the appropriate time of the female's menstrual cycle. After being deposited, sperm must be able to penetrate and be sustained by receptive and supportive cervical mucus. Sperm must undergo capacitation (Chapter 7) to prepare for fertilization. Then they migrate through the uterus to the ampulla of the uterine tube to fertilize a receptive normal ovum.

In the female, a graafian follicle must mature and release a healthy ovum able to be fertilized. The ovum must be drawn by the fimbria into a healthy, patent uterine tube and fertilized within a few hours. The conceptus must migrate down the tube into a well-developed normal uterus. Implantation of the blastocyst must occur within 7 to 10 days in a hormone-prepared endometrium. The conceptus must develop normally, reach viability, and be delivered in good condition for extrauterine life.

An alteration in one or more of these structures, functions, or processes results in some degree of impairment of fertility. Causes of impaired fertility are sometimes difficult to assign to either the male or the female (Willson, Carrington, 1987). A male factor may be solely responsible in 30% of infertile couples, but it may be contributory in another 10%. Tubal factors are identified in about 25% of infertile couples, an ovulatory disorder in about 20%,* or a cervical factor in approximately 15%. Miscellaneous factors (5%) or unknown (unexplained) factors (5%) account for the remaining causes.

Unexplained infertility and recurrent (habitual) abortion may be the result of aberrations of the immune system (e.g., antisperm antibodies, failure of implantation and growth of a blastocyst) (Evans et al, 1989).

■ INVESTIGATION OF FEMALE INFERTILITY

The investigation of impaired fertility is conducted systematically, since multiple factors involving both partners are common. Both partners must be interested in the solution to the problem. The medical investigation requires time and considerable financial expense, as well as causes emotional distress and strain on the couple's interpersonal relationship. Nurses can be instrumental in providing information about the latest tests and treatment (Nero, 1988). A thorough investigation usually requires 3 to 4 months of time.

Investigation of impaired fertility begins with a complete history and physical examination (see box on p. 1283). The history explores the duration of infertility, past obstetric events, and contains a detailed sexual history. Medical and surgical conditions are evaluated. Exposure to reproductive hazards in the home (e.g., mutagens such as plastic-vinyl chlorides, teratogens such as alcohol, and emotional stresses) and workplace are explored.

A complete general physical examination is followed by a specific assessment of the reproductive tract. Evidence of endocrine system abnormalities is sought. Inadequate development of secondary sex characteristics (e.g., inappropriate distribution of body fat and hair) may point to problems with the hypothalamic-pituitary-ovarian axis or genetic aberrations (e.g., Turner's syndrome). Women with Turner's syndrome are typically short, have underdeveloped breasts, and abnormal gonads. These women are infertile. Other women may have an abnormal uterus and tubes as a result of exposure to diethylstilbestrol (DES) in utero. Evidence of past infection of the genital urinary system is sought. Bimanual examination of the internal organs may reveal lack of mobility of the uterus or abnormal contours of the uterus and adnexa.

Laboratory data are assembled. Data from routine urine and blood tests is obtained along with other tests (see box at right).

Tests and Examinations

There are several examinations and tests for impaired fertility. The basic infertility survey involves evaluation of the cervix, uterus, tubes, and peritoneum; detection of ovulation; assessment of immunologic compatibility; and evaluation of psychogenic factors (Scott et al, 1990). Procedures commonly used include the following:

Detection of ovulation: basal body temperature (BBT), cervical mucus characteristics, endometrial biopsy, radioimmunoassays of hormones essential for fertility, laparoscopic and sonographic examination

Assessment of tubal patency and peritoneum: hysterosalpingography, laparoscopic examination, culdoscopy

Assessment of the uterus: hysterosalpingography, timed endometrial biopsy, laparoscopic examination, serum progesterone levels

Evaluation of the vagina and cervix: BBT, cervical mucus characteristics, postcoital test of interaction between sperm and cervical mucus, in vitro test of cervical mucus penetration by sperm

Evaluation of immunologic compatibility: sperm agglutination tests, sperm immobilization tests

Nurses can alleviate some of the mystery associated with impaired fertility by explaining to clients the timing and rationale for each test (Table 42-1).

*Other authors (Evans et al, 1989) suggest that ovulation disorders are implicated in 40% to 50% of infertile couples.

Assessment of the Woman

HISTORY

1. Duration of impaired fertility: length of contraceptive and noncontraceptive exposure
2. Fertility in another sexual relationship
3. Obstetric
   a. Number of pregnancies and abortions
   b. Length of time required to initiate each pregnancy
   c. Complications of any pregnancy
   d. Duration of lactation
4. Gynecologic: detailed menstrual history
5. Previous tests and therapy done for impaired fertility
6. Medical: general medical history including chronic and hereditary disease (e.g., endocrine dysfunction); drug use
7. Surgical: especially abdominal or pelvic surgery
8. Sexual history in detail: libido, orgasm capacity, techniques, frequency of intercourse, and postcoital practices; number of sexual partners
9. Occupational and environmental exposure to chemicals, or x-ray equipment; physical nature of occupation or hobbies; vacations and work habits
10. Personal: motivation for childbearing; attitude toward partner, career aspirations; reason for seeking advice regarding impaired fertility at this time

PHYSICAL EXAMINATION

1. General: complete physical examination
2. Genital tract: state of hymen (full penetration); clitoris; vaginal infection, including trichomoniasis and candidiasis; cervical tears, polyps, infection, patency of os, accessibility to insemination; uterus, including size and position, mobility; adnexae, tumors, evidence of endometriosis

LABORATORY DATA

1. Routine urine, complete blood count, gonorrhea and chlamydia tests, and serologic test for syphilis; additional laboratory studies as indicated
2. Basic endocrine studies in women with irregular menstrual cycles or in amenorrhea, hirsutism, acne, or excessive weight gain
3. For women with irregular menstrual cycles: protein-bound iodine (PBI) or other thyroid tests, 17-ketosteroid assay test, 17-hydroxycorticosteroid test, glucose tolerance test (GTT), endometrial biopsy, and progesterone levels
4. For women with amenorrhea: tomographic x-ray films of skull, T_4 or other thyroid tests, 17-ketosteroid assay test, 17-hydroxycorticosteroid test, GTT, endometrial biopsy, gonadotropin follicle-stimulating hormone (FSH), luteinizing hormone (LH) determination, and buccal smear and chromosomal studies

Other laboratory tests added as desired for a more complete diagnosis of endocrine problems:

5. Rh factor and antibody titer tests—important in abortion and preterm birth problems
6. *Sperm antibody agglutination studies:* special laboratory procedure involves obtaining a fresh semen specimen from the man and a blood sample from the woman; sperm are incubated in the blood serum of the woman and checked at intervals for agglutination; the test is negative if no agglutinated sperm are found
7. Chromosome studies, where indicated

Fertility test findings favorable to fertility are summarized on p. 1290. A discussion of the most common tests follows.

DETECTION OF OVULATION. Documentation of time of ovulation is important in the investigation of impaired fertility. Direct proof of ovulation is pregnancy or the retrieval of an ovum from the uterine tube. There are several indirect or presumptive methods for detection of ovulation. These include assessment of BBT (for discussion of BBT, see p. 1303) and cervical mucus characteristics (for discussion of cervical mucus, see p. 1304), as well as endometrial biopsy. These clinical tests more or less determine whether progesterone is secreted in significant amounts (Table 42-1) (Willson, Carrington, 1987) to accommodate implantation and maintain pregnancy. Occurrence of mittelschmerz and midcycle spotting provides unreliable presumptive evidence of ovulation (Scott et al, 1990).

HORMONE ANALYSIS. Hormone analysis is performed to assess endocrine function of the *hypothalamic-pituitary-ovarian axis*. Blood and urine specimens are obtained at varying times during a woman's menstrual cycle. Blood specimens are drawn to deter-

TABLE 42-1 Tests for Impaired Fertility

Test/Examination	Timing (Menstrual Cycle Days)	Rationale
Hysterosalpingogram	7-10	Late follicular, early proliferative phase will not disrupt a fertilized ovum. May open uterine tubes before time of ovulation.
Postcoital (Huhner test)	Peak cervical mucus flow*	Ovulatory late proliferative phase—look for normal motile sperm in cervical mucus.
Sperm immobilization antigen-antibody reaction		Immunologic test to determine sperm and cervical mucus interaction.
Assessment of cervical mucus		Cervical mucus should have low viscosity, high spinnbarkheit.
Ultrasound observation of follicular collapse	Ovulation	Collapsed follicle is seen after ovulation.
Serum assay of plasma progesterone	20-25	Midluteal midsecretory phase—check adequacy of corpus luteal production of progesterone.
Basal body temperature (BBT)		Elevation occurs in response to progesterone.
Endometrial biopsy	26-27	Late luteal, late secretory phase—check endometrial response to progesterone and adequacy of luteal phase.

*Exogenous estrogen may be given to induce mucus flow if spontaneous and reasonably regular ovulation does not occur.

mine levels of progesterone, estrogen, FSH, and LH. Urine specimens provide information about the levels of 17-ketosteroids and 17-hydroxycorticosteroids.

Blood is drawn late in the woman's menstrual cycle to assess the function of the *corpus luteum*. This test can be done in a serial manner to determine if the levels of plasma progesterone correlate well with the client's BBT and cervical mucus characteristics (pp. 1303 and 1304).

TIMED ENDOMETRIAL BIOPSY. Endometrial biopsy is scheduled after ovulation during the luteal phase of the menstrual cycle. Late in the menstrual cycle, 3 to 4 days before expected menses, a sample of the endometrium is removed for histologic study to assess the function of the corpus luteum and the receptivity of the endometrium for implantation. There are two methods of performing a timed endometrial biopsy; neither method requires hospitalization. The first method is implemented 3 to 4 days before expected menses. With the woman draped and in the lithotomy position, a vaginal speculum is inserted into the vagina. Using a small lumen vabra aspirator, a sample of the endometrium is obtained.

The second method includes the following steps:

1. The couple is cautioned to abstain from intercourse during preceding "fertile" period to avoid dislodging a possible embryo during the procedure.
2. The cervix is dilated with laminaria 4 to 24 hours before the procedure, which requires no analgesia. (**Laminaria** are small, thin inserts of packed seaweed or synthetic osmotic dilators that when inserted into the cervix, absorb moisture, expand, and thus dilate the cervix; see Fig. 42-14).
3. The woman assumes the lithotomy position and is draped, and the speculum is inserted.
4. The laminaria are removed.
5. If not previously dilated with laminaria, the cervix is dilated at this time with metal rod dilators. Analgesia or anesthesia is often necessary.
6. A small specimen of endometrium is removed from the side wall in the fundus to avoid dislodging an embryo should conception have occurred. (When implantation occurs, it is usually high in the fundus, either in the anterior or posterior portion.)

Findings favorable to fertility include an endometrium that is negative for tuberculosis, polyps, or inflammatory conditions and that reflects secretory changes normally seen in the presence of adequate luteal (progesterone) phase.

HYSTEROSALPINGOGRAPHY. Radiographic (x-ray) film allows visualization of the uterine cavity and tubes after the instillation of radioopaque contrast material through the cervix (Fig. 42-1). It is possible to see abnormalities of the uterus such as congenital defects (Fig. 42-2) or defects produced by submucous myomas and endometrial polyps. Distortions of the uterine cavity or uterine tubes as a result of current or past pelvic inflammatory disease (PID) are identified. Scar tissue and adhesions from inflammatory processes can immobilize the uterus and tubes, kink the tubes, and surround the ovaries. PID may

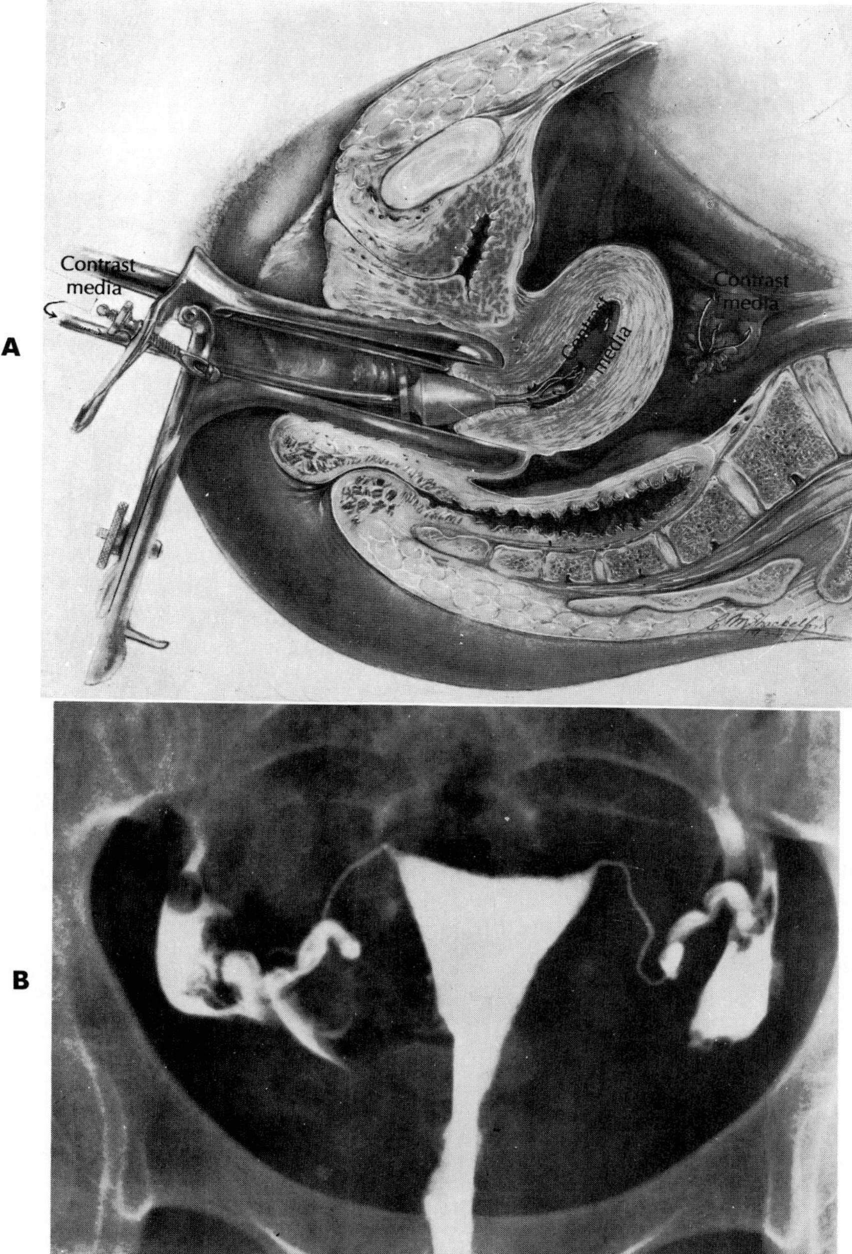

Fig. 42-1 A, Hysterosalpingography. Sagittal section showing technique. Contrast medium flows through intrauterine cannula and out through tubes, the cervix being closed by a rubber stopper. **B,** Normal hysterosalpingogram showing passage of radiopaque material through fimbriated ends of tubes.

A, From Willson JR: *Management of obstetric difficulties*, ed 6, St Louis, 1961, Mosby–Year Book. B, From Willson JR, Carrington ER: *Obstetrics and gynecology*, ed 9, St Louis, 1991, Mosby–Year Book.

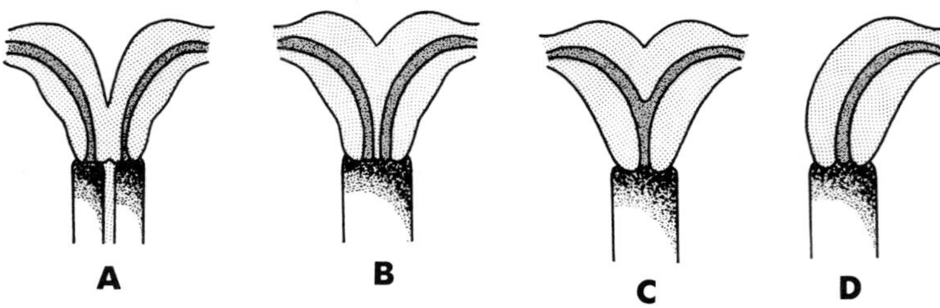

Fig. 42-2 Abnormal uteruses. **A,** Uterus didelphys bicollis (septate vagina). **B,** Uterus bicornis bicollis (vagina simplex). **C,** Uterus bicornis unicollis (vagina simplex). **D,** Uterus unicornis.

Modified from Willson JR, Carrington ER: *Obstetrics and gynecology*, ed 9, St Louis, 1991, Mosby–Year Book.

follow infection from sexually transmitted diseases (STDs) or rupture of an inflamed appendix.

Hysterosalpingography is scheduled 2 to 5 days after menstruation to avoid flushing a potential fertilized ovum out through a tube into the peritoneal cavity. Also at this time there are no open vessels and menstrual debris has all been discharged. This decreases the risk of embolism or of forcing menstrual debris out through the tubes into the peritoneal cavity. If the woman has PID, she is treated with antimicrobials and the test is rescheduled in 2 to 3 months.

Referred shoulder pain may occur during this procedure. The referred pain is indicative of subphrenic irritation from the contrast material if it is spilled out of the patent uterine tubes or if the tubes are occluded. The discomfort subsides with position change. It usually disappears within 12 to 14 hours and can be controlled with mild analgesics.

This procedure may be therapeutic as well as diagnostic. The passage of contrast medium may clear tubes of mucous plugs, straighten kinked tubes, or break up adhesions within the tubes (secondary to salpingitis). The procedure may stimulate cilia in the lining of the tubes to facilitate transport of the sex cells. It also may aid healing as a result of the bacteriostatic effect of the iodine within the contrast medium.

LAPAROSCOPY. Laparoscopy is usually scheduled early in the menstrual cycle. During the procedure, a small telescope is inserted through a small incision in the anterior abdominal wall. Cold fiberoptic light sources allow for superior visualization of the internal pelvic structures (Fig. 42-3). The woman is usually admitted shortly before surgery, having taken nothing by mouth (NPO) for 8 hours. She voids before surgery. A general anesthetic is usually given and the woman is placed in the lithotomy position. Her pubic hair is shaved only if this examination is likely to be followed by laparotomy. A needle is inserted and a pneumoperitoneum with carbon dioxide gas is established to elevate the abdominal wall from the organs, thereby creating an empty space that permits visualization and exploration with the laparoscope. If tubal patency is being assessed, a cannula is used to instill a dye contrast medium through the cervix. Visualization of the peritoneal cavity in infertile women may reveal endometriosis, pelvic adhesions, tubal occlusion, or polycystic ovaries. Fulguration (destruction of tissue by means of electricity) of small endometrial implants, lysis of the adhesions, and taking ovarian biopsies are some of the procedures possible through the use of a laparoscope. After surgery, deflation of most of the gas is done by direct expression. Trocar (and needle) sites are closed with a single subcuticular absorbable suture or skin clip, and an adhesive bandage is applied. Postoperative recovery requires taking of vital signs, assessing level of consciousness, preventing aspiration, monitoring intravenous fluids, and reassuring the client regarding

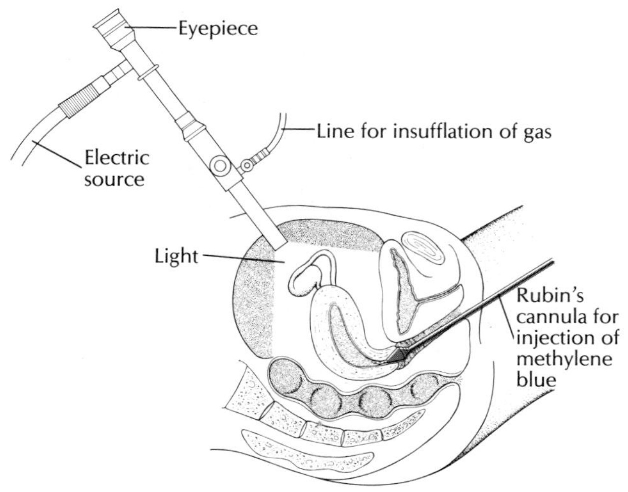

Fig. 42-3 Laparoscopy.

referred shoulder discomfort. Discharge from the hospital usually occurs in 4 to 6 hours. Referred shoulder pain or subcostal discomfort (from pneumoperitoneum) usually lasts only 24 hours and is relieved with a mild analgesic. The woman must be cautioned against heavy lifting or strenuous activity for 4 to 7 days, at which time she is usually asymptomatic.

ULTRASOUND PELVIC EXAMINATION. Abdominal (Chapter 27) or transvaginal ultrasound is also used to assess pelvic structures (Fig. 42-4). This procedure is used to visualize pelvic tissues for a variety of reasons (e.g., to identify abnormalities, to verify follicular development and maturity, or to confirm intrauterine [vs. ectopic] pregnancy).

■ REPRODUCTIVE STRUCTURES AND FACTORS IMPLICATED IN INFERTILITY

Congenital or Developmental Factors

If the woman has abnormal external genitals, surgical reconstruction of abnormal tissue and construction of a functional vagina may permit normal intercourse. If internal reproductive tract structures are absent, there is no hope for fertility. Surgical intervention depends entirely on the anatomic development (Fig. 42-2), the surgical feasibility, and the individual's actual gender role.

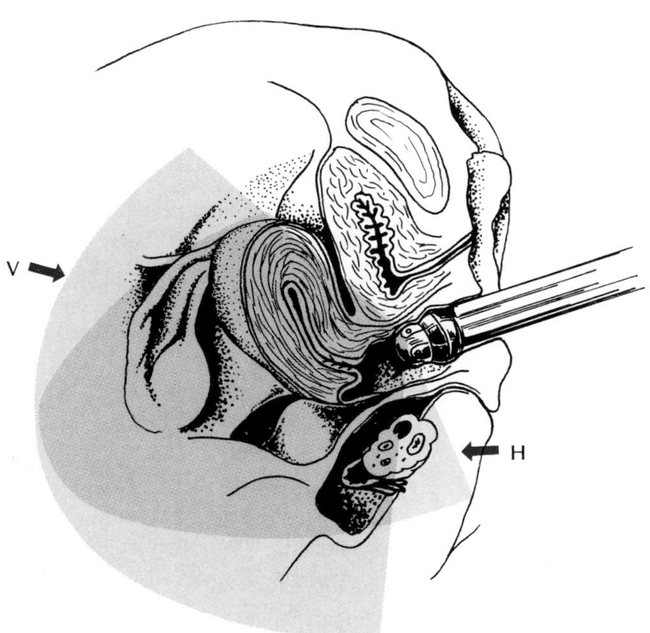

Fig. 42-4 Vaginal ultrasonography. Major scanning planes of transducer: *H*, Horizontal, *V*, vertical.

Vaginal and uterine anomalies and their surgical repair vary from individual to individual. If a functional uterus can be reconstructed, pregnancy may be possible. After surgical repair of the uterus, cesarean birth is necessary to prevent uterine rupture during labor. Women with ovarian agenesis (absence of ovaries) or dysgenesis (abnormal ovaries) are sterile, and no treatment will improve their fertility.

Ovarian Factors

Within healthy ovaries, graafian follicles respond to FSH and LH by the maturation of an ovum and ovulation. The graafian follicle produces estrogen; the empty graafian follicle becomes the corpus luteum and produces estrogen and progesterone.

Anovulation may be primary or secondary. *Primary anovulation* may be caused by a pituitary or hypothalamic hormone disorder or an adrenal gland disorder such as congenital adrenal hyperplasia. *Secondary anovulation* may be caused by ovarian disease. In amenorrheic states and instances of anovulatory cycles, hormone studies usually reveal the problem.

TREATMENT AND PROGNOSIS. Drug therapy is often an important but expensive component of client care. *Ovulatory stimulants* may be warranted. *Clomiphene* (Clomid, Serophene), an oral preparation, is a follicular maturing agent. It is used to treat anovulation caused by hypothalamic suppression when the hypothalamic-pituitary-ovarian axis is intact. *Bromocriptine* (Parlodel), a synthetic ergot alkaloid that inhibits the release of prolactin, is used to treat anovulation caused by elevated levels of prolactin. *Thyroid-stimulating hormone* (TSH) is indicated if the woman has hypothyroidism; *human menopausal gonadotropin* (hMG) (Pergonal), if she has hypogonadotropic amenorrhea. When anovulation is caused by hypothalamic-pituitary dysfunction, hypothalamic failure, or failure to respond to clomiphene, *gonadotropin-releasing hormone* (GnRH) may be prescribed.

Hormone replacement therapy may be indicated. The woman who has low levels of estrogen is a candidate for *conjugated estrogens and medroxy-progesterone*. A hypoestrogenic condition may result from a high stress level or decreased percentage of body fat as a result of an eating disorder (e.g., anorexia nervosa) or excessive exercise. *Hydroxyprogesterone* supplementation with vaginal suppositories or intramuscular injection is used to treat luteal phase defects.

The nurse may encounter other medications as well. In the presence of adrenal hyperplasia, *prednisone*, a glucocorticoid, is taken orally. *Danazol* is the drug of choice in the management of endometriosis. Infections are treated with appropriate antimicrobial formulations.

The nurse's role is that of teacher/counselor. Although the physician is responsible for informing clients fully about the prescribed medications, the nurse must be ready to answer clients' questions. Clients often ask the nurse to confirm their understanding of the drug, its administration, potential side effects, and expected outcomes. Since information varies with each drug, the nurse needs to consult the medication package inserts, pharmacology references, physician, and pharmacist as necessary.

Ovarian tumors must be excised. Whenever possible, functional ovarian tissue is left intact. Scar tissue adhesions caused by chronic infection may cover much or all of the ovary. These adhesions usually necessitate surgery to free and expose the ovary so that ovulation can occur.

Thyroid gland dysfunction may be associated with menstrual abnormalities, impaired fertility, or recurrent fetal wastage. Therapy consists of management of the thyroid condition coupled with careful scrutiny of BBT charts (p. 1304) to promote sperm deposition at the same time as ovulation. Continuous monitoring and management of thyroid function during pregnancy are also carried out.

In the presence of severe emotional problems the woman is referred to a mental health therapist. Her condition may require the teamwork of the mental health therapist, the endocrinologist, and an obstetrician-gynecologist.

Tubal (Peritoneal) Factors

The fingerlike processes of the fimbriated end of the uterine tube and the tube itself need to be freely movable to approach the ovary to "catch" the ovum. The tube must be open, sufficiently long, and capable of ciliary action and peristalsis to carry the ovum into and down the tube. In most cases fertilization occurs in the ampulla of the tube. Some unknown factor, possibly an enzyme, supplied by the ampulla of the tube seems to be required for the physiologic change or "conditioning" of the sperm called capacitation (Chapter 7).

The motility of the tube and its fimbriated end may be reduced or absent as a result of infections, adhesions, or tumors. Chlamydial infection negatively influences tubal function and impedes fertility (Eggert-Kruse et al, 1990). In rare instances there may be congenital absence of one tube. It is also possible to find one tube relatively shorter than the other. This condition is often associated with an abnormally developed uterus.

Inflammation within the tube or involving the exterior of the tube or the fimbriated ends represents a major cause of impaired fertility. Tubal adhesions resulting from pelvic infections (e.g., ruptured appendix) may impair fertility. When infection with purulent discharge eventually heals, scar tissue adhesions form. In the process the tube may be blocked anywhere along its length. It can be closed off at the fimbriated end, or it can be distorted and kinked by adhesions. Adhesions may permit the tiny sperm to pass through the tube but may prevent a fertilized egg from completing the journey into the intrauterine cavity. This results in an ectopic pregnancy that may completely destroy the tube (see discussion of ectopic pregnancy, Chapter 30).

In other cases, adhesions of the tubes to the ovary or bowel may follow *endometriosis* (for further discussion of endometriosis, see Chapter 41). Endometriosis is a disease in which endometrial tissue, ordinarily found only within the uterus, is present outside the uterus attached to other organs or tissue in the woman's body (Fig. 41-2). The ectopic endometrial tissue responds to hormonal stimulation in the way that uterine endometrium does. In endometriosis, periodic monthly bleeding from endometrial implants causes dense adhesions, making pregnancy difficult or impossible.

TREATMENT AND PROGNOSIS. Treatment must include prevention and early adequate management of infection with appropriate antibiotics. Surgery may be necessary when drainage of a serious focus of infection is required. Hysterosalpingography is useful for identification of tubal obstruction and also for the release of blockage. During laparoscopy, delicate adhesions may be divided and removed and endometrial implants may be destroyed by electrocoagulation or Nd:YAG laser. Women with severe endometriosis have an improved chance for pregnancy when treated with GIFT (Yovich, Matson, 1990) (see p. 1298). Laparotomy and even microsurgery may be required to do extensive repair of the damaged tube. Prognosis is dependent on the degree to which tube patency and function can be restored.

Uterine Factors

The uterus must be of sufficient size and shape to permit maintenance of a pregnancy to term gestation. The endometrium must be prepared by estrogen and progesterone and must be healthy for implantation to occur.

Congenital abnormalities of the uterus are far more common than might be expected. Minor developmental anomalies of the uterus are fairly common;

major anomalies occur rarely (see Fig. 42-2). Hysterosalpingography may reveal a double uterus or other anomalous congenital variations. Endometrial and myometrial *tumors* (e.g., polyps or myomas [Chapter 44]) may also be revealed by x-ray studies of infertile women.

Asherman's syndrome, uterine adhesions or scar tissue, is characterized by hypomenorrhea or amenorrhea. The adhesions, which may partially or totally obliterate the uterine cavity, are sequelae to surgical interventions such as too vigorous curettage (scraping) after an abortion (elective or spontaneous). The hysteroscope is useful in the verification of intrauterine anomalies.

Endometritis (inflammation of the endometrium) may result from any of the causes of infection of the cervix or uterine tubes (e.g., chlamydia). Women who have numerous sex partners are more susceptible to endometrial infection than are women in monogamous relationships.

TREATMENT AND PROGNOSIS. A woman with a relatively small uterus may become pregnant, but the uterus may be incapable of accommodating the enlarging fetus, and a spontaneous abortion may result. In such cases recurrent or habitual (three or more) spontaneous abortions often occur. No medical therapy has been effective for the enlargement of an abnormally small uterus. Observation suggests that women who do become pregnant but who miscarry, often abort at a later time with each successive pregnancy. Finally, after two or three pregnancy losses, they may deliver a viable infant. Apparently actual "growth" of the uterus occurs with each pregnancy. Plastic surgery—for example, the unification operation for bicornuate uterus—often improves a woman's ability to conceive and carry the fetus to term.

Surgical removal of tumors or fibroids involving the endometrium or uterus often improves the woman's chance of conceiving and maintaining the pregnancy to viability. Surgical treatment of uterine tumors or maldevelopment that results in successful pregnancy requires birth by cesarean surgery near term gestation. The uterus may rupture as a result of weakness of the area of surgical healing.

Vaginal-Cervical Factors

Vaginal fluid is acidic (pH of 4 or less), whereas cervical mucus is normally alkaline (pH of 7 or more). Ejaculation should place the sperm at or near the cervical os. The alkalinity of cervical mucus helps support sperm and permits the ascending transportation of sperm at the time of ovulation.

In addition, endocervical mucus normally obstructs or plugs the cervix, acting as a barrier against infection. The latter is important because, in the woman, ascending infection to the peritoneum is virtually unimpeded with a normally patent genital tract. Alkaline mucus in the cervix not only controls procreation but also is a specific protection to life and health. The amount of cervical mucus and its characteristics are influenced by the hormones estrogen and progesterone (see Figs. 6-22 and 6-23).

Vaginal-cervical infections (e.g., trichomoniasis vaginitis) increase the acidity of the vaginal fluid and reduce the alkalinity of the cervical mucus. Thus vaginal infection often destroys or drastically reduces the number of viable, motile sperm before they enter the cervical canal. The amount of mucus and its physical changes are influenced by the presence of blood, pathogenic bacteria, and such irritants as an IUD or a tumor. Severe emotional stress, antibiotic therapy, and diseases such as diabetes mellitus alter the acidity of mucus.

About 20% of infertile women have sperm antibodies. The production of antibodies by one member of a species against something that is commonly found within that species is termed **isoimmunization.** Sperm may be immobilized within the cervical mucus, or they become incapable of migration into the uterus (see postcoital test, p. 1292). A greater incidence of sperm agglutination occurs in women with otherwise unexplained impaired fertility. However, the true significance and reliability of tests for sperm immobilization or agglutination are uncertain.

TREATMENT AND PROGNOSIS. Therapy for lower genital factors requires the elimination of vaginitis or cervicitis (Chapter 29). Appropriate antibiotic or chemotherapeutic drugs generally resolve this problem. In addition to antibiotics, radial chemocautery (destruction of tissue with chemicals) or thermocautery (destruction of tissue with heat, usually electrical) of the cervix, cryosurgery (destruction of tissue by application of extreme cold, usually liquid nitrogen), or conization (excision of a cone-shaped piece of tissue from the endocervix) is effective in eliminating chronic inflammation and infection. When the cervix has been deeply cauterized or frozen or when extensive conization has been performed, extreme limitation of mucus production by the cervix may result. Therefore sperm migration may be difficult or impossible because of the absence of a mucous "bridge" from the vagina to the uterus. Therapeutic intrauterine insemination may be necessary to carry the sperm directly through the *internal os* of the cervix.

If the cervical os is unusually small, it is often called a pinhole os. In such cases, gentle dilatation of the cervix or several shallow radial incisions followed by dilatation are often sufficient to open the lower cervix. In contrast, if the cervix is grossly lacerated after birth and widely gaping, suturing the cervix (trachelorrhaphy) or cryosurgery may be required to reduce the size of the external os. Prevention of recurrent infection helps maintain a column of mucus.

Treatment is available for women who have *immunologic reactions to sperm*. Exposure to semen via the orogenital and anal modes is avoided. The use of condoms during genital intercourse for 6 to 12 months will reduce female antibody production in the majority of women who have elevated antisperm antibody titers. After the serum reaction subsides, condoms are used at all times except at the expected time of ovulation. Approximately one third of couples with this problem conceive by following this course of action. A summary of fertility test findings favorable to fertility is outlined in the box below.

The prognosis for the infertile woman is generally good provided a serious genital or inflammatory disorder is not identified. Most women present numerous so-called minor problems that, although compounded, may be relatively easy to correct (e.g., chronic cervicitis, hypothyroidism). If successful treatment has not been achieved after a year, for example, other alternatives may be considered (e.g., adoption, childlessness, therapeutic insemination, or in vitro fertilization).

■ INVESTIGATION OF MALE INFERTILITY

The systematic investigation of impaired fertility in the male, as it does for the female, begins with a thorough history and physical examination (see box on p. 1291). Assessment of the male proceeds in a manner similar to that of the female (p. 1283), starting with

Summary of Findings Favorable to Fertility

1. Follicular development, ovulation, and luteal development are supportive to pregnancy:
   a. BBT (presumptive evidence of ovulatory cycles)
      (1) Is biphasic
      (2) Reveals temperature elevation that persists for 12 to 14 days just before menstruation
   b. Cervical mucus characteristics change appropriately during phases of the menstrual cycle
   c. Findings from endometrial biopsies taken at different times during menstrual cycle are consistent with day of cycle
   d. Laparoscopic visualization of pelvic organs verifies follicular and luteal development
2. The luteal phase is supportive to pregnancy:
   a. Levels of plasma progesterone are adequate
   b. Endometrial biopsy findings indicate a secretory endometrium
3. Cervical factors are receptive to sperm during expected time of ovulation:
   a. Cervical os is open
   b. Cervical mucus is clear, watery, abundant, and slippery and demonstrates good spinnbarkheit and arborization (fern pattern)
   c. Cervical examination is negative for lesions and infections
   d. Postcoital test findings are satisfactory (adequate number of live, motile, normal sperm present in cervical mucus)
   e. No immunity to sperm can be demonstrated
4. The uterus and uterine tubes are supportive to pregnancy:
   a. Uterine and tubal patency is documented by
      (1) Passage of carbon dioxide into peritoneal cavity
      (2) Spillage of dye into peritoneal cavity
      (3) Outlines of uterine and tubal cavities of adequate size and shape with no abnormalities
   b. Laparoscopic examination verifies normal development of internal genitals and absence of adhesions, infections, endometriosis, and other lesions
5. The male's reproductive structures are normal:
   a. There is no evidence of developmental anomalies of the penis, testicular atrophy, and varicocele (varicose veins on the spermatic vein in the groin)
   b. There is no evidence of infection in the prostate, seminal vesicles, and urethra
   c. The testes are more than 4 cm in the largest diameter
6. Semen is supportive to pregnancy:
   a. Sperm are adequate in number per milliliter of ejaculate
   b. Majority of sperm show normal morphology
   c. Sperm are motile, forward moving
   d. No autoimmunity* exists
   e. Seminal fluid is normal

*The production of antibodies against one's own tissues or secretions is termed autoimmunization.

Assessment of the Man

HISTORY

1. Fertility in another sexual relationship
2. Medical: general medical history, including infections (e.g., sexually transmitted diseases, mononucleosis), mumps orchitis, chronic diseases, recent fever, drug use
3. Surgical: herniorraphy, injuries to genitals, or other surgery in genital area
4. Occupational and environmental exposure to chemicals or x-ray equipment; physical nature of occupation and hobbies; vacations and work habits
5. Previous tests and therapy done for study of impaired fertility; duration of impaired fertility
6. Sex history in detail: libido, coital techniques such as frequency and ability to ejaculate, adequacy of erection, number of sex partners
7. Personal: motivation for childbearing; attitude toward partner; career aspirations

PHYSICAL EXAMINATION

1. General: complete physical examination, with special attention given to habitus and fat and hair distribution
2. Genital tract: penis and urethra; scrotal size; position, size, and consistency of testes; epididymides and vasa deferentia; prostate size and consistency
3. Careful search for varicocele, with man in both supine and upright positions

LABORATORY DATA

1. Routine urine test, complete blood count, gonorrhea and chlamydia tests, and serologic test for syphilis
2. Complete semen analysis—essential
   a. Liquefaction: usually complete within 10 to 30 minutes
   b. Semen volume 2-5 mL (range: 1 to 7 mL)
   c. Semen pH 7.2 to 7.8
   d. Sperm density 20 to 200 million/mL
   e. Normal morphology (%) ≥60% normal oval
   f. Motility (important consideration in sperm evaluation); percentage of forward-moving sperm (swim-up test) estimated in relationship to abnormally motile and nonmotile sperm. This requires evaluation by a technician with some degree of experience, but since the test provides a more accurate diagnosis, it is well worth the time involved; ≥50% is normal
   g. Cell count: average normal, 60 million or more per milliliter or a total of 150 to 200 or more million per ejaculate; minimum normal standards: 40 million/mL, with a total count of at least 125 million per ejaculate (average of counts on two or preferably three separate specimens)

NOTE: These values are not absolute, but only relative to the final evaluation of the couple as a single reproductive unit.

   h. Ovum penetration test
3. Additional laboratory studies as indicated
   a. Basic endocrine studies indicated in men with oligospermia or aspermia:
      (1) Tomographic x-ray films of skull
      (2) T_4 or other thyroid tests
      (3) 17-Ketosteroids
      (4) Gonadotropin FSH, LH determination
      (5) 17-Hydroxycorticoids and pregnanediol
      (6) Buccal smear and chromosome studies (e.g., Klinefelter's syndrome, XXY sex chromosomes)
      (7) Test for sperm antibodies; **autoimmunization.** Autoimmune antibodies (produced by the man against his own sperm) agglutinate or immobilize sperm in less than 5% of men with impaired fertility
   b. Testicular biopsy, where correct interpretation is available (may give a more accurate diagnosis and prognosis in cases of azoospermia and severe oligospermia), vasography if indicated and available

noninvasive tests. Male reproductive failure may be caused by many of the difficulties that also affect women, such as nutritional, endocrine, and psychologic disorders. Exposure to reproductive hazards in the workplace and home is evaluated (see Chapter 27).

Substance abuse can be a major factor in male infertility. *Alcohol* consumption causes erectile problems (impotence). Cigarette smoking has been associated with abnormal sperm, a decreased number of sperm, and chromosome damage. The degree of abnormality is related to the number of cigarettes smoked per day (Mattison et al, 1989). *Marijuana (cannabis sativa)* adversely affects spermatogenesis (e.g., it depresses the number and motility of sperm and increases the percentage of abnormally formed sperm). *Monoamine oxidase* (MAO), an antidepressant, adversely affects spermatogenesis. *Amyl ni-*

trate, butyl nitrate, ethyl chloride, and *methaqualone* (used to prolong orgasm) cause changes in spermatogenesis. *Heroin, methadone,* and *barbiturates* decrease libido. Infertile men have reported lower self-esteem, higher anxiety, and more somatic symptoms than have fertile men (Bartov, 1990).

Tests and Examinations

The basic infertility survey of the male includes a semen analysis. The postcoital test evaluates characteristics of the sperm within the cervical mucus of the man's sexual partner.

SEMEN ANALYSIS. Examination of semen is an important part of investigation of impaired fertility, since the male is often at least partially responsible (Willson, Carrington, 1987). A complete **semen analysis,** study of the effects of cervical mucus on sperm forward motility and survival, and evaluation of the sperm's ability to penetrate an ovum provide basic information. Sperm counts vary from day to day and are dependent on emotional and physical status and sexual activity. Therefore a single analysis may be inconclusive (Willson, Carrington, 1987). Usually three specimens taken at monthly intervals are evaluated.

Semen is collected by ejaculation into a clean, wide-mouthed plastic or glass jar with a screw top (Willson, Carrington, 1987). The specimen is usually collected by masturbation following 2 to 5 days of abstinence from ejaculation. Some couples are unable to collect the semen in the manner described. These couples can collect the semen in a special nonrubber, unpowdered condom.

The semen is taken to the laboratory in a sealed container within 1 hour of ejaculation. Exposure to excessive heat or cold is avoided. Normal values for semen characteristics are given in the box on p. 1291.

The fertility potential of sperm is difficult to evaluate solely by semen analysis, which gives little insight into sperm survival, cervical penetration, migration to the uterine tubes, or capacity for ovum penetration and fertilization (Cunningham, MacDonald, Gant, 1989). In addition, there is insufficient knowledge of the method by which male and female antibodies can act to inhibit fertility potential of sperm. An immunologic disorder as yet not identified may be the basis for unexplained infertility (Cunningham, MacDonald, Gant, 1989).

Seminal deficiency may be attributable to one or more of a variety of factors. The male is assessed for these factors (Scott et al, 1990): hypopituitarism, nutritional deficiency, debilitating or chronic disease, trauma, exposure to environmental hazards such as radiation and toxic substances, gonadotropic inadequacy, and obstructive lesions of the epididymis and vas deferens. A genetic basis such as Klinefelter's syndrome is ruled out. Hormone analyses are done for testosterone, gonadotropin, FSH, and LH. Testicular biopsy may be warranted.

POSTCOITAL TEST. The postcoital test is one method used to test for adequacy of coital technique, cervical mucus, sperm, and degree of sperm penetration through cervical mucus. The test is performed within 2 hours after ejaculation of semen into the vagina. A specimen of cervical mucus is obtained. Intercourse is synchronized with the expected time of ovulation (as determined from evaluation of BBT, cervical mucus changes, and usual length of menstrual cycle). It is performed only in the absence of vaginal infection. Couples may experience some difficulty abstaining from intercourse for 2 to 4 days before expected ovulation and then having intercourse with ejaculation "on schedule." Sex "on demand" may strain the couple's interpersonal relationship. A problem may arise if the expected day of ovulation occurs when facilities or the physician are unavailable (such as over a weekend or holiday). If no sperm is found, the coital technique used must be evaluated (e.g., extreme obesity may prevent adequate penile penetration).

General Therapies

The difficulty may be caused by timing and frequency of intercourse. The couple is taught about the menstrual cycle, the peak cervical mucus symptom, and the appropriate timing of intercourse.

Penile intromission is often difficult because of chordee (painful downward curvature on erection) and obesity. The couple is advised to alter positions used for intercourse. Heavy use of alcohol makes penile erection difficult to achieve and maintain until ejaculation. The man is advised to avoid imbibing alcohol during the time of the woman's ovulation.

Medical therapy for male infertility has been disappointing, especially when pituitary or testicular disease is discovered. Occasionally it is possible to suppress the production of sperm with injections of testosterone and in that way cause a reduction in the number of autoimmune antibodies present in the man. Following the reduction in sperm autoantibodies, sperm quality improves, and a pregnancy sometimes occurs.

Drug therapy may be indicated for male infertility. Infections are identified and treated promptly with antimicrobials. Problems with the thyroid or adrenal glands are corrected with appropriate medications.

Testosterone enanthate (Delatestryl) and testosterone cypionate (Depo-Testosterone) by injection are used to stimulate virilization, especially in the adolescent. Human chorionic gonadotropin (hCG) (Pregnyl) given intramuscularly virilizes a hypogonadotropic male to restore Leydig cell function and spermatogenesis. FSH and hMG aid hCG for completion of spermatogenesis. Bromocriptine, an ergot derivative and dopamine agonist, is used to treat hypogonadotropic hypogonadism–associated prolactin-producing hypothalamic or pituitary tumors and may reduce the tumor. Clomiphene may be given for idiopathic subfertility.

Surgical repair of **varicocele** (enlargement of the veins of the spermatic cord) has been relatively successful. A varicocele on the left side is found in a substantial number of subfertile men. Ligation of the varicocele does lead to improvement of the sperm quality and commonly to pregnancy.

Simple changes in life-style may be effective in the treatment of subfertile men. Poor nutritional state is corrected if it exists. High temperatures in the groin area reduce the number of sperm produced. High temperatures may be caused by wearing brief shorts and tight jeans that keep the scrotal sac pressed against the body regardless of environmental temperature changes. The testes are kept at temperatures too high for efficient spermatogenesis. Frequent and prolonged hot tubbing has also been implicated in relative infertility. It must be remembered that these conditions only lead to relative infertility and should not be employed as a means of contraception. Lubricants used during intercourse should not contain spermicides or have spermicidal properties.

NURSING PROCESS

ASSESSMENT

The nurse assists in obtaining data relevant to fertility through interview and physical examination. The data base needs to include information to identify whether infertility is primary or secondary. Religious, cultural, and ethnic data are noted.

Some of the data needed to investigate impaired fertility are of a sensitive, personal nature. Obtaining these data may be viewed as an invasion of privacy. The tests and examinations are occasionally painful and intrusive and can take the romance out of lovemaking. A high level of motivation is needed to endure the investigation.

Many couples have already visited various physicians and have read extensively on the subject. Their previous experiences are recorded. The depth and breadth of their knowledge base are explored.

NURSING DIAGNOSES

Following are examples of nursing diagnoses that may become apparent from the data base.

- Anxiety related to
  - —Unknown outcome of diagnostic workup
- Body image or self-esteem disturbance related to
  - —Impaired fertility
- High risk for impaired individual/family coping related to
  - —Methods used in the investigation of impaired fertility
- Decisional conflict related to
  - —Therapies for impaired fertility
  - —Alternatives to therapy: childlessness or adoption
- Altered family processes related to
  - —Unmet expectations for pregnancy
- Anticipatory grieving related to
  - —Expected poor prognosis
- Acute pain related to
  - —Effects of diagnostic tests (or surgery)
- Powerlessness related to
  - —Lack of control over prognosis
- Altered patterns of sexuality related to
  - —Loss of libido secondary to medically imposed restrictions
- High risk for social isolation related to
  - —Impaired fertility, its investigation and management

PLANNING

Planning requires sensitivity to the client's needs. Based on knowledge of impaired fertility, the nurse is equipped to assist with the development of a plan of care for the couple with impaired fertility. Blenner (1990) developed a theory to facilitate self-care in infertility treatment. It involves the client changing from a passive to an active participant. The four sequential phases experienced by the client include perceiving that physicians lack the complete picture, acquiring knowledge, taking control, and being satisfied with treatment. The plan is developed in collaboration with the physician in light of the nurse's level of expertise and with other members of the health team and the couple to achieve certain mutually determined goals. The *goals* are phrased in client-centered terms and may include the following:

1. Couple understands the anatomy and physiology of the reproductive system

2. Couple undergoes treatment for any abnormalities identified through various tests and examinations (e.g., infections, blocked uterine tubes, sperm allergy, and varicocele)
3. Couple understands their potential to conceive
4. Couple resolves guilt feelings and does not need to focus blame
5. Couple conceives or, failing to conceive, decides on an alternative acceptable to both of them (e.g., childlessness or adoption)
6. Couple finds acceptable methods for handling pressures they may feel from peers and relatives regarding their childless state

---

IMPLEMENTATION

Nursing actions vary with the nurse's level of education, position held, and policies of the agency. Basic to all nursing actions is knowledge of those factors that are essential to or contribute to fertility, of assessment strategies (history, examinations, and tests), and of management and therapy. The nurse acts on the client's readiness to learn and her or his level of understanding of impaired fertility. Although primary responsibility for teaching the client or clients rests with the physician, the nurse assists in the identification of the client's gaps in knowledge, clarifies information, and reinforces the physician's explanations and instructions. Occasionally the nurse acts as the client's advocate by helping the client state a concern or question or request further explanation from the physician or technician.

The nurse's nonverbal behavior before and during the procedure can reassure and support the client. Often the client feels inadequate because of the necessity for testing and the intimidating nature of the tests.

Written and verbal instructions for specific preparation for tests will increase the client's feeling of adequacy. Supportive nursing actions include providing privacy while giving instructions for obtaining specimens and changing clothes, draping, creating a comfortable physical environment, padding the stirrups of the examination table, efficiency in use of equipment, warming the speculum, and coaching for relaxation.

In addition to discussing the specifics of common tests for impaired fertility, nurses can provide sensory information about these future tests. To acquire descriptions of commonly used tests, nurses can interview current clients and ask them to describe their tests in sensory terms. Then nurses can share the most commonly occurring descriptions with future clients. Providing preparatory information can help clients form a mental image of what an experience will include and thus help make the testing experience more tolerable and less distressing.

Women often experience anxiety when undergoing a pelvic examination. After any procedure, after the client is fully dressed and comfortably seated (at the same level as the nurse and physician), she or he benefits from an opportunity to talk about the experience in an unhurried manner. Not only do these behaviors help the client relax, but also they indicate that the recipient of such care is worthy and thus helps build self-esteem. The goal of nursing-medical *care* is to encourage the client to become an active partner in care as well as to establish rapport to ensure that therapy and eventual counseling are facilitated.

The nurse needs to know the correct method for obtaining, labeling, and transporting specimens to the laboratory. A mishandled specimen may lead to misdiagnosis or the need to obtain another specimen. These errors create added expense and stress for the client as well as significant time delays before therapy can be instituted.

Nurses can help clients express and discuss their feelings as honestly as possible. Ventilation may help couples unburden themselves of negative feelings. Current research reveals an infertility strain profile including tension, worry, depressive symptoms, and interpersonal alienation (Berg, Wilson, 1990; Wright et al., 1989). Professional referral may be necessary. A study was conducted to explore the coping strategies of infertile women (see Research Highlight, p. 1295).

The myriad of psychologic responses to a diagnosis of impaired fertility may tax a couple's giving and receiving of physical and sexual closeness. The prescriptions and proscriptions for achieving conception may add tension to a couple's sexual functioning. Couples are instructed about frequency and timing of intercourse as well as use of certain coital positions. It is no wonder that these couples complain of decreased desire for intercourse, orgasmic dysfunction, or midcycle erectile disorders. A once-spontaneous act of expressing love has become a mechanical act for creating a baby.

During evaluation of impaired fertility, the previously private act of intercourse becomes a topic of discussion. Even in the sexually liberated culture of the 1990s, few people eagerly share the frequency of coitus and positions used during intercourse.

To be able to deal comfortably with a couple's sexuality, nurses must be comfortable with their own sexuality. Nurses need to have up-to-date factual knowledge about human sexual practices, be able to accept the preferences and activities of others with-

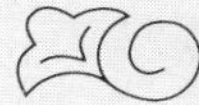 **Research Highlight** 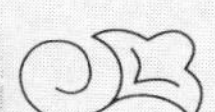

Coping Strategies of Infertile Women

RESEARCH ABSTRACT

This study was undertaken to explore the patterns of coping of women who are infertile. The sample was 30 infertile women who were clients of a physician who specializes in infertility. In a private interview, the subjects were asked to describe what they had done to cope with the feelings and experiences associated with infertility. Interviews were tape-recorded, transcribed, and then analyzed for basic themes. The researchers identified six strategies used by the women to cope with infertility. These categories were labeled: "(1) increasing space between themselves and reminders of infertility, (2) regaining control, (3) being the best, (4) looking for hidden meaning, (5) giving in to feelings, and (6) sharing the burden" (p. 224).

IMPLICATIONS FOR PRACTICE

Nurses caring for infertile couples can use the information about how women cope with infertility to provide more sensitive, informed care. Nurses can provide an atmosphere where the woman can give in to her feelings and share her burden. She can be assured that her feelings are normal and directed to organized support groups of couples experiencing similar difficulties. As the woman seeks to regain control, the nurse can provide an opportunity for the woman to successfully do so. The nurse should be available to listen to concerns.

RELATED RESEARCH QUESTIONS

1. What are coping strategies of infertile men?
2. Are there cultural differences in coping strategies?
3. Is there a relationship between use of coping strategies and rate of conception?
4. Do coping strategies vary with the length of time that treatment for infertility has been pursued?

REFERENCE

Davis DC, Dearman CN: Coping strategies of infertile women, *JOGNN* 20(3):221, 1991.

out being judgmental, acquire skill in interviewing and in therapeutic use of self, develop sensitivity to the nonverbal cues of others, and be knowledgeable of the couple's sociocultural and religious tenets. Once nurses are comfortable with their own sexuality, they can better help couples understand why the private act of lovemaking needs to be shared with health care professionals.

Because of the interference with the spontaneity of coitus, many infertility specialists limit the period of investigation. These specialists have found that the shorter the diagnostic period, the less the disruption of a couple's sexual life-style.

The woman or couple facing impaired fertility exhibits behaviors that resemble the *grieving process* that is associated with loss (Chapter 40). The loss of one's genetic continuity with the generations to come leads to loss of self-esteem, of a sense of adequacy as a woman (or man), of control over one's destiny, and of a sense of self. Infertile individuals experience impaired self-concept and greater dissatisfaction with their marriages (Hirsch, Hirsch, 1989). The investigative process leads to a loss of spontaneity and control over the couple's marital relationship and sometimes over progress toward career and life goals. All people do not experience every one of the reactions described, nor can it be predicted how long any one reaction will last for an individual.

The nurse may feel unsure how to assist. Table 42-2 presents characteristic behaviors of people experiencing the psychologic impact of impaired fertility along with some suggestions for nursing (or other health professionals') actions.

The support systems of the couple with impaired fertility need to be explored. This exploration should include persons available to assist, their relationship to the couple, their ages, their availability, and the cultural or religious support that is available. This type of assessment is suitable for a health team conference in which representatives of several disciplines can share ideas and work cooperatively in developing a plan for management.

TABLE 42-2 Nursing Actions in Response to Behavior Associated with Impaired Fertility

Behavioral Characteristic	Nursing Actions
Surprise: each person assumes she or he is fertile and that pregnancy is an option.	Point out resemblance to grieving process—a normal, expected reaction to loss (Chapter 40). Refer to support group.* Prepare them for length of time it may take to grieve, types of feelings (psychologic, somatic) to expect. Encourage and allow time to talk of past and present feelings of sexuality, self-image, and self-esteem.
Denial: "It can't happen to me!"	Allow time for denial because it gives the body and mind time to adjust a little at a time. Do not feed into the client's denial; instead say, "It must be hard to believe such a devastating report."
Anger: toward others (perhaps even at the nurse) or themselves.	Explain that the reaction to loss of control and to a feeling of helplessness is often anger, which can easily be projected onto another person. Without release, anger can lead to chronic depression. Anger is a natural feeling. Allow time to express anger at losing their sense of control over their bodies and destinies; identify and direct energy directly at the problem. Airing one's own anger often eases the intensity of the emotion. A helpful approach may be, "It's OK to be angry . . . at those who are pregnant, at people who want abortions, at self, at mate, at caregivers, and so forth."
Bargaining: "If I get pregnant, I'll dedicate the child to God."	Accept bargaining statements without comment.
Depression:	
Isolation: personal.	Allow time for both woman and man to talk about how it feels whenever a sight, event, or word serves as a reminder of own state of impaired fertility. Develop role playing situations to practice interactions with others under various circumstances to increase the couple's ability to cope and to problem solve (increases their self-confidence). The nurse may say, "You must feel so terribly alone sometimes."
Guilt or unworthiness.	Allow time to identify feelings that may be based on earlier behaviors (e.g., abortion, premarital sex, contact with sexually transmitted disease [STD]). Couple or person comes to the realization that "unworthiness" and impaired fertility are unrelated.
Acceptance (resolution).	Clients need to know that grief feelings are never laid away forever; they may be activated by special reminders (e.g., anniversaries).

*RESOLVE, Inc, PO Box 474, Boston, Mass, 02178 and 5 Water Street, Arlington, Mass, 02174.

If the couple conceives, nurses need to be aware that the concerns and problems of the previously infertile couple may not be over. Many couples are overjoyed with the pregnancy. However, some are not. Some couples rearrange their lives, sense of self, and personal goals within their acceptance of their infertile state. The couple may feel that those who worked with them to identify and treat impaired fertility expect them to be happy with the pregnancy. The couple may be shocked to find that they themselves feel resentment because the pregnancy, once a cherished dream, now necessitates another change in goals, aspirations, and identities. Bernstein et al (1988) found interpersonal sensitivity, hostility, and depression among previously infertile women. The normal ambivalence toward pregnancy (Chapter 11) may be perceived as reneging on the original choice to become parents. The couple might choose to abort the pregnancy at this time. Other couples worry about spontaneous abortion. If the couple wishes to continue with the pregnancy, they will need the care other pregnant couples need (see Unit 2). The couple may need extra preparation for the realities of pregnancy, labor, and parenthood, because they have developed fantasies about childbearing when they thought it was beyond their reach. *A history of impaired fertility is considered to be a risk factor for pregnancy.* The couple who has a history of impaired fertility before this pregnancy faces another label, that of being at high risk for this pregnancy (see Chapter 27).

The couple too may desire information about contraception after the birth of this baby. If the previously infertile couple desires additional children, the couple is advised about those contraceptive methods that are least likely to cause damage and impair fertility.

If the couple does not conceive, they are assessed regarding their desire to be referred for help with adoption, therapeutic intrauterine insemination, or with choosing childlessness. The couple would find a list of such agencies within their particular community helpful.

EVALUATION

The nurse can be reasonably assured that care was effective when the client-centered goals have been achieved:

1. Couple increases their knowledge of anatomy and physiology of reproduction.
2. Couple collaborates with caregivers during the investigation of impaired fertility.
3. Any abnormalities identified through various tests and examinations are treated successfully.
4. Couple resolves guilt feelings and does not need to focus blame.
5. If the couple conceives, they accept their responses to pregnancy; realign their goals, aspirations, and identities; and are comfortable with their decisions regarding the pregnancy.
6. If the couple does not conceive, they decide on an acceptable alternative and seek support as necessary. They find acceptable methods for handling pressures they may feel from peers and relatives regarding their childless state, and they receive a list of community agencies that assist with adoptions or provide appropriate support.

REPRODUCTIVE ALTERNATIVES

There have been remarkable developments in reproductive medicine (Evans et al, 1989). Alternative birth technologies, heralded by involuntarily childless couples, are creating ethical and legal issues (Chapter 4). The nature of new technologies and the high costs have focused attention on the ethics of provision of services (Ryan, 1989). Several alternatives are presented here in some detail: in vitro fertilization and embryo transfer (IVF-ET), gamete intrafallopian tube transfer (GIFT), and zygote intrafallopian transfer (ZIFT). Other alternatives, including surrogate motherhood, are mentioned.

IN VITRO FERTILIZATION AND EMBRYO TRANSFER. The first successful term delivery of an infant conceived by in vitro fertilization (test-tube pregnancy) in 1978 was the culmination of years of study and experimentation by Robert Edwards and Patrick Steptoe in England. Since then several other "laboratory conceived" and normal-appearing newborns have been delivered.

Many women whose uterine tubes either are obstructed or have been removed are not potential candidates for similar treatment. However, because of the complexity and cost of the procedure, the likelihood is that this approach to impaired fertility must remain limited for the near future. The following steps, ultrasimplified, are necessary for **in vitro fertilization-embryo transplant.**

1. Ovulation is induced by gonadotropin therapy (e.g., clomiphene or menotropin) to ensure as many mature follicles as possible.
2. Mature follicles are identified by laparoscopy, pelvic ultrasound, or transvaginal ultrasound. Needle aspiration may be through the laparoscope, transvaginally, or transurethrally (Seibel, 1988).
3. Ova are examined through a microscope to verify maturity and then transferred to tissue culture media.
4. Before laparoscopy, semen is collected. Freshly ejaculated sperm cannot fertilize an ovum; they must be capacitated. A simple process, capacitation involves only a short incubation period in a culture medium. After capacitation, sperm are added to the ova (Pernoll, Benson, 1987).
5. After fertilization a second tissue culture transfer allows division to approximately a 12-cell blastocyst (3 to 6 days) when it is returned to the uterus.
6. Progesterone therapy in the interval induces a late secretory type of endometrium, whereupon the blastocyst is transferred to the uterus, where the implantation (nidation) of the zygote occurs and embryonic development proceeds. The efficacy of progesterone therapy has not been established but most centers administer it anyway (Seibel, 1988).

Recent figures indicate a pregnancy rate of 11% per treatment cycle for in vitro fertilization (Hatcher et al, 1990). This vast improvement is attributable to increased precision in predicting ovulation and in retrieving the ovum. The conventional methods of predicting ovulation—calendar, BBT, cervical mucus, fertility awareness, and laboratory tests such as vaginal cytology and serum hormone determination—can only approximate the moment of ovulation. The more precise methods are beyond the scope of this text but are mentioned here for interest. These methods are (1) stimulating ovulation with clomiphene or menotropin given at a precise time during the cycle, (2) monitoring ovulatory function with realtime ultrasound, and (3) performing rapid radioimmunoassay for estrogen level. Through a laparoscope or transvaginally, the ovum is retrieved by inserting an aspiration needle into the ripened follicle and removing the ovum. Semen is collected and treated before its use for fertilizing the ovum. In vitro fertilization costs from $5000 to $8000 per treatment in 1991.

Human experimentation and manipulation of this type have been sanctioned by the U.S. Department of Health and Human Services. The Roman Catholic Church is strongly opposed to in vitro fertilization. Legal aspects of in vitro fertilization are discussed in Chapter 4.

GAMETE INTRAFALLOPIAN TUBE TRANSFER. Gamete **intrafallopian (uterine) tube transfer (GIFT)** is similar to IVF-ET. Ovulation is induced as in IVF-ET; a menotropin injection is given; and the oocytes are aspirated from follicles via laparoscopy (Fig. 42-5, *A*) or minilaparotomy (Pernoll, Benson, 1987). A newer approach is the use of ultrasonographic transvaginal ovum retrieval (Rabar et al, 1988). Before laparoscopy, semen is collected. Sperm are capacitated using the same technique as for IVF-ET. The eggs are identified in the laboratory. Capacitated sperm are then mixed with the ova and drawn up into a catheter. The ova and sperm are then transferred to the uterine tubes (Fig. 42-5, *B*) permitting natural fertilization and cleavage, with subsequent successful pregnancies. A 20% to 30% pregnancy rate per cycle has been reported for this technique.

GIFT is only useful for women who have normal tubal function. In fact, a high rate of ectopic pregnancy has been reported in women with underlying tubal disease (Yovich, Matson, 1990). The success of this technique has not been compared with the less complicated technique of simple induced ovulation combined with therapeutic intrauterine insemination. GIFT is more expensive to perform than IVF-ET using ultrasound egg aspiration.

ZYGOTE INTRAFALLOPIAN TRANSFER. A third technique, **zygote intrafallopian transfer (ZIFT)**, combines the advantages of IVF-ET and GIFT (Hamori et al, 1988). Ovulation is induced, the mature follicles are aspirated, and the semen is prepared as with IVF-ET and GIFT. The follicles are inseminated in a petri dish. They are examined 18 hours later for pronuclei (evidence that fertilization has occurred). The zygotes are then transferred back to the uterus via laparoscopy into the fimbriated end of the fallopian tubes. No more than two zygotes are implanted on either side. This technique is possible only for women with at least one patent fallopian tube.

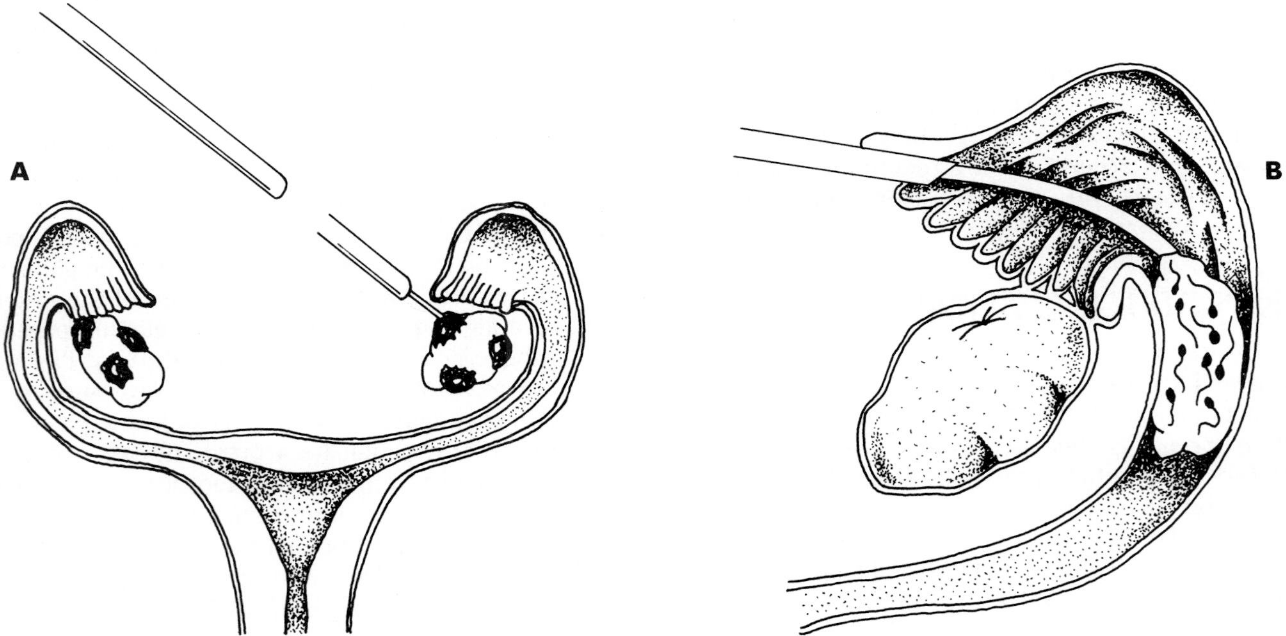

Fig. 42-5 **A,** Via laparoscope, a ripe follicle is located and the fluid containing the egg is removed. **B,** The separated sperm and egg are placed into the uterine tubes, where fertilization occurs.

ZIFT appears to have certain advantages: abnormally fertilized eggs can be rejected, and the zygote follows as close to "natural" a path as possible. However, the success rate is still low (12.1%).

For IVF-ET, GIFT, and ZIFT procedures, the protocols vary from center to center. In any of these procedures, donated sperm, ova, or even embryos may be used.

CARE OF RECIPIENTS. Nurses working in fertility programs serve as consultants to infertile couples (Pace-Owens, 1989). Most of these procedures are done on an out-of-hospital basis. However, a woman may be admitted to the hospital for a few hours to recover after a follicular retrieval or an implantation. These women are generally in good health and have little or no pain. However, they need supportive nursing care. The nurse should remember that the woman may already have a sense of failure because of her inability to get pregnant without intervention.

High-technology infertility treatments offer hope to couples but also cause physical, emotional, and financial stress (Olshansky, 1988). The woman may be tense, irritable, and afraid to urinate or even move. The nurse may feel that because the woman is not ill, may not have been anesthetized, and has voluntarily undergone this procedure, she does not need much nursing care. Actually, the woman would benefit from the nurse sitting with her for a few minutes and talking calmly. After any of these procedures, the woman must be able to walk and urinate before leaving the hospital.

THERAPEUTIC INSEMINATION. During a 12-month interval from 1986 to 1987, 11,000 physicians performed insemination with spousal or donor semen on 172,000 women in the United States (U.S. Congress, 1988). Approximately 30,000 births occurred during that year as a result of therapeutic donor insemination (TDI), previously referred to as artificial insemination donor (AID) (Ory, 1989). Donor semen is subjected to laboratory testing to reduce the possibility of life-threatening illnesses for the recipient and her fetus, as well as for factors that could jeopardize the woman's future fertility or compromise the chance of the success of the procedure (Ory, 1989). Donor semen is tested for serology, serum hepatitis B antigen, *Neisseria gonorrhoeae, Chlamydia trachomatis,* cytomegalovirus (CMV) antibodies, and human immunodeficiency virus (HIV) antibodies (Ory, 1989).

When the husband's sperm has poor quality or motility, several semen samples are collected from him. The samples consist of split ejaculates, that is, the sperm-rich *first portion* only is collected for freezing and later pooling for **therapeutic intrauterine insemination.** Rapid freezing with liquid nitrogen and subsequent thawing do not cause genetic damage even after 10 years' storage using glycerol. Pooling should increase the sperm count and improve the placement of a portion of the total semen specimen at the cervical os.

Assuming normal female fertility, therapeutic intrauterine insemination at or about the time of ovulation has resulted in pregnancy in as many as 70% of cases. Numerous inseminations may be necessary to ensure proper timing of ovulation. Ovulation detection kits using urinary LH or serial ultrasound offer more reliable evidence of impending ovulation than do BBT charts (Ory, 1989).

Insemination directly into the uterine cavity should be avoided because of severe cramping (prostaglandin effect) and possible infection. The recommended procedure is the instillation of about 0.5 mL of the specimen into the cervical canal with the remainder deposited in a cleanly washed contraceptive diaphragm to be worn by the woman for about 1 hour.

Insemination with the husband's semen presents no legal problems, but insemination with donor sperm may involve many legal, ethical, and emotional aspects (Ory, 1989). The couple must know there is no guarantee of pregnancy and that in either case the spontaneous abortion rate is approximately the same as in a control population. There is no increase in maternal or perinatal complications; the same frequency of anomalies (about 5%) and obstetric complications (between 5% and 10%) that accompanies normal insemination applies also to therapeutic insemination.

OTHER TECHNIQUES. *Ovum or embryo transfer* involves inseminating a donor female with semen from the husband of an infertile woman. After 4 days, when the fertilized (or unfertilized) egg reaches the uterus, it is lavaged out of the donor female and placed into the uterus of the infertile wife. The infertile woman carries the pregnancy. Term pregnancy rate is only 3%.

Embryos have been *donated* from one woman to another with resultant live births. These women are not candidates for IVF-ET because of severe pelvic adhesions or absence of functional ovaries. In the latter case, the endometrium must be primed with estrogen and progesterone before transfer of the donated embryo. Progesterone supplementation must be maintained for 10 weeks.

Freezing and preservation of the embryo for thawing and transfer in a later cycle have been successful in cattle but have had limited success in humans. Oocyte cryopreservation has not been successful in any species. No one advocates the discarding of embryos (see ethical issues, Chapter 4). These, as well as the other procedures, have enormous future potential but create many ethical and legal concerns.

COMPLICATIONS. Other than the established risks associated with laparoscopy and general anesthesia, few risks are associated with IVF-ET, GIFT, or other techniques. Transvaginal needle aspiration requires no anesthesia. Congenital anomalies occur no more frequently than in normally conceived embryos. Ectopic pregnancies, however, do occur more frequently, and these carry a significant maternal risk.

SURROGATE MOTHERHOOD. Surrogate motherhood can be achieved by two methods. One way is to have the surrogate mother inseminated with semen from the infertile woman's husband and carry the baby to delivery. Then the baby is formally adopted by the infertile couple. A less common method is to retrieve an ovum from the infertile woman, fertilize it with her husband's sperm, and place it into the uterus of the surrogate mother-to-be. These newer interventions cause some legal and ethical problems (Chapter 4).

ADOPTION. For couples who can give up the quest for biologic parenthood, adoption is also an option (Adoption, 1989). However, with increasing numbers of single mothers keeping their babies, the achievement of this option may take 3 or more years.

The decision to adopt should be mutual. The clients' attitudes and feelings must be examined before they can assume the responsibility for an adopted child. Most adults assume that they will be able to have children of their own. To discover that they are unable to do so is often accompanied by feelings of inferiority, doubts about masculinity or femininity, and feelings of guilt or blame in relation to the spouse. These feelings and frustrations, superimposed on the anxious waiting for pregnancies, feelings of loss, and the endless medical procedures to investigate impaired fertility, provide an adoptive couple with their own unique needs in preparing for parenthood (Whaley, Wong, 1991).

■ CONTROL OF FERTILITY

The combination of traditions and contemporary reproductive health technologies fosters responsibility among women and couples and offers the freedom to choose the number and spacing of their children (Hatcher et al, 1990).

Contraception is the voluntary prevention of pregnancy, having both individual and social implications. It has been established that more than 90% of couples in the United States have used or intend to use some method of contraception (birth control).

The availability of reliable and safe techniques for fertility management has meant that parenthood, with its tasks and responsibilities as well as its pleasures, can be willingly assumed by adults who wish to do so.

Spacing of children is important for promotion of health not only of the mother but also of her children. Quality of the offspring rather than quantity is now emphasized.

The anticipation and preparation for coitus relies on the capability to perceive cause and effect (Norris, 1988). An important health decision is the choice of a contraceptive. This choice changes in the course of one's reproductive life. Nurses can be instrumental in the decision-making process.

Cultural and Religious Considerations

Cross-cultural information about contraceptive practices is limited. Before modern times, probably the most effective contraception resulted from sexual taboos. Postpartum taboos were generally effective. Kay (1982) points out that the Mexican Americans she studied continued to place a 40-day restriction on sexual intercourse after childbirth.

In the past, Native Americans used herbs as oral contraceptives (Vogel, 1973). Information about these herbs was useful in the development of today's oral contraceptives. Some Native American groups today favor the use of contraceptives, but others believe that contraceptives are against God's will. Although the Japanese were one of the earliest cultural groups to accept the use of birth control and abortion (Okamoto, 1978), Japanese couples are reluctant to use contraception until they have borne one child (Bernstein, Kidd, 1982). The use of breast-feeding as a contraceptive among nonWestern cultures is described by Lethbridge (1989).

Fertility management has posed numerous problems for nurses working with persons whose belief systems place a high value on having children. Some subcultural groups in the United States and in third-world countries believe that the great emphasis placed on family planning is based on the desire of the white middle class to limit minority groups. Nevertheless, many persons with these belief systems are interested in learning about contraception and will listen to explanations if they include respect for another's values. Health care innovations are accepted or rejected depending on how they fit into the client's cultural pattern.

To control excessive world population, voluntary limitation of family size is important. Family planning is accepted in principle by all religions. Some strict protestant denominations, Hasidic Jews, and Roman Catholics believe that family planning can be achieved by periodic abstinence alone. Ostling (1987) reported that according to the National Center for Health Statistics many women under age 45 have used contraceptive methods not approved by their religions. Samoans represent a variety of religions, but for them contraceptive practices are not highly valued (Clark, Howland, 1978). Rather, priority is placed on demonstration of male and female fertility through childbirth. In some religious and cultural groups, attitudes regarding menstruation might appear to present a barrier to the use of any agent that alters menstrual function (Kaunitz, 1989). Religion, however, may not be as great a barrier as once believed. For further discussion of cultural and religious aspects of care, see Chapter 3.

■ NURSING PROCESS

ASSESSMENT

A history, physical examination, and laboratory tests precede the initiation of some forms of contraception. A complete gynecologic examination is performed. Menstrual, contraceptive, and obstetric histories are taken. The woman's knowledge about contraception and her sexual partner's commitment to any particular method are determined. Data are required about the frequency of coitus (once every so often or several times per week), whether the woman has one sexual partner or several, the level of involvement the woman wishes to assume, and her (their) objections to any methods. The woman's level of comfort and willingness to touch her genitals and cervical mucus are assessed. Myths are identified. Religious and cultural factors are determined. The woman's verbal and nonverbal responses to hearing about the various available methods are carefully noted. An individual's reproductive-life plan needs to be considered.

NURSING DIAGNOSES

Nursing diagnoses reflect analysis of the assessment findings. Following are examples of nursing diagnoses that may emerge.

- High risk for decisional conflict related to
  —Contraceptive alternatives
- Fear related to
  —Contraceptive method side effects
- High risk for infection related to
  —Being sexually active
  —Use of contraceptive method
- High risk for altered sexuality patterns related to
  —Fear of pregnancy

PLANNING

Planning is a collaborative effort among the woman, her sexual partner (when appropriate), the physician, and the nurse. The *goals* are determined and stated in client-centered terms, and may include the following:

1. The woman verbalizes understanding about contraceptive methods
2. The woman is comfortable and satisfied with the chosen method
3. If further childbearing is desired, the couple achieves pregnancy at the time planned
4. The couple experiences no adverse sequelae as a result of the chosen method of contraception

IMPLEMENTATION

Client teaching (Chapter 1) is fundamental to initiating and maintaining any form of contraception. A careprovider relationship based on trust is an important facet in client compliance. The nurse counters myths with facts, clarifies misinformation, and fills in gaps of knowledge. There are various contraceptive techniques used in North America. The ideal contraceptive should be safe, easily available, economical, acceptable, simple to use, and promptly reversible. Although no means or method may ever achieve all these objectives, impressive progress has been made recently. The woman or couple must be fully informed of the risks, effectiveness, reversibility, and alternatives (see discussion of informed consent, Chapter 4).

Contraception failure rate refers to the percentage of contraceptive users expected to experience an accidental pregnancy during the first year, even when they use a method consistently and correctly. Failure rates decrease over time either because a user will gain experience with and use a method more appropriately or because the less effective users will drop out of the study.

Contraception employs one or more of the following methods:

1. Methods available to people without prescription
   a. Biologic periodic abstinence: natural family planning
   b. Chemical barriers: spermicidal creams, gels, or vaginal suppositories and sponges
   c. Mechanical barrier: condoms or sheaths
2. Methods that require periodic medical examination and prescription
   a. Hormonal therapy: estrogen or progestogen preparations or a combination of these compounds
   b. Mechanical barrier: cervical uterine occlusion by diaphragms or caps
   c. Intrauterine contraceptive devices
3. Methods that require surgical intervention
   a. Female sterilization
   b. Male sterilization

The following discussion of the above methods provides the nurse with information needed for client teaching. After implementing the appropriate teaching for contraceptive use, the nurse supervises return demonstrations and practice to assess client understanding. The client is given written instructions and phone numbers for questions. If the client has difficulty understanding written instructions, the woman (couple) is offered graphic material and a phone number to call as necessary, or an offer to return for further instruction.

Nonprescription Methods for Control of Fertility

Several nonprescription methods for control of fertility (**contraception**) are practiced. Prescription and supervision are unnecessary for barrier methods, that is, condom, foam, spermicide, and vaginal sponges, as well as for periodic abstinence. In 1987, among women age 15 to 44 exposed to the risk of unwanted pregnancy, 92% used some form of contraception (Mishell, 1989). Oral contraception was used by 32%, 17% used the condom, 6% used spermicide, 4% used the diaphragm, 4% used periodic abstinence (i.e., "natural family planning"), and 3% had an intrauterine device (IUD). Two methods were practiced that are *not* recommended: 6% used withdrawal (coitus interruptus), and 1% used douching. The percentages do not add up because some women used more than one method (Mishell, 1989). Coitus interruptus, a method practiced for centuries, requires the man to withdraw before ejaculation. Extreme self-discipline is needed, and the sexual relationship may be strained. The danger of pregnancy from sperm in the pre-ejaculatory drops is ever present. No advantages are given for this method, which has the lowest rate of effectiveness, comparable to the use of no contraceptive method (Lethbridge, 1991).

PERIODIC ABSTINENCE. The term **periodic abstinence** is preferred over "natural family planning" for contraceptive methods that rely on avoidance of intercourse during presumed fertile days of the menstrual cycle. Many couples find abstinence for 7 to 18 or more consecutive days of each menstrual cycle to be quite difficult.

Periodic abstinence methods employ a combination of the following:

1. Rhythm or calendar method
2. BBT method
3. Cervical mucus (Billings or ovulation) method
4. Symptothermal method
5. Fertility awareness method
6. Predictor test for ovulation

These methods depend on the continuous observation and recording of events of the menstrual cycle. The woman or couple must be able to assess hormone-induced signs and symptoms that indicate whether she is in the fertile or infertile part of the menstrual cycle. While teaching a woman about fertility awareness, the nurse uses this opportunity for helping the woman or couple learn a great deal about their bodies.

The *mode of action* for these methods of contraception is the avoidance of intercourse during the presumed fertile period of the menstrual cycle.*

The human ovum can be fertilized no later than 16 to 24 hours after ovulation. Motile sperm have been recovered from the uterus and the oviducts as long as 60 hours after coitus. However, their ability to fertilize the ovum probably lasts no longer than 24 to 48 hours. Pregnancy is unlikely to occur if a couple abstains from intercourse for 4 days before and for 3 or 4 days after ovulation (**fertile period**). Unprotected intercourse on the other days of the cycle (**safe period**) should not result in pregnancy. There are two principal problems with this method: the exact time of ovulation cannot be predicted accurately, and couples may find it difficult to exercise restraint for several days before and after ovulation. Women with irregular menstrual periods have the greatest risk of failure with this form of contraception (*Medi-*

*The World Health Organization (Liskin, Fox, 1981) concluded in 1979 that the cervical mucus and symptothermal methods "had very limited application, particularly in developing countries, and recommended that the World Health Organization Programme devote no further research to measuring their effectiveness." Similarly, the International Planned Parenthood Federation concluded in 1982 that "couples electing to use periodic abstinence should, however, be clearly informed that the method is not considered an effective method of family planning."

cal Letter, 1988). The typical failure rate is 20% during the first year of use (Hatcher et al, 1990).

Ovulation usually occurs about 14 days before the onset of menstruation. Therefore variations in the length of menstrual cycles are usually a result of differences in the length of the preovulatory phases. The fertile period can be anticipated by the following:

1. Calculating the time at which ovulation is likely to occur based on the lengths of previous menstrual cycles *(calendar method)*
2. Recording the rise in basal body temperature (BBT), a result of the thermogenic effect of progesterone *(temperature method)*
3. Recognizing the changes in cervical mucus at different phases of the menstrual cycle *(ovulation or Billings method)*
4. Using a predictor test for ovulation
5. Utilizing a combination of several methods

CALENDAR METHOD. Practice of the **calendar method** is based on a count of the number of days in each cycle counting from the first day of menses (Labbok, Queenan, 1989). With the calendar method the fertile period is determined after accurately recording the lengths of menstrual cycles for 1 year. The first unsafe day (beginning of the fertile period) can be determined by subtracting 18 days from the length of the shortest cycle. The last unsafe day (beginning of postovulatory safe period) can be calculated by subtracting 11 days from the length of the longest cycle. If the shortest cycle is 24 days and the longest is 30 days, application of the formula is as follows:

Shortest Cycle	Longest Cycle
24	30
−18	−11
6th day	19th day

To avoid conception the couple would abstain during the "fertile" period, days 6 through 19.

If the woman has very regular cycles of 28 days each, the formula indicates the fertile days to be:

Shortest Cycle	Longest Cycle
28	28
−18	−11
10th day	17th day

To avoid pregnancy, the couple abstains from day 10 through 17 because ovulation occurs on day 14 ±2 days. A major drawback of the calendar method is that one is trying to predict future events with past data. The predictability of the menstrual cycle to be unpredictable is also not taken into consideration.

The method is most useful as an adjunct to the BBT or cervical mucus method. It is *not* useful in the postpartum period, during lactation, or at extremes of reproductive age when cycles are most variable (Labbok, Queenan, 1989).

BASAL BODY TEMPERATURE. The basal body temperature (BBT) during the menses and for approximately 5 to 7 days thereafter usually varies from 36.2° to 36.3° C (97.2° to 97.4° F) (see Table 6-1, p. 125). If ovulation fails to occur, this pattern of lower body temperature continues throughout the cycle. Infection, fatigue, less than 3 hours of sleep per night, awakening late, and anxiety may cause temperature fluctuations, altering the expected pattern. If a new BBT thermometer is purchased, this fact is noted on the chart because the readings may vary slightly. Jet lag, alcohol taken the evening before, or sleeping in a heated water bed must also be noted on the chart because each will affect the BBT (see box below).

About the time of ovulation, a slight drop in temperature (about 0.05° C [0.1° F]) may be seen; after ovulation, in concert with the increasing progesterone levels of the early luteal phase of the cycle, the BBT rises slightly (about 0.2° to 0.4° C, [0.4° to 0.8° F]) (Fig. 42-6; Table 6-1, p. 125) (Labbok, Queenan, 1989). The temperature remains on an elevated plateau until 2 to 4 days before menstruation. Then it drops to the low levels recorded during the previous cycle unless pregnancy has occurred and temperature remains elevated.

The drop and subsequent rise in temperature are referred to as the **thermal shift.** When the entire month's temperatures are recorded on a graph, the pattern described is more apparent. It is more difficult to perceive day-to-day variations without the entire picture (Fig. 42-6). The BBT alone is not a reliable method to predict ovulation (Labbok, Queenan,

TEACHING Basal ("Resting") Body Temperature

Discuss BBT with the woman.

Show woman a diagram depicting the phases of the menstrual cycle (Fig. 6-21).

Discuss the different hormones in the woman's body that are responsible for her menstrual cycle and ovulation. Leave time for questions.

Show woman a sample BBT graph (Fig. 42-6) and the biphasic line seen in ovulatory cycles.

Show the client the BBT thermometer and how it is calibrated.

Provide a demonstration.

Encourage woman to demonstrate taking and reading the thermometer and how she will graph the temperature while nurse watches.

Encourage woman to start a log at the same time that keeps track of any other activity that might interfere with her true BBT (see Fig. 42-7).

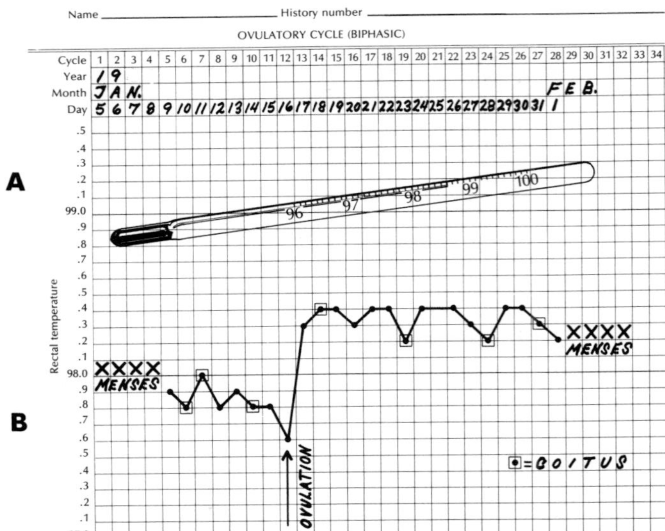

Fig. 42-6 A, Special thermometer for recording BBT, marked in tenths to enable person to read more easily. **B,** Basal temperature record shows drop and sharp rise at time of ovulation. Biphasic curve indicates ovulatory cycle.

1989). To determine if a rise in temperature is indeed the thermal shift, the woman must be aware of other signs approaching ovulation while she continues to assess the BBT. See discussion of symptothermal method for other indicators of ovulation.

Most counselors advise the couple who wish to prevent conception to avoid unprotected intercourse from the day of the drop in the BBT and for 3 days of elevated temperature (Labbok, Queenan, 1989). Others require the woman to abstain for the entire preovulatory period, starting with day 1 of menses until the third consecutive day of elevated BBT (Mishell, 1989).

CERVICAL MUCUS METHOD. The **cervical mucus method,** also called the *Billings method* or the *ovulation method,* requires that the woman recognize and interpret the characteristic cyclic changes in the amount and consistency of cervical mucus (see box above, Table 6-1, and Figs. 6-22 and 6-23). The cervical mucus that accompanies ovulation is necessary for viability and motility of sperm. Without adequate cervical mucus, coitus will not result in conception. These changes are easily learned by most couples (see teaching box). To ensure learning accurate assessment of changes, the cervical mucus should be free of semen, contraceptive gels or foams, and blood or discharge from vaginal infections for at least one full cycle. Other factors that create difficulty in identifying mucus changes include douches and vaginal deodorants, being in the sexually aroused state (which thins the mucus), and medications such as antihistamines, which dry up the mucus. One study found that self-evaluation of cervical mucus was highly accurate (see Research Highlight, p. 1305).

It is difficult to evaluate the mucus in the presence of semen or discharge from vaginal infection. Therefore the woman double checks for fertility by assessing her BBT record and other symptoms of fertility. (NOTE: Each woman has her own unique pattern of mucus changes.)

Some women may find this method unacceptable if they find touching their genitals uncomfortable. Whether or not the individual wants to use this method for contraception, it is to the woman's advantage to learn to recognize mucus characteristics at ovulation. Assessing changes in cervical mucus can be useful diagnostically for any of the following purposes:

1. To alert the couple to the reestablishment of ovulation while breast-feeding and after discontinuation of oral contraception
2. To note anovulatory cycles at any time and at the commencement of menopause
3. To assist couples in planning a pregnancy

TEACHING Cervical Mucus Characteristics

Setting the stage:

Show charts of menstrual cycle along with changes in the cervical mucus (see Figs. 6-22 and 6-23).

Have woman practice with raw egg-white.

Supply her with a BBT log and graph if she doesn't already have one.

Explain that assessment of cervical mucus characteristics is best when mucus is not mixed with semen, contraceptive jellies or foams, or discharge from infections.

Content related to cervical mucus:

Explain to woman (couple) how cervical mucus changes throughout the menstrual cycle.

Right before ovulation, the watery, thin, clear mucus becomes more abundant and thick. It feels like a lubricant and can be stretched 5+ cm; this is called **spinnbarkheit.** This indicates the period of maximum fertility. Sperm deposited in this type of mucus can survive until ovulation occurs.

Assessment technique:

Stress that good hand-washing is imperative to begin and end all self-assessment.

Start observation from last day of menstrual flow.

Assess cervical mucus several times a day for several cycles. Mucus can be obtained from vaginal introitus; no need to reach into vagina to cervix.

Record findings on the same record on which her BBT is entered. Record any other events also.

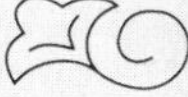 **Research Highlight** 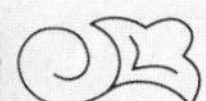

Methods Used to Self-Predict Ovulation

RESEARCH ABSTRACT

The purpose of this study was to compare the time of ovulation detected by a urine self-test of luteinizing hormone (LH) with the time of ovulation determined by the peak day of cervical mucus. Twenty women between the ages of 22 and 41 years with no known fertility problems were selected from a natural family planning clinic to participate in the study. The women had regular reproductive cycles, were nonsmokers, and were taking no medication that would affect the hormonal pattern or cervical mucus of the ovulation cycle. The LH surge in the urine was detected with an ovulation self-test kit. The manufacturer claims that the LH surge can be detected with 98% to 100% accuracy as early as 36 hours before ovulation. The peak day of cervical mucus was determined by the Creighton model VDRS (vaginal discharge recording system). Each subject was given two fertility charts and two ovulation self-test kits. LH surges were detected in 15 of the 20 subjects in the first cycle. Two subjects achieved pregnancy in the first cycle. In the second cycle, LH surges were detected in 14 of 18 subjects. LH surges occurred on or within 3 days of the peak day of mucus in 28 of the 29 cycles. LH surges were detectable in only 77.7% of the cycles, despite the manufacturer's claim of greater than 90% accuracy.

IMPLICATIONS FOR PRACTICE

Self-evaluation of cervical mucus is highly accurate in determining the time of optimal fertility. Predicting ovulation is also critical for couples who use abstinence for family planning. Daily observation of mucus by a woman is an inexpensive and accurate way to determine optimal fertility days. Nurses can use this information to counsel women about detection of mucus or to refer clients to practitioners certified in natural family planning methods.

RELATED RESEARCH QUESTIONS

1. Will an educational program directed at adolescents be successful in teaching self-evaluation of cervical mucus?
2. Will sexually active adolescents use self-evaluation of cervical mucus as a means of preventing pregnancy?
3. What are factors associated with acceptance of self-evaluation of cervical mucus as a means of family planning?
4. What factors affect the consistency of cervical mucus?

REFERENCE

Fehring RJ: Methods used to self-predict ovulation: a comparative study, *JOGNN* 19(3):233, 1990.

SYMPTOTHERMAL METHOD. The symptothermal method combines the BBT and cervical mucus methods with awareness of secondary, cycle phase-related symptoms (see Table 6-1). Both partners take responsibility for assessments, recordings, and evaluation of their findings. Together they determine the days for abstinence. Couples who use the symptothermal method commonly report an improvement in their sexual relationship.

The couple gains fertility awareness as they learn the woman's individual psychologic and physiologic symptoms that mark the phases of her cycle. Secondary symptoms (see Table 6-1) include increased libido, midcycle spotting, mittelschmerz, pelvic fullness, or tenderness, and vulvar fullness. The couple, perhaps using a speculum, looks at the cervix to assess for changes indicating ovulation: that is, the os dilates slightly, the cervix softens and rises in the vagina, and cervical mucus is copious and slippery. To complete their records, the couple notes days on which coitus, changes in routine, illness, and so on have occurred (Fig. 42-7). Calendar calculations and cervical mucus changes are used to estimate the onset of the fertile period; changes in cervical mucus or the BBT are used to estimate its end.

Effectiveness of the symptothermal method with abstinence during the fertile period ranges between 73% and 97%.

FERTILITY AWARENESS METHOD. The fertility awareness method is a combination of menstrual cycle charting based on observable physiologic changes and barrier contraception (Hatcher, et al, 1990). During the fertile period the couple has the choice of either abstinence from genital-genital contact or the use of barrier contraception. After the fertile period the couple may enjoy freedom from contraception for the remaining nonfertile days of the menstrual cycle.

PREDICTOR TEST FOR OVULATION. All of the preceding discussion is about assessments that are indicative of but do not prove the occurrence and exact timing of ovulation. Unique developments of

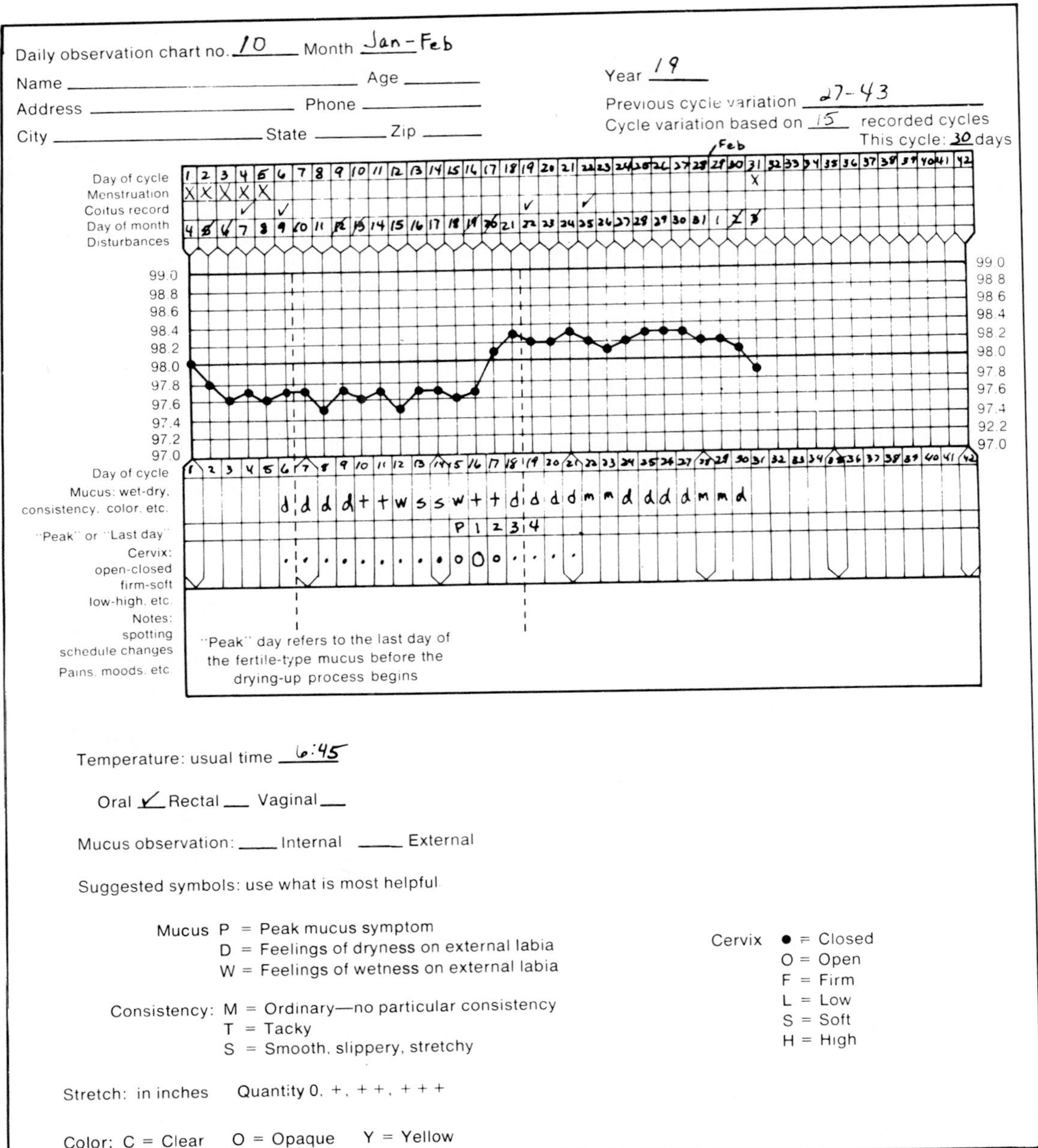

Fig. 42-7 Example of completed symptothermal method chart.
From Fogel C, Woods NF: *Health care of women,* St Louis, 1981, Mosby–Year Book.

monoclonal antibody technology have added the *predictor test* for ovulation. This type of test is a major addition to the periodic abstinence methods to help women who want to plan the time of their pregnancies and those who are trying to conceive. The **predictor test** for ovulation detects the sudden surge of LH that occurs approximately 12 to 24 hours *before* ovulation. Unlike BBT, the test is not affected by illness, emotional upset, or physical activity. Available for home use, a test kit contains sufficient material for several days' testing during each cycle. A positive response indicative of an LH surge is noted by color change that is easy to read. Directions for use of this home test kit vary with the manufacturer.

CHEMICAL AND MECHANICAL CONTRACEPTIVE BARRIERS. Barrier contraceptives are currently receiving great attention and increased use (Connell,

1989). This method has an additional distinct advantage of reducing the spread of sexually transmitted diseases (Mishell, 1989).

SPERMICIDES. A vaginal **spermicide** is a physical barrier to sperm penetration that also has a chemical action on sperm. *Nonoxynol 9* (N-9) and octoxynol 9 are the most commonly used spermicidal chemicals. Intravaginal spermicides are marketed as aerosol foams, foaming tablets, suppositories, creams and gels (Fig. 42-8). Preloaded, single-dose applicators small enough to be carried in a small purse are available (Grimes, 1986). This form of contraceptive must be placed deeply in the vagina in contact with the cervix before each coitus. Special precautions must be taken. The can of foam must be shaken to distribute the spermicide before use. Tablets and suppositories take from 10 to 30 minutes to dissolve. *Maximum spermicidal effectiveness lasts usually no longer than 1 hour.* If intercourse is to be repeated, reapplication of additional spermicide must precede it. Douching must be avoided for at least 6 hours after coitus (Grimes, 1986) (see box at right).

Spermicides provide a physical and chemical barrier that prevents viable sperm from entering the cervix. The effect is local, within the vagina.

Ease of application, safety, low cost, and ready availability without prescription or previous medical examination characterize this method. The delicate vaginal mucosa is not harmed unless the woman is allergic to a particular preparation. Spermicides aid in lubrication of the vagina. Because their effect is local, spermicides offer an alternative to hormonal contraception (e.g., for the nursing mother [to avoid interfering with lactation], for the premenopausal woman [to prevent masking symptoms of onset of the climacterium], and as a backup for the woman who forgets to take her oral contraceptive). There is evidence that *nonoxynol 9 plus a barrier method provide some protection against sexually transmitted disease* through bacteriostatic action (North, 1988; Louv et al, 1988). In the laboratory, it has been shown to have both bactericidal and virucidal activity (Connell, 1989). The addition of spermicides increases the effectiveness of the other forms of contraception (e.g., condoms and diaphragms).

Users of this method may complain of its "messiness," unpleasant "fizz," stickiness, or unpleasant

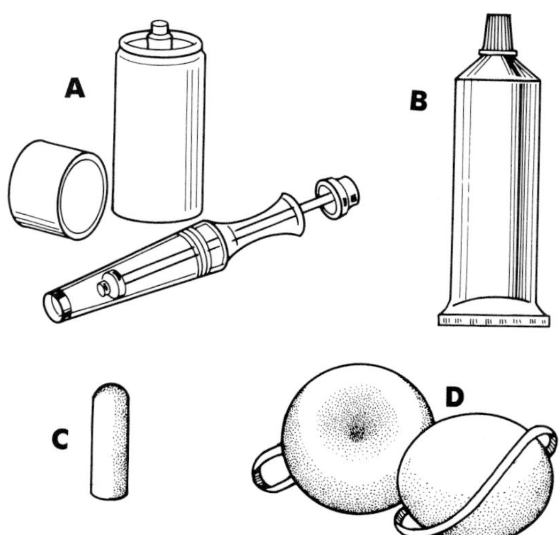

Fig. 42-8 Vaginal spermicides. **A**, Foam with applicator. **B**, Gel or cream. **C**, Suppository, **D**, Sponge.

TEACHING Spermicidal Vaginal Foam

Application (10 to 15 minutes before coitus):

- Shake canister gently
- Screw applicator to tip of canister *(A)*
- Press down until foam fills applicator
- Unscrew applicator from canister
- Insert applicator into vagina *(B)*
- Push plunger to release foam into vagina *(B)*
- Remove applicator from vagina

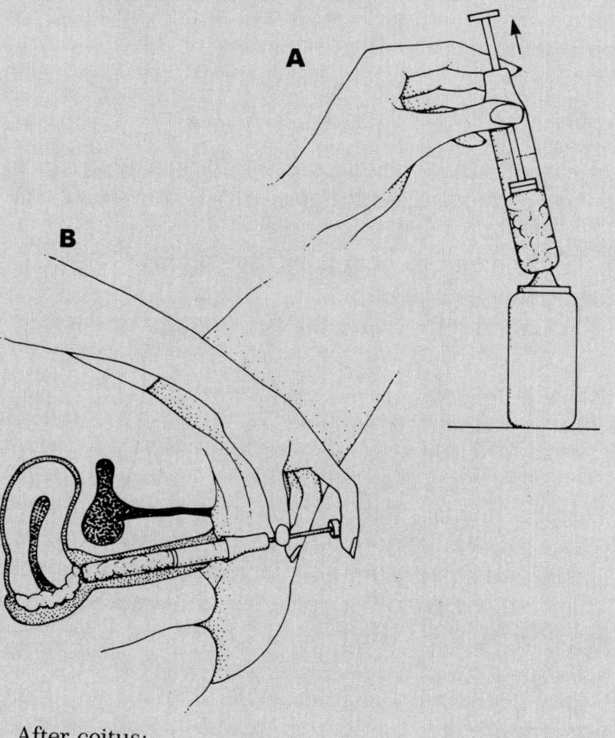

After coitus:

- Wash applicator and plunger with mild soap and warm water
- Dry thoroughly
- Do not boil applicator

taste. Allergic response or irritation of vaginal or penile tissue may occur. Some users experience decreased tactile sensation. The need to wait 10 minutes to 30 minutes before coitus initially and to reapply additional spermicide before repeated intercourse is not acceptable to all people.

According to Cunningham, MacDonald, and Gant (1989), the high pregnancy rate seen with this method is probably the result of inconsistent use of the spermicide. A typical failure rate is 21% (accidental pregnancy rate during the first year of use).

The nurse encourages open communication between the sexual partners to discuss intravaginal contraception. Clients are offered the opportunity to see and handle a variety of samples. To maximize learning, the woman is given the opportunity to insert one application into a medical model of the vagina. The male partner sometimes indicates an interest in learning how to insert the spermicide into his female partner. The nurse needs to feel comfortable teaching him as well.

VAGINAL SPONGE. The polyurethane **vaginal sponge** was approved by the Food and Drug Administration (FDA) in 1983 (see Fig. 42-8). Water is needed to activate the spermicide (nonoxynol 9) and facilitate insertion. Spermicide is released continuously for 24 hours. A woven loop is used for retrieval from the vagina. It is recommended that at least 6 hours lapse between last intercourse and removal (Grimes, 1986). Therefore the sponge has a total allowable wear-time of 30 hours (Connell, 1989). The sponge should be discarded after removal. It must not be washed and reused. Washing removes the spermicide.

The mode of action is the same as that for the spermicides.

Like the other spermicides, the sponge is an over-the-counter (OTC) product. It offers spontaneity and is less "messy" than other spermicide delivery systems. Furthermore, use of the sponge has been found to reduce the risk of chlamydia and gonorrhea (Hatcher et al, 1990). In vitro studies suggest it is effective against *Staphylococcus aureus*, which causes toxic shock syndrome (TSS) (p. 875) (Connell, 1989). Reapplication of spermicide during the 24 hours the sponge is in place is unnecessary.

The only reported side effects were allergic reactions (2% to 3%) or irritation (2% to 3%) that typically occur with all nonoxynol 9 products. There is an increased risk for candidiasis (Rosenberg et al, 1987). Six percent of users reported difficulty in removing the sponge (Grimes, 1986). Water must be available to activate the nonoxynol 9. To decrease the risk of TSS, no obstructive vaginal barrier (i.e., sponge, diaphragm) should be used during menses or soon after childbirth (Connell, 1989).

The first-year failure rates reported for sponge users range from 17 to 24.5 pregnancies per 100 women. Parous users (women who have borne children) are more likely than nulliparous users (women who have not borne children) to become pregnant (Hatcher et al, 1990).

Nursing actions are similar to those for other spermicides. Clients are reminded that each sponge is to be used once, for 24 hours only. It is left in place for 6 hours after coitus, and discarded. The woman is coached to "bear down" to facilitate removal of the sponge.

VAGINAL SHEATH (FEMALE CONDOM). The vaginal sheath of natural latex rubber has flexible rings at both ends (Connell, 1989) (Fig. 42-9). Basically this device is a combination of a diaphragm and a condom. The closed end of the pouch is inserted into the vagina and is anchored around the cervix; the open ring covers the labia. It can be applied well in advance of intercourse so that spontaneity is unaffected. Before intercourse, a spermicide is added. Since it is a relatively loose sheath, it tends to heighten sensation for the man. Both women and men report that intercourse with the sheath is generally about as satisfying as intercourse without the sheath. Application of this disposable barrier requires no special training. It comes in one size and is available over the counter (Greydanus, Lonchamp, 1990). This device may provide more protection against STDs than do condoms. Research is ongoing to produce acceptable mechanical barriers for women (Hatcher et al, 1990; Sakondhavat, 1990).

CONDOM. The **condom** is a thin, stretchable sheath to cover the penis (Fig. 42-10, *A*). In addition to three available sizes, four basic features differ among condoms marketed in the United States. These features are material, shape, lubricants, and spermicides. Ninety-nine percent are made of latex rubber. A functional difference in condom shape is the presence or absence of a sperm reservoir tip. To enhance vaginal

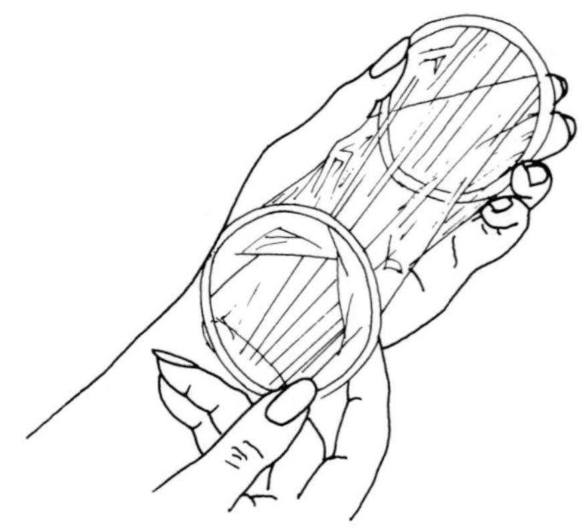

Fig. 42-9 WPC-333 soft polymer vaginal sheath.

stimulation, some condoms are contoured and rippled or have ribbed or roughened surfaces. Thinner construction increases heat transmission and sensitivity; a variety of colors increase their acceptability and attractiveness (Connell, 1989). A wet jelly or dry powder lubricates some condoms. Since 1982, spermicide (0.5 g of nonoxynol 9) has been added to the interior or exterior surfaces of some condoms. The addition of nonoxynol 9 to latex condoms not only increases contraceptive effectiveness, but it also increases protection against transmission of STDs, including HIV (Hatcher et al, 1990).

The sheath is applied over the erect penis before insertion or loss of preejaculatory drops of semen. Conception is made possible even if preejaculatory drops fall around the external vaginal opening because sperm are contained in these drops.

Used correctly, condoms prevent sperm from entering the cervix. Spermicide-coated condoms cause ejaculated sperm to be immobilized rapidly, thus increasing contraceptive effectiveness.

Condoms are safe, without side effects, and are readily available. Premalignant changes in the cervix can be prevented or ameliorated in women whose partners use condoms (Cunningham, MacDonald, Gant, 1989). If the condom is used throughout the act of intercourse and there is no unprotected contact with female genitals, a *latex rubber condom, which is impermeable to viruses,* can act as a protective measure against spread of sexually transmitted diseases (STDs). The STDs include gonorrhea, syphilis, herpes, chlamydia, acquired immunodeficiency syndrome (AIDS), human papillomavirus (HPV), and trichomoniasis (Morbidity Mortality Weekly Report, 1988; Hatcher et al, 1990; Mishell, 1989). The unique feature of this method is **male contraception** (Grimes, 1986).

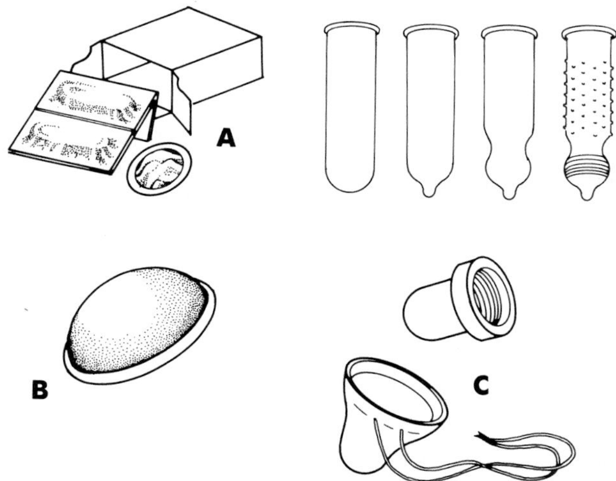

Fig. 42-10 Mechanical barriers. **A**, Types of condoms. **B**, Diaphragm. **C**, Cervical caps.

Some couples object to interrupting lovemaking to apply the sheath or complain that sensation is blunted. If condoms are used improperly, spillage of sperm can result in pregnancy. On occasion, condoms have torn during intercourse (*Consumer Reports*, 1989).

The pregnancy rate can be as low as 2% among correct and consistent users and about 12% among typical users (Hatcher et al, 1990). Condoms with spermicide are highly effective at killing sperm within the condom.

For years, health care providers assumed that everyone knew how to use condoms, so proper instruction was not provided. To prevent unintended pregnancy and the spread of STDs, it is essential that condoms be used correctly. To this end, the FDA has recently suggested instructions (Connell, 1989). Nurses can use these instructions in teaching clients (see box below).

TEACHING Use of Condoms

Use a new condom (check expiration date) for each act of sexual intercourse or other acts between partners that involve contact with the penis.
Place condom after penis is erect and before intimate contact.
Place condom on head of penis *(A)* and unroll it all the way to the base *(B)*.
Leave an empty space at the tip *(A)*; remove any air remaining in the tip by gently pressing air out towards the base of the penis.
If a lubricant is desired, use water-based products such as K-Y jelly.
After ejaculation, carefully withdraw still erect penis, holding onto condom rim; discard.
Store unused condoms in cool, dry place.
Do not use condoms that are sticky, brittle, or obviously damaged.

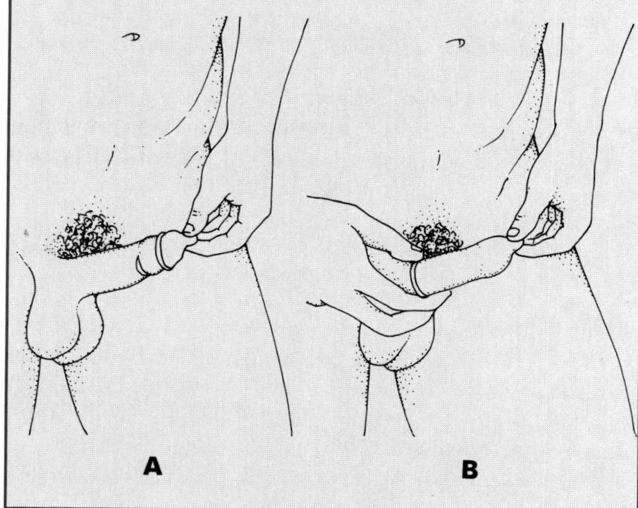

Methods Requiring Prescription

Several methods for the control of fertility require prescription and supervision. Interview, physical examination, and occasionally laboratory tests are prerequisites for some forms of contraception. These methods of contraception include hormonal therapy, use of diaphragms or cervical caps, and IUDs.

HORMONAL CONTRACEPTION. Steroidal contraceptives are available in several dosage forms. General classes are described in Table 42-3, below. Because of the wide variety of preparations available, the woman and nurse need to read the package insert for information about specific products prescribed. Formulations include combined estrogen-progestin steroidal medications, progestational agents, and an estrogenic agent. The formulations are administered orally, subdermally, or by implantation. Combined estrogen-progestin steroidal medications are discussed first.

MODE OF ACTION. The normal menstrual cycle is maintained by a feedback mechanism (Chapter 6). Follicle-stimulating hormone (FSH) and luteinizing hormone (LH) are secreted in response to *fluctuating* levels of ovarian estrogen and progesterone. Regular ingestion of combined estrogen-progestin steroidal medication suppresses the action of the hypothalamus and anterior pituitary leading to inappropriate secretion of FSH and LH. Therefore follicles do not mature; ovulation is inhibited.

Other contraceptive effects are induced by the combined steroids. Maturation of the endometrium is altered, making it a less favorable site for implantation should ovulation and conception occur. It also has a direct effect on the endometrium, so that from 1 to 4 days after the last steroid tablet is taken, the endometrium sloughs and bleeds as a result of hormone withdrawal. The **withdrawal bleeding** usually is less profuse than that of normal menstruation and may last only 2 to 3 days. Some women have no bleeding at all.

The cervical mucus remains thick as a result of the effect of the progestin. Cervical mucus under the effect of progesterone does not provide as suitable an environment for sperm penetration as does the thin, watery mucus at ovulation (Willson, Carrington, 1987).

The possible role, if any, of altered tubal and uterine motility induced by the steroidal hormones is not clear (Cunningham, MacDonald, Gant, 1989). As a consequence of these actions, **oral hormonal contraceptives,** if taken daily for 3 weeks of every 4, provide virtually absolute protection against conception (Cunningham, MacDonald, Gant, 1989).

Phasic pills (e.g., triphasic oral contraceptives) are those in which the amount of progestin, and sometimes the amount of estrogen, varies within each cycle. These preparations reduce the total dosage of steroid hormones in a single cycle without sacrificing contraceptive efficacy or cycle control (Cunningham, MacDonald, Gant, 1989). The theoretic advantage is a reduction in progestin-related metabolic changes and the adverse effects attributed to those metabolic changes. The estrogen dose is also kept low with only 30 to 40 μg of ethinyl estradiol; no tablet sold in the United States contains more than 50 μg (Cunningham, MacDonald, Gant, 1989; FDA Bulletin, 1988).

ADVANTAGES. For motivated women it is easy to take an oral contraceptive (OC) at about the same time each day. Taking the pill does not relate directly to the sexual act; this fact increases its acceptability to some women. Commonly, there is an improvement in sexual response once the possibility of pregnancy is not an issue. For some, it is convenient to know when to expect the next "menstrual" flow.

TABLE 42-3 Hormonal Contraception

Composition	Route of Administration	Duration of Effect
Combination of an estrogen and a progestin	Oral	24 hours
Mini-pill: progestin (norethindrone, 0.35 mg) only	Oral	24 hours
Morning-after pill: estrogen (diethylstilbestrol [DES]) in very high doses—25 mg	Oral	Taken within 72 hours of unprotected coitus during fertile period; because of DES effect on fetus, abortion advised if method fails
Depo-Provera: progestin only (medroxyprogesterone acetate), 150 mg	Intramuscular injection	From 3 to 6 months
Norplant system: progestin (Levonorgestrel) in Silastic containers	Implant, subdermal	Up to 5 years

Oral contraceptives are considered to be a safe option for older, nonsmoking women until menopause. Perimenopausal women can benefit from regular bleeding cycles, a regular hormonal pattern, and the noncontraceptive health benefits of OCs (Contraception, 1992a).

There has been little publicity about the advantages of hormonal contraceptives. Mishell (1989 a, b) and Cunningham, MacDonald, and Gant (1989) list the noncontraceptive health benefits of oral contraceptives. The benefits include decreased menstrual blood loss and resultant decreased iron-deficiency anemia, regulation of menorrhagia and irregular cycles, lowered incidence of dysmenorrhea (menstrual cramps) and premenstrual syndrome (PMS), protection against endometrial adenocarcinoma, reduced incidence of benign breast disease and possibly breast cancer, protection against the development of functional ovarian cysts, protection against acute salpingitis* and pelvic inflammatory disease (PID) caused by gonorrhea, and possible protection against ovarian cancer and postmenopausal osteoporosis. However, there is biologic and epidemiologic evidence that PID caused by *Chlamydia* is enhanced by oral contraceptives (Washington et al, 1985). Combination oral contraceptives have been used to treat such medical conditions as idiopathic thrombocytopenia purpura and endometriosis.

Since ovulation is suppressed, the risk for ectopic pregnancy is about one tenth that of women not using contraceptives. This form of contraception is associated with minimum risk for women aged 15 to 29 years. The mortality is 1.2 and 1.4/100,000 for nonsmoking and smoking women, respectively.

Women taking steroidal contraceptives are examined before the medication is prescribed and yearly thereafter. The examination includes medical and family history, weight, blood pressure, general physical and pelvic examination, screening cervical cytologic analysis (Pap smear), and hemoglobin determination. Consistent medical surveillance is valuable in the detection of noncontraception-related disorders as well, so that timely treatment can be initiated.

Use of oral hormonal contraceptives is initiated on one of the first 7 days of the menstrual cycle (day 1 of the cycle is the first day of menses). Other women start their use after delivery or abortion. If contraceptives are to be started at any time other than during normal menses, or within 3 weeks after delivery or abortion, another method of contraception should be used throughout the first week to avoid the risk of pregnancy if ovulation had already occurred (Cunningham, MacDonald, Gant, 1989). The combined estrogen-progestin pill taken daily 3 weeks out of every 4 is the most effective reversible form of contraception available (Cunningham, MacDonald, Gant, 1989). Taken exactly as directed, OCs prevent ovulation, and pregnancy cannot occur; the overall effectiveness rate is almost 100%. Almost all failures (i.e., pregnancy occurs) are caused by omission of one or more pills during the regimen.

DISADVANTAGES AND SIDE EFFECTS. Since hormonal contraceptives have come into use, the amount of estrogen and progestational agent contained in each tablet has been reduced considerably (Cunningham, MacDonald, Gant, 1989). This is of importance, because adverse effects are, to a degree, dose-related.

Women must be screened for conditions that present absolute or relative contraindications to oral contraceptive use. *Absolute contraindications* include a history of thromboembolic disorders, cerebrovascular or coronary artery disease, breast cancer, estrogenic-dependent tumors, pregnancy, impaired liver function, liver tumor, and previous cholestasis. Strong relative *contraindications* include migraine headaches, hypertension, acute mononucleosis, surgery requiring immobilization for 4 weeks, long-leg cast or major lower leg injury, age of 40 years or older accompanied by a second cardiovascular risk factor, age of 35 years or older and heavy smoking (more than 15 cigarettes per day), and abnormal genital bleeding (Hatcher et al, 1990). The main causes of hospitalization and death are cardiovascular problems (e.g., myocardial infarction [heart attack], cerebrovascular accident [stroke], and thromboembolism) (Grimes, 1986).

The risk of dying as a consequence of using this method of contraception is very low if the woman is less than 35 years of age, has no systemic illness, and is a nonsmoker. The risk of death secondary to use of oral contraceptives is less than that from pregnancy and the risk of dying from pregnancy is quite low (Cunningham, MacDonald, Gant, 1989; Porter, Jick, Walker, 1987). Under careful supervision, women with certain chronic medical conditions (e.g., diabetes mellitus) can take OCs (Carlone, Keen, 1989).

Certain side effects of anovulatory drugs are attributable to estrogen and progestin or both. Side effects of *estrogen excess* include nausea and vomiting, dizziness, edema, leg cramps, increase in breast size, chloasma (mask of pregnancy), visual changes, hypertension, and vascular headache. Side effects of *estrogen deficiency* include early spotting (days 1 to 14), hypomenorrhea, nervousness, and atrophic vaginitis leading to painful intercourse (dyspareu-

*Wolner-Hanssen et al (1985) suggest that this protection may apply to both gonococcal and chlamydial salpingitis. Oral contraceptives provide no protection against HIV transmission.

nia). Side effects of *progestin excess* include increased appetite, tiredness, depression, breast tenderness, vaginal yeast infection, oily skin and scalp, hirsutism, and postpill amenorrhea. Side effects of *progestin deficiency* include late spotting and breakthrough bleeding (days 15 to 21), heavy flow with clots, and decreased breast size. One of the most common side effects is bleeding irregularities (Hillard, 1989).

In the presence of side effects, especially those that are bothersome to the woman, a different product, a different drug content, or another method of contraception may be required. The "right" product for a woman contains the lowest dose of sex steroid hormones that prevents ovulation and that has the fewest and least harmful side effects. There is no way to predict the "right" dose* for any particular woman; trial and error is the main method for prescribing OCs, starting with the lowest possible estrogen dose.

The *changes in glucose tolerance* that occur in some women taking OCs are similar to those changes that occur during pregnancy. The dose, type, and potency of progestin (not estrogen) produce some deterioration of glucose tolerance in normal women, as well as in those with a history of gestational diabetes (Mishell, 1989).

The changes in levels of *nutrients* that have been described for some women who use oral contraceptives are similar to changes induced by normal pregnancy. Some investigators have described lower plasma levels in users compared with nonusers, for ascorbic acid, folic acid, vitamin B_{12}, niacin, riboflavin, and zinc (Cunningham, MacDonald, Gant, 1989). Combined estrogen-progestin oral contraceptives conserve a woman's iron by reducing the amount of blood lost during menstruation.

Women who discontinue oral contraception for a planned pregnancy commonly ask whether they should wait before attempting to conceive. Although data are controversial, studies indicate that these infants have no greater chance of being born with any type of birth defect than do infants born to women in the general population, even if conception occurred in the first month after the medication was discontinued (Mishell, 1989).

After discontinuing oral contraception there is usually a delay before ovulation and menstrual cycles recur, similar to that experienced by a newly delivered mother. However, *postpill amenorrhea* exceeding 6 months should be investigated.

Uncommonly, *hypertension* is first noted after the woman begins oral contraception, especially if she is 30 years of age or older. In some women, higher blood levels of angiotensinogen and plasma renin have been found. It is thought that these factors play a part in the hypertension experienced by some women (Mishell, 1989). After discontinuing oral contraception, hypertension subsides.

Some women complain of *edema,* which is associated with administration of estrogens; however, if the dose of estrogen is sufficiently low, fluid retention is not likely to occur or can be compensated for by decreasing the oral intake of sodium compounds.

Some conditions are aggravated by fluid retention. Women susceptible to *migraine headaches* may notice an increase in headaches when taking the pill. Since headaches are also symptomatic of cerebral thrombosis, there may be confusion with correct diagnosis. Therefore women who experience migraine headaches are counseled to use other forms of contraception. Although many women with *epilepsy* tolerate OCs well, others tend to have an increased incidence of seizures.

More serious *neuroocular lesions* are associated with use of OCs. Optic neuritis, or retinal thrombosis, although rare, has been reported. Symptoms such as sudden or gradual and partial or complete loss of vision and double vision require immediate diagnosis and treatment. *Women must stop taking OCs at the first sign of visual disorders.*

A somewhat increased risk of gallstones and gallbladder disease has been reported. One study (Royal College, 1982) suggests that oral contraceptives may only accelerate the development of gallbladder disease in women who are susceptible; there is no overall increased long-term risk.

The effectiveness of OCs is decreased when the following drugs are taken at the same time:

- Barbiturates (for sedation)
- Phenytoin sodium (for seizure disorders)
- Antibiotics

Also, the use of OCs can decrease the effectiveness of several drugs (e.g., insulin and oral anticoagulants) (Orshan, 1988).

It is unclear whether oral hormonal contraceptives contribute to the development of breast cancer. Four recently published studies fail to clarify the controversy (Meirik et al, 1986; Peterson, Lee, 1989).

The risk of *deep vein thrombosis* and *pulmonary embolism* has been estimated to be 3 to 11 times greater in women who use oral contraceptives than in otherwise apparently similar women who do not (Peterson, Lee, 1989). The risk of postoperative thromboembolism is increased if the woman uses oral hormone contraceptives during the month before the operative procedure. There is a smaller increase

*Warn women, young and old, that using another woman's OCs may not prevent ovulation if the dose is not correct for them.

in risk for women taking preparations containing less estrogen (see box below) (Cunningham, MacDonald, Gant, 1989).

NURSING ACTIONS. There are many different preparations of oral hormonal contraceptives. The nurse reviews the prescribing information in the package insert with the client. Because of the wide variations, each woman must be clear about the unique dosage regimen for the preparation prescribed for her. Directions for care after missing one or two tablets also vary. Recent findings indicate that if one or two tablets are missed, another form of contraception needs to be used until the required regimen is reestablished. Typical counseling regarding missed doses follows:

The woman needs to take the pill at the same time each day to maintain constant blood levels of estrogen and progesterone for 21 days. If one pill is missed, the woman takes that pill as soon as she remembers it. She takes the next pill at the regularly scheduled time. If the woman misses two pills, she takes both as soon as she remembers to do so. A second form of contraception (e.g., condom with spermicide) for the rest of that cycle is advised. If three pills are missed, the remainder of the pills in that packet are discarded and use of a back-up type of contraceptive is advised. A new packet of pills is begun on the first Sunday or the fifth day of the next cycle (bleeding should begin within 2 to 3 days after she misses the pills; day 1 of the new cycle is the first day of bleeding.)

Withdrawal bleeding ("periods") tends to be short and scanty when some combination OCs are taken. A woman may see no fresh blood at all. Some women may have only a drop of blood or a brown smudge on their tampon or underwear. This counts as a period. This fact may explain why some women have difficulty remembering the first day of their last period.

No more than 50% to 70% of women who start taking OCs are still taking them after 1 year. It is therefore important that nurses recommend that all women choosing to use the OC also be provided with a second method of birth control and that women be instructed and comfortable with this backup method. Most women stop taking OCs for nonmedical reasons; that is, they *choose* to stop; not because they develop a complication or a serious side effect.

TEACHING OCs and Reportable Symptoms: ACHES

Before OCs are prescribed and periodically throughout hormone therapy, the woman is alerted to stop taking the pill and to report any of the following symptoms to the physician immediately. The word *aches* helps in retention of this list:

- A—Abdominal pain: may indicate a problem with the liver or gallbladder
- C—Chest pain or shortness of breath: may indicate possible clot problem within lungs or heart
- H—Headaches (sudden or persistent): may be caused by cardiovascular accident or hypertension
- E—Eye problems: may indicate vascular accident or hypertension
- S—Severe leg pain: may indicate a thromboembolic process

PROGESTIN-ONLY CONTRACEPTION

Oral Progestins ("Mini-pill"). The mini-pill of 0.5 mg or less of a progestational agent daily presumably impairs fertility. Ovulation may occur. Progestational impact on cervical mucus decreases sperm penetration and alters endometrial maturation to discourage implantation should conception occur. Users report a higher incidence of irregular bleeding.

Injectable Progestins. The advantages of depo medroxyprogesterone (DMPA, Depo-Provera) include a contraceptive effectiveness comparable to combined oral contraceptives, long-lasting effects, the requirement of injections only 2 to 4 times a year, and lactation not likely to be impaired (Cunningham, MacDonald, Gant, 1989). The modes of action are several and include inhibition of ovulation and alteration in endometrial maturation and cervical mucus. Disadvantages are prolonged amenorrhea or uterine bleeding and increased risk of venous thrombosis and thromboembolism. Medroxyprogesterone is used by millions of women worldwide, but not in the United States. FDA approval has not been granted as yet. "Newer injectable and implantable progestin-only methods should, by the 1990s, expand the selection of these convenient and effective and popular methods of contraception for women worldwide" (Kaunitz, 1989).

Implantable Progestin (Norplant). The **Norplant** system consists of six flexible, nonbiodegradable Silastic capsules. They contain progestin providing up to 5 years of contraception. Insertion and removal of the capsules are minor surgical procedures involving a local anesthetic, a small incision, and no sutures. The capsules are placed subdermally in the inner aspect of the upper arm. The progestin prevents some, but not all, ovulatory cycles and thickens cervical mucus. The effectiveness is greater than 99% over 5 years. Other advantages include long-term continuous contraception, not coitus related, and reversibility. Irregular menstrual bleeding is the most common side effect (Darney et al, 1990). Other side effects, including headaches, nervousness, nausea, skin changes, and vertigo, are less common

(Shoupe, Mishell, 1989; Wyeth Labs, 1990). This method is now approved for use in the United States.

Clinical trials are ongoing for the Capronor (Darney et al, 1989), a biodegradable rod, and for contraceptive pellets. These provide contraception for 1½ and 1 year respectively (Cunningham, MacDonald, Gant, 1989; Kaunitz, 1989).

Vaginal Rings. The World Health Organization (WHO) and the Population Council are conducting research on the Silastic vaginal ring. It releases small amounts of levonorgestrel daily. Women continue to ovulate, but contraception is achieved by making cervical mucus impermeable to sperm. The ring is designed to remain in the vagina for 3 months. One major disadvantage is irregular vaginal bleeding (Monier, Laird, 1989; Hatcher et al, 1990).

DIAPHRAGM WITH SPERMICIDE. The vaginal **diaphragm** is a shallow, dome-shaped rubber device with a flexible wire rim that covers the cervix (Fig. 42-10, *B*). There are three main styles of diaphragms available in a wide range of diameters (50 to 95 mm). Diaphragms differ in the inner construction of the circular rim. The three types of rims are flat spring, coil spring, and arching spring.

The diaphragm should feel comfortable. It should be the largest size the woman can wear without her being aware of its presence. The use of a contraceptive gel or cream with the diaphragm offers both mechanical and chemical barriers to pregnancy.

The diaphragm is a mechanical barrier preventing the meeting of the sperm with the ovum. The diaphragm holds the spermicide in place against the cervix for the 6 hours it takes to destroy the sperm. The *effectiveness* of this combined method is approximately 83% to 90%. Highly motivated women may achieve rates of 99%.

NURSING ACTIONS. The woman is informed that she needs an annual gynecologic examination. The device may need to be refitted after 2 years, the loss or gain of 9 kg (20 lb) or more, term delivery, or second trimester abortion (Kugel Verson, 1986; Connell, 1989). Since there are various types of diaphragms on the market, the nurse uses the package insert for teaching the woman how to use and care for the diaphragm (see box on pp. 1315 and 1316).

Except for occasional allergic responses to the diaphragm or spermicide, there are no side effects from a well-fitted device. The diaphragm can be inserted as long as 6 hours before intercourse to increase spontaneity, but spermicide must be added each time intercourse is repeated (*Medical Letter,* 1988). It must be left in place for at least 6 hours after the last intercourse. The woman who engages in intercourse infrequently may choose this barrier method. The spermicide does offer additional lubrication if it is needed. A decreased incidence of vaginitis, cervicitis (including cervicitis caused by *Chlamydia trachomatis* and *Neisseria gonorrhoeae*), PID, and cervical intraepithelial neoplasia is noted among women who use contraceptive creams, foams, and gels with the diaphragm.

This method is contraindicated for the woman with relaxation of her pelvic support (uterine prolapse) or a large cystocele. It is also not advised for the woman who is "uninformed."

Disadvantages include the reluctance of some women to insert and remove the diaphragm. A cold diaphragm and a cold gel temporarily reduce vaginal response to sexual stimulation if insertion of the diaphragm occurs immediately before intercourse. Some women or couples object to the "messiness" of the spermicide. These annoyances of diaphragm usage, along with failure to insert the device once foreplay has begun, are the most common reasons for failures of this method. Side effects may include irritation of tissues related to contact with spermicides. Urethritis and recurrent cystitis (Strom, 1987) caused by upward pressure of the diaphragm rim against the urethra may be increased by the use of the contraceptive diaphragm.

Toxic shock syndrome (TSS) (Chapter 29), although reported in very small numbers, can occur in association with the use of the contraceptive diaphragm (Connell, 1989). The nurse should instruct the woman about ways to reduce her risk for TSS. These measures include prompt removal 6 to 8 hours after intercourse; not using the diaphragm during menses; and learning and watching for danger signs of TSS. These danger signs include temperature of 38.4° C (101° F), diarrhea, vomiting, muscle aches, and sunburn-like rash (for further discussion, see Chapter 29).

CERVICAL CAP. The Prentif cavity-rim **cervical cap** was approved in the late 1980s for use in the United States (Brokaw, Baker, Haney, 1988; Mishell, 1989; Women's Health, 1989). The cap has a 1¼-to 1½-inch soft natural rubber dome with a firm but pliable rim (see Fig. 42-10, *C*). It fits snugly around the base of the cervix close to the junction of the cervix and vaginal fornices (Hatcher et al, 1990). The device is available in four sizes. It is recommended that the cap remain in place no less than 8 hours and not more than 48 hours at a time (NAACOG 1988; Mishell, 1989). It is left in place 6 to 8 hours after the last act of intercourse. The seal provides a physical barrier to sperm; spermicide inside the cap adds a chemical barrier.

The extended period of wear is an added conve-

TEACHING Use and Care of the Diaphragm

POSITIONS FOR INSERTION OF DIAPHRAGM

Squatting

This is the most commonly used position, and most women find this position satisfactory.

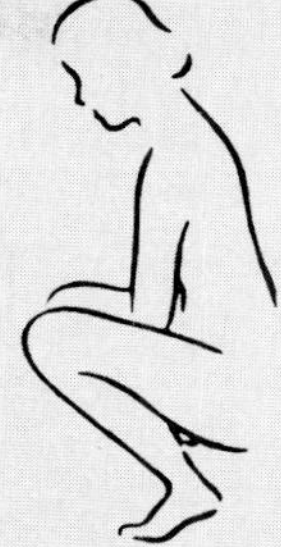

Leg Up Method

A position to suit the convenience of particular women is to raise the left foot (if right hand is used for insertion) on a low stool, and in a bending position the diaphragm is inserted.

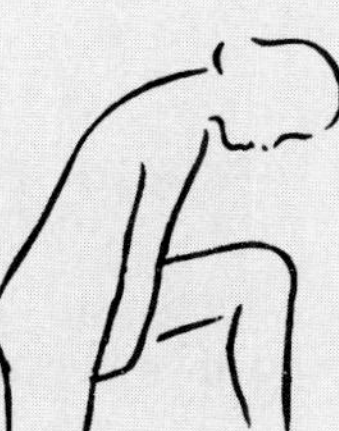

Chair Method

A practical method for diaphragm insertion is for the woman to sit far forward on the edge of a chair.

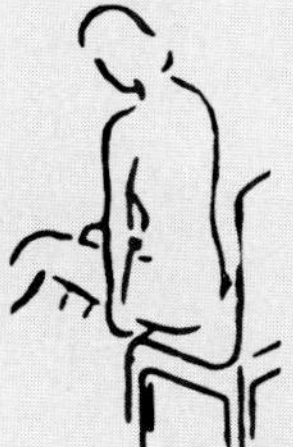

Reclining

In some instances, certain women prefer to insert the diaphragm while in a semi-reclining position in bed.

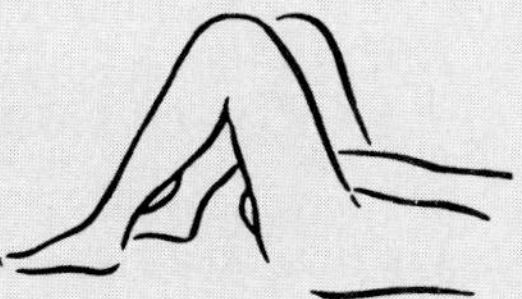

INSPECTION OF DIAPHRAGM

Your diaphragm must be inspected carefully before each use. The best way to do this is:

Hold the diaphragm up to a light source. Carefully stretch the diaphragm at the area of the rim, on all sides, to make sure there are no holes. Remember, it is possible to puncture the diaphragm with sharp fingernails.

Another way to check for pinholes is to carefully fill the diaphragm with water. If there is any problem, it will be seen immediately.

If your diaphragm is "puckered," especially near the rim, this could mean thin spots.

The diaphragm should not be used if you see any of the above; consult your physician.

PREPARATION OF DIAPHRAGM

Your diaphragm must always be used with a spermicidal lubricant to be effective. Pregnancy cannot be prevented effectively by the diaphragm alone.

Always empty your bladder before inserting the diaphragm. Place about 2 teaspoonsful of contraceptive gel, contraceptive jelly, or contraceptive cream on the side of the diaphragm that will rest against the cervix (or whichever way you have been instructed). Spread it around to coat the surface and the rim. This aids in insertion and offers a more complete seal. Many women also spread some gel (jelly) or cream on the other side of the diaphragm (see Fig. A).

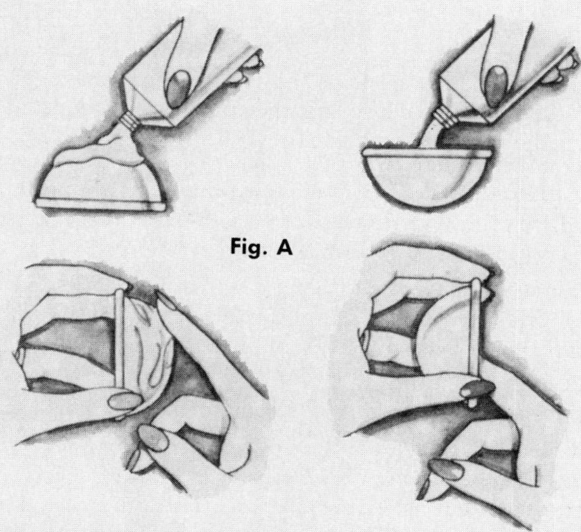

Fig. A

INSERTION OF DIAPHRAGM

The diaphragm can be inserted as much as 6 hours before intercourse. Hold the diaphragm between your thumb and fingers. The dome can either be up or down, as directed by your physician. Place your index finger on the outer rim of the compressed diaphragm (see Fig. B). Use the fingers of the other hand to spread the labia (lips of the vagina). This will assist in guiding the diaphragm into place.

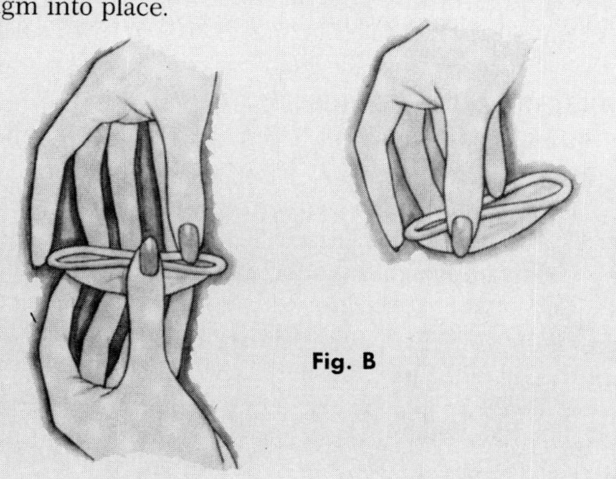

Fig. B

Continued.

TEACHING Use and Care of the Diaphragm—cont'd

Insert the diaphragm into the vagina. Direct it inward and downward as far as it will go to the space behind and below the cervix (see Fig. C).

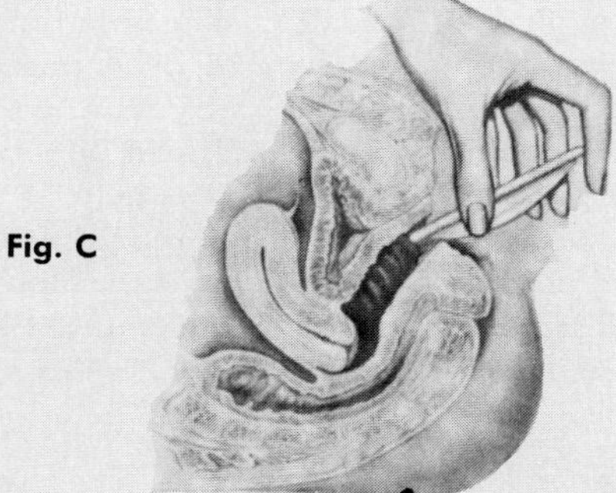

Fig. C

Tuck the front of the rim of the diaphragm behind the pelvic bone so that the rubber hugs the front wall of the vagina (see Fig. D).

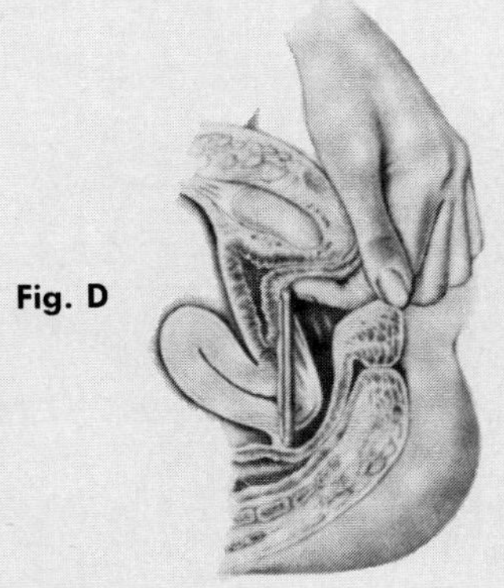

Fig. D

Feel for your cervix through the diaphragm to be certain it is properly placed and securely covered by the rubber dome (see Fig. E).

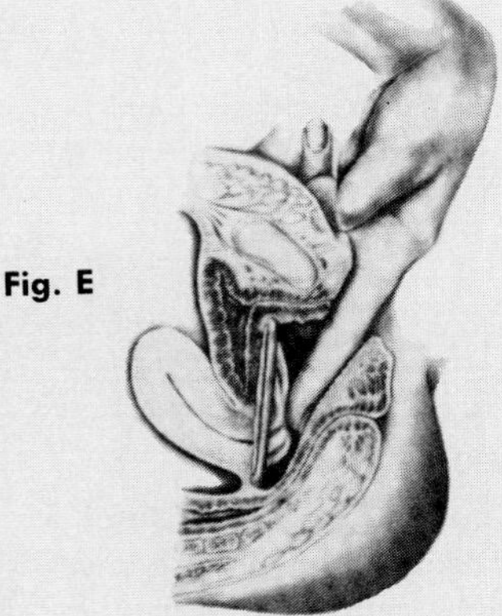

Fig. E

To clean the introducer, wash with mild soap and warm water, rinse and dry thoroughly.

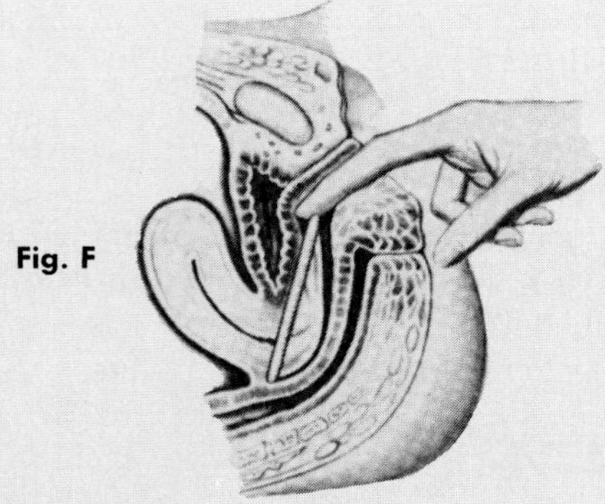

Fig. F

GENERAL INFORMATION

Regardless of the time of the month, this method of contraception must be used each and every time intercourse takes place. Your diaphragm must be left in place for at least 6 hours after the last intercourse. If you remove your diaphragm before the 6-hour period, your chance of becoming pregnant could be greatly increased.

REMOVAL OF DIAPHRAGM

The only proper way to remove the diaphragm is to insert your forefinger up and over the top side of the diaphragm, and slightly to the side.

Next, turn the palm of your hand downward and backward hooking the forefinger firmly on top of the inside of the upper rim of the diaphragm, *breaking the suction.*

Pull the diaphragm down and out. This avoids the possibility of tearing the diaphragm with the fingernails. The diaphragm *should not* be removed by trying to catch the rim from *below* the dome (see Fig. F).

CARE OF DIAPHRAGM

When using a vaginal diaphragm, avoid using products that may contain petroleum, such as certain body lubricants, vaginal lubricants, or vaginitis preparations. These products can weaken rubber.

A little care means longer wear for your diaphragm. After each use the diaphragm should be washed in warm water and mild soap. Do not use detergent soaps, cold cream soaps, deodorant soaps, and soaps containing petroleum, since they can weaken the rubber.

After washing, the diaphragm should be dried thoroughly. All water and moisture should be removed with your towel. The diaphragm should then be dusted with *cornstarch.* Scented talc, body powder, baby powder, and the like should not be used because they can weaken the rubber.

The diaphragm should then be placed back in the plastic case for storage. It should not be stored near a radiator or heat source or exposed to light for an extended period.

nience for women who previously used the diaphragm. Instructions for the actual insertion and use of the cervical cap closely resemble the instructions for use of the contraceptive diaphragm. Some of the differences are that the cervical cap can be inserted hours before sexual intercourse without a need for additional spermicide later, no additional spermicide is required for repeated acts of intercourse when the cap is used, and the cervical cap requires less spermicide than the diaphragm when initially inserted (NAACOG, 1988).

Some women are not good candidates for wearing the cervical cap. They include women with abnormal Pap test results, women who cannot be fitted properly with the existing cap sizes, women who find the insertion and removal of the device too difficult, women with a history of TSS, women with vaginal or cervical infections (NAACOG, 1988), and women who experience allergic responses to the cap or spermicide.

The angle of the uterus, the vaginal muscle tone, and the shape of the cervix may interfere with ease of fitting and use. Correct fitting requires time, effort, and skill from both the client and the clinician (Brokaw, Baker, Haney, 1988). The woman must check the cap's position before and after each act of intercourse.

After 3 months of use; cervical cap users had a higher rate of conversion from class I (no abnormal cells present) to class III (suspicious abnormal cells present) Pap tests when compared with diaphragm users (NAACOG, 1988; Mishell, 1989). These conversions may be manifestations of the human papillomavirus (HPV). Women using the cap should have a Pap test at least every year. If the cap is left in place more than 48 hours, it will produce an odor.

Whereas no link has been discovered between TSS and the use of the cervical cap, such an association remains possible (NAACOG, 1988).

The package insert recommends that another form of birth control be used during menstrual bleeding and up to at least 6 postpartum weeks.

The cap should be refitted after any gynecologic surgery or delivery, and after major weight losses or gains. Otherwise, the size should be checked at least once a year (Women's Health, 1989).

Strong client motivation is the most important criterion for successful cap use. First-year failure rates range from 8 to 27 pregnancies per 100 women who initiate the use of this method (Hatcher et al, 1990, Mishell, 1989; Women's Health, 1989). That failure rating is similar to the one given the diaphragm.

The client must be given the information available for this product as presented above. The nurse needs to assess the woman's understanding and skill in the use of the cervical cap (see box at right).

TEACHING Use and Care of the Cervical Cap

To insert:
Push cap up into vagina until it covers cervix.

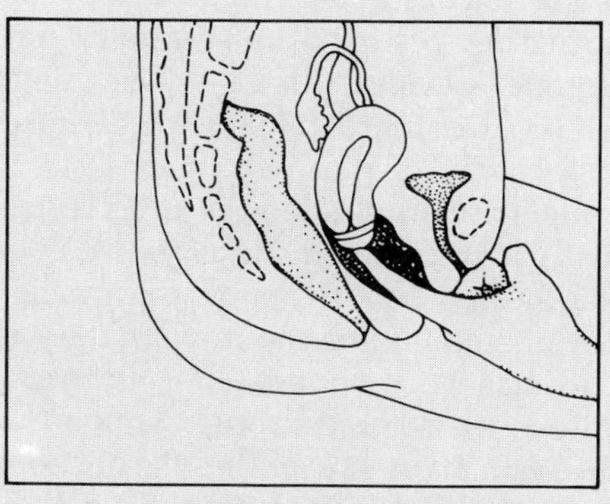

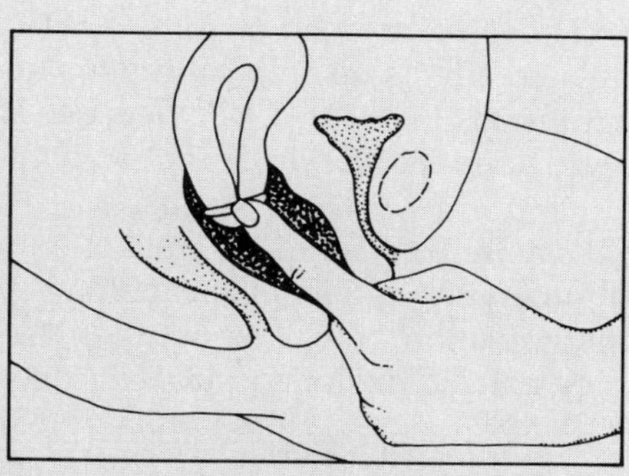

To remove:
Lift rim away from cervix and remove.

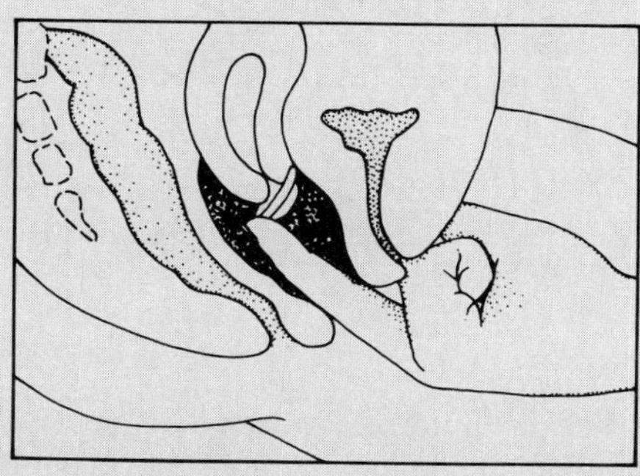

The woman can assume a number of positions to insert the cervical cap, See the four positions shown for inserting the diaphragm, p. 1315.

INTRAUTERINE DEVICES. An **intrauterine device (IUD)** is a small, T-shaped device inserted into the uterine cavity. Medicated IUDs have taken the place of nonmedicated IUDs (Grimes, 1986).* Medicated IUDs are loaded with either copper† (Fig. 42-11) or a progestational agent. These chemically active substances are released continuously; for example, copper-bearing devices for 4 to 8 years (at present) and progesterone devices for 1 year (Contraception, 1992). IUDs are impregnated with barium sulfate for radiopacity.

The mechanism of action is not precisely known. Previously, it was thought that the IUD caused pronounced foreign body reaction that made the endometrium unsuitable for the implantation of fertilized ova. This has been found to be incorrect (Grimes, 1989). Recent evidence strongly supports a true contraceptive effect in preventing fertilization (Contraception, 1992). The copper-bearing IUD damages sperm in transit to the uterine tubes and "interferes with the reproductive process anatomically and temporally before ova reach the uterus" (WHO, 1987; Ortiz Croxatto, 1987; Grimes, 1989) (Fig. 42-11, *A* and *B*). The progesterone-bearing IUD causes progestin-related effects on cervical mucus and endometrial maturation (Fig. 42-11, *C*). Because the effect is local, there is no disruption of the woman's ovulatory pattern.

The IUD offers constant contraception without the need to remember to take pills each day or engage in other manipulation before or between coital acts. If pregnancy can be excluded, an IUD may be placed at any time during the menstrual cycle. An IUD may be inserted immediately after abortion (Liskin, Fox, 1982).

The absence of interference with hormonal regulation of menstrual cycles makes the IUD more appropriate than hormonal contraception for heavy smokers, women over 35, women who have hypertension, or those with a history of vascular disease or familial diabetes. Contraceptive effects are reversible. When pregnancy is desired, the IUD may be removed by the physician.

The Progestasert offers two important noncontraceptive progesterone-related advantages: less blood loss during menstruation and decreased primary dysmenorrhea. The mean blood loss is increased for the copper IUD. This blood loss may be clinically significant in undernourished populations. Because the IUD reduces the absolute number of pregnancies overall, current IUD wearers have only 40% of the risk for ectopic pregnancy experienced by women not using contraception (Grimes, 1989).

The use of an IUD is contraindicated for women with a history of PID, known or suspected pregnancy, undiagnosed genital bleeding, suspected genital malignancy, or a distorted intrauterine cavity. Early IUD warning signs should be taught to each woman (see box below).

When compared with contraceptive methods that protect against PID, the risk of infection with an IUD seems high. Earlier studies did not take into consideration the number of sex partners and exposure to STDs (Grimes, 1989). There is no increased risk of PID among IUD users who reported having only one sex partner (Cramer et al, 1985; Grimes, 1989; Lee, Rubin, Borucki, 1988). The risk of IUD-related PID clusters around the time of insertion. The endometrium is contaminated with bacteria during insertion and rids itself of these bacteria soon thereafter. Women may benefit from prophylactic antimicrobial medication taken 1 hour before insertion (Grimes, 1989). The two monofilament tails on contemporary IUDs are *not* associated with an increased risk of PID.

The presence of the IUD thread must be checked after menstruation and at the time of ovulation as

*The last nonmedicated plastic IUD (the Lippes loop) was discontinued by its manufacturer in 1985.

†Searle and Company removed CU-7 and TATUM-7 from the United States market on February 1, 1986.

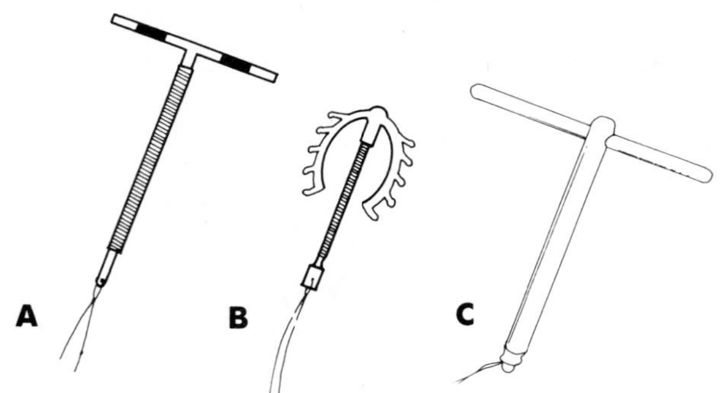

Fig. 42-11 Intrauterine devices. **A**, Copper-T 380A. The "380" signifies the total of 380 mm^2 of copper (mounted on polyethylene) exposed to the endometrium; the "A" refers to the copper on the arms (approved by FDA). **B**, Multiload devices come in different sizes and are prepared with different loads of copper. Not yet available in the United States, they are widely available outside of the United States. **C**, Progestasert.

TEACHING **IUD Warning Signs**

Early IUD danger signs can be remembered in this manner (Hatcher et al, 1990):

- P Period late, abnormal spotting or bleeding
- A Abdominal pain, pain with coitus
- I Infection exposure, abnormal vaginal discharge
- N Not feeling well, fever, or chills
- S String missing

well as before coitus to rule out expulsion of the device. If pregnancy occurs with the IUD in place, it should be removed immediately, if possible (Grimes, 1986). Retention of the IUD during pregnancy increases the risk of septic spontaneous abortion (Liskin, Fox, 1982). Some women allergic to copper develop a rash, necessitating the removal of the copper-bearing IUD.

The use of medical diathermy (shortwave and microwave) in a woman with a metal-containing IUD may cause heat injury to surrounding tissue. Therefore medical diathermy to the abdominal and sacral areas should not be used on women using copper-bearing IUDs.

Because of the litigious nature of contemporary American society, most health care providers are requiring lengthy, detailed consent forms to be signed by any woman requesting an IUD. In 1988 a new copper IUD was released on the U.S. market (see Fig. 42-11, *A*). Family planning experts recommend that only women who are involved in stable, monogamous relationships and who have at least one child are appropriate candidates for IUDs. The manufacturer does not recommend women using the Copper-T 380A if they are under 25, have never had children, or are involved in anything but an exclusive, monogamous relationship (Medical Letter, 1988; Mishell, 1989; ParaGard, 1988).

According to Hatcher et al (1990), the first-year failure rate is 3% in typical IUD users.

Contemporary IUDs provide highly effective contraception that is superior to use-effectiveness of combined oral hormonal contraceptives (Grimes, 1989). The efficacy of the Copper-T 380A is greater than that of the Progestasert.

VACCINE TO BLOCK PREGNANCY. An experimental birth control vaccine shows promise for blocking pregnancy for 6 months without significant side effects, a preliminary study suggests. The vaccine was designed to spur the immune system into making antibodies that block the action of human chorionic gonadotropin, which is produced during pregnancy.

POSTCOITAL CONTRACEPTION. Diethylstilbestrol (DES) provides postcoital contraception (see Table 42-3). It is also known as the "morning-after" pill. This preparation must be started within 3 days after intercourse. DES, 25 mg, is taken twice daily for 5 days. The mechanism of action is not understood (Cunningham, MacDonald, Gant, 1989). Nausea and vomiting are common effects.

Another method is to use Ovral, a birth control pill containing ethinylestradiol and norgestrel. Two tablets are taken within 72 hours after coitus and 2 tablets 12 hours later (Greydanus, Lonchamp, 1990).

FUTURE TRENDS. The dramatic reduction of the pharmaceutical industry's research and development of contraception has severely limited potential new and improved methods (Djerassi, 1989). Changes in American society's litigious climate and increased funding can reverse this trend. The state of contraception directly influences the incidence of unintended pregnancies. Djerassi (1989) formulated a priority list of new methods, which includes an antiviral spermicide, a once-a-month pill that induces a menses, a reliable ovulation predictor, a male contraceptive pill, and an antifertility vaccine. The development of these new products is dependent on the social and political climate in the United States.

EVALUATION

The nurse can be reasonably assured that care was effective if the goals of care have been achieved: the woman (couple) learns about the various methods of contraception; the couple achieves pregnancy only when it has been planned; and they experience no adverse sequelae as a result of the chosen method of contraception. A case study and nursing plan of care follows this section.

■ STERILIZATION

Sterilization refers to surgical procedures intended to render the person infertile. Most procedures involve the occlusion of the passageways for the ova and sperm (Fig. 42-12). For the female the oviducts (uterine tubes) are occluded; for the male the sperm ducts (vas deferens) are occluded. Only surgical removal of the ovaries (oophorectomy) or uterus (hysterectomy) or both will result in absolute sterility for the woman. All other operations have a small but definite failure rate; that is, pregnancy may result.

Since 1950, voluntary sterilization has grown rapidly in acceptance and is currently the most prevalent method of contraception in the world (Hatcher et al, 1990). A recent study documented widespread satisfaction with sterilization for both women and men (Kjersgaard et al, 1989). In the United States, voluntary sterilization is the most common choice of contraception for couples who are 30 years of age or older.

MOTIVATION FOR STERILIZATION. Motivation for elective sterilization includes personal preference; obstetric reasons, such as multiparity; medical reasons, such as hypertensive, cardiovascular, or renal disease in the woman or recurrent acute epididymitis in the man; and diagnosis of inheritable disease.

CASE STUDY

Sexually Active 22-Year-Old Woman

Jayne is a 22-year-old woman who has just become sexually active. She and her partner are high school graduates with 1 year of education at a community college.

ASSESSMENT

The interview reveals that Jayne has not previously used any method of contraception. She and her partner want to choose a reliable method before they have coitus again. She expresses concern about the ease of use and possible side effects of the different methods. The nurse-practitioner found the physical examination to be within normal limits. The Pap smear and STD tests are negative.

NURSING DIAGNOSIS

Because Jayne verbalizes concern over her choice of contraceptive method, the nurse identifies the following diagnosis: decisional conflict related to contraceptive alternatives.

PLANNING

A plan of care is developed with Jayne's input. The mutually agreed-on *goal* is to review the alternatives and make an informed choice. *Expected outcomes* set by the nurse to be met by the end of the visit include a thorough discussion of the most commonly used methods. In addition to the contraceptive benefit, the chosen method(s) will also reduce the potential for STD transmission.

IMPLEMENTATION

Nursing actions are derived from current concepts of contraceptive technology and Jayne and her partner's choice. This couple chooses oral hormonal contraception and condoms. Specific interventions include counseling and teaching regarding the advantages, disadvantages, mode of action, effectiveness, and proper use of their chosen method. The nurse discusses and demonstrates how to use both methods. The clients are referred to the written instructions and illustrations that accompany these methods. A return demonstration of both methods (using a plastic model and a birth-control pill container) is performed. The couple is given a phone number to use for any questions that may arise before the follow-up visit. Jayne is scheduled for a following visit in 3 months for blood pressure reading and counseling.

EVALUATION

The couple stated satisfaction with their choices of contraceptive methods. The couple could accurately state the advantages, disadvantages, mode of action, effectiveness, and proper use of their methods. The return demonstrations were accurate.

CARE PLAN Sexually Active 22-Year-Old Woman

GOALS	IMPLEMENTATION	RATIONALE	EVALUATION
Nursing diagnosis: Fear related to contraceptive method side effects.			
Jayne and George no longer feel fearful.	The nurse discusses potential side effects for the chosen methods.	Knowledge of information reduces fear of the unknown. Knowledge strengthens one's ability to cope.	Jayne and George verbalize reasonable comfort with the knowledge.
Nursing diagnosis: High risk for infection related to being sexually active.			
Jayne and George will suffer no STDs.	The nurse discusses safer sex and barrier methods.	Couples in monogomous relationships are at least amount of risk for STDs. Certain barrier methods can reduce the risk of STD transmission.	Jayne and George exhibit no signs and symptoms of STDs at this time and at subsequent visits.

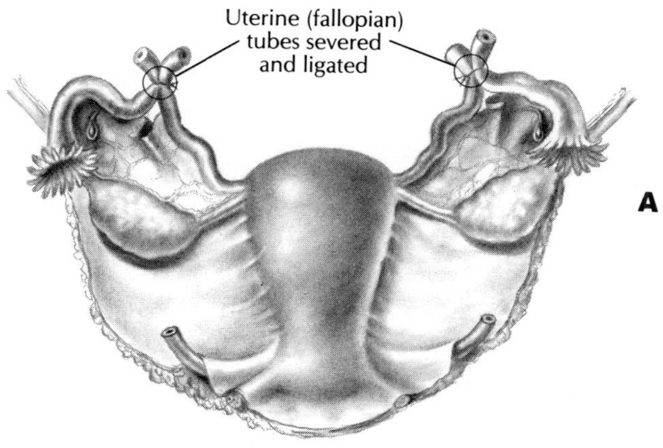

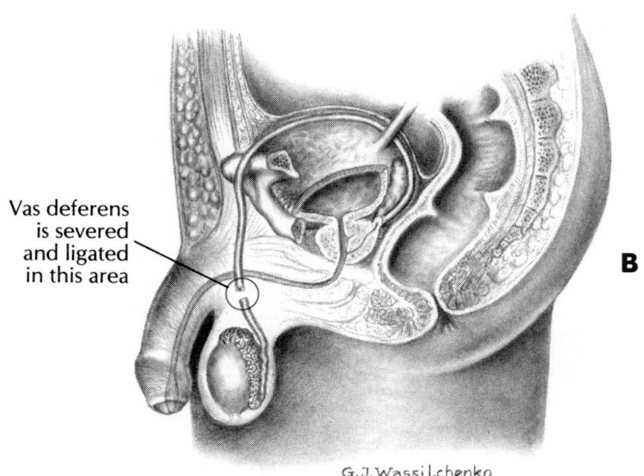

Fig. 42-12 Sterilization. **A,** Oviduct ligated and severed (tubal ligation). **B,** Sperm duct severed (and ligated) (vasectomy).

Sterilization as a means of contraception may be requested by couples who have almost come to the end of their childbearing years and have the desired number of children. It is also chosen by young adults who have decided not to bear children. Persons in the first group are generally receptive to the procedure even though there may be some feelings of regret because one of life's phases is over. Persons in the second group need the opportunity to explore the consequences of their choice. See surgical interruption of pregnancy (p. 1325) for values clarification and counseling techniques helpful in implementing the nursing process with clients seeking sterilization.

LAWS AND REGULATIONS. All states have strict regulations for informed consent (see Chapter 4). Many states in the United States permit voluntary sterilization of any mature, rational woman without reference to her marital or pregnancy status. Although the partner's consent is not required, the client is encouraged to discuss the situation with her or his partner.

Sterilization of minors or mentally incompetent females is restricted by most states. The operation often requires the approval of a board of eugenicists or other court-appointed individuals.

If federal funds are used, the person must be at least 21 years of age and mentally competent. Some state and federal regulations govern medicaid funds for elective sterilization; for example, counseling and a waiting period after the decision is made are mandatory.

NURSING PROCESS

ASSESSMENT

Motivation for sterilization and the result of exploration of alternatives are explored. The client's knowledge of the sterilization methods and of the chosen method is assessed. Gaps in knowledge and misinformation are noted.

History, physical examination, and laboratory data are collected. The record is reviewed for the signed informed consent, and the client's understanding is verified. General preoperative, operative, and postoperative assessments are performed.

NURSING DIAGNOSES

After analyzing the data, nursing diagnoses are identified. Examples of nursing diagnoses for the woman undergoing surgical sterilization include the following:

- Decisional conflict related to
  - —Alternative methods of surgical sterilization
  - —Readiness for permanent termination of fertility
- High risk for infection related to
  - —Broken skin or mucous membrane secondary to surgery
- Pain related to
  - —Postoperative recovery
- Spiritual distress related to
  - —Discrepancy between religious or cultural beliefs and choice of sterilization

PLANNING

Planning is a collaborative effort among the woman, her sexual partner (if appropriate), the physician, and the nurse. Depending on the motivation for sterilization, other physicians may need to be part of the health care team. *Goals* are determined and stated in client-centered terms and may include the following:

1. Client has received and understood all information necessary to give informed consent.
2. Client experiences a successful procedure and uneventful recovery.
3. Client continues to be satisfied with the decision for sterilization, the procedure, and the experience with the health care team.

IMPLEMENTATION

The nurse plays an important role in assisting people with decision making so that all requirements for informed consent are met. People seek information about the various methods of sterilization. Clinical information about the various procedures follows the evaluation section. The nurse also provides information about alternatives to sterilization (e.g., contraception).

The nurse acts as a sounding board for people who are exploring the possibility of choosing sterilization and their feelings about and motivation for this choice. The nurse records this information, which may be the basis for referral to a family planning clinic, a psychiatric social worker, or another professional health care provider.

Information must be given about what is entailed in various procedures, how much discomfort or pain can be expected, and what type of care is needed. Many individuals fear sterilization procedures because of the imagined effect on their sexual life. They need reassurance concerning the hormonal and psychologic basis for sexual function and the fact that uterine tube occlusion or vasectomy has no biologic sequelae in terms of sexual adequacy. The psychosocial and physical effects of tubal sterilization and vasectomy were studied (see Research Highlight below).

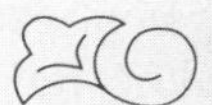 **Research Highlight** 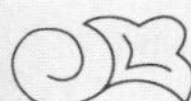

Impact of Tubal Sterilization and Vasectomy on Sexuality

RESEARCH ABSTRACT

Surgical sterilization is a common method for contraception among married women in the United States. Despite the popularity of the procedure, there is limited information available about psychosocial and physical effects of sterilization on sexuality. In this study, changes in the frequency of coitus, desire for coitus, satisfaction with the sexual relationship, and sexual response over 5 years were compared among three groups of women: 152 sterilized women, 106 women married to men with vasectomies, and 83 women who chose not to be sterilized. Baseline information was collected before sterilization for women in the sterilization and vasectomy groups and soon after being recruited for the others. Follow-up interviews were conducted yearly for 5 years. There were no differences among groups in satisfaction with the sexual relationship. There was a time effect; all groups declined in satisfaction over time. There were no differences in satisfaction with sexual response among groups or over time. There were no group differences in coital desire or coital frequency, but all groups exhibited a decline in both over time. Women in the sterilization group had an increase in coital frequency at the first year and a decrease the second year. No detrimental effects on female marital sexuality related to the procedures were detected.

IMPLICATIONS FOR PRACTICE

Nurses can assure women that sterilization removes the possibility of pregnancy but does not adversely affect sexuality. Good communication between partners is to be encouraged.

RELATED RESEARCH QUESTIONS

1. What are the effects of tubal ligation and vasectomy on the marital satisfaction of men?
2. Does a man's own sexual satisfaction change over time?
3. Do factors associated with sexual satisfaction differ for men and for women?
4. Are there cultural variations in sexual satisfaction?

REFERENCE

Shain RN et al: Impact of tubal sterilization and vasectomy on female marital sexuality: results of a controlled longitudinal study, *Am J Obstet Gynecol* 164(3):763, 1991.

PREOPERATIVE PREPARATION. Printed instructions are usually available for clients from the physician. The physician performs the preoperative health assessment, which includes a psychologic assessment, physical examination, and laboratory tests. The nurse assists with the health assessment, answers questions, and confirms the client's understanding of printed instructions (e.g., nothing by mouth [NPO] after midnight). Ambivalence and extreme fear of the procedure are reported to the physician.

POSTOPERATIVE CARE. Postoperative care depends on the procedure performed, for example, laparoscopy (p. 1286) or laparotomy for tubal occlusion, or vasectomy. General care includes recovery after anesthesia, vital signs, fluid-electrolyte balance (intake and output, laboratory values), prevention of or early identification and treatment for infection or hemorrhage, control of discomfort, and assessment of emotional response to the procedure and recovery.

DISCHARGE PLANNING. Discharge planning depends on the type of procedure performed. In general, the client is given written instructions about observing for and reporting symptoms and signs of complications, the type of recovery to be expected, and the date and time for a follow-up appointment.

Female Sterilization

Female sterilization may be done immediately after delivery (within 24 to 48 hours), concomitantly with abortion, or as an interval procedure (during any phase of the menstrual cycle). Most sterilization procedures are performed immediately after a pregnancy, probably because of heightened motivation or increased practicality. Usually the woman is already in the hospital, and all preoperative preparations (blood work, physical examination, etc.) have been completed.

However, all sterilization procedures have the lowest morbidity and failure rates when performed at a time other than immediately after a pregnancy. Tissue edema continues during the early postpartum period, which may permit the sutures to cut through the tubal wall and leave an opening into the uterine tube.

TUBAL OCCLUSION. The operation used commonly is the laparoscopic tubal fulguration (destruction of tissue by means of an electric current [electrocoagulation]). See p. 1286 for laparoscopy examination, a procedure of entering the abdomen for access to the uterine tubes. A minilaparotomy may be used for tubal ligation (Fig. 42-13) or for the application of

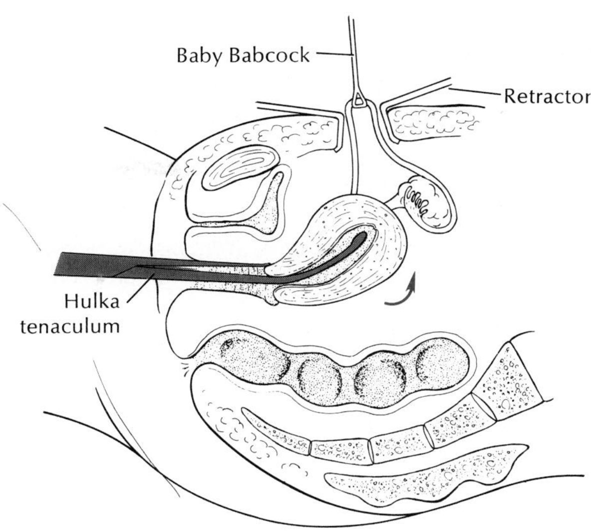

Fig. 42-13 Use of minilaparotomy to gain access to oviducts for tubal occlusion procedures. Tenaculum is used to lift uterus upward *(arrow)* toward incision.

bands or clips. Bands (e.g., Falope ring) and clips (e.g., Hulka-Clemens) are placed around the tubes to block them (Cunningham, MacDonald, Gant, 1989). Fulguration and ligation are considered to be permanent methods. Use of the bands or clips has the theoretic advantage of possible removal and return of tubal patency. Transcervical approaches to inject occlusive material into the tubes are being investigated (Hatcher et al, 1990; Shuber, 1989).

For the minilaparotomy approach the woman is admitted the morning of surgery, having received nothing by mouth (NPO) since midnight. Preoperative sedation is given. The procedure may be carried out with a local anesthetic, but a regional or general anesthetic may also be used. A small vertical incision is made in the abdominal wall below the umbilicus. The woman may experience sensations of tugging but no pain, and the operation is completed within 20 minutes. She may be discharged several hours later if she has recovered from anesthesia. Any abdominal discomfort usually can be controlled with a mild analgesic (e.g., Acetaminophen), although Fraser et al (1989) found that 85% of their sample reported that pain or fatigue hindered recovery and delayed resumption of normal activities by 4½ days. Within 10 days the scar is almost invisible. (see box on p. 1324)

A recent study reported that out-of-hospital minilaparotomy under local anesthesia is both safe and effective (Nisanian, 1990). Major medical complications after elective sterilization are rare. Dysfunctional uterine bleeding or ovarian cyst formation

TEACHING **What to Expect after Tubal Ligation**

No change in hormones and their influence
Menses should not be affected
Woman may feel pain at ovulation
Ovum disintegrates within abdominal cavity
No more pregnancies
Woman should not experience a change in sexual functioning; in fact, her libido may improve because of reduced fear of pregnancy

may occur after tubal surgery, presumably because of disturbance of the utero-ovarian circulation. As occurs with any surgery, there is always a possibility of complications of anesthesia, infection, hemorrhage, and trauma to other organs.

TUBAL RECONSTRUCTION. Restoration of tubal continuity (reanastomosis) and function is technically feasible except after laparoscopic tubal fulguration. Sterilization reversal, however, is costly, difficult (requiring microsurgery), and uncertain (Cunningham, MacDonald, Gant, 1989). The success rate varies with the extent of tubal destruction and removal. The incidence of successful pregnancy after reanastomosis is only about 15%. The loss of a segment of tube necessary for sperm capacitation and fertilization is the probable reason for low pregnancy rates.

Male Sterilization

Vasectomy is the easiest and most commonly employed operation for male sterilization. In the United States one-half million men undergo vasectomy each year (Cunningham, MacDonald, Gant, 1989). Vasectomy can be carried out with local anesthesia and on an out-of-hospital basis.

In vasectomy, short right and left incisions are made into the anterior aspect of the scrotum above and lateral to each testis over the spermatic cord (Fig. 42-12, *B*). Each vas deferens is identified and doubly ligated with fine, nonabsorbable sutures. Then each vas deferens is incised between the ligatures. Occasionally the surgeon fulgurates the cut stumps of the sperm ducts. Many surgeons bury the cut ends into scrotal fascia to lessen the chance of reunion. Then the skin incisions are closed. Usually one nonabsorbable suture is used for closure of each skin incision. A dressing is applied.

The man is instructed in self-care to promote a safe return to routine activities. To reduce swelling and relieve discomfort, ice packs are applied to the scrotum intermittently for a few hours postoperatively. A suspensory, or bandage, is applied to decrease discomfort by supporting the scrotum. Moderate inactivity for about 2 days is advisable because of local scrotal tenderness. The skin suture can be removed 5 to 7 days postoperatively. Sexual intercourse may be resumed as desired.

Sterility is not immediate. Some sperm will remain in the proximal portions of the sperm ducts after vasectomy. One week to several months are required to clear the ducts of sperm (i.e., after approximately 15 ejaculations). Therefore some form of contraception is needed until the sperm count in the ejaculate on two consecutive tests is down to zero (Cunningham, MacDonald, Gant, 1989).

Vasectomy has no effect on potency (ability to achieve and maintain an erection) or volume of ejaculate. Endocrine production of testosterone continues so that secondary sex characteristics are not affected. Sperm production continues. Men occasionally may develop a hematoma, infection, or epididymitis (Hatcher et al, 1990). Less common are painful granulomas from accumulation of sperm. Sperm unable to leave the epididymis are lyzed by the immune system.

Complications after bilateral vasectomy are uncommon and usually not serious (Giovannucci, 1992). They include bleeding (usually external), suture reaction, and reaction to anesthetic agent. Sterilization failures, usually caused by a recanalization, are rare, occurring in about 2 per 1000 men.

TUBAL RECONSTRUCTION. Microsurgery to reanastomose (restoration of tubal continuity) the sperm ducts can be accomplished successfully in 90% of cases (i.e., sperm in the ejaculate) (Jarow, 1987). However, the fertility (pregnancies) rate is much lower (40% to 60%). The rate of success decreases as the time since the procedure increases. The vasectomy may result in permanent changes in the testes that leave men unable to father children. The changes are those ordinarily seen only in the elderly (e.g., interstitial fibrosis [scar tissue between the seminiferous tubules]). Some men develop antibodies against their own sperm (**autoimmunization**). The role of antisperm antibodies in fertility after vasectomy reversal has not been completely determined.

EVALUATION

The nurse can be assured that care was effective when the goals of care are achieved: the client has received and understood all information necessary to give informed consent; the procedure was successful, and recovery was uneventful; and the client continues to be satisfied with the decision for sterilization, the procedure, and the experience with the health care team.

■ SURGICAL INTERRUPTION OF PREGNANCY

Elective abortion is the purposeful interruption of a previable pregnancy. Indications for elective abortion are as follows:

1. Preservation of the life or health of the mother (e.g., class III or IV heart disease)
2. Avoidance of the birth of an offspring with a serious developmental or hereditary disorder (e.g., Tay-Sachs disease)
3. Inability of the parents to support or care for the child
4. Rape, incest, or various personal reasons

Many women report more than one factor contributing to the decision (Torres, Forrest, 1988).

The control of birth, dealing as it does with human sexuality and the question of life and death, is one of the most emotionalized components of health care. Abortion as one of the surgical alternatives to contraception is regulated in most countries (Cohen, 1990; Henshaw, 1990). Regulations exist presumably to protect the mother from the complications of abortion or because of religious constraints. The U.S. Supreme Court set aside previous antiabortion laws in January 1973, holding that first-trimester abortion is permissible inasmuch as the mortality from interruption of early gestation is now less than the mortality after normal term delivery. Second-trimester abortion was left to the discretion of the individual states (Annas, 1989; Chavkin, Rosenfield 1990; Rhodes, 1988, 1989, 1990; Rogers et al, 1991). Roman Catholic hospitals and some of those maintained by strict fundamentalists forbid abortion (and often sterilization) despite legal challenge.

Before the legalization of abortion, many illegal abortions took place, with little-documented sequelae other than death from infection or hemorrhage or both. Although studies indicate that biologic sequelae do occur after abortion (e.g., ectopic pregnancy) rates of biologic complications tend to be low, especially if the woman aborts during the first trimester (Holt et al, 1989; Seidman et al, 1988). Studies related to psychologic sequelae (e.g., anxiety) suggest that they are short lived (Adler et al, 1990; Llewelyn, Putches, 1988; Roger et al, 1989). Sequelae are related to circumstances surrounding the abortion, such as rape or the attitudes reflected by friends, family, and health workers. It must be remembered that the woman facing an abortion is pregnant and will exhibit the emotional responses shared by all pregnant women, including postdelivery depression.

In an attempt to regulate the conflict between professional responsibilities and personal ethics, the Nurses' Association of the American College of Obstetricians and Gynecologists (NAACOG) published a position paper on the nurse's role with the abortion client in December 1989, in which the simultaneous rights of each are described (NAACOG, 1989). Women have the right to expect and receive supportive, nonjudgmental care. Nurses have the right to refuse to assist with abortions or sterilizations in keeping with their own moral or religious beliefs, unless the woman's life is in danger. Many nurses have written about these issues (Doe, 1988; Frye, 1989; Kennedy, 1988; Nagle, 1988).

The values and moral convictions of the nurse are involved to the same extent as those of the pregnant woman. The conflicts and doubts of the nurse can be readily communicated to women who are already anxious and overly sensitive. Health professionals need assistance to identify and come to terms with their own feelings. It is not uncommon for confusion to arise as beliefs are challenged by the reality of care. A nursing student reacted to learning experiences associated with in-hospital abortions in the following manner:

> I really feel I believe in the rightness of elective abortion, but when I watched the physician insert the needle and then inject the dose of prostaglandin, I felt an unreasoning rage sweep over me. I could have attacked him. Funny, I felt no anger toward the woman at all. I really need to rethink my beliefs.

Responses can also change with life experiences. A nurse who before her marriage had worked as a counselor in a municipal clinic established a reputation as a supportive and concerned counselor of young persons with regard to birth control. Four years later she remarked:

> I've been trying to get pregnant for the past 3 years. I didn't realize how important it would be to me. You know I can't counsel about abortion any more. I can't be objective. I keep feeling, "Have your baby and please give it to me." I am more concerned about myself now, not them [the pregnant women], and counseling won't work that way.

■ NURSING PROCESS

ASSESSMENT

A thorough assessment is conducted through history, physical examination, and laboratory tests. If the woman is Rh negative and the pregnancy is greater than 8 weeks' gestation, she is a candidate for prophylaxis against Rh isoimmunization (p. 1154). She receives Rh_0 (D) immune globulin within 72 hours after the abortion if she is D^u negative and if Coombs' test results are negative (if she is unsensitized or has not developed isoimmunization). Compelling medical, surgical, or psychiatric indications for elective abortion, though not numerous, are possible factors. The following conditions probably would qualify: class III coronary heart disease; fulminating (pelvic) Hodgkin's disease; stage 1B carcinoma of the cervix; and Marfan's syndrome with early aortic aneurysm. The length of pregnancy and the condition of the woman need to be determined to select the appropriate type of abortion procedure.

The woman's understanding of alternatives, the types of abortions, and expected recovery is assessed. Misinformation and gaps in knowledge are identified and corrected. The record is reviewed for the signed informed consent, and the client's understanding is verified. General preoperative, operative, and postoperative assessments are performed.

NURSING DIAGNOSES

Analysis of data leads to the identification of the appropriate nursing diagnoses. Following are examples of nursing diagnoses for the woman undergoing interruption of pregnancy:

- Decisional conflict related to
  - —Perceived threat to value system
- Fear related to
  - —The abortion procedure
  - —Potential complications
  - —Implications for future pregnancies
- Anticipatory grieving related to
  - —Distress at loss and/or feelings of guilt
- High risk for infection related to
  - —Effects of the procedure
  - —Lack of understanding of preoperative and postoperative self-care
- Acute pain related to
  - —Effects of the procedure and/or postoperative events

PLANNING

Planning is a collaborative effort among the woman, her sexual partner (as appropriate), the physician, and the nurse. Depending on the motivation for elective abortion, other physicians may need to be part of the health care team. *Goals* are established collaboratively, should be stated in client-centered terms, and may include the following:

1. Client understands all information necessary to give informed consent.
2. Client experiences a successful procedure, and recovery is uneventful.
3. Client continues to be satisfied with the decision for elective abortion, the procedure, and the experience with the health care team.

IMPLEMENTATION

Counseling about abortion includes help for the woman in identifying how she perceives the pregnancy; information about the choices available (i.e., having an abortion or carrying the pregnancy to term and then either keeping the child or giving the child up for adoption); and information about types of abortion procedures. *The goal is to assist the woman in making an informed decision.*

First-Trimester Abortion

Methods for performing early **elective abortion** (EAB) (sometimes called therapeutic abortion [TAB]) include the following:

1. Menstrual extraction—early aspiration of the endometrium in women who have not yet missed a period
2. Surgical D&C when newer aspiration equipment is unavailable
3. Uterine aspiration after one or two missed periods

Surgical D&C refers to cervical **dilatation and curettage(D&C)** of the uterine endometrium. Curettage is the scraping of the uterine lining with a metal curette or a flexible aspiration tip to remove the products of conception implanted in the endometrium. The procedure is similar to that of uterine aspiration. Cervical trauma and uterine perforation, infection, or hemorrhage are possible through rare complications.

Uterine aspiration (**vacuum or suction curettage**) abortion is the most common procedure. The insertion of a small laminaria tent retained by a vaginal tampon for 4 to 24 hours usually will facilitate the purposeful interruption of a first-trimester pregnancy greater than 10 weeks' gestation by dilating the cervix atraumatically (see Fig. 42-14). On removal of the moist, expanded laminaria, the cervix will have dilated two or three times its original (dry) diameter. Rarely will further mechanical dilatation of the cervix be required. The insertion of an adequate-sized aspiration cannula (8.5 to 10.5 mm) is almost always possible. Cervical laceration and bleeding are reduced by the use of laminaria. A disadvantage is the delay nec-

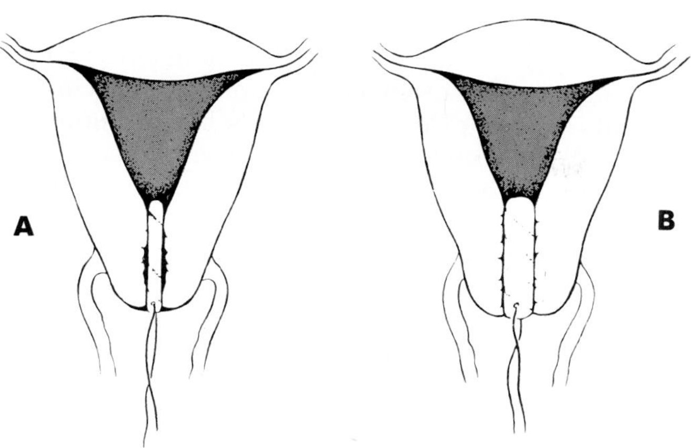

Fig. 42-14 Laminaria. **A,** Inserted through narrow cervical canal beyond the internal os. **B,** Cervix dilated 4 to 12 hours later.
From Sanberg EC: *Synopsis of obstetrics,* ed 10, St Louis, 1978, Mosby–Year Book.

essary and the need for an additional visit to the physician's office or clinic.

The woman comes to the clinic or physician's office the day before the abortion procedure. An antiseptic solution is used to prepare the pelvic area. A vaginal speculum is inserted, and the vaginal canal and cervix are cleansed. Injection of a local anesthetic agent into the cervix may follow (see paracervical block, Chapter 15, p. 385). Again the area is cleansed, and the laminaria tent is inserted into the endocervical canal. Prophylactic use of an antibiotic is usually begun. Some women experience a mild cramping or have light spotting from the anesthetic injection. Discomfort can usually be controlled with mild analgesics (e.g., acetaminophen).

Aspiration abortion may be performed in the physician's office, clinic, or in the hospital setting. If the woman chooses a hospital setting, she is admitted the day after insertion of the laminaria tent and is given preoperative sedation. The vaginal area is cleansed (shaving is not necessary). The suction procedure for accomplishing an early elective abortion (ideal time is 8 to 12 weeks since last menstrual period) usually requires less than 5 minutes and can easily be effected under paracervical block anesthesia and single sedation. Independent nursing interventions have the potential to reduce pain during the procedure (Wells, 1989). During the procedure the nurse or physician keeps the woman informed about what to expect next; for example, menstrual-like cramping and sounds of suction machine. The nurse assesses the woman's vital signs. The aspirated uterine contents must be carefully inspected to ascertain whether all fetal parts and adequate placental tissue have been evacuated. A single dose of oxytocin is used occasionally to control bleeding. The woman may remain in the health care facility for 1 to 3 hours for detection of excessive cramping or excessive bleeding; then she is discharged. If the procedure is done in the physician's office, preoperative sedation is usually not given, and the anesthetic of choice is usually paracervical block. After the abortion the woman rests on the table until she is ready to stand. Then she remains in the waiting room until she feels she can travel. She may be discharged alone or in the company of a relative or friend, depending on the anesthetic used.

Bleeding after the operation is normally about the equivalent of a heavy menstrual period, and cramps are rarely severe. Infection such as endometritis or salpingitis occurs in about 8% of women. Subsequently, a D&C procedure for bleeding or sepsis caused by retained placental tissue is necessary in about 2% of women. A recent study reported an overall complication rate of less than 1% (Hakim-Elahi et al, 1990). Serious depression or other psychiatric problems are rare.

Postabortal instructions differ among health care providers (e.g., use of tampons may be denied for only 3 days or for up to 3 weeks, and resumption of sexual intercourse may be permitted within 1 week or discouraged for 3 weeks). The woman may shower daily. Instruction is given to watch for excessive bleeding (i.e., more than one large pad per hour for 4 hours), cramps, or fever and to avoid douches of any type. The woman may expect her menstrual period to resume 4 to 6 weeks from the day of the procedure. The nurse offers information about the birth control method the woman prefers, if this has not been done previously during the counseling interview that usually precedes the decision to have an abortion. The woman must be strongly encouraged to return for her follow-up visit so that complications can be avoided and an acceptable contraceptive method prescribed.

Second-Trimester Abortion

There are several techniques used for second-trimester abortions:

TRANSABDOMINAL INTRAUTERINE INJECTION OF HYPERTONIC SODIUM CHLORIDE. The woman is admitted to the hospital for this procedure. Amniocentesis is performed. The physician determines where the needle (an 18-gauge, 7.5 cm [3 in] spinal needle) will be inserted. The area is cleansed, and if desired, a local anesthetic agent is given. Approximately 200 mL of amniotic fluid is withdrawn, and a similar amount of sterile 20% to 25% sodium chloride is injected. The woman is instructed to report to the nurse when uterine contractions begin—generally, within 8 to 48 hours. In most cases augmentation with oxytocin is necessary to effect uterine evacuation in a reasonable time. Occasionally reinjection is required. Labor begins, in theory at least, because the hypertonic saline solution releases the placental uterine progesterone blockade that normally prevents the onset of labor. The same careful monitoring of uterine contractions is as necessary as for a term delivery. Instruction in relaxation and breathing techniques is indicated, and an analgesic can be administered for discomfort. The assistance of a supportive person at the time of birth of the dead fetus is essential. If the woman wishes to see the fetus, emotional support should be provided before and after the procedure. Many woman are relieved to find the fetus normal and commonly inquire as to its sex. After the delivery the standard observations and postpartum care are carried out (see Chapters 23 and 25). Contraceptive counseling is given before discharge. The woman is advised to return should excessive bleeding occur.

Complications of hypertonic saline injection for second-trimester abortion may occur. Complications with the approximate frequency of their occurrence include infection (10%), need for D&C to remove retained tissue (15%), failure to abort (10%), and excessive bleeding, necessitating transfusion (2%). Symptomatology related to saline solution (hypernatremia) includes tinnitus, tachycardia, and headache; that of water intoxication, edema, oliguria ($\leq$200 mg/8 hours), dyspnea, thirst, and restlessness. Rarely, disseminated intravascular coagulation (DIC) or expulsion of the fetus through the uterine isthmus occurs.

DILATATION AND EVACUATION (D&E). This procedure extends the D&C and vacuum curettage up to 20 weeks of gestation (Hatcher et al, 1990). The cervix requires more dilatation because the products of conception (POC) are larger. Often laminaria are inserted on the 2 preceding days of the procedure (i.e., two to three may be inserted on the first day; on the second day these are removed, and four to six may be inserted). This allows slow dilatation of the cervix. The procedure is performed on the third day. Larger instruments are employed and additional anesthetic is required. Nursing care includes monitoring vital signs, providing emotional support, administering analgesics, and postoperative monitoring.

INJECTION OF UREA SOLUTION AFTER AMNIOCENTESIS. After the removal of about 200 mL of amniotic fluid, 200 mL of 30% solution of urea in 5% dextrose in water is introduced into the uterus by gravity drip. After 1 hour a solution of 5 units of oxytocin in 500 mL of 5% dextrose in water is started intravenously. Fetal death occurs, and delivery ensues in most cases within 12 hours. Complications are less common and are less serious than with hypertonic saline solution.

PROSTAGLANDIN E2. A vaginal suppository of prostaglandin E2 (20 mg) can be used to induce a second-trimester abortion (Hatcher et al, 1990). High incidences of gastrointestinal side effects (e.g., nausea, vomiting, and diarrhea) have been reported.

ABDOMINAL HYSTEROTOMY. Hysterotomy may be chosen after more than 14 to 16 weeks of pregnancy, after failure of intrauterine injection of saline solution or $PGF_{2\alpha}$, and when sterilization is desired. The management is comparable to that of cesarean delivery.

COMPLICATIONS FOLLOWING ABORTION. The most common complications following abortion include infection, retained products of conception or intrauterine blood clots, continuing pregnancy, cervical or uterine trauma, and excessive bleeding (Hatcher et al, 1990). Women are advised to report fever, pelvic pain, and excessive bleeding. Prophylactic chlamydia and gonorrhea treatment and the use of an oral ergotrate postoperatively may reduce the incidence of infection and retained products of conception.

RU 486 (Mifepristone)

Progesterone is essential for maintaining pregnancy. RU 486 (mifepristone) is a progesterone antagonist that prevents implantation of a fertilized egg. It is most effective in early gestation, during the luteal phase, within 10 days of the expected onset of what would be the first missed period after conception. It can be taken up to 5 weeks after conception. The effectiveness of RU 486 is inversely related to gestational age as determined by β-hCG levels and duration of amenorrhea (Grimes et al, 1988). However, it is considered to be an effective and safe method for termination of early pregnancy. The medication should be used only under close medical supervision (Couzinet et al, 1986).

Uterine bleeding begins within 4 days of administration of the first dose. Usually a period of painless, heavy bleeding is reported. Termination of pregnancy occurs for most women. For the woman in whom abortion does not occur, evacuation of the uterus by aspiration is facilitated by the softening of the uterine cervix. RU 486 is responsible for cervical softening. Some women experience slight nausea and fatigue during the period of bleeding.

The present results are similar to those reported in investigations in which prostaglandin analogs were used to terminate early pregnancy. Although the success rate with prostaglandins also approaches 85%, this method is associated with painful uterine contractions and gastrointestinal side effects in approximately 50% of subjects. In contrast, RU 486 is well tolerated. Supporters of this method feel that even with known disadvantages, RU 486 offers a reasonable alternative to surgical abortion, which carries the risks of anesthesia, surgical complications, infertility, and psychologic sequelae (Couzinet et al, 1986; Debate 1987a). Others have taken a strong stand against the use of RU 486 (Debate, 1987b). Regelson et al (1990) maintain that women's health care needs are being limited by a political and economic battle regarding the unborn. Other possible roles are emerging for RU 486 (Hodgen, 1988; Spitz, Bardin, 1989; Ulmann et al, 1990). It opens, softens, and dilates the cervix; suppresses breast tumors; opposes proliferation of endometrial tissue (as seen in endometriosis); and blocks ovulation. It may have a future application for uterine evacuation following fetal death. RU 486 may be considered as a "transitional" contraceptive pill for women age 35 to 50.

The woman will need help to explore the meaning of the various alternatives and consequences to herself and her significant others. It is often difficult for a woman to express her true feelings (e.g., what abortion means to her now and in the future, and what support or regret her friends and peers may demonstrate). A calm, matter-of-fact approach on the part of the nurse can be helpful (e.g., "Yes, I know you are pregnant, I am here to help. Let's talk about alternatives.") Listening to what the woman has to say and encouraging her to speak are essential. Neutral responses such as "Oh," "Uh-huh," and "Umm" and nonverbal encouragement such as nodding, maintaining eye contact, and use of touch are helpful in setting an open, accepting environment. Clarifying, restating, and reflecting statements, use of open-ended questions, and giving feedback are communication techniques that can be used to maintain a reality focus on the situation and bring the woman's problems into the open. Once a decision has been made, the woman must be assured of continued support. Information about what is entailed in various procedures, how much discomfort or pain can be expected, and what type of care is needed must be given. If family or friends cannot be involved, scheduling time for the nursing personnel to give the necessary support is an essential component of the care plan.

Preoperative preparation, postoperative care, and discharge planning parallel the methods used for sterilization (see p. 1323).

EVALUATION

The nurse can be reasonably assured that care was effective when the goals of care have been met: the client understands all information necessary to give informed consent; the procedure is successful, recovery is uneventful, and the client continues to be satisfied with the decision for elective abortion, the procedure, and the experience with the health care team.

■ ANESTHESIA FOR GYNECOLOGIC PROCEDURES

Paracervical block anesthesia is used for a variety of obstetric (Chapter 15) and gynecologic procedures (see Fig. 15-8). Tests for infertility such as endometrial biopsy and aspiration abortion are two such procedures. Complications may include vasovagal syncope and intravascular injection.

The procedure is explained to the woman. She is asked to void if her bladder is full. Her vital signs are checked and recorded. The sight of the long needle used to inject the anesthesia may be frightening (see Fig. 15-8). The woman can be reassured that only the tip of the needle will be inserted. For this sterile procedure the physician or anesthesiologist will need the nurse's assistance in positioning the woman (dorsal recumbent position with knees flexed), handling supplies, and helping the woman remain immobile while the injection is made.

■ SUMMARY

The roles of the nurse vary in the care of clients requiring treatment for impaired fertility, control of fertility, termination of fertility, and interruption of pregnancy. A solid knowledge base of anatomy and physiology, mastery of nursing skills, and the nurse's self-awareness are all essential factors in meeting client needs. Professional satisfaction is the reward for the nurse who is able to assist clients coping with reproductive issues. Seeking help for impaired fertility and fertility control is commonly the only contact some people have with the health care system. Positive perceptions of the interest, concern, and technical skill of health care providers may induce wider use of health facilities and care in the future.

REFERENCES

Adler NE et al: Psychological responses after abortion, *Science* 248(4951):41, 1990.

Adoption services for your pregnant patient, *Contemp OB/GYN* 33(3):114, 1989.

Annas GJ: The supreme court, privacy, and abortion, *N Engl J Med* 321(17):1200, 1989.

Berg BJ, Wilson JF: Psychiatric morbidity in the infertile population: a reconceptualization, *Fertil Steril* 53(4):654, 1990.

Bernstein JL, Kidd YA: Childbearing in Japan. In Kay MA, editor: *Anthropology of human birth,* Philadelphia, 1982, FA Davis.

Brokaw AK, Baker NN, Haney SL: Fitting the cervical cap, *Nurse Pract* 13(7):49, 1988.

Brownlee AT: *Community, culture, and care: a cross-cultural guide for health workers,* St Louis, 1978, Mosby–Year Book.

Can you rely on condoms? *Consumer Reports* 54(3):135, 1989.

Carlone JP, Keen PD: Oral contraceptive use in women with chronic medical conditions, *Nurse Pract* 14(9):9, 1989.

Chavkin W, Rosenfield A: A chill wind blows: Webster, obstetrics, and the health of women, *Am J Obstet Gynecol* 163(2):450, 1990.

Clark AL, Howland IH: The American Samoan. In Clark AL, editor: *Culture/childbearing/health professionals,* Philadelphia, 1978, FA Davis.

Clark M: *Health in the Mexican-American culture: a community study,* Berkeley, 1970, University of California Press.

Cohen SS: Health care policy and abortion: a comparison, *Nurs Outlook* 38(1):20, 1990.

Connell EB: Barrier contraceptives, *Clin Obstet Gynecol* 32(2):377, 1989.

Contraception choices for women over age 35: Focus on benefits and risks, *The Contraception Report* 3(2):4, May 1992.

Coughlin R: Pregnancy and birth in Vietnam. In Hart D et al, editors: *Southeast Asian birth customs: three studies in human reproduction,* New Haven, Conn, 1965, Human Relations Area Files.

Couzinet B et al: Termination of early pregnancy by the progesterone antagonist RU 486 (mifepristone), *N Engl J Med* 315(25):1565, 1986.

Cramer DW et al: Tubal infertility and the intrauterine device, *N Engl J Med* 312:941, 1985.

Cunningham FG, MacDonald PC, Gant NF: *Williams obstetrics,* ed 18, Norwalk, Conn, 1989, Appleton & Lange.

Darney PD et al: Acceptance and perceptions of Norplant® among users in San Francisco, USA, *Stud Fam Plann* 21(3):152, 1990.

Darney PD et al: Clinical evaluation of the Capronor contraceptive implant: preliminary report, *Am J Obstet Gynecol* 160(5):Part 2, 1989.

The debate: abortion pill (RU 486): we should test this drug in the USA, *USA Today,* p. 10A, Jan 15, 1987a.

The debate: abortion pill: keep this chemical killer out of the USA (an opposing view), *USA Today,* p. 10A, Jan 15, 1987b.

Djerassi C: The bitter pill, *Science* 245(4916):356, 1989.

Doe J: There to comfort, not to judge, *Nursing* 18(9):82, 1988.

Eggert-Kruse W et al: Chlamydial infection—a female and/or male infertility factor? *Fertil Steril* 53(6):1037, 1990.

Examining the IUD: Highlights from a recent international conference, *The Contraception Report* 3(3):4, July 1992.

Evans MI et al, editors: *Fetal diagnosis and therapy: science, ethics and the law,* Philadelphia, 1989, JB Lippincott.

Food and Drug Administration: Data inconclusive on birth control pills and ovarian cysts, *FDA Talk Paper,* June 15, 1988.

Fraser RA et al: The prevalence and impact of pain after day-care tubal ligation surgery, *Pain* 39(2):189, 1989.

Frye B: Nurses and abortion, *JOGNN* 18(3):193, 1989.

Giovannucci E et al: Vasectomy and its effects of lifespan, *N Engl J Med* 326:1392, 1992.

Greydanus DE, Lonchamp D: Contraception in the adolescent: preparation for the 1990s, *Med Clin North Am* 74(5):1205, 1990.

Grimes DA: Reversible contraception for the 1980s, *JAMA* 255(1):69, 1986.

Grimes DA: Whither the uterine device? *Clin Obstet Gynecol* 32(2):369, 1989.

Grimes DA et al: Early abortion with a single dose of the antiprogestin RU 486, *Am J Obstet Gynecol* 138(6):1307, 1988.

Hakim-Elahi et al: Complications of first-trimester abortion: a report of 170,000 cases, *Obstet Gynecol* 76(1):129, 1990.

Hamori MH et al: Zygote intrafallopian transfer (ZIFT): evaluation of 42 cases, *Fertil Steril* 50(3):519, 1988.

Hatcher RA, et al: *Contraceptive technology: 1990-1992,* ed 15, New York, 1990, Irvington Publishers.

Henshaw SK: Induced abortion: a world review, *Fam Plan Perspectives* 22(2):76, 1990.

Hillard PA: The patient's reaction to side effects of oral contraceptives, *Am J Obstet Gynecol* 161(5):1412, 1989.

Hirsch AM, Hirsch SM: The effect of infertility on marriage and self concept, *JOGNN* 18(1):13, 1989.

Hodgen GD: Progesterone antagonists (RU 486), *Contemp OB/GYN* 32(special issue):65, Sept, 1988.

Holt VL et al: Induced abortion and the risk of subsequent ectopic pregnancy, *Am J Public Health* 79(9):1234, 1989.

Jarow JP: Vasectomy: autoimmunity and reversal, *JAMA* 257(15):2087, 1987.

Kaunitz AM: Injectable contraception, *Clin Obstet Gynecol* 32(2):356, 1989.

Kay MA, editor: *Anthropology of human birth,* Philadelphia, 1982, FA Davis.

Kedem P et al: Psychological aspects of male infertility, *Br J Med Psychol* 63:73, 1990.

Kennedy BJ: I'm sorry, baby, *AJN* 88(8):1067, 1988.

Knersgaard AG et al: Male or female sterilization: a comparative study, *Fertil Steril* 51(3):439, 1989.

Kugel C, Verson H: Relationship between weight change and diaphragm size change, *JOGNN* 15:123, March/April 1986.

Labbok M, Queenan JT: The use of periodic abstinence for family planning, *Clin Obstet Gynecol* 32(2):387, 1989.

Lee NC, Rubin GL, Borucki R: The intrauterine device and pelvic inflammatory disease revisited: new results from the Women's Health Study, *Obstet Gynecol* 72:1, 1988.

Lethbridge DJ: Coitus interruptus—considerations as a method of birth control, *JOGGN* 20(1):80, 1991.

Lethbridge DJ: The use of breastfeeding as a contraceptive, *JOGNN* 18(1):31, 1989.

Liskin LS, Fox G: Periodic abstinence: how well do new approaches work, *Popul Rep* (I), no 3, 1981.

Liskin LS, Fox G: IUDs: an appropriate contraceptive for many women, *Popul Rep* (B), no 4, 1982.

Llewelyn SP, Putches R: An investigation of anxiety following termination of pregnancy, *J Adv Nurs* 13(4):468, 1988.

Mattison DR et al: Effects of drugs and chemicals on the fetus, *Contemp OB/GYN* 33(3):164, 1989.

Mattison DR et al: Reproductive toxicity: male and female reproductive systems as targets for chemical injury, *Med Clin North Am* 74(2):391, 1990.

Medical Letter: Choice of contraceptives, *Med Lett* 30(779) whole issue, Nov 18, 1988.

Meirik O et al: Oral contraceptive use and breast cancer in young women: a joint national case—control study in Sweden and Norway, *Lancet* 1:650, 1986.

Menning B: *Infertility: a guide for the childless couple,* Englewood Cliffs, NJ, 1977, Prentice-Hall.

Mishell DR: Contraception, *N Engl J Med* 320(12):777, 1989a.

Mishell DR: Optimizing contraceptive decisions: clinical implications of the triphasic randomized clinical trial, *Am J Obstet Gynecol* 161(5):1385, 1989b.

Monier M, Laird M: Contraceptives: a look at the future, *AJN* 89(4):496, 1989.

Morbidity, Mortality Weekly Report: Sexually transmitted diseases, *MMWR* 37:133, 1988.

NAACOG: Cervical cap enters North American market, *NAACOG Newsletter,* 15(9):1, 1988.

NAACOG: *Statement: abortion,* The Organization, 1989.

Nagle S: Abortion: one question clearly answered, *RN* 51(10):69, 1988.

Nero FA: When couples ask about infertility, *RN* 51(11):26, 1988.

Nisanian A: Outpatient minilaparotomy sterilization with local anesthesia, *J Reprod Med* 35(4):380, 1990.

Norris AE: Cognitive analysis of contraceptive behavior, *Image J Nurs Sch* 20(3):135, 1988.

North BB: Spermicides, *J Reprod Med* 33:307, 1988.

Okamoto NJ: The Japanese American. In Clark A, editor: *Culture/childbearing/health professionals,* Philadelphia. 1978, FA Davis.

Orshan SA: The pill, the patient, and you, *RN* 51(7):49, 1988.

Ortiz MF, Croxatto HB: The mode of action of IUDs, *Contraception* 36:37, 1987.

Ory SJ: Keeping up to date on donor insemination, *Contemp OB/GYN* 33(3):88, 1989.

Ostling RN: A bold stand on birth control. In Haas K, Haas A: *Understanding sexuality,* ed 3, St Louis, 1993, Mosby–Year Book.

Pace-Owens S: Gamete intrafallopian transfer (GIFT), *JOGNN* 18(2):93, 1989.

ParaGard Intrauterine Copper Contraceptive model T-3804, Somerville, NJ, 1988, Gyno Pharm.

Pernoll ML, Benson RC, editors: *Current obstetric and gynecologic diagnosis and treatment,* ed 6, Los Altos, Calif, 1987, Appleton & Lange.

Peterson HB, Lee NC: The health effects of oral contraceptives: misperceptions, controversies, and continuing good news, *Clin Obstet Gynecol* 32(2):309, 1989.

Porter JB, Jick H, Walker AM: Mortality among oral contraceptive users, *Obstet Gynecol* 70:29, 1987.

Rabar FG et al: Ultrasonographic transvaginal ovum retrieval: a new approach to in vitro fertilization, *AORN J* 48(1):36, 1988.

Regelson W et al: Beyond "abortion": RU 486 and the needs of the crisis constituency, *JAMA* 264(8):1026, 1990.

Rhodes AM: Options and issues for pregnant adolescents, *MCN* 13:427, 1988.

Rhodes AM: Issue update: Abortion, *MCN* 15:289, 1990.

Rogers JL et al: Impact of the Minnesota parental notification law on abortion and birth, *Am J Public Health* 81(3):294, 1991.

Rogers JL et al: Psychological impact of abortion: methodological and outcomes summary of empirical research between 1968 and 1988, *Health Care Women Int* 10(4):347, 1989.

Rosenberg MJ et al: Effect of the contraceptive sponge on chlamydial infection, gonorrhea, and candidiasis, *JAMA* 257(17):2308, 1987.

Royal College of General Practitioners' Oral Contraceptive Study: Oral contraceptives and gallbladder disease, *Lancet* 2:957, 1982.

Ryan KJ: Ethical issues in reproductive endocrinology and infertility, *Am J Obstet Gynecol* 160(6):1415, 1989.

Sakondhavat C: The female condom, *Am J Public Health* 80(4):498, 1990.

Scott JR et al: *Danforth's obstetrics and gynecology,* ed 6, Philadelphia, 1990, JB Lippincott.

Seibel MM: A new era in reproductive technology: in vitro fertilization, gamete intrafallopian transfer, and donated gametes and embryos, *N Engl J Med* 318(13):828, 1988.

Seidman DS: Childbearing after induced abortion: reassessment of risk, *J Epidemiol Comm Health* 42(3):294, 1988.

Shoupe D, Mishell DR: Norplant: subdermal implant system for long-term contraception, *Am J Obstet Gynecol* 160(5): Part 2, 1286, 1989.

Shuber J: Transcervical sterilization with use of methyl 2-cyanoacrylate and a newer delivery system, *Am J Obstet Gynecol* 160(4):887, 1989.

Speroff L et al: *Clinical gynecologic endocrinology and infertility,* Baltimore, 1983, Williams & Wilkins.

Spitz IM, Bardin CW: Progesterone antagonists on the horizon, *Clin Obstet Gynecol* 32(2):403, 1989.

Strom BL et al: Diaphragms, *Ann Intern Med* 107:816, 1987.

Torres A, Forrest JD: Why do women have abortions? *Fam Plann Perspect* 20(4):169, 1988.

Ulmann A et al: RU 486, *Sci Am* 262(6):42, 1990.

US Congress, Office of Technology Assessment, Artificial Insemination: *Practice in the United States: summary of a 1987 survey—background paper, OTA-BP-BA-48,* Washington, DC, 1988, US Government Printing Office.

Veevers JE: The social meaning of parenthood, *Psychiatry* 36:291, 1973.

Vogel G: *American Indian medicine,* New York, 1973, Ballantine Books.

Washington AE et al: Oral contraceptives: *Chlamydia trachomatis'* infection, and pelvic inflammatory disease, *JAMA* 253:2246; 1985.

Wells N: Management of pain during abortion, *J Adv Nurs* 14:56, 1989.

Whaley LF, Wong DL: *Nursing care of infants and children,* ed 4, St Louis, 1991, Mosby–Year Book.

Willson JR, Carrington ER: *Obstetrics and gynecology,* ed 9, St Louis, 1991, Mosby–Year Book.

Wolner-Hanssen P et al: Laparoscopic findings and contraceptive use in women with signs and symptoms suggestive of acute salpingitis, *Obstet Gynecol* 66:233, 1985.

Women's Health: Cervical cap approved for marketing, *AJN* 89(2):165, 1989.

World Health Organization: *Mechanism of action, safety, and efficacy of intrauterine devices, Technical Report Series 753,* Geneva, 1987, World Health Organization.

Wright J et al: Psychological distress and infertility: a review of controlled research, *Int J Fertil* 34(2):126, 1989.

Wyeth Laboratories, Inc: *The Norplant system: instructions for insertion and removal,* Philadelphia, Penn, 1990, Wyeth-Ayerst.

Yovich JL, Matson PL: The influence of infertility etiology on the outcome of IVF-ET and GIFT treatments, *Int J Fertil* 35(1):26, 1990.

References—Nursing Research

Bernstein et al: Psychological status of previously infertile couples after successful pregnancy, *JOGNN* 17(6):404, 1988.

Blenner JL: Attaining self-care in infertility treatment, *Appl Nurs Res* 3(3):98, 1990.

Frank DI: Factors related to decisions about infertility treatment, *JOGNN* 19(2):162, 1990a.

Frank DI: Gender differences in decision making about infertility treatment, *Appl Nurs Res* 3(2):56, 1990b.

Olshansky EF: Responses to high technology infertility treatment, *Image* 20(3):128, 1988.

BIBLIOGRAPHY

Adler NE et al: Adolescent contraception behavior: an assessment of decision processes, *J Pediatr* 116(3):463, 1990.

American Academy of Pediatrics, Committee on Bioethics: Sterilization of women who are mentally handicapped, *Pediatrics* 85(5):868, 1990.

Baulieu EE: Contragestion and other clinical applications of RU 486, an antiprogesterone at the receptor, *Science* 245:1351, 1989.

Baulieu EE: RU 486 as an antiprogesterone steroid, *JAMA* 262(13):1808, 1989.

Cates W Jr, Stone KM: Family planning, sexually transmitted diseases and contraceptive choice: A literature update—Part I, *Fam Plann Perspect* 24:75-84, 1992.

Coker AL et al: Barrier methods of contraception and cervical intraepithelial neoplasia, *Contraception* 45:1-10, 1992.

Clinical News: Cervical cap approved for marketing, *AJN* 89(2):165, 1989.

Daniels KR: Psychosocial factors for couples awaiting in vitro fertilization, *Soc Work Health Care* 14(2):81, 1989.

Dunnington R, Glazer G: Maternal identity and early mothering behavior in previously infertile and never infertile women, *JOGNN* 20(4):309, 1991.

Dunphy BC et al: Is routine examination of the male partner of any prognostic value in the routine assessment of couples who complain of involuntary infertility? *Fertil Steril* 52(3):454, 1989.

Eschenbach DA: The IUD and infertility, *Fertil Steril* 57:1177, 1992.

Farley TMM et al: Intrauterine devices and pelvic inflammatory disease: an international perspective, *Lancet* 339:785-788, 1992.

Francis G, Nosek J: Ethical considerations in contemporary reproductive technologies, *J Perinat Neonat Nurs* 1(3):37, 1988.

Gerstman BB et al: Oral contraceptive estrogen dose and the risk of deep venous thromboembolic disease, *Am J Epidemiol* 133(1):32, 1991.

Gerstmann BB et al: Trends in the content and use of oral contraceptives in the United States, 1964-88, *Am J Public Health* 81(1):90, 1991.

Goldzeiher JW: Pharmacology of contraceptive steroids: a brief review, *Am J Obstet Gynecol* 160(5) Part 2:1260, 1989.

Griffith CS, Grimes DA: The validity of the postcoital test, *Am J Obstet Gynecol* 162(3):615, 1990.

Hill NCW: The efficacy of oral Mifepristone (RU38, 486) with a prostaglandin E_1 analog vaginal pessary for the termination of early pregnancy: complications and patient acceptability, *Am J Obstet Gynecol* 162(2):414, 1990.

Hovatta O et al: Direct intraperitoneal or intrauterine insemination and superovulation in infertility treatment: a randomized study, *Fertil Steril* 54(2):339, 1990.

Kaeser L: Contraceptive development: why the snail's pace? *Fam Plann Perspect* 22(3):139, 1990.

Landry E: How and why women choose sterilization: results from six follow-up surveys, *Stud Fam Plann* 21(3):143, 1990.

Louchs A: A comparison of satisfaction with types of diaphragms among women in a college population, *JOGNN* 18(3):194, 1989.

Lutwak RA, Ney AM, White JE: Maternity nursing and Jewish law, *MCN* 13(1):44, 1988.

McClure RD: New hope for subfertile men, *West J Med* 151(3):333, 1989.

Milne BJ: Couples' experiences with in vitro fertilization, *JOGNN* 17(5):347, 1988.

Mosher WD, Pratt WF: Use of contraception and family planning services in the United States, 1988, *Am J Public Health* 80(9):1132, 1990.

Mukhtar Q, Addy C, Macera C: Contraception and HIV prevention among women in public health clinics, *Health Values* 16(1):3, 1992.

Nader S: Prostaglandin inhibitors in the management of premenstrual syndrome, *The Female Patient* 17(8):38, Aug 1992.

Niruthisard S et al: Nonoxynol-9 and bacterial STDs, *Lancet* 339:1371, 1992.

Oakley D et al: Expanded nursing care for contraceptive use, *Appl Nurs Res* 2(3):121, 1989.
Opsahl MS, Klein TA: Tubal and peritoneal factors in the infertile woman: use of patient history in selection of diagnostic and therapeutic surgical procedures, *Fertil Steril* 53(4):632, 1990.
Palca J: The pill of choice? *Science* 245:1319, 1989.
Pool TB et al: Zygote intrafallopian transfer with "donor rescue": a new option for severe male factor infertility, *Fertil Steril* 54(1):166, 1990.
Sandelowski M et al: Mazing: infertile couples and the quest for a child, *Image* 21(4):220, 1989.
Sherrod RA: Coping with infertility: a personal perspective turned professional, *MCN* 13(3):191, 1988.
Sise BC: Maternal rights versus fetal interests: an ethical issue with nursing implications, *J Prof Nurs* 4(4):262, 1988.
Strader MK, Beaman ML: College students' knowledge about AIDS and attitudes toward condom use, *PHN* 6(2):62, 1989.
Stubblefield PG: Choosing the best oral contraceptive, *Clin Obstet Gynecol* 32(2):316, 1989.
Swanson JM et al: Readability of commercial and generic contraception instructions, *Image* 22(2):96, 1990.
The polyurethane vaginal pouch: new barrier contraceptive may give women more control over STD prevention, *The Contraception Report* 3(2):12, May 1992.
Thomas JA, Ballantyne B: Occupational reproductive risks: sources, surveillance, and testing, *J Occup Med* 32(6):547, 1990.
Tyrer LG, Salas JE: Contraceptive problems unique to the United States, *Clin Obstet Gynecol* 32(2):307, 1989.
Zion AB: Resources for infertile couples, *JOGNN* 17(4):255, 1988.

chapter 42 review

Key Concepts

- Impaired fertility is the inability to conceive and carry a child to term gestation at a time the couple has chosen to do so.
- Impaired fertility affects between 15% and 20% of otherwise healthy adults.
- Male and female factors each separately account for 40% of impaired fertility. Factors from both partners are responsible for the remaining 20%.
- Common etiologic factors of impaired fertility include decreased sperm production, interference with hypothalamic-pituitary-ovarian axis, tubal occlusion, and varicocele.
- It is estimated that 40% to 50% of couples with impaired fertility who seek assistance will be able to become pregnant and carry the child to viability.
- Reproductive alternatives to achieve parenthood include IVF-ET, GIFT, ZIFT, therapeutic insemination, surrogate motherhood, and adoption.
- There are a variety of contraceptive methods and various effectiveness ratings, advantages, and disadvantages.
- Nurses need to help couples choose the contraceptive method or methods best suited to them.
- Proper concurrent use of spermicides and latex condoms provides protection against AIDS.
- Tubal ligations and vasectomies are permanent sterilization methods used by increasing numbers of women and men.
- Elective abortion accomplished in the first trimester is 10 times safer than carrying a pregnancy to term.

Key Terms

- autoimmunization (p. 1324)
- basal body temperature (BBT) (p. 1303)
- calendar method (p. 1303)
- cervical cap (p. 1314)
- cervical mucus method (p. 1304)
- condom (p. 1308)
- contraception (p. 1302)
- dilatation and curettage (D&C) (p. 1326)
- diaphragm (p. 1314)
- elective abortion (p. 1325)
- fertile period (p. 1302)
- GIFT (p. 1298)
- impaired fertility (p. 1280)
- intrauterine device (IUD) (p. 1318)
- in vitro fertilization/embryo transplant (p. 1297)
- isoimmunization (p. 1289)
- laminaria (p. 1284, 1291)
- male contraception (p. 1309)
- Norplant (p. 1313)
- oral hormonal contraceptives (p. 1310)
- periodic abstinence (p. 1302)
- predictor test (p. 1304)
- referred shoulder pain (p. 1286)
- safe period (p. 1302)
- semen analysis (p. 1292)
- spermicide (p. 1307)
- spinnbarkheit (p. 1304)
- therapeutic intrauterine insemination (p. 1299)
- thermal shift (p. 1303)
- vacuum or suction curettage (p. 1326)
- vaginal sponge (p. 1308)
- varicocele (p. 1293)
- withdrawal bleeding (p. 1310)
- ZIFT (p. 1298)

Critical Thinking Exercises

1. You are assigned to the infertility clinic. A couple has arrived to begin diagnostic workup for infertility.
   a. Interview the couple to determine how infertility has affected their lives.
   b. Examine what your feelings would be if you were told that you were infertile.
   c. Identify ways you can assist the couple in coping with the diagnosis of infertility. Justify your interventions.
   d. Discuss in your clinical group the ethical issues resulting from treatment of infertility (i.e., *in vitro* fertilization, surrogate motherhood, and artificial insemination by donor).
2. You are working in a family planning clinic. A seventeen-year-old single woman and a 35-year-old married mother of two children are requesting birth control information.
   a. Examine your beliefs about who should have access to birth control and which methods are perceived by you to be acceptable. How might these beliefs affect your ability to provide birth control information?
   b. What client information is needed as you assist these two women in making a decision about a birth control method?
   c. What information is needed by the women in order for them to make an informed decision about a method of contraception?
   d. Select one method for each of the above women; justify your choices.
   e. Write a teaching plan to provide specific instructions for each method.

Topics for Nursing Research

Infertility

- Which nursing interventions promote comfort during infertility tests?
- What are the components of grieving in relation to the diagnosis of infertility?
- What anticipatory guidance is most effective for couples facing infertility?

Control of fertility and sterilization

- Is there regret after sterilization?
- What coping strategies are effective for oral hormonal contraceptive side effects?
- What strategies enhance knowledge about methods of birth control that also inhibit the transmission of STDs?

Interruption of pregnancy

- Is there guilt following elective abortion?
- What factors affect the decision to have an elective abortion?
- Which pain-relief measures are most effective during abortion procedures?
- What positive factors are derived from making the decision to terminate a pregnancy?

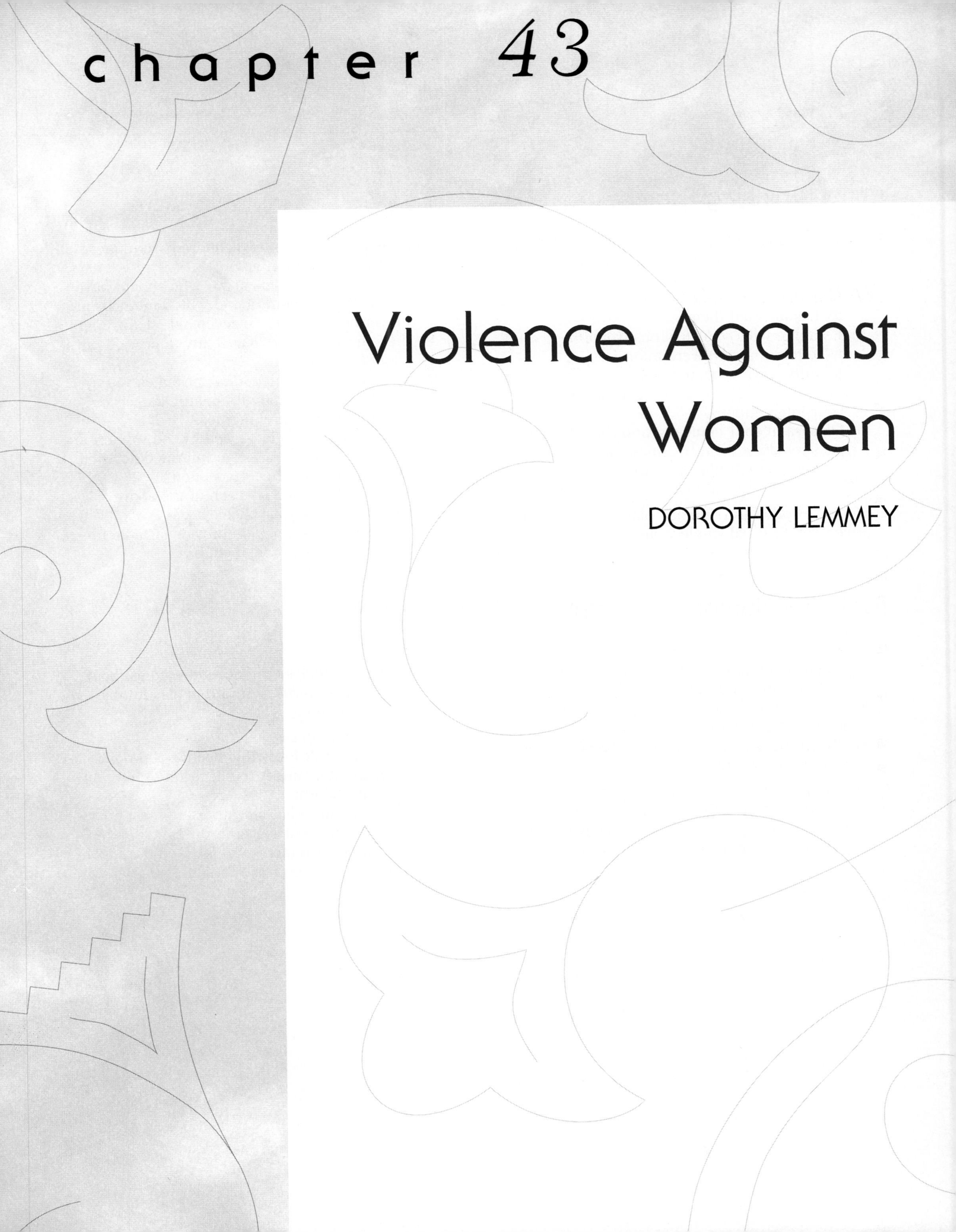

chapter 43

Violence Against Women

DOROTHY LEMMEY

LEARNING OBJECTIVES

- Define the key terms listed.
- Describe the historic events that have perpetuated violence against women.
- Identify behaviors associated with children who experience sexual assault.
- Identify behaviors associated with women who experience sexual assault as children.
- Discuss the nursing process surrounding care of a survivor of childhood sexual abuse.
- Describe types of rape.
- Describe the rape trauma syndrome.
- Develop a nursing plan of care for the immediate care and follow-up care of rape survivors.
- Explain the cycle of violence and its use in assessment and intervention for battered women.
- Describe characteristics of survivors and abusers in battering relationships.
- Develop a plan of care for a battered woman.
- Identify topics of nursing research related to violence against women.

Violence against women includes battering, sexual assault, rape and incest. These are significant problems, each carrying the potential for serious physical, psychologic, and emotional injury or impairment.

Battery of women refers to assault, a violent physical attack. Clinical findings include bruises, lacerations, burns, hematomas, and fractures. A **sexual assault** is any aggressive or violent act involving sexual intimacy performed by one person on another without that person's consent. **Abuse** of women is defined as physical, emotional, or sexual mistreatment: aggressive behavior, including acts of a sexual or physical nature, verbal belittling, or intimidation. Battery, abuse, and assault are often used interchangeably.

Violence against women is prevalent worldwide, although accurate statistics are not always available. Levinson (1989) studied 90 cultures around the world and found family violence in almost all cultures and violence against women the most common form of violence reported. For example, in Papua, New Guinea, a law reform committee reports that 67% of rural women and 56% of urban women were battered by their husbands (Heise, 1989). In Ecuador, more than 80% of women interviewed were beaten by their mates (Heise, 1989). One in 10 married Canadian women is physically abused each year (Delgaty, 1985). A comparison of wife abuse between two cultures was studied (see Research Highlight, p. 1339).

The statistics regarding violence against American women reveal a serious and growing problem. In the United States as many as 50% of families may experience violence (Stenchever, Stenchever 1991). Approximately one third of the women in the United States experience sexual violence in their lifetimes (Sampselle 1991). Since 1974, reports of assaults against women, particularly young women (ages 20-24), have increased by almost 50% (Senate Judiciary Committee, 1990). According to Federal Bureau of Investigation (FBI) estimates, 25 million wives are abused by their husbands each year (Witkin-Lanoil, 1987). It is estimated that in the United States, one woman is beaten every 18 seconds (Senate Judiciary Committee, 1990). Pregnancy is a time of increased battering episodes, with a reported incidence of 40% to 60% (Helton, McFarlane, Anderson, 1987; Parker, 1991). These numbers are impressive despite the fact that assault within families is the most underreported of all crimes (Hillard, 1986; Klaus, 1984).

An estimated 25% to 50% of females are victims of sexual abuse before their eighteenth birthday (Bagley, 1991; Wyatt, 1990; McCarthy, 1989; Brown, 1990; Koss, 1990).

Although the incidence of rape can only be approximated, the Senate Judiciary Committee (1990) reports that a woman is raped every 6 minutes in the United States. However, less than 10% of rape victims report the attack in spite of the fact that most occurrences (80%) of rapes are perpetrated by someone the woman knows (Gibbs, 1991). Many of the victims do not seek health care.

An estimated 100,000 cases or more of incest occur per year; 12% to 24% of the female victims become pregnant (Zdanuk, Harris, Wisian, 1987). The overwhelming physical evidence of the prevalence of these serious crimes precludes the need to identify them as major issues in current society.

Although both women and men may take on either role or both roles—abuser and/or victim—this chapter focuses only on women (from adolescence through old age) as victims of violence. Child abuse and molestation and men as victims of spouse battering and rape are beyond the scope of this text.

Nurses will see victims in all age groups and in every area of their practice. Because of the magnitude of the problems of violence against women, maternity and gynecologic nurses cannot ignore this reality of client care. There is a need to focus on prevention, effective nursing actions, and long-term counseling of victims. See discussion of preventive measures included in each section.

FACTORS THAT INFLUENCE VIOLENCE AGAINST WOMEN

Effective prevention requires an understanding of societal factors that foster destructive behaviors against women. Some of these factors are devaluation of women, power imbalance, viewing women as property, sex role stereotyping, and a culture in which aggressive behavior is held in high esteem (Walker, 1984; Koop, 1985; Yllo, 1988; Kodd, 1990; Sampselle, 1991). In prehistoric times, it was thought that women were the creators of life and men made no contribution. There was no need to control the woman or her sexuality because she was the creator of life. Approximately 3500 years ago it was discovered that men were essential to fertilization, and culture began to change (Stephenson, 1988). In order to ensure paternity, women and their sexuality had to be controlled. Name, property, legal rights, money, and power were taken by males; women became possessions (Miles, 1989). This new order robbed women of freedom and of control over their bodies; it dehumanized females. As females were divested of human qualities, the inhumane treatment recorded by history became acceptable.

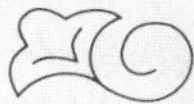 **Research Highlight** 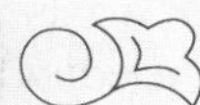

A Comparison of Wife Abuse Between Two Cultures

RESEARCH ABSTRACT

This study identified women's perceptions of wife abuse and attitudes toward abuse. It compared the nature, severity, and frequency of wife abuse in 25 Anglo-American and 25 Mexican-American women over the age of 18 who had been abused by their husbands at least twice and had lived in a shelter for battered women. Data were collected during interviews. The majority of the women were between the ages of 18 and 30; 80% were from the lower socioeconomic class, and 20% were from the middle class. Mexican-American women averaged one more child than Anglo-American women. Mexican-American women stayed in the relationship longer than Anglo-American women. Almost half of the women reported abuse in the home of origin. The conflicts that led to battering were husband domination, jealousy, and drinking. Forty percent of the Mexican-American women reported not knowing when they were going to be battered. On the average, batterings lasted from 1 to 15 minutes; however, some episodes lasted as long as 2 hours. All of the women were physically injured; injuries included bruises, scars, burns, cuts, fractured bones, and broken teeth. Battering occurred during pregnancy in 60% of the Anglo-American women and 72% of the Mexican-American women. Anglo-American women perceived more incidents as abusive and emotional abuse as more serious than did Mexican-American women. Mexican-American women were more likely to be beaten in front of relatives than were Anglo-American women, suggesting that wife-battering is more acceptable in Mexican-American families.

IMPLICATIONS FOR PRACTICE

Nurses working with women should incorporate questions about abuse in their assessment interviews. The incidence and response to wife abuse may differ in cultural groups. Nurses need culturally relevant education in the prevention and treatment of family abuse. Families and the community need to be educated about family violence and ways to deal with stress that may precipitate abuse.

RELATED RESEARCH QUESTIONS

1. What are the attitudes toward family violence in families in which abuse does not occur?
2. What are the attitudes of African-American families toward family violence?
3. Does the incidence of and attitudes toward family violence differ among cultural groups?
4. Is there a difference in attitudes toward family violence between Anglo-American and Mexican-American men?

REFERENCE

Torres S: A comparison of wife abuse between two cultures: perceptions, attitudes, nature and extent, *Issues Mental Health Nurs* 12(1):113, 1991.

Sex role stereotyping begins in childhood. Male children are often socialized to be aggressive, competitive, and able to maintain power over themselves and their environment (Lipman-Blumen, 1984). Female children are socialized differently. They are taught to be dependent, helpless, timid, fearful, and controlled (i.e., **learned helplessness**). This training prevents pursuit of self-interests and perpetuates dependence on the "powerful" male (Lipman-Blumen 1984).

■ BATTERED WOMEN

Women should have the right to move about within the confines of their homes among those persons with whom they share the most intimate, interpersonal relationships without fearing for their safety and well-being, or for life itself. In general, women accept and expect that right as a given (Drake, 1982). Battering is a criminal act; in a marriage, it is a fundamental betrayal of trust (Delgaty, 1985).

The abuse of spouses occurs at all socioeconomic levels, as well as all educational levels. The myth that only persons in the low socioeconomic classes or only those with little education are the primary perpetrators of wife abuse has been refuted. Wives are more likely to be abused than are husbands, although it is not entirely unknown for a man to report physical or emotional abuse by his spouse.

Since nurses come from the general population, how many have themselves been abused (or have been abusers)? What effect has the experience had on their ability to cope with the crisis state presented by victims who have come for medical care?

Wife battering, spouse abuse, and domestic (family) violence are all terms applied to forceful physical, social, and/or psychologic trauma inflicted by the male partner on the female partner in a marriage or marital-like relationship. An extraordinary variety of other definitions have been formulated for this behavior. Some common elements in these definitions are (1) repetition of episodes, (2) some demonstrable injury or injuries resulting from the violence, and (3) violence that is deliberate and severe.

These elements preclude the occasional physical acts of shoving, shaking, or restraining that occur in some marriages. At present, family violence generally is considered a part of family life by both the law and large numbers of women. Some people are socialized to believe that domestic violence is an acceptable way of dealing with the stresses of family life (Mandel, 1986; Stuart, Sundeen, 1987; Battered, 1987); for example, women have reported that they believe it is acceptable for a husband to beat his wife "every once in a while."

Initial studies of wife abuse began in the early 1970s. Several disciplines approached the problem from different viewpoints. For example, researchers in *psychiatry* were concerned with the causative factors that drive a man to beat his wife and the reasons that women who are repeatedly beaten will stay with the spouse. Researchers in *sociology* looked at the factors in society and the institution of marriage that would keep a woman captive in a violent marriage. The *health care providers* were concerned with case finding, documentation, physical care of victims, and developing preventive measures through education, research, and political activism.

Characteristics of Victims and Abusers

Every socioeconomic group is represented among abused wives. As noted earlier in this chapter, race, religion, social background, age, and educational level are not significant factors in differentiating women at risk.

Battered wives may feel they are to blame for their situation because they are "not good-enough wives." These women blame themselves for bringing on the violent behavior in their relationship because they believe they need to "try harder" to do better in pleasing the abuser. In many cases, there is a traumatic bonding with the man that hinges on loyalty, fear, terror, and learned helplessness. Many women suffer from low self-esteem and may have histories of domestic violence in their families of origin. They fear societal rejection if they discuss their problem openly. This fear is justified in many cases, because society has stereotyped these women as masochistic. It is difficult for many people to comprehend why a woman would remain in a situation where she is repeatedly beaten and injured.

Elbow (1977) has identified four types of men who become abusive husbands and has categorized them as the Controller, the Defender, the Approval Seeker, and the Incorporator.

CONTROLLER. The Controller strives for autonomy through the control of others. He is not emotionally reciprocal in his relationships; he usually gets his way and is never to blame when things go wrong. He sees other people in terms of what they can do for him. When the Controller feels he can no longer dominate, he will use violence as an attempt to regain control. It is possible that his wife represents his extremely domineering parent(s), who did not permit him to be autonomous as a child.

DEFENDER (PROTECTOR). Having a spouse to harm, love, and forgive is a fundamental need of the Defender. His fear is that he will be harmed, and he strikes out before he is struck. He needs a wife who is totally dependent on him, clings to him, and is defenseless so that he can protect her. He believes, however, that his wife will try to punish him for being assertive or sexual. He tries, through violence, to keep his wife powerless, thereby reducing his own vulnerability.

APPROVAL SEEKER. Continued reaffirmation of self-esteem is required by the Approval Seeker. He has a low self-image and expects rejection. He may even precipitate rejection by his mate through his behavior. Violence occurs when he feels the most criticized.

INCORPORATOR. The need of the Incorporator is to draw another individual's strengths into his own psyche to fill his emotional gaps. His desperation can be observed in several ways. He may cling to his mate, have public displays of anger, and have suicidal ideation. Any attempt by the wife to withdraw from the situation increases his desperation and may lead to violence.

This discussion focuses on abuse within a marital or a marital type of relationship. There is also an increase in the number and severity of abuse incidents inflicted on women in dating situations. These incidents and sexual harassment have been reported as occurring in the workplace, in colleges and universities, and even in high school relationships. Complementary personality characteristics and childhood influences are found in couples who are susceptible to development of abuser/victim relationships (Table 43-1).

Myths About Battered Women

Health professionals often become frustrated by women who remain in battering relationships. As with other human dynamics that are not easily explained, a number of myths have emerged to account for this perceived self-destructive behavior (Collier, 1987; Griffith-Kenney, 1986). Table 43-2 lists a series of myths and facts about abuse and battering.

Cycle of Violence: The Dynamics of Battering

Lenore Walker pioneered the cause of women as victims of violence in United States when she published her research in a book, *The Battered Woman* (1979). Using the qualitative research method, she recorded results from interviews with 120 battered women. Their accounts of the progress of the abuse were remarkably similar; the resulting pattern is now recognized as the theory of the **cycle of violence.** According to this theory, battering is neither random nor constant, but rather it occurs in repeated cycles (Fig. 43-1). A cyclic pattern to the battering behavior has been described as a period of increasing tension leading to the battery, followed by an aftermath characterized by kind, loving behavior and a plea for forgiveness by the husband/partner (Hillard, 1986).

PHASE I: THE TENSION-BUILDING STATE. There is a gradual escalation of tension. The batterer expresses dissatisfaction and hostility without violent outbursts. He may be angered because the food is too cold, his socks are not to be found, or the children are unruly. The woman senses the danger and anxiously tries to placate him. These tactics work for awhile but only reinforce the woman's unrealistic belief that she can control his violent behavior. Eventually, she can no longer control his anger, and she withdraws to cope. He senses this withdrawal and becomes angrier until the violent outburst occurs. ***The woman suppresses the knowledge of the impending abuse from her mate.***

PHASE II: THE ACUTE BATTERING INCIDENT. This phase is characterized by the man's uncontrollable discharge of the tension that has been building for

TABLE 43-1 Characteristics of Victim and Abuser

Victim	Abuser
CHILDHOOD INFLUENCES	CHILDHOOD INFLUENCES
Many raised to be submissive, passive, and dependent Likely to accept traditional female role in marriage Accepts female sex-role stereotypes	Raised in family where males reign supreme As children may have used violence to problem-solve Accepts "macho" values
PERSONALITY CHARACTERISTICS	PERSONALITY CHARACTERISTICS
Attributes beating to some personal inadequacy Low self-esteem and feelings of worthlessness Learned helplessness reduces problem-solving ability Low tolerance for frustration Easily upset, critical, aloof, and reserved Severe stress reactions and psychophysiologic symptoms Can't trust anyone Some attempt suicide Punishment justified if marriage fails Unable to make "I" statements or maintain eye contact and denies and/or minimizes abuse	Feelings of inadequacy, inferiority, and insecurity Emotionally immature and/or aggressive Extremes in behavior and overreacting are typical Low self-esteem with high degree of self-loathing Intolerant of having masculinity threatened Lacks respect for women Poor impulse control Excessive possessiveness and jealousy Some use aggressive sexual attacks to punish and enhance own self-esteem Alcohol or substance abuse may be present
LIFE-STYLE FACTORS	LIFE-STYLE FACTORS
Isolated from family and friends Totally dependent on husband for financial and emotional support	No particular profession, occupation, or socioeconomic group Often has difficulties at work Severely restricts freedom and mobility of wife

TABLE 43-2 Myths and Facts About Abuse and Battering

Myth	Fact
Battering occurs in a small percentage of the population.	Physical assault reportedly occurred in 28% of all American homes in 1976 (Strauss et al, 1980).
Battering occurs only in lower-class families.	Although lower-class families have a higher incidence of battering (Gelles, 1979), it also occurs in middle- and upper-income families. Incidence not really known because of tendency of middle- and upper-income families to hide their battering.
Battered women like to be beaten and deliberately provoke the attack. They are masochistic.	Women are terrified of their assailants and go to great lengths to avoid a confrontation. In some cases the woman may provoke her husband to release tension that, if left unchecked, might lead to a more severe beating and possible death.
Batterers are uneducated men who are unable to cope with the world.	Many batterers are successful professionals, including politicians, ministers, physicians, and lawyers.
Men who batter their wives also beat their children.	One half of wife-batterers do not beat their children.
Battered women were battered children.	This myth holds true in only a few cases. Most battered women report that their husbands were the first person to beat them.
Alcohol and drug abuse causes battering.	Gelles (1976) and Delgaty (1985) proposed that batterers use alcohol as an excuse to batter and shift the blame from themselves to the alcohol.
Once a battered wife, always a battered wife.	Many women who have battering relationships do not marry again. Those who stay in the relationships do so out of fear and financial dependence. Shelters have long waiting lists.
Batterers and battered women cannot change.	Counseling can effectively help resocialize both batterers and battered women.

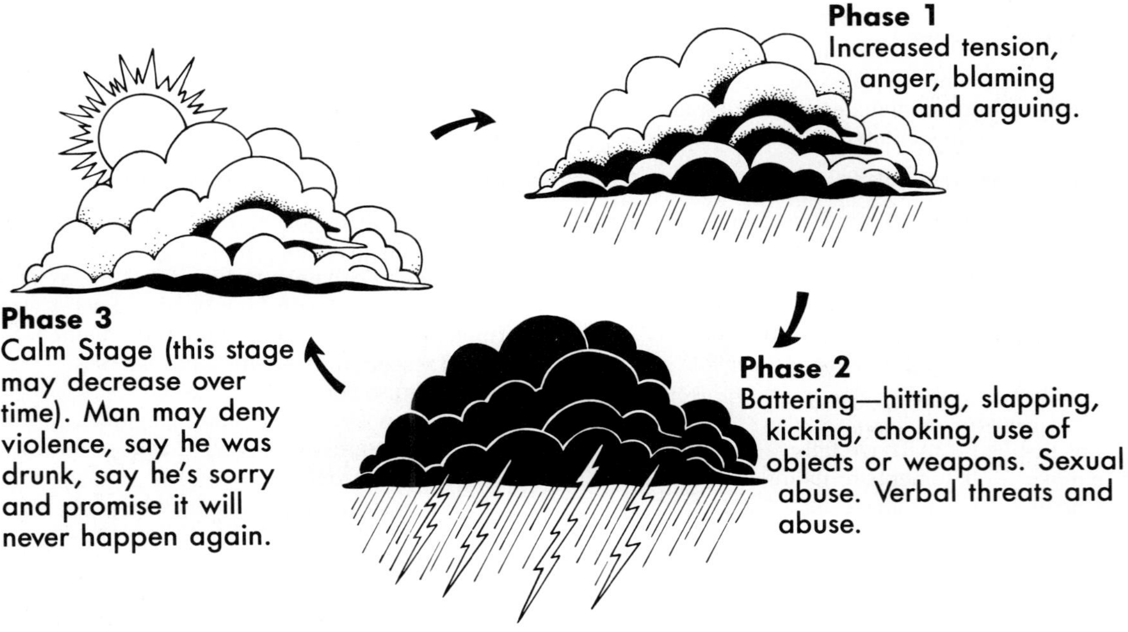

Fig. 43-1 Cycle of violence.
From Helton A: *A protocol of care for the battered woman,* White Plains, NY, 1987, March of Dimes Birth Defects Foundation.

the purpose of "teaching her a lesson." The phase can last hours to several days. The woman's injuries are usually to her face, buttocks, and hands and forearms as she tries to protect herself. The types of behaviors are slaps, punches to face and head, kicking, stomping, punching, choking, pushing, breaking of bones, burns from irons, and mutilation from knives and guns. ***The woman denies to herself and others the severity of the damage.***

PHASE III: KINDNESS AND CONTRITE, LOVING BEHAVIOR. This "honeymoon" phase is characterized by the batterer apologizing profusely. He may try to help her, take her to the hospital, or shower her with gifts they may not be able to afford. He promises it will never happen again, and he may believe at that time it will not. She desperately wants to believe him, and this behavior restores her hope that he will change. This stage is the positive reinforcement for remaining in the relationship. ***The woman denies the inevitable reoccurrence of the abuse.***

Over time, the tension and battering phase get longer and the honeymoon phase gets shorter until there is no honeymoon phase (Walker, 1984).

Power and control are again at the core of the perpetuation of battering against women (Fig. 43-2 illustrates a model of how the man maintains power and control over his mate). Power and control are the driving force of the behavior and are depicted as the axle of the wheel. The spokes are tactics used to maintain power and control, and the circular ring is the pervasive threat of physical harm that holds the wheel together.

Battery during Pregnancy

Many women report that they were first beaten when their husbands learned of their pregnancy

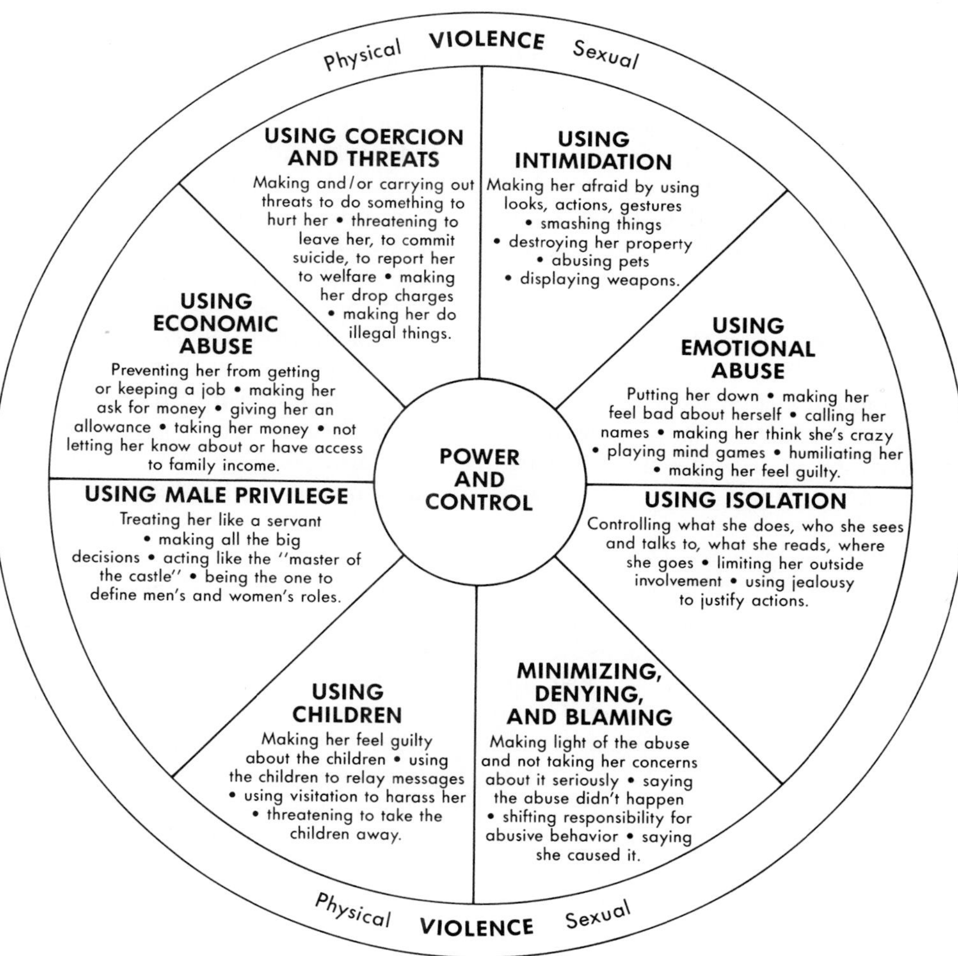

Fig. 43-2 Model of how power and control issues perpetuate battering.
From Domestic Violence Intervention Project: *Power and Control: Tactics of Men Who Batter.*

(Walker, 1984). Studies of battered women report that 40% to 60% of pregnant women admit battering during pregnancy (Parker McFarlane, 1991). Studies have demonstrated that battery during pregnancy results in a higher rate of births of low-birth-weight newborns (Bullock, 1989; Satin et al, 1991). Sexual assault also increased the rate of births of preterm infants (Satin et al, 1991). For a discussion of low-birth-weight and preterm infants, see Chapter 37.

The blows are often directed toward the breasts, abdomen, and genitals. It has been hypothesized that jealousy of the baby's intrusion on the couple's relationship and the increased strain on the marriage either triggers or exacerbates abuse.

The battered pregnant woman should be treated as a high-risk obstetric client because she often has more medical, social, or psychologic needs (Gelles, 1988) that require special attention. She is at additional risk for repeated physical trauma and for psychologic trauma because of a deficient support system.

Pregnancy is a time of increased battering episodes for a variety of reasons: (1) The biopsychosocial stresses of pregnancy may strain the relationship beyond the couple's ability to cope; frustration is followed by violence. (2) The man may be jealous of the fetus, resenting its intrusion into the couple's relationship. As one expectant father succinctly stated, "I don't get the TLC I got before that thing came along." (3) The beating may be the man's conscious or subconscious attempt to end the pregnancy. After birth the mother may be so physically and emotionally drained that she may have difficulty bonding with her infant. She is considered at risk of becoming an abusive mother whether she chooses to stay in the abusive relationship or not. If she remains with her husband, the chances are 1 in 2 that he will batter the child as well (de Lang, 1986).

Reaching Out for Help

Battered women are reluctant to seek help for various reasons: the need to avoid the stigma associated with the nature of the family violence, the fear that they will not be believed, the fear of reprisal from their husbands, and in some states in which battering is a reportable crime, the wish to avoid involvement with police.

Exactly what drives a woman to seek assistance is not clear, but apparently it may be the result of a behavioral change in the woman. The women who display any of the following three characteristics are more likely to seek assistance:

1. Women who are beaten frequently and severely
2. Women who have not experienced or witnessed family violence in their family of origin
3. Women who see an alternative to life in their marriages—specifically, women with jobs

■ NURSING PROCESS

ASSESSMENT

Health care providers are often the first and only contact with "outsiders" that a severely isolated woman will make. Therefore it is important that nurses assess all women entering the health care system for potential abuse. Identification of women who are experiencing abuse is the first step in effecting change. Failure to identify spousal abuse and to recognize the risk of serious injury or even death further endangers lives of women and their children.

The nurse performs a health history and physical examination to identify the following cues that may point to abuse: delay in seeking medical assistance (hours or days); nonspecific psychosomatic complaints; social isolation; injuries to face, breasts, abdomen, and buttocks; no eye contact; vague explanation of injuries; a husband/partner who does not want to leave client alone with the health care provider; old and new injuries; abdominal injuries with pregnancy; spontaneous abortion; abruptio placentae; missed appointments; and presence of drug abuse (Hartman, 1987; Chez, 1988; Follingstad et al, 1991; Chez, 1990). Pregnancy in girls under 15 years of age is frequently the result of sexual abuse (Butler, Burton, 1990).

A suspected assaulted woman should be examined and interviewed in private. The abused woman may feel safer and more comfortable with a female health care provider. She should be asked directly if she has been injured by her husband/partner. A history form should be developed that includes at least the following two questions: (1) "Are you with a spouse/partner who physically/psychologically hurts you?" and, (2) "Are you afraid of your spouse/partner?" These questions give a woman permission to disclose sensitive information (Chez, 1990).

If she does disclose this information, believe her. Remember, the coping mechanism most used by battered women is denial: denial of impending abuse, denial of severity of injury, denial of future recurrence, and denial of possible death. Often, women are embarrassed and believe the abuse relates to their inadequacies. By asking a woman directly, telling her that similar injuries are common in women who have been abused, and pointing out that ***she (the victim) is not responsible for another's violent behavior,*** the nurse may help her disclose what is happening to her.

Nursing Diagnoses

Assessment findings may give rise to several nursing diagnoses. Examples of potential nursing diagnoses for battered women may include the following:

- Hopelessness related to
  —Prolonged exposure to physical, mental, social, and sexual abuse.
- Knowledge deficit related to
  —Phenomenon of battering
  —Cycle of violence
  —Community resources for protection and support
- Ineffective individual and family coping related to
  —Persistence of victim-abuser relationship
- Physical injury related to
  —Battering episode
- Self-esteem disturbance related to
  —Continuing victim-abuser relationship
- Spiritual distress related to
  —Continuing victim-abuser relationship

Planning

To develop an effective plan, the caregiver must be comfortable working with the victim and her family. In addition, the caregiver must have a broad knowledge base of this phenomenon, excellent communication skills, and access to appropriate community resources. If possible, continuity of care is planned with the health care provider(s) with whom the woman develops a relationship of trust.

Goals are formulated in client-centered terms. Following are examples of goals for care.

1. The battered woman is identified
2. The woman is protected from further abuse
3. The woman perceives herself as deserving of respect and not as "deserving" to be victimized
4. The woman reestablishes a feeling of control
5. The woman identifies her areas of strength and develops goals for herself
6. The woman increases her knowledge of:
   a. Alternatives, options, and choices
   b. Community resources (shelters, financial aid, child care, education, etc.)
   c. Roles of members of the health care team
7. Her physical injuries are treated promptly
8. If the woman is pregnant or has children, the fetus and children are protected from abuse.

Implementation

Skillful interview techniques help women disclose and describe abuse. Some nurse (helper) responses facilitate discussion of her abuse; others may inhibit the victim (see box below).

During assessment, the nurse-client relationship is initiated. A battered woman has often experienced years of powerlessness and rigid control. Nursing practice that empowers women can help them gain a personal sense of control. The nurse provides options, explains procedures, asks permission, and conveys trust in a woman's ability to make the right decision for herself and her children.

If the woman is pregnant, a support network is developed with the other maternity nurses who will be involved in her care during the peripartum period. Each nurse can plan care that will point out the woman's strengths and raise her self-esteem. The husband/partner is welcomed to attend prenatal visits and classes and is included in other ways if the woman chooses to stay with him. Counseling services are offered to both spouses. The first days after birth are particularly crucial—the mother is physi-

Helper Responses

FACILITATIVE

- Ask woman if abuse is occurring.
- Identify described behavior as abusive.
- Acknowledge seriousness of abuse.
- Express belief in woman's description of abuse.
- Acknowledge that woman does not deserve the abuse.
- Be directive in exploring resources.
- Tell the man to stop the abuse.
- Aid woman to consider full range of available options.
- Avoid telling woman what to do.
- Aid woman to assess her internal strengths.
- Suggest tangible resources (e.g., shelters and financial aid).
- Offer support groups with other abused women.
- Be active in listening and empathizing.

INHIBITIVE

- Demonstrate irritation/anger with woman.
- Blame woman.
- Advise woman to accept abuse as better than nothing.
- Refuse to help until woman leaves abuser.
- Align with abuser.
- Disbelieve woman.
- Avoid responding to abuse disclosure.
- Advise woman to leave abuser.

From Limandri B: The therapeutic relationship with abused women, *J Psychosoc Nurs* 25(2):9, Feb 1987.

cally and emotionally vulnerable and usually tired, and the baby's crying may be intolerable to both the father and the mother. The danger of abuse to mother and child is acute during this time. A support network of maternity and pediatric staff, community health nurses, and parental crisis center personnel is needed to coordinate efforts to provide support during this crucial period.

The nurse *does* do the following:

1. Treat the woman with dignity and concern to help her reduce her feelings of isolation, embarrassment, shame, and guilt.
2. Encourage the woman to refer to herself specifically, using statements such as "I am" rather than referring to herself in general terms (Finley, 1981).
3. Indicate sensitivity to and acceptance of the woman's state of confusion.
4. Indicate that hope exists. As the woman develops a sense of hope, her ability to formulate realistic goals increases.
5. Help the woman identify and explore her options; for example, remaining in the relationship is one option among several. The woman's feeling of being controlled by the situation may be reduced as she considers her choices.
6. Offer family planning counseling, since unplanned or unwanted pregnancy is a precipitating factor in wife abuse.
7. Offer referrals for treating substance abuse and for learning problem-solving behaviors and techniques for "fighting fair" to replace violence.

The nurse *does not* do the following:

1. Berate the woman's husband/partner. The woman may be very protective of him, and negative input from the nurse may force her to sever therapeutic ties.
2. Urge or encourage the woman to leave home. She alone must make this decision. Leaving before a commitment to a different way of life is firm can bring the woman back into the situation. Studies indicate that this is a high-risk time for homicide (Elbow, 1977).

A woman indicates her readiness to leave the relationship when she indicates she is capable of planning for herself, investing in herself as a person, recognizing that the abuse is part of a continuing pattern, and when she is able to express the desire to leave when no abuse is occurring at the moment.

When the battered woman decides to leave her situation, she will benefit from the nurse's assistance. A nurse can provide her with phone numbers of shelters, support groups, legal aid, financial services, and employment training programs, if these are needed. Most cities have a Battered Women's Hotline listed in the business section of the phone book. The YWCA provides free counseling for battered women in or out of the battering relationship. A list of organizations that can be called for information on setting up a protocol for treatment and for referral of battered women can be found in Appendix H. Typical shelters provide women and children with rooms, beds, food, clothing, and other basic supplies. The woman's length of stay may be limited by the shelter to 30 to 90 days.

Anticipatory guidance is imperative. The battered woman needs help to realize that violence will recur. She needs to decide what she will do the next time (e.g., use an exit plan). An **exit plan** includes the phone numbers for the police and a battered women's hotline; where she will run to for safety; a suitcase packed ahead of time with birth certificates, marriage license, bank accounts, copy of deed and will, toys, clothes, insurance papers, and an extra set of house and car keys.

Many nurses become frustrated when a battered woman returns to a previously abusive situation. Nurses as caregivers need to feel that they have made a difference. It is important to remember that many victims have been abused for a long time, making it difficult for them to seek and accept help. Goodman (1990) found that more than 50% of battered women return to the environment that perpetuates the abuse even when they are provided with shelter facilities.

Prevention measures need to be identified and implemented. Parents should be encouraged to teach their children more androgynous sex roles (e.g., both sexes are equal; both sexes can be nurturing; neither needs to engage in violent behavior). Health care workers should encourage/reinforce nurturing behaviors in male clients. Assertiveness training and self-defense courses should be offered to help women become more assertive and confident.

EVALUATION

The nurse can be reasonably assured that care was effective to the extent that goals and expected outcomes for care have been achieved. That is: the battered woman is identified, she is protected from further abuse, she perceives herself as deserving of respect, she reestablishes a feeling of control, she identifies her areas of strength and develops goals for herself, she increases her knowledge of options and community resources, her physical injuries are treated promptly, and if she is pregnant, her fetus and children are protected from abuse.

■ SEXUAL ABUSE

Childhood sexual abuse is defined as (1) a child less than 18 years old at the time of the first molestation, (2) at least a 3-year age difference between the victim and perpetrator, and (3) the presence of physical contact of a sexual nature between the victim and the perpetrator (e.g., fondling of the genitalia, buttocks, or breasts; oral or anal sodomy; and attempted or actual genital intercourse) (Hunter, 1991). Childhood sexual abuse acts, according to law, are acts perpetrated by someone responsible for care of the child, such as the parents, grandparent, day care provider, or babysitter. If a stranger commits sexual abuse, it is considered **sexual assault** (National Center on Child Abuse and Neglect, 1989). **Incest** is sexual abuse by a father, mother, stepparent, or significantly older sibling (Tower, 1989). The peak abuse ages are between 7 and 12 years of age (Hunter, 1991; Koop, 1985).

Historically, the numbers of reported cases of sexual abuse are believed to be much lower than the actual incidence. Psychologic constraints such as guilt, repression, and shame have prevented victims from revealing their experiences (Kinzl, 1991). The passage of the 1974 Child Abuse Prevention and Treatment Act and the women's movement have facilitated public acknowledgment of the prevalence of childhood sexual abuse (Hurley, 1991).

Childhood sexual abuse is associated with delayed onset, post-traumatic stress disorder (p. 1350) (Elliott, 1991; Kinzl, 1991; Petit, 1991). Sexual assault in pregnancy also has been studied (see Research Highlight below).

■ NURSING PROCESS

ASSESSMENT

Female sexual abuse and assault victims appear to be the largest single group to experience post-traumatic stress disorder (Koss, 1990). Therefore

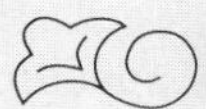 **Research Highlight** 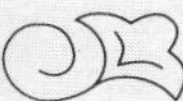

Sexual Assault in Pregnancy

RESEARCH ABSTRACT

There is little known about the effects of sexual assault on pregnant women and the outcomes of their pregnancies. A retrospective review of records of sexual assault victims during a 5-year period was conducted. There were 5734 sexual assaults; 114 (2%) of the victims were pregnant. The demographics, patterns of injury, and forensic evidence in the pregnant victims were compared with 114 matched nonpregnant victims of sexual assault. Pregnancy outcome was compared with that of the hospital obstetric population. The typical victim was an African-American multigravida in her twenties with no prenatal care. Mean gestational age at time of assault was 15 weeks. Type of penetration was similar in both groups: vulvar (85%), oral (27%), and anal (6%). Nonpregnant victims experienced more physical trauma, especially genital trauma. There were more injuries to the head, neck, and extremities than to the abdomen, chest, or back. Low-birth-weight and preterm births were common, but there were no births or spontaneous abortions within 4 weeks of the assault.

IMPLICATIONS FOR PRACTICE

The frequency of sexual assault is increasing in the United States. It is likely that nurses will come in contact with victims of sexual assault in the emergency room or in the maternity unit. Nurses need special training in dealing sensitively with the victims of such assault. Since the majority of sexual assaults are never reported, nurses can participate in educational programs about the prevention of sexual assault and the importance of reporting assaults if they occur. Nurses can work for legislative reform that ensures protection of victims and with community agencies that work with assault victims.

RELATED RESEARCH QUESTIONS

1. Is maternal-infant interaction affected by sexual assault during pregnancy?
2. Will an educational program in prevention of sexual assault decrease the incidence of rape?
3. Are the psychologic sequelae of sexual assault during pregnancy different from the sequelae of sexual assault in a nonpregnant victim?
4. Will an educational program directed at adolescents result in an increase in the number of sexual assaults that are reported?

REFERENCE

Satin AJ et al: Sexual assault in pregnancy, *Obstet Gynecol* 77(5):710, 1991.

nurses and all health care providers must assess for the physical and psychosocial signs and symptoms typical of incest survivors. With open discussion of sexual abuse, marked changes have been observed in survivors with mental disorders (Kinzl, 1991).

The history obtained from an interview and review of medical records may reveal cues suggestive of sexual abuse. A history of self-inflicted injuries may be indicative of post-traumatic stress disorder: cutting oneself, nail biting, hair pulling, broken bones, recurrent nightmares, and substance abuse (Muhovich, 1990). Long-term symptoms are found in some incest survivors. These include sexual dysfunction or maladjustment, difficulty with interpersonal relationships, avoidance of intimacy, low self-esteem, and anti-male feelings (Coker, 1990). Suicidal ideation, chronic depression, and guilt feelings have also been identified in adult incest survivors (Brown, Garrison, 1990). Clients may exhibit feelings of self-blame, shame, body rejection, anxiety, fear, mistrust, and hatred.

A thorough physical examination may be anxiety-provoking and/or physically uncomfortable. Scalp hair is examined for bald spots; eyes for scleral hemorrhages, detached retina, or ecchymoses; skin for bruises in various stages of healing, cuts, scars, human bites, burns, or evidence of substance abuse (see Chapter 33); fingernails for biting to the raw flesh; and vaginal discharge for STDs (see Chapter 29). Posture, grooming, and general nutritional state (see Chapter 9) add to the data base for level of self-esteem.

Laboratory and diagnostic test results add to the diagnosis. STDs, substance abuse, and x-ray evidence of fractures in various stages of healing may be found.

NURSING DIAGNOSES

Nursing diagnoses are based on analysis of the assessment findings. Potential diagnoses may include:

- Self-esteem disturbance
- Sexual dysfunction
- Sleep pattern disturbance
- Anxiety
- Decisional conflict
- High risk for self- or other-inflicted injury

PLANNING

Planning for the adult incest survivor includes *goals* for the survivor to be able to recognize that abuse occurred, to share the story, and to begin a growth process. *Outcome criteria* may include that the survivor, with the assistance of the nurse, psychologist, and/or counselor, will be able to:

- Remove blocks to memory of the sexual abuse.
- Describe the personal history of the abuse.
- Participate in a group therapy process.
- Identify fears and anxieties.
- Express a sense of hope.
- Reminisce and review life positively.
- Express confidence in self and others.
- Verbalize realistic goals.
- Discuss effect past had on present behaviors and feelings.
- Demonstrate initiative, self-direction, and autonomy in decision making.

IMPLEMENTATION

Many authors and researchers support the use of group therapy for incest survivors in decreasing depression, anger and guilt, reducing isolation, improving self-esteem, and developing effective coping mechanisms (Axelroth, 1991; Alexander, 1991; Coker, 1990; Petit, 1991; Tower, 1989). Al-Anon provides groups specific to incest survivors at no cost. Al-Anon is based on the 12-step program of Alcoholics Anonymous.

Keeping a diary often helps survivors connect with repressed feelings. This technique can be a safe way to describe the abuse and to explore their lives.

Another therapeutic action is to encourage survivors to spend time with children who are the same age as they were at the time they experienced the abuse. This therapeutic action provides a basis for understanding that children are not capable of thinking logically or refusing the perpetrator (Coker, 1990). Looking at pictures of themselves as children, survivors can reflect on their innocence and powerlessness at that level of development.

Nursing can facilitate healing and growth by providing education on the effects of sexual abuse of children, power differences of age and gender, current issues for women, assertive behaviors, and constructive ways to handle anger. The need for affection is differentiated from sexual desires (Petit, 1991). With open discussion of the abuse, marked changes have been observed in survivors with mental disorders (Kinzl, 1991).

Some form of confrontation with the perpetrator and caretakers is necessary for recovery to be complete (Coker, 1990; Kinzl, 1991). Confrontation helps to place the anger where it belongs and gives survivors a sense of personal power. However, survivors must identify what they hope to accomplish by the confrontation. If they hope to get an apology or validation from the perpetrator, then the confrontation will more than likely be unsuccessful. The survivor must focus on her own change and validate her experience for herself by the confrontation.

Most prevention programs are directed at teaching children to recognize inappropriate behavior from adults. Children can participate in games to explore potentially dangerous situations and the importance of saying "no." Studies are needed to determine if these programs are effective in preventing sexual abuse.

EVALUATION

Evaluation may be somewhat difficult because some changes are hard to evaluate objectively or because the woman (family) may not return for care. Intervention can be considered effective to the extent that goals for care have been met. That is: the survivor removes blocks to memory of the sexual abuse, describes the personal history of the abuse, participates in a group therapy process, identifies fears and anxieties, expresses a sense of hope, reminisces and reviews life positively, expresses confidence in self and others, verbalizes realistic goals, discusses the effect her past had on present behaviors and feelings, and demonstrates initiative, self-direction, and autonomy in decision making.

■ RAPE

"For any person who has been raped, I want them to know that they can get better. You can take power and control over your life again . . . having something like this happen in your life can make you evaluate many other things. There's a chance for real personal growth. You can actually make positive things come out of it. All it takes is time." (Words of a 21-year-old female student who had been raped by 5 men at the age of 16.)

Forcible rape is a crime that women may fear more than any other. **Rape,** a legal and not a medical entity, is defined differently from state to state. In many jurisdictions, rape, in its strictest sense, is the penile penetration of the female sex organ, or labia in some states, without her consent. Rape is also defined as an act of sexual intercourse committed by a man with a woman not his wife and without her consent, committed when the woman's resistance is overcome by force or fear, or under other prohibitive condition (Black, 1990). As of 1989, legislators in 11 out of 50 states have eliminated the "with a woman not his wife" clause (Weingourt, 1990). Penetration by any other male appendage or other object or penile penetration of any other orifice constitutes **sexual assault,** another legal term. Hymenal penetration or ejaculation does not have to occur. The key feature to establish rape is the *absence of consent:* threat or coercion implies the lack of consent. The victim who is mentally retarded, is unconscious or otherwise physically unable to move, has been drugged without her knowledge, or is a minor (statutory rape) is not capable of giving consent. It is up to the court to prove absence of consent; hence the term *alleged rape* or *alleged sexual assault* is used in medical records.

Several states have laws defining rape in terms of a perceived threat to the victim's well-being. Sometimes the threat is simple to describe. If the rapist uses a weapon such as a gun or knife, the threat is obvious; if he first engages the intended victim in conversation or is admitted by her into her home and then rapes her without a weapon, the threat she perceives may be more difficult to prove. Defense attorneys have used the argument that the woman gave implicit consent for intercourse by the fact that she let the rapist into her apartment, engaged in conversation with him in a bar, or made no attempt to get help during the attack. In court, the victim had to prove "utmost" resistance to successfully prosecute. However, "utmost" resistance may place her life in jeopardy (NOW Legal Defense, 1987).

Some couples willingly engage in violent sexual acts, considered perverse by many; legal defense could focus on showing that the victim gave consent to enter into sexual behaviors in spite of the risk for injury.

Rape is a violent crime on the increase. Since there are many reasons that deter a woman from reporting the crime, accurate statistics concerning psychosocial and demographic variables relating to rape are not available.

Women do not report rape because of the associated stigma or out of embarrassment; guilt that in some way they provoked the assault; fear of retribution from the rapist or his friends; dread of being humiliated and figuratively "raped" again by the police, the court, or the publicity; and discouragement generated by the dismally small number of convictions, to name a few reasons. Victims often fear the reactions of husbands, lovers, friends, family, and children, and they prefer to suffer alone.

Most men are not aware of the effort that women must exert to avoid becoming victims. In a criminal law class at the University of Kentucky, a professor asked the male students to share what they do every day to prevent sexual assault. There was no response. However, after hearing how the females in the class must continually protect themselves from sexual assault, they were astounded (Goldfarb, 1991). The anticipatory fear of rape in women, the trauma experienced during an attack, and the terror that persists after the attack are all damaging to women's lives (Krall, 1990).

Dynamics of Rape

Power and control surface as explanations for the perpetuation of rape in our society (Koss, 1990; Sampselle, 1991; Walker, 1989). Stets (1991) suggests men's use of physical aggression reflects and reinforces a societal norm to maintain power and control in a patriarchal system. In an aggressive society the stronger member is permitted the use of his strength to satisfy desires. The convenient myth that the female secretly desires to be raped makes the use of force more acceptable. For example, a survey of college-age men found that 51% would rape a woman if they thought they would not be punished; furthermore, they felt the woman would enjoy it (Sampselle, 1991). Other myths that continue to exist are: "there is no such thing as a *real* rape," or women "ask for it" by dressing and acting in a sexually provocative way (Stuart, Greer, 1984).

Rape is not an act of lust, nor is it an overzealous release of passion. Rape is a violent, aggressive assault on the body and integrity of the victim. As one victim said: "No matter how terrible people think rape is, it's worse than they know. It's like a bomb going off at the center of your soul."

The rapist has no regard for his victim's age, race, sexual attraction, or physical condition—10-day-old infants, as well as handicapped elderly women confined to wheelchairs, have been raped. Most rapes occur *intra*racially rather than *inter*racially. The victim often knows her attacker as a casual acquaintance or as a friend of long standing, or he may be a complete stranger to her.

Types of Rape

Two main types of rape have been identified. **Acquaintance rape** involves a perpetrator with whom the victim had a previous nonviolent relationship, but who uses deceit and coercion to obtain sex from a nonconsenting partner (Warshaw, 1988). Two types of acquaintance rape are wife rape and date rape. **Wife rape** is the sexual experience with a man the victim was either legally married to or considered married under common law. Wife rape has three characteristics: (1) attempted or actual vaginal, digital, anal, or oral sexual activity; (2) use of force or threat to use force; and (3) absence of freely given consent (Weingourt, 1990). **Date rape** refers to forced sexual contact within the context of what could be construed as a date or the preliminaries of what could possibly lead to a date (McIvor, Harting, 1990). The second main type of rape is **Blitz** (stranger) **rape,** which occurs when the victim and assailant are strangers and the rape is sudden and often involves weapons (Nichaus, 1986).

Nichaus (1986) describes four other categories of rape:

Confidence rape: deceit is the major characteristic of confidence rape; for example, the date who uses coercion to obtain sex when the partner is a reluctant, unconsenting acquaintance. This kind of rape is common and seldom reported because the woman is afraid of being considered an accomplice to the rape.

Power rape: the man's victims are usually strangers attacked in a blitz rape. By dominating his victim, the man places the woman in the powerless position he experiences and despises. He fantasizes sexual conquest as a demonstration of his strength and potency. He believes that the woman enjoys the experience.

Anger rape: this is a revenge rape. The assailant uses rape to symbolically punish a significant woman in his life. These are impulse rapes characterized by considerable brutality and trauma.

Sadistic rape: sadism usually characterizes all of the sadistic rapist's relationships. They eroticize their aggression. They abuse and torture the woman until they are completely out of control. In a frenzy, he may commit a "lust murder."

Rape Trauma Syndrome

In order to assess and provide care to a woman who experiences a rape, a nurse must first understand the psychologic effect of **rape trauma syndrome.** This syndrome is marked by confusion and disorder immediately following an attempted or forcible sexual assault. It includes a process of reorganization that is long term. Rape trauma syndrome is experienced by all survivors of sexual assault (Gulanick et al, 1990). Rape is a realization of a woman's worst nightmare, and the rape survivor needs the acceptance and anticipatory guidance of a caring nurse. Table 43-3 shows the phases and responses related to rape trauma syndrome. It should be understood that the phases overlap, and individual responses are varied.

Post-traumatic stress disorder (PTSD) is similar to the rape trauma syndrome in many respects. It is

TABLE 43-3 Phases and Responses Related to Rape Trauma Syndrome

Phase	Response
Acute	Anxiety Hostility Aggression Denial Withdrawal Guilt Emotional outbursts Abrupt changes in relationships with men Sense of humiliation
Long-term	Repetitive nightmares Reliving assault Phobias, including fear of being indoors or outdoors, fear of being alone or in crowds, and fear of men or spouse Reactivated life problems (i.e., physical or psychiatric illnesses) Alcohol or drug abuse Sleep disturbances Eating disturbances GI irritability Sexual dysfunctioning Depression or loss of self-esteem

From Michael Reese Hospital: *Nursing care plans: diagnosis and intervention,* ed 2, St Louis, 1990, Mosby–Year Book.

defined as the development of physiologic or behavioral signs and symptoms following a psychologically traumatic event that is generally outside the range of usual human experience. There are three types of traumatic events: (1) natural, (2) accidental, and (3) intentional (Lancaster, 1988). Three main symptom clusters associated with post-traumatic stress disorder include recurrent nightmares or recollection of the event, numbing of responsiveness or reduced interaction with the external world, and symptoms of anxiety (Lancaster, 1988; McLeer, 1988).

ACUTE PHASE: DISORGANIZATION. The assault itself marks the beginning of this phase of rape trauma syndrome, which can last for several days or up to 3 weeks (Gordon, Riger, 1989). Reactions such as shock, denial, and disbelief are similar to those described by Kübler-Ross in grief and dying (for a discussion of loss and grief, see Chapter 40). In addition, the rape survivor is embarrassed, degraded, fearful, angry, vengeful, and usually blames herself. She feels unclean and wants to bathe and douche despite the fact she may be destroying evidence. Her affect may change rapidly from crying to being calm and controlled. She relives the scene over and over in her mind and considers things she "should have done." Physiologically she may be uncomfortable, experiencing skeletal muscle pain or tension, gastrointestinal irritability, sighing respirations, hyperventilation, flushing, and/or a sense of feeling too hot or too cold.

LONG-TERM PROCESS: REORGANIZATION. This phase has been described as consisting of three phases (Beebe, 1990). During the *adjustment phase,* the survivor may appear to have resolved her crisis. She may return to a job or to maintaining a household, or both, but she is denying and suppressing her thoughts and feelings. She needs this time to regain some control in her life. She may move, change jobs, buy a weapon to protect herself, or install an alarm system in her home. She becomes less interested in discussing the rape.

The second reorganization phase is that of *integration.* Denial and suppression cannot be maintained forever. Pennebaker (1990) states that the more people try to suppress thoughts and feelings, the stronger those thoughts and feelings get, and the more power and control they have over people's lives. Disclosing personal thoughts and feelings has a profound effect in improving health and reducing stress (Pennebaker, 1990). As a rape survivor's suppression of feelings and emotions starts to deteriorate, she becomes depressed and anxious. Her own healthy spirit pressures her to discuss the rape with someone. Since she is losing her control of denial, her fears start to surface; she may be afraid to be alone or to be in a crowd, or may fear being attacked from behind.

The last reorganization phase is that of *recovery.* During this phase, which may take weeks to years, the survivor returns to her previous level of functioning (Rowland, 1985). The victim has progressed through recovery when the physical distress and the constant memories of the rape have diminished.

Nightmares and eating disorders are very common in these last two phases. If the woman has been prepared by a sensitive nurse or counselor during this phase, the outcome may be a new self-concept and an awareness of how reorganization has helped her to grow.

Rape affects everyone who comes in contact with the victim. The family also experiences the acute phase of disorganization and the long-term process of reorganization (Burgess, Holmstrom, 1974a). Nursing care and counseling should include the family and close friends of the victim.

■ NURSING PROCESS

ASSESSMENT

Since rape is a crime, nursing care must be guided by the need to preserve evidence. However, preservation of evidence should not overshadow a survivor's rights (see box below). Women tend not to report forced sex unless questioned carefully and sensitively (Weingourt, 1990). To assist the nurse with a comprehensive assessment, most sexual assault treatment centers have standard assessment guidelines for obtaining and recording pertinent data.

Consent forms must be signed before evidence can be collected and released to the police and before photographs can be taken. If the victim is under 16 years of age, a pediatrician is notified. A parent or guardian is required to sign the consent forms. The children's protective service may need to be called to facilitate consent.

HISTORY. The history includes the client's age, allergies, and *menstrual* history, including the age of menarche, date of last menstrual period (LMP), and menstrual pattern. If LMP was not normal, the woman is asked to describe it. Her *obstetric* history is determined: gravidity, parity, date of termination of last pregnancy, and, if she thinks she may be pregnant now, symptoms she is experiencing. She is asked to describe her *sexual* history: the date and

The Rights of the Rape Survivor

The rape victim has the right:

1. To transportation to a hospital when incapacitated.
2. To emergency room care with privacy and confidentiality.
3. To be listened to carefully and treated as a human being, with respect, courtesy, and dignity.
4. To have an advocate of choice accompany her through the treatment process.
5. To be given as much credibility as a victim of any other crime.
6. To have her name kept from the news media.
7. To be considered a victim of rape regardless of the assailant's relationship to her.
8. Not to be exposed to prejudice against race, age, class, life-style, or occupation.
9. Not to be asked questions about prior sexual experience.
10. To be treated in a manner that does not usurp her control but enables her to determine her own needs and how to meet them.
11. To be asked only those questions that are relevant to a court case or to medical treatment.
12. To receive prompt medical and mental health services, regardless of whether the rape is reported to the police.
13. To be protected from future assault.
14. To accurate collection and preservation of evidence for court in an objective record that includes the signs and symptoms of physical and emotional trauma.
15. To receive clear explanations of procedures and medication in language she can understand.
16. To know what treatment is recommended, for what reasons, and who will administer the treatment.
17. To know any possible risks, side effects, or alternatives to proposed treatments, including all drugs prescribed.
18. To ask for another physician, nurse practitioner, or nurse.
19. To consent to or refuse any treatment, even when her life is in serious danger.
20. To refuse to be part of any research or experiment.
21. To make reasonable complaints, and to leave a care facility against the physician's advice.
22. To receive an explanation of and understand any papers she agrees to sign.
23. To be informed of continuing health care needs after discharge from the emergency room, hospital, physician's office, or care facility.
24. To receive a clear explanation of the bill and review of charges and to be informed of available compensation.*
25. To have legal representation and be advised of her legal rights, including the possiblity of filing a civil suit.

From Foley TS, Davies MA: *Rape: nursing care of victims*, St Louis, 1983, Mosby–Year Book.

*A bill for treatment, sent to the victim, adds insult to injury. Many municipalities have funds to cover these costs (see p. 1355).

time of the most recent coitus before the alleged assault and whether a condom was used, her current mode of contraception, whether she was a virgin before the assault, whether she uses tampons, whether she uses douches, and the date of the last douche.

The woman is asked to describe the *assault* (she may need support and assistance in verbalizing the offender's acts): Did the penis enter the vagina? Did he have an orgasm? Was there oral or anal penetration? Did he wear a condom? She is asked to recount her *activity since the assault;* Did she douche, bathe or shower, or defecate or urinate? How, when, and from whom did she seek assistance afterward?

PHYSICAL EXAMINATION AND LABORATORY TESTS. The physical examination is conducted after the procedure is explained to the woman. She remains clothed* while her vital signs and blood pressure are determined, and her clothing is inspected for stains, tears, and foreign material. She is assisted to undress and is draped; a female attendant, rape counselor, or other person of her choice may remain with her during the examination. The physician informs her of every step of the procedure. Her body is inspected for bruises, swelling, scratches, lacerations, stab wounds, and body lice. A head-to-toe examination is performed. Special attention is given to the area assaulted (e.g., pelvic structures and genitals).

External genitals, thighs, buttocks, and lower abdomen are assessed, and if there are injuries, photographs may be taken or drawings made. A new test, not yet acceptable to the courts, is toluidine blue staining; a positive toluidine blue staining of the vulva occurs in a significant percentage of rape victims but rarely in women who have coitus with consent (Lauber and Souma, 1982; Shepard, 1983).

A speculum examination (no lubricant is used) is performed gently to detect tears or bruises and to collect appropriate specimens. The cervix is scraped for *Neisseria gonorrhoeae* culturing, and vaginal fluid is obtained for analysis. One slide is fixed and dried to be stained and examined for sperm, a swab of fluid is placed in saline solution for potential sperm serovaring and a sample is assayed for acid phosphatase.†

A bimanual pelvic examination is performed carefully to determine the size and position of the uterus and adnexa. If a pelvic mass is palpated, it may be caused by bleeding into the broad ligament. If pregnancy is a possibility, a pregnancy test is done. Internal pelvic assessment is ended with a rectovaginal examination.

Blood is drawn for a Venereal Disease Research Laboratory (VDRL) test and antibodies for HIV. Any x-ray films or photographs that were taken are noted at this time.

Additional specimens are obtained for evidence to document the identity of the offender.

1. Swabs are taken from all orifices if she is unconscious, or as deemed appropriate from the woman's history. Slides are prepared from the material on the swabs and allowed to air-dry. The slides are placed into mailers; the swabs are put into one test tube.
2. Contents of the vaginal vault are aspirated and put into another test tube.
3. The woman's pubic hair is combed; the comb and adhering hair are placed into an envelope, sealed, and labeled "combings." At least 12 of her pubic hairs are pulled out by the roots (or hair is clipped very close to the skin), placed into an envelope, and labeled "pubic hair samples."
4. Fingernail scrapings are placed into a separate envelope and labeled.

All slides, envelopes, test tubes, and slide mailers must be labeled personally by the examining physician with a Carborundum pencil, with the woman's name, the date and time, and the site from which the specimen was taken. Her clothes are put into a paper bag, sealed, and labeled. All transactions—obtaining her specimens, packaging them, labeling them, and giving them over to either the police or a laboratory technician—are witnessed and signed by both the giver and the receiver; the time and date are also noted.

During the examination the woman's *emotional status* is assessed and findings are recorded; which impact reactions she is exhibiting, her orientation to time and place, and her attention span, affect, and verbal description and feelings about the assault. The availability of family or peer support systems is assessed. She is asked about her plans to report or not report the crime to the police.

Nursing Diagnoses

Following are nursing diagnoses for the immediate and later posttrauma periods.

Immediate posttrauma period:

- Anxiety/fear related to
  —The experience itself
- —The interactions with police and caregivers
- —The physical examination to assess injury and collect evidence

*An ultraviolet light (Wood's lamp) will cause semen to fluoresce even if the man has had a vasectomy. The fluorescent areas of the body and clothing can then be identified for further examination and for sources of specimens for acid phosphatase determination. Specimens can be aspirated or scraped off, appropriately packaged, and labeled.

†Acid phosphatase is an enzyme found in high concentrations in seminal fluid.

- Pain related to
  - —The experience itself
  - —The examination
- Rape trauma syndrome, silent or compound reaction, related to
  - —The experience
- High risk for injury related to
  - —The experience
- Self-esteem disturbance related to
  - —Post-trauma syndrome
- High risk for decisional conflict related to
  - —Possible pregnancy

Later post-trauma period:

- Post-trauma response (phobias) related to
  - —Post-trauma syndrome
- High risk for infection with sexually transmitted diseases (STDs) related to
  - —The experience
- High risk for impaired social interaction related to
  - —Rape trauma syndrome

PLANNING

Planning for care for victims of rape, sexual assault, or incest requires the same sensitivity, understanding, and knowledge as that needed for the care of the battered woman.

Priorities of personnel who provide care to victims of rape or sexual assault in hospital-based sexual assault centers or in community-based rape crisis centers should include the following (Klingbeil et al, 1976):

1. An emotional support system for the family, friends, and parents, as well as for the victim
2. A sensitive health care system to provide optimum care and to document objective data
3. Presentation of information and education sessions to health care providers, educators, students, members of criminal justice systems, and community groups
4. Interaction and effective communication with the criminal justice system at all levels
5. Involvement with community interest groups concerned with the problems of sexual assault

GOALS

1. The woman's care is provided in a nonjudgmental, caring, and unhurried manner
2. All evidence is collected during the examination, and all laboratory specimens are individually packaged and carefully labeled, dated, and sealed; receipts are obtained from the laboratory technicians and police
3. The woman does not perceive herself to be victimized by the health care providers
4. The woman understands the phases of the rape trauma syndrome
5. The woman's antimicrobial prophylaxis for infection (e.g., for STD following rape; for tetanus or other infection following trauma from assault) is successful in preventing infection
6. Pregnancy is prevented, or if pregnancy occurs, the woman is able to make an informed decision about its management
7. The woman's physical injuries heal without disfigurement or loss of function
8. The woman participates in scheduled follow-up care
9. The woman successfully passes through all the stages in the rape trauma syndrome
10. Family bonds are strengthened; family members are supportive of each other

IMPLEMENTATION

Medical management includes (1) treating the physical injuries, (2) providing prophylaxis for infection (e.g., gonorrhea, tetanus) and (3) providing prophylaxis for pregnancy if the woman is not pregnant already. If physical trauma is life-threatening, appropriate intervention takes precedence over collecting evidence.

IMMEDIATE CARE. If the victim is menarchal, is using no contraception, and is at a time of high risk for pregnancy in her cycle, hormonal therapy may be prescribed for her. Hormonal therapy such as ethinyl estradiol (Estinyl) may be prescribed for 5 days to prevent pregnancy if the assault occurred within the previous 48 hours. She is told that the drug can cause nausea and that she should expect withdrawal bleeding shortly after finishing the therapy. Antinauseant therapy in the form of a prochlorperazine preparation (Compazine) is also prescribed to counter the side effects of high doses of estrogens. She is apprised of the availability of abortion or menstrual extraction as a backup measure. If she misses a menstrual period in spite of therapy or if she fails to have withdrawal bleeding from the estrogens, she is assessed for the β-subunit of human chorionic gonadotropin in 2 to 3 weeks (a highly accurate test for pregnancy). She has the option of continuing a pregnancy if pregnancy does occur but is warned about the teratogenic effects of estrogen in these doses.

If the woman is pregnant at the time of the assault, she should be observed for several hours for uterine contractility.

Psychologic support is provided by the manner in which the woman is signed into the emergency room, the respect she is shown, the privacy that is provided for the examination and consultation, and the manner in which the examination is carried out. Access to supplies (including mouthwash) and facilities in which to clean up, clothes to wear home, money as needed, and transportation to wherever she is staying (an alternate place may need to be found for her) add to the woman's comfort and perception of being in control.

In some facilities the social worker is notified the moment a victim is admitted; other facilities contact local rape crisis centers, usually staffed by specially trained volunteers on 24-hour call for just these types of emergencies. Some hospitals have rape trauma teams in the emergency room. The victim needs to be informed of all the steps involved in the rape examination and follow-up. Rape counselors provide ongoing support in a variety of ways. In addition to providing emotional support, transportation, etc., the counselor helps her interact with her family, friends, and various authorities, informs her of the rape trauma syndrome, and finds other resources for her as needed. Male volunteers help to counsel male members of the victim's family and peers.

DISCHARGE. The woman is discharged with medications and printed instructions about their use, printed instructions for self-care, and names and phone numbers of resource people should she require assistance. Medical follow-up in the gynecology or pediatric clinic is scheduled for 1 week for a repeat culture for gonorrhea, at 6 weeks for assessment of healing of injuries, and at 8 weeks for a repeat VDRL test and test for acquired immune deficiency syndrome (AIDS) antibodies. Repeat tests are rescheduled as necessary (Chapter 29). The woman and her counselor determine whether there is a need for additional medical or psychologic follow-up between the scheduled visits. The woman has a choice of site for follow-up—some women choose to continue with the physician who first performed the examination, others prefer their private physician, and still others need referral to a clinic in the area (city, state) to which they may have moved.

AFTER DISCHARGE. Because of the phases of recovery, follow-up telephone contact is continued until the woman has no further need of such help.

A bill for laboratory work and treatment, if sent to the victim, adds insult to injury. Not only can the bill impose a financial burden, but it is a tangible reminder of the assault and adds the indignity of having to pay a financial penalty for being a victim. Today, many municipalities are assuming the cost of examination and treatment for rape.

Education in *prevention* strategies is often offered by community agencies or rape awareness groups. The focus of the classes is usually on increasing women's awareness of situations that put them at high risk for rape or sexual assault. Other courses may teach self-defense methods or how to change personal behaviors to reduce the risk of being victimized (Warshaw, 1988). Still other courses may focus on changing societal attitudes about rape. Nurses can have a role in preventive education by offering courses or participating in courses offered by community or health care groups.

EVALUATION

The nurse can be reasonably assured that care was effective when priorities of care have been met. The woman receives care that is nonjudgmental and caring. The examination is accomplished in a nonhurried manner and meets all legal specifications. The woman does not perceive herself as a victim; she receives anticipatory guidance regarding delayed reactions; STDs and pregnancy are prevented: and family bonds are supported and strengthened. Later the woman has no adverse physical, psychologic, or emotional sequelae. See the related case study and nursing plan of care for a woman who has been raped (p. 1356).

■ JOINT COMMISSION ABUSE GUIDELINES

In its 1992 guidelines, the Joint Commission on the Accreditation of Health Care Organizations (JCAHO) now requires emergency and ambulatory care departments to have protocols on physical assault; rape or other sexual molestation; and domestic abuse of elders, spouses, partners, and children (Limandri, 1992).

These protocols must address client consent, examination, and treatment guidelines and the health care facility's responsibility for collecting evidence, photographing injuries, and releasing evidence to law enforcement officials. In addition, the emergency and ambulatory care departments must provide to victims a referral list of community-based and private family violence service agencies (Limandri, 1992).

The medical records of victims of family violence must now include detailed documentation of the examination, treatment, referral, and mandated reporting of known and/or suspected cases of abuse throughout the life cycle. JCAHO member organizations also must implement a plan for educating appropriate staff about identifying, treating, and referring abuse victims.

The specific guidelines are in the *AMH Accredita-*

CASE STUDY

Rape Trauma Syndrome: Acute Phase

Georgette Cline is a 23-year-old Caucasian woman who states she was dragged from her car and raped. She arrived at the emergency room alone, looking disheveled.

ASSESSMENT

The interview with Georgette reveals that according to her LMP, she is at midcycle, which puts her at risk for pregnancy. She asks, "He couldn't have made me pregnant, could he?" Further questioning reveals that it has been a year since her last voluntary coitus. Georgette says her side hurts where he kicked her, her left wrist is sore where he twisted it and her rectum hurts because he performed sodomy. The physical examination of Georgette reveals that she has scratches from the knife the rapist used and a right periorbital bruise where he hit her. A microscopic examination of vaginal and rectal smears indicates motile sperm. At the end of the examination Georgette states, "I thought I was going to die," and then she begins to cry.

NURSING DIAGNOSIS

Because Georgette has just been raped, the nurse identifies the following nursing diagnosis: rape trauma syndrome, acute phase.

PLANNING

A plan of care is developed with Georgette's input. One mutually defined *goal* takes priority: Georgette's physical trauma will be assessed and treated. The nurse sets *expected outcomes:* Georgette will recover from physical injuries; she will not develop STDs or become pregnant.

IMPLEMENTATION

Nursing actions are based on the nursing diagnosis, medical orders, and standards of care. Specific interventions include providing care for Georgette's physical injuries as ordered by her physician, obtaining specimens for initial assessment for STDs and pregnancy, and providing emotional support during the examination and the interview process.

EVALUATION

The extent to which goals and expected outcomes are met is used to evaluate the effectiveness of care provided. Georgette's physical injuries were examined and treated, and total recovery from these injuries was estimated to take 2 weeks. Cultures for STDs and tests for pregnancy remained negative.

CARE PLAN Rape Trauma Syndrome: Acute Phase

GOALS	INTERVENTIONS	RATIONALE	EVALUATION*
Nursing diagnosis: Rape trauma syndrome, acute phase, physical injuries.			
Georgette's physical trauma will be assessed and treated. She will not develop STDs or become pregnant.	Assess, record findings, and photograph injuries.	Findings determine appropriate therapy; careful documentation meets legal requirement.	Georgette's injuries are assessed and documented.
	Treat injuries per physician's orders. Provide comfort measures as ordered/needed.	Prevents infection, supports immune system functioning; reduces physical pain, which facilitates emotional coping.	Her injuries are treated and pain relieved.
	Obtain specimens for diagnosis of STDs and pregnancy. Administer medications per physician's order (e.g., antibiotics, analgesics.)	Establishes baseline information regarding current status of STDs/pregnancy and choice of present and future therapy.	Her test results indicate no STD or pregnancy at this time.

*May take weeks/months for evaluation to be made with certainty. Evaluation may be difficult and may need to be redone by the community health nurse or rape counselor at a later time to determine just how effective interventions have been.

CARE PLAN **Rape Trauma Syndrome: Acute Phase—cont'd**

GOALS	INTERVENTIONS	RATIONALE	EVALUATION*
Nursing diagnosis: Ineffective coping (survivor) related to sexual assault trauma.			
Georgette will verbalize feelings. She will get anticipatory guidance. She will be able to use support system.	Provide calm, supportive, safe environment. Allow time, encourage, validate her feelings.	Allows time for her to feel safe, in control of the situation, and not alone in the way she is reacting.	Georgette expresses feelings, states she feels "more in control for now."
	Explain procedures, examinations. Provide anticipatory guidance regarding the feelings or thoughts she may experience.	Provides reassurance when she actually experiences these thoughts or feelings; it is ego-strengthening to be prepared.	She states she understands but requires repetition.
	Help her determine where she will go immediately after leaving ER, (e.g., to call friend/family/community resource).	Helps her with decision making about her options for care.	A friend and a rape counselor come to be with her, arrange for a place for her to stay, and arrange future counseling/support.
Nursing diagnosis: Self-concept/body image disturbance related to sexual assault trauma.			
Georgette will make positive expressions of self-worth.	Show respect, warmth, nonjudgmental attitude; avoid accusatory or negative questions.	Relieves self-blame, guilt for happening; erases belief that rape is a sexual act—rape is a crime of violence, not passion.	Georgette expresses negative feelings toward assailant, not herself.
	Listen attentively, convey belief in what she is saying; acknowledge her feelings as valid.	Gives her feelings that she is worthy of being listened to and believed.	She states she feels more in control for now.
	Encourage presence of supportive person of her choosing, PRN.	Gives her sense of control and safety.	
	Provide anticipatory guidance to her and significant other/family. Address her special concerns (e.g., infection or pregnancy).	Alerts her and family/significant other that she and they will have reactions that are normal and may require some counseling to resolve. Preparation for possible reactions increases one's ability to cope, to make decisions, to integrate and resolve the event.	Her family/significant other express desire to help her and confirm that she is not to blame. She and family/significant other arrange for counseling.

tion Manual for Hospitals (1992), pp. 22-24, 33 and 34. Copies of this manual are usually available through hospital or health care organization quality assurance offices or through administration. All Nursing Network on Violence Against Women (NNVAW) members should obtain a copy of these guidelines and, whenever possible, work with administration to develop guidelines that are appropriate, sensitive, and accurate and do not blame the victim (Limandri, 1992).

■ SUMMARY

Violence against women is a major social problem. Society and health professionals must move beyond mere recognition of the problem to understand the dynamics of violence against women. Nurses as client advocates can intervene in the cycle of violence by helping victimized women recognize their options and take appropriate action.

REFERENCES

Axelroth E: Retrospective incest group therapy for university women, *J College Student Psychotherapy* 5(2):81, 1991.

Bagley C: The prevalence and mental health sequels of child sexual abuse in a community sample of women aged 18 to 27, *Can J Commun Mental Health* 10(1):103, Spring 1991.

Battered wives testify—no legal recourse, *San Francisco Chronicle,* p A18, Sept 17, 1987.

Beebe D: Emergency management of the adult female rape victim, *Am Fam Physician* 43(6):2041, June 1991.

Black H: *Black's law dictionary,* p 1260, St Paul, Minn, 1990, West Publishing.

Chez R: Battering in pregnancy, *National Perinatal Association* 5(2):5, 1990.

Chez R: Woman battering, *Am J Obstet Gynecol* 158(1):1, Jan 1988.

Coker L: A therapeutic recovery model for the female adult incest survivor, *Issues Mental Health Nurs* 11:109, 1990.

Collier JA: When you suspect your patient is a battered wife. *RN* 50(5):33, May 1987.

deLang C: The family place: children's therapeutic program, *Children Today,* March/April, p. 12, 1986.

Delgary K: Battered women: the issues for nursing, *NAACOG Newsletter* 12(10):9, 1985.

Drake VK: Battered women: health care problem in disguise. *Image* 14:40. June 1982.

Elbow M: Theoretical considerations of violent marriages. *Social Casework,* p 515. Nov 1977.

Elliott D: *The effects of a childhood sexual abuse on adult functioning in a national sample of professional women,* Biola University, 1991, Rosemead School of Psychology.

Finley B: Nursing process with the battered woman. *Nurse Pract* 6(4):11, 1981.

Foley TS, Davies MA: *Rape: nursing care of victims,* St Louis, 1983, Mosby–Year Book.

Follingstad D: Identification of patterns of wife abuse, *J Interpersonal Violence* 6(2):187, June 1991.

Follingstad D: Factors moderating physical and psychological symptoms of battered women, *J Fam Violence* 6(1):81, 1991.

Gelles RJ: Violence and pregnancy: are pregnant women at greater risk of abuse? *J Marriage Fam* p 841, 1988.

Gibbs N: When is it rape? *Time,* p. 48, June 3, 1991.

Goldfarb S: Violence against women: the need for a federal response, *National NOW Times* 9, Mar/April 1991.

Goodman M: Pattern changing: an approach to the abused woman's problem, *Research and Treatment Issues* 6(4):14, Winter 1990.

Gordon MT, Riger S: *The female fear,* New York, 1989, Free Press.

Griffith-Kinney J: *Contemporary women's health nursing advocacy approach,* Menlo Park, Calif, 1986, Addison-Wesley Publishing.

Michael Reese Hospital: *Nursing care plans: diagnosis and intervention,* ed 2, St Louis, 1990, Mosby–Year Book.

Hartman D: Battered women: the fight you can help them win, *Nursing Life* 37, Sept/Oct 1987.

Heise L: Crimes of gender, *World Watch* 12, March/April 1989.

Hillard PJ: Physical abuse and pregnancy, *Fam Prac Recertification* 8(9):89, 1986.

Hunter J: A comparison of the psychological maladjustment of adult males and females sexually molested as children, *J Int Violence* 6(2):205, June 1991.

Hurley D: Women, alcohol, and incest: an analytical review, *J Studies Alcohol* 52(3):253, 1991.

Kinzl J, Biebl W: Sexual abuse of girls: aspects of the genesis of mental disorders and therapeutic implications, *Acta Psychiatr Scand* 83:427, 1991.

Klaus PA, Rand MR: *Family violence, Bureau of Justice statistics (special report),* Washington, DC, 1984.

Klingbeil KS et al: Multidisciplinary care for sexual assault victims, *Nurs Pract* 1(6):21, 1976.

Koop C: *Surgeon general's workshop on violence & public health report,* Washington, DC, 1985, U.S. Department of Health & Human Services.

Koss M: The women's mental health research agenda, *Am Psychol* 45(3):374, March 1990.

Krall R: *Rape's power to dismember women's lives: personal realities and cultural forms,* 1990, School of Theology at Claremont.

Lancaster J: *Adult psychiatric nursing,* ed 3, New York, 1988, Medical Examiners Publishing.

Lauber AA, Souma ML: Use of toluidine blue for documentation of traumatic intercourse, *Obstet Gynecol* 60:644. 1982.

Levinson D: *Family violence in a cross cultural perspective,* Newbury Park, Calif, 1989, Sage.

Limandri B: The therapeutic relationship with abused women, *J Psychosoc Nursing* 25(2):9, February 1987.

Limandri B: Joint commission sets abuse guidelines, *Nursing Network on Violence Against Women Newsletter* 3(1), March 1992.

Lipman-Blumen J: *Gender roles and power,* New Jersey, 1984, Prentice-Hall.

Mandel B: Woman victimized twice—by her ex-lover and the system, *San Francisco Examiner,* Nov 2, 1986.

Martin D: *Battered wives,* New York, 1976, Pocket Books (also published by New Glide Publications).

McIvor D, Harting C: Working with female adolescent date-rape victims, *Psychiatr Nurs* 31(3):8, 1990.

McLeer S: Post-traumatic stress disorder in sexually abused children, *J Am Acad Child Adolesc Psychiatry* 27(5):650, 1988.

Miles R: *Women of the world,* Topsfield, Mass, 1989, Salem House.

Muhovich M: Clinical diagnostic signs associated with adult female incest victims, *Dissertation Abstracts International* 51(8):406, Feb 1991.

Nichaus MA: Rape In Griffith-Kenney J: *Contemporary women's health,* Menlo Park, Calif, 1986, Addison-Wesley Publishing.

NOW/Legal Defense and Education Fund, Cherow-O'Leary R: *The state-by-state guide to women's legal rights,* New York 1987, McGraw-Hill.

Parker B, Ulrich Y: A protocol of safety: research on abuse of women, *Nursing Research Consortium on Violence and Abuse* 39(4):248 July/Aug 1990.

Parker B, McFarlane J: Identifying and helping battered pregnant women, *MCN* 16:161, May/June 1991.

Pennebaker J: *Opening up: the healing power of confiding in others,* New York, 1990, William Morrow.

Petit M: Recognizing post-traumatic stress, *RN,* Vol. 54 March 1991.

Sampselle C: The role of nursing in preventing violence against women, *JOGNN* 20(6):481, Nov/Dec 1991.

Shepard M: Guide to managing the victim of rape. *Contemp OB/GYN* 22(3):253, 1983.

Stenchever M, Stenchever D: Abuse of women: an overview, *WHI* 1(4):187, Fall 1991.

Stephenson J: *Woman's roots,* 1988, Napa, Calif, Diemer, Smith Publishing.

Stets J: Psychological aggression in dating relationships: the role of interpersonal control, *J Fam Violence* 6(1):97, 1991.

Stuart GW, Sundeen SJ: *Principles and practice of psychiatric nursing,* ed 4, St Louis, 1991, Mosby–Year Book.

Stuart I, Greer J: *Victims of sexual aggression: treatment of children, women and men,* New York, 1984, Van Nostrand Reinhold.

Tower C: *Secret scars: a guide for survivors of child sexual abuse,* New York, 1988, Penguin Books.

Walker L: *The battered woman,* NY, 1979, Harper & Row.

Walker L: Psychology and violence against women, *Am Psychol* 44(4):695 April 1989.

Walker L: *The battered woman syndrome,* vol 6, New York, 1984, Springer Publishing.

Warshaw R: *I never called it rape: the Ms. report on recognizing, fighting and surviving date and acquaintance rape,* Grand Rapids, 1988, Harper & Row.

Weingourt R: Wife rape in a sample of psychiatric patients, *J Nurs Sch* 22(3):144, Fall 1990.

Whaley L, Wong D: *Nursing care of infants and children,* ed 4, St Louis, 1991, Mosby–Year Book.

Witkin-Linoil G: Too close to home, *Health,* p. 6, Jan 1987.

Wyatt G, Newcomb M: Internal and external mediators of women's sexual abuse in childhood, *J Consult Clin Psychol* 58(6):758, 1990.

Yllo K, Bogard M, editors: *Feminist perspectives on wife abuse,* London, 1988, Sage.

Zdanuk JM, Harris CC, Wisian NL: Adolescent pregnancy and incest: the nurse's role as counselor, *JOGNN* 16(2):99, 1987.

References: Nursing Research

Brown B, Garrison C: Patterns of symptomatology of adult women incest survivors, *West J Nurs Res* 12(5):587, 1990.

Bullock L, McFarlane J: birthweight/battering connection, *AJN,* p. 153, Sept 1989.

Helton A, McFarlane J, Anderson E: Battered and pregnant: a prevalence study, *Am J Public Health* 77(10):1337, Oct 1987.

BIBLIOGRAPHY

Brendtro M, Bowker L: Battered women: how can nurses help? *Issues Mental Health Nurs* 10(2):169, 1989.

Bullock L: Battering among pregnant teenagers: a unique role for the school nurse, *School Nurse,* Feb 1990.

Butler J, Burton L: Rethinking teenage childbearing: is sexual abuse a missing link? *Fam Relations* 39:73, 1990.

Campbell J: The second national nursing conference on violence against women, *Response* 10(2):27, 1987.

Campbell J, Alford P: The dark consequences of marital rape, *AJN* 89(7):946, July 1989.

Campbell J: Women's responses to sexual abuse in intimate relationships, *Health Care for Women International* 10:335, 1989.

Copenhaver S, Grauerholz E: Sexual victimization among sorority women: exploring the link between sexual violence and institutional practices, *Sex Roles* 24(1/2), 1991.

Erickson R, Drenovsky C: The decision to leave an abusive relationship: the testing of an alternate methodological approach, *J Fam Violence* 5(3):237, 1990.

Finklehor D: Sexual abuse in a national survey of adult men and women: prevalence, characteristics, and risk factors, *Child Abuse and Neglect* 14:19, 1990.

Furby L, Weinrott M, Blackshaw L: Sex offender recidivism: a review, *Psychol Bull* 105(1):3, 1989.

Geffner B: Family abuse and ethical issues, *Family Violence Bulletin* 6(4), Winter 1990.

Hughes H: Psychological adjustment of children of battered women: influences of gender, *Family Violence Bulletin* 7(1):15, Spring 1991.

Humphreys J: Children of battered women: worries about their mothers, *Pediatr Nurs* 17(4):342, July/Aug 1991.

Kleinke C, Meyer C: Evaluation of rape victim by men and women with high and low belief in a just world, *Psychol Women Quarterly* 14:343, 1990.

Kramer T, Green B: Post-traumatic stress disorder as an early response to sexual assault, *J Interpersonal Violence* 6(2):160, June 1991.

Langford D: Consortia: a strategy for improving the provision of health care to domestic violence survivors, *Response* 13(1):17, 1990.

McLeer S, Anward R: A study of battered women presenting in an emergency department, *Am J Public Health* 79(1), Jan 1989.

Perry B, Conroy L, Ravitz A: Persisting psychophysiological effects of traumatic stress: the memory of "states," *Violence Update* 1(8):1, April 1991.

Satin A: Sexual assault in pregnancy, *Obstet Gynecol* 77(5):710, 1991.

Simons R, Whitbeck L: Sexual abuse as a precursor to prostitution and victimization among adolescent and adult homeless women, *J Family Issues* 12(3):361, Sept 1991.

chapter 43 review

Key Concepts

- One out of every three women will experience some form of violence.
- Perpetuation of violence against women is influenced by the historical and societal norm of valuing women.
- Nurses must explore their values and beliefs concerning violence against women in order to identify and intervene effectively.
- The true incidence of childhood sexual abuse, rape, and battering will not be known until women feel free to report the crime and are not revictimized by the system.
- The abuse of spouses/partners occurs at all socioeconomic levels as well as all educational levels.
- Pregnancy is often a time of initial or increased battering incidences.
- The rapist has no regard for his victim's age, race, sexual attraction, or physical condition.
- Rape is not just a woman's problem; it is a community problem.

Key Terms

- abuse (p. 1338)
- acquaintance rape (p. 1350)
- battery (p. 1338)
- blitz rape (p. 1350)
- childhood sexual abuse (p. 1347)
- cycle of violence (p. 1341)
- date rape (p. 1350)
- exit plan (p. 1346)
- incest (p. 1347)
- learned helplessness (p. 1339)
- post-traumatic stress disorder (PTSD) (p. 1350)
- rape (p. 1349)
- rape trauma syndrome (p. 1350)
- sexual assault (p. 1338, 1349)
- wife rape (p. 1350)

Critical Thinking Exercise

You are observing the care given to a rape victim in the Emergency Room.

1. Describe your feelings regarding the victim.
2. What feelings do you think the victim might have about herself and about seeking care?
3. How can the nurse demonstrate a supportive role to the victim?
4. Examine newspaper reports of alleged rape attacks and rape trials. What are your feelings about how the victim is viewed by the media and by the legal system?
5. What role do you think nurses have in educating the public about violence against women?
6. Design an educational strategy for rape prevention.

Topics for Nursing Research

- Develop instruments that can screen for the long-term sequelae of sexual abuse in childhood.
- Study treatment methods and outcomes of victims currently found in the community.
- Identify methods of prevention, specifically the sexual education of children, and their effect on decreasing sexual abuse of children.
- Examine reasons some incest-surviving women become substance abusers and some do not.
- Examine reasons some incest-surviving women become prostitutes and some do not.
- Study the cumulative effects of chronic sexual assaults on post-traumatic stress disorder (PTSD) symptoms.
- Study how supportive vs. nonsupportive environments affect those symptoms.
- Investigate the effects of providing anticipatory guidance on PTSD to survivors of sexual assault.
- Investigate the impact of rigid sex-role socialization on gender behavior.
- Measure both individual and situational variables that have been identified by survivors of abuse.
- Perform longitudinal studies to measure the impact of sexual violence on the child's subsequent behavior.
- Compare current aggressive family relations and the historical patterns of aggression found in the family of origin.

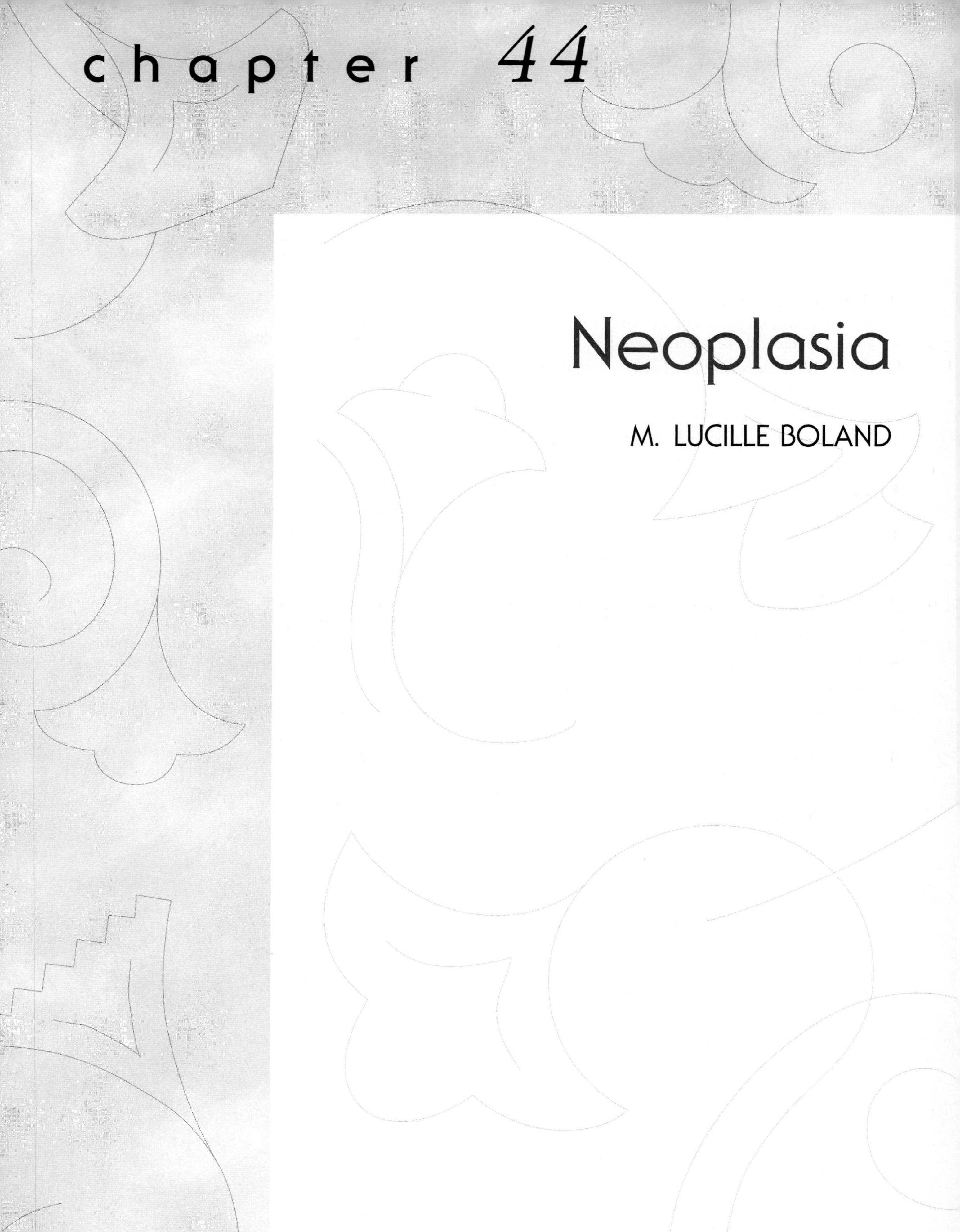

chapter 44

Neoplasia

M. LUCILLE BOLAND

LEARNING OBJECTIVES

- Define the key terms listed.
- Discuss the pathophysiology of selected benign and malignant neoplasms of the female reproductive tract.
- Identify the common medical therapies for selected conditions.
- Discuss the emotional impact of benign and malignant neoplasms.
- Develop a nursing plan of care for the woman with a lump in her breast.
- Develop a nursing plan of care for a woman with endometrial cancer, having undergone radical hysterectomy.
- Explain diagnostic procedures in client-centered terms.
- Explain treatments for preinvasive and invasive conditions.
- Review health-promoting behaviors that reduce cancer risk.
- Assess the impact of benign and malignant neoplasms on pregnancy.
- Discuss the development and sequelae of gestational trophoblastic neoplasia.
- Identify critical elements for teaching clients with selected benign or malignant neoplasms.
- Identify topics for nursing research related to gynecologic neoplasia.

Neoplasia refers to the growth of new tissue, also known as a tumor, that serves no physiologic function. These tumors can be either benign or malignant. **Benign** tumors usually do not endanger life, tend to grow slowly, and are not invasive. **Malignant** tumors grow rapidly in a disorganized manner and invade surrounding tissues. When this occurs, the common term used to describe this phenomenon is **cancer.**

When neoplasias occur in the female reproductive system, they may involve both the primary and secondary sex organs. The impact of the development of benign or malignant neoplasms can have far-reaching effects for the woman and her family. Beyond the obvious physiologic alterations, the woman also experiences threats to her self-concept and her ability to cope. A woman's concept of herself as a sexual being can be affected by the condition and its treatments. A woman's family is also challenged in the way it responds to her diagnosis of neoplasia. When neoplasia occurs with pregnancy, it adds to the complexity of both physical and emotional responses to childbearing.

Nurses have important roles in teaching women about early detection and treatment and in providing supportive care to clients and their families. This chapter presents information that will assist the nurse in providing care for women with benign or malignant neoplasias. Nursing care concepts related to early detection, treatment methods and education are included.

■ BREAST NEOPLASIAS

Benign Conditions of the Breast

The most common of the benign breast lesions is the formation of multiple cysts in the breast tissue. Medical terms for this are **mammary dysplasia, fibrocystic disease,** or chronic cystic mastitis. Multiple cysts occur in approximately 1 in 3 premenopausal women. The incidence peaks among women 30 to 50 years of age. Since the formation of new cysts after menopause is rare, it is thought that ovarian hormones may be a causative factor. Some women experience premenstrual pain or tenderness of the breasts. However, most women are asymptomatic and seek medical advice only after they palpate a lump.

CLINICAL MANIFESTATIONS AND DIAGNOSIS. The usual clinical presentation is bilateral multiple cysts. However, single simple cysts may also occur. When symptoms do occur, they include dull heavy pain and a sense of fullness and tenderness that increases premenstrually (DiSaia, Creasman, 1992). The cysts are soft to palpation, well differentiated, and movable. Deeper cysts, especially aggregations of cysts, are indistinguishable by palpation from **carcinomas,** which are malignant growths that infiltrate surrounding tissue. Surgical **biopsy,** a procedure in which tissue is removed for diagnostic examination, is required in this case to differentiate the malignant from the benign condition. Generally, a diagnosis is based on history and physical examination. **Mammography,** the visualization of breast tissue by x-ray examination, and ultrasonography are also used to differentiate cysts from solid tumors. Needle aspiration may help in forming a differential diagnosis.

THERAPEUTIC MANAGEMENT. Treatment for fibrocystic breast disease is usually conservative and follows a two-pronged approach. Diet changes and vitamin supplements comprise the first therapy. Although still controversial, some advocate eliminating dimethylxanthines (e.g., caffeine and theophylline) and nicotine from the diet. Clients are encouraged to stop consuming coffee, cola, tea, and chocolate and taking certain respiratory drugs. Stopping smoking is also advocated. Many women report a lessening of symptoms after adopting these measures. Increasing vitamin E intake to between 400 and 600 units daily has been reported to reduce symptoms (Beare, Myers, 1990).

Hormonal therapy is the other approach to treatment. Currently, the most commonly used medications in treating fibrocystic disease are danazol (Danocrine), tamoxifen, or oral contraceptives. Pregnancy should be ruled out before initiating any of the hormonal therapies, and a nonhormonal contraceptive should be recommended since ovulation may not be suppressed.

Although the hormones are effective in diminishing the symptoms of fibrocystic breast disease, they may produce side effects that are more traumatic than the symptoms. Danazol (an anterior pituitary suppressor) can cause weight gain, hot flashes, menstrual irregularities, hirsutism, and deepening of the voice. Tamoxifen (an antiestrogen) may cause vaginitis, decreased libido, nausea, or anorexia (Beare, Myers, 1990).

Surgical removal of nodules is attempted only in selected cases. In the presence of multiple nodules, the surgical approach would involve multiple incisions and tissue manipulation and may not prevent the development of more nodules.

The next most common benign condition of the breast that occurs is a **fibroadenoma.** It is the single most common lump seen in the adolescent population, although it can also occur in women in their

30s. Fibroadenomas are characterized by a firm, painless, well-defined mass that is mobile. *The upper outer quadrant of the breast is the usual site of detection.* Diagnosis is made by reviewing client history and by physical examination. Fibroadenomas do not respond to either dietary changes or hormonal therapy. Mammography may be helpful in following the mass for changes. Surgical excision may be necessary if the lump is suspicious or if the symptoms are severe.

Mammary duct ectasia is an inflammation of the ducts behind the nipple. It is characterized by a nipple discharge that is thick, sticky, and multicolored. Frequently the client will experience a burning pain, itching, or a palpable mass behind the nipple. Generally no treatment is required for this condition unless complications arise. Development of an infection in the inflamed area would require antibiotic therapy, and incision and drainage would be necessary should an abscess develop.

Intraductal papilloma is a rare, benign condition that develops within the terminal nipple ducts. Usually too small to be palpated, the characteristic sign is nipple discharge that is serous, serosanguinous, or bloody. After malignancy is ruled out, the affected segments of the ducts and breasts are surgically excised.

Lipoma is a common benign tumor that may resemble a malignant lesion because of its firm consistency and poor encapsulation. After biopsy confirmation of lipoma, surgical excision is the only therapy needed.

NURSING PROCESS. As with all nursing care, using the nursing process will assist the nurse in developing the most comprehensive approach to care for the individual client.

Assessment should include a careful client history and physical examination. The nurse should document the following client information: pain, whether or not symptoms increase with menses, dietary habits, regular performance of self–breast examination, and the examination technique used. The client's emotional status, including her fears and concerns and her ability to cope, should also be assessed.

Nursing Diagnoses of the client with benign breast disease would of course be specific to the individual client, but general diagnoses might include:

Knowledge deficit related to benign breast disease and its treatment.

Fear/anxiety related to concerns about the development of cancer.

Pain related to symptoms of the condition.

Planning involves establishing realistic goals in collaboration with the client. The criteria used in identifying the client goals should also be measurable and should relate to the already established nursing diagnoses. Examples of client goals based on the previously identified nursing diagnoses might include:

Client will demonstrate appropriate breast self-examination technique.

Client will verbalize a decrease in anxiety.

Client will identify and report any changes in breast mass.

Client will verbalize a decrease in physical discomfort.

Implementation involves selecting those nursing actions that will best assist the client in achieving the established goals. Nursing actions that would complement the previous example might include:

Demonstrating correct breast self-examination technique (see Chapter 41).

Encouraging the verbalization of fears and concerns.

Providing specific information regarding the client's condition and treatment.

Describing pain-relieving strategies in detail.

Evaluation consists of taking the client-centered goals that have been established and determining whether or not the client has been able to meet them. In the previous example, it would be important to evaluate the technique and consistency of the client's performance of the breast self-examination. The client's coping ability and adherence to any therapeutic regimen should also be evaluated.

Malignant Conditions of the Breast

The United States has one of the highest rates of breast carcinoma in the world. Statistics released from the American Cancer Society indicate that 175,000 new cases are diagnosed, and approximately 44,500 deaths occur yearly from breast cancer (Boring, Squires, Tong, 1991). The specific risk to American women of developing a breast carcinoma in her lifetime is one in nine. It is the leading cause of death in American women between 35 and 54 years of age. Although the exact cause of breast cancer continues to elude investigators, certain risk factors have been identified that increase a woman's risk for developing a malignancy. These factors include a history of breast cancer, family history (especially in first-degree female relatives [i.e., mother or sisters), age older than 40 years, and no children or experiencing a first pregnancy after age 30. Other factors being investigated as having a potential link to the development of breast cancer include dietary habits (particularly those diets high in fats), obesity, history of benign breast disease, oral contraceptive use, radiation exposure, and hormones. The link between estrogen replacement therapy and breast cancer remains under investigation. However, to date most studies do not substantiate a significant link between exogenous estrogen therapy and the development of breast cancer. Even with the identification of some risk factors, the fact remains that risk factors help identify only 25% of women who will eventually develop breast cancer. Two problems prevent a clear understanding of the risk factors of breast cancer. One is the long latent period, 15 to 25 years, before the development of clinically recognizable carcinoma. The other is consideration both of the duration and the intensity of factors that may induce or promote cancer. Many risk factors are additive. Although there are limits in the clinical applicability of risk factors, women at increased risk should be screened at more frequent intervals.

PATHOPHYSIOLOGY. Breast carcinomas usually arise from epithelial cells with the origin being either the ductal or lobular tissue (Baird, McCorkle, Grant, 1991). These cancers can be either invasive (infiltrating) or noninvasive **(in situ)**. By far, the most commonly occurring cancer of the breast is invasive ductal carcinoma, followed by invasive lobular carcinoma; noninvasive (in situ) carcinoma comprises the smallest incidence.

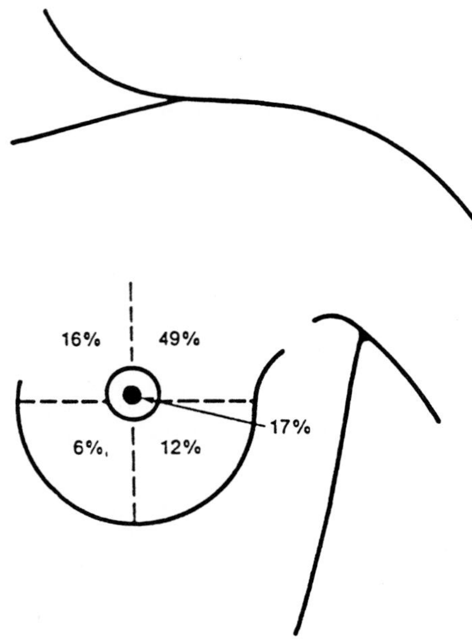

Fig. 44-1 Relative location of malignant lesions of the breast.
From DiSaia PF, Creasman WT: *Clinical gynecologic oncology*, ed 4, St Louis, 1992, Mosby–Year Book.

CLINICAL MANIFESTATIONS AND DIAGNOSIS. It is estimated that 90% of all breast lumps are detected by the client. Of this 90%, only 20% to 25% are malignant. The most common presenting symptom is a lump or thickening of the breast. The lump may feel hard and fixed or soft and spongy. It may have well-defined or irregular borders. It may be fixed to the skin, thereby causing dimpling to occur. A nipple discharge that is bloody or clear also may be present. *About half of all breast cancers occur in the upper outer quadrant of the breast*. The second most common location is under the nipple or around the areolar area (Baird, McCorkle, Grant, 1991) (Fig. 44-1).

Since early detection and diagnosis reduce mortality because cancers are smaller, lesions are more localized, and there tends to be a lower percentage of positive nodes, it becomes imperative that other protocols for assessment and diagnosis be established. In addition to regular breast self-examination (BSE) from midadolescence on, the use of screening mammography may aid in the early detection of breast cancers. The American Cancer Society's recommendations for screening mammography are as follows (Beare, Myers 1990):

1. Baseline mammogram for women between 35 and 39 years of age.
2. Every 1 to 2 years for women between 40 and 49 years of age.
3. Yearly for women age 50 and older.

In addition to the above, a practitioner should annually perform a breast examination and assess a woman's BSE technique and frequency. Transillumination, thermography, and ultrasound breast imaging are unproven as methods to detect early breast carcinoma and should be considered experimental. Research with magnetic resonance imaging (MRI) is just beginning. New investigative serum assay, breast cancer radioimmunoassay (RIA) is being used in research for detecting and monitoring breast cancer. This development is part of the emerging technology involving monoclonal antibodies (for a discussion of monoclonal antibodies see Chapter 8).

When a suspicious mammogram is noted or a lump detected, diagnosis is confirmed by needle aspiration when a cyst is suspected or by a needle localization biopsy. The latter procedure requires the collaborative efforts of both the radiologist and the surgeon. It often requires that the procedure take place in two different environments (radiology and surgery). Therefore clients need specific information regarding procedures, duration, and outcomes.

Analysis of cells from breast fluid may offer a way to predict the likelihood of breast cancer many years before the first symptoms are detected in mammograms or physical signs of lumps (Wrensch et al, 1992). Researchers at the University of California at San Francisco obtained the fluid by nipple aspiration. The technique takes 15 seconds; cells in the fluid are examined microscopically for abnormal shapes (Wrensch et al, 1992). Research into the use of tamoxifen (a synthetic nonsteroidal antiestrogen) continues for primary prevention of breast cancer for at-risk women (Bernstein, Ross, Henderson, 1992). The effects of body size, parity, and menstrual events on breast cancer incidence in seven countries has been studied (Pathak, Whittemore, 1992).

THERAPEUTIC MANAGEMENT. Major advances in the understanding of the biology of cancer have occurred in the past 10 years. Many studies now support the theory that ***breast cancer is a systemic disease,*** which means that micrometastases could be present at the initial presentation with or without nodal involvement (Baird, McCorkle, Grant, 1991). Nodal involvement, however, remains the single most significant prognostic criterion for long-term survival (Fig. 44-2).

More recently, hormone receptor studies such as the estrogen receptor (ER) assay also have been used as a prognostic factor and are being used in planning treatment for breast cancer (Baird, McCorkle, Grant, 1991; Beare, Myers, 1990; DiSaia, Creasman, 1992).

SURGICAL APPROACHES. The most common surgical approach in recent years has been the modified radical **mastectomy,** which involves the removal of the breast tissue and axillary lymph nodes, leaving the pectoralis major muscle intact. This surgery has all but replaced the Halsted procedure, which involved the removal of the pectoral muscles as well as the breast tissue and lymph nodes. There has been no difference in the survival rate between the two procedures, and the modified radical mastectomy has fewer postoperative complications.

In addition to the removal of the breast, breast reconstruction during or after initial surgery offers the woman an alternative to achieve symmetry and preserve body image (Fig. 44-3). Reconstruction involves creating a breast mound, which can be accomplished with either the implantation of a prosthesis* or a tissue expander that is placed under the pectoralis muscle. The tissue expander is used to gradually stretch the skin until the desired symmetry is attained. At this point a permanent prosthesis is inserted. As with all implantation procedures, risks of

*The FDA restricted the use of breast implants filled with silicone gel (1992) to women participating in research on their safety.

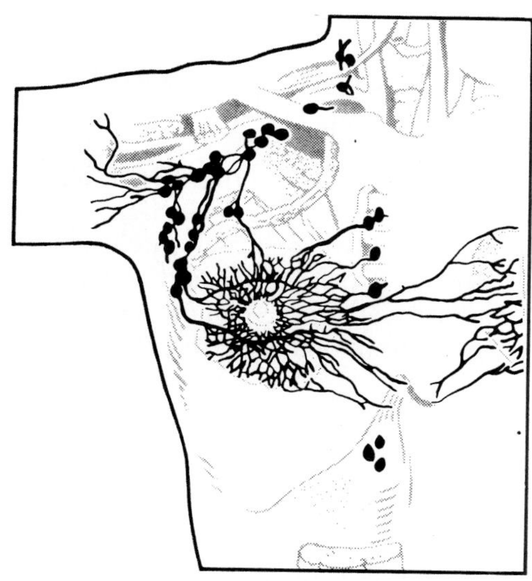

Fig. 44-2 Lymphatic spread of breast cancer.

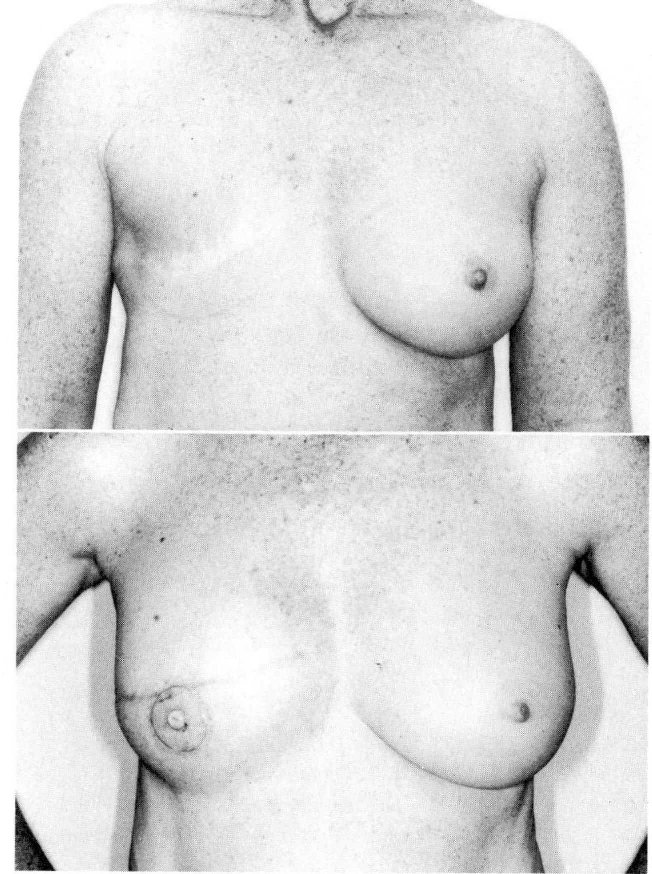

Fig. 44-3 Latisimus dorsi reconstruction following radical mastectomy.

surgical complications such as hematoma, infection, and delayed wound healing are possible, as well as the possibility of capsular contractions from or leakage of the implant (Baird, McCorkle, Grant, 1991).

A somewhat more controversial and conservative approach to treatment involves excising and radiating the tumor and surrounding normal tissue (known as lumpectomy, tylectomy, partial mastectomy, or segmental mastectomy). It should be noted that not all women are candidates for this approach. At this time it is reserved for women whose tumors are small (≤4 cm) and who have stage I or II disease. For these women, the lumpectomy with radiation has demonstrated the same survival rate as other surgical techniques while preserving the breast tissue. Fig. 44-4 identifies the different types of breast surgery in current use.

Since removal of the breast is a significant loss, the impact on the woman's ability to cope is a tremendous challenge. Having a choice of surgical approach appears to have a positive influence on the woman's ability to cope and retain her self-concept (Leinster et al, 1989; Morris, Ingham, 1988).

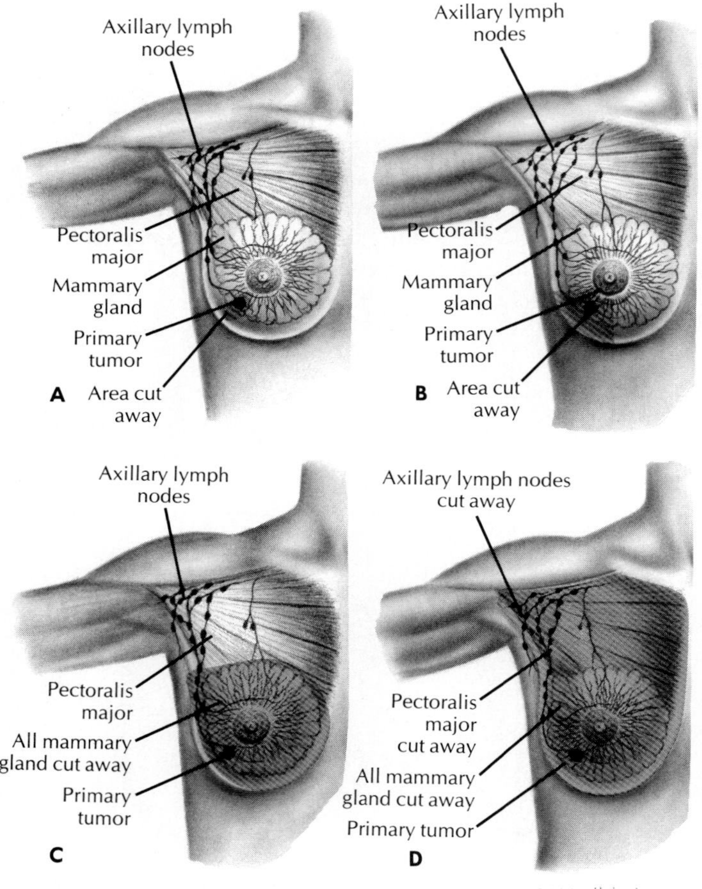

Fig. 44-4 Four ways to deal surgically with cancer of breast: **A**, lumpectomy (tylectomy), **B**, quadrectomy (segmental resection), **C**, total (simple) mastectomy, and **D**, radical mastectomy.

MEDICAL THERAPY. Hormone therapy is used when the cancer is sensitive to estrogen or progesterone (i.e., estrogen or progesterone receptor-positive). Bilateral oophorectomy is common in a premenopausal woman; tamoxifen, an oral antiestrogen, is an alternative to oophorectomy (castration). Oral estrogens, depo-medroxyprogesterone, androgens, and danazol also have been used to treat breast carcinoma.

Combined hormonal therapy and chemotherapy (the treatment of disease by means of clinical substances or drugs) may improve the cytotoxicity of chemotherapy (Levine Lippman, 1984; Levine et al, 1988). Combinations of cytotoxic drugs are superior to a single agent. The chemotherapeutic agents chosen most often for breast cancer are cyclophosphamide, methotrexate, doxorubicin (Adriamycin), 5-fluorouracil, and vinblastine. In addition to their antineoplastic qualities, these cytotoxins have some immunosuppressive side effects. Episodes of thrombosis can be expected to occur in women undergoing chemotherapy for breast cancer (Levine et al, 1988).

The 5-year survival of a woman whose breast carcinoma is believed to be localized to the breast with negative axillary nodes is 85%; when axillary nodes are positive, 5-year survival is 53%. Chemotherapy substantially prolongs survival (Henderson, 1988).

With the advance in monoclonal antibody technology, it is now possible to test for residual disease with a serum tumor marker, CA 125. This technology is used to determine effectiveness of therapy for cancer without the need for second-look diagnostic surgery.

THE EMOTIONAL IMPACT OF A DIAGNOSIS OF CANCER. When a woman is confronted with a diagnosis of cancer that is a potentially chronic illness or potentially lethal, it challenges the coping ability of both the woman and her family. The stigma of cancer still exists in that many people associate it with suffering, disfigurement, hopelessness, and certain death.

A diagnosis of breast cancer carries with it not only a threat to life but a tremendous change in appearance that can affect at the deepest level the client's self-image and self-esteem. The feelings generated by a diagnosis of cancer are always intense, and the manifold disruptions caused by the disease, such as the large expense, the loss of usual work and recreation patterns, changes in body functions or appearance, and prolonged disability or pain, challenge the ability to cope. Despair, fear, and shame may be difficult to discuss and manage. Yet failure to examine these deep feelings or share them with others can only increase the sense of isolation, loneliness, and confusion. When the emotional turmoil is not recognized by the woman and those around her, associated "negative" behaviors may be misinterpreted and condemned, and the woman may alienate her loved ones and lose the support she so desperately needs.

Reaction to cancer can have positive effects as well. Today, more and more people are accepting and adjusting to cancer. They are finding that many kinds of cancer are compatible with career, marriage, and parenthood and that a full, productive, and happy life is possible with a diagnosis of cancer. For some, having cancer gives them a greater appreciation of the experiences of daily life and encourages them to focus on what is most important and meaningful.

Alternative therapies may be used concurrently with medical regimens to augment healing and assist the client in coping with the diagnosis of cancer. The nurse should be knowledgeable of these alternatives and support the client and family if they choose to participate. Alternative therapies can include progressive relaxation, meditation, visualization, hypnosis, support groups, and healthful life-style changes such as regular exercise, balanced diets, vitamin supplements, and rest. Many oncologists recognize the importance of these alternatives to the emotional and physical well-being of their clients and regularly refer them for these adjunct therapies (Siegal, 1989).

■ NURSING PROCESS

ASSESSMENT

The nurse takes a client history of symptoms including timing of detection of lump, size, changes, location, pain, nipple discharge, and breast symmetry. Review of physical examination, laboratory results, mammography, and other imaging diagnostic procedures is necessary. Psychosocial assessment should include not only this client's present emotional state but the reaction of her family and significant others and history of handling crises. The nurse needs to identify what the diagnosis of cancer means to her and her family.

It is also important to remember that the initial reaction is generally anguish and shock followed by disbelief and denial. During this time, processing information is difficult, and the nurse needs to be sensitive to how this may affect decision-making abilities. When the client has to relinquish her denial or disbelief, it is often replaced by anger, grief, or depression. Being able to assess the woman's emotional state will assist the nurse in selecting the most appropriate support.

At the time of the diagnosis the woman is distracted by worry, and yet this is the time when hospital personnel want her to plan for her future. Obviously, treatment decisions must be made immediately, but many other decisions can wait and, in fact, will be sounder if the woman is rested and relatively unshaken as she considers them.

Families often suffer as much or more than the woman herself. Those who never enjoyed warm relationships may be consumed with remorse over past injustices or missed opportunities, or their rancor may be so deep that the thought of investing time, money, and emotion in the care of the woman is intolerable. Some relatives are jealous of the attention the sick person receives, and many, exhausted by the responsibilities the illness places on them, are angry and resentful. Other families, bound by affection, may deplore the present, dread the future, and set impossible standards of care based on self-abnegation.

Some families facing cancer, while crushed by the initial blow, are united and strengthened by all of their resources, and together they find support and meaning in adversity. Positive family attitudes can be cultivated by the nurses's strong assurance that family members are very important to the woman, and by acceptance of their feelings as natural rather than either admirable or repugnant.

NURSING DIAGNOSES

Nursing diagnoses for women with a diagnosis of breast cancer might include:

- Fear/anxiety related to
  — The diagnosis of breast cancer
- High risk for decisional conflict related to
  —Inability to choose a treatment option
- High risk for sexual dysfunction related to
  — Altered body image and reaction of significant other
- High risk for ineffective family coping related to
  — Diagnosis

PLANNING

Planning realistic goals in collaboration with the woman might include these *goals*/expected outcomes:

- The client will verbalize acceptance of her diagnosis and elicit appropriate support from significant others.

- The client will choose among alternative treatment options and verbalize satisfaction with the decision-making process.
- The client will report resuming satisfactory sexual function after surgery.
- The family will accept the diagnosis and provide appropriate support through all stages of treatment.

IMPLEMENTATION

Nursing actions are selected that will best assist the client in achieving her goals. For example:

- Provide time to discuss the diagnosis, answer questions, and listen to concerns.
- Encourage ventilation of feelings by client and family in a nonjudgmental atmosphere.
- Validate and reinforce accurate information processing by client and family.
- Suggest approaches the client might take to deal with the sexual concerns of her significant other.
- Discuss the application of alternative therapies to alleviate stress and promote healing.
- To assist in client decision making, arrange for the client to speak with others with similar diagnoses who have chosen a variety of treatment options.

In addition to assisting the client with accepting the diagnosis and obtaining support, nursing care in the preoperative, postoperative, and convalescent period must be considered. The discussion that follows is pertinent to the care required by a woman after a modified radical mastectomy.

PREOPERATIVE CARE. General preoperative teaching and care are given, including expectations regarding physical appearance, pain management, equipment to be used (IV therapy, drain, etc.), and emotional support. Some emotional support may be obtained by arranging for a visit from a member of an organization such as Reach for Recovery, Inc. The woman is reminded that when she awakens after surgery, her arm on the affected side will feel tight.

IMMEDIATE POSTOPERATIVE CARE. After recovery from anesthesia, the woman is returned to her room. Special precautions must be observed to prevent or to minimize lymphedema of the affected arm. When vital signs are taken, the blood pressure cuff is never applied on the affected arm. The affected arm is elevated with pillows above the level of her right atrium. Blood is not drawn from nor are parenteral fluids given in this arm. Early arm movement is encouraged. Any increase in the circumference of that arm is reported immediately.

Nursing care of the wound involves observation for signs of hemorrhage (dressing, drainage tubes, and Hemovac or Jackson-Pratt drainage reservoirs are emptied at least every 8 hours and more frequently as needed), shock, and infection. Dressings are reinforced as necessary. Since the nipple may be "stored" on another body site (abdomen) pending future reimplantation over the reconstructed breast, this site is observed for hemorrhage and infection every hour and care is given exactly as ordered.

The woman is asked to turn (alternating between unaffected side and back), cough (while nurse or woman applies support to chest), and deep breathe every 2 hours. Breath sounds are auscultated every 4 hours. Active range-of-motion exercise of legs is encouraged. Parenteral fluids are given until adequate oral intake is possible. Emotional support is continued.

CONVALESCENT CARE. Care given during the immediate postoperative period is continued as necessary. Early ambulation is encouraged not only to improve circulation and ventilation and prevent loss of calcium from bone but also for the psychologic benefits of the upright position (e.g., mood elevation, decrease of perception of self as continuing in the sick role). Arm exercises are encouraged at least 4 times daily (see box on p. 1371). Exercise is increased as tolerated and is stopped at the point of pain. Initially, the woman alternately clenches and extends her fingers, then progresses to wrist and elbow exercises, gradually abducting her arm and raising it up to and over her head. She is encouraged to exercise by assisting with her care—washing her face, brushing teeth, eating with her hand and arm on the affected side. Physical therapy is usually prescribed. A representative of Reach for Recovery, Inc., often visits, reinforces the woman's exercise efforts, assists with providing emotional support relating to her change in body image (anatomic, physiologic, sexual), and may assist with teaching wound care.

DISCHARGE PLANNING. Before discharge, considerable time should be spent counseling the woman (and her family) about the aspects of self-care (printed instructions should be available) (see box on p. 1371).

EVALUATION

Evaluation is based on the client-centered goals. The nurse can be assured that care was effective to

TEACHING Postmastectomy Arm Exercises*

EXERCISE: CLIMBING THE WALL

1. Stand facing wall with toes close to wall
2. Bend elbows and place palms of hands against wall at shoulder level
3. Move both hands parallel to each other up the wall as far as possible until incisional pull or pain occurs
4. Move both hands down to starting position
5. Goal is complete extension with elbow straight
6. Activities that use the same action: reaching top shelves, hanging out clothes, washing windows, hanging curtains, setting hair

EXERCISE: ARM SWINGING

1. Bend forward from waist, permitting both arms to relax and hang naturally
2. Swing arms together left-to-right (motion comes from shoulder)
3. Swing arms in circles parallel to floor, clockwise and counterclockwise
4. Stand up slowly

EXERCISE: ROPE PULL

1. Attach a rope over a shower rod or hook
2. Grasp each end of rope, alternately pulling on each end, raising arm on affected side to a point of incisional pull or pain
3. Shorten rope over time until arm on affected side is raised almost directly overhead

EXERCISE: ELBOW SPREAD

1. Clasp hands behind neck
2. Raise elbows to chin level, holding head erect; move slowly and rest when incisional pull or pain occurs
3. Gradually spread elbows apart; rest when pull or pain occurs

*From American Cancer Society: *Reach to Recovery*, New York, The Society.

the extent that the goals for care have been met. That is, the client verbalizes acceptance of her diagnosis and elicits appropriate support from significant others; chooses among alternative treatment options and verbalizes satisfaction with the decision-making process; reports resuming satisfactory sexual function after surgery; and the family accepts the diagnosis and provides appropriate support through all stages of treatment (see case study (p. 1372) and care plan for a single woman with breast cancer (p. 1373).

TEACHING Discharge Teaching for the Client With a Mastectomy

1. Perform arm exercises as indicated
2. Call physician if inflammation of incision or swelling of the incision or the arm occurs
3. Wash hands well before touching incision area
4. Avoid constriction of circulation in affected area
5. Contact Reach for Recovery regarding external prosthesis
6. Avoid depilatory creams, strong deodorants, and shaving of affected axilla
7. Empty reservoir every 8 hours, and record amounts
8. Shower after reservoir removed, sponge bath until drains are removed.
9. Continue with monthly BSE on unaffected side
10. Note that sensation around the wound and the affected area may be diminished or absent.
11. Resume sexual intercourse as desired.

UTERINE NEOPLASIAS

Benign Conditions of the Uterus

Leiomyomas, also known as fibroid tumors, fibromas, myomas, or fibromyomas, are benign tumors arising from the muscle tissue of the uterus (Beare, Myers, 1990). It is estimated that 20% to 25% of women over the age of 30 develop uterine fibroids. They tend to occur more often in African-American women or women who have never been pregnant. They rarely become malignant. Because their growth is influenced by ovarian hormones, these benign tumors can become quite large when they coexist with pregnancy, and they can spontaneously seem to disappear after menopause when circulating ovarian hormones are diminished.

Cervical **polyps** are pedunculated (footed) tumors that usually originate from the lining of the cervical canal but may arise from the external cervical mucosa as well. Usually these reddish or purplish growths occur singly and remain relatively small. Occasionally, they may grow so long that they will protrude from the vagina. Polyps are often asymptomatic and are found on routine examination. Sometimes

CASE STUDY

Single Woman With Breast Cancer

Mary L. is a 35-year-old single woman who has been teaching elementary school for the past 10 years. She is engaged to be married to a 36-year-old insurance agent whose job requires out-of-town travel approximately 2 weeks a month. She discovered a hard lump in her right breast in the upper outer quadrant while showering 2 months ago. She delayed contacting her physician out of fear. When she did come to the office, a biopsy was scheduled that confirmed a diagnosis of cancer. The recommended course of treatment is a modified radical mastectomy with possible chemotherapy. Her other family includes a 70-year-old mother from whom she is estranged and one sister who lives out of state.

ASSESSMENT

The nurse's interview with Ms. L revealed fear and extreme anxiety, making information processing difficult. Her fiance appears supportive, as does her sister. Her mother has been unable to acknowledge Mary's diagnosis, and Mary herself has been experiencing physical symptoms associated with stress (e.g., nausea, diarrhea, and weight loss).

NURSING DIAGNOSIS

Mary's emotional status leads the nurse to give priority to the following *nursing diagnosis:* Fear/anxiety related to a diagnosis of breast cancer.

PLANNING

A plan of care is developed with Mary's input. One mutually identified *goal* for Mary is that she will exhibit a decrease in physical signs of stress. The *expected outcomes* are that the symptoms of nausea and diarrhea will decrease and that Mary's weight will stabilize.

IMPLEMENTATION

Nursing actions are based on medical management, physician orders, and nursing diagnosis. Specific interventions that will best assist Mary in achieving her goal include providing an opportunity for Mary to discuss her feelings about her diagnosis, teaching Mary stress-relieving exercises, and suggesting dietary changes such as eating smaller, more frequent meals.

EVALUATION

The expected outcomes are used to determine the effectiveness of the interventions. Mary was able to begin to express her feelings about her diagnosis. She learns to use guided imagery and breathing exercises for stress reduction. She spaces her small meals at frequent intervals throughout the day, and the symptoms of nausea and diarrhea have abated. She has regained 2 pounds. Based on these findings, the goal set for Mary was met. See the related plan of care.

they are the cause of intermenstrual bleeding, bleeding after coitus, or bleeding while straining at stool. Biopsy confirms their benign nature. These growths can be removed by tying them off and allowing them to necrose and slough away. Rarely are they malignant.

CLINICAL MANIFESTATIONS AND DIAGNOSIS. The cause of leiomyomas remains unknown. Most of the tumors are found in the body of the uterus. However, some tumors can occur in the cervix or broad ligament. Depending on the location, fibroid tumors can cause uterine enlargement or bleeding. In some instances, submucous tumors can produce pedicles that may protrude through the vagina or cervix, resulting in infection or ulceration (Beare, Myers, 1990).

Menorrhagia (excessive bleeding) is the most common symptom of fibroids. If the tumor is very large, pelvic circulation may be compromised, and surrounding viscera may be displaced. A client may complain of backache, low abdominal pressure, constipation, or dysmenorrhea (painful menstruation). Since the tumors appear to be influenced by the presence of estrogen, during pregnancy the tumors may produce complications such as preterm labor, spontaneous abortion, or dystocia (difficult labor). The severity of the symptoms seems to be directly related to the size and location of the tumors. By and large however, most women are asymptomatic. Diagnosis is usually accomplished by a process of elimination. Pregnancy tests will rule out pregnancy as the cause of the symptoms. Cervical dilatation and uterine curettage will detect submucosal fibroids, and laparoscopy visualizes subserous fibroids. Ultrasound can differentiate between inflammatory masses or endometriosis and subserous fibroids.

THERAPEUTIC MANAGEMENT. Treatment for benign tumors of the uterus depends on the severity of the symptoms and the age of the client. If symptoms are mild, regular checkups may suffice. If the tumor is

CARE PLAN Single Woman With Breast Cancer

GOALS	IMPLEMENTATION	RATIONALE	EVALUATION
Nursing diagnosis: Fear/anxiety related to a diagnosis of breast cancer			
Mary will verbalize acceptance of her diagnosis and elicit support from her fiance and sister.	Review the information from the physician.	Identifies what information has already been given to the client.	Mary begins to accept diagnosis and actively seeks support from her fiancé and sister.
	Assess client's perception of physician's information.	Gives information about accuracy of interpretation as well as areas of information not processed.	
	Provide time to discuss diagnosis, answer questions, and listen to concerns.	An unhurried environment and good listening skills will promote processing of information.	Mary reports a positive discussion with significant others regarding her diagnosis.
	Suggest approaches Mary might take to ascertain the feelings of her support person.	Providing suggestions gives the client a starting point and facilitates goal attainment.	Mary reports every-other-day phone contact with her sister and daily contact with her fiancé.
	Encourage frequent contact and open discussion with support person.	Prevents isolation and promotes functional communication.	
Mary will verbalize her feelings regarding her mother's lack of support.	Provide a nonjudgmental atmosphere in which to discuss feelings.	Feelings are best expressed when acceptance is present.	Mary identifies mother's behavior with common reactions to stress.
	Describe the various reactions people have to crisis situations.	Provides insight and promotes acceptance.	Mary reports her mother will attend the next physician's visit.
	Encourage Mary to have her mother visit the physician with her.	Facilitates acceptance of the diagnosis and promotes contact with the mother.	Mary reports relief at being able to discuss her feelings regarding her mother.
Mary will cease to exhibit physical symptoms of stress.	Demonstrate stress-relieving exercises such as conscious breathing techniques and relaxation	Use of relaxation and breathing techniques can reduce physical symptoms.	Mary will report a cessation of nausea and diarrhea.
	Suggest smaller meals more frequently.	Small, frequent feedings buffer acidic content and decrease over-distention.	Mary's weight will stabilize.
	Refer for counseling if symptoms persist.	More frequent intensive counseling is often needed to reduce stress when in crisis.	
Nursing diagnosis: Decisional conflict related to knowledge deficit regarding options			
Mary will decide on immediate or postpone breast reconstruction until after postoperative recovery.	Review the therapies being considered by the physician.	Identifies the options open to the client.	Mary will choose an option for or against breast reconstruction that she feels is good for her.
	Provide written materials from the American Cancer Society regarding options.	Written materials help client to focus on specific options and provide another medium in which to learn.	
	Provide time to discuss the feelings and review materials.	Feelings need to be worked through before options can be processed.	
	Arrange for Mary to speak with women who have chosen various options.	Provides additional information to facilitate decision making.	

near the outer wall of the uterus and symptoms are significant, myomectomy (surgical removal of the tumor) may be performed. This technique leaves the uterine muscle walls relatively intact, thereby preserving the uterus and allowing future pregnancies. **Hysterectomy** (removal of the uterus) is the treatment of choice if bleeding is severe or if obstruction occurs. An abdominal or vaginal surgical approach depends on the size and location of the tumors.

NURSING PROCESS. *Assessment* should include a history of symptoms, which might include abnormal bleeding, abdominal pain, dysmenorrhea, pelvic fullness or heaviness, or problems with elimination. A differential diagnosis would be made using the diagnostic tests described above.

Nursing Diagnoses are determined from the client's assessment data and might include:

- Anxiety related to uncertain diagnosis and fear of malignancy.
- Pain related to leiomyomas.
- High risk for sexual dysfunction related to dyspareunia.

Planning measurable mutually determined goals for the above diagnoses might include:

- Client will be able to demonstrate two pain-relieving techniques to counteract the symptoms.
- Client will report no compromise in sexual functioning as a result of the therapeutic intervention.
- Client will verbalize a decrease in anxiety related to the diagnosis and therapeutic regimen.

Implementation of nursing actions might include reinforcing the physician's therapeutic plan, demonstrating pain-relieving techniques, encouraging the verbalization of fears and concerns, and providing anticipatory guidance with regard to possible changes in sexual functioning. Much will depend on the medical treatment indicated. If surgery is required, nursing interventions would be similar to those discussed under radical hysterectomy on p. 1376.

Evaluation involves the client's ability to achieve the collaborative goals that have been established. Using the previously stated goals, the following outcome would be anticipated: the client's pain will be relieved, sexual functioning will be maintained at the presurgery level, and anxiety will be decreased.

Malignant Conditions of the Uterus

CANCER OF THE ENDOMETRIUM

Endometrial cancer is the most common malignancy of the reproductive system. The American Cancer Society estimates that approximately 33,000 new cases will be reported this year, and 5500 women will die this year as a result of endometrial cancer (Boring, Squires, Tong, 1991). It is most commonly seen in mature women with the mean age at diagnosis being between 50 and 64 years. It is being seen in younger women, however, with increasing frequency. Certain risk factors have been associated with the development of endometrial cancer, including obesity, nulliparity, late onset of menopause, diabetes mellitus, and hypertension. Hormone imbalance however, seems to be the most significant risk factor. Unopposed estrogen stimulation (i.e., absence of progesterone) may set up an environment conducive to the development of uterine cancer. The incidence of endometrial cancer among Caucasian women is approximately twice the rate in African-American women (Herbst et al, 1991). Diabetes increases the risk by 2.8%.

THERAPEUTIC MANAGEMENT. For adenocarcinoma of the endometrium, in its early stages, total abdominal hysterectomy (TAH) and bilateral salpingo-oophorectomy (BSO) are the usual treatments of choice. Abdominal lymphadenectomy and peritoneal washing is also commonly performed depending on the stage of the disease. For women at high risk for postoperative complications of thromboembolism (e.g., the obese client, the client with a bleeding disorder) preoperative heparin therapy and the use of antiembolism stockings will minimize the risk of thrombus formation. The woman who is given the diagnosis and a thorough examination of the proposed surgery in a caring and personalized manner is more likely to experience an uncomplicated recovery physically and emotionally.

For more extensive disease, steroid hormones, chemotherapy, and **radiotherapy** are used singly or in combination or as adjunctive therapy to surgery. Radiotherapy is the use of electromagnetic or particular radiation to treat a disease. This therapy uses precise doses of radiation projected directly into affected tissues in tumors with the projected outcome being the eradication of the tumor and the preservation of surrounding tissue.

NURSING PROCESS

ASSESSMENT

Assessment includes a history of physical symptoms. The ***cardinal sign of endometrial cancer is abnormal uterine bleeding*** (e.g., postmenopausal bleeding and premenopausal recurrent metrorrhagia). Thirty percent of postmenopausal bleeding is caused by carcinoma. After **metastasis** to the vagina, a mucosanguineous discharge may be seen. Local extension of endometrial tumors may involve the myometrium, paravaginal tissues, and paracervical tissues. Lymph node involvement usually indicates advanced disease.

Histologic examination is used for diagnosis. Papanicolaou smear of cellular material obtained by aspiration of the endocervix will identify one third to one half of cases. The woman is instructed not to douche during the 24 hours preceding the tests. Fractional curettage or endometrial biopsy yields the most accurate results. Fractional curettage involves scraping the endocervix and endometrium for histologic evaluation to determine the grade of neoplasm and its stage (extent). Perforation of the uterus is a possible complication. Endometrial biopsy will identify about 90% to 92% of cases. The FIGO (International Federation of Gynecology and Obstetrics) classification system is used to describe the stages of endometrial carcinoma (Table 44-1).

Acceptable miscellaneous methods include palpation, inspection of uterus (laparoscopy) and vagina, **colposcopy** (the examination of the vagina and cervix by means of an endoscope), hysteroscopy, cystoscopy, intravenous pyelogram (IVP [intravenous pyelography]), proctosigmoidoscopy, barium enema, bone and liver scans, arteriography, venography, lymphangiography, and biopsy of areas suspected to have been invaded.

TABLE 44-1 FIGO Classification of Endometrial Carcinoma*

Stage	IA G123	Tumor limited to endometrium
	IB G123	Invasion of less than half of the myometrium
	IC G123	Invasion of more than half of the myometrium
	IIA G123	Endocervical glandular involvement only
	IIB G123	Cervical stromal invasion
	IIIA G123	Tumor invades serosa and/or adnexae and/or positive peritoneal cytology
	IIIB G123	Vaginal metastases
	IIIC G123	Metastases to pelvic and/or paraaortic lymph nodes
	IVA G123	Tumor invasion of bladder and/or bowel mucosa
	IVB	Distant metastases including intraabdominal and/or inguinal lymph node

Histopathology: Degree of differentiation

Cases of carcinoma of the corpus should be grouped according to the degree of differentiation of the adenocarcinoma as follows:

G1 = 5% or less of a nonsquamous or nonmorular solid growth pattern

G2 = 6% to 50% of a nonsquamous or nonmorular solid growth pattern

G3 = more than 50% of a nonsquamous or nonmorular solid growth pattern.

*Approved by FIGO, October 1988, Rio de Janeiro. From DiSaia PF, Creasman WT: *Clinical gynecologic oncology*, ed 4, St Louis, 1992, Mosby–Year Book.

NURSING DIAGNOSES

Nursing diagnoses that would apply to a woman having a *radical* hysterectomy might include:

- Fear/anxiety related to
  —The surgical procedure and anticipated outcome
- Knowledge deficit related to
  —Preoperative procedures and postoperative outcomes
- Pain related to
  — Surgical procedure

Other nursing diagnoses related to specific postoperative care are not discussed here.

PLANNING

Planning for care of the client experiencing radical hysterectomy would change depending on which phase of the operative experience she is in. However, some overall goals would remain the same throughout. Goals would relate to the nursing diagnoses that had been established. Whenever possible, goals are mutually determined, stated in client-centered terms, and measurable. Examples of such *goals* would be:

- The client will understand information related to surgery and diagnosis.
- The client will describe a decrease in anxiety related to surgery and its outcome.
- The client will set realistic expectations for the postsurgical period.
- The client will describe a relief of pain.

IMPLEMENTATION

Nursing care again is individualized to the client and her specific situation and diagnosis. Interventions are directed by assessment of the client's perception of the anticipated surgery, her knowledge of what to expect after surgery, and any preoperative special procedures, such as cleansing enemas or douches. In today's practice of short hospital stays even for radical surgery, many of these preoperative procedures are performed at home before admission, so assessment of understanding becomes a critical nursing action.

PREOPERATIVE CARE. The nurse working with the client preparing for a radical hysterectomy needs to explain any preoperative procedures to be done as described above. Teaching also continues regarding postsurgical events; for example, intravenous fluids, pain management, drainage tubes, dressings, indwelling urinary bladder catheter, breathing exercises, coughing, turning, and early ambulation. The woman needs to be prepared to see a suprapubic drain with a reservoir that will remain in place several days to a week.

POSTOPERATIVE CARE. Vital signs usually follow a postanesthesia protocol, gradually decreasing in frequency to 4 times a day. IV fluids are maintained at a rate rapid enough to maintain hydration and electrolyte balance. Diet is gradually resumed as bowel sounds are heard and flatus is passed. A nasogastric tube may be in place to prevent distention. Intake and output are monitored.

The woman will need to be reminded to turn and deep breathe: assistance is given as needed. Breath sounds are assessed and any deviations from normal reported immediately. The most significant single cause of morbidity and prolonged hospitalization after major procedures is respiratory complications. Anesthesia and surgery alter breathing patterns and

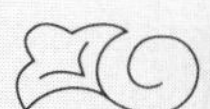 **Research Highlight** 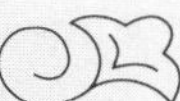

Effect of Massage on Cancer Pain

RESEARCH ABSTRACT

This pilot study was conducted to determine the effect of massage on pain for people with cancer. Twenty-eight participants were selected randomly from an oncology unit in a private hospital. In the sample, there were 10 women and 18 men (6 African Americans and 22 Caucasians). Clients were paired based on past frequency of medications given for pain, anxiety, or nausea and then assigned randomly to a treatment or a control group. Pain was measured with a visual analog scale, which is a line with end points of *no pain* and *pain as bad as it could possibly be*. Subjects placed a mark on the line that best indicated how much pain they were experiencing at that time. The distance from the *no pain* end to the point is measured and used as a pain score. After a training session, senior nursing students provided a 10-minute Swedish massage to the back of each subject in the experimental group. Students sat and visited with subjects in the control group for 10 minutes to control for the effects of the researcher's presence and interest. Pain was measured immediately after the massage or the visit and again at 1 and 2 hours after the massage or the visit. Information on medications taken during the study was obtained from clients' charts. The researchers found that pain before the procedure averaged 2.6 with a range of 0 to 9. Subjects in the experimental group had higher levels of pain initially (mean = 3.1) than the subjects in the control group (mean = 2.2). Men reported higher levels of pain (mean = 4.19). Men had a significant decrease in level of pain immediately after massage; however, for women there was no difference. There was no difference in pain at 1 or 2 hours after the massage. Age was not related to pain. Medication was not effective in pain reduction for any subject for more than 2 hours after receiving the medication.

IMPLICATIONS FOR PRACTICE

Massage is effective in reducing pain for a short time in men. Pain reduction was noted for those who experienced more pain. The finding that medication was not effective in reducing pain needs to be examined. According to the literature, nurses frequently undermedicate clients in pain. Nurses need to be encouraged to assess the pain and offer appropriate interventions; massage and analgesics are two effective means of reducing pain. Discussion of pain and its relief with clients and their families is warranted.

RELATED RESEARCH QUESTIONS

1. Does the effectiveness of massage in reducing pain vary with the gender of the person administering the massage?
2. Does the effectiveness of massage in reducing pain vary with the length of time the massage is administered?
3. Is one type of massage better than another in effecting pain relief?
4. Is massage combined with visualization more effective in pain reduction than massage alone?

REFERENCE

Weinrich SP, Weinrich MC: The effect of massage on pain in cancer patients, *Appl Nurs Res* 3(4):140, 1990.

ability to cough. Atelectasis, pneumonia, and pulmonary embolus may occur.

Hemorrhage is always a possible complication after surgery. The Hemovac is emptied every 1 to 2 hours and the amount and character of drainage is recorded. Drainage from any tubes is also assessed for bleeding. Vaginal drainage, if any, should be serosanguineous. Hematuria is noted and recorded. The physician is kept apprised of any deviations from normal expectations.

Paralytic ileus may occur after surgery in which the intestinal tract has been manipulated. A nasogastric tube, limiting oral fluids, and early ambulation all support the return of gastrointestinal function. An enema or suppository may bring relief of flatus and stimulate the return of bowel function. Oral laxatives should not be given until lower bowel function has returned.

Sitting may result in pelvic congestion so that the high Fowler's position is avoided. Pelvic congestion is discouraged by putting the bed flat for 10 minutes every 2 hours for the first 24 hours and avoiding the use of the knee gatch (or pillow).

Nursing measures such as massages, repositioning, fresh linen, regular perineal care, and emotional support are all helpful adjuncts to pharmacologic control of discomfort (see related Research Highlight, p. 1376).

CONVALESCENT CARE. Since the in-hospital convalescent period is generally short, close observation by the nurse and attention to detail becomes critical. Nursing actions appropriate to this period include monitoring for urinary retention after the catheter is removed, monitoring the woman's appetite and diet, monitoring bowel function, and encouraging progressive ambulation and self-care.

Some women benefit from an abdominal binder especially when walking, but this is no longer a routine measure: the woman is encouraged to use her own abdominal muscles to support her abdomen.

Estrogen therapy is usually started as soon as the woman can take oral fluids. The nurse can take this opportunity to remind the woman she will no longer have menstrual periods and to encourage her to verbalize questions or concerns she may have about hormone replacement therapy (see discussion of hormone replacement therapy, p. 1261).

The woman needs continuous emotional support. She may have fears of death; permanent disfigurement and change in functioning; altered feelings of self as a woman; concerns regarding her femininity, sexuality, and loss of reproductive capacity; and questions arising from things she has heard about posthysterectomy changes (e.g., facial hair, going mad, or becoming depressed).

Discharge planning and teaching is done throughout the preoperative and postoperative phases and culminates during the convalescent phase. Discharge teaching topics for the woman with a radical hysterectomy can be found in the box below.

EVALUATION

The nursing care of a woman with a radical hysterectomy is evaluated by returning to the goals and using measurable criteria to ascertain the degree to which the goals were met. For example, using the goal of relief from pain, evaluation might include:

- The woman verbalized satisfactory pain control with prescribed analgesics.
- The woman stated she used comfort measures with success in pain control.

CANCER OF THE CERVIX

Cancer of the cervix is the sixth most common cancer in women, ranking behind cancer of the breast, colon and rectum, endometrium, lung, and ovary (Silverberg, 1990). The accessible location of the cervix to both cell and tissue study and direct examination have led to a refinement of diagnostic techniques. Cytology to identify neoplasia and use of the colposcope to localize the site of change and allow directed biopsy are two procedures that have contributed to improved management of these disorders. The squamocolumnar junction is an important landmark identified with neoplastic changes of the cervix (Fig. 44-5).

TEACHING The Client With a Radical Hysterectomy

1. Eat three well-balanced meals per day, including 6 to 8 8-oz. glasses of water.
2. Rest when you are tired, resume activities as comfort level permits. Avoid heavy lifting for 6 weeks, and avoid sitting for long periods. Resume driving when comfort allows, at approximately 3 weeks.
3. Avoid tub baths, intercourse, and douching until after the follow-up examination. Alternative methods of achieving sexual satisfaction are permissible.
4. Report the following symptoms to the physician: vaginal bleeding, gastrointestinal changes, persistent postoperative symptoms (cramping, distention, change in bowel habits), and signs of wound infection (redness, swelling, heat, or pain at incision site).
5. Take estrogen replacement therapy (ERT) and other medications as prescribed.

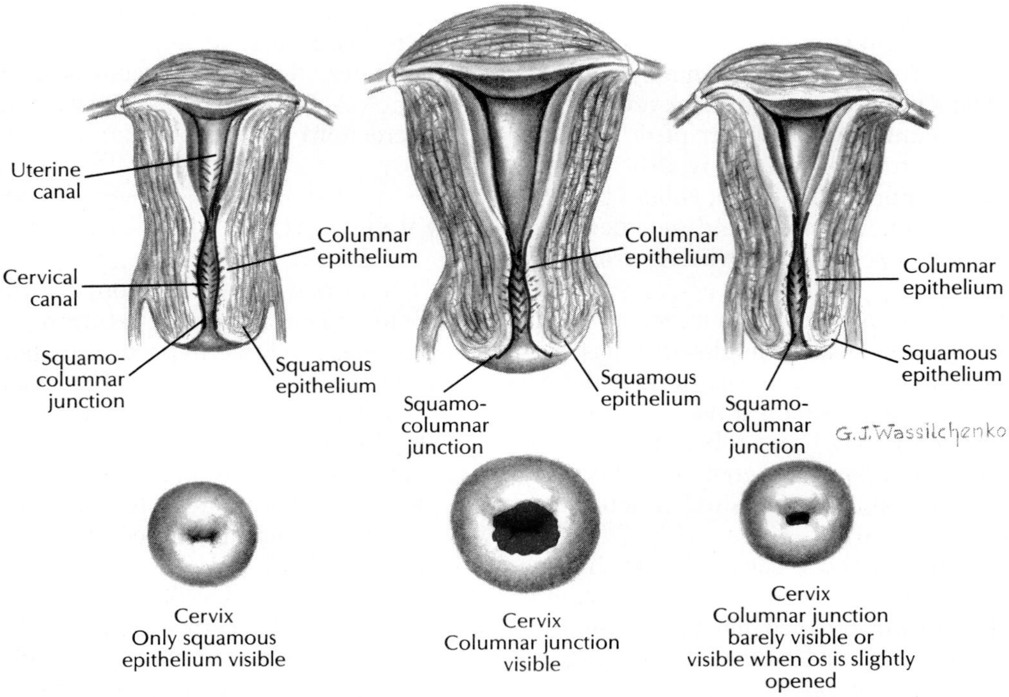

Fig. 44-5 Uterine and cervical canals and the squamocolumnar junction. Color denotes columnar epithelium.

Intensive study of the cervix and the cellular changes that take place has shown that most cervical tumors have a gradual onset rather than an explosive one. Preinvasive conditions may exist for years before the development of invasive disease. These preinvasive conditions are also highly treatable in many cases.

The average age range for the occurrence of cervical cancer is 40 to 50 years. However, preinvasive conditions may exist for 10 to 15 years before the development of an invasive carcinoma. There has been a strong link established between human papillomavirus (HPV) types 16 and 18 and **cervical intraepithelial neoplasia (CIN).** This is an updated inclusive term used to describe all epithelial abnormalities of the cervix (DiSaia, Creasman, 1992).

Other common risk factors include early age at first coitus (less than age 20); history of sexually transmitted diseases, especially HPV, herpesvirus, and possibly cytomegalovirus; multiple sexual partners (more than two); abnormal Pap smears; a sexual partner with a history of multiple sexual partners; addiction to cigarettes; exposure to DES (diethylstilbestrol) in utero; and belonging to a lower socioeconomic group (Beal, 1990; Baird, McCorkle, Grant, 1991; Beare, Myers, 1990).

Typically women report a history of cervical infections. Infections most commonly linked to subsequent cervical carcinoma are caused by herpes simplex virus 2; human papillomavirus types 16, 18, and 31; and perhaps cytomegalovirus. These viruses alter the deoxyribonucleic acid (DNA) of nuclei of immature cervical cells. The addition of semen (sperm) from many different partners promotes the initiation of a process that ends in dysplasia; years later, carcinoma results.

Some women have been exposed to **diethylstilbestrol (DES)** in utero. Administration of DES or another nonsteroidal estrogen to a pregnant woman may be followed by developmental or functional genital problems in both female and male progeny (see Fig. 6-2). The abnormalities are rare, when one considers the estimate that about 500,000 pregnant women received DES between 1940 and 1970. Single or multiple abnormalities may be noted. Some abnormalities develop or are recognized after puberty. Curiously, most individuals who were exposed prenatally appear to have been unaffected. Hence, an association rather than an actual cause-and-effect relationship is likely, and a trigger factor or factors are being sought.

In DES-exposed girls the following developmental or functional disorders have been described: circumferential vaginal ridges; cervical deformity, for example, "cock's comb" cervix, hooding, clefts, or pseudopolyps; hypoplastic or T-shaped uterus; constricting bands within the uterus; tubal anomalies; vaginal or cervical adenosis; dysplasia; and cervical incompetence. There appears to be an increased frequency of oligomenorrhea and a lower incidence of pregnancy in these women also. Most critical is the assessment that about 1 out of 1000 women exposed to DES prenatally develop vaginal or cervical clear-cell adenocarcinoma, usually during adolescence.

Approximately 90% of cervical malignancies are squamous cell carcinomas; 10% are adenocarcinomas.

In DES-exposed males the most common gross lesions reported are epididymal cysts, hypotrophic testes, or testicular capsular thickening. In addition, sperm analyses have revealed low volume of ejaculate, oligospermia, diminished sperm density, and the lower motile sperm count per milliliter. No equivalent of female clear-cell carcinoma or increase in male genitourinary cancer has been noted, however.

PREINVASIVE CANCER OF THE CERVIX

CLINICAL MANIFESTATIONS AND DIAGNOSIS. Cervical intraepithelial neoplasia (CIN) is the term now used to encompass all epithelial abnormalities of the cervix. The older classification system, **dysplasia** and carcinoma in situ, indicate two separate entities that in the past have affected treatment approaches. The newer classification, while still having subgroups, indicates more of a single neoplasia continuum.

This updated classification is as follows:

CIN I	Mild dysplasia
CIN II	Moderate dysplasia
CIN III	Severe dysplasia, and carcinoma in situ

The single most reliable method to detect CIN is the **Papanicolaou (Pap) test.** The Papanicolaou test will detect 90% of early cervical dysplasia. Early detection and treatment of preinvasive neoplasia is responsible for reducing deaths from this cause by 50% (Herbst et al, 1991). However, 2 out of 5 women do not have routine Papanicolaou tests. The American College of Obstetricians and Gynecologists (ACOG) currently recommends annual Pap tests for all sexually active women. The American Cancer Society recommends annual Pap tests for all sexually active women or for those who have reached 18 years of age or less frequently if three negative Pap tests at discretion of health care provider (ACS, 1992; Moore, 1990). Women in high-risk categories should have more frequent Pap tests.

Papanicolaou test results in the past have been recorded in one of five categories. Since some laboratories still use these categories they are presented here.

Class I	No abnormal cells present
Class II	Atypical cells are identified; inflammation must be ruled out
Class III	Suspicious abnormal cells present
Class IV	Malignant cells present—carcinoma in situ
Class V	Malignant cells present—invasive cancer

Current practice utilizes a descriptive classification. The descriptive terminology is as follows:

Normal
Metaplasia
Inflammation
Minimal atypia—koilocytosis
Mild dysplasia
Moderate dysplasia
Severe dysplasia—carcinoma in situ
Invasive carcinoma

Reexamination is warranted following treatment for infection. Additional diagnostic procedures (e.g., biopsy) are advised as necessary.

Biopsy. The value of the cervical Papanicolaou cytologic test is not in diagnosis, but in screening; diagnosis rests with a *tissue biopsy*. Pathologic areas are identified for biopsy by colposcopic inspection in 85% of cases. If colposcopy is unavailable, abnormal areas may be identified by staining the cervix with an iodine solution, for example. Lugol's (strong iodine) or Schiller's (potassium iodide 2 g, iodine 1 g, and water 3000 mL).

Cervical Conization. Histologic study of tissue obtained by cervical conization (Fig. 44-6) or amputation assists in the staging of cervical carcinoma. *Minimal* cervical dysplasia refers to abnormal cellular proliferation in the lower one third of the epithelium; this dysplasia tends to be self-limiting and generally regresses to normal. *Severe* cervical dysplasia involves the lower two thirds of the epithelium and often progresses to carcinoma in situ. *Carcinoma in situ (CIS)* is diagnosed when the full thickness of epithelium shows abnormal cells. *Invasive carcinoma* is the diagnosis when abnormal cells penetrate the basement membrane and invade the stroma. Invasive carcinoma spreads via the lymphatics to distant tissues and by direct extension to surrounding structures.

There are two advantages to a cone biopsy. It can be used (1) to establish the diagnosis and (2) to effect a cure. If carcinoma in situ is diagnosed, and if the woman wishes to retain her childbearing capacity, conization removes the abnormal tissue: further treatment is unnecessary. The woman is monitored with Papanicolaou tests every 3 months to ensure

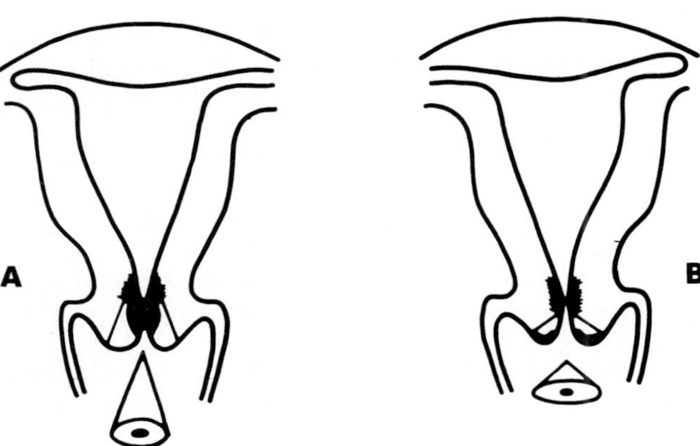

Fig. 44-6 **A**, Cone biopsy for endocervical disease. Limits of lesion were not seen colposcopically. **B**, Cone biopsy for CIN of the exocervix. Limits of lesion were identified colposcopically.
From DiSaia PJ, Creasman WT: *Clinical gynecologic oncology*, ed 4, St Louis, 1992, Mosby–Year Book.

that all abnormal tissue has been removed and that there is no recurrence.

Fractional Curettage. Out-of-hospital *cervical punch biopsy* and *endocervical curettage* accurately identify about 90% of cases. In-hospital *cold knife cone biopsy* and *fractional curettage* with anesthesia may be necessary if results from other methods are inconclusive. *Fractional curettage* consists of an endocervical canal scrape followed by an endometrial curettage; the two specimens are submitted to the laboratory separately. This test serves to detect an occult endocervical carcinoma or to determine if the endometrial carcinoma has extended from the corpus into the cervix.

Ultrasound. *Ultrasonography* contributes to the recognition, staging, and assessment of recurrence in carcinoma of the uterus, ovary, and cervix (Herbst et al, 1991). Ascites is easily recognized with ultrasound. For a discussion of ultrasound, see Chapter 27.

THERAPEUTIC MANAGEMENT. Once a diagnosis has been identified, a course of treatment is planned. For preinvasive lesions, several techniques are currently being used. As stated earlier, since many preinvasive conditions are detected in younger women who may wish to continue childbearing, treatment is geared toward eradicating abnormal cells while attempting to preserve the structure of the cervix. The techniques currently available are electrocautery, cryotherapy, and laser therapy. Electrocautery destroys abnormal cells using a heat source. **Cryosurgery** uses a freezing technique that freezes abnormal cells, and when sloughing occurs, regeneration of tissue is normal.

Side effects occurring after treatment are usually few and not of a serious nature. The profuse watery discharge that persists for 2 to 4 weeks is usually viewed only as a nuisance. Follow-up examination and a Papanicolaou test is scheduled in 4 months. Because repair may still be in progress, the finding of "abnormal" cells should be reassessed at 6 months. Persistent abnormal cells require reevaluation, and plans are made for repeat cryosurgery or other therapy. Rarely, spotting or cervical stenosis are complications.

Endocervical cells seem to regenerate, leaving a normal cervical canal in most instances. Surveillance with frequent Papanicolaou tests and colposcopic examination must continue indefinitely after this type of conservative therapy.

Laser* surgery is the newest technique. This technique allows for precise direction of a beam of light. Unlike healing after cryosurgery, cervixes treated with CO_2 laser show epithelial regrowth beginning by 2 days. Cervixes are reepithelialized within 3 weeks, with healing complete by 6 weeks. The original architecture of the cervix is preserved, and the squamocolumnar junction remains visible. For treatment of the cervix (relatively insensitive tissue), the woman may need no anesthesia. Some women complain of a burning or cramping sensation that is tolerable for most women.

The treated vulva and vagina also heal rapidly. Vulvar healing is painful however, especially during urination. Pain intensifies for about 3 to 4 days postoperatively and usually disappears by 2 weeks. Sitz baths, whirlpool baths, soaking, and local anesthetic/antibiotic creams bring relief from discomfort and aid healing. A squeeze bottle can be used to spray water over the perineum *during* urination to decrease discomfort. Also, the woman can urinate through the cardboard tube from toilet tissue held up around the meatus and in this way keep the urine off the perineum. Hair dryers are used to dry the area.

The CO_2 laser may be used for several lesions on the cervix: CIN, chronic cervicitis, condylomata, cysts, hemangiomas, polyps; and to relieve stenosis. The following lesions in the vagina may be treated with the laser: adenosis, condylomata, DES lesions, endometriosis, granuloma, herpesvirus infection, and vaginal intraepithelial neoplasia (VAIN). A vaginal speculum designed for laser therapy is seen in Fig. 44-7. The vulva may be treated for the following: benign nevi, carbuncles, condylomata, dystrophy, hemangioma, herpesvirus infection, molluscum contagiosum, and vulvar intraepithelial neoplasia (VIN).

The CO_2 laser may also be used for internal le-

*LASER: *l*ight *a*mplification by *s*timulated *e*mission of *r*adiation.

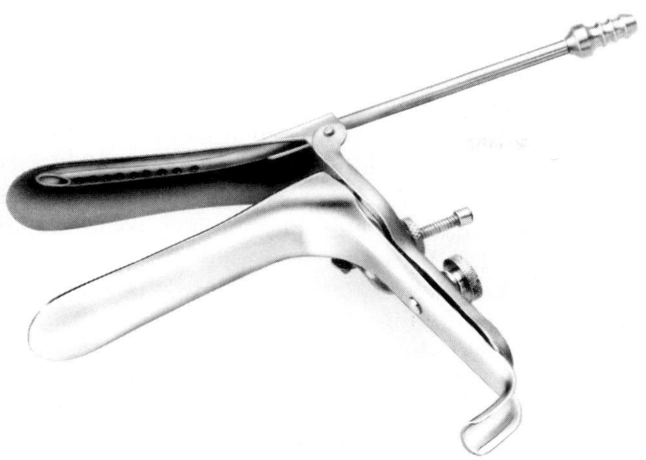

Fig. 44-7 Smoke caused by laser-induced tissue vaporization can be drawn out of the vagina with an instrument such as the Smoke Removal Tube (SRT), a malleable stainless steel tube permanently fixed to the speculum blade. The SRT is open at the distal end and has a number of holes along the length of the tube for gathering the smoke. Its proximal end has a standard hose fitting for connection to a suction machine.
Courtesy Amko Manufacturing Co, Bellmawr, NJ.

sions during hysteroscopy and laparoscopy and for infertility surgery (lysis of adhesions and endometriosis), among others.

However, experience has shown that the most effective treatment with the laser requires obliteration of the whole transformation zone to a depth of 5 to 7 mm. The effectiveness of this technique has not proven to be significantly better than cryosurgery. With no difference in clinical results, the limitations of increased pain for the client, and increased time for the physician to perform the procedure, the cost effectiveness of this technique needs to be considered. (DiSaia, Creasman, 1992).

With cervical **conization,** the extent of epithelial involvement is determined on the ectocervix and clearly delimited by colposcopy or Schiller's staining. The incision is made to include all the abnormal and some normal surrounding tissue (Fig. 44-6). Bleeding can be lessened by a prior injection of a dilute solution of phenylephrine (Neo-Synephrine) along the proposed incision line. Hemorrhage, uterine perforations, and anesthesia present immediate risks; rare complications include delayed bleeding, cervical stenosis, cervical incompetence, or impaired fertility.

To retain optimum fertility, cryosurgery, laser surgery, or local excision is indicated. If multiple lesions are present, therapeutic conization is preferred. Once a woman has had carcinoma in situ, she will always be at greater risk and needs to be monitored carefully. Removal of the cervix or uterus continues to be the definitive therapy in women who do not wish to retain their reproductive capacity.

INVASIVE CANCER OF THE CERVIX

CLINICAL MANIFESTATIONS AND SYMPTOMS. Currently there are two types of invasive carcinoma of the cervix, microinvasive and invasive. There has been much confusion surrounding microinvasive carcinoma because of variation in terminology and lack of agreement in anatomic description. In 1974 the Society of Gynecologic Oncology accepted a statement identifying microinvasive carcinoma as one or more lesions that penetrate no more than 3 mm into the stroma below the basement membrane with no areas of lymphatic or vascular invasion (Baird, McCorkle, Grant, 1991; DiSaia, Creasman, 1992). Invasive carcinoma is invasion that goes beyond the above identified parameters. The staging of invasive carcinoma extends from Stage 0 (carcinoma in situ) to Stage IVB (distant metastasis or disease outside the true pelvis). A number of substages within each stage also exist.

No single symptom occurs that specifically identifies invasive cervical cancer. Contact bleeding that occurs from touch, such as during coitus or physical examination, is the most common symptom. The bleeding can vary from a thin watery pink to a continuous bloody discharge to frank hemorrhage. Late symptoms include referred pain to the flank or leg from sciatic nerve involvement, hematuria and renal failure from bladder invasion and obstruction, and rectal bleeding and bowel obstruction from rectal invasion. Once the disease is staged, treatment is begun.

THERAPEUTIC MANAGEMENT. The choice of treatment is between surgery and radiotherapy. In most institutions, the initial treatment is radiotherapy; both intracavitary radium and external radiotherapy are used. The controversy between surgery and radiotherapy surrounds the treatment of Stages I and IIA. Chemotherapy has not proven to be a significant treatment for cervical carcinoma, since 95% of these cancers are squamous cell carcinomas and are less responsive to most chemotherapeutic agents.

Radiotherapy. Radiation may be delivered by radium applications to the cervix followed by external radiation therapy that includes lymphatics of the pelvic side wall. Major complications include radiation cystitis and proctitis and rectovaginal and vesicovaginal fistula formation (see Fig. 41-11).

The use of hydroxyurea as a radiosensitizer may improve survival for those treated for cervical carcinoma with radiation (Piver, 1984). In preparation for radiotherapy, the woman needs to maintain good nutritional status and a high protein-vitamin and high caloric diet. Anemia, if present, should be corrected before the initiation of radiotherapy.

External irradiation and intracavitary radium therapy is used in various combinations for the best results, and tailored to each woman and her particular lesion. Megavoltage machines such as cobalt, linear accelerators, and the betatron have the distinct advantage of providing a more homogeneous dose to the pelvis. The hard, short rays of megavoltage pass through the skin without much absorption by the skin and therefore cause little dermal injury.

Radium is the isotope that has traditionally been used in the treatment of cancer of the cervix; cesium and cobalt have been added to therapy regimens. There are three intracavitary techniques using specially designed applicators (Fig. 44-8) and the fourth technique involves the application of radium in the form of needles directly into the tumor.

In advanced carcinoma of the cervix, conventional intracavitary applicators are not applicable. Interstitial therapy employs a template to guide the insertion of a group of 18-gauge hollow steel needles into the lesion transperineally (Fig. 44-9). After the needles are placed, the iridium wires are inserted when the woman is returned to her hospital room.

Complications of Radiation Therapy. Morbidity as a direct result from properly conducted therapy is usually minimal. Some of the morbidity seen may be caused by the uncontrolled tumor and not by the therapy. Acute treatment complications occurring during or shortly following therapy, include irritation of the rectum, small bowel, and bladder, reactions in the skin folds, and mild bone marrow suppression. Dysuria and frequency may occur. Late irradiation sequelae, including damage to the rectum and bladder, are less common. Symptoms of radiation proctitis may follow an asymptomatic interval of many months to years after treatment. The symptoms of small bowel injury (post-prandial crampy abdominal pain and anorexia) should not be confused with recurrence of the tumor; diversion surgery yields good results.

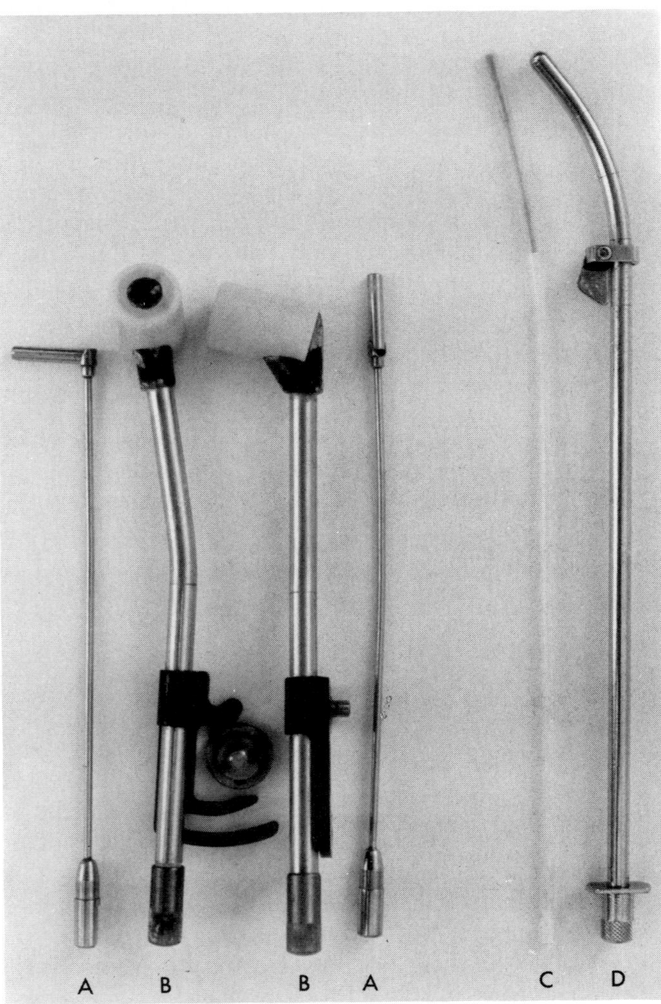

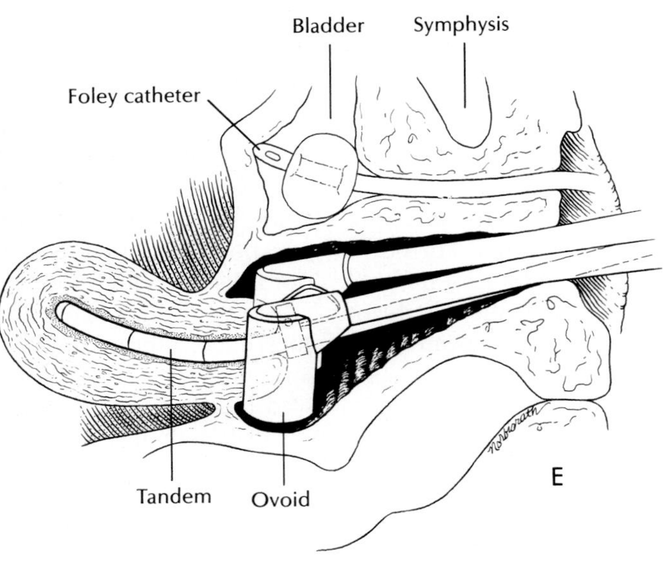

Fig. 44-8 Intracavitary implant. **A,** Inserts for colpostats to insert radium or cesium. **B,** Colpostats. **C,** Teflon tubing to insert radium or cesium into tandem. **D,** Tandem. **E,** Placement of tandem and colpostats before vaginal packing.

From Phipps WJ et al, editors: *Medical-surgical nursing: concepts and clinical practice,* ed 4, St Louis, 1991, Mosby–Year Book.

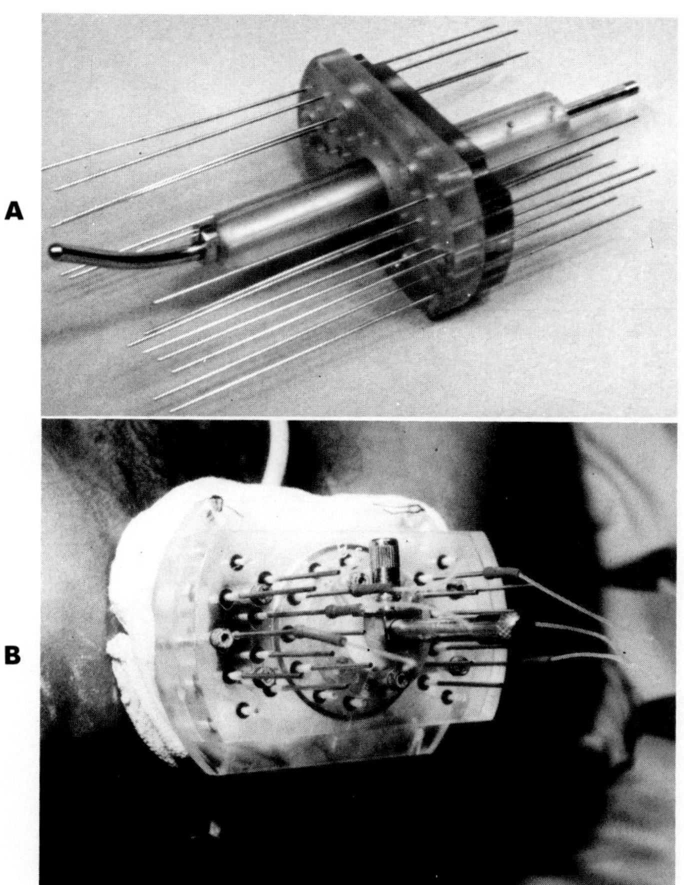

Fig. 44-9 **A,** Interstitial-intracavitary implant (Syed/Neblett applicator). **B,** Implant procedure completed.
From DiSaia PJ, Creasman WT: *Clinical gynecologic oncology,* ed 4, St Louis, 1992, Mosby–Year Book.

Radical Hysterectomy. In early stages, comparable survival rates are obtained by both radiotherapy and surgery. Radiotherapy is applicable to virtually all clients; radical surgery excludes certain medically inoperable clients. Surgery may be the method of choice for those women with stage I and stage IIA disease for whom preservation of ovarian function is desired. Complications of less than 1% can be expected postoperatively. Surgery is necessary when radiation is contraindicated, for example, in the presence of pelvic inflammatory disease (PID) or inflammatory disease of the bowel, concurrent pregnancy, and client preference. Some lesions are not radiosensitive.

With modern techniques of surgery, anesthesia, antibiotics, and electrolyte balance, morbidity after radical hysterectomy is between 1% and 5%. Radical hysterectomy involves removal of the uterus, tubes, ovaries, upper third of the vagina, entire uterosacral and uterovesicle ligaments, and all of the parametrium on each side, along with pelvic node dissection encompassing the four major pelvic lymph node chains: ureteral, obturator, hypogastric, and iliac. Dissection serves to preserve the bladder, rectum, and ureters while removing as much of the remaining tissue of the pelvis as is feasible.

Women with positive pelvic nodes usually receive postoperative whole-pelvis irradiation, although there is no evidence that it alters the incidence of recurrence in the pelvic area. However, there does seem to be a lesser incidence of distant metastases in the irradiated group.

Major complications following radical hysterectomy are formation of ureteral fistulas and lymphocysts, pelvic infection, and hemorrhage; the incidence of complications is decreasing steadily.

RECURRENT AND ADVANCED CANCER OF THE CERVIX. Approximately 1 of 3 women with invasive cervical cancer will have recurrent or persistent disease after therapy; prognosis is discouraging with a survival rate of between 10% and 15% for 1 year. Irradiation of mestastatic areas is commonly successful in providing local control and symptomatic relief; irradiation for recurrent disease is usually not considered.

Once treatment by radiation therapy has failed, selected clients may be considered for **pelvic exenteration.** In women, a total exenteration involves removal of the perineum, pelvic floor, levator muscles and all reproductive organs. Additionally, pelvic lymph nodes, rectum, sigmoid colon, urinary bladder, and distal ureters are removed, and a colostomy and ileal conduit are constructed (Fig. 44-10). In very select cases, the procedure can be modified to either an anterior or posterior exenteration. In anterior pelvic exenteration, all of the above-mentioned pelvic viscera are removed except the rectosigmoid, which is preserved. Urine is rerouted via an ileal conduit. In the posterior pelvic exenteration procedure, all pelvic viscera with the exception of the bladder are removed. The feces is rerouted via a colostomy (Fig. 44-10).

Women are carefully selected for this procedure; 5-year survival rates average around 20% to 35%. Many of the complications that follow this surgery are those that follow any form of major surgery, for example, pulmonary embolism, pulmonary edema, myocardial infarction, and cerebrovascular accidents. These complications are seen immediately after surgery. Infection originating in the pelvic cavity usually occurs later, if it occurs.

One of the most serious postoperative complications is small bowel obstruction related to the denuded pelvic floor; about 50% of these women need repeat surgery for this complication, and about half of them die as a result.

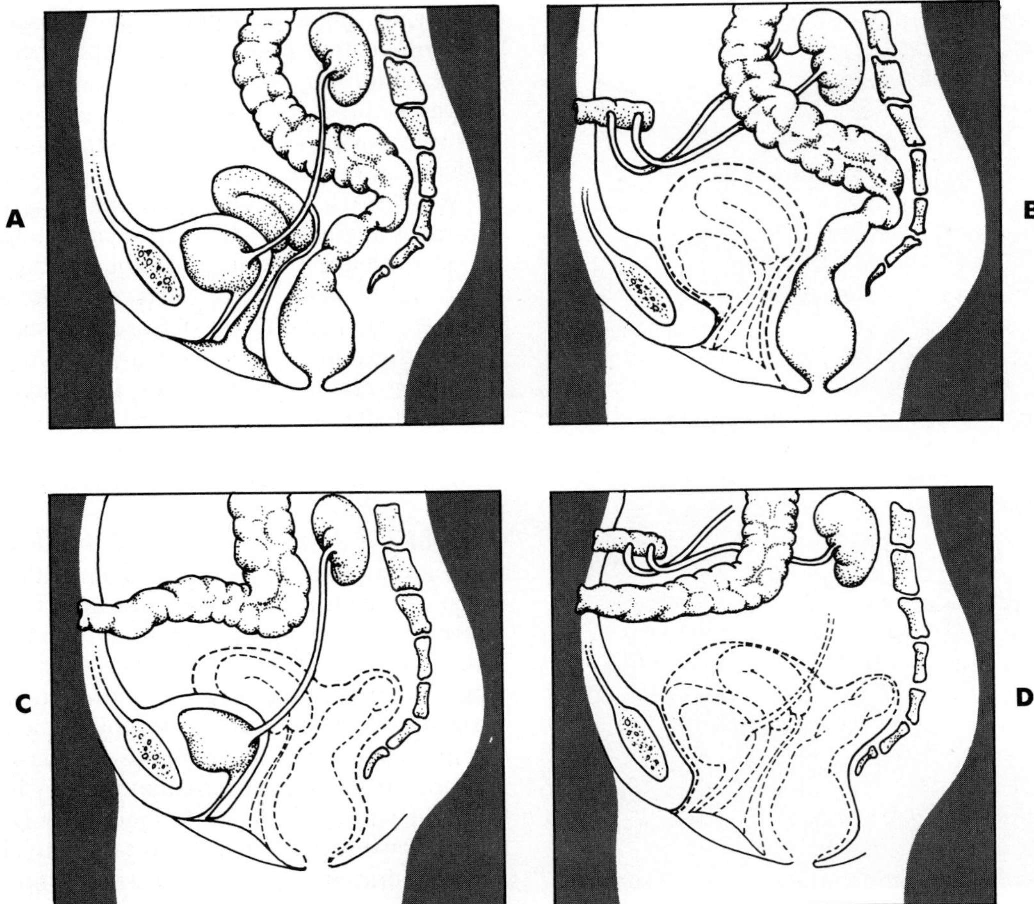

Fig. 44-10 Pelvic exenteration procedures. **A**, Natural. **B**, Anterior. **C**, Posterior. **D**, Total.

Courtesy P. Townsend, graphic artist. From Baird SB, McCorkle R, Grant M: *Cancer nursing: a comprehensive textbook*, Philadelphia, 1991, WB Saunders Co.

NURSING PROCESS

ASSESSMENT

For the client diagnosed with invasive carcinoma of the cervix, pretherapy assessment includes physical, psychologic, and educational components. Physical assessment includes a review of current medications, because medications for other medical problems may need to be continued. Skin is assessed to identify potential pressure points; respiratory and gastrointestinal status and state of nutrition are all important systems to assess. Urinalysis and complete blood count are also commonly performed. An ECG and chest x-ray examination may be done if use of a general anesthetic is anticipated for placement of internal applicators.

Psychologic assessment is important because frequently these women are emotionally distressed about the diagnosis and anticipated treatment (fear of being radioactive and fear of pain) and fear that family and/or significant others will become distant.

Educational assessment involves identifying the client's current knowledge base regarding the diagnosis and proposed therapeutic regimen.

NURSING DIAGNOSES

Nursing diagnoses that might arise from such an assessment might include:

- Knowledge deficit related to
  - —Treatment procedures
- Fear/anxiety related to
  - —Diagnosis
  - —Anticipated pain
  - —Concerns about radioactivity
  - —The response to the significant other/family

- Sensory deprivation related to
  - Treatment
  - Restricted contact with visitors and nursing staff
- Altered skin integrity related to
  - External radiation exposure
  - Immobility and bed rest
- High risk for injury related to
  - Dislodgment of radiation source.
- High risk for pain related to
  - Internal applicators
- High risk for alteration of sexual function related to
  - Treatment and/or concerns of significant other

PLANNING

Mutually determined *goals* for this type of client related to the identified nursing diagnoses above might include:

- Client will verbalize an understanding of the proposed treatment and accompanying procedures.
- Client will verbalize her fears regarding diagnosis, treatment, and response of significant others/family.
- Client will maintain contact with family and friends through short visitations and by telephone.
- Client will remain free from skin breakdown.
- Client will identify methods to maintain skin hygiene.
- Client will remain on strict bedrest on her back to prevent dislodgment of the internal applicators.
- Client will verbalize control of pain.
- Client will resume satisfactory sexual functioning.

IMPLEMENTATION

Nursing actions for external and internal radiation differ, so they will be separated here to preserve clarity.

External Radiation Therapy

PRETREATMENT CARE. The client's anxiety may be so high that information given by the radiologist may not be processed. The nurse needs to reinforce or fill in gaps, especially related to the following: the equipment, which is like that used for x-ray examination except larger; the hyperbaric oxygen chamber, which may be used to increase cellular oxygen and thus make tumor cells more radiosensitive; the radiotherapist, who will be behind a shield, but still close by and in communication with her; the position she will be put in and asked to maintain for some minutes; and the therapy, which is painless.

DURING THERAPY. The woman is counseled regarding maintaining general good health. She is more vulnerable to infection; therefore she is reminded of general measures to avoid infection (e.g., practice good hygiene, avoid people with infection, avoid large crowds, keep environment clean). To maintain good skin care the woman is taught to assess her skin often; avoid soaps, ointments, cosmetics, deodorants if axilla is being irradiated, etc., because these may contain metals that would alter the dose she receives and could lead to skin breakdown; wear loose clothing over the area; use air mattress or cover mattress with foam pads or sheep skin; and of course, avoid removing the markings made by the radiologist. If her skin becomes red or itchy, it is treated with remedies prescribed by the radiologist (e.g., sprays, A & D ointment, or lanolin). To treat skin that is broken or desquamating, the woman is shown how to use remedies prescribed by the radiologist (e.g., irrigation with equal parts peroxide and saline; application of antibiotic or lanolin ointment; exposure to air; and application of loose dressing but avoiding use of adhesive [or any] tape directly on the target area of skin).

To maintain good nutrition the woman is reminded to maintain a daily record of weight; use high-protein supplements; eat small, attractive, appetizing meals, probably bland in nature; take vitamins; and keep environment light, airy, clean, and quiet (especially before and after meals). If the woman is ill enough to be hospitalized, she may need total parenteral nutrition or tube feedings. Nausea interferes with adequate intake; therefore the woman may take antiemetics, as necessary. Maintain high daily fluid intake (2000 to 3000 mL) as suggested if not contraindicated. To increase her comfort, minimize infection, and promote adequate food intake, the woman is encouraged to perform frequent oral hygiene.

The nurse explains, as necessary, the need for blood studies to monitor white blood cell count (to determine degree of immunosuppression).

POSTTREATMENT CARE. Before discharge (if the woman is in the hospital during treatment) or the posttherapy care, the woman's need for information is met. The woman has a continued need to avoid infection and to report symptoms of infection to her physician immediately. She will need to maintain good nutrition and fluid intake. She and her family are forewarned of the persistence of radiation effects for 10 to 14 days after last treatment and to expect signs of healing in about 3 weeks. Good skin and mouth care are needed to support a sense of well-being and prevent infection. The woman and her family are informed of symptoms to report to the physician: continued gastrointestinal symptoms (nausea, vomiting, anorexia, diarrhea) and increasing skin irritation at the site of therapy (redness, swelling, pain, pruritis). She will need clear, explicit instructions about the medications she is to take (name, dose, times, purpose, side effects) and instructions to avoid any medications not prescribed by her physician. The woman and her family are reassured that she is not "radioactive"!

Internal Radiation Therapy

GENERAL NURSING CONSIDERATIONS. Internal radiotherapy requires hospitalization. The radiation safety officer determines the precautions to be observed in each situation. Printed instruction sheets are usually available stating precautions to be followed for each type of radiation substance used. A precaution sign is placed on the door to the person's room. Personnel who come in direct contact with anyone receiving radiotherapy may be required to wear isolation gowns, rubber gloves, and a film badge (worn under the gown) to monitor the amount of exposure received.

If no contact is permitted, the room must be equipped with an intercom, a telephone, and a radio and television set. Food and other articles are given to the woman through a special porthole.

Nurses and those receiving radiotherapy need to know how unsealed radioactive substances are eliminated so that the woman does not get the impression that she will be a danger to others indefinitely. An unsealed radioactive substance such as iodine–131 or phosphorus—32 are placed in a colloidal suspension and applied directly to the tissues involved. If the isotope is systemically administered, one half of the isotope is excreted in the first 2 days. During this time, rubber gloves should be worn while providing direct care (Baird, McCorkle, Grant, 1991).

Misconception could increase her feelings of isolation and cause her to be fearful of returning to her family. Before therapy is begun, the woman's room is prepared; that is, it is stocked with linens, extra pillows and blankets, and equipment, and everything (including the window blinds) is checked for workability.

Nurses must protect themselves from overexposure to radiation. Precautions include the following behaviors:

1. Careful isolation techniques: avoiding putting one's possibly contaminated hands into the mouth, carefully handling the woman's secretions and excrement (if she is receiving unsealed radioactive chemotherapy), and observing good hand-washing technique. These behaviors reflect knowledge that alpha and beta rays cannot pass through skin but may be in body fluids and excrement.
2. Careful planning of nursing activity to limit time (to 30 minutes or less per shift) spent in close proximity to the woman (Fig. 44-11) to avoid exposure to gamma rays, which can penetrate several inches of lead.

Exposure to radiation is controlled in three ways—distance, time and shielding (with lead). Increasing the distance from the source decreases exposure. Brief communication from an open doorway is permissible and reassures the woman (Baird, McCorkle, Grant, 1991).

Familiarity with applicators is a *must* for all nurses working with people receiving radiotherapy so that if a "strange object" is found in the linen or on the floor, it is not touched.

Today most hospital protocols include having a lead container and forceps in the room for use should a radioactive implant become dislodged. For the person with sealed radiotherapy, a movable lead screen is available that can be placed between the area in which the therapeutic applicator is located and the personnel. The lead screen is also used to protect visitors from radiation. Refer to medical-surgical nursing texts for more extensive discussion.

Orientation to this type of unit mandates thorough orientation to safety precautions to be implemented at all times by all personnel.

PREINSERTION CARE. The woman is prepared for insertion with the following care, which is accompanied by an explanation for each activity. To reduce the need for an enema or attention to bowel elimination for a few days, the gastrointestinal tract is prepared using low-residue diet, enemas, and sometimes bowel sedation. The vaginal vault is prepared with an antiseptic douche such as povidone-iodine. The woman may be asked to prepare the vaginal vault by douching before admission. A vaginal douche is usually ordered after hospital admission.

An indwelling urinary bladder catheter is inserted, as ordered, to prevent urinary distention that could dislodge the applicator. Nothing is taken by mouth the night before the procedure in anticipation of gen-

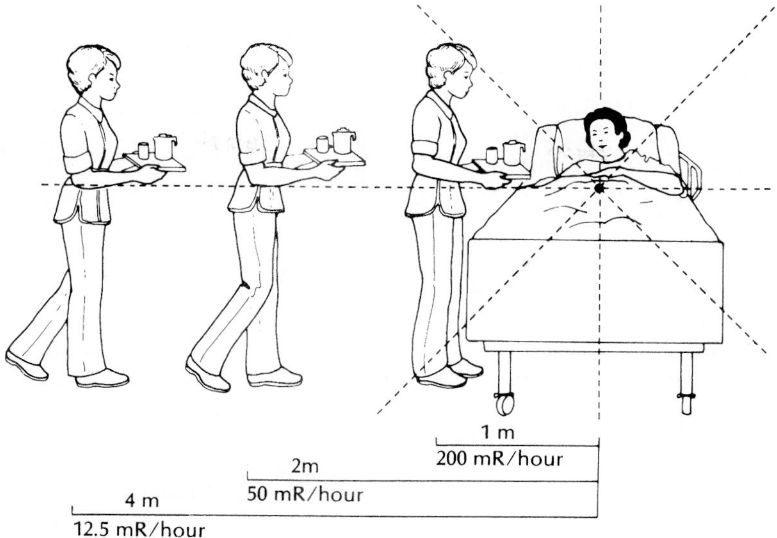

Fig. 44-11 Nurse nearest source of radioactivity (woman) is exposed to more radioactivity. Some hospitals have movable shield that can be placed between care provider and source of radioactivity.
Modified from Bouchard-Kurtz R, Speese-Owens N: *Nursing care of the cancer patient,* ed 4, St Louis, 1981, Mosby–Year Book.

eral anesthesia. Preoperative medications may be ordered for the morning of the procedure. Deep-breathing exercises, range-of-motion exercises, and positioning are all demonstrated before the procedure to minimize the effects of immobilization afterward. An IV solution will likely be started before the procedure, and IV therapy may be continued if nausea prevents good oral intake of fluids. The woman is assured that pain will be managed.

Explanations about restricted visitation of personnel and visitors is also given in the preinsertion phase. Women are often encouraged to bring reading materials or other hobbies such as crossword puzzles to the hospital to combat the boredom that isolation imposes upon them (Lowdermilk, 1990).

DURING RADIATION THERAPY. The applicator is inserted in surgery with the woman under general anesthesia if necessary to facilitate vaginal examination and ease of placement. The usual postanesthesia recovery care follows, and she is returned to her room. The woman is positioned on her back. There the applicators are loaded with the radioactive substance.

A lead shield is placed next to the woman's pelvic area. Vital signs are monitored every 4 hours. Active range-of-motion exercises and deep breathing are encouraged every 2 hours; she is not permitted to turn from side to side. The head of the bed is elevated about 20 degrees.

Her diet is progressed from clear liquid to low residue, as ordered.

Many women have difficulty eating while lying flat or even if the bed is elevated slightly. The nurse arranges the food so that it is easy to reach. Finger foods or liquids are generally more manageable. Parenteral or oral fluids are given up to 3000 mL daily. The urinary catheter remains in the bladder while the implant is in place. However, no perineal or catheter care is given. Intake and output are measured. The woman is given a partial bath, washing only above her waist. Massage is restricted to her shoulders and neck. Linen is changed only as absolutely necessary. Any linen or equipment used is retained in the room until therapy is complete to prevent loss of an applicator or seed.

If vaginal or rectal bleeding or hematuria occurs, the physician is notified immediately.

Emotional support is provided by planning to be with her for short periods, encouraging her to verbalize concerns and needs, encouraging family members, clergy, or others to visit for short periods daily or to communicate by phone. Pregnant women and children are not permitted to visit.

Many women undergoing internal radiation treatment are given medication to prevent complications and to promote comfort during the procedure. Such medications might include antibiotics to prevent bladder infections, heparin injections to prevent thrombophlebitis, sedatives for relaxation, antiemetics for nausea, and narcotics for pain. Usually the length of treatment is two applications, 2 weeks apart for 36 to 50 hours each, given after completion of external radiation therapy. The woman is considered radioactive during the time the internal sources are in place (Baird, McCorkle, Grant, 1991).

POSTTREATMENT CARE. Posttreatment complications range from those arising from immobilization such as thrombophlebitis, pulmonary embolism, and pneumonia to those arising from the treatment itself such as hemorrhage, skin reactions (rashes or inflammation), diarrhea, cramping, dysuria, and vaginal stenosis. The woman is assessed for any of these complications before discharge.

After the radium is removed, bladder function is monitored, oral fluid intake is encouraged at least to 3000 mL daily, douches and enemas are given as needed, and the woman is allowed to shower.

Progressive ambulation is encouraged, and the woman and her family are assured that she is not radioactive. She is usually discharged the same day. Discharge teaching can be found in the accompanying box.

TEACHING Discharge Teaching for the Client Undergoing Internal Radiation

1. Eat three balanced meals a day, and increase fluid to 3000 mL daily.
2. Rest when tired, and resume normal activities as comfort permits.
3. Maintain good hygiene (e.g., daily showers and daily douches until discharge stops).
4. Resume sexual intercourse in 7 to 10 days or as recommended by physician. Use vaginal dilator if needed for vaginal stenosis. Understand that sterilization and cessation of menstruation usually occur with this procedure.
5. Report any of the following to the physician: bleeding (vaginal, rectal, or in the urine), foul-smelling vaginal discharge, fever, abdominal distention or pain.
6. Take any prescribed medications as directed.
7. Do not hesitate to call the physician or clinic if there are concerns or problems.
8. Plan follow-up visits to determine emotional as well as physical recovery.

EVALUATION

The nurse can be reasonably assured that care was effective to the extent that the goals of care have been met. That is, everyone maintains radiation precautions; the woman verbalizes her fears and concerns, maintains contact with family and significant others, identifies and initiates appropriate skin care, maintains restricted mobility during internal radiation therapy, and verbalizes understanding regarding resumption of sexual activity and the use of vaginal dilators; and the woman's skin remains intact and her pain is adequately controlled.

■ OTHER PELVIC MALIGNANCIES

Cancer of the Uterine Tubes

Primary carcinoma of the uterine (fallopian) tube (usually the distal one third) is rare, with a peak incidence between the ages of 50 and 60. The cause is unknown. Vaginal bleeding is the most common symptom of tubal carcinoma and is present in more than 50% of cases. Because of this and other vague symptoms such as vague abdominal discomfort (from pressure on the bladder or rectum) and an enlarging unilateral pelvic mass or ascites are often misdiagnosed as ovarian carcinoma or endometrial carcinoma. Differential diagnosis of tubal carcinoma is usually made postoperatively. It is currently recommended that therapy guidelines parallel those established for ovarian carcinoma. Therefore a total abdominal hysterectomy with bilateral salpingo-oophorectomy is the minimal therapy. Even with apparent early-stage disease, it may exist bilaterally. An omentectomy should also be performed. Postoperative therapy consists of radiation therapy if the disease is limited to the tube, ovary, and uterus. The role of chemotherapy has not been well studied and is only speculative at this time.

Cancer of the Vagina

Vaginal carcinomas account for only 1% of gynecologic malignancy, with a peak incidence between the ages of 45 and 65. Almost all (95%) are squamous cell carcinomas; 5% are primary and secondary adenocarcinomas, secondary squamous cell carcinomas (older women), clear cell adenocarcinomas (young women, especially following intrauterine exposure to DES), and sarcoma botryoides (embryonal rhabdomyosarcoma) in infants and children. The lesion, usually seen in the upper one third of the vagina, often extends into the bladder and rectum.

Bleeding after coitus or examination, dyspareunia, and watery discharge are characteristic of vaginal cancer. Bladder involvement results in urinary frequency or urgency; rectal extension causes painful defecation.

Papanicolaou test and biopsy of Schiller-stained areas disclose the diagnosis.

Therapy for vaginal cancer is directed by the extent of the lesion and the age and condition of the client; radical hysterectomy and removal of the upper vagina with dissection of the pelvic nodes or radium and external radiation are the usual options. Radiation therapy is the usual treatment of choice. Survival rates have improved in recent years. In early stages 5-year survival rates approach 90%, with all stage survival rates falling in the 50% to 60% range.

Cancer of the Vulva

INCIDENCE AND ETIOLOGY. Vulvar carcinoma accounts for 3% to 5% of all female genital malignancies. It appears most frequently in older women in their middle 60s to 70s. However, up to 25% of cases may be found in younger women less than 40 years of age. The disease has been linked to the presence of condylomata acuminata (genital warts) caused by the human papillomavirus (HPV) and also to herpes simplex 2 virus (HSV).

By far the majority (90%) of vulvar carcinoma is squamous cell; 6% are attributed to Paget's disease, adenocarcinoma of Bartholin's glands, fibrosarcoma and melanoma; and 4% are basal cell carcinoma.

Prognosis depends on the size of the lesion and the tumor grade at the time of diagnosis. Fifty percent of clients have had symptoms for 2 to 16 months before seeking treatment. Fortunately, vulvar cancer grows slowly, extends slowly, and metastasizes fairly late. Even with a pattern of delayed diagnosis, survival rates approach 90% for stage I and II disease. Survival rates plummet, however, if lymph node metastasis has occurred.

CLINICAL MANIFESTATIONS AND DIAGNOSIS. The vulvar lesion is usually asymptomatic until it is 1 to 2 cm in diameter. Carcinoma in situ (CIS) is usually pruritic (itchy). Necrosis and infection of the lesion result in ulceration with bleeding or watery discharge.

Vulvar intraepithelial neoplasms are usually multifocal. Initially, growth is superficial but later extends into the urethra, vagina, and anus. In approximately 50% of late cases, superficial inguinal and femoral lymph nodes become involved.

Simple biopsy with histologic evaluation reveals the diagnosis. The areas of pathologic involvement are identified by staining the vulva with toluidine blue (1%), allowing an absorption time of 3 to 5 minutes, then washing with acetic acid (2% to 3%); abnormal tissue retains the dye. Biopsy is necessary to rule out such conditions as STD (e.g., chancroid, granuloma inguinale, syphilis), basal cell carcinoma, and CIS. In situ malignancies are initially small, red, white, or pigmented friable papules. In Paget's disease, the lesions are red, moist, and elevated. Melanomas appear as bluish-black, pigmented, or papillary lesions. Melanomas metastasize through the blood stream and lymphatics.

THERAPEUTIC MANAGEMENT. One method of treatment has been the **radical vulvectomy** (removal of the labia majora, labia minora, clitoris, part of vagina, and sometimes part of the rectum) plus inguinal and pelvic lymphadenectomy. Current surgical practice defers deep pelvic lymphadenectomy unless metastasis to the inguinal lymph nodes is found. An investigational procedure using inguinal "sentinel" nodes for sampling and wide excision of the lesion in the absence of metastasis to the nodes is currently being explored. If effective, this technique would do much to preserve the body image and sexual functioning of the client. A technique of vulvar self-examination similar to that of breast self-examination has shown some promise for early detection and diagnosis leading to definitive treatment and vulvar conservation (Lawhead, Majmudar, 1990). In any event, this type of surgery does not affect fertility.

Laser therapy used in the treatment of HPV* (human papillomavirus), a virus associated with the development of vulvar and cervical carcinoma, has shown some success in preventing the development of this type of cancer. One study by Reid et al (1990) indicated that extended laser ablation (vaporization of both clinically apparent and adjacent subclinical changes) in dysplastic vulvar diseases produced excellent primary results. However, they also stated that adjuvant therapy with a chemotherapeutic agent such as 5-fluorouracil would be a valuable addition.

NURSING PROCESS. A client history of symptoms and a physical examination should be done. An *assessment* of the client's understanding of the surgical procedure and her emotional state should also be done.

Possible *nursing diagnoses* include:

- High risk for infection related to surgical incision
- Sexual dysfunction related to vulvectomy
- Body image disturbance related to loss of sexual organ

*Laser therapy may *not* be the treatment of choice for HPV; see p. 860 in Chapter 29.

- Altered patterns of elimination, urinary and bowel, related to surgery

Planning goals are again based on the nursing diagnoses established, mutually determined, measurable, and stated in client-centered terms. A plan of care is developed based on the following goals:

- Client will remain free of infection at the operative site.
- Client will demonstrate positive adaptation to altered body image.
- Client with significant other will discuss altered sexuality and identify alternative means to achieve sexual satisfaction.
- Client will maintain adequate elimination.

Implementation for the woman undergoing radical vulvectomy requires some special nursing actions in addition to the routine postoperative care given. Additional nursing actions focused on the prevention of infection would include:

- Irrigate the surgical site after each elimination.
- Dry area thoroughly, using a hair dryer on cool setting or a heat lamp.
- Give stool softeners to decrease straining and disruption of suture line.
- Note any change in color of surgical site.
- Note any drainage or foul odor and notify physician.
- Perform catheter care as needed.
- Provide and instruct client in the use of sitz baths.

The client is at high risk for sexual dysfunction related to the effects of the surgery. Nursing actions that focus on minimizing these risks include:

- Encouraging verbalization of feelings.
- Providing privacy for discussion.
- Encouraging open communication between client and significant others.
- Providing resources for counseling if necessary.
- Discussing when sexual activity can be safely resumed.
- Discussing alternative methods to achieve sexual satisfaction.

See box above for additional information.

Using the goals set with the client, *evaluation* is based on the complete or partial achievement of those goals. Evaluative statements for the above goals might include:

- The client exhibits normal inflammation of tissue.
- The client's verbal statements indicate appropriate acceptance of the altered body image.
- The client expresses her fears and concerns and reports open discussion with significant other.
- The client and the significant other agree on alternative techniques to achieve sexual satisfaction.
- The client is able to void without difficulty and defecates soft-formed stools.

TEACHING Home Care of the Client Undergoing a Radical Vulvectomy

1. Avoid sexual activity for 4 to 6 weeks or as physician directs.
2. Rest frequently.
3. Avoid crossing legs, sitting, or standing for long periods.
4. Avoid tight, constricting clothing and synthetic underwear.
5. Keep perineal area clean and dry. Wash perineum with a solution of peroxide and water after each elimination, and pat dry.
6. Report to the physician any swelling, redness, unusual tenderness, drainage, or foul odor of incision site.
7. Report any temperature over 101° F.
8. Eat a well-balanced diet to promote healing.
9. Take all medications as prescribed.
10. Elevate legs periodically to prevent pelvic congestion (see Fig. 12-4).
11. When in doubt, call the physician or clinic.

Cancer of the Ovary

Neoplasia of the ovary causes more deaths than any other female genital tract cancer. It is estimated that 20,500 new cases will be diagnosed each year, and 12,400 women will die of the disease each year (Silverberg, 1990). When ovarian cancer is diagnosed and treated early, 85% of the women live 5 years or longer. However, because the symptoms of this type of cancer are vague and definitive screening tests do not exist, ovarian cancer is often diagnosed in an advanced stage. When this occurs, the survival rate falls to 23%. The overall survival rate for this type of cancer is 38% (Boring, Squires, Tong, 1991). The incidence in the United States is 1 in 70 women. Malignant neoplasia of the ovaries occurs at all ages, including infants and children. However, the greatest number of cases are found in the 50 to 59 age group.

Major histologic cell types occur in different age groups, with malignant germ cell tumors most common in women in the 20 to 40 age groups and epithelial cancers occurring in the perimenopausal age groups.

A number of theories have been proposed to explain the pathogenesis of ovarian cancer. Theories of environmental stimulants such as exposure to asbestos and talc have been suggested, but definite correlations between specific substances in the environment and ovarian cancer have yet to be established. However, since the highest ratio of ovarian cancers occur in highly industrialized countries (Japan being the exception), an environmental connection seems likely.

Hormonal factors also seem to influence the incidence of ovarian cancer. An increased incidence is noted in women with poor functioning status of the ovary, i.e., before menarche, older than 18 years, menopause occurring before 45 years, nulliparity, and infertility. Another documented risk factor is a genetic predisposition. The risk increases if a mother or sister has had ovarian cancer.

Other risk factors have included life-style behaviors such as ingesting a diet high in saturated fats or using chemicals or carcinogens in the genital area with ascending migration and absorption of the toxins into the tubes and ovaries. Because of its gonadotropic potential, exposure to the mumps virus has also been postulated.

CLINICAL MANIFESTATIONS AND DIAGNOSIS. Ovarian cancer has been called a silent disease because early warning symptoms that would send a woman to her physician are absent (e.g., no bleeding or other discharge and no pain). Vague lower abdominal discomfort and mild digestive complaints are the early symptoms for some. An ovary enlarged to 5 cm or more found during routine examination requires careful diagnostic workup. The accompanying increase in abdominal girth (caused by ovarian enlargement or ascites) is usually attributed to an increase in weight, or a shift in weight that is seen commonly in women entering their middle years. Pelvic pain, anemia, and cachexia are late findings.

Ovarian cancer is rarely diagnosed early. Seventy percent of all women have metastasis outside of the pelvis at the time of diagnosis. Attempts at early detection have not proven to be reliable so far. Pelvic ultrasound, CA-125 antigen (a tumor-associated antigen) and frequent pelvic examinations have all been used without a great deal of success because these tumors grow quickly and painlessly. Any ovarian enlargement should be considered highly suspicious and in need of further evaluation by laparoscopy or laparotomy. Responsibility for diagnosis rests with the pathologist. The size of the tumor is not indicative of the severity of disease. A positive Papanicolaou test of vaginal, pleural, or peritoneal fluids and lung and bone scans also contribute to a differential diagnosis. Clinical staging is done surgically and gives direction to treatment and prognosis (DiSaia, Creasman, 1992; Baird, McCorkle Grant, 1991).

THERAPEUTIC MANAGEMENT. Treatment is dictated by the stage of the disease at the time of initial diagnosis. Surgical removal of as much of the tumor as possible is the first step in therapy. This may involve just the removal of one ovary and tube or radical excision of uterus, ovaries, tubes, and omentum. Cytoreductive surgery (the debulking of the poorly vascularized larger tumors) is also done. The smaller the volume of tumor remaining, the better the response to adjuvant therapy. Since almost two thirds of women are in stage II or IV disease at the time of diagnosis, surgical cure is not possible. Therefore, after tumor reduction surgery is performed, women with epithelial cell carcinoma will receive chemotherapy. Many institutions use a multiagent approach. Combinations of neoplastic drugs such as cyclophosphamide (Cytoxan) and cisplatin or cisplatin and doxorubicin (Adriamycin) are common.

The efficacy of intraperitoneal installation with radioactive phosphorus (^{32}P) is currently being investigated at a number of institutions.

The role of radiation in treating ovarian carcinoma is unclear. Although radiation has been used in the past, its use has decreased as the effectiveness of chemotherapy has increased. More study is needed to determine the role of radiation in earlier-stage ovarian cancer.

Second-look surgery is a technique used to determine the response of the disease to chemotherapy and to determine whether treatment should be continued.

NURSING IMPLICATIONS. Ovarian carcinoma carries with it a poor prognosis because of the advanced stage at initial diagnosis. When a cure or remission cannot be achieved, palliative measures that alleviate symptoms of the progressing disease and provide comfort and maximum function during the woman's remaining time are initiated. The goal is maintaining quality of life.

Because the period between a focus on cure and a focus on palliation is often prolonged, the woman with cancer is apt to experience most of the stages described by Kübler-Ross and to require support through each.

After diagnosis, the woman experiences denial, then anger. As treatment begins, she may "bargain" for a cure. If treatment is successful and death is forestalled by remission or cure, the process of adjustment to terminality ceases and the woman again focuses on life and its challenges. When treatment fails to secure a cure or remission ends, the woman must turn again to the task of adjustment.

Grieving for relatives, friends, possessions, and all of the familiar and pleasant aspects of living that are to be lost, the woman is profoundly depressed. She may regret unaccomplished tasks, unfulfilled dreams, mistakes, and marred relationships, and she may be deeply frustrated. Time has run out for her, and it is likely that there will be no second chances. Starting alone on a long journey to the unknown, she is afraid. Seeing healthy people all about her apparently destined for a long life, she may be angry and jealous. Sometimes, in approaching death, she finds greater meaning in life and gains much strength, communicating this to others. Many finally accept dying as an inevitable, sad, but meaningful final phase of living.

Family and friends also experience diverse feelings. When grieving is prolonged, as it often is when the woman has cancer, the stress can be enormous and can interfere with other interpersonal relationships. The hospital environment may further intrude on relationships, limiting privacy and access to the woman and hindering opportunities for caring gestures (for further discussion of loss and grief, see Chapter 40).

Because these factors may diminish the woman's chances for a dignified and peaceful death, alternative modes of health care delivery for the terminally ill are being explored. These approaches include home care, with provisions for supportive medical and nursing services as needed, and hospice care, where the woman is not abandoned once cure is no longer the focus of medical intervention. Hospice care may take place in a specific institutional setting, bringing together dying people in a single building or building complex, or it may exist within an acute care facility. Regardless of setting, the principles of care include support of normalcy for as long as possible, adequate relief of pain and other discomforts, removal of barriers to interaction with family and loved ones, and sustained emotional and spiritual support.

CANCER AND PREGNANCY

Cancer occurs with relative infrequency during the reproductive years. Approximately one of each 118 women of childbearing age diagnosed with cancer will be pregnant at the time. This translates into the fact that for each 1800 pregnant women, one will also have cancer (Donegan, 1983). Although all forms of neoplasms have been documented in conjunction with pregnancy, the most frequently occurring types are breast cancer, leukemia and lymphomas as a group, melanomas, gynecologic (cervical and ovarian), and bone tumors, in that order. Some sources also include colorectal (Donegan, 1983). When pregnancy and cancer coincide, therapeutic issues are complex, and intense reactions occur in the client, her family, and the health care team. Clients are confronted with issues such as continuing or terminating the pregnancy, and the selection and timing of therapies such as chemotherapy, radiation, and surgery are all affected by the pregnancy. Add to this the conflicting feelings the client has (i.e., the joy of pregnancy vs. the fear and anxiety associated with cancer), and the task of providing comprehensive care for the client and her family presents a formidable challenge to the health care team.

A brief discussion of the most frequent types of cancers that occur during pregnancy and the current therapies associated with them follows.

CANCER OF THE BREAST. Approximately 1% to 2% of women are pregnant or lactating at the time of diagnosis of cancer of the breast (Pernoll, Benson, 1987). Breast cancer complicates about 1 in 3000 pregnancies. The prognosis for women who are diagnosed with breast cancer while pregnant is some 15% to 20% below the overall survival rate of 50% because the disease is generally in the advanced stages when first diagnosed (DiSaia, Creasman, 1992). Diagnosis is often delayed because breast engorgement may obscure the mass from palpation and increased density of the tissue makes mammographic visualization more difficult. In addition, increased vascularity and lymphatic drainage in the breast of a pregnant client may increase the speed of metastasis. Pregnancy or lactation is not a contraindication to surgery. Surgery is usually the treatment of choice for breast cancer in pregnancy. If an invasive tumor is found, it must be determined whether the tissue is estrogen receptor (ER) positive or negative. ER-negative tumors spread more rapidly than ER-positive tumors and are more common in pregnancy.

Termination of the pregnancy in early stages of the disease appears to have no impact on survival. Therapeutic abortion may become an issue in the presence of advanced disease and may be deemed necessary to achieve effective palliation. For advanced disease in the second or third trimester, alkylating agents, 5-fluorouracil, and vincristine are relatively safe for the fetus (DiSaia, Creasman, 1992). Chemotherapy may significantly improve the survival of these women.

Radiation therapy is avoided if at all possible because, even with careful shielding, the fetus may still receive sufficient radiation to produce detrimental effects.

After diagnosis, breast-feeding is contraindicated on two counts: (1) if one of the oncogens for breast cancer is a virus, as many have postulated, then the remaining breast may be contaminated and the virus may be passed to the newborn and may act as a latent inducer of breast carcinoma, and (2) lactation increases vascularity in the remaining breast, which may contain a neoplasm.

The question of subsequent pregnancies depends on the disease-free interval and the status of the lymph nodes (Morrow, Townsend, 1987). A disease-free interval of 2 years, no evidence of metastatic disease, and negative nodes are good prognostic signs. That is, prognosis is not adversely affected by a subsequent pregnancy (Harris, 1990; Morrow, Townsend, 1987).

A 70% 5-year survival rate is anticipated after therapy when the neoplasm is confined to the breast. If axillary metastases are present, the 5-year survival rate after therapy is 30% to 40%. Earlier diagnosis in pregnant women and improved therapy underlie the improvement in the overall survival rate.

LEUKEMIA. The average age for pregnant women with acute leukemia is 28; incidence during pregnancy is not specified, but the incidence in the general population in the United States is 10 in 100,000.

Pregnancy seems to have no specific effect on the course of the disease except that vigorous therapy is detrimental to early gestation. Preterm labor and postpartum hemorrhage are associated with acute leukemia. Acute myelocytic leukemia (90% of cases) has a more fulminant course and requires immediate therapy; in the presence of chronic myelocytic leukemia, therapy can be delayed somewhat. Some pregnant women with the chronic form of the disease who had chemotherapy and radiotherapy directed at the spleen have given birth to apparently healthy infants. The decision to terminate the pregnancy rests with the woman and her family: however, prompt, aggressive therapy is always advisable if remission is to be achieved. Decisions may be influenced by the aggressiveness of the disease.

HODGKIN'S DISEASE (LYMPHORETICULOMA). Hodgkin's disease is a malignant lymphoma that affects many younger people and complicates about one in 6000 pregnancies. Younger women (under 40) have a better prognosis.

Pregnancy appears to have no effect on the disease and vice versa, other than those effects resulting from therapy. Radiotherapy and chemotherapy now are responsible for the care or control of Hodgkin's disease for long periods. Unless gestation is well into the third trimester, delay in initiating therapy should be minimal, which brings up the dilemma of therapeutic abortion. Radiotherapy to diseased areas above the diaphragm can be initiated during the third trimester with proper shielding of the fetus. Chemotherapy is strongly contraindicated during the first trimester and is relatively contraindicated in the second and third trimesters.

If the woman and her family refuse any therapy until pregnancy terminates naturally, the physician has no choice. However, termination of the pregnancy before initiating radiotherapy or chemotherapy is most desirable (DiSaia, Creasman, 1992).

MELANOMA. Malignant melanoma may be one of the rare cancers that can be affected by pregnancy. This is suggested by many reports in which pregnancy has been shown to induce or exacerbate a melanoma. During pregnancy the following changes occur naturally:

1. Melanocyte-stimulating hormone (MSH) increases after 8 weeks' gestation.
2. Adrenocorticotropic production increases, and ACTH heightens MSH activity.
3. Estrogen, which is produced in enormous amounts during pregnancy, has been shown to control melanocyte activity in the guinea pig model (DiSaia, Creasman, 1992).

Although pregnancy has been implicated in the more rapid metastases to regional lymph nodes, stage for stage, there does not seem to be a significant difference in the survival of pregnant and nonpregnant women. As a result, most authorities recommend that women who have histories of malignant melanoma delay pregnancy for about 3 years after surgical excision, since this is the period of highest risk for recurrence.

Diagnosis is established by biopsy. Therapy consists of radical local excision. For most other malignancies, the placenta is unexplainably resistant to invasion by maternal cancer. Though melanoma accounts for few cases of malignant disease during pregnancy, almost 50% of the *placental metastases* and almost 90% of *fetal metastases* occur from maternal melanoma.

BONE TUMORS. Ewing's sarcoma and osteogenic sarcoma and osteocystoma are the most common primary malignant bone tumors seen in pregnancy. Usually the areas involved are the clavicle, sternum, spine, humerus, and femur. A lump or mass, local pain, and disability are characteristic manifestations.

Osteogenic sarcoma affects areas of high bone turnover (during growth spurts especially): Ewing's sarcoma is a rare condition that develops within bone marrow. Pregnancy does not affect nor is affected by the disease.

Surgical excision is usually well tolerated during pregnancy; adjuvant chemotherapy is delayed until after birth if the cancer is diagnosed near term. With prompt chemotherapy (within a few weeks of diagnosis), 50% to 70% (compared with 5% before the advent of chemotherapy) of affected women are disease-free at 5 years. If the disease recurs, it usually does so within 3 years. Therefore women are counseled to defer pregnancy during this time.

CANCER OF THE VULVA. The diagnosis of preinvasive (vulvular intraepithelial neoplasia) disease during pregnancy is not uncommon. Therapy is postponed until the postpartum period.

If invasive disease is diagnosed during the first trimester, vulvectomy with bilateral groin dissection may be done after the fourteenth week. When it is diagnosed in the third trimester, local wide excision is done, deferring definitive surgery until after birth. Pregnancy does not alter the course of the disease.

After radical vulvectomy and bilateral inguinal lymphectomy, several women who have become pregnant again carried the pregnancies to term and gave birth vaginally. If local fibrosis is present and could impede birth, abdominal birth is advisable.

CANCER OF THE VAGINA. Except for clear-cell adenocarcinoma of DES-exposed women, cancer of the vagina is not common. If clear-cell adenocarcinoma of the cervix and vagina or sarcoma is found in the upper vagina, the preferred surgery is radical hysterectomy, upper vaginectomy, and bilateral pelvic lymphadenectomy, followed by chemotherapy. If disease is advanced, the preferred treatment is to empty the uterus and begin radiotherapy.

CANCER OF THE CERVIX. A tremendous diversity of opinion can be found in the literature regarding the cause and effect of carcinoma of the cervix and pregnancy. Some believe that carcinoma of the cervix prevents pregnancy, and others believe pregnancy prevents carcinoma of the cervix. Some reports argue that pregnancy accelerates cervical cancer while others propose that it actually slows the growth of cancer in the cervix. Consensus has yet to be achieved. Fortunately, the incidence of cervical cancer in the pregnant population is low. The incidence of cervical cancer concurrent with pregnancy is generally reported to be around 1%. Birth can be accomplished by either vaginal or cesarean routes. However, there is some concern regarding vaginal birth in the presence of invasive disease because the risk of hemorrhage and metastatic seeding from local trauma may be increased (DiSaia, Creasman, 1992; Harris, 1990).

The cancer itself does not harm the pregnancy: stage for stage, the outcome for the woman with cervical cancer is roughly the same as for the nonpregnant woman (DiSaia, Creasman, 1992; Herbst et al, 1991). Carcinoma of the cervix is curable if diagnosed and treated in its early stages.

A diagnosis of microinvasion made by colposcopy-directed biopsy must be followed by cone biopsy to rule out frankly invasive disease. This is the only absolute indication for conization during pregnancy. Because cervical hemorrhage is a concern during a biopsy, some authors recommend using hemostatic sutures in the cervix before the conization.

Fortunately in pregnancy the squamocolumnar junction is everted, so a deep tissue sample is not necessary; rather, a shallow cone biopsy or "coin" biopsy can be done.

The therapy of invasive carcinoma of the cervix during pregnancy is affected by many factors. The stage of the disease and the trimester in which the cancer is diagnosed are important. Equally important are the beliefs and desires of the woman and her family in terms of initiating therapy that can interrupt the pregnancy as opposed to postponing the therapy until fetal viability is achieved. If the carcinoma is diagnosed in the first trimester or early in the second trimester (before 20 weeks), treatment is preferably undertaken immediately. The main concern is that a delay of over 4 months would lead to tumor progression or spread.

One source reports that the survival rate for the mother may decrease 15% for every month of delay before initiating therapy (Harris, 1990).

For pregnancies beyond the twentieth week of gestation, a decision regarding initiating therapy immediately or delaying until fetal viability must be made. If it is desired to continue the therapy, the health of the fetus and its maturity is assessed. Appropriate ultrasound studies and amniotic fluid analyses are used to ensure fetal lung maturity. After cesarean birth, therapy is completed by surgery, radiation, or chemotherapy with the same considerations of tumor size, stage, and invasiveness for any woman who is treated before the twentieth week of pregnancy. If immediate treatment is to be undertaken, hysterotomy is first performed and then surgery or radiation therapy completed. The woman who is diagnosed during the first trimester has a better prognosis than those diagnosed during the third trimester.

CANCER OF THE UTERUS. Endometrial carcinoma during pregnancy is rare; only a few cases have been documented since 1900. Diagnosis was usually an incidental finding after therapeutic abortion or surgery, and the lesions were minimally or not invasive. Recommended therapy is total abdominal hysterectomy and bilateral salpingo-oophorectomy (TAH-BSO) and adjuvant radiotherapy.

CANCER OF THE UTERINE TUBE. With a peak incidence between 50 and 55 years, concurrent pregnancy is only a remote possibility. Should it occur, the recommended therapy (TAH-BSO with postoperative radiotherapy or chemotherapy) is the same as for the nonpregnant woman. A few cases have been first diagnosed following tubal ligation during routine histologic evaluation of the small resected segment.

CANCER OF THE OVARY. Cancer of the ovary is the third most frequent cancer that occurs with pregnancy. Still, ovarian malignancy is relatively rare, being reported to occur in one per 9000 to 25,000 births (Harris, 1990).

Ovarian masses occur frequently during pregnancy. Since corpus luteum cysts account for a high percentage of these masses and because 99% of these resolve by the 14th week, any mass <5 cm may simply be observed until the end of the first trimester. Any mass >5 cm, one that is growing, or one that does not resolve after the 14th week warrants further investigation. Abdominal palpation and ultrasound are the diagnostic tools of choice during pregnancy. However, in many cases laparotomy is necessary to confirm the diagnosis. Laparotomy after 16 weeks' gestation has negligible fetal wastage associated with the procedure and is therefore considered safe. The most common complication is torsion, which occurs most often when the uterus is rising rapidly (8 to 16 weeks) or involuting during the puerperium. Indicators of torsion are lower abdominal pain, tense and tender abdomen with guarding, nausea, vomiting, and shocklike symptoms.

An ovarian tumor may be first diagnosed at birth because the enlarged uterus obscured its presence. If it falls back into the cul-de-sac, it may obstruct the birth canal and during labor may be traumatized. Hemorrhage into the tumor is followed by necrosis and suppuration (pus formation).

Cancer Therapy and Pregnancy

Decisions about the type and timing of therapy for cancer in the pregnant woman evoke moral and philosophic dilemmas as well as complex medical judgments and intense emotional responses. The fetus is at risk with either chemotherapy or radiation therapy. The impact of cancer therapy on the fetus can include death, spontaneous abortion, teratogenesis, alteration in growth and development, alterations in function, and mutagenesis. The long-term effects on the fetus are unknown. However, the long-term experiences of young women exposed to DES in utero make the possibility of long-term effects associated with cancer therapy very real. These theoretic dangers must be weighed against the potential detrimental effects to the mother if treatment is withheld.

Timing of therapy is also an important issue to discuss. Since most cancer therapy (except surgery) is geared toward having a differential and noxious effect on rapidly growing tissue, the fetus is most at risk during the first trimester when organogenesis and rapid tissue growth occurs.

Chemotherapy is avoided in the first trimester if at all possible. Although most chemotherapeutic agents have had isolated reports of fetal abnormalities associated with them, data on the agents used after the first trimester have recorded surprisingly few fetal abnormalities. Therefore, while risk still exists, the judicious use of chemotherapy after the first trimester can result in live births with few congenital abnormalities.

Radiation therapy presents its own set of issues. During embryonic development, tissues are extremely radiosensitive. If cells are genetically altered or killed during this time, the child either will fail to survive or will be deformed. From a radiologic stance there are three significant periods in embryonic development (for further discussion, see Chapter 7):

1. *Preimplantation:* If irradiation does not destroy the fertilized egg, it probably does not affect it significantly.
2. *Critical period of organogenesis:* During this period, especially between days 18 and 38, the organism is most vulnerable; microcephaly, anencephaly, eye damage, growth retardation, spina bifida, and foot damage may occur.
3. *After day 40:* Large doses may still cause observable malformation and damage to the central nervous system.

Irradiation of gonads involves genetic damage—gene mutation and chromosome breakage—even at relatively low doses. Most mutations are recessive so that mutant effects may not surface for many generations.

Pregnancy After Cancer Treatment

If cancer therapy has not included the removal of the uterus, ovaries, or uterine (fallopian) tubes, there is a possibility that the woman may still be able to become pregnant. Although a woman's menstrual cycle may have resumed, successful pregnancy may be difficult to achieve. Therapy that has affected the pituitary or thyroid gland may make conception difficult. Radiation appears to have the most deleterious effects on the endocrine system (Harris, 1990). If ovarian function is desired after treatment, single-agent chemotherapy is preferred if an effective agent is available (Harris, 1990).

In order for recovery from the disease and treatment to be complete, a delay of at least 2 years from the end of therapy to conception is advised. An exception is the women who has had ovarian cancer, who because of a high incidence of a second primary tumor, is advised to complete her childbearing as soon as possible (Harris, 1990).

Before conception, women who have had cancer should have a complete physical examination to rule out complications that may place her or a fetus in jeopardy. Cardiac, pulmonary, hematologic, neurologic, renal, or gonadal function may be impaired.

■ GESTATIONAL TROPHOBLASTIC DISEASE

Gestational Trophoblastic Disease (GTD), more recently termed **Gestational Trophoblastic Neoplasia (GTN)**, is a term that encompasses a spectrum of disorders arising from the placental trophoblast. It includes hydatidiform mole (see Chapter 30), invasive mole, and choriocarcinoma. Before the middle 1950s, the prognoses of these neoplasias, especially end-stage choriocarcinoma, were dismal. Today, however, GTN is recognized as the most curable gynecologic malignancy. The reasons for this change in thinking are related to several factors: (1) a sensitive marker is produced by the tumor (human chorionic gonadotropin [hCG]); (2) the tumor is extremely sensitive to various chemotherapeutic agents; (3) high-risk factors in the disease process can be identified, allowing for individualized therapy; and (4) the aggressive use of multiple treatment methods is possible.

The incidence and etiology of the hydatidiform mole are discussed in Chapter 30. However, the clinical classification of benign or malignant indicates that 80% to 85% of clients will have the benign form, and the remaining 15% to 20% have a malignant form requiring further treatment.

Passage of vascular tissue is often the first symptom suggesting hydatidiform mole (Fig. 44-12). Bleeding in the first trimester is also a common symptom. The diagnosis is usually confirmed by ultrasound, beta-hCG levels, and sometimes amniography. Thecal luteal cysts of the ovaries, caused by excessive amounts of hCG, may also be present. Clients with associated thecal luteal cysts appear to have a higher incidence of developing malignant sequelae of GTN.

Once diagnosis is confirmed, evacuation of the intact mole is the initial therapy. The uterus is evacuated with a cervical dilatation and uterine curettage (D & C) accompanied by oxytocin infusion to stimulate uterine contractions that facilitate emptying the uterus. Hysterectomy is an option if retention of reproductive capacity is not an issue. This procedure results in a cure rate of 90%.

Follow-up care requires close monitoring of hCG levels, since hCG is a sensitive marker to trophoblastic cells in the body. Initially beta-hCG levels are monitored every 1 to 2 weeks until there are two normal determinations. The hCG level should then be monitored bimonthly for 1 year. During this time pregnancy is contraindicated since normal pregnancy cannot be differentiated from GTN by monitoring hCG levels. An initial chest x-ray film is also recommended to rule out metastasis and is repeated only if hCG levels reach a plateau or rise. Physical examination including pelvic examination is performed every 2 weeks until hCG levels return to normal and continue every 3 months thereafter for 1 year.

The use of single-agent or combination drug chemotherapy depends on the classification of the disease as either metastatic or nonmetastatic. Clients with nonmetastatic disease can be treated with single-agent chemotherapy. Methotrexate has been the treatment of choice for years. However, it is contraindicated in the presence of abnormal liver function. Dactinomycin has also been used with equally good results. Recent studies using methotrexate with folinic acid rescue have also shown excellent results. Because of the lower toxicity and high rate of remission, this latter combination has become the first-line treatment in the United States (DiSaia, Creasman, 1992). Clients with GTN who are found to have metastasis are classified as having either good or poor prognosis depending on the absence or presence of brain or liver metastasis, unsuccessful prior chemotherapy, symptoms lasting longer than 4 months, and serum beta-hCG levels greater than 40,000 mIU/mL. Treatment progresses from single-agent chemotherapy in the good prognosis category to multiple-agent chemotherapy and multiple methods of treatment for the poor-prognosis group.

Because hysterectomy is no longer a standard therapy for GTN, subsequent pregnancy is a possibility for many women, even those who have received chemotherapy. However, the risk of developing another molar pregnancy is increased 5 to 10 times in these women (Huff, 1990). It is therefore important that a pregnant woman with a history of GTN receive early prenatal care and careful monitoring to ensure prompt intervention should another molar pregnancy occur.

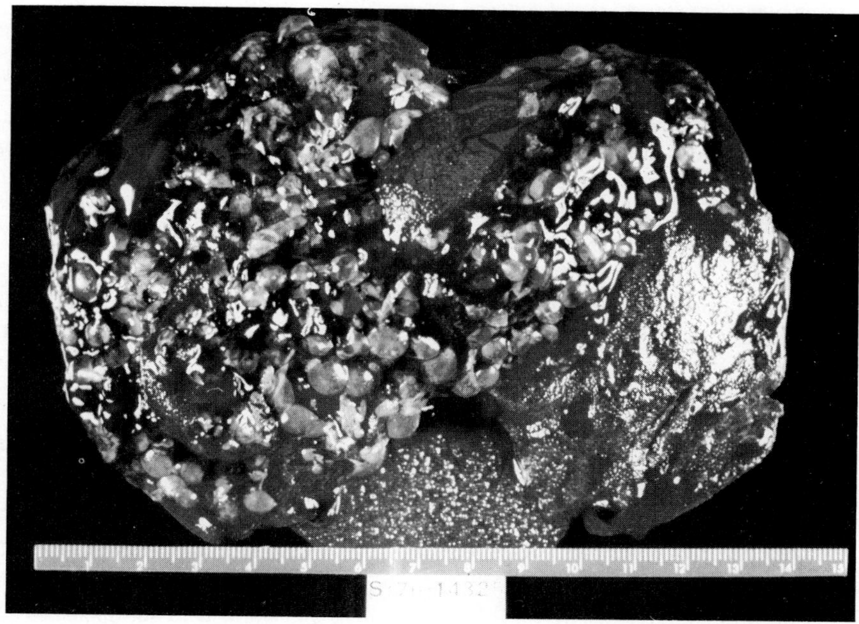

Fig. 44-12 Typical enlarged cystic villi are apparent in this molar pregnancy. Courtesy Department of Pathology, Duke University Medical Center. From DiSaia PJ, Creasman WT: *Clinical gynecologic oncology,* ed 4, St Louis, 1992, Mosby–Year Book.

EXPERIMENTAL THERAPIES FOR GYNECOLOGIC CANCER

Prostaglandins (PGs), their metabolites, and related compounds have a vital function in almost every aspect of human physiology. The biosynthesis, mode of action, and pharmacologic configuration of these compounds have important implications in cell biology and clinical medicine. Their possible role in cancer may be related to biologically important interactions in carcinogenesis, the rate of proliferation and differentiation of tumor cells, tumor cell metastasis, the host-tumor relationship, and cancer therapy (Karmali, 1983).

Two processes are identified in chemical carcinogenesis: initiation by chemical reactive carcinogens, and promotion by a promoting agent. PGs may be implicated in both processes. Excessive PGs have been found in several types of malignant neoplasias. PGE_2 has been associated with symptoms commonly seen with breast cancer, for example, metastatic spread to bone and hypercalcemia. Carcinomas of the breast and lung produce more PG-like material than do normal tissues. In some people with cancer, PG production by tumor cells causes immunosuppression.

Research continues on the role of PGs in neoplasia and drugs that may influence the synthesis and action of PGs in such a way as to suppress carcinogenesis and metastasis.

WORKING WITH THE WOMAN WITH CANCER

Many health professionals find cancer depressing, viewing it as a hopeless disease. These professionals are trained to promote healthfulness and cure disease, but the nature of cancer thwarts their self-image as helping, healing persons. Unfortunately, in dismissing the disease as hopeless, they are dismissing the woman, too.

Others view cancer as a challenge to be combated with all the treatment possibilities medical technology can provide. The danger here is that the woman becomes a casualty in the battle, an interesting specimen upon which to test new or radical treatments long after hope of cure has been abandoned.

Still others see cancer care as an opportunity to fully use their knowledge and skills in the care of a complex disease. For these professionals, hope is always present, advanced therapies are administered within a framework of total nursing care, and palliative measures are offered when oppressive therapy is no longer appropriate.

Caring for women with cancer on an ongoing basis can be emotionally draining. It is to nurses that desperate family members and women with cancer turn with their pleas and complaints. Sometimes, nurses identify closely with the woman with cancer; having cared for her through many devastating episodes, the final loss is severe and personal. Nurses are particularly taxed when groups of people on the hospital unit or in the nurse's case load compete for attention and energies. Nurses must seek emotional support from peers, superiors, and others within and outside the hospital or clinic to regain emotional strength.

■ SUMMARY

Cancer, neoplasia, and tumor are words that evoke a multitude of images, mostly negative, in all who hear them. It is devastating to hear these words used in relation to oneself. The context of this chapter provides the nurse with an overview of neoplasia (both benign and malignant) of the breast, the reproductive organs, and perineum and of gestational trophoblastic neoplasia. The effects of various cancers on the pregnant woman are also included. Nursing care for women who have selected cancers is discussed, providing suggestions for nurses who work with these women and their families.

Care of the woman with cancer and her family presents the nurse with energy-draining challenges. This challenge also offers the potential for fulfillment on both professional and personal levels.

REFERENCES

American Cancer Society: *1992 Facts and Figures,* New York, NY, 1992, ACS.

American Cancer Society: *Reach to recovery,* New York, The Society.

Baird SB, McCorkle R, Grant M: *Cancer nursing: a comprehensive textbook,* Philadelphia, 1991, WB Saunders Co.

Beal MW: Cervical cytology, *Clin Issues Perinat Women's Health Nurs* 1(4):470, 1990.

Beare PG, Myers JL: *Principles and practice of adult health nursing,* St Louis, 1990, Mosby–Year Book.

Bernstein L, Ross RK, Henderson BE: Prospects for the primary prevention of breast cancer, *Am J Epidemiol* 135(2):142, 1992.

Boring CC, Squires TS, Tong T: Cancer statistics, 1991, *CA Cancer J Clin* 41(1):19, 1991.

DiSaia PF, Creasman WT: *Clinical gynecologic oncology,* ed 4, St Louis, 1992, Mosby–Year Book.

Donegan WL: Cancer and pregnancy, *Cancer* 33:194, 1983.

Herbst AL et al: *Comprehensive gynecology,* ed 2 St Louis, 1991, Mosby–Year Book.

Harris BG: Issues in nursing care of pregnant patients with cancer, *Clin Issues Perinat Women's Health Nurs* 1(4):423, 1990.

Henderson IC: Adjuvant therapy for breast cancer, *N Engl J Med* 318(7):443, 1988.

Huff BC: Gestational trophoblastic disease, *Clin Issues Perinat Women's Health Nurs* 1(4):453-458, 1990.

Karmali RA: Prostaglandins and cancer, *CA Cancer J Clin* 33:322, 1983.

Grover ST et al: Factors influencing serum CA 125 levels in normal women, *Obstet Gynecol* 70(4):511, April 1992.

Lawhead RA, Majmudar B: Early diagnosis of vulvar neoplasia as a result of vulval self-examination, *J Reprod Med* 35(12):1134, 1990.

Leinster SL et al: Mastectomy versus conservative surgery: psychosocial effects of the patient's choice of treatment, *J Psychosoc Oncol* 7:179, 1989.

Levine RM, Lippman ME: Breast cancer management: recent advances and recommendations, *Adv Intern Med* 29:215, 1984.

Levine MN et al: The thrombogenic effect of anticancer drug therapy in women with stage II breast cancer, *N Engl J Med* 318(7):404, 1988.

Lowdermilk DL: Nursing care update: internal radiation therapy, *Clin Issues Perinat Women's Health Nurs* 1(4):532, 1990.

Moore MD: Precursor lesions of the cervix, *Clin Issues Perinat Women's Health Nurs* 1(4):513, 1990.

Morris J, Ingham R: Choice of surgery for early breast cancer: psychosocial considerations, *Soc Sci Med* 27:1257, 1988.

Morrow CP, Townsend DE: *Synopsis of gynecologic oncology,* ed 3, New York, 1987, John Wiley & Sons.

Pathak DR, Whittemore AS: Combined effects of body size, parity, and menstrual events on breast cancer incidence in seven countries, *Am J Epidemiol* 135(2):153, 1992.

Pernoll, ML, Benson, RC, editors: *Current obstetric and gynecologic diagnosis and treatment,* Los Altos, Calif, 1987, Lange Medical Books.

Piver MS: The promise of hydroxyurea for cervical Ca, *Contemp Obstet Gynecol* 23:45, 1984.

Reid R, et al: Superficial laser vulvectomy, IV: extended laser vaporization and adjunctive 5-fluorouracil therapy of human papillomavirus associated vulval disease, *Obstet Gynecol* 76(3):439, 1990.

Siegel BS: *Peace, love and healing,* New York, 1989, Harper & Row.

Silverberg E: Cancer statistics, *Cancer* 40(9):1990.

Wrensch MR et al: Breast cancer incidence in women with abnormal cytology in nipple aspirates of breast fluid, *Am J Epidemiology,* 135(2):158, 1992.

BIBLIOGRAPHY

Austin D, Davis P: Valvular disease in pregnancy, *J Perinat Neonat Nurs* 5(2):13, 1991.

Berek JS, Bagshawe KD, Bast RC: Monoclonal antibodies' role in combating gynecologic malignancies. *Contemp OB/GYN* 35(2), Feb 1990.

Bergkwist L et al: The risk of breast cancer after estrogen and estrogen-progestin replacement, *N Engl J Med* 321(5):293, 1989.

Berkowitz RS et al: Chemoprophylaxis: still controversial for molar pregnancy, *Contemp OB/GYN* 32(4):27, 1988.

Bornstein BA et al: Results of treating ductal carcinoma in situ of the breast with conservative surgery and radiation therapy, *Cancer* 67(1):7, 1991.

Bourne TH et al: Ultrasound screening for familial ovarian cancer. *Gynecol Oncol* 43:92, 1991.

Boyages J, Harris JR: Local therapy of invasive disease, *Hematol Oncol Clin North Am* 3(4):675, 1989.

Brand E: Photodynamic therapy pinpoints cancer cells, *Contemp OB/GYN* 33(1):30, 1989.

Brumsted JR, Shirk GJ, Gimpleson RJ: Expanding gyn applications of the Nd:YAG laser, *Contemp OB/GYN,* 34 (Technology):31, 1990.

Carter CL: A prospective study of reproductive, familial, and socioeconomic risk factors for breast cancer using NHANES I data, *Publ Health Rep* 104(1):45, 1989.

Cawley MM: Recent advances in chemotherapy: administration and nursing implications, *Adv Oncol Nurs* 25(2):377, 1990.

DePrec N, Wils J: Long term survival of patients with advanced ovarian carcinoma treated with cisplatin-based chemotherapy regimen, *Anticancer Res* 9:1869, 1989.

Doane LS, Fischer LM, McDonald TW: How to give peritoneal chemotherapy, *AJN* 58-66, April 1990.

Elliott EA et al: Body fat patterning in women with endometrial cancer, *Gynecol Oncol* 39:253, 1990.

Fanning J et al: Prognostic significance of the extent of cervical involvement by endometrial cancer, *Gynecol Oncol* 40:46, 1991.

Feldman JE: Ovarian failure and cancer treatment: incidence and intervention for the premenopausal woman, *Oncol Nurs Forum* 16(5), 651, 1989.

Ginsberg AD et al: Systemic adjuvant therapy for node-negative breast cancer, *Can Med Assoc J* 141:381, 1989.

Greifzer S, Radjeski D, Winnick B: Oral care is part of cancer care, *RN* 53:43-46, June 1990.

Harris RE, Wynder EL: Breast cancer and alcohol consumption: a study in weak association, *JAMA* 259(19):2867, 1988.

Heaps JM, Nieberg RK, Berek JG: Malignant neoplasms arising in endometriosis, *Obstet Gynecol* 75(6):1023, 1990.

Henderson IC: Adjuvant systemic therapy: state of the art 1989, *Breast Cancer Res Treat* 14:3, 1989.

Jones MW, Durman RJ: New ways of managing endometrial hyperplasia, *Contemp OB/GYN* 35(12):36, 1990.

Jotti GS: New prognostic indicators in resectable breast cancer, *Anticancer Res* 9:1227, 1989.

Knobf MT: Early-stage breast cancer: the options, *AJN* 90:28, Nov 1990.

Koss LG: The Papanicolaou test for cervical cancer detection: a triumph and a tragedy, *JAMA* 261(5):737, 1989.

Kwikkel HJ: Treating CIN—laser vaporization or cryotherapy, *Contemp OB/GYN* 33(3):29, 1989.

Lawhead RA: Vulvar self-examination, what your patients should know, *The Female Patient* 15:33, Jan 1990.

Loomer L et al: Postoperative follow-up of patients with early breast cancer: pattern of care among clinical oncologists and a review of the literature, *Cancer* 67(1):55, 1990.

Louden S, Willett W: Diet and the risk of breast cancer, *Hematol Oncol Clin North Am* 3(4):559, 1989.

Love RR et al: Side effects and emotional distress during cancer chemotherapy, *Cancer* 63:604, 1989.

Lucas VA: Human papillomavirus infection: a potentially carcinogenic sexually transmitted disease (condylomata acuminata, genital warts), *Nurs Clin North Am* 23(4):917, 1988.

Lungu O et al: Relationship between human papillomavirus type and grade of CIN, *JAMA* 267(18):2493, 1992.

Maass H et al: New trends in the endocrine treatment of breast cancer, *Recent Results Cancer Res* 118:225, 1990.

Mack E: Most breast lumps aren't cancer, *RN* 53:20-23, Dec 1990.

McClay EF, Howell SB: A review: intraperitoneal cisplatin in the management of patients with ovarian cancer, *Gynecol Oncol* 36:1, 1990.

McGowan KL: Radiation therapy: saving your patients' skin, *RN* 52:24-27, June 1989.

Monga M et al: Surgery without adjuvant chemotherapy for early epithelial ovarian cancer, *Gynecol Oncol* 43:195, 1991.

Monk BJ, Montz FJ: Invasive cervical cancer complicating intrauterine pregnancy: treatment with radical hysterectomy, *Obstet Gynecol* 80(2):199, August 1992.

Moore J: Vaginal hysterectomy: its success as an outpatient procedure, *AORN J* 48(6):1114, 1988.

Nielsen BB, East D: Advances in breast cancer; implications for nursing care, *Nurs Clin North Am* 25(2):365, 1990.

Noguchi M, Miyazaki I: The surgical management of breast cancer, *Int Surgery* 75:8, 1990.

Norwood SL: Fibrocystic breast disease: an update and review, *JOGNN* 19(2):116, 1990.

Ollendorff DA, et al: Markedly elevated material serum alpha-fetoprotein associated with a normal fetus and choriocarcinoma of the placenta, *Obstet Gynecol* 76(3):494, 1990.

Papatestas AE: Breast disease in pregnancy, *Contemp OB/GYN,* 34 (Special Issue), 79-88.

Pritchard KI, Sutherland DJ: The use of endocrine therapy, *Hematol Oncol Clin North Am* 3(4):765, 1989.

Richard RM, Townsend DE: A new technique for ablating the endometrium, *Contemp OB/GYN* 33(4):90, 1989.

Richard RM et al: Endometrial cancer: state of the art, *Contemp OB/GYN* 31(6):107, 1988.

Rubin MM, Lawler D: Assessment and management of cervical intraepithelial neoplasia, *Nurse Pract* 15(9):23, 1990.

Schnitt SJ et al: Ductal carcinoma in situ (intraductal carcinoma of the breast), *N Engl J Med* 318(14);898, 1988.

Seibel MM: Does minimal endometriosis always require treatment, *Contemp OB/GYN* 34(1):27, 1989.

Smith DB: Pelvic exenteration: a historical overview, *J Enterostomal Therapy* 16(5):195, 1989.

Sparks JM, Varner RE: Ovarian cancer screening, *Obstet Gynecol* 77(5):787, 1991.

Young-McCaughan S, Sexton DL: Exercise: working out with cancer, *Oncol Nurs Forum* 18(4):751, 1991.

Zemlickis D, et al: Breast cancer during pregnancy—maternal and fetal outcomes, *Am J Obstet Gynecol* 166:781, 1992.

BIBLIOGRAPHY—NURSING RESEARCH

Albrecht SA, London WP: Season of birth and laterality of breast cancer, *Nurs Res* 39(2), March/April 1990.

Bruera E et al: Asthenia in breast cancer, *AJN* 89:737, May 1989.

Lauver D, Barsevick A, Rubin M: Spontaneous causal searching and adjustment to abnormal Papanicolaou test results, *Nurs Res,* 39(5), Sept/Oct 1990.

Mishel MH, Sorenson DS: Uncertainty in gynecological cancer: a test of the mediating functions of mastery and coping, *Nurs Res,* 40(3), May/June 1991.

chapter 44 review

Key Concepts

- The development of neoplasms, whether benign or malignant, can have a significant physical and emotional impact on the woman and her family.
- The risk of American women developing cancer of the breast is 1 in 9.
- An estimated 90% of all breast lumps are detected by the woman during breast self-examination.
- Monthly breast self-examination, routine screening mammography, and yearly breast examinations by practitioners are recommended for early detection of breast cancer.
- The modified radical mastectomy is the most common surgical procedure for breast cancer, although lumpectomy and radiation may be an alternative for stage I and II disease and tumors less than or equal to 4 cm.
- Menorrhagia is the most common symptom of leiomyomas or fibroid tumors.
- Endometrial cancer is the most common reproductive system malignancy.
- Hysterectomy is the usual treatment for early-stage endometrial cancer.
- Infections such as herpes simplex virus 2 and human papillomavirus types 16 and 18 have been linked to subsequent cervical cancer.
- The squamocolumnar junction is an important landmark identified with neoplastic changes of the cervix.
- Preinvasive cancer of the cervix may be treated with techniques such as electrocautery, cryotherapy, and laser therapy to save the structure of the cervix, particularly in women who desire to retain childbearing ability.
- External and internal radiation therapy in combination are as successful as surgery in treating cancer of the cervix.
- The Papanicolau test will detect approximately 90% of early cervical dysplasias.
- Cancer of the ovary causes more deaths than any other female genital tract cancer.
- Treatment of the pregnant woman who has cancer with radiation or chemotherapy places the fetus at risk for death, spontaneous abortion, teratogenesis, and/or alterations in growth and development.
- Nurses can control their exposure to radiation in three ways—increasing the distance from the radiation source, limiting the time of exposure, and using lead shielding.
- Cancer is relatively infrequent during the reproductive years, occurring about once in every 1800 pregnancies.
- Gestational trophoblastic neoplasms are highly curable but require close monitoring of hCG levels for at least 1 year after treatment.

Key Terms

- benign (p. 1364)
- biopsy (p. 1364)
- cancer (p. 1364)
- carcinoma (p. 1364)
- cervical intraepithelial neoplasia (CIN) (p. 1378)
- colposcopy (p. 1375)
- conization (p. 1381)
- cryosurgery (p. 1380)
- diethylstilbestrol (DES) (p. 1378)
- dysplasia (p. 1379)
- fibroadenoma (p. 1364)
- fibrocystic disease (p. 1364)
- gestational trophoblastic neoplasia (GTN) (p. 1396)
- hysterectomy (p. 1374)
- in situ (p. 1366)
- laser surgery (p. 1380)
- leiomyomas (p. 1371)
- malignant (p. 1364)
- mammary duct ectasia (p. 1365)
- mammary dysplasia (p. 1364)
- mammography (p. 1364)
- mastectomy (p. 1367)
- metastasis (p. 1375)
- neoplasia (p. 1364)
- Papanicolaou (PAP) test (p. 1379)
- pelvic exenteration (p. 1383)
- polyps (p. 1371)
- prostaglandins (PGs) (p. 1397)
- radical vulvectomy (p. 1389)
- radiotherapy (p. 1374, 1381)

Critical Thinking Exercises

1. You are assigned to a woman preparing for surgery for breast cancer.
   a. Identify your feelings regarding breast cancer or other female reproductive malignancy. How might these feelings affect your ability to provide effective nursing care?
   b. What kind of support system do you believe is needed by the woman experiencing surgery for breast cancer? What might be special needs of her family?
   c. Develop a plan of care for the above woman and her family. Incorporate your responses to female malignancy in your plan of care.
2. Interview nursing students and other students regarding the knowledge and use of screening methods for cancer detection.
   a. Analyze your findings to determine the degree of awareness among non-nursing students and nursing students.
   b. Examine reasons for the differences and similarities.
   c. Propose an educational strategy to increase awareness of resources for cancer detection and prevention.

Topics for Nursing Research

- What is an effective intervention for increasing client motivation for performing monthly breast self-examinations?
- What will be the impact of the breast implant controversy on women seeking reconstructive surgery after mastectomy?
- How do different health care settings affect the nurse's knowledge and beliefs about breast cancer and its prevention?
- What are effective nursing interventions for preventing complications related to surgery, radiation therapy, and chemotherapy for gynecologic cancers?
- What are effective nursing interventions for preventing psychologic complications after hysterectomy?
- What are the long-term effects of cancer therapy during pregnancy on the fetus?

Glossary

Abdominal Belonging or relating to the abdomen and its functions and disorders.

A. delivery Birth of a child through a surgical incision made into the abdominal wall and uterus; cesarean birth.

A. gestation Implantation of a fertilized ovum outside the uterus but inside the peritoneal cavity.

A. hysterectomy Surgical removal of the uterus through an abdominal wall incision.

A. pregnancy See *abdominal gestation*.

Ablatio placentae See *abruptio placentae*.

ABO incompatibility Occurs when the mother's blood type is O and the newborn's is A, B, or AB.

Abortion Termination of pregnancy before the fetus is viable and capable of extrauterine existence. See *abortus* below.

Complete a. Abortion in which fetus and all related tissue have been expelled from the uterus.

Criminal a. Termination of pregnancy performed by unqualified people usually under septic conditions. Women may resort to this if elective abortions are unavailable.

Elective a. Termination of pregnancy chosen by the woman that is not required for her physical safety.

Habitual (recurrent) a. Loss of three or more successive pregnancies for no known cause.

Incomplete a. Loss of pregnancy in which some but not all the products of conception have been expelled from the uterus.

Induced a. Intentionally produced loss of pregnancy by woman or others.

Inevitable a. Threatened loss of pregnancy that cannot be prevented or stopped and is imminent.

Missed a. Loss of pregnancy in which the products of conception remain in the uterus after the fetus dies.

Septic a. Loss of pregnancy in which there is an infection of the products of conception and the uterine endometrial lining, usually resulting from attempted termination of early pregnancy.

Spontaneous a. Loss of pregnancy that occurs naturally without interference or known cause.

Therapeutic a. Pregnancy that has been intentionally terminated for medical reasons.

Threatened a. Possible loss of a pregnancy; early symptoms are present (e.g., the cervix begins to dilate).

Voluntary a. See *abortion, elective*.

Abortus An embryo/fetus that is removed or expelled from the uterus at 20 weeks' gestation or less, or weighing 500 g or less, or measuring 25 cm or less.

Abruptio placentae Partial or complete premature separation of a normally implanted placenta.

Abstinence Refraining from sexual intercourse periodically or permanently.

Accreta, placenta See *placenta accreta*.

Acculturation Process of adopting the cultural traits or social patterns of another group.

Acetonuria Presence of acetone and diacetic bodies in the urine.

Acidosis Increase in hydrogen ion concentration resulting in a lowering of blood pH below 7.35.

Metabolic a. Increase in hydrogen ion concentration caused by increased acids from (1) abnormal metabolism (too many acids produced), (2) renal malfunction (acids not being excreted), or (3) excessive loss of base (diarrhea).

Acini cells Milk-producing cells in the breast.

Acme Highest point (e.g., of a contraction).

Acrocyanosis Peripheral cyanosis; blue color of hands and feet in most infants at birth that may persist for 7 to 10 days.

Acromion Projection of the spine of the scapula (forming the point of the shoulder); used to explain the presentation of the fetus.

Adenomyoma Type of tumor affecting glandular and smooth muscle tissue, such as uterine musculature.

Adjuvant therapy Treatment given in addition to primary treatment.

Adnexa Adjacent or accessory parts of a structure.
Uterine a. Ovaries and fallopian tubes.

Adult respiratory distress syndrome (ARDS) Set of symptoms including decreased compliance of lung tissue, pulmonary edema, and acute hypoxemia. The condition is similar to respiratory distress syndrome of the newborn.

Afibrinogenemia Absence or decrease of fibrinogen in the blood such that the blood will not coagulate. In obstetrics, this condition occurs from complications of abruptio placentae or retention of a dead fetus. See *DIC*.

Afterbirth Lay term for the placenta and membranes expelled after the birth of the child.

Afterpains Painful uterine cramps that occur intermittently for approximately 2 or 3 days after birth and that result from contractile efforts of the uterus to return to its normal involuted condition.

AGA Appropriate (weight) for gestational age.

Agalactia Absence or failure of milk secretion after childbirth.

Agenesis Failure of an organ to develop.

Alae nasi Nostrils.

Albuminuria Presence of readily detectable amounts of albumin in the urine; proteinuria.

Alkalosis Abnormal condition of body fluids characterized by a tendency toward an increased pH, as from an excess of alkaline bicarbonate or a deficiency of acid.

Alveoli, fetal Terminal pulmonary sacs that in fetal life are filled with fluid. This fluid is a transudate of fetal plasma.

Ambient Surrounding; around.

Amenorrhea Absence or suppression of menstruation.

Amnesia Loss of memory.

Amniocentesis Procedure in which a needle is inserted through the abdominal and uterine walls into the amniotic fluid; used for assessment of fetal health and maturity and for elective abortion.

Amniography Procedure used primarily to detect placenta previa by x-ray examination, entailing injection of radiopaque dye into amniotic fluid.

Amnion Inner membrane of two fetal membranes that form the sac and contain the fetus and the fluid that surrounds it in utero.

Amnionitis Inflammation of the amnion, occurring frequently before or after early rupture of membranes.

Amniotic Pertaining or relating to the amnion.
A. fluid Fluid surrounding fetus derived primarily from maternal serum and fetal urine.
A. sac Membrane "bag" that contains the fetus before birth.

Amniotomy Artificial rupture of the fetal membranes (AROM).

Analgesia Lack of pain without loss of consciousness.

Analgesic Any drug or agent that will relieve pain.

Androgen Substance that produces masculinizing effects (e.g., testosterone).

Androgynous personality Having some characteristics of both sexes.

Android pelvis Male type of pelvis.

Anencephaly Congenital deformity characterized by the absence of cerebrum, cerebellum, and flat bones of skull.

Anesthesia Partial or complete absence of sensation with or without loss of consciousness.

Aneuploidy Having an abnormal number of chromosomes.

Anomaly Organ or structure that is malformed or in some way abnormal with reference to form, structure, or position.

Anovular menstrual period Cyclic uterine bleeding not accompanied by the production and discharge of an ovum.

Anovulatory Failure of the ovaries to produce, mature, or release eggs.

Anoxia Absence of oxygen.

Antenatal Occurring before or formed before birth.

Antepartal Before labor.

Anterior Pertaining to the front.
A. fontanelle See *fontanelle, anterior*.

Anteroposterior repair Operation in which the upper and lower walls of the vagina are reconstructed to correct relaxed tissue.

Anthropoid pelvis Pelvis in which the anteroposterior diameter is equal to or greater than the transverse diameter.

Anthropometry Study of human body measurements.

Antibody Specific protein substance developed by the body that exerts restrictive or destructive action on specific antigens, such as bacteria, toxins, or Rh factor.

Anticipatory grief Grief that predates the loss of a beloved person or object.

Antigen Protein foreign to the body that causes the body to develop antibodies. Examples: bacteria, dust, Rh factor.

Apgar score Numeric expression of the condition of a newborn obtained by rapid assessment at 1, 5, and 15 minutes of age; developed by Dr. Virginia Apgar.

Apnea Cessation of respirations for more than 10 seconds associated with generalized cyanosis.

Apt test Differentiation of maternal and fetal blood when there is vaginal bleeding. It is performed as follows: Add 0.5 mL blood to 4.5 mL distilled water. Shake. Add 1 mL 0.25N sodium hydroxide. Fetal and cord blood remains pink for 1 or 2 minutes. Maternal blood becomes brown in 30 seconds.

Areola Pigmented ring of tissue surrounding the nipple.

Secondary a. During the fifth month of pregnancy, a second faint ring of pigmentation seen around the original areola.

Arthralgia Any pain that affects a joint.

Articulation Fastening together or connection of the various bones of the skeleton; a joint. The articulations of the bones are classified as (1) immovable (synarthrosis), (2) slightly immovable (amphiarthrosis), and (3) freely movable (diarthrosis).

Artificial insemination Introduction of semen by instrument injection into the vagina or uterus for impregnation. Preferred term: *therapeutic insemination.*

Asherman's syndrome Intrauterine adhesions following inflammation and infection; one cause of impaired fertility.

Asphyxia Decreased oxygen and/or excess of carbon dioxide in the body.

A. livida Condition in which the infant's skin is characteristically pale, pulse is weak and slow, and reflexes are depressed or absent; also known as *blue asphyxia.*

A. pallida Condition in which the infant appears pale and limp and suffers from bradycardia (80 beats/min or less) and apnea.

Fetal a. Condition occurring in utero, with the following biochemical changes: hypoxemia (lowering of Po_2), hypercapnia (increase in Pco_2), and respiratory and metabolic acidosis (reduction of blood pH).

Aspiration pneumonia Inflammatory condition of the lungs and bronchi caused by the inhalation of vomitus containing acid gastric contents.

Aspiration syndrome See *meconium aspiration syndrome.*

Asynclitism Oblique presentation of the fetal head at the superior strait of the pelvis; the pelvic planes and those of the fetal head are not parallel.

Ataractic Drug capable of promoting tranquility; a tranquilizer.

Atelectasis Pulmonary pathosis involving alveolar collapse.

Athetosis Neuromuscular condition characterized by slow, writhing, continuous, and involuntary movement of the extremities, as seen in some forms of cerebral palsy and in motor disorders resulting from lesions in the basal ganglia.

Atony Absence of muscle tone.

Atresia Absence of a normally present passageway.

Biliary a. Absence of the bile duct.

Choanal a. Complete obstruction of the posterior nares, which open into the nasopharynx, with membranous or bony tissue.

Esophageal a. Congenital anomaly in which the esophagus ends in a blind pouch or narrows into a thin cord, thus failing to form a continuous passageway to the stomach.

Attachment A feeling of affection or loyalty that binds one person to another, which occurs at critical periods, such as birth or adoption; it is unique, specific, and enduring.

Attitude Body posture or position.

Fetal a. Relation of fetal parts to each other in the uterus (all parts flexed, all parts flexed except neck is extended, etc.).

Autoimmunization Development of antibodies against constituents of one's own tissues (e.g., a man may develop antibodies against his own sperm).

Autosomal inheritance Characteristics transmitted by genes on the autosomes, not the sex chromosomes.

Autosomes Any of the paired chromosomes other than the sex (X and Y) chromosomes.

Axis Line, real or imaginary, about which a part revolves or that runs through the center of a body.

Pelvic a. Imaginary curved line that passes through the centers of all the anteroposterior diameters of the pelvis.

Azoospermia Absence of sperm in the semen.

Back labor Uncomfortable labor that occurs when fetus, in occiput posterior position, presses on sacral nerves during contractions.

Bacteremic shock Shock that occurs in septicemia when endotoxins are released from certain bacteria in the blood stream.

Bag of waters Lay term for the sac containing amniotic fluid and fetus.

Ballottement (1) Movability of a floating object (e.g., fetus). (2) Diagnostic technique using palpation: a floating object, when tapped or pushed, moves away and then returns to touch the examiner's hand.

Bandl's ring Abnormally thickened ridge of uterine musculature between the upper and lower segments that follows a mechanically obstructed labor, with the lower segment thinning abnormally.

Barr body (sex chromatin) Chromatin mass located against the inner surface of the nucleus in females, possibly representing the inactive X chromosome.

Basal body temperature (BBT) Lowest temperature of a healthy person when awake.

Basalis, decidua See *decidua basalis.*

Battery Repeated beating of or use of force on a person without regard to personal rights; may be physical, sexual, psychologic, or social.

Bell's palsy See *palsy, Bell's.*

Bicornuate uterus Anomalous uterus that may be either a double or single organ with two horns.

Biliary atresia See *atresia, biliary.*

Bilirubin Yellow or orange pigment that is a breakdown product of hemoglobin. It is carried by the blood to the liver, where it is chemically changed and excreted in the bile or is conjugated and excreted by the kidneys.

Billings method See *ovulation method.*

Bimanual Performed with both hands.

B. palpation Examination of a woman's pelvic organs done by placing one hand on the abdomen and one or two fingers of the other hand in the vagina.

Biopsy Removal of a small piece of tissue for microscopic examination and diagnosis.

Birth plan Plan or list of options designed by a woman (couple) regarding the type of childbirth preferred (minimal medical intervention, home birth, etc.)

Birthing chair Chair designed so that a woman can labor and/or give birth in an upright position.

Blastocyst The stage in development of an embryo following the morula, made of an outer layer of trophoblast and an inner cell mass.

Blastoderm Germinal membrane of the ovum.

B. vesicle Stage in the development of a mammalian embryo that consists of an outer layer, or trophoblast, and a hollow sphere of cells enclosing a cavity.

Blood-brain barrier Obstruction that prevents passage of certain substances from blood into brain tissue.

Bloody show Vaginal discharge that originates in the cervix and consists of blood and mucus; increases as cervix dilates during labor.

Body image Person's subjective concept of his or her physical appearance.

Bonding Describes the initial mutual attraction between people, such as between parent and child, at first meeting. Also see *attachment*.

Bradley method Preparation for parenthood with active participation of father and mother.

Braxton Hicks sign Mild, intermittent, painless uterine contractions that occur during pregnancy. These contractions occur more frequently as pregnancy advances but do not represent true labor.

Braxton Hicks version One of several types of maneuvers designed to turn the fetus from an undesirable position to a more acceptable one to facilitate birth.

Brazelton assessment Criteria for assessing the interactional behavior of a newborn.

Breakthrough bleeding Escape of blood occurring between menstrual periods; may be noted by women using chemical contraception (birth control pill).

Breast milk jaundice See *jaundice, breast milk*.

Breech presentation Presentation in which buttocks and/or feet are nearest the cervical opening and are born first; occurs in approximately 3% of all births.

Complete b.p. Simultaneous presentation of buttocks, legs, and feet.

Footling (incomplete) b.p. Presentation of one or both feet.

Frank b.p. Presentation of buttocks, with hips flexed so that thighs are against abdomen.

Bregma Point of junction of the coronal and sagittal sutures of the skull; the area of the anterior fontanelle of the fetus.

Brim Edge of the superior strait of the true pelvis; the inlet.

Bronchopulmonary dysplasia Emphysematous changes caused by oxygen toxicity.

Brown fat Source of heat unique to neonates that is capable of greater thermogenic activity than ordinary fat. Deposits are found around the adrenals, kidneys, and neck, between the scapulas, and behind the sternum for several weeks after birth.

Bruit, uterine Sound of passage of blood through uterine blood vessels, synchronous with fetal heart rate.

Caked breast See *engorgement*.

Candida vaginitis Vaginal, fungal infection; moniliasis.

Capacitation Enzymatic process resulting in removal of plasma protein over acrosome of sperm; prerequisite for sperm to fertilize an ovum.

Capsularis, decidua See *decidua capsularis*.

Caput Occiput of fetal head appearing at the vaginal introitus preceding birth of the head.

C. succedaneum Swelling of the tissue over the presenting part of the fetal head caused by pressure during labor.

Carcinoma Malignant, often metastatic epithelial neoplasm; cancer.

Cardinal movements of labor Typical sequence of positions assumed by the fetus as it descends through the pelvis during labor and birth, usually designated as engagement, flexion, descent, internal rotation, extension, and external rotation or restitution.

Carrier Individual who carries a gene that does not exhibit itself in physical or chemical characteristics but that can be transmitted to children (e.g., a female carrying the trait for hemophilia, which is expressed in male offspring).

Caudal anesthesia Type of regional anesthesia used in childbirth in which the anesthetic agent is injected into the caudal area of the spinal canal through the sacral hiatus, affecting the caudal nerve roots and thereby anesthetizing the cervix, vagina, and perineum. Medication does not mix with cerebrospinal fluid (CSF).

Caul Hood of fetal membranes covering fetal head during birth.

Cautery Method of destroying tissue by the use of heat, electricity, or chemicals.

Centesis Suffix pertaining to a surgical puncture or perforation.

Cephalhematoma Extravasation of blood from ruptured vessels between a skull bone and its external covering, the periosteum. Swelling is limited by the margins of the cranial bone affected (usually parietals).

Cephalic Pertaining to the head.

C. presentation Presentation of any part of the fetal head.

Cephalocaudal development Principle of maturation that development progresses from the head to the feet.

Cephalopelvic disproportion (CPD) Condition in which the infant's head is of such a shape, size, or position that it cannot pass through the mother's pelvis.

Cerclage Use of nonabsorbable suture to keep an incompetent cervix closed; released when pregnancy is at term to allow labor to begin.

Cervical cap (custom) Individually fitted contraceptive covering for the cervix.

Cervical cauterization Destruction (usually by heat or electric current) of the superficial tissue of the cervix.

Cervical conization Excision of a cone-shaped section of tissue from the endocervix.

Cervical erosion Alteration of the epithelium of the cervix caused by chronic irritation or infection.

Cervical mucus method See *ovulation method.*

Cervical os "Mouth" or opening to the cervix.

Cervical polyp Small tumor on a stem (pedicle) attached inside the cervix.

Cervical stenosis Narrowing of the canal between the body of the uterus and the cervical os.

Cervicitis Cervical infection.

Cervix Lowest and narrow end of the uterus; the "neck." The cervix is situated between the external os and the body or corpus of the uterus, and its lower end extends into the vagina.

Cesarean delivery Birth of a fetus by an incision through the abdominal wall and uterus.

Cesarean hysterectomy Removal of the uterus immediately after the cesarean birth of an infant.

Chadwick's sign Violet color of mucous membrane that is visible from about the fourth week of pregnancy; caused by increased vascularity of the vagina.

Change of life See *climacterium.*

Chemotaxis Response involving movement that is positive (toward) or negative (away from) to a chemical stimulus.

Chloasma Increased pigmentation over bridge of nose and cheeks of pregnant women and some women taking oral contraceptives; also known as *mask of pregnancy.*

Choanal atresia See *atresia, choanal.*

Cholecystitis Acute or chronic inflammation of the gallbladder.

Cholelithiasis Presence of gallstones in the gallbladder.

Choreoathetoid cerebral palsy Condition characterized by both choreiform (jerky, ticlike twitching) and athetoid (slow, writhing) movements.

Chorioamnionitis Stimulated by organisms in the amniotic fluid, which then become infiltrated with polymorphonuclear leukocytes.

Chorioepithelioma Carcinoma of the chorion; rapid malignant proliferation of the epithelium of the chorionic villi.

Chorion Fetal membrane closest to the intrauterine wall that gives rise to the placenta and continues as the outer membrane surrounding the amnion.

Chorionic villi See *villi, chorionic.*

Chromosome Element within the cell nucleus carrying genes and composed of DNA and proteins.

Circumcision

- **Male** Excision of the prepuce (foreskin) of the penis, exposing the glans.
- **Female** Religious or cultural removal of a portion of the clitoris and labia.

Cleavage Cell division following the fertilization of an ovum.

Cleft lip Incomplete closure of the lip; harelip.

Cleft palate Incomplete closure of the palate or roof of mouth; a congenital fissure.

Climacterium (change of life) Period when the human body undergoes significant psychologic and physiologic changes, such as the termination of reproductive function in the woman.

Clitoris Female organ analogous to male penis; a small, ovoid body of erectile tissue situated at the anterior junction of the vulva.

- **Prepuce of the c.** See *prepuce of the clitoris.*

Coccyx Small bone at the base of the spinal column.

Coitus Penile-vaginal intercourse.

- **C. interruptus** Intercourse during which penis is withdrawn from vagina before ejaculation.

Colostrum Yellow secretion from the breast containing mainly serum and white blood corpuscles preceding the onset of true lactation 2 or 3 days after birth.

Colpectomy Surgical excision of the vagina.

Colporrhaphy (1) Procedure of suturing the vagina. (2) Procedure whereby the vagina is denuded and sutured for the purpose of narrowing the vagina.

Colpotomy Any surgical incision into the wall of the vagina.

Complement Naturally occurring blood component that is a factor in the destruction of bacteria.

Complementary feeding Supplemental feeding given to the infant if he is still hungry after breast-feeding.

Complete abortion See *abortion, complete.*

Complete breech presentation See *breech presentation, complete.*

Compliance, lung Degree of distensibility of the lung's elastic tissue.

Conception Union of the sperm and ovum resulting in fertilization; formation of the one-celled zygote.

Conceptional age In fetal development, the number of completed weeks since the moment of conception. Because the moment of conception is almost impossible to determine, conceptional age is estimated at 2 weeks less than gestational age.

Conceptus Embryo or fetus, fetal membranes, amniotic fluid, and the fetal portion of the placenta.

Condom Mechanical barrier worn on the penis for contraception; "rubber"; also provides some protection against transmission of STDs.

Condylomata accuminata Wartlike growth on the skin usually seen near the anus or external genitals caused by human papillomavirus (HPV); genital warts. (Must be differentiated from condyloma latum seen in secondary syphilis.)

Confinement Period of childbirth and early puerperium.

Congenital Present or existing before birth as a result of either hereditary or prenatal environmental factors.

Conjoined twins See *twins, conjoined.*

Conjugate

Diagonal c. Radiographic measurement of distance from *inferior border* of SP to sacral promontory; may be obtained by vaginal examination; 12.5 to 13 cm.

True c. (c. vera) Radiographic measurement of distance from *upper margin* of symphysis pubis (SP) to sacral promontory; 1.5 to 2 cm less than diagonal conjugate.

Conjunctivitis Inflammation of the mucous membrane that lines the eyelids and that is reflected onto the eyeball.

Consanguinity Existing blood relationship between persons.

Contraception Prevention of impregnation or conception.

Contraction ring See *Bandl's ring.*

Coombs' test Indirect: determination of Rh-positive antibodies in maternal blood; direct: determination of maternal Rh-positive antibodies in fetal cord blood. A positive test result indicates the presence of antibodies or titer.

Coping mechanism Any effort directed at stress management. It can be task oriented and involve direct problem-solving efforts to cope with the threat itself or be intrapsychic or ego defense oriented with the goal of regulating one's emotional distress.

Copulation Coitus; sexual intercourse.

Corpus Discrete mass of material; body

C. cavernosum Term referring to one of two cylinders of spongy tissue within the penis or tissue within the clitoris that engorges with blood during sexual excitement, resulting in erection.

C. luteum Yellow body. After rupture of the graafian follicle at ovulation, the follicle develops into a yellow structure that secretes progesterone in the second half of the menstrual cycle, atrophying about 3 days before sloughing of the endometrium in menstrual flow. If impregnation occurs, this structure continues to produce progesterone until the placenta can take over this function.

C. spongiosum One of the spongy cylinders of tissue within the penis; has a protective function.

Cotyledon One of the 15 to 28 visible segments of the placenta on the maternal surface, each made up of fetal vessels, chorionic villi, and an intervillous space.

Couvade Custom whereby the husband goes through mock labor while his wife is giving birth.

Couvelaire uterus See *uterus, Couvelaire.*

CPAP Continuous positive airway pressure.

Cradle cap Common seborrheic dermatitis of infants consisting of thick, yellow, greasy scales on the scalp.

Craniotabes Localized softening of cranial bones.

Creatinine Substance found in blood and muscle; measurement of levels in maternal urine correlates with amount of fetal muscle mass and therefore fetal size.

Crib death Unexpected and sudden death of an apparently normal and healthy infant that occurs during sleep and with no physical or autopsic evidence of disease. Also referred to as sudden infant death syndrome (SIDS).

Cri-du-chat syndrome Rare congenital disorder recognized at birth by a kittenlike cry, which may prevail for weeks, then disappear. Other characteristics include low birth weight, microcephaly, "moon face," wide-set eyes, strabismus, and low-set misshaped ears. Infants are hypotonic; heart defects and mental and physical retardation are common. Also called cat-cry syndrome.

Critical path The exact timing of all key incidents that must occur to achieve the standard outcomes within the DRG-specific length of stay.

Crowning Stage of birth when the top of the fetal head can be seen at the vaginal orifice.

Cryo- Prefix meaning cold, freezing.

Cryosurgery Local freezing and removal of tissue without injury to adacent tissue and with minimum blood loss, done with special equipment.

Cryptochidism Failure of one or both of the testicles to descend into the scrotum. Also called undescended testis.

Cul-de-sac of Douglas Pouch formed by a fold of the peritoneum dipping down between the anterior wall of the rectum and the posterior wall of the uterus; also called *Douglas' cul-de-sac, pouch of Douglas,* and *rectouterine pouch.*

Culdocentesis Use of needle puncture or incision to remove intraperitoneal fluid (blood, purulent material) by way of the vagina.

Culdotomy Incision or needle puncture of the cul-de-sac of Douglas by way of the vagina.

Cullen's sign Faint, irregularly formed, hemorrhagic patches on the skin around the umbilicus. The discolored skin is blue-black and becomes greenish brown or yellow. Cullen's sign may appear 1 to 2 days after the onset of anorexia and the severe, poorly localized abdominal pains characteristic of acute pancreatitis. Cullen's sign is also present in massive upper gastrointestinal hemorrhage, ruptured ectopic pregnancy.

Culture The total learned way of life of a society.

Curettage Scraping of the endometrium lining of the uterus with a curet to remove the contents of the uterus (as is done after an inevitable or incomplete abortion) or to obtain specimens for diagnostic purposes.

Cutis marmorata Transient vasomotor phenomenon occurring primarily over extremities when the infant is exposed to chilling. It appears as a pink or faint purple capillary outline on the skin. Occasionally it is seen if the infant is in respiratory distress.

Cycle of violence Pattern of three phases: period of increasing tension, the abusive episode, and a period of contrition and kindness.

Cyesis Pregnancy.

Cystitis Inflammatory condition or infection of urinary bladder and ureters.

Cystocele Bladder hernia; injury to the vesicovaginal fascia during labor and birth may allow herniation of the bladder into the vagina.

Cytology The study of cells, including their formation, origin, structure, function, biochemical activities, and pathology.

Death Cessation of life; mortality.

Decidua Mucous membrane, lining of uterus, or endometrium of pregnancy that is shed after giving birth.

- **D. basalis** Maternal aspect of the placenta made up of uterine blood vessels, endometrial stroma, and glands. It is shed in lochial discharge after birth.
- **D. capsularis** That part of the decidual membranes surrounding the chorionic sac.
- **D. vera** Nonplacental decidual lining of the uterus.

Decrement Decrease or stage of decline, as of a contraction.

Deletion Loss of a piece of a chromosome that has broken off.

Delivery Expulsion of the child with placenta and membranes by the mother or their extraction by the obstetric practitioner.

- **Abdominal d.** See *abdominal birth.*

ΔOD_{450} (read delta OD_{450}) Delta optical density (or absorbance) at 450 nm, obtained by spectral analysis of amniotic fluid. This prenatal test is used to measure the degree of hemolytic activity in the fetus and to evaluate fetal status in women sensitized to Rh(D).

Deoxyribonucleic acid (DNA) Intracellular complex protein that carries genetic information, consisting of two purines (adenine and guanine) and two pyrimidines (thymine and cytosine).

Dermatoglyphics Study of skin ridge patterns on fingers, toes, palms of hands, and soles of feet.

DES Diethylstilbestrol, used in treating menopausal symptoms. Exposure of female fetus predisposes her to reproductive tract malformations and (later) dysplasia.

Desquamation Shedding of epithelial cells of the skin and mucous membranes.

Developmental crisis Severe, usually transient, stress that occurs when a person is unable to complete the tasks of a psychosocial stage of development and is therefore unable to move on to the next stage.

Developmental task Physical or cognitive skill that a child must accomplish during a particular age period in order to continue developing, as walking, which precedes the development of sense of autonomy in the toddler period.

Diaphragmatic hernia Congenital malformation of diaphragm that allows displacement of the abdominal organs into the thoracic cavity.

Diastasis recti abdominis Separation of the two rectus muscles along the median line of the abdominal wall. This is often seen in women with repeated childbirths or with a multiple gestation (triplets, etc.). In the newborn it is usually due to incomplete development.

DIC Disseminated intravascular coagulation.

Dick-Read method An approach to childbirth based on the premise that fear of pain produces muscular tension, producing pain and greater fear. The method includes teaching physiological processes of labor, exercise to improve muscle tone, and techniques to assist in relaxation and prevent the fear-tension-pain mechanism.

Dilatation of cervix Stretching of the external os from an opening a few millimeters in size to an opening large enough to allow the passage of the infant.

Dilatation and curettage (D and C) Vaginal operation in which the cervical canal is stretched enough to admit passage of an instrument called a *curet*. The endometrium of the uterus is scraped with the curet to empty the uterine contents or to obtain tissue for examination.

Dilatation and evacuation (D and E) A surgical method of pregnancy interruption between weeks 15 and 24; requires extreme cervical dilatation and evacuation of uterine contents using large-bore suction equipment and crushing instruments.

Diploid number Having 2 sets of chromosomes; found normally in somatic (body) cells; 23 pairs or 46 chromosomes.

Discordance Discrepancy in size (or other indicator) between twins.

Disparate twins See *twins, disparate.*

Disseminated lupus erythematosus Chronic inflammatory disease affecting many systems of the body. Also called systemic lupus erythematosus (SLE).

Diverticulum Pouch-like herniation through muscular wall of a tubular organ. A diverticulum may be present in the stomach, small intestine, or, most commonly, in the colon.

Dizygotic Related to or proceeding from two zygotes (fertilized ova).

Dizygotic twins See *twins, dizygotic*

Döderlein's bacillus Gram-positive bacterium occurring in normal vaginal secretions.

Dominant trait Gene that is expressed whenever it is present in the heterozygous gene state (e.g., brown eyes are dominant over blue).

Doppler velocimetry Use of ultrasound to study blood flow noninvasively.

Douglas' cul-de-sac See *cul-de-sac of Douglas*.

Doula A lay person who provides support during labor.

Down syndrome Abnormality involving the occurrence of a third chromosome, rather than the normal pair (trisomy 21), that characteristically results in a typical picture of mental retardation and altered physical appearance. This condition was formerly called *mongolism* or *mongoloid idiocy*.

Dry labor Lay term referring to labor in which amniotic fluid has already escaped. A "dry birth" does not exist.

Dubowitz assessment Estimation of gestational age of a newborn, based on criteria developed for that purpose.

Ductus arteriosus In fetal circulation, an anatomic shunt between the pulmonary artery and arch of the aorta. It is obliterated after birth by a rising Po_2 and change in intravascular pressures in the presence of normal pulmonary function. It normally becomes a ligament after birth but in some instances remains patent.

Ductus venosus In fetal circulation, a blood vessel carrying oxygenated blood between the umbilical vein and the inferior vena cava, bypassing the liver. It is obliterated and becomes a ligament after birth.

Duncan's mechanism Delivery of placenta with the maternal surface presenting, rather than the shiny fetal surface.

Dura (dura mater) Outermost, toughest of the three meninges covering the brain and spinal cord.

Dynamic ileus Spastic ileus; intestinal obstruction characterized by recurrent and continuous spasms (sudden muscular contractions).

Dys- Prefix meaning abnormal, difficult, painful, faulty.

Dyscrasia Incompatible mixture (e.g., fetal and maternal blood incompatibility).

Dysfunctional uterine bleeding Abnormal bleeding from the uterus for reasons that are not readily established.

Dysmaturity See *intrauterine growth retardation (IUGR)*.

Dysmenorrhea Difficult or painful menstruation.

Dysmorphogenesis Development of ill-shaped or malformed structures.

Dyspareunia Painful sexual intercourse.

Dystocia Prolonged, painful, or otherwise difficult birth because of mechanical factors produced by either the passenger (the fetus) or the passageway (the pelvis of the mother) or because of inadequate powers (uterine and other muscular activity).

Placental d. Difficulty in the delivery of the placenta.

Ecchymosis Bruise; bleeding into tissue caused by direct trauma, serious infection, or bleeding diathesis.

Eclampsia Severe complication of pregnancy of unknown cause and occurring more often in the primigravida; characterized by tonic and clonic convulsions, coma, high blood pressure, albuminuria, and oliguria occurring during pregnancy or shortly after birth.

ECMO Extracorporeal membrane oxygenation used primarily for newborns suffering refractory respiratory failure or meconium aspiration syndrome.

Ectoderm Outer layer of embryonic tissue giving rise to skin, nails, and hair.

Ectopic Out of normal place.

E. pregnancy Implantation of the fertilized ovum outside of its normal place in the uterine cavity. Locations include the abdomen, fallopian tubes, and ovaries.

EDC Expected date of confinement; "due date."

Effacement Thinning and shortening or obliteration of the cervix that occurs during late pregnancy or labor or both.

Effleurage Gentle stroking used in massage.

Ejaculation Sudden expulsion of semen from the male urethra.

Elective abortion See *abortion, elective*.

Electroshock (therapy) Induction of a brief convulsion by passing an electric current through the brain for the treatment of affective disorders, especially in clients resistant to psychoactive drug therapy. Also called electroconvulsive therapy (ECT).

Embolus Any undissolved matter (solid, liquid, or gaseous) that is carried by the blood to another part of the body and obstructs a blood vessel.

Embryo Conceptus from the second or third week of development until about the eighth week after conception, when mineralization (ossification) of the skeleton begins. This period is characterized by cellular differentiation and predominantly hyperplastic growth.

Empathy Projection of one's own consciousness and awareness onto that of another so as to obtain an objective awareness of and insight into the emotions, feelings, and behavior of another person and their meaning and significance. Empathy may be distinguished from sympathy in that sympathy is usually nonobjective and noncritical, whereas the state of empathy includes relative freedom from emotional involvement.

Endocervical Pertaining to the interior of the canal of the cervix of the uterus.

Endocrine glands Ductless glands that secrete hormones into the blood or lymph.

Endometriosis Tissue closely resembling endometrial tissue but aberrantly located outside the uterus in the pelvic cavity. Symptomatology may include pelvic pain or pressure, dysmenorrhea, dyspareunia, abnormal bleeding from the uterus or rectum, and sterility.

Endometrium Inner lining of the uterus that undergoes changes caused by hormones during the menstrual cycle and pregnancy; decidua.

En face Position in which neonate is held 8 inches (20 cm) away facing the observer to allow for direct eye contact.

Engagement In obstetrics, the entrance of the fetal presenting part into the superior pelvic strait and the beginning of the descent through the pelvic canal.

Engorgement Distention or vascular congestion. In obstetrics, the process of swelling of the breast tissue brought about by an increase in blood and lymph supply to the breast, which precedes true lactation. It lasts about 48 hours and usually reaches a peak between the third and fifth postpartum days.

Engrossment Sustained involvement of a parent with an infant.

Entoderm Inner layer of embryonic tissue giving rise to internal organs such as the intestine.

Entrainment Phenomenon observed in the microanalysis of sound films in which the speaker moves several parts of the body and the listener responds to the sounds by moving in ways that are coordinated with the rhythm of the sounds. Infants have been observed to move in time to the rhythms of adult speech but not to random noises or disconnected words or vowels. Entrainment is thought to be an essential factor in the process of maternal-infant bonding.

Epidural anesthesia See *peridural anesthesia.*

Epicanthus Fold of skin covering the inner canthus and caruncle that extends from the root of the nose to the median end of the eyebrow; characteristically found in certain races but may occur as a congenital anomaly.

Episiotomy Surgical incision of the perineum at the end of the second stage of labor to facilitate birth and to avoid laceration of the perineum. (See also *perineotomy.*)

Epispadias Defect in which the urethral canal terminates on dorsum of penis or above the clitoris (rare).

Epstein's pearls Small, white blebs found along the gum margins and at the junction of the soft and hard palates. They are a normal manifestation and are commonly seen in the newborn. Similar to Bohn's nodules.

Epulis Tumorlike benign lesion of the gingiva seen in pregnant women.

Equilibrium A state of balance or rest owing to the equal action of opposing forces, as calcium and phosphorus in the body. In psychiatry, a state of mental or emotional balance.

Erb-Duchenne paralysis Paralysis caused by traumatic injury to the upper brachial plexus, occurring most commonly in childbirth from forcible traction during birth. The signs of Erb's paralysis include loss of sensation in the arm and paralysis and atrophy of the deltoid, the biceps, and the brachialis muscles. Also called Erb's palsy.

Ergot Drug obtained from *Claviceps purpurea,* a fungus, which stimulates the smooth muscles of blood vessels and the uterus, causing vasoconstriction and uterine contractions.

Erythema toxicum Innocuous pink papular neonatal rash of unknown cause, with superimposed vesicles appearing within 24 to 48 hours after birth and resolving spontaneously within a few days.

Erythroblastosis fetalis Hemolytic disease of the newborn usually caused by isoimmunization resulting from Rh incompatibility or ABO incompatibility.

Erythropoiesis Erythrocyte (RBC) production, which involves the maturation of a nucleated precursor into a hemoglobin-filled, nucleus-free erythrocyte regulated by erythropoietin, a hormone produced by the kidney.

Escutcheon Pattern of distribution of pubic hair.

Esophageal atresia See *atresia, esophageal.*

Estradiol An estrogen.

Estrangement, psychologic Reaction to the birth of and subsequent separation from a sick and/or preterm infant, whereby the mother is diverted from establishing a normal relationship with her baby.

Estriol Major metabolite of estrogen that increases during the second half of pregnancy with an intact fetoplacental unit (normal placenta, normal fetal liver and adrenals) and normal maternal renal function.

Estrogen Female sex hormone produced by the ovaries and placenta.

Estrus Cyclic period of sexual activity in mammals other than primates; state of being in heat.

Ethnocentrism Belief in the inherent superiority of the race or group to which one belongs. Also a proclivity to consider other ethnic groups in terms of one's own racial origins.

Eu- Prefix meaning normal, good, well, easy.

Eugenics Science that deals with the improvement of the human race through control of hereditary (genetic) factors by voluntary social action.

Euthenics Science that deals with the improvement of the human race through the control of environmental factors (pollution, drug abuse, malnutrition, and disease).

Eutocia Normal or natural labor or birth.

Exchange transfusion Replacement of 75% to 85% of circulating blood by withdrawing the recipient's blood and injecting a donor's blood in equal amounts, the purposes of which are to prevent an accumulation of bilirubin in the blood above a dangerous level, to prevent the accumulation of other by-products of hemolysis in hemolytic disease, and to correct anemia.

Exocervix Outer layer of the portion of the cervix that protrudes into the vagina; ectocervix.

Exostosis Benign cartilage-covered hump on the surface of a bone, often resulting from chronic irritation.

Expulsive Having the tendency to drive out or expel.

E. contractions Labor contractions that are characteristic of the second stage of labor.

Exstrophy Eversion; the turning inside out of a part.

Extension Straightening of a body part; opposite of flexion.

Extraperitoneal Occurring or located outside the peritoneal cavity.

Extrauterine Occurring outside the uterus.

E. pregnancy Ectopic pregnancy in which the fertilized ovum implants itself outside the uterus.

Facies Pertaining to the appearance or expression of the face; certain congenital syndromes typically present with a specific facial appearance.

FAD Fetal activity determination.

Failure to thrive Condition in which neonate's or infant's growth and development patterns are below the norms for age.

Fallopian tubes Two canals or oviducts extending laterally from each side of the uterus through which the ovum travels, after ovulation, to the uterus; uterine tubes.

False labor Uterine contractions that do not result in cervical dilatation, are irregular, are felt more in front, often do not last more than 20 seconds, and do not become longer or stronger.

False pelvis The part of the pelvis superior to a plane passing through the linea terminalis.

Ferguson's reflex Reflex contractions of the uterus after stimulation of the cervix.

Ferning (arborization) test The appearance of a fernlike pattern in dried smears of uterine cervical mucus, indicating the presence of estrogen.

Ovulation f. t. Test in which cervical mucus, placed on a slide, dries in a branching pattern in the presence of high estrogen levels at the time of ovulation.

Pregnancy f. t. Test in which cervical mucus, placed on a slide, does not dry in a branching pattern because of high levels of progesterone along with estrogen.

Fertility Quality of being able to reproduce.

Fertility rate Number of births per 1000 women aged 15 through 44 years.

Fertilization Union of an ovum and a sperm.

Fetal Pertaining or relating to the fetus

F. alcohol syndrome Congenital abnormality or anomaly resulting from maternal alcohol intake. It is characterized by typical craniofacial and limb defects, cardiovascular defects, intrauterine growth retardation, and developmental delay.

F. alveoli See *alveoli, fetal.*

F. attitude See *attitude, fetal.*

F. asphyxia See *asphyxia, fetal.*

F. biophysical profile Noninvasive dynamic assessment, employing ultrasound and external fetal monitoring, of several parameters: breathing movements, movements, tone, amniotic fluid volume, NST, and often placental grading.

F. distress Evidence such as a change in the fetal heartbeat pattern or activity indicating that the fetus is in jeopardy.

F. lie Relation of the fetal spine to the maternal spine; i.e., in vertical lie, maternal and fetal spines are parallel and the fetal head or breech presents; in transverse lie, fetal spine is perpendicular to the maternal spine and the fetal shoulder presents.

F. presentation The part of the fetus that presents at the cervical os.

Fetofetal transfusion See *parabiotic syndrome.*

α-Fetoprotein (AFP) Fetal antigen; elevated levels in amniotic fluid associated with neural tube defects.

Fetotoxic Poisonous or destructive to the fetus.

Fetus Child in utero from about the eighth week after conception, until birth.

Fibroid Fibrous, encapsulated connective tissue tumor, especially of the uterus.

Fimbria Structure resembling a fringe, particularly the fringe-like end of the fallopian tube.

FiO_2 (fraction of inspired oxygen) Percentage of oxygen a person is receiving.

Fissure Groove or open crack in tissue.

Fistula Abnormal tubelike passage that forms between two normal cavities, possibly congenital or caused by trauma, abscesses, or inflammatory processes.

Flaccid Having relaxed, flabby, or absent muscle tone.

Flaring of nostrils Widening of nostrils (alae nasi) during inspiration in the presence of air hunger; sign of respiratory distress.

Flexion In obstetrics, resistance to the descent of the baby down the birth canal causes the head to flex, or bend, so that the chin approaches the chest. Thus the smallest diameter (suboccipitobregmatic) of the vertex presents.

Fluid, amniotic See *amniotic fluid.*

Follicle Small secretory cavity or sac.

Graafian f. Mature, fully developed ovarian cyst containing the ripe ovum. The follicle secretes estrogens, and after ovulation, the corpus luteum develops within the ruptured graafian follicle and secretes estrogen and progesterone.

Follicle-stimulating hormone (FSH) Hormone produced by the anterior pituitary during the first half of the menstrual cycle. Stimulates development of the graafian follicle.

Fomites Nonliving material on which disease-producing organisms may be conveyed (e.g., bed linen).

Fontanelle Broad area, or soft spot, consisting of a strong band of connective tissue contiguous with cranial bones and located at the junctions of the bones.

Anterior f. Diamond-shaped area between the frontal and two parietal bones just above the baby's forehead at the junction of the coronal and sagittal sutures.

Mastoid f. Posterolateral fontanelle usually not palpable.

Posterior f. Small, triangular area between the occipital and parietal bones at the junction of the lambdoidal and sagittal sutures.

Sagittal f. Soft area located in the sagittal suture, halfway between the anterior and posterior fontanelles; may be found in normal newborns and in some neonates with Down syndrome.

Sphenoid f. Anterolateral fontanelle usually not palpable.

Footling (incomplete) breech presentation See *breech presentation, footling.*

Foramen ovale Septal opening between the atria of the fetal heart. The opening normally closes shortly after birth, but if it remains patent, surgical repair usually is necessary.

Foreskin Prepuce, or loose fold of skin covering the glans penis.

Fowler's position Posture assumed by client when head of bed is raised 18 or 20 inches and individual's knees are elevated.

Frank breech presentation See *breech presentation, frank.*

Fraternal twins Nonidentical twins that come from two separate fertilized ova.

Frenulum Thin ridge of tissue in midline of undersurface of tongue extending from its base to varying distances from the tip of the tongue.

Friedman's curve Labor curve; pattern of descent of presenting part and of dilatation of cervix; partogram.

Frigidity Archaic term designating a woman's inability to achieve orgasm; orgasmic dysfunction.

FSH See *follicle-stimulating hormone.*

Fulguration Destruction of tissue by means of electricity.

Fundus Dome-shaped upper portion of the uterus between the points of insertion of the fallopian tubes.

Funic Souffle See *souffle, funic.*

Funis Cordlike structure, especially the umbilical cord.

Galacto-, galact- Combining form denoting milk.

Galactorrhea Excessive flow or secretion of milk.

Galactosemia Inherited, autosomal recessive disorder of galactose metabolism, characterized by a deficiency of the enzyme galactose-1-phosphate uridyl transferase.

Gamete Mature male or female germ cell; the mature sperm or ovum.

Gametogenesis Development of gametes; ova or sperm.

Gastroschisis Abdominal wall defect at base of umbilical stalk.

Gastrostomy Surgical creation of an artificial opening into the stomach through the abdominal wall, performed to feed a client when oral feeding is not possible.

Gate control theory Proposed in 1965 by Melzack and Wall, this theory explains the neurophysical mechanism underlying the perception of pain.

Gavage Feeding by means of a tube passed to the stomach.

Gender identity The sense or awareness of knowing to which sex one belongs. The process begins in infancy, continues throughout childhood, and is reinforced during adolescence.

Gene Factor on a chromosome responsible for hereditary characteristics of offspring.

Genetic Dependent on the genes. A genetic disorder may or may not be apparent at birth.

Genetic counseling Process of determining the occurrence or risk of occurrence of a genetic disorder within a family and of providing appropriate information and advice about the courses of action that are available, whether care of a child already affected, prenatal diagnosis, termination of a pregnancy, sterilization, or artificial insemination is involved.

Genitalia Organs of reproduction.

Genotype Hereditary combinations in an individual determining physical and chemical characteristics. Some genotypes are not expressed until later in life (e.g., Huntington's chorea); some hide recessive genes, which can be expressed in offspring; and others are expressed only under the proper environmental conditions (e.g., diabetes mellitus appearing under the stress of obesity or pregnancy).

Gestation Period of intrauterine fetal development from conception through birth; the period of pregnancy.
Abdominal g. See *abdominal gestation.*

Gestational age In fetal development, the number of completed weeks counting from the first day of the last normal menstrual cycle.

GIFT Gamete intrafallopian transfer of ova and washed sperm into uterine tubes.

Glabella Bony prominence above the nose and between the eyebrows.

Glans penis Smooth, round head of the penis, analogous to the female glans clitoris.

Glomerulonephritis Noninfectious disease of the glomerulus of the kidney, characterized by proteinuria, hematuria, decreased urine production, and edema.

Glycosuria Presence of glucose (a sugar) in the urine.

Gonad Gamete-producing, or sex, gland; the ovary or testis.

Gonadotropic hormone Hormone that stimulates the gonads.

Goodell's sign Softening of the cervix, a probable sign of pregnancy, occurring during the second month.

Gossypol Oral contraceptive for males produced from cotton plants; not available in the United States.

Graafian follicle (vesicle) See *follicle, graafian.*

Gravid Pregnant.

Grieving process A complex of somatic and psychologic symptoms associated with some extreme sorrow or loss, specifically the death of a loved one.

Grunt, expiratory Sign of respiratory distress (hyaline membrane disease [respiratory distress syndrome, or RDS] or advanced pneumonia) indicative of the body's attempt to hold air in the alveoli for better gaseous exchange.

Gynecoid pelvis Pelvis in which the inlet is round instead of oval or blunt; heart shaped. Typical female pelvis.

Gynecology Study of the diseases of the female, especially of the genital, urinary, and rectal organs.

Habitual (recurrent) abortion See *abortion, habitual.*

Habituation An acquired tolerance from repeated exposure to a particular stimulus. Also called negative adaptation; a decline and eventual elimination of a conditioned response by repetition of the conditioned stimulus.

Habitus Indications in appearance of tendency or disposition to disease or abnormal conditions.

Harlequin sign Rare color change of no pathologic significance occurring between the longitudinal halves of the neonate's body. When infant is placed on one side, the dependent half is noticeably pinker than the superior half.

Haploid number Having half the normal number of chromosomes found in somatic (body) cells; 23 chromosomes.

Hawthorne effect A general beneficial effect on a person or group of people as a result of a therapeutic encounter with a health care provider or as a result of a change in the environment (lighting, temperature, or type of room [family-centered versus four-bed unit]).

Hegar's sign Softening of the lower uterine segment that is classified as a probable sign of pregnancy and that may be present during the second and third months of pregnancy and is palpated during bimanual examination.

HELLP syndrome Condition characterized by hemolysis, elevated liver enzymes, and low platelet count (it is *not* DIC).

Hematocrit Volume of red blood cells per deciliter (dL) of circulating blood; packed cell volume (PCV).

Hematoma Collection of blood in a tissue; a bruise or blood tumor.

Hematopoiesis The production of blood cells.

Hemizygous Having only one of a gene pair that determines a particular genetic trait.

Hemoconcentration Increase in the number of red blood cells resulting from either a decrease in plasma volume or increased erythropoiesis.

Hemoglobin Component of red blood cells consisting of globin, a protein, and hematin, an organic iron compound.

- **H. electrophoresis** Test to diagnose sickle cell disease in newborns. Cord blood is used.
- **H. F** Hemoglobin of fetal RBCs having greater affinity for O_2 than adult hemoglobin A; helps to ensure adequate fetal tissue oxygenation.

Hemorrhagic disease of newborn Bleeding disorder during first few days of life based on a deficiency of vitamin K.

Hereditary Pertaining to a trait or characteristic transmitted from parent to offspring by way of the genes; used synonymously with *genetic.*

Hermaphrodite Person having genital and sexual characteristics of both sexes.

Heterologous insemination Insemination in which the semen specimen is provided by an anonymous donor. The procedure is used primarily in cases where the husband is sterile.

Heterozygous Having two dissimilar genes at the same site, or locus, on paired chromosomes (e.g., at the sites for eye color, one chromosome carrying the gene for brown, the other for blue).

High risk An increased possibility of suffering harm, damage, loss, or death.

Hirsutism Condition characterized by the excessive growth of hair or the growth of hair in unusual places.

Hoffman's exercises Areola-stretching exercise to break adhesions, allowing inverted nipples to become more everted (protractile).

Homans' sign Early sign of phlebothrombosis of the deep veins of the calf in which there are complaints of pain when the leg is in extension and the foot is dorsiflexed.

Homoiothermic Referring to the ability of warm-blooded animals to maintain internal temperature at a specified level regardless of the environmental temperature. This ability is not fully developed in the human neonate.

Homologous Similar in structure or origin but not necessarily in function.

Homologous insemination Insemination in which the semen specimen is provided by the husband. The procedure is used primarily in cases of impotence or when the husband is incapable of sexual intercourse because of some physical disability.

Homozygous Having two similar genes at the same locus, or site, on paired chromosomes.

Hormone Chemical substance produced in an organ or gland that is conveyed through the blood to another organ or part of the body, stimulating it to increased functional activity or secretion. See specific hormones.

Hot flash (flush) Transient sensation of warmth experienced by some women during or after menopause, resulting from autonomic vasomotor disturbances that accompany changes in the neurohormonal activity of the ovaries, hypothalamus, and pituitary gland.

Hourglass uterus Uterus in which a segment of circular muscle fibers contracts during labor. The resultant "constriction ring" dystocia is characterized by lack of progress in spite of adequate contractions; by pain experienced before palpation of a uterine contraction and persisting after the observer feels the contraction end; and by recession of the presenting part during a contraction, instead of descent of the presenting part.

Hyaline membrane disease (HMD) Disease characterized by interference with ventilation at the alveolar level, theoretically caused by the presence of fibrinoid deposits lining alveolar ducts. Membrane formation is related to prematurity (especially with fetal asphyxia) and insufficient surfactant production (L/S ratio less than 2:1). Now known as *respiratory distress syndrome (RDS)*.

Hydatidiform mole Abnormal pregnancy characterized by a degenerative process in the chorionic villi that produces high levels of human chorionic gonadotropin (hCG), multiple cysts, and rapid growth of the uterus with hemorrhage. Signs and symptoms include vaginal bleeding, the discharge containing grapelike vesicles. Sequela may be chorioadenoma, a highly malignant neoplasm.

Hydramnios (polyhydramnios) Amniotic fluid in excess of 1.5 L; often indicative of fetal anomaly and frequently seen in poorly controlled, insulin-dependent, diabetic pregnant women even if there is no coexisting fetal anomaly.

Hydrocele Collection of fluid in a saclike cavity, especially in the sac that surrounds the testis, causing the scrotum to swell.

Hydropic Dropsical or pertaining to edema; abnormal accumulation of serous fluid in the body tissues and cavities.

Hydrops fetalis Most severe expression of fetal hemolytic disorder, a possible sequela to maternal Rh isoimmunization; infants exhibit gross edema (anasarca), cardiac decompensation, and profound pallor from anemia and seldom survive.

Hymen Membranous fold that normally partially covers the entrance to the vagina in the virgin.

Hymenal caruncles Small, irregular bits of tissue that are remnants of the hymen.

Hymenal tag Normally occurring redundant hymenal tissue protruding from the floor of the vagina that disappears spontaneously in a few weeks after birth.

Hymenotomy Surgical incision of the hymen.

Hyperbilirubinemia Elevation of unconjugated serum bilirubin.

Hyperemesis gravidarum Abnormal condition of pregnancy characterized by protracted vomiting, weight loss, and fluid and electrolyte imbalance.

Hyperesthesia Unusual sensibility to sensory stimuli, such as pain or touch.

Hyperplasia Increase in number of cells; formation of new tissue.

Hyperreflexia Increased action of the reflexes.

Hypertrophy Enlargement, or increase in size, of existing cells.

Hyperventilation Rapid, shallow (or prolonged, deep) respirations resulting in respiratory alkalosis: a decrease in H^+ concentration and Pco_2 and an increase in the blood pH and the ratio of $NaHCO_3$ to H_2CO_3. Symptoms may include faintness, palpitations, and carpopedal (hands and feet) muscular spasms. Relief may result from rebreathing in a paper bag or into one's cupped hands to replace the CO_2 "blown off" during hyperventilation.

Hypofibrinogenemia Deficient level of a blood clotting factor, fibrinogen, in the blood; in obstetrics, it occurs following complications of abruptio placentae or retention of a dead fetus.

Hypogastric arteries Branches of the right and left iliac arteries carrying deoxygenated blood from the fetus through the umbilical cord, where they are known as *umbilical arteries*, to the placenta.

Hypoglycemia Less-than-normal amount of glucose in the blood, usually caused by administration of too much insulin, excessive secretion of insulin by the islet cells of the pancreas, or by dietary deficiency.

Hypospadias Anomalous positioning of urinary meatus on undersurface of penis or close to or just inside the vagina.

Hypotensive drugs Drugs that lower the blood pressure.

Hypothalamus Portion of the diencephalon of the brain forming the floor and part of the lateral wall of the third ventricle. It activates, controls, and integrates the peripheral autonomic nervous system, endocrine processes, and many somatic functions, as body temperature, sleep, and appetite.

Hypothenar Fleshy elevation on the ulnar (little finger) side of the palm of the hand. Also called *hypothenar eminence*.

Hypotonia Reduced tension; relaxation of arteries. Also, loss of tonicity of the muscles or intraocular pressure.

Hypoxemia Reduction in arterial Po_2 resulting in metabolic acidosis by forcing anaerobic glycolysis, pulmonary vasoconstriction, and direct cellular damage.

Hypoxia Insufficient availability of oxygen to meet the metabolic needs of body tissue.

Hysterectomy Surgical removal of the uterus.

- **TAH-BSO** Transabdominal hysterectomy and bilateral salpingo-oophorectomy. Removal of uterus, both tubes, and both ovaries.
- **TVH** Transvaginal hysterectomy.

Hysterosalpingography X-ray of the uterus and uterine tubes after filling them with radiopaque material.

Hysterotomy Surgical incision into the uterus.

Iatrogenic Caused by a physician's words, actions, or treatment.

Icterus neonatorum Jaundice in the newborn.

IDM Infant of a diabetic mother.

IgA Primary immunoglobulin in colostrum.

IgG Transplacentally acquired immunoglobulin that confers passive immunity against the infections to which the mother is immune.

IgM Immunoglobulin neonate can manufacture soon after birth. Fetus produces it in the presence of amnionitis.

Iliopectineal line Bony ridge on the inner surface of the ilium and pubic bones that divides the true and false pelves; the brim of the true pelvic cavity; the inlet.

Implantation Embedding of the fertilized ovum in the uterine mucosa; nidation.

Impotence Archaic term designating a man's inability, partial or complete, to perform sexual intercourse or to achieve orgasm; erectile dysfunction.

Inborn error of metabolism Hereditary deficiency of a specific enzyme needed for normal metabolism of specific chemicals (e.g., deficiency of phenylalanine hydroxylase results in phenylketonuria [PKU]; a deficiency of hexosaminidase results in Tay-Sachs disease).

Incompetent cervix Cervix that is unable to remain closed until a pregnancy reaches term.

Incomplete abortion See *abortion, incomplete.*

Increment An increase, or buildup, as of a contraction.

Induced abortion See *abortion, induced.*

Induction Artificial stimulation or augmentation of labor.

Inertia Sluggishness or inactivity; in obstetrics, refers to the absence or weakness of uterine contractions during labor.

Inevitable abortion See *abortion, inevitable.*

Infant A child who is under 1 year of age.

Infertility Decreased capacity to conceive.

Infiltration Process by which a substance such as a local anesthetic drug is deposited within the tissue.

Inhalation analgesia Reduction of pain by administration of anesthetic gas. Occasionally given during the second stage of labor. Consciousness is retained to allow the woman to follow instructions and to avoid the adverse effects of general anesthesia.

Inlet Passage leading into a cavity.

Pelvic i. Upper brim of the pelvic cavity.

Internal os Inside mouth or opening.

Interstitial cell-stimulating hormone (ICSH) Hormone that stimulates production of testosterone; analogous to LH in the female.

Intertuberous diameter Distance between ischial tuberosities. Measured to determine dimension of pelvic outlet.

Intervillous space Irregular space in the maternal portion of the placenta, filled with maternal blood and serving as the site of maternal-fetal gas, nutrient, and waste exchange.

Intrapartum During labor and birth.

Intrathecal Within the subarachnoid space.

Intrauterine device (IUD) Small copper- or progesterone-containing form used for contraception.

Intrauterine growth retardation (IUGR) Fetal undergrowth of any etiology, such as deficient nutrient supply or intrauterine infection, or associated with congenital malformation.

Introitus Entrance into a canal or cavity such as the vagina.

Intromission Insertion of one part or object into another (e.g., introduction of penis into vagina).

Intussusception Prolapse of one segment of bowel into the lumen of the adjacent segment.

In utero Within or inside the uterus.

In vitro fertilization Fertilization in a culture dish or test tube.

Inversion Turning end for end, upside down, or inside out.

I. of the uterus Condition in which the uterus is turned inside out so that the fundus intrudes into the cervix or vagina; may be caused by a too vigorous removal of the placenta before it is detached by the natural process of labor.

Involution (1) Rolling or turning inward. (2) Reduction in size of the uterus after birth and its return to its normal size and condition. See *retraction.*

Isoimmune hemolytic disease Breakdown (hemolysis) of fetal/neonatal Rh-positive RBCs because of Rh antibodies formed by an Rh-negative mother who had been previously exposed to Rh-positive RBCs.

Isoimmunization Development of antibodies in a species of animal with antigens from the same species (e.g., development of anti-Rh antibodies in an Rh-negative person).

ITP Idiopathic thrombocytopenic purpura.

Jaundice Yellow discoloration of the body tissues caused by the deposit of bile pigments (unconjugated bilirubin); icterus.

Breast–feeding j. Appearing about day three, this jaundice is related to the number of feedings; the greater the number, the lower the bilirubin level (feedings should be ≥ 8 every 24 hr).

Breast milk j. Yellowing of infant's skin from pregnanediol (in mother's milk) inhibition of enzyme (glucuronyl transferase) necessary for conjugation of bilirubin.

Pathologic j. Jaundice usually first noticeable within 24 hours after birth; caused by some abnormal condition such as an Rh or ABO incompatibility and resulting in bilirubin toxicity (e.g., kernicterus)

Physiologic j. Jaundice usually occurring 48 hours or later after birth, reaching a peak at 5 to 7 days, gradually disappearing by the seventh to tenth day, and caused by the normal reduction in the number of red blood cells. The infant is otherwise well.

Jet hydrotherapy Use of warm water under pressure to relax muscles and promote comfort.

Kahn test Precipitation or flocculation test for the diagnosis of syphilis.

Karyotype Schematic arrangement of the chromosomes within a cell to demonstrate their numbers and morphology.

Kegel exercises Exercises to strengthen the pubococcygeal muscles.

Kernicterus Bilirubin encephalopathy involving the deposit of unconjugated bilirubin in brain cells, resulting in death or impaired intellectual, perceptive, or motor function, and adaptive behavior.

Kin group People related by blood, marriage, or mutual agreement.

Klumpke's palsy Atrophic paralysis of forearm.

Labor Series of processes by which the fetus is expelled from the uterus; parturition; childbirth.

Labor-delivery-recovery room (LDR) Unit in which a woman labors, gives birth, and recovers during the fourth stage of labor.

Labor-delivery-recovery-postpartum room (LDRP) An LDR in which a woman continues to stay after recovery until discharge home.

Laceration Irregular tear of wound tissue; in obstetrics, it usually refers to a tear in the perineum, vagina, or cervix caused by childbirth.

Lactase Enzyme necessary for the digestion of lactose.

Lactation Function of secreting milk, or period during which milk is secreted.

Lactogenic Stimulating the production of milk.

- **L. hormone** Gonadotropin produced by anterior pituitary and responsible for promoting growth of breast tissue and lactation; prolactin; luteotropin.

Lactose intolerance Inherited absence of the enzyme lactose.

Lactosuria Presence of lactose in the urine during late pregnancy and during lactation. Must be differentiated from glycosuria.

Lamaze method Method of psychophysical preparation for childbirth developed in the 1950s by a French obstetrician, Fernand Lamaze. It requires classes, practice at home, and coaching during labor and birth.

Lambdoid Having the shape of the Greek letter lambda (λ).

- **L. suture** Suture line extending across the posterior third of the skull, separating the occipital bone from the two parietal bones, and forming the base of the triangular posterior fontanelle.

Laminaria tent Cone of dried seaweed that swells as it absorbs moisture. Used to dilate the cervix nontraumatically in preparation for an induced abortion or in preparation for induction of labor.

Lanugo Downy, fine hair characteristic of the fetus between 20 weeks' gestation and birth that is most noticeable over the shoulder, forehead, and cheeks but is found on nearly all parts of the body except the palms of the hands, soles of the feet, and the scalp.

Laparoscopy Examination of the interior of the abdomen by inserting a small telescope through the anterior abdominal wall.

Large for dates (large for gestational age [LGA]) Exhibiting excessive growth for gestational age.

Learned helplessness Belief that one is powerless and unable to act independently; the result of socialization.

Lecithin A phospholipid that decreases surface tension; surfactant (i.e., surface-active agent).

Lecithin/sphingomyelin ratio Ratio of lecithin to sphingomyelin in the amniotic fluid. This is used to assess maturity of the fetal lung.

Leopold's maneuver Four maneuvers for diagnosing the fetal position by external palpation of the mother's abdomen.

Let-down reflex Oxytocin-induced flow of milk from the alveoli of the breasts into the milk ducts.

Leukorrhea White or yellowish mucous discharge from the cervical canal or the vagina that may be normal physiologically or caused by pathologic states of the vagina and endocervix (e.g., *Trichomonas vaginalis* infections).

LH See *luteinizing hormone (LH).*

Libido Sexual drive.

Lie Relationship existing between the long axis of the fetus and the long axis of the mother. In a longitudinal lie, the fetus is lying lengthwise or vertically, whereas in a transverse lie the fetus is lying crosswise or horizontally in the mother's uterus.

Ligation Act of suturing, sewing, or otherwise tying shut.

- **Tubal l.** Abdominal operation in which the fallopian tubes are tied off and a section is removed to interrupt tubal continuity and thus sterilize the woman.

Lightening Sensation of decreased abdominal distention produced by uterine descent into the pelvic cavity as the fetal presenting part settles into the pelvis. It usually occurs 2 weeks before the onset of labor in nulliparas.

Linea nigra Line of darker pigmentation seen in some women during the latter part of pregnancy that appears over the midline of the abdomen and extends from the symphysis pubis toward the umbilicus.

Linea terminalis Line dividing the upper (false) pelvis from the lower (true) pelvis.

Lithotomy position Position in which the woman lies on her back with her knees flexed and abducted thighs drawn up toward her chest.

Live birth Birth in which the neonate, regardless of gestational age, manifests any heartbeat, breathes, or displays voluntary movement.

Lochia Vaginal discharge during the puerperium, consisting of blood, tissue, and mucus.

- **L. alba** Thin, yellowish to white, vaginal discharge that follows lochia serosa on about the tenth postpartum day and that may last from the end of the third to the sixth postpartum week.
- **L. rubra** Red, distinctly blood-tinged vaginal flow that follows birth and lasts 2 to 4 days.
- **L. serosa** Serous, pinkish brown, watery vaginal discharge that follows lochia rubra until about the tenth postpartum day.

L/S ratio (lecithin/sphingomyelin ratio) Test for fetal lung maturity.

Lumpectomy Excision of a breast lump, usually followed by radiation and chemotherapy.

Lunar month Four weeks (28 days).

Lutein Yellow pigment derived from the corpus luteum, egg yolk, and fat cells.

L. cells Ovarian cells involved in the formation of the corpus luteum and that contain a yellow pigment.

Luteinizing hormone (LH) Hormone produced by the anterior pituitary that stimulates ovulation and the development of the corpus luteum.

Luteotropin (LTH) Lactogenic hormone; prolactin; an adenohypophyseal hormone.

Lymphedema Collection of excessive fluid in tissue when lymph nodes or vessels have been removed.

Lysis of adhesions Operation to free adhesions (bands of scar tissue) that have caused organs to be abnormally drawn or tied to each other.

Lysozyme Enzyme with antiseptic qualities that destroys foreign organisms and that is found in blood cells of the granulocytic and monocytic series and is also normally present in saliva, sweat, tears, and breast milk.

Maceration (1) Process of softening a solid by soaking it in a fluid. (2) Softening and breaking down of fetal skin from prolonged exposure to amniotic fluid as seen in a postterm infant. Also seen in a dead fetus.

Macroglossia Hypertrophy of tongue or tongue large for oral cavity; seen in some preterm neonates and in neonates with Down syndrome.

Macrophage Any phagocytic cell of the reticuloendothelial system, including Kupffer cell in the liver, splenocyte in the spleen, and histocyte in the loose connective tissue.

Macrosomia Large body size as seen in neonates of diabetic or prediabetic mothers; macrosomatia.

Malpractice Professional negligence that is the proximate cause of injury or harm to a client, resulting from a lack of professional knowledge, experience, or skill that can be expected in others in the profession or from a failure to exercise reasonable care or judgment in the application of professional knowledge, experience, or skill.

Mammography X-ray examination technique used to screen for and evaluate breast lesions.

Manic depressive psychosis Major affective disorder characterized by episodes of mania and depression. One or the other phase may be predominant at any given time; one phase may appear alternately with the other; or elements of both phases may be present simultaneously. Also called bipolar disorder.

Mask of pregnancy See *chloasma*.

Mastalgia Breast soreness or tenderness.

Mastectomy Excision, or removal, of the mammary gland.

Mastitis Inflammation of mammary tissue of the breasts.

Maternal mortality See *mortality, maternal*

Maturation (1) Process of attaining maximum development. (2) In biology, a process of cell division during which the number of chromosomes in the germ cells (sperm or ova) is reduced to one half the number (haploid) characteristic of the species.

Maturational crisis Crisis that arises during normal growth and development, e.g., puberty.

Meatus Opening from an internal structure to the outside (e.g., urethral meatus).

Meconium First stools of infant: viscid, sticky; dark greenish brown, almost black; sterile; odorless.

M. aspiration syndrome Function of fetal hypoxia: with hypoxia, the anal sphincter relaxes and meconium is released; reflex gasping movements draw meconium and other particulate matter in the amniotic fluid into the infant's bronchial tree, obstructing the air flow after birth.

M. ileus Lower intestinal obstruction by thick, putty-like, inspissated meconium that may be the result of deficiency of trypsin production in the newborn with cystic fibrosis.

M.-stained fluid In response to hypoxia, fetal intestinal activity increases and anal sphincter relaxes, resulting in the passage of meconium, which imparts a greenish coloration.

Meiosis Process by which germ cells divide and decrease their chromosomal number by one half.

-Melia Pertaining to a limb or part of a limb or extremity, as in amelia (absence of a limb) or phocomelia (absence of part of arms or legs).

Membrane Thin, pliable layer of tissue that lines a cavity or tube, separates structures, or covers an organ or structure; in obstetrics, the amnion and chorion surrounding the fetus.

Menarche Onset, or beginning, of menstrual function.

Meningomyelocele Saclike protrusion of the spinal cord through a congenital defect in the vertebral column.

Menopause From the Greek words *men* (month) and *pausis* (to stop), the actual permanent cessation of menstrual cycles.

Menorrhagia Abnormally profuse or excessive menstrual flow.

Menses (menstruation) Periodic vaginal discharge of bloody fluid from the nonpregnant uterus that occurs from the age of puberty to menopause.

Mentum Chin, a fetal reference point in designating position (e.g., "Left mentum anterior" [LMA], meaning that the fetal chin is presenting in the left anterior quadrant of the maternal pelvis).

Mesoderm Embryonic middle layer of germ cells giving rise to all types of muscles, connective tissue, bone marrow, blood, lymphoid tissue, and all epithelial tissue.

Metritis Inflammation of the endometrium and myometrium.

Metrorrhagia Abnormal bleeding from the uterus, particularly when it occurs at any time other than the menstrual period.

Microcephaly Congenital anomaly characterized by abnormal smallness of the head in relation to the rest of the body and by underdevelopment of the brain, resulting in some degree of mental retardation.

Micrognathia Abnormal smallness of mandible or chin.

Midwife One who practices the art of helping and aiding a woman to give birth.

Milia Unopened sebaceous glands appearing as tiny, white, pinpoint papules on forehead, nose, cheeks, and chin of a neonate that disappear spontaneously in a few days or weeks.

Milk-leg See *phlegmasia alba dolens.*

Miscarriage Spontaneous abortion; lay term usually referring specifically to the loss of the fetus between the fourth month and viability.

Misogyny Hatred of women.

Missed abortion See *abortion, missed.*

Mitleiden Suffering along with.

Mitral valve prolapse Protrusion of mitral valve leaflets into atrium during ventricular systole.

Mitosis Process of somatic cell division in which a single cell divides, but both of the new cells have the same number of chromosomes as the first.

Mittelschmerz Abdominal pain in the region of an ovary during ovulation, which usually occurs midway through the menstrual cycle. Present in many women, mittelschmerz is useful for identifying ovulation, thus pinpointing the fertile period of the cycle.

Molding Overlapping of cranial bones or shaping of the fetal head to accommodate and conform to the bony and soft parts of the mother's birth canal during labor.

Mongolian spot Bluish-gray or dark, nonelevated pigmented area usually found over the lower back and buttocks present at birth in some infants, primarily nonCaucasian. The spot fades by school age in African-American or Oriental infants and within the first year or two of life in other infants.

Mongolism See *Down syndrome.*

Moniliasis Infection of the skin or mucous membrane by a yeastlike fungus, *Candida albicans;* see *thrush.*

Monitrice One trained in psychoprophylactic methods and in supporting women during labor.

Monosomy Chromosomal aberration characterized by the absence of one chromosome from the normal diploid complement.

Monozygotic Originating or coming from a single fertilized ovum, such as identical twins.

Monozygotic twins See *twins, monozygotic*

Mons veneris Pad of fatty tissue and coarse skin that overlies the symphysis pubis in the woman and that, after puberty, is covered with short curly hair.

Montgomery's glands, tubercles Small, nodular prominences (sebaceous glands) on the areolas around the nipples of the breasts that enlarge during pregnancy and lactation.

Morbidity (1) Condition of being diseased. (2) Number of cases of disease or sick persons in relationship to a specific population; incidence.

Morning sickness Nausea and vomiting that affect some women during the first few months of their pregnancy; may occur at any time of day.

Moro's reflex Normal, generalized reflex in a young infant elicited by a sudden loud noise or by striking the table next to the child, resulting in flexion of the legs, an embracing posture of the arms, and usually a brief cry. Also called startle reflex.

Mortality (1) Quality or state of being subject to death. (2) Number of deaths in relation to a specific population; incidence.

- **Fetal m.** Number of fetal deaths per 1000 births (or per live births).
- **Infant m.** Number of deaths per 1000 children 1 year of age or younger.
- **Intrauterine m.** Death of a fetus weighing 500 g or more, of 20 weeks' gestation or more.
- **Maternal m.** Number of maternal deaths per 100,000 births during the childbearing cycle.
- **Neonatal m.** Statistical rate of infant death during the first 28 days after live birth, expressed as the number of such deaths per 1000 live births in a specific geographic area or institution in a given time.
- **Perinatal m.** Combined fetal and neonatal mortality.

Morula Developmental stage of the fertilized ovum in which there is a solid mass of cells resembling a mulberry.

Mosaicism Condition in which some somatic cells are normal, whereas others show chromosomal aberrations.

Mourning Expressions and behaviors of grief.

Mucous membrane Specialized thin layer of tissue lining certain cavities and passages that is kept moist by the secretion of mucus.

Multigravida Woman who has been pregnant two or more times.

Multipara Woman who has carried two or more pregnancies to viability, whether they ended in live infants or stillbirths.

Multifetal pregnancy Pregnancy in which there is more than one fetus in the uterus at the same time; multiple pregnancy.

Mutation Change in a gene or chromosome in gametes that may be transmitted to offspring.

Nägele's rule Method for calculating the estimated date of confinement (EDC), or "due date."

Natal Relating or pertaining to birth.

Navel Depression in the center of the abdomen, where the umbilical cord was attached to the fetus; umbilicus.

Necrotizing enterocolitis (NEC) Acute inflammatory bowel disorder that occurs primarily in preterm, low-birth-weight, or cocaine-exposed neonates. It is characterized by ischemic necrosis (death) of the gastrointestinal mucosa that may lead to perforation and peritonitis.

Negligence Commission of an act that a prudent person would not have done or the omission of a duty that a reasonably prudent person would have fulfilled, resulting in injury or harm to another person.

Neonatal hypovolemic shock Cardiovascular collapse resulting from a diminished volume of circulating fluid in the cardiovascular system.

Neonatal mortality See *mortality, neonatal.*

Neonatology Study of the neonate.

Neoplasia Growth of new tissue; tumor that serves no physiologic function; may be benign or malignant.

Neural tube Tube formed from fusion of the neural folds from which develops the brain and spinal cord.

Neutral temperature range That grouping of environmental conditions in which the neonate's oxygen consumption is at a minimum and temperature is within normal limits.

Nevus Natural blemish or mark; a congenital circumscribed deposit of pigmentation in the skin; mole.

- **N. flammeus** Port-wine stain; reddish, usually flat, discoloration of the face or neck. Because of its large size and color, it is considered a serious deformity.
- **N. vasculosus (strawberry hemangioma)** Elevated lesion of immature capillaries and endothelial cells that regresses over a period of years.

Nidation Implantation of the fertilized ovum in the endometrium, or lining, of the uterus.

Nondisjunction Failure of homologous pairs of chromosomes to separate during the first meiotic division or of the two chromatids of a chromosome to split during anaphase of mitosis or the second meiotic division. The result is an abnormal number of chromosomes in the daughter cells.

Nonshivering thermogenesis Infant's method of producing heat by increasing metabolic rate.

Nonstress test (NST) Evaluation of fetal response (fetal heart rate) to natural contractile uterine activity or to an increase in fetal activity.

Nosocomial Pertaining to a hospital.

Nulligravida Woman who has never been pregnant.

Nullipara Woman who has not yet carried a pregnancy to viability.

Nurse practitioner Registered nurse who has additional education to practice nursing in an expanded role.

Obstetrix Midwife; from *obstare,* to stand before.

Occipitobregmatic Pertaining to the occiput (the back part of the skull) and the bregma (junction of the coronal and sagittal sutures) or anterior fontanelle; the smallest diameter of the fetal head.

Occiput Back part of the head or skull.

Oligohydramnios Abnormally small amount or absence of amniotic fluid; often indicative of fetal urinary tract defect.

Oliguria Diminished secretion of urine by the kidneys.

Omphalic Concerning or pertaining to the umbilicus.

Omphalitis Inflammation of the umbilical stump characterized by redness, edema, and purulent exudate in severe infections.

Omphalocele Congenital defect resulting from failure of closure of the abdominal wall or muscles and leading to hernia of abdominal contents through the navel.

Oogenesis Formation and development of the ovum.

Oophorectomy Excision or removal of an ovary.

Operculum Plug of mucus that fills the cervical canal during pregnancy.

Ophthalmia neonatorum Infection in the neonate's eyes, usually resulting from gonorrheal or other infection contracted when the fetus passes through the birth canal (vagina).

Opisthotonos Tetanic spasm resulting in an arched, hyperextended position of the body.

Oral GTT Test for blood sugar following oral ingestion of a concentrated sugar solution.

Orchitis Inflammation of one or both of the testes, characterized by swelling and pain, often caused by mumps, syphilis, or tuberculosis.

Organogenesis Period of embryonic development (between weeks 3 to 4 and 8) during which all major organ systems are formed. Period of extreme vulnerability to teratogens (e.g., environmental hazards and toxic substances).

Orgasmic platform Congestion of the lower vagina during sexual intercourse.

Orifice Normal mouth, entrance, or opening, to any aperture.

Os Mouth, or opening.

- **External o.** External opening of the cervical canal.
- **Internal o.** Internal opening of the cervical canal.
- **O. uteri** Mouth, or opening, of the uterus.

Ossification Mineralization of fetal bones.

Osteoporosis Deossification of bone tissue resulting in structural weakness.

-Otomy Combining form meaning cutting, incision, section.

Outlet Opening by which something can exit.

- **Pelvic o.** Inferior aperture, or opening, of the true pelvis.

Ovary One of two glands in the female situated on either side of the pelvic cavity that produce the female reproductive cell, the ovum, and two known hormones, estrogen and progesterone.

Ovulation Periodic ripening and discharge of the unimpregnated ovum from the ovary, usually 14 days before the onset of menstrual flow.

- **O. method** Evaluation of cervical mucus throughout the menstrual cycle; ovulation occurs just after the appearance of the peak mucus sign; Billings method.

Ovum Female germ, or reproductive cell, produced by the ovary; egg.

Oxygen toxicity Oxygen overdosage that results in pathologic tissue changes (e.g., retinopathy of prematurity, bronchopulmonary dysplasia in the neonate).

Oxytocics Drugs that stimulate uterine contractions, thus accelerating childbirth and preventing postbirth hemorrhage. They may be used to increase the let-down reflex during lactation.

Oxytocin Hormone produced by the posterior pituitary gland that stimulates uterine contractions and the release of milk in the mammary gland (let-down reflex).

O. challenge test (OCT) Evaluation of fetal response (fetal heart rate) to contractile activity of the uterus stimulated by exogenous oxytocin (Pitocin).

$Paco_2$ Partial pressure of carbon dioxide in arterial blood.

Palsy Permanent or temporary loss of sensation or ability to move and control movement; paralysis.

Bell's p. Peripheral facial paralysis of the facial nerve (cranial nerve VII), causing the muscles of the unaffected side of the face to pull the face into a distorted position.

Erb's p. See *Erb-Duchenne paralysis.*

Pao_2 Partial pressure of oxygen in arterial blood.

Papanicolaou (Pap) test Microscopic examination using scrapings from the cervix, endocervix, or other mucous membranes that will reveal, with a high degree of accuracy, the presence of premalignant or malignant cells.

Para Term used to refer to past pregnancies that reached viability regardless of whether the infant(s) was dead or alive at birth.

Parabiotic syndrome Fetofetal blood transfer caused by placental vascular anastomoses occurring in a small plethoric twin (polycythemia) and one pale twin (anemia).

Parity Number of pregnancies that reached viability.

Parturient Woman giving birth.

Parturition Process or act of giving birth.

Patent Open.

Pathogen Substance or organism capable of producing disease.

Pathologic hyperbilirubinemia High (toxic) levels of serum bilirubin resulting from a disease process causing hemolysis (e.g., Rh incompatibility); jaundice apparent within first 24 hours.

Pathologic jaundice See *jaundice, pathologic.*

Patulous Open or spread apart.

Peak mucus sign Lubricative, cloudy-to-clear-egg white cervical mucus occurring under high estrogen levels close to time of ovulation; ferns; good spinnbarkheit.

Peau d'orange "Orange-peel"-like skin secondary to cancerous lesions and seen over edematous breasts.

Pedigree Shorthand method of depicting family lines of individuals who manifest a physical or chemical disorder.

Pelvic Pertaining or relating to the pelvis.

P. axis See *axis, pelvic.*

P. inflammatory disease (PID) Infection of internal reproductive structures and adjacent tissues usually secondary to STD infection.

P. inlet See *inlet, pelvic.*

P. outlet See *outlet, pelvic.*

Pelvimetry Measurement of dimensions and proportions of the pelvis to determine its capacity and ability to allow the passage of the fetus through the birth canal.

Pelvis Bony structure formed by the sacrum, coccyx, innominate bones, and symphysis pubis, and the ligaments that unite them.

Android p. See *android pelvis.*

Anthropoid p. See *anthropoid pelvis.*

False p. Pelvis above the linea terminalis and symphysis pubis.

Gynecoid p. See *gynecoid pelvis.*

Platypelloid p. See *platypelloid pelvis.*

True p. Pelvis below the linea terminalis.

Penis Male organ used for urination and copulation.

Peridural anesthesia Injection of anesthetic outside the dura mater (anesthetic does not mix with spinal fluid); epidural anesthesia.

Perinatal Of or pertaining to the time and process of giving birth or being born.

Perinatal period Period extending from the twentieth or twenty-eighth week of gestation through the end of the twenty-eighth day after birth.

Perinatologist Physician who specializes in fetal and neonatal care.

Perineum Area between the vagina and rectum in the female and between the scrotum and rectum in the male.

Periodic breathing Sporadic episodes of cessation of respirations for periods of 10 seconds or less not associated with cyanosis; commonly noted in preterm infants.

Periods of reactivity (newborn infant) *First period* (within 30 minutes after birth): brief cyanosis, flushing with crying; rales, nasal flaring, grunting, retractions; heart sounds loud, forceful, irregular; alert; mucus; no bowel sounds; followed by period of sleep. *Second period* (4 to 8 hours after birth): swift color changes; irregular respiratory and heart rates; mucus with gagging; meconium passage; and temperature stabilizing.

Pessary Device placed inside the vagina to function as a supportive structure for the uterus or a contraceptive device.

Petechiae Pinpoint hemorrhagic areas caused by numerous disease states involving infection and thrombocytopenia and occasionally found over the face and trunk of the newborn because of increased intravascular pressure in the capillaries during birth.

pH Hydrogen ion concentration.

Phenotype Expression of certain physical or chemical characteristics in an individual, resulting from interaction between genotype and environmental factors.

Phenylketonuria (PKU) Recessive hereditary disease that results in a defect in the metabolism of the amino acid phenylalanine caused by the lack of an enzyme, phenylalanine hydroxylase, that is necessary for the conversion of the amino acid phenylalanine into tyrosine. If PKU is not treated, brain damage may occur, causing severe mental retardation.

Phimosis Tightness of the prepuce, or foreskin, of the penis.

Phlebitis Inflammation of a vein with symptoms of pain and tenderness along the course of the vein, inflammatory swelling and acute edema below the obstruction, and discoloration of the skin because of injury or bruise to the vein, possibly occurring in acute or chronic infections or after operations or childbirth.

Phlebothrombosis Formation of a clot or thrombus in the vein; inflammation of the vein with secondary clotting.

Phlegmasia alba dolens Phlebitis of the femoral vein with thrombosis leading to a venous obstruction, causing acute edema of the leg, and occurring occasionally after birth; also called *milk-leg.*

Phocomelia Developmental anomaly characterized by the absence of the upper portion of one or more limbs so that the feet or hands or both are attached to the trunk of the body by short, irregularly shaped stumps, resembling the fins of a seal.

Phosphatidylglycerol A phospholipid, a component of pulmonary surfactant; its presence in amniotic fluid is considered a sign of fetal lung maturity when the pregnancy is complicated by maternal diabetes.

Phototherapy Utilization of lights to reduce serum bilirubin levels by oxidation of bilirubin into water-soluble compounds that are then processed in the liver and excreted in bile and urine.

Physiologic hyperbilirubinemia Hemolysis of excessive fetal RBCs in the early neonatal period; jaundice not apparent during first 24 hours. Levels are nontoxic to the individual.

Physiologic jaundice See *jaundice, physiologic.*

Pica Unusual craving during pregnancy (e.g., for laundry starch, dirt, or red clay).

Pinna Ear cartilage.

Placenta Latin, flat cake; afterbirth; specialized vascular disc-shaped organ for maternal-fetal gas and nutrient exchange.

Abruptio p. See *abruptio placentae.*

Battledore p. Umbilical cord insertion into the margin of the placenta.

Circumvallate p. Placenta having a raised white ring at its edge.

P. accreta Invasion of the uterine muscle by the placenta, thus making separation from the muscle difficult if not impossible.

P. previa Placenta that is abnormally implanted in the thin, lower uterine segment and that is typed according to proximity to cervical os: total—completely occludes os; partial—does not occlude os completely; and marginal—placenta encroaches on margin of internal cervical os.

P. succenturiata Accessory placenta.

Placental Pertaining or relating to the placenta.

P. dysfunction Failure of placenta to meet fetal needs and requirements; placental insufficiency.

P. dystocia See *dystocia, placental.*

P. infarct Localized, ischemic, hard area on the fetal or maternal side of the placenta.

P. souffle See *souffle, placental.*

Platypelloid pelvis Broad pelvis with a shortened anteroposterior diameter and a flattened, oval, transverse shape.

Plethora Deep beefy red coloration ("boiled lobster" hue) of a newborn caused by an increased number of blood cells (polycythemia) per volume of blood.

Podalic Concerning or pertaining to the feet.

P. version Shifting of the position of the fetus so as to bring the feet to the outlet during labor.

Polycythemia Increased number of erythrocytes per volume of blood, which may be caused by large placental transfusion, fetofetal transfusion (in twin pregnancy), or maternal-fetal transfusion, or it may be due to hypovolemia resulting from movement of fluid out of vascular into interstitial compartment.

Polydactyly Excessive number of digits (fingers or toes).

Polygenic Pertaining to the combined action of several different genes.

Polyhydramnios See *hydramnios.*

Polyuria Excessive secretion and discharge of urine by the kidneys.

Position Relationship of an arbitrarily chosen fetal reference point, such as the occiput, sacrum, chin, or scapula, on the presenting part of the fetus to its location in the front, back, or sides of the maternal pelvis.

Positive sign of pregnancy Definite indication of pregnancy (e.g., hearing the fetal heartbeat, visualization and palpation of fetal movement by the examiner, sonographic examination).

Posterior Pertaining to the back.

P. fontanelle See *fontanelle, posterior.*

Postmature infant Infant born at or after the beginning of week 43 of gestation or later and exhibiting signs of dysmaturity.

Postnatal Happening or occurring after birth (newborn).

Postpartum Happening or occurring after birth (mother).

Precipitate delivery Rapid or sudden labor of less than 3 hours' duration beginning from onset of cervical changes to completed birth of neonate.

Preeclampsia Disease encountered during pregnancy or early in the puerperium characterized by increasing hypertension, proteinuria, with or without generalized edema; pregnancy-induced hypertension (PIH): toxemia.

Pregnancy Period between conception through complete delivery of the products of conception. The usual duration of pregnancy in the human is 280 days, 9 calendar months, or 10 lunar months.

Ectopic p. See *ectopic pregnancy.*

Extrauterine p. See *extrauterine pregnancy.*

Premature infant Infant born before completing week 37 of gestation, irrespective of birth weight; preterm infant.

Premenstrual syndrome (PMS) Syndrome of nervous tension, irritability, weight gain, edema, headache, mastalgia, dysphoria, and lack of coordination occurring during the last few days of the menstrual cycle preceding the onset of menstruation.

Premonitory Serving as an early symptom or warning.

Prenatal Occurring or happening before birth.

Prepartum Before delivery; prior to giving birth.

Prepuce Fold of skin, or foreskin, covering the glans penis of the male.

P. of the clitoris Fold of the labia minora that covers the aroused glans clitoris.

Presentation That part of the fetus which first enters the pelvis and lies over the inlet: may be head, face, breech, or shoulder.

Breech p. See *breech presentation.*

Cephalic p. See *cephalic presentation.*

Presenting part That part of the fetus which lies closest to the internal os of the cervix.

Presumptive signs Manifestations that suggest pregnancy but that are not absolutely positive. These include the cessation of menses, Chadwick's sign, morning sickness, and quickening.

Preterm infant See *premature infant.*

Previa, placenta See *placenta previa.*

Primigravida Woman who is pregnant for the first time.

Primipara Woman who has carried a pregnancy to viability without regard to the child's being dead or alive at the time of birth.

Primordial Existing first or existing in the simplest or most primitive form.

Probable signs Manifestations or evidence which indicates that there is a definite likelihood of pregnancy. Among the probable signs are enlargement of abdomen, Goodell's sign, Hegar's sign, Braxton Hicks' sign, and positive hormonal tests for pregnancy.

Prodromal Serving as an early symptom or warning of the approach of a disease or condition (e.g., prodromal labor).

Progesterone Hormone produced by the corpus luteum and placenta whose function is to prepare the endometrium of the uterus for implantation of the fertilized ovum, develop the mammary glands, and maintain the pregnancy.

Prolactin See *lactogenic hormone.*

Prolapsed cord Protrusion of the umbilical cord in advance of the presenting part of the fetus.

Proliferative phase of menstrual cycle Preovulatory, follicular, or estrogen phase of the menstrual cycle.

Promontory of the sacrum Superior projecting portion of the sacrum at the junction of the sacrum and the L5 vertebrae.

Prophylactic Pertaining to prevention or warding off of disease or certain conditions; condom, or "rubber."

Proscription See *taboo.*

Prostaglandin (PG) Substance present in many body tissues; has a role in many reproductive tract functions.

Proteinuria Excretion of protein into urine.

Pruritus Itching.

Pruritus gravidarum Itching of the skin caused by pregnancy.

Pseudocyesis Condition in which the woman has all the usual signs of pregnancy, such as enlargement of the abdomen, cessation of menses, weight gain, and morning sickness, but is not pregnant; phantom or false pregnancy.

Pseudopregnancy See *pseudocyesis.*

Psychoprophylaxis Mental and physical education of the parents in preparation for childbirth, with the goal of minimizing the fear and perception of pain and promoting positive family relationships.

Ptyalism Excessive salivation.

Puberty Period in life in which the reproductive organs mature and one becomes functionally capable of reproduction.

Pubic Pertaining to the pubis.

Pubis Pubic bone forming the front of the pelvis.

PUBS (Percutaneous umbilical blood sampling) Fetal blood sampling obtained by inserting a needle through the maternal abdominal wall into the umbilical cord.

Pudendal block Injection of a local anesthetizing drug at the pudendal nerve root in order to produce numbness of the genital and perianal region.

Pudendum External genitalia of either sex; Latin, "that of which one should be ashamed."

Puerperal sepsis Infection of the pelvic organs during the postbirth period; childbed fever.

Puerperium Time following the third stage of labor and lasting until involution of the uterus takes place, usually about 3 to 6 weeks.

Quickening Maternal perception of fetal movement; usually occurs between weeks 16 and 20 of gestation.

Rape trauma syndrome Characteristic symptoms seen in victims of rape, consisting of several phases; similar to posttraumatic stress syndrome.

RDS See *respiratory distress syndrome (RDS).*

Recessive trait Genetically determined characteristic that is expressed only when present in the homozygotic state (e.g. blue eyes, blond hair).

Reasonably prudent nurse Person who acts with the average degree of skill, care, and diligence as those with similar background, training, and experience. One who acts wisely and judiciously. See *negligence.*

Reasonably prudent person Person who demonstrates the external code of behavior or expected performance (average degree of skill, care, and diligence) exercised by any other person with similar background, training, and experience.

Rectocele Herniation or protrusion of the rectum into the posterior vaginal wall.

Reflex Automatic response built into the nervous system that does not need the intervention of conscious thought (e.g., in the newborn, rooting, gagging, grasp).

Regional block anesthesia Anesthesia of an area of the body by injecting a local anesthetic to block a group of sensory nerve fibers.

Regurgitation Vomiting or spitting up of solids or fluids.

Residual urine Urine that remains in the bladder after urination.

Respiratory distress syndrome (RDS) Condition resulting from decreased pulmonary gas exchange, leading to retention of carbon dioxide (increase in arterial PCO_2). Most common neonatal causes are prematurity, perinatal asphyxia, and maternal diabetes mellitus; hyaline membrane disease (HMD).

Restitution In obstetrics, the turning of the fetal head to the left or right after it has completely emerged from the introitus as it assumes a normal alignment with the infant's shoulders.

Resuscitation Restoration of consciousness or life in one who is apparently dead or whose respirations or cardiac function or both have ceased.

Retained placenta Retention of all or part of the placenta in the uterus after birth.

Retraction (1) Drawing in or sucking in of soft tissues of chest, indicative of an obstruction at any level of the respiratory tract from the oropharynx to the alveoli. (2) Retraction of uterine muscle fiber. After contracting, the muscle fiber does not return to its original length but remains slightly shortened, a unique attribute of uterine muscle that aids in preventing postbirth hemorrhage and results in involution.

Retroflexion Bending backward

R. of the uterus Condition in which the body of the womb is bent backward at an angle with the cervix, whose position usually remains unchanged.

Retrolental fibroplasia (RLF) *Retinopathy of prematurity* associated with hyperoxemia, resulting in eye injury and blindness.

Retroversion Turning or a state of being turned back.

R. of the uterus Displacement of the uterus; the body of the uterus is tipped backward with the cervix pointing forward toward the symphysis pubis.

Retrovirus A single piece of RNA surrounded by a protein coat, or envelope. A unique enzyme, reverse transcriptase, allows this RNA retrovirus to go backward, *against the "flow of life."* The RNA becomes a piece of DNA, which infects the cell's DNA nucleus and remains in the cell until its death (e.g., HIV). (The normal flow of genetic information in life is from DNA to RNA to protein.)

Rh factor Inherited antigen present on erythrocytes. The individual with the factor is known as *positive* for the factor.

Rhythm method Contraceptive method in which a woman abstains from sexual intercourse during the ovulatory phase of her menstrual cycle and at least 3 days before and 1 day after the ovulation date.

Ribonucleic acid (RNA) Element responsible for transferring genetic information within a cell; a template, or pattern.

Risk factors Factors that cause a person or a group of people to be particularly vulnerable to an unwanted, unpleasant, or unhealthful event.

Risk management Actions taken to eliminate or minimize either the chance of injury to a client or the harm that occurs.

Ritgen maneuver Procedure used to control the birth of the head.

Role playing Psychotherapeutic technique in which a person acts out a real or simulated situation as a means of understanding intrapsychic conflicts.

Rooming-in unit Maternity unit designed so that the newborn's crib is at the mother's bedside or in a nursery adjacent to the mother's room.

Rooting reflex Normal response in newborns when the cheek is touched or stroked along the side of the mouth to turn the head toward the stimulated side, to open the mouth, and to begin to suck. The reflex disappears by 3 to 4 months of age but in some infants may persist until 12 months.

Rotation In obstetrics, the turning of the fetal head as it follows the curves of the birth canal downward.

Rubin's test Transuterine insufflation of the fallopian tubes with carbon dioxide to test their patency.

Rugae Folds of vaginal mucosa; creases in scrotum.

Sac, amniotic See *amniotic sac*.

Sacroiliac Of or pertaining to the sacrum and ilium.

Sacrum Triangular bone composed of five united vertebrae and situated between L5 and the coccyx; forms the posterior boundary of the true pelvis.

Saddle block anesthesia Type of regional anesthesia produced by injection of a local anesthetic solution into the cerebrospinal fluid intrathecal (subarachnoid) space in the spinal canal; "low spinal" anesthesia.

Sagittal suture Band of connective tissue separating the parietal bones, extending from the anterior to the posterior fontanel.

Salpingo-oophorectomy Removal of a fallopian tube and an ovary.

Scaphoid abdomen Abdomen with a sunken interior wall.

Schultze's mechanism Delivery of the placenta with the fetal surfaces (shiny in appearance) presenting (archaic).

Sclerema Hardening of skin and subcutaneous tissue that develops in association with such life-threatening disorders as severe cold stress, septicemia, and shock.

Scrotum Pouch of skin containing the testes and parts of the spermatic cords.

Sebaceous glands Oil-secreting glands found in the skin.

Secondary areola See *areola, secondary*.

Secretory phase of menstrual cycle Postovulatory, luteal, progestational, premenstrual phase of menstrual cycle; 14 days in length.

Secundines Fetal membranes and placenta expelled after childbirth; afterbirth.

Semen Thick, white, viscid secretion discharged from the urethra of the male at orgasm; the transporting medium of the sperm.

Sensitization Development of antibodies to a specific antigen.

Septic abortion See *abortion, septic*.

Sex chromosome Chromosome associated with determination of gender: the X (female) and Y (male) chromosomes. The normal female has two X chromosomes, and the normal male has one X and one Y chromosome.

Sexual assault Penetration of any orifice by the penis, other male appendage, or object without the victim's consent; achieved through use of actual or implied threats, force, intimidation, or deception.

Shake test "Foam" test for lung maturity of fetus; more rapid than determination of L/S ratio.

Sims' position Position in which the client lies on the left side with the right knee and thigh drawn upward toward the chest.

Singleton Pregnancy with a single fetus.

Situational crisis Crisis that arises suddenly in response to an external event or a conflict concerning a specific circumstance. The symptoms are transient, and the episode is usually brief.

Small for dates (small for gestational age [SGA]) Refers to inadequate growth for gestational age.

Smegma Whitish secretion around labia minora.

Somatic Pertaining to the body, not reproductive cells.

Souffle Soft, blowing sound or murmur heard by auscultation.

Funic s. Soft, muffled, blowing sound produced by blood rushing through the umbilical vessels and synchronous with the fetal heart sounds.

Placental s. Soft, blowing murmur caused by the blood current in the placenta and synchronous with the maternal pulse.

Uterine s. Soft, blowing sound made by the blood in the arteries of the pregnant uterus and synchronous with the maternal pulse.

Sperm Male sex cell. Also called spermatozoon.

Spermatogenesis Process by which mature spermatozoa are formed, during which the diploid chromosome number (46) is reduced by half (haploid, 23).

Spermicide Chemical substance that kills sperm by reducing their surface tension, causing the cell wall to break down by a bactericidal effect or by creating a highly acidic environment.

Spina bifida occulta Congenital malformation of the spine in which the posterior portion of laminas of the vertebras fails to close but there is no herniation or protrusion of the spinal cord or meninges through the defect. The newborn may have a dimple in the skin or growth of hair over the malformed vertebrae.

Spinnbarkheit Formation of a stretchable thread of cervical mucus under estrogen influence at time of ovulation.

Splanchnic engorgement Excessive filling or pooling of blood within the visceral vasculature that occurs following the removal of pressure from the abdomen, e.g., birth of a child, removal of an excess of urine from bladder (≥1000 mL), removal of large tumor.

Spontaneous abortion See *abortion, spontaneous*.

Square window Angle of wrist between hypothenar prominence and forearm; one criterion for estimating gestational age of neonate.

Standards of care Actions that a reasonably prudent person would have performed or omitted under specific conditions; conduct against which the defendant's actions are judged in a malpractice/negligence case. See *Nurse Practice Act* and *ANA and NAACOG standards of care*.

Station Relationship of the presenting fetal part to an imaginary line drawn between the ischial spines of the pelvis.

Sterility (1) State of being free from living microorganisms. (2) Complete inability to reproduce offspring.

Sterilization Process or act that renders a person unable to produce children.

Stillborn Born dead.

Stork bites See *telangiectatic nevi*.

Striae gravidarum ("stretch marks") Shining reddish lines caused by stretching of the skin, often found on the abdomen, thighs, and breasts during pregnancy. These streaks turn to a fine pinkish white or silver tone in time in fair-skinned women and brownish in darker-skinned women.

Subinvolution Failure of a part (e.g., the uterus) to reduce to its normal size and condition after enlargement from functional activity (e.g., pregnancy).

Supine hypotension Shock; fall in blood pressure caused by impaired venous return when gravid uterus presses on ascending vena cava, when woman is lying flat on her back; vena caval syndrome.

Surfactant Phosphoprotein necessary for normal respiratory function that prevents the alveolar collapse (atelectasis). See also *lecithin* and *L/S ratio*.

Suture (1) Junction of the adjoining bones of the skull. (2) Operation uniting parts by sewing them together.

Symphysis pubis Fibrocartilaginous union of the bodies of the pubic bones in the midline.

Syndactyly Malformation of digits, commonly seen as a fusion of two or more toes to form one structure.

Synostosis Articulation by osseous tissue of adjacent bones; union of separate bones by osseous tissue.

Taboo Proscribed (forbidden) by society as improper and unacceptable.

Tachypnea Excessively rapid respiratory rate (e.g., in neonates, respiratory rate of 60 breaths/min or more).

Talipes equinovarus Deformity in which the foot is extended and the person walks on the toes.

Telangiectasia Permanent dilatation of groups of superficial capillaries and venules.

Telangiectatic nevi ("stork bites") Clusters of small, red, localized areas of capillary dilatation commonly seen in neonates at the nape of the neck or lower occiput, upper eyelids, and nasal bridge that can be blanched with pressure of a finger.

Teratogenic agent Any drug, virus, or irradiation, the exposure to which can cause malformation of the fetus.

Teratogens Nongenetic factors that cause embryonic/fetal malformations and disease syndromes in utero.

Teratoma Tumor composed of different kinds of tissue, none of which normally occur together or at the site of the tumor.

Term infant Infant born between weeks 38 and 42 of completed gestation.

Testis One of the two glands contained in the male scrotum that produce the male reproductive cell, or sperm, and the male hormone testosterone; testicle.

Tetany, uterine Extremely prolonged uterine contractions.

Tetralogy of Fallot Congenital cardiac malformation consisting of pulmonary stenosis, intraventricular septal defect, dextroposed aorta that receives blood from both ventricles, and hypertrophy of the right ventricle.

Therapeutic abortion See *abortion, therapeutic.*

Thermogenesis Creation or production of heat, especially in the body.

Thermoneutral environment Environment that enables the neonate to maintain a body temperature of 36.5° C (97.7° F) with minimum use of oxygen and energy.

Threatened abortion See *abortion, threatened.*

Thrombocytopenia Abnormal hematologic condition in which the number of platelets is reduced, usually by destruction of erythroid tissue in bone marrow owing to certain neoplastic diseases or to an immune response to a drug.

Thrombocytopenic purpura Hematologic disorder characterized by prolonged bleeding time, decreased number of platelets, increased cell fragility, and purpura, which result in hemorrhages into the skin, mucous membranes, organs, and other tissue.

Thromboembolism Obstruction of a blood vessel by a clot that has become detached from its site of formation.

Thrombophlebitis Inflammation of a vein with secondary clot formation.

Thrombus Blood clot obstructing a blood vessel that remains at the place it was formed.

Thrush Fungal infection of the mouth or throat characterized by the formation of white patches on a red, moist, inflamed mucous membrane and caused by *Candida albicans.*

Toco- (toko-) Combining form that means childbirth or labor.

Tocolytic drug Drug used to suppress preterm labor.

Tocotransducer Electronic device for measuring uterine contractions.

Tongue-tie Congenital shortening of the frenulum, which, if severe, may interfere with sucking and articulation; a rare condition.

TORCH organisms Organisms that damage the embryo or fetus; acronym for *t*oxoplasmosis, *o*ther (e.g., syphilis), *r*ubella, *c*ytomegalovirus, and *h*erpes simplex.

Torticollis Congenital or acquired stiff neck caused by shortening or spasmodic contraction of the neck (sternocleidomastoid) muscles that draws the head to one side with the chin pointing in the other direction; wryneck.

Toxemia Term previously used for hypertensive states of pregnancy.

Tracheoesophageal fistula Congenital malformation in which there is an abnormal tubelike passage between the trachea and esophagus.

Transition Last phase of first stage of labor; 8 to 10 cm dilatation.

Translocation Condition in which a chromosome breaks and all or part of that chromosome is transferred to a different part of the same chromosome or to another chromosome.

Trait A distinguishing feature or characteristic.

Trauma Physical or psychic injury.

Trichomonas vaginitis Inflammation of the vagina caused by *Trichomonas vaginalis,* a parasitic protozoan and characterized by persistent burning and itching of the vulvar tissue and a profuse, frothy, white discharge.

Trimester Period of 3 months.

Trisomy Condition whereby any given chromosome exists in triplicate instead of the normal duplicate pattern.

Trophoblast Outer layer of cells of the developing blastodermic vesicle that develops the trophoderm or feeding layer which will establish the nutrient relationships with the uterine endometrium.

TSS Toxic shock syndrome.

Tubal ligation See *ligation, tubal.*

Tubercles of Montgomery Small papillae on surface of nipples and areolae that secrete a fatty substance that lubricates the nipples.

Twins Two neonates from the same impregnation developed within the same uterus at the same time.

- **Conjoined t.** Twins who are physically united; Siamese twins.
- **Disparate t.** Twins who are different (e.g., in weight) and distinct from one another.

Dizygotic t. Twins developed from two separate ova fertilized by two separate sperm at the same time; fraternal twins.

Monozygotic twins Twins developed from a single fertilized ovum; identical twins.

Ultrasonography High-frequency sound waves to discern fetal heart rate or placental location or body parts.

Umbilical cord (funis) Structure connecting the placenta and fetus and containing two arteries and one vein encased in a tissue called *Wharton's jelly*. The cord is ligated at birth and severed; the stump falls off in 4 to 10 days.

Umbilicus Navel, or depressed point in the middle of the abdomen that marks the attachment of the umbilical cord during fetal life.

Urachus Epithelial tube connecting the apex of the urinary bladder with the allantois. Its connective tissue forms the median umbilical ligament.

Urethra Small tubular structure that drains urine from the bladder.

Urinary frequency Need to void often or at close intervals.

Urinary meatus Opening, or mouth, of the urethra.

Uterine Referring or pertaining to the uterus.

U. adnexa See *adnexa, uterine*.

U. bruit Abnormal sound or murmur heard while auscultating the uterus.

U. ischemia Decreased blood supply to the uterus.

U. prolapse Falling, sinking, or sliding of the uterus from its normal location in the body.

U. souffle See *souffle, uterine*.

Uterus Hollow muscular organ in the female designed for the implantation, containment, and nourishment of the fetus during its development until birth.

Couvelaire u. Interstitial myometrial hemorrhage following premature separation (abruptio) of placenta. A purplish-bluish discoloration of the uterus and board-like rigidity of the uterus are noted.

Inversion of the u. See *inversion of the uterus*.

Retroflexion of the u. See *retroflexion of the uterus*.

Retroversion of the u. See *retroversion of the uterus*.

Vagina Normally collapsed musculomembranous tube that forms the passageway between the uterus and the entrance to the vagina.

Vaginismus Intense, painful spasm of the muscles surrounding the vagina.

Varices (varicose veins) Swollen, distended, and twisted veins that may develop in almost any part of the body but are most commonly seen in the legs, caused by pregnancy, obesity, congenitally defective venous valves, and occupations requiring much standing.

Vascular spiders See *telangiectasia*.

Vasectomy Ligation or removal of a segment of the vas deferens, usually done bilaterally to produce sterility in the male.

VBAC Vaginal birth after cesarean.

VDRL test Abbreviation for Venereal Disease Research Laboratory test, a serologic flocculation test for syphilis.

Velocimetry See *Doppler velocimetry*.

Vernix caseosa Protective gray-white fatty substance of cheesy consistency covering the fetal skin.

Version Act of turning the fetus in the uterus to change the presenting part and facilitate birth.

Podalic v. See *podalic version*.

Vertex Crown or top of the head.

V. presentation Presentation in which the fetal skull is nearest the cervical opening and born first.

Viable Capable of living, such as a fetus that has reached a stage of development, usually 24 weeks, which will permit it to live outside the uterus.

Villi Short, vascular processes or protrusions growing on certain membranous surfaces.

Chorionic v. Tiny vascular protrusions on the chorionic surface that project into the maternal blood sinuses of the uterus and that help to form the placenta and secrete hCG.

Voluntary abortion See *abortion, elective*.

Vulva External genitalia of the female that consist of the labia majora, labia minora, clitoris, urinary meatus, and vaginal introitus.

Wharton's jelly White, gelatinous material surrounding the umbilical vessels within the cord.

Witch's milk Secretion of a whitish fluid for about a week after birth from enlarged mammary tissue in the neonate, presumably resulting from maternal hormonal influences.

Womb See *uterus*.

X chromosomes Sex chromosome in humans existing in duplicate in the normal female and singly in the normal male.

X linkage Genes located on the X chromosome.

X-linked inheritance Characteristics transmitted by genes on the X chromosome.

Y chromosome Sex chromosome in the human male necessary for the development of the male gonads.

Zona pellucida Inner, thick, membranous envelope of the ovum.

Zygote Cell formed by the union of two reproductive cells or gametes; the fertilized ovum resulting from the union of a sperm and an ovum.

Appendices

A *NAACOG Standards for the Nursing Care of Women and Newborns*
B *NANDA-Approved Nursing Diagnoses (Through the 10th Conference, 1992)*
C *Nursing Responsibilities in Implementing Intrapartum Fetal Heart Rate Monitoring*
D *Standard Laboratory Values: Pregnant and Nonpregnant Women*
E *Human Fetotoxic Chemical Agents*
F *Standard Laboratory Values in the Neonatal Period*
G *Relationship of Drugs to Breast Milk and Effect on Infant*
H *Resources*

appendix A

NAACOG Standards for the Nursing Care of Women and Newborns

■ I: NURSING PRACTICE

Comprehensive nursing care for women and newborns focuses on helping individuals, families, and communities achieve their optimum health potential. This is best achieved within the framework of the nursing process.

The nurse is responsible for decisions and actions within the domain of nursing practice, which may include

- integration of the nursing process components of assessment, planning, implementation, and evaluation in all areas of nursing practice;
- individualization and prioritization of nursing care to meet the physical, psychological, spiritual, and social needs of patients;
- collaboration with the individual, family, and other members of the health-care team;
- promotion of a safe and therapeutic environment for both the recipients and providers of nursing care;
- demonstration and validation of competence in nursing practice;
- acquisition of specialized knowledge and skills and additional formal education to provide specialized care; and
- provision for complete and accurate documentation of care.

From NAACOG: *Standards for the nursing care of women and newborns,* ed 4, Washington, D.C., 1991, NAACOG.

The written or computerized patient record is the documented means of communication among all members of the health-care team. It also promotes continuity of care and provides a mechanism for evaluating care. The record should contain accurate and complete recordings of the patient's history and physical examination as well as the nursing plan of care, including goals, interventions, health education, and evaluation of patient and family responses. Additional documentation may include planned follow-up and appropriate referrals. All information contained in the patient record and related to the care of the patient and family is confidential and should be released only according to institutional policy.

Note: To apply this universal standard to a specific area of gynecologic, obstetric, or neonatal nursing practice, refer directly to the specialty-specific nursing practice standards section.

■ II: HEALTH EDUCATION AND COUNSELING

Health education for the individual, family, and community is an integral part of comprehensive nursing care. Such education encourages participation in, and shared responsibility for, health promotion, maintenance, and restoration.

Comprehensive health education includes

- identification of the needs and abilities of the learner;

- collaboration with the patient and other health-care providers in design, content, and follow-up of the educational plan;
- provision of accurate and current information;
- provision of information based on educationally sound principles of teaching and learning;
- recognition of patient rights, responsibilities, and alternative choices;
- utilization of available educational resources in the practice environment;
- utilization of available educational resources to provide health education information to individuals/families in the community; and
- documentation and evaluation of health education including patient response.

The nurse participates in and/or coordinates the health education and counseling process. It begins with the initial patient contact or admission to the unit or service and is an ongoing, continuous process.

Note: To apply this universal standard to a specific area of gynecologic, obstetric, or neonatal nursing practice, refer directly to the specialty-specific nursing practice standards section.

III: POLICIES, PROCEDURES, AND PROTOCOLS

Written policies, procedures, and protocols clarify the scope of nursing practice and delineate the qualifications of personnel authorized to provide care to women and newborns within the health-care setting.

The components of policies, procedures, and protocols are based on

- recognition of the organization's philosophy;
- recognition of the unit's philosophy;
- coordination with the overall mission of the organization;
- assessment of the practice setting and determination of types of services to be provided;
- incorporation of a multidisciplinary approach in their development;
- identification of specific areas of practice to be addressed;
- reflection of current practice, standards, and local regulations; and
- anticipated use as references for health-care providers, orientation of new personnel and students, quality assurance activities, and/or guiding nursing actions in emergency situations.

The development of policies, procedures, and protocols should include consideration of staff availability, skill, and licensure; the physical plant and equipment; effects on other departments; and fiscal impact. Policies, procedures, and protocols should be reviewed and revised at least on an annual basis or more frequently as science/technology changes.

Note: To apply this universal standard to a specific area of gynecologic, obstetric, or neonatal nursing practice, refer directly to the specialty-specific nursing practice standards section.

IV: PROFESSIONAL RESPONSIBILITY AND ACCOUNTABILITY

Comprehensive nursing care for women and newborns is provided by nurses who are clinically competent and accountable for professional actions and legal responsibilities inherent in the nursing role.

Responsibility and accountability for newborns include

- awareness of changing practices and professional and ethical issues;
- knowledge and clinical skills gained through in-service education, professional continuing education, research data, and professional literature;
- implementation of newly acquired knowledge and skills;
- collaboration through networking and sharing with other professionals;
- participation in the development of standards and policies, procedures, and protocols;
- participation in periodic peer and self-evaluations; and
- recognition of certification as one mechanism for the demonstration of special knowledge within a specialty area of practice.

Legal accountability extends to the

- nurse practice acts;
- parameters of professional practice established by professional organizations;
- institutional standards;
- legislative changes that affect practice; and
- policies, procedures, and protocols within the practice environment.

V: UTILIZATION OF NURSING PERSONNEL

Nursing care for women and newborns is conducted in practice settings that have qualified nursing staff in sufficient numbers to meet patient-care needs.

Each practice setting should have sufficient nursing personnel to meet patient-care requirements. Nursing staff who provide direct care to women and newborns should be supervised by registered nurses who are clinically proficient in the specialty area of practice. The patient-care unit or service is managed by a professional nurse who is prepared educationally and clinically to assume a leadership position. In all practice settings, the nurse may practice independently or collaboratively with other health-care team members. It is essential that nurses know both the responsibilities and the limitations of professional nursing practice specific to the practice setting.

Many variables are considered in determining both the number and type of nursing staff needed for a practice setting. Among these variables are those related to the patient, practice, organization, and personnel. Patient-related variables may include

- patient demographics and acuity of patients served;
- length of stay;
- educational needs;
- cultural factors and level of comprehension;
- communication barriers; and
- discharge or home-care needs.

Practice-related variables may include

- difference in educational and experiential level of nursing staff;
- nursing philosophy;
- type of nursing-care delivery system;
- use of assistive personnel;
- use of nurses in expanded roles; and
- participation in teaching programs.

Organizational variables may include

- scope of services provided;
- availability of support services;
- patient volume;
- mission or philosophy of the organization;
- risk-management concerns;
- quality assurance programs;
- policies, procedures, and protocols;
- physical plant;
- marketing strategies; and
- fiscal considerations.

Personnel variables relate to the type and number of professional and nonprofessional staff and may include

- education, skill, and experience of the nursing leadership;
- educational preparation, skill, and experience of staff;
- types and mix of nursing staff;
- availability of qualified alternative staff to deal with emergencies or unanticipated volumes;
- distribution of staff, e.g., temporary reassignment, floating, on-call, cross-training, and supplemental staffing;
- responsibilities for orientation, precepting, or students;
- turnover rates; and
- clinical and technical support.

Competency-based job descriptions should be available for each level of nursing staff. Orientation for all personnel should include a general overview of the organization and specific information about the individual practice setting. Performance evaluations for all personnel should be conducted, documented, and discussed on a regular basis with input from the individual, colleagues, and supervisory staff.

VI: ETHICS

Ethical principles guide the process of decision making for nurses caring for women and newborns at all times and especially when personal or professional values conflict with those of the patient, family, colleagues, or practice setting.

The nurse should have the opportunity to participate in the ethical decision-making process. To participate actively, nurses should

- clarify their own personal and professional values;
- recognize the difficulty in selecting a course of action that is morally and ethically acceptable to all parties;
- communicate openly and assertively;
- identify options; and
- seek consultations.

Nurses must carefully examine their own value systems, since values influence the decision-making process. Opportunities should be provided in the practice setting for discussion of potential ethical issues. Each practice setting should have a framework for decision making regarding bioethical dilemmas. Ethical dilemmas generally arise when there is a conflict between loyalties, rights, duties, or values.

For nurses, most ethical dilemmas occur when there is a real or perceived requirement to act in a manner contrary to personal values or when care ordered or provided does not seem compatible with the best interest of the patient. Common areas of concern may include

- nursing autonomy and decision making;
- maternal interests versus fetal interests;
- issues of duty, obligation, and loyalty (for example, employer to employee, professional to public, professional to professional);
- patients' rights to resources, privacy, confidentiality, information, participation in decision making, and refusal of therapy;
- the right to live or die;
- life cycle concerns, including contraception, sterilization, pregnancy termination, genetic ma-

nipulation, infanticide, sexuality and choices of life-style, and euthanasia;
- fetal or neonatal conditions incompatible with life;
- fetal tissue use; and
- biomedical intervention.

The bioethics literature can provide nurses with strategies to cope with or resolve decisions in situations when conflicts of values occur. For ethical decision-making frameworks to be applied to practice situations, working relationships must be established in which individuals may express their own points of view. All persons potentially affected by an ethical decision have the right to participate in the decision-making process.

■ VII: RESEARCH

Nurses caring for women and newborns utilize research findings, conduct nursing research, and evaluate nursing practice to improve the outcomes of care.

Knowledge of the research process and participation in scientific inquiry are necessary to

- conduct or participate in the conduct of research according to ethical guidelines;
- use research findings to provide appropriate and safe nursing care;
- use research findings as a basis for validating standards of nursing care;
- evaluate the relevance and application of research findings from nursing and related disciplines; and
- validate the effect of nursing practice on patient outcomes.

■ VIII: QUALITY ASSURANCE

Quality and appropriateness of patient care are evaluated through a planned assessment program using specific, identified clinical indicators.

Each unit or service should have a written quality assurance plan that reflects a philosophy that is coordinated with the organization's mission and overall quality assurance program. Objectives of the unit-based or service-based quality assurance plan should include

- assurance of consistent quality patient outcomes;
- identification and correction of potential nursing practice deficiencies;
- promotion of professional nursing practice based on appropriate nursing standards; and
- education and participation of staff in quality assurance activities.

The unit nurse manager is responsible for developing and implementing the unit-based quality assurance plan. The plan should include

- responsibilities of all personnel in the quality assurance process;
- the scope of service provided;
- important aspects of care or service involving high-risk, high-volume, and problem-prone patients or activities;
- clinical indicators or measurable standards that affect the aspects of care and service that have been identified as important;
- specific criteria and thresholds for use in monitoring clinical indicators;
- methods for the collection and analysis of data, including reference to collection tools, sample size, time frame, and staff responsibility;
- determination of appropriate corrective action, when indicated, that will fall into one of three categories; educational, organizational, or behavioral change;
- follow-up assessment of identified problems;
- documentation of all aspects of the quality assurance program, including results; and
- a process for communication related to quality assurance activities within the total organization.

appendix B

NANDA-Approved Nursing Diagnoses

Activity intolerance
Activity intolerance, high risk for
Adjustment, impaired
Airway clearance, ineffective
Anxiety
Aspiration, high risk for
Body image disturbance
Body temperature, altered, high risk for
Bowel incontinence
Breast-feeding, effective
Breast-feeding, ineffective
Breast-feeding, interrupted
Breathing pattern, ineffective
Cardiac output, decreased
Caregiver role strain
Caregiver role strain, high risk for
Communication, impaired verbal
Constipation
Constipation, colonic
Constipation, perceived
Coping, defensive
Coping, family, potential for growth
Coping, ineffective family, compromised
Coping, ineffective family, disabling
Coping, ineffective individual
Decisional conflict (specify)
Denial, ineffective
Diarrhea
Disuse syndrome, high risk for
Diversional activity deficit
Dysfunctional ventilatory weaning response (DVWR)
Dysreflexia
Family processes, altered
Fatigue
Fear
Fluid volume deficit (1)
Fluid volume deficit (2)
Fluid volume deficit, high risk for
Fluid volume excess
Gas exchange, impaired
Grieving, anticipatory
Grieving, dysfunctional
Growth and development, altered
Health maintenance, altered
Health-seeking behaviors (specify)
Home maintenance management, impaired
Hopelessness
Hyperthermia
Hypothermia
Incontinence, functional
Incontinence, reflex
Incontinence, stress
Incontinence, total
Incontinence, urge
Infant feeding pattern, ineffective
Infection, high risk for
Injury, high risk for
Knowledge deficit (specify)
Mobility, impaired physical
Noncompliance (specify)
Nutrition, altered, less than body requirements
Nutrition, altered, more than body requirements
Nutrition, altered, high risk for more than body requirements
Oral mucous membrane, altered
Pain
Pain, chronic
Parental role conflict
Parenting, altered
Parenting, altered, high risk for
Peripheral neurovascular dysfunction, high risk for
Personal identity disturbance
Poisoning, high risk for
Post-trauma response
Powerlessness
Protection, altered
Rape-trauma syndrome
Rape-trauma syndrome, compound reaction
Rape-trauma syndrome, silent reaction
Role performance, altered
Self-care deficit, bathing/hygiene
Self-care deficit, dressing/grooming
Self-care deficit, feeding
Self-care deficit, toileting
Self-esteem disturbance
Self-esteem, chronic low
Self-esteem, situational low
Self-mutilation, high risk for
Sensory/perceptual alterations (specify) (visual, auditory, kinesthetic, gustatory, tactile, olfactory)
Sexual dysfunction
Sexuality patterns, altered
Skin integrity, impaired
Skin integrity, impaired, high risk for
Sleep pattern disturbance
Social interaction, impaired
Social isolation
Spiritual distress (distress of the human spirit)
Stress syndrome, relocation
Suffocation, high risk for
Swallowing, impaired
Therapeutic regimen (individual), ineffective management of
Thermoregulation, ineffective
Thought processes, altered
Tissue integrity, impaired
Tissue perfusion, altered (specific type) (renal, cerebral, cardiopulmonary, gastrointestinal, peripheral)
Trauma, high risk for
Unilateral neglect
Urinary elimination, altered patterns
Urinary retention
Ventilation, inability to sustain spontaneous
Violence, high risk for, self-directed or directed at others

(Through the 10th Conference, 1992)

appendix C

Nursing Responsibilities in Implementing Intrapartum Fetal Heart Rate Monitoring

With the publication of the new position on fetal heart rate monitoring from The American College of Obstetricians and Gynecologists (ACOG), as reflected in the 1988 *Guidelines for Perinatal Care,*[1] NAACOG finds it necessary to clarify the nursing responsibilities in implementing intrapartum fetal heart rate monitoring.

The primary goal of perinatal care is to ensure optimal maternal and neonatal outcomes. The intrapartum period represents a time of risk for the parturient and the fetus. An assessment of fetal heart rate (FHR) has long been recognized as a vital aspect of evaluating fetal well-being during the stresses of labor and birth. Two techniques of fetal heart rate assessment are auscultation and electronic fetal heart monitoring. Each method has its advantages and limitations necessitating individualized decision-making for appropriate use. The method of fetal heart rate monitoring selected and the frequency of FHR evaluation should be based on consideration of maternal-fetal risk factors and the availability of nursing personnel skilled in the monitoring techniques. The client's preference should be carefully considered.

Nurses who perform fetal heart rate monitoring are responsible for their actions and will be held to the established standards of care as defined by their professional organizations, the standards of practice in their institutions, and the laws governing practice in their states.

METHODOLOGY

AUSCULTATION. Auscultation of the fetal heart rate is an auditory assessment procedure that, when properly performed, allows the evaluation of the FHR both during and immediately following the stress of a uterine contraction. Further, auscultation between contractions establishes the baseline FHR. Auscultation as a primary technique of fetal heart rate surveillance requires a thorough knowledge of the basic principles of fetal heart and uterine physiology and pathophysiology. Clinical experience in recognizing and responding to significant FHR changes is required. The validation of competency in using this technique must be in accordance with established institutional policy.

Recently ACOG indicated that auscultation of the fetal heart at 15-minute intervals during the active phase of the first stage of labor and at 5-minute intervals during the second stage is equivalent to electronic fetal monitoring (EFM) when risk factors are present during labor or when intensified monitoring is elected. For low-risk clients, the suggested auscultation frequency remains unchanged at 30 minutes in active first stage labor and 15 minutes in second stage labor. Therefore, for the high-risk client, and for the low-risk client in the second stage of labor, if auscultation is prescribed as the primary technique of fetal heart rate surveillance, a minimum of a 1:1 nurse-fetus ratio is required.

ELECTRONIC FETAL MONITORING. EFM is an auditory and visual assessment procedure that provides continuous data for evaluating uterine activity and fetal heart responses, including baseline heart rate, variability, and fetal heart rate change over time. Further, EFM produces a continuous printed record. The use of EFM requires knowledge of its equipment and thorough knowledge of the basic principles of fetal heart and uterine physiology and pathophysiology. Nurses who use EFM must be able to recognize fetal heart rate patterns, beat-to-beat variability, and uterine activity. Fetal monitoring patterns have been given descriptive names (e.g., accelerations and early, late, or variable decelerations). Nurses should use these terms in written chart documentation and verbal communication. When a change in fetal heart rate patterns is noted, the nurse should also document a subsequent return to normal patterns.

The client medical record should include observations and assessments of fetal heart rate and characteristics of uterine activity as well as specific actions taken when changes in fetal heart rate patterns are observed. The monitor tracing is a legal part of the medical record and should include identifying information about the client as well as times and events related to the client's ongoing care.

After identifying a nonreassuring pattern, the nurse is responsible for initiating appropriate nursing interventions, as indicated by the pattern identified, and for notifying a physician. Once the physician is notified of a nonreassuring pattern, the nurse can expect the physician to respond. An institutional policy should be established for the nurse to follow in the event the physician is unable to respond in a timely fashion.

Core competencies in fetal heart rate monitoring have been published by NAACOG.[2] Competency validation of this expertise must be in accordance with established institutional policy.[3] Standards for staffing when EFM is the primary method of monitoring are found in the NAACOG OGN Nursing Practice Resource *Considerations for Nurse Professional Staffing in Perinatal Units* and in AAP/ACOG *Guidelines for Perinatal Care*.[1,4]

EVALUATION AND DOCUMENTATION. The institution should establish policies and procedures that define evaluation and documentation of fetal heart rate monitoring. In developing policies and procedures, the institution should address the following:

- Method(s) for assessment (EFM, auscultation, or a combination of both)
- Maternal-fetal risk factors
- Stage of labor
- Frequency of assessment
- Qualifications of health-care providers performing assessments
- Nurse-fetus ratios
- Methods of documentation

Documenting the evaluation of FHR monitoring information during labor is applicable regardless of the method of monitoring selected and may be accomplished in narrative nurses' notes and/or by using comprehensive flow sheets at the time of assessment. Documentation may also be achieved by using abbreviated nurses' notes with follow-up summary nurses' notes at intervals specified by institutional policy. The format for abbreviated notes may include initialing the EFM tracing, annotating the EFM tracing, or annotating basic flow sheets.

Suggested frequencies for interval evaluation of FHR information have been addressed in the recent ACOG position. For the high-risk clients being monitored with auscultation during the active phase of the first stage and during the second stage of labor, suggested intervals for both evaluating and recording FHR information are at 15 and 5 minutes, respectively. For the same group of clients being monitored electronically, evaluation of the tracing is suggested at the same intervals.

For low-risk clients being monitored with auscultation, the suggested intervals for evaluating and recording remain unchanged at 30 and 15 minutes in the first and second stages of labor, respectively. An interval frequency for evaluation of the tracing for this same group of clients being monitored electronically was not suggested.

Evaluation of FHR information may take place at the intervals suggested above or more frequently as necessitated by the individual client care situation. Written documentation of these FHR evaluations, however, may occur at longer intervals in narrative, abbreviated, and/or summary formats in accordance with institutional policy and procedure.

CONFLICT RESOLUTION. The potential for conflict exists in terms of professional judgment and decision making regarding which method of monitoring is best for a particular client in a given situation. Institutional policies and procedures must provide a mechanism that will allow nurses the flexibility to decline to implement the prescribed method of fetal heart rate monitoring if any question exists regarding the ability to meet the required staffing ratios or if the methodology is beyond the individual nurse's expertise. Ultimately, the responsibility for implementing the prescribed method of fetal heart rate monitoring remains with the prescriber. In the event of differences of opinion among professionals regarding the ability to implement the prescribed method, the established institutional policy for the resolution of the conflict should be followed.

REFERENCES

[1]American Academy of Pediatrics and The American College of Obstetricians and Gynecologists: *Guidelines for perinatal care*, ed 2, Washington, DC, 1988.

[2]NAACOG: *Electronic fetal monitoring: nursing practice competencies and educational guidelines*, Washington, DC, 1986.

[3]NAACOG: *Competency validation: Resource book from Essentials of electronic fetal monitoring*, (videotape), Washington, DC, 1988, NAACOG.

[4]NAACOG: OGN Nursing Practice Resource. *Considerations for professional nurse staffing in perinatal units*, Washington, DC, 1988, NAACOG.

This statement replaces the Joint ACOG/NAACOG Statement on Electronic Fetal Monitoring published in January 1986 by NAACOG.

appendix D

Standard Laboratory Values: Pregnant and Nonpregnant Women

	Nonpregnant	Pregnant
HEMATOLOGIC VALUES		
Complete Blood Count (CBC)		
Hemoglobin, g/dL	12-16*	10-14*
Hematocrit, PCV, %	37-47	32-42
Red cell volume, mL	1600	1900
Plasma volume, mL	2400	3700
Red blood cell count, million/mm^3	4-5.5	4-5.5
White blood cells, total per mm^3	4500-10,000	5000-15,000
Polymorphonuclear cells, %	54-62	60-85
Lymphocytes, %	38-46	15-40
Erythrocyte sedimentation rate, mm/h	≤	30-90
MCHC, g/dL packed RBCs (mean corpuscular hemoglobin concentration)	30-36	No change
MCH/(mean corpuscular hemoglobin per picogram [less than a nanogram])	29-32	No change
MCV/μm^3 (mean corpuscular volume per cubic micrometer)	82-96	No change
Blood coagulation and fibrinolytic activity†		
Factors VII, VIII, IX, X		Increase in pregnancy, return to normal in early puerperium; factor VIII increases during and immediately after birth
Factors XI, XIII		Decrease in pregnancy
Prothrombin time (PT)	12-14 sec	Slight decrease in pregnancy
Partial thromboplastin time (PTT)	60-70 sec	Slight decrease in pregnancy and again decrease during second and third stage of labor (indicates clotting at placental site)
Bleeding time	1-3 min (Duke) 2-4 min (Ivy)	No appreciable change
Coagulation time	6-10 min (Lee/White)	No appreciable change

*At sea level. Permanent residents of higher levels (e.g., Denver) require higher levels of hemoglobin.
†Pregnancy represents a hypercoagulable state.

	Nonpregnant	Pregnant
Platelets	150,000 to 350,000/mm^3	No significant change until 3 to 5 days after birth, then marked increase (may predispose woman to thrombosis) and gradual return to normal
Fibrinolytic activity		Decreases in pregnancy, then abrupt return to normal (protection against thromboembolism)
Fibrinogen	250 mg/dL	400 mg/dL
Mineral/vitamin concentrations		
Vitamin B_{12}, folic acid, ascorbic acid	Normal	Moderate decrease
Serum proteins		
Total, g/dL	6.7-8.3	5.5-7.5
Albumin, g/dL	3.5-5.5	3.0-5.0
Globulin, total, g/dL	2.3-3.5	3.0-4.0
Blood sugar		
Fasting, mg/dL	70-80	65
2-hour postprandial, mg/dL	60-110	Under 140 after a 100 g carbohydrate meal is considered normal
CARDIOVASCULAR DETERMINATIONS		
Blood pressure, mm Hg	120/80*	114/65 during midtrimester, then return to usual value by end of third trimester
Pulse, rate/min	70	80
Stroke volume, mL	65	75
Cardiac output, L/min	4.5	6
Circulation time (arm-tongue), sec	15-16	12-14
Blood volume, mL		
Whole blood	4000	5600
Plasma	2400	3700
Red blood cells	1600	1900
Chest x-ray studies		
Transverse diameter of heart	—	1-2 cm increase
Left border of heart	—	Straightened
Cardiac volume	—	70 mL increase
HEPATIC VALUES		
Bilirubin total	Not more than 1 mg/dL	Unchanged
Serum cholesterol	110-300 mg/dL	↑ 60% from 16-32 weeks of pregnancy; remains at this level until after birth
Serum alkaline phosphatase	2-4.5 units (Bodansky)	↑ from week 12 of pregnancy to 6 weeks after birth
Serum globulin albumin	1.5-3.0 g/dL 4.5-5.3 g/dL	↑ slight ↓ 3.0 g by late pregnancy
RENAL VALUES		
Bladder capacity	1300 mL	1500 mL
Renal plasma flow (RPF), mL/min	490-700	Increase by 25%, to 612-875
Glomerular filtration rate (GFR), mL/min	105-132	Increase by 50%, to 160-198
Nonprotein nitrogen (NPN), mg/dL	25-40	Decreases
Blood urea nitrogen (BUN), mg/dL	20-25	Decreases
Serum creatinine, mg/kg/24 hr	20-22	Decreases
Serum uric acid, mg/kg/24 hr	257-750	Decreases
Urine glucose	Negative	Present in 20% of pregnant women
Intravenous pyelogram (IVP)	Normal	Slight-to-moderate hydroureter and hydronephrosis; right kidney larger than left kidney

*For the woman about 20 years of age; 10 years of age: 103/70; 30 years of age: 123/82; 40 years of age: 126/84.

appendix E

Human Fetotoxic Chemical Agents

Maternal Medication	Reported Effects on Fetus or Neonate
ANALGESICS	
Indomethacin (Indocin)	Prolongs gestation (monkey); in neonates, used to close patent ductus arteriosus
Narcotics	70% of maternal level; death, apnea, depression, bradycardia, hypothermia
Salicylates	Death in utero; hemorrhage, methomoglobinemia, ↓ albumin-binding capacity, salicylate intoxication, difficult birth, (?) prolonged gestation
ANESTHESIAS	
Conduction	Indirect effect of maternal hypotension; direct effect—convulsions, death, acidosis, bradycardia, myocardial depression, fetal hypotension, methemoglobinemia
Paracervical	Methemoglobinemia, fetal acidosis, bradycardia, neurologic depression, myocardial depression
ANTICOAGULANTS	
Coumarins	Fetal death, hemorrhage, calcifications
ANTICONVULSANT AGENTS	
Barbiturates	Irritability and tremulousness 4 to 5 months after birth, hemorrhage, enzyme inducer
Phenytoin and barbiturate	Congenital malformations, cleft lip and palate, congenital heart disease (CHD), CNS and skeletal anomalies, failure to thrive, enzyme inducer, hemorrhage
ANTIMICROBIALS	All antimicrobials cross placenta
Ampicillin	↓ Maternal urinary and plasma estriol levels
Chloramphenicol	Crosses placenta with no reported effect; interferes with biotransformation of tolbutamide, phenytoin, biohydroxycoumarin (i.e., hypoglycemia may occur if used in combination)
Chloroquine	Death, deafness, retinal hemorrhage
Erythromycin	Possible hepatic injury
Nitrofurantoin	Megaloblastic anemia, G6PD deficiency
Novobiocin	Hyperbilirubinemia
Streptomycin	Therapeutic levels reached, nerve deafness
Sulfonamides	Icterus, hemolytic anemia, kernicterus, growth retardation (?), thrombocytopenia

Modified from Babson SG et al: *Diagnosis and management of the fetus and neonate at risk: a guide for team care,* ed 4, St Louis, 1980, Mosby–Year Book.

Maternal Medication	Reported Effects on Fetus or Neonate
Tetracycline	Placental transfer after 4 months' gestation; enamel hypoplasia, delay in bone growth, congenital cataract (?)
ANTITUBERCULOSIS	
Isoniazid	Toxic blood level in fetus; no reported effect; mother should be on pyridoxine supplement
Pyridoxine	*See* vitamins
CANCER CHEMOTHERAPEUTIC AGENTS	
Aminopterin 6-Mercaptopurine Methotrexate	Abortion, congenital anomalies (first trimester); combination of drugs detrimental to fetus; skeletal and cranial malformations, hydrocephalus; questionable long-term effects such as slow somatic growth; ovarian agenesis; ↓ immune mechanisms
CARDIOVASCULAR AGENTS	
Digitoxin	Placental transfer, no reported effect
Propranolol	Indirect effect of delay in cervical dilatation
CHOLINESTERASE INHIBITORS	Myasthenia-like symptoms for 1 week; muscle weakness in 10% to 20% of infants
Cigarette smoking	Effect equal to number of cigarettes smoked; ↑ incidence of stillbirth; low birth weight; effect on later somatic growth and mental development (?); reduction in O_2 transport to fetus
DIURETICS	
Ammonium chloride Thiazide	Maternal and fetal acidosis; thrombocytopenia, hemorrhage, hypoelectrolyemia, convulsions, respiratory distress, death, hemolysis
DRUGS OF ABUSE (usually multiple drugs consumed)	
Alcohol	Blood level equal to mother's; convulsions, withdrawal syndrome, hyperactivity, crying, irritability, poor sucking reflex, low birth weight; cleft palate, ophthalmic malformation, malformation of extremities and heart; poor mental performance, microencephaly, small for dates, growth deficiency
Barbiturates	Withdrawal symptoms, convulsions, onset immediately after delivery or at 2 weeks of age
Cocaine	Abruptio placentae, preterm labor
"Ice"—methamphetamine	Preterm labor, IUGR, abnormal sleep patterns, poor feeding, tremors, hypertonia.
LSD (lysergic acid diethylamide)	Chromosome breakage, limb and skeletal anomalies
Narcotics Heroin Methadone	Small for dates, 4% to 10% mortality, habituation, withdrawal symptoms, convulsions, sudden infant death syndrome (SIDS), indirect effect of maternal complications (i.e., infection, hepatitis, STD), permanent effect on somatic growth (?)
HORMONES	
Androgens Estrogens Progestins	Labioscrotal fusion before week 12; after 12 weeks, phallic enlargement; other anomalies (?); ↑ bilirubin (?), vaginal cancer; cleft lip and palate, CHD; tracheoesophageal fistula and atresia; cancer of prostate, testes, and bladder
Corticosteroids	Adrenal insufficiency, cleft palate, small-for-dates infant
Ovulatory agents	Anencephaly (?), chromosomal abnormalities in abortus (?), multiple pregnancy
PSYCHOTROPIC DRUGS	
Diazepam (Valium)	High fetal levels; hypotonia, poor sucking reflex, hypothermia; ↑ low Apgar score; ↑ resuscitation, ↑ assisted deliveries; dose related
Lithium carbonate	Neonatal serum levels reach adult toxic range; lethargy, cyanosis for 10 days; teratogenic—dose related
RADIATION	Microencephaly, mental retardation, many unknown effects; nondisjunction of chromosomes

Maternal Medication	Reported Effects on Fetus or Neonate
SEDATIVES	
Barbiturate	Apnea, depression, depressed EEG, poor sucking reflex, slow weight gain; concentration of drug in brain; enzyme inducer, lower bilirubin level
Bromides	Growth failure, lethargy, dilated pupils, dermatitis, hypotonia, ? effect on mental development
Magnesium sulfate	Neonatal blood level does not correlate with clinical condition; respiratory depression, hypotonia, convulsions, death; exchange transfusion may be required
Paraldehyde	Apnea, depression
Thalidomide	Administered between days 34 and 50 of gestation causes phocomelia, malformation of cord, angiomas of face, CHD, intestinal stenosis, eye defects, absence of appendix
TOXINS	
Carbon monoxide	Stillbirth, brain damage equal to anoxia
Heavy metals	
Arsenic	Concentrated in brain
Lead	Abortion, growth retardation, congenital anomalies, sterility
Mercury	Cerebral palsy, mental retardation, convulsions, involuntary movements, defective vision; mother asymptomatic
Naphthalene	Hemolysis
VITAMINS	
A and D	Congenital anomalies
K (water-soluble analogs)	Icterus, anemia, kernicterus
Pyridoxine	Withdrawal seizures

appendix *F*

Standard Laboratory Values in the Neonatal Period

1. HEMATOLOGIC VALUES		Neonatal	
Clotting factors			
Activated clotting time (ACT)		2 min	
Bleeding time (Ivy)		1-8 min	
Clot retraction		Complete 1-4 hr	
Fibrinogen		150-300 mg/dL*	
	Term		Preterm
Hemoglobin (g/dL)	17-19		15-17
Hematocrit (%)	57-58		45-55
Reticulocytes (%)	3-7		Up to 10
Fetal hemoglobin (% of total)	40-70		80-90
Nucleated RBC/mm^3 (per 100 RBC)	200(0.05)		(0.2)
Platelet count/mm^3	100,000-300,000		120,000-180,000
WBC/mm^3	15,000		10,000-20,000
Neutrophils (%)	45		47
Eosinophils and basophils (%)	3		
Lymphocytes (%)	30		33
Monocytes (%)	5		4
Immature WBC (%)	10		16

2. BIOCHEMICAL VALUES		Neonatal
Bilirubin, direct		0-1 mg/dL
Bilirubin, total	Cord:	<2 mg/dL
	Peripheral blood: 0-1 day	6 mg/dL
	1-2 day	8 mg/dL
	3-5 day	12 mg/dL
Blood gases	Arterial:	pH 7.31-7.45
		Pco_2 33-48 mm Hg
		Po_2 50-70 mm Hg
	Venous:	pH 7.28-7.42
		Pco_2 38-52 mm Hg
		Po_2 20-49 mm Hg
α_1-fetoprotein		0
Fibrinogen		150-300 mg/dL

3. URINALYSIS

Volume: 20-40 mL excreted daily in the first few days; by 1 week, 24-hr urine volume close to 200 mL
Protein: may be present in first 2-4 days
Casts and WBCs: may be present in first 2-4 days
Osmolarity (mOsm/L); 100-600

*dL refers to deciliter (1 dL = 100 mL); this conforms to the SI system: international measurements that have been standardized.

Urinalysis	Normal Ranges	
	Adult	Newborn
Color	Clear, amber	Clear, straw
Specific gravity	1.001-1.040	1.001=1.018
pH	4.5-8	5-7
Protein	Negative	Negative
Glucose	Negative	Negative
Ketones	Negative	Negative
RBC	1-2	Rare
WBC	3-4	0-4
Casts	Occasional	Rare
17-Ketosteroids	Male 8-25 Female 5-15	Under 1
17-Hydroxycorticosteroids	3.1-10.0	Same
Urinary calcium	50=300 mg/dL depending on dietary intake	5 mg/kg body weight
Urinary sodium	40-220 mEq/24 hr.	20% of adult values
Urinary vanillymandelic acid (VMA)	1.5-7.5 mg/24 hr.	1.40-15.0

4. CARDIORESPIRATORY DETERMINATIONS

Blood pressure at birth
- Term: systolic, 78 mm Hg; diastolic, 42 mm Hg
- Preterm: Systolic, 50-60 mm Hg; diastolic 30 mm Hg

Respiratory rate: 30-60 min

Heart rate, fetus
- Baseline: 120-160/min
  - Tachycardia: >160 bpm (with maternal complications)
  - Bradycardia: <120 bpm (with maternal hypotension and hypoxia)
  - Acceleration: tachycardia >160 bpm with uterine contractions—normal (usually)
- Beat-to-beat variability: disappears with fetal distress
- With uterine contraction
  - Early deceleration: bradycardia with onset of contraction—benign
  - Variable deceleration: bradycardia due to cord compression—usually benign
  - Late deceleration: bradycardia after lag period due to fetal hypoxia—ominous sign

Heart rate, term infant: 140 ± 20 bpm

5. URINE SCREENING TESTS FOR INBORN ERRORS OF METABOLISM

Benedict's test: for reducing substances in the urine—glucose, galactose, fructose, lactose; phenylketonuria, alkaptonuria, tyrosyluria, and tryosinosis may give a positive Benedict's test result.

Ferric chloride test: an immediate, green color for phenylketonuria, histidinemia, and tyrosinuria, a gray to green color for presence of phenothiazines, isoniazid, red to purple color for presence of salicylates or ketone bodies.

Dinitrophenylhydrazine test: for phenylketonuria, maple syrup urine disease, Lowe's syndrome.

Cetyltrimethyl ammonium bromide test: for mucopolysaccharides: immediate positive reaction in gargoylism (Hurler's syndrome); delayed, moderately positive reaction for Marfan's, Morquio-Ullrich, and Murdoch syndromes.

Metachromatic stain (or *urine sediment*): Granules (free or as inclusion bodies in cells) are seen in metachromatic leukodystrophy; may also be seen rarely in Tay-Sachs and other lipid diseases of the central nervous system.

Amino acid chromatography: Aminoaciduria may be normal in newborns; chromatography may be helpful to detect hypophosphatasia and argininosuccinicaciduria.

Diaper test, Phenistix test, and *Dinitrophenyl-hydrazine (DNPH) test:* simple, inexpensive tests for PKU (phenylketonuria): used for screening; most useful when infant is at least 6 weeks of age.

6. BLOOD SERUM PHENYLALANINE TESTS

Guthrie inhibition assay methods: drops of blood placed on filter paper; laboratory uses bacterial growth inhibition test; phenylalanine level above 8 mg/dL blood: diagnostic of PKU. Effective in newborn period; used also to monitor PKU diet; blood easily obtained by heel or finger puncture; inexpensive; used for wide-scale screening appendix G

Relationship of Drugs to Breast Milk and Effect on Infant

Drug	Excreted in Milk	Amount in Milk After Therapeutic Dose	Effect on Infant
ANALGESICS AND ANTIINFLAMMATORY DRUGS (NONNARCOTIC)			
Acetaminophen (Datril, Tylenol)	Yes		Detoxified in liver. Avoid in immediate postbirth period; otherwise no problems with therapeutic dose.
Aspirin	Yes	1-3 mg/dL*	Long history of experience shows complications rare. Can cause interference with platelet aggregation and diminished factor XII (Hageman factor) at birth. When mother requires high, continuing level of medication for arthritis, aspirin is drug of choice. Observe infant for bruisability. Platelet aggregation can be evaluated. Salicylism only seen in maternal overdosing. Mother should increase vitamin C and vitamin K intake.
Indomethacin (Indocin)	Yes		Convulsions in breast-fed neonate (case report). Used to close patent ductus arteriosus. Insufficient data as to effect on other vessels. May be nephrotoxic.
Mefenamic acid (Ponstel)	Yes	Trace amounts†	No apparent effect on infant at therapeutic doses; infant able to excrete via urine.
Naproxen (Naproxyn, synaxyns, naprosine, naxen, proxen)	Yes	1% of maternal plasma; binds to plasma protein	Less toxic in adults than some other organic derivatives.
Propoxyphene (Darvon)	Yes	0.4% of maternal‡ dose	Only symptoms detectable would be failure to feed and drowsiness. On daily, around-the-clock dosage, infant could consume 1 mg/day.

Modified from Lawrence RA: *Breastfeeding: a guide for the medical profession,* ed 3, St Louis, 1989, Mosby—Year Book.

*Plasma level was 1-5 mg/dL.

†0.91 μg/mL mean maternal plasma level showed 0.21 μg/mL mean milk level. Mean infant plasma level was 0.08 μg/mL and mean urine level, 9.8 μg/mL.

‡Shown by animal experiments. Milk plasma ratio (M/P) = ½.

Drug	Excreted in Milk	Amount in Milk After Therapeutic Dose	Effect on Infant
ANTIBIOTICS			
Ampicillin (Polycillin, Amcill, Omnipen, Penbritin)	Yes	0.07 μg/mL	Sensitivity resulting from repeated exposure; diarrhea or secondary candidiasis.
Carbenicillin (Pyopen, Geopen)	Yes	0.265 μg/mL 1 hr after 1 g given	Levels not significant. Drug is given to neonate.
Cefazolin (Ancef, Kefzol)	Yes	1.5 μg/mL (0.075% of dose)	Probably not significant.
Cephalexin (Keflex)	No		
Cephalothin (Keflin)	No		
Chloramphenicol (Chloromycetin)	Yes	Half blood level; 2.5 mg/dL	Gray syndrome. Infant does not excrete drug well, and small amounts may accumulate. Contraindicated. May be tolerated in older infant with mature glycuronide system.
Colistin (Colymycin)	Yes	0.05-0.09 mg/dL	Not absorbed orally.
Demeclocycline (Declomycin)	Yes	0.2-0.3 mg/dL	Not significant in therapeutic doses. Can be given to infants.
Erythromycin (Ilosone, E-Mycin, Erythrocin)	Yes	0.05-0.1 mg/dL; 3.5-6.2 μg/mL	Higher concentrations have been reported in milk than in plasma. Should not be given under 1 month of age because of risk of jaundice. Dose in milk higher when given IV to mother.
Gentamicin	Unknown		Not absorbed from gastrointestinal tract, may change gut flora. Drug is given to newborns directly.
Isoniazid (Nydrazid)	Yes	0.6-1.2 mg/dL*	Infant at risk for toxicity, but need for breast milk may outweigh risk.
Kanamycin (Kantrex)	Yes	18.4 μg/mL after 1 g given IM	Infant absorbs little from gastrointestinal tract. Infants can be given drug.
Lincomycin (Lincocin)	Yes	0.5-2.4 mg/dL	Not significant in thrapeutic doses to affect child.
Mandelic acid	Yes	0.3 g/24 hr after dose of 12 g/day	Not significant in therapeutic doses to affect child.
Methacycline (Rondomycin)	Yes	½ plasma level; 50-260 μg/dL	Same precautions as with tetracycline.
Metronidazole (Flagyl)	Yes	Level comparable to serums†	Caution should be exercised because of its high milk concentrations. Contraindicated when infant under 6 months; may cause neurologic disorders and blood dyscrasia.
Nitrofurantoin (Furadantin)	Yes	Trace to 0.5 μg/mL	Not significant in therapeutic doses to affect child except in G6PD deficiency.
Novobiocin (Albamycin, Cathomycin)	Yes	0.36-0.54 mg/dL	Infant can be given drug directly.
Nystatin (Mycostatin)	No	Not absorbed orally	Can be given to infant directly.
Oxacillin (Prostaphlin)	No		
Para-aminosalicylic acid	No		
Penicillin G, benzathine (Bicillin)	Yes	10-12 units/dL	Clinical need should supersede possible allergic responses.
Penicillin G, potassium	Yes	Up to 6 units/dL; 1.2-3.6 μg/dL	Infant can be given penicillin directly. Parents should be told to inform physician that infant has been exposed to penicillin because of potential sensitivity.
Streptomycin	Yes	Present for long periods in slight amounts when given as dihydrostreptomycin	Not to be given more than 2 weeks. Ototoxic and nephrotoxic with long use. Is given to infants directly.

*Same concentration in milk as in maternal serum.
†Gives serum levels in infants of 0.05 to 0.4 μg/mL.

Drug	Excreted in Milk	Amount in Milk After Therapeutic Dose	Effect on Infant
Sulfisoxazole (Gantrisin)	Yes	Concentration similar to plasma level	To be avoided during first month after birth; may cause kernicterus.
Tetracycline HC1 (Achromycin, Panmycin, Sumycin)	Yes	0.5-2.6 μg/mL after dose of 500 mg four times a day	Not enough to treat an infection in an infant. May cause discoloration of the teeth in the infant; the antibiotic, however, may be largely bound to the milk calcium. Do not give longer than 10 days or repeatedly.
ANTICOAGULANTS			
Coumarin derivatives Dicumarol (bishydroxycoumarin) Warfarin (Panwarfin)	Yes	Probably little but may be cumulative*	Monitor prothrombin time. Give vitamin K to infant. Discontinue if surgery or trauma occurs. Drug of choice if mother to continue breast-feeding.
Heparin	No		Heparin ineffective orally.
ANTICONVULSANTS AND SEDATIVES†			
Barbital (Veronal)	Yes	8-10 mg/L after 500 mg dose	May produce sedation in infant, in general, barbiturates pass into milk but do not sedate infant. Watch for symptoms.
Phenytoin (Dilantin)	Yes	1.5 to 2.6 μg/mL after 300 mg/24 hr dose	One case of hemolytic reaction reported. Other infants appear to tolerate the small doses. Therapeutic plasma level 10-20 μg/mL.
Pentobarbital (Nembutal)	Yes		Depends on liver for detoxification so may accumulate in first week of life until infant is able to detoxify. No problem for older infant in usual doses.
Phenobarbital (Luminal)	Yes	0.1-0.5 mg when plasma level 0.6-1.8 mg	Sleepiness and decreased sucking possible. On usual analeptic doses infants alert and feed well. On hypnotic doses infants depressed and difficult to rouse.
Sodium bromide (Bromo-Seltzer and across-the-counter sleeping aids)	Yes	Up to 6.6 mg/dL	Drowsy, decreased crying, rash, decreased feeding.
ANTIHISTAMINICS Brompheniramine (Dimetane) Diphenhydramine (Benadryl)	Yes	No specific data available; all pass into milk	Drug is used in neonates. May cause sedation, decreased feeding, or may produce stimulation and tachycardia. Should avoid long-acting preparations, which may accumulate in infant. When combined with decongestants, may cause decrease in milk.
AUTONOMIC DRUGS			
Atropine sulfate‡	Yes	0.1 mg/dL	Hyperthermia, atropine toxicity, infants especially sensitive; also inhibits lactation. Infant dose 0.01 mg/kg.
Ergot (Cafergot)	Yes	Unknown	90% of infants had symptoms of ergotism: vomiting and diarrhea to weak pulse and unstable blood pressure. Short-term therapy for migraine should not exceed 6 mg. Cafergot also contains 100 mg caffeine.

*Reports conflict.
†All barbitals appear in breast milk.
‡Ingredient in many prescription and nonprescription drugs.

Drug	Excreted in Milk	Amount in Milk After Therapeutic Dose	Effect on Infant
Neostigmine	No		No known harm to infant.
Propranatheline bromide (Pro-Banthine)	No	Uncontrolled data indicate no measurable levels	Drug rapidly metabolized in maternal system to inactive metabolite. Mother should avoid long-acting preparations, however.
Scopolamine (Hyoscine)	Yes		Usually given as single dose and of no problem to neonate. No data on repeated doses.
CARDIOVASCULAR DRUGS			
Diazoxide (Hyperstat)			Arteriolar dilators and antihypertensive, only given IV, not active orally.
Digoxin	Yes	0.96-0.61 ng/mL*	Dixogin 20% bound to protein; infant receives <1/100 of dose. If mother at toxic level of 5 ng/mL, milk would have a 4.4 ng/mL and infant would receive only 1/20 daily dose.
Hydralazine (Apresoline)	Yes		Jaundice, thrombocytopenia, electrolyte disturbances possible.
Methyldopa (Aldomet)†	Yes		Galactorrhea. No specific data except as affects mother's milk production.
Propranolol (Inderal)‡	Yes	40 ng/mL of maternal plasma§	Insignificant amount. Infants reported had no symptoms noted. Should watch for hypoglycemia and/or "β-blocking" effects.
Quinidine	Yes		Arrhythmia may occur.
Reserpine (Serpasil)‖	Yes		May produce galactorrhea, lethargy, diarrhea, or nasal stuffiness.
CATHARTICS			
Cascara	Yes	Low	Caused colic and diarrhea in infant.
Milk of magnesia	No	None	No effect.
Mineral oil	No	None	No effect.
Phenolphthalein	Unknown	Unknown¶	Reported to cause symptoms in some.
Rhubarb	Unknown	None	None in syrup form. Fresh rhubarb may give symptoms of colic and diarrhea.
Saline cathartics	No	None	No effect.
Senna	No	None	None.
Stool softeners and bulk-forming laxatives	No	None	No effect.
Suppositories (for constipation)	No	None	Not absorbed
DIURETICS			
Acetazolamide (Diamox)	Probable	No specific data available but probably similar to sulfonamide	Acts as enzyme inhibitor on carbonic anhydrase non-bacteriostatic sulfonamide. Observe only for dehydration and electrolyte loss by monitoring urine and turgor.
Furosemide (sulfamoylanthranilic acid) (Lasix)	No		Drug is given to children under medical management.
Spironolactone (Aldactone)	Yes	Canrenone, a metabolite, appears	Acts as antagonist of aldosterone; causes sodium excretion and potassium retention. The metabolite apparently has some activity.

*Peak level occurs 4-6 hr after dose given. Maternal plasma level was higher, M/P = 0.9 and 0.8; infant's plasma level was 0.
†Adrenergic blocking agent.
‡β-blocking agent.
§Total daily dose to infant via milk is 15-20 μg.
‖Adrenergic blocking agent.
¶Reports differ.

Drug	Excreted in Milk	Amount in Milk After Therapeutic Dose	Effect on Infant
Thiazides (Diuril, Enduron, Esidrix, Hydrodiuril, Oretic, Thiuretic tablets)	Yes	>0.1 mg/dL*	Risk of dehydration and electrolyte imbalance, especially sodium loss, which would require monitoring. Watching weight and wet diapers and taking an occasional specific gravity reading of the urine and serum sodium would indicate status of infant. Risk, however, is extremely low, May suppress lactation because of dehydration in mother.
ENVIRONMENTAL AGENTS			
Benzene hexachloride (BHC)	Yes	Varies by location	Not a reason to wean from breast. No need to test milk unless inordinate exposure.
Dichlorodiphenyltrichloroethane (DDT or DDE)	Yes	Varies by location	Not a reason to wean from breast. No need to test milk unless inordinate exposure.
Methyl mercury	Yes	500-1000 ng/mL†	Infant blood level 600 ng mL in heavy exposure. Only in excessive exposure is testing and/or weaning necessary.
Polybrominated biphenyl (PBB)	Yes	Varies by location	If mother at high risk from the environment or the diet, milk sample should be measured. If level in milk is high, then breast-feeding should be discontinued. Those at risk are (1) workers who handle PBB/PCB and (2) individuals who eat game fish from contaminated waters. Crash diets mobilize fats and should be avoided especially if PBB or PCB present.
Polychlorinated biphenyl (PCB)	Yes	Varies by location	
^{99}Sr, ^{89}Sr (strontium)	Yes	1/10 of that in maternal diet	Cow's milk has six times as much as human milk. Cow's milk-fed infant doubles amount in body in 1 month.
HEAVY METALS			
Arsenic	Yes	Can be measured for given woman	Can accumulate. Check infant's blood level if there is reason to suspect exposure.
Fluorine	Yes		Monitor for excessive dose.
Iron	Yes		
Lead	Unknown		Nursing contraindicated if maternal serum 40 μg; conflicting reports, breast milk not always cause of lead poisoning in breast-fed infant.
Mercury	Yes		Hazardous to infant.
HORMONES AND CONTRACEPTIVES			
Chlorotrianisene (Tace)	Yes		Has estrogenic effect although does not change consistency of milk. May have feminizing effect on infant.
Contraceptives (oral) Ethinyl estradiol Mestranol 19-Nortestosterone Norethindrone (Norlutin) Norethynodrel (Enovid)	Yes		May diminish milk supply. May decrease vitamins, protein, and fat in milk. One author showed no difference when mothers took norethindrone. Most significant concern is long-range impact of hormone on young infant, which is not certain. Reports of feminization of infant.
Corticotropin	Yes		Destroyed in gastrointestinal tract of infant. No effect.

*Linear relationship between plasma and milk. In 1 L of milk at 0.1 mg/dL there would be 1 mg/24 hr. Infant dose is 20 mg/kg/24 hr.
†M/P = 8.6% in heavy exposure.

Drug	Excreted in Milk	Amount in Milk After Therapeutic Dose	Effect on Infant
Cortisone	Yes		Animal studies show 50% lower weight than controls and retarded sexual development and exophthalmos.
Epinephrine (Adrenalin)	Yes		Destroyed in gastrointestinal tract of infant.
Estrogen	Yes	0.17 μg/dL after 1 g	Risks as with oral contraceptives.
Insulin	Unknown		Destroyed in intestinal tract.
Medroxyprogesterone acetate (Provera)	No		Destroyed in intestinal tract.
Prednisone	Yes	0.07-0.23% dose/L after 5 mg dose*	Minimum amount not likely to cause effect on infant in short course.
Pregnanediol	Yes		Unknown risk as with other female hormones over a long time.
Tolbutamide (Orinase)	Yes		Not recommended in the childbearing years.
NARCOTICS			
Codeine		0 to trace after 32 mg every 4 hr (6 doses)	No effect in therapeutic level and transient usage. Can accumulate. Individual variation. Watch for neonatal depression.
Heroin	Yes		13 of 22 infants had withdrawal. Historically breast-feeding had been used to wean addict's infant. This is no longer recommended.
Marijuana (*Cannabis*)	Yes		Shown in laboratory animals to produce structural changes in nursling's brain cells; impairs DNA and RNA formation. Infant at risk of inhaling smoke during feeding or when held by person who is smoking.
Meperidine (Demerol)	Yes	>0.1 mg/dL†	Trace amounts may accumulate if drug taken around the clock when infant is neonate. Watch for drowsiness and poor feeding.
Methadone	Yes	0.03 μg/mL or 0.023-0.028 mg/24 hr*	When dosage not excessive, infant can be breast-fed if monitored for evidence of depression and failure to thrive.
Morphine	Yes	Trace	Single doses have minimum effect. Potential for accumulation. May be addicting to neonate. Breast-feeding no longer considered appropriate means of weaning infant of an addict.
Percodan (oxycodone [derived from opiate thebaine] aspirin, phenacetin, caffeine)	Yes		Consider for its component parts. In neonatal period sleepiness and failure to feed, which increase maternal engorgement and neonatal weight loss, have been observed, probably caused by oxycodone.
PSYCHOTROPIC AND MOOD-CHANGING DRUGS			
Alcohol	Yes	Similar to plasma level	Ordinarily no problem and can be therapeutic in moderation, infants are more susceptible to effects. Chronic drinking reported to cause obesity in infant. Ethanol in doses of 1-2 g/kg to mother causes depression of milk-ejection reflex (dose dependent). No acetaldehyde found in infants.
Amphetamine	Yes		Has caused stimulation in infants with jitteriness, irritability, sleeplessness. Long-acting preparations cumulative.

*0.16 μg/mL after 10 mg dose; 2.67 μg/mL after 2 hr.
†Plasma 0.07-0.1 mg/dL.
*Mother received 50 mg/24 hr; M/P = 0.83. Peak level 4 hr after oral dose. Results obscured if addict also taking the herbal root golden seal.

Drug	Excreted in Milk	Amount in Milk After Therapeutic Dose	Effect on Infant
Benzodiazepines*	Yes		Not sufficient to affect infant first week when glucuronyl system needed for detoxification. May accumulate. Older infant, no apparent problem.
Chlordiazepoxide (Librium)			
Diazepam (Valium)	Yes	90 μg/L†	Detoxified in glucuronyl system. In first weeks of life may contribute to jaundice. Metabolite active. Effect on infant: hypoventilation, drowsiness, lethargy, and weight loss. Single doses over 10 mg contraindicated during breastfeeding. Accumulation in infant possible.
Haloperidol (Haldol)	Yes	Unknown	A butyrophenone antidepressant: animal studies in nurslings show behavior abnormalities.
Lithium carbonate (Eskalith, Lithane, Lithonate)	Yes	⅓-½ maternal plasma level‡	Measurable lithium in infants' serum. Infant kidney can clear lithium; however, lithium inhibits adenosine 3′:5′-cyclic monophosphate, significant for brain growth. Also affects amine metabolism. Real effects not measurable immediately. Report of cyanosis and poor muscle tone and ECG changes in nursing infant.
Monomine oxidate (MAO) inhibitors (Eutonyl, Nardil)			Inhibits lactation.
Meprobamate (Miltown, Equanil)	Yes	2-4 times maternal plasma level	If therapy continued, infant should be followed closely.
Phenothiazines			
Chlorpromazine (Thorazine)	Yes	⅓ plasma level§	Can be safely nursed; minimum in milk. Increase maternal prolactin. No symptoms in infants reported; 5-year follow-up showed infants normal.
Piperacetazine (Quide)	Yes	Minimum	Probably no effect.
Thioridazine (Mellaril)	Yes	No information	Thioridazine is less potent in general than other phenothiazines. Probably safe.
Trifluoperazine (Stelazine)	Yes	Minimum	
Tricyclic antidepressants	Yes		Apparently no accumulation. No infants that have been observed showed symptoms. Watch for depression or failure to feed. Increase maternal prolactin secretion.
Amitriptyline (Elavil)	Yes	Minimum amounts	
Desipramine (Norpramin, Pertofrane)		Minimum amounts	
Imipramine (Tofranil)	Yes	0.1 mg/dL‖	

*Alcohol enhances effect of this group.

†10 mg or less yields 45 mg of diazepam/mL and 85 ng of metabolite/mL. P/M ratio is variable. Mean P/M ratio of diazepam is 6.14; of metabolite is 3.64. Effect lasts about 4 days.

‡0.030 mmol/L in infant's serum, 0.57 mmole/L in infant's urine. Milk level was half of maternal serum level in one case report.

§If dose <200 mg, milk contains bare trace. Dose of 1200 mg showed trace.

‖Plasma level 0.2-1.3 mg/dL.

Drug	Excreted in Milk	Amount in Milk After Therapeutic Dose	Effect on Infant
STIMULANTS			
Caffeine	Yes	1% of dose	Accumulates when intake moderate and continual. Causes jitteriness, wakefulness, and irritability. Caffeine present in many hot and cold drinks. Consider if infant very wakeful.
Theobromine	Yes	3.7-8.2 mg/L after 240 mg dose*	No adverse symptoms observed in the infants. Chocolate most common cause of exposure.
Theophylline	Yes	10% of maternal dose†	Irritability, fretfulness.
THYROID AND ANTITHYROID MEDICATIONS			
Thiouracil	Yes	9-12 mg/dL‡	Same as for propylthiouracil.
Thyroid and thyroxine	Yes		Does not produce adverse symptoms on long-range follow-up. Noted to improve milk supply of hypothyroid mothers. No contraindication.
MISCELLANEOUS			
DPT	Yes	Minimum	Does not interfere with immunization schedule.
Methotrexate	Yes	Minor route of excretion: M/P = 0.08/1.0	Antimetabolite. Infant would receive 0.26 μg/dL, which researchers consider nontoxic for infant.
Nicotine	Yes	Mean 91 ppb (20-512 ppb)§	Decreases milk production. No apparent effect on infant—perhaps a tolerance is developed in utero. Smoking may interfere with let-down reflex if smoking started before onset of a feeding.
Poliovirus vaccine	No		Live vaccine taken orally. Not necessary to withhold nursing 30 min before and after dose. Provide booster after infant no longer nursing.
Rh antibodies	Yes		Destroyed in gastrointestinal tract; not effective orally.
Rubella virus vaccine	Yes	Minimum	Will not confer passive immunity. Mother should not be given vaccine when at risk for pregnancy.
Tuberculin test	No		Tuberculin-sensitive mothers can adaptively immunize their infants through breast milk, and that immunity may last several years.
Chest x-ray films			No effect.

*113 g chocolate bar.
†M/P = 0.7.
‡Maternal plasma level was 3.4 mg/dl after a 1 g dose; M/P = 3.
§At ½-1½ packs/day. Large variation from single donor.

appendix H

Resources

This Appendix includes community and national resources, national clearinghouses, journals, and nursing organizations of interest to the maternity nurse.

■ COMMUNITY AND NATIONAL RESOURCES

AASK (Aid to the Adoption of Special Kids)
3530 Grand Avenue
Oakland, CA 94610
(415) 451-1748

AIDS Medical Foundation
10 East 13th Street, Suite LD
New York, NY 10003
(212) 206-0670

AMEND
Aiding a Mother Experiencing Neo-Natal Death
4324 Berrywick Terrace
St. Louis, MO 63141
(314) 487-7582

American Academy of Husband-Coached Childbirth
P.O. Box 5224
Sherman Oaks, CA 91413
(818) 788-6662

American Cancer Society, Inc.
1599 Clifton Road, NE
Atlanta, Georgia 30329
1-800-ACS-2345

American Cleft Palate Association
331 Salk Hall
Pittsburgh, PA 15261
(412) 681-9620

American Diabetes Association
Diabetes Information Service Center
1660 Duke Street
Alexandria, VA 22314
1-800-ADA-DISC

American Fertility Foundation
2131 Magnolia Avenue
Suite 201
Birmingham, AL 35256
(205) 251-9764

American Foundation for Maternal and Child Health, Inc.
(research on the perinatal period)
30 Beekman Place
New York, NY 10022
(212) 759-5510

American Red Cross
17th and E Streets
Washington, DC 20006
(202) 737-8300

American Society for Psychoprophylaxis in Obstetrics (ASPO)
1840 Wilson Boulevard
Suite 204
Arlington, VA 22201
(703) 524-7802

Association for the Aid of Crippled Children
345 East 46th Street
New York, NY 10017

Association of Birth Defects in Children
3201 E. Crystal Lake Avenue
Orlando, FL 32806

Association for the Care of Children's Health
7910 Woodmont Avenue, Suite 300
Bethesda, MD 20814
(301) 654-6549

Association for Childbirth at Home, International
P.O. Box 39498
Los Angeles, CA 90039
(213) 667-0839

Association of Voluntary Sterilization, Inc. (AVS)
122 E. 42nd Street
New York, NY 10168
(212) 351-2500

Black Male Youth Health Enhancement Project
Family Life Center
Shiloh Baptist Church
Washington, DC

Boston Women's Health Book Collective
47 Nichols Avenue
Watertown, MA 02172
(617) 921-0271

Centers for Disease Control
1600 Clifton Road, N.E.
Atlanta, GA 30333
(404) 329-1819, (404) 329-3286

Child Study Association of America
9 East 89th St.
New York, NY 10028
Provides parent education materials.

Cleft Palate Foundation
1218 Grandview Avenue
Pittsburgh, PA 15211
1-800-24-CLEFT

Compassionate Friends
(Following death of an infant)
P.O. Box 1347
Oak Brook, IL 60521
(312) 990-0010

COPE (Coping with the Overall Pregnancy/Parenting Experience)
37 Clarendon Street
Boston, MA 02116
(617) 357-5588

C/SEC, Inc. (Cesarean/Support Education and Concern)
22 Forest Road
Framingham, MA 01701
(617) 877-8266

DES Action USA
Long Island Jewish Medical Center
New Hyde Park, NY 11040

ECMO Moms and Dads
c/o Blair and Gayle Willson
HCR1, Box 108
Plainview, TX 79072
(806) 889-3877

Ed-U-Press
760 Ostrum Ave.
Syracuse, NY 13210
Offers series of excellent cartoon books for adolescents and parenting classes.

Educational and Scientific Plastics, Ltd.
76 Holmethorpe Avenue
Holmethorpe, Red Hill Surrey, RH1, 2PF, England
Offers numerous plastic models.

Endometriosis Association
238 West Wisconsin Avenue
P.O. Box 92187
Milwaukee, WI 53202
(414) 962-8972

Environmental Protection Agency (EPA)
Public Information Center
Room PM 211-B
401 M Street, SW
Washington, DC 20460
(202) 382-7550

Equal Rights for Fathers
P.O. Box 90042
San Jose, CA 95109-3042
(415) 848-2323

Florence Crittenton Association of America
608 South Dearborn Street
Chicago, IL 60605
Assists in bringing about a greater understanding of factors relating to unmarried mothers and adolescent girls with other problems in adjustment.

International Childbirth Education Association (ICEA)
P.O. Box 20048
Milwaukee, WI 55420

La Leche League
P.O. Box 1209
Franklin Park, IL 60131-8209
(312) 455-7730 (24-hour line)

March of Dimes See *National Foundation/March of Dimes*

Maternal Health Society
Box 46563, Station G
Vancouver, BC V6R 4G8

Maternity Center Association, Inc.
48 East 92nd Street
New York, NY 10028
(212) 269-7300

NAACOG, the Organization for Obstetric, Gynecologic, and Neonatal Nurses
Name change: The Association of Women's
Health, Obstetric, and Neonatal Nurses
(AWHONN). Department 3299
Washington, DC 20042-3299
1-800-673-8499 (USA)
1-800-245-0231 (Canada)

National Abortion Rights Action League
1101 14th Street, NW
Washington, DC 20005
(202) 371-9779

National Association of Childbirth Education, Inc. (NACE)
3940 Eleventh Street
Riverside, CA 92501

National Association for Sickle Cell Disease
3345 Wilshire Blvd., Suite 1106
Los Angeles, CA 90010-1880
(213) 736-5455; 1-800-421-8453

National Childbirth Trust
9 Queensborough Terrace
London, W2, England
Offers books, films, and other aids for use in classes or in labor.

National Coalition Against Domestic Violence
Suite 305
2401 Virginia Avenue, NW
Washington, DC 20037
24-hour Toll-free line 1-800-333-SAFE

National Coalition Against Sexual Assault
c/o Fern Ferguson, President
Volunteers of America of Illinois
8787 State Street, Suite 202
East St. Louis, IL 62203

The National Coalition of Hispanic Health and Human Services Organizations (COSSMHO)
1030 15th Street, N.W. Suite 1053
Washington, DC 20005
(202) 371-2100

National Conference of Catholic Charities
1346 Connecticut
Washington, DC 20036
Service for children and youth; i.e., foster care, counseling, adoption services, short-term counseling to families and youth, emergency material assistance.

National Down Syndrome Congress
1800 Dempster Street
Park Ridge, IL 60068-1146
1-800-232-6372

National Down Syndrome Society
141 Fifth Avenue
New York, NY 10010

National Foundation/March of Dimes
1275 Mamaroneck Avenue
White Plains, NY 10605
(914) 428-7100

National Foundation for Jewish Genetic Diseases, Inc.
250 Park Avenue, Suite 1000
New York, NY 10177

National Institute of Child Health and Human Development (NICHD)
National Institutes of Health
9000 Rockville Pike
Bldg 31, Room 2A32
Bethesda, MD 20892
(301) 496-4000

National Organization of Mothers of Twins Clubs, Inc.
12404 Princess Jeanne, NE
Albuquerque, NM 87112-4640
(505) 275-0955

National Right to Life Committee
419 7th Street, NW
Suite 402
Washington, DC 20004
(202) 626-8800

National Sudden Infant Death Syndrome Foundation
10500 Little Patuxent Parkway
Suite 420
Columbia, MD 21044
800-221-7437
(301) 964-8000 (in Maryland)

Office of Minority Health Resource Center
P.O. Box 37337
Washington, DC 20013-7337
(301) 587-1938

Parent Care, Inc. (neonatal intensive care unit family support)
101-½ South Union
Alexandria, VA 22314
(703) 836-4678

Parenthood After Thirty
451 Vermont
Berkeley, CA 94707
(415) 524-6635

Parents of Prematures
℅ Houston Organization for Parent Education, Inc.
2990 Richmond
Suite 204
Houston, TX 77098
(713) 524-3089

Parents Without Partners
8807 Colesville Road
Silver Spring, MD 20910
(301) 588-9354

Patient Counseling Library
Budlong Press Co.
5428 N. Virginia Avenue
Chicago, IL, 60625
(312) 541-7800
Provides videotapes covering topics such as pregnancy, infant care, sexuality, breast-feeding, and weight control.

Planned Parenthood Federation of America, Inc.
810 Seventh Avenue
New York, NY 10019

Pregnancy and Infant Loss
1421 East Wayzata Boulevard
Suite 40
Wayzata, MN 55391
(612) 473-9372

Premenstrual Syndrome Action
P.O. 16292
Irving, CA 92713
(714) 854-4407

Reach to Recovery (breast cancer)
American Cancer Society

Resolve, Inc. (impaired fertility)
5 Water Street
Arlington, MA 02174
(617) 643-2424

Resolve Through Sharing
(R.T.S.) (Perinatal Bereavement)
Lutheran Hospital—La Crosse
1910 South Ave.
La Crosse, WI 54601
(608) 791-4747

Save the Children Federation, Inc.
345 East 46th Street
New York, NY 10017

SHARE (Source of Help in Airing and Resolving Experiences) for parents who have suffered loss of newborn baby
% St. John's Hospital
800 E. Carpenter Street
Springfield, IL 62760
(217) 544-6464

SIECUS
Human Science Press
72 Fifth Avenue
New York, NY 10011
Provides publications (e.g., "Sexual relations in pregnancy and postpartum") and teaching aids.

Spina Bifida Association of Ameria
1700 Rockville Pike
Suite 250
Rockville, MD 20852
800-621-3141
(301) 770-7222

Teen Obstetrical Perinatal Parenting Services Clinic (TOPPS)
University of Arkansas College of Medicine
Little Rock, AR

Twins Magazine,
P.O. Box 12045
Overland Park, KS 66212
1-800-821-5533

Victims Anonymous
9514-9 Reseda Blvd. #607
Northridge, CA 91324
(818) 993-1139

VBAC (Vaginal Birth After Cesarean)
10 Great Plain Terrace
Needham, MA 01292

Women Against Rape
P.O. Box 02084
Columbus, OH 43202
(614) 291-9751

Women Against Violence Against Women (WAVAW)
543 North Fairfax Avenue
Los Angeles, CA 90036

■ NATIONAL CLEARINGHOUSES

American Foundation for Maternal and Child Health
(research on the perinatal period)
300 Beekman Place
New York, NY 10022
(212) 759-5510

Food and Drug Administration (FDA)
Office of Consumer Affairs
Public Inquiries
5600 Fishers Lane (HFE-88)
Rockville, MD 20857
(301) 443-3170

National AIDS Information Clearinghouse
1-800-458-5231 (English and Spanish)

National Maternal and Child Health Clearinghouse
3520 Prospect St., N.W., Ground Floor
Washington, DC 20057

Sudden Infant Death Syndrome Clearinghouse
8201 Greensboro Dr., Suite 600
McLean, VA 22102

■ NURSING JOURNALS

Birth: Issues in Prenatal Care and Education (formerly **Birth and Family Journal**)
110 El Camino Real
Berkeley, CA 94705
(415) 658-5099

Bookmarks
ICEA Supplies Center
P.O. Box 20048
Minneapolis, MN 55420
Complimentary annotated catalogue of book reviews.

Canadian Nurse
The Canadian Nurses Association
50 The Driveway
Ottawa, Canada K2P1E2

NAACOG's
Clinical Issues in Perinatal and Women's Health Nursing
JB Lippincott
East Washington Square
Philadelphia, PA, 19105

The Female Patient
Division Excerpta Medica
301 Gibraltar Drive
P.O. Box 528
Morris Plains, NJ 07950

Journal of Nurse-Midwifery
Editor
82 Willow Ln.
Tenafly, NJ 07670

Journal of Obstetric, Gynecologic and Neonatal Nursing (JOGNN)
Harper & Row, Publishers
Medical Department
2350 Virginia Avenue
Hagerstown, MD 21740

Journal of Perinatal and Neonatal Nursing
Aspen Publishers, Inc.
7201 McKinney Circle
Frederick, MD 21701

Maternal/Newborn Advocate
The National Foundation/March of Dimes
P.O. Box 2000
White Plains, NY 10602

MCN The American Journal of Maternal Child Nursing
555 W. 57th Street
New York, NY 10019

Nursing Network on Violence Against Women Newsletter
Trauma Program, UHN-66
Oregon Health Sciences University
3181 SW Sam Jackson Pk Rd
Portland, OR 97201-3098
Fax: (503) 494-4357

Nurse Practitioner: A Journal of Primary Nursing Care
3845 42nd Ave., N.E.
Seattle, WA 98105

Nursing Research
555 W. 57th Street
New York, NY 10019

Perinatal Press
Perinatal Press Subscriptions
The Perinatal Center
Sutter Memorial Hospital
52nd and F Sts.
Sacramento, CA 95819

Women's Health Nursing Scan
J.B. Lippincott Co.
Downsville Pike, Rte 3, Box 20-B
Hagerstown, MD 21740

Loss and Grief

"Bereavement" Magazine
305 Gradle Dr.
Carmel, IN 46032
(317) 846-9429

Our Newsletter
(a Multiple Birth Loss Support Network)
P.O. 1064
Palmer, AK 99645
(907) 745-2706

■ NURSING ORGANIZATIONS

American College of Nurse Midwives
1522 K Street, NW
Suite 1120
Washington, DC 20005
(202) 347-5445

American Nurses Association
1101 14th Street, NW
Suite 200
Washington, DC 20005
(202) 789-1800;
Head office
600 Maryland Ave. SW
Washington, DC

Canadian Nurses Association
50 The Driveway
Ottawa, Ont. K2P 1E2

Midwives Alliance of North America
United States and Canada
℅ Concord Midwifery Service
30 South Main Street
Concord, NH 03301
(603) 225-9586

NAACOG: The Organization for Obstetric, Gynecologic, and Neonatal Nurses
Name change: The Association of Women's
Health, Obstetric, and Neonatal Nurses
(AWHONN). Department 3299
Washington, DC 20042-3299
1-800-673-8499 (USA)
1-800-245-0231 (Canada)

National League for Nursing (NLN)
Ten Columbus Circle
New York, NY 10019
(212) 582-1022

■ ORGANIZATIONS INVOLVED IN PARENT EDUCATION

American Academy of Husband-Coached Childbirth (AAHCC)
P.O. Box 5224
Sherman Oaks, CA 91413

American Society for Psychoprophylaxis in Obstetrics (ASPO)
1411 K Street N.W., Suite 200
Washington, DC 20005

Council of Childbirth Education Specialists, Inc. (CCES)
168 West 86th Street
New York, NY 10024

International Childbirth Education Association (ICEA)
P.O. Box 20048
Minneapolis, MN 55420

Maternity Center Association
48 East 92nd St
New York, NY 10028

National Association of Childbirth Education, Inc. (NACE)
3940 11th Street
Riverside, CA 92501

NAACOG: The Organization for Obstetric, Gynecologic, and Neonatal Nurses
409 12th Street, S.W.
Washington, DC 20024-2188

Read Natural Childbirth Foundation, Inc.
1300 S. Elisco Drive, Suite 102
Greenbrae, CA 94904

Index

D

E

F

N

V

Temperature Equivalents

Celsius	Fahrenheit	Celsius	Fahrenheit
34.0	93.2	38.6	101.4
34.2	93.6	38.8	101.8
34.4	93.9	39.0	102.2
34.6	94.3	39.2	102.5
34.8	94.6	39.4	102.9
35.0	95.0	39.6	103.2
35.2	95.4	39.8	103.6
35.4	95.7	40.0	104.0
35.6	96.1	40.2	104.3
35.8	96.4	40.4	104.7
36.0	96.8	40.6	105.1
36.2	97.1	40.8	105.4
36.4	97.5	41.0	105.8
36.6	97.8	41.2	106.1
36.8	98.2	41.4	106.5
37.0	98.6	41.6	106.8
37.2	98.9	41.8	107.2
37.4	99.3	42.0	107.6
37.6	99.6	42.2	108.0
37.8	100.0	42.4	108.3
38.0	100.4	42.6	108.7
38.2	100.7	42.8	109.0
38.4	101.1	43.0	109.4

To convert Fahrenheit to Celsius:
(Temperature minus 32) $\times \frac{5}{9}$
Example: To convert 98.6 degrees Fahrenheit to Celsius:
$98.6 - 32 = 66.6 \times \frac{5}{9}$
$= 37$ degrees

To convert Celsius to Fahrenheit:
$\frac{9}{5} \times$ temperature $+ 32$
Example: To convert 40 degrees Celsius to Fahrenheit:
$\frac{9}{5} \times 40 = 72 + 32$
$= 104$ degrees

Conversion of Pounds and Ounces to Grams for Newborn Weights*

Pounds	Ounces 0	1	2	3	4	5	6	7	8	9	10	11	12	13	14	15	Pounds
0	—	28	57	85	113	142	170	198	227	255	283	312	430	369	397	425	0
1	454	482	510	539	567	595	624	652	680	709	737	765	794	822	850	879	1
2	907	936	964	992	1021	1049	1077	1106	1134	1162	1191	1219	1247	1276	1304	1332	2
3	1361	1389	1417	1446	1474	1503	1531	1559	1588	1616	1644	1673	1701	1729	1758	1786	3
4	1814	1843	1871	1899	1928	1956	1984	2013	2041	2070	2093	2126	2155	2183	2211	2240	4
5	2268	2296	2325	2353	2381	2410	2438	2466	2495	2523	2551	2580	2608	2637	2665	2693	5
6	2722	2750	2778	2807	2835	2863	2892	2920	2948	2977	3005	3033	3062	3090	3118	3147	6
7	3175	3203	3232	3260	3289	3317	3345	3374	3402	3430	3459	3487	3515	3544	3572	3600	7
8	3629	3657	3685	3714	3742	3770	3799	3827	3856	3884	3912	3941	3969	3997	4026	4054	8
9	4082	4111	4139	4167	4196	4224	4252	4281	4309	4337	4366	4394	4423	4451	4479	4508	9
10	4536	4564	4593	4621	4649	4678	4706	4734	4763	4791	4819	4848	4876	4904	4933	4961	10
11	4990	5018	5046	5075	5103	5131	5160	5188	5216	5245	5273	5301	5330	5358	5386	5415	11
12	5443	5471	5500	5528	5557	5585	5613	5642	5670	5698	5727	5755	5783	5812	5840	5868	12
13	5897	5925	5953	5982	6010	6038	6067	6095	6123	6152	6180	6209	6237	6265	6294	6322	13
14	6350	6379	6407	6435	6464	6492	6520	6549	6577	6605	6634	6662	6690	6719	6747	6776	14
15	6804	6832	6860	6889	6917	6945	6973	7002	7030	7059	7087	7115	7144	7172	7201	7228	15
	0	1	2	3	4	5	6	7	8	9	10	11	12	13	14	15	
	Ounces																

*To convert pounds and ounces to grams, multiply the pounds by 453.6 and the ounces by 28.35; add the totals.
To convert grams into pounds and decimals of a pound, multiply the grams by 0.0022
To convert grams into ounces, divide the grams by 28.35 (16 oz = 1 lb).